BRIEF CONTENTS

PEDIATRIC NURSING
Caring for Children and Their Families

About the ONLINE COMPANIONS™

Delmar offers a series of Online Companions™. Through the Delmar site on the World Wide Web, the Online Companions™ let readers access online companions that update the information in the books.

To access the *Pediatric Nursing: Caring for Children and Their Families* site, simply point your browser to:

www.delmarnursing.com/olcs/potts

Online Services

Delmar Online
To access a wide variety of Delmar products and services on the World Wide Web, point your browser to:

http://www.delmarnursing.com
or email info@delmar.com

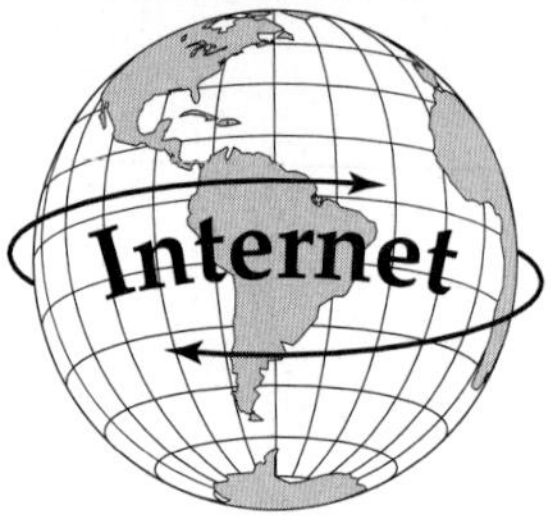

A service of Thomson Learning™

PEDIATRIC NURSING
Caring for Children and Their Families

Nicki L. Potts RN, PhD
Former Associate Professor
School of Nursing, Austin Community College
Austin, Texas
Former Assistant Professor
School of Nursing, University of Texas at Austin
Austin, Texas

and

Barbara L. Mandleco, RN, PhD
Associate Professor
Associate Dean of Research and Scholarship
Brigham Young University
Provo, Utah

DELMAR
THOMSON LEARNING
Australia Canada Mexico Singapore Spain United Kingdom United States

DELMAR

THOMSON LEARNING

Pediatric Nursing: Caring for Children and Their Families

Nicki L. Potts, RN, PhD
Barbara L. Mandleco, RN, PhD

Health Care Publishing Director:
William Brottmiller

Executive Editor:
Cathy L. Esperti

Acquisitions Editor:
Matthew Kane

Developmental Editor:
Marah E. Bellegarde

Executive Marketing Manager:
Dawn F. Gerrain

Channel Manager:
Jennifer McAvey

Project Editor:
David Buddle

Editorial Assistant:
Shelley Esposito

Technology Project Manager:
Laurie Davis

Technology Project Specialist:
Joe Saba

Art/Design Coordinator:
Jay Purcell

Production Coordinator:
Anne Sherman

Production Assistant:
Sherry McGaughan

Printed in the United States of America
2 3 4 5 XXX 07 06 05 04 03 02

For more information, contact Delmar,
5 Maxwell Road, P.O. Box 8007,
Clifton Park, NY 12065-8007

Or find us on the World Wide Web at http://www.delmar.com

Library of Congress Cataloging-in-Publication Data
Pediatric nursing : caring for children and their families / [edited by]
Nicki L. Potts, Barbara L. Mandleco.
p. ; cm.
Includes bibliographical references and index.
ISBN 0-8273-8148-4
1. Pediatric nursing. I. Potts, Nicki L. (Nicki Lee) II. Mandleco, Barbara Hartwig.
[DNLM: 1. Nursing Care—methods—Child. 2. Pediatric Nursing—methods. WY 159 P37332 2002]
RJ245 .P4185 2002
610.73'62—dc21 2001054804

NOTICE TO THE READER

The publisher does not warrant or guarantee any of the products described herein or perform any independent analysis in connection with any of the product information contained herein. The publisher does not assume, and expressly disclaims, any obligation to obtain and include information other than that provided to it by the manufacturer.

The reader is expressly warned to consider and adopt all safety precautions that might be indicated by the activities herein and to avoid all potential hazards. By following the instructions contained herein, the reader willingly assumes all risks in connection with such instructions.

The publisher makes no representation or warranties of any kind, including but not limited to, the warranties of fitness for particular purpose or merchantability, nor are any such representations implied with respect to the material set forth herein, and the publisher takes no responsibility with respect to such material. The publisher shall not be liable for any special, consequential, or exemplary damages resulting, in whole or part, from the readers' use of, or reliance upon, this material.

CONTENTS

CONTRIBUTORS

Stephanie Rockwern Amlung, PhD, RN
Clinical Director of Research
Hill-Rom Company
Batesville, Indiana

Natalie Annen-Ricks, BSN
Charge Nurse
Neonatal Critical Care Unit
Primary Children's Medical Center
Salt Lake City, Utah

Phyllis Augspurger, PhD, RN
Associate Professor
Xavier University
Cincinnati, Ohio

Patricia Becker, RN, MSN, JD
Attorney
Akin, Gump, Strauss, Hauer & Feld, LLP
Austin, Texas

Barbara Caldwell, RN, PhD, CNS-C
Associate Professor
School of Nursing
University of Medicine and Dentistry
of New Jersey
Newark, New Jersey

Susan Chasson MSN, CNM, JD
Lecturer
College of Nursing
Lecturer
J. Reuben Clark School of Law
Brigham Young University
Provo, Utah

Bonnie Clay, RN, MS, CCRN, PNP
Pediatric Nurse Practitioner
Pediatric Critical Care
Primary Children's Medical Center
Salt Lake City, Utah

Janet Craig, RN, MS, CCRN, PNP
Pediatric Nurse Practitioner
Pediatric Cardiology
Primary Children's Medical Center
Salt Lake City, Utah

Frances Dotton, RN, PhD
Faculty
Excelsior College
Albany, New York
Retired Associate Professor
College of Nursing
Niagara University
Niagara University, New York

Mary L. Dowell, PhD, RNC
Associate Professor of Pediatric Nursing
School of Nursing
The University of Mary Hardin-Baylor
Belton, Texas

Susan G. Fister, PhD, RN
Associate Professor
Eastern Kentucky University
Richmond, Kentucky

Shirley Goodman, BSN, RN, CDE
Diabetes Education Program Coordinator
Endocrine-Diabetes Nurse Clinician
Children's Memorial Medical Center
Chicago, Illinois

Elaine R. Graf, PhD, PNP, CS
Clinical Education Research and
Funding Coordinator
Children's Memorial Medical Center
Chicago, Illinois

Carole Gutt, RN, EdD
Associate Professor and Department Chair
Department of Nursing
D'Youville College
Buffalo, New York

Helene Harris, MSN, RN
Clinical Research Coordinator
Tampa Bay Medical Research
Temple, Texas

Sharon Horner, RN, PhD
Associate Professor
School of Nursing
The University of Texas at Austin
Austin, Texas

Janet Ihlenfeld, RN, PhD
Professor
Department of Nursing
D'Youville College
Buffalo, New York

Lisa Nicole Sessoms Kaplan, RN, MSN
Former Professor of Nursing
Valencia Community College
Orlando, Florida
Professional Sales Representative
Reliant Pharmaceuticals
Bridgewater, New Jersey

Barbara J. Keating, RN, MS
Clinical Educator, Ambulatory Surgical Services
Children's Memorial Medical Center
Chicago, Illinois

Carole Kenner, RNC, DNS, FAAN
Associate Dean for Academics Advancement
College of Nursing
University of Illinois at Chicago
Chicago, Illinois

Barbara S. Kiernan, PhD, RN, CS, PNP
Assistant Professor of Nursing
School of Nursing
Medical College of Georgia
Augusta, Georgia

Patricia King, RN, FNP
President
ABC Pediatrics
Dudley, North Carolina

Lauri A. Linder, MS, RN
Assitant Professor (Clinical)
College of Nursing
University of Utah
Salt Lake City, Utah

Christina P. Linton, RN, MSNc
Family Nurse Practitioner Program
Brigham Young University
Provo, Utah

J. Kelly McCoy, PhD
Assistant Professor
School of Family Life
Brigham Young University
Provo, Utah

Maureen Meyer, RN, MS, CSN
School Nurse
Instructor for EMSC School Nurse Emergency Care Course
School District U46
Elgin, Illinois

Debra Ann Mills, RN, MS
Assistant Teaching Professor
College of Nursing
Brigham Young University
Provo, Utah

Angela Ciolfi Murphy, PhD, RN
Professor of Pediatric Nursing
Department of Nursing
Rhode Island College
Providence, Rhode Island

Kathy Murphy, MSN, RN, CS
Clinical Nurse Specialist
Sibley Heart Center
Children's Healthcare of Atlanta-Egleston
Atlanta, Georgia
The Emory Clinic
Atlanta, Georgia

Jennifer Obrecht, RN, MS
Advanced Practice Nurse
Pain Management Team
Children's Memorial Medical Center
Chicago, Illinois

Karen D. Peterson, MSN, RN, CPNP
Pediatric Nurse Practitioner
Division of Endocrinology, Formerly of
Immunology/Rheumatology
Children's Memorial Medical Center
Chicago, Illinois

Carolyn C. Reynolds, APRN, MS
Pediatric Clinical Nurse Specialist
Primary Children's Medical Center
Salt Lake City, Utah

Linda S. Rieg, PhDc, RN
Associate Professor
Xavier University
Cincinnati, Ohio

Hazel M. Sanderson, EdD, RN
Associate Professor
School of Nursing
Long Island University
Brooklyn Campus
Brooklyn, New York

Pam Schlomann, PhD, RN
Professor
Department of Baccalaureate and Graduate Nursing
Eastern Kentucky University
Richmond, Kentucky

Joan Schmitke, DSN, RN, CS, FNP
Associate Professor
Department of Baccalaureate and Graduate Nursing
Eastern Kentucky University
Richmond, Kentucky

E. Ann Sheridan, RN, MS, EdD
Professor Emerita
University of Massachusetts, Amherst
Amherst, Massachusetts

Kimberly A. Stieglitz, DNSc, RN, CS
Director of Youth Services
Pediatric Nurse Practitioner
Howard Brown Health Center
Chicago, Illinois

Suzanne Sutherland, RN, PhD
Professor, Division of Nursing
California State University
Sacramento, California
Staff Nurse II
University of California Davis Medical Center
Sacramento, California

Mary Tiedeman, PhD, RN
Assistant Professor
College of Nursing
Brigham Young University
Provo, Utah

Jo Trilling, RNC, MS
Staff Nurse
Sacred Heart Medical Center
Spokane, Washington

Janice L. Vincent, DSN, RN
Assistant Professor
University of Alabama School of Nursing
Birmingham, Alabama

Susan O'Connor Von, DNS, RNC
Assistant Professor
Department of Nursing
The College of St. Catherine
St. Paul, Minnesota

Robert F. Wayner, MD
Neurosurgeon, The Neurological Clinic
Chief of Surgery
Saddleback Memorial Medical Center
Laguna Hills, California

Marcia C. Wellington, RNC, MS
Clinical Manager
Children's Hospital of Orange County
Mission Viejo, California

Ellen M. White, ARNP, MSN, OCN
Advanced Registered Nurse Practitioner
University of Miami
Miami, Florida

Barbara C. Woodring, RN, EdD
Professor and Associate Dean
University of Alabama School of Nursing
Birmingham, Alabama

Mary N. Yeaney, RN, MSN, CPNP
Pediatric Nurse Practitioner
Georgetown University Hospital
Washington, D.C.

Kerry Fitzgerald Zebold, RN, MSN
Pediatric Urology Clinical Nurse Specialist
Children's Memorial Medical Center
Chicago, Illinois

REVIEWERS

Marty Bachman, RN, CNS, MSN, PhD
Associate Professor, Nursing Department
Fort Range Community College,
Larimer Campus
Fort Collins, Colorado

Marion E. Broome, RN, FAAN, PhD
Associate Dean and Professor, Center for Nursing Research
University of Alabama at Birmingham
Birmingham, Alabama

Vera V. Cull, RN, DSN
Assistant Professor of Nursing
School of Nursing
University of Alabama at Birmingham
Birmingham, Alabama

Karen D'Apolito, BSN, MSN, PhD
Assistant Professor, School of Nursing
Vanderbilt University
Nashville, Tennessee

Betty Davis, RN, MS
Associate Professor
Mary Black School of Nursing
University of South Carolina—Spartanburg
Spartanburg, South Carolina

Judith Herrman, MS, RNC
Undergraduate Clinical Coordinator
Department of Nursing
University of Delaware
Newark, Delaware

Barbara R. Kelley, MS, MPH, EdD, PNP
Associate Professor, School of Nursing
Northeastern University
Boston, Massachusetts

Lynn E. Kelly, RN, MSN, PhD
Associate Professor, School of Nursing
Widener University
Chester, Pennsylvania

Katherine Pearson, FNP, RN, CS
Instructor, Nursing Division
Temple College
Temple, Texas

Linda Pehl, RNC, PhD
Associate Dean and Professor
School of Nursing
University of Mary Hardin-Baylor
Belton, Texas

Melanie S. Percy, RN, PhD, CPNP
Assistant Professor, School of Nursing
University of Texas at Austin
Austin, Texas

Kathleen D. Pickrell, RN, MSN
Chairperson
Associate Degree Nursing Program Department
Associate Professor, School of Nursing
Indiana State University
Terre Haute, Indiana

Ann Quinn-Wallace
Professor
School of Health Sciences and Community Services
Canestoga College
Kitchener, Ontario

Regina D. Reed, RN
Assistant Professor, Associate Degree Nursing
School of Nursing
Washington State Community College
Marietta, Ohio

Antonia M. Scacco-Neumann, RN, MSN, PhDc
Lecturer, College of Nursing
Kent State University
Kent, Ohio

Shirley R. Schantz, MSN, EdD, ARNP
Associate Professor, School of Nursing
Director, Primary Care Nursing Center
Barry University
Miami Shores, Florida

Janice A. Selekman, DNSc, RN
Chairperson, Department of Nursing and Professor
University of Delaware
Newark, Delaware

Lynn M. Stover, DSN, MSN, RNC
Instructor, Capstone College of Nursing
University of Alabama
Tuscaloosa, Alabama

Carolyn L. Walker, PhD, RN, CPON
Professor, School of Nursing
San Diego State University
San Diego, California

William Wojociechowski, MS, RRT
Chairman and Associate Professor
Department of Cardiorespiratory Care
University of South Alabama
Mobile, Alabama

Michele Woodbeck, MS, RN
Associate Professor, School of Health Sciences
Hudson Valley Community College
Troy, New York

JoAnne Youngblut, RN, FAAN, PhD
Professor, Frances Payne Bolton School
of Nursing
Case Western Reserve University
Cleveland, Ohio

PREFACE

Pediatric Nursing: Caring for Children and Their Families is a comprehensive text for undergraduate nursing students that approaches the topic of children's health care from a holistic and family-centered perspective. It provides a learner-oriented, visually attractive approach to understanding and retaining the vast amount of information required to become a safe and caring practitioner.

Caring for children and their families has always been challenging but has become increasingly more complex at the dawn of the 21st century. Technologic advances, reform in the delivery of health care, and efforts to control costs have greatly influenced the method and settings in which pediatric nursing care is provided. Hospital stays have shortened, acuity levels have increased, and more children are treated and cared for in settings other than acute care. A significant amount of care occurs in ambulatory, outpatient, and home settings. Increasing numbers of families are caring for children with complex health problems in their homes, therefore requiring families to be familiar with the caring and medical techniques their children need. Nursing educators must prepare students for these changes.

As the new century begins, many children and their families are still feeling the impact of poverty, drug abuse, the cycle of physical, emotional, and sexual abuse, and violence. To this we add the aftermath of terrorism in the United States and the sequelae it brings to the impressionable child.

Pediatric Nursing: Caring for Children and Their Families addresses these changes and realities with a perspective of children as evolving human beings in their family, home, school, community, country, and world. The contemporary social and cultural influences on children and their families is emphasized in addition to the more traditional areas of assessment, disease processes, and health promotion. Providing nursing care to children will be more effective when nursing students are aware of the pressures and problems confronting children and their families.

CONCEPTUAL APPROACH

The idea for this text arose from the authors' years of experience teaching nursing students and observing their difficulty with reading and comprehending greater amounts of content in shorter periods of time. A major goal of this text is to present the material in depth and breadth using simple-to-understand language as succinctly as possible. Additionally, each student has her or his own learning style. Some students require more than text to learn and assimilate what they read. Full-color pages, a visually appealing design, boxes that emphasize important points, and original photography engage the learner and create a reader-friendly approach.

The nursing process provides the organizational framework for the discussion of nursing care. Applicable nursing research has also been incorporated throughout the text to reflect the latest in evidence-based practice. The enhancement of student critical thinking skills is encouraged throughout. Emphasis on health and health promotion is reflected in comprehensive growth and development sections and in the alteration chapters. Anticipatory guidance is stressed throughout the text.

ORGANIZATION OF THE TEXT

Pediatric Nursing: Caring for Children and Their Families consists of 36 chapters, organized into 8 units. Each chapter has special features allowing the student to approach the content from a variety of perspectives. Specific information about these features is presented later in the preface.

Unit I: Pediatric Nursing in a Changing Society (Chapters 1 through 5) These five chapters introduce the student to pediatric nursing and set the stage for the remainder of the book. The first chapter discusses societal trends affecting children, their health, and their families, as well as the *Healthy People 2000, 2010*, and *Healthy Children 2000* documents and recent statistics relative to children's health. The various roles a nurse might accept as well as the diverse settings he or she might practice in relation to children and families are also covered. Chapter 2 describes legal and ethical issues nurses working with children and their families might face, including confidentiality. The third chapter provides information about the family and describes its significance to children. Family theories, assessment models, types, and forms are discussed in relation to their impact on individual members. The fourth and fifth chapters describe the pediatric nurses' role in the community, home, and school.

Unit II: Growth and Development of Children (Chapters 6 through 12) These seven chapters review theories of human development (Chapter 6) and discuss the major developmental milestones and characteristics of the newborn, infant, toddler, preschooler, school-aged child, and adolescent (Chapters 7, 8, 9, 10, 11, and 12). Each of these chapters has a summary table of important developmental indicators, as well as a discussion of the physiological, psychosexual, cognitive, psychosocial, and moral development occurring during that particular stage. Health promotion strategies are also presented that relate to nutrition, sleep, rest, activity, dental health, safety, and injury prevention. Also found is a discussion of health screenings for each age group.

Unit III: Unique Considerations in Children (Chapters 13 through 20) These eight chapters contain content that is unique in relation to caring for children rather than adults, and are devoted to discussing information needed to appropriately care for children and their families in a variety of settings. To provide a high level of care, the nurse needs to know how to communicate effectively with children and families (Chapter 13). Following communication are assessment strategies with normal and abnormal findings (Chapter 14), infectious diseases (Chapter 15), interaction with children who are ill or hospitalized (Chapter 16), and caring for children with chronic conditions (Chapter 17). Managing pain (Chapter 18) and administering medication (Chapter 19) are presented next. Caring for children experiencing loss and/or bereavement (Chapter 20) completes the unit.

Unit IV: Alterations in Nutrition and Elimination (Chapters 21 through 23) The body system alteration chapters in this unit as well as in the units to follow have a similar format. They describe the anatomy and physiology of the child's body system. The disorders discussed at length in each chapter are those that commonly occur or are frequently seen in the pediatric population. Although some alterations may also be seen in adults, the material is centered on information relevant to the child. For each disorder, the incidence, etiology, pathophysiology, clinical manifestations, diagnosis, treatment, nursing management, and family teaching are clearly presented. Nursing management for the most common disorders in each body system follows the five steps in the nursing process. All body system alteration chapters also have a case study scenario that introduces the student to real-life elements of the particular disorder, followed by the nursing process in care plan format, including assessment, nursing diagnosis, expected outcomes, interventions with rationales, and evaluation.

The chapters in this unit describe common pediatric physiological alterations related to nutrition and elimination. Chapter 21 presents fluid and electrolyte alterations, whereas Chapters 22 and 23 discuss genitourinary and gastrointestinal alterations, respectively. The unit organization is logically presented; one needs to have information about fluid and electrolyte imbalances and know what those imbalances mean before entertaining possible causes such as genitourinary (glomerulonephritis, nephrotic syndrome, renal failure) and gastrointestinal (gastroenteritis, pyloric stenosis, gastroesophageal reflux) alterations.

Unit V: Alterations in Oxygen Transport (Chapters 24 through 26) These three chapters cover respiratory, cardiovascular, and hematologic alterations frequently identified in children. Although presented separately, the three body systems are interrelated and dependent upon one another for oxygen transport. Alterations discussed include anemia, sickle cell disease (hematologic system); congenital cardiac anomalies, rheumatic fever, shock (cardiovascular system); and asthma, bronchiolitis, otitis (respiratory system).

Unit VI: Alterations in Protective Mechanisms (Chapters 27 through 30) These four chapters discuss alterations related to the immune system (HIV, rheumatoid arthritis, systemic lupus erythematosus), endocrine system (growth hormone deficiency, thyroid disorders, diabetes), and integumentary system (impetigo, tinea infections, pediculosis) that serve to protect the body from illness, as well as cellular alterations (childhood cancer) that may occur when there are problems in the body's ability to protect itself from illness or injury.

Unit VII: Alterations in Sensorimotor Function (Chapters 31 through 34) These four chapters discuss alterations related to the sensory system (hearing, sight), the neurological system (neural tube defects, meningitis, hydrocephalus, cerebral palsy), cognition (mental retardation, autism), and the musculoskeletal system (fractures, congenital hip dysplasia, scoliosis, muscular dystrophy).

Unit VIII: Other Alterations to Children's Health (Chapters 35 and 36) These final two chapters explain psychosocial alterations (attention deficit-hyperactivity disorder, depression, eating disorders) and child abuse and neglect (physical, psychological, and sexual abuse; abandonment).

Appendices: Eleven appendices augment *Pediatric Nursing: Caring for Children and Their Families.* They include a family assessment model, growth charts, the recommended childhood immunization schedule, recommended dietary allowances, the Denver II, sexual maturity ratings, pediatric cardiopulmonary resuscitation, common laboratory tests and normal values, temperature and weight conversions, NANDA diagnoses, and abbreviations.

SPECIAL FEATURES

- *Short vignettes*, written by a child or family member, promote thoughts from the client's perspective in every chapter.
- *Competencies*, found at the beginning of each chapter, introduce the main areas targeted for mastery and provide a checkpoint for study.
- *Family Teaching* sections, specific to each chapter, highlight the significance of keeping family members involved in the caring process and offer them the tools to continue the caring at home.
- *Nursing Management* sections provide the student with the information needed to successfully help the family manage a health alteration.
- *Case Study/Care Plans* are provided throughout the book to provide the student a glimpse of clinical situations and to walk them through a nursing plan of care.
- *Nursing Tips* help the student apply basic knowledge to practice by offering hints and shortcuts useful to both new and experienced nurses.
- *Nursing Alerts* highlight serious or life-threatening information that the nurse needs to be aware of.
- *Kids Want to Know* presents children's questions and suggested nursing responses to help the student consider children's needs, concerns, and fears.
- *Eye On* presents content in areas including complementary/alternative therapies; cultural, international, and spiritual perspectives; and new and controversial treatments related to chapter content.
- *Reflective Thinking* boxes encourage students to examine their own personal views on particular issues and understand the varying viewpoints they may encounter in clients and coworkers. These boxes encourage reflection on issues from a personal context, raise awareness of the diversity of opinions, and foster empowerment.
- *Critical Thinking* boxes stimulate the thought process, as students digest material related to the technical or clinical aspects of the chapter content.
- *Research Highlights* outline current research pertinent to pediatric clients and their families and stress the significance of evidence-based action by linking theory to practice. Systematic format promotes organized and focused student research.
- *Reflections from Families* are writings by the child or family member that encourage the nurse's understanding and sensitivity to the feelings of the clients in their care.
- *In the Real World* is found at the end of each chapter. Perspectives on nursing care from the viewpoint of the student or experienced practicing nurse are presented.
- *Key Concepts* highlight the main points of the chapter and are ideal to use as a starting point of study.
- *Review Questions* provide students with a way to self-assess their comprehension and retention of chapter material.

EXTENSIVE LEARNING PACKAGE FOR THE STUDENT

Pediatric Nursing Skills and Student Tutorial CD-ROM

Free with textbook package, this CD-ROM contains illustrated **pediatric nursing skills** for basic- and intermediate-level procedures to print out and use as a reference in clinical use or practice. The skills are presented in a step-by-step approach with rationale, equipment required, safety information, and documentation instruction. A highly interactive and enjoyable study tool, the CD-ROM also contains activities to learn terminology of pediatric nursing. The flashcard program tests level of knowledge, accuracy, and speed. It also has an option of one or two players for joint study.

Student Study Guide

(Order 0-8273-8150-6)

The *Student Study Guide to Accompany Pediatric Nursing: Caring for Children and Their Families* provides multiple choice, true-false, and fill-in questions, as well as case studies with critical thinking scenarios (answers appear at the end of the book).

The Pediatric Nurse's Survival Guide, 2nd edition by Lisa Rebeschi and Mary Brown

(Order 0-7668-4952-X)

This pocket-sized clinical guide provides necessary information in a convenient format. Information includes physical assessment hints, common childhood medications, drug administration, and tips to recognize and treat common childhood illnesses. It is an essential companion for the student and practicing nurse.

Online Resource

Go to *www.delmarnursing.com/olcs/potts* for author information, content updates, and text description.

EXTENSIVE TEACHING PACKAGE FOR THE INSTRUCTOR

Electronic Classroom Manager

(Order 0-7668-4547-8)

With everything an instructor needs to organize and run a class on pediatrics, this two-CD-ROM comprehensive resource includes:

Instructor's Manual

- Chapter competencies
- Key terms
- Instructional strategies for classroom use, including a detailed outline of each chapter
- Suggested answers to critical thinking and review questions found in the text

Computerized Testbank

The computerized testbank contains approximately 2,000 multiple choice questions and answers. The instructor can also add his or her own questions or let the software create tests in less than 5 minutes. Instructors can print out quizzes and tests in a variety of layouts. Innovative electronic "take-home testing" (put test on disk) and Internet-based testing capabilities are perfect for distance learning. Additionally, the software allows the user to include video or audio in the electronic tests.

PowerPoint Presentation

A vital resource for instructors, this PowerPoint presentation parallels the content found in the book and serves as a foundation on which instructors may customize their own unique presentations.

Image Library

The Image Library is a software tool that includes an organized digital resource of approximately 600 illustrations and photographs from the text. A Microsoft Windows 3.1 and Windows 95 application, it can be used with the most common graphics file formats (BMP, TIFF, GIF). This software also allows instructors to add new images.

With the Image Library you can:

- Sort art by desired categories
- Create hyperlinks in PowerPoint that point to images or collections in the Image Library
- Create additional libraries
- Print selected pieces

The Image Library works in combination with:

- Microsoft PowerPoint for Windows 95, version 7.0 and higher
- Other Delmar image collections

Conversion Grids

Changing your class notes from a competitor's text to *Pediatric Nursing: Caring for Children and Their Families* is made simple with our conversion grids. All the work has been done in advance, including page number references, to save you valuable time and energy. These grids can be found at our Online Resource: *www.delmarnursing.com/olcs/potts*.

Online Resource

Go to *www.delmarnursing.com/olcs/potts* for author information, content updates, and conversion grids.

ACKNOWLEDGMENTS

The creation of this textbook represents the efforts of many knowledgeable, hard-working, and dedicated individuals who supported us. First and foremost, I *(Nicki Potts)* want to thank my husband, Stan, and my daughter, Jennifer, for their encouragement, support, and sacrifices during the years required to complete this project. Stan stood by me and never failed in his loyalty and dedication; thanks for always being there. You graciously took on the responsibilities of rearing our daughter and managing our household when I was absorbed in this book. Jennifer has grown up with her mother in school or writing, among other things, a doctoral program and dissertation, then this textbook. When it is published, she will be 18 years old; she was 12 when this adventure started. Jennifer, I could not have survived this project without your smiles, hugs, and kisses. You are the light of my life.—Nicki

Many individuals are responsible for the completion of this book. Initially, I *(Barbara Mandleco)* express deep appreciation and gratitude to Dr. Elaine Sorenson Marshall, colleague, dear friend, and dean of Brigham Young University College of Nursing. Not only did Elaine provide me the support and assistance needed to pursue this project, but her genuine interest and concern motivated and encouraged my efforts. I also thank my faculty colleagues, who were a frequent source of support and help, and my secretary, Wendy Berry, who was always there to check references and resources as well as retype edited chapters, sometimes at the shortest notice. Most importantly, I wish to express sincere thanks and gratitude to my husband, Carl, our children, Luke and Sarah, and their spouses, Christine and Chad. Without their devotion, patience, understanding, love, and support, I would not have been able to complete this project.—Barbara

Delmar has provided us with its best in Beth Williams and Marah Bellegarde, our developmental editors. Beth was there at the beginning, helping us crystalize our ideas and clarify the chapter format. Her knowledge, attention to details, and resources were invaluable. With her help, we were able to get this project up and running. Marah has taken us to completion. She was encouraging, supportive, and prodded us when we were not sure we could complete the daunting task of producing a textbook. She urged us on when our energies and motivation flagged. Her weekly repetition of "you're almost finished" kept us going, and we thank her for that. She obtained artwork and often clarified what we had written on short notice. Without her the book would not be the high quality that it is. A heartfelt thank you to Shelley Esposito for her assistance with procuring permissions. Kudos to the production and technology staff at Delmar including David Buddle, Anne Sherman, Jay Purcell, Sherry McGaughan, Laurie Davis, and Joe Saba and to the staff of Argosy.

We acknowledge and thank Primary Children's Medical Center in Salt Lake City, Utah, for allowing us to take photographs of children receiving care. We are grateful to Bonnie Midget, from PCMC Public Relations, for arranging and coordinating these photo sessions. We sincerely thank you, Bonnie, for your assistance. We would also like to extend our gratitude to the children and families who participated in the photo shoots.

A textbook of this magnitude, depth, and breadth would not be possible without the expertise of contributing authors. They have shared their ideas and expert knowledge. We especially thank them for their perseverance and willingness when more work and rewriting was required as the book evolved. Their professional experience and standards of excellence are reflected in the chapters they researched, wrote, and revised.—Nicki and Barbara

ABOUT THE AUTHORS

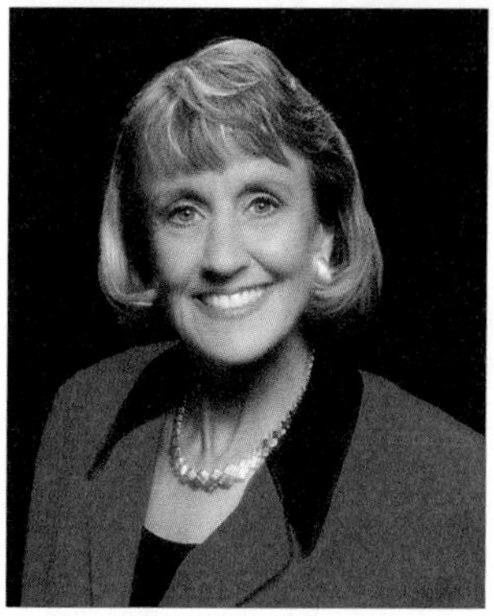

Nicki Lee Warren Potts

Nicki Lee Warren Potts is a second-generation registered nurse who earned her bachelor of science in nursing from Texas Christian University, Fort Worth, Texas. She first practiced her profession as an assistant head nurse in medical surgical nursing and public health nursing, and she discovered her true passion in nursing education in Nashville at Tennessee State University. She continued her preparation for a career in education by obtaining a master of science in nursing from the University of Texas at Austin's College of Nursing. Texas Woman's University College of Nursing conferred her doctor of philosophy in nursing research and theory.

With over 30 years as a clinician and academician, Dr. Potts has taught psychiatric/mental health nursing and pediatric nursing in associate degree and baccalaureate schools of nursing. The majority of her teaching career has been at Texas Woman's University in Houston, Texas; the University of New Mexico in Albuquerque, New Mexico; the University of Texas in Arlington, Texas; and the University of Texas in Austin, Texas. Other areas of professional experience include Assistant Director for Education, Texas Nurse's Association, and Nursing Consultant for Advanced Practice at the Board of Nurse Examiners for the State of Texas.

Dr. Potts's professional development and contributions are well documented at the local and national levels. She has delivered numerous presentations throughout the country based on her special interest and research in females with eating disorders. She is a member of Sigma Theta Tau, Society of Pediatric Nurses, American Nurses Association, Texas Nurses Association, and the Southern Nursing Research Society. Dr. Potts has numerous journal, textbook, and abstract publications to her credit.

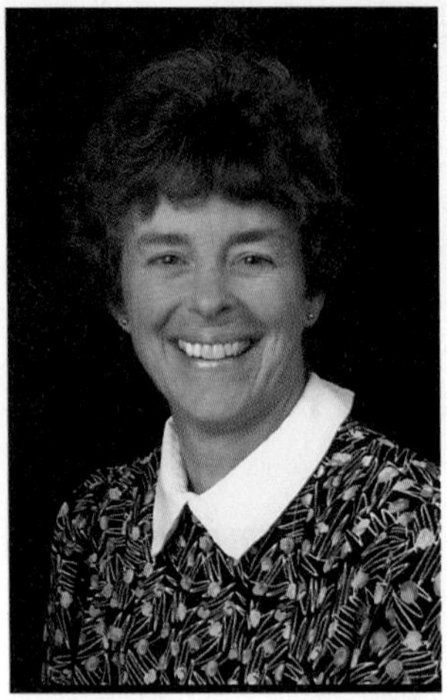

Barbara Hartwig Mandleco

Barbara Hartwig Mandleco received her bachelor of science degree in nursing from the University of Wisconsin–Madison, her master's degree in pediatric nursing from the University of Florida–Gainesville, and her doctor of philosophy in family sciences with an emphasis in human development from Brigham Young University. She has been a staff nurse on pediatric and adult medical surgical nursing units, and a nursing educator for over 30 years. She has taught advanced human development and pediatric nursing, fundamentals of nursing, nursing research, and family nursing to undergraduate and graduate students at the University of Utah and Brigham Young University Colleges of Nursing. Currently, Dr. Mandleco is an associate professor and associate dean for research and scholarship at Brigham Young University College of Nursing.

Dr. Mandleco is a member of Sigma Theta Tau International, the Utah Nurses Association, the American Nurses Association, the Western Institute of Nursing, the Western Academy of Nursing, the American Nurses Foundation, Phi Kappa Phi, Sigma Xi, and the National Council on Family Relations. She has served as an officer locally and nationally in Sigma Theta Tau International and the National Council on Family Relations. She currently serves as abstract and collateral reviewer (grants, scientific sessions, podium presentations) for Sigma Theta Tau International and the National Council on Family Relations, as a manuscript reviewer for *MCN (Maternal Child Nursing)*, the *Journal of Family Nursing*, and the *Journal of Nursing Scholarship*, and is a program evaluator for the CCNE.

Dr. Mandleco has given numerous professional presentations at the local, regional, national, and international levels, and published in several peer-reviewed journals. She also has written several book chapters and was co-author of a pediatric nursing student study guide published in the 1980s. Her research interests include families adapting to a child with a special need or chronic illness, children's resilience, social development and family processes, and developing innovative methods of teaching.

HOW TO USE THIS TEXT

The following are suggestions on how you can use the features of this text to gain competence and confidence in nursing practice of pediatric clients and their families.

SHORT VIGNETTES

Read these short stories before your begin to read a chapter to gain perspective of the feelings of the child and family. Once you have completed the chapter, go back and re-read the story. Ask yourself if you have a better comprehension and sensitivity of how the child and family feel.

Mama has been sad since my baby sister died. It has been hard for me and my brother, Will, too. Our daddy left us when Mama told him she was going to have another baby. Mama had to work real hard at her job to take care of us then. She tried to get us food stamps, but they said no because she had her job. Her job didn't have insurance, so she couldn't go to the doctor about the baby. She got real tired and sick a lot. When my baby sister came, she was very small and wasn't very strong. They kept her in the baby intensive care at the hospital for two weeks, but then she died. Mama is too sick to go back to work now, and she thinks it is her fault the baby died. When I grow up, I am going to be a doctor and help take care of mamas and their babies, so they can get stronger. I miss my baby sister so much too.

COMPETENCIES

Read the chapter competencies before reading the chapter content to set the stage for learning. Return to the competencies when the chapter study is complete to see which entries you can respond with, "Yes, I can do that."

COMPETENCIES

Upon completion of this chapter, the reader will be able to:

- *Identify differences among adults, children, and infants related to fluid requirements, fluid therapy, and electrolytes.*
- *Calculate daily maintenance fluid requirements for children of various ages.*
- *Explain the principles of acid-base imbalances.*
- *Explain the causes and clinical manifestations of the four major types of acid-base imbalances.*
- *Compare mild, moderate, and severe dehydration.*
- *Describe the treatment of the child with gastroenteritis based on the degree of dehydration.*
- *Discuss common types of burn injuries in children and their prevention.*
- *Describe the treatment and nursing management of the child with a major burn injury.*

CASE STUDY/CARE PLANS

Walk through the process of assessment, diagnosis, planning care, performing interventions, and evaluating the success of the course of care. These are helpful in strengthening the understanding of the nursing process through a case study approach and in exercising critical thinking skills.

Case Study/Care Plan

Infant with Surgical Repair of Ventricular Septal Defect

Jack is an eight-month-old infant who was noted to have a murmur at two months of age. He was not cyanotic, he fed well, and was gaining weight appropriately. Echocardiogram demonstrated a large VSD, CXR showed cardiomegaly and increased pulmonary blood flow, and ECG demonstrated ventricular hypertrophy. Over the ensuing couple of months he developed tachypnea, retractions, diaphoresis, poor feeding, and poor weight gain. His physical exam and CXR were consistent with congestive heart failure. He was placed on lasix, aldactone, and digoxin. In addition caloric density of his formula was slowly increased to 30 cal/oz. Nighttime continuous feedings were implemented so that his total caloric intake was 150 cal/kg/day. In spite of these interventions he did not gain weight, and his symptoms were only moderately controlled, so captopril was added. The decision to close his VSD was made.

He underwent patch closure of his VSD; the surgery went well without complications. He was in the PICU for three days after which he was transferred to a pediatric unit.

Nursing Care Plan

Assessment Accurate and frequent ongoing assessment of the cardiovascular system in the postoperative child is an essential part of care. Nurses should monitor for signs of decreased cardiac output such as tachycardia, poor perfusion, mottling of the skin, decreased or absent distal pulses, and poor urine output. Listen to the child's heart sounds to note changes in heart tones or murmurs. Assess the rhythm strip for arrhythmias.

Nurses should auscultate breath sounds bilaterally. Listen to the quality of the breath sounds; listen for rales, coarse rhonchi. Observe the child's color and work of breathing either spontaneously or while on mechanical ventilation. Monitor for tachypnea, retractions, and nasal flaring. Monitor oxygen saturations, keeping in mind the child's anatomy. It is essential that the nurse understand the surgical repair and the expected norm for each defect. When the child has awakened from anesthesia, the nurse assesses the neurologic function by noting equal movement of all extremities, absence of any signs of seizures, and pupillary function. Pain in the nonverbal child is expressed by an increase in heart rate and blood pressure and by grimacing and crying. Older children can convey their degree of pain by verbalization or through the use of one of the multiple pain scores and charts available to nurses. Refer to Chapter 18 for more information about pain assessment.

Many cardiac repairs involve multiple suture lines in and around a very small heart. These sutures combined with the destruction of platelets secondary to cardiopulmonary bypass can lead to excessive bleeding in the postoperative period. The child is monitored for signs of bleeding from surgical incisions and intravenous insertion sites.

Nursing Diagnosis #1

Ineffective breathing pattern related to pulmonary edema, pleural effusions, poor respiratory effort, atelectasis and/or phrenic nerve damage, as indicated by prolonged intubation, tachypnea, increased work of breathing.

Expected Outcomes

1. Child will have adequate respiratory function as evidenced by respiratory rate normal for age and comfortable respiratory pattern.
2. Child will have no increased work of breathing.

Interventions/*Rationales*

1. Provide analgesia and sedation. *A child who is in pain related to a sternal or thoracotomy incision is unlikely to take deep breaths.*
2. Frequently reassess breath sounds. *Unequal aeration may signal pleural effusion, pneumothorax, or damage to the phrenic nerve.*
3. Obtain chest X-ray as ordered. *To evaluate for presence of pneumothorax or pleural effusion.*
4. Administer scheduled diuretics. *To prevent interstitial fluid from accumulating in the lungs.*
5. Provide good pulmonary toilet (i.e., deep breathing, coughing, head of bed elevated, early ambulation) to prevent atelectasis. *Will assist in establishing good respiratory function.*
6. Provide supplemental oxygen as needed. *To maintain oxygen saturations in desired range.*
7. Obtain arterial blood gases as ordered. *To evaluate for CO_2 retention and hypoxia.*

Evaluation

Supplemental oxygen is weaned over the expected time period. Oxygen saturations are within normal limits for child's physiology. There is no increased work of breathing, and arterial blood gases are within normal limits.

NURSING TIPS

In any profession there are many helpful hints that can assist you to perform more efficiently. In nursing, you need to be able to practice sensitivity in the process. The wide variety of hints, tips, and strategies presented here help as you work toward professional advancement. Study, share, and discuss with your fellow students.

Nursing Tip:

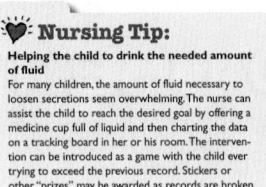

Helping the child to drink the needed amount of fluid

For many children, the amount of fluid necessary to loosen secretions seem overwhelming. The nurse can assist the child to reach the desired goal by offering a medicine cup full of liquid and then charting the data on a tracking board in her or his room. The intervention can be introduced as a game with the child ever trying to exceed the previous record. Stickers or other "prizes" may be awarded as records are broken.

NURSING ALERTS

As a professional, you will need to be able to react immediately in some situations to ensure the health and safety of your clients. Pay careful attention to this feature, as it helps you to begin to identify and effectively respond to critical situations on your own.

Nursing Alert:

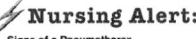

Signs of a Pneumothorax

A pneumothorax is suspected if a child with CF experiences acute signs of respiratory distress such as tachypnea, tachycardia, dyspnea, and pallor or cyanosis.

KIDS WANT TO KNOW

This feature is designed to enhance the communication between you and the pediatric client, since responses to children's questions about care may differ from those given to adults. Read the questions that have been posed by children and think about what your response would be. Then go ahead and read the suggested nursing responses. Ask yourself, "How do mine compare with the suggested answers?" Would you alter your response based on the suggested responses? Was your response developmentally appropriate for the child?

Kids Want To Know

Do I really have to check my blood sugars so often?

The 10-year-old child you are caring for has been diagnosed with type 1 diabetes and is preparing to be discharged home. In preparing for her discharge, she asks "Do I really have to check my blood sugars so often? Can't I just test them in the morning and then test my urine the rest of the day? Every time I test, it hurts so much!"

A child of 10 has not developed an abstract cognitive thought process and may not understand the relationship between the blood glucose testing and the ongoing evaluation of the success of diabetes management. Additionally, blood glucose testing does require a small lancing of the skin, which can be uncomfortable. Review with her the techniques for doing less painful blood testing, using the sides of her upper fingers, not the tips or the pads, or using a meter that allows for less painful testing sites like the forearm. Reassure her that over the next several weeks, the discomfort will ease a bit as her fingers become slightly callused.

EYE ON

Throughout your nursing practice, you are going to be exposed to a myriad of cultures, beliefs, and value systems. Read the information found in this feature to get extra information on various issues. Those presented will include complementary and alternative therapies; cultural, spiritual, and international perspectives; and new and controversial treatments. After you have completed the readings, consider how you feel about the topic discussed. How can you incorporate this information into your nursing care?

Eye On:

Health care providers also need to be sensitive to cultural and ethnic variations when comparing children to preestablished norms. For instance, attention should be given to the height/weight assessment of Asian children. A single evaluation of a child of Asian ancestry, compared to standard U.S. Caucasian norms, may lead to an inaccurate judgment that the child is short in stature or malnourished for age, when actually this should be attributed to genetic makeup.

REFLECTIVE THINKING

This feature can help you to develop or enhance sensitivity to ethical and moral issues. You may choose to read through each one and explore issues before reading the chapter. After reading through the chapter, re-address each Reflective Thinking item and evaluate your original thoughts. If you choose to read them as you go through the chapter, perhaps write your thoughts down to look at them at a later time.

Reflective Thinking

Jumping the Gun

Active listening takes conscious effort, time, and practice. When nurses listen, they are able to convey in their own words what children and their caregivers have said and the feelings that were expressed. If nurses construct responses before children or caregivers finish speaking, or answer questions while they are being asked, listening isn't occurring. Can you in your own words express the thoughts and feelings of the children and caregivers? If you cannot, you are not listening. Evaluate yourself. How well do you listen?

CRITICAL THINKING

This feature is designed to guide you to think analytically in clinical situations and be active in problem solving. As you go through the chapters, consider the questions posed and provide answers. Discuss your answers with other students to promote the exchange of ideas.

Critical Thinking

A Toddler Who Is Immobilized

Andrew, a healthy, active child of 20 months, has been admitted to the hospital and is placed in traction for treatment of a fractured femur. A hip spica cast will be applied within a few days, and a clinical pathway has been determined regarding care in traction, care after the cast is applied, and discharge instructions. He is the youngest of four children and is rarely cared for by adults other than parents. His mother plans to stay with him throughout the hospital stay except for brief periods of a few hours each day.

What kind of assessment data at the time of admission would assist the nurse in understanding the effects of this child's experience on the child and family? What strengths of a child of this age would facilitate coping? What strengths of the family would facilitate coping?

What are ways of helping this child to manage immobility, diminished control, and brief separations?

RESEARCH HIGHLIGHT

This feature emphasizes the importance of clinical research in nursing by linking findings to practice. This useful learning tool focuses attention on current issues and trends in nursing, stresses the significance of evidence-based practice, and illustrates the correct way to write an abstract for a research project.

Research Highlight

Children and Families Affected by HIV/AIDS

Study Purpose

To explore goals and the strategies families use to reach these goals when raising a child with HIV.

Methods

This ethnographic study used semi-structured and open-ended interviews. Five uninfected adult family member caregivers, nine children between 7 and 15 who were diagnosed with HIV infection, and six mothers and one father with HIV infection participated. Families were asked to talk about their family composition, symptom management, and how they disclosed information about the disease to others.

Findings

The three goals that helped families maintain stability and establish normalcy included (1) facilitating their child's participation in social and school activities, (2) staying healthy, and (3) enhancing emotional and social well-being of family members. Strategies included a balanced diet and exercise, active participation in treatment, juggling multiple responsibilities so they could care for family members, allowing and encouraging children to attend and participate in school activities, being selective about disclosing information about the infection to those outside the family group, so their children would be treated normally, having other family members help care for the child, having spiritual and religious beliefs and practices, and using supportive professionals.

Implications

Nurses should (1) be aware that families might limit information they share with others about their child's illness, (2) encourage children and families to establish goals and strategies that will help them achieve their goals, and (3) help parents raising children with HIV/AIDS realize most families impacted by chronic illness such as HIV/AIDS are able to set and meet their goals of living a "normal" life.

Citation

Rehm, R., & Franck, L. (2000). Long-term goals and normalization strategies of children and families affected by HIV/AIDS. *Advances in Nursing Science, 23*, 69–82.

REFLECTIONS FROM FAMILIES

Read these as glimpses into a family's mindset and feelings about the loved one in your care before reading the chapter. After you have finished the chapter, go back and revisit your own feelings. Consider if your feelings have changed and examine why.

REFLECTIONS FROM FAMILIES

Having a seven-year-old child who moves around slowly and painfully is heartbreaking. Arthritis always seemed like something you get when you are old. Emily had not been able to jump rope, play tag,, or swing on the swing set. She was sad and angry. The doctors put her on ibuprofen. I can't believe what a difference putting Emily on ibuprofen has made. Now after taking her morning dose, she is able to be much more active and can join her friends in their play. A normal childhood is what I pray for every day.

IN THE REAL WORLD

These short musings from the student or professional nurse are intended to provide a snapshot of actual practice. They are included as a reality check as you read through the text. It may be helpful for you to keep a running journal of your own experiences—Did a certain child and family affect you in some way? Did you work with a practicing pediatric nurse who is a wonderful mentor? Journal writing is a good way to begin to examine your own responses and provide other aspiring nurses the wisdom of your experiences.

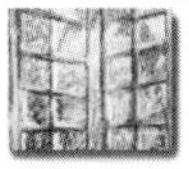

In the Real World

This past week I cared for 16-year-old Morgan, who had had a ureteral resection. Rebecca (the other nurse) and I and spoke with him frankly about procedures, care plans, and equipment. At one point I explained how a pulse oximeter worked to measure oxygen-carrying productivity. This 6-foot, 90-kg young man did not need to be babied, but he did need to be respected and supported in his recovery. Recognizing adolescents' general desire for privacy and sensitivity about anatomy, I tried to keep him well-covered and work as professionally as possible. Morgan was appreciative, polite, and cooperative.

KEY CONCEPTS

Review these main points of the chapter and use them for a beginning point of study and review.

Key Concepts

- The function of the immune system is to prevent or ameliorate infections, recognize self from nonself, and maintain homeostasis.
- Immune system alterations are almost always chronic illnesses that are managed rather than cured; health care is best delivered by a multidisciplinary team.
- Immune system dysfunction demonstrates a wide variety of clinical manifestations not confined to the immune system.
- Juvenile rheumatoid arthritis, an autoimmune disorder involving joints and occasionally the eyes or heart, affects mobility and activities of daily living and has multiple psychosocial consequences.
- Systemic lupus erythematosus, a lifelong autoimmune disorder characterized by multiple system involvement, requires a delicate balance between symptoms of the disease, side effects of medication and treatment, and psychosocial aspects of both.
- HIV/AIDS is an infectious disease known for affecting primarily the immune system, but demonstrates multiple clinical manifestations directly related to its multiorgan system involvement.
- Drug reactions may vary from a mild rash to a serious systemic reaction.
- Nursing care of children with immune system alterations involves knowing about the etiology, treatment, medications, management, and educational needs of children and their families.

REVIEW QUESTIONS

Review questions in each chapter assist you with the learning process and help you assimilate the information presented in the text.

Review Questions

1. Describe a feedback loop system characteristic of an endocrine system.
2. Discuss the relationship between the clinical manifestations and pathophysiology of diabetes insipidus.
3. Describe the impact of neonatal screening on congenital hypothyroidism.
4. Differentiate the symptoms of hypothyroidism and hyperthyroidism.
5. List the clinical manifestations of type 1 diabetes.
6. Identify the clinical manifestations of diabetic ketoacidosis (DKA).
7. What is the most serious complication of the treatment of DKA?
8. Describe the difference in time action of Lispro, Regular, NPH, and Ultra Lente insulin.
9. Differentiate the symptoms of hypoglycemia and hyperglycemia.
10. Differentiate the diagnosis of type 1 diabetes from type 2 diabetes.

UNIT I

Pediatric Nursing in a Changing Society

CHAPTER 1

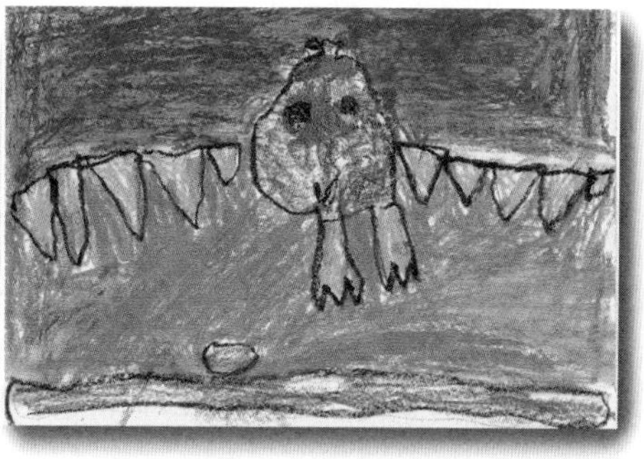

Mama has been sad since my baby sister died. It has been hard for me and my brother, Will, too. Our daddy left us when Mama told him she was going to have another baby. Mama had to work real hard at her job to take care of us then. She tried to get us food stamps, but they said no because she had her job. Her job didn't have insurance, so she couldn't go to the doctor about the baby. She got real tired and sick a lot. When my baby sister came, she was very small and wasn't very strong. They kept her in the baby intensive care at the hospital for two weeks, but then she died. Mama is too sick to go back to work now, and she thinks it is her fault the baby died. When I grow up, I am going to be a doctor and help take care of mamas and their babies, so they can get stronger. I miss my baby sister so much too.

OVERVIEW OF PEDIATRIC NURSING

Nicki L. Potts, PhD, RN
Barbara L. Mandleco, PhD, RN

COMPETENCIES

Upon completion of this chapter, the reader will be able to:

- *Discuss current societal trends and describe their influence on children in the United States.*
- *Identify the effects of immigration, poverty, homelessness, migrant farm work, and violence on children and their health.*
- *Discuss the current status of children's physical and social health.*
- *Identify five strategies to prevent unintentional childhood injuries.*
- *Discuss the effects of problems with access to health care and lack of health insurance on children's health status.*
- *Identify elements of family-centered care.*
- *Discuss the influence of professional standards on pediatric nursing.*
- *Describe and discuss the importance of each role of the pediatric nurse.*

During the 20th century, amazing progress has been made in scientific and technological fields. The genetic code has been discovered, people are living longer than ever before, and very low birth weight infants have survived. However, the status of children and their health has not kept pace with these accomplishments. For example, one in two children live in a single parent family at some point in their childhood; one in three is a year or more behind in school; one in eight is born to a teenage mother; and one in 60 sees his or her parents divorce in any given year (Children's Defense Fund, 2000). Box 1-1 and Table 1-1 provide a view of the reality for American children today.

On the positive side, child health care has changed from a strictly curative approach to a disease prevention and health promotion model. The role of the pediatric nurse has expanded from child caretaker to child advocate. Today, pediatric nursing focuses on preventing acute and chronic illness while promoting normal growth and development. This focus requires a broad knowledge base consisting of an understanding of the culture at large, a host of health and illness issues, and a wide range of clinical competencies.

This chapter begins with an overview of social changes as they affect children. It describes the status of children's health, their health problems, and their care. The focus of the chapter then turns to a discussion of the roles of pediatric nurses and concludes with a discussion of differentiated practice roles and advanced practice.

BOX 1-1 Children's Defense Fund: Key facts on youth 2000 in the U.S.

- In 1997, firearms killed 4,205 children age 19 and under; of these, 2,562 were murdered, 1,262 committed suicide, and 306 were victims of accidental shootings.
- In 1997, there were approximately 984,000 confirmed victims of maltreatment (physical abuse, neglect, sexual abuse, medical neglect, psychosocial abuse, other abuses); three-fourths of the perpetrators of child maltreatment were parents; an additional one-tenth were relatives.
- In 1998, 5.4 million children lived in households headed by a relative other than a parent.
- In 1999, 1.2 million children (one in six) were poor; of these, 33.1% were African American; 30.3% were Hispanic; 13.5% were Caucasian; and 11.8% were Asian and Pacific Islanders.
- In 1999, 10.8 million children 18 and under lacked health coverage; of these, 4.4 million were Caucasian; 3.4 million were African American; and 2.1 million were Hispanic.
- In 1999, an estimated 547,000 children were in foster care; of these, 117,000 were waiting for permanent adoptive families.

Children's Defense Fund. (2000). *The state of America's children yearbook.* Washington, DC: Author.

TABLE 1-1 Moments in America for All Children

Time Frame	Experience
Every 1 second	A public high school student is suspended*
Every 9 seconds	A high school student drops out*
Every 10 seconds	A public school student is corporally punished*
Every 17 seconds	A child is arrested
Every 37 seconds	A baby is born to a mother who is not a high school graduate
Every 56 seconds	A baby is born into poverty
Every 1 minute	A baby is born to a teen mother
Every 2 minutes	A baby is born at low birth weight (less than 5 lbs., 8 oz.)
Every 4 minutes	A baby is born to a mother who had late or no prenatal care; a child is arrested for drug abuse
Every 7 minutes	A child is arrested for a violent crime
Every 10 minutes	A baby is born at very low birth weight (less than 3 lbs., 4 oz.)
Every 19 minutes	A baby dies
Every 41 minutes	A child or youth under 20 dies from an accident
Every 2 hours	A child or youth under 20 is killed by a firearm or is a homicide victim
Every 4 hours	A child or youth under 20 commits suicide
Every 19 hours	A young person under 25 dies from HIV infection

** Based on calculations per school day (180 days; 7 hours/day).*

Children's Defense Fund. (2000). The state of America's children yearbook. *Washington, DC: Author.*

SOCIETAL TRENDS IMPACTING CHILDREN

Children are members of families, communities, populations, and overall society, which shapes the context, experiences, and opportunities of their lives. Their well-being is inextricably linked to the well-being of their families, communities, and the society in which they live. In a world that is continually changing, emergent societal trends have profound effects on the environment surrounding children and their families, and now pose formidable challenges to children, their families, and their health. These trends include immigration, poverty, homelessness, migrant farm workers, and violence.

Immigration

Currently in the United States, one in five children under the age of 18 (14 million) is either an immigrant or a member of an immigrant family (Children's Defense Fund, 2000). The reasons that people are coming to the United States are many: freedom, economic opportunity, political asylum, graduate education, specialized medical care, or to give birth to an infant in the United States, thereby granting the child automatic citizenship. Sometimes these children are welcomed into well-functioning communities, and many become valuable members of society. However, they face many challenges related to health status and education, because they often have difficulty speaking English. This lack of skill in English has a direct impact upon their educational attainment, economic viability, and ability to enter the mainstream of U.S. society.

With each new wave of immigrants comes debate about whether they contribute to the economy or create a drain on public and private resources. Concerns also include perceived threats to the public health and order from infectious diseases, increased crime, and diverse social mores (American Academy of Pediatrics [AAP] Committee on Community Health Services, 1997). These debates have raised the issue of eligibility of immigrants for health, educational, and social services. Some have argued that this group should not be entitled to any local, state, or federal benefits. States that have a large number of immigrants (California, Texas, Florida) have proposed removing eligibility for these services. Opponents of these efforts counter that denying children access to services is unwise public policy. For example, in health care, denial of preventive services such as prenatal and dental care and immunizations eventually results in spiraling costs for emergency medical services (for which immigrants are eligible).

The health status of immigrant children can be compromised due to intestinal parasites, poor diets, dental problems, tuberculosis, hepatitis A, hepatitis B (particularly in those children from Southeast Asia), and other conditions originating in their country of origin (Worley, Worley, & Kumar, 2000). They are also at risk because of significant language, cultural, financial, and legal barriers to receiving health care. Their families often delay seeking care for minor conditions until they become more serious. Another factor affecting their underutilization of health services is the possibility that family members may have different immigration statuses. When one member is an illegal (undocumented) immigrant, the entire family may limit access to care for fear of an investigation (AAP, 1997).

The immigrant population's access to health care services also affects their psychological well-being. For many children and their families, the immigration process poses unique stresses. Individuals may be torn by conflicting social and cultural demands while trying to adapt to an unfamiliar environment. Other stresses include differences between social and economic status in their country of origin and the United States, separation from support systems, and, for illegal immigrants, fear of deportation (Hulewat, 1996).

Poverty

Families are classified as being in poverty if their annual income falls below official poverty thresholds (Table 1-2). In 1999, the poverty rate for all Americans was 11.8%, the lowest rate since 1979. For children under age 18, the poverty rate was 16.9%, again the lowest rate since 1979 (U.S. Census Bureau, 2000). Although the rates have improved, one in five children still lives in poverty. Rates of poverty, including childhood poverty, are highest for minority groups. However, the majority of poor children are white because whites are the largest population group in the United States (Children's Defense Fund, 2000).

Family structure has an important bearing on child poverty. Poverty rates for children in married couple families are much lower than for those in families headed by a single parent. The explanation for this fact is that when both spouses are present, there are two potential (and, frequently, actual) breadwinners. Almost half of all poor children live in single parent households. The risk of poverty in these households is high for several reasons, including low wages for women, the low educational attainment of many single mothers, and low rates and levels of child support from fathers (McLoyd, 1998).

Several factors are at the root of child poverty. Slow growth in wages, the rising inequality in earnings, significant loss of low-skill, high-wage jobs due to a decline in manufacturing industries, and workers' lack of education and skills account for much of the increase in child poverty in recent years. In the past two decades, average earnings have not

TABLE 1-2 Preliminary Estimates of the U.S. Poverty Threshold for 2000

Size of Family Unit	Estimated Threshold
1 person	$8,787
2 people	$11, 234
3 people	$13,737
4 people	$17,601
5 people	$20,804

U.S. Census Bureau. (2000). Preliminary estimates of poverty threshold for 2000 *[On-line]. Available: http://www.census.gov/hhes/poverty/ threshld/00prelim.html*

grown much. At the same time, there has been an increase in the inequality of earnings among workers. Today, the top 5% of American families make nearly 20 times the average income of the bottom 20% of families (Betson & Michael, 1997). This gap is the widest it has been in the 52 years for which annual income statistics exist (Children's Defense Fund, 2000). Educational level is an indicator of market skills that yield higher earnings. The education of the adults in the family is critical for the family income. As education rises, the number of adults who are not in the labor force and who experience a period of unemployment during the year declines dramatically.

Family income also has significant effects on the well-being of children and adolescents. Poor children are at greatest risk for the physical, social, and emotional effects of living in poverty (Sidel, 1996) (Figure 1-1). Some of the effects of living in poverty are listed in Figure 1-2. Compared with nonpoor children, poor children experience diminished physical health. They have higher than average rates of death and illness from almost all causes except suicide and motor vehicle accidents, which are most common among white, nonpoor children (Behrman, 1996). They also have a higher prevalence of illnesses such as asthma, respiratory infections, anemia, and gastrointestinal infections. Infant mortality rate is closely linked to poverty, and children born to poor families are at great risk of infant death (Annie Casey Foundation, 2000). Deficits in children's nutritional status are associated with poverty. Stunted growth (low height for age), a measure of nutritional status, is more prevalent among poor than nonpoor children (Brooks-Gunn & Duncan, 1997).

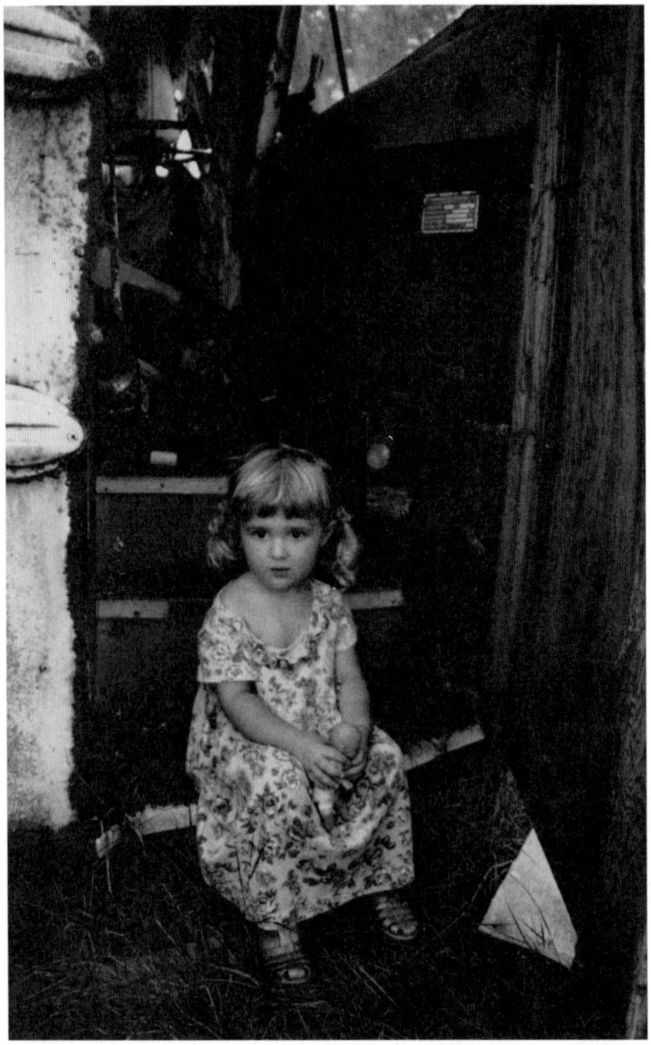

Figure 1-1 Poor children are at greatest risk for the physical, social, and emotional effects of living in poverty. Source: Photodisc.

Poverty also affects children's cognitive abilities and achievement. A child's poverty status at 3 years of age predicts the child's IQ at age 5, and persistent poverty has more adverse effects on a child's cognitive functioning than transitory poverty. In addition, children from lower socioeconomic status perform less well than nonpoor children and middle class children on test scores, grade retention, course failures, placement in special education, high school graduation rates, high school drop-out rates, and the completed numbers of years of schooling. School achievement also declines with the time spent in poverty, and the chance a child will be retained in a grade or placed in special education increases 2%–3% for every year that the child lives in poverty. In fact, long-term poverty is associated with deficits in verbal, mathematical, and reading skills that are two to three times greater than those associated with current poverty status. Poverty also affects a child depending on when, during the child's life, poverty is experienced; poverty during the first five years of life will affect the completed years of schooling more than if poverty occurs during middle childhood and adolescence (Brooks-Gunn & Duncan, 1997; McLoyd, 1998).

There is a higher prevalence of emotional and behavioral problems (e.g., externalizing, internalizing) among poor and low socioeconomic status children and adolescents than among children from families where there is higher income. The externalizing behavior problems include disobedience, fighting, difficulty getting along with others, and impulsivity, which become more prevalent the longer the children live in poverty. The internalizing behavior problems include anxiety, sadness-depression, and dependency (Brooks-Gunn & Duncan 1997; McLoyd, 1998).

Homelessness

An increasing number of children and families in all communities in the United States are homeless. Traditionally, the homeless population has been composed of single adults, mostly men. However, families with children are the fastest growing segment of the homeless population, accounting for more than one-third (Weinreb, Goldberg, Bassuk, & Perloff, 1998). Today, homeless families generally are headed by women with two or three children. Although

Low-income children are:

- Two times more likely than other children to die from accidents.
- Three times more likely to die from all causes combined.
- Four times more likely to die from fires.
- Five times more likely to die from infectious diseases and parasites.
- Six times more likely to die from other diseases.

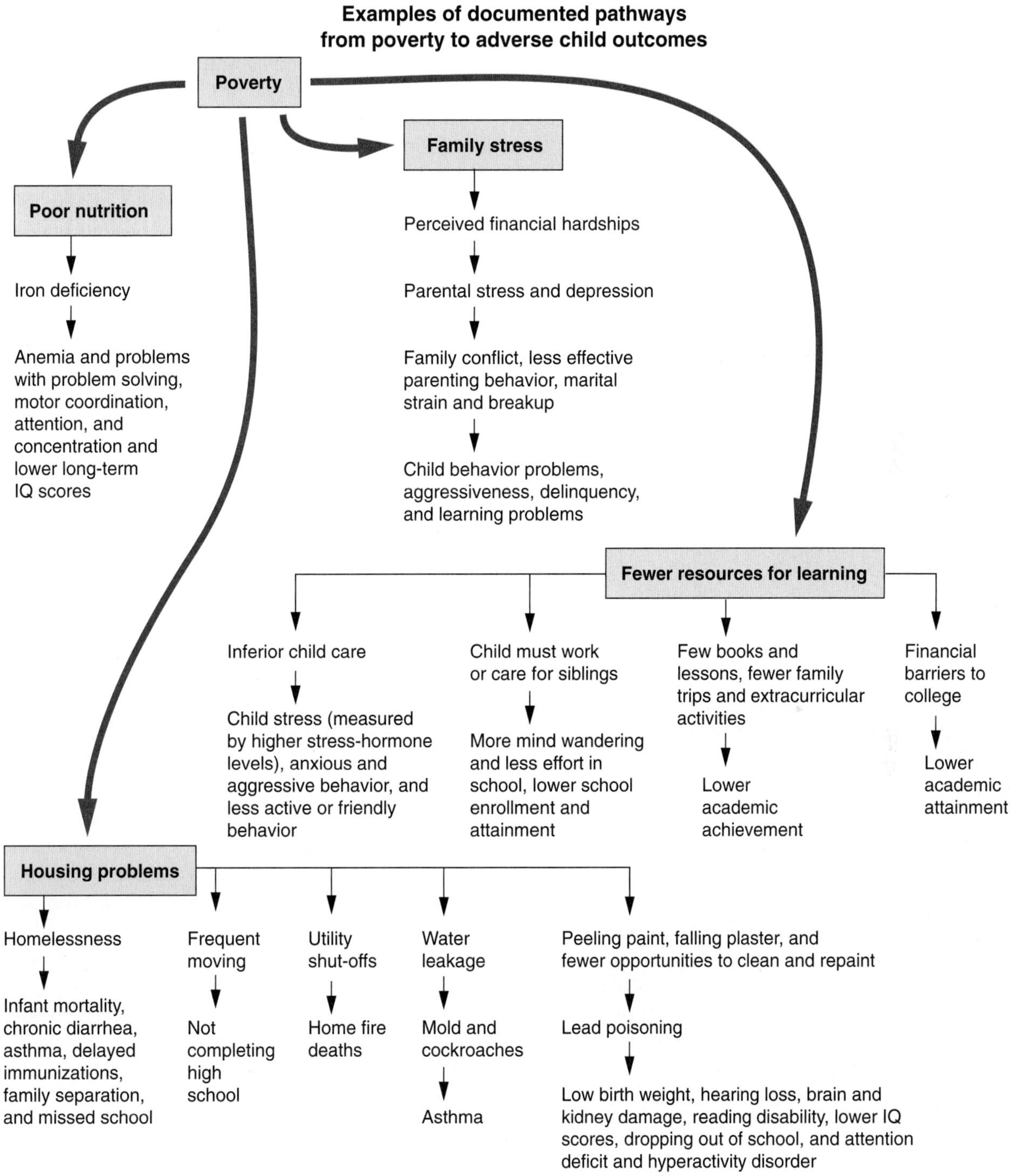

Figure 1-2 Adverse Outcomes for Children Living in Poverty. *Source:* Sherman, A. (1994). *Wasting America's Future: The Children's Defense Fund report on the costs of child poverty.* Boston: Beacon. Used with permission of the Children's Defense Fund, Washington, DC.

there is disagreement concerning the exact number of homeless persons, there is a consensus that the numbers are large and continuing to grow.

Homelessness was initially a phenomenon of large urban areas but more recently has swept across the nation, affecting midsize cities as well as suburban and rural areas. Contributing to the rise of homelessness in midsize cities is the migration of disadvantaged families from large urban settings to smaller towns and cities in search of a safer environment and a better life for their children. The homeless population is disproportionately represented by African-Americans (U.S. Department of Housing and Urban Development [HUD], 1999).

Several societal problems contribute to the increasing rate of homelessness among American families, including the following (AAP, 1996):

- Increases in poverty
- Lack of affordable housing
- Decreases in availability of rent subsidies
- Unemployment, especially among those who have held only marginal jobs
- Personal crises such as divorce, domestic violence, and substance abuse
- Cutbacks in public welfare programs
- Deinstitutionalization of the mentally ill

Having been abused or neglected by a household member as a child is a risk factor for homelessness. Another factor is living in a foster home, a group home, or other out-of-home placement as a child, such as a residential treatment center or juvenile detention (HUD, 1999).

Homeless children experience the specific health effects directly related to homelessness, as well as the effects of poverty, the umbrella issue of homelessness. The most common physical health problems include upper respiratory, ear, and skin infections, gastrointestinal disorders (diarrhea), and infestations (scabies, lice) (AAP, 1996). Compared with housed children, homeless youth have a higher incidence of chronic health problems such as asthma, anemia, visual and neurological deficits, eczema, and trauma-related injuries (Weinreb, et al., 1998). The conditions in many private and public shelters place children at risk of lead poisoning and other environmental hazards. Many health problems may predate shelter entry, including crowding in doubled-up housing situations, or exposure to the elements and lack of sanitary facilities in public places. Access to health care, especially preventive care (immunizations, well child services), is impaired for homeless families. Because caregivers are struggling to meet the family's basic demands for food and shelter, health becomes a lower priority. When they do seek health care, they are more likely to use emergency services for preventive and sick care than housed families (Ensign & Santelli, 1998).

To date, the struggle to provide adequate food and nutrition to homeless families has proven to be an overwhelming task. Homeless families have little access to cooking facilities, and families living in shelters report having less access to food than they previously had, with more children going hungry or eating once per day. The children are especially at risk for malnutrition. Inadequate benefits and difficulties in accessing food and entitlements are the major mediators of hunger and poor nutrition in the homeless. The vast majority of homeless families are headed by women who rely on Aid to Families with Dependent Children (AFDC) as their primary source of income, and problems are often compounded by failure to receive benefits to which they are entitled, erroneous case closings, and benefit reductions. Loss of these benefits has been shown to have directly contributed to loss of housing. In addition, the children of these women who are eligible to receive benefits under the federally funded Special Supplemental Food Program for Women, Infants, and Children (WIC) often do not receive benefits. Families with limited resources are often left with no other alternative than emergency food assistance facilities, and in many cities, such facilities have reported having to turn away people in need because of lack of resources.

Psychological problems identified most often among homeless children include depression, anxiety, and behavioral problems. Homeless children are more likely to exhibit poor attention span, trouble sleeping, delayed speech, aggressive behaviors, shyness, and withdrawal (HUD, 1999). Poor school attendance resulting from family transience is also a serious concern. Enrollment in school may be delayed for weeks because of lack of immunizations and records.

Nurses, together with other service providers such as physicians, psychologists, and teachers can increase the local and national awareness of the effects of homelessness on children and bring political attention to the underlying causes of widespread poverty.

Nurses are in a unique position to advocate for homeless children within the social services system concerning access to health care, mental health care, and essential housing, nutritional, and educational needs. Nurses can also advocate for making prenatal care available to homeless mothers. Lack of such care places unborn homeless children at risk of low birth weight, subsequent health problems, chronic diseases, and cognitive and developmental problems. In addition, health problems are associated with psychological problems, classroom performance, and drop-out rates, all of which, gone unaddressed, can seriously compromise the future of homeless children.

Migrant Farm Workers

Migrant and seasonal farm workers constitute a major portion of the labor force in the U.S. agricultural industry, and children make up almost one-fourth of all farm labor in the United States (Gwyther & Jenkins, 1998). The majority of adult workers are married and have children. Children of migrant workers constitute a population at high risk for many health problems because of their living conditions and limited access to health care (Wilson, Wold, Spencer, & Pittman, 2000). They suffer from many of the problems seen in homeless children: gastroenteritis, dental caries, inadequate immunizations, intestinal parasites, infestations, skin infections, pesticide exposure, and infectious diseases (AAP, 1995; Bechtel, 1998; Wilson, Pittman, Wold, 2000).

Agriculture surpasses mining and construction as the most hazardous occupation in the United States. Children of migrant families often are involved in farm work and, being physically weaker and less experienced with farm operations and machinery than their adult counterparts, are more at risk for injury. Each year some 24,000 children working in agriculture experience nonfatal trauma, and nearly 300 children die, primarily as a result of accidents involving farm machinery (Gwyther & Jenkins, 1998). Children are also at risk for pesticide exposure both in the fields where they work and play, and at home, where they can be exposed through pesticide drift. Although research on childhood exposures is limited, it is believed that children are at greater risk than adults for pesticide-related illnesses because of their higher metabolism, increased body surface area, and potential for long-term chemical exposure. Long-term exposure to pesticides has been implicated in several types of cancer, birth defects, sterility, spontaneous abortion, and cognitive deficits (Gwyther & Jenkins, 1998).

The conditions of migrant life place families, and especially children, at increased risk for contracting a variety of viral, bacterial, and fungal infections, including rabies, anthrax, Rocky Mountain spotted fever, tetanus, plague, typhoid, tuberculosis, HIV, and hepatitis. Crowded, unsanitary living conditions create the opportunity for rapid disease spread. Lack of access to health care services results in a high incidence of preventable disease in the migrant population. The high incidence of tuberculosis in this population has been linked with high rates of infection in migrant's countries of origin, substandard housing and overcrowding, poor baseline health status, malnutrition, and lack of access to preventive health care services. There are high rates of HIV infection in the migrant population. Specifically, the number of women with HIV is rising, putting children at risk for contracting the virus *in utero* or at birth. Migrant women are particularly at risk because of their lack of access to educational counseling, prevention, and treatment services.

Migrant children are frequently at risk nutritionally. Migrant communities often have limited choices for the purchase of food, and their low incomes may preclude them from receiving adequate amounts of nourishment. Furthermore, they often lack the means for properly storing or preparing foods (e.g., lack of refrigeration, impotable water). Though many are eligible for supplementation through programs such as WIC and food stamps, many do not participate because of multiple barriers to these services. Iron-deficiency anemia is a common diagnosis reported by clinics serving migrant children. Child obesity is also raised as a major clinical concern given the link of obesity to diabetes and hypertension in adult Hispanics (Gwyther & Jenkins, 1998).

The health status of these children is further threatened because of barriers to health care such as family mobility, financial constraints, and legal (fear of immigration penalties), language, and cultural barriers. The mobility of the families impedes adequate follow-up and referral for health problems for the children. Financial constraints stemming from being in a low-wage work group, being paid according to how much is harvested, and lack of health insurance hinder migrant farm workers from seeking health care for their children. Language is a major cultural barrier for Hispanic workers who speak little English and for health care providers who do not speak Spanish (Wilson, et al., 2000).

There is a critical need for nurses working with migrants to advocate for the health of migrant children. Nurses must not only act as health educators for migrant families, but they must also aid them in negotiating a complex and dynamic health care system that is unfamiliar. It is equally important that those familiar with the lives of migrant families educate the public and its leaders about the significant contributions of these workers to the economy. Further, the research literature on migrant children has many critical gaps. Basic information on the number and distribution of migrant children in the United States, prevalence rates for common causes of morbidity and mortality in this group, and measures of the impact of the migrant health system on child health status are lacking. Nurses and other clinicians are in key positions to fill these gaps and thus expand the knowledge base from which further target interventions may be developed (Gwyther & Jenkins, 1998).

Violence

As the 20th century ended, violence by and against children declined. Yet it still occurs. Today children and adolescents are more likely to be the victims of violent crime than the offenders. **Violent crimes** include murder, forcible rape, robbery, and aggravated assault. Although the number of children injured by violent crime has declined significantly, the level of violence in the U.S. surpasses those in any other developed country. For example, the rate of death by homicide among U.S. males aged 15 to 24 is 10 times higher than that in Canada and 28 times higher than that in France or Germany (Danielsen, 1998).

An examination of other statistics on juvenile violence is alarming. One statistical trend to consider is the numbers of juveniles arrested for violent crimes. In 1999, 5% of juvenile arrests were for violent crimes. Comparing racial groups indicates that, although African-American youths accounted for 15% of the juvenile population, they were involved in more than 50% of arrests for murder and rape. Another trend to examine is juveniles who are victims of homicide, which indicates a positive trend in 1998. The homicide rate fell an estimated 14%, the fifth straight year of decline. However, it still remains a major cause of death among 10–19-year-olds and the leading cause of death for black males 15–24 years of age (Snyder & Sickmund, 1999).

In recent years, injuries and deaths among children and adolescents from firearms, specifically handguns, have increased. In 1998, firearms were involved in 85% of all homicides, and 60% of all suicides in adolescents were committed with a firearm (Snyder, 1999). The presence of a gun in the home increases the risk of homicide, suicide, and injury to family and friends (Laraque, Spivak, & Bull, 2001). Recent evidence suggests that the majority of firearms used in suicide attempts and accidental shootings are stored in the home of the victim or in the home of a relative or friend (Grossman, Reay, & Baker, 1999).

Reflective Thinking

Inquiring about Guns in the Home

Some families may not want to reveal the fact that they have guns in their homes. How can you approach the topic? How could you ask the family about ways that they keep themselves and their children safe?

REFLECTIONS FROM FAMILIES

My family has been devastated ever since my 12-year-old son, Johnny, was shot in our home. But we were more fortunate than most. He survived. Johnny was seriously injured when his best friend Bill, also aged 12, and he were playing and found my husband's loaded revolver on the shelf of our closet. They began playing with it, and the gun went off in Bill's hand, hitting Johnny in the shoulder at close range. Johnny's doctors say the outlook is good and that he will regain full use of his arm, though he will require extensive medical care and long-term physical therapy. But the trauma of that night will never leave us. My husband and I blame ourselves for the shooting and want to do something to prevent other families from going through what we have. We have started working with the schools to help teach gun safety to parents and children. We could have lost our son simply because we didn't take responsibility for owning and keeping a gun in our home. No parent should ever have to find out what that feels like, especially too late.

Family Teaching

Firearm Injury Prevention

Home:

1. Communicate the risks of keeping a firearm in the home.
2. Advise that it's safest not to keep a firearm in the home.
3. Review safe methods of storage.
4. Educate caregivers to teach children not to touch or handle firearms.
5. Explain that handguns and semiautomatic weapons pose the greatest risk of intentional and unintentional injury for children. The reason for this is because they are more often stored unsafely and are more often involved in serious injuries and deaths.
6. Explain to caregivers that it is easier to keep guns away from adolescents than to keep adolescents away from guns, which are often glamorized in the media. Caregivers should watch for signs of depression or changes in behavior since teens feeling this way are at increased risk for suicide.

School:

1. Incorporate violence prevention programs in school curricula at an early age, including firearm violence. Examples of such programs include conflict resolution, alternatives to violence, anger management, risk awareness, and coping skills.
2. Have after-school programs for youths, and obtain community support for such programs.

Community:

1. In an effort to reduce the romaticization of guns in the popular media, urge the development of violence-free programming among child health and education advocates, and the television and motion picture industries.
2. Support legislation that regulates the manufacture and importation of classes of guns, such as handguns and assault weapons, and that requires background checks for weapons purchased at gun shows.
3. Improve playgrounds and parks to make safe play areas for children.

Kids Want To Know

I'm afraid that someone will bring a gun to school.

What should I do if I know someone has brought a gun to school?

- Report any guns brought by classmates to a principal, teacher, or a school nurse.
- When you report guns brought by classmates, your identity does not need to be revealed.
- Many schools have metal detectors so that guns cannot be brought to school without being detected.

Although, in recent years, a great deal of attention has understandably been focused on tragic school shootings and homicides, school violence rates are declining overall (Children's Defense Fund, 2000). In fact, school-associated violent deaths are rare occurrences. Students are much more likely to be the victims of violent crimes away from school than at school (Snyder & Sickmund, 1999). Even though violent crimes in schools have decreased, physical fights, thefts, weapon carrying, teacher victimization, and fear of school environments have increased. The most effective strategies for reducing violence in schools involve coordination among education, law enforcement, social service, and mental health systems.

Nurses must become involved in responding to the increases in firearm-related deaths in children by encouraging gun control legislation. Laws to hold gun owners responsible for how their guns are stored in the event a child is injured may lead to decreases in rates of accidental firearm deaths. A number of gun design options have been proposed to decrease the likelihood of unintentional injury. These include trigger locks, lock boxes, personalized safety mechanisms, and trigger pressures that are too high for young children. However, it is not conclusive if these measures will decrease injuries and deaths (AAP, 2000). Until guns are no longer accessible to children, education should inform all adults about gun hazards and safety. Nurses can be involved in this education process by teaching families about firearm safety.

CURRENT STATUS OF CHILDREN'S HEALTH

In January 2000, the U.S. Department of Health and Human Services (DHHS) launched *Healthy People 2010: National Health Promotion and Disease Prevention Objectives*, a comprehensive, nationwide health promotion and disease prevention agenda. The document contains 28 focus areas and 467 objectives designed to serve as a guide for improving the health of all people in the United States during the first decade of the 21st century (DHHS, 2000). Most of the objectives target the lifestyle choices and environmental conditions that cause 70% of premature deaths in this country. The overarching goals are to increase the quality and years of healthy life, and eliminate health disparities between ethnic groups. The Healthy People framework allows governments to focus resources in the right place. A variety of indicators reflect the health status of Americans. Health status can be measured by birth and death rates, life expectancy, morbidity from specific diseases, and many other factors. Box 1-2 lists the 10 leading health indicators.

Because Healthy People (HP) 2010 emphasizes health promotion and prevention, almost all of it pertains to nursing. Health promotion and education are central to nursing practice; therefore, nurses need to develop an awareness of the HP 2010 program and incorporate it as a benchmark for their interventions. Nurses are well educated and prepared

BOX 1-2 Leading health indicators

- Physical activity
- Overweight and obesity
- Tobacco use
- Substance abuse
- Responsible sexual behavior
- Mental health
- Injury and violence
- Environmental quality
- Immunizations
- Access to health care

Critical Thinking

Healthy People 2010

From the 10 leading health indicators found in Box 1-2, choose four that you think would have objectives pertaining to children aged 1–18 years and list them. For each one of the four you have chosen, write down an idea for the specific area that the objective should address. For example, if you were to choose priority areas for adults, one area would be cancer, and the specific area the objective could address is to increase the number of adults who receive a colorectal screening exam each year.

to work with individuals, families, and communities to meet the special needs of vulnerable populations and to eliminate health disparities. The public, by and large, trusts nurses and is receptive to their teaching and intervention. Nurses can use their unique position to help meet the goals of HP 2010 and, in doing so, can improve the health of all Americans: adults, children, and adolescents.

Infant Mortality

Infant mortality is an important measure of a nation's health and a worldwide indicator of health status. The **infant mortality rate** (IMR) is the number of infant deaths during the first year of life per 1,000 live births. IMR has shown an exponential decline in the 20th century from 200 per 1,000 live births in 1900 to a record low of 7.2 per 1,000 live births in 1998 (Martin, Smith, Matthews, & Ventura, 1999). Figure 1-3 demonstrates IMR by race from 1915 to 1998. The low overall IMR in 1998 was the same as the record low reported in 1997. It is the first time that there has been no improvement in this measure in nearly four decades. The IMR in 1998 for white infants was 6.0 and for black infants, 14.3—a figure more than twice the rate for white infants. This racial difference is a major national concern because the ratio of black to white infant deaths has remained unchanged from 1990 to 1998. One reason for this disparity in IMR is the high rate of **low birth weight** (LBW) infants born to minority mothers, which suggests a decrease in the overall health status or health care access of these women. IMRs were also higher for infants whose mothers were teenagers or 40 years of age or older, did not complete high school, were unmarried, began prenatal care after the first trimester of pregnancy, or smoked during pregnancy (Guyer, Hoyert, Martin, Ventura, MacDorman, & Strobino, 1999).

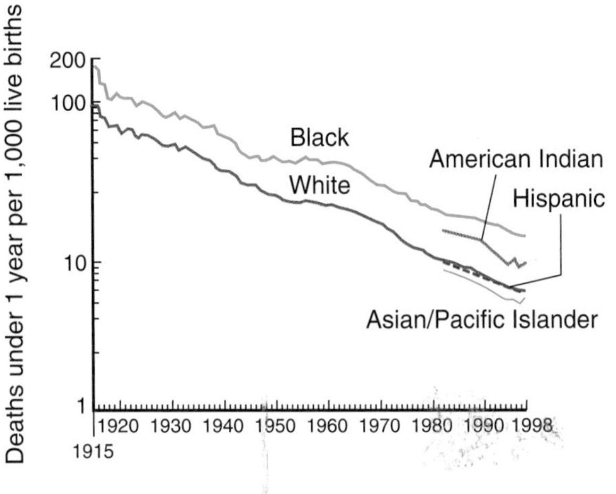

Figure 1-3 Infant Mortality Rates by Race, United States, 1915–1998. Source: Guyer, B., Freedman, M., Strobino, D., & Sondik, E. (2000). Annual summary of vital statistics: Trends in the health of Americans during the 20th century. *Pediatrics, 106*(6), 1307–1317.

The upward trend in infant survival has been due to improvements in perinatal care, such as high frequency ventilation, use of surfactant therapy for the neonate, and improved public education efforts (Figure 1-4). In spite of these improvements in infant mortality, the United States ranks 23 among the 24 nations that have the lowest infant mortality rates (Department of Economic and Social Affairs, 1999). The unfavorable birth weight distribution in this country continues to be one reason for its unenviable IMR, and the proportion of the smallest and most vulnerable infants increased during the 1990s. The IMR target goal for the year 2010 is 4.5 deaths per 1,000 live births. To achieve further reductions in infant mortality, the public health community, health care providers, and individuals must focus on modifying the behaviors, lifestyles, and conditions that affect birth outcomes. These include smoking, substance abuse, poor nutrition, lack of prenatal care, medical problems, chronic illness, and other psychosocial problems (e.g., stress, domestic violence). Additionally, the financial, educational, social, and logistic barriers to receiving prenatal care in the first trimester for all women must be removed.

Low Birth Weight

One reason for the racial disparity in IMRs and the poor ranking of the United States is the high rate of LBW (weight of less than 2,500 grams, or 5 pounds, 8 ounces at birth). The rate of LBW was 7.6% in 1998, up from 7.5% in 1997. This percentage has been increasing fairly steadily from the low of 6.7% reported in 1984 (Guyer, et al., 1999). Infants with a LBW have a six times higher risk of death during their first year of life. Those weighing less than 1,500 grams have an 89 times higher risk of death than do babies having a normal birth weight. Figure 1-5 shows trends in LBW since 1950 for white and black infants, since 1970 for American Indians, and since 1980 for infants born to women of Hispanic and Asian/Pacific Island descent. The LBW rate is much higher for black infants than for any other group for all years for which data are shown. The reasons for this higher rate are the same as for high IMR in this group.

Figure 1-5 also shows an increase between 1990 and 1999 in the LBW rate for infants born to white, American Indian, and Asian/Pacific Islander women. The increase among white women has been shown to be attributable to an increase in multiple births (Guyer, Freedman, Strobino, & Sondik, 2000). The increase in multiple births has been associated with an increase in assisted reproductive technologies such as *in vitro* fertilization and, to a lesser extent, with the rising age of childbearing. If this increase continues, it is unlikely that there will be much improvement in the position of the nation in infant mortality relative to other developed countries (Guyer, et al., 2000).

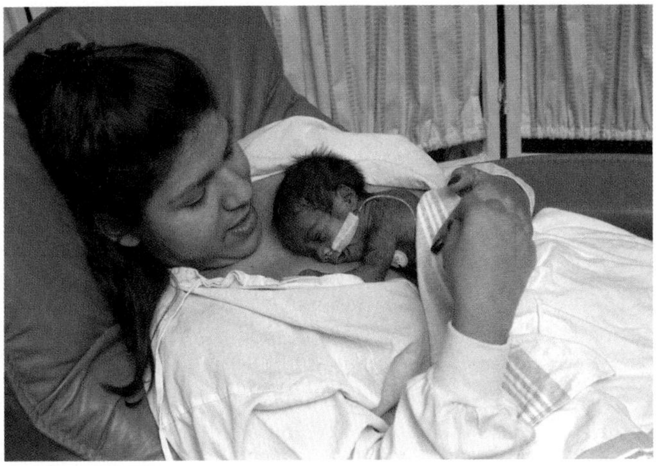

Figure 1-4 Although advances in perinatal care during the last 20 years have led to dramatic increases in survival of extremely small and immature infants, low birth weight remains a major contributor to infant mortality.

Reflective Thinking

The Cost of Keeping LBW Infants Alive

Hospitals and health care delivery systems have poured substantial amounts of money into neonatal intensive care units to care for LBW infants. These babies are usually technology dependent and often require extensive medical equipment and nursing care in their homes. How do you feel about this emphasis on high-tech solutions versus allocating some resources to preventive services?

LBW infants are at risk for impaired health, developmental delay, neurosensory deficits, cognitive delays, and school and behavioral difficulties. The most common major neurologic abnormality seen in these infants is cerebral palsy, which increases with decreasing birth weight. Additionally, deafness, blindness, seizures, and hydrocephalus are all found more commonly in LBW infants.

Immunization Rates

The reduction in incidence of vaccine-preventable diseases is one of the most significant public health achievements of the 20th century. The global eradication of smallpox in 1977 is an illustration of this success (DHHS, 1999). Not only are immunized individuals themselves protected from developing a potentially serious illness, but, also, if enough of the

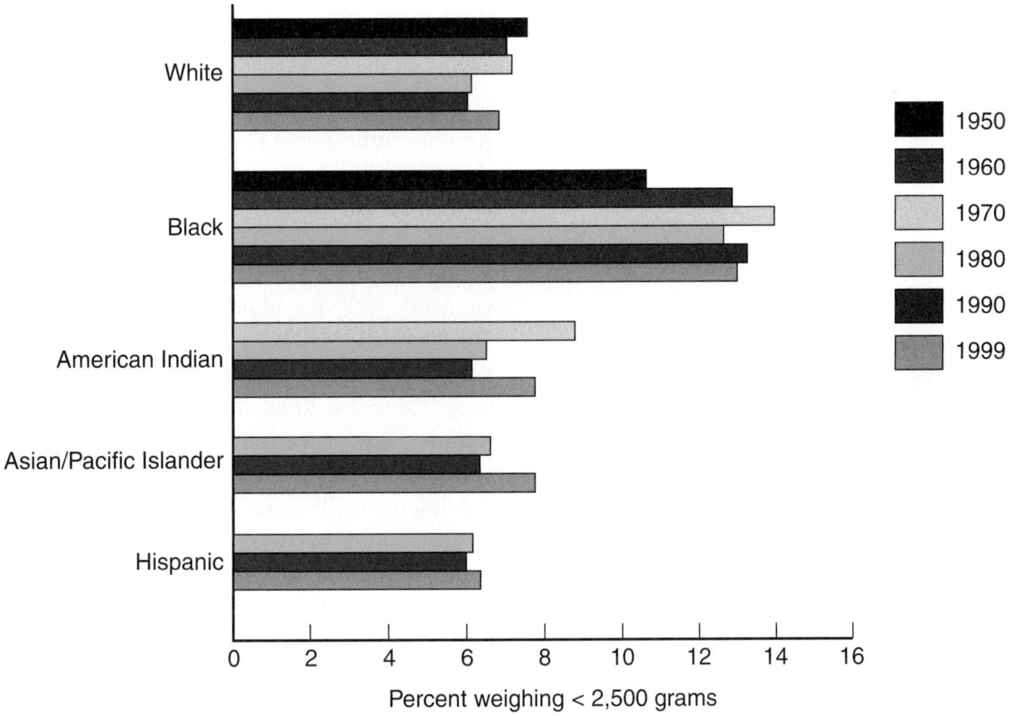

Figure 1-5 Percent Low Birth Weight by Race, United States, Selected Years, 1950–1999. Source: Guyer, B., Freedman, M., Strobino, D., & Sondik, E. (2000). Annual summary of vital statistics: Trends in the health of Americans during the 20th century. *Pediatrics, 106*(6), 1307–1317.

population is immunized, transmission of the disease in a community may be interrupted. This concept is known as **herd immunity,** i.e., the reduction of the number of persons susceptible to a communicable disease by immunization, thus preventing the spread of disease in epidemic proportions. Immunization rates should be at least 80% to provide herd immunity. The increasing number of safe and effective vaccines has improved the health status of millions of U.S. children. In 1999, the highest rates of childhood immunization were achieved. The overall rate for children of preschool age increased to a record of 80%. Three vaccines—polio, measles, and *Haemophilus influenza* type b (Hib)—had a coverage rate at or above 90% (Centers for Disease Control, National Center for Health Statistics, 1999). Figure 1-6 illustrates the childhood vaccination coverage for 1999 by race. Rates are for 19–35-month-old children who have received at least four doses of DTP (diptheria, tetanus, pertussis), three polio, one MMR (measles, mumps, rubella), three Hib, and three hepatitis B. The Healthy People 2010 target is 90% coverage for all recommended vaccines in all populations.

Although immunization coverage is high in almost all states, areas within each state and within major cities persist where substantial numbers of underimmunized children reside. Significant segments of this population are minority children. These areas are of great concern because there is a potential for outbreaks and epidemics of vaccine-preventable diseases. Another challenge is the emergence of a vocal movement resisting childhood immunization requirements. All 50 states have immunization requirements for entrance into school; however, some groups are seeking changes in these state laws. They want to enable caregivers to choose how and if their children are vaccinated. Exemptions are allowed from immunization requirements for medical reasons in all states and for religious reasons in 48 states, and 15 states allow exemptions for philosophical reasons (National Vaccine Advisory Committee, 1998). Children who are not immunized may create health risks if they contract a vaccine-preventable disease because they can transmit it to other family members, peers, friends, and neighbors. Yet, vaccinations are among the safest and most effective preventive measure, and, in general, a child is more likely to suffer complications from the disease than from immunizations.

Kids Want To Know

Why do I have to get shots when I go to the doctor even when I'm not sick?

The nurse can assist the school-aged child to develop an early concept of preventive health care and to form a more positive view of the helping role of health care personnel. Taking into consideration the child's developmental level, explain that in the past these diseases made children very sick and that many of them died. Give the child a clear explanation of what each immunization is for and how often it will be needed. Tell the child which immunizations must be injected and which can be taken in oral form. Also, clarify that the shot will hurt for only a second. Introducing immunizations to young children in this positive perspective will help emphasize the role of prevention at an early age.

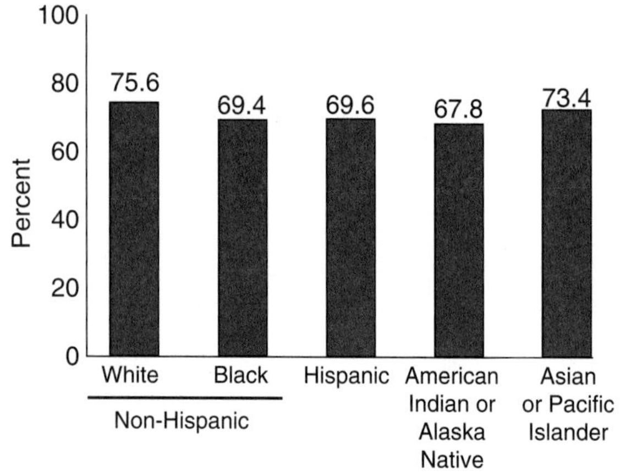

Figure 1-6 Childhood Vaccination Coverage by Race, 1999. Source: Department of Health and Human Services. (1999). [On-line]. Available: http://raceandhealth.hhs.gov/3rdpgBlue/Immuno/k21.gif

Child Mortality

Another indicator of children's health status is child mortality. For children over 1 year of age, the overall decline in mortality during the 20th century has been impressive (Figure 1-7). In 1900, the death rate for children 1–4 years of age was about 2,000 per 100,000 population, 460 for 5–9-year-olds, 300 for children 10–14 years old, and 500 for 15–19-year-olds. By 1998, the death rates in these age groups had declined by 98%, 96%, 93%, and 85%, respectively (Murphy, 2000). The decline in deaths for adolescents has plateaued since the 1960s. At the beginning of the 20th century, the major cause of child mortality for 1–19-year-olds was infectious diseases. However, the mortality and morbidity from all of these diseases are dwarfed by the numbers of children who die or who are disabled as the result of unintentional injuries. Until recently, injuries were commonly termed "accidents," suggesting that they were unpredictable and unavoidable events affecting unlucky children. Today, the term "injury" is favored because it more accurately suggests that the problem can be averted and prevented.

Injury is defined as damage or harm to an individual resulting in destruction of health, disability, or death (Deal, Gomby, Zippiroli, & Behrman, 2000). An injury is classified

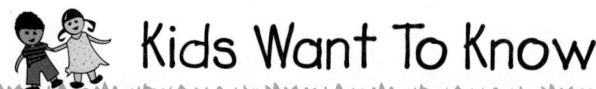

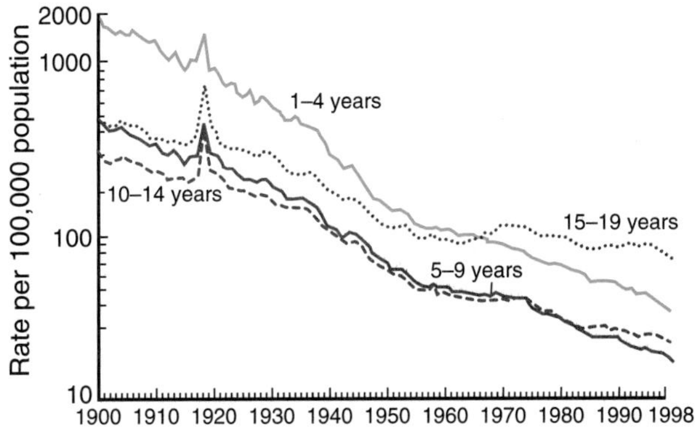

Figure 1-7 Childhood Mortality Rates by Age at Death, United States, 1900–1998. *Source:* Guyer, B., Freedman, M., Strobino, D., & Sondik, E. (2000). Annual summary of vital statistics: Trends in the health of Americans during the 20th century. *Pediatrics, 106*(6), 1307–1317.

as intentional or unintentional, denoting whether or not it was meant to harm the victim. Box 1-3 shows those typically included in each category.

Among children aged 1–19, unintentional injuries are responsible for more deaths each year than homicide, suicide, congenital anomalies, cancer, heart disease, respiratory illness, and HIV combined (CDC, National Center for Injury Prevention and Control, 1999a). Although unintentional injuries are the leading cause of death for all children over 1 year of age, the incidence varies by age. More than one-half of all unintentional injury-related deaths occur in the 15–19-year-old group due to motor vehicle–related injuries. Common subcategories of motor vehicle injuries include (1) occupant (drivers and passengers), (2) bicycle-related, (3) motorcycle, and (4) pedestrian injuries.

There is considerable variation in injury rates among children depending on their age group. Among children under 1 year of age, suffocation is the leading cause of unintentional injury-related death, followed by motor vehicle occupant injury, choking, drowning, and fires or burns. Some suffocation deaths in infants are due to entrapment of the head and neck in cribs. Another cause is choking on food or an object, leading to airway obstruction. For children aged 1–4 years, drowning is the leading cause of injury death, followed by motor vehicle occupant injury, fires or burns, and airway obstruction. Infants often drown in bathtubs, usually as a result of poor supervision or neglect, whereas toddlers and young children fall into a body of water such as a swimming pool, lake, or river, usually while unsupervised. Among children aged 5–14, motor vehicle occupant–related injury is the leading cause of death, followed by drowning, pedestrian injury (i.e., motor vehicle collisions with the child), bicycle injury, and fires or burns (National SAFE KIDS Campaign, 1998). Pedestrian injury often occurs when a child darts out

BOX 1-3 Categories of injuries

Unintentional Injuries	Intentional injuries
Injuries due to motor vehicles	Homicide
Bicycle injuries	Suicide
Boating injuries	Rape
Choking and suffocation	Assault and battery
Falls	Domestic violence
Drowning	Child abuse and neglect
Near-drowning	Any other injury caused on purpose
Fires and burns	
Firearm injury	
Poisoning	
Occupational injuries	
Farm injuries	
Sports injuries	
Injuries due to toys and recreational equipment	
Any other injury that was not intended to harm the victim	

Children's Safety Network. (1991). *A data book on child and adolescent injury.* Washington, DC: National Center for Education in Maternal and Child Health.

between parked cars or into the street to get a ball or another object. During adolescence (14–19 years), motor vehicle occupant injuries are the primary cause of injury-related deaths. Driver inexperience and alcohol use are key contributors to the high rate of fatal crashes in adolescents (Grossman, 2000).

Rates of unintentional injury deaths among children have declined by 43% over the past several decades. Decreases in injury deaths have been observed for every age group and for nearly all causes. Reductions have been most evident among adolescents and for poisoning deaths (CDC, National Center for Injury Prevention and Control, 1999b). Additionally, most unintentional injury deaths to children can be prevented. Simple proven interventions such as using child car seats and bicycle helmets, requiring that prescription medications have child-resistant caps, installing smoke detectors in homes, requiring that children's sleep wear be flame retardant, and enclosing swimming pools with fences have saved the lives of thousands of children each year.

The key approaches to injury prevention are education, changes in the environment and in products, and legislation or regulation. Education to promote changes in individual's behaviors has reduced the risk of childhood injuries. Education by health care professionals has increased individual safety behaviors, including seat belt and car seat use, smoke detector ownership, and safe hot water temperature. Nurses and other health care providers should incorporate education about safety practices into routine health visits. Pediatric nurses can play an important educational role by teaching caregivers about expected behaviors for their child's upcoming developmental stage. This alerts them to the types of injuries common to that age group and to potential environmental hazards. Nurses can initiate safety programs in schools, neighborhoods, and cities (Figure 1-8).

Changes in the environment and in products can make children's physical surroundings, toys, and clothing safer. Strategies that make children's environments safer such as traffic calming to reduce or slow the speed of traffic in neighborhoods and fencing to enclose swimming pools on all sides should be implemented in all communities and be mandated by law. Legislation and regulation are among the most effective tools to reduce injuries, and most environment and product modifications require legal action. However, some laws have not been adopted in every state, e.g., 35 states lack bicycle helmet laws (Bicycle Helmet Safety Institute, 2000), and most states do not require appropriate protection in automobiles for children between the ages of 4 and 8. For maximum effectiveness, laws, regulations, and policies must be supported by the public and enforced at the community level. A major challenge is to coordinate all groups involved in unintentional injury prevention to create a critical mass for action (Schieber, Gilchrist, & Sleet, 2000). Safety information is discussed in detail in chapters 7–12.

REFLECTIONS FROM FAMILIES

Whenever I heard people say that the leading cause of death in teenagers is in car accidents, I never thought it would happen to me. I am only 17, but I feel that my life is over since the day my best friend, Andy, was killed in the car I was driving. I was driving too fast, and we had the music on real high. We had just left a friend's house, where we had been drinking beer. We were just having fun, we thought, but suddenly when a car turned in front of us too fast, I lost control of my car, and we ended up rolled over in a ditch. Andy is gone, and his family will never be the same. Neither will mine. I just keep wishing I had one more chance to go back to that day and do it over again.

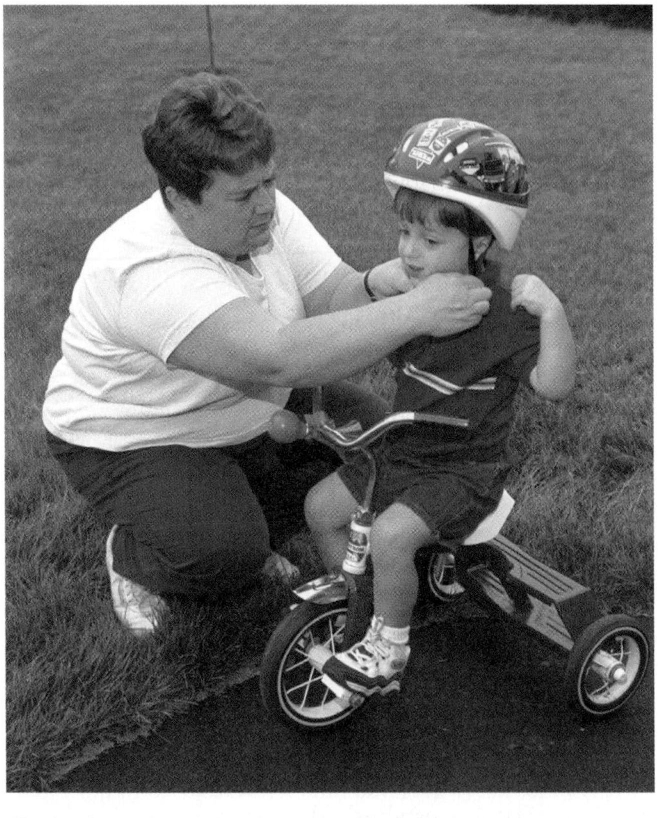

Figure 1-8 The use of safety equipment such as safety helmets helps to protect children from injury. What other measures can nurses implement and promote to help children protect themselves from harm?

Access to Health Care

For a growing number of children, access to health care is hampered by lack of health insurance. The number of uninsured children has been growing at an alarming rate. In 1999, approximately 11.9 million children (one in seven) under the age of 19 lacked health insurance (U.S. Census Bureau, 1999). Ethnic minority children are overrepresented among the uninsured. They account for more than half of uninsured children. Three-quarters of uninsured children are among the working poor, that is, in families in which the head of the household is employed full time for all or part of the year (Office of the Assistant Secretary for Planning and Evaluation [OASPE], 1998).

Socioeconomic status largely dictates the source of children's health insurance. Those from higher income families are more likely to have private health insurance (90%) than are children from lower income families (40%) (Brennan, Holahan, & Kenney, 1999). Uninsured children in low-income families experience substantial difficulties in accessing health care. They tend to lack (1) the usual sources of routine and sick care, (2) a primary care provider, and (3) recent visits to health care providers. Uninsured children are more likely to be underimmunized and to go without needed medical services due to the costs of care (Newacheck, Halfon, & Inkelas, 2000).

Despite high employment and a robust economy during the previous 8 years, the number of uninsured children continued to grow. Several factors have contributed to this situation, predominately welfare reform. Between 1995 and 1997, 1.25 million individuals lost Medicaid coverage due to welfare-to-work initiatives (Families USA, 1999). Many families who left the welfare roles obtained low-paying jobs for which their employer did not offer health insurance coverage or could not afford to pay the contributions toward the insurance premiums. Although many adult members of families were no longer eligible for Medicaid due to reforms, most of the children in these families were and are still eligible for its benefits; however, many of these families are unaware that their children continue to be eligible. Additionally, some children lost their coverage because welfare administrators failed to inform families of their continuing eligibility. Other families lost coverage because of state administrative errors, barriers, and misunderstandings. Finally, in some states, efforts were made to deter individuals from applying for Medicaid (Sochalski & Villarruel, 1999).

In response to the growing problem of uninsured children and to expand health insurance coverage for them, Congress enacted the State Children's Health Insurance Program (SCHIP) as part of the Balanced Budget Act of 1997. SCHIP was established as Title XXI of the Social Security Act. Not since the enactment of Medicaid in 1965 has there been greater funding for children's health insurance coverage. The purpose of SCHIP is to provide health insurance coverage for children through 18 years of age who are uninsured or ineligible for Medicaid. More than $40 billion in federal grants will be allocated to states over a 10-year period. States must contribute a defined share of funds to obtain federal matching grants (American Academy of Pediatrics Committee on Child Health Financing, 2001). By October 2000, 3.3 million children were enrolled in SCHIP programs (Health Care Financing Administration, 2001).

The success of SCHIP will depend heavily on getting caregivers to enroll their children in the program. Nurses must assume responsibility for helping to facilitate access to health care for families with children. First, they need to be aware of their state health insurance coverage's eligibility requirements and procedures for enrollment. Nurses should work with community agencies in developing mechanisms for identifying children eligible for federal and state programs. Then, they must refer families to available resources and intervene if necessary to help them navigate through the system.

Beyond the barriers created by lack of health insurance, there are other factors involved in access to and use of care. Demographic factors such as family income, race/ethnicity, place of residence, and type of insurance have been identified as barriers to access of care (Sochalski & Villarruel, 1999). Institutional factors such as gate keeping by health plans, distance from families' homes to health site, availability of transportation, and waiting times are other factors. Nurses need to assess barriers for families in accessing health care beyond their insurance status in order to ensure that children will receive needed health care.

PERSPECTIVES ON PEDIATRIC NURSING

Family-Centered Care

All health care professionals recognize that quality health care of children must extend to the entire family. Thus, the focus of pediatric nursing must be on the child as well as the family. The term **family-centered care** describes a philosophy of care that recognizes the centrality of the family in the child's life and inclusion of the family's contribution and involvement in the plan for care and its delivery. It is a health care delivery model that seeks to fully involve families in the care of children. Family-centered care evolved in response to the critical need to maintain the relationship between hospitalized children and their families. Previously this relationship had been neglected or disrupted because of forced separation by the health care system.

In 1987, a revolutionary document that defined the elements of family-centered care was published by the Association for the Care of Children's Health (ACCH). Family-centered care was defined by this group as including eight equally important elements (Box 1-4). Meeting the ever-changing needs of *all* family members, not just those of

BOX 1-4 The key elements of family-centered care

1. Incorporating into policy and practice the recognition that the family is *the constant* in a child's life, whereas the service systems and support personnel fluctuate.
2. Facilitating family/professional collaboration at all levels of hospital, home, and community care: care of an individual child; program development, implementation, and evaluation; and policy formation.
3. Exchanging complete and unbiased information between families and professionals in a supportive manner at all times.
4. Incorporating into policy and practice the recognition and honoring of cultural diversity, strengths, and individuality within and across all families, including ethnic, racial, spiritual, social, economic, educational, and geographic diversity.
5. Recognizing and respecting different methods of family coping and implementing comprehensive policies and programs that provide developmental, educational, emotional, environmental, and financial supports to meet the diverse needs of families.
6. Encouraging and facilitating family-to-family support and networking.
7. Ensuring that hospital, home, and community services and support systems for children needing specialized health and developmental care and their families are flexible, accessible, and comprehensive in responding to diverse family-identified needs.
8. Appreciating families as families and children as children, recognizing that they possess a wide range of strengths, concerns, emotions, and aspirations beyond their need for specialized health and developmental services and support.

From Shelton, T. L., & Stepanek, J. S. (1994). *Family-centered care for children needing specialized health and developmental services*. Association for the Care of Children's Health. Copyright Child Life Council, 11820 Parklawn Drive, Suite 202, Rockville, Maryland 20814, (301) 881-7090.

the child, is paramount to the concept of family-centered care. When families are incorporated into the care of their children, the physical and psychosocial health of the child improves and accelerated rates of progress have been seen. Additionally, these families have demonstrated enhanced learning, less stress, and more satisfaction with care (Heller & McKlindon,1996).

The elements of family-centered care are based on principles that are designed to promote greater family self-determination, decision-making capabilities, control, and self-efficacy. Collectively, these attributes are said to reflect a sense of empowerment. In contrast, the medical model directs health care professionals to assume the roles of evaluator and controller of treatment interventions. This approach results in child and caregiver dependence on the health care providers (Dunst & Trivette, 1996). This position is in direct conflict with the conditions necessary for more active involvement of caregivers in the care of their health-impaired children.

Many health care providers respect and support the idea of family-centered care; however, the practice of this type of care has not been fully actualized (Ahmann, 1994). This discrepancy between their support and actual practice of family-centered care may be attributed in part to the model they employ (family empowerment versus medical approach). Additionally, professionals often inadvertently foster family dependency, alienation, and helplessness by taking control and administering care without family input for the convenience and expediency of the staff and the institution. However, in order to facilitate family-centered care, health care providers must seek caregiver input, suggestions, and advice; incorporate this information into the plan of care; and teach the family the appropriate health care interventions. By providing education and knowledge to the family, caregivers can be empowered to make informed decisions about their child's care (Dunst & Trivette, 1996). Other strategies that enhance family-centered care include no limits on the ages or number of visitors (unless directed otherwise by the family); adequate sleeping facilities for caregivers in the child's room; meals or discounts in cafeterias for caregivers; free parking or a discount for caregivers; and family attendance at interdisciplinary conferences regarding the child's care.

Atraumatic Care

Atraumatic care is a philosophy of providing care that minimizes or eliminates physical and psychological distress for children and their families in the health care environment. In pediatric care, many interventions are traumatic, stressful, and painful; therefore, it is important for nurses to be cognizant of these situations and provide care that minimizes distress. Three principles provide the basis for atraumatic care: (1) identifying stressors for the child and family,

(2) minimizing separation of the child from caregivers, and (3) minimizing or preventing pain (Furdon, Pfell, & Snow, 1998). Examples of atraumatic interventions include:

- Preparing the child prior to every procedure using age-appropriate explanations
- For the child scheduled for surgery, preparing her or him prior to hospital admission (encourage child and caregivers to visit the hospital, allow the child to play with equipment and items such as a stethoscope, blood pressure cuff, IV equipment, masks and gowns)
- Allowing caregivers to be involved and physically present as much as possible to provide support and comfort for the child
- Controlling pain by administering analgesics freely
- Using a euteric mixture of local anesthetics (EMLA) cream at least 1 hour prior to blood draws, insertion of IV needles, and injections

Roles of the Pediatric Nurse

The professional pediatric nurse has the responsibility to provide high-quality care no matter the setting nor the role practiced. Settings where pediatric nurses are involved in caring for children include schools (see Chapter 5), acute care settings, clinics, physician's offices, home health agencies, rehabilitation centers, hospice programs, day care centers, psychiatric centers, and summer camps. Nurses may also work as administrators or nurse executives. Although each setting may have separate roles and responsibilities, the roles that nurses take are universal. Specifically, the primary roles include caregiver, advocate, educator, researcher, and manager/leader. Secondary roles include behaviors related to coordinating, collaborating, communicating, and consulting, and are embedded within the primary roles. Other roles seen in the acute care setting involve **differentiated practice** (a philosophy that delineates a nurse's role and functions according to experience, competence, and education) and include the clinical care coordinator, care manager, and clinical nurse. In addition to these, nurses function in expanded roles as pediatric nurse practitioners, clinical nurse specialists, and case managers. For the most part, these expanded roles require advanced preparation. See Box 1-5 for a listing of the various roles of the nurs[...] practice.

The roles that the nurse takes in these setti[...] on the level of performance expected by practice [...]ines. *The Standards of Maternal and Child Health Nursing Practice* as developed by the American Nurses' Association describe these standards and set expectations for the general behaviors of pediatric nurses while caring for children and their families. These standards were developed in 1983 and are out of print; therefore, they are not included in this textbook.

Caregiver

Patricia Benner (1984) identified several domains of nursing practice that are inherent in the **caregiver** role. They include helping, patient diagnosing/monitoring, administering/monitoring therapeutic interventions/regimens, monitoring/ensuring the quality of health care practices, organizational and work role competencies, and effectively managing rapidly changing situations. More specifically, the caregiver delivers direct nursing care to children and their families that is based on the nursing process. This requires skills in critical thinking, coordinating, collaborating, and consulting, as well as the ability to incorporate and integrate knowledge of pathophysiology, pediatric illness, human growth and development, and the biological sciences, and findings from the physical/cultural/spiritual assessment into a plan that accurately reflects child and family needs. Care provided also should demonstrate knowledge of pediatric pharmacology, including methods of administration, dosage,

Reflective Thinking

Caregiver

Describe the responsibilities of caregivers you see on the pediatric unit where you have experience. Of all the responsibilities nurses have as caregivers for children and their families, which are the most important? Why?

BOX 1-5 Roles of the pediatric nurse

Primary Roles	Secondary Roles	Differentiated Practice Roles	Advanced Practice Roles
Caregiver	Coordinator	Clinical Care Coordinator	Nurse Practitioner
Advocate	Collaborator	Care Manager	Clinical Nurse Specialist
Educator	Communicator	Clinical Nurse	Case Manager
Researcher	Consultant		
Manager/Leader			

and side effects, and the ability to accurately administer medication by various routes to children of all ages.

Advocate

The **advocate** pleads causes for and assists others in making informed decisions that are in the child and family's best interest (Rushton, 1993; Rushton, Armstrong, & McEnhill, 1996). Generally, pediatric nurses acting as advocates inform clients and families of their rights and options as well as the consequences of those options. Pediatric nurse advocates function by allowing clients/families to make their own informed decisions and then supporting those decisions. Even though advocates do not need to approve the decision, they do need to respect that decision and the right to make that decision. In fact, advocates shouldn't make decisions for their clients, but rather should facilitate decision making.

Typically, advocates in pediatrics are concerned with informing children and their families about their health care decisions, and providing information about research, experimental protocols, and alternative treatments. They also provide complete, clear, concise, understandable, and accurate information concerning treatment and procedures as well as inherent risks, provide for privacy and respect, and allow clients/families to refuse a drug, treatment, test, or procedure. Advocates also need to be careful not to impose their own personal values and standards, but to allow the child and family to make autonomous decisions.

Nurses also advocate for clients and families who are vulnerable or cannot speak for themselves; for those who do not know how to speak for themselves because of lack of knowledge, difficulty articulating needs/ideas, fear, physical or mental disability, or perceived lack of power; and for those who are afraid to speak out. The more dependent the client is on the system, the more diligent the advocate should be on his or her behalf. Effective advocates should be assertive, attentive, knowledgeable, and trustworthy, and have the ability to openly communicate with members of the health care team and remain educated about current legal and ethical trends.

Educator

One of the most important roles the pediatric nurse takes is that of **educator,** or teacher, because education is one of the major avenues that the nurse uses to enable clients and families to make informed decisions. In fact, Florence Nightingale emphasized the role of the nurse as an educator, and today, nurses spend most of their time teaching, informally and formally. Nurses teach children and their families in a variety of settings, on a fairly wide range of topics, and in many circumstances (Wilkey & Gardner, 1999). Although discussed as a separate role, teaching is inherent in the caregiver role (Figure 1-9).

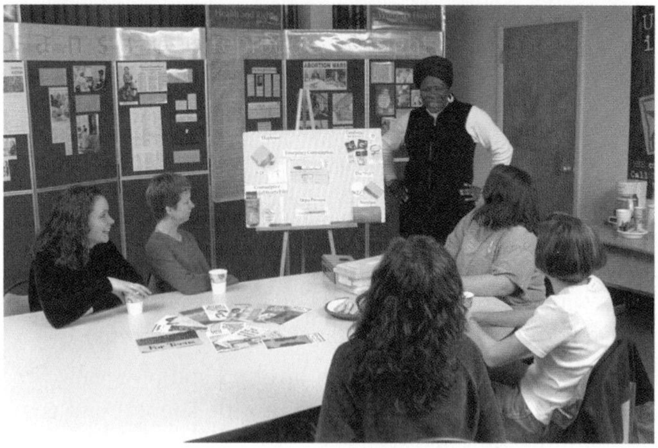

Figure 1-9 Pediatric nurses have many opportunities to teach, including teaching adolescents about contraception.

To be an effective educator, the nurse must initially have knowledge of cognitive development since teaching a preschool child and family about an experience will be different than teaching an adolescent and family about the same experience (see Chapters 7–12). Techniques based on developmental levels include imitation, repetition, association, trial and error, conditioning, and the development of concepts. Each developmental level requires particular strategies. For example, infants and toddlers are best taught by their caregiver, and prefer to explore their environment or handle equipment. If toddlers are not interested in learning, it would be better to just delay the session. Most preschool children want to learn, and even though they might have limited verbal abilities, they do like to practice and manipulate equipment. Preschoolers will ask many questions, and answers should be short, be at an understandable level, and not imply punishment. Since young children often imitate others, imitation would be an appropriate method of teaching this age group. School-aged children have a short attention span and learn best in brief stages and at frequent intervals where they can handle objects, draw pictures, and color in books. Since the school-aged child asks many "why" questions, explanations should meet their needs and should involve only words at their level of comprehension. Adolescents often learn by associating new information with what they already know and may not want parents present during educational sessions.

Critical Thinking

Advocate

What would you do if the client/family has values and beliefs different than yours regarding treatment decisions? How would you respond?

Adolescents also learn best when they see an immediate personal benefit. For example, if they understand that taking medicine regularly will permit continuation of current activities, they often will comply.

Typically, the nurse working with children and families will act in the educator role as they prepare children and families for procedures, surgery, or the hospitalization experience itself. Educators will also answer questions about experiences and treatments, help interpret and integrate information received from the health care team, and assist parents in learning how to care for their child. They also will be called on to provide information related to childrearing; to answer questions about human development; to discuss injury/illness prevention, health promotion and maintenance, and immunization schedules; to clarify diagnoses or treatment plans; to supply children and their families with appropriate literature; and to refer to lay or professional groups that might be helpful.

Since learning takes place in three domains—cognitive, affective, and psychomotor—the nurse educator must integrate all domains into teaching if it is to be effective. **Cognitive learning** is concerned with intellectual activities, can be compared to thinking, and involves describing or explaining something, or answering questions. **Affective learning** is learning that takes place in relation to feelings and emotions; as for example in role playing, modeling, or one-to-one discussion where learners are asked to share their feelings and ideas about the information taught. **Psychomotor learning** is concerned with physical skills; as when the opportunity to actually practice what is being taught is offered. Often psychomotor learning is accompanied by explanation, demonstration and then practice with "hands on" experiences, repetition, and immediate feedback.

An example of these types of learning could be applied to a situation involving learning how to use an inhaler. Cognitive learning would include information about when to use the inhaler, how much medicine to use in the inhaler, and how to evaluate the effectiveness of the treatment. Affective learning occurs when the child recalls feelings before and after the treatment and the effects of using the inhaler. Psychomotor skills are needed to correctly administer the inhaler therapy and encouraged by allowing practice in front of the nurse.

Nurses may also be responsible for teaching their colleagues. For example, they may need to teach other nurses or health care providers about new information relative to a specific disease/condition or treatment, or how to improve their skills and troubleshoot when things go wrong.

Critical Thinking

Teaching a 4-Year-Old

A 4-year-old boy has been admitted to the same day surgery department for a tonsillectomy and adenoidectomy. How would you prepare him for the experience both prior to surgery and after surgery?

Researcher

One criteria for a profession is the existence of a body of knowledge that is distinct from other disciplines. Nursing has traditionally borrowed from the natural and social sciences, and has only recently begun to concentrate on establishing a unique body of knowledge allowing clear identification as a distinct profession. Scientific research is a valid way to develop this knowledge, and pediatric nurses are in an important position to improve this knowledge. Nurse researchers have a responsibility to identify problems that warrant scientific investigation and integrate into their practice, evidence-based research. In fact, professional accountability demands nurses utilize research findings and determine the usefulness of these findings in practice. Pediatric nurses are also called upon to evaluate the methods used to carry out research projects, and estimate how confident they are in the results.

The ANA has differentiated the investigative function of nurses at various educational levels, from the associate degree graduate, through the doctorate. Although certain responsibilities have been spelled out specifically, it is not uncommon for

Reflective Thinking

Educator

How often do you see pediatric nurses teach their clients? Families? Other staff? What can we do to improve teaching effectiveness? What needs to be done to increase client/family teaching opportunities?

Reflective Thinking

Researcher

Think of a project you might become involved in that would improve pediatric client outcomes. Describe three different reasons why nursing research is difficult for staff nurses to integrate into their role at the bedside.

Research Highlight

Preparing Mothers for Children's Posthospital Adjustment

Study Purpose

To determine if mothers' participation in an intervention program about common behavioral and emotional responses young children typically display during and following hospitalization made a difference in their anxiety level and their child's posthospital adjustment.

Methods

Forty-nine mothers whose young children (mean age = 41 months) were unexpectedly admitted to the pediatric units of two acute care hospitals were either assigned to the intervention ($n = 25$) or control group ($n = 24$). Twelve hours after their child was admitted to the hospital, both groups of mothers completed a demographic questionnaire and the State-Trait Anxiety Inventory (Spielberger, Gorsuch, & Lushene, 1983). Those mothers in the experimental group then listened to a 7-minute audiotape informing them of the most common emotional and behavioral responses displayed by young children during and after hospitalization. The mothers in the control group listened to a 7-minute audiotape describing hospital policies and services. Both groups then answered questions to determine whether or not they had processed the information on the tapes. Between 48 and 72 hours after admission, mothers in both groups again completed the State-Trait Anxiety Inventory and the Index of Parent Participation (Melnyk, 1994), which measures self-reported parenting behaviors during childhood hospitalization. From 10 to 14 days after the child was discharged from the hospital, mothers were mailed the Post Hospital Behavior Questionnaire (Vernon, et al., 1966), which asks parents to compare their child's typical behaviors during and following hospitalization on a 5-point Likert scale, ranging from much less than before, to much more than before.

Findings

Mothers who participated in the experimental intervention had less anxiety than mothers who did not participate in the intervention, and also participated more in the care of their hospitalized child. These mothers also reported that their children had less posthospital negative behavioral change than did mothers who listened to the audiotape about hospital policies and procedures.

Implications

Encouraging caregivers to participate in the care of their hospitalized children and educating them about how they might participate and the kinds of negative behaviors their children might demonstrate after hospitalization would not only help caregivers cope with the stresses of the experience, but also help their children.

Citation

Melnyk, B., & Feinstein, N. (2001). Mediating functions of paternal anxiety and participation in care on young children's posthospital adjustment. *Research in Nursing and Health, 24*, 18–26.

nurses at all levels to work together on teams investigating a particular practice problem. In fact, involving all levels of education in a research study improves the project since each nurse brings different knowledge and skills to the team. More specifically, nurses can be a principal investigator on a research project, although special preparation is often necessary (usually a doctorate), or a member of a research team. As a team member they could be involved as a data collector; responsible for administering a new nursing intervention; create, manage, and analyze data files; develop questionnaires; interview and observe subjects; transcribe and analyze audio tapes and interviews; analyze diaries, journals, photographs, and drawings; conduct literature searches; synthesize and critique articles; or assist in writing proposals and editing manuscripts. Being a member of a team may also raise interest and enthusiasm for nurses to conduct their own research (LoBiondo-Wood & Haber, 1997) and should be encouraged.

Manager/Leader

Another role discussed is manager/leader. A **manager/leader** includes management of one's own clients if caring for more than one client, as well as managing staff. Typically, managing requires prioritizing, planning, and organizing comprehensive and accountable nursing care for a group of clients. It also requires one to differentiate care that is important from care that is urgent, so that children and their families have needs met in a timely fashion.

Managing also means delegating aspects of care to others in the nursing staff consistent with their level of expertise and education. However, the nurse is always held accountable for delegated tasks to be sure that there is adherence to ethical and legal standards. Managing also requires that one assume a leadership role in health care management (AACN, 1995). Therefore, effective pediatric nurse managers need to have knowledge of the care requirements of children and their families even though they may not be personally delivering the care in order to efficiently and effectively supervise the care given by others. Effective nurse managers interact with clients and their families both directly and indirectly by visiting clients on rounds, reviewing records, receiving reports on client status, and answering questions from staff and requests from clients and families.

Nurse managers are also responsible for representing the institution to the client/family and the client/family to the institution, and must also work within the bureaucratic environment, which sometimes means subordinating the needs of individuals to the needs of the institution. This may cause serious conflicts for professionals attempting to give individualized care and may require the manager to step in to help staff deal with the conflict. Finally, nurse managers determine the character of the unit, attitudes and behavior of staff, and relationships with other professionals at the agency. If the manager's interactions with physicians, radiology, pharmacy, and housekeeping for example, are professional, the relationships these departments have with the staff will also be professional. The atmosphere of the unit also mirrors the manager's. That is, if the manager is quiet and efficient, those feelings will be communicated to children and their families; if the manager is stressed and seemingly unorganized, this too will be communicated.

Differentiated Practice Roles

Differentiated practice, a nursing practice model currently being implemented in some care settings, refers to a philosophy that delineates a nurse's role and functions according to experience, competence, and education (Boston, 1990). It also promotes contributions, and recognizes and values all nursing personnel delivering care to clients regardless of their role, position, or educational preparation (Fosbinder, Ashton, & Koerner, 1997). The integrated care delivery system was developed to improve use of resources, care quality, and career satisfaction (Koerner, 1992), and seeks to divide work responsibilities according to educational preparation. For example, the clinical nurse (who holds an associate degree in nursing) provides care for clients in structured settings where procedures and policies are established and followed (Koerner, 1992). Specifically, that means being responsible for managing the care of pediatric clients for one shift; monitoring, evaluating, and documenting responses to treatments and the plan of care; performing nursing skills within the scope of practice; delegating aspects of care to other team members according to their role/responsibilities; actually implementing the individualized plan of care; assessing clients to determine needs and learning readiness; and networking with team members to enhance continuity of care (Baker, et al., 1997).

The care manager (who holds a baccalaureate degree in nursing) is responsible for integrating client care from preadmission to post discharge and uses independent nursing judgment. This nurse may or may not work in a structured environment, where there may or may not be established procedures/policies (Koerner, 1992). Specifically, this means assessing and developing a plan of care reflecting client discharge needs; designing, implementing, and evaluating teaching plans that restore, maintain, and/or promote health; determining long-term goals for clients in collaboration with the family; collaborating with health care team members to implement care plans both within and outside the acute care setting; assuming responsibility for care plan outcomes; completing discharge planning assessment; and collaborating with other disciplines as needed to facilitate referrals to other agencies within the community (Parkin & Dumas 1995).

The clinical care coordinator (who holds a master's degree in nursing) provides leadership, functions in a variety of settings, uses independent nursing judgment based on specialized knowledge, research, and theory, and promotes health care outcomes for clients (Koerner, 1992). Specifically, this means assessing nursing resources and staffing needs, and then implementing a staffing plan reflective of this assessment; facilitating communication within the health care team; serving as a resource to clients, families, and the health care team; fostering development and education of students and staff; using unit resources effectively; and providing administrative and clinical assistance as needed (Parkin & Dumas 1995).

Advanced Practice Roles

Advanced practice or expanded roles include the pediatric nurse practitioner, clinical nurse specialist, and case manager.

Eye On:

Alternative Treatment Modalities

Many pediatric nurse practitioners use alternative or complementary modalities, either by themselves or in conjunction with conventional medical therapies. One example is herbal therapy, which uses plant extracts for therapeutic outcomes. In pediatrics, infants who are teething may experience pain, fever, diarrhea, and inflamed gums. Traditional medical treatment involves medications such as analgesics, sedatives, or local anesthetics. Many PNPs utilize herbs such as chamomile in conjunction with medications and have found this therapy effective.

For the most part, these roles require a master's degree and additional skills in assessing and managing children.

Pediatric Nurse Practitioners

The **pediatric nurse practitioner** (PNP) role evolved to meet the need in the 1960s and 1970s for primary care providers of routine health maintenance and preventative services in ambulatory settings (Brush & Capezuti, 1996; Cukr, 1996). The PNP usually is a registered nurse who has received advanced education (often a master's degree) and has graduated from a nurse practitioner program. In the past, the PNP traditionally worked in ambulatory/clinic settings and focused on disease prevention, minor disease management, and well children and families. Today, the PNP may be employed in acute care settings and focus on management of particular disease entities (Callendar-Price, 1996), or partner with physician groups, HMOs, or other types of managed care organizations (Cohen & Juszczak, 1997).

Practitioners are independent, autonomous, and highly skilled at performing nursing assessments and physical examination, counseling, treating minor health problems, and teaching. The PNP also is able to order, carry out, and evaluate laboratory studies; discriminate between normal and abnormal findings that require treatment, referral, or collaboration with other health care professionals; serve as a consultant to other health care professionals; and identify topics, interpret results, and implement evidence-based findings into practice.

Clinical Nurse Specialist

The **clinical nurse specialist** (CNS) "provides an expert approach to health focused on a refined body of knowledge and specialized practice competencies" (ANA, 1980) and usually has a master's degree in nursing. When initially developed, the CNS role was seen as a way for the nurse who wanted to maintain direct client contact to remain at the bedside and still advance in the profession. The CNS provides expert physical, social, and psychological support and care, consults with nursing staff and other health care personnel, educates clients and families in health care management, conducts practice outcome research, serves as a role model for staff, and validates the nursing observations and interventions that staff make (Wilkey & Gardner, 1999). It is not unusual for the CNS to be competent in providing care during all stages of an illness, and function in any setting where clients are found, for example, clinics, community agencies, or long-term care facilities. Many work in acute care facilities and have prescriptive practice privileges (Gaddis, 1996; Page & Mackowiak, 1997). Others are used as staff educators/consultants to the health care team, managers, expert clinicians, or researchers (Naylor & Brooten, 1993).

Case Management

Case management is a practice model initially developed to minimize fragmentation of services and maximize individualization of care. It uses a systematic approach ensuring optimal outcomes by developing **clinical pathways** that are designed to achieve specific patient outcomes in a defined time frame. Length of hospital stay can be reduced when this method is used (Ignatavicius & Hausman, 1995; Strong, 1992). Case management also allocates and coordinates services for individuals who cannot manage their own care or cannot negotiate the health system. Typically, the case manager obtains services that the client needs and then monitors the effectiveness of the interventions provided to meet those needs (Epstein, Nelson, Polsgrove, Coutinho, Cumblad, & Quinn, 1993). The plans developed are based on evidence-based research and past medical decisions, so the most effective practices, considering the client's condition, are used (Merritt, Palmer, Bergman, & Shiono, 1997; Turley, Higgens, Archer-Duste, & Cafferty, 1995). These critical pathways guide the team through the client's course of therapy, indicating key events that must occur each day in order to achieve an appropriate length of stay (Turley et al., 1995).

STANDARDS OF CARE AND STANDARDS OF PROFESSIONAL PERFORMANCE

Professional nurses, as well as all health care professionals, are being held more accountable for their actions. This change is translating into more emphasis on adherence to standards of care. The **standard of care** is the accepted action expected of an individual of a certain skill or knowledge level. It is considered the minimal level of functioning and what a reasonable and prudent person would do in a similar situation. Standards are a tool for determining if the

BOX 1-6 ANA-SPN standards of care and standards of professional performance for pediatric nurses

Standards of care for the pediatric nurse:

- Collects health data
- Analyzes the assessment data in determining diagnoses
- Identifies expected outcomes individualized to the client
- Develops a plan of care that prescribes interventions to attain expected outcomes
- Implements the interventions identified in the plan of care
- Evaluates the child's and family's progress toward attainment of outcomes

Standards of professional performance for the pediatric nurse:

- Systematically evaluates the quality and effectiveness of pediatric nursing practice
- Evaluates her or his own nursing practice in relation to professional practice standards and relevant statutes and regulations
- Acquires and maintains current knowledge in pediatric nursing practice
- Contributes to the professional development of peers, collegues, and others
- Makes decisions and takes actions on behalf of children and their families that are determined in an ethical manner
- Collaborates with the child, family, and health care providers in providing client care
- Uses research findings in practice
- Considers factors related to safety, effectiveness, and cost in planning and delivering care

American Nurses Association and the Society of Pediatric Nurses. (1996). *Statement on the scope and standards of pediatric clinical practice.* Washington, DC: American Nurses Publishing.

care provided was adequate or negligent (less than adequate). Professional standards are derived from regulatory agencies, nursing practice acts, professional nursing organizations, and state or federal laws. Additionally, they come from scientific literature, which is typically research-based or evidence-based, and from health care institutions' policies and procedures. Standards are used not only to evaluate the effectiveness of nursing care provided, but also are used in litigation as a legal yardstick to determine if care can be considered acceptable nursing practice.

Specific standards of care and professional performance have been developed for pediatric clinical nursing practice by the American Nurses Association (ANA) and the Society of Pediatric Nurses (SPN) (Box 1-6). Other standards of practice have been developed by pediatric nursing specialty groups, such as oncology and emergency nursing.

STANDARDS AND GUIDELINES FOR PRELICENSURE AND EARLY PROFESSIONAL EDUCATION

Caring for children and their families has always been challenging, but has become increasingly more complex as technology advances. This complexity has resulted in challenges for nursing educators, one of which is an expanded and more complex amount of knowledge in pediatric nursing. Also, with increased attention to family-centered and community-based care, all nurses will care for children and their families at some point during their nursing career. Thus, the Standards and Guidelines for Prelicensure and Professional Education for the Nursing Care of Children and Their Families were developed to support the education of prelicensure students and the professional development of new graduates for the nursing of children and their families (Box 1-7). These standards and guidelines are based on (1) child, family, and societal factors, (2) clinical problems or areas, and (3) care delivery.

The intent is that the goals will be implemented across all settings where prelicense and early professional education occur. Resources and circumstances unique to each education situation will influence how the goals are implemented, how teaching-learning processes are chosen and applied, and the outcomes that are selected as the main aims of the education. Additionally, it is expected that the standards and guidelines will be integrated throughout the entire curriculum rather than only in one course.

MEETING THE CHALLENGES OF THE 21ST CENTURY

Child health care has changed considerably over the past 20 years. Health care systems were previously focused on the treatment of disease. Health care personnel placed a greater emphasis on treating disease while neglecting early detection and treatment of illness as well as health promotion and maintenance. Disease treatment usually involved invasive procedures through medical technology in acute care set-

BOX 1-7 Standards and guidelines for prelicensure and early professional education for the nursing care of children and their families

I. Child, family, and societal factors
   1. *Concept:* Anatomic structures and physiologic and psychologic processes in neonates, infants, children, and adolescents
      Goal The nurse will integrate knowledge of the unique anatomic structures, physiologic and psychologic processes of children from birth through adolescence to make assessments, plan, implement, and evaluate care.
   2. *Concept:* Health behaviors
      Goal The nurse will use opportunities to positively influence the health behaviors of children and their families.
   3. *Concept:* Separation, loss, and bereavement
      Goal The nurse will provide supportive care for children and families experiencing separation, loss, and/or death.
   4. *Concept:* Economic, social, and political influences
      Goal The nurse will use knowledge of how the larger environment influences the child's health and development and the family's care to (a) make assessments, plan strategies, and implement approaches that are in accord with the family's economic and social situation and available resources, and (b) work with others in the community to make and implement plans for the health care needs of children.

II. Clinical problems or areas
   1. *Concept:* Safety and injury prevention
      Goal The nurse will provide and promote safety in order to prevent injuries and support the development of the child.
   2. *Concept:* Children with chronic conditions or disabilities and their families
      Goal The nurse will make assessments, plan strategies of care, and intervene in ways that promote the growth and development of the child with a chronic condition or disability. Additionally, the nurse will support the child's and family's management of care and promote a healthy family lifestyle. Evaluation of nursing care is a part of this process.
   3. *Concept:* Children with acute illness or injuries and their families
      Goal When providing care to children with acute illness or injuries and their families, the nurse will make assessments, plan strategies of care, and intervene in ways that promote the growth, development, and safety of the child. Evaluation of nursing care is a part of this process.

III. Care delivery
   1. *Concept:* Family-centered care
      Goal A The nurse will use the family-centered approach to: (a) assess needs, plan and implement interventions, and evaluate outcomes relevant to the health care needs of children in partnership with them and their families; (b) work with other health care providers and the family to promote coordinated service delivery; and (c) advocate for family-centered care of children.
      Goal B The nurse will participate in developing and working within service delivery systems to support practice that is consistent with principles of a family-centered approach.
   2. *Concept:* Cultural competence
      Goal The nurse will acknowledge and integrate into health care the beliefs, practices, and values of cultural groups defined by geography, race, ethnicity, religion, or socioeconomic status.
   3. *Concept:* Communication
      Goal The nurse will communicate effectively with the child, family, and others who participate in the care and education of the child and family.
   4. *Concept:* Values and moral and ethical reasoning
      Goal The nurse will respond to ethical, moral, or legal health-related dilemmas in ways that promote the development of families and children, assist them in making decisions, and support them in implementing the decisions.

Pridham, K., Broome, M., Woodring, B., & Baroni, M. (1996). Education for the nursing of children and their families. Standards and guidelines for pre-licensure and early professional education. *Journal of Pediatric Nursing, 11,* 273–280.

tings, a costly approach. Financing and reorganization of services has changed to a managed care system. With managed care, the traditional physician-oriented focus has shifted to a payer-oriented focus emphasizing health promotion, disease prevention, and cost containment. Cost cutting in health care institutions is currently pervasive in the market-driven system of the United States, resulting in a move from inpatient acute care or more ambulatory and community-based care. Health promotion has always been an area of strength for nursing practice. Nurses are in an excellent position to be leaders in today's health care market. Additional major shifts have occurred in providing health care, including:

- Children in inpatient facilities having conditions that are more acute
- Shorter length of stay in these facilities
- Increased incidence of chronic illnesses
- Constraints on delivery of care, including reduced human and material resources
- Advances in telecommunications and information technology

These changes in the health care delivery system have resulted in unprecedented challenges for nurses who care for children and their families.

Telecommunications and the Internet have made available vast amounts of health information for health care providers as well as the consumer. The public is becoming so well informed about their health problems that the mystique, and therefore, the power of medical providers are disappearing. Clients are challenging clinicians with information obtained on the Internet, and the increasing available health information is changing nurses' role from health expert to information broker (Clark, 2000). Yet, this information is of variable quality. Nurses caring for children will need to be able to use critical appraisal skills to evaluate health information and to help caregivers interpret it. They can direct families to valid websites, identify reliable sources of information, and teach them evaluation skills.

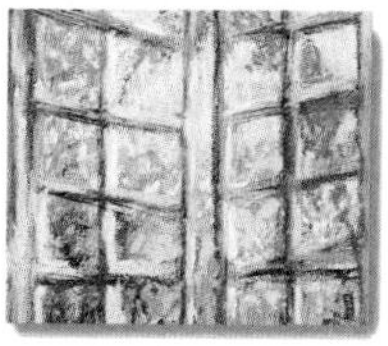

In the Real World

I have been so impressed with the attention paid to the prevention of disease and the promotion of health here at the hospital even though many children have an already existing disease like diabetes. I also have begun to realize that when working with children who have a disease like diabetes as much, if not more, attention is directed toward teaching and advocating for the patient and family than toward administering medications and performing other nursing activities. Yes, I know that medical expertise is important, but the teaching from nursing staff and the encouraging of the family to ask questions of the staff and give input regarding what will work for them in managing the disease is so important. Physicians and nurses must realize that patients (and their families) who do not understand how to control their disease will have problems and may return to the hospital for care. Taking the time to answer questions over and over again is so important. Indeed, being and educator and an advocate are important roles for the nurse when working with children and their families.

Key Concepts

- Current societal trends affecting children, their health, and their families include immigration, poverty, homelessness, migrant farm work, and violence.
- *Healthy People 2010* sets forth national health goals and objectives for adults and children, and focuses on disease prevention and health promotion.
- The aggregate health status of infants, children, and adolescents is determined statistically by keeping records of indicators such as infant mortality rate, low birth rate, and immunization rate.
- The infant mortality rate is the lowest ever recorded in the United States, and low birth weight is considered the leading cause of infant mortality in the United States.
- The leading cause of death in children 1–19 years of age is unintentional injuries, with the majority of deaths resulting from motor vehicle occupant injury.
- Family-centered care is based on principles that are designed to promote greater family self-determination, decision-making capabilities, control, and self-efficacy.
- The primary roles of pediatric nurses include caregiver, advocate, educator, researcher, and manager/leader.
- Diversity of pediatric health care settings and a shift in focus of health care from treatment of disease to promotion of health have led to nurses functioning in advanced practice or expanded roles such as pediatric nurse practitioners, clinical nurse specialists, and case managers.

Review Questions

1. Describe how poverty affects children.
2. Define infant mortality.
3. What can nurses do to prevent firearm-related injuries and deaths in the home, school, and community?
4. Which of the following is the leading cause of death in children under 19 years of age?
   a. cancer
   b. heart disease
   c. congenital anomalies
   d. injuries
5. What major health protection measure has reduced the incidence of poisoning from prescription drugs?
6. What strategies can nurses include in their practice that relate to family-centered care?
7. Describe each of the roles that nurses take when interacting with children and their families, and explain how they are connected to one another.
8. Define differentiated practice, and describe why it was developed.
9. Discuss the differences between the pediatric nurse practitioner and the pediatric clinical specialist.
10. Describe case management, and discuss why it was developed.

References

Ahmann, E. (1994). Family-centered care: Shifting orientation. *Pediatric Nursing 20*(2), 113–117.

American Academy of Pediatrics Committee on Child Health Financing. (2001). Implementation principles and strategies for the state's children's health insurance program. *Pediatrics, 107*(5), 1214–1220.

American Academy of Pediatrics Committee on Community Health Services. (1995). Health care for children of farmworker families. *Pediatrics, 95*(6), 952–953.

American Academy of Pediatrics Committee on Community Health Services. (1996). Health needs of homeless children and families. *Pediatrics, 98*(4), 351–353.

American Academy of Pediatrics Committee on Community Health Services. (1997). Health care for children of immigrant families. *Pediatrics, 100*(1), 153–156.

American Academy of Pediatrics Committee on Injury and Poison Prevention. (2000). Firearm-related injuries affecting the pediatric population. *Pediatrics, 105*(4), 888–895.

American Association of Colleges of Nursing (AACN), American Organization of Nurse Executives. (1995). *A model for differentiated nursing practice.* Washington, DC: AACN.

American Nurses Association. (1980). *Nursing: A social policy statement.* Kansas City: Author.

American Nurses Association and the Society of Pediatric Nurses. (1996). *Statement on the scope and standards of pediatric ethical practice.* Washington, DC: American Nurses Publishing.

Annie E. Casey Foundation. (2000). *Kids count data book.* Baltimore, MD: Author.

Baker, C., Lamm, G., Winter, A., Robbeloth, A., Ransom, C., Conly, F., Carpenter, K., & McCoy, L. (1997). Differentiated nursing practice: Assessing the state of the science. *Nursing Economics,15*(5), 253–261.

Bechtel, G. (1998). Parasitic infections among migrant farm families. *Journal of Community Health Nursing, 15*(1), 1–7.

Behrman, R. (1996). Children at special risk. In R. Behrman, R. Kliegman, & A. Arvin (Eds.), *Nelson textbook of pediatrics* (15th ed, pp. 134–140). Philadelphia: W. B. Saunders.

Betson, D., & Michael, R. (1997). Why so many children are poor. *The Future of Children, 7*(2), 25–39.

Bicycle Helmet Safety Institute. (2000). Mandatory helmet laws: A summary [On-line]. Available: http://www.helmets.org/webdocs/mandator.htm

Boston, C. (1990). Introduction. In C. Boston (Ed.), *Current issues and perspectives on differentiated practice.* Chicago: American Organization of Nurse Executives.

Brennan, N., Holahan, J., & Kenney, G. (1999). Snapshots of American families: Health insurance coverage of children. [On-line]. Available: http://www.newfederalism.urban.org/nsaf/childhealth.html.

Brooks-Gunn, J., & Duncan, G. (1997). The effects of poverty on children. *The Future of Children, 7*(2), 55–71.

Brush, B., & Capezuti, E. (1996). Revisiting "a nurse for all settings": The nurse practitioner movement, 1965–1995. *Journal of the American Academy of Nurse Practitioners, 8*(1), 5–11.

Callender-Price, N. (1996). Nurse practitioners move into acute care. *Nurseweek, 9*(15), 1–7.

Centers for Disease Control and Prevention, National Center for Heath Statistics. (1999). National vaccination coverage levels among children aged 19–35 months—United States, 1998. *Morbidity and Mortality Weekly Report, 48*(37), 829–830.

Centers for Disease Control and Prevention, National Center for Injury Prevention and Control. (1999a). *Ten leading causes of death, United States, 1999, all races, both sexes* [On-line]. Available at http://www.cdc.gov/ncip/osp/states.htm

Centers for Disease Control and Prevention, National Center for Injury Prevention and Control. (1999b). *U.S. injury mortality statistics* [On-line]. Available: http://www.cdc.gov/ncipc/osp/usmort.htm

Children's Defense Fund. (2000). *The state of America's children yearbook.* Washington, DC: Author.

Children's Safety Network. (1991). *A data book on child and adolescent injury.* Washington, DC: National Center for Education in Maternal and Child Health.

Clark, D. (2000). Old wine in new bottles: Delivering nursing in the 21st century. *Image Journal of Nursing Scholarship, 32*(1), 11–15.

Cohen, S., & Juszczak, L. (1997). Promoting the nurse practitioner role in managed care. *Journal of Pediatric Health Care, 11*(1), 3–11.

Cukr, P. (1996). Viva la difference: The nation needs both types of advanced practice nurses: Clinical nurse specialists and nurse practitioners. *Online Journal of Issues in Nursing,* [On-line] *June 15.* Available: http://www.nursingworld/tpc/tpc1 4.htm

Danielsen, R. (1998). Adolescent violence in America. *Clinical Reviews, 8*(5), 167–184.

Deal, L., Gomby, D., Zippirolli, L., & Behrman, R. (2000). Unintentional injuries in childhood: Analysis and recommendations. *The Future of Children, 10*(1), 4–22.

Department of Economic and Social Affairs. (1999). *1997 demographic yearbook.* New York: United Nations.

Dunst, C., & Trivette, C. (1996). Empowerment, effective helpgiving practices and family centered care. *Pediatric Nursing, 22*(4), 334–337, 343.

Epstein, M., Nelson, C., Polsgrove, L., Coutinho, M., Cumblad, C., & Quinn, K. (1993). A comprehensive community-based approach to serving students with emotional and behavioral disorders. *Journal of Emotional and Behavioral Disorders, 1,* 127–133.

Ensign, J., Santelli, J. (1998). Shelter-based homeless youth: Health and access to care. *Archives of Pediatric and Adolescent Medicine, 151*(8), 817–823.

Families USA. (1999). *Losing health insurance: The unintended consequences of welfare reform* (Publication No. 99-103). Washington, DC: Author.

Fosbinder, D., Ashton, C., & Koerner, J. (1997). The national healing web partnership: An innovative model to improve health. *Journal of Nursing Administration, 27*(4), 37–41.

Furdon, S., Pfell, V., & Snow, K. (1998). Operationalizing Donna Wong's principle of traumatic care: Pain management protocol in the NICU. *Pediatric Nursing, 24*(4), 336–342.

Gaddis, M. (1996). Clinical nurse specialist and nurse practitioner role merger. *Central Lines, 12*(1), 14–17.

Grossman, D. (2000). The history of injury control and the epidemiology of child and adolescent injuries. *The Future of Children, 10*(1), 23–52.

Grossman, D., Reay, D., & Baker, S. (1999). Self-inflicted and unintentional firearm injuries among children and adolescents: The source of the firearm. *Archives of Pediatric and Adolescent Medicine, 155,* 875–878.

Guyer, B., Freedman, M., Strobino, D., & Sondik, E. (2000). Annual summary of vital statistics: Trends in the health of Americans during the 20th century. *Pediatrics, 106*(6), 1307–1317.

Guyer, B., Hoyert, D., Martin, J., Ventura, S., MacDorman, M., & Strobino, D. (1999). Annual summary of vital statistics—1998. *Pediatrics, 104*(6), 1229–1246.

Gwyther, M., & Jenkins, M. (1998). Migrant farmworkers' children: Health status, barriers to care, and nursing innovations in health care delivery. *Pediatric Health Care, 12,* 60–66.

Health Care Financing Administration. SCHIP Aggregate Enrollment Statistics for the 50 states and the District of Columbia for Federal fiscal year 1999 and 2000 [On-line]. Available: http://www. hcfa.gov/init/fy99-00.pdf

Heller, R., & McKlindon, D. (1996). Families as "faculty": Parents educating caregivers about family centered care. *Pediatric Nursing, 22*(5), 428–431.

Hulewat, P. (1996). Resettlement: A cultural and psychological crisis. *Social Work, 41,* 129–135.

Ignatavicius, D., & Hausman, K. (1995). *Clinical pathways for collaborative practice.* Philadelphia: Saunders.

Koerner, J. (1992). Differentiated practice: The evolution of professional nursing. *Journal of Professional Nursing, 8*(6), 335–341.

Laraque, D., Spivak, H., & Bull, M. (2001). Serious firearm injury prevention does make sense. *Pediatrics, 107*(2), 408–410.

LoBiondo-Wood, G., & Haber, J. (1997). *Nursing research: Methods, critical appraisal, and utilization.* St. Louis: Mosby.

Martin, J., Smith, B., Matthews, T., & Ventura, S. (1999). Births and deaths: Preliminary data for 1998. *National vital statistics reports.* Hyattsville, MD: National Center for Health Statistics.

McLelland, D., Thompson, P., Piete, S., & Hatcher, P. (1996). Assessing firearms safety in inner-city homes. *Nursing and Health Care (N&HC): Perspectives on Community, 17*(4), 174–178.

McLoyd, V. (1998). Socioeconomic disadvantage and child development. *American Psychologist, 53*(2), 185–204.

Melnyk, B., & Feinstein, N. (2001). Mediating functions of paternal anxiety and participation in care on young childrens posthospital adjustment. *Research in Nursing and Health, 24,* 18–26.

Merritt, T., Palmer, D., Bergman, D., & Shiono, P. (1997). Clinical practice guidelines in pediatric and newborn medicine, implications for their use in practice. *Pediatrics, 99*(1), 100–114.

Murphy, S. (2000). Deaths: Final data for 1998. *National Vital Statistics Report, 48*(11). Hyattsville, MD: National Center For Health Statistics.

National SAFE KIDS Campaign. (1998). *Injury facts: Childhood injury* [On-line]. Available: http://www.safekids.org

National Vaccine Advisory Committee. (1998). Report of the NVAC working group. *Minutes of the National Vaccine Advisory Committee (NVAC), January 13, 1998.* Atlanta: National Vaccine Program Office.

Naylor, M. & Brotten, D. (1993). The roles and functions of clinical nurse specialists. *Image, the Journal of Nursing Scholarship, 25*(1), 73–78.

Newacheck, P. Halfon, N., & Inkelas, M. (2000). Monitoring expanded health insurance for children: Challenges and opportunities. *Pediatrics, 105*(4), 1004–1007.

Office of the Assistant Secretary for Planning and Evaluation. (1998). Chartbook on children's insurance status [On-line]. Available: http://www.aspe.os.hns.gov/health/98Chartbk/98-chtbk.htm

Page, N.D., & Mackowiak, L. (1997). The clinical nurse specialist and nurse practitioner: Complementary roles. *Journal of the Society of Pediatric Nurses, 2*(4), 188–190.

Parkin, S., & Dumas, K. (1995). Differentiated practice: The model, role development and implementation. *Communicating Nursing Research, 28*(3), 93.

Pridham, K.F., Broome, M., Woodring, B., & Baroni, M. (1996). Education for the nursing of children and their families: Standards and guidelines for pre-licensure and early professional education. *Journal of Pediatric Nursing, 11,* 273–280.

Rushton, C. H. (1993). Child/family advocacy: Ethical issues, practical strategies. *Critical Care Medicine, 21*(9), S387.

Rushton, C. H., Armstrong, L., & McEnhill, M. (1996). Establishing therapeutic boundaries as patient advocates. *Pediatric Nursing, 22*(3), 185–189.

Schieber, R., Gilchrist, J., & Sleet, D. (2000). Legislative and regulatory strategies to reduce childhood unintentional injuries. *The Future of Children, 10*(1), 111–136.

Shelton, T., & Stepanek, J. (1994). *Family-centered care for children needing specialized health and developmental services.* Bethesda, MD: Association for the Care of Children's Health.

Sherman, A. (1994). *Wasting America's future: The Children's Defense Fund report on the costs of child poverty.* Boston: Beacon.

Sidel, R. (1996). *Keeping women and children last: America's war on the poor.* New York: Penguin Books.

Snyder, H. (1999). *Juvenile justice bulletin: Juvenile arrests 1998.* Washington, DC: Office of Juvenile Justice and Delinquency Prevention, U.S. Department of Justice.

Snyder, H., & Sickmund, M. (1999). *Juvenile offenders and victims: 1999 national report.* Washington, DC: Office of Juvenile Justice and Delinquency Prevention, U.S. Department of Justice.

Sochalski, J., and Villarruel, A. (1999). Improving access to health care for children. *Journal of the Society of Pediatric Nurses, 4*(4), 147–154.

Strong, A. (1992). Case management and the CNS. *Clinical Nurse Specialist, 6*, 64.

Turley, K.J., Higgins, S.S., Archer-Duste, Y., & Cafferty, P. (1995). Role of the clinical nurse coordinator in successful implementation of critical pathways in pediatric cardiovascular surgery patients. *Progress in Cardiovascular Nursing, 10*(1), 22–26.

U.S. Census Bureau. (1999). *Current population survey.* Washington, DC: Author.

U.S. Census Bureau. (2000). *Preliminary estimate of poverty thresholds for 1999* [On-line]. Available: http://www.census.gov/hhes/poverty/threshld/00prelim.html

U.S. Department of Health and Human Services. (1999). *The initiative to eliminate racial and ethnic disparities in health*[On-line]. Available: http://raceandhealth.hhs.gov

U.S. Department of Health and Human Services. (2000). *Healthy people 2010: National health promotion and disease prevention objectives*: Washington, DC: Author.

U.S. Department of Housing and Urban Development. (1999). Homelessness: Programs and the people they serve: *Findings of the national survey of homeless assistance providers and clients.* Washington, DC: Author.

Weinreb, L., Goldberg, R., Bassuk, E., & Perloff, J. (1998). Determinants of health and service use patterns in homeless and low-income housed children. *Pediatrics, 102*(3), 554–562.

Wilkey, S., & Gardner, S. (1999). The varied roles of community health nursing. In J. Hitchcock, P. Schubert, & S. Thomas (Eds.), *Community health nursing: Caring in action.* Albany, NY: Delmar.

Wilson, A., Pittman, K., & Wold, J. (2000). Listening to the quiet voices of Hispanic migrant children about health. *Journal of Pediatric Nursing, 15*(3), 137–147.

Wilson, A., Wold, J., Spencer, L., & Pittman, K. (2000), Primary health care for Hispanic children of migrant farm workers. *Journal of Pediatric Health Care, 14*, 209–215.

Worley, C., Worley, K., & Kumar, L. (2000). Infectious disease challenges in immigrants from tropical countries. *Pediatrics, 106*(1), e3.

Suggested Readings

American Association of Colleges of Nursing. (1998). *Nurse practitioners: The growing solution in health care delivery.* Washington, DC: Author.

Azrael, D., Miller, M., & Hemenway, D. (2000), Are household firearms stored safely? It depends on whom you ask. *Pediatrics, 106*(3), e31.

Bissinger, R., Allred, C., Arford, P., & Bellig, L. (1997). A cost-effective analysis of neonatal nurse practitioners. *Nursing Economics*, 15(2). 92–96.

Campbell, D. (1997). Prognosis of very low-birthweight babies. *Pediatrics in Review, 18*, 99–100.

Finkleman, A. (2001). *Managed care: A nursing perspective.* Upper Saddle River, NJ: Prentice Hall.

Gaedeke, N., & Blount, K. (1995). Advanced practice in pediatric acute care. *Critical Care Nursing Clinics of North America, 7*(1), 61–70.

Haas, D. (1996). Managed care. *Journal of the Society of Pediatric Nurses, 1*(2), 95.

Johnston, B. (2000). High-risk periods for childhood injury among siblings. *Pediatrics, 105*(3), 562–568.

Kowalski, K., MacMullen, N.M. Sifter, J., Brundage, J., Slack, J., Strodtbeck, F., & Broome, M. (1996). The high-touch paradigm: A 21st century model for maternal child nursing. *MCN, 21*, 43–51.

Laraque, D., Barlow, B, & Durkin, M. (1999). Prevention of youth injuries. *Journal of the National Medical Association, 91*(10), 557–571.

May, C., Schraeder, C., & Britt, T. (1997). *Managed care and case management: Roles for professional nursing.* Washington, DC: American Nurses Association.

Miles, M. (1996). A historical perspective. *Journal of the Society of Pediatric Nurses, 1*(1), 46–47.

Page, N., & Arena, D. (1994). Rethinking the merger of the clinical nurse specialist and the nurse practitioner roles. *Image, 26*(4), 315–318.

Polit, D., Beck, C., & Hungler, B. (2001). *Essentials of nursing research.* Philadelphia: J.B. Lippincott.

Rankin, S., & Stallings, K. (1996). *Patient education: Issues, principles, and ethics in nursing.* Philadelphia: J.B. Lippincott.

Schuster, M., Franke T., Bastian, A., Sor, S., & Halfon, N. (2000). Firearm storage patterns in U.S. homes with children. *American Journal of Public Health, 90*(4), 588–594.

Sparacino, P., Cooper, D., & Minarik, P. (Eds.). (1990). *The clinical nurse specialist.* Norwalk, CT: Appleton & Lange.

Stennies, G., Ikeda, R., Leadbetter, S., Houston, B, & Sacks, J. (1999). Firearm storage practices and children in the home, United States, 1994. *Archives of Pediatric and Adolescent Medicine, 153*(6), 586–590.

Sullivan, E., & Decker, P. (1997). *Effective leadership in management in nursing* (4th ed.). Menlo Park, CA: Addison-Wesley-Longman.

Villareal, A. (2001). Eliminating health disparities for racial and ethnic minorities: A nursing agenda for children. *Journal of the Society of Pediatric Nurses, 6*(1), 32–38.

Resources

Organizations and Websites

American Academy of Nurse Practitioners
179 Princeton Boulevard
Lowell, MA 01851
(617) 937-7343

American Academy of Pediatrics
141 Northwest Point Blvd.
Elk Grove, IL 60009-0927
www.aap.org

American Nurses' Association
600 Maryland Avenue, S.W., Suite 100 West
Washington, DC 20024-2571
(202) 651-7000
www.ana.org

Annie E. Casey Foundation
701 Saint Paul Street
Baltimore, MD 21202
(410) 547-6600
www.aecf.org

Agency for Health Care Policy and Research
2101 East Jefferson Street
Rockville, MD 20852
(301) 594-1364
www.ahcpr.gov

The Brady Center to Prevent Gun Violence
1225 Eye Street, N.W., Suite 1100
Washington, DC 20005
(202) 289-7319
www.bradycenter.org

Case Management Society of America
8201 Cantrell Road, Suite 230
Little Rock, AR 72227
(501) 225-2229
www.cmsa.org

Centers for Disease Control and Prevention
1600 Clifton Road, N.E.
Atlanta, GA 30306
(404) 639-3311
www.cdc.gov

Center for the Future of Children
The David and Lucile Packard Foundation
300 Second Street, Suite 102
Los Altos, CA 94022
www.futureofchildren.org

Children's Defense Fund
25 E. Street, N.W.
Washington, DC 20001
(202) 628-8787
www.childrensdefense.org

Maternal and Child Health Bureau
National Institutes of Health
Bethesda, MD
(301) 443-5720

National Alliance of Nurse Practitioners
P.O. Box 44707 L'Enfant Plaza, S.W.
Washington, DC 20006

National Association of Pediatric Nurse Associates and Practitioners
1101 Kings Highway North, Suite 206
Cherry Hill, NJ 08034
(609) 667-1773

National Safety Council
11221 Spring Lake Drive
Itasca, IL 60143
(800) 621-7619
www.nsc.org

Office of Juvenile Justice and Delinquency Prevention (OJJDP)
U.S. Department of Justice
810 7th Street, N.W.
Washington, DC 20531
(202) 307-5911
www.usdoj.gov

Society of Pediatric Nurses
2170 South Parker Road, Suite 350
Denver, CO 80231-5711
(800) 723-2902
www.pednurse.org

U.S. Department of Health and Human Services
200 Independence Ave., S.W.
Washington, DC 20201
(202) 619-0257
www.hhs.gov

CHAPTER 2

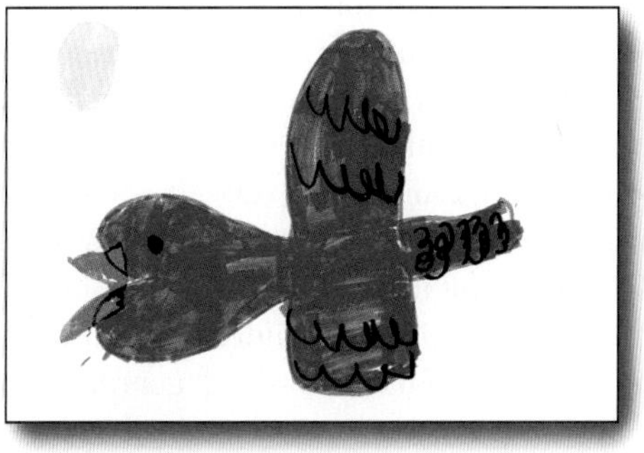

Mrs. Brown is on the telephone, upset about finding a package of birth control pills in her daughter Amy's purse. Amy is 16 years old, and she came to the clinic with her mother last Tuesday for an annual checkup. When her mother was not in the room, Amy informed the nurse practitioner she was sexually active and wanted birth control pills to prevent pregnancy. The nurse practitioner counseled the client about the risks of early sexual activity and encouraged Amy to discuss these issues with her mother. The nurse practitioner then gave Amy a 3-month supply of birth control pill samples and the name and number of a free clinic where she could receive confidential follow-up care. Mrs. Brown is now threatening to sue the clinic because she did not give permission for Amy to receive birth control pills.

LEGAL AND ETHICAL ISSUES

Susan Chasson, MSN, CNM, JD
Carole Gutt, RN, EdD
Janet T. Ihlenfeld, RN, PhD

COMPETENCIES

Upon completion of this chapter, the reader will be able to:

- *List sources of law, including state, federal, and judicial.*
- *Identify the elements of informed consent.*
- *Describe a situation in which a minor can consent to health care or refuse medical care.*
- *Identify situations in which a nurse can breach confidentiality.*
- *List the elements of negligence, and describe nursing practices that can reduce the risk of malpractice claims.*
- *Discuss the concepts of ethics.*
- *Identify major ethical theories and principles.*
- *Explain the process of ethical decision making.*
- *Discuss several ethical dilemmas and how these influence children, their caregivers and families, and health care professionals.*
- *Discuss the relationship of ethics committees to nursing practice.*

Pediatric nursing spans a broad developmental spectrum within a narrow age range. This developmental spectrum presents a challenge for pediatric nurses not only in the delivery of health care, but also in legal and ethical decision making. Whether or not a minor can consent to confidential health care is one of the many legal issues faced by pediatric nurses.

Nurses are confronted every day with situations in which difficult decisions must be made based on the determination of right and wrong. Technological advances have created unprecedented choices not only for society at large, but specifically for nurses and their clients. Nurses caring for children in critical care areas encounter ethical dilemmas such as whether or not to resuscitate a dying child whose quality of life may be bleak or which treatment option will provide the most benefit and do the least harm for a child. Therefore, it is important for nurses to have a basic understanding of the laws that affect their practice and the ethical guidelines that can be used to resolve dilemmas. This chapter explores pediatric legal topics, along with the concept of ethics, ethical theories and principles, and the process of ethical decision making.

LEGAL CONSIDERATIONS

It is essential for nurses to understand that the same legal problem may be solved differently in different states. Health care is often controlled by state laws and regulations. The answers to many questions will vary from state to state, depending on both the specific laws of each state and how the state courts interpret those laws. It is difficult for a textbook to provide answers to specific legal questions. In dealing with actual legal problems, it is important for the nurse always to consult with someone who is familiar with the laws of the state where the individual is licensed. Table 2-1 lists the different sources of law.

INFORMED CONSENT AND ASSENT FOR HEALTH CARE

In 1914, Justice Benjamin Cardozo stated, "Every human being of adult years and sound mind has a right to determine what shall be done with his own body . . ." *Schloendorff v. Society of N.Y. Hospital* (1914). This famous court case created the legal foundation for requiring informed consent prior to medical treatment. **Informed consent** is the duty of a health care provider to discuss the risks and benefits of a treatment or procedure with a client prior to giving care. Informed consent must include the following: the nature of the procedure, the risks and hazards of the procedure, the alternatives to the procedure, and the benefits of the procedure (Box 2-1). After receiving informed consent, the client has the right to accept or refuse any health care. If a hospital or health care provider treats a client without proper consent, they may be charged with assault and held liable for any damages. While pediatric clients are entitled to informed consent, it is usually the role of the child's parent or legal guardian to give informed consent. In most cases, a child is asked to give assent prior to receiving a treatment or a procedure. **Assent** means the pediatric client has been informed about what will happen during the treatment or procedure, and is willing to permit a health care provider to perform it.

For example, a 10-year-old boy comes into the office to have stitches placed in his right hand. The health care provider asks the child's parent for informed consent after the parent has been provided information about the risks and benefits of local anesthesia and the placement of sutures. Alternatives to suturing and the risks of leaving the wound open are discussed. Once the parent provides informed consent, the boy is asked to assent to the proce-

TABLE 2-1 Sources of Law

Sources of Law	Example
Constitutional law (uphold Constitution, Bill of Rights, and other 16 Constitutional amendments	The U.S. Supreme Court has interpreted the Constitution to include the right of privacy. The right of privacy is fundamental to the Supreme Court's decisions involving the right to die and access to contraception and abortion.
Federal laws and regulations (congressional laws or federal statutes, Health Care Financing Administration [HFCA], Occupational Safety and Health Administration [OSHA], Food and Drug Administration [FDA])	*Law:* Emergency Medical Treatment and Active Labor Act requires all hospitals that accept payment for Medicaid and Medicare to follow specified procedures before transferring a client from an emergency room to another hospital. *Regulations:* OSHA-developed regulations
State laws and regulations	*Laws:* Nurse Practice Acts; Good Samaritan Acts; Mandatory Reporting Laws (child or elder abuse). *Regulations:* Nurses Practice Act can state a nurse needs to graduate from an approved nursing program, yet board of nursing will determine by regulation what is an approved nursing program.
Case law (laws that result from judicial decision)	Judicial interpretation of Americans with Disabilities Act (ADA) of 1990 (federal law). The act states that "reasonable accommodation" must be made for handicapped employees. The ADA does not define reasonable accommodation. In the case of *Howell v. Michelin Tire Corporation* (1994) the court decided that it would be "reasonable accommodation" to reassign an employee with a disability to an existing light-duty job that was vacant. Once a case is decided by a judge, attorneys use these legal decisions to help their clients understand how to interpret and follow the law.

BOX 2-1 Elements of informed consent

1. A statement that the study involves research.
2. An exploration of the purpose of the research, delineating the expected duration of the subject's participation.
3. A description of the procedures to be followed and identification of any procedures that are experimental.
4. A description of any reasonably foreseeable risks or discomforts to the subject.
5. A description of any benefits to the subject or to others that may reasonably be expected from the research.
6. A disclosure of appropriate alternative procedures or courses of treatment, if any, that might be advantageous to the subject.
7. A statement describing the extent to which anonymity and confidentiality of the records identifying the subjects will be maintained.
8. For research involving more than minimal risk, an explanation as to whether any medical treatments are available if injury occurs and, if so, what they consist of or where further information may be obtained.
9. An explanation about who to contact for answers to questions about the research and subject's rights, and who to contact in the event of a research-related injury to the subject.
10. A statement that participation is voluntary, that refusal to participate will not involve any penalty or loss of benefit to which the subject is otherwise entitled, and that the subject may discontinue participation at any time without penalty or loss of otherwise entitled benefits.

From: Code of Federal Regulations: Protection of human subjects, 45 CFR, 46, *OPPR Reports*. Revised March 8, 1983.

dure. The boy is told that a tiny needle will be used to put a little numbing medication in the skin. When the skin is numb, the health care provider will place some stitches to close the cut. If the child agrees to having stitches, he has given assent to the procedure. While assent is not legally required, it is always better to have the cooperation of the child prior to giving care (Pieranunzi & Freitas, 1992). Assent from the child may maximize success of the procedure and minimize trauma to the child.

When Informed Consent Is Not Required

Most health care facilities will provide care to a minor or an adult in an emergency situation if they cannot obtain prior informed consent. A **minor** is defined as a person who has not yet obtained the age at which she or he is considered to have the rights and responsibilities of an adult. When consent is not obtained for an adult client, it is usually because the individual is unconscious or physically unable to consent. The care given under these circumstances is usually an emergency lifesaving procedure. Health care providers may provide emergency care to a child if they have made a reasonable attempt to contact the child's parent or legal guardian. When that person cannot be located, especially in the case of an adolescent, it is prudent to obtain informed consent from the child (Abbott, 1996). Many states allow the evaluation and treatment of a child for suspected physical or sexual abuse without the informed consent of a parent or guardian. In Utah, physicians can take photographs or X rays of a child without parental consent if they suspect child abuse (Utah Code Annotated 62A-4a-406).

Legally, it may not be necessary to obtain parental consent prior to performing a sexual assault or other forensic examination, but it is important to have the assent of the child or adolescent prior to starting an examination. A **forensic examination** is performed for the purpose of collecting medical evidence when the health care provider suspects the client may be the victim of a crime. In cases of sexual assault or abuse, a child should never be forcibly restrained for a genital or rectal examination (Wissow, 1990). Forcing a child to participate in a forensic examination may damage the child's ability to testify in a criminal case, especially if the child perceives the medical examination as another episode of abuse (Figure 2-1).

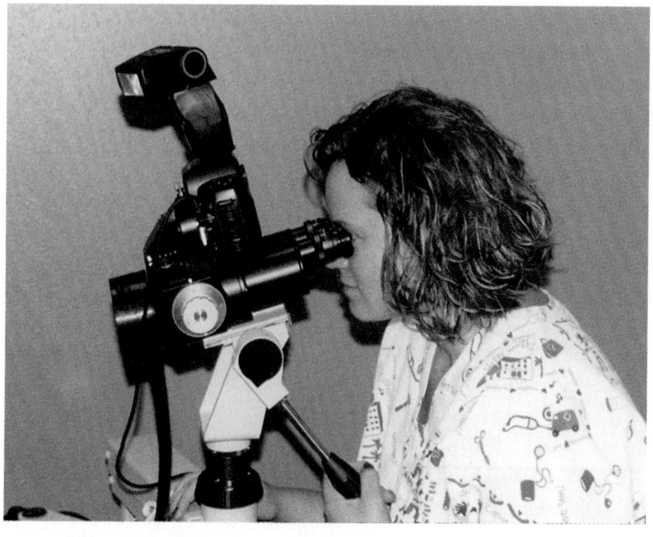

Figure 2-1 Sexual Abuse Examination

When a Minor Can Consent for Care

In all but three states, a minor is a person under the age of 18. In Alabama, Nebraska, and Wyoming, the age of majority is 19 (Jacobstein & Baren, 1999). In many states, a child under the age of 18 can consent to specialized types of care without the notification or consent of parents. In most states, care involving pregnancy, contraception, or treatment of sexually transmitted diseases does not require either consent from or notification of parents. Children may also seek drug and alcohol treatment without the consent of a caregiver. The purpose of these laws is to encourage children to seek help in situations in which they might avoid care if they were required to inform their caregivers (Abbott, 1996).

Some states allow minors to make medical decisions if, under the laws of the state, the minor is considered to be emancipated. **Emancipation** is the legal recognition that a minor lives independently and is legally responsible for his or her own support and decision making. Emancipation can occur through an official court proceeding. During the proceeding, the judge will establish whether the minor is living on his or her own and no longer requires the financial support of parents. In some states, a minor may become automatically emancipated by marrying, joining the military, or becoming a parent before the **age of majority** (the age, determined by state law, at which a person is considered to have all the legal rights and responsibilities of an adult). Emancipation laws vary from state to state, and some states do not officially recognize any form of emancipation.

A minor who has not achieved emancipation may be able to consent to medical care in some states following the **mature minor doctrine,** under which a minor can consent to care as long as the individual demonstrates the maturity to understand the risks and benefits of the treatment (Nixon, 1992). The mature minor doctrine is another example of how the courts create laws through decisions made by judges. Unless the definition of a mature minor is defined by a law or statute, appellate courts in each state have the ability to define the legal requirements for a mature minor. This definition can be created only when a case that disputes the ability of a child to make a health care decision is brought to court. In Illinois, the Supreme Court decided, "To permit a minor to make her own health care decisions a court must find, by clear and convincing evidence, that a minor is mature enough to appreciate consequences of actions and mature enough to exercise the judgment of an adult . . ." (*E.G. v. E.G.,* 1989). In Tennessee "Whether a minor has capacity to consent to medical treatment depends upon age, ability, experience, education, degree of maturity or judgment obtained by the minor . . ." (*Caldwell v. Bechtol,* 1987).

Critical Thinking

Hospital Policy and Procedure

You are the nurse risk manager for a hospital. Your hospital is in a state that does not have any statutes or court decisions determining when a minor can consent for health care. It is your job to create a hospital policy defining when a child can consent for care.

1. Does the Illinois Supreme Court provide a definition that would allow your hospital to create precise guidelines for when a minor can consent to care? Why?
2. Does the Tennessee court provide a better definition for deciding when a minor can give consent for health care? Why?
3. If a U.S. Supreme Court decision conflicts with your state statute, which rule would you follow, the state law or the Supreme Court ruling?

Parental Consent after Divorce

After divorce, the ability to consent for medical care rests with the parent who has been granted legal custody by the **divorce decree** (the legal document approved by the court that grants divorce, divides marital property, and specifies child custody). In order to serve the best interests of the child, the court will often grant both parents legal custody of the child. This means that both parents will be able to give consent for medical care. Even when one parent has legal custody, the parent who has physical custody of the child may be able to give informed consent for emergency care (Veilleux, 1989). For example, if a child is visiting the parent who does not have legal custody, the one who is physically present with the child may be able to consent for emergency care. If parents have joint legal custody and disagree on whether or not a child needs medical care, it may be necessary to obtain a court order before providing care.

Refusal of Medical Care by Parent or Child

What are the rights of the child when a parent refuses health care that could benefit the child? In most situations, a parent will seek appropriate medical care for an ill child. However, there are cases in which an individual refuses to give consent for potentially lifesaving medical care when it conflicts with her or his religious beliefs. If a parent refuses to act in the best interests of the child, the state may step in and make legal decisions for the child. Under the theory of parens patrie, the state has an overriding interest in the health and welfare of a child. **Parens patrie** is a legal rule that allows the state to make decisions in place of parents when they are unable or unwilling to provide for the best interests of the child.

In certain situations, adolescents have been able to refuse medical care without notifying or obtaining consent from their parents. Using the mature minor doctrine, some courts have allowed older adolescents to refuse lifesaving medical treatment or to refuse medical care that prolongs a terminal illness (Wadlington, 1994).

Some states use child abuse statutes that make medical neglect a form of abuse as legal justification to take custody of a child who needs medical care. While many of these abuse statutes include an exemption for religious practices, the court will still take custody of an endangered child. The religious exemption clause only prevents the parents from being prosecuted for medical neglect. However, religious exemptions do not protect parents when medical neglect has resulted in the death of a child (Wadlington, 1994). The ability of the state to take legal custody or guardianship of a child is usually limited to circumstances in which the life of a child is endangered.

OBTAINING INFORMED CONSENT UNDER SPECIAL CIRCUMSTANCES

Advances in medical and nursing science create both new opportunities and new legal conflicts. Often the legal implications of new technologies are not anticipated until a conflict occurs. Legislation is often created after a problem is given a legal interpretation by the courts.

Consent for Donation of Tissue or Organs

The improved availability of transplant technology has increased the demand for suitable donors of tissue and organs. An organ or tissue from a living child may be the only hope of survival for a terminally ill sibling or other family member. When a child is too young to give informed consent for organ or tissue donation, the parent or legal guardian may consent for the child. Usually, a court hearing will be required to establish whether the individual providing consent is acting in the best interests of the child who is donating the tissue or organ. In the case of *Curran v. Bosze* (1990), the Supreme Court of Illinois decided that for a minor child to donate tissue, three requirements must be met. First, the parent who is consenting must be aware of the risks and benefits. Second, the child's primary caregiver must be able to provide emotional support for the child. Third, there must be a close relationship between the donor and the recipient (Dufault, 1991). It is important to realize that other state courts may require different standards to be met before allowing a minor to participate in tissue or organ donation.

> **Reflective Thinking**
>
> **Organ Donation**
>
> You are a registered nurse and your 17-year-old son is the star quarterback for his high school football team. He is an average student, and a football scholarship may be his only hope for a college education. Your 13-year-old daughter is in renal failure and her only chance for long-term survival is a kidney transplant. Her brother is a perfect match for a transplant. If your son donates a kidney, he will be advised not to participate in contact sports, including football, due to the possibility of injuring his one remaining kidney. How would you approach your children and talk to them about choices that will determine their futures?

Consent for Genetic Testing

Another dilemma created by new technology is genetic testing of children. While a parent or guardian can consent to genetic testing for the child, as in the case of all diagnostic tests, the benefits and the risks should be discussed with the child when appropriate. Since most genetic testing requires only a blood sample, there is usually no physical risk to the child. At the same time, there can be psychological risks to the child that include decreased sense of self-worth, anxiety, and disruption of family bonds (Lessick & Faux, 1998).

Overall, the best interests of the child should be evaluated before any genetic testing is ordered. A health care facility that offers genetic testing should be able to provide appropriate counseling both before testing and after results are received. The facility should also establish policies for advocating for the best interests of the child. When possible, informed consent should be obtained from both the parent and the child. Finally, there needs to be a process by which a mature adolescent can receive test results without the consent or notification of the parent (Lessick & Faux, 1998).

Children and Medical Experimentation

Medical research is an important part of improving health care. Since there are many diseases and physical conditions that have an impact on the lives of children, there is often a need for them to participate in research studies. Many researchers believe that children should not be used as research subjects unless there is a benefit to the child participating in the study or to children in general (Rowell &

Research Highlight

Informed Consent in Children and Adolescents

Study Purpose

The purpose of this study was to determine if there are factors that increase a child's ability to understand participation in a research project. The factors studied included the child's age, cognitive development, anxiety level, and perception of control of his or her life.

Methods

Pediatric clients ranging from 7 to 20 years of age were interviewed to assess 12 elements of knowledge of research participation of a medical protocol. The interview was coded for: (1) *Knowledge of research participation score.* This score determined the level of knowledge the individuals had about their participation in a research project. (2) *Weighted knowledge of participation score.* In this test physicians rated what was most-to-least important for children and adolescents to know about an experimental procedure. (3) *Global control score.* This score measured perceived control over subjects' life, illness and treatment. (4) *Anxiety score.* (5) *Cognitive development score.*

Findings

Emotional factors were more frequently related to understanding of research participation than to age or cognitive development. Individuals with high global control scores had a better understanding of the research project in which they were going to participate than those with low scores.

Implications

Providing medical environments that decrease anxiety and increase control may enhance a pediatric client's understanding of a research project no matter what the age or cognitive development of the child.

Citation

Dorn, L. D., Susman, E. J., & Fletcher, J. C. (1995). Informed consent in children and adolescents: Age, maturation, and psychological state. *Journal of Adolescent Health, 16,* 185–190.

Zlotkin, 1997). All research facilities that receive federal funds must comply with federal regulations that require review of all experimental protocols by an Institutional Review Board (IRB) (Code of Federal Regulations, 1983). An IRB is a group of professionals that reviews research proposals for an institution to make sure that the research does not cause undue harm to subjects. The IRB also makes sure that all state and federal regulations are followed by researchers at the institution. Federal regulations require the consent of one or both parents and the assent of the child, depending on the amount of the potential risk and benefit associated with the treatment or procedure (Glantz, 1998). As client advocates, nurses who are involved in pediatric experimental protocols should make sure that all efforts are made to acquire appropriate consent and assent from study participants. Further discussion of children and medical experimentation can be found in the ethical section of this chapter.

CONFIDENTIALITY

The right to confidential health care is protected by the U. S. Constitution, federal and state laws, and the ethical codes of health care professionals. Confidentiality is an essential part of the relationship between client and health care provider. If clients do not feel secure about divulging their medical information to a provider, their care becomes restricted. Most nurse practice acts define a nurse's duty of confidentiality. If a nurse breaches confidentiality, she or he can be held responsible for any damages that result. The nurse may also be disciplined by both the employer and the state board of nursing.

When a Minor Can Receive Confidential Care

As stated earlier, some states allow children to access confidential care for contraception, treatment of sexually transmitted diseases, drug and alcohol treatment, and mental health care. Some states also provide access to confidential human immunodeficiency virus (HIV) testing. It is important for nurses to be familiar with the laws and regulations concerning confidentiality in the state where they practice.

When a Health Care Provider Can Breach Confidentiality

There are four recognized exceptions when a provider can breach client confidentiality. The first is mandatory reporting laws for child abuse. All 50 states have these laws. If a health care provider fails to report suspected abuse, the individual may be liable for criminal charges. Most mandatory reporting laws carry the possibility of both fines and a term of imprisonment for failure to make a report. If a child receives additional injuries after the health care provider should have reported suspected abuse, the provider may be liable for civil damages to compensate the child.

The second exception is mandatory injury reporting laws that apply to all clients who are injured by a weapon or criminal act. If a client is given care for a gunshot or stab wound, the provider may be required to breach confidentiality and report that information to law enforcement.

A provider may also be required to follow public health laws that require reporting infectious diseases to the local health department. Many states require providers to report cases of tuberculosis, HIV, hepatitis, and sexually transmitted diseases. Some states also require reporting of poisonings by pesticides or other agricultural products.

Finally, providers may be required to breach confidentiality when there is a duty to warn third parties. In the case of *Tarosoff v. The Regents of the University of California* (1976), a psychiatrist was held liable for the death of a woman who was murdered by her boyfriend. The boyfriend, a client of the psychiatrist, had disclosed during a therapy session his intent to kill his girlfriend. The family of the murdered woman sued the psychiatrist and won on the grounds that the physician had a duty to warn the woman about the threat to her life. In this case, the court decided that the risk of harm to a third party outweighed the client's right to confidential health care. The duty to breach confidentiality by warning a third party is required only when there is a specific threat to an identifiable person.

There is new case law that may extend the duty to warn to persons who may have a genetically inherited disease risk.

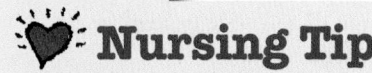

Nursing Tip

Mandatory reporting laws

When an adolescent is diagnosed with a sexually transmitted disease, it is important to explain to the client that you have an obligation to report the infection to the local health department. If the adolescent understands that the report is required by law and that the information will be handled in a sensitive and appropriate manner, there is a better chance for maintaining a relationship of trust between you and your client.

In the case of *Safer v. Estate of Pack* (1996), a physician failed to warn the child of a client that she could have a higher risk of colon cancer and should receive early and frequent screening. When colon cancer developed in the daughter, the physician was sued for failure to warn.

Role of Nurses in Maintaining Confidentiality

Nurses play an important role in maintaining client confidentiality. They are legally and ethically responsible for keeping medical records and other types of client communications confidential. They need to be especially cautious about giving client information over the phone or releasing information to the news media. Prior to releasing any confidential health information, the nurse should always receive written permission from the client.

Nurses also need to be aware of the need to keep electronic medical records confidential and secure. Proper use of passwords and screen savers can prevent unauthorized access to computerized medical records. As more medical records and client interactions are transmitted electronically, nurses will need to develop strategies for maintaining privacy in this rapidly changing area of health care.

MALPRACTICE IN THE PEDIATRIC SETTING

Anyone who works in the field of health care is constantly faced with the issue of negligence or malpractice. **Negligence** is defined as an occasion when a person owes a duty to another and, through failure to fulfill that duty, causes harm. **Malpractice** is professional negligence. It is important to understand that a bad outcome for a client in the hospital or clinic setting is not automatically malpractice. Even when a nurse or physician makes a mistake while providing care to a client, a malpractice lawsuit may not be a possibility. For a court to recognize a claim of malpractice or negligence, four legal elements must be present.

1. There must be a duty owed to the client by the nurse.
2. The nurse must breach that duty.
3. The breach of duty must be the cause of the damage.
4. There must be actual damage to the client.

When a claim of malpractice is made, the person making the claim (client) is the plaintiff. The nurse who is being accused of causing the injury is the defendant. Using the example of a medication error, let us look at the four elements required to prove a case of malpractice.

Duty

Duty is the special relationship created when a person agrees to provide care to a client. The amount of time the duty is owed to the client will depend on the setting in which the care is given. When a nurse accepts an assignment of clients at the beginning of the morning shift, under the laws of negligence, the nurse is considered to have a legal duty to provide care for those clients. After the shift is completed and the evening shift nurse accepts the assignment of those clients, the first nurse is relieved of his or her duty to them. If the evening shift nurse gives a child gentamicin instead of the ampicillin that was ordered and the child suffers an anaphylactic reaction, the duty of the morning nurse is not extended to the actions of the evening nurse. The nurse from the morning shift will not be held responsible for this medication error because that individual no longer owed a duty of providing the child with medication after the shift was completed.

Breach of Duty

When a nurse fails to meet the standard of care, he or she has breached the duty to the client. In medical administration the standard of care is the right client, the right medication, the right dosage, the right time, by the right route. By giving the wrong medication in the example above, the nurse breached the standard of care. Most malpractice cases require testimony from a nurse who is familiar with the particular area of nursing in question to determine whether the standard of care was breached. In other words, a labor and delivery nurse would not be able to testify about the standard of care for a pediatric client unless the individual could show prior experience in that area of nursing. Both the plaintiff and the defendant may each have a nurse testify about what is considered to be the standard of care.

Causation

The injury to the client must be the result of the breach of the standard of care. If the child actually died because of respiratory failure that was unrelated to the medication error, malpractice did not occur. Causation is sometimes a difficult element to prove in a malpractice case. It may be impossible to determine whether the injury was the result of care given or if the client had a preexisting problem that caused the injury. Often medical expert testimony is required to establish causation.

Damages

Unless there are damages when an error is made, there is no malpractice. If the nurse gave the antibiotic 2 hours late but the child had no adverse affects, the client would have no claim for malpractice. Damages in a malpractice case may include lost wages, pain and suffering, and actual medical expenses. When a child is injured by malpractice, the actual cost of treating the injury is not the only money awarded. Costs will be awarded to pay for any care that will be required in the future because of the malpractice injury. An infant with severe brain damage will recover more money than an 80-year-old man because the cost of providing total care for the child will be multiplied by the child's life expectancy. A child with a 40-year life expectancy will be compensated more than an 80-year-old man with a 1-year life expectancy.

Malpractice Prevention

Caring for pediatric clients can create situations that increase the risk for allegations of malpractice or negligence. Using the weight of a child to confirm a dosage can decrease

Reflective Thinking

Does the Threat of Malpractice Improve the Quality of Health Care?

A private health care provider can refuse to accept any client. In a small community, there was a law firm that had represented several clients in malpractice lawsuits against local health care providers. The lawyers and all of their employees were refused as clients by the local providers and forced to travel to another community for health care.

1. Would you refuse to provide care to these lawyers and their employees if you were a health care provider in this community? Why?
2. Does the ability to sue a health care provider improve the quality of care received by clients? Why?
3. What would happen to the quality of health care if physicians and nurses were immune to medical malpractice suits?

Nursing Tip

What do you do when a client is injured?

It is very frightening when a client has a problem as the result of nursing care. Get immediate help for the client to prevent further injury. Document exactly the facts of the situation. Try not to discuss with other persons what happened. Notify appropriate personnel, including the client's physician, the nursing supervisor, and the hospital risk manager. Do not alter or falsify any medical records.

medication errors, which are an area of special concern. Pediatric medications come in several forms, including elixir, pill, parenteral, and suspension; therefore, it is important to make sure any medication is given by the correct route (Hamlin & Coplein, 1998). It is especially important to give accurate amounts of intravenous solutions, since a small volume can create significant problems in a child or infant.

Child safety is another area of concern when caring for the pediatric client. It is important to keep side rails elevated to prevent small children from falling out of bed. Children are also more susceptible than adults to burns. Hot water bottles, heating pads, and heat lamps should be avoided or used only with extreme caution. Children are considered to be a vulnerable population; therefore, the nurse has a heightened duty of care with pediatric clients (Hamlin & Coplein, 1998).

Medical Records

The client's chart is usually the most important document in a malpractice case. Charting is the nurse's opportunity to document the care given. This medical record will be the best evidence of both the chronology of events and what actually happened during a critical event. Always chart legibly and completely. When charting, avoid using judgmental terms—describe rather than label behavior. An example would be to chart that the caregiver has not performed the exercises that were prescribed by the physical therapist, rather than saying a caregiver is not cooperating with physical therapy. Never alter a medical record. In some states, altering a medical record is considered unprofessional conduct and can result in a formal complaint against a nurse's license. If you forget to chart an important detail, date and time a late entry.

LEGAL RESOURCES FOR PEDIATRIC NURSES

Every nurse should read and understand the Nurse Practice Act in the state where he or she is licensed to practice nursing. This act describes the scope of nursing practice and defines both illegal and unprofessional conduct for nurses. The state board of nursing is an excellent resource for assisting nurses with the resolution of legal issues. The board of nursing can provide valuable guidance if there is a particular legal concern involving nursing practice in the state.

Nurses also need to be aware of other state laws that affect nursing practice. Does your state have a Good Samaritan Act that protects a nurse from liability when care is rendered voluntarily at the scene of the accident? Nurses also need to know their duty under the mandatory reporting laws of the state. All states require reporting child abuse. Your state may also require reporting of other types of abuse or injuries, including gunshot or stab wounds.

Find out if your hospital or health care facility employs a risk manager. In many health care facilities, the risk manager is a nurse with specialized training or a nurse who is also an attorney. The risk manager is responsible for making sure the facility conforms to state and federal laws. A risk manager should also review policies and procedures, which affect both client care and the legal rights of clients. Your facility should have policies and procedures dealing with informed consent, confidentiality, refusal of care, and other important legal issues (Figure 2-2).

If you work at a large health care institution, your hospital may have an ethics committee. The role of this committee is to provide a team of both professionals and laypersons to discuss and provide guidance when an ethical conflict arises. The ethics committee may also facilitate communication between clients and health care providers when there is an ethical conflict. As with other aspects of health care, nurses should update their knowledge of legal issues on a regular basis. The law is constantly changing, and in order to provide appropriate care, a nurse must keep up with the changes that affect both nursing practice and the rights of clients.

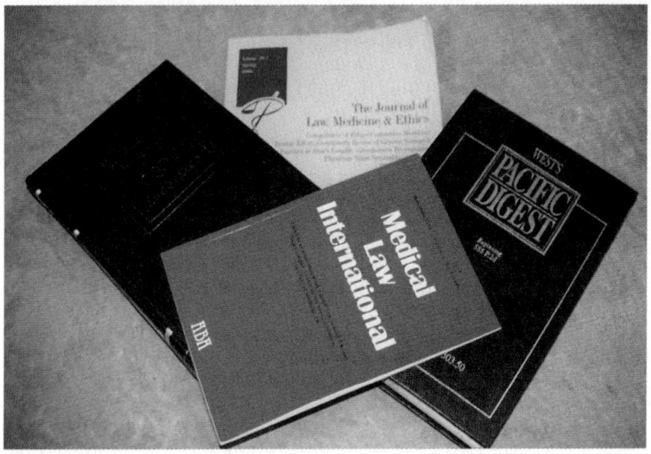

Figure 2-2 Legal Resources

CONCEPTS OF ETHICS

Pediatric nursing practice today occurs in a multitude of settings, including acute care facilities and community-based agencies. Nurses are most often the primary care providers whatever the setting and are, therefore, the first health care group to become aware of an ethical issue. In addition to understanding the legal parameters of safe practice, the professional nurse must ground her or his daily activities in a solid ethical foundation. It is important, then, for the nurse to understand basic terms relevant to ethics. **Ethics** is the study of the nature and justification of principles that guide human behaviors and that are applied when moral problems arise. It is the study of the rightness of conduct. As children develop, they learn and internalize standards of right and wrong. Religion, culture, and society all influence the formation of **morals** (principles of right or wrong in behavior).

Morality is behavior in accordance with custom or tradition that usually reflects personal or religious beliefs. An example of a moral belief is a person's desire to maintain her or his right to die. **Values** are the constructs used to give meaning to our lives. These are also influenced greatly by the religion, family, and society into which one is socialized. Values are motivational preferences. When one assesses what is beautiful, it is considered an aesthetic value. Monetary preferences reflect economic values. Judgments on what is good or bad, right or wrong reflect our moral values (Omery, 1995). It is important for nurses to assess their own values and prioritize them. A student nurse in a pediatric clinical rotation might feel that the priority value for the mother of a 4-year-old boy recovering from a vehicular accident is to be at her child's bedside rather than to continue to work and see the child for a limited time in the evening. He calls out for his mother continuously.

The student in this situation has given "family" a higher priority than economic considerations and is conveying her value judgment to the parent. Education in the nursing profession and the effects of role modeling by significant others in our lives are also key factors in the acquisition of values. Most of us, consciously or unconsciously, make small daily decisions, as well as more monumental ones, based on our values. The employment setting sought by new nurses entering the field reflects a value in the sense that the setting is one that the individual prizes and chooses above others.

Values and ethics have an obvious relationship, and the intermingling of the two can complicate the nurse's role in an increasingly complex health care system. Today's health care practitioners are faced with a vast array of situations for which they have no past experience or tradition on which to base a moral judgment or ethical choice. Moral values are evaluated in terms of positive or negative effects. If the choice between good or bad results is very clear, no confusion or ethical dilemma will ensue. If, however, the good and bad effects are blended or the choice is between two evils, the moral choices for the nurse and the health care team become more difficult.

High-tech care of an infant born prematurely seems to be an obviously good choice in that it saves the infant's life. The converse side of that situation requires evaluation of the possible long-term negative consequences to the infant and family, such as the development of cerebral palsy. This result, with the accompanying lifelong disability, medical, social, and emotional consequences, may become a burden to the family unit (Merenstein & Gardner, 1993).

Knowledge of the major ethical theories and principles are of benefit to the nurse because they can be used to develop a theoretical framework for nursing practice. The following section will present ethical theories and principles relevant to contemporary practice.

REFLECTIONS FROM FAMILIES

When Omar first got hit by the car, I thought I would die of fright. They rushed him to the ER and then hospitalized him in traction. They had to check for internal bleeding. I took a day off, but just couldn't stay out of work any longer. I'm a single parent, and I just started this new job. I sense that the young nurse assigned to him feels that I should be there a lot more because he cries for me all the time. But what can I do? I know family should come first, but someone has to pay these bills and feed us. She doesn't understand our life.

ETHICAL THEORIES

Ways of thinking about ethical problems and issues are represented in a variety of theoretical positions or frameworks. Each framework has something to offer and should not be viewed as being in conflict with the others. **Normative ethics** provides the standards to justify our moral actions and choices. Ethical issues in health care generally involve normative ethics. **Descriptive ethics** differs from normative in that it "seeks to identify actual preferences or dispositions in ethical situations as they occur" (Omery, 1995, p. viii). Descriptive ethics looks at what is actually done in any given ethical situation, whereas normative ethics looks at what "ought" to be done.

Most situations encountered by the nurse in practice involve normative ethics. Four main groups of theory fall under the umbrella of normative ethics: deontologic theory, teleologic theory, virtue theory, and care theory. These guides are useful in providing meaning for moral experiences. They serve to justify human actions, maybe right or wrong, and present obligations or "ought to" statements (Bandman & Bandman, 1995).

Deontologic theory uses principles or rules to guide the decision-making process. The rightness or wrongness of acts is clear-cut regardless of the consequences. Duty to others is emphasized. This theory is regarded by some as the key theory to be used for ethical decision making in health care (Loeb, 1992). The American Nurses Association *Code for Nurses* (1985) can be classified as a document based in deontologic theory, as it delineates rules and standards of behavior for nurses (Omery, 1995). This code is a guideline for ethical conduct and delineates the nurse's obligation to clients.

Teleologic theory uses the consequentialist approach to set criteria for justifying any moral action. The desired outcome serves as the basis for the moral action rather than examining what should be done. For example, rationing of health care may deprive some vulnerable groups, such as developmentally disabled children, of the full array of health care services, but it would serve the greater good by providing health care to larger, broader segments of the general population (Kjervik, 1996).

Virtue theory looks at the intent of the moral agent. Development of traits of character such as excellence, truthfulness, gentleness, politeness, and trustworthiness lead to appreciation of a situation and the resulting appropriate decisions (Beauchamp, 1991). An example would be the general public's response to nurses belonging to unions, asking for contracts, or going on strike. It may be particularly offensive to some to think that nurses would abandon pediatric clients to go on strike. This perspective is based on the public's trust in nurses and its expectation that they will sublimate their desires for a just wage to the children's needs for care.

Care theory incorporates advocacy or acting on the client's behalf based on empathy and caring (Cameron, 1993). It tends to use the individual's needs or concerns as the framework for ethical decision making and essentially rejects objective-based rules or criteria for these decisions. An example of care theory is when a nurse practitioner employed in a school setting advocates for a teenage victim of sexual abuse to obtain counseling and protection.

Frequently, the terms *ethics* and *bioethics* are used interchangeably, but there is a distinction in meaning. **Bioethics** refers to "the application of moral reasoning to the life sciences, medicine, nursing, and health care" (Rachels & Callahan, 1995). Nurses are faced with a vast array of bioethical issues, including allocation of health care resources, prolongation of life, euthanasia, genetic engineering, abortion, and research involving fetal life. It is important to remember that the personal perspectives of the nurse and other health care professionals also enter into moral judgments because they all have biases that color the way they view any given ethical situation (Devettere, 1995).

ETHICAL PRINCIPLES

Knowledge of the following key ethical principles can assist the nurse when confronted with dilemmas of ethics: autonomy, justice, beneficence, nonmaleficence, veracity, and fidelity. Table 2-2 presents definitions and examples of these major principles.

TABLE 2-2 Ethical Principles Influencing Health Care

Ethical Principle	Definition	Example
Autonomy	The right of the client to freedom and self-determination. As health care providers, nurses may not always agree with clients' decisions, but must respect the clients' right to make these choices (Aiken & Catalano, 1994).	Allowing a teen to refuse a home visit.
Justice	Treating individuals equally or with fairness regardless of gender, ethnicity, culture, or socioeconomic status (Aiken & Catalano, 1994).	Providing care to children regardless of the family's ability to pay for services.
Beneficence	Doing good for and to others. In health care, competent care is the primary goal of health care providers and is thus viewed as the "good" (Aiken & Catalano, 1994).	Teaching a school-aged child about sports safety.
Nonmaleficence	Doing no harm to the client. It also involves preventing harm to clients who are underage, incompetent, nonresponsive, or unable in any way to protect themselves (Pence, 1998).	Not leaving a pediatric client in acute distress.

continues

TABLE 2-2 *Continued*

Ethical Principle	Definition	Example
Veracity	Telling the truth, particularly in health care, regarding diagnosis, treatment, or prognosis. Clients cannot be misled or intentionally deceived under this principle (Aiken & Catalano, 1994).	Answering a terminally ill child's questions about his or her condition.
Fidelity	Keeping one's promise or word (Pence, 1998).	Taking a pediatric client to the playroom on a promised day and time.

Adapted from Aiken, J., & Catalano, H. (1994). Legal, ethical, and political issues in nursing. *Philadelphia: F. A. Davis; and Pence, G. (1998).* Classic works in medical ethics. *Boston: McGraw-Hill.*

ETHICAL DECISION MAKING

Ethical reasoning is the process of thinking through what you ought to do in an orderly, systematic manner to provide justification for your actions based on principles. Ethical decision making is a rational way of resolving ethical dilemmas in nursing practice. It is used in situations in which the right decision is not clear or in which there are conflicts of rights and duties. Figure 2-3 presents a model for the ethical-decision-making process.

This five-step process is one model of a framework for resolving ethical issues (Aiken & Catalano, 1994). Step 1 involves collecting information about the situation, including client and family wishes and the biopsychological problems and circumstances. Step 2 entails stating the dilemma, which should be done as succinctly as possible in a brief statement of the main ethical issues. Step 3 consists of listing all possible courses of action to resolve this dilemma, though results of these options are not considered at this point; input from colleagues and experts is helpful at this "brainstorming" stage. Step 4 involves analysis of the advantages and disadvantages of each course of action. Enumeration of the advantages and disadvantages of each action must be considered in detail along with an evaluation of each course of action. Realistic choices can then be arrived at within, for example, a framework such as the ANA Code of Ethics. Step 5 consists of making the decision. Consequences of the decision must be accepted and framed within the client's wishes and a collaborative health team perspective.

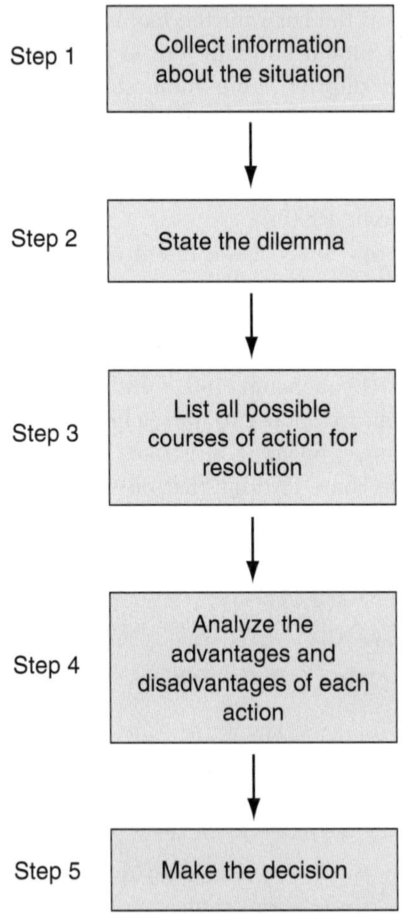

Figure 2-3 The Ethical-Decision-Making Process

Nursing Tip

Ethical decision making

Use of an ethical-decision-making model is helpful when confronted with complex ethical situations in the pediatric setting. A sample format to be followed would include the following questions:

1. Has all the relevant information been gathered?
2. Has the ethical dilemma been clearly identified?
3. Have all options or possible courses of action been determined?
4. Has the best alternative been selected?
5. What information does evaluation of the actions give us?

Case Study/Care Plan

ETHICAL DECISION MAKING

Jennifer is a 10-year-old autistic child living in a rural suburb with her father and mother. The local school district recently announced its decision to purchase a large tract of land near Jennifer's home to be used as an athletics practice field and an outdoor football field. Jennifer, as part of her autism, has an increased sensitivity to any type of loud noise. It triggers increased hyperactivity, crying, and sometimes screaming behavior. Her parents purchased their home in a quiet country setting to accommodate this problem. They have offered to buy the tract of land themselves by taking out a loan against their home, which has been paid for. The school district emphatically states that this parcel of land is the only available property of sufficient size to accommodate the athletic needs of the students. It is felt by the town board that this project is of benefit to a large high school student population. Jennifer's parents are concerned about the needs of their child.

It is helpful to take this situation through the five steps of the ethical-decision-making process to arrive at a moral/ethical judgment.

Step 1. Collect Information about the Situation.

In looking at the key players in this case study, you would need to ask the following: Who has the ultimate decision-making ability in this situation? Have all other options been explored by the school district? By Jennifer's parents? Do the family and concerned public groups have the power to override the district's decision?

Step 2. State the Dilemma.

In this situation does the greater good (the needs of the student athletes) outweigh the needs of one individual (Jennifer)? If so, how would this affect the school district's decision?

Step 3. List All Possible Courses of Action for Resolution.

Is it feasible to delay this decision? Can additional medical consultation be sought to deal with Jennifer's symptoms? Can the family be assisted in relocating?

Step 4. Analyze the Advantages and Disadvantages of Each Action.

What advantage is there to the school district in pursuing this action? Does the negative public image outweigh the positive gains? If the family seeks legal resolution, will the financial costs outweigh the gain? What about the community goodwill factor?

Step 5. Make the Decision.

Alternatives should be evaluated as to least harm or greatest good and follow-up evaluation done. An interdisciplinary perspective is paramount here to respect the needs and wishes of both parties.

Although use of the ethical-decision-making model does not provide easy answers to every solution, it provides a framework for guiding nurses and the health care team through the dilemmas encountered in everyday practice.

ETHICAL DILEMMAS

Ethical dilemmas are part of nursing practice. Nurses find themselves in situations every day that are difficult both ethically and morally (Hagedorn, Gardner, Laux, & Gardner, 1997). No two situations or circumstances are ever the same. Each client, parent, legal guardian, caregiver, and family is different and poses different ethical concerns. The nurse with skill, knowledge, and caring can help families cope with these situations. Many of the circumstances surrounding illness in children are tragic. Many are sudden and due to unforeseen events; others are slow and insidious.

When identifying the ethical dilemma in a situation, the nurse must look closely at the issues involved. These may include, but are not limited to, issues such as conflicting rights, conflict between duties and outcomes, withholding truth versus informed consent, powerlessness versus authority, freedom versus submission, and client autonomy versus safety/welfare concerns. It is also important to note the legal/ethical rights of each person and whose "best interests" are being served (Alberta Association of Registered Nurses, 1987). The following sections give examples of situations in which the nurse may be presented with an ethical dilemma.

Withholding and Termination of Life-Sustaining Treatment

Many ethical dilemmas develop within the confines of the pediatric intensive care unit. Severely ill premature infants, newborns, and children present significant moral concerns to their caregivers and the entire health care team, including cardiopulmonary resuscitation orders or "do not resuscitate" orders, limiting treatment, withdrawing treatment, and definitions of brain death (Nelson, 1997). Parents need to be given the best information possible by health care professionals; however, they must still grapple with heart-wrenching decisions about health care for their child.

Children born extremely prematurely or with congenital defects or genetic disorders that are incompatible with life become clients in the pediatric or neonatal intensive care unit. It is the responsibility of the physician to carefully diagnose the child's health problems so that decisions can be made with all of the appropriate information available. Once these diagnoses are made, it becomes a case of acting in the best interests of the child. This issue concerns itself with providing optimal life opportunities in addition to valuing the life and health of that child. Discussions about the absolute value of life, the authority of the parent, and the degree to which the child will contribute to society need to take place (Bagwell & Goodwin, 1992; Geddes, Pace, & Hallworth, 1992).

The highly technological intensive care unit has many advanced and sophisticated technologies that can sustain life regardless of the eventual outcome. Aggressive treatment of all defects in children must be weighed against the long-term goal of success, quality of life, and/or a life of dependence or disability. There must be discussion about whether the child's illness is terminal and whether treatment is only prolonging the process of dying (Saal, 1995).

Nurses and physicians need to support the caregivers of children whose life expectancy is short. Giving correct information about the eventual outcomes of treatment may help them see the reality of the situation. They also need to understand that the purpose of the treatment may be palliative or life sustaining (Mims & Crisham, 1996). Parents who decide to withdraw treatment from their critically ill child are faced with the most heart-breaking decision of their lives—to let their child die. Because the health care system cannot repair all congenital defects or injuries, the caregiver, family, and health professional need to continue to keep in mind what is in the best interest of the child and their lives together (Geddes et al., 1992). Allowing a child to die by withdrawing treatment could be deemed the use of **passive euthanasia,** i.e., deciding not to treat and to let "nature take its course."

Parents may also be faced with making decisions based solely on the results of diagnostic tests performed while the woman is pregnant. These include the determination of severe spinal cord abnormalities such as spina bifida, **anencephaly** (congenital absence of major portions of the brain and malformation of the brainstem), or trisomy disorders—all diagnosed from an amniocentesis or an ultrasound. Both the mother and the father must decide whether they will consent to aggressive treatment in the delivery room upon the birth of their child, who they know will be impaired and disabled. They are often given the option to abort the fetus, decline treatment for the infant, or consent to aggressive treatment (Bagwell & Goodwin, 1992). They may hope that the diagnosis was incorrect or further hope that a miracle will save their child (Purcell, 1997). In addition, they need to weigh what the potential outcome of treatment will be.

Another issue arises when the child is treated against the will of the parents or legal guardians. It is possible that physicians and nurses can be held responsible for the "wrongful life" of a disabled child. In these instances, the decision to treat the child was taken out of the legal consent

Reflective Thinking

Survivability of Multiple Births

Through advances in the science of *in vitro* fertilization and the use of medications to stimulate ovulation, multiple births are becoming more commonplace. When a woman becomes pregnant with a large number of fetuses following the use of fertility drugs, the chances that these babies will be born prematurely and seriously ill are increased. Is it appropriate for the health care team to offer treatments that will provide increased opportunities for life and healthy survival to some of the fetuses while terminating the others? How would you respond to parents who are pregnant with six fetuses who desire to selectively reduce the number of fetuses so that healthy twins survive?

process of the parents and usurped by the health care team and/or the courts (Bagwell & Goodwin, 1992).

Euthanasia (ending life by passive or active means) is an open practice within the health system of the Netherlands. Clients can decide for themselves whether to be part of active euthanasia and may request life-terminating treatments such as overdoses of medication. In a research study of pediatricians and neonatologists in that country, it was found that in the case of children these end-of-life decisions were never undertaken without the approval of the parents or legal guardians. However, **active euthanasia,** or intentionally causing death by giving a lethal treatment, did occur with the parents' consent in hopeless cases (van der Heide, van der Maas, van der Wal, Kollee, de Leeuw, & Hall, 1998). While this is not legal in the United States or Canada, the debate continues about who should decide whether a child should live or die.

Genetic Testing

Technology has allowed scientists to map the human genome. Genetic testing is determining whether or not individuals have genes that predispose them to a particular disease. It is already standard practice to routinely test newborns for phenylketonuria (PKU), sickle cell disease, hypothyroidism, and other disorders. However, there is an ethical concern as to whether or not determination of the potential for disease through genetic testing may limit a child's future ability to seek employment or obtain health insurance. This controversy is sure to grow in the future as more diseases are found to have a genetic basis that can be identified early in life (Cline, 1999; Lessick & Forsman, 1995).

Autopsies of Children

Caregivers are in a state of shock and disbelief when they are informed that their child has died. Often, they refuse to believe the news, accuse the health professional of lying, or emotionally strike out at the nurse or other health care professional. In other situations, the caregivers of a seriously ill child may express relief that death has occurred and may respond stoically to the news.

In instances in which the death of a child has occurred suddenly, state laws govern whether an autopsy will be required. An **autopsy** is a surgical procedure designed to determine the cause of death. When death is due to homicide, suicide, mysterious circumstances, and, possibly, accident, an autopsy will be performed regardless of the wishes of the parents or legal guardians. In other situations when a child dies, an autopsy may be suggested and encouraged by the health care professionals. For example, when a child dies from an illness that was not diagnosed prior to the death, the actual cause of death may be unknown. When death cannot be attributed to a particular cause, an autopsy may give a clearer picture about the child's illness. In this case, parents or legal guardians must give written consent before an autopsy can be performed.

Parents may also object to autopsy by saying that they do not want their child to have to endure any more pain or suffering. This may indicate that they are still in shock and have not been able to realize that the child is dead and cannot feel the autopsy. The nurse can help them cope with the death of their child when an autopsy is suggested by reassuring them that the results of the procedure will help define the cause of death and possibly may help other children and families. Some families find reassurance in the knowledge that the death of their child helped the health care profession in its quest to help others.

REFLECTIONS FROM FAMILIES

I was so shocked after my baby daughter died, supposedly from sudden infant death syndrome (SIDS). I wanted the autopsy done to find out what really happened. Even though the diagnosis still came out as SIDS, it was comforting to know that nothing could have predicted her death. It wasn't my fault after all.

Eye On:

Religious Preferences

You should be aware of the religious faith of children and their families because their faith will influence their ethical decision making in areas such as autopsy, organ transplantation, and treatment decisions. You should encourage families to consult with clergy in making such decisions.

Reflective Thinking

Palliative Care

Parents or legal guardians of children with cancer whose prognosis is terminal face the dilemma of continuing future oncologic treatments or ending treatments and instead pursuing palliative care. How would you respond when asked your opinion on changing the focus of care? What would you take into consideration?

Organ Donation and Transplantation

Organ transplantation is another situation in which ethical considerations develop. The parents or legal guardians of a child who needs a transplant are usually desperate to find a suitable organ that matches the improperly functioning one in their child. On the other hand, another child has to die before that happens. State laws often require that family members be approached about donating organs after every death. This is particularly important for transplants in children because there are so few organs available. Organs can be obtained from dead or brain-dead individuals. **Brain death** is an irreversible form of unconsciousness characterized by complete loss of brain function while the heart continues to beat. Brain-dead individuals are kept alive by ventilators, without which there would be no breathing (Loewy, 1996).

Do parents have the right to sign a consent form allowing their child's organs to be donated? This has been made legal by the courts, but what is the ethical standpoint for a child who was not of sufficient age to consent beforehand to

Research Highlight

Children Donating Organs

Study Purpose

This research was undertaken to determine whether transplantation centers in the United States sought compatible organs from children for siblings when no other suitable organs were available for transplantation.

Methods

A questionnaire was sent to 259 transplantation centers to determine their policies on approaching siblings to donate kidneys for transplantation, the preferred donor source of transplants, and the minimum age required to donate for such a transplantation. Of the 161 centers who responded, only 117 performed renal transplantations in children.

Findings

The results showed that 33% of the centers used childhood twin sibling donors and 21% used other siblings as donors. They indicated that parental permissions, and donor consents as well were required in over 75% of the pediatric transplant procedures. The centers that did not use children as donors cited the failure of children to be able to give legal informed consent as donors in this situation. Because of this, 68% of the centers required that all donors had to be 18 years of age or older.

Implications

The best organ source for a transplant is often an adult family member. If a suitable organ cannot be found in the family or in the community, siblings may be approached to be donors. The implication of this is the minor age of the donor sibling and the possibility of coercion in this life-threatening situation. Nurses need to be careful to help families weigh the benefits of sibling organ transplantation because of the legal requirement of donor consent. There may be legal implications for the nurse who witnesses the consent if the child is too young to give consent and the legal guardian has the right to impose this painful procedure on the child. Also if the child is going to be the donor, the nurse must prepare the child for surgery and recovery with all of the preoperative and postoperative health teaching necessary for the child.

Citation

Spital, A. (1997). Should children ever donate kidneys? Views of U.S. transplant centers. *Transplantation*, *64*(2), 232–236.

REFLECTIONS FROM FAMILIES

Our 4-year-old son was critically injured in a car accident. When faced with the decision to donate his organs, our answer was "yes." We knew our baby would not recover; death was only a short time away. We knew our decision would allow another child a chance at a full life and would prevent another family from having to bury a child.

Kids Want To Know

Since I'm getting a bone marrow transplant, did the other person give permission for me to get it or will the doctors just take it for me?

You should tell the child that the person is giving bone marrow voluntarily. The child should be told that the bone marrow is a gift to him to help him get better.

organ donation? In addition, what ethical dilemmas are posed when a child is the perfect match for a family member for the donation of a kidney or bone marrow? In these instances, the courts have allowed the organ donation since the legal consents were signed. However, is it proper for the child to undergo painful procedures in order to save the life of another person?

Another dilemma arises regarding who should receive the transplanted organs. Since human organs are scarce, value judgments are made as to which person is the best individual to receive a particular organ when several people all have appropriate tissue matches for that same organ. This dilemma is a concern for children because their social worth is only a potential since they have not yet contributed to society. However, decisions about which child receives the organ are still made according to who will receive the most benefit from the new organ (Loewy, 1996).

In some instances, organs such as kidneys and bone marrow can be obtained from living persons. One example of an ethical dilemma regarding bone marrow transplantation in children was the Ayala family. Their teenage daughter needed a bone marrow transplantation to treat her rapidly progressing chronic myelogenous leukemia. No suitable matches were found in the donor registry so the parents decided to have a baby, taking a chance that the child's bone marrow could be a perfect match. The baby was a match, and the transplant was performed successfully, saving the teenage daughter's life. Ethicists are still debating the appropriateness of this case despite its success (Films for the Humanities & Sciences, Inc., 1991).

Another situation may develop when a brain-damaged child is the perfect match to donate an organ to another child. This has caused considerable debate when children born with significant birth defects that were incompatible with life were kept alive until the organs could be transplanted. In some states (e.g., Florida) transplantation from an anencephalic child (a child born without a cerebrum or other higher brain organs) is prohibited by the courts (Rhodes, 1996).

Using Children as Subjects in Research

Research into health care for children is undertaken to learn more about treatments or new procedures and is conducted in order to provide more information to help science advance. However, when a child is the subject in a research study, it is most important that steps are taken to make sure that the proper consent and assent for the child is voluntarily obtained. This is especially true when researchers give experimental drugs to children, such as when investigating new therapies for childhood leukemia.

Following the development of the Nuremberg Code in 1949, which required the voluntary consent of individuals to be part of research studies, the National Commission for the Protection of Human Subjects of Biomedical and Behavioral Research (1979) issued the *Belmont Report*, in which guidelines were proposed for research involving human subjects. Informed consent and the voluntary agreement to be in a study were essential in these guidelines. Several groups of individuals were determined to be vulnerable as subjects, including prisoners, mentally ill and mentally disabled individuals, pregnant women, and children. It was determined that, whenever possible, adults would be the subjects of research before children were used (U.S. Department of Health and Human Services [DHHS], 1994).

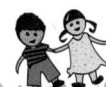

In 1994, the latest version of the *Code of Federal Regulations, Title 45* related to the protection of human subjects was issued. In this document children were determined to be individuals who had not yet reached the legal age (18 years) to consent to treatment. The policy required that children who are developmentally able to decide for themselves must assent, or give their permission, to be in a research study. In addition, their parents or legal guardians must also voluntarily consent for their child to be in the study. Research cannot be done unless both parties assent and consent to being in the study. If either the child or the parent declines, the child will not be in the study. The age and physical condition of the child must be also be taken into account. In instances in which the child is unable to give assent because of very young age and/or health conditions, only consent from the parent or legal guardian is required (DHHS, 1994).

Ethical dilemmas in research arise when children are not asked for their assent to be in the study despite these guidelines. In addition, it is possible for one parent to sign a consent for their child to be a human subject in an investigational study, while the other parent declines. In this case, the study can still proceed since only one signature is required. Furthermore, caregivers who are not the legal guardians sometimes refuse to allow a researcher to approach the parent or legal guardian about research when they have no legal right to prevent it.

Children's Assent to Treatment

The rights of children to health care have been established worldwide. An ethical dilemma develops when that child refuses health care. From a practical standpoint, it is obvious that health care workers would not refrain from giving care to a 4-year-old child who refuses an intramuscular injection because it is painful. However, would that same nurse withhold care at the request of an intelligent, competent 16-year-old who is dying of leukemia? It is generally established that the parents or legal guardian makes all consent decisions for their minor children. As assent to research participation is paramount, so is assent to treatment for children, or specifically, to refuse to receive care. The developmental abilities of the child must be considered first. If the child is capable of abstract thinking and can understand the consequences of the refusal to receive what would be life-saving care, then the wishes of the child may be granted (Kline, 1995). The maturity level of the child and his or her understanding of the situation must be taken into account along with the wishes of the parents so that a mutual decision is reached (Loewy, 1996). Great Britain has a law that requires that the wishes of the child be incorporated into the decision-making process (Devereux, Jones, & Dickenson, 1993). In these instances, the values of the entire family, including the pediatric client, are the primary focus of the ethical-decision-making process. The consent and assent of parents and children for treatment remain an area of concern based on the child's ethical and legal rights (Loewy, 1996). Every situation will be resolved differently.

Positive Toxicology Screening in Infants

An increase in substance abuse by women during pregnancy has resulted in greater numbers of infants born with drug tests positive for cocaine, marijuana, heroin, morphine, methadone, or other narcotic substances. A dilemma develops when the positive test reveals that, not only was the infant exposed to the drugs during labor, but also throughout pregnancy. Some governmental jurisdictions view this situation as child abuse and arrest the mother. This may result in the child, who is withdrawing from the drug, being placed in foster care away from his or her biological mother. The ethical dilemma comes from the paradox between the potential criminalization of the mother and the breakup of the family by the state (Burns, 1997). Nurses need to be aware of their legal obligations regarding notification of authorities in these instances. However, they also must be aware of their obligation to care for both the mother and the infant in the best possible way. The nurse must nonjudgmentally care for the mother and infant, knowing that willful actions of the mother have harmed the infant (Caitlin, 1997). For more information, see Chapter 36.

ETHICS COMMITTEES

Ethics committees have come to play a key role in resolving such dilemmas. The complexity and multitude of ethical situations confronting nursing and health care with the increase in technology and new treatments is staggering. When an individual nurse, health team member, or group is faced with difficult decisions, these situations are increasingly being reviewed by ethics committees at the hospital or agency in question. These ethics committees can assist the involved parties in achieving resolution in the ethical-decision-making process. Several basic roles for these committees have emerged and are listed in Box 2-2.

Ethics committees are usually made up of professional experts, community representatives, and those who bring a broad values perspective. Medical staff from the major specialty areas—e.g., obstetrics, neurology, and psychiatry—are needed. Nursing staff representation will usually include the director of nursing and major department supervisors. Social services representatives, a bioethicist or member of the

BOX 2-2 Roles of ethics committees

1. To educate the hospital staff on utilization of the ethics committee and basic issues involved in ethical decision making.
2. To lead multidisciplinary discussion involving the team versus specific disciplines in ways to resolve conflict and clarify values.
3. To allocate resources so quality outcomes are cost effective.
4. To document and disseminate the hospital's mission, philosophy, image, and community identity.
5. To formulate policies related to ethical issues.
6. To consult and assist medical and other health care providers in difficult decisions.

clergy, an attorney, and a hospital board member are included to provide knowledge of the broader community and its needs as well as a moral, theological, and legal perspective.

Ethics committees are generally organized in one of three basic structures. They can be developed as a committee of the hospital's governing board, a committee that reports to the hospital's chief executive officer, or a committee responsible to the medical staff executive committee (Monagle & Thomasma, 1998) (Figure 2-4).

The consultation provided by an ethics-advisory group can vary from actual decision making to input and advice on specific ethical situations. Client and family input is presented as part of the discussion of any ethics committee if the issue is client-focused; their concerns would be represented by the nurse, social worker, and/or physician. Although the final decisions related to diagnosis and treatment have always rested with the physician, the emergence of managed care has greatly altered the practice of medicine. Increasingly, diagnostics and procedures are strictly regulated by the health maintenance organizations (HMOs), preferred provider organizations (PPOs), and other provider groups. In light of these changes, the role of an ethics committee is even more imperative in ensuring that decisions and judgments will be made that provide quality care based on moral principles rather than on economics.

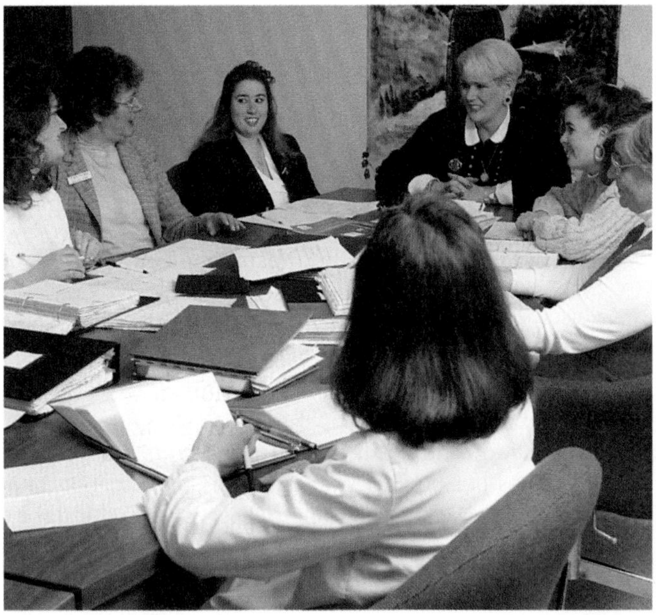

Figure 2-4 A hospital ethics committee of an attorney, social worker, physician, clinical nurse specialist, medical ethicist, chaplain, and hospital administrator (left to right) are discussing a pediatric case. Photo Credit: Michael Morin, used with permission.

Reflective Thinking

Maintaining Life

Mrs. Smith's 13-year-old son was injured in a head-on car collision. He has remained in a vegetative state since the accident. Life support systems are maintaining his vital functions. She wants to stop life support but is encountering resistance from the health care team. What role could an ethics committee play in this situation? What are your feelings regarding her position in this situation? Is there a right or wrong answer to this issue?

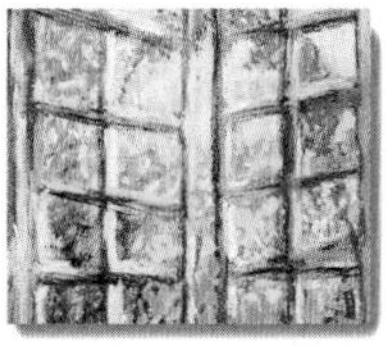

In the Real World

When asked by a family what I thought about continuing life support for their son, I yearned to say they shouldn't continue life support. However, I told them that this was a choice they had to make based on what they were told about his medical condition and what they believed was right for their son and their family. I assured them that whatever decision they made our staff would support them and provide whatever counseling they required.

Key Concepts

- Sources of law include state and federal legislation, agency regulations, and case law made by judges.
- Informed consent is the process used by health care providers to inform a client about the risks and benefits of a medical treatment or procedure in order to get permission from the client to provide care. In most cases involving pediatric clients, the caregiver or legal guardian provides informed consent for the child.
- State and federal laws often allow children to give their own informed consent when they seek certain specialized care, such as treatment for pregnancy, sexually transmitted diseases, or drug abuse.
- If a caregiver or legal guardian refuses needed medical care for a child, the state may take custody of the child and obtain medical care against the wishes of the child's caregivers or legal guardian.
- Genetic testing should not be performed on a child unless the results of the test will serve the best interests of the child.

- Federal law provides strict guidelines for using children as subjects of medical experiments.
- Nurses owe a duty of confidentiality to their clients to safeguard private health information from other persons unless the nurse has the consent of the client to divulge confidential information.
- Nurses may breach confidentiality when mandated by laws that require the disclosure of child abuse, infectious diseases, and situations in which one or more persons are at risk.
- Key ethical theories include deontology, teleology, care theory, and virtue theory.
- Use of an ethical-decision-making process is of value in organizing thinking and clarifying issues in difficult moral situations.
- Organ donation by children is contingent on the written permission of the caregiver or legal guardian.
- Children, based on their developmental level, must give assent to be a participant in research, or to assent to or refuse treatment.
- Ethics committees can assist health care personnel in resolving difficult ethical situations since they offer a broad, community representation of viewpoints on the issue.

Review Questions

1. A nurse is volunteering at a community clinic. Where can she find out whether she is legally responsible if she does not provide the correct treatment to a child at the clinic?
2. If a nurse is permitted to give intravenous narcotics in Idaho, should she assume that she can legally give intravenous narcotics in New Hampshire?
3. The Stone Drug Company wants to study a new antidepressant to see if it decreases sexual drive in teenagers. Would this study receive approval by an institutional review board? Why or why not?
4. You are taking care of a 3-year-old child who climbs out of the crib and falls and breaks her arm. List the steps you would take to protect yourself from a possible malpractice suit.
5. A 14-year-old with osteosarcoma (bone cancer) wants to receive an experimental chemotherapy treatment that the parents refuse. How would the nurse approach this situation?
6. The caregivers of a child who has been declared brain-dead following a skiing accident must be approached with information about donating the child's organs. Who would give permission for the organ donation?
7. A physician opts to treat a developmentally "slow" teenager seen in the clinic for a sexually transmitted disease (STD) without telling her or her parents of the diagnosis. How could the nurse use an ethics committee in this situation? What must the ethics committee consider?
8. The charge nurse in the intensive care unit (ICU) chastises her nursing staff regarding participation in a strike proposed by their union. Discuss the ethical theories relevant to this situation.

References

Abbott, K. M. (1996). Minors and consent to treatment: A policy proposal for the health care provider. *Journal of Nursing Law, 3*(2), 45–55.

Aiken, T., & Catalano, H. (1994). *Legal, ethical, and political issues in nursing*. Philadelphia: F. A. Davis.

Alberta Association of Registered Nurses. (1987). *Guidelines for bioethical decision making in nursing*. Edmonton: Author.

American Nurses Association. (1985). *Code for nurses with interpretive statements*. Kansas City, MO: Author.

Americans with Disabilities Act of 1990, 42 U.S.C.A. § 12101 *et seq*. (West 1993).

Bagwell, C. E., & Goodwin, S. R. (1992). Spinning the wheels: A CAPS survey of ethical issues in pediatric surgery. *Journal of Pediatric Surgery, 27*(11), 1385–1390.

Bandman, E. L., & Bandman, B. (1995). *Nursing ethics through the life span*. Norwalk, CT: Appleton & Lange.

Beauchamp, T. L. (1991). Aristotle and virtue ethics. In T. L. Beauchamp (Ed.), *Philosophical ethics: An introduction to moral philosophy*. New York: McGraw-Hill.

Burns, D. L. (1997). Positive toxicology screening in newborns: Ethical issues in the decision to legally intervene. *Pediatric Nursing, 23*(1), 73–75.

Caitlin, A. J. (1997). Commentary on Deborah L. Burns' article, Positive toxicology screening in newborns: Ethical issues in the decision to legally intervene. *Pediatric Nursing, 23*(1), 76–78, 86.

Caldwell v. Bechtol, 724 S.W.2d 739 (Tenn. 1987).

Cameron, M. E. (1993). *Living with AIDS: Experiencing ethical problems*. Newbury Park, CA: Sage.

Cline, H. S. (1999). Genetic testing of children: An issue of ethical and legal concern. *Pediatric Nursing, 25*(1), 61–65, 68.

Curran v. Bosze, 566 N.E.2d 1319 (Ill. 1990).

Devereux, J. A., Jones, D. P. H., & Dickenson, D. L. (1993). Can children withhold consent to treatment? *BMJ, 306*, 1459–1561.

Devettere, R. (1995). *Practical decision making in health care ethics*. Washington, DC: Georgetown University Press.

Dorn, L. D., Susman, E. J., & Fletcher, J. C. (1995). Informed consent in children and adolescents: Age, maturation and psychological state. *Journal of Adolescent Health, 16*, 185–190.

Dufault, R. M. (1991). Bone marrow donations by children: Rethinking the legal framework in light of Curran v. Bosze. *Connecticut Law Review*, 24, 211–246.

E.G. v. E.G., 549 N.E.2d 322 (Ill. 1989).

Emergency Medical Treatment and Active Labor Act, 42 U.S.C.A. § 1395dd.

Films for the Humanities & Sciences, Inc. (1991). *Leukemia* [Videotape]. Princeton, NJ: Author.

Geddes, S., Pace, N., & Hallworth, D. (1992). Selectively withholding treatment from newborn babies. *British Journal of Hospital Medicine, 47*(4), 280–283.

Glantz, L. H. (1998). Research with children. *American Journal of Law and Medicine, 24*, 213–244.

Hagedorn, M. I. E., Gardner, S. L., Laux, M. G., & Gardner, G. L. (1997). A model for professional nursing practice. In S. L. Gardner & M. I. E. Hagedorn (Eds.), *Legal aspects of maternal child nursing practice: Concepts and strategies in risk management* (pp. 67–94). Menlo Park, CA: Addison-Wesley.

Hamlin, J. J., & Coplein, G. E. (1998). Legal risks of pediatric nursing care and guidelines for documentation. *Journal of Nursing Law, 5*(3), 7–24.

Jacobstein, C. R., & Baren, J. M. (1999). Emergency department treatment of minors. *Emergency Medical Clinics of North America, 17*(2), 341–352.

Kjervik, D. K. (1996). Legal and ethical issues. In J. M. Cookfair (Ed.), *Nursing care in the community* (2nd ed.), (pp. 664–680). St. Louis, MO: Mosby–Year Book.

Kline, N. E. (1995). A minor's consent to treatment: An ethical dilemma. *Journal of Pediatric Health Care, 9*(6), 282–284.

Lessick, M., & Faux, S. (1998). Implications of genetic testing of children and adolescents. *Holistic Nurse Practice, 12*(3), 38–46.

Lessick, M., & Forsman, I. (1995). Advances in genetic health care: New challenges for pediatric nursing. *Capsules & Comments in Pediatric Nursing, 1*(3), 3–12.

Loeb, S. (Ed.). (1992). *Nurses' handbook of law and ethics*. Springhouse, PA: Springhouse.

Loewy, E. H. (1996). *Textbook of healthcare ethics*. New York: Plenum Press.

Merenstein, G. B., & Gardner, S. L. (1993). *Handbook of neonatal intensive care* (3rd ed.). St. Louis, MO: Mosby–Year Book.

Mims, J., & Crisham P. (1996). Health care management of children with cognitive and physical disabilities: To treat or not to treat. *Journal of Neuroscience Nursing, 28*(1), 238–251.

Monagle, J., & Thomasma, D. (1998). *Health care ethics: Critical issues for the 21st Century*. Gaithersburg, MD: Aspen.

National Commission for the Protection of Human Subjects of Biomedical and Behavioral Research. (1979). *Belmont report: Ethical principles and guidelines for research involving human subjects*. Washington, DC: Government Printing Office. Available: http//www.nih.gov/grants/oprr/belmont.htm

Nelson, R. M. (1997). Ethics in the intensive care unit: Creating an ethical environment. *Critical Care Clinics, 13*(3), 691–701.

Nixon, M.W. (1992). Mental health rights of adolescents: What mental health nurses need to know. *Journal of Child and Adolescent Psychiatric and Mental Health Nursing, 5*(2), 14–20.

The Nuremberg Code. (1949). In *Trials of war criminals before the Nuremberg Military Tribunals under Control Council Law, 2*(10) (pp. 181–182). Washington, DC: Government Printing Office. Available: http://www.med.umich.edu/irbmed/ethics/Nuremberg/NurembergCode.html.

Omery, A. (1995). Care: The basis for a nursing ethic? *Journal of Cardiovascular Nursing, 9*(3), 1–10.

Pence, G. (1998). Classic works in medical ethics. Boston: McGraw-Hill.

Pieranunzi, V. R., & Freitas, L. G. (1992). Informed consent with children and adolescents. *Journal of Child and Adolescent Psychiatric and Mental Health Nursing, 5*(2) 21–27.

Purcell, C. (1997). Withdrawing treatment from a critically ill child. *Intensive and Critical Care Nursing, 13*, 103–107.

Rachels, J., & Callahan, S. (1995). Can ethics provide answers? In J. H. Howell & W. F. Sale (Eds.), *Life choices* (pp. 3–23). Washington, DC: Georgetown University Press.

Rhodes, A. M. (1996). Anencephalic organ donation. *MCN, 21*(1), 15.

Rowell, M., & Zlotkin, S. (1997). The ethical boundaries of drug research in pediatrics. *Pediatric Clinics of North America, 44*(1) 27–40.

Saal, H. M. (1995). Neonatal intensive care as a locus for ethical decisions. *Cleft Palate-Craniofacial Journal, 32*(6), 500–503.

Safer v. Estate of Pack, 677 A.2d. 1188 (N.J. Sup. Ct. App. Div. 1996).

Schloendorff v. Society of N.Y. Hosp., 105 N.E. 93 (N.Y. 1914).

Spital, A. (1997). Should children ever donate kidneys? Views of U.S. transplant centers. *Transplantation, 64*(2), 232–236.

Tarasoff v. Regents of the University of California, 551 P.2d. 334 (Cal. 1976).

U.S. Department of Health and Human Services (1994). *Code of Federal Regulations, Title 45, Public Welfare*. Department of Health and Human Services. Part 46—Protection of Human Subjects (45 CFR 46). Washington, DC: Government Printing Office. Available: http://www.med.umich.edu/irbmed/Federal Documents/hhs/HHS45CFR46.html.

Utah Code Annotated, 62A-4a-406.

van der Heide, A., van der Maas, P. J., van der Wal. G., Kollee, L. A. A., de Leeuw, R., & Holl, R. A. (1998). The role of parents in end-of-life decisions in neonatology: Physician's views and practice. *Pediatrics, 101*(3), 413–418.

Veilleux, D. R. (1989). Medical practitioner's liability for treatment given child without caregiver's consent. *American Law Reports*, 4th ed., vol. 67, p. 511.

Wadlington, W. (1994). Medical decision making for and by children: Tensions between caregiver state and child. *University of Illinois Law Review*, pp. 311–336.

Wissow, L. S. (1990). *Child advocacy for the clinician: An approach to child abuse and neglect*. Baltimore: Williams & Wilkins.

Suggested Readings

American Academy of Pediatrics Committee on Bioethics. (1996). *Ethics and the care of critically ill infants and children (RE9624). Policy statement.* Available: http://www.aap.org/policy/01460.html.

Beauchamp, T. L., & Childress, J. F. (1994). *Principles of biomedical ethics* (4th ed.). New York: Oxford University Press.

Canadian Nurses' Association. (1994). *Ethical guidelines for nurses in research involving human participants* (2nd ed. revised). Ottawa, ON: Author.

Chambliss, D. F. (1996). *Beyond caring: Hospitals, nurses and the social organization of ethics.* Chicago: University of Chicago Press.

Levine C. (1995). *Taking sides: Clashing views on controversial bioethical issues* (6th ed.). Guilford, CT: Dushkin.

McKenzie, N. F. (Ed.). (1990). *The crisis in health care: Ethical issues.* New York: Meridian.

Neisser, J. (1993). Disclosing adolescent suicide impulses to caregivers: Protecting the child or confidence? *Indiana Law Review, 26,* 433–468.

Sharpe, C. C. (1999). *Nursing malpractice: Liability and risk management.* Westport, CT: Auburn.

Society for Adolescent Medicine. (1997). Confidential health care for adolescents: Position paper of the Society for Adolescent Medicine. *Journal of Adolescent Health, 21,* 408–415.

Taylor, B. (1999). Parental autonomy and consent to treatment. *Journal of Advanced Nursing, 29*(3), 570–576.

Trandel-Korenchuk, D. M., & Trandel-Korenchuk, K. M. (1997). *Nursing and the law* (5th ed.). Gaithersburg, MD: Aspen.

Resources

Organizations and Websites

The American Association of Nurse Attorneys
7794 Grow Drive
Pensacola, FL 32514
(877) 538-2262
www.taana.org

American Nurses Association
600 Maryland Avenue, SW
Suite 100 West
Washington, DC 20024-2571
(202) 651-7000
www.ana.org

Findlaw.com
www.findlaw.com
This website provides access to state and federal statutes and case law.

The Hastings Center Studies in Ethics
Route 9D
Garrison, NY 10524
(914) 424-4040
Fax (914) 424-4545

Health Privacy Project
Institute for Health Care Research and Policy
Georgetown University
2233 Wisconsin Avenue NW, Suite 525
Washington, DC 20007
(202) 687-0880
www.healthprivacy.org
This website provides information about health privacy statutes in each state.

International Association of Forensic Nurses
E. Holly Avenue, Box 56
Pitman, NJ 08071
(856) 256-2425
www.forensicnurse.org

National Clearinghouse on Child Abuse and Neglect Information
www.calib.com/nccanch
This website allows an individual to search all child abuse reporting statutes by state.

National Council State Boards of Nursing
676 N. St. Clair Street, Suite 550
Chicago, IL 60611
(312) 787-6555
www.ncsbn.org/files/boards/boardswebsites.asp
This organization's website provides access to every state board of nursing and nurse practice act.

National Institutes of Health
Office for Protection from Research Risks
Division of Human Subject Protections
6100 Executive Boulevard, Suite 3B01
Rockville, MD 20892-7507
(301) 496-7041
Fax (301) 402-0527

CHAPTER 3

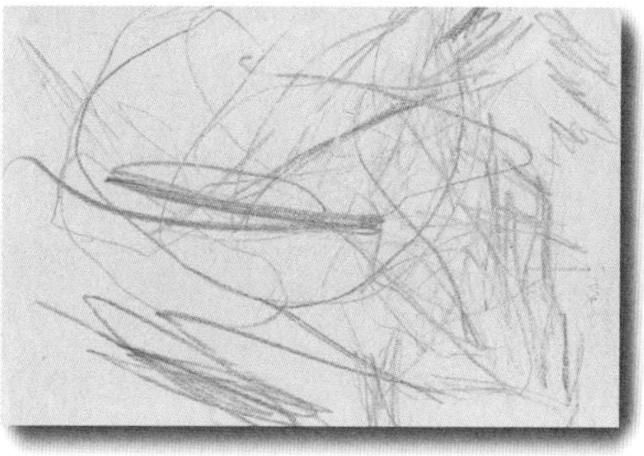

You'll never know what it is like to want a child of your own so much. My husband and I had been trying to have a baby for 5 years and had gone through so many tests and procedures . . . and the questions and comments that friends, family, and neighbors would make. I always felt so sad. When we tried to adopt through the state division of family services, they told us we were too old. That's when we contacted an attorney our friend recommended. He was so helpful and understanding and gave us hope again. Six months later, we got a phone call telling us there was a baby available. We picked up Chad the next day. He is beautiful and such a good baby . . . we are so happy.

THE CHILD IN CONTEXT OF THE FAMILY

Nicki L. Potts, PhD, RN
Sharon D. Horner, PhD, CNS, RN

COMPETENCIES

Upon completion of this chapter, the reader will be able to:

- *Discuss definitions of family, including one that encompasses the changing family structure.*
- *State some nursing theories that provide guidance for understanding families.*
- *Discuss social science theories that explain family dynamics, processes, and tasks.*
- *Identify family assessment tools that can be used in clinical practice, and state the advantages and disadvantages of each.*
- *Describe different types of family structures.*
- *Identify parenting tasks for the various stages of child development.*
- *Discuss the impact of various parenting styles on children and caregivers.*
- *Discuss the role of the nurse in supporting caregivers and their child-rearing practices.*

No other factor in a child's life has a greater influence than the family, which is the first and generally, the most important socializing agent in one's life. Successful socialization is the process by which children acquire the beliefs, values, and behaviors deemed significant by society and is, to a large degree, a function of parenting and other familial interactions. The family's organization, structure, and function have significant impacts on children during growth and development. Nurses caring for children must consider the entire family, rather than just the child, as the client.

This chapter reviews several family theories relevant to pediatric nursing, discusses the various family structures in today's society, and concludes with a discussion of parenting.

DEFINITION OF THE FAMILY

The family, despite its changing and increasingly diverse nature, remains the basic social unit. Two ways that nurses identify families have been described by Gilliss (1993). The first views the family as context; the second sees the family as a client. When families are treated as the context within which individuals are assessed, the emphasis is on the individual (**family as context**).

Conversely, when the nurse treats the family as a set of interacting parts and emphasizes assessment of the dynamics among these parts rather than the individual parts themselves (family members), the family as a whole, rather than the individual members, becomes the client (**family as client**). In either case, the nurse must grasp the interacting aspects of the family, to understand the context within which the individual lives and to which she or he reacts, or to work with the family as client (Hitchcock, 1999).

Definitions of the family differ depending on one's discipline and theoretical orientation. The legal definition emphasizes relationships through blood ties, adoption, guardianship, or marriage. The biological definition focuses on perpetuating the species. Sociologists define the family as a group of people living together; psychologists define it as a group with strong emotional ties.

Traditional definitions usually include a legally married woman and man with their children. This narrow definition is reflected in the U.S. Bureau of the Census (2000) definition of family as a group of two or more persons related by birth, marriage, or adoption and residing together. The Census Bureau has used this same definition for years. However, this traditional definition fails to address the diversity of family structures present in U.S. society today. A broader definition of **family** is two or more persons who are joined by bonds of sharing and emotional closeness, and who identify themselves as members of the family (Friedman, 1998). Another definition that reflects contemporary society is that a family is what the client says it is (Patterson, 1995). Nurses working with families should first ask their clients whom they consider to be in their family and then include those individuals in their health care planning.

THEORETICAL FOUNDATIONS OF FAMILY NURSING

Nursing has consistently had an interest in families and has acknowledged its importance in relation to health. A number of theories of families in nursing and social sciences give insight into understanding its dynamics and processes.

Nursing Theories

Early nursing theories focused on the individual and considered the family only as part of the client's context. However, some theorists have enlarged their perspectives to include the family as the client.

Neuman's System Theory

Neuman's (1983) theory is consistent with a family systems approach. Originally, her theory did not discuss the family as such, but it was later expanded to include the family as the recipient of nursing care (Neuman, 1972). The family is described as an appropriate target for both assessment and nursing interventions. The way each member expresses self influences the whole and creates the basic structure of the family. The major goal of the nurse is to help keep the structure stable within its environment.

> **Reflective Thinking**
>
> **Family and Nursing Theory**
>
> Choose a nursing theory. How would you explain your family in terms of that theory? Do some theories fit your family life better than others? Or do they all seem to have relevance to your life experience?

King's Open Systems Theory

King viewed the family as a social system that influences the growth and development of individuals (King, 1981). The family is seen as both context (environment) and client. Her theory of goal attainment is useful for nurses when assisting families to set goals to maintain their health or cope with problems or illness. She believes that nurses are partners with families. The role of nursing is to help members become healthy enough to function in their roles.

Roy's Adaptation Theory

In Roy's (1983) theory, the client is an individual, family, group, or community in constant interaction with a changing environment. The family system is continually changing and attempting to adapt. When the family is confronted with unusual stresses and coping patterns are ineffective, problems in family functioning occur. The goal of nursing is to promote adaptation and minimize ineffective responses.

Social Sciences Theories

A number of theories from the social sciences help to explain families; however, there is little consensus about which are the major ones. Therefore, for the purpose of this chapter, three will be examined: structural-functional, developmental, and general systems.

Structural-Functional Theory

The structural-functional theory emphasizes the organization or structure of the family and how this structure facilitates its functioning. It characterizes the family as a social system and examines the relationship between the members as they carry out family functions (Friedman, 1998).

Basic assumptions of this theory are as follows:

- The family is viewed as part of the social system, with individuals being parts of the family system.
- The family, as a social system, performs functions that serve both the individual and society.
- Individuals act in accordance with a set of internalized norms and values that are learned primarily in the family through socialization.

Family structure refers to the ordered set of relationships among the parts, and between the family and other social systems. Family structure or organization is evaluated based on how well it fulfills its functions, and the goals important to its members and society. The structure serves to facilitate the achievement of the functions. To determine family structure, the nurse must identify the individuals that make up the family, their relationships to each other, and the relationships between the family and other social systems.

Five functions of the family have been identified that are important for nurses to understand (Friedman, 1998):

- Affective
- Socialization and social placement
- Reproductive
- Economic
- Health care

The affective function is one of the most vital functions for the formation and continuation of the family unit. This function refers to the family meeting the needs for love and belonging of each member. The family is a home base where the individuals can express their true feelings and thoughts without fear of rejection. The family is the social milieu for the generation and maintenance of affection, where one is first loved and given to, and learns to love and give in return. Although the affective function is important for all families, those that must focus on providing the basic physical necessities of life have minimal energy remaining to meet the affective needs.

Socialization and social placement function refers to teaching children how to function and assume adult social roles. This function involves the acquisition of internal controls needed for self-discipline and values such as what is right and wrong according to society. Socialization occurs predominately in the family, and caregivers are the primary agent (Gelles, 1995).

The continuity of both the family and society continues to be ensured through the reproductive function. In the past, marriage and the family were designed to control sexual behavior as well as reproduction. Individuals considered it their responsibility to marry, have many children, and rear those children within the bounds of marriage. The reproductive function is carried out very differently today. Many single people are having children, including adolescents, and many married couples are remaining childless. Reproduction has also been influenced by technological advances such as artificial insemination, *in vitro* fertilization, and surrogate mothers.

The economic function involves the family's provision of sufficient resources and their effective allocation. An assessment of the family's economic resources provides the nurse with information about their ability to appropriately allocate these resources to meet needs such as food, shelter, clothing, and health care. By gaining an understanding of how a family distributes its resources, the nurse can also obtain a perspective about their value system. One responsibility of the nurse is to assist families in obtaining appropriate community resources to meet their needs.

The health care function includes provision of physical necessities to keep the family healthy, such as food, clothing, and shelter as well as health care (Friedman, 1998). The family keeps its members well by passing on attitudes, values, and behaviors that promote health and by caring for them in times of illness.

The structural-functional approach is very useful for assessing family life because it enables the nurse to examine the family system holistically, in parts, and interactionally with other institutions and the wider society. A limitation of this theory is that it tends to present a static view of the family and minimizes the importance of growth and change (Friedman, 1998).

Developmental Theory

The developmental or life-cycle theory is based on the premise that families evolve through predictable developmental stages, and experience growth and development in much the same way as individuals. Stages begin with marriage followed by childbirth and child rearing. Each stage is characterized by specific issues and tasks. Developmental theories explain the changes that occur in human organisms or groups over time. This approach is based on the following assumptions (Duvall, 1977):

- Critical role transitions of individual members, such as birth, retirement, and death of a spouse, are viewed as resulting in a distinct change in the family life patterns.
- Families develop and change over time in predictable ways.
- Families and their members perform certain time-specific tasks that are decided upon by themselves, within their cultural and societal context.
- Family behavior is the sum of the previous experiences of its members as incorporated in the present and in their expectations for the future.

The best known formulation of the developmental stages comes from Duvall (1977; Duvall & Miller, 1985), who identified eight chronological stages through which the family passes. Each stage includes predictable tasks that the family must master prior to proceeding to the next one.

Table 3-1 delineates the stages of family development and tasks of each stage.

An advantage of the developmental approach is that it provides nurses with information about what to expect of families at different points in their life cycle and, thus, what teaching and counseling services may be needed. This theory also provides criteria for assessing a family's current stage and its ability to accomplish the tasks of this stage. The nurse is then able to support the family in order to progress smoothly from one stage to another.

There are several limitations of the developmental theory. It has a middle class bias and it assumes homogeneity

TABLE 3-1 Duvall's Developmental Stages and Tasks of the Family

Stage	Task
Beginning family	**1.** Establish couple identity and a mutually satisfying marriage **2.** Realign relationships with extended family to include spouse **3.** Make decisions about parenthood
Childbearing family	**1.** Integrate infant into family **2.** Find mutually satisfying ways to deal with child care responsibilities **3.** Expand relationships with extended family by adding parenting and grandparenting roles
Families with preschool children	**1.** Socialize the children **2.** Integrate new children while still meeting needs of the other children **3.** Maintain healthy relationships within the family (marital and parent-child) and outside the family (extended family and community)
Families with school-aged children	**1.** Promote school achievement and foster the healthy peer relations of children **2.** Maintain a satisfying marital relationship **3.** Meet the physical health needs of family members
Families with teenagers	**1.** Balance freedom with responsibility as teenagers mature and become more autonomous **2.** Refocus on marital and career issues
Families launching young adults	**1.** Develop adult–adult relationships with grown children **2.** Expand family circle to include new members acquired by the marriage of grown children **3.** Assist aging and ill parents of husband and wife **4.** Renew and renegotiate marital relationship
Middle-aged parents	**1.** Strengthen marital relationship **2.** Provide health-promoting lifestyle **3.** Sustain satisfying relationships with aging parents and children
Families in later years	**1.** Maintain satisfying living arrangement **2.** Adjust to reduced income **3.** Maintain marital relationship **4.** Continue to make sense of one's existence **5.** Maintain intergenerational family ties **6.** Adjust to loss of spouse

Friedman, M. M. (1998). Family nursing theory and practice. *Stamford, CT: Appleton & Lange; Duvall, E. M. & Miller, B. (1985).* Marriage and family development. *New York: Harper & Row.*

Reflective Thinking

Family Development

Did you have an opportunity to live and learn as a single young adult, or did you move directly into a committed relationship? How have choices in this regard affected your life?

(two caregivers, nuclear family) and that young adults marry in their early twenties before they develop a career. Additionally, this theory views the family from a traditional perspective. It does not take into consideration the diversity of family forms found in today's society, such as divorced, remarried, single-parent, and gay or lesbian families. The focus of the developmental approach is primarily child rearing; however, today this activity occupies less than half of a woman's adult life span. Thus, child rearing is no longer the central focus of the life cycle.

Family Systems Theory

The family systems approach is based on the general systems theory developed by von Bertanlanffy (1968), which describes principles that govern all living systems. One of the central propositions of the general systems theory is that the system is not the total sum of its parts but is characterized by wholeness and unity. Family theorists have applied these principles to explain how families interact with their members and with society. The family is defined as a system characterized by continual interaction between its members and with the environment. The interrelationships in a family system are closely tied together so that a change in one member results in a change in the other members. Therefore, one cannot understand the family as a whole by only knowing each of its members. The interrelationships of the members with each other and with the larger society must be analyzed.

FAMILY ASSESSMENT

Family assessment is the process of collecting data about the family structure, and the relationships and interactions among individual members. It is a continuously evolving process of data collection. Data about the family are systematically collected using predetermined guidelines or questions, and then classified and analyzed according to their meaning. Nursing diagnoses can then be generated, with goals and interventions for care created in collaboration with the child and caregivers.

Assessment Instruments

Two of the most commonly used instruments for developing a family database are the genogram and the ecomap. Neither requires the purchase of a standardized assessment instrument; yet, both have the advantage of providing a means for interacting with children and their family members in a nonthreatening way to obtain data about potentially complex and difficult issues (Kodadek, 2000).

A **genogram** is a format for drawing a family tree that records information about family members and their relationships over a period of time, usually three generations. It is a method of mapping the structure of the family and to record the health history of all members (morbidity, mortality, and onset of illnesses), thus revealing information about genetic and familial diseases. The genogram displays the family visually and graphically in a way that provides a quick overview of family complexities. It is also an efficient and nonjudgmental way to convey information about a family to other health care providers. Figure 3-1 is an example of a genogram/family tree.

An **ecomap** is a visual representation of a family in relation to the community. It demonstrates the nature and quality of family relationships and what kinds of resources or energies are going in and out of the family. Figure 3-2 shows a family ecomap. This assessment instrument is useful in identifying the strengths of family networks and what resources they have available during stressful times or crises.

An in-depth family assessment requires a significant amount of time, and every family does not need a comprehensive assessment. However, when a nurse identifies a family at risk for dysfunction, such an assessment may be required. Referral to other health care professionals and community organizations is appropriate in these situations. Assessment information can be obtained through interviewing and questioning, observing interactions between members, and utilizing a family assessment instrument. Ideally, all family members are included in the interview, and it takes place in the child's home. At a minimum, the child and primary caregivers are assessed.

Several family assessment instruments are available. Criteria for the selection of an instrument are listed in Box 3-1.

Many assessment instruments have been developed by family theorists, mostly nonnurses, and are used by the health care team to obtain information about family systems. Nurses have created some instruments, two of which will be presented: the Calgary Family Assessment Model (Wright & Leahey, 1994) and the Friedman Family Assessment Model (Friedman, 1998).

The Calgary Family Assessment Model

The Calgary Family Assessment Model (CFAM) combines nursing and family therapy concepts and is based on systems,

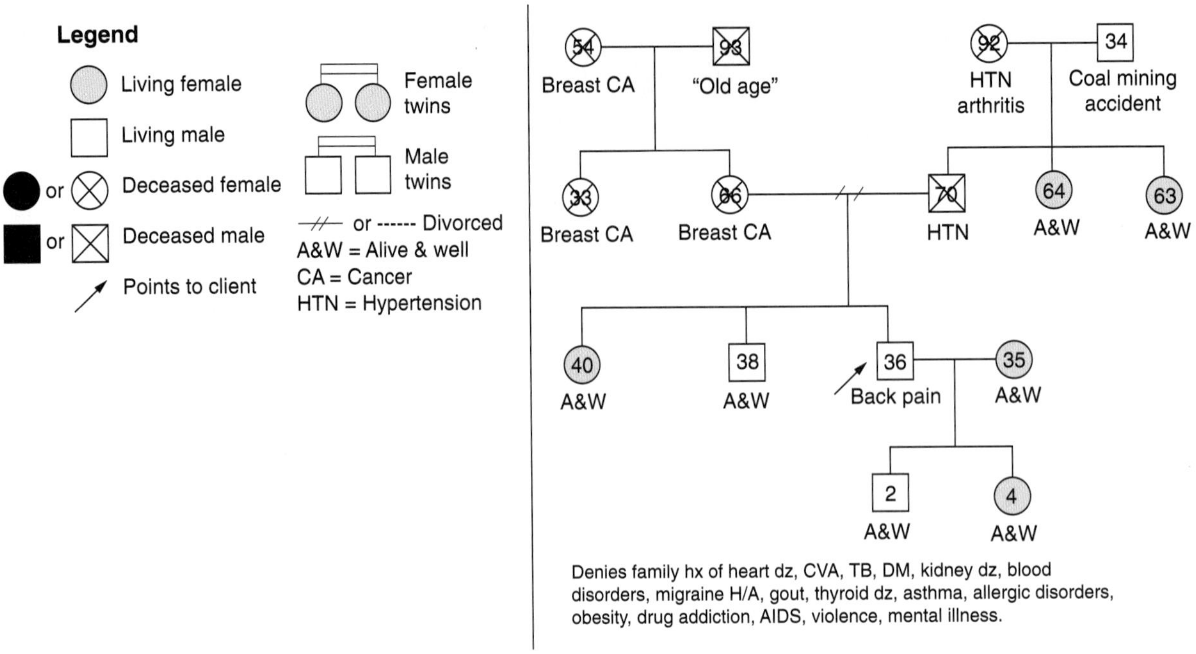

Figure 3-1 Family Genogram

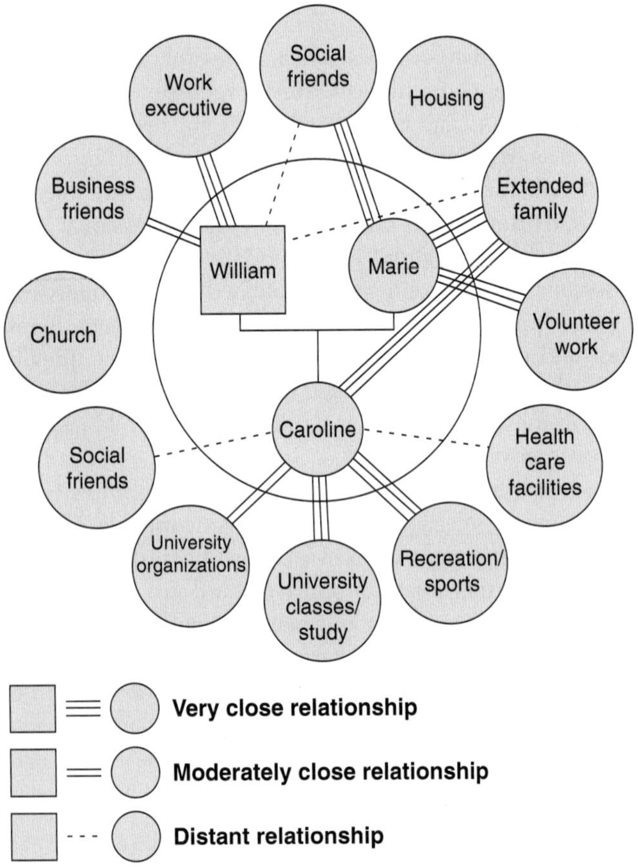

Figure 3-2 Family Ecomap

BOX 3-1 Criteria for selecting family assessment instruments

1. It is clear, uncomplicated, and easily understood.
2. Questions are worded at an appropriate grade level so that family members with poor reading skills and/or limited vocabulary can comprehend them.
3. It can be administered in a short period of time and scored easily.
4. It is reliable and valid.
5. Questions are appropriate for the majority of families; i.e., they are not geared to a particular social class, age group, or ethnic background.
6. It is clinically relevant; i.e., it focuses on family needs for which nursing interventions can be planned.

Bomar, P. (1996). *Nurses and family health promotion: Concepts, assessment, and interventions* (2nd ed., p. 170). Philadelphia: Saunders.

cybernetics, communication, and change theories. As illustrated in Figure 3-3, the model consists of three major categories: structural, developmental, and functional. The assessment questions are organized into these groupings. The first major category is the family structure, which has internal, external, and contextual components. Structure

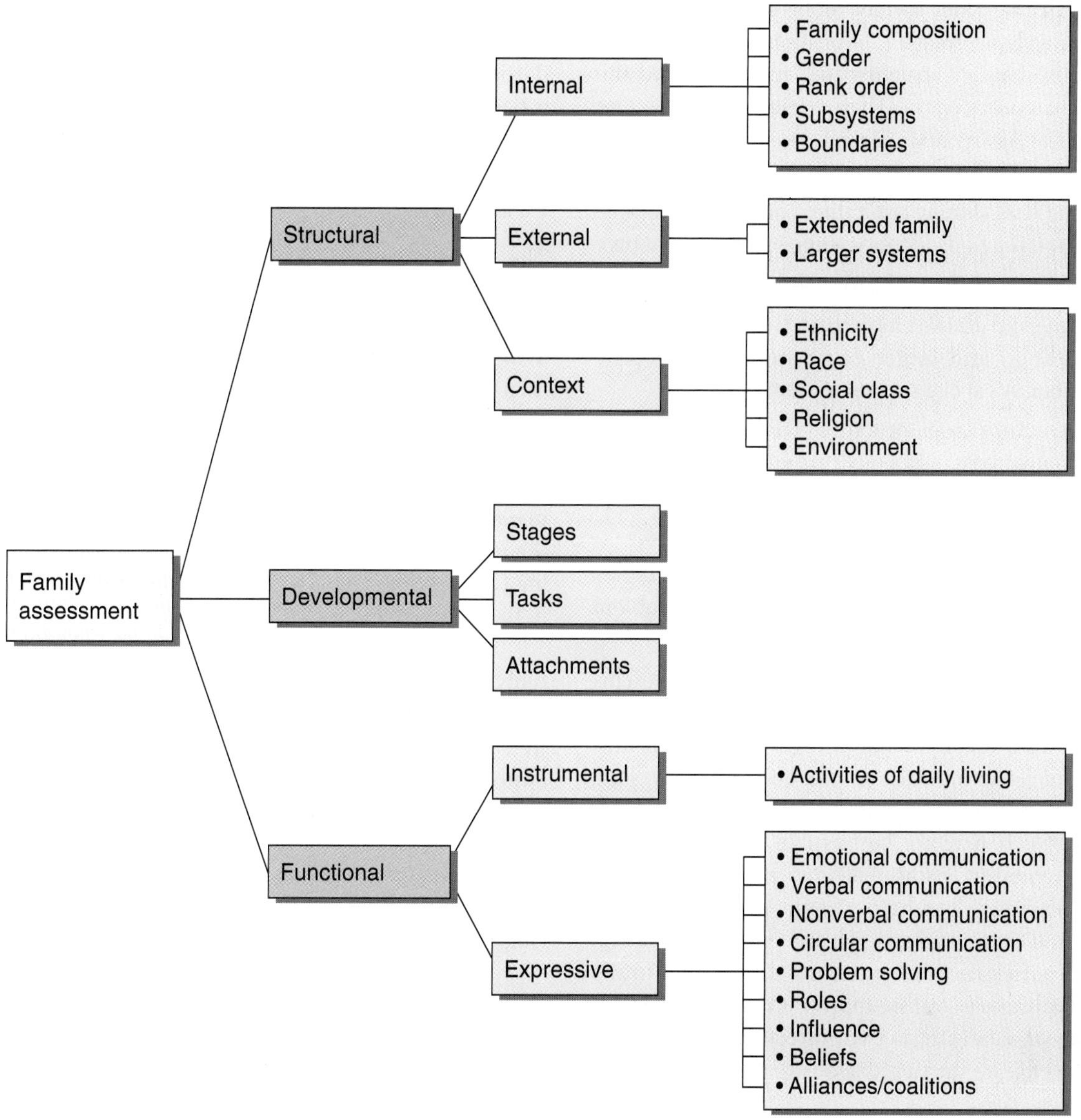

Figure 3-3 The Calgary Family Assessment Model. From *Nurses and Families: A guide to family assessment and intervention*, by L. M. Wright and M. Leahy. (1994). Philadelphia: F. A. Davis. Used with permission.

includes the composition of the family, the connection among family members, and the family's context. The genogram and ecomap are appropriate instruments to assess the external structure of the family. Family development, the second major category, includes assessment of family stages, tasks, and attachments. There are no specific tools for assessing family development; however, developmental tasks can be used as guidelines (Hanson, 1996). The third area for assessment is family functioning, which includes instrumental and expressive subcategories. Instrumental aspects of family functioning are activities of daily living such as sleeping, eating, meal preparation, etc. Expressive areas include emotional functioning, communication patterns, problem-solving methods, beliefs, and alliances. The CAFM is broad in perspective, though it focuses on internal relations within the family rather than on the family's relationship with the community. Although assessment of every element is not always necessary, following this guide ensures that data about the family are not presented as isolated facts. The nurse is able to develop an integrated picture of the many dimensions of the family.

Friedman Family Assessment Model

The Friedman Family Assessment Model is based on the structural-functional theory, as well as on developmental and systems theory. This model views the family as just one of the basic units of the wider society, along with such institutions as those involving religion, education, and health. Its main focus is the family's structure and functions, and the family's relationships with other social systems. The Friedman Family Assessment Model consists of six broad categories of interview questions:

1. Identifying data (family last name, composition, ethnic background, religious identification, social class status)
2. Developmental stage and history of the family
3. Environmental data (characteristics of the home, neighborhood and larger community, geographic mobility, family's social support system)
4. Family structure (role structure, family values, communication patterns, and power structure)
5. Family functions (affective, socialization, reproductive, economic, health care)
6. Family coping (current stressors, coping strategies used, dysfunctional adaptive strategies used, problem areas in which family has achieved mastery)

Each category contains numerous subcategories. This instrument exists in a short and a long form. The short form in Appendix A lists the six major categories and subcategories about which the interviewer asks questions. The long form is quite extensive, providing nine pages of questions (Friedman, 1998). It may not be possible to collect all the data in one encounter. Additionally, all the categories of information listed may not be pertinent for every family. This instrument is broad and general, and is especially useful for viewing families in the context of their community. However, a disadvantage of this approach is that it provides large quantities of data with no clear direction about how to utilize it in developing nursing diagnoses, plans, and interventions (Hanson, 1996).

FAMILY STRUCTURE

The structure of the family refers to how it is organized—i.e., the manner in which members relate to one another, and the form it takes, such as nuclear or blended. During the past 40 years, U.S. society has undergone vast economic and social changes that have transformed the structure of the family, and the roles and responsibilities of women and men. Some of these societal changes are the increase in rates of divorce and remarriage, an increase in the number of mothers employed outside the home, the incidence of more adults waiting until they are older to marry or choosing to remain single, lower birth rates, and a longer life expectancy. Today, society is composed of a greater multiplicity of values, lifestyles, and family forms than ever before. The two-parent nuclear family consisting of a mother and father bonded by marriage with one or more children no longer reflects contemporary lifestyles. Knowledge of a child's family structure helps the nurse to determine the communication patterns and decision-making authority within the family unit (Grossman, 1996). Such information is vital when the nurse is deciding who will be involved in making decisions related to heath care.

Nuclear Family

The nuclear family is defined as a husband, wife, and their children—biological, adopted, or both (Friedman, 1998) (Figure 3-4). No other individuals, relatives or nonrelatives, live in the household. The nuclear family form became common after World War II, and, until recently, it was considered the most common family form. However, with the increase in divorce rates, nonmarital childbearing, and cohabitation outside of marriage, family forms other than the nuclear family have proliferated. Currently, in the United States in 2001, families in the traditional pattern of a working father, homemaker mother, and one or more children are in the minority.

The nuclear family has been credited with providing stability for children. However, concern has been raised about the limited number of adult role models in this type of family structure. Additionally, in the nuclear family, the two adults have many expectations placed on them, such as working to meet the financial needs, rearing the children, meeting the emotional needs of all members, and maintaining a home. In situations where both parents are employed, managing all of these responsibilities often results in significant stress in the family.

Extended Family

The extended family consists of those members of the nuclear family and other blood-related persons such as

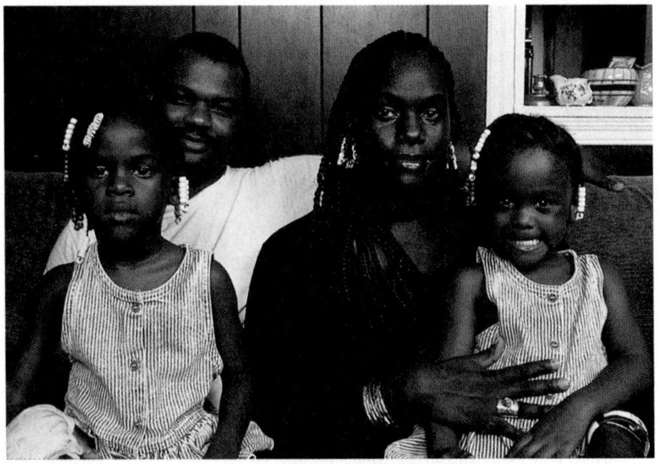

Figure 3-4 Family structure is different for every family; thus the nurse needs to understand this structure to determine communication patterns and decision-making authority.

grandparents, aunts, uncles, and cousins (Figure 3-5). This family structure was prominent in the 1800s in the United States because the family was the main unit of economic production. Several generations of a family lived together, worked together, and shared resources and responsibilities. Children were reared by not only their parents but also by grandparents, aunts, and uncles and had a choice of adult role models after which to pattern their behavior and personalities. With the advent of the Industrial Revolution, families were forced to move and seek employment in urban areas, and the nuclear family became more common. Extended family situations are still seen. Situations include elderly parents moving in with adult children or an adult child and/or their spouse and children moving back into the home of their older parents for financial reasons.

Blended (or Step) Family

A blended or stepfamily occurs when a divorced, widowed, or never-married single parent forms a household with a new partner; both partners or only one may have children. The formation of a stepfamily can present many stresses for the parent, stepparent, and children. In the new stepfamily, there has been no time to blend family styles and traditions, or to negotiate parenting. Additionally, there has not been time to establish or nurture the marriage. A remarried parent must deal with many strong emotions, and feeling a special loyalty to one's own biological children may create conflicts with the new spouse. The remarried couple may be unable to form a new spousal relationship because to do so would appear to be a betrayal of the intimacy between parent and child. This issue frequently conflicts with the needs of the new spouse, who may feel like an outsider in an established household. Stepfamilies in which both adults have children from a previous marriage living with them have the greatest incidence of redivorce (Witrak, 1997). Divorces occur more frequently and rapidly in remarriages than in first marriages, with one-fourth of remarriages being disrupted within 5 years (Hetherington & Stanley-Hagan, 1999).

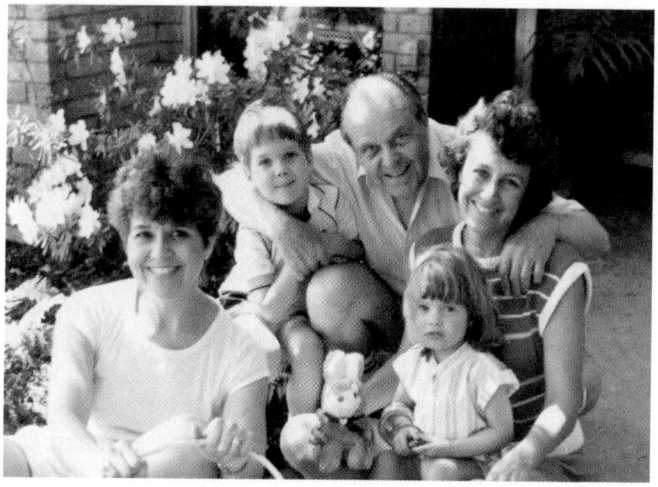

Figure 3-5 Members of an extended family benefit from the sharing of responsibilities and resources. Courtesy of Nicki Potts.

Stepparents and biological parents often believe that the growth of the new family will be instantaneous. The time required to create the stepfamily is usually longer than the adults expect. The stepparent should make clear to the children that she or he does not consider herself or himself to be a replacement for a dead or absent parent. Instead, the stepparent is another adult who can meet some of the child's needs for closeness and love. Parental relationships need time to build. With older children, they may never fully materialize (Visher & Visher, 1995).

The transition to a stepfamily is also stressful for the children. Having suffered the loss of one of their parents and typically the loss of familiar surroundings, children may encounter a new series of losses, and suffer loyalty conflicts and loss of control. The adults have chosen to make major changes in their lives; the children have had those changes imposed on them. Feelings of sibling rivalry are more intense in the stepfamily as the children feel jealousy, insecurity, and a fear that a new sibling is more loved.

Children's responses to stepfamilies vary depending on their age. The stress of a remarriage often causes preschoolers to cling to parents and to regress behaviorally. With their magical thinking, preschoolers may believe that their angry thoughts or behaviors led to the family disruption. They may also believe that they can magically reunite the divorced parents. School-aged children are often angry about their powerlessness to stop the dissolution of the family. Children at this stage are rarely able to express their feelings verbally and are likely to act out their anger. They may have fights with siblings or classmates, develop psychosomatic symptoms, become accident prone, perform poorly in school, or even try to break up the new marriage. On the other hand, they may act "angelic," thus hiding their inner turmoil. Adolescents are dealing with their own issues of identity and autonomy, making the new relationships even more difficult to accept. Additionally, they are dealing with their own sexuality at a time when the addition of a stepsibling or stepparent of the opposite sex can create sexual tensions. Divided loyalties may cause them to act out in a negative way toward the stepparent (Visher & Visher, 1995).

Single Parent Family

While there has been a variety of shifts in family structures, none has been more dramatic than the shift toward families headed by a single parent. Single parenting occurs by means of divorce, separation, death of a spouse, or choice. A single parent family can be created when a single person acquires a child through birth or adoption, however, most single parent households have been created by divorce, and 90% of them are comprised of single mothers and their children (Lamb,

1999). It is estimated that 50% of all children born in the 1990s will spend some time in a single parent household (Tanner, 1995).

Major concerns of single parents are limitations of available resources such as money, time, and physical and emotional energy. Increasingly, two incomes are needed to raise children at a decent standard of living. Single mothers are three times as likely to be poor compared with other adults, and almost half of all poor children live in single parent families. Poverty for a three-person family is defined as an annual income of $13,003 (Children's Defense Fund, 2000). Single parents who are employed often feel overwhelmed in an attempt to provide adequate time for the family, the job, and the endless details of daily life. The single parent must also provide the majority of emotional support and sustenance for the children. Managing all of these responsibilities leaves little time for the parent's social or personal needs (Figure 3-6).

Single parent status is often born out of crisis such as separation or divorce. Such events have different meanings for the child than for the parent. For example, the parent may feel independence and relief due to the separation and divorce; however, the child may experience a sense of uncertainty, instability, and loss. There may be changes in the family home, the child's school, friends, and community. The subsequent transitional period is likely to be disorganized and tumultuous until a realignment of roles, schedules, and expectations can permit a new and stabilized family life (Tanner, 1995). Chapter 20 offers more discussion on the feelings a child may experience due to separation and divorce.

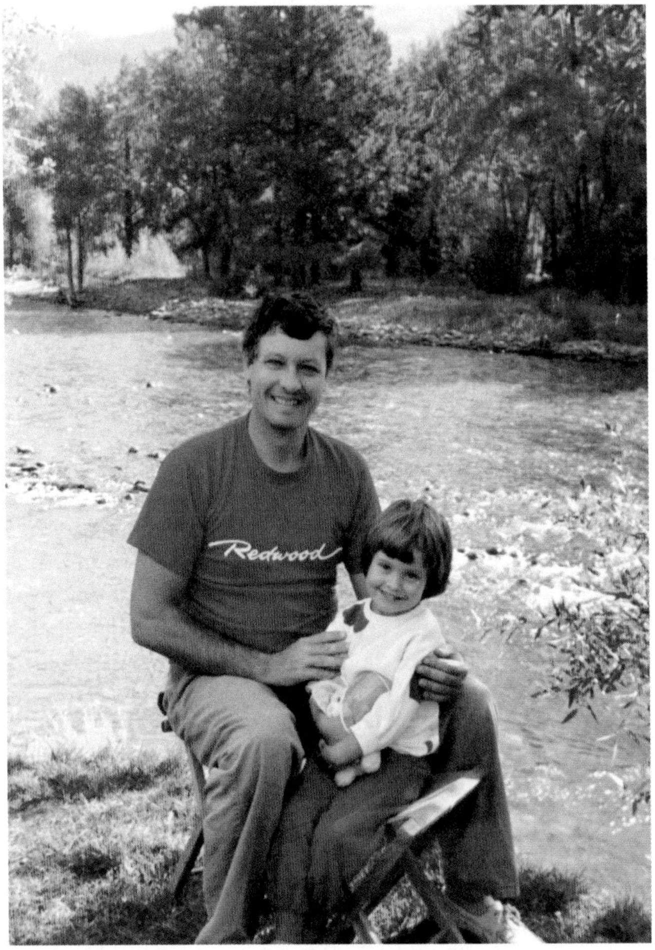

Figure 3-6 Major concerns of single parents are limitations of available resources such as money, time, and physical and emotional energy. Courtesy of Nicki Potts.

Gay and Lesbian Families

Gay and lesbian families are increasing in numbers. Because homosexuality is stigmatized in our society, many of these parents are not open about their sexual orientation. Thus, good estimates of their numbers are not available. However, the estimates that exist suggest there are 1–3 million gay fathers and 1–5 million lesbian mothers. Estimates of the numbers of children of gay and lesbian parents range from 8 to 10 million (Gershon, Tschann, & Jemerin, 1999). Such families can be defined by the presence of two or more persons of the same sex, or by the presence of at least one gay or lesbian adult rearing a child (Allen & Demo, 1995). The structure of these families is quite variable. Many lesbians, single or in a relationship, are giving birth through artificial insemination. Gays are increasingly becoming parents through adoption or the use of a surrogate mother.

Many legal barriers exist for lesbian and gay families. Some of these include:

1. Same-sex relationships are often denied the legal benefits of marriage.
2. Gay and lesbian parents who were married are often denied custody and/or visitation with their children following divorce because of their sexual orientation.
3. In many states, regulations governing adoption and foster care make it difficult for lesbians and gays to adopt children or become foster parents.
4. Medical procedures often require approval of the biological parent, meaning that a durable power of attorney might be necessary for the nonbiological parent to legally authorize health services.

Contrary to common opinion, no significant differences have been found in gender identity and sex role behaviors among children of gay and lesbian parents compared to children of heterosexual parents. Such children are no more likely to be lesbian or gay than are children with heterosexual parents (Patterson & Chan, 1999). Another common misconception is that children raised by gay men and lesbians have psychological problems. However, such children do not differ from children with heterosexual parents in terms of psychological health (Gershon, Tschann, & Jemerin, 1999).

Nursing Alert:

Working with Gay and Lesbian Families

When working with families, do not assume that all parents are heterosexual. In obtaining the family history, the following questions may be asked: (1) Who makes up your family? (2) Do you have a partner? (3) Do you share parenting responsibilities with anyone else? (4) Who else is responsible for the child's care if you are not available?

Kids Want To Know

Will I grow up to identify as a lesbian since both of my parents are lesbians?

The nurse can answer this 10-year-old girl's question by stating that having lesbian parents does not mean she is more or less likely to be lesbian. This is a sensitive issue in U.S. society today because some conservative individuals maintain that homosexuals should not rear children because they will likely follow their parents' lifestyle. Children reared in a gay and lesbian family who discover they are homosexual often have fears of revealing this to their parents. Many feel they have failed their parents, who may believe their children's lives would be easier and less frustrating if they were straight. It is important to explain that gay/lesbian people do not make others gay/lesbian.

REFLECTIONS FROM FAMILIES

Because of my sexual orientation, people think of me as a lesbian, but I think mostly of myself as a woman and, now, a mother. I have been in a close and loving committed relationship with my partner for 10 years. After living together for 6 years, we both realized that we very much wanted a child in our lives. We decided to try to have a baby through artificial insemination, but after many unsuccessful tries at getting pregnant, we found that we only wanted a child that much more. So we adopted our precious little son Brandon, who is now 6 years old and beginning public school.

When his classmates told him he was different because he had two mothers instead of a mother and a father, he was very confused. Yet, the children and teachers all like him so much because of his happy nature and pleasant attitude towards school, and he rapidly adjusted to the school and socialization process much like all the other first graders. In fact, he has proven to be much better adjusted than some of them who do not come from such loving homes. We have gotten involved in school activities, and most of the other parents are now at ease with our parenting arrangement. Brandon has lots of friends, going often to visit at their homes or having them over here. In fact, some of the mothers we have gotten to know the best, after seeing how well two mothers can create a loving and nurturing home for a child, often ask us to care for their own children when they go out for an evening.

CULTURAL INFLUENCES ON THE FAMILY

Because of growing proportions of ethnic minorities, the United States is becoming more culturally diverse. This diversity brings with it many challenges for health care providers. All families are shaped by their surrounding culture, which provides them with social norms. Some families are strongly influenced by their original culture, whereas others are more assimilated to the homogenous "American" culture. Many factors influence the extent to which families identify with a given culture and incorporate its customs and traditions into their daily lives: country of origin, language, level of education, religion, socioeconomic status, number of generations in this country, and urban versus rural lifestyle (Kohlenberg, Joseph, Prudent, & Richardson, 1995) (Figure 3-7). Each culture has its own values, attitudes, and practices with regard to families and child rearing; yet, there can be a wide range of beliefs and practices among families from the same cultural background.

For nurses working with families from cultures other than their own, the development of cultural sensitivity is paramount in order to respond accurately and sensitively to their needs and to provide care. **Cultural sensitivity** means having an awareness and appreciation of cultural influences in health care and being respectful of differences in cultural belief systems and values. Nurses can be most effective in their work if they adopt a multicultural perspective, which means using appropriate aspects of the family's cultural orientation to

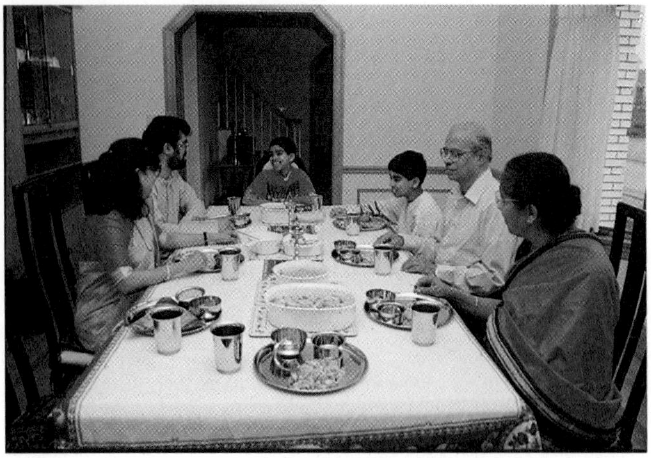

Figure 3-7 Respect for a family's cultural values and practices is important in providing culturally sensitive nursing care.

Critical Thinking

Culturally Sensitive Care

You are assigned to care for a Vietnamese boy hospitalized for a fractured femur who is in traction. He speaks his native language as well as English. His caregivers, who also speak both languages, are present in the child's room when you enter to perform an initial nursing assessment. What considerations are important in order to provide culturally sensitive care?

develop health care interventions. To provide culturally sensitive care to children and their families, nurses must first be aware of their own values and beliefs and recognize how they influence their attitudes and actions. Additionally, they should be knowledgeable about the different cultural groups they encounter in practice. Then they are able to determine whether a certain behavior is peculiar to the individual or characteristic of the culture.

PARENTING

Parenting is a dynamic process that evolves over time as parents acquire experience and mature as individuals. The social goal of parenting is to guide and nurture children so that they become productive members of society. The personal goal of parenting is far more individualized, but, in general, it reflects a desire to raise a child, see aspects of oneself continue to exist such as perpetuating the family line, upholding family traditions, or in some cases, the fulfilling of personal dreams through the child's accomplishments. Individuals approach the topic of parenting from a unique, experiential base: each has been parented. In the parenting role, women and men create models incorporating those elements that they believe comprise "good" parenting. Whether this personal model is congruent with or antithetical to the parenting they received while growing up, it is nevertheless founded upon personal experiences, acquired knowledge, and beliefs about parents and children.

Social changes have influenced the timing of childbearing, so that large numbers of young people are delaying the start of families to meet other social expectations. The need to complete one's education, initiate a career track, establish financial security, and build a committed relationship are fast becoming benchmarks to be achieved before one takes on the responsibility of raising a child. Parental roles are shaped by socially ascribed expectations for enacting the role; by family traditions, values, and cultural beliefs, which shape one's personal perceptions; and by legal and ethical role sanctions and expectations. Principle among these expectations is the responsibility for preparing the child to become a productive member of society. Children learn from their parents how to behave in a manner consistent with their role in the family and appropriate to their culture (Gross, 1996). While family traditions dictate much of the child-rearing strategies used by parents, they do engage in a process of adapting their actions to fit their personal model of parenting. Such a reflective adaptation of child-rearing strategies may be stimulated when the traditional strategies are not effective, when the parent is confronted with new situations, or when the traditional strategy is incongruent with the parent's "good parent" model.

Parenting by Developmental Stage

Parenting is an evolving process that changes as parents and children grow and mature. Parents must actively adapt their parenting strategies to meet the needs of the growing child. The work of parenting is sustained by the attachment that develops between parents and their children—the strongest of all human relationships. Parents and children develop deep, personal attachments that enable them to care for and about each other, even when families experience great stress or the family system structure changes through divorce, death, or the addition of new family members. Such caring is essential for human survival. Indeed, small children cannot grow and thrive without care activities, including technical tasks like diapering and feeding, as well as those emotive, cognitive responses that support the growth of a centered well-integrated person.

In order to parent, individuals fulfill certain tasks. These parenting tasks are designed to both support the child's development as well as maintain family functioning. As children and their parents grow and develop as individuals, these parenting tasks change to reflect family development. See Table 3-2 for a listing of developmental-related parenting tasks. The growth and development chapters (7–12) in this text contain more detailed information on parenting by developmental stage.

Parenting Styles

Each child is unique in her or his own temperament and basic personality. Birth order, gender, and personality traits are a few of the characteristics a child brings to a family. The way caregivers respond to these attributes and interact with the child are related to the individual's style of parenting. Four styles have been identified: (1) authoritarian or autocratic,

Reflective Thinking

What Kind of Parent Are You or Do You Want to Be?

Consider the following questions as you clarify your personal view of parenting.

What are the sources of parenting that shape your ideal view of what it means to be a parent? Are there role models available who model the kind of parenting you give or want to give to your child? Which of your parents' strategies do you want to retain, and which do you want to avoid using?

TABLE 3-2 Development-Related Parental Tasks

Stage	Parental Tasks
Infancy	**1.** Establish routines in daily care activities. **2.** Foster trust by maintaining consistency in interactions. **3.** Modify the home environment to meet the growing infant's needs. **4.** Discuss the division of labor among family members in providing for the infant's needs. **5.** Develop effective communication patterns to accommodate emerging differences in parental role expectations and enactment.
Toddlerhood	**1.** Support the child's growing autonomy in a safe environment. **2.** Role model appropriate behavior for the toddler to imitate. **3.** Initiate discipline that is congruent with family beliefs. **4.** Help the child adjust to temporary separations from the parents.
Preschool	**1.** Support the development of creativity and problem-solving skills. **2.** Help the child to understand another's viewpoint. **3.** Define socially acceptable behaviors. **4.** Teach safety around the home and neighborhood. **5.** Begin sex education.
School age	**1.** Promote cognitive development. **2.** Maintain discipline. **3.** Foster a sense of social responsibility. **4.** Learn to accept rejection as the child assumes greater self-sufficiency. **5.** Encourage involvement in appropriate interests and activities outside the family.
Adolescence	**1.** Maintain open lines of communication. **2.** Grant greater responsibilities. **3.** Negotiate and consistently apply house rules. **4.** Affirm the adolescent's developing sense of self and identity.

Friedman, M. (1998). Family nursing theory and practice. *Stamford, CT: Appleton & Lange; Duvall, E. M. & Miller, B. (1985).* Marriage and family development. *New York: Harper & Row.*

(2) authoritative or democratic, (3) indulgent or permissive, and (4) indifferent or uninvolved (Macoby & Martin, 1983). Authoritarian caregivers value obedience over independence and favor punitive measures, harsh disapproval, and withdrawl of love when children question authority or disobey. They are likely to be less emotionally expressive and to use power to assert their will on their children. Deference and respect for authority are expected. They establish strict and rigid rules, which they don't discuss with their child. Children whose caregivers are authoritarian tend to be dependent, passive, and less intellectually curious. They usually lack social competence and spontaneity, and have low self-esteem.

Authoritative or democratic caregivers are warm but firm. They provide opportunities for their children to develop a sense of autonomy and allow active involvement in decisions that affect them. They are consistent and clear about the expectations they have for their children and are firm when they are disobedient. They guide children's behavior by sharing reasons for their decisions, rules, and standards. Independence is valued, and they are receptive to the child's needs and desires. Children reared in this type of environment have self-control and high self-esteem, and are socially competent and self-reliant.

Indulgent or permissive caregivers are interested and involved in their children's lives but place few demands on them and rarely attempt to control their behavior. With the indulgent style, there is an absence of restraints and maximum freedom for the child. Caregivers provide little input or direction, and seldom punish their children because they are encouraged to develop their own standards of behavior (most of their behavior is considered acceptable by the caregivers). Although children are allowed freedom to set their own limits, most do not feel comfortable with this lack of direction. Additionally, the caregivers' permissiveness doesn't usually foster the development of internal control in these children, who tend to be disrespectful, defiant of authority, and irresponsible.

Indifferent or uninvolved caregivers attempt to minimize the amount of time and energy they must invest in their children's lives. They tend to be very self-centered and structure their home life primarily around their own needs and interests. They are rejecting of and unresponsive to their child's needs. The child receives little guidance, and discipline is inconsistent. Children from indifferent homes are often more impulsive, demonstrate disregard for other's rights, and are more likely to be involved in delinquent behavior (Macoby & Martin, 1983).

Parental Role in Socialization of Children

Socialization is a process of learning the rules and expected behaviors of a society. Expectations for a child's behavior depend not only on the society and culture, but also on the child's developmental stage, and physical and cognitive capabilities, and on the values and beliefs of the family and home. One goal of parenting is to socialize children, which includes teaching which behaviors are expected and appropriate, and fostering the development of self-control. Initially, during infancy and early childhood, caregivers provide external controls. Gradually and eventually, children guided by caregivers take responsibility for that control and integrate the adults' values, attitudes, and expectations into their behavior.

Thus, caregivers nurture their children so that they will achieve self-control, competence, and self-direction in order to be a productive individual in society. It could be said that this is also the goal of discipline, which comes from the root word *disciplinare*—to teach or instruct (American Academy of Pediatrics [AAP] Committee on Psychosocial Aspects of Child and Family Health, 1998). Discipline should be approached in the broadest sense of helping the child learn rules, regulations, and goals of living in a world with others—and not just as setting limits and punishing (Murphy, 2000). The AAP (1998) suggests that effective discipline should include three components: (1) a positive, supportive, nurturing caregiver–child relationship, (2) positive reinforcement techniques to increase desirable behaviors, and (3) removal of reinforcement or use of punishment to reduce or eliminate undesirable behaviors.

Increasing Desirable Behavior

Many desirable behaviors occur as part of a child's normal development; however, others need to be taught such as empathy, sharing, telling the truth (not lying), and good study habits. Family members can teach these behaviors by role modeling since children naturally learn through imitation. Other strategies that help children learn positive behaviors are listed in Box 3-2. By implementing these strategies, the desired behavior is more likely to become internalized by the child, and the new behaviors will become a foundation for other desirable ones.

Reducing or Eliminating Undesirable Behaviors

When undesirable behaviors occur, discipline strategies are necessary to reduce or eliminate such behaviors. Undesirable behaviors are those that put the child or others in danger, do not comply with expectations of caregivers or other appropriate adults (e.g., teachers), and interfere with social interactions and self-discipline (AAP, 1998). However, effective discipline cannot occur if caregivers do not develop their abilities to be positive and rewarding. An important quality of discipline is that the consequences are effective, constructive, and not unduly harsh (Box 3-3) (Wolraich, 1997).

BOX 3-2 Positive discipline guidelines

- Misbehaving children are "discouraged children" who have mistaken ideas about ways to achieve their primary goal–to belong. Their mistaken ideas lead them to misbehavior. We cannot be effective unless we address the mistaken beliefs rather than just the misbehavior.
- Use encouragement to help children feel that they "belong" so that the motivation for misbehaving is eliminated. Celebrate each step in the direction of improvement rather than focusing on mistakes.
- A great way to help encourage children is to spend special time "being with them." Many teachers have noticed a dramatic change in "problem" children after spending five minutes simply sharing those things that they both like to do for fun.
- When tucking children into bed, ask them to share with you their "saddest time" and their "happiest time" of the day. Then share yours with them. You will be surprised what you learn.
- Have family meetings or class meetings to solve problems via cooperation and mutual respect. This is the key to creating a loving, respectful atmosphere while helping children develop self-discipline, responsibility, cooperation, and problem-solving skills.
- Give children meaningful jobs. In the name of expediency, many parents and teachers do things that children could do for themselves and for one another. Children feel that they belong when they know they can make a real contribution.
- Decide together those jobs that must be done. Put them all in a jar and let each child draw out a few each week; that way, no one is stuck with the same jobs all the time. Teachers can invite children to help them make class rules and list these rules on a chart titled "We decided." Children feel ownership, motivation, and enthusiasm when they are included in decisions.
- Take time for training. Make sure children understand what "clean the kitchen" means to you; to them, it may mean simply putting the dishes in the sink. Parents and teachers may ask, "What is your understanding of what is expected?"
- Punishment may "work" if all you are interested in is stopping misbehavior for the moment. Sometimes, we must beware of what works in the present when the long-range results are negative–resentment, rebellion, revenge, or retreat.
- Teach and model mutual respect. One way is to be kind and firm at the same time: kind to show respect for the child, and firm to show respect for yourself and "the needs of the situation." This is difficult during conflict, so use the next guideline whenever you can.
- Proper timing will improve your effectiveness tenfold. It does not "work" to deal with a problem at the time of conflict: Emotions get in the way. Teach children about cooling-off periods. You (or the child) can go to a separate room and do something to make yourself feel better and then work on the problem via mutual respect.
- Abandon the crazy idea that in order to make children do better, you must first make them feel worse. Do you feel like doing better when you feel humiliated? This suggests a whole new approach to "time out." Tell children in advance that we all need time out sometimes when we are misbehaving, so when they are asked to go to their room or to a time-out area they can do something to make themselves feel better. "When you are ready, come back and we will work together on solutions."
- Use logical consequences when appropriate. Follow the Three Rs of Logical Consequences: ensure that consequences are (1) *r*elated, (2) *r*espectful, and (3) *r*easonable.
- During family or class meetings, allow children to help decide on logical consequences for not keeping their agreements. (Remember not to use the word *punishment*, which does not foster long-range "good" results.)
- Teach children that mistakes are wonderful opportunities to learn. A great way to do so is to model this yourself by using the Three Rs of Recovery after you have made a mistake: (1) *R*ecognize your mistake with good feelings, (2) *r*econcile by being willing to say "I'm sorry, I didn't like the way I handled that," and (3) *r*esolve by focusing on solutions rather than blame.
- Ensure that the message of love and respect gets through. Start with "I care about you. I am concerned about this situation. Will you work with me on a solution?"
- Have fun! Bring joy into homes and classrooms.

BOX 3-3 Characteristics of appropriate discipline

- Set clear, reasonable, and developmentally appropriate rules.
- Explain the consequences that the child can expect when the problem behavior occurs.
- Develop consequences that are appropriate to the child's level of development and sufficient to be considered negative without being unduly harsh.
- Administer consequences as soon after the infraction occurs as possible.
- Administer consequences calmly without becoming angry.
- Praise the child when she or he behaves appropriately.

Several disciplinary strategies are used by caregivers to deal with undesirable or unacceptable behaviors, including disapproval, verbal reprimands, time-out, and corporal punishment. **Disapproval** can be verbal or nonverbal, and can be very effective. Tone of voice, facial expressions, and gestures often convey the caregiver's disapproval of a specific behavior. Even young children can learn when a their caregiver is irritated by observing and responding to voice inflections, facial expressions, and gestures.

Many caregivers use disapproving **verbal statements** to alter undesired behavior. Such reprimands may be effective in immediately stopping or reducing the behavior when used infrequently and targeted toward specific behaviors. However, if caregivers use verbal reprimands frequently and indiscriminately, they may reinforce the undesired behavior because the child gets attention. It is important that reprimands should refer to the child's behavior rather than him or her as a person. They should not slander the child's character.

Time-out is an effective discipline strategy that involves removing positive reinforcement for unacceptable behavior. It is a defined period of time in which the child is removed from activities and social interactions. The goal of time out is to interrupt a pattern of negative behavior. The child should be placed in an area that is unstimulating and safe for a given amount of time (usually 1 minute per year of age). A timer can be used so the child knows when time is up. Verbal or physical interaction with the child tends to negate the effects of time-out because the child is given attention for unacceptable behavior. It is important to determine the behaviors that warrant a time out, and to provide the child with this information. The child should also be aware of the procedure to be followed and the "rules." Each time the child misbehaves, the time-out should take place. The use of time-out is advocated by many child care experts because it avoids the problems of other discipline methods such as corporal punishment. The advantage of time-out strategies is that they reduce direct confrontations between parent and child and allow for a "cooling off" period. Additionally, this technique has shown to increase compliance with caregiver expectations from 25% to 80% (AAP, 1998).

One cannot overlook the fact that many families believe that **corporal punishment** is the only means for ensuring that children behave as instructed. Corporal punishment involves the application of some form of physical pain in response to undesired behavior. Concerns have been raised about its negative effects, however. Still, one form of corporal punishment, spanking, remains a strategy commonly used to reduce undesirable behaviors (AAP, 1998). Additionally, it continues to be sanctioned by many states in public schools in the United States (American Academy of Pediatrics Committee on School Health, 2000).

Corporal punishment may inhibit misbehavior, but at great cost. Its effectiveness decreases with subsequent use. The child becomes habituated to this strategy, and its intensity must be systematically increased each time it is used, which can quickly escalate into abuse. Further, corporal punishment increases the chance of physical injury, especially for infants and young children. It leads to altered caregiver–child relationships, making other forms of discipline more difficult when corporal punishment is no longer an option (e.g., with adolescents). Thus, because of the negative consequences of this type of punishment, caregivers should be encouraged and assisted to develop alternative methods in response to undesired behavior, such as using time-out and verbal reprimands. This is especially important for foster families, where caregivers may be prohibited from using corporal punishment but not know other strategies.

SPECIAL PARENTING SITUATIONS

A variety of special family situations can increase the complexity of parenting and present different issues. These situations include adolescent parents, adoption, grandparents as parents, and foster parents.

Adolescent Parenting

Adolescence is a time of considerable growth and development, with progression toward taking on adult roles and responsibilities. For some adolescents, this includes taking on the task of parenting at a time when they are still shaping their own identities. Most pregnancies occur in girls 18–19 years old (Figure 3-8). Fifty-one percent of adolescent pregnancies end in a live birth, 35% are aborted, and 14% are miscarriages or still births (American Academy of Pediatrics, 1999). Although birth rates to women under 20 have declined since the 1970s, the United States continues to

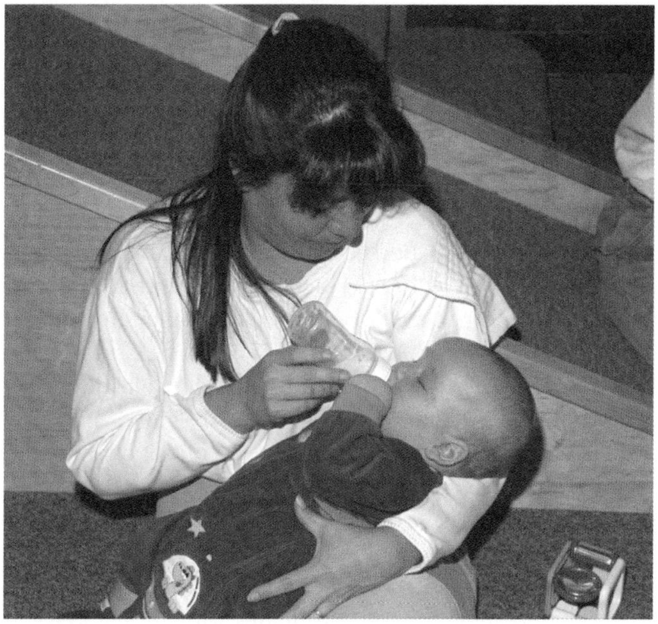

Figure 3-8 The adolescent parent and child face many challenges, yet some of these families have positive outcomes.

have one of the highest adolescent pregnancy rates among developed countries (Ventura, Peters, Martin, & Mauer, 1997). African-American adolescent pregnancy rates are higher than rates in Caucasians, and continue to increase (Murray & Zentner, 2000). Most teenage mothers are unmarried. The resulting unplanned pregnancy affects not only the mother and child, but also the child's father and their respective families because adolescents are often not socially, emotionally, educationally, economically, or physically ready for pregnancy and/or parenthood. Several societal factors influencing the incidence of adolescent pregnancy have been identified. These include implied acceptance of intercourse outside marriage, a variety of adult behavioral values, media pressure, inadequate access to contraception, and the availability of public assistance/welfare for single young mothers (American Academy of Pediatrics Committee on Adolescence, 1999; Dworetzky,1995).

There are risks associated with adolescent pregnancies—medical and psychosocial. Medical risks include low birth weight (more than double the rate for adults) and neonatal death (almost three times as high as in adults). The mortality rate for the mother is twice as high as for adult pregnant women. Other problems include poor maternal weight gain, pregnancy-induced hypertension, sexually transmitted diseases, anemia, and premature births. Psychosocial problems include failure to complete school, persistent poverty, separation from the child's father, repeat pregnancy, limited vocational opportunities, and nonnurturing parenting strategies (Thompson, Powell, Patterson, & Ellerbee, 1995).

Children of adolescent mothers have an increased risk of developmental delay, academic difficulties, substance abuse, and behavioral problems. They are also at risk of dropping out of school and becoming adolescent parents themselves. It is hypothesized that these children do not fare as well as do children of adult mothers because teenagers do not possess the same level of parenting skills and maturity as do adults. Additionally, poverty and frequent changes of caregivers seem to play as much a role as the adolescent's parenting style. The two strongest predictors of school and behavioral problems in these children are the mother's prolonged dependence on public assistance and an unstable relationship between the mother and father (Kohlenberg, 1995).

Despite these difficulties, some adolescents and their children have positive outcomes. Some studies have presented a more positive, hopeful view of adolescent mothers. Early parenthood enhances their personal strength and feelings of hope about the future, increases their motivation to improve their position in life, and improves their ability to bond to their family. Other mothers form a stronger identity and express more confidence in themselves and more engagement with their children (SmithBattle, 1995). Several factors have been associated with improved outcomes for adolescent mothers (Box 3-4).

When a pregnant adolescent is identified, comprehensive prenatal care is essential even if she decides to terminate the pregnancy. She should also receive information about available options, including continuing the pregnancy, keeping and parenting the infant, creating an adoption plan, or terminating the pregnancy via abortion. The nurse can fulfill an important role in assisting the pregnant adolescent by promoting effective parenting skills through education, providing feedback for positive efforts, and providing referrals to community agencies, such as parenting classes, support groups, school-based programs, and infant stimulation programs.

BOX 3-4 Factors associated with improved outcomes for adolescent mothers

- Completion of high school before becoming pregnant
- Active participation in a program for pregnant teens
- Support from her family (financial assistance or child care) that allows her to finish school
- Little social isolation
- A sense of control over her life

American Academy of Pediatrics Committee on Adolescence and Committee on Early Childhood, Adoption, and Dependent Care, 2001.

Additionally, all health care professionals who work with teenage parents need to understand not only adolescent development and child development, but the factors that make teenaged parenting particularly challenging. The primary source of support and advice for these parents is often their family of origin (Wayland & Rawlins, 1997). In the event of a discrepancy or a difference of opinion about a child care issue between the professional and the family, the teenaged parent will almost always adhere to the family's advice. To successfully support teenagers in the parenting role, it is necessary to clarify their knowledge and perceptions of child care issues. It is important to remember that it is the teenaged parent who will make decisions for the child's care. The teenaged parent needs information in order to arrive at an informed decision. In fact, the teenaged parent may need more information than an older parent.

When caring for a child of a teenaged parent who does not seem to adhere to professional advice, it is imperative that family health beliefs and strategies be explored. Although the teenaged parent is the legal guardian and primary caretaker of the child, it may be necessary to encourage other family caregivers to participate in health visits so that all persons who have a significant role to play in the care of the child are involved. In this way, issues can be openly discussed among all parties rather than having the teenaged parent serve as the "go-between."

Parenting the Adopted Child

Adoption is a legal procedure in which a relationship is established between a child and parents who are not related by birth. This process severs all legal ties between the adopted child and his or her biological parents, and establishes such ties between the adoptee and the adoptive parents. The adopted child has the same legal status with respect to his or her adoptive parents as do any biological children (Lobar, Phillips, & Simunek, 1997).

Estimates are given that, in the United States, there are 1 million adopted children living with adoptive parents, that 2%–4% of families include an adopted child, and that there are 5 million adopted individuals of all ages. These figures are gross estimates, most extending back to 1986, and are of questionable reliability. The only current, reliable information appears to be that related to international adoption, which is collected by the U.S. Immigration and Naturalization Service. Since 1975, the federal government has had no system in place for collecting comprehensive national data on adoption (American Academy of Pediatrics Provisional Section on Adoption, 2000).

Several types of adoption exist: agency, independent or private, international, and transracial. Agency adoptions can be public or private, for profit or nonprofit. Costs of agency adoptions vary; however, public agency adoptions are usually less expensive or free. Independent adoptions (also known as private) are usually accomplished through individuals, such as physicians, attorneys, or social workers. Internationally adopted children may have incomplete information about health and medical histories. Because of their diverse origins, unknown backgrounds before adoption, and the inadequacy of health care in many developing countries, these children may be at risk for medical problems. Transracial adoptions of children from minority backgrounds continues to be challenging because of the limited availability of adoptive parents from the same race or ethnic group or caregivers from another race or ethnic group willing to adopt a transracial child (Brady, 2000).

Adoptions may also be open or closed. A **closed adoption** is when there is no contact between biological and adoptive parents. In **open adoption**, there is contact between the birth parents and adoptive parents and possibly between the child and his or her birth parents as well. Advocates of open adoption believe it will aid in lessening the identity struggles that some teenage adoptees go through by having knowledge of their biological past. Additionally, the communication between both sets of parents provides better genetic, medical, and mental health background information for caring for the adopted child. Opponents argue, generally on privacy grounds for birth parents, that the effects on both adoptee and birth mother are not helpful, healthy, or positive, and can seriously threaten vital bonds of the adoptee with adoptive parents. It is agreed that a system of long-term follow-up on the impact of open adoption should be put in place before more meaningful conclusions pro or con may be drawn (American Academy of Pediatrics, 1994).

Individuals who adopt a child in order to become parents are faced with the same tasks in child rearing as biological parents. However, the point at which they begin building an interdependent connection with their adoptive child presents distinctly unique challenges for these new parents. Unlike the biological parents, who begin developing connections with their child throughout pregnancy, adoptive parents do not have this particular experience. They are presented with a stranger with whom they must build a loving, interdependent relationship. For a growing number of these families, the adoptive children are not infants; rather they are older children who have already experienced some form of parenting/caretaking, which will influence their responses to their new adoptive parents. However, since most adoptions frequently take a long time to execute, adoptive parents can go through their own transitional period of beginning the definition of "self-as-parents."

Unique to adoptive parents are the decisions of what and when to tell their child about the adoption. Parents now are advised to openly discuss adoption from the beginning, keeping in mind the child's developmental stage, cognitive abilities, and emotional needs. The child's understanding of the adoption will change with each stage. At the infant/toddler stage, when both the parents and child are adjusting to a changed environment and forming secure attachments, nurses can assist parents in the following ways: (a) allow them to discuss the actual adoption process with the provider; (b) encourage parents to discuss the process with relatives and close friends; (c) suggest or provide resources such as support groups, newsletters, or books; and (d) prepare them for the possibility of insensitive or unenlightened comments from other people (Lears, Guth, & Lewandowski, 1998).

The preschool years produce typical questions such as "Where do babies come from?" and "Where did I come from?," but also render adoption-specific questions such as "Why or how did you choose me?," "Why don't I look like you?," and "Can my birth parents or another family take me away?," Nurses can assist in the following ways: (a) remind parents that preschool children are preoperational and egocentric thinkers who can understand adoption only on a concrete level and not as an abstract concept (e.g., the adoptee may believe that if he or she was adopted, then all children must be adopted); (b) encourage parents to talk openly about

Research Highlight

Outcomes for Adopted Children and Their Adoptive Parents

Study Purpose

The purpose of this study was to investigate whether adopted children and adoptive parents are at greater risk for negative outcomes than biological children and non-adoptive parents.

Methods

The adopted and biological groups were selected from the National Survey of Families and Households data. Data were collected from randomly selected adults in 13,017 households. Seventy-two adopted children (43 boys, 29 girls) and their parents (28 fathers, 44 mothers) were chosen. Of these children, 28 had adopted siblings, 21 had biological siblings, and three had step siblings. A matched group of biological-parent child dyads was created. This was accomplished by selecting parents who had a biological child similar to the adoptive counterpart in gender, age, birth order, and parent's race and educational level. The parents' well being, attitudes toward family life, parenting behaviors and values, and perceptions of their child's adjustment were measured using various instruments.

Findings

The results revealed no significant difference between the parents of adopted and those of biological children in areas of depression, overall happiness, sense of overall health, and self-esteem. Similar findings occurred in the areas of attitudes toward family life, parenting values and behaviors, and parents' view of children's adjustment.

Implications

These results based on nationally matched groups are in contrast with previous studies that used local and clinical samples. The adopted children were not found to be at additional risk of any of the variables measured. Additionally, their adoptive parents did not believe them to be less socially capable and responsible in their behaviors than biological parents about their children. Thus, these results present a consistent view of adopted children and their parents as functioning quite well, at least as well as their biological counterparts. Health care professionals need to be aware of the growing evidence of the successes of adoptive children and their families. They need to view the developmental tasks unique to these families (e.g., telling the child about her/his adoption) as normal events which they handle relatively well. Professionals can begin to challenge negative attitudes about adoption whenever possible.

Citation

Borders, L., Black, L., & Pasley, B. (1998). Are adopted children and their parents at greater risk for negative outcomes? *Family Relations, 47*(3), 237–243.

the process of bringing the child into the family; (c) advise them to answer only the specific questions asked by the child and to answer questions truthfully; (d) emphasize similarities between the child and the family; and (e) reassure the child that the adoption is permanent (Lears et al., 1998).

In the middle childhood stage, questions posed by adoptees include such difficult topics as: "Why was I placed for adoption?," "If you're adopted, can you be unadopted?," and "Who do I look like?" Children at this age may begin searching for answers regarding their origins and reasons for relinquishment. Coping with the public stigma of adoption, peer reactions to adoption, and adoption related losses and reactions (such as grief, sadness, or anger over the loss of biological parents) are key tasks for this age group. Nurses can help by (a) reminding parents to verbally acknowledge the loss adoptees may feel; (b) reassuring them that the child's feelings of grief, sadness, and anger typically dissipate with time; (c) supporting them in their own feelings that may arise as the child expresses thoughts and feelings about their origins; (d) encouraging them to continue to share factual information about the child's adoption; (e) proposing that they work with the school to educate others about adoption; (f) advising them to refrain from making negative comments about biological family since the child does integrate some of their identity into self; and (g) suggesting support groups and services for the parents and child (Lears et al., 1998).

In the adolescent stage, the prevailing question—"Who am I?"—assumes a different or additional meaning for adoptees. Adolescent adoptees have to deal with identity issues regarding both their adoptive parents as well as their biological parents. Since adolescents can now understand abstract processes, the implications and meaning of being adopted is a key area of exploration. Nurses can (a) remind parents that all adolescents deal with identity issues, but that adopted adolescents must deal with integration of both adopted and biological parent identities; (b) suggest that they share the actual adoption papers with the adolescent; (c) prepare them for the possibility that the child may search for the biological family; and (d) suggest that both child and parent continue to use support groups (Lears et al., 1998).

Parenting by Grandparents

An increasing number of grandparents are raising their grandchildren with 6% of children in the United States under 18 years (3.9 million) living in homes of their grandparents. (Figure 3-9). The majority of these grandparents are under the age of 65, with almost half between 50 and 64 years of age (U.S. Bureau of the Census, 1998). There are grandparent-headed households in every socioeconomic and ethnic group and geographic area. However, these families are more likely to be poor. African-American children are more likely to live with a grandparent (13%) than Hispanic (6%) or Caucasian (4%) children (Saluter, 1996).

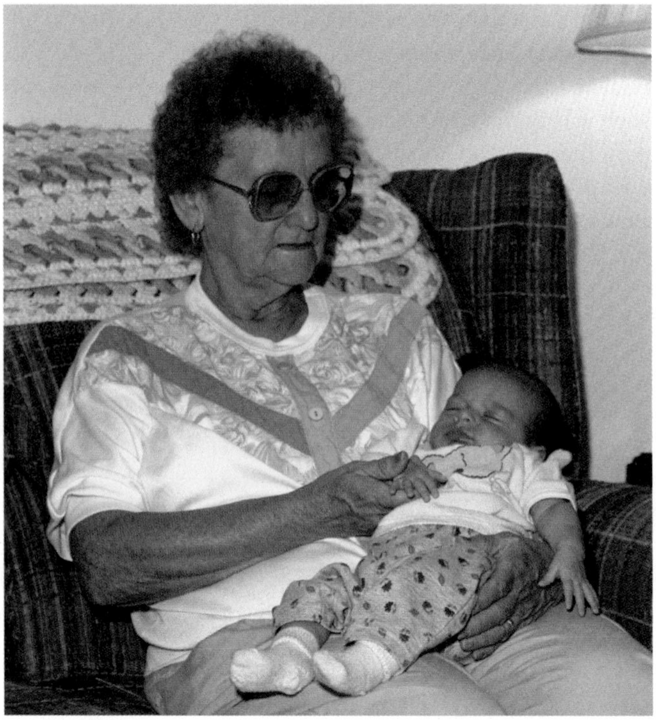

Figure 3-9 Grandparents may assume care of grandchildren because of problems of the parents.

Grandparents assume a parenting role for a variety of reasons, most of which revolve around problems related to the child's biological parent (Morrow-Kondos, Weber, & Hesser, 1997) (Box 3-5). Regardless of the reason, all result in a great deal of responsibility for those who take on the task.

Grandparent caregivers face a myriad of challenges and difficulties in almost all aspects of their lives when they assume the role of surrogate parent (Kelley & Damato, 1995). For many, their physical health is an issue. Health problems begin to emerge in later years, and this can compromise the grandparent's ability to provide care for grandchildren. Some experience deterioration in health once they

BOX 3-5 Antecedents to grandparents raising grandchildren

- Child abuse and/or neglect
- Divorce
- Substance abuse
- Death
- Adolescent pregnancy
- Unemployment
- Mental illness
- Incarceration

become primary caregivers. Closely related to health is the issue of stamina. Many report feeling physically and emotionally drained and fatigued from caring for young children. They fear that, as a result of their tiredness and health problems, they may be unable to meet the demands of parenting.

Grandparents often experience emotional difficulties such as psychological distress, depression, disappointment, guilt, anger, and resentment. Social isolation and restrictions of the parenting role are related to psychological distress and depression. Disappointment, guilt, anger, and resentment are common feelings they have toward their own child. Many feel disappointed with the person their child has become as an adult and guilt about having raised a child that is incapable of being a competent parent. Anger and resentment are associated with having to assume the parent role because of their adult child's problems and incompetencies (Morrow-Kondos et al., 1997). The grandparents' lifestyle and relationships with family and friends are changed. They may become isolated from other members of their family, who may resent the role they have taken on.

Economic difficulties are common due to taking on the care of a child at a time in their lives when their income is dramatically decreased. Many grandparents are denied the financial benefits of foster parents because of their blood relation to the child, though some states have "Kinship care" programs. Some financial assistance is available through the federal government (Medicaid, Social Security, Food Stamps, and Head Start programs).

Despite the negatives, there are also benefits to grandparents parenting a grandchild. Many experience a greater purpose for life and some feel young and alive (Jendrek, 1994). Raising a grandchild in a safe, nurturing environment and helping the child grow to be a productive person is rewarding. They are able to draw upon their own parenting experiences with the wisdom and knowledge they've accumulated over the years.

Grandparents and grandchildren need significant support for health care providers and social service agencies. Nurses can be instrumental in providing referrals to available services and supports (see Resources). Nurses who encounter grandparent-headed families in their practice should assess and intervene when problems such as physical and mental health problems are identified.

Foster Parenting

Children in foster care are rapidly increasing in numbers, and meeting their psychosocial needs is a significant challenge. More than 500,000 children are in foster care in the United States (American Academy of Pediatrics Committee on Early Childhood, Adoption, and Dependent Care, 2000). African-American children are disproportionately represented in the foster care system, followed by Caucasians and Latinos. The majority of children are placed in foster care as a result of neglect, physical abuse, parental substance abuse, or abandonment. In many cases, the caregiver is unable or unwilling to care for them because of substance abuse, mental illness, or major physical illness such as HIV infection. The majority of children in out-of-home placements are living with relatives. The next largest percentage are in residential group care, followed by licensed foster homes and other facilities such as emergency shelters and psychiatric hospitals (Scahill, 2000).

Children in foster care are at risk in many ways: having chronic health deficits, experiencing the trauma of abuse and neglect, and suffering from emotional challenges (Rosenfeld et al., 1997). They usually have experienced significant psychological stress during their early years and have not had a nurturing, stable home environment, which is necessary for the development of optimal cognitive, language, and socialization skills. Additionally, multiple placements and interruptions in the continuity of caregivers are often detrimental to the child's well-being (American Academy of Pediatrics Committee on Early Childhood, Adoption, and Dependent Care, 2000). Foster children are more likely to have unmet health needs and chronic health problems because they are often in and out of the health care system. Frequent changes in health care providers occur without the necessary transfer of medical information and records.

Health care providers can be effective advocates for children in foster care in several ways. Those with expertise in child development and parenting can provide advice and support for foster and biological families. Caseworkers may need assistance in obtaining records from previous health care providers and interpreting the information. Individuals responsible for the child's care need an understanding of her or his physical and emotional problems. Providers can be proactive advisors for social services and the judicial system in determining what is in the best interest of the child and whether these interests can be met within the biological family or another family.

IMPLICATIONS FOR NURSING

Parenting is a highly valued activity both on a personal as well as a societal level. Good parenting is necessary for the healthy functioning of children and to produce successful members of society. Parenting is learned through imitation, acquired knowledge, and practice. Nurses can play a vital role in supporting parenting as they work with families. This work must be done in collaboration with parents if positive results are to be achieved. Too often health care providers talk to parents rather than with them. Merely giving advice based on the providers' background and knowledge may fail to address the parents' personal and cultural beliefs. If the advice given is not congruent with the parents' valued beliefs, then it will be ignored.

Assessment of parenting includes:

- The parent's views on parenting
- Clarifying cultural and social expectations for parenting
- Identifying issues or children's behaviors that are of concern to parents
- Evaluating the interactions between children and their parents during health care encounters

Potential sources of problems can be identified from the assessment data. The identified problems should:

- Be confirmed or clarified with parents
- Be mutually agreed upon as the priority issues parents wish to address

When a problem is identified, then the parents and nurse can collaborate on creating a plan of care. Collaboration with parents can improve the success of the plan as parents will be involved with identifying:

- Resources for implementing the plan
- Strategies that are congruent with parental beliefs
- Outcomes for determining effectiveness of the plan

The nurse will need to follow up with the parents at subsequent encounters to determine:

- How effective the plan of care was in achieving the stated outcomes
- Any adaptations the family made in the plan of care
- The parent's satisfaction with this format for reducing or resolving the identified problem

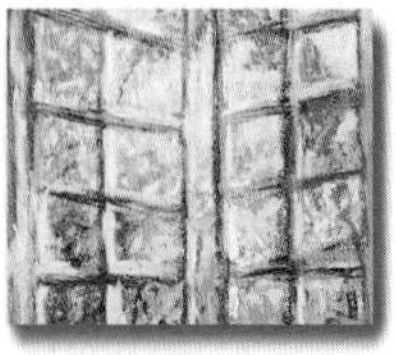

In The Real World

Heather, 12 years old, is my client at the mental health mental retardation (MHMR) clinic. When she was 8, her parents divorced, and she has been living with her mother since that time. Based on my conversation with her, I considered more deeply the profound effects that divorce and single parenting can have on a child and the family. I realized that some of my assumptions about them were not correct. As Heather talked, I realized that, more than anything else at the moment, she probably needed someone to just listen and empathize. She didn't need me to tell her what I thought. She just wanted me to listen. As she expressed feelings common to children whose parents divorced, my assumptions about her family changed. In other words, she allowed me to refine my perceptions of her family's experiences and thereby understand her situation and how she felt.

It is crucial that nurses work with parents rather than against them if parenting is to be supported. Nurses should continually ask themselves whether they are imposing their personal beliefs about parenting when they evaluate others' parent–child relationships. Parenting issues or problems will not be resolved in a single encounter. The work of parenting is ongoing and dynamic. It will take weeks or months for a problem to be resolved. By establishing an open exchange of ideas, and respecting parents' personal and cultural values, nurses can support the work of parenting.

Key Concepts

- The definition of family varies widely. The most inclusive definition of family is when two or more persons are joined by bonds of sharing and emotional closeness and who identify themselves as members of the family (Friedman, 1998).
- The three family theories from the social sciences that have major relevance to nursing are the structural-functional, the developmental, and the systems theories.
- The process of family assessment includes data collected in a systematic fashion using a family assessment tool in which information is then classified and analyzed as to its meaning.
- The traditional nuclear family structure no longer reflects contemporary U.S. lifestyles. Other forms such as the single parent, blended, and gay and lesbian families have emerged in recent years.
- Nurses have a responsibility to understand the influence of the cultural framework on a family's child-rearing practices and attitudes about health and illness.
- As children grow and develop, parenting tasks change to both support their development and maintain family functioning.
- Parenting styles have an effect on the child's personality outcomes.
- A variety of special parenting situations can further increase the complexity of child rearing: adolescent parents, adoption, grandparents as surrogate parents, and foster care.
- Nurses can play a vital role in supporting parents as they work with families. This work must be done in collaboration with parents if positive results are to be achieved.

Review Questions

1. How is the family conceptualized in various nursing theories?
2. How is the family conceptualized in the following frameworks: (1) structural-functional, (2) developmental, and (3) systems theory?
3. Identify the strengths and limitations of the three frameworks in question #2.
4. According to Duvall's developmental stages, what are the tasks for each of these families: (1) parents of an infant, (2) parents of an adolescent, and (3) a retired couple?
5. According to the structural-functional theory, what are four functions of the family?
6. Why is the view of the nuclear family not representative of contemporary families?
7. Discuss salient characteristics of the following types of family structure: (1) extended, (2) blended, (3) single parent, and (4) gay/lesbian.
8. Discuss the importance of culture to nurses providing multicultural health care.
9. How can parents support the child's developing problem-solving skills at different developmental stages?
10. What is the role of family time in successful parenting?
11. Discuss the impact of the following parenting situations on the child and parents: (1) adolescent parents, (2) adoption, (3) grandparent as surrogate parents, and (4) foster parents.

References

Allen, K. R., & Demo, D. H. (1995). The families of lesbian and gay men: A new frontier in family research. *Journal of Marriage and the Family, 57*, 111–127.

American Academy of Pediatrics. (2000). Health care needs of children in the foster care system. *Pediatrics, 106*(4), 909–918.

American Academy of Pediatrics Committee on Adolescence. (1999). Adolescent pregnancy—Current trends and issues. *Pediatrics, 103*(2), 516–520.

American Academy of Pediatrics Committee on Adolescence and Committee on Early Childhood, Adoption, and Dependent Care. (2001). Care of adolescent parents and their children. *Pediatrics, 107*(2), 429–434.

American Academy of Pediatrics Committee on Early Childhood, Adoption, and Dependent Care. (2000). Developmental issues for young children in foster care. *Pediatrics, 106*(5), 1145–1150.

American Academy of Pediatrics Committee on Early Childhood, Adoption and Dependent Care. (1994). Issues of confidentiality in adoption: The role of the pediatrician. *Pediatrics, 93*(2), 339–341.

American Academy of Pediatrics Committee on Psychosocial Aspects of Child and Family Health. (1998). Guidance for effective discipline. *Pediatrics, 101*(4), 723–728.

American Academy of Pediatrics Committee on School Health (2000). Corporal punishment in schools. *Pediatrics, 106*(2), 343.

Bomar, P. (1996). *Nurses and family health promotion: Concepts, assessment, and interventions* (2nd ed., p 170). Philadelphia: W.B. Saunders.

Borders, L., Black, L., & Pasley, B. (1998). Are adopted children and their parents at greater risk for negative outcomes? *Family Relations, 47*(3), 237–243.

Brady, M. (2000). Role relationships. In C. Burns, M. Brady, A. Dunn, & N. Starr (Eds.), *Pediatric primary care: A handbook for nurse practitioners* (2nd ed., pp. 435–472). Philadelphia: W. B. Saunders.

Children's Defense Fund. (2000). *Yearbook 2000: The state of America's children.* Washington, DC: Author.

Duvall, E. M. (1977). *Marriage and family development* (5th ed.). Philadelphia: J. B. Lippincott.

Duvall, E. M. & Miller, B. (1985). *Marriage and family development* (6th ed.). New York: Harper and Row.

Dworetzky, J. (1995). *Human development: A lifespan approach* (6th ed.). St. Paul, MN: West Publishing.

Friedman, M. M. (1998). *Family nursing: Theory and practice* (4th ed.). Stamford, CT: Appleton & Lange.

Frisch, N., & Frisch, L. (1998). *Psychiatric mental health nursing.* Albany, NY: Delmar.

Gelles, R. (1995). *Contemporary families: A sociological view.* Thousand Oaks, CA: Sage.

Gershon, T., Tschann, J., & Jemerin, J. (1999). Stigmatization, self-esteem, and coping among the adolescent children of lesbian mothers. *Journal of Adolescent Health, 24*, 437–445.

Gilliss, C. L. (1993). Family nursing research, theory, and practice. In G. D. Wegner & R. J. Alexander (Eds.), *Readings in family nursing* (pp. 34–42). Philadelphia: J. B. Lippincott.

Grossman, D. (1996). Cultural dimensions in home health nursing. *American Journal of Nursing, 96*(7), 33–36.

Hanson, S. (1996). Family assessment and intervention. In S. Hanson & S. Boyd (Eds.), *Family health care nursing: Theory, practice, and research* (pp. 147–172). Philadelphia: F. A. Davis Co.

Hetherington, E., & Stanley-Hagan, M. (1999). Stepfamilies. In M. Lamb (Ed.), *Parenting and child development in "nontraditional" families* (pp. 137–159). Mahwah, NJ: Lawrence Erlgbaum Associates, Inc.

Hitchock, J., Schubert, P., & Thomas, S. (1999). Frameworks for assessing families. In J. Hitchcock, P. Schubert, & S. Thomas (Eds.), *Community health nursing: Caring in action* (pp. 407–437). Albany, NY: Delmar.

Jendrek, M. P. (1994). Grandparents who parent their grandchildren: Circumstances and decisions. *The Gerontologist, 34*, 206–216.

Kelley, S. J., & Damato, E. G. (1995). Grandparents as primary caregivers. *Maternal Child Nursing, 20*, 326–332.

King, I. (1981). *A theory for nursing: Systems, concepts, process.* New York: John Wiley.

Kodadek, S. (2000). Family assessment in pediatric primary care. In C. Burns, M. Brady, A. Dunn, & N. Starr (Eds.), *Pediatric primary care: A handbook for nurse practitioners* (2nd ed., pp. 41–52). Philadelphia: W. B. Saunders.

Kohlenberg, T. (1995). Teen mothers. In S. Parker & B. Zuckerman (Eds.), *Behavioral and developmental pediatrics* (pp. 396–401). Boston: Little, Brown.

Kohlenberg, T., Joseph, H., Prudent, N., & Richardson, V. (1995). Cultural responses to behavioral problems. In S. Parker & B. Zuckerman (Eds.), *Behavioral and developmental pediatrics* (pp. 396–401). Boston: Little, Brown.

Lamb, M. (1999). Parental behavior, family processes, and child development in nontraditional and traditionally understudied families. In M. Lamb (Ed.), *Parenting and child development in "nontraditional" families* (pp. 1–14). Mahwah, NJ: Lawrence Erlgbaum Associates, Inc.

Lears, M., Guth, K., & Lewandowski, P. (1998). International adoption: A primer for pediatric nurses. *Pediatric Nursing, 24*(6), 578–586.

Lobar, S., Phillips, S., & Simunek, L. (1997). Legal issues in nonrelated infant adoption: Nursing implications. *Journal of the Society of Pediatric Nurses, 2*, 116–124.

Macoby, E. E. & Martin, J. A. (1983). Socialization in the context of the family: Parent-child interaction. In P. H. Mussen (Ed.), *Handbook of child psychology* (4th ed., vol. 4, p. 37–56) New York: Wiley.

Morrow-Kondos, D., Weber, J., Cooper, K., & Hesser, J. (1997). Becoming parents again: Grandparents raising grandchildren. *Journal of Gerontological Social Work, 28*(112), 35–45.

Murphy, M. (2000). Developmental management of toddlers and preschoolers. In C. Burns, A. Dunn, & N. Starr (Eds.), *Pediatric primary care: A handbook for nurse practioners* (2nd ed., pp. 114–141). Philadelphia: W.B. Saunders.

Murray, R., & Zentner, J. (2000). *Health assessment and promotion strategies throughout the lifespan* (7th ed.). Upper Saddle River, NJ: Prentice Hall.

Nelson, J. (1996). *Positive discipline.* New York: Ballantine Books, a Division of Random House.

Neuman, B. (1972). The Betty Neuman model: A total person approach to patient. *Nursing Research, 21*(3), 264–269.

Neuman, B. (1983). Family intervention using the Betty Neuman health care systems model. In J. Clements & F. Roberts (Eds.), *Family health: A theoretical approach to nursing care.* (pp. 161–175). New York: John Wiley.

Patterson, J. (1995). Promoting resilience in families experiencing stress. *Pediatric Clinics of North America, 42*(1), 47–63.

Patterson, C., & Chan, R. (1999). Families headed by lesbian and gay parents. In M. Lamb (Ed.), *Parenting and child development in "nontraditional" families* (pp. 191–219). Mahwah, NJ: Lawrence Erlgbaum Associates, Inc.

Rosenfeld, A., Pilowsky, D., Fine, P., Thorpe, M., Fein, E., Simms, M., Halfon, N., Irwin, M., Alfaro, J., Saletsky, R., & Nickman, S. (1997). Foster care: An update. *Journal of the American Academy of Child & Adolescent Psychiatry, 36*(4), 448–457.

Roy, Sr., C. (1983). Roy adaptation model. In I. Clements & F. Roberts (Eds.), *Family health: A theoretical approach to nursing care* (pp. 161–175). New York: John Wiley.

Saluter, A. (1996). Marital status and living arrangements. *Current Population Series.* Washington, DC: National Center for Health Statistics.

Scahill, M. (2000). The healthcare needs of children in foster care. *Journal of the Society of Pediatric Nurses, 5*(4), 183–184.

SmithBattle, L. (1995). Teenage mothers' narratives of self: An examination of risk the future. *Advances in Nursing Science, 27*(4), 22–36.

Tanner, J. L. (1995). Single parents. In S. Parker & B. Zuckerman (Eds.), *Behavioral and developmental pediatrics* (pp. 387–390). Boston: Little, Brown.

Thompson, P. J., Powell, J., Patterson, R. J., & Ellerbee, S. M. (1995). Adolescent parenting: Outcomes and maternal perceptions. *Journal of Gynecological and Neonatal Nursing, 24*, 713–718.

U.S. Bureau of the Census. (1998). Co-resident grandparents and their grandchildren: Grandparent maintained families. *Working paper no. 27, March.* Washington, DC: Population Division.

Ventura, S. J., Peters, K. D., Martin, J. A., & Maurer, J. D. (1997). Births and deaths: United States 1996. *Monthly vital statistics report, 46*(1), Supplement 2. Atlanta: National Center for Health Statistics, CDC, USDHH.

Visher, J. S., & Visher, E. B. (1995). Beyond the nuclear family. *Pediatric Clinics of North America, 42*(1), 31–43.

Von Bertalanffy, L. (1968). *General systems theory.* London: Penguin Press.

Wayland, J., & Rawlins, R. (1997). African American teen mothers perceptions of parenting. *Journal of Pediatric Nursing, 12*, 13–20.

Witrak, M. (1997). The stepfamily. In J. Fox (Ed.), *Primary health care of children* (pp. 353–356). St. Louis: Mosby.

Wolraich, M. (1997). Addressing behavior problems among school-aged children: Traditional and controversial approaches. *Pediatrics in Review, 18*, 266–270.

Wright, L., & Leahey, M. (1994). *Nurses and families: A guide to family assessment and intervention.* Philadelphia: F. A. Davis.

Suggested Readings

Barnhill, S. (1996). Three generations at risk: Imprisoned women, their children, and grandmother caregivers. *Generations, 20*, 39–40.

Berrick, J. (1998). When children cannot remain home: Foster family care and kinship care. *Future of Children, 8*(1), 72–87.

Brazelton, T. B. (1992). *Touchpoints, the essential reference: Your child's emotional and behavioral development.* Reading, MA: Addison-Wesley.

Brazelton, T. B. (1994). Touchpoints: Opportunities for preventing problems in the parent-child relationship. *Acta Pediatrica Supplement, 394*, 35–39.

Castiglia, P. (1999). Growth and development. Extended families! Social support systems for children. *Journal of Pediatric Health Care, 13*(3 part 1), 139–141.

Emick, M., & Hayslip, B. (1996). Custodial grandparenting; New roles for middle-aged and older adults. *International Journal of Aging and Human Development, 43*(2), 135–154.

Fuller-Thomson, E., Minkler, M., and Driver, D. (1997). A profile of grandparents raising grandchildren in the United States. *The Gerontologist, 37*(3), 406–411.

Gerris, J. M., Dekovic, M., & Janssens, J. M. (1997). The relationship between social class and childrearing behaviors: Parents' perspective taking and values orientations. *Journal of Marriage and the Family, 59*, 834–847.

Gross, D. (1996) What is a "good" parent? *Maternal Child Nursing, 21*, 178–182.

Hernandez, D. J. (1995). Changing demographics: Past and future demands of early childhood. *The Future of Children, 5*, 145–160.

Hetherington, E., Bridges, M., & Insabella, G. (1998). What matters? What does not? Five perspectives on the association between marital transitions and children's adjustment. *American Psychologist, 53*(2), 167–184.

Riesch, S., Bush, L., Nelson, C., Ohm, B., Portz, P., Abell, B., Wightman, M., & Jenkins, P. (2000). Topics of conflicts between parents and young adolescents. *Journal of the Society of Pediatric Nurses, 5*(1), 27–40.

Russell, K. M., & Champion, V. L. (1996). Health beliefs and social influence in home safety practices of mothers with preschool children. *Image: Journal of Nursing Scholarship, 28*, 59–64.

Stevens-Simon, Kelly, L., Singer, D., & Nelligan, D. (1998). Reasons for first teen pregnancies predict the rate of subsequent teen conceptions. *Pediatrics, 101*(1), e8.

Yau, J., & Smetana, J. G. (1996). Adolescent-parent conflict among Chinese adolescents in Hong Kong. *Child Development, 67*, 1262–1275.

Resources

Organizations and Websites

Adoptive Families
3333 Highway 100 North
Minneapolis, MN 55422
(800) 372-3300

Child Welfare League of America
444 First Street, N.W.
Washington, DC. 20001-2085
(202) 638-2952

Families Adopting Children Everywhere Inc. (FACE)
P.O. Box 28058
Northwood Station
Baltimore, MD 21239
(410) 488-2656

Families Like Mine
1730 New Brighton Blvd., #175
Minneapolis, MN 55413
(612) 362-3389
www.familieslikemine.com

Grandparent Information Center
American Association of Retired Persons (AARP)
601 E. Street NW
Washington, DC 20049
(202) 434-2296
www.aarp.org

National Organization of Adolescent Pregnancy, Parenting, and Prevention (NOAPPP)
4421-A East/West Hwy.
Bethesda, MD 20814
(301) 913-0378

Parents Without Partners
1650 South Dixie Hwy., Suite 510
Boca Raton, FL 33432
(561) 391-8833
www.parentswithoutpartners.org

Stepfamily Association of America
650 J Street, Suite 205
Lincoln, NE 68508
(402) 477-7837

CHAPTER 4

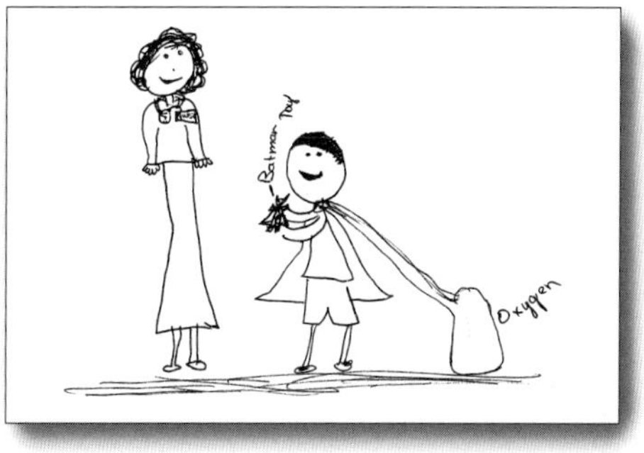

I began pediatric home health nursing after I had been practicing as a pediatric nurse in the acute care setting. I wasn't sure what taking care of pediatric patients in their own environment was going to be like. I vividly remember going to the home of my first home health case, a 7-year-old boy who was dependent on a ventilator. The child and his caregiver were very receptive to my visit. I found that all the skills I had used in the acute care setting came in handy while providing the care this child needed and the teaching his caregiver required. As I made more visits I began to realize that I was getting to know this child better because I was seeing and caring for him in his own familiar environment. I discovered he enjoyed playing with Batman action toys and indeed had a whole collection of action figures with all the accessories needed to play Batman and Robin. I began to incorporate this knowledge into my nursing plan of care. For instance, we played many games of "eating special Batman-type lunches" to increase caloric intake and pretending that the pulse oximeter light was a special Batman laser light. Being in the home really allowed me to use the child's own familiar environment to improve the nursing care I was delivering. The chapter opening picture was drawn for me by one of my own children who thought I was pretty lucky to get to play Batman and Robin while I was working as a nurse.

COMMUNITY AND HOME HEALTH NURSING

Mary L. Dowell, RNC, MN

COMPETENCIES

Upon completion of this chapter, the reader will be able to:

- *Review the history of community health nursing as it relates to children and their families, including the role government has played.*
- *Discuss how* Healthy People *objectives (health promotion, health protection, and disease prevention) relate to community health nursing care of children and their families.*
- *Describe the role of the community health nurse as it relates to assessment of the child, family, community, and environmental toxins.*
- *Compare types of home care agencies.*
- *Describe the role of the home health care nurse as it relates to skills, case management, and the home visit.*
- *Examine future trends in the area of community and home health care nursing for children and their families.*
- *Identify community resources that are available to help maintain the strength of the family and promote the child's health.*

This chapter will discuss community and home health nursing care as it relates to children and their families. Community health nursing is a broad category of nursing that can be defined by the area and focus of practice and by the population it serves. Home health nursing is one of the specialty areas under the umbrella of community health nursing and is defined as a variety of services provided to people, in this instance children, in their place of residence (Smith & Maurer, 2000).

According to a report by the U.S. Department of Health and Human Services (DHHS, 1997), in 1996 there were 362,600 community health nurses practicing in a variety of settings. These 362,600 nurses constituted 17% of all employed registered nurses. Approximately one in four community health nurses were employed by local and state health departments or community health centers. The largest percentage of community health nurses worked in home health. School health, occupational health, hospice, and other settings make up the remaining areas where community health nurses are employed. School health nursing is discussed in Chapter 5. This chapter will focus on a broad discussion of community health nursing and home health nursing for children and their families.

COMMUNITY HEALTH NURSING

Community health nursing is defined as "the care provided by educated nurses in a particular place and time directed toward promoting, restoring, and preserving the health of the total population or community" (Smith & Maurer, 2000, p. 7). The community health nurse has a focus on health promotion and disease prevention. While that focus may be on the individual or family, the well-being of the community as a whole is the final objective. The community health nurse can focus on health promotion at an individual (child) or family level while promoting the well-being of the community by conducting well-child assessments, giving immunizations, conducting screening tests, teaching, and making referrals for the child and family to other health care associates and resources. The community nurse also has an instrumental role in immunization programs. "Community health nursing, with its population-based focus and emphasis on health promotion and disease prevention, has a unique opportunity to play a central leadership role in meeting the national health objective of increasing the number of children under age 2 who receive basic immunizations to 90%" (Moore, Fenlon, & Hepworth, 1996, p. 22).

Community health nurses who care for children and their families practice in a variety of settings that teach

TABLE 4-1 Various Roles of the Community Health Nurse

Roles	Functions	Examples
Clinician	Combines nursing, epidemiology, case management, resource coordination, expertise in working with families, into formulating health policy, assessing communities, and carrying out all phases of population-focused programs.	Provides information to a group of teenagers regarding safe sex practices. Plans, implements, and evaluates a program to decrease drug use by adolescents.
Advocate	Advocates for the child and their family by promoting their needs and desires.	Speaks for the needs of a family with a child who is dependent on technology who are facing homelessness.
Collaborator	Collaborates with other health care members, social service agencies, judicial systems, and schools to ensure holistic care.	Works with a caregiver, teacher, principal, physician, and social worker to develop a plan to faciliate the successful integration of a child with a disability into a public school setting.
Consultant	Serves as an expert (teacher, leader, resource person) who is able to propose solutions for identified problems.	Organizes a child and family health fair.
Counselor	Helps clients choose appropriate solutions to their problems.	Works with caregivers to decide if their child who is dependent on technology should attend school or be tutored at home.
Educator	Teaches health promotion and disease prevention activities as well as maintains optimal levels of health and wellness.	Teaches a prenatal class on nutrition and healthy habits.
Researcher	Participates in research that will be of benefit to the community. Should include identifying problem areas; collecting, analyzing, and intrepreting data; applying findings; and evaluating, designing, and conducting research.	Identifies an area where environmental toxins near a popular playground are jeopardizing the health of children and develops solutions that will promote health and well-being.
Case manager	Develops and coordinates services for a selected client and family.	Coordinates all the services needed by a child recuperating from a hospital stay to ensure a healthy recovery: occupational therapy, physical therapy, tutoring, as well as financial resources for the caregivers.

Adapted from Hitchcock, J., Schubert, P., & Thomas, S. (1999). Community health nursing: Caring in action. *Albany, NY: Delmar.*

health promotion and disease prevention, including the child's home, well-child clinics, migrant health clinics, neighborhood health centers, and centers that implement federally mandated or specific state-funded programs (Stanhope & Lancaster, 1996). The nurse may have a primary or team role during the delivery of services. Table 4-1 lists the various roles of community health nurses.

Governmental Influence

The government has influenced community health nursing for children and their families through federal programs such as Medicaid, public laws, and the *Healthy People* documents. The role of the community health nurse includes implementation of government-supported programs and referral of families who are eligible for these services. Children with disabilities and those with chronic conditions can receive assistance with health care services through the Title V Children with Special Health Care Needs (CSHCN) programs. Community health nurses can be instrumental in referring children and families for services under this program. Promotion of adequate nutrition for poor families is important for growth and development and functioning in school (Smith & Maurer, 2000). Community and school nurses can assist families in obtaining services through the supplemental food program for Women, Infants, and Children (WIC) and the federally funded school breakfast and lunch programs.

In the mid-1980s, federal amendments to Medicaid expanded services to low-income pregnant women. As part of case management for these women, many states now reimburse for home visits by nurses employed by local health departments or health centers. Nurses who make home visits focus on teaching caregivers to implement measures to promote growth, development, and safety; ensuring that the child is being provided with proper nutrition; and assessing the child's and family's health care for its adequacy and accessibility (Smith & Maurer, 2000).

The Early and Periodic Screening, Diagnosis, and Treatment (EPSDT) program entitles qualified children to having their medical histories taken, physical examinations, immunizations, screening tests, nutrition assessment, and education at specified age levels from birth to 18 years. Nurses in well-child clinics and on home health visits can perform screenings. These include vision and hearing screening, lead detection, developmental assessments, and routine physical examinations (Bryan & Wirth, 1995).

REFLECTIONS FROM FAMILIES

I was a single mother with two small children. I felt embarrassed to go to the grocery store and use the coupons I had received from WIC. The nurse at WIC was always supportive and constantly focused on the importance of using the coupons, not because I wanted to get free food, but because I wanted to give my children nutritious meals. Thanks to her, I quit feeling so embarrassed when I went to the store.

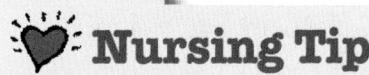

Nursing Tip

Optional services covered by Medicaid

Medicaid covers optional services determined by individual states, such as dental care; speech, hearing, and language disorder services; and eyeglasses. You can be instrumental in helping the family access optional care if covered. Staying informed about the services covered by Medicaid in the state where you practice can be invaluable.

Healthy People 2010 Objectives

Changes and additions to the *Healthy People 2000* national health objectives, which were reflected in *Healthy People 2010* (DHHS, 2000), will specifically affect community health care of children and their families. These include (a) adding some new focus areas such as Medical Products Safety and Access to Quality Health Services and Programs, (b) combining violence and abusive behavior with unintentional injuries to become Injury/Violence Prevention, and (c) adding children to the maternal and infant priority area, becoming Maternal, Infant, and Child focus area. Some of the primary goals of community health nursing are also goals of *Healthy People 2010*. These are health promotion, health protection, and disease prevention.

Health Promotion

Health promotion is defined as "activities or interventions that identify risk factors related to disease; the lifestyle changes related to disease prevention; the process of enabling individuals and communities to increase control over and improve their health; these activities or strategies are directed toward developing the resources of clients to maintain or enhance their physical, social, emotional, and spiritual well-being" (Hitchcock, Schubert, & Thomas, 1999, p. 891). Health promotion is a major goal of community health nursing practice. Community health nurses facilitate health in the population through direct nursing interventions for health promotion and disease prevention with individuals, families, groups, and populations. The community health nurse develops, implements, and evaluates health promotion programs in schools, work sites, hospitals, faith communities, prisons, and community settings

REFLECTIONS FROM FAMILIES

I went to a baby-care workshop after I had my first baby that was taught by a nurse from the local health department. I learned well-child care (e.g., bathing, feeding, holding, and diapering) as well as interpreting communication cues and average ages for achieving certain developmental milestones. My mother-in-law insisted that if a child was not rolling over by 2 months of age there was something wrong with him. Because of the workshop I could feel assured that my 3-month-old baby was not "slow" just because he was not rolling over yet. I offered to take my mother-in-law to the next class so she could learn about the average ages for achieving developmental milestones and she happily accepted.

(Smith & Maurer, 2000). These health promotion strategies are implemented by nurses through counseling, education, and anticipatory guidance.

Health Protection

Health protection is defined as "activities designed to maintain the current level of health, actively prevent disease, detect disease early, thwart disease processes or maintain functioning within constraints of disease" (Hitchcock et al., 1999, p. 891). Screening programs for infants, children, and adolescents include blood lead levels, phenylketonuria (PKU), growth and development, hearing and vision, dental health, scoliosis, and testicular and breast self-examination. Screening programs are conducted by nurses through health departments, clinics, schools, health fairs, community centers, and well-child clinics.

Firearm and playground safety and car-seat loan programs are other examples of health protection programs. Community health nurses can assess these areas and provide guidance and educational resources for families who have needs in these areas. In 1997, firearm-related deaths accounted for 23% of all injury-related deaths in children and adolescents aged 1–19 (National Center for Injury Prevention and Control, CDC, 2000). Firearm-related injuries to children occur when children are left at home alone and firearms are kept in readily accessible places (McClelland, Thompson, Piete, & Hatcher, 1996). Community nurses need to routinely inquire about the presence of firearms.

Disease Prevention Services

"Disease prevention refers to those activities designed to protect persons from disease and its consequences" (Hitchcock et al., 1999, p. 13). Programs included in the area of preventive services for children and their families include immunization programs, environmental screening programs, hearing and vision screening programs, and screening programs for children at risk for developmental delay. Community health nurses have a major role in administration of immunizations to children at well-child clinics, at immunization clinics, and during special immunization days at schools. They also assist in measuring serum lead levels, performing vision and hearing screenings, and administering assessments to screen for developmental delays. Once an area of risk is identified, the community health nurse follows through by making referrals as needed, following up with home visits, or arranging return visits to the clinic. These interventions may be initiated through community health centers, school-based clinics, home health programs, public health departments, or health maintenance organizations. Some federally and state-funded programs can provide these services.

Standards

Standards have been developed by the American Nurses Association (ANA) (1986a) that guide the practice of community health nurses (Box 4-1).

These standards reflect the steps of the nursing process and indicate that community health nurses are to apply this process to individuals, families, and groups to promote health and wellness throughout life. These standards provide guidelines for competent levels of practice and behavior for the community health nurse. They also help to define the scope and quality of community health nursing care (Smith & Maurer, 2000).

Community Assessment

The community health nurse's assessment should also be conducted at the community level. (Family assessment is discussed in Chapter 3.) This assessment should include information regarding economic, social, and political influences on the child, and his or her family. Some questions to be included are (Pridham, Broome, & Woodring, 1996):

- What is the child's neighborhood, school, and peer group like?
- Are there adequate community resources and agencies available?
- What is the availability and funding of health care resources, including managed care models?

The nurse's goal is to use knowledge gained during the community assessment to determine how the larger

Research Highlight

Reversing Growth Deficiency in Children

Study Purpose

The goal of the study was to investigate the effectiveness of nursing interventions on health outcomes of growth deficiency in children receiving care through public health clinics.

Methods

The sample consisted of 39 children (ages 3 months to 3 years) with growth deficiency in weight or height for age or weight for height or a decrease in growth across two percentiles. The children were enrolled in Special Supplemental Feeding Programs for Women, Infants, and Children (WIC) clinics in county health departments and were randomly assigned to experimental or control groups. After preliminary data were collected for the entire sample, a community-based intervention was administered to the experimental group during home visits. The intervention included education about nutrition and about parenting and community skills.

Results

After the intervention was implemented by a research assistant blind to group assignment, the data indicated positive changes ($p = 0.05$) in the experimental group's growth quotients, home environments, and their mothers' perceived stress.

Implications

This study supports the community health nursing practice of teaching nutrition and child care during home visits to families of children with growth deficiency.

Citation

Reifsnider, E. (1998). Reversing growth deficiency in children: The effect of a community-based intervention. *Journal of Pediatric Health Care, 12* (6 Pt. 1), 305–311.

BOX 4-1 American Nurses Association standards of community health nursing practice

Standard I: Theory
The nurse applies theoretical concepts as a basis for decisions in practice.

Standard II: Data Collection
The nurse systematically collects data that are comprehensive and accurate.

Standard III: Diagnosis
The nurse analyzes data collected about the community, family, and individual to determine diagnoses.

Standard IV: Planning
At each level of prevention, the nurse develops plans that specify nursing actions unique to client needs.

Standard V: Intervention
The nurse, guided by the plan, intervenes to promote, maintain, or restore health, to prevent illness, and to effect rehabilitation.

continues

BOX 4-1 *Continued*

Standard VI: Evaluation
The nurse evaluates responses of the community, family, and individual to interventions to determine progress toward goal achievement and to revise the data base, diagnosis, and plan.

Standard VII: Quality Assurance and Professional Development
The nurse participates in peer review and other means of evaluation to assure quality of nursing practice. The nurse assumes responsibility for professional development and contributes to professional growth of others.

Standard VIII: Interdisciplinary Collaboration
The nurse collaborates with other health care providers, professionals, and community representatives in assessing, planning, implementing, and evaluating programs for community health.

Standard IX: Research
The nurse contributes to theory and practice in community health nursing through research.

From ANA (1986). *Standards of community health nursing practice.* Washington, DC: Author. Reprinted with permission.

environment influences the child's and family's health and development.

Another community assessment the nurse can perform is a windshield survey. A **windshield survey** is a systematic assessment that is performed while the nurse travels through the community (Lindell, 1997) (Figure 4-1).

All of the senses should be used to look closely at the community and note housing, environment, common areas, and community development. The findings that have an impact on the health of children from the windshield survey could include safety hazards, loud sounds and noxious odors, unsafe air and water quality, lack of green space, homeless individuals or families, stray animals, limited public services, and inadequate public education systems. Attention should be paid to the environment in order to assess risk factors for safety and to prevent injury.

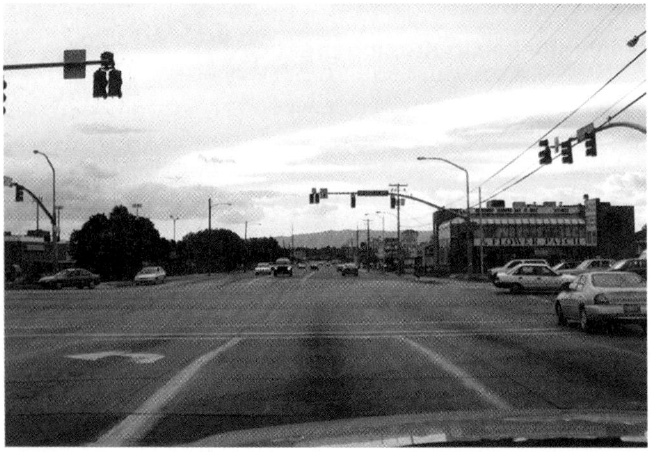

Figure 4-1 From the car, the nurse can directly observe a community and gain valuable assessment data.

Environmental Toxins

The community health nurse can have an instrumental role in providing information and promoting safety and injury prevention. This role is especially important when assessing the child's environment. Community health nurses need to have a knowledge of how children, because of their unique physical, biologic, and social characteristics, are especially vulnerable to the adverse effects from interaction with polluted environments (Bearer, 1995). The illnesses caused by environmental hazards include asthma exacerbated by air pollution and second-hand cigarette smoke, developmental delays caused by lead in paint and contaminated drinking water, and increased respiratory symptoms from exposure to radon (a radioactive gas caused by the decaying of uranium that can enter homes through floors, cracks, and walls) (Smith & Maurer, 2000). Early recognition and prevention of exposure to environmental toxins is a goal of the community health nurse.

Assessment of the environment is the first step toward recognizing and preventing exposure to environmental toxins. Stanhope and Lancaster (1996) suggest use of a site assessment checklist that prompts the nurse to assess groundwater use, surface water use, soil use, ambient air quality, food chain use, and physical hazards (Figure 4-2). The family should be taught about the key areas to assess for potential exposures to environmental toxins. Teaching should focus on both the home and the school and community environments.

Families should be encouraged to minimize the use of household chemicals and pesticides, and to ensure safe (locked cabinet, out of reach) storage when they are not in use. Proper ventilation should be ensured when chemicals are used within the house. Families should be taught about the effects that second-hand smoke can have on children.

Source of environment pollution:
Location:

Regulatory status: [ ] Federal _____
[ ] State _____
[ ] Local _____
[ ] Unregulated _____

(Assess by contacting EPA or state environment department)

Closest resident / residential area:

Closest school / daycare / youth club:

	Past	Present	Future
Groundwater use (within a mile) [ ] Private well use/number			
[ ] Drinking/cooking			
[ ] Outdoor/yard			
[ ] Irrigation			
[ ] Industrial			
[ ] Abandoned			
[ ] Public/municipal well			
Surface water use (within a mile) Description:			
[ ] Swimming/recreation			
[ ] Drinking water source			
[ ] Health advisories			
[ ] Fishing			
[ ] Water contact			
Soil use (within a mile) [ ] Parks/play areas for children			
[ ] Trespassing in restricted areas			
[ ] Gardening			
Ambient air quality (within a mile) Prevailing wind direction:			
[ ] Frequent air inversions			
[ ] Odors			
[ ] Visual emission			
Food chain use (within a mile) [ ] Game animal hunting			
[ ] Farming			
[ ] Gardening			
[ ] Fishing			
[ ] Subsistence			
[ ] Sport			

Physical hazards (on or near the site)

[ ] Equipment _____
[ ] Storage containers _____
[ ] Debris _____
[ ] Fire _____
[ ] Lagoons, ponds, impoundments _____

[ ] Confined spaces _____
[ ] Asphyxiation _____
[ ] Acid conditions _____
[ ] Caustic conditions _____

[ ] Unstable structures _____
[ ] Waste piles _____
[ ] Mine shafts _____
[ ] Explosive conditions _____
[ ] Pits _____

Figure 4-2 Environmental Site Assessment Checklist. From Stanhope, M., & Lancaster, J. (2000). *Community health nursing: Promoting health of aggregates, families, and individuals.* (4th ed). St. Louis: Mosby. Used with permission.

Nursing Alert

Lead Poisoning

The effects of lead on the central nervous system are significant because they are believed not to be reversible. In the central nervous system, lead causes an increase in membrane permeability, which causes a fluid shift into brain tissue, producing increased intracranial pressure, ischemia, and cellular destruction. Acute encephalopathy, manifested by hypertension, intellectual deficits, seizures, cerebral edema, coma, and even death may result. The nurse or family should seek immediate medical attention if the child has been exposed and lead levels are elevated, because lead can be removed from the body only by chelation therapy, which requires that the child be under the care of a health care provider.

Teaching about the prevalence of lead poisoning in children between the ages of 6 months and 6 years should also be conducted.

Follow-up evaluation of teaching should be conducted. Referrals to the appropriate resources must be instituted. Resources in the area of environmental health can be found at the end of this chapter. Community health nurses who work in clinics can assist in obtaining blood for lead-level screenings (in high-risk communities, routine screening is done by a fingerstick). When the blood lead level exceeds 10 mg/100 mL, further studies are indicated.

Future Trends

The care provided by community health nurses will continue to focus on promoting, restoring, and preserving the health of the total population or community. In the future, how this care is delivered and the role of the community nurse in delivering this care will change. This change will be in response to four major change drivers that are altering the nature of health care delivery (Hitchcock et al., 1999). The four major change drivers are market-driven economic policy, technology, demographics, and science. Each of these changes will have an impact on the future of community health care for children and their families.

First, the market-driven economic policy has prompted a change in the health delivery system of community health for children and their families. Many of the services provided by the health department are being shifted to managed care systems or not-for-profit and proprietary home care agencies (Erickson, 1996). Second, technology is changing the promotion, preservation, and restoration of health. For example, new immunizations are being introduced that can change the preservation of health for a large number of children. Third, population demographics have changed. Some of these demographic changes have meant that there are more children living in poverty and without health insurance than in the past. Lastly, science is making an impact on poorly understood diseases. This has an impact on the community health nurse caring for children and their families because more will be known about the prevention of disease and the preservation of health.

Models of future community health care practice for children may include community-based nursing centers, school-based family health centers, health ministries, and neighborhood nursing. The role of the community health nurse will be one of independent functioning, interdependence with flexible role boundaries, and a focus on health promotion (Hitchcock et al., 1999).

HOME HEALTH NURSING

Stanhope and Lancaster (1996) define **home health care** as "an arrangement of health-related services provided to people in their place of residence" (p. 1094). The health-related services provided for children and their families range from providing direct hourly nursing care to children who are dependent on technology, to intermittent visits from nurses, home health aids, physical therapists, occupational therapists, speech therapists, or social workers. Home care for children is growing in the area of referrals for home antibiotic therapy, pediatric hospice programs, nursing care for children who are dependent on technology, home phototherapy, private-duty nursing, and home visits to new mothers who are discharged with their babies after brief, routine hospital stays because of uncomplicated deliveries.

Home care services can be provided for either short-term or long-term needs. Referrals for home antibiotic therapy, home phototherapy, and home visits to new mothers are examples of children and families needing short-term home care services. The focus for short-term care is on primary and secondary prevention of disease. **Primary prevention** involves interventions for children that promote health and prevent disease processes from developing. Teaching new mothers how to perform infant care is one example of a home care service that is primary prevention. **Secondary prevention** aims to detect disease in the early stages before clinical signs and symptoms manifest in order to intervene with early diagnosis and treatment. The goal is to reverse or reduce the severity of the disease or provide a cure. Home phototherapy or short-term nursing visits to teach diabetes care would be examples of home care services that would provide secondary prevention (Stanhope & Lancaster, 1996). **Tertiary prevention** is directed toward children with clinically apparent disease. The aim is to ameliorate the course of disease, reduce disability, or rehabilitate. Examples of tertiary prevention include services provided by home care agencies that are long term, such as provision of care for a child who is dependent on technology, or hospice care (Smith & Maurer, 2000).

Many different factors have an impact on home care for children and their families. The three factors this section will focus on include (1) types of agencies and the impact of managed care on these agencies, (2) family needs (family and nurse interactions, respite care), and (3) the scope of nursing care (skills, case management, and the home visit).

Home Care Agencies and Managed Care

Home care agencies that provide care for children and their families fall into five categories: official, voluntary, combined, private, and hospital-based agencies. An explanation of these types of agencies is found in Table 4-2.

Managed care refers to cost-effective delivery of health care services. Home health care services are supported by managed care organizations in situations where they will result in shortened hospital stays. Caring for children at home with the assistance of home care services continues to be cost effective as compared with prolonged hospital stays. Early-discharge programs are encouraged by managed care organizations because of their cost effectiveness. Children with acute and chronic illnesses are being affected by early-discharge protocols. Managed care, by supporting these early discharges, has created a need for comprehensive home care programs for children. Children are going home sicker, and families are required to assume more responsibility for their care. These children and families have special needs and require comprehensive nursing care and teaching.

Critical Thinking

Problems with Managed Care Systems

Managed care programs are concerned with cost containment. How will this concern with cost containment affect the quality of home care for children?

Family Needs

Children who are dependent on technology and those who need hospice care receive the majority of home care nursing hours. The other home care hours consist of teaching caregivers how to use apnea monitors, initiating short-term phototherapy, and administering medications through intravenous lines, or performing dressing changes or teaching the caregiver how to administer tube feedings. Leonard, Brust, and Sielaff (1991) evaluated the nursing hours received by children who were dependent on technology. They found that most families with a child who was dependent on technology received some nursing care each day (96.8%), and 16.1% received 24-hour care. During the evaluation, they found that factors such as hours that the caregivers worked outside the home and support systems influenced the number of hours a professional was needed more heavily than the child's medical condition.

Advantages and disadvantages of having an ill child at home, rather than in a hospital, have been identified by families. Advantages include a less-threatening environment, easier access to the child's loved ones, decreased need for

TABLE 4-2 Types of Home Health Agencies

Type of Agency	Explanation
Official or public agencies	Receive power through statutes enacted by legislation, Early and Periodic Screening, Diagnosis, and Treatment (EPSDT) Program. Care includes well-child visits.
Voluntary agencies	Receive funds from contributions, fees for service, united community funds, contracts for services, and grants. Provide skilled nursing care in the home.
Combined governmental and voluntary agencies	Receive funds from official and nonofficial sources. Provide both health promotion/disease prevention services in addition to home health services.
Private agencies	Function as either for-profit or not-for-profit. Provide hourly nursing care for acutely or chronically ill children, as well as intermittent visits for short-term needs. Do not necessarily provide health promotion/disease prevention services.
Hospitial-affiliated agencies	Receive majority of referrals from sponsoring hospital.
Specialty agencies	Specialize in particular population care (pediatric care or geriatric care).

travel to and from the hospital, strengthening of the family unit, and restoration of control of the child's care to the family (Krepper, Young, & Cummings, 1994). The disadvantages include intrusion of professionals on the family's privacy, financial pressures, and the impact on siblings of having the ill child at home. Another disadvantage reported by families is the stress of taking care of a child with special needs at home (Ahmann, 1994). Home health care nurses have an important role in alleviating the disadvantages families can experience with having the ill child at home. Healthy interpersonal relationships between the nurse and family can improve the family's adjustment to having home health care for their child. Nurses can provide referrals if the family is experiencing financial strain, and they can assist the siblings in adjusting to having an ill brother or sister at home.

Kids Want To Know

Why can't my home care nurse skip some of my treatments?

Sometimes I want my home care nurses to play games with me and skip some of my respiratory treatments. Why won't they do that?

Home care nurses are professionals who are there to help you maintain health. If the home care nurse can set up a schedule that ensures treatment protocols are being carried out, she or he may have time to play a game with you.

Interpersonal Relationships

Interpersonal relationships among the home care nurse, the child, and family can be described as **collaborative**—in other words, where mutual sharing and working together help to achieve common goals such that all persons or groups are recognized and growth is enhanced (Ahmann, 1994). During this collaborative relationship, the nurse should maintain professional boundaries. **Professional boundaries** are defined as the space between the nurse's power and the client's vulnerability. The power of the nurse comes from the professional position and the access to private knowledge about the client. Establishing boundaries allows the nurse to control this power differential and allows a safe connection to meet the client's needs (National Council of State Boards of Nursing, 1996). Krepper et al. (1994) discuss how the child's caregivers need to have home care nurses listen to them and respect their knowledge and feelings because they are involved in care on a 24-hour, 7-day-a-week basis. These researchers discuss how caregivers felt it was important when the home care nurse respected the family's wishes, was flexible, allowed them to participate in the child's care, communicated with the family, and talked on the caregiver's level. Clarifying roles can assist the home care nurse to maintain professional boundaries. For instance, establishing house rules such as where to park and where to store belongings and defining issues such as routines, discipline, mealtime, and homework can help to clarify roles. Having professional support through nursing supervisors will also help the home care nurse to define appropriate family roles. Blurring of nurse–patient/family boundaries can be a significant problem. Caregivers may possess significant knowledge of their child's illness/needs from past experience, the library, and Internet resources. Including caregivers in the care plan and considering their judgment can facilitate or maintain a professional working relationship. Home health care nurses should recognize signs that they have crossed boundaries, including excessive self-disclosure, secretive behavior, "super nurse" behavior, selective communication, flirtations, and failure to protect the client (National Council of State Boards of Nursing, 1996).

The Council of State Boards of Nursing (1996) states that every nurse–client relationship can be plotted on a continuum of professional behavior. This continuum ranges from underinvolvement (distancing, disinterest, and neglect) to overinvolvement (boundary crossings and boundary violations). The zone of helpfulness is in the center of the professional behavior continuum. This zone is where the majority of child and family interactions should occur to ensure effective nursing care. Home health care nurses are at risk of becoming overinvolved with the family because of the informal home environment, casual, social conversations that occur with family members throughout the day, participation by family members in the care of the child, and attempts by some families to reduce the stress of having a stranger in the home by incorporating the nurse as a member of the family (Ahmann, 1994). Guidelines to determine professional boundaries and the continuum of professional behavior for the nurse are given by the National Council of State Boards of Nursing (1996) (Box 4-2).

Guidelines important to the home health care nurse caring for children and their families are delineation and maintenance of boundaries, examination of boundary crossings, variables of the care setting, actions that overstep established boundaries, and post-termination relationships. The nurse and family should be cognizant of feelings and behaviors and the nurse should always act in the best interests of the child and family.

By maintaining collaboration and professional boundaries, the home care nurse can begin to develop a trusting therapeutic relationship with the child and the family. Family caregivers report that nurses who come into the home offer them support for the physical and emotional challenges of caring for a child with a chronic illness at home. Without this support, caregivers are at risk for burnout and may need respite care.

BOX 4-2 Principles to determine professional boundaries and professional behavior

- Be responsible for delineating and maintaining boundaries.
- Examine any boundary crossing, be aware of its potential implications, and avoid repeated crossings.
- Be aware of the care setting, community influences, client needs, and the nature of therapy since they affect the delineation of boundaries.
- Avoid actions that overstep established boundaries to meet the needs of the nurse.
- Avoid dual relationships, in other words, where the nurse has a personal or business relationship as well as the professional one.
- Be aware of the complexity of post-termination relationships in which the client needs additional services. It may be difficult to determine when the nurse–client relationship is truly terminated.

National Council of State Boards of Nursing (1996). *Professional boundaries: A nurse's guide to the importance of appropriate professional boundaries.* Chicago: National Council of State Boards of Nursing, Inc. Reprinted by permission of the National council of State Boards of Nursing, Inc. Chicago, IL.

Critical Thinking

Collaboration with the Family

You routinely perform home care for a child who has a tracheostomy and is dependent on oxygen. You prefer to do the bath and tracheostomy care in the early morning, but the child's caregivers prefer after lunch because this fits their afternoon and early evening schedule. How will you determine when the bath should be given? What factors will you consider?

Respite Care

Respite care is short-term, temporary care that is normally provided in the home for a child who requires specialized care; it provides relief for the caregivers, which may help to prevent burnout and increase the caregiver's ability to cope with stress. The home care nurse may provide this relief or may be instrumental in referring the family to sources for this care (Mausner, 1995). Unfortunately, respite care has often been viewed as a luxury rather than a necessity, and it has been arranged only after the family exhibits significant stress (Mausner, 1995). Families taking care of children at home who have medical complications have complex and conflicting feelings about using respite care services if they are unfamiliar with the caretakers who will provide the respite care. Families want to be familiar with the person to whom they are entrusting the care of their child. When caretakers begin to think in terms of their need for a break, it is natural for them to turn to the home health care nurse to assist them in making arrangements.

Some agencies have successfully developed formal programs of respite care that are available to families taking care of children with a chronic illness at home. The agency ensures that if the child is to remain at home under the care of a nurse, and the caregiver is absent overnight, a designated substitute caretaker with power of attorney is appointed (Hogue, 1993). When respite time is well planned, it can be therapeutic for the family and the child. Refer to Chapter 17 for additional information about respite care.

Scope of Nursing Practice

Nurses have many responsibilities when they care for the child and the family in the home. The scope of nursing practice will be discussed as it relates to these many responsibilities in the area of nursing skills, case management, and the home visit.

Home health care nurses provide direct care, assessments, instruction, support, screening, referrals, and case management (Ahmann, 1996). The characteristics necessary for home care nurses to work effectively with children and families are flexibility, creativeness, sensitivity, and professionalism (Peirson, 1993). Although both hospital-based nurses and home health care nurses use acute care and high tech skills, the home visit requires nursing practice that is very different from the hospital setting. The home health care nurse must take into consideration the family's psychosocial resources, the neighborhood, and the presence or absence of community services (Clemen-Stone, McGuire, & Eigsti, 1998).

Skills

The dimensions of home care for children are becoming more complex, requiring nurses to be competent in high tech care. Krepper and associates (1994) found that families of children who were dependent on technology and had home health care nurses felt nursing skill competency was a critical issue. Families repeatedly stated that nurses must have "good judgment skills, particularly respiratory skills" (p. 17). Even nurses who are experienced in these technological skills in the hospital may encounter new challenges in the home setting (O'Neill & Pennington, 1996). Competency-based curricula have been developed for home care nurses and caregivers to update or learn these skills and are now a part of the home care agency's orientation program for nurses. An example of such a curriculum has been developed for tracheostomy and ventilator care for caregivers, hospital-based nurses, home care nurses, nurse educators, school health nurses, educators, early intervention specialists, and training coordinators of home care agencies (Dougherty, Parrish, & Hock-Long, 1995).

Standards

Along with competency-based standards, the American Nurses Association (1986b) has developed practice standards for home health care nurses that provide guidelines for competent levels of skills and practice behaviors, as shown in Box 4-3.

The emphasis is on theory, data collection, diagnosis, planning, intervention, evaluation, continuity of care, professional development, research, and ethics. These standards guide all facets of home health nurses' practice as they care for children and their families. The case management role of the home health care nurse is delineated in standard VIII.

Case Management

Home health agencies may use nurses as case managers for children and their families. The home care nurse is concerned with providing continuous, comprehensive, cost-effective, quality care. Case management includes comprehensive nursing assessment of the child and family needs, coordination of the level of support needed for the

BOX 4-3 American Nurses Association standards of home health nursing practice

Standard I: Organization of Home Health Services
All home health services are planned, organized, and directed by a master's-prepared professional nurse with experience in community health and administration.

Standard II: Theory
The nurse applies theoretical concepts as a basis for decisions in practice.

Standard III: Data Collection
The nurse continuously collects and records data that are comprehensive, accurate, and systematic.

Standard IV: Diagnosis
The nurse uses health assessment data to determine nursing diagnoses.

Standard V: Planning
The nurse develops care plans that establish goals. The care plan is based on nursing diagnoses and incorporates therapeutic, preventive, and rehabilitative nursing actions.

Standard VI: Intervention
The nurse, guided by the care plan, intervenes to provide comfort; to restore, improve, and promote health; to prevent complications and sequelae of illness; and to effect rehabilitation.

Standard VII: Evaluation
The nurse continually evaluates the client's and family's responses to interventions in order to determine progress toward goal attainment and to revise the data base, nursing diagnoses, and plan of care.

Standard VIII: Continuity of Care
The nurse is responsible for the client's appropriate and uninterrupted care along the health care continuum, and therefore uses discharge planning, case management, and coordination of community resources.

Standard IX: Interdisciplinary Collaboration
The nurse initiates and maintains a liaison relationship with all appropriate health care providers to assure that all efforts effectively complement one another.

Standard X: Professional Development
The nurse assumes responsibility for professional development and contributes to the professional growth of others.

Standard XI: Research
The nurse participates in research activities that contribute to the profession's continuing development of knowledge of home health care.

Standard XII: Ethics
The nurse uses the code for nurses established by the American Nurses Association as a guide for ethical decision making in practice.

From ANA. (1986). *Standards of home health nursing practice.* Washington, DC: Author. Reprinted with permission.

care needs identified, and evaluation of the effectiveness of the coordination of care.

The case management approach includes a collaborative effort that takes place among the physician, family, home care providers, and case managers. The approach builds on the nursing process in order to assess, plan, implement, coordinate, monitor, and evaluate options and services specifically designed to meet children's and families' health needs to promote quality, cost-effective outcomes. As case manager, the nurse will be responsible for coordinating the care the child receives. As coordinator of care, the home care nurse must be knowledgeable about the availability of community resources not provided by the primary home care agency. Refer to the "Resources" section at the end of the chapter.

Case management nursing interventions frequently involve providing direct care, sharing community resource information with families, coordinating multidisciplinary care management and discharge planning efforts, and alleviating the family's anxiety about continuing care needs. These interventions are often implemented during the home visit. The kind of relationship that the nurse builds will often depend on how the nurse conducts the home visit.

The Home Visit

Reifsnider (1996) describes how therapeutic relationships are developed between the nurse and caregivers when home visits are planned and implemented in phases. The phases of the home visit are:

- Preinteraction—meeting the child and family and performing the assessments
- Engagement/active participation—outlining plans and initiating interventions
- Termination—evaluating the interventions and determining future rehabilitative needs

These phases can be generalized to most children who require home care nursing for either a short or long time.

Preinteraction Phase

The preinteraction phase includes activities performed prior to the first home visit. Before making the home visit the nurse will benefit from collaborating with the physician either through direct contact or through the physician's report sent to the agency. Physician's orders and the medical plan of care should be reviewed. Contact should be made with other interdisciplinary team members involved in the child's care.

The home health care nurse should review available family data, including referral information and previous records, and establish a plan for the visit. The family should be contacted by telephone and services briefly discussed. The nurse should prepare for a safe visit (e.g., identify exact location of home, consider safety issues in relation to the neighborhood being visited, and request escort or shared visit services if needed) (Clemen-Stone et al., 1998). The neighborhood should also be assessed for environmental factors that may affect personal safety, including location of the home in relation to high crime areas and known drug and gang areas.

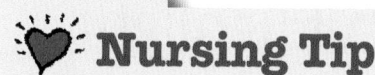

> **Nursing Tip**
>
> **Safety during the home visit**
>
> When traveling to make a home visit keep valuables, including any medical supplies, locked in the trunk of your car, out of sight. Carry a cellular phone in the car at all times, and ensure that it is in working order. Avoid dimly lit areas/streets/hallways, give travel route and arrival/departure times to your supervisor, and don't enter a situation you feel is unsafe. Dress professionally, avoid wearing expensive jewelry, and park near the home.

Engagement/Active Participation Phase

During this phase the home health care nurse begins to build the nurse–client relationship (Figure 4-3). The nurse carries out an initial client, family, and environmental assessment (see accompanying Family Teaching Box). Thorough assessments should be conducted. Collaboration with the child and caregivers and clarification of roles are done in the active participation phase (Reifsnider, 1996). Refer to Chapter 3 for a discussion of family assessment.

Assessment of the adequacy and safety of the general living environment should be conducted. Some important

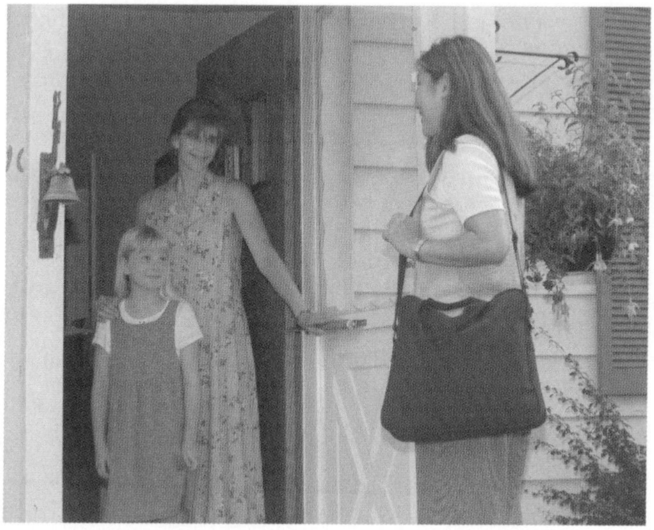

Figure 4-3 The nurse begins to build a relationship with the family on the first home visit.

Research Highlight

Personal Safety, Violence, and Home Health

Study Purpose

A critical issue facing the health care industry today is the potential impact of community and interpersonal violence on home health care. The purposes of this study were to (1) serve as a source for understanding the personal safety risk issues facing home care staff in a large Midwest region and its surrounding rural areas; (2) provide an understanding of how perceived threats to personal safety may have an impact on patient care and patient outcomes; (3) identify strategies for increasing the personal safety of direct care staff; and (4) identify organizational, educational, and procedural issues that impede or enhance staff safety.

Methods

Data were collected by a qualitative method of focus groups, in-depth individual interviews, critical event narratives, and a participant self-report form. The study used a purposive sample consisting of five men and 56 women who were either administrators or direct-care staff from 13 home health agencies.

Findings

Seven major themes emerged: (1) unsafe conditions that direct care staff must face; (2) organizational and administrative issues that impede or promote the personal safety of staff; (3) ethical issues that staff face daily; (4) protective factors associated with maintaining safety; (5) issues of gender, race, age, and experience; (6) education and training; and (7) the potential impact that staff's fear of interpersonal and community violence can have on patient care and patient outcomes.

Implications

Home health agencies need to have ongoing education and training programs that are specific to home health situations and made equally available to professional and nonprofessional staff. Comprehensive personal safety policies and procedures relevant to home health care should be developed and implemented. Administrators should have the knowledge, skills, organizational structure, and process to support and guide staff through frightening experiences in the field. More research should be done to see what effects threats to staff safety have on patient care.

Citation

Fazzone, P., Barloon, L., McConnell, S., & Chitty, J. (2000). Personal safety, violence, and home health. *Public Health Nursing, 17*(1), 43–52.

areas to assess are (Ahmann, 1996; Stanhope & Knollmueller, 1992):

- Adequacy of physical space, cooking facilities, and heating
- Accessibility of the home environment for the child who may be wheelchair-bound.
- Presence and functioning of smoke detectors.
- Adequacy of electrical sources and back-up electrical source if the child has a respiratory ventilator that requires electricity.
- Condition of electrical cords and outlets. (Does the equipment require a three-pronged outlet but the outlets are two-pronged?)
- Functioning of telephones.
- Presence of rodents, roaches, loose plaster, and paint chips.
- Education about age-specific safety measures followed in a child's home (i.e., gates on stairs for an active 15-month-old).

Family Teaching

Key Areas to Assess for Potential Exposure to Environmental Toxins

Home

Exposure

If there was an exposure to a toxic substance, family should note:

- Location
- Name of hazardous substance
- Route into body (ingestion, inhalation, absorption)
- Contact time
- Frequency
- Dose

Homes can be a Source of Environmental Toxin Exposure

Families should assess:

- Water source
- Use of fertilizers or pesticides
- Home insulating
- Heating and cooling
- Age of the home and general state of repair (recent renovation/remodeling)
- Air pollution (exposure to second-hand cigarette smoke)
- Use of home cleaning agents

School/Community

Schools and Communities Can Be Sources of Exposure to Environmental Toxins.

The family should assess:

- Proximity to industry, highways, or landfills
- Population density (urban, suburban, rural)
- Age of the school the child attends

Stanhope, M., & Lancaster, J. (1996). *Community health nursing: Promoting health of aggregates, families, and individuals* (4th ed.). St. Louis: Mosby

Documentation of assessment findings is necessary through all phases of the visit. Home care equipment should be assessed during the initial visit and reassessed periodically for adequacy of routine and emergency maintenance and replacement, and the presence of explicit instructions about the care and operation of the equipment.

In the home, the family may initially view the nurse as a stranger or intruder since the nurse is basically a guest in their home. An awareness of and respect for the cultural and ethnic diversity of families is essential to gaining their trust. The family may have specific beliefs and practices about health and healing that the nurse should help them integrate into the treatment plan.

The nurse should inquire about social customs usually practiced, such as removing shoes before entering the house or avoiding eye contact when talking, which may be considered impolite behavior. If these customs are breached, it may prevent the nurse from being able to interact effectively with the child and family. Box 4-4 provides guidelines for providing culturally sensitive nursing care for children in the home.

Eye On:

Cultural Assessment in the Home

Caring for a child with a cultural or ethnic background different from that of your own can be challenging, especially when you enter a family's home. For instance, it is important to know if a Jewish family observes Kosher dietary laws. The Kosher household will have different silverware for dairy and meat products.

BOX 4-4 Providing culturally sensitive nursing care in the home

- Remember that the setting for care is controlled by the family and not by the health care provider.
- Engage in social conversation to facilitate rapport since the nurse is often viewed as a guest by the child and family.
- Be nonjudgmental about the condition of the home (e.g., presence of clutter or disarray).
- Show respect and consideration for the child and family. For example, wipe your feet, or take off your shoes if it is a family custom, before entering the home; ask permission before moving items in the child's room, and replace them after you have finished a task.
- Take advantage of the home environment to assess cultural values and norms. Cultural clues may include:
  - Orderliness and decor of the home
  - Assignment of family roles and tasks
  - Types of family interactions
  - Presence of religious objects in the home
  - Value placed on privacy and possessions

Children who have complex medical conditions, are dependent on technology, and are being cared for in the home may be at risk for developmental delays and problems. A developmental assessment should be performed by the home health care nurse initially and periodically. When the child is assessed at regular intervals, objective data can be obtained so small developmental changes can be noticed. When problems are detected, the nurse can either provide treatment or, more likely, refer the child for early intervention services. The nurse needs to provide feedback to families about their child's developmental level, strengths, and deficits. Caregivers need this information in order to meet the developmental needs of the child.

The home health care nurse should assess the appropriateness of third-party reimbursement systems and discuss with the caregivers the estimated length of service, including limits set by third-party payers. The home care nurse should become familiar with financial resources and therapeutic programs. Financial resources include private insurance, health maintenance organizations (HMOs), Medicaid, Supplemental Security Income (SSI), Women, Infants, and Children (WIC) programs, food stamps, and state Crippled Children's services. Therapeutic programs include infant stimulation, educational, occupational, physical, audiologic, and speech programs (Scher & Ahmann, 1996). Many of these therapeutic programs are mandated under the Early Intervention Service Program (P.L. 94-142 and its subsequent amendments 98-199, 99-457, and 101-476 [Individuals with Disabilities Education Act {IDEA}]).

REFLECTIONS FROM FAMILIES

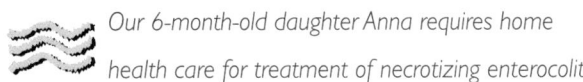

Our 6-month-old daughter Anna requires home health care for treatment of necrotizing enterocolitis. She is being treated by hyperalimentation, a process of feeding her nutrients through a central line to her heart. Anna's father and I find this treatment very frightening. It requires the presence of a home health nurse, as well as various technical personnel in our home at various times. Because Anna's condition is so delicate, we have moved her crib into our dining room so that we are able to watch her continually. It has been hard for our family to adjust to the loss of privacy and the disruption of routine. My two older daughters have begun to display behavioral problems because my husband and I have not been able to give them the time and attention they need. We have both become exhausted, which has been compounded by the fact that both of us are too anxious most of the time to get much sleep. We have tried getting out of the house for a little break, but respite care is very expensive, and it is hard to find anyone to care for a baby as sick as Anna, even for a little while.

Reflective Thinking

Third-Party Payment Systems

Third-party payments for home care services may run out before the child is rehabilitated fully or the family is ready to assume full responsibility for the child's care. What are your feelings on this discontinuation of services? What are the family's options?

Termination Phase

The home health care nurse evaluates the child's status and the caretakers' ability to assume responsibility for the child's total care. Part of the termination process involves collaboration and coordination with other disciplines involved in the care of the child. Plans for terminating home care should begin during the engagement and active participation phase so that the continuity of care that was started can be maintained. During the termination phase, it may be necessary to continue with some rehabilitative services, such as speech, physical, or occupational therapies. Allowing for the family to evaluate the home care services is important at this time. The home care agency should have standard forms that are sent to families that allow them to routinely evaluate the home care service received.

Future Trends

Home health care nursing for children and their families has grown significantly within the past decade, and it is predicted that this area of nursing will continue to grow. The cost of taking care of a child with chronic illness in the home is less than it would be in the hospital. However, in the future, cost containment for home care will become an issue, as insurance companies and the government try to manage the spiraling increase in medical care, whether inpatient or home care. Competition in home health care for children and their families will increase as more home health care agencies offer pediatric care. The quality of service will

Case Study/Care Plan

Home Care for a Child

Ryan is a child who receives 12 hours of nursing home care a day. He is 2 years old and was born prematurely with a tracheoesophageal fistula (TEF) and ventricular septal defect (VSD), both of which were repaired at birth. The repair for the TEF required him to have a tracheostomy, and he has not been able to be decannulated yet. Ryan is oxygen-dependent because of bronchopulmonary dysplasia (BPD) that developed while he was on the ventilator because of his prematurity. Necrotizing enterocolitis (NEC; see Chapter 23) also developed within the first 5 months of his life; it required surgery that removed a portion of his bowel. Since that time Ryan has needed total parenteral nutrition (TPN) through a central line and feedings through a gastrostomy button in order to achieve optimal nutritional status. Ryan's family consists of his mother, father, and two older sisters, ages 10 and 12. Ryan's father works, while his mother stays home and cares for him when there is no nursing coverage. Insurance coverage for Ryan is through his father's work, and the plan has been changed so that some of the expenses of Ryan's care are not covered. Ryan's paternal grandparents live nearby, but have not had any instruction in caring for Ryan. Lately, Ryan's mother has expressed concern that the older girls feel like he takes up too much of their mother's time and there is not enough time left for her to help them with homework and to attend school functions. Ryan's mother is also expressing feelings of being overwhelmed and depressed with the constancy of his care.

Nursing Care Plan

Assessment You need to assess the family's knowledge of the child's medical condition and the necessary home treatment. Inquiring about their ability and willingness to assume the child's care is essential for home care to be effective. The physical resources of the family need to be evaluated, such as the appropriateness of the physical environment of the home. The adequacy of the caregivers' physical and psychic energy for providing long-term care also needs to be assessed. Assessment of the family's financial resources for home care should include the cost to implement the treatment plan (e.g., equipment, supplies, medications), insurance coverage, and changes in work situations outside the home.

Nursing Diagnosis #1

High risk for feeling of powerlessness (family) related to financial stress.

Expected Outcome

The family will verbalize feelings of having control over the financial situation.

Interventions/*Rationales*

1. Assess family's ability to understand financial changes associated with the new insurance carrier. *Determines family's understanding of the current situation.*

2. Inform the family of additional avenues for financing care of the child's illness such as Aid to Families with Dependent Children (AFDC) and Supplemental Security Income (SSI). *Information can increase family's feeling of being proactive in this situation.*

3. Explore ways to implement cost-containing measures, such as disinfecting equipment that can be reused instead of using disposable equipment. *Helps the family to take control of the situation.*

4. Encourage family to discuss feelings of powerlessness over the change in insurance companies. *Allows the family to vent feelings of powerlessness and identify positive ways of coping.*

continues

continued

Evaluation

The family verbalizes they are exploring avenues of additional financing to help with the costs of caring for the child at home, and they are planning to implement cost-containing measures.

Nursing Diagnosis #2

High risk for interrupted family processes related to the strain of caring at home for a child who is chronically ill.

Expected Outcome

The family will regain ability to care for their chronically ill child and to meet the needs of all its members.

Interventions/*Rationales*

1. Assess the family dynamics (use a family assessment tool) and coping skills. *Assessment of these skills will allow the nurse to capitalize on the family's strength.*

2. Allow the family to verbalize feelings of guilt and inadequacy and stress the normalcy of these feelings. *Family will recognize the impact caring for a chronically ill child at home has on all family members.*

3. Discuss acceptable ways to modify the ill child's care to accommodate the usual family lifestyle. *Maintenance of a routine is important for family processes.*

4. Reinforce the importance of planning time for self, spouse, and the other children. *Allows family members to plan time away from the ill child without feeling guilty.*

5. Suggest that siblings be allowed to help in age-appropriate ways as family responsibilities are shifted to accommodate home care. *Sibling involvement can give them a feeling of worth and a sense of importance at a time when they might otherwise feel insecure.*

Evaluation

The family is using appropriate coping skills, and they have worked out a schedule so that each family member can have some time away from caring for Ryan. The siblings have agreed to take on some family responsibilities that they feel they can handle.

Nursing Diagnosis #3

High risk for delayed growth and development related to chronic illness and prolonged hospitalization.

Expected Outcome

The child will display growth and development that, as much as possible, meets age-appropriate norms.

Interventions/*Rationales*

1. Assess current developmental level. *To determine if there is a delay in growth and development.*

2. Provide opportunities to enhance development (i.e., play that encourages motor development, contact with other children to encourage social development). *Providing opportunities allows the child chances to improve developmental level.*

3. Refer to the Early Childhood Intervention (ECI) program for assistance from the child development team. *This community resource is skilled in improving the developmental level of a delayed child.*

4. Teach the caregivers strategies to foster improvement of developmental level. *Caregivers have the best opportunity for consistent interaction with the child.*

Evaluation

The child is making progress in meeting growth and developmental norms.

continues

continued

Nursing Diagnosis #4

Strain on the caregiver related to the requirements of caring for a child with a chronic illness.

Expected Outcome

Caregiver will plan time away from the ill child.

Intervention/*Rationales*

1. Identify support systems available, especially additional family members who can provide care for the child. *Provides respite care for the primary caregiver.*

2. Encourage the primary caregiver to express feelings and suggest joining a support group. *Helps the caregiver to vent and to recognize that feelings of strain are normal.*

3. Assist the primary caregiver to organize care, thereby reducing time spent on routine tasks. *Helps caregiver to manage time and to have more time for other activities.*

Evaluation

Caregiver is planning to go to the beauty shop during the time the home care nurse is with the child.

continue to increase in response to this competition (Taylor & Rawson, 1997).

The home health care nurse will continue to care for the child who is dependent on technology. In addition to providing illness care, the nurse, increasingly, will provide health promotion and disease prevention care to children and their families. This is already beginning to happen as home health care nurses are providing home antibiotic therapy, home phototherapy, and home visits to children who are enrolled in early childhood intervention programs. The home health care nurse who cares for children and their families will need to have knowledge of acute care, community health, mental health, management, and pediatric acute and chronic illnesses (Ahmann, 1996).

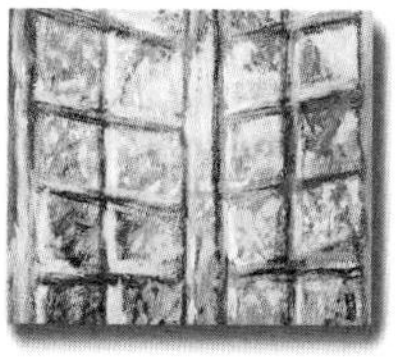

In the Real World

I am a home health care nurse and have been caring for Mary Xu, who is 4 years old and is dependent on a ventilator. For the past 3 months, I have visited Mary and her family four times a week. They have welcomed me into their home and are appreciative of everything I do for Mary. However, as time goes on, I have found it more and more difficult to maintain professional boundaries. I feel like they're beginning to see me as a family member. It's so easy for the boundaries to become blurred because of the informality of the home setting, the social conversation that occurs, and the involvement of the family in the child's care. But I know the signs of boundary crossing and will make changes if necessary.

Key Concepts

- Community health nursing is a broad category of nursing that can be defined by the focus of practice and by the population it serves; home health nursing is a specialty of community health nursing and is defined as a variety of services provided to children in their place of residence.
- Activities that the community health nurse conducts to promote child and family wellness include well-child assessments, administering immunizations, screening, teaching, referring, and providing direct care under federally mandated programs.
- The government has influenced public health for children and their families through Medicaid, public laws, and outlining goals for health promotion, protection, and illness prevention through the publication of *Healthy People 2010*.
- The community health nurse assesses, intervenes, teaches, and refers families for health promotion, protection, and illness prevention services.
- The community health nurse who cares for children and their families has a variety of roles, including clinician, advocate, collaborator, consultant, counselor, educator, researcher, and case manager.

- Home health care nurses who care for children and their families provide direct care, assessments, instruction, support, screening, referrals, and case management.
- The types of home care agencies that provide services to children and their families are official, voluntary, combined, private, and hospital-based.
- Children who are dependent on technology and those who receive hospice care receive the majority of home health care nursing hours.
- The home health nurse must establish a therapeutic relationship with the child and family while at the same time respecting professional boundaries.
- The three phases of the home visit are preinteraction, engagement/active participation, and termination.
- Home health care for children and their families will continue to grow in the future.

Review Questions

1. How does the community health nurse promote health for children and their families?
2. What role does the government play in community health for children and their families?
3. Describe some of the resources that the community health nurse may use to promote and protect health and prevent illness for children and their families.
4. What role does the community health nurse have in promoting firearm safety, immunization programs, and environmental assessments?
5. What is the purpose of standards for community health nursing practice?
6. What is included in the assessment the community health nurse conducts for children and their families?
7. What is included in an environmental assessment?
8. What are some of the roles the home care nurse assumes when caring for children and their families?
9. Why has there been an increase in the need for home care for children and their families?
10. What are the types of home care agencies for children and their families?
11. How does the home care nurse relate therapeutically to children and their families?
12. What are some of the skills the home care nurse demonstrates?
13. How does a home care nurse conduct a home visit?
14. What are future trends for community health and home care nursing for children and their families?

References

Ahmann, E. (1994). Thinking critically about family-centered home care nursing. *Pediatric Nursing, 20*(6), 588–590.

Ahmann, E. (1996). Family-centered home care. In E. Ahmann (Ed.), *Home care for the high-risk infant: A family-centered approach* (2nd ed., pp. 29–35). Gaithersburg, MD: Aspen.

American Nurses Association. (1986a). *Standards of community health nursing practice*. Washington, DC: Author.

American Nurses Association. (1986b). *Standards of home health nursing practice*. Washington, DC: Author.

Association of Community Health Nursing Educators Task Force on Basic Community Health Nursing Education [ACHNF]. (1990). *Essentials of baccalaureate nursing education for entry level community health nursing practice*. Louisville, KY: Author.

Bearer, C. (1995). Environmental health hazards: How children are different from adults. *The Future of Children: Critical Issues for Children and Youths, 5*(2) 11–26.

Bryan, A., & Wirth, D. (1995). Birth to three early intervention: Nursing's role on the interdisciplinary team. *Journal of Community Health, 12*(2), 73–88.

Clemen-Stone, S., McGuire, S., & Eigsti, D. (1998). *Comprehensive community health nursing: Family, aggregate, & community practice* (5th ed.). St. Louis: Mosby.

Dougherty, J., Parrish, J., & Hock-Long, L. (1995). Part 1: Developing a competency-based curriculum for tracheostomy and ventilator care. *Pediatric Nursing, 21*(6), 581–584.

Erickson, G. (1996). To pauperize or empower: Public health nursing at the turn of the 20th and 21st century. *Public Health Nursing, 13*(3), 163–169.

Fazzone, P., Barloon, L., McConnell, S., & Chitty, J. (2000). Personal safety, violence, and home health. *Public Health Nursing, 17*(1), 43–52.

Hitchcock, J., Schubert, P., & Thomas, S. (1999). *Community health nursing: Caring in action*. Albany, NY: Delmar.

Hogue, E. (1993). Care in the absence of primary caregivers. *Pediatric Nursing, 19*(1), 49–50.

Krepper, R., Young, A., & Cummings, E. (1994). Pediatric home healthcare: A paradox. *Home Healthcare Nurse, 12*(4), 15–19.

Leonard, B., Brust, J., & Sielaff, B. (1991). Determinants of home care nursing hours for technology-assisted children. *Public Health Nursing, 8*(4), 239–244.

Lindell, D. (1997). Community assessment for the home healthcare nurse. *Home Healthcare Nurse, 15*(9), 618–626.

Mausner (1995). Families helping families: An innovative approach to the provision of respite care for families of children with complex medical needs. *Social Work in Health Care, 21*(1), 95–106.

McClelland, C., Thompson, P., Piete, S., & Hatcher, P. (1996). Assessing firearms safety in inner-city homes. *N&HC: Perspectives on Community, 17*(4), 174–178.

Moore, P., Fenlon, N., & Hepworth, J. (1996). Hispanic infants in a Medicaid managed care system. *Public Health Nursing, 13*(1), 21–30.

National Center for Injury Prevention and Control, Centers for Disease Control. (2000). [On-line] Available: http://www.cdc.gov/ncipc/osp/usmort.htm.

National Council of State Boards of Nursing (1996). *Professional boundaries: A nurse's guide to the importance of appropriate professional boundaries*. Chicago: National Council of State Boards of Nursing, Inc.

O'Neill, E., & Pennington, E. (1996). Preparing acute care nurses for community-based care. *N&HC Perspectives on Community, 17*(2) 62–65.

Peirson, G. (1993). What pediatric home care offers the nurse. *MCN: American Journal of Maternal Child Nursing, 18*(6), 306–308.

Pilliteri, A. (1999). *Maternal & child health nursing: Care of the childbearing & childrearing family* (3rd ed.). Philadelphia: Lippincott.

Pridham, K., Broome, M., & Woodring, B. (1996). Education for the nursing of children and their families: Standards and guidelines for prelicensure and early professional education. *Journal of Pediatric Nursing, 11*(5), 273–280.

Reifsnider, E. (1996). Helping children grow: A home-based intervention protocol. *Journal of Community Health Nursing, 13*(2), 93–106.

Reifsnider, E. (1998). Reversing growth deficiency in children: The effect of a community-based intervention. *Journal of Pediatric Health Care, 12*(6 Pt. 1), 305–311.

Scher, A. & Ahmann, E. (1996). Community resources for the family. In E. Ahmann (Ed.), *Home care for the high-risk infant: A family-centered approach* (2nd ed., pp. 77–80). Gaithersburg, MD: Aspen.

Smith, C., & Maurer, F. (2000). *Community health nursing theory and practice* (2nd ed.). Philadelphia: Saunders.

Stanhope, M., & Knollmueller, R. (1992). *Handbook of community and home health nursing: Tools for assessment, intervention, and education*. St. Louis: Mosby.

Stanhope, M., & Lancaster, J. (1996). *Community health nursing: Promoting health of aggregates, families, and individuals* (4th ed.). St. Louis: Mosby.

Taylor, G. & Rawson, R. (1997). Providing high-quality care for children. *Caring, 16*(8), 50–51.

U.S. Department of Health and Human Services. (1997). *Registered nurse population 1996: Findings from the national sample survey of registered nurses*. Washington, DC: Division of Nursing, Bureau of Health Professions, Health Resources and Services Administration.

U.S. Department of Health and Human Services. (2000). *Healthy people 2010*. Washington, DC: Government Printing Office.

Suggested Readings

American Public Health Association. (1991). *Healthy community 2000: Model standards* (3rd ed.). Washington, DC: American Public Health Association.

Benefield, L. (1996). Component analysis of productivity in home care RNs. *Public Health Nursing, 13*(4), 233–243.

Benefield, L. (1996). Making the transition to home care nursing. *American Journal of Nursing, 96*(10), 47–49.

Dougherty, J., Parrish, J., Parra, M., Kinney, Z., & Kandrak, G. (1996). Part 2: Using a competency-based curriculum to train experienced nurses in ventilator care. *Pediatric Nursing, 22*(1), 47–50.

Hill, D. (1993). Coordinating a multidisciplinary discharge for the technology-dependent child based on parental needs. *Issues in Comprehensive Pediatric Nursing, 16*(4), 229–237.

Kendra, M., Weiker, A., Simon, S., Grant, A., & Shullick, D. (1996). Safety concerns affecting delivery of home health care. *Public Health Nursing, 13*(2), 83–89.

Landrigan, P., & Carlson, J. (1995). Environmental policy and children's health. *The Future of Children: Critical Issues for Children and Youths, 5*(2), 34–52.

Reiss, J., Cameon, R., Matthews, D., & Shenkman, E. (1996). Enhancing the role public health nurses play in serving children with special health needs: An interactive videoconference on public law 99-457 Part H. *Public Health Nursing, 13*(5), 345–352.

Scannel, S., Gillies, D., Biordi, D., & Child, D. (1993). Negotiating nurse-patient authority in pediatric home health care. *Journal of Pediatric Nursing, 8*(2), 70–78.

Resources

Organizations and Websites

Access to Respite Care Help (ARCH)
800 Easttowne Dr.
Chapel Hill, NC 27514
(800) 473-1727

Centers for Disease Control and Prevention (CDC)
Morbidity and Mortality Weekly Report (MMWR)
www.cdc.gov

Division of Immunization, Centers for Disease Control and Prevention
1600 Clifton Rd. NE
Altanta, GA 30333
(800) 311-3435
www.cdc.gov

March of Dimes Birth Defects Foundation
1275 Mamaroneck Ave.
White Plains, NY 10016
(888) MODIMES
www.modimes.org

National Center for Environmental Health (CDC) Lead Poisoning Prevention
(404) 488-7330
National Lead Information Center (800) LEAD-FYI

National Center for Farmworker Health, Inc.
1770FM967
Buda, TX 78610
(512) 312-2700
www.ncfh.org

National Clearinghouse on Child Abuse and Neglect Information
P.O. Box 1182
Washington, DC 20013
(800) FYI-3366
www.nccanch@calid.com

National Coalition of Hispanic Health & Human Services Organizations (COSSMHO)
1501 16th Street, NW
Washington, DC 20036-1401
(202) 387-5000

National Council on Child Abuse and Family Violence
1155 Connecticut Ave. NW, Ste. 400
Washington, DC 20036
(202) 429-6695
www.nccafv.org

National Hotlines for Child Abuse
(800) 421-0353—Parents Anonymous
(800) 422-4453—National Abuse Hotline

National Information Center for Children and Youth with Disabilities
P.O. Box 1492
Washington, DC 20013
(800) 999-5599

National Rifle Association of America, The Eddie Eagle Gun Safety Program, NRA Safety and Education Division
11250 Waples Mill Rd.
Fairfax, VA 22030
(800) 231-0752
www.nrahq.org

Office on Smoking and Health, Centers for Disease Control and Prevention
Mailstop K-50
4770 Buford Highway NE
Atlanta, GA 30341-3724
(800) CDC-1311 (copies of action guide on second-hand smoke)
www.cdc.gov/tobacco

Olney Foundation (parenteral/enteral feedings)
124 Hun Memorial A-23
Albany Medical Center
Albany, NY 12208
(518) 262-5079

Sibling Information Network
1776 Ellington Rd.
South Windsor, CT 06074
(860) 648-1205

Sick Kids Need Involved People (SKIP)
216 Newport Dr.
Severna Park, MD 21146
(301) 621-7830

U.S. Environmental Protection Agency
1200 Pennsylvania Ave., NW
Washington, DC 20460
(202) 260-2080
www.epa.gov

CHAPTER 5

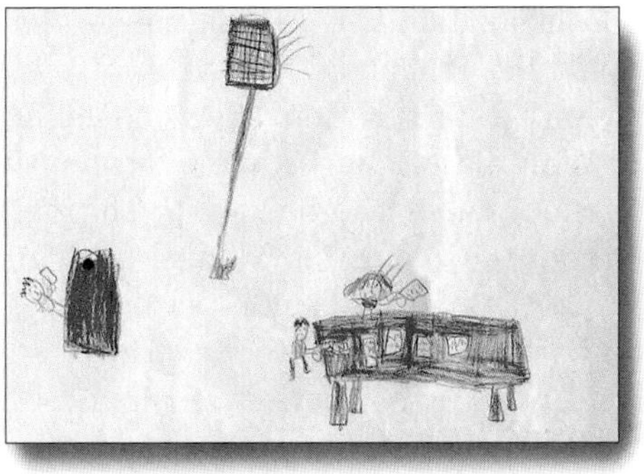

SCHOOL NURSING

Maureen L. Meyer, MS, CSN

As summer comes to an end, every parent feels many emotions as their child heads off to school the first day. When that child has a medical condition or chronic illness, there are additional concerns. As a mother of a child with insulin-dependent diabetes, I wanted the school administrator and nursing staff to understand that communication was of the utmost importance. Providing for the well-being of a child with diabetes requires planning and cooperation among parents and school nurses. When caregivers communicate the child's needs to the school nurse, it is easier to provide a safe and healthy atmosphere in the school setting.

COMPETENCIES

Upon completion of this chapter, the reader will be able to:

- *Describe how political and social changes in history affected the development of the school nurse's role.*
- *Describe three screenings often performed by nurses in the school setting.*
- *List common immunization requirements for children entering school, and explain strategies the school nurse employs for communicable disease control.*
- *Describe the school nurse's role in emergency care of children at school.*
- *Discuss the individual health plan and the role of the school nurse in its development.*
- *Identify and explain five content areas for health education the school nurse might teach.*
- *Describe the differences between school-based and school-linked health centers.*
- *Discuss two current issues affecting school nurses.*

In 1999, 46 million children attended public schools in the United States (Thompson, 1999). Their caregivers sent them off to school to learn to read and write, and develop social skills such as sharing, friendship, and respect for others. Once most children had their physical examination and immunizations, contact with the school nurse was minimal. However, this is not the case for children who have a chronic illness or need medication during the day. To the caregivers of some of these children, the school nurse's role is as important as the teacher's. For students with a chronic condition or for those who need medication, the school nurse can make the transition from home to school smoother; for some children, it would be impossible to attend school without this individual.

What does the nurse do all day in the school? In a place where children are supposed to sit in class and learn all day, why would a nurse be needed? This chapter will provide a brief review of the history of school nursing; types of health services, including the various screenings performed by the nurse; health education programs taught; and psychological services offered in which the nurse may be involved. The need for health services to be more accessible to children has led to the development of school-based and school-linked health centers. Both models will be discussed and their similarities and differences explored. Finally, the current roles of the school nurse will be described, as well as future issues facing her or him.

HISTORY OF SCHOOL NURSING

School nursing owes its beginnings in both the United States and Europe to the field of Community/Public Health Nursing (see Chapter 4). Public health nurses in England and France began extending their services to the schools in the mid-1800s. Social factors in the United States such as an increase in immigrants, overcrowded living conditions in urban areas, and activities of the reformists of the World War I era played a role in calling attention to the need for social services in schools (Passarelli, 1994; Wold, 1981). However, it was a public health nurse, investigating the number of children absent from school due to infectious diseases, who formulated the plan that led to school nursing in the United States.

Lillian Wald, a pioneer in community nursing and founder of the Henry Street Settlement, was astonished by the number of children who never returned to school after being excluded for a communicable disease. In 1893, she convinced the New York Board of Health to try an experiment: place a nurse in selected schools in New York City to screen for infectious diseases, provide education regarding their control, and follow up by visiting the homes of children who had been excluded. The Board agreed, and in 1902 Lina Rogers became the first school nurse in the United States (Thomas, 1998; Wold, 1981). Amazingly, exclusion rates dropped from 10,567 students in 1902 to just 1,101 in 1903 (Thomas, 1998). The Board of Health was convinced that the program was helpful, and 25 more public health nurses were hired. Absentee rates continued to drop after this, and the role of the school nurse expanded from identifying, educating, and following up on communicable diseases to health and wellness education and disease prevention (Wold, 1981). The shift in focus from secondary to primary prevention had begun.

During the 1920s, school nurses continued to identify children with communicable diseases and to provide home follow-up care to educate the students and their families about treatment. The role then expanded to identifying physical defects in children and providing referrals for their correction. By the 1930s, the school nurse worked as part of a team with physicians and school personnel to develop educational programs, including not only communicable disease prevention and treatment, but health-promotion topics such as hygiene, nutrition, and other basic needs of children. The growth and development of the student and their effects on the child's ability to learn became the focus of school nurses at this time. These changes in the duties of the school nurse also brought some role confusion. Cutbacks in funding due to World War II led nurses to delegate tasks to teachers and other school personnel. The school nurse was consequently caught between the roles of education and health professional.

After World War II, the focus in the United States changed and, again, so did the role of the school nurse. By 1945, teacher involvement in the health of the child was increased. Health education became a subject in and of itself in school curricula. Collaboration between the nurse, the student, the school, and the community was stressed, and the relationship between health behaviors at school and at home was explored. With these changes, the educational preparation of the school nurse also needed to change. Nurses now needed more technical knowledge, a wider background in education and family health, better-developed leadership skills, and the ability to work as part of an interdisciplinary team. At this time, 16 states required special education courses and certification to become a school nurse (Wold, 1981).

The 1960s again brought about many changes in the United States. Social attitudes across the nation as well as financial changes in the schools affected the school nurse. Services not deemed essential were cut back, and the school nurse become a luxury, not a need. Changes in society brought about an increase in drug use and chemical dependence, sexual relations, and teen pregnancy. Students had new educational needs, and there was no one to address them.

Help came from professional nurses' organizations such as the American Nurses Association (ANA) and the American School Health Association (ASHA). The ANA formulated a broad definition of nursing in 1965, and in the 1970s it formulated minimum standards of practice for nurses. These guidelines helped better define the role of the nurse in various settings, including school nursing. In 1974, a philosophy of practice for school nurses was developed and endorsed by both the ANA and the ASHA, and guidelines for school nurses were developed (Box 5-1). Professional nursing organizations became further involved in the educational preparation of the school nurse. Both the ANA and the ASHA recommended a minimum of a baccalaureate degree. By 1976, mandated certification requirements were in place in 23 states (Wold, 1981).

During the 1970s, the federal government also played a part in the changing role of the school nurse. Although some federal laws addressing the educational needs of children with mental and physical handicaps were in place, it wasn't until 1975 that their education was guaranteed. The Education for All Handicapped Children Act (P.L. 94-142), renamed the Individuals with Disabilities Education Act (IDEA) in 1990, required that all states provide a free and appropriate education in the least restrictive environment to children with handicaps (Drew, Hardman, & Logan, 1996). Table 5-1 provides information on some laws affecting education and children with disabilities.

With special education now a right of students, schools found themselves responsible for educating children and adolescents with a multitude of physical, medical, and mental disabilities. Children began school at an earlier age and often had complex medical conditions needing specialized equipment and care (Passarelli, 1994). School nurses needed

BOX 5-1 ASHA guidelines for school nurses

- Every child is entitled to educational opportunities that allow each to reach full capacity as an individual and to prepare him or her for responsibility as a citizen.
- Every child is entitled to a level of health that permits maximum utilization of educational opportunities.
- Every school has a legal and moral obligation to provide a school health program that will promote and protect the health of its children.
- The school health program should be consistent with the philosophy and objectives of the school program.
- The school health program, through the components of health services, health education, and concern for the environment, provides the knowledge and understanding on which to base decisions for the promotion and protection of individual, family, and community health.
- A dual preparation in health and education best qualifies professional personnel for participation in the intraprofessional and interdisciplinary approach to school health.
- Activities of the school health program play a primary role in establishing a viable working relationship with home and community.
- Parents have the basic responsibility of providing comprehensive health and related services; the school health program will assist parents and youth in carrying out their responsibilities.
- The community has the responsibility of providing comprehensive health and related services; the school health program will assist parents and youth to utilize such community services effectively.
- School health program activities should include participation in regional, state, and local comprehensive health planning to identify and interpret health needs, and to coordinate health services for children.

From American School Health Association (1974). *Guidelines for the school nurse in the school health program.* Kent, OH: ASHA.

TABLE 5-1 Laws Affecting Education

Year	Public Law	Name and Summary
1965	89-10	Elementary and Secondary Education Act—Addressed inequality of education for economically disadvantaged children.
1973	93-112	Rehabilitation Act of 1973—Provided for rehabilitation services to all individuals regardless of severity of disability. Civil rights enforced under Section 504.
1975	94-142	Education for All Handicapped Children Act—Mandated free appropriate education for all children with disabilities. Mandated due process, least restrictive environment, and Individual Educational Plans for children 3–18 years old.
1978	95-602	Comprehensive Rehabilitation Service Amendment—Provided definition of developmental disability.
1986	99-457	Education of the Handicapped Act Amendment—Mandated services for preschoolers with disabilities ages 3–5 years and provided early intervention services from birth to 3 years.
1990	101-392	Carl D. Perkins Vocational and Applied Technology Education Act—Guaranteed vocational education for youths with disabilities.
1990	101-476	Individuals with Disabilities Education Act (IDEA)—Mandated transition services and assistive technology. Added autism and traumatic brain injury as disabilities. Extended services to 21 years.

Adapted from Chauvin, V. (1994). Students with special health care needs: A manual for school nurses. *Scarborough, ME: National Association of School Nurses.*

additional education and expertise in caring for children with specialized needs and in securing appropriate education placement.

In 1992, there were approximately 26,000 registered professional nurses working in schools across the United States (Passarelli, 1994). Six years later there were approximately 60,000 school nurses, serving 46 million children, in the United States (Thompson, 1999). Advances in medicine have improved the survival rates of premature infants and extremely sick children, which, in turn, have further increased the number of children with special needs served by the public school system. Approximately 20 million children have chronic illnesses (Ludder-Jackson & Vessey, 1996) and 1 to 2 children per 1,000 are dependent on some form of medical technology (Palfrey, Haynie, McManus, Fenton, & Shaw, 1995). Because of the passage of federal laws such as the Individuals with Disabilities Education Act, children with disabilities now have the same right to an education as every other child in the United States, causing the role of the school nurse to continue to evolve and adapt. In fact, new guidelines have been developed by ASHA (1998) to address the changing needs of children enrolled in today's schools (Box 5-2).

Staffing ratios and educational requirements for school nurses continue to vary from state to state, as does the availability of such nurses in schools (Fryer & Igoe, 1995). For example, only 17 states currently require school districts to provide certified school nurses (Thompson, 1999); registered nurses are usually used when students have special medical needs.

The role of the school nurse continues to include identifying communicable diseases and enforcing immunization requirements. Preventive procedures such as vision and hearing screening; education in nutrition, healthy lifestyle, and safety practices; and a curriculum on drug-use and violence prevention have been added. In addition, the nurses' duties may now include activities such as ventilator care, gastrostomy feedings, and clean intermittent catheterization (Porter, Haynie, Bierle, Heinz-Caldwell, & Palfrey, 1997). Financial constraints continue, and many school nurses must cover several schools even as their responsibilities have increased. In some states, the future of the school nurse as a certified professional is uncertain, although the need is greater than ever. Clarifying the importance of the nurse's role can assist in securing school nurses' positions now and in the future. The National Association of School Nurses provides standards of school nursing practice to assist the nurse in her role (Box 5-3). Before others can see the need and value of nurses in the school, the individual must be confident about her or his worth in the health and education of today's children.

BOX 5-2 ASHA recommendations, 1998

- One certified registered nurse to every 750 regular education students
- One nurse to every 225 mainstreamed students
- One nurse to every 125 severely/profoundly handicapped students

Critical Thinking

Too Many Schools, Too Few Nurses

Recommended staff ratios are not possible in all areas, and some school nurses are responsible for several schools. You are the only school nurse in a district with seven elementary schools. Six of the seven buildings have children on medication, and two have children with complex medical needs. How would you manage? What skills would you need? How would you prioritize your duties?

SCHOOL HEALTH SERVICES

The school nurse is involved in many school health services, including direct or indirect nursing care. **Direct services** include providing nursing procedures or care to individual students; **indirect services** include consulting with staff on behalf of a child's health needs and providing community referrals and health education. Health services also include screening programs, communicable disease control, emergency care, and medication administration. Education and health promotion activities include presenting subjects such as personal care, sex education, substance abuse, and violence prevention programs. The school nurse may also collaborate with social workers and school psychologists to provide services to families after unusual events in a child's life.

Screenings

One task of the school nurse is organizing and performing a variety of screening programs for school children. These screening programs assist in the early identification of possible problems related to children's health. When abnormalities are noted, the nurse plays a vital role in referring the child for further evaluation and/or correction. Traditional screening programs offered in the school include vision and hearing testing, height and weight measurement, scoliosis and pediculosis screening, immunizations, and, in some districts, dental and tuberculosis screening (Adams, 1992; Kane, 1994).

BOX 5-3 Standards of professional school nursing practice

Standards of Care

The School Nurse:

- Collects client data
- Analyzes the assessment data in determining nursing diagnoses
- Identifies expected outcomes individualized to the client
- Develops a plan of care/action that specifies interventions to attain expected outcomes
- Implements the interventions identified in the plan of care/action
- Evaluates the client's progress toward attainment of outcomes

Standards of Professional Performance

The School Nurse:

- Systematically evaluates the quality and effectiveness of school nursing practice
- Evaluates one's own nursing practice in relation to professional practice standards and relevant statutes, regulations, and policies
- Acquires and maintains current knowledge and competency in school nurse practice
- Interacts with and contributes to the professional development of peers and school personnel as colleagues
- Makes decisions and actions on behalf of clients determined in an ethical manner
- Collaborates with the student, family, school staff, community, and other providers in providing student care
- Promotes the use of research findings in school nursing practice
- Considers factors related to safety, effectiveness, and cost when planning and delivering care
- Uses effective written, verbal, and nonverbal communication skills
- Manages school health services
- Assists students, families, school staff, and the community in achieving optimal levels of wellness through appropriately designed and delivered health education

From National Association of School Nurses. (1999). *Standards of professional school nursing practice.* Scarborough, ME: NASN. Reprinted with permission.

Vision and Hearing Screening

Vision screening, one of the most common procedures performed in the school (Fryer, Igoe, & Miyoshi, 1997), is recommended by the American Academy of Ophthalmology and the American Academy of Pediatrics as part of routine school programs (Fryer et al., 1997). The purpose of vision screening is to identify children with potential problems in visual acuity and muscle balance so treatment can begin as soon as possible. Early vision screening can assist in detecting conditions such as strabismus, or lazy eye.

Screening also often includes inspecting the eye and evaluating visual acuity, muscle balance (phoria), excessive farsightedness (hyperopia), and color vision. Ideally, all students should be screened annually. A school-aged child who does not have visual acuity of at least 20/30 should normally be referred for further evaluation; however, the school nurse must verify the state's referral criteria before referring children since all states do not follow the same criteria. Numerous instruments are available for assessing vision in children, and the school nurse needs to be familiar with these products. The traditional Snellen chart, which uses letters in various sizes, is also available in tumbling letters and pictures to match the age and ability level of the child being screened. Stereoscopic instruments, which use mirrors, lenses, and occluders to screen for vision problems and require special training, are also used in mass screening programs.

Hearing screening is another responsibility of the school nurse (Figure 5-1). Hearing difficulties can have an impact on the child's ability to learn. If the child cannot hear adequately, directions and important information may be missed, speech development impaired, and reading affected. The nurse can help prevent or limit this problem by annually testing the child's hearing at 500, 1,000, 2,000, and 4,000 hertz in both ears at a fixed decibel (dB) level. Children with hearing loss between 70 and 90 dB are considered hard of hearing, and those with hearing loss greater than 90 dB are defined as having a severe or profound hearing loss

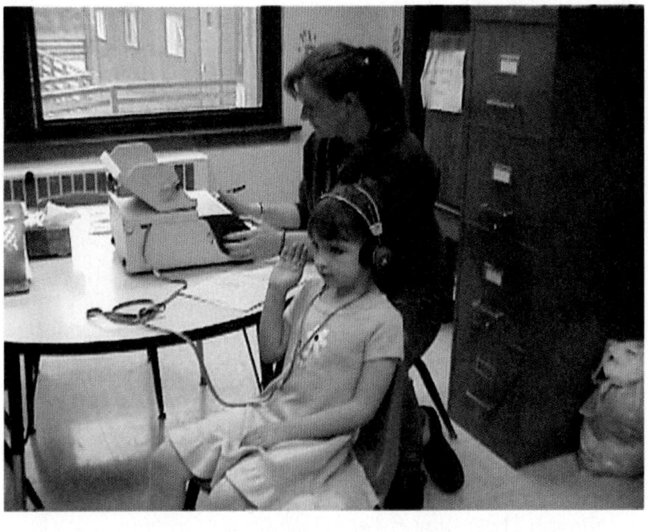

Figure 5-1 Hearing tests are part of screening programs carried out by school nurses.

(Copmann, 1996). (Refer to Chapter 31 for more information on hearing.)

Identification is only the beginning of vision and hearing screening programs; the screening itself is of limited value without referral and follow-up care (Yawn, Kurkland, Butterfield, & Johnson, 1998). Statistics show that 1 in 5 children will need corrective lenses by the time they graduate from high school (Yawn et al.,1998), and the prevalence of deafness and hearing loss is estimated at 15.3 per 1,000 children (Ludder-Jackson & Vessey, 1996). Studies on follow-up care after a failed vision screening revealed that the time from identifying a vision problem until treatment averaged about 18 months (Mark & Mark, 1999; Yawn et al., 1998). In the school setting, that equals about a grade level and a half without proper treatment. The nurse can play a vital role in speeding up this process by consistently following up on students who failed screenings and knowing about existing local resources to share with caregivers. The school nurse also needs to be aware of organizations that can assist families in obtaining vision and hearing services for their children. If a permanent vision or hearing loss is detected, the nurse can assist in obtaining specialized services or needed adaptations.

Height and Weight Measurement

Height and weight measurements are usually taken at the physician's office as part of a physical exam. However, some states require these measurements only on entry to kindergarten and 9th grade. Unless the child receives a yearly exam, height and weight can go unchecked for several years. A school nurse's annual measurements of a student's height and weight can provide valuable information for the health care provider, especially if a growth abnormality or weight problem is suspected. For further information on normal height and weight measurements in children, see Chapter 14.

Kids Want To Know

Getting Glasses

"My mom said I need to get glasses. It's been hard to see the chalkboard for awhile, but I was afraid to tell her. I don't want to get glasses. What if the kids laugh at me and call me names? I don't want to be different."

To help the child with this transition you can explain, in developmentally appropriate terms, why the child is getting glasses and how they will help him or her; point out other children and adults in the child's life who have glasses; encourage the parents to allow the child some choice in selecting the glasses, as appropriate; and supply developmentally appropriate books and videos to the student's family and teacher such as *Blueberry Eyes,* by M. Driscoll Beatty (1996); *Glasses for D.W.,* by M. Brown (1996); *Ben's Glasses,* by D. Johnson (1996); and *Let's Talk About Getting Glasses*, by D. Shaughnessy (1997).

REFLECTIONS FROM FAMILIES

Diane was in the 4th grade. We had just moved to a new neighborhood, a new school for the kids. Our previous school district did not have the resources to do annual vision and hearing testing on all the students. We really didn't think anything of it when Diane failed the hearing screening, thinking it was probably due to a cold. At the recommendation of the school nurse, we took her to our family physician, who then referred us to a specialist. We were shocked to learn that Diane had a 40% hearing loss and that hearing aids were recommended. The specialist said it had probably been present at birth and had gone undetected. Testing children's vision and hearing every year is an important part of school services.

Scoliosis Screening

Scoliosis is defined as a lateral curvature of the spine (Ludder-Jackson & Vessey, 1996), which occurs spontaneously or is associated with other diseases. It can cause gait disturbances, inflexibility, and back pain, and can affect posture. Scoliosis affects 0.5% to 2% of the population and is most often seen in the preadolescent or early adolescent because this is a period of rapid growth (NASN, 1995; Ludder-Jackson & Vessey, 1996). School nurses participating in scoliosis screening usually provide this service between 5th and 9th grades (NASN, 1995). Treatment options for scoliosis depend on the type of scoliosis diagnosed and are aimed at straightening and realigning the spine with exercise, external bracing, or surgical intervention. Because treatment/intervention may extend over several years, screening for scoliosis is considered less cost effective than other school screening programs, and in some cases, inadequate training in screening techniques may result in overreferral. For more information on scoliosis, see Chapter 34.

Immunization Monitoring

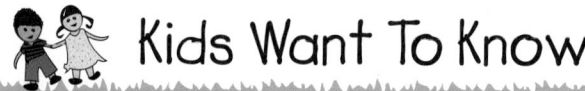

Another important role of the school nurse is monitoring student immunization records. Since the introduction and use of vaccines, the occurrence of communicable diseases such as diphtheria, tetanus, polio, and measles has decreased (Selekman, 1998). Immunizations are now available for hepatitis B, *Haemophilus influenzae* type b (HiB), chickenpox, and Lyme disease (Centers for Disease Control, 1999; Selekman, 1998). The school nurse is responsible for knowing about current immunizations, protocols, and schedules, and should also know when communicable disease outbreaks occur that may affect children.

By 1997, almost all 50 states had written policies excluding children from school without proper immunizations (Vernon, Bryan, Hunt, Allensworth, & Bradley, 1997). Depending on individual state guidelines, a student could be denied entrance to school or be required to obtain a physician-approved schedule for immunization when there is no verification of completed immunizations or a statement of religious or medical objection. Different states enforce different immunization requirements (Boyer-Chuanroong & Deaver, 2000). For further information and recommended schedules on childhood immunizations and communicable diseases, see Appendix C.

Communicable Disease Control

Communicable disease control has been a major factor in developing school health services and the nurse's role in these services (Constante & Smith, 1997; Wold, 1981). Specifically, the nurse's role in communicable disease control revolves around the three factors necessary for spread of disease: transmission, susceptibility, and a favorable environment.

An infectious agent is an organism, such as a virus or bacteria, capable of producing an infection (Benenson, 1995). It may be spread by direct contact with an infected person, indirect contact with contaminated objects, or transmission by air, a vehicle, or a vector. Knowledge of how common childhood diseases are spread can assist the nurse in keeping transmission to a minimum since many illnesses seen in students are spread by direct contact. Handwashing has been shown to be an effective way to decrease the spread of communicable diseases (Kimel, 1996). The school nurse can provide valuable and creative ideas for educating children about the importance and correct method of washing hands. Participating in programs to ensure clean air and water and decreasing exposure to possible hazardous materials are other ways that the school nurse can decrease children's potential for contact with infectious agents.

School nurses can also help decrease the school child's susceptibility to communicable diseases by confirming whether a child's health record indicates whether he or she is up-to-date on all required immunizations. When a child's immunization status does not show adequate protection, referral is necessary. Some school districts provide this service directly if they have established school-based or school-linked clinics, and the nurse may be responsible for administering the immunizations (Figure 5-2). The nurse can also help decrease susceptibility to disease by providing education about health issues and promoting healthy living habits in students, especially in the early grades. Nutrition, exercise, adequate rest, and personal care can affect one's ability to fight off infectious diseases; these are possible topics for health promotion classes.

Lastly, the school nurse can help contain the spread of communicable diseases by providing a less favorable environment for their growth. By identifying children with communicable diseases and excluding them from school as policies dictate, the number of other children exposed can be decreased. Almost all states have laws requiring exclusion of students and mandatory reporting of certain communicable diseases; the school nurse needs to check with local or state health departments to determine which diseases are reportable.

Although the incidence of serious communicable diseases has decreased because of vaccination, other illnesses, such as strep throat, scabies, and lice, still need to be moni-

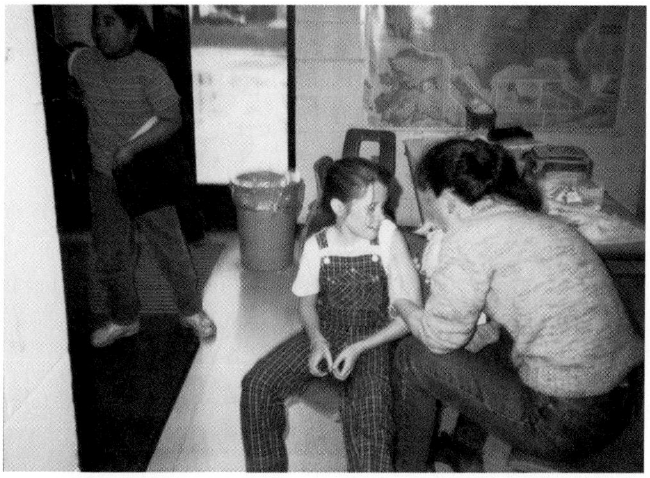

Figure 5-2 To assist parents in keeping their children up to date on immunizations, some school nurses administer immunizations in traveling clinics.

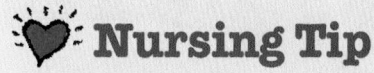

Nursing Tip

Communicable disease exclusion

Keeping a list of students enrolled in your school with medical or religious objections to immunizations or those with special health concerns that lessen their immunity makes exclusion of students easier in the event of an outbreak of a serious communicable disease such as measles.

tored. Even though these diseases are less serious than measles, they can spread quickly through the classroom and lead to complications in some children. For children who are immunosuppressed, caregivers must be notified if these diseases occur in classmates because of the need for special monitoring or prophylactic treatment to prevent serious complications. Further information on communicable disease can be found in Chapter 15.

Emergency Care

Emergency care of the child at school centers on two main concerns: (1) basic first aid care for a child with an illness or injury and (2) emergencies requiring transport and more extensive treatment at a hospital (see Figure 5-3). Because the school nurse is often the only health professional in the school, that individual must have excellent physical assessment skills and be able to make quick and accurate decisions regarding the extent of illnesses or injuries. Education in triage skills, including classification of illnesses/injuries as emergent, urgent, or nonurgent will assist in making these decisions (University of Connecticut Health Center, Department of Pediatrics, 1997).

When a student comes into the nurse's office, an across-the-room assessment of the child is necessary in order to decide on the best course of action. The nurse must think:

- How does the child look and act?
- Are there visible signs of illness or injury?
- Does the child say one thing, but body language or physical signs say another?
- What brought this student to the nurse's office; what is his or her chief complaint?

Then the nurse should:

- Assess the child from head to toe while the child talks about the reason for seeking out the nurse.
- Check vital signs such as temperature, pulse, and respiration, as appropriate.
- Look for signs of bruising or bleeding if an injury was the cause for the visit.

Allow the child to rest quietly, observe changes, or assist the child in washing a cut and applying a bandage or an ice pack, and always watch for signs of a more serious problem or complaint that is not relieved with these measures. This information can assist in deciding if the child's caregiver needs to be notified. Most school districts have developed a policy on specific instances when children need to be sent home. These policies may include a temperature over 100°F, an undiagnosed rash, and a constant productive cough. Sometimes physicians' standing orders allow the nurse to treat minor illnesses at school with medications such as acetaminophen or cough syrup. However, before dispensing any medications, the nurse must know the district medication policy. See Box 5-4 for a list of first aid supplies the school nurse should have readily available.

One would think that school is the safest place for a child to be, but the potential for injuries in a school is nearly endless. Playground equipment, participation in gym and sports, and injuries in classes such as metal shop and chemistry can all lead to serious accidents. In the case of more serious injuries such as a fall with a possible head injury or broken bone, additional assessment is essential. If the child has fallen in gym and is complaining of ankle pain and difficulty walking, the nurse should look for swelling, bruising, deformities, and decreased movement, circulation, and sensation in the extremity. If abnormalities are found the extremity should be splinted as necessary. If there is a head injury, the child should never be left alone. Any bleeding

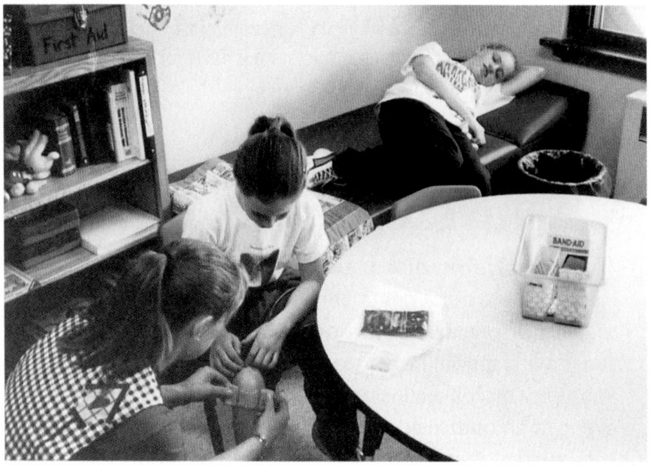

Figure 5-3 A school nurse is responsible for administering emergency first aid.

Kids Want To Know

An Ambulance Ride

"What happens if I get hurt at school and have to go to the hospital? What's it like to ride in an ambulance? How will my parents find me?"

To help lessen the fears of students, the school nurse can:

- Arrange a visit from the local fire department so children can tour the ambulance
- Provide various equipment the children may see in the ambulance/emergency room for hands-on experiences
- Have a familiar staff person from the school ride in the ambulance with the child if possible and, if appropriate, reassure the child that caregivers will meet them at the hospital

BOX 5-4 First aid supplies

Soap and accessibility to running water
Ice packs
Thermometer
Bandage scissors
Tweezers
Penlight
Blanket
Mouth-to-mask resuscitator
Blood pressure cuff (adult and pediatric)
Stethoscope
Dressing supplies:
- Bandages (a variety of sizes)
- Sterile gauze pads/dressings (a variety of sizes)
- Medical tape
- Triangle bandages
- Elastic bandages (a variety of sizes)
- Splints (magazines can be used as splints if needed)
- Eye pads/eye flush kit

Protective equipment:
- Gloves
- Goggles
- Sharps container

If allowed by school district (and standing orders are present):
- Acetaminophen
- Bee sting pads
- Diphenhydramine
- EpiPen

should be controlled, and vital signs as well as vision disturbances, headaches, nausea, vomiting, and changes in level of consciousness or seizure activity should be noted. The caregiver should be notified and emergency services contacted as the assessment dictates. Knowing when to call for help when a child is injured is the most important aspect of caring for an injured child. Since extensive medical supplies and equipment are not always available in schools, help from paramedics who are often only minutes away can be essential.

Even though some days are filled with taking care of children with stomach aches and scraped knees, there is more to school nursing than just taking temperatures and supplying bandages. When the nurse assesses the child's illness or injury, she can also teach children to care for themselves, promote self-esteem, and encourage healthy habits.

Ongoing Health Situations

An increasingly common school emergency today is a child experiencing difficulty breathing due to an asthma attack. Asthma is a chronic disease characterized by reversible airway narrowing, inflammation of the airway, and hyperresponsiveness of the airway to stimuli (McEwen, Johnson, Neatherlin, Millard, & Lawrence, 1998). Symptoms vary in severity and can include wheezing, cough, difficulty breathing, prolonged expiration, chest tightness, tachypnea, and excessive mucosal secretions. (For more information on the diagnosis and treatment of asthma, see Chapter 24.)

The number of children diagnosed with asthma has risen in recent years and is estimated at 4.8 million (McEwen et al., 1998; Meurer, McKenzie, Mischler, Subichin, Malloy, & George, 1999). In the United States, asthma is the most common cause of school absence; McEwen et al., 1998).

Case Study/Care Plan

Asthma

Jimmy is a 8-year-old African American student. He was diagnosed at 4 years of age and currently attends 3rd grade. Jimmy's current medications include montelukast (Singulair) and albuterol (Proventil) inhaler as needed. He has a nebulizer machine at home but has not needed regular treatments for over a year. On entry to school the school nurse obtained an allergy and asthma assessment, and discovered Jimmy had made several trips to the emergency room when he was first diagnosed with asthma, but he has never been hospitalized overnight. His last trip to the ER was over 2 years ago. Jimmy's mother reports his asthma is often triggered by an infection, season changes, and exposure to cats and some cleaning supplies. Every 6 months he sees a pediatrician who specializes in the care of children with asthma. Jimmy has a peak flow meter at home but has not been using it recently. A Proventil inhaler has been prescribed prn and is available at school. Today Jimmy came to the office for his inhaler at 9:30AM. His complaint was of

continues

continued

some difficulty breathing. No audible wheeze was noted, but a faint expiratory wheeze was noted on auscultation. Other vital signs were within normal limits. He self-administered his inhaler, rested, improved, and returned to class.

At 10:25AM, Jimmy is brought to the office by his teacher. The class had been outside for recess when he came to the teacher complaining of difficulty breathing. He is sitting in a chair, leaning forward, slightly gray in color, and an audible wheeze is heard on expiration. His heart rate is 84 and the respiratory rate 28. No retractions are seen but Jimmy appears worried. He remains calm and is attempting to control his breathing. The nurse assists him in administering his inhaler while the secretary attempts to reach his parents. Within a few minutes after using his inhaler, Jimmy's wheeze is less audible, his face has relaxed, and his color has improved. The secretary has been unable to reach a parent. Jimmy is resting in the office. Within 10 minutes, he again begins having difficulty. Slowly the audible wheeze reappears and can be heard on both inspiration and expiration. His color again begins to take on a gray hue. The school nurse recognizes that Jimmy's condition is emergent, instructs the secretary to call for emergency services, and continues to monitor Jimmy's vital signs. Paramedics arrive as Jimmy shows signs of suprasternal retractions. They administer oxygen by mask and start a nebulizer treatment with albuterol. His oxygen saturation is 92%. Jimmy requires an additional nebulizer treatment as he is transported to the hospital. He is discharged later that night on antibiotics, prednisone, and nebulizer treatments every 6 hours.

Nursing Diagnosis #1

Ineffective breathing pattern related to inflammatory process.

Expected Outcome

Child's breathing will return to normal.

Interventions/*Rationales*

- Assess respiratory status, including rate, depth, use of accessory muscles, positioning, cough, mental status. *To determine severity of asthma attack.*
- Assist in positioning. *For optimal chest expansion and comfort of child.*
- Administer medication as prescribed. *Bronchodilators assist in opening airway to relieve dyspnea.*
- Contact EMT/paramedics as needed. *For unimproved or deteriorating status.*

Evaluation

Child's breathing pattern became more effective.

Nursing Diagnosis #2

Deficient knowledge about disease process and treatment.

Expected Outcome

Child/family will describe asthma signs and symptoms and treatment as related to his disease process.

Interventions/*Rationales*

- Assess child/family's understanding of asthma and treatment. *To determine further information needs.*
- Determine developmental level of child. *To present information at level the child can understand.*
- Provide clear simple information on the disease, signs and symptoms, and treatment. *Based on determined needs.*

continues

continued

Evaluation

Child/family knowledge increased, but they will need continued reinforcement.

Nursing Diagnosis #3

Fear/anxiety related to difficulty breathing.

Expected Outcome

Child has decreased anxiety.

Interventions/*Rationales*

- Provide care during acute attack in calm, reassuring manner. *Anxiety is communicated interpersonally.*
- Assess developmental level of child. *Signs of anxiety can be reflected differently in children of various ages.*
- Encourage child to verbalize feelings related to disease process. *Allows acknowledgment of feelings and promotes positive coping.*

Evaluation

Child/family fear and anxiety decreased.

Individualized Health Plan

When a child returns to school after having had a health problem, the school nurse must evaluate the incident and develop a plan for the child while at school. Since nurses are not always present when needed in an emergency, other school personnel may become responsible for administering first aid care and deciding when and if to transport a child to an acute care facility. Having a written plan available to assist in emergency situations can be invaluable. In the hospital, this is called the nursing care plan. In the school, this is known as the **Individual Health Plan (IHP).** An IHP is a document, based on the health assessment of a child, that outlines the special health needs, goals, and strategies necessary to improve/maintain the health of the child and allow full participation in school experiences. The IHP can consist of a brief health history, base-line assessment data, medications, nutritional considerations, specialized equipment, possible problems, and interventions, and an emergency plan individualized for each child with a health problem (Porter, et al., 1997). Box 5-5 provides an example of an Individualized Health Plan that could be used for Jimmy, the boy described in the case study.

Since plans can be developed for the student with any health problem, school personnel should be educated on the IHP and how it works. In fact, the best health plan is of little use if others responsible for first aid are unable to follow it. By taking the time early in the year to provide the staff with a list of students with special health needs and to familiarize them with emergency procedures, health care can be delivered to students quickly and competently, and problems avoided.

Injuries and Accidents

According to a report from the Children's Safety Network (U.S. Department of Health and Human Services, 1997), injuries are one of the most frequent conditions cared for by school health personnel, with falls being the most frequent cause of injury (43%). Sports activities cause 34% of school injuries. The school nurse can be instrumental in developing programs for students and staff related to injury prevention in the school. If a student or staff member needs to leave school because of an injury, it should be recorded on a standardized injury report form. These records can be important when examining data on injuries, looking for patterns, and developing plans to eliminate potential injuries. Curricula can include information on playground safety, the use of seat belts, school bus safety rules, bike helmet use (Figure 5-4), and injury prevention tips for sports activities. By becoming aware of legislation and policies on injury prevention within the school district and community, the nurse can help to decrease injuries and accidents.

BOX 5-5 Individual health plan

Student Information Jimmy Miller **DOB** 8/11/87

Grade 3 **Teacher** Miss Smith

Physical Education Schedule: Mondays 1:10 PM to 1:50 PM

Emergency Information

Parents' Names John and Nancy Miller

Telephone Numbers:

Home: 847-555-6943

Mother's work: 630-555-3456

Father's work: 847-555-9843

Physician's Name: Dr. R. Lung

Telephone: 847-555-8890

Current Medications:

At school: Proventil inhaler 2 puffs as needed every 4 hours for wheezing

At home: Singulair 1 tab q day

Proventil inhaler with spacer as needed every 4 hours

Proventil per nebulizer as needed for wheezing

Allergies: cats, ragweed, pollen, seasonal allergies

Brief History: diagnosed with asthma at age 4 years, no overnight hospitalizations, several ER trips for asthma attacks. Nebulizer at home, has not needed scheduled treatments for over a year, parents use for emergency or bas attacks. Last emergency room trip over $1^1/_2$ years ago. Peak flow meter at home, has not used for a while.

Known Asthma Triggers: cats, cleaning products, seasonal allergies, infections

Plan of Care

If having difficulties breathing measure peak flow:

Green zone: 300 and above – allow to rest

Yellow zone: 270 to 300

symptoms (wheezing, resp rate increased, shortness of breath)

_____ no–rest and retest peak flow in 5 minutes

_____ yes–administer medication Proventil inhaler 2 puffs reevaluate in 5 minutes:

improved?_____ yes–rest, return to class as allowed

_____ no

other symptoms?

_____ no–notify nurse/parent

_____ yes (difficulty breathing, chest tightness, wheezing, tripod positioning)–call Emergency Medical Service (EMS)

Red zone: 270 and under – Call nurse

Administer medication Proventil inhaler 2 puffs; allow to rest; reevaluate in 5 minutes:

Recheck peak flow

Improved? _____ yes

_____ no:

Symptoms? _____ no–rest

_____ yes–notify parents

Call EMS if continued difficulty breathing or talking, positioning, chest tightness, wheezing, pale, ashen or color change

To Activate EMS from School

Call: 911

My name is__________________. I am calling from (name of school).

A child is having an asthma attack.

(Give directions for which school entrance to use. Arrange for someone to meet EMS at door.)

EMS dispatch may ask if nurse is in building, if child has had medications, and symptoms.

Answer questions as possible, stay with the child.

Adapted from U.S. Department of Health and Human Services (1995). *Asthma and physical activity in the school*; and National Asthma Education Program (1991). *Managing asthma: A guide for schools.*

Source: National Heart, Lung, and Blood Institute.

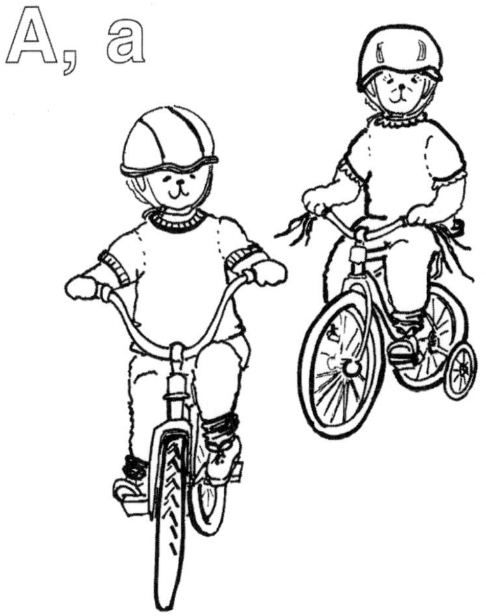

Figure 5-4 Coloring pages can be given to young children to reinforce safety concepts. Used with permission of the Brain Injury Association (BIA). For further information, contact BIA at www.biausa.org or at (703) 236-6000.

Medication Administration/Monitoring

Another important service the school nurse provides is the monitoring and administration of medication children receive while at school (Figure 5-5). Although most children will not need to take medication during school hours, there are circumstances when it is necessary, as with chronic illnesses such as seizure disorder, diabetes, attention deficit/hyperactivity disorder (ADHD), and asthma. The nurse is responsible for making sure that children who must receive medication at school have written orders from their physicians and written permissions from their caregivers to receive the medication at school. All medications should be stored in a locked cabinet, and if the principal or another designated staff member is to administer medications in the nurse's absence, the nurse should train these personnel and provide information on the medication itself and the five rights (right patient, right medication, right dose, right route, right time). All medication must be labeled by a pharmacy with the child's name, medication name, dose, and time to be administered.

Many children attending school are taking stimulant medications such as methylphenidate (Ritalin) or dextroamphetamine (Dexedrine) for attention deficit disorder/attention deficit hyperactivity disorder (ADD/ADHD). In fact, an estimated 3% to 5% of school-aged children have ADD/ADHD, with boys being affected almost six times as often as girls (Borowsky, 2000). The school nurse must be knowledgeable about the assessment procedures that accompany the evaluation of ADD/ADHD and the various medications prescribed for children with these conditions. Many medications are controlled substances (Ritalin, Dexedrine) and must be treated as such. However, medication is not the only treatment these children receive. Other measures include behavior modification, psychological counseling, and classroom intervention. By being knowledgeable about all medications and interventions, the school nurse can assist students, families, and teachers in delivering appropriate care. For more information on ADD/ADHD, refer to Chapter 33.

HEALTH EDUCATION AND PROMOTION

Health education and health promotion principles have existed for many years, but how they have been defined has

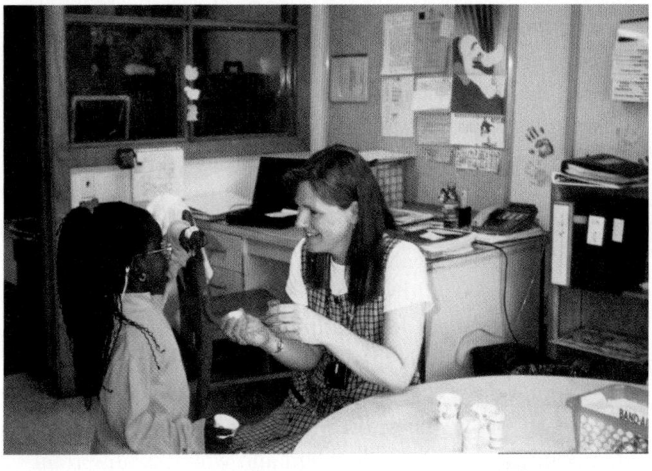

Figure 5-5 The school nurse often administers medications to children during school days.

Eye On:

The Use of Herbal Therapies

In schools across the United States, children with a variety of diagnosed conditions are receiving prescription medications at school. Caregivers who worry about their child receiving Ritalin or psychotropic drugs are exploring the possibility of alternative treatments such as herbal therapies. Most school districts still require caregiver and physician permission for the use of herbal therapies at school even if they can be purchased over the counter. For the safety of students, you must remain current on popular herbal preparations and their side effects and contraindications.

changed over time. For example, Green, Krueter, and Deeds (1980) described health education as a combination of learning experiences intended to help an individual change behaviors to be more favorable to health. The National Task Force on the Preparation and Practice of Health Educators (1983) described health education as assisting individuals to make informed decisions about matters affecting their personal health, which can include disease prevention, promoting optimal health, and illness treatment. Nolte (1994) defines health education as:

> A planned, sequential, K–12 curriculum that addresses the physical, mental, emotional, and social dimensions of health. The curriculum is designed to motivate and assist students to maintain and improve their health-related risk behaviors. It allows students to develop and demonstrate increasing sophisticated health-related knowledge, attitudes, skills, and practices. The curriculum is comprehensive and includes a variety of topics such as personal health, family health, community health, consumer health, environmental health, family life, mental and emotional health, injury prevention and safety, nutrition, prevention and control of disease, and substance use and abuse. Health education is taught by qualified personnel who have been trained to teach the subject (Nolte, 1994, p. 5152).

His definition is based on the Centers For Disease Control and the National Center for Chronic Disease Prevention and Health Promotion Division of Adolescent and School Health (CDC, 1991).

One of the *Healthy People 2010* goals is planned health education for grades kindergarten through 12 (U.S. Department of Health and Human Services, 2000). Studies have shown that health attitudes developed when young influence morbidity and mortality later in life (Kann et al., 1998; Vernon et al., 1997). In addition, increased knowledge about health-related topics can influence attitudes and behaviors in health. The certified school nurse, with her background in health and additional preparation in education, can present this information to students or act as a resource for teachers who are planning lessons in health-related topics.

A health education curriculum should include information about these five preventative behaviors that often cause intentional or unintentional injury and increased morbidity in children (Vernon et al., 1997): (1) tobacco use, (2) alcohol and drug use, (3) sexual behaviors that lead to sexually transmitted diseases and pregnancy, (4) unhealthy diet, and (5) physical inactivity. Other important topics include personal and dental hygiene, safety, first aid, anger management, and conflict resolution. Since not all topics are appropriate for children of all ages, it is important to be sure the information presented is age-appropriate. The most common topics school nurses are involved in are personal and dental hygiene, sex education, antismoking campaigns, alcohol and drug prevention, and violence prevention instruction.

Personal and Dental Hygiene

Personal and dental hygiene information can be easily adapted for preschool through elementary levels and is a nice way for the school nurse to introduce herself to younger children. Many large companies offer free videos, supplies, and educational materials to schools, which can be useful in presenting information. If the budget allows, there are also numerous books, tapes, and instructional materials that can be purchased from medical supply catalogs, book stores, and teacher centers.

One important personal hygiene topic to discuss is handwashing since it helps prevent the spread of infection. Instructions about handwashing can be presented by reading stories about cartoon germs, providing coloring books and activity sheets, viewing videotapes, using puppets, and making take-home charts. Presenting material in a variety of creative ways on how and when to wash one's hands and how germs are spread can hold young children's interest and make learning fun. For example, *Germs, Germs, Germs* by Katz (1996) is an excellent story about germs. Information on what germs are, how they get into one's body, how one can protect oneself from them, and the proper technique for washing hands should also be provided. The *Scrubby Bear Handwashing* program, developed by the American Red Cross, is an example of a creative multimedia method of instruction. A videotape with a friendly singing bear provides information to preschool and kindergarten children on handwashing. Colorful posters, a take-home handwashing chart, and a bear puppet reinforces learning.

Another favorite is the *Glo-germ* (1997) program. A nontoxic oil or powder, which is purchased from the Glo-Germ Company, is sprinkled on children's hands, after which anywhere the child touches will light up when you shine a black light on the area. For example, children who have put their fingers in their mouth will have a glow around their lips, and table tops will show glowing fingerprints. The students can then wash their hands with soap and water and see if all the "germs" have disappeared. Whatever program is chosen, physically involving the child in the learning increases understanding.

Dental hygiene is another topic the school nurse can discuss with young children, since dental disease remains a major health problem for children and tooth decay is one of the most preventable diseases in our society (Peterson, Niessen, & Lopez, 1999). Education on the correct way to brush teeth should begin in preschool, and as children get older, education can include when and why it is important to brush, how to floss, the importance of proper nutrition for dental health, and visiting a dentist. School nurses can request free dental education material from toothpaste companies and local dentists' offices. Children's books telling stories of favorite characters visiting the dentist are available in bookstores and libraries. A favorite method of teaching dental hygiene to young children is to use a giant set of teeth and a big toothbrush for demonstration or practice (Figure 5-6).

A take-home chart showing how often the child has brushed provides reinforcement and gets the family involved. Another method is to let the children show what they have learned by writing a story or drawing a picture (Figure 5-7). Hanging these pictures on the bulletin board is a great way to celebrate Dental Health month during February.

REFLECTIONS FROM FAMILIES

I have two children, Luke is in 2nd grade and Sarah is in 4th. It's a daily battle to get them to brush their teeth before they leave for school. One day, Luke came home with a new toothbrush. Not only does he brush his teeth twice a day but he's been correcting Sarah's brushing techniques. He told me his school nurse came in the classroom with a set of really big teeth and showed him "the right way to brush his teeth." He even asked to bring his toothbrush to school.

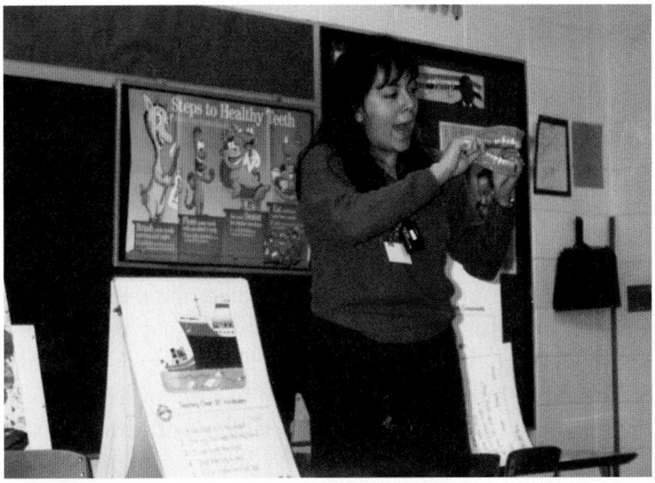

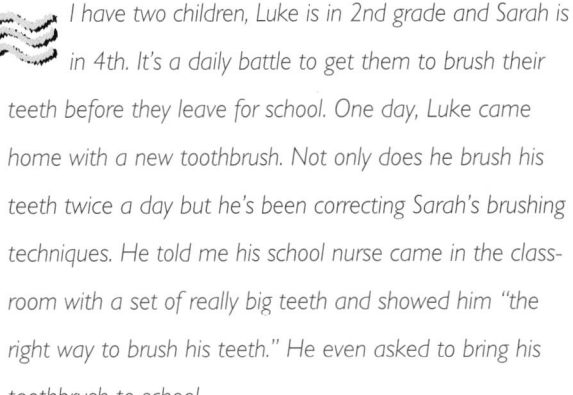

Figure 5-6 School nurses provide health education classes for students. Here, how to properly brush your teeth is being demonstrated.

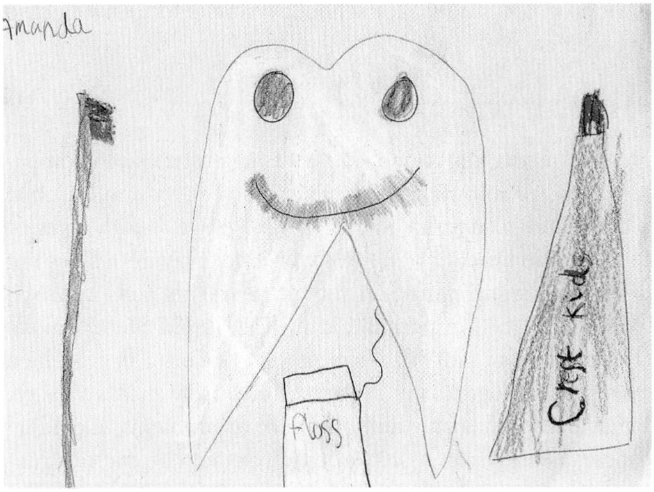

Figure 5-7 Children's Drawing after Dental Health Education Class

As children progress through elementary school, they grow physically, emotionally, socially, and cognitively (Muscari, Phillips, & Bears, 1997). Topics in health education must grow with them. Personal attitudes and behaviors related to diet, safety, sex, and alcohol or drug use often develop during this period. As children reach the intermediate grades (4th, 5th, and 6th), health education can focus on these health habits and their short- and long-term implications. Personal hygiene and programs that enhance self-esteem provide a good beginning for health education before discussing more serious topics such as sexually transmitted diseases and teen pregnancy.

Sex Education

As children reach preadolescence, the school nurse is often asked by teachers or the parent–teacher organization to provide classroom materials or instruction on human growth and development and sex education. Finding materials and resources that are developmentally appropriate for this group of students is important. Since 9% of students under 13 years of age have already experienced sexual intercourse, providing accurate information on this topic needs to be addressed at an early age. By the 9th grade, approximately 40% of boys and 31% of girls have had intercourse, and by 17 years of age, 50% of both boys and girls have had intercourse (Allensworth, 1994; Robinson, Price, Thompson, & Schmalzried, 1998). Two of the more serious implications of teenage sex are sexually transmitted diseases (STDs) and teenage pregnancy. The school nurse can be helpful in planning preventive programs and teaching these topics to students. In the past, having an STD meant living with the physical complications and psychological stigma of diseases such as herpes or gonorrhea. Today, the outcome can be far more serious.

When preparing sex education curricula, the primary goal is to increase knowledge and encourage the student to make positive health choices. Programs designed to increase knowledge alone are not enough. Students also need instruction on values, decision making, and communication skills; risk reduction programs should also be considered (Hubbard, Geise, & Rainey, 1998). Since sexuality is influenced by cultural, societal, physiologic, and psychological factors, all must be considered when planning a sex education program. Finding creative ways to reinforce material or opportunities for application of knowledge can foster healthy lifestyle choices. See Chapter 12 for more information on adolescent sexuality.

Sex education regarding STDs needs to be focused on several areas. Teens need information on how STDs are spread, precautions they can take, and treatments for the various diseases. Box 5-6 provides a quick HIV/AIDS fact sheet that can be used as an ice breaker for opening discussions with students.

Decision-making skills also need to be discussed and cultural and social values explored. Remembering the developmental level of the students is important. Many teens feel nothing bad can happen to them; bad things happen only to other people. Students need to know that if they are participating in unprotected sex, they may contract an STD; although abstinence can be encouraged, education aimed only at this option is less effective (Lindley, Reininger, Vincent, Richter, Saunders, & Shi, 1998; Swartwout & Russell, 1999).

BOX 5-6 HIV/AIDS: Did you know?

- Every state and most cities have reported cases with HIV. It's not just in a few places in the United States.
- In the United States, deaths from HIV/AIDS have increased in young adults.
- You do not have to have AIDS if you are HIV-positive, but you can still spread HIV to others.
- In day-to-day contact, people with AIDS are more likely to pick up an infection from you, than you are to get AIDS from them. However, sexual intercourse with a person with HIV/AIDS does put you at risk for contracting HIV/AIDS.
- A negative serum test does not guarantee you do not have HIV. It can take 6 weeks to several months before antibodies are detected, and during that time a person can pass HIV to others.
- To date there is no cure for AIDS–only treatments that slow the progression in people infected with HIV.

Adapted from Minor, K. (1994). Educating about HIV/AIDS. In P. Cortese & K. Middleton (Eds.), *The comprehensive school health challenge.* Santa Cruz, CA: ETR.

Sex education would not be complete without providing information on preventing pregnancy. However, there is controversy regarding teaching the use of contraception, so before developing or implementing an education program, the nurse must be familiar with the policies of the school district and the values of the community. Negative attitudes can be a barrier to sex education, so being aware of these attitudes and providing instruction with a nonjudgmental attitude are critical. Discussing sensitive information in an open, relaxed manner and letting students know the hours the school nurse is available is helpful. Helping students share personal information regarding sexual practices or possible pregnancies is challenging, and client confidentiality is of utmost importance. A student coming for help needs to know the school nurse is able and willing to help without notifying guardians. This presents a moral dilemma for some nurses. Answering questions and referring the student to appropriate resources is the key. For more information on confidentiality and ethics, see Chapter 2.

The nurse must also be prepared to assist a pregnant teen who remains in school until her baby is delivered. The nurse can provide instruction in prenatal care and assist in securing community medical services. It is not uncommon for the school nurse to be the first contact the teen has with a health professional, and in some cases it may be the only health care she receives. The nurse can develop and provide classes for a student so she can learn to care for herself during pregnancy as well as instruct her on infant care and parenting skills. The nurse can also be instrumental in helping the pregnant student to stay in school and obtain community resources after giving birth. Finally, the nurse must be prepared if students go into labor at school. Any school where a pregnant student is enrolled should have an emergency delivery kit available. An IHP should also be developed for each pregnant student for school personnel to follow in case of emergency.

Antismoking Education

Despite media attention on lawsuits against tobacco companies, laws prohibiting smoking in many private and public places, and research showing the negative health risks of tobacco, the number of people who smoke cigarettes has not decreased significantly in recent years. In fact, approximately 25% of the population in the United States smoke (Robinson et al., 1998). Nicotine is a powerful drug, which causes physiologic dependence and adversely affects all ages. It has been linked to multiple medical problems, including cancer, heart disease, stroke, emphysema, chronic obstructive pulmonary disease, infertility, low-birth-weight infants, and drug interactions (Matza & Loya, 1994). Because of its high addiction potential, tobacco has been called a "gateway" drug; it is associated with experimentation and the use of alcohol and illegal substances (Matza & Loya, 1994; VanAntwerp, 1995). Research shows that 90% of current tobacco users started smoking in their teens (Office of Smoking & Health, 1996; Perry-Casler, Price, Telljohan, & Chesney, 1997; VanAntwerp, 1995); over 2 million adolescents are regular smokers (Perry-Casler et al., 1997). Therefore, health education programs in school regarding tobacco misuse is important, and it needs to be taught before adolescents start smoking because every day 3,000 children try smoking their first cigarette (Denehy, 1999; Hahn, Hall, Rayens, Burt, Corley, & Sheffel, 2000). To be effective, antismoking education must begin before children form habits and are swayed by peers. Many education programs are targeted for the middle- or high-school level, with more recent programs developed for fourth through sixth grades. Antismoking education, however, needs to be incorporated into health promotion and wellness education beginning in kindergarten and continuing through high school. Education regarding smoking should include the short- and long-term effects of tobacco, the social implications of smoking, and how tobacco industries glorify smoking in advertisements. Decision-making skills and peer-relation workshops can be helpful, as well as information on the use of smokeless tobacco, which has recently increased in prevalence among adolescents (Price, Beach, Everett, Telljohan, & Lewis 1998).

For teaching to be effective, it cannot be simply lecturing on the risks of smoking. It must be interactive, with the teacher facilitating small student-led discussion groups. Peer teaching with older teens grouped with younger teens is recommended (Robinson et al., 1998). Material should be current and presented annually. Antismoking groups such as "Doctors Ought to Care" (DOC) or the American Lung Association can serve as valuable resources. DOC, founded by a group of physicians, focuses its education efforts on the effects of smoking and calls attention to strategies the tobacco industry uses in advertising cigarettes (Mahoney, Costley, Cain, Zaiger, & McMullen, 1998).

TAR WARS, developed by DOC, is one antitobacco program designed for 5th grade students. Its goal is to discourage tobacco use in school-aged children by increasing their awareness about attitudes and the effects of tobacco. The program itself is divided into three sections, each with objectives and activities. Key activities, such as examining magazine ads and running in place while breathing through a straw, are designed to physically involve and mentally motivate the student. Involvement in the community is encouraged; the American Academy of Family Physicians sponsors a national poster contest every June (Figure 5-8). The free curriculum can be requested by educators and school nurses (Mahoney et al., 1998).

Providing education is not enough. To see a significant decrease in the number of people who smoke, additional support is necessary. Teachers need to be trained if they also provide antismoking instruction and follow-up to ongoing programs. Cessation programs need to be developed for students and staff who need help quitting. Local school policies regarding smoking must be in place and enforced. Ways to involve the family and the community need to be explored. Despite laws prohibiting the sale of cigarettes to minors, adolescents have little difficulty purchasing them. Making cigarettes less easy to obtain by enforcing these laws can help. The school nurse can become involved with organizations such as the American Cancer Society or DOC and help promote antitobacco education at the state and local level, while always evaluating existing programs and looking for ways to improve or expand antismoking education.

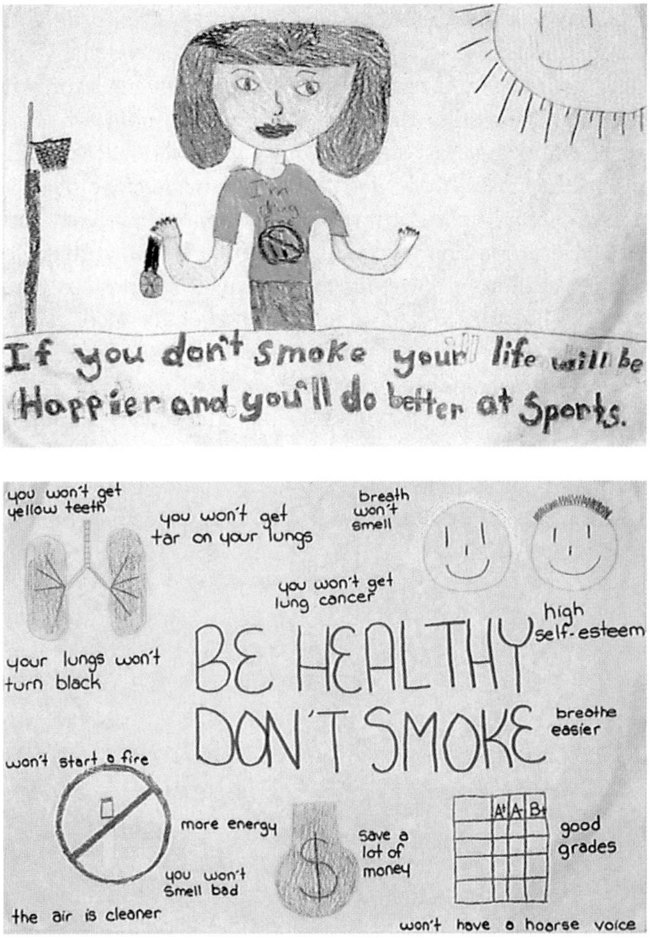

Figure 5-8 Reasons not to smoke are shown in drawings by students after TAR WARS presentation.

Alcohol and Drug Abuse Prevention

From smoking cigarettes, adolescents may progress to risk-taking behaviors such as alcohol use, drug use (Copeland, Shope, & Waller, 1996; Lowry, Holtzman, Truman, Kann,

Collins, & Kolbe, 1994), and/or inhaling aerosol products. Kandal and Logan's (1984) 20-year study on the stages of drug use suggested that tobacco use is one of the strongest predictors for other drug use. Pesa (1998) indicates cigarette smoking has been found to coexist with other unhealthy lifestyle behaviors. It must be made clear that *use* and *abuse* are different terms, but both are a problem and can have serious long-term effects. Research shows that the earlier adolescents regularly use illegal substances, the greater the risk for later abuse and addiction. Alcohol use and drug use have been associated with truancy, poor academic performance, higher dropout rates, and low self-esteem (Treiman & Beck, 1996). One 8th-grade student out of every six is reported to have consumed over five drinks in a row (Wynn, Schulenberg, Kloska, & Laetz, 1997). Forty-seven percent of youths reported having tried marijuana, 8.2% had tried cocaine, and 16% had used inhalants (Kann et al., 1998).

Although risk-taking and experimentation are considered a normal part of the developmental stage adolescents go through on their way to independence, the long-term effects of experiences that lead to the regular use or abuse of alcohol and drugs can be serious. The best way to educate youths on the dangers of alcohol and drug use has been debated over the years. Curricula that present drug information, how to resist peer pressure, and social and communication skills have been incorporated into various programs. The goal of these programs is the prevention of drug and alcohol use. However, the reality of achieving that goal has been questioned.

Research on how prevention programs influence adolescent behavior is not abundant, and studies showing specific

Research Highlight

The Mediating Influence of Refusal Skills in Preventing Adolescent Alcohol Misuse

Study Purpose

Alcohol is the most frequently used substance in the adolescent population. Misuse puts this group at risk for serious social and psychological consequences. Several approaches to alcohol prevention education have been implemented, including teaching refusal skills, but evaluation of the programs is lacking. This study investigates the relation of teaching refusal skills to alcohol use.

Methods

Data were collected from 3,704 6th grade students in a Midwestern state. Random selection for refusal-skill intervention was done, and self-reports of drinking behaviors were obtained over several grade levels.

Findings

The refusal-skill curriculum showed a significant positive effect in lowered alcohol use in students.

Implications

Teaching refusal skills to these 6th grade children showed positive results; self-reported alcohol use was lower in the group that received instruction. Although 6th grade may be considered young for teaching about alcohol use, this is a time when lifestyle decisions are being made and peer influence occurs. The school nurse can assist teachers in planning and implementing these programs and continually evaluating and following up their effectiveness.

Citation

Wynn, S., Schulenberg, J., Kloska, D., & Laetz, V. (1997). The mediating influence of refusal skills in preventing adolescent alcohol misuse. *Journal of School Health, 67*(9), 390–395.

program effects may not be true across different groups of teens. When a teen makes the decision whether or not to try alcohol or drugs, multiple variables such as parental attitudes, support, and use; school policies and how they are enforced; geographic location; socioeconomic issues; and even friends or associates of the child come into play. The particular prevention program attended is also important.

When planning or being part of a drug/alcohol prevention program the school nurse needs to consider the developmental level of the students being instructed, local district policy, and the community where the school is located. Knowledge of illegal drugs, how they are used, and their effects is important. A chart showing some of the various categories of drugs, symptoms of use, and how they are taken is provided in Table 5-2.

The U.S. Department of Education has developed grade-specific curricula for drug prevention education that provide a sound framework for the nurse to use or expand on when developing a more individualized program for particular students. It, along with a multitude of resources and information, is available free of charge from the National Clearinghouse for Drug and Alcohol Information. Many state and local governments have also developed educational programs and activities, and coordinating the school program with these community resources is ideal. No single program has proven superior in all groups of children, but interactive, peer-led, small-group instruction appear to be better accepted by students (Black, Tobbler, & Sciacca, 1998). Like antismoking education, other skills that improve self-esteem and communication and increase knowledge are the focus.

TABLE 5-2 Frequently Abused Drugs

Drug	Symptoms of Use	Route	Medical Use
Narcotics (heroin, morphine, codeine, meperidine [Demerol], oxycodone/aspirin [Percodan], methadone)	Lethargy, drowsiness, euphoria, nausea, constricted pupils	oral, injected	Pain medication (except heroin and methadone)
Hallucinogens (LSD, PCP, DMT, MDA)	Trancelike, euphoria, excitation, insomnia, increased heart rate, hallucinations, altered perceptions	Oral, smoked, injected	None
Depressants (tranquilizers, diazepam [valium], choral hydrate, barbiturates)	Slurred speech, uncoordinated movements, drowsiness, disorientation	Oral, injected	Anesthetic, sedative, antianxiety
Stimulants (cocaine, amphetamines, methylphenidate [Ritalin])	Restlessness, talkative, excitation, euphoria, exaggerated reflexes, dilated pupils	Sniffed, injected, smoked, oral	Local anesthetic, weight control, ADD/ADHD
Cannabis (marijuana, hashish)	Euphoria, increased appetite, relaxed inhibitions	Smoked, oral	None

Adapted from Drug Enforcement Administration (1996). Drugs of abuse; *and U.S. Department of Health and Human Services (1997).* Keeping youth drug free.

The use of inhalants among children and teens has been an increasing concern for school nurses. More than 1,400 aerosol products such as cleaners, solvents, adhesives, hair spray, or even whipped cream are being misused by students to get a high (Cook, 1999). In fact, because they are legal to purchase, they have become more popular with younger students than marijuana, with one in five students below 8th grade having tried inhalants (Cook, 1999; Harrison, 1999). Parents are often unaware of how these products are being misused, and children can be unaware of the dangers. "Sniffing" or "huffing" these products to get high is dangerous, as the chemicals dissolve the protective myelin around brain cells. This can result in personality changes, mental impairment, hallucinations, learning disabilities, or damage to vital organs and even death due to a sudden disturbance in the heart rhythm (Cook, 1999; Harrison, 1999). School nurses need to be aware of the signs of inhalant use and be prepared to act in an emergency. When planning any drug prevention program, the dangers of inhalants must be included.

Statistics can be startling when the percentages of youths who use alcohol or take drugs are laid out in black and white. Alcohol and drug use in teens is not just a school problem but a problem that has an ongoing impact on society. Experimentation with these substances is starting at a younger age than any parent, educator, or health professional wants to believe. Providing children with the skills to make healthy choices and the ability to resist pressures must begin early. The school is the logical place for learning and practicing these skills. The nurse can be a resource, instructor, or coordinator for these programs and assist schools in meeting this important need. (See Chapter 12 for additional information on this topic.)

Violence Prevention

(For additional information on violence, refer to Chapter 12.) The United States has more violent crimes than any other industrial nation (Dusenbury, Falco, Lake, Brannigan, & Bosworth, 1997; Fry-Bowers, 1997). In Chicago 75% of 10- to 19-year-olds had witnessed a shooting, stabbing, robbery or killing, and in Washington, DC, 61% of first- and second-graders had witnessed a violent crime (Fry-Bowers, 1997). However, violence is not seen only in inner-city schools, it is also seen nationwide in suburban schools.

Newspaper headlines across the United States shock us with reports of school violence. Americans have read about children not only bringing guns to school but opening fire on classmates and staff. In 1998, we read about a student in Pennsylvania shooting a teacher, two Arkansas boys killing four girls and a teacher, a 15-year-old Oregon student opening fire in a cafeteria, killing 2 and wounding 22 students, and an Illinois student gunned down at an alternative school by a rival gang member; in 1999, we read about two Colorado students killing 15 and injuring many more in a shooting rampage that involved guns and explosives (National Education Association, 1999). These are the extremes of violence in the school. But violence also includes bullying and intimidation, which have been around for a long time and are not confined to school property.

Long-term exposure to violence affects the cognitive, psychological, and moral development of children. Some researchers believe children who have experienced violence are prone to difficulties in concentrating, mental impairment, uncaring behavior, powerlessness, aggressive play, and lasting symptoms of stress (Fry-Bowers, 1997). Media attention focuses on violence at school, but children experience violence at home and in the community as well.

There are many types of violence prevention programs. Some are designed for specific grade levels; others provide instruction for grades kindergarten through 12 (Haynie, Alexander, & Russell-Walter, 1997). Only recently has research begun evaluating the effectiveness of these programs. For violence prevention programs to be effective, they must be matched to the developmental level of the child. Although violence prevention needs to begin in the early grades, teaching strategies and interventions that work in primary grades do not necessarily meet the needs of middle- or high-school students. Teaching needs to be interactive, allowing group work, role playing, and practice time for skills across multiple environments. Curricula that provide information alone or aim solely at enhancing self-esteem have not been very effective. Rather, instruction combining information on the negative consequences of violence, anger-management skills, decision making, development of prosocial skills, communication, and resisting peer pressure has had greater success (Dusenbury, et al., 1997).

Training of school staff is crucial to the success of any prevention program. Teachers and nurses may be uncomfortable with the topic, but they need to learn how to help students handle violence. The school must make violence prevention a priority. Education provided by a handful of teachers is less effective than education in a school system where the program starts early and builds through the grade levels. Having strategies available in class and during less structured times and having teachers and staff as role models is more effective. Developing a curriculum with culture and ethnic sensitivity is important but difficult to implement in schools with an interracial mix of students; it is better to stress that every child deserves courtesy and respect no matter their background. Lastly, schools must develop set rules and policies on how violence will be dealt with on school grounds. Schools with less formal policies and wavering guidelines of what is tolerated have increased violence as compared with schools where known consequences are established (Dusenbury, et al., 1997).

Second Step, a successful violence prevention education program used in many schools, is an integrated program with specific curricula for grade levels kindergarten through third, fourth and fifth, and sixth through eighth grades. The goal of Second Step is to assist children in becoming independent problem solvers, targeting skill deficits that put kids at risk for violence. Three main components are covered: empathy training, impulse control, and anger management (Committee for Children, 1992). The empathy training unit focuses on identifying feelings of others through verbal, physical, and situational clues. It assists the child to realize people may have conflicting feelings and perceptions at different times and in different situations. In the impulse control unit, the goal is to decrease aggressive and impulsive behavior by practicing problem solving strategies. The key points discussed are how to identify the problem, choose a solution, and evaluate the consequences before acting. Friendship skills, conversation and social skills, and taking responsibility for oneself are also included in this unit. The last unit, anger management, focuses on how to recognize triggers and angry feelings, what to do with put-downs and criticism, and assertiveness training.

The classroom teacher should be the primary presenter of this information, with other school personnel (social worker, school nurse) playing a supporting role. To be most effective, the curriculum is designed in sequenced lessons, each building on the previous section, and used throughout the entire school. Large lesson cards are designed with a photograph of children on one side and a story on the reverse. Questions and key points are provided for discussion and role playing. Follow-up activities and suggestions on applying the skills in real-life situations are included. Optimally, lessons take 30 to 45 minutes, with two lessons presented per week; however, the schedule can be tailored to classroom needs. The Second Step kit provides a teacher's guide, lesson plans (cards), classroom posters for reinforcement, parent letters, and additional resources.

PSYCHOLOGICAL SERVICES

School psychological services focus on issues such as child abuse, crisis intervention, and disaster preparedness. Child abuse includes physical, sexual, and emotional abuse, and emotional or physical neglect. The school nurse's main focus in child abuse or neglect issues is awareness. It is necessary to recognize the signs of abuse and report them to the appropriate authorities. Documenting assessment and history, if abuse is suspected, is extremely important since health records from the school can be admissible in court. Before taking photographs of the child to document observable signs of abuse, it is important to check with local and state laws. A report from a child indicating abuse must be documented in the child's exact words. The nurse can also be instrumental in prevention activities by either teaching or referring parents to local resources for improving parenting practices. For more information about child abuse and neglect see Chapter 36 and contact the National Committee to Prevent Child Abuse at 1-800-CHILDREN or the National Clearinghouse on Child Abuse at 1-800-FYI-3366.

Disaster Preparedness in the School

As the only health professional on staff, the school nurse must be ready in case a crisis or traumatic event occurs. Traumatic events include natural disasters such as fires, tornadoes, hurricanes, and earthquakes, and acts of violence such as riots or random shootings similar to those reported in the media. In any of these situations, the nurse's role involves planning, training, and resources for referral. Every school should have an emergency plan for natural and human-made disasters that has been practiced so it can quickly and efficiently be put into action. The school nurse can be part of the team that develops, practices, and evaluates these plans and must also be prepared to handle all possible emergency situations. This requires training in emergency procedures and knowing triage and methods of handling mass trauma since school personnel may expect the nurse to direct and lead them in such situations.

Finally, the school nurse can be an excellent resource for staff, parents, and students when handling the aftermath of disasters since children and adults may be affected after the actual crisis has passed. They may have seen a classmate severely injured or killed, have been injured themselves and unable to attend a friend's funeral, or simply not know what to do with the feelings they are experiencing when a friend commits suicide. Working closely with crisis counselors and social workers, the nurse can assist students and staff through this difficult period or provide referrals as appropriate.

However, psychological services do not have to be related to a crisis event that the whole school experiences. The school nurse may be needed to provide psychological services to students experiencing emotional stress due to a family situation such as separation, divorce, or death. Other students may be diagnosed with depression. The nurse may also learn about individual situations through a concerned teacher. In all these situations the nurse's focus should be on identifying signs of

Reflective Thinking

After a Crisis

A child from the school where you work was reported missing several days ago. Her body was recently found. As the school nurse and a member of the community, how do you help deal with this loss in the school, the fear of parents and staff, and your own fears?

REFLECTIONS FROM A TEACHER

Jim is on multiple medications at home and at school. I know he has ADHD and sees a psychiatrist. Recently, I heard that he has been diagnosed with depression. Sometimes around 10 AM he just gets too antsy sitting in the classroom. I know he has established a relationship with our school nurse. When his frustration level is about ready to top off, he asks to go to see her for an illness of some sort. I know he is not sick, but I allow him to go. The school nurse told me he comes in and just sits and talks about home, class, TV, whatever he wants, and she just sits and listens. Within 5 or 10 minutes, he's ready to come back to class. The simple act of walking to the nurse's office and expressing his frustrations or thoughts to someone he believes cares about him calms him down. He's more productive in his schoolwork when he returns.

stress in the child and working closely with the child, teacher, and social worker to provide support. If the child is under the care of a physician or psychiatrist, the nurse's role is to act as a liaison between the school and other health professionals and to monitor the administration and effects of prescribed medication. Of course, referral to appropriate community agencies is always part of the nurse's job.

SCHOOL HEALTH SERVICES MODEL

Schools are changing quickly, and the one-room schoolhouse is long gone. Today's Americans expect schools to provide more than just basic education; they expect services such as nursing care, social work referral, speech and language programs, special education classes, occupational and physical therapy, counseling, early childhood interventions, and transition services. The services provided by school nurses are being expanded as well, and two models of expansion are **school-based health clinics (SBHCs)** and **school-linked health clinics (SLHCs)**. SBHCs are health centers set up and staffed by health care professionals other than the school nurse but are within a school building (Figure 5-9). SLHCs are also staffed by separate health care professionals and centrally located, sometimes within a school, but serve several schools and service students and other family members. The goal of both is to provide a level of extended health services to children. In addition, access to services is needed for the underserved and unserved children in America. These clinics can help provide care by eliminating barriers to health care, such as lack of transportation or inability of the parent to take time off from work. SBHCs and SLHCs are funded from various sources, including local hospitals, community groups, health departments, and in some cases school district funds. Funding is complicated because money comes from multiple sources and the cash flow is not necessarily consistent.

The first SBHCs started in the 1960s in Texas and Massachusetts (Barnett, Niebuhr, & Baldwin, 1998). By 1990 there were approximately 150 clinics in schools. By 1997, that number increased to over 900, and currently there are more than 1,200 SBHCs nationwide (Dryfoos, 1998). Although SBHCs and SLHCs have a similar goal (increased accessibility of health care to children), they are different in how they provide services. Ninety percent of SBHCs are offered in the actual school building to ensure that school-aged children have access to health care (Yates, 1994). SLHCs on the other hand, are a collaborative effort among schools, local health professionals, and social service agencies providing services to children and their families. SBHCs usually serve children only at the school where they are located, but some SBHCs are shared by a selected group of schools. SLHCs, on the other hand, are usually located outside the school building, and provide services to schools of several areas and the youths who have been suspended from them or who have dropped out. Being located outside the school building also allows the SLHCs to have hours that extend beyond traditional school hours and continue throughout the summer, when many SBHCs are closed. SLHCs are often managed by someone outside the school district and may have more flexibility in the services provided. Because many SBHCs are managed by the district they are often unable to provide reproductive health care, sexually transmitted disease management, or contraception, which can be provided by SLHCs (Yates, 1994).

Physicians and nurse practitioners at SBHCs and SLHCs have the ability to diagnose health conditions of children and adolescents. Common childhood diseases such as otitis media, strep throat, and undiagnosed rashes can be treated easily. Antibiotics can be prescribed and follow-up provided without the child missing another day of school. Staff at both SBHCs and SLHCs are trained in growth and development and the physical and emotional needs of children. Social workers and mental health counselors may be on site depending on the community's needs. The school nurse may act as the triage nurse for both health centers and can continue to be the liaison between the school and the family. Some SBHCs and SLHCs have the ability to provide adolescents with reproductive health services such as routine gynecologic exams, pap smears, contraceptives, diagnosis

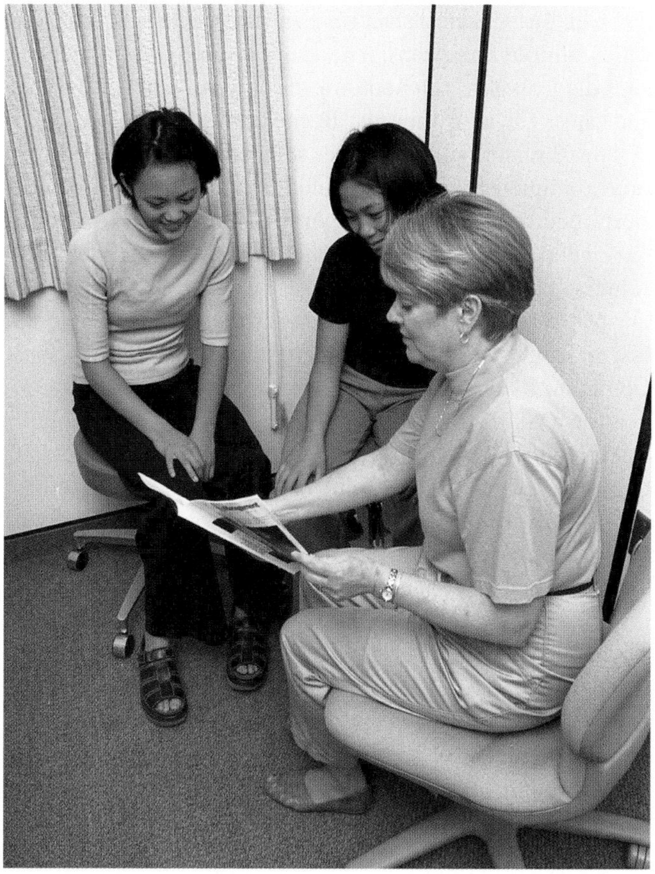

Figure 5-9 Nurse practitioners often staff the SBHC, where they provide information to teens on sex education.

and treatment of sexually transmitted diseases, and pregnancy tests, referral, and counseling; however, 71% of SBHCs do not provide any form of contraceptive services (Swartwout & Russell, 1999). SLHCs are more likely to provide these types of services (Yates, 1994) because they are often off-site and managed by personnel separate from the school. Controversy exists in many communities, however, about whether these services should be provided.

Some school nurses are concerned about SBHCs and SLHCs entering their district. Most school nurses agree that children with health care needs not met at other facilities need services, but they feel threatened by a clinic based at their schools. However, once they gain information on how SBHCs and SLHCs are used, fears often subside. Since school nurses are used to working independently, clear guidelines stating roles and responsibilities of both the school nurse and the clinic nurse or nurse practitioner are helpful. If boundaries are unclear, a strain in the professional relationships between school and clinic nurses can develop, leading to internal conflict. (Hacker & Wessel, 1998). In most cases where SBHCs/SLHCs are used, the school nurse provides basic first aid for student/staff illnesses and injuries and refers children needing more advanced care to the clinic. The nurse also acts as a liaison between clinic, families, and community resources and provides the link between health care and education as the child progresses through the school years. With training, professional courtesy, shared ownership, mutual respect, and creative compromise, SBHCs and SLHCs can provide children what they need: quality heath care that is accessible and affordable.

SCHOOL NURSING TODAY

Multidisciplinary Teams

Besides giving first aid care, overseeing various screening services, and health promotion education, the school nurse plays an important role as part of a multidisciplinary team assessing and evaluating children for special education services. The **pupil personnel team,** or **service team,** is a team of professionals who work together with teachers to provide interventions for students having difficulties. The team may consist of the principal, social worker, school psychologist, speech therapist, regular education teacher, special education teacher, special education supervisor, and school nurse. Other specialists participate as appropriate. If a teacher feels a student is having trouble learning or concentrating or is displaying other difficulties, the situation may be informally discussed with colleagues in searching for different approaches. If these approaches do not work, the teacher asks the caregiver or guardian for permission to discuss the child with the team. The teacher then shares with the team the concerns and what has been used in the past. The team brainstorms, offering additional information they may have about the student. Interventions are suggested and a date is set for the team to reconvene to determine if progress has been made. Before the team reconvenes, members may observe the child in various class situations, provide screenings, and gather more information. When the team meets again, they determine whether the problem has been resolved. If the problem has been resolved, the teacher continues to monitor the child as needed. If difficulties are still present, special testing, often called a full case study, is needed. Permission from the child's guardian is necessary for this extensive evaluation, and specific guidelines for testing must be followed.

Once permission is obtained, each team member has specific assessments or tests to perform, including IQ tests, processing tests, speech and language screenings or evaluations, adaptive skills and social developmental histories, and an in-depth health history. This health history can include information on prenatal complications, developmental milestones, past hospitalizations, past and current medical conditions, allergies, medications, and information on diet, sleep, fine and gross motor skills, and activities of daily living. A recent vision and hearing screening must be on file or be completed before other testing is begun. The idea is to rule out health-related issues that adversely affect the child's ability to learn. In addition, screening tools for ADHD may be included if that is a concern. The school nurse can obtain written permission for the release of records from physicians' offices or medical testing if appropriate and can often provide additional information if the child has a diagnosed medical condition.

On completion of testing, the team sets up a meeting with the child's caregivers. All results are presented and explained, and eligibility for special education is determined using federal, state, and district guidelines. If the child needs special services an **Individualized Educational Plan (IEP),** a written plan spelling out the type and amount of services needed for that particular child, is developed.

Children with Unique Health Problems

For some school nurses, an increasing amount of the day is committed to the specialized care of students with unique health needs. Public schools are now providing education to children with complex medical diagnoses who a decade ago would not have lived or been able to attend their neighborhood school. In 1984, the U.S. Supreme Court ruled in favor of an 8-year-old girl, named Amber Tatro, who had spina bifida. The court ruling stated that the Irving Independent School District had to provide supportive services to Amber so she could attend school, including providing nursing services in the form of clean intermittent catheterization (CIC). Even though the school district argued that CIC was a medical service and too expensive to be provided at school (Vitello, 1988), Amber won the case. Other cases followed, but children who needed more extensive care were denied admission to school. In 1987, a Pennsylvania court ruled in favor of the school district in the case of a 7-year-old boy with multiple handicaps. The boy required extensive care, including oxygen, tracheotomy care, gastrostomy feedings, and chest physical therapy. Because a mucous plug could clog his breathing at any time, someone was needed at his side continuously. The court ruled that, in this case, services were medically extensive, expensive, and beyond the ordinary related services of a school nurse (Vitello, 1988). Admission to school was denied.

More recently, however, things have changed. In 1999, Garret Frey won his case against the Cedar Rapids Iowa Community School District. Garret is a teen who is dependent on a ventilator and who has a tracheotomy and requires gastrostomy feeding, tracheal suctioning, and catheterization. The U.S. Supreme Court ruled that the school district had to provide nursing services to carry out Garret's extensive daily care. Without nursing care, he would be unable to attend school (Greenburg, 1999).

This case has an impact on children with disabilities across the nation, because ruling in Garret's favor could force school districts to expand their definition of related services and pay for nursing care for children with extensive health needs. With advances in technology and medical breakthroughs, premature babies are surviving at younger and younger gestational ages. Previously fatal childhood illnesses are controlled with extensive treatments and medications, and children who survived major traumas and head injuries are receiving rehabilitation services and recovering to their fullest potential. These children are entering or returning to school, and school nurses are extremely important in supporting their education. In fact, many would not be able to attend school without the services of a nurse. All of these children may not have health needs as complex as Garret's, but their cases are no less important. School nurses will need to organize their day so they are available to provide services like CIC or gastrostomy feedings. These additional responsibilities may mean traveling to several buildings in one day and keeping up to date with advances in direct services.

With this increase in children with special needs, some school districts are also looking for new ways to provide these services (Brandt, 1999). Either because there are not enough school nurses employed or the school's financial situation does not allow employing more nurses, some districts are training **unlicenced assistive personnel (UAP)** to perform direct services, such as first aid, medication administration, tube feedings, and catheterizations. UAPs are individuals trained to work in an assistive role to the licensed registered nurse to provide patient care as directed by and under the supervision of the nurse (Luckenbill, 1996). The legal definition of *delegation* is the "transferring to a competent individual the authority to perform a selected nursing task in a selected situation with the registered professional nurse retaining the accountability for the delegation."

Reflective Thinking

Special Services

You have been employed as a school nurse in a small school district for several years.

Just recently, your district has begun to return special needs students to their home schools. Your new case load will include daily tube feedings for a student in one building and catheterization assistance in another. How do you feel about providing such services? How do you balance taking care of these students and the needs of the rest of the students? Should the district be required to pay additional money for these services, or should insurance or the government provide assistance?

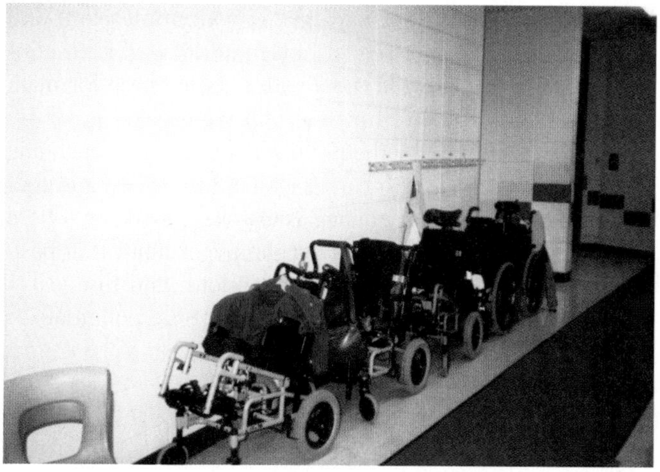

Figure 5-10 Meeting the needs of special education students has brought changes to the role of the school nurse. Can you list some of the special challenges that a school nurse may face?

Nursing Alert

Delegation to Unlicensed Assistive Personnel

When unlicenced assistive personnel are assigned to provide services to children in the school, you remain accountable for the service. It is your responsibility to see that the UAP is properly trained and competent in the assigned skill before delegating the task. Written instructions, documentation of training, and ongoing supervision are important in delegation.

Kids Want To Know

Why are some kids in my school in wheelchairs?

As the school nurse in a building with children with special needs, you can help by providing information appropriate to the developmental level of the children regarding disabilities and what they mean and why children use wheelchairs. It would also be helpful to allow time for questions, to read and have available books about children with disabilities, and to encourage teachers to include special education students in class time.

(National Council of State Boards of Nursing, 1995). Different states' Nurse Practice Acts have different regulations for delegation, and the school nurse must be sure the UAP's function is within the scope of practice. The primary consideration in the decision to delegate is the health, safety, and welfare of the student (Luckenbill, 1996). Before delegating a task, the school nurse must ask if the procedure can be legally delegated, who is available to perform the task, what the level of their training is, and whether or not the student's medical condition is stable. After deciding delegation is appropriate, the school nurse remains responsible for the initial assessment, care plan, training, and supervision of the UAP.

School nurses remain apprehensive about the widespread use of UAPs. The reasons for this apprehension are not clearly established, but many factors could contribute. First, there is the perceived threat that with budget cuts through school districts, the UAP will become the primary school health provider. School nurses may fear that by opening the door a little for the additional help, most UAPs will take over all nursing duties. Another reason may be that some school districts do not have clear policies regarding the use of UAPs, causing confusion for the school nurse and the UAPs. School personnel other than the school nurse may also be making decisions on the delegation of nursing tasks without knowing that the nurse remains responsible for the care. Third, some nurses may be concerned they are delegating duties to persons not qualified to perform them, but are feeling pressure from administration to delegate the duties against their better judgment. This can be especially important, since procedures delegated to UAPs are still the responsibility of the nurse (Josten, Smoot, & Beckley, 1995). If UAPs are used in the school setting, the school nurse must be involved in developing their role and determining district policies regarding delegation and the UAP's role. Legal ramifications regarding delegation and supervision procedures need to be explored before policies are formalized. If UAPs will be used, additional training on delegating and supervising may

In the Real World

I had been a pediatric nurse for 11 years. When I went back to school and became a school nurse, I admit I was looking forward to a slower pace. My nurse friends laughed at me and told me it would be a boring job. When I spent my first day in an elementary school building with 700 children, I realized this job was not what others believed. There was no sitting around giving out Band-Aids. In fact, there was no sitting around, period. There were tube feedings, asthma attacks, falls from playground equipment, hockey stick injuries, health classes to teach, medications to give, families in need of help getting their child glasses, blood sugars to check, multidisciplinary conferences to attend, and special education rules and regulations to learn. Yes, I gave out my share of Band-Aids, but with them came the opportunity to care for children, to teach them to care for themselves, to let them know someone cared about them. The best part of my job is when I'm out somewhere, maybe shopping, and hear a child call out, "Hey Mom, that's my nurse!"

be needed by nurses to increase their confidence in deciding how to delegate safely. For further information on delegation and UAPs, see Chapter 2.

The school nurse's role has changed and grown since its experimental beginnings in New York. What started as a way to control communicable diseases in children has evolved into a complicated role that encompasses many different responsibilities and requires a variety of skills. This chapter has reviewed the technical components of the nurse's role and looked at the wide variety of topics included in health promotion education. Today's school nurse must have excellent skills in assessment and triage, communication, and diplomacy. In addition, school nurses must be able to educate children and provide them with a strong base for making healthy lifestyle choices. School nurses must be committed to continuing their education in the ever-changing world of children's health care, technical advances, and federal regulations. School nursing is a well-kept secret, where the responsibilities are endless but the opportunities for positively influencing children are tremendous, and the goal—enabling children to reach their full academic potential—is rewarding.

Key Concepts

- The role of the school nurse, established to decrease the number of children out of school due to infectious diseases is influenced by societal, political, economic, and educational changes.
- The school nurse provides vision/hearing/scoliosis screening, height/weight measurement, as well as health education, which includes personal and dental hygiene, sex education, antismoking programs, and alcohol, drug use, and violence prevention information.
- Emergency care of children in the school includes basic first aid, deciding when to transport to a hospital, and the development of emergency plans.
- An Individual Health Plan—including goals, how they will be met, expected outcomes, and types of services needed—is developed and updated annually and as needed for students with special medical conditions.
- School-based health clinics and school-linked health clinics are located within or near schools to provide health services to children and families unable to secure health care.
- School nurses work as part of a multidisciplinary team, provide direct care to children with complex medical needs in a school setting, and delegate tasks, such as medication administration, to unlicenced assistive personnel.

Review Questions

1. What changes in society and government have influenced the role of the school nurse? How has it evolved over time?
2. Vision and hearing screenings are mandated in selected grade levels in many states. What other examples of secondary prevention are part of the school nurse's duties?
3. A first-grader falls from the playground equipment. A group of children are around him with a teacher's assistant. He is crying loudly. Think of the order in which you would proceed as you come upon the scene. What would you include in your initial assessment and interventions?
4. A 9-year-old child with diabetes has transferred into your school. Although he tests his own blood sugar, he has not yet learned to administer his own insulin. The personnel in the building are anxious because you are in the building only 2 days a week. How would you handle monitoring his blood sugar and the need for intermittent administration of insulin when you are not in the building?
5. Health education is an important aspect of the school nurse's role. What information would you include when teaching 2nd graders about dental health? What teaching strategies would be appropriate for this group's developmental level? What outside activities could you tie into the lesson? How would you evaluate the teaching?
6. Distinguish between school-based health centers and school-linked health centers. What are the advantages and disadvantages of each?
7. You are the only school nurse covering four elementary schools. Your first priority is a student who needs a tube feeding, but several students in another building need medication at the same time. You have been asked to train the principal of the building to administer medications. What assessments are needed before delegating this task? What would you include in the training? How would you continue to supervise this procedure? What is your liability?

References

Adams, M. (1992). Screening programs. In H. Wallace, K. Patrick, G. Parcel, & J. Igoe (Eds.), *Principles and practices of student health* (pp. 329–335). Oakland, CA: Third Party.

Allensworth, D. (1994). School health services: Issues and challenges. In P. Cortese & K. Middleton (Eds.), *The comprehensive school health challenge* (pp. 179–212). Santa Cruz, CA: ETR.

American School Health Association. (1974). *Guidelines for the school nurse in the school health program.* Kent, OH: ASHA.

American School Health Association. (1998). ASHA board pass new, revised resolutions. *The Pulse of American School Health Association, 18*(4), p. 8.

Barnett, S., Niebuhr, V., & Baldwin, C. (1998). Principles for developing interdisciplinary school-based primary care centers. *Journal of School Health, 68*(3), 99–104.

Benenson, A. (1995). *Control of communicable diseases manual.* Washington, DC: American Public Health Association.

Black, D., Tobbler, N., & Sciacca, J. (1998). Peer helping/involvement: An efficacious way to meet the challenge of reducing alcohol, tobacco, and other drug use among youths. *Journal of School Health, 68*(3), 87–93.

Borowsky, I. (2000). Attention deficit/hyperactivity disorder. In C. Berkowitz (Ed.), *Pediatrics: A primary care approach,* 2nd ed. pp. 469–473.

Boyer-Chuanroong, L., & Deaver, P. (2000). Meeting the preteen vaccine law: A pilot program in urban middle school. *Journal of School Health, 70*(2), 39–44.

Brandt, C. (1999). Creating a living document: Developing the NASN mission statement for the new millennium. *Journal of School Nursing, 15* (5), 30–32.

Centers for Disease Control and Prevention. (1999). Recommended childhood immunization schedule: US—1999. *Morbidity and Mortality Weekly Report, 48*(1), 12–15.

Centers for Disease Control and Prevention, National Center for Chronic Disease Prevention and Health Promotion, Division of Adolescent and School Health. (1991). *Developing comprehensive school health programs to prevent important health problems and improve educational outcomes: A guide for state and local education agencies.* Atlanta: CDC.

Chauvin, V. (1994). Students with special health care needs: A manual for school nurses. Scarborough, ME: National Association of School Nurses.

Committee for Children. (1992). *Second Step: A violence prevention curriculum,* 2nd ed. Seattle, WA: Author.

Constante, C., & Smith, E. (1997). Beyond band aids: School health nurses as program developers and coordinators. *Journal of School Health, 67*(7), 290–291.

Cook, K. (1999). Assessment of potential inhalant use by students. *Journal of School Nursing, 15*(5), 20–23.

Copeland, L., Shope, J., & Waller, P. (1996). Factors in adolescent drinking/driving: Binge drinking, cigarette smoking and gender. *Journal of School Health, 66*(7), 254–259.

Copmann, K. (1996). The audiological assessment. In S. Schwartz, (Ed.), *Choices in deafness: A parents' guide to communication options.* Bethesda, MD: Woodbine.

Denehy, J. (1999). Health promotion: A golden opportunity for school nurses. *Journal of School Nursing, 15*(5), 4–5.

Drew, C., Hardman, M., & Logan, D. (1996). *Mental retardation: A life cycle approach* (6th ed.). Englewood Cliffs, NJ: Prentice Hall.

Drug Enforcement Administration. (1996). *Drugs of abuse.* [Online.] Available: http://www.usdoj.gov/dea/concern/abuse/contents.htm.

Dryfoos, J. (1998). School-based health centers in the context of education reform. *Journal of School Health, 68*(10), 404–407.

Dusenbury, L., Falco, M., Lake, A., Brannigan, R., & Bosworth, K. (1997). Nine critical elements of promising violence prevention programs. *Journal of School Health, 67*(10), 409–414.

Fry-Bowers, E. (1997). Community violence: Its impact on the development of children and implications for nursing practice. *Pediatric Nursing, 23*(2), 117–121.

Fryer, G., & Igoe, J. (1995). A relationship between availability of school nurses and child well being. *Journal of School Nursing, 11*(3), 12–17.

Fryer, G., Igoe, J., & Miyoshi, T. (1997). Considering school health program screening services as a cost offset: A comparison of existing reimbursement in the states. *Journal of School Nursing, 13*(2), 18–21.

Glo-Germ Journal. (1997). Spring, UT: Glo-Germ.

Green, L., Krueter, M., & Deeds, S. (1980). *Health education planning: A diagnostic approach.* Palo Alto, CA: Mayfield.

Greenburg, J. (1999, March 4). One-on-one care ordered for paralyzed student. *Chicago Tribune,* section 1, p. 3.

Hacker, K., & Wessel, G. (1998). School-based health centers and school nurses: Cementing the collaboration. *Journal of School Health, 68*(10), 409–413.

Hahn, E., Hall, L., Rayens, M., Burt, A., Corley, D., & Sheffel, K. (2000). Kindergarten children's knowledge and perceptions of alcohol, tobacco and other drugs. *Journal of School Health, 70*(2), 51–55.

Harrison, V. (1999). A whiff of growing abuse. *NEA Today, 17*(6), 24.

Haynie, D., Alexander, C., & Russell-Walter, S. (1997). Considering a decision-making approach to youth violence prevention programs. *Journal of School Health, 67*(5), 165–170.

Hubbard, B., Geise, M., & Rainey, J. (1998). A replication study of reducing the risk, a theory-based sexuality curriculum for adolescents. *Journal of School Health, 68*(6), 243–247.

Josten, L., Smoot, C., & Beckley, S. (1995). Delegation to assistive personnel by school nurses: One state's experience. *Journal of School Nursing, 11*(2), 8–16.

Kandal, D., & Logan, J. (1984). Patterns of drug use from adolescence to young adulthood: Periods of risk for initiation, continued use and discontinuation. *American Journal of Public Health, 74*(4), 600–605.

Kane, W. (1994). Planning for a comprehensive school health program. In P. Cortese & K. Middleton (Eds.), *The comprehensive school health challenge* (pp. 83–120). Santa Cruz, CA: ETR.

Kann, L., Kinchen, S., Williams, J., Ross, J., Lowry, R., Hill, C., Grunbaum, J., Blumson, P., & Collins, J. (1998). Youth risk behavior surveillance—United States, 1997. *Journal of School Health, 68*(9), 355–369.

Katz, B. (1996). *Germs, germs, germs.* New York: Scholastic.

Kimel, L. (1996). Hand washing education can decrease illness absenteeism. *Journal of School Nursing, 12*(2), 14–18.

Lindley, L., Reininger, B., Vincent, M., Richter, D., Saunders, R., & Shi, L. (1998). Support for school-based sexuality education among South Carolina voters. *Journal of School Health, 68*(5), 205–211.

Lowry, R., Holtzman, D., Truman, B., Kann, L., Collins, J., & Kolbe, L. (1994). Substance use and HIV-related sexual behaviors among US high school students: Are they related? *American Journal of Public Health, 84,* 1116–1120.

Luckenbill, D. (1996). *The school nurse's role in delegation of care: Guidelines and compendium.* Scarborough, ME: NASN.

Ludder-Jackson, P., & Vessey, J. (1996). *Primary care of the child with a chronic condition* (2nd ed.). St. Louis: Mosby.

Mahoney, M., Costley, C., Cain, J., Zaiger, D., & McMullen, S. (1998). School nurses as advocates for youth tobacco education programs: The TAR WARS experience. *Journal of School Health, 68*(8), 339–341.

Mark, H., & Mark, T. (1999). Parental reasons for non-response following a referral in vision screening. *Journal of School Health, 69*(1), 35–38.

Matza, N., & Loya, R. (1994). Tobacco use prevention. In P. Cortese & K. Middleton (Eds.), *The comprehensive school health challenge* (pp. 331–349). Santa Cruz, CA: ETR.

McEwen, M., Johnson, P., Neatherlin, J., Millard, M., & Lawrence, G. (1998). School-based management of chronic asthma among inner-city African American school children in Dallas, Texas. *Journal of School Health, 68*(5), 196–201.

Meurer, J., McKenzie, S., Mischler, E., Subichin, S., Malloy, M., & George, V. (1999). The Awesome Asthma School Days program: Educating children, inspiring a community. *Journal of School Health, 69*(2), 63–68.

Minor, K. (1994). Educating about HIV/AIDS. In P. Cortese & K. Middleton (Eds.), *The comprehensive school health challenge.* Santa Cruz, CA: ETR.

Muscari, M., Phillips, C., & Bears, T. (1997). Health beliefs and behaviors in rural high school juniors. *Pediatric Nursing, 23*(4), 380–389.

National Association of School Nurses. (1995). *Postural screening guidelines for school nurses.* (Publication no. S013.) Scarborough, ME: NASN.

National Association of School Nurses. (1999). *Standards of professional school nursing practice.* Scarborough, ME: NASN.

National Asthma Education Program. (1991). *Managing asthma: A guide for schools.* Bethesda, MD: Author.

National Council of State Boards of Nursing (NCSBN). (1995). *Delegation and decision making process.* Chicago: Author.

National Education Association. (1999). Safe schools. *NEA Today, 17*(7), 4–6.

National Task Force on the Preparation and Practice of Health Educators, Inc. (1983). *A guide for the development of competency-based curricula for entry-level health educators.* New York: National Center for Health Education Credentialing.

Nolte, A. (1994). School health education today: Highlights and milestones. In P. Cortese & K. Middleton (Eds.), *The comprehensive school health challenge.* Santa Cruz, CA: ETR.

Office of Smoking and Health, Division of Adolescent and School Health and National Center for Chronic Disease Prevention and Health Promotion. (1996). Tobacco use and usual sources of cigarettes among high school students. *Journal of School Health, 66*(6), 222–224.

Palfrey, J., Haynie, M., McManus, M., Fenton, T., & Shaw, D. (1995, May). A study of financing of services for children with complex medical conditions. Paper presented at the Annual Ambulatory Pediatric Association Meeting, San Diego, CA.

Passarelli, C. (1994). School nursing: Trends for the future. *Journal of School Health, 64*(4), 141–150.

Perry-Casler, S., Price, J., Telljohan, S., & Chesney, B. (1997). National assessment of early elementary teachers' perceived self-efficacy for teaching tobacco prevention based on the CDC guidelines. *Journal of School Health, 67*(8), 348–354.

Pesa, J. (1998). The association between smoking and unhealthy behaviors among a national sample of Mexican-American adolescents. *Journal of School Health, 68*(9), 376–380.

Peterson, J., Niessen, L., & Lopez, N. (1999). Texas public school nurses' assessment of children's oral health status. *Journal of School Health, 69*(2), 69–72.

Porter, S., Haynie, M., Bierle, T., Heinz-Caldwell, T., & Palfrey, J. (1997). *Children and youth assisted by medical technology in educational settings: Guidelines for care* (2nd ed.). Baltimore: Brooks.

Price, J., Beach, P., Everett, S., Telljohann, S., & Lewis, L. (1998). Evaluation of a three-year urban elementary school tobacco prevention program. *Journal of School Health, 68*(1), 26–31.

Robinson, K., Price, J., Thompson, C., & Schmalzried, H. (1998). Rural junior high school students' risk factors for and perceptions of teen-aged parenthood. *Journal of School Health, 68*(8), 334–338.

Selekman, J. (1998). Infectious diseases and the immunizations of today and tomorrow. *Pediatric Nursing, 24*(4), 309–315.

Swartwout, K., & Russell, J. (1999). A successful strategy: Garnering community support for contraceptive services to be provided in a school based health center. *Journal of School Nursing, 15*(5), 36–38.

Thomas, S. (1998). Historical development of community health nursing. In Hitchcock, J., Schubert, P., & Thomas, S. (Eds.), *Community health nursing: Caring in action* (pp. 17–38). Albany, NY: Delmar.

Thompson, A. (1999). In depth: Playing doctor. In *Nightly News with Tom Brokaw.* New York: NBC.

Treiman, K., & Beck, K. (1996). Adolescent gender differences in alcohol problem behaviors and the social contexts of drinking. *Journal of School Health, 66*(8), 299–304.

U.S. Department of Health and Human Services. (1995). *Asthma and physical activity in the school.* Washington, DC: NIH Publication No. 95-3651.

U.S. Department of Health and Human Services. (1997). *Keeping youth drug free.* Available: http://www.health.org/govpubs/phd711/intro.htm and http://www.health.org/govpubs/phd711/five.htm.

U.S. Department of Health and Human Services. (2000). *Healthy people 2010.* Washington, DC: Government Printing Office.

University of Connecticut Health Center, Department of Pediatrics. (1997). *School nurse emergency care course: School nurse manual.* (Project MCH-094992-01-0.) Farmington, CT: Author.

VanAntwerp, C. (1995). The lifestyle questionnaire for school-aged children: A tool for primary care. *Journal of Pediatric Health Care, 9*(6), 251–255.

Vernon, M., Bryan, G., Hunt, P., Allensworth, D., & Bradley, B. (1997). Immunization services for adolescents within comprehensive school health programs. *Journal of School Health, 67*(7), 252–255.

Vitello, S. (1989). The Detsel case: Limitation of school health services for special education students. *Journal of School Health, 59*(1), 37–38.

Wold, S. (1981). *School nursing: A framework for practice.* St. Louis: Mosby.

Wynn, S., Schulenberg, J., Kloska, D., & Laetz, V. (1997). The mediating influence of refusal skills in preventing adolescent alcohol misuse. *Journal of School Health, 67*(9), 390–395.

Yates, S. (1994). The practice of school nursing: Integration with new models of health service delivery. *Journal of School Nursing, 10*(1), 10–19.

Yawn, B., Kurkland, M., Butterfield, L., & Johnson, B. (1998). Barriers to seeking care following school vision screening in Rochester, Minnesota. *Journal of School Health, 68*(8), 319–323.

Suggested Readings

American Red Cross. (1991). *Don't get sick, wash up quick with Scrubby Bear.* Santa Ana, CA: American Red Cross.

Beatty, M. D. (1996) *Blueberry eye.* Santa Fe, NM: Health Presses.

Boynton, R., Dunn, E., & Stephens, G. (1994). *Manual of ambulatory pediatrics.* Philadelphia: Lippincott.

Brenner, N., Krug, E., Dahlberg, L., & Powell, K. (1997). Nurses' logs as an evaluation tool for school-based violence prevention programs. *Journal of School Health, 67*(5), 171–174.

Brown, M. (1996). *Glasses for D.W.* West Minister, MD: Random House.

Cortese, P., & Middleton, K. (Eds.). (1994). *The comprehensive school health challenge: Promoting health through education.* Santa Cruz, CA: ETR.

Council for Exceptional Children Today. (1997, September). *New developments in ADD/ADHD,* pp. 12–13. Arlington, VA: Author.

Graff, J., Mulligan, M., Guess, D., Taylor, M., & Thompson, B. (1990). *Health care for students with disabilities: An illustrated medical guide for the classroom.* Baltimore: Brookes.

Johnson D. (1996). *Ben's glasses.* Rutherford, NJ: Penguin Platinum Books.

National Association of School Nurses. (1994). *Students with special health care needs: A manual for school nurses.* Scarborough, ME: Author.

National Heart, Lung, and Blood Institute (NHLBI), National Institutes of Health, U.S. Department of Health and Human Services and the Fund for the Improvement and Reform of Schools and Teaching. (1991). *Asthma: A guide for schools.* Washington, DC: Government Printing Office. (NIH publication no. 91-2650.)

Rose, S. (1998). Ambloypia: The silent thief. *Journal of School Health, 68*(2), 76–79.

Shaughnessy, D. (1997). *Let's talk about getting glasses.* New York: Rosen.

Vessey, J. (1997). School services for children with chronic conditions. *Pediatric Nursing, 23*(5), 507–510.

Vincent, M., Geiger B., & Willis, S. (1994). Preventing teenage pregnancy: The necessity for school and community collaboration. In P. Cortese & K. Middleton (Eds.), *The comprehensive school health challenge* (pp. 289–330). Santa Cruz, CA: ETR.

Resources

Organizations and Websites

American Academy of Family Physicians
11400 Tomahawk Creek Pky.
Leawood, KS 66211-2672
(913) 906-6000
fp@aafp.org
www.aafp.org

American School Health Association
7263 State Route 43
P.O. Box 708
Kent, OH 44240
(330) 678-1601
www.ashawen.org

National Association of School Nurses
P.O. Box 1300
Scarborough, ME 04070-1300
(207) 883-2117
www.nasn.org

National Clearing House for Drug and Alcohol Information
P.O. Box 2345
Rockville, MD 20847-2345
(800) 729-6686
info@health.org
www.health.org

National Clearinghouse on Child Abuse
(800) FYI-3366
www.calib.com/nccanch

National Committee to Prevent Child Abuse
332 S. Michigan Ave., #1600
Chicago, IL 60604
(312) 663-3520
(800) CHILDREN

UNIT II

Growth and Development of Children

CHAPTER 6

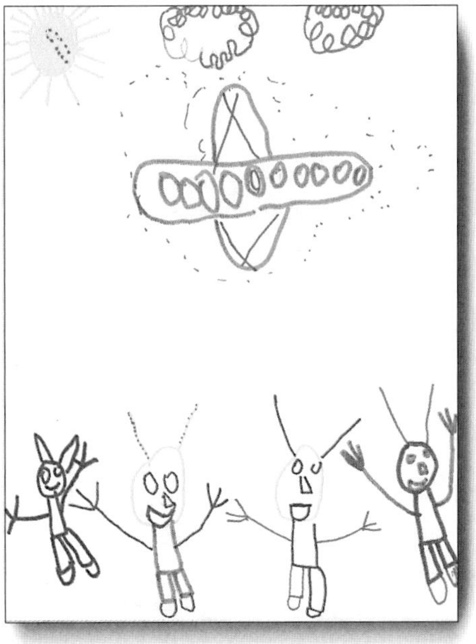

I can't believe how fascinating, different and marvelous children are. They grow so fast, and yet each is so unique. Luke was such a good baby—happy and always smiling. As a youngster, he always was building things with his Lego blocks and Tinker toys. Sarah was also a good baby, but much more content to watch others instead of jumping into activities. She spoke in complete sentences much earlier than her brothers and sister. Teachers always remarked on what a good student she was. Christine loved books. She would always climb on to her dad's lap with a book for him to read . . . and it was always the same book! I wondered why she never tired of hearing the story. Then there was Chad. He too was a busy child and always had friends over. When he was about 8, I think his friend Ronnie and he were either at our house or Ronnie's house for dinner every night during the summer months.

THEORETICAL APPROACHES TO THE GROWTH AND DEVELOPMENT OF CHILDREN

Barbara L. Mandleco, PhD, RN

COMPETENCIES

Upon completion of this chapter, the reader will be able to:

- *Identify and describe eight principles of human development.*
- *Explain how these principles are applied to the various theories of human development.*
- *Compare and contrast the major theories of human development.*
- *Describe, compare, and contrast the major issues of human development.*
- *Explain how the major developmental issues can be applied to the theories of human development.*
- *Apply theories of human development to pediatric nursing practice.*

Understanding human development is an essential part of the nursing process. Knowledge of normal behavior for specific age groups allows for individualizing assessments and care plans. Emphasis on promoting and maintaining health, anticipatory guidance related to human development, and assisting children and families to achieve optimal development are all important aspects of pediatric nursing. Knowledge of several principles, issues, and theories help us to understand holistic optimal development and care. This chapter will describe the various principles and issues that are interwoven within the major developmental theories discussed. Each theory will be fully explained and analyzed. The discussion will also include ideas on how the nurse can apply the theories to practice.

GROWTH, MATURATION, AND DEVELOPMENT

Growth, maturation, and development are common terms used to describe human development. An explanation of these terms and of the age ranges associated with child development is needed before principles, issues, and theories can be understood. **Growth** refers to a physiologic increase in size through cell multiplication or differentiation. This is most obviously seen in weight and height changes occurring during the first year of life. **Maturation** refers to changes that are due to genetic inheritance rather than life experiences, illness, or injury. These changes allow children to function at increasingly higher and more sophisticated levels as they get older. **Development** refers to the physiological, psychosocial, and cognitive changes occurring over one's life span due to growth, maturation, and learning, and assumes that orderly and specific situations lead to new activities and behavior patterns (Figure 6-1).

The five stages and age ranges of human development relating specifically to pediatric nursing are found in Table 6-1.

PRINCIPLES OF GROWTH AND DEVELOPMENT

At least eight principles providing a framework for studying human development are embedded within the issues and theories discussed in the following pages. Although not all of these principles are proven by research, they are often observed in children and generally assumed to be true (Hetherington & Parke, 1993; Murray & Zentner, 2001).

1. *Development is orderly and sequential.* This principle suggests that maturation follows a predictable and universal timetable. For example, children learn to crawl before they learn to walk, and they learn to walk before they learn to run. These changes occur rapidly during the first year of life and slow during middle and late childhood. Even though the onset and length of each developmental change vary among children, the basic sequence is the same, allowing comparison to norms.
2. *Development is directional.* Skill development proceeds along two different pathways: cephalocaudal and proximodistal. **Cephalocaudal** development proceeds from the head downward. Therefore, areas closest to the brain or head develop first, followed by the trunk, then legs and feet. For example, head control is followed by sitting, then crawling, and then walking. **Proximodistal** development proceeds from the inside out. Controlled movements closest to the body's center (trunk, arms) develop before controlled movements distant to the body (fingers). For example, grasping changes from using the entire hand to just the fingers as infants get older (Figure 6-2).

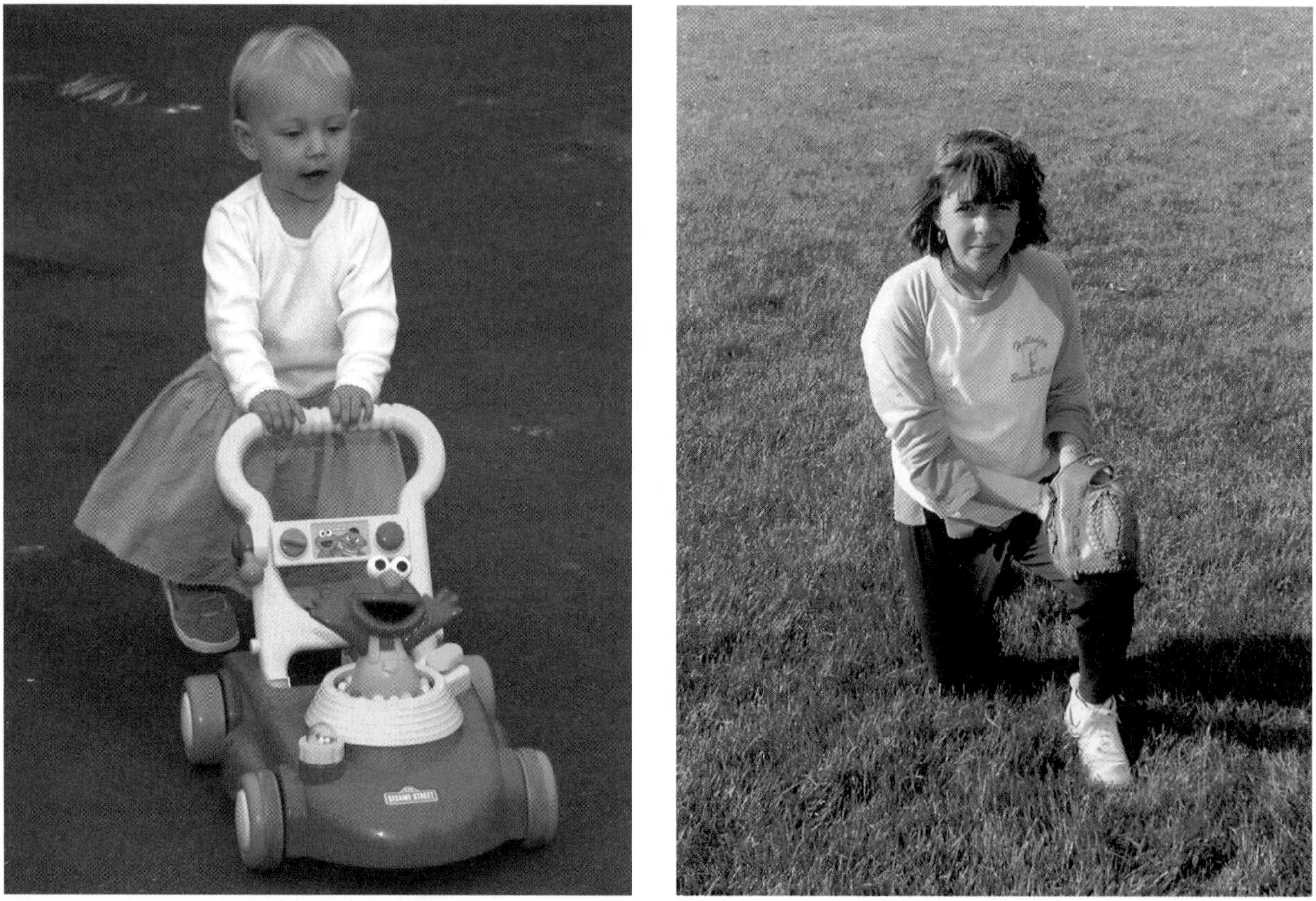

(A) (B)

Figure 6-1 (A) Toddlers are developing their gross motor skills. (B) School-aged children often become involved in physical activities and team sports.

TABLE 6-1 Stages, Age Ranges, and Characteristics of Human Development Related to Pediatric Nursing

Stage	Age	Characteristics
Infant	Birth to 1 year	Period of rapid growth and change; attachments to family members and other caregivers are formed; trust develops.
Toddler	1 to 3 years	Motor ability, coordination, sensory skills developing; basic feelings, emotions, a sense of self, and being independent become important.
Preschooler	3 to 6 years	Continued physiological, psychological, and cognitive growth; better able to care for selves, interested in playing with other children; beginning to develop a concept of who they are.
School age	6 to 12 years	Interested in achievement; ability to read, write, and complete academic work advances; understanding of the world broadens.
Adolescent	12 to 19 years, or later	Transition period between childhood and adulthood; physiological maturation occurs, formal operational thought begins; preparation for becoming an adult takes place.

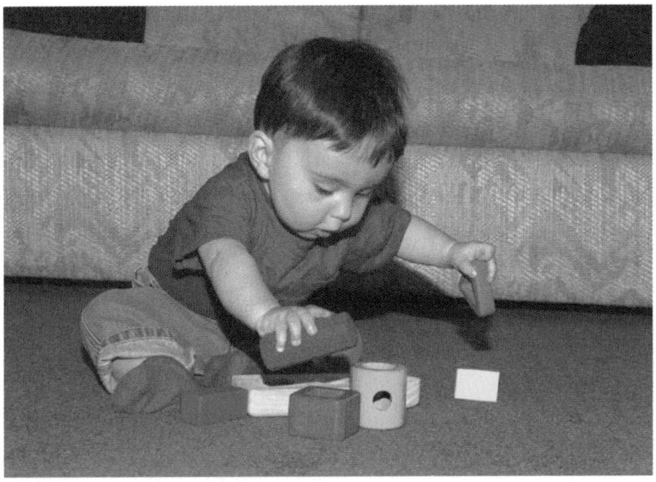

Figure 6-2 Infants' motor development improves with practice.

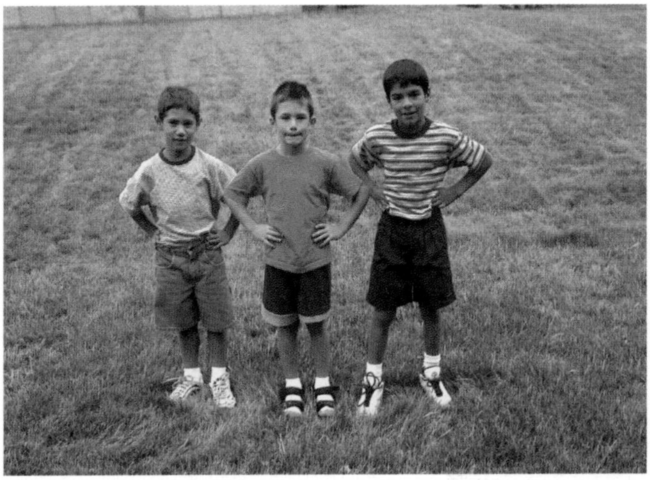

Figure 6-3 These children are the same age yet of different heights.

3. *Development is unique for each child.* Every child has a unique timetable for physiological, psychosocial, cognitive, and moral development (Figure 6-3). For example, some children can name four colors by the time they are 3 years old, whereas others cannot name four colors until they are $4^1/_2$ years old. Some children walk well at 11 months; others do not walk well until they are 14 months old.
4. *Development is interrelated.* Physiological, psychosocial, cognitive, and moral aspects of development affect and are affected by one another. For example, central nervous system maturation is necessary for cognitive development. Children cannot be independent in toileting if they are not aware of the urge to void and cannot independently remove clothing.
5. *Development becomes increasingly differentiated.* This means responses become more specific and skillful as the child grows. Young infants respond to stimuli in a generalized way involving the entire body, whereas older children respond to specific stimuli in a more refined and specialized way. For example, infants will react with their entire body to pain by crying and withdrawing, whereas a child is able to localize the pain, can often identify its source, and may only withdraw the extremity experiencing the pain. An infant will use the entire hand to grab a toy before developing the fine motor ability necessary for the pincer grasp.
6. *Development becomes increasingly integrated and complex.* This means, as new skills are gained, more complex tasks are learned. For example, learning to

drink from a cup initially requires eye–hand coordination, then grasping, and then hand–mouth coordination. Infants' cooing is followed by babbling, before these sounds are refined into the understandable speech of a child.

7. *Children are competent.* They possess qualities and abilities ensuring their survival and promoting their development. For example, newborns can cough, sneeze, suck, swallow, digest, breathe, and elicit caretaking responses from adults. Children make their needs known to caregivers in increasingly sophisticated ways so that others know if they are cold, hungry, or in pain.
8. *New skills predominate.* This occurs because of the strong drive to practice and perfect new abilities, especially early in life, when the child is not capable of coping well with several new skills simultaneously. For example, when children are learning to walk, talk, or feed themselves with utensils, their attention and effort is focused on developing that one skill; they do not usually learn to walk, talk, and feed themselves at the same time.

Reflective Thinking

Principles of Development

Do you agree that development is orderly, sequential, directional, unique, and interrelated? Do you think development becomes increasingly differentiated, integrated, and complex as children get older? Are children competent? Do new skills predominate? Why? Provide examples other than those suggested in the text.

Family Teaching

Principles of Development

- Teach caregivers that development, although orderly and sequential, may vary in individual children, so that some preschoolers may have advanced language skills and others may not.
- Remind caregivers of the importance of connections that exist among physiological, psychosocial, and cognitive development. Therefore, children need to know what it feels like to have a wet diaper and to be able to tell the caregiver that they are wet before they can be successfully toilet trained.

ISSUES OF HUMAN DEVELOPMENT

Theories on growth and development are often considered from the perspective of seven issues. These issues help explain how development occurs and what humans are like and can be applied to theories of human development. These issues answer questions related to the importance of biology or the environment on development, whether children are inherently good, bad, or actively involved in their own development, if development occurs gradually or abruptly, if children are more similar than different from one another, or if one's personality or way of interacting with others remains stable throughout life. The issues discussed include nature versus nurture, continuity versus discontinuity, passivity versus activity, critical versus sensitive periods, universality versus context specificity, assumptions about human nature, and behavioral consistency (Parke, Ornstein, Riesser, & Zahn-Waxler, 1994; Sigelman, 1999).

Nature Versus Nurture

One of the more important and oldest issues discussed in human development is the nature/nurture controversy. This debate concerns the influence that biology (nature) and the environment (nurture) have on an individual. **Nature** describes genetically inherited traits such as eye color or body type, or disease such as cystic fibrosis or hemophilia. This view sees development as predetermined by genetic factors and not altered by the environment. A person believing in the principle of nature would suggest that all normal children achieve identical developmental milestones at a similar time due to maturational forces. If children differed in achieving these milestones, it would be because of differences in their genetic makeup. **Nurture** refers to the influences that the environment has on development, and includes the influences that child-rearing methods, culture, learning experiences, and society have on development. A person believing in the principle of nurture would suggest that development can take different paths depending on the experiences that an individual has over a lifetime.

Today, most developmentalists believe that both nature and nurture are important, and that the relative contribution of each depends on the aspect of development studied. Developmentalists today are also more concerned about how biological and environmental factors interact to produce developmental differences and changes, rather than the importance of one over the other (Figure 6-4).

Continuity Versus Discontinuity

This issue addresses the nature of change across development. **Continuity** suggests that change is orderly and built upon earlier experiences. Development is a gradual and

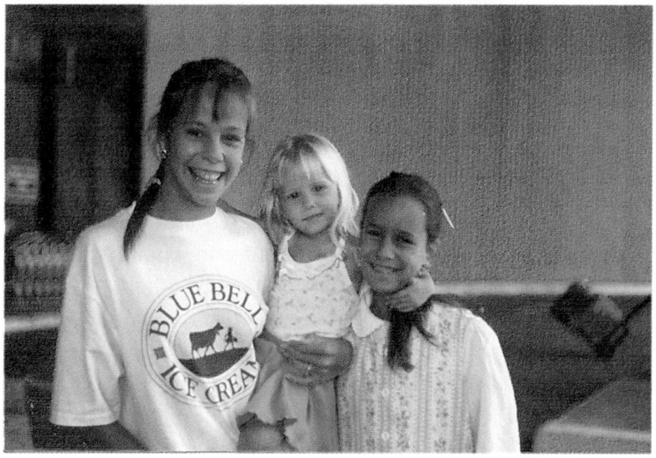

Figure 6-4 Which of these children are sisters? Why do you think so?

smooth process without abrupt shifts; the course of development looks like a smooth growth curve. This issue also suggests early and late development are connected; aggressive toddlers become aggressive adults, curious infants become creative adolescents, and shy preschoolers become introverted adults. Finally, continuity proposes that changes occur quantitatively, or in degrees. For example, when children grow older, they become taller, run faster, and learn more about the world around them.

Discontinuity suggests development is a series of discrete steps or stages that elevate the child to a more advanced or higher level of functioning with increased age. The course of development looks like a flight of stairs. There is no connection between early and later development; behavior seen later in life has replaced behavior seen earlier in life. For example, infants once comfortable around strangers may come to fear them as they get older; a shy and introverted preschooler may become an outgoing, extroverted adolescent. Discontinuity would also argue that adult behavior cannot be predicted by knowing what the person was like as a child. Finally, discontinuity implies qualitative change, or changes that make the individual different as growth occurs, as when a nonverbal infant becomes a toddler using language, or when a prepubertal child becomes a mature adolescent.

Passivity Versus Activity

This issue views the child as either a passive recipient shaped by external environmental forces, or as internally driven and actively participating in development. The passive view suggests that child-rearing beliefs, practices, and behaviors cause children to be either shy or assertive. Children become delinquent because of their association with an antisocial peer group. Talented and creative teachers deserve credit for a child's interest in mathematics or literature. Those disagreeing with this view believe children purposefully, creatively, and actively seek experiences to control, direct, and shape their development. Active children also modify caregiver, peer, and teacher behavior (Figure 6-5). For example, an inquisitive, friendly child may encourage that same behavior in an otherwise indifferent or unfriendly peer or adult.

Critical Versus Sensitive Period

This issue concerns the importance of different time periods in development, and asks if some phases are more important than others in developing particular abilities, knowledge, or skills. The **critical period** refers to a limited time span when a child is biologically prepared to acquire certain behaviors, but needs the support of a suitably stimulating environment. Indeed, there are some periods during development when children need to experience certain sensory and social input if their development is to proceed normally. The first 3 years of life are important for developing language, social, and emotional responsiveness. If there is little or no opportunity for these experiences during this time, children may have difficulty learning language, developing close friendships, or having an intimate emotional relationship later in life.

The **sensitive period,** on the other hand, is a time span that is optimal for certain capacities to emerge when the individual is especially receptive to environmental influences (Bornstein, 1989). Supporters of this view believe some behaviors can be modified during early development. For example, infants reared in an impoverished orphanage grew up without identifiable intellectual deficits if they were placed in a stimulating and nurturing adoptive home (Skeels, 1966). The fact that early experiences can be modified suggests humans are malleable and adaptable and, for some areas of development, there are sensitive rather than critical periods.

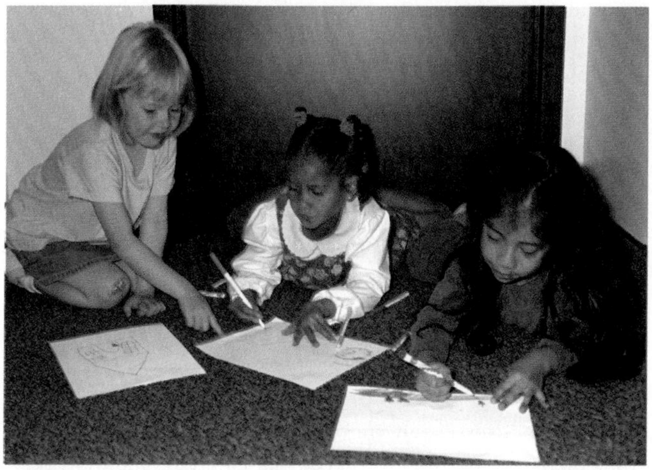

Figure 6-5 Active children are interested in learning about other children's projects and art work.

Universality Versus Context Specificity

The importance of culture to development is embedded within this issue. Some theorists believe an individual's culture has a profound influence on development. Others suggest there are culture-free laws of development that apply to all children in all cultures. For example, universality would say humans follow similar developmental pathways regardless of their culture: language is acquired and used at 11–14 months of age, cognitive changes preparing children for school or higher learning occur during 5–7 years of age, and sexual maturity is reached during the preteen or teenage years. **Context specificity** on the other hand, would suggest there are differences in children related to cultural values, beliefs, and experiences. For example, some societies encourage early walking by providing opportunities to exercise and practice these new skills, whereas in other societies carrying or swaddling infants is the norm, thereby reducing the chance of walking until older.

Assumptions about Human Nature

The doctrine of **original sin** used by Thomas Hobbes (1588–1679) to describe a child's nature, suggests children are inherently evil and selfish egotists who must be controlled by society. The doctrine of **innate purity,** proposed by Jean Jaques Rousseau (1712–1778), suggests children are inherently good and born without an intuitive sense of what is right and wrong. The doctrine of **tabula rasa,** proposed by John Locke (1632–1704), suggests children are neither good nor evil, but rather enter the world as a blank slate without inborn tendencies, and are molded through life experiences. These assumptions are based on 17th and 18th century social philosophers and rarely addressed directly in theories of human development today. However, emphasis on positive or negative aspects of a child's character and a particular theorist's belief reflect an individual's orientation and assumptions about human nature. For example, if one believes children are inherently caring and helpful, or on the other hand, innately selfish, child-rearing practices would vary. Permissive parents may believe children should be allowed to develop without interference (innate purity), whereas authoritarian parents may take an approach that would combat and control their child's selfish and aggressive impulses so they would develop positive behaviors.

Behavioral Consistency

This issue addresses whether or not a child's basic behavioral traits change according to the setting (school, neighborhood, family). Some theorists suggest individual personality characteristics and predispositions cause children to behave similarly no matter the setting. Others suggest children's behavior changes from one setting to another. Those supporting the former view would say a particular child can always be described as honest, helpful, aggressive, or independent, no matter the situation. The latter view would argue children's behavior shifts according to the situation and who/what is present—friend in need, angry caregiver or teacher, competitive game, or a difficult test.

> **Reflective Thinking**
>
> **Experiences and the Child**
>
> What do you think the impact of providing young children with experiences formerly reserved for older children (academic preschool, computer technology) has on developing specific skills, habits, or relationships? What impact does political and social change have on a child's development in countries experiencing loss of traditional cultural values?

THEORIES OF HUMAN DEVELOPMENT

The following theoretical views present various ways of examining human development during childhood and adolescence. Although each theory may describe only one aspect of development, holistic pediatric care assumes that all are important and need consideration when providing nursing interventions. Each theory focuses on particular areas of human development and has underlying assumptions, principles, strengths, and weaknesses that can help guide practice. Figure 6-6 provides a visualization of all theories discussed. Even though the figure is portrayed as a circle, consider it a sphere, with each part of the sphere a three-dimensional necessary part of the whole.

Psychoanalytic Perspective

The psychoanalytic perspective focuses on the emotional forces reflected in the individual's personality. These theories describe and define motivations and inner workings of the human mind during development, and answer questions related to the origin and development of personality and the outward expression of the inner self (mood, character traits, temperament, interaction patterns, behaviors). Stages of development, unconscious motivation for behavior, and conflicts within the personality are emphasized (Sigelman, 1999). The psychoanalytic perspective is divided into the psychosexual (Freud), psychosocial or epigenetic (Erikson), and interpersonal (Sullivan) theories of development.

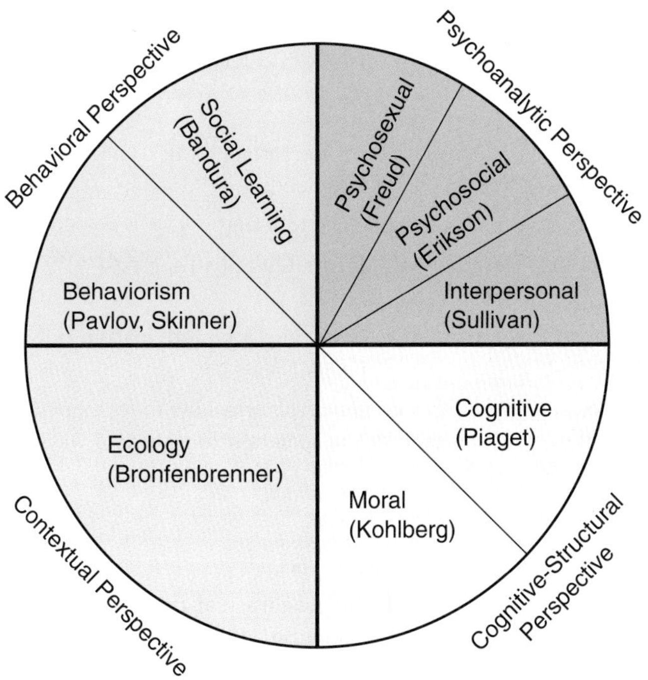

Figure 6-6 The Eclectic Nature of Human Development

Freud and Psychosexual Development

Sigmond Freud (1856–1939), a Viennese physician, originated the **psychosexual** theory emphasizing the importance of unconscious motivation and early childhood experiences in influencing behavior, and describing concepts related to personality and stages of development (Freud, 1933). His ideas, considered radical when proposed early in the twentieth century, became popular in the United States during the 1930s and continue to influence thinking about human development today.

Central to Freudian theory is the notion that two basic biological instincts (life and death) motivate behavior, must be satisfied, and compete for supremacy (Freud, 1933). The life instinct aims for survival and is responsible for such life sustaining activities as eating, breathing, copulation, and behavior that expresses self preservation, love, and constructive conduct. The death instinct on the other hand, is a destructive force expressed by self centered and cruel behavior, hate, aggression, and destructive conduct. These instincts, the source of psychic energy that drives human behavior, have three components: id, ego, and superego. As the child matures, these components of personality become more rational and reality bound (Freud, 1933).

During infancy, all psychic energy resides in the **id,** the inborn element of personality that is driven by selfish urges. The id obeys the "pleasure principle," oriented toward maximizing pleasure and immediately satisfying needs, even when biologic needs cannot be appropriately or realistically met. The id is manifest as the irrational, selfish, impulsive part of personality (Freud, 1933).

As the infant develops, the **ego** or rational and controlling part of the personality emerges. The ego operates according to the "reality principle" as realistic ways of gratifying instinctual drives are discovered. Ego functions allow individuals to be successful and include memory, cognition, intelligence, problem solving, compromising, separating reality from fantasy, and incorporating experiences and learning into future behavior. Ego development continues during childhood and throughout the life span (Freud, 1933).

The third component of personality is the **superego** or conscience, which emerges when the child internalizes caregiver or societal values, roles, and morals. Superego development begins in infancy, and becomes apparent in the preschool and school-aged years when the child learns socially acceptable behavior. The superego strives for perfection rather than for pleasure or reality. After the superego emerges, children have a conscience that tells them the difference between right and wrong, and which behaviors are socially acceptable outlets for the id's undesirable impulses. The superego also serves as a disciplinarian by creating feelings of remorse and guilt for transgressing rules, and self praise and pride for adhering to rules (Freud, 1933).

Conflict among the id, ego, and superego is inevitable throughout life. Mature, healthy personalities, however, are in a dynamic balance, with the id communicating its basic needs, the ego restraining the id until realistic ways are found to satisfy these needs, and the superego determining whether or not the ego's problem-solving strategies are morally acceptable. Freud believed defense mechanisms, such as regression, displacement, projection, and sublimation were created as escape valves to repress painful experiences or threatening thoughts coming from the id's unsatisfied needs that were not managed by the ego or superego (Freud, 1933).

To Freud, the most important life instinct was the sex instinct, which changed its character and focus according to biological maturation. (Freud's concept of sex and sexuality was broader than what is implied in the use of these words today, and indicates sexuality in its genital manifestations as well as any kind of pleasure seeking.) As the sex instinct's psychic energy (**libido**) shifts from one part of the body to another, the child passes through five stages of development: oral, anal, phallic, latency, and genital (Table 6-2). Each stage is related to a specific body part (erogenous zone) that brings primary pleasure to the child during that stage. According to Freud, adult personality is profoundly impacted by how each stage is managed.

Stages of Psychosexual Development

During the **oral stage** (birth to 1 year), the infant is preoccupied with activities associated with the mouth such as sucking, biting, chewing, and satisfying hunger. Freud

TABLE 6-2 Stages of Freud's Psychosexual Development

Stage	Age	Characteristics
Oral	Birth to 1 year	Receives satisfaction from oral needs being met; attachment to mother important because she usually meets infant's needs
Anal	1 to 3 years	Learning to control body functions, especially toileting
Phallic	3 to 6 years	Fascinated with gender differences, childbirth; Oedipus/Electra complex
Latency	6 to 11 years	Sexual drives submerged; appropriate gender roles adopted; learning about society
Genital	12 years and older	Sexual desires directed toward opposite gender; learns how to form loving relationships and manage sexual urges in societally appropriate ways

believed infants received satisfaction and enjoyment from these oral behaviors and later development was affected by how well oral needs were met as well as how closely attached the infant was to the mother who usually met these needs. Children whose oral needs were not met appropriately could become thumb suckers, nail biters, or pencil chewers in childhood, and compulsive eaters or smokers later in life. They also could become overly dependent or have difficulty developing mature relations later if they were weaned too early or fed on a rigid schedule thereby depriving them of oral gratification (Freud, 1933).

During the **anal stage** (1–3 years), sphincter muscles are maturing and children develop the ability to eliminate and retain fecal material. Sexual urges are gratified primarily by learning to voluntarily defecate. Freud suggested methods caregivers use to toilet train children during this period may have long lasting effects on personality. For example, children who were products of rigid, severe toilet training could become obsessive about routines and schedules, or very meticulous and hypercritical. Children whose caregivers were overly attentive and concerned about success during this time could hoard possessions or use material objects to demonstrate love and affection when they are adults (Freud, 1933).

During the **phallic stage** (3–6 years), the child's psychic energy is redirected to the genitals. Children are curious about childbirth, fascinated with anatomic differences, and find pleasure in their own genitals. The phallus (penis) assumes a critical role in the development of both boys and girls. Girls wish they had a penis (penis envy) and occasionally believe they once had one that was removed by a jealous, hostile mother. Boys fear losing their penis due to an attack or injury by others (castration anxiety). During these years, children also develop a strong incestuous desire for the caregiver of the opposite gender. The **Oedipal complex** (attachment of a boy to his mother) and **Electra complex** (attachment of a girl to her father) produce anxiety that must be resolved and controlled. Resolution and control allows children to identify with the caregiver of the same gender and fosters male and female identity (Freud, 1933).

At about age 6, children realize a sexual relationship with caregivers is impossible, and their energies and attention turn to the task of socialization. During this **latency stage** (6–11 years), sexual drives are submerged, appropriate gender roles are adopted, and the Oedipal/Electra conflicts are resolved. Since by now the superego has developed sufficiently to keep the id under control, children in this period rapidly learn about society and themselves while developing useful skills. They increasingly identify with the same-gender caregiver and become intensely involved with their same-gender peers. Energies are directed toward school, play, and increasing their problem-solving abilities (Freud, 1933) (Figure 6-7).

Freud's last period, the **genital stage,** begins at puberty (about age 12) and lasts throughout adulthood. Sexual desires reemerge due to physiological changes, fluctuating hormone levels, and changing social relationships (Figure 6-8). Before

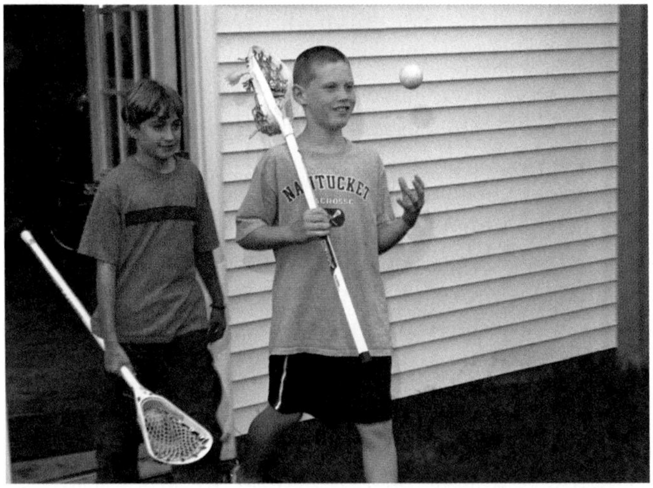

Figure 6-7 School-aged children actively engage in a variety of activities.

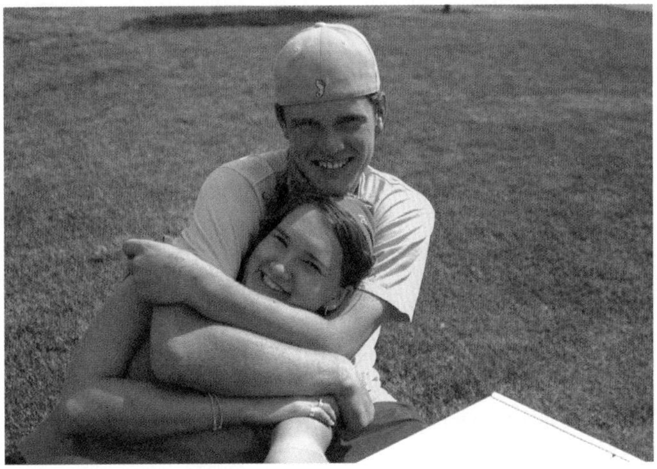

Figure 6-8 Relationships with the opposite gender change during adolescence.

mature adult adjustment is possible however, turmoil and adaptation are necessary. The adolescent vacillates between dependence/independence from parents, learns how to form loving relationships, and manages sexual urges in societally appropriate ways. Some adolescents struggle with their sexuality, reexperience earlier conflicting feelings toward caregivers, and may consequently distance themselves from their caregivers as they defend against anxiety. These psychic conflicts are necessary for fully functioning and mature adult personality development (Freud, 1933).

Evaluation

Freud has been criticized for developing a theory that is difficult to test, too narrow and simple, and based primarily on biological drives rather than sociocultural influences and learning. In addition, some of his theories are not always supported (Crain, 2000; Fisher & Greenberg, 1977); many preschoolers are ignorant of anatomical differences between genders. Freud's theory may also not be scientifically valid because it depends on instincts, defense mechanisms, and the unconscious, is based on retrospective memories of maladjusted adult clients, many of whom were women, and was not tested on children (Crain, 2000; Sigelman, 1999).

Reflective Thinking

Psychosexual Development

Which points of Freud's theory of psychosexual development do you agree or disagree with? Provide examples. How relevant and current is Freud's theory today? Explain your thinking.

On the other hand, Freud's theory did describe the concept of unconscious motivation for behavior and the importance of early family experiences on later development. Freud has also explored the emotional side of development (fear, anxieties, love), and has made us realize people are individuals who place meaning on different life experiences (Emde, 1992). His theory is also well developed and virtually unlimited in explaining a variety of behaviors from mate selection, habits, and art, to adversity and the meaning of dreams (Crain, 2000; Sigelman, 1999).

Application

Freud provides insight into human actions, and helps us understand others by realizing all behavior is meaningful and may hide inner needs or conflicts. Therefore, it is especially important to teach this information as well as normal behavior for the various stages to parents. Since during infancy comfort and pleasure are obtained through the mouth, it is important to offer babies a pacifier if they are NPO, or a bottle, pacifiers, or the breast after painful procedures. When hungry, they should be promptly fed (if not NPO). Providing plastic or rubber rings or other toys suitable for teething infants are also appropriate.

Toddlers are gratified by controlling body excretions. Therefore, when caring for children between 1 and 3 years of age, asking about the status of toileting and words and rituals used for elimination is important. It is wise to provide a child-sized potty chair and avoid starting toilet training during periods of illness or stress. In addition, toddlers should be reprimanded carefully if toilet training is difficult or if the child has accidents. Finally, parents need to be flexible and patient in toilet training and begin when the toddler indicates readiness.

Preschool children are concerned about sexuality and initially identify with the parent of the opposite gender. Nurses should teach parents that curiosity about gender differences and masturbation is normal. In addition, nurses should be aware of preschoolers who appear more comfortable with a particular nurse (no matter the gender), attempt to accommodate that situation, and encourage parents to participate in the care of their child. School-aged children and adolescents should be encouraged to have contact with friends, and their questions answered honestly. Privacy for both school age and adolescent clients should be ensured during physical examinations or when they are changing clothes or showering in gym class.

Erikson and Psychosocial Development

Erik Erikson (1902–1994) acknowledged the contribution of biologic factors to development, but felt that the environment, culture, and society were also important. His **psychosocial** (epigenetic) **theory** of development stresses the complexity of interrelationships existing between emotional and physical variables during one's lifetime (Erikson, 1963). Erikson agreed with many of Freud's ideas regarding basic instincts and the three components of personality (id, ego, superego). In addition, he believed development was stage-like, and conflict resolution was necessary at each stage in order for the individual to successfully advance to the next stage. In fact, Erikson's first five stages of development and the approximate ages of each stage correspond closely with those outlined by Freud (Table 6-3). Erikson differs from Freud, however, in that he believes children actively adapt and explore their environment instead of being passively controlled and molded by caregivers and society. Erikson also assumes humans are rational creatures whose actions, feelings, and thoughts are controlled primarily by the ego instead of the id, superego, or conflicts between the three components of personality.

For Erikson, lifespan development consisted of eight sequential stages. Five of these stages describe infants through adolescents (Table 6-4). Each stage is dominated by major developmental conflicts or crises related to societal demands and expectations that must be addressed or resolved before the individual can progress to the next stage. The resolution of each conflict or crisis might be positive (favorable and growth enhancing), or negative (unfavorable, frustrating, and making later development difficult). Erikson believed major conflicts occurring during each stage are rarely completely resolved. Instead, they are of primary or dominant importance during a particular stage and then become less important or dominant as other conflicts arise in later stages. In addition, he suggests conflict is rarely completely resolved positively. Rather, the positive resolution predominates over the negative resolution during a particular stage. Failure to successfully master a crisis or developmental task does not destine the child to failure since delayed mastery is possible. It is true, however, that difficulty at one stage may affect progress through later stages (Erickson, 1963).

Stages of Psychosocial Development

Erikson's first stage, **trust versus mistrust**, occurs during infancy (1 month to $1^1/_2$ years) when the basic task is to establish trust rather than mistrust in relation to oneself and others. Infants whose needs for comfort, food, and warmth are effectively and consistently met by a nurturing caregiver learn that the world is not only predictable, but safe, reliable, and can be trusted. If caregivers are unpredictable,

TABLE 6-3 Comparison of Stage Theories of Human Development

Age Period	Freud	Erikson	Sullivan	Piaget	Kohlberg
Infancy (Birth to 1 year)	Oral (Birth to 1 year)	Trust/Mistrust (Birth to $1^1/_2$ years	Infant (Birth to $1^1/_2$ years)	Sensorimotor (Birth to 2 years)	Preconventional (Birth to 7 years)
Toddler (1 to 3 years)	Anal (1 to 3 years)	Trust/Mistrust (continued)	Infant (continued)	Sensorimotor (continued)	Preconventional (continued)
		Autonomy/ Shame-Doubt ($1^1/_2$ to 3 years)	Early Childhood ($1^1/_2$ to 6 years)	Preoperational (2 to 7 years)	
Preschool (3 to 6 years)	Phallic (3 to 6 years)	Initiative/Guilt (3 to 6 years)	Early Childhood (continued)	Preoperational (continued)	Preconventional (continued)
School age (6 to 12 years)	Latency (6 to 12 years)	Industry/Inferiority (6 to 12 years)	Late Childhood (6 to 9 years) Preadolescence (9 to 12 years)	Concrete Operations (7 to 11 years)	Conventional (7 to 12 years)
Adolescence (12 to 19 years)	Genital (12 years and older)	Identity/Role Confusion (12 to 18 years)	Early Adolescence (12 to 15 years) Late Adolescence (15 to 19 years)	Formal Operations (12 years and older)	Postconventional (12 years and older)

TABLE 6-4 Stages of Erikson's Psychosocial Theory of Development

Stage	Age	Characteristics
Trust versus Mistrust	1 month to $1\frac{1}{2}$ years	Learns world is good and can be trusted as basic needs are met
Autonomy versus Shame and Doubt	$1\frac{1}{2}$ to 3 years	Learns independent behaviors regarding toileting, bathing, feeding, dressing; exerts self; exercises choices
Initiative versus Guilt	3 to 6 years	Goal directed, competitive, exploratory behavior; imaginative play
Industry versus Inferiority	6 to 11 years	Learns self worth as gains mastery of psychosocial, physiological, and cognitive skills; becomes society/peer focused
Identity versus Role Confusion	12 to 18 years	Develops sense of who I am; gains independence from parents; peers important

inconsistent, inadequate, or convey a sense of confusion or chaos, the child learns to view the environment with mistrust or wariness, and may demonstrate restlessness, crying, whining, or physiological dysfunctions such as sleep disturbances, vomiting, or diarrhea (Erikson, 1963).

During the toddler years ($1\frac{1}{2}$ to 3 years), **autonomy versus shame and doubt** occurs. Autonomy develops as children discover their new mental and physical abilities while improving language and motor skills and learning competencies related to bathing, eating, toileting, and dressing. Shame occurs if assertiveness and independence are considered unacceptable or ineffective by caregivers. Doubt occurs if children learn to mistrust not only themselves, but also others in the immediate environment. Children demonstrating dependency and constantly needing approval for their actions have not resolved this conflict (Erikson, 1963).

The third developmental stage (3–6 years) is **initiative versus guilt.** Initiative refers to a person's independently beginning an activity rather than merely responding to or imitating others. It occurs when a child tries out new ways of combining activities, invents creative ways to use skills and abilities, imagines what other people or things are like, and takes responsibility for one's own actions. Guilt occurs when caregivers frequently reprimand behaviors reflecting initiative. Children experiencing severe restrictions and belittling feel guilty about their actions and thoughts, and may become passive, reluctant, or refuse to participate in activities (Erikson, 1963).

The major developmental task of the school age years (6–11 years) is **industry versus inferiority.** Industry involves mastery of social, physical, and intellectual skills, and orientation toward and competition with peers. No longer interested in merely participating, school-aged children in many western countries are interested in being best, first, fastest, or smartest as they complete projects and compare their efforts to others. Attention and energy now are turned to learning academic skills and social roles, as the child becomes less family focused and more society and peer focused (Figure 6-9). Inferiority develops when school-aged children are ridiculed by peers, don't measure up to adult or their own expectations, or lack certain skills so they are not always the best, first, fastest, or smartest (Erikson, 1963).

Adolescence (12 to 18 years) is characterized by **identity versus role confusion.** Identity involves achieving a sense of who one is intellectually, cognitively, behaviorally, and emotionally, as emerging physical and sexual maturity is integrated with already existing skills and abilities. Erikson believed identity is attained as the young person's view of who one is becomes consistent with others' views. Identity achievement also requires resolution of subconflicts, including finding

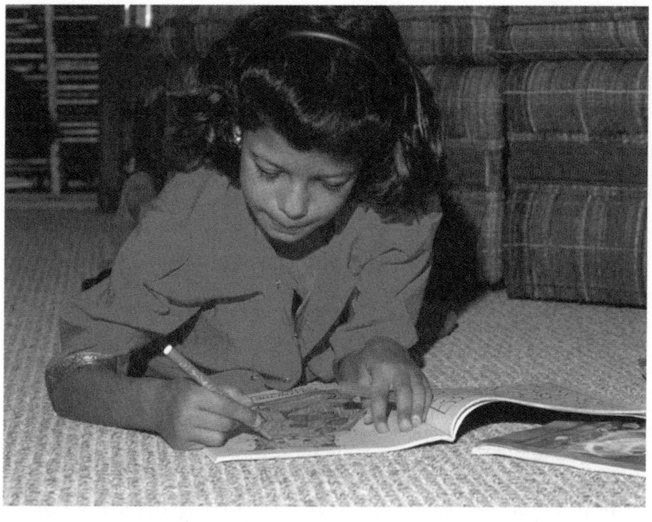

Figure 6-9 Industry is a task of school-aged children.

one's own political, social, economic, and religious ideology, adopting an appropriate gender identity, making an occupational or vocational choice, and adopting behaviors consistent with one's own self concept. Considered a crucial stage in development, identity formation affects commitments and decisions made later in life. Role confusion occurs when the adolescent is unable to acquire a sense of direction, self, or place within the world (Erikson, 1963).

Erikson identified three other stages beyond identity versus role confusion that occur during adulthood. They are intimacy versus isolation, generativity versus stagnation, and integrity versus despair. In each of these stages, as with the earlier stages, conflict needs to be resolved before the next stage is reached.

Evaluation

Erikson's theory is broader than Freud's and focuses on the importance of a variety of psychological motivations for behavior and the influence of both environmental and maturational factors on development. His theory also encompasses the entire life span and emphasizes the importance of assuming responsibility for self development and methods of achieving healthy resolution of each stage.

Those criticizing Erikson believe he is biased against women and does not consider the differences between men and women in relation to social and cultural influences or experiences. In addition, he is criticized for being imprecise about the causes of psychosocial development, not able to articulate specifically how outcomes of one stage impact development at another stage, or specify the kinds of experiences needed to resolve or cope with conflicts. Instead, he describes development socially and emotionally, but does not explain well, how or why development occurs. He also does not discuss observable behaviors indicating that trust, autonomy, initiative, industry, or identity has been achieved (Crain, 2000; Sigelman, 1999).

Application

Erikson's theory provides us with a means of assessing and gaining insight into five developmental crises children and adolescents face, and allows us to use this knowledge to teach caregivers behaviors they can expect to see in their children. It also helps us realize the importance of societal influences on health and behavior, and that psychosocial development is a lifelong process.

Erikson's theory is easy to apply to practice. Health care provides a variety of situations and opportunities where a child's progression through stages can be facilitated, and caregivers taught how to encourage positive resolution of each developmental crisis. Since meeting basic needs (feeding, bathing, changing) in a timely and appropriate fashion during infancy results in the development of trust, it is critical that feeding and hygiene needs be met promptly. When an infant is ill, parents should be encouraged to spend as much time as possible with their infant.

For toddlers, independence is increasing and self control gained by maintaining familiar daily routines. Allowing opportunities for the child to independently dress, feed, and do self-hygiene care is important (Figure 6-10). If restraint

Critical Thinking

Using Psychosocial Development in Practice

How would you identify children having difficulty developing trust, autonomy, initiative, industry, or identity? What suggestions would you give parents to help them help their children positively resolve each developmental crisis?

Eye On:

Psychosocial Development

The culture and beliefs that a person grows up with will affect how they trust and express autonomy, initiative, industry, and identity. Examine how you demonstrate(d) these elements, then compare your findings to someone else's who comes from a different cultural background.

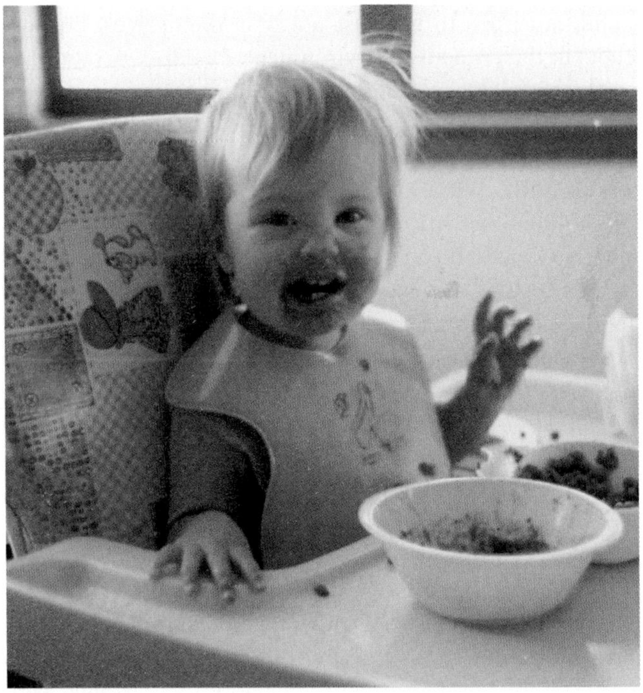

Figure 6-10 Letting toddlers feed themselves is important.

Research Highlight

Erikson's Theory

Study Purpose

To discover if adolescent identity exploration was associated with fluctuations in ego strength, mood swings, rebelliousness, and increased physical complaints.

Methods

Eighty-two high school students between 14 and 17 years of age completed the Minnesota Multiphasic Personality Inventory (MMPI), an empirically based assessment of adult psychopathology to determine symptomatology, and the Ego Identity Interview (EII). The EII provided information relative to commitment to and exploration of six domains commonly associated with adolescence: religion, friendships, politics, dating, occupation, and sex roles, and is based on Marcia's operationalization of Erikson's theory.

Findings

Factor analysis revealed seven scales from the MMPI consistent with Erikson's theory of adolescent crisis (self doubt, disturbed thinking, conflicts with parents and other authority figures, increased physical symptoms, reduced ego strength, impulsivity, confusion), explained 39% of the variance in active identity exploration of the six domains.

Implications

Nurses need to realize when interacting with adolescents, that identity formation includes periods of confusion, vulnerability, and conflict. Nurses need to be aware of the importance of encouraging and providing supportive interactions with adolescents that facilitate growth and build strength needed to overcome the dark side of forming identity.

Citation

Kidwell, J. S., Dunham, R. M., Bacho, R., Pastorino, E., & Portes, P. (1995). Adolescent identity exploration: A test of Erikson's theory of transitional crisis. *Adolescence, 30*(120), 785–793.

for procedures or treatments is necessary, explanations and comfort should be provided and caregivers encouraged to participate. Love, approval, and praise are important for toddlers and children in all stages.

Preschoolers like to initiate activities and remain curious and interested in the world around them. Opportunities to explore, ask questions, and create should be provided (Figure 6-11). Nurses should accept children's choices and negative expression of feelings, answer their questions, and allow them to play with medical equipment so their curiosity is satisfied and their knowledge about experiences broadened.

For school-aged children, involvement and success in a variety of activities provide a sense of self-worth and value. Nurses should provide the school-aged child with opportunities for continuing school work if hospitalized or ill, maintaining hobbies or activities, interacting with their peers, and adjusting to limitations imposed by illness or hospitalization.

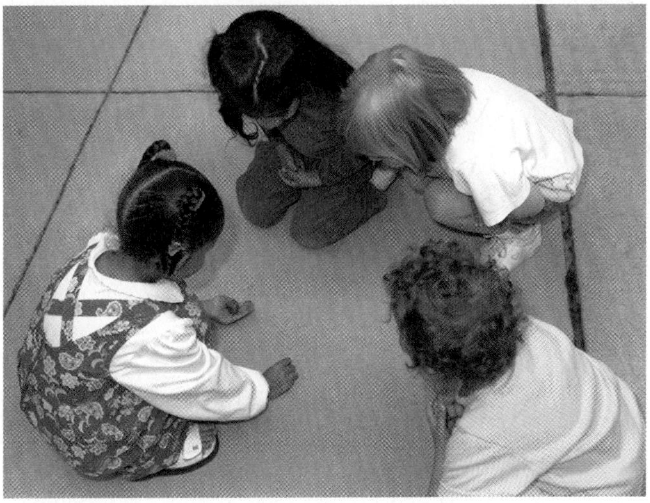

Figure 6-11 Children are curious about nature.

Family Teaching

Erikson's Theory

- Teach parents to meet infant's basic needs in a timely and appropriate manner.
- Allow opportunities for toddlers to be independent.
- Provide preschoolers with a variety of experiences where they can explore, ask questions, and create.
- Encourage school-aged children to interact with peers.
- Support adolescents' choices, be available to listen, and offer guidance.

Primary care nurses need to be in touch with school nurses when a child with a chronic condition is hospitalized and when this child is ready to return home and to school.

Adolescents are searching for who they will become independent from their parents. Nurses should allow adolescent clients to be as autonomous as possible, encourage them to take responsibility for their own actions, support their life choices, introduce them to other teens, and provide them with a separate recreation or activity area if in an acute care setting. Parental involvement in the care of adolescents is still important.

Sullivan and Interpersonal Development

Harry Stack Sullivan (1892–1949) focused on interpersonal relations as important behavioral motivators and the source of psychological health. His **interpersonal theory** posits that the self concept is the key to personality development. He acknowledged the importance of the environment (especially the home), and also emphasized the role of social approval and disapproval in forming a child's self concept. Sullivan believed personality development was largely the result of childhood experiences, interpersonal encounters, and the mother–child relationship. How well physiological needs were met in an interpersonal situation affected not only one's sense of satisfaction and security, but also allowed anxiety to be avoided. Poor environmental interactions caused anxiety and tension; a positive social relationship resulted in security, a major life goal (Sullivan, 1953).

Stages of Interpersonal Development

Sullivan describes seven stages of interpersonal development (Sullivan, 1953); six relate specifically to infants through adolescents (Table 6-5). Sullivan believed each stage prepared the personalty for the next stage and failure to successfully achieve stage activities limited personality development and opportunities for a successful life. Refer to Table 6-3 for a comparison of Sullivan's first six stages with Freud's and Erikson's stages.

The first stage (infant) encompasses birth to when the child is able to use words that convey the same meaning to the child as they do to others (18 months). The primary task of this stage revolves around learning to rely on others, especially the primary caregiver to gratify physiological needs and achieve satisfaction, When basic needs are met, infants are in a state of well being. If these needs are not met, a fear-like state occurs, manifested by excessive crying or difficulties eating or sleeping. Infants are sensitive to other's negative and positive attitudes and emotions while these needs are being met. Sullivan felt one's self image emerged according to how the infant interpreted the mother (primary care-

TABLE 6-5 Stages of Sullivan's Interpersonal Theory of Development

Stage	Age	Characteristics
Infant	Birth to 18 months	Learns to rely on others, especially mother; "good me/bad me" emerges
Early Childhood	18 months to 6 years	Learns to clarify communication; recognizes approval/disapproval; delays gratification
Late Childhood	6 to 9 years	Increasing intellectual abilities; learns to control behavior and own place in the world
Preadolescence	9 to 12 years	Vulnerable to teasing; "chum" important
Early Adolescence	12 to 15 years	Mastering independence; develops relationships with persons of opposite gender
Late Adolescence	15 to 19 years	Masters expression of sexual impulses; forms responsible and satisfying relationships with others

giver)–infant relationship when these needs were met. "Good me" feelings occur when acceptance is sensed; "bad me" feelings occur when the infant experiences anxiety while interacting with caregivers. Excessive anxiety may cause children to believe they are bad, leading to feelings of inferiority or depression. "Good me" and "bad me" fuse around 18 months of age; but the dominant "me" can change with situational or maturational crises (Sullivan, 1953).

During the early childhood stage (18 months to 6 years), children are able to communicate better with others, thereby facilitating interpersonal relationships (Figure 6-12). As children learn to recognize signs indicating approval/disapproval of their behavior, they learn about controlling personal desires, delaying gratification, and accepting interference from others. Excess parental disapproval during this time may cause children to view themselves and the world as negative and/or hostile.

The third stage, late childhood (6–9 years), is characterized by increasing intellectual ability and developing internal control over behavior. Children learn to pay attention to others' wishes, form satisfying relations with peers of both genders, and sometimes oppose rules. They also learn to accept subordination from authority figures (parents, teachers, other adults) and develop a sense of their own status and role in society (Sullivan, 1953).

During preadolescence (9–12 years), children participate in an expanding world that provides confrontation with rules and knowledge about themselves. They realize their status within the peer group is based on performance, are vulnerable to teasing, and become interested in relating closely to a peer of the same gender, which Sullivan calls the "chum." This special friend allows the 9–12-year-old to participate in a genuine love relationship with another, furthers self identity, and helps develop concern for others. "Chums" may share secrets, fantasies, dreams, and realities of life, and often collaborate, experiment, explore, and manipulate people and the environment. Preadolescents who do not have a chum may experience difficulty with relationships later (Sullivan, 1953).

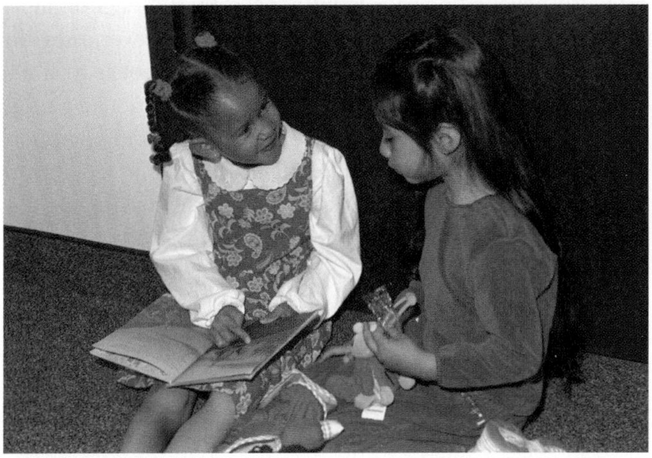

Figure 6-12 During childhood, children learn to communicate with others.

During early adolescence (12–15 years), independence is mastered and satisfying relations with members of the opposite gender are established as attempts are made to integrate sexual urges with other aspects of personal relationships. Early adolescents may demonstrate a variety of behaviors including rebellion, dependence, cooperation, and collaboration as they become independent.

The sixth stage is termed late adolescence (15–19 years). Sullivan believes initial feelings of love for the opposite gender emerge here, as the individual learns to master expression of sexual impulses, form responsible and satisfying relationships, and use communication skills in interactions.

Evaluation

There is little criticism of Sullivan's theory because most of his work (lectures, papers) was published after he died, was not systematic, and did not lead to replication. However, his view that social interactions are essential for personality development, and suggestions that personality can and does change are meaningful contributions. Like Erikson, he emphasized the importance of caregivers, peers, other adults, and the wider social environment in shaping a child's self concept.

Application

Sullivan also has relevance to the nursing care of children. Perhaps the two most important points he made is to emphasize the significance of interpersonal relations with others on personality development, and meeting the child's basic needs in a timely and appropriate fashion. This does not mean, however, that caregivers protect children from all discomforts or meet needs before they are expressed. The key is to relieve unpleasant feelings associated with basic needs so feelings of security and attachment result in a "good me" rather than a "bad me." Sullivan also has helped us realize the important place chums have in a school-aged child's life, and how this experience is critical for developing interpersonal relationships later in life.

Family Teaching

Sullivan

- Teach caregivers that their interactions with children should be positive, nurturing, and consistent.
- Remind caregivers that children need special friends during the school age years to share experiences, secrets, and dreams.

Reflective Thinking

Contributions of the Psychoanalytic Perspective

Consider the contributions the psychoanalytic perspective makes to the study of human development. Do you think that caregivers influence young children as much as Freud, Erikson, and Sullivan suggest? Why or why not? How would you explain children who grow up in dysfunctional environments but who overcome adversity and become well-adjusted and psychologically healthy adults?

Therefore, when children of any age are ill it is important to meet their basic needs and provide an opportunity for school-aged children and adolescents to interact with others their same age. If children are hospitalized or have a chronic illness, caregivers should be involved in their child's care. Nurses also need to teach caregivers about Sullivan's theory so they may help their child develop a healthy personality, and realize the importance they have in a child's life.

Behavioral Perspective

The **behavioral perspective** posits that human actions and interactions come from learned responses to environmental stimuli. Behavioral theorists study human behavior in a laboratory setting and then apply this information to the general population, and look for ways to alter or control the environment to change, modify, or teach desired behaviors. The past or unconscious motives are not the root of behavior and learning does not depend on maturation. These theorists believe children randomly respond to the environment consistent with developmental capabilities, and rewards and/or punishment influence behavior. Behavior resulting in punishment, pain, disappointment, or frustration often is discontinued, whereas behavior that is rewarded or viewed positively is retained and repeated in similar situations. The behavioral perspective is divided into behaviorism (classical and operant conditioning) and social learning (Crain, 2000; Sigelman, 1999).

Pavlov and Classical Conditioning

Ivan Pavlov (1849–1936), a Russian physiologist, initially discovered linkages between a stimulus and a response while studying a dog's response to food. He learned a dog would respond (salivate) not only when he saw food (unconditioned stimulus), but also when he saw the person who fed him or heard a bell ring just before the food appeared (conditioned stimulus), because the dog had learned that the bell or appearance of the man meant food would follow. This learning to respond to a new stimulus the same way a familiar stimulus was responded to is called **classical conditioning,** and suggests learning occurs when a response that is already part of the organism's normal activities (salivating) can be reproduced by an associated stimulus that previously would not have produced it—for example, the presence of a person or the sound of a bell (Crain, 2000; Murray & Zentner, 2001). Another example of classical conditioning would be when an infant, seeing the spoon used for feeding, becomes excited (waving hands and arms, kicking legs, making babbling sounds) because the spoon is associated with being fed and the infant knows that feeding time is coming soon.

Skinner and Operant Conditioning

Operant conditioning, a term originated by B. F. Skinner (1904–1990), involves behavioral changes due to either negative (punishment) or positive (reinforcers) consequences rather than just the occurrence of a stimuli. If behavior is rewarded, the likelihood of it reoccurring increases; if behavior is punished, chances are it will not reoccur. Positive reinforcement includes friendly smiles, praise, or special treats/privileges; punishment includes criticism, a frown, or withdrawal of privileges. Skinner discovered behavioral change became more permanent when consequences were provided intermittently rather than continuously, and believed the essence of development involved constantly acquiring new behaviors or habits due to reinforcing or punishing stimuli. He emphasized why behaviors occur rather than simply describing the behavior seen (Skinner, 1953).

Bandura and Social Learning

A third kind of behaviorism is **social learning,** proposed by Albert Bandura (b. 1925). According to this view, children learn by imitating and observing others (a model), as well as by classical and operant conditioning. Social learning theorists also believe behavior is influenced by the environment and learned through various experiences. However, they do not believe behavioral change is a mindless response to stimuli. Rather, they suggest personality, past experiences, relationships with the model, the situation itself, and cognition also impact behavioral change (Bandura, 1977). Cognition plays a part because to successfully imitate behavior, a child must be capable of remembering, rehearsing, and organizing the behavior seen. Children often will think about connections between behavior and consequences and will likely be affected more by what they believe will be the consequences rather than what the consequences actually are. For example, learning to play a musical instrument is expensive for families, and demanding and time consuming for children. However, children and their parents continually tolerate the cost and inconvenience because they are anticipating rewards once the child learns to play the instrument.

Bandura also believes modeled behavior can be weakened or strengthened depending on whether it is punished or rewarded. Bandura suggests observational learning (learning that results from merely watching others), where children acquire a variety of new behaviors when "models" are merely pursuing their own interests and not attempting to teach, reward, or punish, is another important method of learning behaviors. For example, research has shown children who watch television violence frequently are more aggressive than those children who do not watch very much television violence (Murray & Zentner, 2001). Finally, Bandura found children tend to model behavior of children and adults of their same gender more often than not, and males model behavior of others more often than females do (Crain, 2000; Sigelman, 1999) (Figure 6-13).

Evaluation

Behavioral/learning theories are precise and testable since they can be replicated and observed; principles from these theories operate across the entire life span. They have practical applications, have been used to effectively treat developmental problems, and assist in optimizing development. They are also credited with introducing concepts of programmed instruction and computer learning, and emphasize the role of environmental influences in shaping behavior. They make adults aware of the example their behavior sets for children of all ages (Gewirtz & Pelaez-Nogueras, 1992; Horowitz, 1992) since it is not unusual for children to adopt behavior seen in their caregivers (smoking, crude language) even if these same caregivers talk to their children about not smoking, using crude language, or imitating their behavior.

However, critics say the behavioral perspective oversimplifies development by downplaying biological influences and places too much emphasis on environmental experiences. Children cannot achieve certain milestones until they are maturationally or developmentally ready. In addition, the perspective only examines one or two aspects of development instead of examining how all aspects fit together and misses spontaneity often seen in young children. Finally, the theory is viewed as too simplistic and unconnected; isolated aspects of behavior are described rather than examining how feelings, the unconscious, and psychodynamic factors fit into the holistic view of the child (Sigelman, 1999).

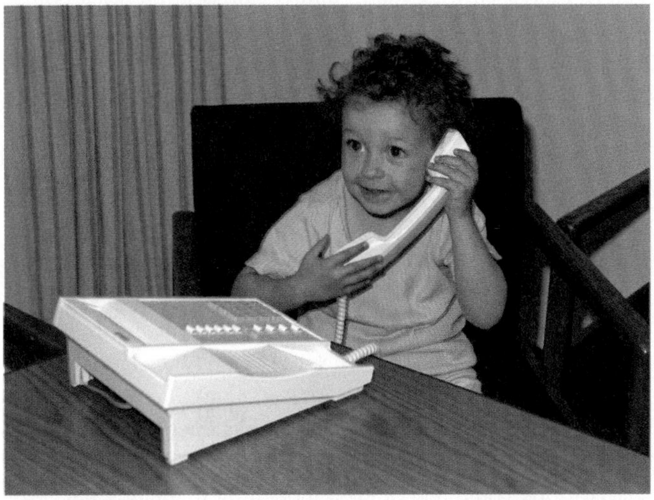

Figure 6-13 It is not uncommon for children to model the behavior they observe in others.

Application

Although behaviorism has been criticized for denying the inherent capabilities of persons to willfully respond to environmental situations and its relative elementary nature, it is useful in health care. Positive behaviors can be reinforced by encouragement, praise, and other rewards, and behaviors needing to be altered or removed from a child's repertoire can be extinguished by either ignoring or punishing. Parents commonly use these concepts when toilet training or teaching their children cooperation, compromise, helpfulness, and empathy. Some academic and preschool programs and parents use behavior modification and time-out activities to modify and change undesirable behavior in children. Operant conditioning can also help plan new or extinguish undesirable behavior by providing specific guidelines, determining available reinforcers, identifying responses acceptable for reinforcement, and planning how reinforcers will be scheduled so behavior is repeated.

Family Teaching

Behavioral Perspective

- Reprimanding children for their unacceptable behavior should be consistent and appropriate.
- Children will model behavior they see in their parents even if parents talk to children about not modeling that same behavior.

Critical Thinking

Children and the Media

How would the behavioral perspective explain the effect that the media (television, movies, videos, newspapers, the Internet) has on children and adolescents relative to violence, drug use, and promiscuity? What might you do to help caregivers concerned about this issue?

Reflective Thinking

Behavioral Perspective

How would you use social learning and conditioning to change your child's behavior and attitudes toward responsibility and accountability?

Social learning theory is also readily applicable to health care. Children often will cooperate with procedures (blood draws, X rays) if they see other children or adults they emulate cooperating for the same procedure. Nurses can help parents realize that their appearance and behavior is often imitated by their children, and determine who might be significant role models for their children to emulate. Finally, nurses need to demonstrate nurturing approaches or discipline methods so parents learn effective parenting practices.

REFLECTIONS FROM FAMILIES

I never realized the impact I have on my children until I heard 14-year-old Sarah tell 5-year-old Luke to "sit down and be quiet" when she was trying to study for a test she had the next day. She sounded just like me when I do not want to be bothered by one of the kids.

Cognitive-Structural Perspective

Cognitive-structural theorists are concerned with how children learn to reason, use language, and think, rather than what they learn. These theorists believe cognitive development is the result of the interaction between central nervous system maturation and active involvement with the environment. They also believe children constantly adapt to their world by integrating new knowledge with existing knowledge. The most significant cognitive-structural theorists are Jean Piaget and Lawrence Kohlberg.

Piaget and Cognitive Development

Jean Piaget (1896–1980) began studying children's intellectual development during the 1920s. He was fascinated by the process and steps children took as they discovered, reinvented, understood, and acquired knowledge of the world around them. He felt that from the moment of birth, children not only acted upon and transformed their environment, but also were shaped by the consequences of their actions. This constant interplay was responsible for intellectual growth.

Piaget believed intellectual growth followed an orderly progression based on the child's maturational level, experiences with physical objects, interactions with caregivers, other adults and peers, and an internal self-regulating mechanism that responded to environmental stimuli. He used several terms (schema, assimilation, accommodation, equilibrium) to describe cognitive development (Piaget, 1963).

To Piaget, interactions with the environment caused people to organize patterns of thought (**schema**), which they used to interpret or make sense of their experiences. For example, young children who believe the sun is alive because it moves are operating on the schema that moving things are alive. As children develop, they may regard other moving objects they see (wind up toy, animals) as alive as well, thereby demonstrating **assimilation,** or interpreting new information in terms of existing information. As they get older, children continually encounter animate and inanimate objects, and learn all objects are not alive. For example, trees do not move from one area of the yard to another even though they are alive. This more adequate understanding of differences between nonliving and living objects reflects **accommodation,** or revising, readjusting, or realigning existing schema to accept this new information. Assimilation and accommodation result in **equilibrium,** or harmonious relationships between thought processes and the environment (Piaget, 1963; Wadsworth, 1989).

Stages of Cognitive Development

According to Piaget, cognitive development occurs gradually, sequentially, and without regression. He postulated development moves from simple to complex, begins with concrete situations and objects, and proceeds to abstraction. Piaget suggested cognitive development passes through four stages and several phases within some of these stages. Stages represented increased integration and organization, and although sequential, children could pass through them at different rates. Table 6-6 presents Piaget's stages of cognitive development. Refer back to Table 6-3 to compare Piaget's stages with Freud, Erikson, and Sullivan.

During the **sensorimotor stage** (birth to age 2), the foundation of future cognitive functioning is established and sensory and motor capabilities are used to gain a basic understanding of the world. Infants learn goal-directed behavior, alternate ways of achieving a goal, the connection between cause and effect, and that they can make things happen. Infants also acquire a primitive sense of who they are and their relation to others, and realize objects continue to exist even after they are out of sight (object permanence). For example, 6-month-old infants will continue to look for a rattle that has been dropped on the floor even though they cannot see it.

The sensorimotor stage is divided into six phases. The **reflexive phase** (birth to 1 month) is characterized by pre-

TABLE 6-6 Stages of Piaget's Theory of Cognitive Development

Stage/Phase	Age	Characteristics
Sensorimotor	Birth to 2 years	
Reflexive	Birth to 1 month	Predictable, innate survival reflexes
Primary Circular Reactions	1 to 4 months	Responds purposefully to stimuli; initiates, repeats satisfying behaviors
Secondary Circular Reactions	4 to 8 months	Learns from intentional behavior; motor skills/vision coordinated; recognizes familiar objects
Coordination of Secondary Schemes	8 to 12 months	Develops object permanence; anticipates others' actions; differentiates familiar/unfamiliar
Tertiary Circular Reactions	12 to 18 months	Interested in novelty, repetition; understands causality; solicits help from others
Mental Combinations	18 to 24 months	Simple problem solving; imitates
Preoperational	2 to 7 years	
Preconceptual	2 to 4 years	Egocentric thought; mental imagery; increasing language
Intuitive	4 to 7 years	Sophisticated language; decreasing egocentric thought; reality-based play
Concrete operations	7 to 11 years	Understands relationships, classification, conservation, seriation, reversibility; logical reasoning limited; less egocentric thought
Formal operations	11 years and older	Capable of systematic, abstract thought

dictable, innate survival reflexes (sucking, grasping) becoming more efficient and generalized. During the **primary circular reaction phase** (1–4 months), the infant performs more complex, repetitive behaviors that appear to be responses to initial chance events centering on the infant's own body (following objects that disappear, expecting disappeared objects to reappear). They initiate and repeat satisfying behavior, and learn how their body feels. Infants during this phase commonly look and reach for objects in their environment. From 4 to 8 months, (**secondary circular reaction phase**), the infant learns from intentional behavior (shaking rattle to hear sound), usually explores the world from a sitting position, and begins to show some understanding of objects (recognizes familiar objects, searches for objects at the point they disappear). Motor skills and vision become further coordinated and interest in the environment increases. The **coordination of secondary schemes phase** (8–12 months) occurs when the infant understands concepts of space and object permanence, learns to direct actions toward an intended goal (searches for hidden objects; drops, throws, examines objects), and anticipates actions of others (caregiver comes with crying). They can differentiate objects (caregiver and stranger; familiar toy and unfamiliar toy), and begin developing individual habits or ways of learning about the world. The **tertiary circular reactions phase** (12–18 months) is characterized by interest in novelty and repetition (continually hitting toy hammer on variety of surfaces or objects), awareness that objects which are out of sight continue to exist, understand causality (if I throw my toy out of the crib, I cannot reach it), and can solicit help (obtain an unreachable toy). Between 12 and 18 months, solutions to problems will be discovered, objects will be increasingly explored to learn how they work, and new behaviors developed. During the **mental combinations phase** (18–24 months), young children are able to think before acting and use memory for simple trial and error problem solving. They can name and locate familiar objects, predict effects when observing causes, imitate behavior, and demonstrate symbolic and ritualistic play (Piaget, 1963).

During the **preoperational stage** (2–7 years), children use language and have a growing understanding of the past, present, and future. However, they have not yet developed the concept of irreversibility. That is, if one of two clay balls that are the same size is flattened in front of the child, the child will not believe the two clay balls still contain the same amount of clay. They do not fully grasp the relationship between objects and events, and do not understand the process of transition (if A is less than B, and B is less than C, then A is less than C). Their thought is egocentric (unable to take another's perspective), are easily fooled, respond to events and objects according to how they appear, are not able to understand the fundamental relationships among and between phenomena, and intermingle fantasy with reality. By the end of the stage they begin to realize others do not always perceive the world as they do (Piaget, 1963).

Piaget divides the preoperational stage into two phases, the preconceptual and intuitive phases. The **preconceptual phase** (2-4 years) is characterized by increasing use of language, egocentric thought, symbolic play, and mental imagery. During the **intuitive phase** (4–7 years), the child demonstrates more sophisticated language development, decreasing egocentrism, incessant questioning, and more reality-based play. Children during this phase are black/white in their thinking (cannot focus on more than one aspect of a situation at the same time, easily deluded by appearances, every question has a simple and direct answer), can concentrate either on the parts or the whole of an object but cannot relate to both at the same time, and cannot reverse actions, situations or physical properties of objects (i.e., wide and tall containers do not contain the same amount of water even if the child is shown that the containers have the same volume). They also believe inanimate objects have human feelings and are capable of human actions, assume everything has been created either by humans or a supernatural force, use symbolic play (pieces of wood become boats, trucks, cars, animals), and play-act events experienced in their everyday life (Piaget 1963).

Children acquire and use mental activities in the **concrete operations stage** (7–11 years) and begin understanding the basic properties of and relationships between objects and events (Figure 6-14). Their capability for logical reasoning is limited to their experiences. However, they are able to classify objects into several categories (size, shape, color), and understand the principle of conservation (things are the same even though shape or arrangement changes). They can also understand seriation according to a principle (arrange buttons according to size). Children in this stage tend to solve practical problems through trial and error, understand reversibility (a lump of clay contains the same volume when it is shaped into a ball or rolled into a rope), focus on several dimensions at the same time (color, size, shape), develop intricate rules, see others' viewpoints, and understand others' intentions (Piaget 1963).

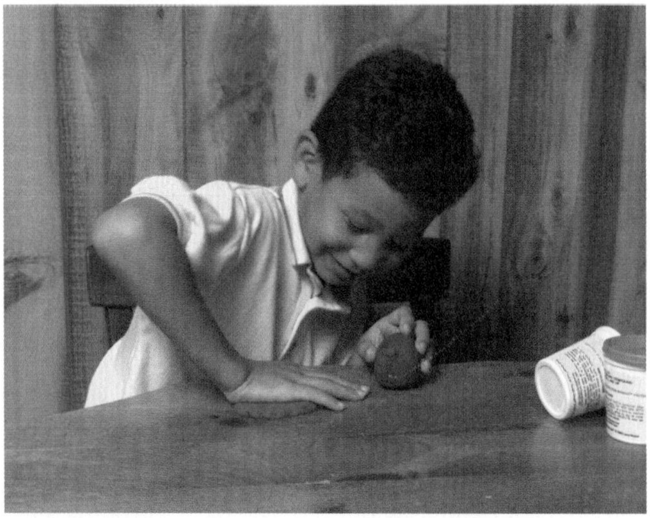

Figure 6-14 During concrete operations, children begin to understand the principle of conservation.

The **formal operations stage** (12 years and older) is characterized by systematic and abstract thought. Because they may enjoy thinking about hypothetical issues, children and adolescents in this stage may become idealistic. Their developing deductive reasoning abilities allows them to consider alternate solutions before choosing the correct answer. Their developing inductive reasoning ability allows them to organize and construct theories about their ideas. Children and adolescents in this stage move from what is real to what is possible, and can project themselves into and plan for the future. Finally, they have a better understanding of mathematics and scientific principles (proportion, variables) and are able to establish personal values and rules (Piaget, 1963).

Evaluation

Piaget has had a major influence on cognitive theory and caused developmental psychologists to focus on mental processes and their role in behavior. Today, most developmentalists accept Piaget's beliefs and have tested many of his propositions. They have demonstrated cognitive development is discontinuous and progresses through a series of different and increasingly complex stages. We now know children think differently than adults, and can only learn and do what they understand. Piaget's ideas influence child rearing and education by encouraging caregivers and teachers to be sure their efforts are understandable and children have first-hand experiences when learning about their world.

Those criticizing Piaget mention he defines his concepts rather loosely, pays little attention to the influences of emotions and motivation on learning, and underestimates the importance of adult interactions as a source of cognitive growth. They also suggest he does not fully explain how children progress from one stage to another and makes no allowance for cognitive growth continuing on through adulthood. Finally, Piaget does not acknowledge that people may advance to a certain cognitive level in one aspect of their lives but not in others, nor accept the idea that some people never reach the higher stages of abstract thought (Crain, 2000; Sigelman, 1999).

Application

Piaget's theory is especially important whenever communicating and interacting with children. This holds true not only when talking about health- and illness-related topics but also in any interactions at home, in the school, or in a community setting (Figure 6-15).

During the sensorimotor stage infants use sight and motor skills to learn about the environment and become familiar with their abilities. Manipulative toys, mobiles, and bright pictures or photographs are helpful since young children in this stage receive comfort from these objects. The environment should be safe, and opportunities provided for exploring and manipulating objects. During the preoperational stage children become more verbal but are limited in thought processes. They may often believe they are the cause of illness in themselves or someone they love. Therefore, careful explanations of experiences in language the child will understand are important. Children also need to be reassured that they are not responsible for illnesses in themselves or others.

School-aged children are in the concrete operations stage. This means they are capable of mature thought, but need to manipulate or see objects to understand how they are related, change, or interact. Details are important when providing explanations, but care should be taken so the child understands the discussion. Allowing children to manipulate or at least see equipment used in treatments and procedures or items talked about in classes will help them understand their experiences better.

Adolescents are capable of abstract thought (formal operations). Therefore, providing complete and clearly understood information, both verbally and in writing, is important. If adolescents have a chronic, long-term illness such as diabetes or cystic fibrosis, reeducation or clarification may help them learn more about their disease and its care. However, since all adolescents may not have developed mature abstract thought, parents, nurses, and teachers should always be prepared to provide information at a more concrete or individualized level.

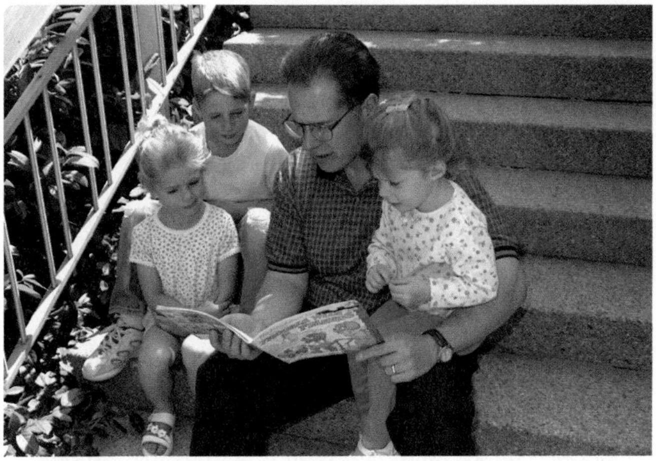

Figure 6-15 Reading to children is important in teaching them how things relate, change, and interact.

Kohlberg and Moral Development

Lawrence Kohlberg (1927–1987), inspired by Piaget, formulated a theory of moral development that described changes in thinking about moral judgments and reflected societal norms and values. In developing his theory, he asked children and

Family Teaching

Cognitive Development

- Remind caregivers their children may learn at different rates and in different ways. Even though adolescents are capable of formal operational thought, some still may use concrete operations.
- Encourage caregivers and family members to use simple language when talking with young children and help them understand directions may need to be repeated several times, or paired with a demonstration. Encourage family members to be patient with a child's questions as that is the way they learn about the world.

Reflective Thinking

Cognitive Development

Think about experiences in your own life that provide examples of Piaget's concepts of assimilation and accommodation. Describe them. Provide examples of formal and concrete operational thought. Do you use concrete operational thought more or less than formal operational thought? Explain your position.

Kids Want To Know

Helping with Homework

"How come Ryan doesn't understand the math problem? I've told him how to do it many times. It was easy for me" (question of a 13-year-old sibling when helping his 6-year-old bother with his homework).

Six-year-olds need lots of practice and explanations whenever you are helping them with homework. Some children catch on easily, but others need more time. Try to be patient and remember we all learn at our own pace.

Research Highlight

How Children Cope with Disasters

Study Purpose

To increase awareness of preschoolers', school-aged childrens', and adolescents' reactions to disasters in relation to Piaget's theory, describe behavioral symptoms signaling coping difficulties, and suggest effective nursing interventions.

Methods

Three case studies (a preschool child, a school-aged child, an adolescent) from the author's volunteer work among flood victims are discussed in relation to Piaget's theory.

Findings

Four-year-old Tameka illustrated sharks and monsters swimming around her house when asked to draw a picture of the flood disaster. The girl's view of the flood attacking her house is personified through Piaget's concept of animism. Tameka also demonstrated increased sleep problems after the flood, including sleepwalking to stranger's cots. John, age 9, demonstrated concrete operations as he recalled the events of the flood and analyzed the dangers and implications involved. John was also influenced by observing cues from others, including his parents and the media: he lost his dog in the flood and was afraid it had died after watching the news report of an animal shelter whose inhabitants had drowned. John misperceived his parents as "not caring" for his dog and therefore thought they did not care about him. Denise, a 13-year-old, demonstrated formal operations and, specifically, projection by directing her anger concerning the flood on her mother for not immediately replacing her clothes; she was concerned about her appearance and felt she was ugly. Denise also illustrated counterdependence by maturely caring for her grandmother, yet at the same time denying her own wish to be cared for. She also experienced separation anxiety from her mother and some regression.

Implications

Children at different ages react uniquely to disasters based on their cognitive development. Understanding and applying Piaget's theory to children in disasters can aid in appropriate interventions.

Citation

Deering, C. G. (2000). A cognitive developmental approach to understanding how children cope with disasters. *Journal of Child and Adolescent Psychiatric Nursing, 13*(1), 7–16.

adults to resolve a series of moral dilemmas, thereby challenging them to choose between obeying a rule, law, or authority figure and taking action to serve a human need that conflicts with these rules, laws, or authority figures. For example, should a mother who cannot afford an expensive drug that would save the life of her child steal the drug from a pharmacy? Kohlberg was interested in the underlying rationale for the moral decisions rather than the decision itself (Kohlberg, 1963).

He also believed the process of moral development was influenced by internal and external factors. Internal factors included empathy, intelligence, impulse control, and the ability to judge behavior. External factors included rewards, punishment, family structure, and parent/peer contacts (Lewis & Volkmar, 1990). Finally, he suggests moral growth progressed through universal and invariant sequences of three broad levels, each containing several stages. The stages cannot be skipped, and regression is not possible (Kohlberg, 1963). Table 6-7 presents Kohlberg's stages of moral development. Refer back to Table 6-3 for a comparison of Kohlberg's stages with Freud, Erikson, Sullivan, and Piaget.

TABLE 6-7 Stages of Kohlberg's Theory of Moral Development

Stage/Level	Age	Characteristics
Preconventional Level	Birth to 7 years	
Premoral Stage	Birth to 2 years	Cannot differentiate right from wrong
Punishment and Obedience Orientation Stage	2 to 3 years	Conforming behavior based on fear of punishment
Instrumental Realistic Orientation Stage	4 to 7 years	Conforming behavior based on rewards
Conventional Level	7 to 12 years	
Interpersonal Concordance Orientation Stage	7 to 10 years	Behavior evaluated on intent and other's reactions
Authority and Social Order Maintaining Orientation Stage	10 to 12 years	Obeys out of respect for laws, authority
Postconventional Level	12 years and older	
Social Contract/Legalistic Orientation Stage	12 years through adolescence	Believes laws should further human values and express majority views
Universal Ethical Principles Orientation Stage	Adolescence through adulthood	Right/wrong defined on universal, comprehensive, and consistent, yet personal ethical principles

Stages of Moral Development

The first level (**preconventional morality**), characterized by an egocentric focus, is divided into three stages. During stage 0 (**premoral stage;** birth to 2 years), impulses rule behavior. Infants and young children are unable to differentiate right from wrong. What is good is pleasant or exciting; what is bad is painful or feared. Stage 1 (2–3 years) is the **punishment and obedience orientation stage.** During this stage, behaviors, decisions, and conformity to rules are based on fear of punishment rather than respect for authority ("I do it because you tell me to and I don't want to be punished"). A child's "goodness" and "badness" are defined by consequences; the more severe the punishment, the more "bad" the act. During stage 2, called the **instrumental realistic orientation stage** (4–7 years), rules are obeyed to gain rewards or satisfy personal objectives. Sometimes the child does something to please others, but other times, children will make decisions and behave out of self satisfaction and self concern; something is done to get something in return ("I do it because it makes me feel good"). There is no feeling of gratitude, loyalty, or justice (Kohlberg, 1963).

The second level (**conventional morality**) is seen in the school years. Here, the individual is concerned with maintaining and valuing the rules and expectations of the family, group, or society. Conformity and loyalty are reflected in good behavior and societal approval. Stage 3 is **interpersonal concordance orientation,** or the "good boy," "good girl" orientation (7–10 years). Here, behavior and decisions are evaluated on the basis of one's intent ("he means well") and concerns about others' reactions ("I'll do it because you expect it and will give me something"). Behavior may also be evaluated on the basis of how the other person feels ("I know what its like to be cold, so I'll give you my sweater"). Stage 4 (10–12 years), **authority and social order maintaining orientation,** is characterized by believing laws should be obeyed because they are the laws and take precedence over any personal wishes, good intentions, or group beliefs. People conform to societal expectations because they want to preserve the social order, rather than because they are afraid of being punished (Kohlberg, 1963).

The third level is **postconventional morality** (12 years and older), with a universal focus where right, wrong, and moral values are defined autonomously and in terms of broad principles of justice that may conflict with authority figures or written laws. Stage 5 (**social contract legalistic orientation**) reflects awareness that just laws should be followed because they further human values and express the majority will. On the other hand, laws compromising human rights or dignity are unjust and should be challenged. Social rules are not the only reason for behavior and decisions; there are higher moral principles (equality, justice, due process) which also need consideration. Stage 6 (**universal ethical principle orientation**) is attained by few. Considered the highest moral state, right and wrong are defined on universal, comprehensive, and consistent, yet personal ethical principles. These ethical principles are abstract moral guidelines that include respect for individual rights and that transcend any law or social contract. People at this stage are able to see the perspective of anyone affected by a moral decision and can make a decision considered fair for everyone. They believe there is a higher order than the social order, and accept pain, death, and injustice as an integral part of existence (Kohlberg, 1963).

Research Highlight

Nursing Students' Moral Reasoning

Study Purpose

To explore the changes occurring in moral reasoning and the relationship between student characteristics and moral reasoning at admission (entry) and graduation (exit) from a baccalaureate nursing program.

Methods

A descriptive longitudinal and cross-sectional study involving a sample of 348 students who entered the upper division nursing program at the University of Minnesota in 1989, 1990, and 1992 served as subjects. Student characteristics including age at entry, gender, prior college credits, and grade point average (GPA) at entry were taken into consideration when examining moral reasoning scores at entry and exit. Students were administered the Defining Issues Test (DIT), which contains six brief moral dilemma stories; three from Kohlberg's instrument and three from Lockwood's instrument. After each story, subjects rated the items representing different ways of stating the critical issue described in the story on a five-point scale anchored by 1 = no importance and 5 = great importance. Subjects also ranked the four most important items. The P% score (which represented principled reasoning), calculated by summing all the item points including the rankings, and then dividing the score by 0.6, is considered the most useful of the scores and used in further analysis.

Findings

Women, older students, those with more college credits, and those with higher admission GPAs tended to have higher moral reasoning scores at entry to the nursing program. Higher DIT P% at graduation was seen more often in students of the female gender, students with higher admission GPAs, and those with more prior credits at admission. All students made significant improvement in moral reasoning scores between entry into and graduation from the program. Those students with lower scores at entry improved the most, and students in the highest scoring bracket at admission showed a negative mean gain. Correlations of DIT P% gain scores (the difference of P% scores at entry and exit) with admission GPA, prior college credits, and age at entry were all close to zero. Mean gain scores did not differ between men and women.

Implications

The overall trend in the improvement of DIT scores from entry to exit is encouraging and supports effectiveness of the baccalaureate nursing education. However, since the experience of higher education provides stimulation of moral reasoning development, the specific influence of the nursing program on moral reasoning is not known.

Citation

Duckett, L., Rowan, M., Ryden, M., Krichbaum, D., Miller, M., Wainwright, H., & Savik, K. (1997). Progress in moral reasoning of baccalaureate nursing students between program entry and exit. *Nursing Research, 46*(4), 222–229.

Evaluation

Kohlberg's theory is important, and offers a detailed stage sequence for moral thinking (Crain, 2000). However, Kohlberg's stages seem more helpful in describing the moral reasoning of adolescents and adults rather than young children. The stages are also clearly related to a person's level of cognitive development. In addition, proficiency at role taking may be necessary for conventional morality since reasoning here requires the ability to recognize another's point of view before being able to evaluate intentions capable of winning approval. Kohlberg also suggests intellectual growth does not guarantee moral development since those able to achieve the highest level of intellect may continue to reason about moral issues at the preconventional or conventional level.

Another criticism of Kohlberg's theory is its bias against women because his subjects were all male (Gilligan, 1977). Gilligan (1977) argues that women develop a different moral orientation than men because of how they are raised. Men are raised to consider moral dilemmas as inevitable conflicts between individuals that laws and other social conventions are designed to resolve (**morality of justice**). Women, on the other hand, are taught to be empathetic, nurturant, and concerned about others, and often define their sense of "goodness" in terms of their interpersonal relations (**morality of care**). However, there is little scientific evidence that women emphasize morality of care more than men do and that they travel different moral paths. Both men and women are concerned with issues of individual rights, justice, and the law, and raise issues of compassion and interpersonal responsibility when reasoning about real-life moral dilemmas (Smetana, Killen, & Turiel, 1991; Walker, de Vries, & Trevethan, 1987).

Family Teaching

Moral Development

- Explain to caregivers and other family members how moral development changes during childhood and why children of certain ages respond the way they do.
- Teach caregivers appropriate ways to help children learn ethical behavior.
- Provide examples of appropriate disciplinary practices caregivers can use for children of various ages based on their level of moral development.

Reflective Thinking

Moral Standards

Think about a moral dilemma that has affected you. Why do some people have higher moral standards than others? Apply your answer to Kohlberg's theory. How can you assist children and adolescents to develop high moral standards?

Application

Although Kohlberg offered age guidelines for his stages, they are approximate and many people do not reach the highest stage (Crain, 2000; Sigelman, 1999). Therefore, adults including nurses, teachers, and parents need to understand the stage a particular child is in relative to moral development. Parents need to be educated about normal behavior at each stage so behavioral expectations are appropriate and discipline is fair. For example, young children may stop hitting each other because of fear of being punished rather than because it is morally wrong, and show no remorse for their behavior. Parents also need to know that only when young children show interest in another's well being will they truly understand why it is wrong to hit others. In addition, children may participate in an activity for the wrong reason (to please others, to avoid punishment), and not fully understand the decisions they are making. In addition, whether or not rules are internalized may affect how well a new regime of care is accepted. Therefore it is important to give clear and specific reasons for requests or treatment regimes and be patient if there are questions or more information is needed. When moral dilemmas arise (should I do it if it is against my parent's wishes? will the new treatment really help or just prolong a painful condition?), clarifying, explaining, and validating concerns may help contribute to moral development.

Contextual Perspective

The contextual perspective adopts a broader focus by viewing human development as a lifelong process affected by other individuals or groups of individuals, and the historical, cultural, political, and economic context one lives in. Ecological theory is an example of the contextual perspective.

Ecological theory stresses the importance of understanding how relationships between the individual and a variety of environmental systems affect human development. The theory proposes changes in the environment produce changes in the individual, and changes in the individual produce changes in the environment. These interchanges occur simultaneously and continuously. Children are seen as active participants in creating their environments, and though biology is important, the main emphasis is on environmental systems. Development is viewed as continuous; experiences throughout the life span are important. However, situational influences have more impact on development than individual characteristics, and there are culture-bound principles explaining differences between individuals raised in different cultures (Asian, Italian, Swedish) and at different historical time periods (1920s, 1950s, 1980s).

Bronfenbrenner and Ecological Theory

Urie Bronfenbrenner (b. 1917) offers an organizational framework for examining the environmental systems' influences on human development (Bronfenbrenner, 1979). For him, the child's world is like a set of nested Russian dolls, with these systems (microsystem, exosystem, macrosystem) ranging from the most immediate setting or context (family, peer group), to the more remote setting or context (the government). The developing individual, embedded within the center of these systems, has a unique heritage (physical appearance, maturation rate, emotionality, innate intelligence, physical health, gender), which is different from any other person. As individuals mature, they impact and are impacted by these changing systems and relationships differently.

The broadest context or system affecting development is the **macrosystem.** This system is large, enduring, and contains cultural and subcultural ideologies and beliefs, hazards, resources, or lifestyles. Although macrosystem effects may not be obviously apparent in the life of any one individual, the macrosystem profoundly affects development (Bronfenbrenner, 1979). For example, children living in poverty or an inner city ghetto (the macrosystem) are exposed to beliefs and values that are different than those of children living in an affluent suburb.

The **exosystem,** or middle system, indirectly affects development. It includes social settings the individual never directly experiences even though these experiences provide an important influence (Bronfenbrenner, 1979). Examples of the exosystem are caregiver work settings, social networks, or educational level; one's neighborhood (including environmental noise or pollution); and community decision-making bodies. For example, when a caregiver travels a great deal or works different shifts, the child's family life may change. Children can be affected by whether or not a caregiver's work is satisfying or stressful, or if the caregiver has supportive social relationships. If a planning and zoning commission decides to build a highway through a neighborhood playground, the child's recreational life changes.

The **microsystem** is the child's immediate environment and includes daily interactions with others (family, peers, teachers, neighbors, religious leaders) or community resources (school, church) (Bronfenbrenner, 1979). The importance of the microsystem changes across development; during infancy, the family and home are of primary importance, whereas in middle childhood and adolescence, the peer group and school becomes more important (Figure 6-16).

The **mesosystem** is the interrelationship among two or more microsystems. For example, the interrelationship among the home, school, and peer group make up a child's mesosystem. For an adult, the mesosystem typically consists of family, employment situations, and friends. If the mesosystem has positive interrelationships, development will progress normally and optimally. If the mesosystem has negative interrelationships, development may not progress normally or optimally.

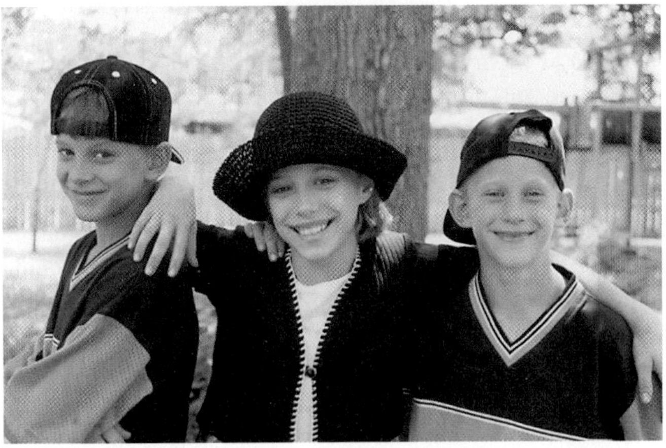

Figure 6-16 Family is important, and the connections made in childhood last throughout adulthood.

Evaluation

Bronfenbrenner brings a unique and essential perspective to the study of human development; the importance of analyzing relationships between the child and environmental systems. He also has emphasized the importance of examining connections between systems, and reminds us that children and their environments are always changing and influencing one another. One weakness of ecological theory is that it does not discuss the influence of biology or cognitive processes on development, and does not describe how these processes influence and are influenced by environmental systems. The theory also provides a limited view of development since it does not give a clear picture of the course of human development over the life span. Initially, it is difficult to generate principles about development that would be true for most people (Sigelman, 1999).

Reflective Thinking

Family Experiences

Is personality shaped by family experiences? If so, why are children from the same family often so different from one another?

Research Highlight

The Importance of Parents' Past Childhood Experiences on Current Parent–Infant Interactions

Study Purpose

To determine the relationship between the quality of interactions between infants and their parents, the current level of marital support for parents, and childhood experiences in the parents' families of origin.

Methods

When their infant was 12 months old, 66 mothers and fathers between 19 and 46 years of age completed a demographic questionnaire, the Dyadic Adjustment Scale, a self-report instrument with four subscales (affectional expression, dyadic consensus, dyadic satisfaction, dyadic cohesion), and the adult version of the Parental Acceptance-Rejection Questionnaire (PARQ). The PARQ measured parents' perceptions of feeling accepted by their own parents when they were between 7 and 12 years of age. The scale subscores are warmth/affection, aggression/hostility, neglect/indifference, and undifferentiated rejection. The quality of parent–infant interactions was measured by using the Nursing Child Assessment Teaching Scale, a standardized observational measure of parent teaching interactions. High scores in the subscales (sensitivity to cues, response to distress, social emotional growth fostering, cognitive growth fostering) indicate more responsive parenting interactions.

Findings

No relationship was found between mothers' childhood experiences, marital support, and the quality of their parenting interactions. Socioeconomic status did, however, predict mother–infant interactions; higher socioeconomic status was associated with more optimal parenting interactions. Fathers on the other hand, who perceived less positive childhood experiences (especially less acceptance) and had higher levels of marital support, were more responsive to infants in interactions.

Implications

Nurses need to remember that parents transfer, use, or modify experiences from their own childhood when interacting with their children, a child's family environment is important, and humans are malleable and can overcome adversity in the right situation. Nurses also need to remember that men and women have different childhood experiences that affect who they are, so our interventions need to be individualized.

Citation

Onyskiw, J., Harrison, M., & Magill-Evans, J. (1997). Past childhood experiences and current parent-infant interactions. *Western Journal of Nursing Research, 19*(4), 501–518.

Application

Bronfenbrenner provides a view of the child impacted by his environment in a way that is different from the behavioral perspective. In the ecological theory, the child is viewed holistically, as a member of a unique family, neighborhood, and cultural belief system, that impact development. The behavioral perspective on the other hand, proposes behavior is impacted by the environment consisting of models, rewards, or punishment only. Ecological theory also suggests the important influence parents have on their children, it reminds us home and cultural environments are not the same, and why those home resources and facilities must be assessed before discharge or prescribing home treatment/procedures.

Finally, ecological theory helps us understand that human development can proceed along several different pathways depending on the interplay of internal/external forces within the individual. All children in the same family really may come from different families, since a first child's experiences with parents may be different than a second or third child's experiences in the same family. Bronfenbrenner also reminds us the influence children have on parents and other family members is as important as the effect family members and parents have on children. It also teaches us to realize stress or illness in one family member will affect the entire family system. Parents with a hospitalized or ill child cannot always be at home with siblings or spouses; siblings may worry about, miss, or feel responsible for the ill child or, on the other hand, resent the attention the ill child receives.

Therefore, nurses implementing Bronfenbrenner's perspective in acute care and in the community will need to understand children in their environmental context, teach this information to parents, and allow for family differences. Other nursing considerations include educating parents and other family members (especially siblings), and appropriately conveying understanding and support of parents struggling with setting priorities relative to family and work commitments. Finally, nurses need to encourage sibling visits and contact with peers and extended family members.

There is no single principle, issue, or theory capable of holistically explaining human development. Therefore, it is important nurses be aware of the contribution each makes to understanding development and apply each in context. For example, behaviorists and social learning theorists help us understand how various stimuli, reinforcers, and models influence behavior. Psychoanalytic theory helps us understand the unconscious mind, reasons for abnormal behaviors, and the importance of the past in influencing present behavior. Erikson helps us realize the best solution to a stage crisis is not always positive; exposure to the negative conflict is sometimes inevitable and helpful. The cognitive theories, oriented toward explaining how we acquire and process information and become knowledgeable about the world, help us learn not only what to expect cognitively from children of all ages, but also help us understand how to challenge and stimulate learning at any age. Ecological theories remind us of the importance of the family, culture, and society in development. Therefore, it is essential that nurses develop an eclectic approach to human development, borrowing and using whatever is appropriate with individual children and their families as they practice holistic care.

Critical Thinking

Developmental Theories

How do the issues discussed in the early part of the chapter relate to the theories described in the later part of the chapter? That is, how does Freud or Erikson or Bandura or Piaget view the child—active or passive; innately pure or of original sin? How would Bronfenbrenner view the impact culture has on a child?

Reflective Thinking

Theory of Human Development

If you could develop a theory of human development, what would you propose? Upon which theoretical orientation do you lean most heavily in constructing your theory? What personal experiences have you had that might influence the developmental theory you would construct?

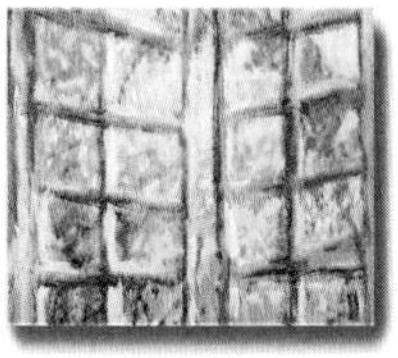

In the Real World

I never realized how important understanding the theories of human development was when I was in school. The all were so confusing and abstract. They didn't make any sense. I didn't understand why I needed to learn them. But now I know I cannot effectively care for children unless I use that knowledge. It is important to know that a 3-year-old needs to be encouraged to learn about the world, a 7-year-old needs friends to visit, an infant needs a primary nurse who meets needs promptly, and an adolescent may have many questions about their care and treatment regime. Now I know why we learn about the important influence parents have on their children and why siblings need to be included in care. I use those theories every day. I always did, I just didn't know it.

Key Concepts

- Principles providing a framework for studying humans suggest that development is orderly, sequential, directional, and interrelated; becomes increasingly differentiated, integrated, and complex as the child grows; and is unique for each child. Also, children are competent and possess qualities and abilities ensuring their survival and promoting their development, and children tend to learn one new skill at a time.
- Seven issues related to human development include nature versus nurture, continuity versus discontinuity, passivity versus activity, cultural versus sensitive periods, assumptions of human nature, universality versus context specificity, and behavioral consistency.
- The psychoanalytic perspective of human development is divided into the psychosexual, psychosocial, and

interpersonal theories. Major theorists are Freud, Erikson, and Sullivan.

- Behaviorism (classical and operant conditioning) and social learning emphasize the importance of the environment on human development. Major theorists include Pavlov, Skinner, and Bandura.
- Cognitive-structural theorists (Piaget, Kohlberg) are concerned about how children learn to think, use language, and develop moral reasoning.
- The contextual perspective suggests a variety of systems (microsystem, exosystem, macrosystem, mesosystem) and historical, cultural, political, and economic environments interact to impact human development. One major theorist is Bronfenbrenner.
- Each theory of human development contributes to our understanding of human behavior. Whenever caring for an individual child, the ecelctic approach to human development will help provide holistic care.

Review Questions

1. List the eight principles characteristic of human development and explain what each means.
2. List the seven issues characteristic of human development and explain each.
3. Summarize the main points of each theory. Which theorists describe life-span development?
4. Suppose a caregiver comes to you with questions regarding sibling rivalry. Using Piaget's theory, what advice would you offer?
5. Using the stages of moral development, provide examples of children's actions or behaviors that would be indicative of each stage.
6. Compare and contrast the theories discussed in the chapter.

References

Bandura, A. (1977). *Social learning theory.* Englewood Cliffs, NJ: Prentice-Hall.

Bornstein, M. H. (1989). Sensitive periods in development: Structural characteristics and causal interpretations. *Psychological Bulletin, 105*, 179–197.

Bronfenbrenner, U. (1979). *The ecology of human development.* Cambridge, MA: Harvard University Press.

Colby, A., Kohlberg, L., Gibbs, J., & Lieberman, M. (1983). A longitudinal study of moral judgement. *Monographs of the Society for Research in Child Development, 48*(1-2), Serial No. 200.

Crain, W. (2000). *Theories of development: Concepts and applications*, (4th ed.). Upper Saddle River, NJ: Prentice Hall.

Deering, C. G. (2000). A cognitive developmental approach to understanding how children cope with disasters. Journal of Child and Adolescent Psychiatric Nursing, 13(1), 7–16. Draucker, C. (1997). *Early family life and victimization in the lives of women. Research in Nursing and Health, 20*, 399–412.

Duckett, L., Rowan, M., Ryden, M., Krichbaum, D., Miller, M., Wainwright, H., & Savik, K. (1997). Progress in moral reasoning of baccalaureate nursing students between program entry and exit. *Nursing Research, 46*(4), 222–229.

Emde, R. N. (1992). Individual meaning and increasing complexity: Contributions of Sigmund Freud and Rene Spitz to developmental psychology. *Developmental Psychology, 28*, 347–359.

Erikson, E. (1963). *Childhood and society* (2nd ed.). New York: Norton.

Fisher, S., & Greenberg, R. (1977). *The scientific credibility of Freud's theories and therapy.* New York: Basic Books.

Freud, S. (1933). *New introductory lectures in psychoanalysis.* New York: Norton.

Gewirtz, J. L., & Pelaez-Nogueras, M. (1992). Skinner, B.F.: Legacy to human infant behavior and development. *American Psychologist, 47*, 1411–1422.

Gilligan, C. (1977). In a different voice: Women's conceptions of self and of morality. *Harvard Educational Review, 47*(4), 481–517.

Hetherington, M., & Parke, R. (1993). *Child psychology: A contemporary viewpoint* (4th ed.). New York: McGraw Hill.

Horowitz, F. D. (1992). John B. Watson's legacy: Learning and environment. *Developmental Psychology, 28*, 360–367.

Kidwell, J. S., Dunham, R. M., Bacho, R., Pastorino, E., & Portes, P. (1995). Adolescent identity exploration: A test of Erikson's theory of transitional crisis. *Adolescence, 30*(120) 785– 793.

Kohlberg, L. (1963). The development of children's orientation toward a moral order: I Sequence in the development of moral thought. *Vita Humana, 6*, 11–33.

Lewis, M., & Volkmar, F. (1990). *Clinical aspects of child and adolescent development* (3rd ed.). Philadelphia: Lea and Febiger.

Murray, R., & Zentner, J. (2001). *Health assessment and promotion strategies through the life span* (7th ed.). Upper Saddle River, NJ: Prentice Hall.

Onyskiw, J., Harrison, M., & Magill-Evans, J. (1997). Past childhood experiences and current parent-infant interactions. *Western Journal of Nursing Research, 19*(4), 501–518.

Parke, R., Ornstein, P., Rieser, J., & Zahn-Waxler, C. (1994). The past as prologue: An overview of a century of developmental psychology. In R. Parke, P. Ornsstein, J. Rieser, & C. Zahn-Waxler (Eds.), *A century of developmental psychology.* Washington, DC: American Psychological Association.

Piaget, J. (1963). *The origins of intelligence in children.* New York: Norton.

Sigelman, C. (1999). *Life-span human development* (3rd ed.). Pacific Grove, CA: Brooks/Cole.

Skeels, H. (1966). Adult status of children with contrasting early life experiences. *Monographs of the Society for Research in Child Development, 31*(9).

Skinner, B. F. (1953). *Science and human behavior.* New York: Macmillan.

Smetana, J. G., Killen, M., & Turiel, E. (1991). Children's reasoning about interpersonal and moral conflicts. *Child Development, 62,* 629–644.

Sullivan, H.S. (1953). *The Interpersonal Theory of Psychiatry.* New York: Norton.

Wadsworth, B. (1989). *Piaget's theory of cognitive and affective development* (4th ed.). New York: Longman.

Walker, L. J., De Vries, B., & Trevethan, S. D. (1987). Moral stages and moral orientations in real-life and hypothetical dilemmas. *Child Development, 58,* 842–858.

Suggested Readings

Angoff, W. (1988). The nature-nurture debate, aptitudes, and group differences. *American Psychologist, 43,* 713–720.

Bandura, A. (1986). *Social foundations of thought and action.* Englewood Cliffs, NJ: Prentice Hall.

Bem, S. (1989). Genital knowledge and gender constancy in preschool children. *Child Development, 60,* 649–662.

Berk, L. (1994). *Child development* (3rd ed.). Boston: Allyn & Bacon.

Bronfenbrenner, U. (1986). Ecology of the family as a context for human development: Research perspectives. *Developmental Psychology, 22,* 723–742.

Brooks-Gunn, J., Duncan, G., & Aber, L. (Eds.). (1997). *Neighborhood poverty: Context and consequences for children.* New York: Russell Sage Foundation.

Buckley, K. W. (1989). *Mechanical man: John Broadus Watson and the beginnings of behaviorism.* New York: Guilford Press.

Child Development and *Developmental Psychology*. These journals are two leading research journals in the field of child development and discuss the research interests of developmentalists over the years.

Colby, A., & Kohlberg, L. (1987). *The measurement of moral judgement. Vol 1: Theoretical foundations and research validation.* Cambridge, U.K.: Cambridge University Press.

Collins, W., Macoby, E., Steinberg, L., Hetherington, E., & Bornstein, M. (2000). Contemporary research on parenting: The case for nature and nurture. *American Psychologist, 55*(2), 212–232.

Cooper, M. (1989). Gilligan's different voice: A perspective for nursing. *Journal of Professional Nursing, 5*(1), 10–16.

Crews, F. (1996). The verdict on Freud [*Review of Freud evaluated: The completed arc*]. *Psychological Science, 7,* 63–68.

Harris, J. (1998). *The nurture assumption: Why children turn out the way they do.* New York: Free Press.

Kohlberg, L. (Ed). (1973). *Collected papers on moral development and moral education.* Cambridge, MA: Moral Educational Research Foundation.

Louv, R. (1990). *Childhood's future.* Boston: Houghton.

Mullahy, P. (1970). *Psychoanalysis and interpersonal psychiatry: The contributions of Harry Stack Sullivan.* New York: Science House.

Peter, E., & Gallop, R. (1994). The ethic of care: A comparison of nursing and medical students. *Image: Journal of Nursing Scholarship, 26*(1), 47–51.

Santrock, J. W., & Yussen, S. R. (1992). *Child development: An introduction* (5th ed.). Dubuque, IA: W. C. Brown.

Schuster, C., & Ashburn, S. (1992). *The process of human development: A holistic life-span approach* (3rd ed.). Philadelphia: Lippincott.

Walker, L. (1989). A longitudinal study of moral reasoning. *Child Development, 60*(1), 157–166.

Watson, J. B. (1928). *Psychological care of infant and child.* New York: Norton.

Whitener, L., Cox, K., & Maglich, S. (1998). Use of theory to guide nurses in the design of health messages for children. *Advances in Nursing Science, 20*(3), 21–35.

Resources

Organizations and Websites

American Academy of Pediatrics
141 Northwest Point Blvd.
Elk Grove Village, IL 60007-1098
(847) 228-5005
www.aap.org

American Academy of Family Physicians
11400 Tomahawk Creek Parkway
Leawood, KY 66211-2672
www.aafp.org

American Association for Maternal and Child Health, Inc.
P.O. Box 965
Los Altos, CA 94022

American Pediatric Society
P.O. Box 1487
St. Louis, MO 63178

American Psychological Association
1200 17th St. NW
Washington, DC 20036
(202) 955-7600
www.apa.org

Pediatrics
www.pediatrics.org

Society for Research in Child Development
505 E. Huron # 301
Ann Arbor, MI 48104-1567
www.srcd.org

The Children's Defense Fund
122 C Street, N.W.
Washington, DC 20001
(800) 424-9602
www.childrensdefense.org

The Children's Foundation
1420 New York Ave. NW, 8th Floor
Washington, DC 20005

CHAPTER 7

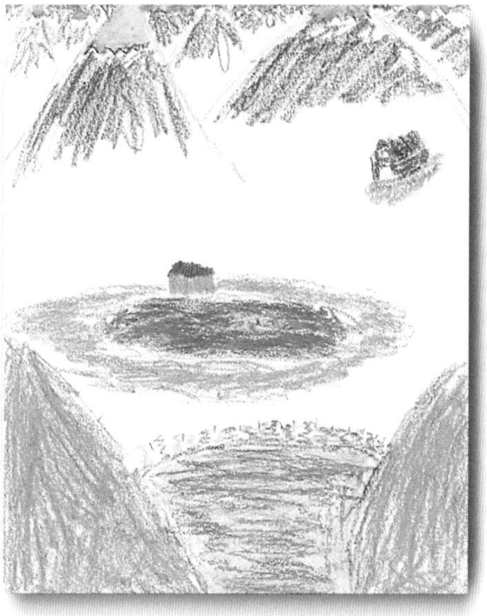

GROWTH AND DEVELOPMENT OF THE NEWBORN

Patricia King, RN, FNP
Natalie Annen-Ricks, BSN

I was so frightened when the nurse brought Ahmed in to my room a few hours after he was born. She said that he was beautiful baby and I must be very happy. She also told me that, since I was a pediatric nurse, I probably already knew how to take care of newborn babies and also how to breastfeed. She was wrong! I had never been a mother before and even though I'd worked for a few years in pediatrics, it was different when you are the mother not the nurse. I wanted her to teach me everything new mothers are taught and to assume that I was just like any other new mother.

COMPETENCIES

Upon completion of this chapter, the reader will be able to:

- *Identify the adaptive changes that occur during the transition to extrauterine life.*
- *Describe the normal physiological development of the newborn.*
- *Discuss the psychosexual, cognitive, and psychosocial development of the newborn.*
- *Identify and explain aspects of health promotion and maintenance pertinent to the newborn.*
- *Describe family educational needs regarding health promotion of the newborn.*
- *Explain the etiology and treatment of the high-risk newborn.*
- *Discuss the nurse's role in caring for healthy and high-risk newborns.*

The neonatal or newborn period is defined as the first 28 days, or 4 weeks, of life. This chapter will present the normal changes that occur during the transition to extrauterine life and the normal physiological, psychosexual, cognitive, and psychosocial development that occurs during the newborn period as well as information related to the high-risk newborn. Nursing care of the normal and high-risk newborn will also be presented.

EXTRAUTERINE TRANSITION

Fetal circulation is different from neonatal circulation due to structural differences that include the (1) placenta, (2) umbilical arteries and veins, (3) ductus venosus, (4) foramen ovale, and (5) ductus arteriosus. The placenta provides oxygen and nutrients for the fetus, and removes carbon dioxide and other waste products. The umbilical cord connects the fetus to the placenta, and contains two arteries and one vein. Blood from the placenta flows through the umbilical vein to the abdominal wall of the fetus. The umbilical vein then divides into two branches. A small portion of the blood flows through one branch and to the liver, sinusoids, and hepatic vein before entering the inferior vena cava. Sixty percent of the blood flows through the **ductus venosus** (a shunt in the fetus that carries oxygenated blood from the umbilical veins) and directly enters the inferior vena cava (Moller & Dwan,

1992a). The blood then enters the right atrium. Most blood will bypass the fetal lungs via the **foramen ovale** (an opening between the right and left atria) and enter the left atrium. From the left atrium, the blood enters the left ventricle and is pumped into the aorta to the hypogastric arteries. The small amount of blood that does pass from the right atrium to the right ventricle will pass into the pulmonary artery. From the pulmonary artery, a small amount will go to the nonfunctional lungs into the pulmonary vein, left atrium, left ventricle, and to the aorta. The remainder of the blood will pass through the **ductus arteriosus** (channel between the main pulmonary artery and the aorta) to the aorta. The hypogastric arteries lead to the iliac arteries, which give rise to the umbilical arteries, which then return the blood to the placenta. Figure 7-1 represents fetal blood flow.

The transition to extrauterine life begins with the loss of the umbilical cord and the initiation of respirations. With the initiation of respirations, the PaO_2 levels are increased, and several changes occur. Decreased pulmonary vascular resistance results in increased pulmonary blood flow, causing an increase in the pressure of the left atrium, a decrease in pressure of the right atrium, and closure of the foramen ovale. The foramen ovale closes shortly after birth and then undergoes fusion of the tissue margins during early childhood. Increased PaO_2 levels also lead to an increase in systemic vascular resistance, a decrease in systemic venous return, cessation of umbilical venous return, and closure of the ductus venosus. The closure of the ductus venosus occurs gradually over a period of about 2 weeks. Since systemic resistance is greater than pulmonary resistance, a left-to-right shunt occurs within the heart, resulting in closure of the ductus arteriosus (usually within 24 hours of birth) and gradual obliteration over the next month (Moller & Dwan, 1992b). Figure 7-2 represents transition to extrauterine life.

The average period of transition is 6–12 hours, but may be shorter or longer depending on the neonate's ability to adjust to the stresses of labor, delivery, and a new environment (Kelly, 1994). Therefore, during this transition period, the neonate needs to be closely observed for any difficulties so that appropriate interventions can be offered.

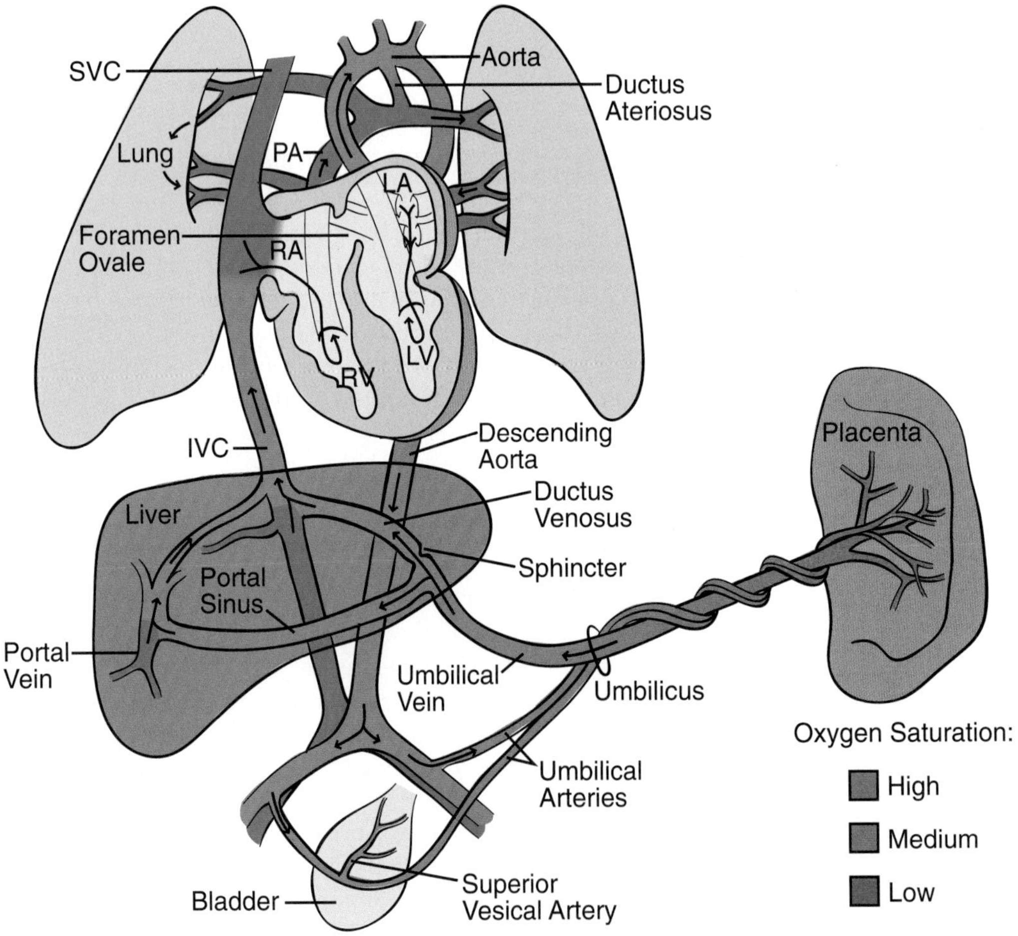

Figure 7-1 Fetal Circulation

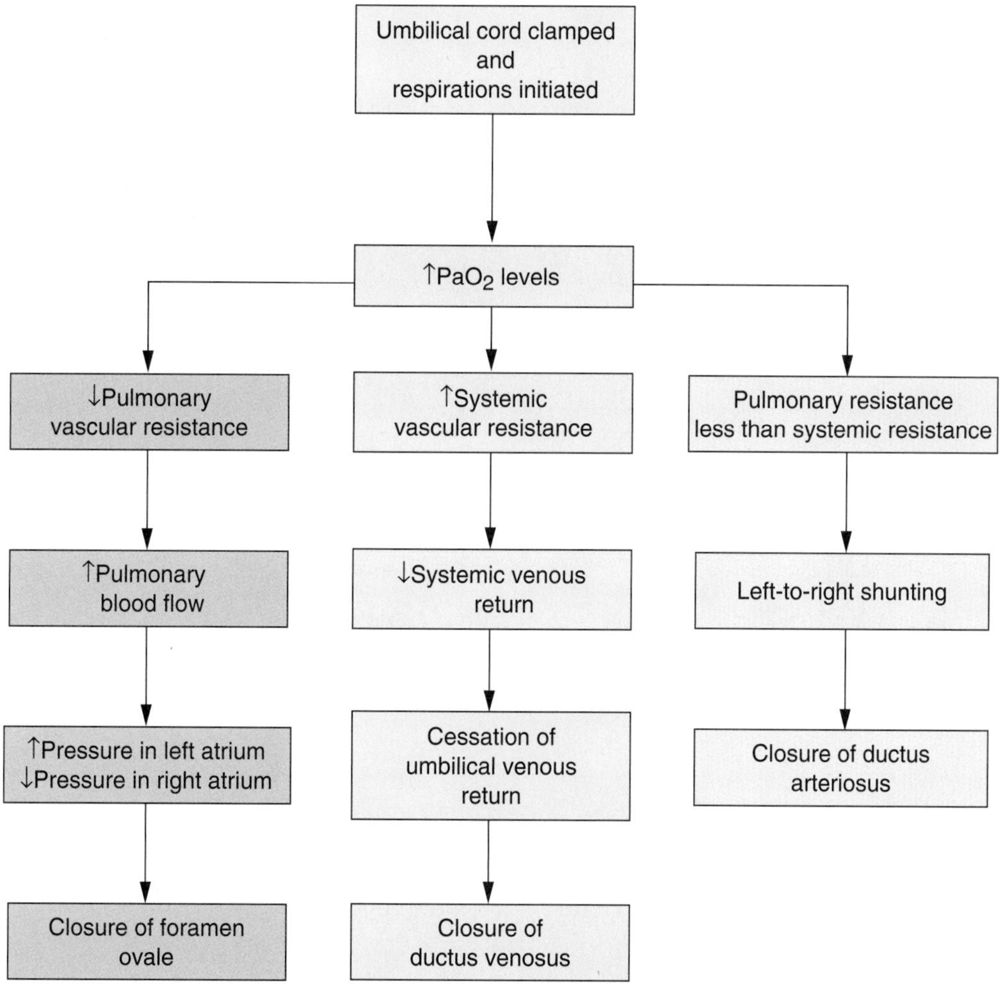

Figure 7-2 Transition to Extrauterine Life

PHYSIOLOGICAL DEVELOPMENT

General Appearance

Most people visualize a newborn as the baby seen in advertisements (Figure 7-3); however, the actual appearance may be a surprise to caregivers. The newborn's head, which is one-quarter of the total body size, may appear out of proportion to the body and be misshapen due to the labor and delivery process (**molding;** Figure 7-4). A **caput succedaneum** may be present as well, especially after a long labor. A caput is the swelling of the soft tissues of the scalp. The swelling may extend across the suture lines, is evident within 24 hours after birth, and usually resolves within a few days. The collection of blood between the skull bone and the periosteum as a result of the rupture of blood vessels secondary to head trauma from the birth process may result in a **cephalhematoma.** A cephalhematoma develops 24–48 hours after birth and does not cross the suture lines (Figure 7-5). A cephalhematoma may take 2–3 weeks to resolve. Reassurance to the caregivers is needed that many of these characteristics will change over the future weeks and months and that the

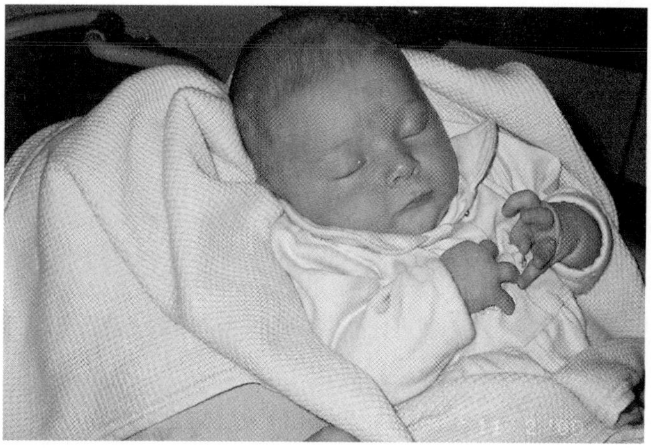

Figure 7-3 Newborns spend many hours of the day sleeping.

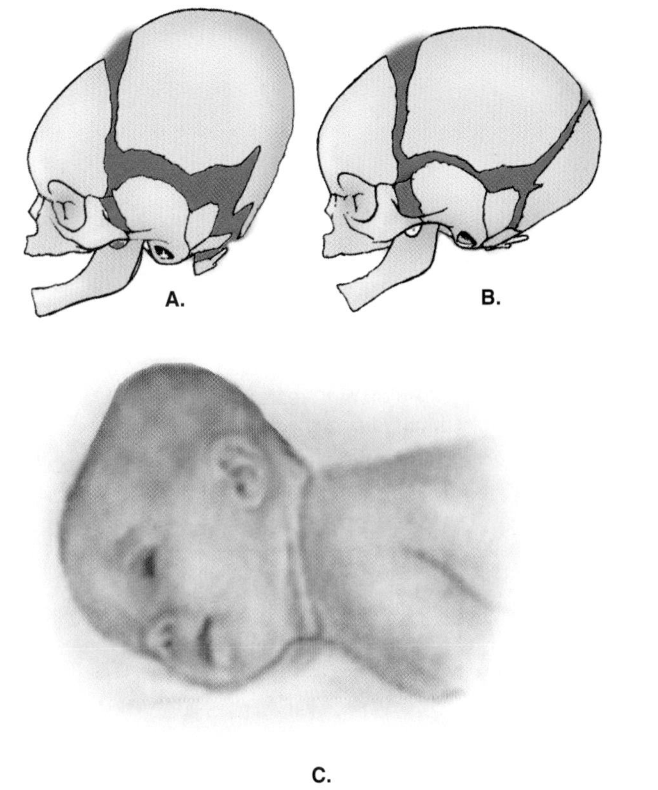

Figure 7-4 Molding. (A) Movement of Cranial Bones During Labor. (B) Cranial bones return to their proper placement in 2 to 3 days. (C) Infant Exhibiting Molding.

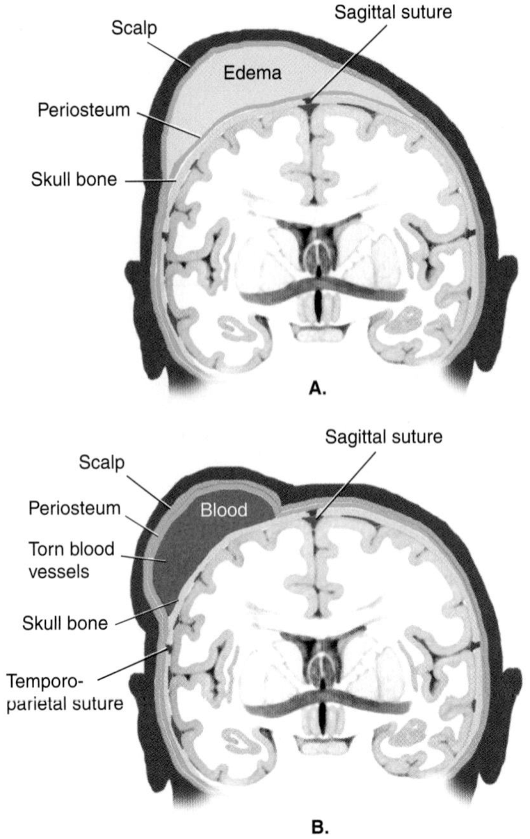

Figure 7-5 (A) Caput Succedaneum and (B) Cephalhematoma

newborn will then begin to take on the appearance of a "normal" baby.

Eyelids may be puffy and eye color indistinguishable. In addition, the newborn has a large, round abdomen with an umbilical area that may protrude for several weeks until the cord stump falls off. The caregiver should be instructed on appropriate umbilical cord care.

The extremities may appear short in comparison to the body, but hands should be able to touch the upper thighs when extended. The legs may appear to be bowed and the newborn typically remains in a position with the extremities flexed. The skin is delicate, often mottled, or **acrocyanosis** may be present. Acrocyanosis is the bluish discoloration of the hands and feet caused by the instability of the peripheral circulation system.

Many caregivers are afraid to touch the baby's head or "soft spot" due to the fear of causing damage. The soft spots, or **fontanels,** occur at junctions or suture lines of the skull bones, allowing for adaptation to the pelvis shape during delivery and growth of the brain over the coming year (Figure 7-6). The posterior fontanel typically closes by 3 months of age, while the anterior fontanel closes around 8–18 months of age. Caregivers need reassurance that many of these characteristics will change during these time periods

Family Teaching

Cord Care

- The diaper needs to be folded or diapers with a notch may be used to provide air circulation to the cord.
- Cord care with 70% isopropyl alcohol or hydrogen peroxide should be performed during diaper changes. It is important to make sure the substance is applied to the base, next to the skin. A small amount of blood may appear on the diaper when the cord falls off.
- Continue to provide cord care after the cord falls off until the skin appears normal.
- Never pull the cord off or attempt to loosen it.

and the newborn will then begin to take on the appearance of a "normal" baby.

Neurological System

The initial neurological examination should include observation of the newborn's position and response to handling

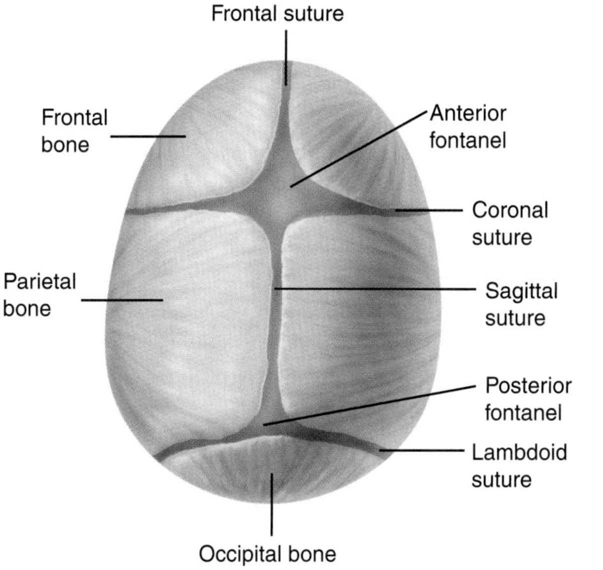

Figure 7-6 Placement of Sutures and Fontanels

and stimulation, as well as a determination of gestational age. The use of the Ballard score assists in determining the gestational age of the newborn. For accuracy and validity the examination should be completed within the first 12 hours of life (Ballard, Khoury, Wedig, Wang, Eilers-Walsman, & Lipp, 1991); (refer to Figure 7-7 for the Ballard Assessment Scale of Gestational Age). After the determination of gestational age, the newborn can be classified as (1) **large for gestational age (LGA),** (2) **appropriate for gestational age (AGA),** or (3) **small for gestational age (SGA).** Newborns who are above the 90th percentile are classified as LGA. The AGA newborn is one who lies between the 10th and 90th percentile. The SGA newborn will fall below the 10th percentile. How the newborn is classified will assist in determining appropriate care, since immaturity may influence the newborn's optimal neurological development and functioning. Refer to the high-risk section of this chapter for more information on LGA and SGA newborns.

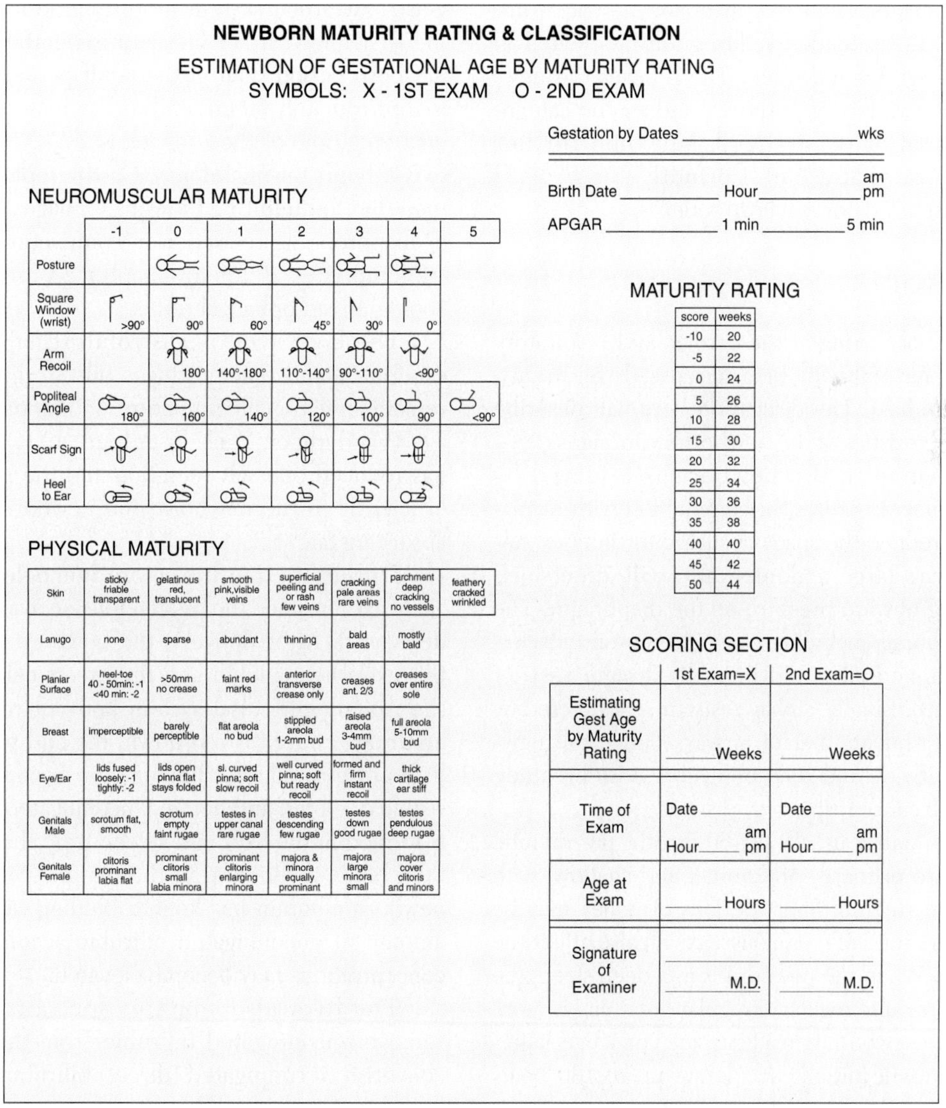

Figure 7-7 Ballard Assessment Scale

Kids Want To Know

How come Maggie always has such funny positions and always grabs my finger?

Those are reflexes that all newborns have. They will disappear within the next few months.

Nursing Tip:

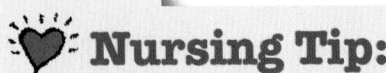

Infant immunity

The newborn immune system is very immature. Some immunity is passed transplacentally from the mother (Behrman and Kliegman, 1990). Additonal immunity is transferred in breast milk.

Most of time the newborn is in a sleep state with short periods of wakefulness between those sleep states. These times provide for caregiver interaction. As the newborn advances to the infant stage, the periods of wakefulness will increase, allowing for more interactions. The newborn is able to respond to the environment and stimulation by changing expression (smiling, grimacing, crying). The caregivers may need assistance in deciphering these signals into a specific meaning for their baby.

Primitive, innate behaviors seen in the newborn are known as reflexes. Deep tendon reflexes can be elicited in the newborn but have limited value. The reflexes the newborn exhibits serve a variety of purposes, and can be categorized into localized or generalized, and then further separated into those that are of a primitive or survival nature. Refer to Table 7-1 for newborn reflexes.

Cardiorespiratory System

The major changes occurring in the cardiac and respiratory system after birth have already been discussed (see transition to extrauterine life). The discussion here will describe and focus on characteristics of the newborn's vital signs.

Lung compliance in the newborn is affected by anatomy. Mediastinal structures, in conjunction with a relatively large heart, reduce the space available for lung expansion. The newborn's large abdomen also will affect lung space by increasing upward pressure on the diaphragm. The structures of the thorax, including weak intercostal muscles, horizontally positioned ribs, and high diaphragm restrict lung expansion space. Finally, airway resistance is affected by the length, radius, and number of airways. Since the newborn has smaller airways and is an obligatory nose breather, any obstruction will cause respiratory distress.

The respiratory rate is usually 30–60 breaths per minute. The respirations are primarily abdominal and shallow, with irregular depth and rhythm. Short periods of apnea may be seen. The newborn's state of consciousness will also affect the respiratory pattern. When the newborn is in a deep sleep, the respiratory pattern is quite regular. Irregular breathing is more noticeable when the newborn is in a light sleep or active state.

The heart rate will initially accelerate up to 180 beats per minute following the first breath. This increase is for a brief period and after 4 hours of life, stroke volume and heart rate decrease and approximate normal ranges (Walther, Benders, & Leighton, 1993). The heart rate will range from 100 beats per minute while asleep to 150 beats per minute while awake. The blood pressure is affected by the changes in blood volume that occur during transition, and the newborn's birth weight and activity state.

Gastrointestinal System

Gastrointestinal system motility gradually matures during the first few years of life, and is significantly slower in the newborn period than in the adult period. Stomach capacity is approximately 60 mL and will increase during infancy. The emptying time of the stomach is $2\frac{1}{2}$–3 hours, and increases to 3–6 hours during infancy. Gastroesophageal reflux is common due to diminished lower esophageal sphincter function or inappropriate relaxation in conjunction with delayed gastric emptying. Refer to Chapter 23 for more information about gastroesophageal reflux.

The liver, from a gastrointestinal standpoint, is an exocrine gland that produces bile to digest fats. The liver remains functionally immature until approximately 1 year of age (Vanderhoof, Zach, & Adrian, 1994). Because the liver has reduced bile salt secretion and the pancreas works less efficiently in the newborn, the newborn is less capable of absorbing fat.

During uterine life, more hemoglobin is required to carry oxygen since the oxygen tension available to the fetus is decreased. After delivery, the newborn no longer requires this extra hemoglobin and the excess cells are destroyed by the reticuloendothial system and not replaced. When the erythrocytes are broken down, the end products of metabolism are formed, and hemoglobin becomes a protein, consisting of globin and heme. Unconjugated (indirect) bilirubin is formed in the liver and spleen from these byproducts, and then binds to albumin in the plasma (Maisels, 1994). Since newborn albumin has limited binding capacity, a significant amount of unconjugated bilirubin accumulates and plasma concentrations may become elevated.

The liver also contains specialized cells that will remove unconjugated bilirubin from the bloodstream and convert it to conjugated (direct) bilirubin. Since conjugated bilirubin is water soluble, it can then be excreted through the stool as bile (Maisels, 1994). However, the newborn's

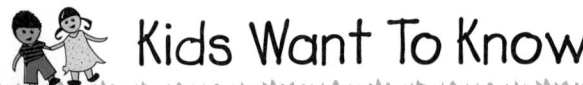

TABLE 7-1 Neonatal Reflexes

Reflex	Stimuli	Response	Disappears	Pathology If Abnormal
LOCALIZED REFLEXES				
Eyes				
Blinking or corneal reflex*	Sudden appearance of a bright light or approach of an object toward cornea	Infant blinks	Persists throughout life	Neurological damage
Doll's eye	Head moved slowly to right or left	Eyes lag behind and do not immediately adjust to new position of head	As ability to fixate develops	Neurological damage
Pupillary*	Bright light shines toward pupil	Pupil constricts	Persists throughout life	Neurological damage
Nose				
Sneeze*	Irritation or obstruction in nasal passages	Sneezing	Persists throughout life	Neurological damage
Mouth and throat				
Cough	Irritation of laryngeal or tracheo-bronchial tree mucous mem-branes	Coughing	Persists throughout life	Neurological damage
Extrusion	Depressing or touching the tongue	Tongue is forced outward	4 Months	
Gag*	Food, suction, or passing a tube stimulating the posterior pharynx	Gagging	Persists throughout life	Neurological damage
Rooting* 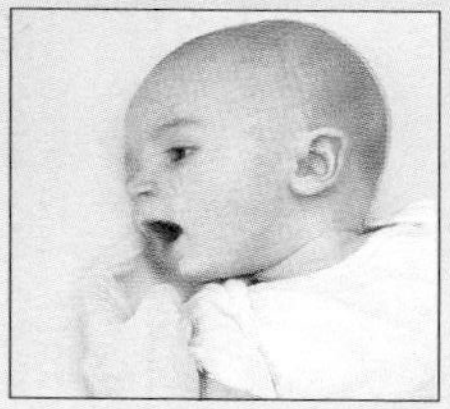	Stroke or touch cheek	Head turns toward stimuli	Approximately 4 months	Central neurological system disease (frontal lobe lesion)
Sucking* 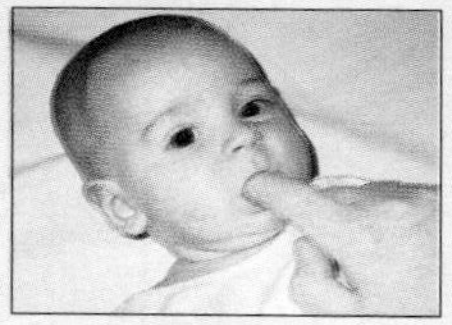	Object touching lips or placed in mouth	Sucking	7 Months	Prematurity; CNS depres-sion in full-term breastfed newborn whose mother has ingested barbiturates

* Survival reflex

continues

TABLE 7-1 *Continued*

Reflex	Stimuli	Response	Disappears	Pathology If Abnormal
Yawn	Decreased oxygen	Baby yawns	Persists throughout life	
Extremities				
Babinski† 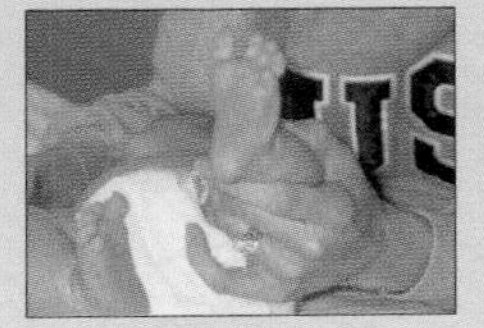	Lateral aspect of the sole is stroked from heel upward and across ball of foot	Hypertension of the toes	1 Year	Cerebral palsy
Grasp†	Palms of hands or soles of feet are touched near base of digits	Flexion of hands and toes	8 Months	
Palmar grasp† 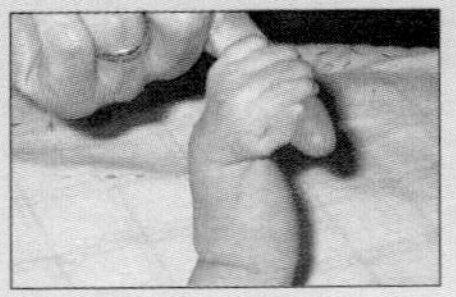	Stimulate the palm	Object is grasped	4 Months	Frontal lobe lesions
Plantar grasp† 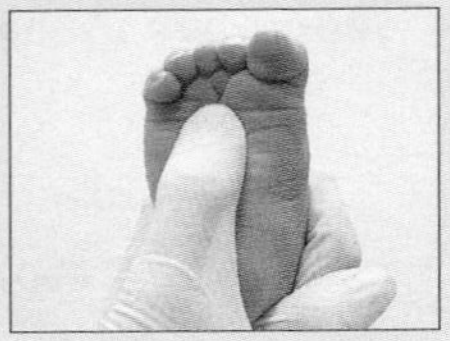	Place the thumb at the base of the newborn's toes	Toes will curl downward	8 Months	Cerebral palsy; obstructive CNS lesion (abscess, tumor)
MASS REFLEXES				
Crawl	Infant placed on abdomen	Makes crawling movements with arms and legs	6 Weeks	Neurological damage
Dance or step† 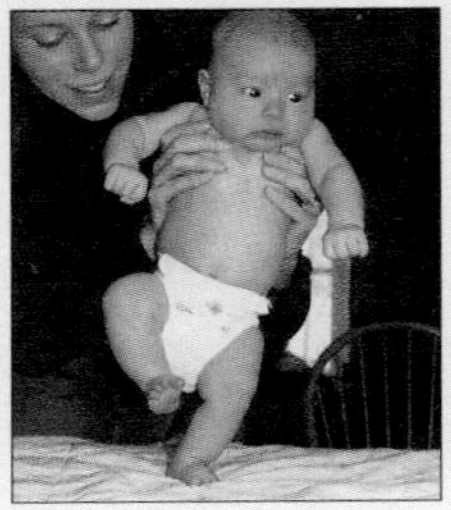	Newborn is held upright, one foot is allowed to touch a flat surface	Alternate stepping movements	4 Months	Cerebral palsy

TABLE 7-1 *Continued*

Reflex	Stimuli	Response	Disappears	Pathology If Abnormal
Moro† 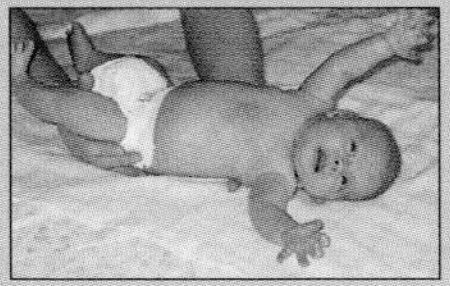	Sudden changes in position or jarring	Arms extend, head moves back, fingers spread apart with thumb and forefinger forming a "c" followed by arms being brought back to center with hands clenched, spine and lower extremities extended	3–4 Months	Neurological damage
Placing 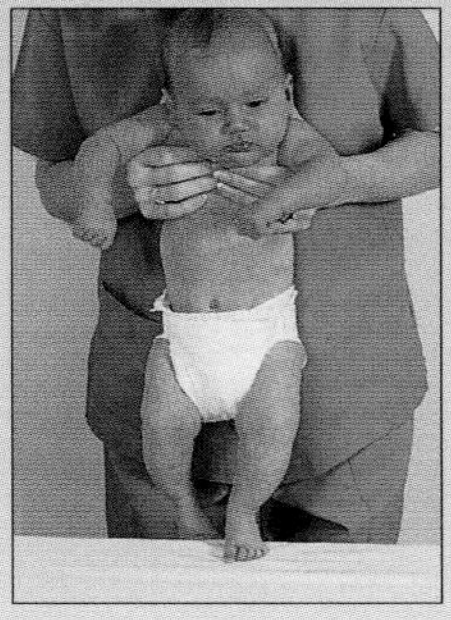	Held upright; dorsal surface of the feet touch the edge of the table	Flexion of the knees and hips and movement of the legs up the table surface	4 Months	Breech paralysis; cerebral cortex abnormalities
Tonic neck 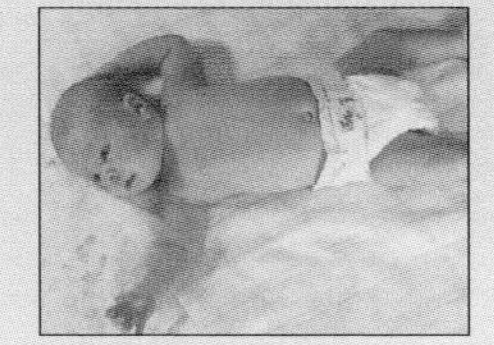	Head turned to one side when supine	Arm and leg extend on the side head is turned toward; arm and leg flexed on opposite side	3–4 Months	Neurological damage
Trunk incurvation (Galant) 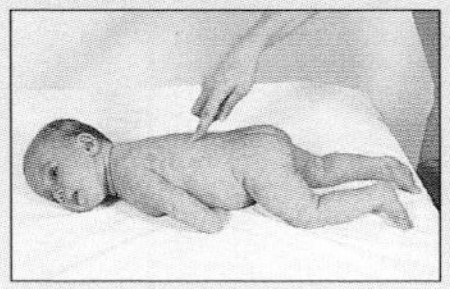	Firmly stroke the back in a downward motion for about 5 cm (2 in.) when in prone position	Body curves to the side of the stimulus. Important to check both sides.	2–3 Months	Spinal cord lesion

† Primitive reflex

immature liver is not always able to adequately alter and remove the excess bilirubin, and as the amounts accumulate, visible **jaundice** (the yellowish discoloration of the skin and eyes caused by excess bilirubin) occurs. Visible jaundice in a normal newborn should be investigated per hospital protocol, such as obtaining blood levels for the total and direct bilirubin.

Physiologic or normal jaundice shows a gradual rise in bilirubin of 8 mg/dL at 3–5 days after birth. The level falls to normal the second week of life. Pathologic or abnormal jaundice is seen with an extreme elevation in bilirubin within the first 24 hours of life. If the unconjugated level is >12 mg/dL when the baby is formula-fed, >14 mg/dL if the baby is breast-fed, or if the jaundice is persistent past 2 weeks of age further evaluation is warranted. Causes of pathologic jaundice may include fetal–maternal blood group incompatibility, nonspecific hemolytic anemias, sepsis, polycythemia, or infants of diabetic mothers.

Kernicterus is a form of newborn jaundice where nuclear masses of the brain and spinal cord undergo pathologic changes accompanied by deposition of bile pigments within them; it can occur when levels of bilirubin reach toxic levels. Kernicterus can lead to permanent brain damage since the lipid-rich nervous system is susceptible to toxicity caused by increasing levels of unconjugated bilirubin.

Phototherapy, or the use of special high-intensity fluorescent lights, is generally an effective method of reducing serum bilirubin levels and preventing kernicterus. The phototherapy light oxidizes the unconjugated bilirubin in the skin, which then becomes soluble in water and is excreted in the stool and urine. The use of phototherapy, ordered by the primary care provider, may be administered in the newborn nursery or at home. The newborn's eyes should be shielded with special patches to prevent possible retinal damage when undergoing phototherapy, and the genital area covered with a surgical mask to provide protection to the gonads, since maximum exposure is accomplished when the newborn is unclothed (Figure 7-8).

Nursing Alert:

Eye and Skin Care During Phototherapy

The eyes of the newborn need to be protected while under phototherapy. The patches should be removed periodically, and the eyes and skin under the patches observed for irritation and breakdown. The skin should be examined for pressure areas and evidence of breakdown. The newborn should be repositioned every 2 hours. The newborn may experience loose stools and increased urine output, which may lead to dehydration and excoriation of the skin in the perianal area.

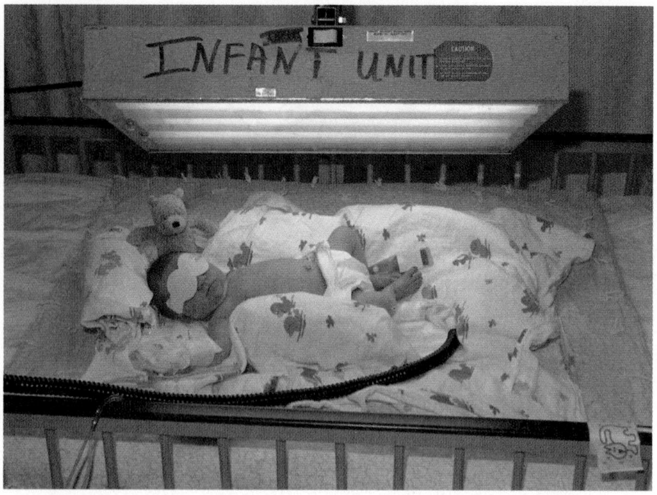

Figure 7-8 Newborn with Jaundice Receiving Phototherapy

Serial serum bilirubin levels, obtained every 8–12 hours while under phototherapy, may be used to assess treatment effectiveness. When the level returns to the normal range, phototherapy may be discontinued. Sometimes a rebound elevation of bilirubin occurs initially after phototherapy has been discontinued, but it should soon return to an acceptable level.

Genitourinary System

The kidneys are responsible for the regulation of fluid and electrolyte balance, arterial blood pressure, and the removal of some toxins. The fetus does not begin urine production with glomerular filtration until 9–12 weeks' gestation, with renal development continuing until 36 weeks' gestation (Bissinger, 1995; Brion, Satlin, & Edelmann, 1994). The term newborn's kidneys have a full complement of nephrons and even though the glomeruli are small, the surface area for filtration, in respect to body weight, is higher than the adult's. Since the glomeruli's full function is lacking, glomerular filtration rate is lower than in the adult. The newborn's renal tubules are short, narrow, and less able to concentrate urine due to the inability to reabsorb water, sodium, glucose, and other solutes back into the blood; the ability to concentrate urine completely will not be achieved until 3 months of age.

Urine output depends on the glomerular filtration rate and tubular reabsorption of water. Normal urinary output for a newborn is 1–3 mL/kg/hour (Brion, Satlin, & Edelmann, 1994). This is equivalent to approximately 2–6 voidings per day. The urine output is typically low during the first day of life and increases as daily intake increases. Renal function should be evaluated in a newborn that does not void in the first 24 hours of life. Normal newborn urine values are identified in Table 7-2.

TABLE 7-2 Normal Values for Newborn Urine

Color	Pale yellow
Glucose	Negative
pH	4.5–8
Protein	<5–10 mg/dL
RBC	Negative
Specific gravity	1.001–1.020
WBC	Negative

Male genitals are evaluated for the presence of testes and the appearance of the rugae on the scrotal sac. Prior to 36 weeks' gestation, the scrotum is small with few rugae (folds), the testes have not descended to the scrotum, and remain in the inguinal canal. The term newborn, however, will demonstrate a pendulous scrotum covered with rugae, with testes palpable in the lower portion of the scrotal sac. If the scrotum is distended, the use of a transilluminator may reveal a **hydrocele** or a collection of fluid between the parietal and visceral layers of the tunica vaginalis, the outermost covering of the testes. No treatment is usually necessary unless the hydrocele persists beyond the first year of life. Caregivers may need reassurance that this is normal and will soon disappear.

Circumcision is the surgical removal of the foreskin, the skin that covers the glans, or head, of the penis. When performed on the newborn this is considered an elective procedure. Circumcisions were initially based on a ritual from religious practices or "rites of passage" to manhood. This ritual continues in some religions today.

The decision to have the newborn male circumcised is left up to the parents. Factors that may affect their decision include cleanliness, tradition, possible prevention of cancer, and personal preference. As with any surgery there are risks involved when a circumcision if performed. Although rare, they may include hemorrhage, infection, injury to the penis, urethra, and scrotum, deformity, and scarring. Newborns that warrant a circumcision not being performed or delaying the procedure include those who are premature, ill, distressed at birth, or have hemophilia or any genitourinary abnormality. If circumcision is done, procedural anethesia should be used (AAP, 1999a).

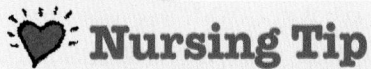

Reflective Thinking

Is circumcision necessary?

If the parents were undecided about having their newborn circumcised and asked you what you would do if you were them—how would you respond?

Family Teaching

Circumcision Care

The immediate care of the circumcised newborn is dependent on the procedure performed. *If the Plastibell was utilized*, it is left on the penis. Instruct the caregiver to gently lift the ring and squeeze warm water from a cotton ball on to the tip when changing the diaper. The ring will fall off in 7–10 days when the circumcision has healed—do *not* pull it off. *If the ring was not used*, there may be gauze on the penis. This may or may not be replaced depending on the person who performed the circumcision. Diapers should be changed often so urine and stool do not irritate the site. A thin layer of petroleum jelly may be applied to prevent the diaper from adhering to the circumcision site. Yellow exudate may be seen on the second day after the circumcision. This is granulation tissue and is normal and should not be removed.

Nursing Tip

Care of the uncircumcised newborn

The caregiver should be instructed to wash the outside of the penis to decrease the chance of odor and infection. **Smegma**, a collection of cells that shed from the outer layer of skin, gathers under the foreskin. Odor and infection may develop if the smegma is not removed. In the uncircumcised male the foreskin remains intact. The foreskin may not be retractable until the child is around 3 years of age. The caregiver must be cognizant of this so that they do not attempt to retract the foreskin and cause damage.

Eye On:

Circumcision

Male Jewish newborns may be circumcised on the 8th day of life at a religious ceremony. The circumcision is performed by a mohel, a person trained on performing circumcisions. Parents should be taught circumcision care prior to leaving the hospital even though the circumcision is done in the home. Anesthesia is not used. The infant is often give a bit of wine as part of the ceremony.

The appearance of female genitalia depends on subcutaneous fat deposition and gestational age. The newborn less than 36 weeks' gestation has a prominent clitoris with the labia majora small and widely separated. The term newborn will have the clitoris and labia minora covered by the labia majora. Vernix caseosa may be present between the labia. Occasionally, the hymenal tag may protrude from the floor of the vagina. Blood may be observed on the diaper due to the withdrawal of the maternal hormones at the time of delivery. This is called **pseudomenstruation,** and caregivers may need reassurance that this is normal and will soon disappear. See Box 7-1 for a description of stools produced by infant (Figure 7-9).

Musculoskeletal System

The term newborn exhibits hypertonic flexion of all extremities. Flexion development occurs in the lower extremities first; therefore, during examination, the legs should be assessed first. To assess flexation, place the newborn on a flat surface with the legs in flexion while manipulating the hip joint and placing a hand on the newborn's knees. After flexing the legs, extend them onto the flat surface and release. The full-term newborn's legs should recoil and quickly return to a flexed position. When examining the elbows, flex them by holding them for 5 seconds and then extending them. The term newborn's elbows form an angle of less than 90° and rapidly recoil back to a flexed position. Because a healthy but fatigued newborn may elicit a slower response, this test should be delayed for the first hour after birth.

Muscles in the extremities are not well defined, and muscle tone is not fully developed. Therefore, the newborn cannot support the full weight of the head, and head lag is seen if the newborn is pulled from a supine to a sitting position (Figure 7-10). However, in the prone position, the newborn is able to slightly raise the head (Figure 7-11). In addition, the hands should reach to the upper thighs when the upper extremities are extended. The legs should be equal length with symmetrical gluteal skin folds.

BOX 7-1 Stool patterns of newborn

Meconium–First bowel movement; black and tarry; usually occurs with 24–48 hours of birth

Transitional–Usually occurs by third day; green brown–yellow brown in color

Breastfed–Yellow to golden, pasty, sour-milk odor

Formula-fed–Pale to light yellow, firmer, strong odor

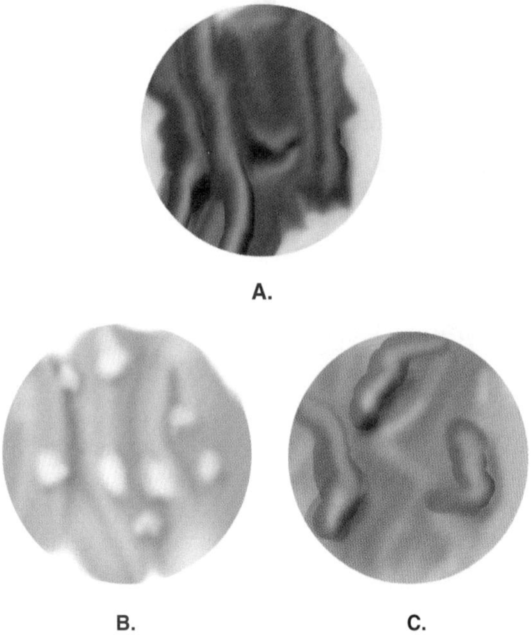

A.

B.

C.

Figure 7-9 (A) Meconium (B) Stool of Breastfed Infant (C) Stool of Formula-fed Infant

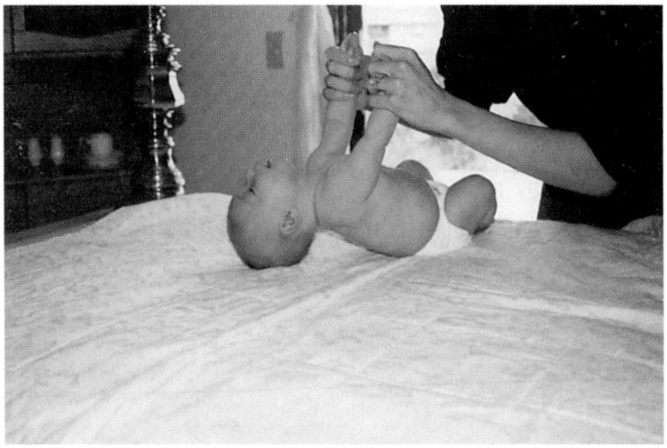

Figure 7-10 Head lag is seen when the newborn is supine and the body lifted.

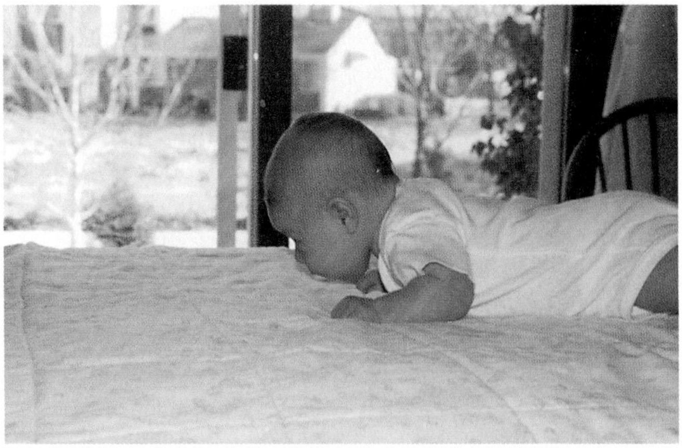

Figure 7-11 Newborns can hold their heads up when placed in a prone position.

Intrauterine positioning of the newborn's feet may result in a talipes deformity or clubfoot. Usually, no treatment is needed if the foot can easily be manipulated to midline. When the foot cannot be aligned readily, an orthopedic consult should be considered. The spine, examined with the newborn in a prone position, should be straight and flat. The lumbar and sacral curves do not develop until the infant begins to sit (refer to Chapter 34 for more information on these conditions). The base of the spine should be closely observed for any deformities such as **spina bifida** (a congenital defect in the walls of the spinal cord caused by a lack of union between the laminae of the vertebrae). Refer to Chapter 32 for more information on this condition. The newborn will gain approximately 5–7 ounces per week, and head circumference and length will increase 1 inch per month.

Integumentary System

The skin is delicate and often mottled, or acrocyanosis may be present. The skin should be observed for other characteristics such as color and color change that may occur during activity, racial features, rashes, milia, birthmarks, and petechiae. **Milia** are small white papules on the nose, face, forehead, and upper torso caused by the plugging of the sebaceous gland. **Petechiae** are small, pinpoint, nonraised, perfectly round, purplish red spots, which are a result of an intradermal or submucosal hemorrhage. Petechiae may be a normal finding if located in the area of the presenting part. If found elsewhere, an investigation of possible causes, such as sepsis, should be pursued. A **mongolian spot** is an irregularly dark pigmented area on the posterior lumbar region. They have no clinical significance but may be noted in newborns of various racial backgrounds such as African American, Asian, and Native Americans. **Desquamation,** or peeling of the skin, may also be present. The degree of peeling depends on the maturity of the newborn with preterm newborns experiencing less and postterm newborns experiencing more. **Telangiectatic nevi** are capillary hemangiomas commonly called "stork bites," which are sometimes found on the nape of the neck and the bridge of the nose. These will disappear with time. **Nevus flammeus,** or port wine stain, is a hemangioma or vascular tumor that will not disappear with time. Some newborns may experience a transient newborn rash that is characterized by a red macular base with a white vesicular center, referred to as **erythema toxicum.**

Table 7-3 provides a summary of the normal and acceptable variations found when performing a newborn assessment.

TABLE 7-3 Summary of Newborn Physical Assessment

Area Assessed	Normal Findings	Acceptable Variances
Head	Anterior fontanel diamond-shaped, soft/flat Posterior fontanel triangle-shaped Head circumference 33–35 cm (13–14 in)	Molding Caput succedaneum Cephalhematoma Puncture mark from internal scalp electrode Head circumference 32.5–37.5 cm (12.5–14.5 in)
Face/Eyes	Symmetrical facial features/movement Eyes symmetrical in shape, placement and movement	Eyelid edema Subconjunctival hemorrhage
Thorax	Symmetrical movement Circumference equal to or less than head circumference Nipples symmetrical Breath sounds clear and equal bilaterally Heart with regular rate and rhythm S2 split	Breast engorgement Supernumerary nipples Noticeable ribs on deep inspiration *Functional* heart murmur
Abdomen	Soft, nondistended Umbilical cord with two arteries and one vein Bowel sounds present	Irregular bowel sounds Reducible umbilical hernia
Genitalia	**Male** • Meatal opening in center of glans • Strong, arching urinary stream • Penile erection when voiding or with stimulation	Hydrocele (accumulation of fluid in the scrotal sac) Testes at external inguinal ring

continues

TABLE 7-3 *Continued*

Area Assessed	Normal Findings	Acceptable Variances
Genitalia	**Male** • Scrotum with rugae and pink or dark brown in color (depends on ethnic background) • Both testes descended **Female** • White or pink vaginal discharge • Edematous clitoris and labia majora • Increased pigmentation	Vaginal/hymenal tag Fusion of labia minora
Anus/rectum	Patent anus Meconium passage by 24 hours	Meconium within 48 hours
Extremities	Flexed position Symmetrical and equal movement Full range of motion Hands reach upper thighs when upper extremities are extended	Extended knees if breech
Spine	Straight Moves head from side to side when prone Can lift head when prone	

PSYCHOSEXUAL DEVELOPMENT

At the time of conception, the gender of the fetus is biologically determined. However, the primitive gonads that develop by the fifth or sixth week of gestation are bipotential, containing both ovarian and testicular components (Mosyang & Thornton, 1994). This genetic information directs development of either ovaries or testes, and in the presence of a Y chromosome, the bipotential primitive gonads develop into testes by 6–7 weeks of gestation. In the presence of two X chromosomes and the absence of a Y chromosome, the primitive gonads will develop into ovaries by 10 weeks of gestation. Psychosexual development continues after birth as the newborn finds satisfaction from oral stimuli, from physical contact with the caregiver, and from being held and cuddled (Figure 7-12).

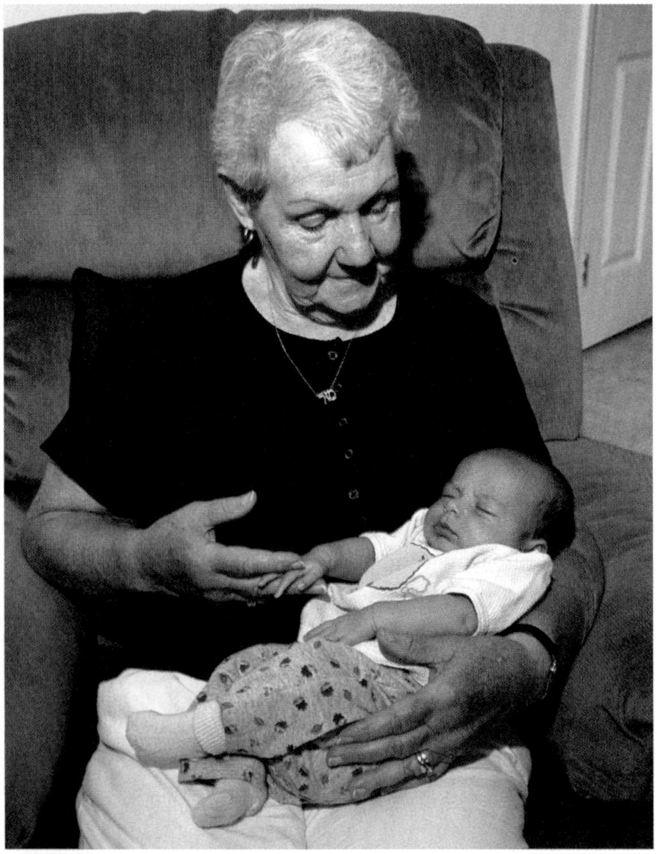

Figure 7-12 All family members, including grandmothers, are important to newborns.

COGNITIVE DEVELOPMENT

Cognitive development refers to the development of thinking and to gaining and using knowledge (Kalat, 1993). T. Berry Brazelton (1994) has shown that the newborn has the ability to interact with the environment and signal needs and gratitude when those needs are met. Learning, which is a function of the cerebral cortex, occurs through imitation and habituation. The newborn as young as 12 days of age is able to imitate facial and manual gestures of adults and prefers sharply contrasting colors, large squares, medium-bright objects, and ovoid objects with eyes and a mouth.

The newborn also has the ability to respond to auditory stimuli by turning the head and "looking" with the eyes to find the source. The frequency and intensity of the auditory stimulus, however, affect the response. High-frequency signals are more likely to produce a response, but it may be a distress response whereas lower intensity signals inhibit distress.

In addition, the newborn is sensitive to touch and handling. If a newborn is quiet, a rapid, intrusive touch will elicit an alert state. When the newborn is upset and crying, a slow soft touch will be calming. If some form of central nervous system irritation exists, there is increasing irritability with stimuli (especially tactile stimulation), and further evaluation is required.

The newborn's response to various stimuli affects the caregiver–infant bond. Since nonverbal communication between caregiver and infant are the initial stages of attachment, caregivers should provide the newborn with stimuli that evoke a response, thus enhancing attachment. Caregivers should also be taught to look for cues that the infant may be overstimulated or becoming habituated.

Habituation, the ability to decrease responses to disturbing stimuli, is a defensive state that the newborn may enter in response to noxious stimuli. Habituation protects the newborn from overstimulation and frees energy to meet physiologic demands. A newborn who cannot habituate will continue to react vigorously to repeated stimuli.

PSYCHOSOCIAL DEVELOPMENT

Child psychoanalyst Erik Erikson has divided the human life span into eight stages. In each of these stages, a human is faced with social and emotional conflicts. The first stage, infancy, which includes the newborn, is trust versus mistrust. Here, the newborn relies on others to fulfill needs, and develops basic trust when the caregivers meet these needs. Through a supportive, nurturing, and loving environment, the newborn will form an attachment to the caregiver and develop positive relationships (refer to Chapter 6 for more information).

However, the development of attachment between the newborn and caregiver requires more than just being fed and having biological needs met. Attachment depends on emotional responses as well. For example, reports from various orphanages and foundling homes from the early 1900s showed that infants who lacked interaction were retarded in physical growth, language, and intellectual development (Kalat, 1993). These infants were also socially inept and unresponsive to their environment. Twenty minutes of extra handling per day has been reported to result in earlier exploring and grasping behavior by the infant (Murray & Zenter, 2001).

HEALTH PROMOTION AND MAINTENANCE

Shortly after birth, all newborns receive ophthalmic drops or ointment. Even though the incidence of mothers infected with gonorrhea at the time of delivery is less than 3%, the importance of preventing blindness makes this procedure mandatory for all newborns (Murray & Zentner, 2001).

Hemorrhagic disease of the newborn due to vitamin K deficiency may be prevented by administering phytonadione within 1 hour of birth. The dosage is usually 1 mg intramuscularly for the full-term newborn or 0.5 mg for preterm infants (Pilliteri, 1999). Prior to discharge from the hospital, the newborn should have a screening blood test to rule out the presence of phenylketonuria (PKU) and hypothyroidism.

Immunizations to promote disease resistance and prevention are also essential for all newborns and infants. Caregivers should be informed of the importance of obtaining recommended immunizations and should receive a written schedule of when immunizations are due (see Appendix C for immunization schedule). Recommendations for routine well baby check-ups vary among practitioners. Some primary care providers will see the breastfed newborns at 1 week of age to check their weight; others will have all newborns return to the office at 2 weeks of age. Finally, caregivers should receive a recommended schedule for follow-up care.

ANTICIPATORY GUIDANCE

Nutrition

The American Academy of Pediatrics (AAP) recommends breastfeeding for the first 6–12 months of life (AAP, 1997). Breast milk has many advantages over formula such as (1) requiring no mixing; (2) being the correct temperature; (3) requiring no sterilization; (4) being easily digested; (5) its fats being well absorbed; (6) having antibodies and immunoglobulins to many types of microorganisms, which are passed from mother to baby; and (7) being cost effective. Many women, however, choose not to breastfeed for a variety of reasons. The mother who chooses not to breastfeed should not be made to feel guilty because of her decision. If breastfeeding is not selected, commercial formulas are available that attempt to mimic human milk. However, most commercial formulas have a slightly higher renal load and higher protein intake that may alter the blood urea nitrogen level and serum or urine level of amino acids (Murray & Zentner, 2001). Cow's milk should not be used to feed infants until recommended by the primary care provider since the composition of cow's milk is designed for a rapidly

Family Teaching

Colostrum

Explain to the mother that breast milk does not come in until the 2nd or 4th day. Until then, the newborn gets nutrients from colostrum, a product the breast produces prior to milk.

Critical Thinking

I Don't Think I Can Do It

Christine, the first-time mother of a 4-hour-old infant says she wants to breastfeed her baby. However, she does not think that she can do it because her milk has not "come in" yet, and her mother and sisters were not able to breastfeed their infants. What would you tell her?

growing animal and differs significantly from human milk or commercial formula. Cow's milk contains more protein, fat, sugar, calcium, sodium, potassium, magnesium, sulfur, and phosphorous than human milk or commercial formulas. The caregivers should be instructed on these differences and the importance of maintaining the newborn and infant on breast milk or commercial formula.

Soy protein may be substituted for milk protein for those newborns with a milk (lactose) intolerance, symptoms of which include abdominal pain, diarrhea, distension, and flatus after ingesting milk products. Special formulas have also been developed to meet the needs of babies with PKU,

Family Teaching

Breastfeeding

1. Breasts may be firm but feel softer after nursing.
2. Nurse at least 10–15 minutes on each side.
3. To prevent nipple tenderness, hold infant correctly: cradle hold, football hold, or side-lying down.
4. Make sure the newborn's lips are behind the nipple, encircling the areola.
5. Release the suction before the newborn is removed from the breast by placing a finger in the side of the mouth and between the jaws.
6. After nursing, express a little breast milk, massage into the nipples and areola, and allow to air dry.
7. Do not use soap or alcohol on breasts or nipples. Clean with water during showering or bathing.
8. Baby's urine should be light yellow with soft yellow stools.
9. Burp baby between breasts and at the end of feeding.

Bottle Feeding

1. Formula should be iron-fortified.
2. All the newborn's nutritional needs are met by formula. Cereal, juice, or other baby foods are not necessary.
3. Formula comes in three forms: ready to feed, concentrated liquid, and powdered.
4. Be sure formula is diluted correctly if in concentrated or powder form. Never add more or less water to the formula than is recommended by the manufacturer because this can be very dangerous for the newborn.
5. Once opened or mixed, a can of formula or prepared bottle should be refrigerated and used within 48 hours.
6. If the newborn drinks part of a bottle, it can be left at room temperature, but it must be used within 1 hour.
7. Do not add fresh formula to a partially used bottle or reuse a bottle that has been out for longer than 1 hour.
8. Do not heat bottles in a microwave. This leads to uneven heating and can cause severe burns to the newborn's mouth and throat.
9. Most babies are satisfied in about 20 minutes. Feedings should not last longer than 30 minutes.
10. Burp after half of the feeding and again at the end of the feeding.
11. Never prop the bottle or leave the newborn unattended.
12. Do not allow the newborn to drink from a bottle for long periods, especially when sleeping. This practice can cause "nursing bottle syndrome" or the development of dental caries and has also been linked to an increased incidence of otitis media.

fat malabsorption problems, or those requiring increased calories (e.g., preterm infants). The choice of formula is often decided by the pediatrician and hospital staff unless the caregivers request a specific formula.

The method of feeding is important, but the procedure for feeding may also have a significant impact on the newborn. Feeding time is crucial to the development of the caregiver–newborn attachment, since it is a time for the newborn and caregiver to interact and learn about each other. If the newborn remains in the crib or in an infant seat with the bottle propped, the attachment process can be delayed. If the newborn is held and cuddled during feeding, both caregiver and newborn experience a feeling of closeness as well as close eye contact.

In past years, newborns were placed on a specific feeding schedule. However, current practice is **on-demand feeds.** This involves feeding the newborn when hungry instead of according to a prearranged time schedule. Because formula is digested more slowly, formula-fed newborns will go longer between feedings and usually establish a pattern of feeding every 3–4 hours, whereas a breastfed newborn may nurse every 1½–3 hours. For the first few feedings, the newborn may only consume ½–1 ounce, and progresses to 6–8 feedings of 2–3 ounces per feeding after the first week of life. By 1 month of age, the newborn is eating 5–6 feedings per day and taking 3–4 ounces per feeding (Figure 7-13).

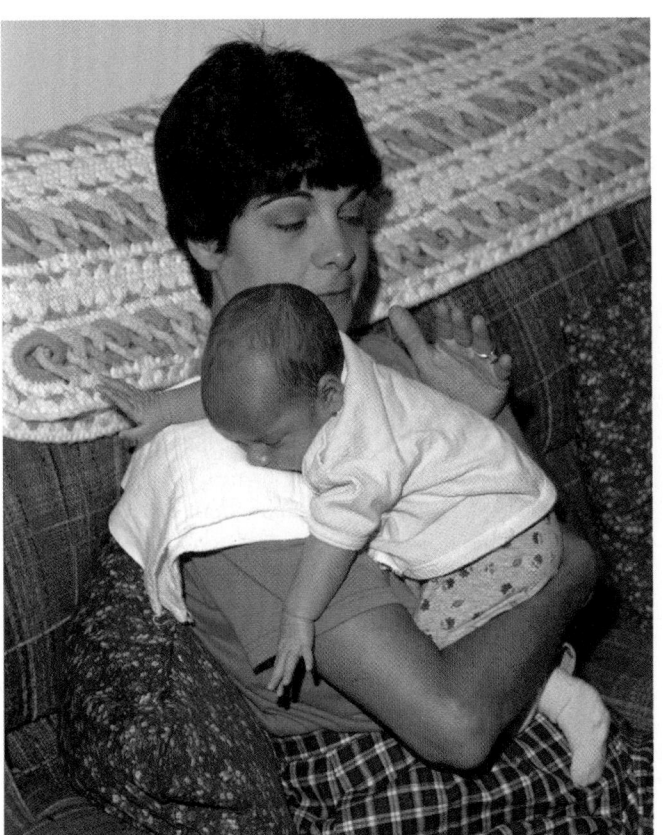

Figure 7-13 Burping after feeding is important.

Thermoregulation

Temperature regulation, or thermoregulation, is controlled by the hypothalamus. Body temperature is altered by changes in metabolism, motor tone and activity, vasomotor activity, and sweating (Thomas, 1994). The adult human is capable of maintaining a constant body temperature over a wide range. The newborn is also capable of maintaining body temperature but not as effectively as a more mature person. Therefore, the newborn is more vulnerable to underheating and overheating because of a relatively large body surface area, poor thermal insulation, limited shivering response, and increased metabolic rate.

Heat exchange occurs through convection, conduction, radiation, evaporation, and over a heat gradient, or from a higher to lower temperature. The transfer of heat between a solid surface and air or liquid is convection. This type of heat exchange would occur between the newborn and liquid during a bath or when exposed to drafts. Conduction of heat occurs between two solid objects that come in contact with each other. For example, when the infant's body comes in contact with a cold scale or counter, heat loss results. The transfer of heat between solid objects that are not in contact is radiation. Placing the newborn next to a cold window, despite the room being warm, will cause heat loss through radiation. Evaporative heat loss occurs when water on or in the body changes from a liquid to a gas. If an infant is not

Family Teaching

Keeping the Newborn Warm

1. Explain how the newborn loses heat:
   a. Convection
   b. Conduction
   c. Radiation
   d. Evaporation
2. Provide information on how to reduce heat exchange:
   a. Reduce the area exposed during a bath.
   b. Limit exposure to drafts created by doors, ventilation systems, and traffic flow around the newborn's bed.
   c. Warm solid surfaces between the newborn by placing a blanket on the scale or counter.
   d. Place the newborn's crib on an inside wall in the room, away from the window.
   e. Block sunlight on the newborn in the car to prevent overheating.

Reflective Thinking

Overdressing

You enter a room to find the thermostat set at 80°F. The newborn is dressed in a t-shirt, sleeper, socks, and bundled in a quilt. How do you approach the mom to explain how overdressing and overbundling can affect the newborn's temperature? What if the mom states she's doing this because of her cultural background?

dried thoroughly after birth or a bath, the body temperature will drop secondary to evaporation.

If the newborn is exposed to temperature variations, multiple physiological responses occur. An increase in environmental temperature may cause vasodilation of the skin arterioles, resulting in increased blood flow from the body core to the periphery in an attempt to dissipate the heat and produce a cooling effect. A decrease in environmental temperature will result in vasoconstriction of the skin arterioles and reduction of heat from the body core. Shivering, a specialized muscular response that increases oxygen consumption and muscle metabolic rate, is limited in the newborn.

The primary form of heat production in the newborn is through brown adipose tissue metabolism. This **brown fat** is found primarily in the subscapular, axillary, adrenal, and mediastinal regions, and increases cellular metabolic rates and oxygen consumption, resulting in heat. Brown fat cells differ from other adipose tissue because of the fat vacuoles, number of mitochondria, and glycogen stores, and enhance the responsiveness of brown fat to thermal stimuli.

Sleep

Term newborns have two sleep states: deep and light. During deep sleep, the eyes are firmly closed and still, no rapid eye movements occur, and little or no motor activity is present, except for occasional startles. During light sleep, rapid eye movements occur during a 10-second interval, and activity ranges from stretching to minor twitches. The newborn will sleep between 16 and 19 hours a day, with sleep cycles averaging 45–50 minutes. The term newborn begins and ends in light sleep (Brazelton, 1994).

Circadian rhythm, the cyclic variations in bodily functions that occur in a 24-hour period, is controlled by the central nervous system. Often the newborn's "clock" will not coincide with the family's and can result in conflict and disruption. This discrepancy may lead the family to perceive the newborn as "difficult." However, through alterations in care giving and patience, the infant's schedule can become synchronous with the family's rhythms.

Family Teaching

Sleeping

1. Explain the American Academy of Pediatrics recommendation for "back to sleep":
   a. Do not position newborn prone.
   b. Position newborn supine or side-lying.
2. Provide information on the type of bedding to avoid:
   a. Soft bedding
   b. Pillows
   c. Comforters
   d. Sheepskin
   e. Water beds
3. Explain that overswaddling or increased room temperature, in combination with the prone position, may increase the likelihood of SIDS threefold.

In 1992, the AAP recommended the supine or side-lying position for sleep for infants (2000). However, newborns with craniofacial abnormalities and gastroesophageal reflux should be positioned prone. In recent studies from various countries, the side or back sleeping position has shown a large and sustained decrease in the incidence of sudden infant death syndrome (SIDS). The type of bedding the newborn is placed on has also been implicated in SIDS with a higher incidence occurring on soft bedding such as pillows, comforters, blankets, or sheepskin (Willinger, Hoffman, & Hartford, 1994). Refer to Chapter 8 for more information about SIDS.

Diaper Care

When changing the diaper of a female, instruct caregivers to wipe from front to back. This will control feces contamination of the vaginal area. Keeping the diaper clean and dry is the best prevention against diaper rash. The AAP recommends using plain water and absorbent cotton or fresh washcloth. There is no need to use commercial wipes. However, if they are used, the wipes should be designed for babies not adults. The adult wipes contain alcohol that can dry babies' skin.

The causes of diaper rash include:

- Too much moisture next to skin
- Chafing or rubbing
- Prolonged skin contact with urine, feces, or both
- Use of antibiotics (yeast infection)
- Allergic reaction to diaper material

Symptoms of diaper rash can be mild to severe and include red skin; painful open sores; and rash around abdomen, genital area, or inside the skin folds of thighs and buttocks. Treatment includes changing diaper often, using clear water to clean diaper area, and applying a thick layer of protective ointment or cream (zinc oxide or petrolatum). Caregivers should contact a health care practioner if the rash doesn't go away within 48–72 hours or gets worse, including open sores and blisters (AAP, 2000).

Newborn Screening

Required screening for newborns differs from state to state. The most common requirements involve phenylkentonuria and congenital hypothyroidism; galactosemia; and sickle cell disease (Galvis, 2000). Check with your institution regarding screenings mandated in your state.

The AAP suggests that all newborns go through a hearing screen to identify possible hearing loss. The AAP and the Joint Committee on Infant Hearing (1995) suggest the goal of universal detection of hearing loss before 3 months of age and appropriate intervention at no more than 6 months of age (AAP, 1999b).

SAFETY PROMOTION AND INJURY PREVENTION

Contrary to popular belief, a newborn is not immobile. Newborns can wiggle themselves into a variety of positions, which can become a safety hazard. The caregivers should be cognizant of this. Therefore, the only place to leave a newborn unattended is in the crib with side rails up. The caregiver should always keep one hand on the newborn when newborn is on top of any object, since he/she can quickly roll off. The greatest risk of injury for the newborn is from drowning, suffocation, burns, falls, or motor vehicle accidents (Gardner, 1992).

Bathing can be a fun time for caregiver and the newborn, but the newborn should never be left unattended for any reason. Therefore, parents should be taught to not answer the phone or door bell when bathing the newborn, unless the newborn is bundled up and taken with the caregiver.

Nursing Alert

Pacifiers for Newborns

When a pacifier is used, it should be of solid, one-piece construction. It should not be tied to a string or rope and placed around the newborn's neck as this poses a strangulation hazard.

Motor vehicle accidents can plague every age group, and all children need to be properly restrained. Recent information has shown the front passenger seat is a dangerous place; so the neonate should be secured in a car seat in the rear, facing backward. Caregivers should know how their car seat should be installed and how it works prior to using it. If the family is involved in an accident, the car seat needs to be removed from service, even if there is no visible damage. Placing the crib away from heat sources, using warm-air vaporizers cautiously, covering unused electrical outlets, and not holding the newborn while drinking hot coffee or other hot liquids will also help prevent injuring or accidents.

Since the incidence of recurrent otitis media and respiratory infections has been linked to secondhand smoke, smoking around the newborn should be avoided. If family members need to smoke, they should go outside, and avoid smoking in the car if a newborn or older infant is present.

Nursing Alert

Water Temperature for Bathing

Water heaters should be set no higher than 120°F. Exposure to hot water for even a brief time may result in second or third degree burns. At a water temperature of 155°F, a burn can occur in 1 second. At a temperature of 120°F, a burn occurs in 5 minutes. After filling the bath tub, turn the hot water off first and then the cold. The water temperature should always be checked before the newborn is placed in the tub.

Case Study/Care Plan

Nursing Care Plan: Newborn

Joshua is a 2-hour-old male newborn who was delivered vaginally after an uneventful term pregnancy. Joshua's mother is a 23-year-old gravida 1 para 1. This a study of his first hours and days.

Nursing Diagnosis #1

Ineffective peripheral tissue perfusion, related to decreased thermoregulation

continues

continued

Expected Outcome

Joshua's skin will be pink in room air and be normothermic (normal body temperature).

Interventions/*Rationale*

1. Place under radiant warmer on servo control until temperature stable (>97.7° axillary). *The newborn's ability to regulate temperature is immature.*
2. Place newborn in t-shirt and diaper, and bundle in a blanket when temperature stable. *The newborn's ability to regulate temperature is immature.*
3. Keep ambient temperature of room at approximately 70°F, and keep newborn out of drafts. *The newborn's ability to regulate temperature is immature.*

Evaluation

Joshua's color will be pink (acrocyanosis may be present) and his temperature will be 97.7–99.5°F (axillary).

Nursing Diagnosis #2

Imbalanced nutrition: less than body requirements, related to limited nutritional/fluid intake

Expected Outcome

Joshua will lose less than 10% of birth weight by 4 days of age.

Interventions/*Rationale*

1. Obtain weight on admission to nursery. *To obtain a baseline measurement.*
2. Begin feedings as soon as newborn is stable and able to eat. *To limit weight loss.*
3. Instruct caregivers on proper feeding techniques and cues that newborn is feeding appropriate amounts. *To minimize weight loss.*
4. Weigh newborn prior to discharge. *To determine amount of weight loss.*
5. If weight gain is questionable, have caregivers return to nursery or primary care provider's office within one week for weight check. *To determine if weight loss is transient and whether or not infant has regained amount lost earlier.*

Evaluation

Joshua will lose less than 10% of birth weight and will begin to gain weight appropriately.

Nursing Diagnosis #3

Potential for ineffective airway clearance, related to secretion obstruction

Expected Outcome

Joshua will maintain patent airway.

Interventions/*Rationale*

1. Position newborn on back or side. *To prevent and/or treat aspiration.*
2. Have bulb syringe readily available in crib. *To treat aspiration.*
3. Teach caregivers on the proper use of the bulb syringe. *So they are prepared in case child aspirates.*
4. Assess for signs/symptoms of airway obstruction. *To determine whether or not airway is patent.*

continues

continued

Evaluation

Joshua will remain pink in room air.

Joshua will not demonstrate signs/symptoms of airway obstruction.

Nursing Diagnosis #4

Deficient caregiver knowledge, related to lack of experience with newborn

Expected Outcome

Caregiver will verbalize or demonstrate appropriate newborn care.

Interventions/*Rationale*

1. Assess caregiver educational needs. *To determine what needs to be taught.*
2. Adjust teaching technique to caregiver needs. *So caregiver is able to learn.*
3. Discuss major aspects of newborn care (safety measures, feeding techniques, bathing and general care, when to call the pediatrician/primary care provider. *Education on care of the normal newborn will help caregivers become more confident and knowledgeable so they are able to provide effective and appropriate care.*

Evaluation:

Caregivers will demonstrate appropriate newborn care.

Caregivers will verbalize when to contact the pediatrician/primary care provider.

NURSE'S ROLE IN FOSTERING HEALTHY NEWBORNS

Although the time allowed for mothers and newborns to remain in the hospital following delivery has decreased in recent years, nurses can still have an impact on their care, as they are in an excellent position to teach parents about their newborn, and what to expect in the coming months. Education should begin early in the hospital stay not the day of discharge, with frequent reinforcement, and in a variety of formats to accommodate various learning styles. One-on-one or classroom instruction, videotapes, written handouts, and/or demonstration are appropriate methods. Information needs to be individualized for each newborn and caregiver considering cultural and religious beliefs, and educational levels.

The nurse is also in an excellent position to ensure caregivers feel comfortable before the newborn is sent home and are provided with information about community resources that may be helpful (Figure 7-14). The nurse should also instruct caregivers on the importance of follow-up care including well-baby check-ups and routine immunizations.

THE HIGH-RISK NEWBORN

The high-risk newborn is SGA, LGA, premature (<37 weeks' gestation), or postmature (>42 weeks' gestation). Unfortunately, these situations cannot always be determined before the birth of the baby, and each condition requires special consideration in care and assessment abilities. It is important to determine the risk factors for each condition as soon as possible so appropriate care can be provided.

Large for Gestational Age (LGA)

A variety of obstetrical situations can result in an LGA infant, including maternal disease such as diabetes, genetic predisposition for largeness, or genetic aberrations such as Beckwith Wiedeman Syndrome (refer to Figure 7-7, the Ballard Assessment Scale). As compared with an AGA infant, an LGA infant has an increased potential for neonatal morbidity since a frequent complication is birth trauma, especially caput succedaneum or cephalhemotoma (refer to Figure 7-5). However, more serious injury such as a subgaleal

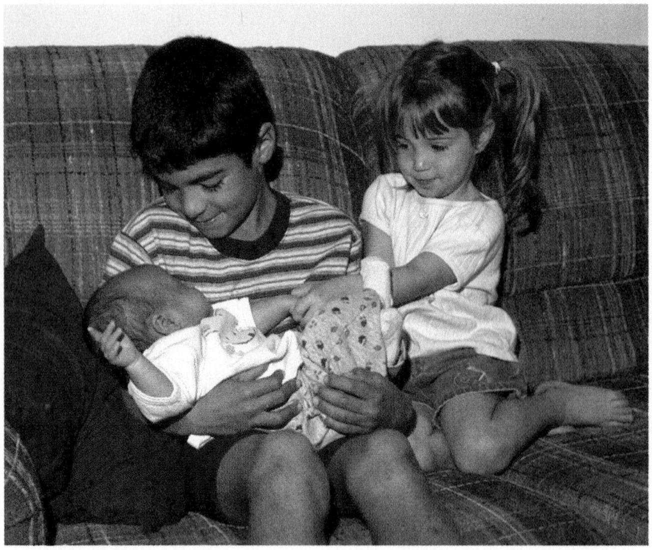

Figure 7-14 Young children love to hold their newborn sibling.

hemorrhage, asphyxia, and even death can occur. The neonatal neurological examination is therefore important to determine to what extent the neurological system is affected if there is a concern the LGA infant suffered birth trauma.

Other injuries that LGA newborns may be at risk for developing include a broken clavicle or a fractured humerus. A broken clavicle is suspected if there is swelling, pain, or tenderness in the affected area, or a reluctance to use the affected extremity. Care should be taken to not manipulate the extremity, though splinting or complete immobilization is rarely needed. A humerus fracture will present similarly, with pain, tenderness, edema, and decreased movement. However, the humerus will need to be immobilized upon diagnosis. These diagnoses can be verified through radiological imaging (Seidel, et al. 1997).

Hypoglycemia is also commonly seen in the LGA infant. Oftentimes, diabetic mothers have LGA infants who are either insulin-dependent or gestational diabetics. These infants develop hyperinsulinemia in response to maternal hyperglycemia and respond by increasing production of their own insulin. After birth, this infant will continue overproducing insulin and can be at risk for developing hypoglycemia for up to 6 hours of age. To prevent neonatal hypoglycemia, it is important to monitor serum glucose, initiate early oral feedings, and supplement as necessary with an IV glucose solution. Twelve percent of LGA infants born of normoglycemic mothers also have hypoglycemia and need close monitoring (Klaus, et al., 1993).

Small for Gestational Age (SGA)

An SGA infant is defined as an infant who has a weight to gestational age ratio that is below the 10th percentile (Seidel, et al., 1997). Assessment may show a baby who is lacking subcutaneous fat, has a scaphoid abdomen, and a head that is disproportionally large for the body (asymmetric intrauterine growth retardation). (An asymmetric intrauterine growth–retarded infant has a head that, although of normal size, appears larger because of the small body size.)

Maternal history of an SGA infant could show cardiovascular or renal disease, diabetes, medication, recreational drug or cigarette use, or placental insufficiencies due to infarction or separation. The neonate may also be small due to an inborn error of metabolism, congenital anomalies, or multiple gestation. Postnatal complications increase the infant's susceptibility to infection, respiratory compromise, neurological challenges, or death. Hypoglycemia can also be present and continue for up to four days. It is therefore important to monitor serum glucose until adequate oral feedings are tolerated. Temperature instability is secondary to the lack of stored fat, which serves as both an insulator and a heat producer. Therefore, the SGA newborn should be monitored closely for hypothermia, dressed warmly, and placed in an artificial heat source such as an isolette or radiant warmer as necessary. Supplemental oxygen or assisted ventilation may also be necessary (Klaus, et al., 1993).

The Premature Infant

The premature infant is born earlier than 37 weeks' gestation (Kenner, Lott, & Flandemeyer, 1998). Preterm deliveries, 8%–10% of live births in the United States, account for roughly 75%–80% of neonatal morbidity and death. Factors precipitating a premature birth can include maternal hypertension, preeclampsia, multiple gestation, renal disease, cardiac disease, and a history of preterm pregnancies and/or labor. Also, late initiation of prenatal care, a lower socioeconomic level, and substance use and abuse can contribute to a preterm delivery. Complications for the preterm infant are similar to those of the SGA infant, and include hypoglycemia, respiratory instability, hypothermia, neurological problems, and necrotizing enterocolitis. The severity as well as the outcome depends on the gestational age and size of the infant.

If an extremely preterm baby is anticipated, maternal transport or immediate neonatal transport to a tertiary center will be attempted. At times, however, the infant will be cared for in the well-baby nursery until relocation to a tertiary center is possible.

A common condition seen in the premature infant is respiratory distress syndrome (RDS), which is defined as an inadequate production of surfactant, a mixture of phospholipids and apoproteins that adhere to the internal surfaces of the alveoli, reduce the surface tension of these surfaces, and improve the lung's ability to remain inflated during exhalation (Deacon & O'Neill, 1999). Without adequate production of this substance, respiratory difficulty increases. Though primarily seen in the preterm infant, RDS is also seen in more mature infants. Precipitating factors include prematurity, cesarean delivery without labor, maternal diabetes, and multiple gestation. Symptoms of RDS include tachypnea (>60 breaths per minute), intercostal, subcostal and sternal retractions, nasal flaring, and audible grunting. Poor aeration of the lung fields despite great respiratory effort will be heard upon auscultation. Symptoms can worsen to the point where supplemental oxygen or assisted ventilation is required. Other systems may also become involved, and are manifested as hypotension, oliguria, acidosis, and hypoglycemia. In these situations, surfactant replacement can be administered, but the infant will need to receive ventilatory support until able to adequately assume respiratory and other functions independently (Deacon & O'Neill, 1999). Figure 7-15 illustrates the size of a premature infant in comparison to an adult hand. Figure 7-16 mentions other situations that place premature infants at risk.

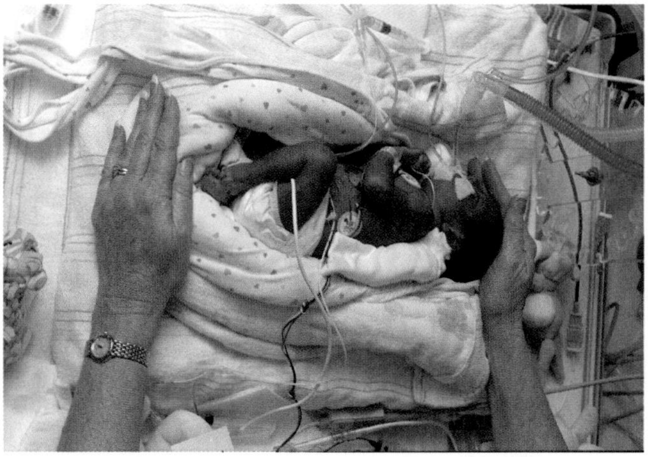

Figure 7-15 Premature Infant. Note how small he is compared to hand.

The Postmature Infant

The postmature infant is greater than 42 weeks' gestation. Since by this date, a significant portion of the placenta has lost its ability to transport nutrients, oxygen, and waste products, the increase in neonatal morbidity and mortality in the postmature infant may be secondary to this placental insufficiency (Divon, et al., 1998). Problems of postmature infants

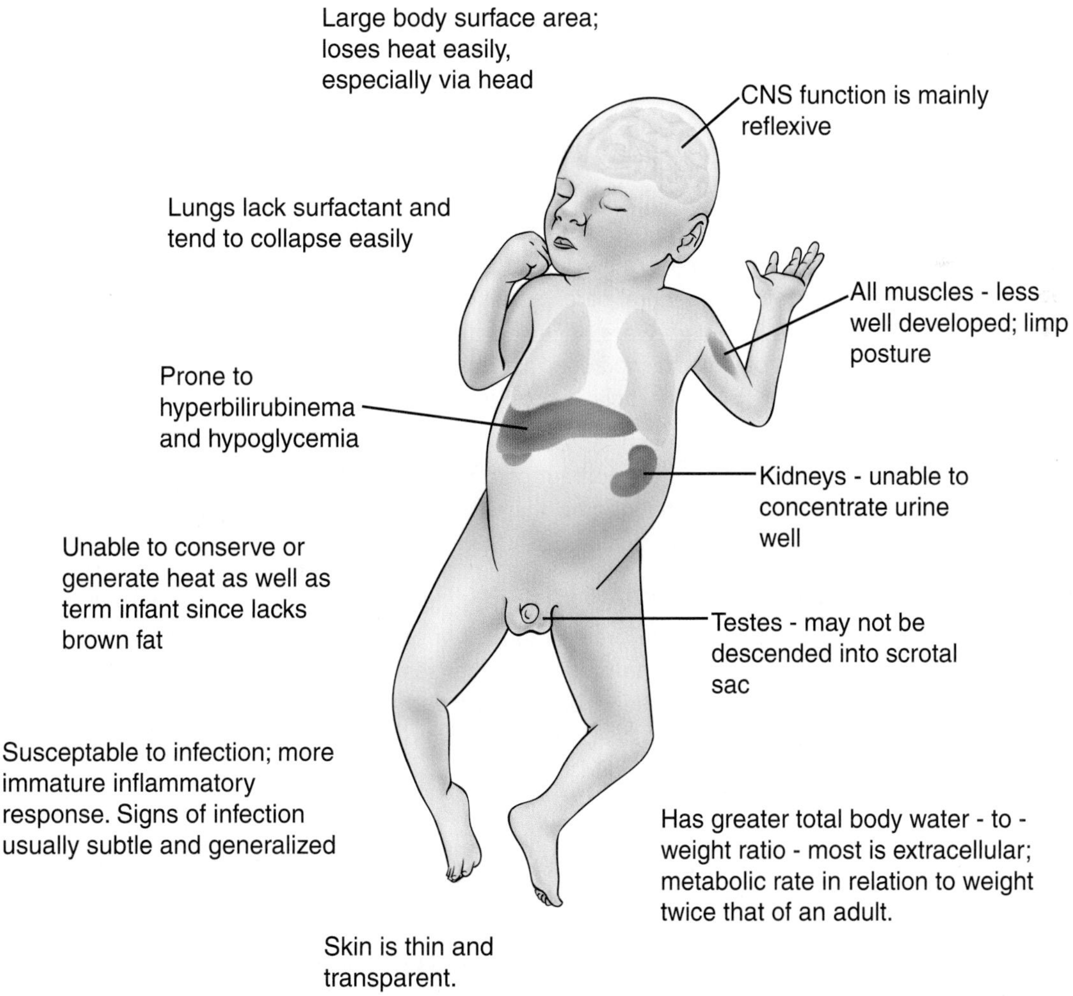
Large body surface area; loses heat easily, especially via head
CNS function is mainly reflexive
Lungs lack surfactant and tend to collapse easily
All muscles - less well developed; limp posture
Prone to hyperbilirubinema and hypoglycemia
Kidneys - unable to concentrate urine well
Unable to conserve or generate heat as well as term infant since lacks brown fat
Testes - may not be descended into scrotal sac
Susceptable to infection; more immature inflammatory response. Signs of infection usually subtle and generalized
Has greater total body water - to - weight ratio - most is extracellular; metabolic rate in relation to weight twice that of an adult.
Skin is thin and transparent.

Figure 7-16 Premature Infant and Associated Problems

Research Highlight

Nursing Care and Preterm Infant Sleep-Wake Behaviors

Study Purpose

To examine the relationship between nursing care and the development of sleep-wake behaviors and related infant behaviors in high-risk preterm infants.

Methods

Seventy-one preterm infants were observed once a week for approximately 4 hours while actions by the nursing and medical staff and parents were allowed as if the observer were not there. The infants' behaviors were recorded by one of two observers every 10 seconds. Five infant characteristics (covariates) were taken into account: race, gender, days of mechanical ventilation, postconceptional age, and theophylline treatment. *Six sleep-wake states* were defined and measured: active waking, drowsiness, alert, sleep-wake transitions, active sleep, and quiet sleep. *Infant behaviors* included jitters and negative facial expressions. Two measures were taken according to the nursing care given: *nurse caregiving contexts*: contact care, routine care, and procedural care; and *nurse interactive behaviors*: move, positive touch, hold, and talk.

Findings

Effects of infant context: When the infant was alone both alertness and active waking occurred infrequently and did not change over time. Drowsiness and jitters decreased over time. Quiet sleep increased over time. When the infant was with the caregiver, alertness, active waking, and drowsiness increased as age increased. Quiet sleep occurred infrequently when the infant was with the caregiver and did not change with increasing gestational age. Regardless of whether the infant was alone or with the caregiver sleep-wake transitions and negative facial expressions increased, while active sleep decreased over time. Covariates had few effects on these developmental patterns.

Effects of nursing caregiving contexts: Active waking was greater in procedural care than in contact care or routine care. Drowsiness increased over time during routine and procedural care, and there was more drowsiness in routine care than in either contact or procedural care. Alertness was greater during contact care than either routine or procedural care. Negative facial expressions were greater in procedural care than routine care. Fewer jitters were observed during routine care than contact and procedural care. Covariate effects showed that increased length of mechanical ventilation resulted in less drowsiness, more jitters, and more negative facial expressions during routine care.

Nursing interactive behaviors: Positive touch increased over time regardless of the nurse caregiving context, and there was more positive touch in contact care than routine or procedural care. Moving during procedural care increased to a greater degree than the increase in contact care with increasing postconceptional age, while moving during routine care (feeding, bathing, diaper change) decreased.

Implications

The development of sleeping and waking in preterm infants appears to depend not only on biological maturation but also nursing stimulation. In the presence of nurses, the normal developmental decrease in active sleep was replaced by an increase in drowsiness and sleep-wake transition, but when the infant was alone it was replaced with quiet sleep. As long-term developmental effects of nursing caregiving are unknown, additional research is needed.

Citation

Brandon, D. H., Holditch-Davis, D., & Beylea, M. (1999). Nursing care and the development of sleeping and waking behaviors in preterm infants. *Research in Nursing & Health, 22*, 217–229.

include meconium aspiration, malnutrition, asphyxia, and death. Physical exam will show a child with dry, cracking skin, and the absence of vernix and Lanugo; the extremities may be long and thin, and the skin may appear green if meconium was passed *in utero* (Kenner, et al., 1998). See Figure 7-17.

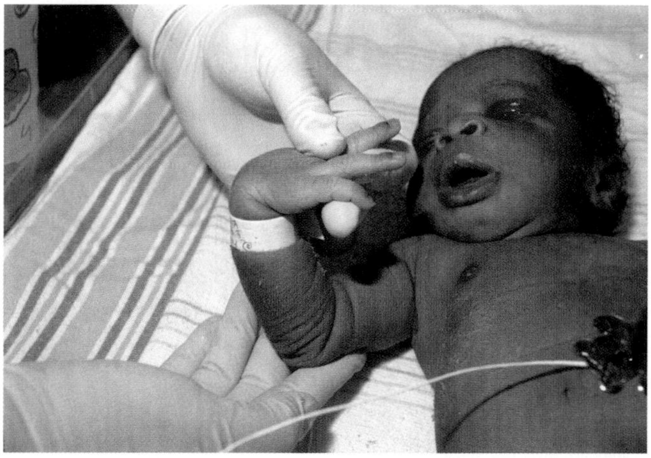

Figure 7-17 Post-term Infant with Peeling Skin

CARE OF THE HIGH RISK NEWBORN

Early intervention in any high-risk situation is essential. This begins by first recognizing the high-risk pregnancy and asking for additional medical staff to attend the delivery. After delivery, nurses should be prepared to perform or initiate assisted ventilation, cardiopulmonary resuscitation, and establish vascular access, while not forgetting to dry and keep the baby warm. The baby will then need to be transported from the delivery room to the nursery; a detailed exam will determine cardiovascular stability, neurological appropriateness, respiratory status, and temperature stability. It will also be necessary to determine if the infant needs to be transferred to a tertiary center.

REFLECTIONS FROM FAMILIES

I was in labor with my second child. I was very excited because my first child was born cesarean, but this time I was having a vaginal delivery. As my daughter Heather was delivered she aspirated fluid. Needless to say she spent the first few days of her life hooked up to a respirator and on antibiotics. This was a very difficult time. I was discharged from the hospital within two days. But every day I would go to the hospital and feed her and hold her. Heather was discharged, and is none the worse for wear. Now she is a healthy 4-year-old who has had no repercussions from her first week of life.

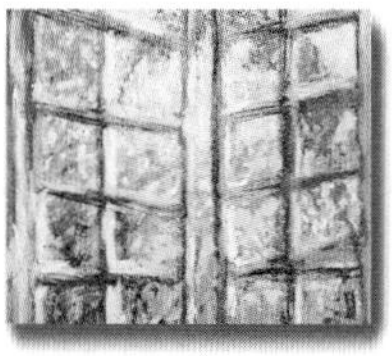

In the Real World

Those babies are so small and fragile, one wonders how they could possibly survive. When I first began to work in the newborn intensive care unit, I was very anxious and afraid that I would hurt them whenever I cared for them. I learned however that although small, and indeed fragile, they are also resilient and many are really strong. I know that the care I give makes a difference, and I really love what I do. I would not want to work on another unit.

Key Concepts

- The transition to extrauterine life involves changes in the cardiovascular and respiratory systems.
- A variety of reflexes are present during the newborn period that can be separated into primitive, survival, localized, or generalized.
- The newborn's musculoskeletal, gastrointestinal, integumentary, and renal systems are immature at birth.
- The newborn can interact with the environment and, within 2 weeks of birth, is able to imitate facial and manual gestures of adults.
- Education on the care of the newborn should begin at birth and include positioning, nutrition, safety, bathing, immunizations, normal growth and development, and schedules for well-baby examinations.
- High-risk newborns (LGA, SGA, premature, postmature) need careful monitoring and interventions.

Review Questions

1. Describe the principal cardiorespiratory changes that occur during the transition to extrauterine life.
2. Discuss the immature physiologic functioning of the neurological, cardiorespiratory, gastrointestinal, genitourinary, and musculoskeletal system in the newborn, and their relationship to the nursing care of the neonate.
3. Describe the expected normal findings of a newborn physical assessment.
4. Discuss the prominent anticipatory guidance concerns for caregivers during the neonatal period.
5. Describe areas addressed in teaching caregivers about safety promotion and injury prevention for the neonate.
6. Describe the etiology and care of the high-risk newborn.

References

American Academy of Pediatrics. (1997). Breastfeeding and the use of human milk. Policy Statement. *Pediatrics, 100*(6), 1035–1039. Available: www.aap.org/policy/re9729.html.

American Academy of Pediatrics. (1999a). *Circumcision policy statement* [On-line]. Available: www.medem.com

American Academy of Pediatrics. (1999b). *Newborn and infant hearing loss: Detection and intervention* [On-line]. Available: www.medem.com

American Academy of Pediatrics. (2000). *Treating diaper rash* [On-line]. Available: www.medem.com

American Academy of Pediatrics Joint Committee on Infant Hearing. (1995). Joint committee on infant hearing 1994 position statement. *Pediatrics, 95*, 152–156.

American Academy of Pediatrics Task Force on Infant Positioning and SIDS. (1992). Positioning and SIDS. *Pediatrics, 89*(6), 1120–1126.

American Academy of Pediatrics Task Force on Infant Sleep Position and Sudden Infant Death Syndrome. (2000). Changing concepts of sudden infant death syndrome: Implications for infant sleeping environment and sleep position. Policy Statement. *Pediatrics, 105*(3), 650–656. Available: www.aap.org/policy/re9946.html.

Bissinger, R. L. (1995). Renal physiology. Part I: Structure and function. *Neonatal Network, 14*(4), 9–19.

Brandon, D. H., Holditch-Davis, D., & Beylea, M. (1999). Nursing care and the development of sleeping and waking behaviors in preterm infants. *Research in Nursing & Health, 22*, 217–229.

Brazelton, T. B. (1994). Behavioral competence. In G. B. Avery, M. A. Fletcher, & M. G. MacDonald (Eds.), *Neonatology: Pathophysiology and Management of the Newborn* (4th ed., pp. 289–300). Philadelphia: Lippincott.

Brion, L. P., Satlin, L. M., & Edelmann, C. M. (1994). Renal disease. In G. B. Avery, M. A. Fletcher, & M. G. MacDonald (Eds.), *Neonatology: Pathophysiology and management of the newborn* (4th ed., pp. 792–836). Philadelphia: Lippincott.

Deacon, J., & O'Neill, P. (1999). *Core curriculum for neonatal intensive care nursing* (2nd ed.). Philadelphia: Saunders.

Dovin, M. Y., Haglund, B., Nisell, H., Otterblad, P. O., & Westgren, M. (1998). Fetal and neonatal mortality in the post-term pregnancy: The impact of gestational age and fetal growth restriction. *American Journal of Obstetrics and Gynecology, 178*(4), 726–731.

Galvis, S. (2000). *Newborn screening for metabolic disorders* [On-line]. Available: www.neonatology.org

Gardner, M. (1992). New treatment for pediatric trauma: Prevention. *Rescue-EMS, 10*(1), 22–25.

Kalat, J. W. (1993). *Introduction to psychology* (3rd ed.). Pacific Grove, CA: Brooks/Cole Publishing Company.

Kelly, J. M. (1994). General care. In G. B. Avery, M. A. Fletcher, & M. G. MacDonald (Eds.), *Neonatology: Pathophysiology and management of the newborn* (4th ed., pp. 301–311). Philadelphia: Lippincott.

Kenner, C., Amlung, S. R., & Flandermeyer, A. A. (1998). *Protocols in neonatal nursing.* Philadelphia: Saunders.

Kenner, C., Lott, J. W., & Flandermeyer, A. A. (1998). *Comprehensive neonatal nursing: A physiological perspective* Philadelphia: Saunders.

Klaus, M. H., & Fanaroff, A. A. (1993). *Care of the high risk neonate* (4th ed.). Philadelphia: Saunders.

Maisels, M. J. (1994). Jaundice. In G. B. Avery, M. A. Fletcher, & M. G. MacDonald (Eds.), *Neonatology: Pathophysiology and management of the newborn* (4th ed., pp. 630–725). Philadelphia: Lippincott.

Moller, J. H., & Dwan, P. F. (1992a). Fetal circulation. In *Ross Laboratories clinical education aid.* Columbus, OH: Ross Laboratories.

Moller, J. H., & Dwan, P. F. (1992b). Congenital heart abnormalities. In *Ross Laboratories clinical education aid.* Columbus, OH: Ross Laboratories.

Moshang, T., & Thornton, P. (1994). Endocrine disorders. In G. B. Avery, M. A. Fletcher, & M. G. MacDonald (Eds.), *Neonatology: Pathophysiology and management of the newborn* (4th ed., pp. 764–791). Philadelphia: Lippincott.

Murray, R. B., & Zentner, J. P. (1993). Assessment and health promotion for the infant. In *Nursing assessment and health promotion: Strategies through the lifespan* (5th ed., pp. 206–252). Norwalk, CT: Appleton & Lange.

Pilliter, A. (1999). *Maternal and Child Health Nursing* (3rd ed). Philadelphia: Lippincott.

Seidel, H. M., Rosenstein, B. J., & Pathak, A. (1997). *Primary care of the newborn.* (2nd ed.) St. Louis, MO: Mosby.

Thomas, K. (1994). Thermoregulation in neonates. *Neonatal Network, 13*(2), 15–25.

Vanderhoof, J. A., Zach, T. L., & Adrian, T. E. (1994). Gastrointestinal disease. In G. B. Avery, M. A. Fletcher, & M. G. MacDonald (Eds.), *Neonatology: Pathophysiology and management of the newborn* (4th ed., pp. 605–629). Philadelphia: Lippincott.

Walther, F. J., Benders, M. J., & Leighton, J. O. (1993). Early changes in the neonatal circulatory transition. *Journal of Pediatrics, 123*(4), 625–632.

Willinger, M., Hoffman, H., & Hartford, R. (1994). Infant sleep position and risk for sudden infant death syndrome: Report of meeting held January 13 and 14, 1994, National Institutes of Health, Bethesda, MD. *Pediatrics, 93*(5), 814–819.

Suggested Readings

Alexander, G., de Caunes, F. L., Hulsey, T., Tompkins, M., & Allen, M. (1992). Validity of postnatal assessments of gestational age: A comparison of the method of Ballard et al. and early ultrasonography. *American Journal of Obstetrics & Gynecology, 166*(3), 891–895.

Arlotti, J. P., Cottrell, B. H., Lee, S. H., & Curtin, J. J. (1998). Breastfeeding among low-income women with or without peer support. *Journal of Community Health Nursing, 15*(3), 163.

Bellig, L. L. (1989). A window on the neonate's brain. *Neonatal Network, 7*(4), 13–20.

Braveman, P., Egerter, S., Pearl, M., Marchi, K., & Miller, C. (1995). Problems associated with early discharge of newborn infants. *Pediatrics, 96*(4.1), 716.

Brooks, C. (1997). Neonatal hypoglycemia. *Neonatal Network, 16*(2), 15–21.

Cheng, T. L., & Partridge, J. C. (1993). Effect of bundling and warm environments on neonatal temperature. *Pediatrics, 92*(2), 238–240.

Chessare, J., Hunt, C., Bourguignon, C., & the Pediatric Research in Office Practices Network. (1995). A community-based survey of infant sleep position. *Pediatrics, 96*(5), 893–896.

Cornell, S. (1997). Understanding infant jaundice. A normal but potentially complicated condition. *Advances for Nurse Practitioners, 5*(2), 71–72.

Curz, E., Perrin, D., Hackman, R., & Czegledy-Nagy, E. (1996). Maternal smoking and pulmonary neuroendocirne cells in sudden infant death syndrome. *Pediatrics, 98*(4), 668–672.

Dodd, V. (1996). Gestational age assessment. *Neonatal Network, 15*(1), 27–36.

Harrison, L. (1997). Research utilization: Handling preterm infants in the NICU. *Neonatal Network 16*(3), 65–69.

Hill, A. S., Kurkowski, T. B., & Garcia, J. (2000). Oral support measures used in feeding the preterm infant. *Nursing Research, 49*(1), 2–10.

Locklin, M. (1987). Assessing jaundice in full-term newborns. *Pediatric Nursing, 13*(1), 15–19.

Messmer, P. R., Rodriguez, S., Adams, J., Wells-Gentry, J., Washburn, K., Zabaleta, I., & Abreu, S. (1997). Effect of kangaroo care on sleep time for neonates. *Pediatric Nursing, 23*, 408–414.

Neu, M., Browne, J. V., & Vojir, C. (2000). The impact of two transfer techniques used during skin-to-skin care on the physiologic and behavioral responses of preterm infants. *Nursing Research, 49*(4), 215–223.

Schraeder, B. D., Heverly, M. A., O'Brien, C., & Goodman, R. (1997). Academic achievement and educational resource use of very low birth weight (VLBW) survivors. *Pediatric Nursing, 23*, 21–25.

Shield-Poe, D., Pinelli, J. & Steinhausen, H. (1993). Prenatal alcohol exposure and long-term developmental consequences. *Lancet, 341*, 907–910.

VandenBerg, K. A. (1997). Basic principles of developmental caregiving. *Neonatal Network, 16*(7), 69–71.

Resources

Organizations and Websites

American Academy of Pediatrics
Division of Public Education
141 Northwest Point Blvd
P.O. Box 927
Elk Grove Village IL 60009-0927
www.aap.org/family/thumbs.htm

The Annual Review of Research for Neonatal Nurses
1304 Southpoint Boulevard, Suite 240
Petaluma, CA 94954-6861
(707) 762-2646

Association of Women's Health, Obstetric, and Neonatal Nurses (AWHONN)
700 14th Street NW, Suite 600
Washington, DC 20005-2019
(202) 662-1600

La Leche League International
P.O. Box 1209
Franklin Park, IL 60131-8209
(800) 525-3243

National Association of Neonatal Nurses
1304 Southpoint Boulevard, Suite 280
Petaluma, CA 94954-6859

CHAPTER 8

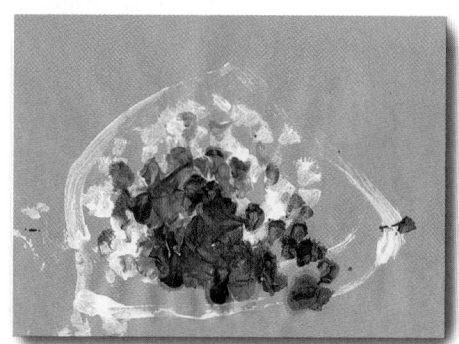

You have a healthy baby boy! How wonderful those words sound, but little do you know what they really mean!

The birth of our son Ronnie was such an exciting time, and we got advice from everyone. He was a great baby!

Once we got him home, we realized he was really ours for the rest of his life. I don't believe we ever thought about it in those terms—"the rest of his life." So many questions came to our minds about this small human and his care, not to mention his future.

- *How are we going to care for him?*
- *Will we do the right things?*
- *What kind of parents are we going to be?*
- *What do parents do?*
- *Who is going to care for him while we are at work?*

As a pediatric nurse, I had cared for children every day of my professional life. I knew what an infant needed. But in reality, what I knew was how to care for a sick child who did not belong to me.

Well, Ronnie belonged to me. He was completely dependent on me for everything. At his birth, I was no longer a pediatric nurse but his mother, with all the normal concerns about his growth and development, care, health, and safety.

GROWTH AND DEVELOPMENT OF THE INFANT

Janice L. Vincent, DSN, RN

COMPETENCIES

Upon completion of this chapter, the reader will be able to:

- *Discuss physiological growth and developmental milestones of infants.*
- *Discuss the process of infant fine and gross motor development, including the principles associated with them.*
- *Describe infant psychosexual, cognitive, and psychosocial development.*
- *Describe health promotion and maintenance activities for infants.*
- *Discuss caloric and fluid requirements for infants.*
- *Describe play activities of infancy.*
- *Discuss educational strategies for caregivers of infants as related to nutritional needs, growth and development patterns, stranger and separation anxiety, and safety.*

The miracle of life begins at conception and continues throughout the life span. The magnificence of this miracle is encountered during infancy and is the focus of this chapter. The first section focuses on the physiological growth patterns and psychosexual, cognitive, and the psychosocial development of an infant. The second section discusses health promotion activities, including health screening, dental care, and nutrition. Educational strategies for promoting an infant's optimal development will then be presented.

Infants are defined as 1 month to 1 year old. Rapid growth and development enables maturation to unfold in a relatively short time, and health status is based on the infant's ability to adapt to these rapid changes. As a health care provider, the nurse must have an understanding of these changes to ensure that the infant and his or her family maintain an optimal level of health.

The nurse can help the family integrate the infant into the family unit. The nurse also has the opportunity to educate the family, assist in problem identification, and facilitate decision making. By asking questions, interpreting feelings, and providing information to the family, the nurse is able to reinforce the self-confidence of each member of the family in caring for the infant.

Eye On:

Cultural Weight Differences

Birth weights differ among ethnic groups. For instance, Native American infants are often heavier at birth than European American infants. Infants of Asian descent are typically shorter and lighter than European American infants.

Critical Thinking

Posterior Fontanel

During 4-month-old Tommy's assessment, the nurse notes that his posterior fontanel is closed. What would be the most appropriate action for the nurse to take at this time? Why?

PHYSIOLOGICAL DEVELOPMENT

The rapid changes seen during infancy will never be encountered again throughout the life span. As the body matures, skill development progresses in an orderly fashion to enable the infant to respond to and cope with the world. Gross and fine motor skills develop in a cephalocaudal (head-to-toe) and proximal–distal (central-to-peripheral) fashion; gross motor abilities develop before fine motor abilities.

The infant's physical growth is influenced by genetics, the environment, ethnic background, and biology (Secker, 1999). Physical growth patterns include weight, height, and head circumference changes. The infant's growth measurements should be plotted on a growth chart and, over time, compared to the infant's own growth curve (see Appendix B for growth charts).

Weight and Height

During the first 6 months of life, the infant's birth weight typically doubles. The approximate weight gain is 1.5 lb per month, or 5–7 oz per week. In the second 6 months of life, the infant will gain about 3–5 oz per week (less than 1 lb per month). By 12 months of age, the infant's birth weight will have tripled.

Height increases during the first 6 months by approximately 1 inch per month. The rate of growth in height slows to approximately 0.5 inch (1.5 cm) per month by 12 months of age, resulting in almost a 50% increase in height from the birth length.

Head Growth

The size of the head changes rapidly during infancy, reflecting rapid brain growth. By the age of 12 months, the infant's brain will be two-thirds the size of an adult. During the first 6 months of life, head circumference will increase by approximately 0.5 inch (1.3 cm) per month. During the second 6 months of life, head circumference will slow to approximately 0.25 inch (0.6 cm) per month. As the head grows, the fontanels gradually close, with the posterior fontanel closing by 2 months of age and the anterior fontanel closing by 12–18 months of age.

Motor Development

Motor development is strongly related to physical, cognitive, and social development. Motor growth includes gross and fine motor development, which provides the infant with the means and freedom to explore the environment. Chapter 6 discusses growth and development in detail. General principles associated with motor development include:

- Voluntary behaviors follow the disappearance of primitive reflexes. To be able to willingly grasp an object, the infant must first lose the involuntary grasp reflex.
- Pronation occurs before supination. The infant must be able to pick up an object (pronation) before being able to put the object in the mouth (supination).
- The ability to grasp an object precedes the ability to release it (Dixon & Stein, 2000).

Gross Motor

Gross motor development is the ability to use large muscle groups to maintain balance and postural control or locomotion. A major task for the infant in obtaining postural control is head control, which is mastered in the prone as well as the upright positions, e.g., standing and sitting. By the age of 1 month, the infant can turn the head to the side while prone and, at 4 months of age, can hold the head up and use the forearms for support (Figure 8-1). At 5 to 6 months of age, the infant has the ability to hold the head, chest, and abdomen up by bearing weight with the hands (Figure 8-2). Once weight bearing with the hands has occurred, the infant will have the ability to turn readily from a prone to a supine position and, 1 month later, will be able to turn from a supine position to a prone position.

Infant head control is judged by the presence or absence of head lag. The amount of head lag can be determined when the infant is pulled by the arms from a supine to a sitting position. At 1 month of age, the infant's back is completely rounded while in a sitting position, with the head

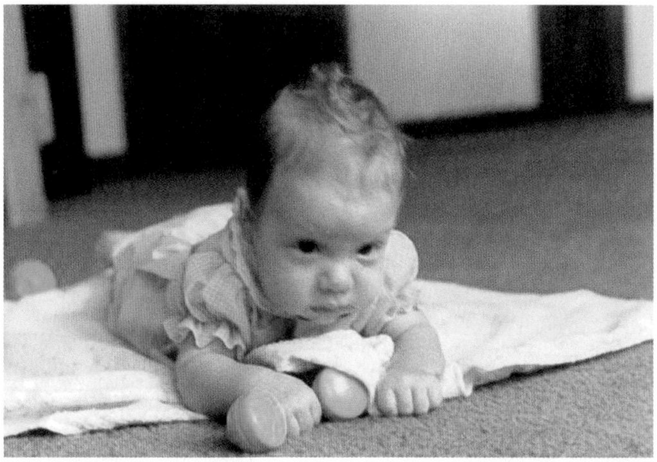

Figure 8-1 Four-month-old infant can lift head and support self on forearms.

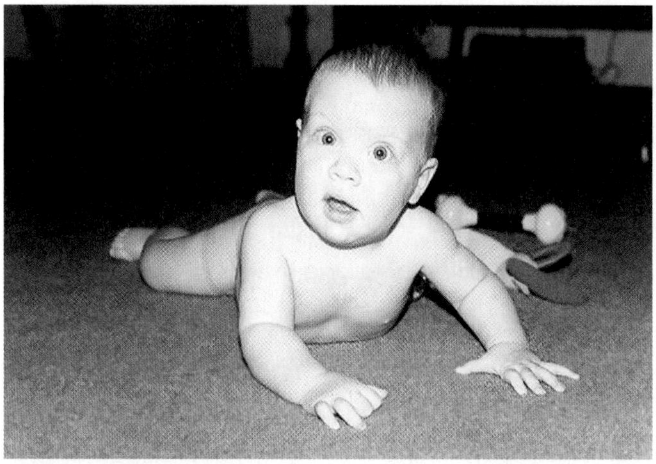

Figure 8-2 At 5–6 months of age, infant can bear weight on arms, and lift head, chest, and abdomen.

falling forward. By 2 months, partial head lag is evident, and the infant can hold the head erect with minimal head bobbing while sitting. At 4 months, the infant has no head lag and good head control while sitting (Figure 8-3).

Once head control is established, the infant begins to sit without support. At 4 months of age, the infant can sit only with support. By 6 months of age, the infant can sit alone while using the hands for support. Between 7 and 8 months, the infant is able to sit alone steadily without any support and, by 12 months, sits alone well (Figure 8-4). When the infant is able to sit alone without support, then he or she can explore the environment by scooting or moving on the floor while sitting.

Locomotion, the ability to move from place to place without assistance, is dependent on head control and sitting without support. A variety of skills such as rolling over, bearing weight, moving forward on all extremities, and standing upright without assistance are also necessary for locomotion (Figure 8-5). Once these skills are developed,

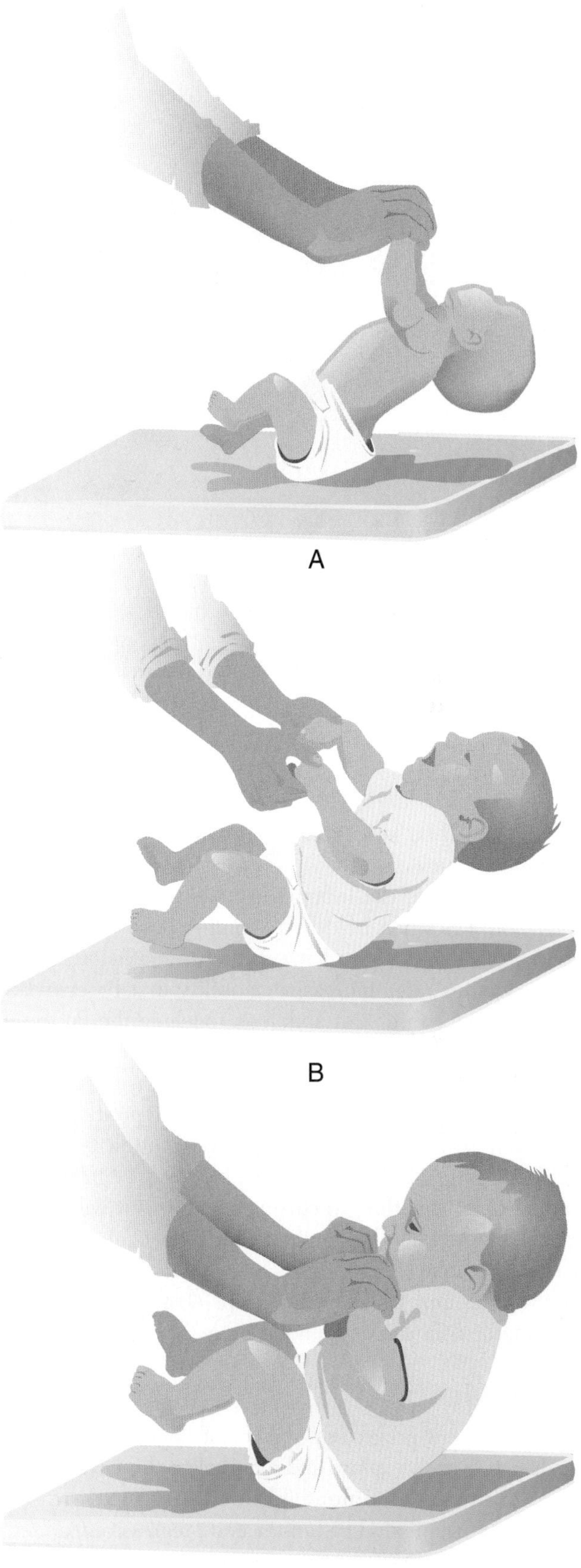

Figure 8-3 Head Lag at (A) 1 Month Old, (B) 2 Months Old, and (C) 4 Months Old

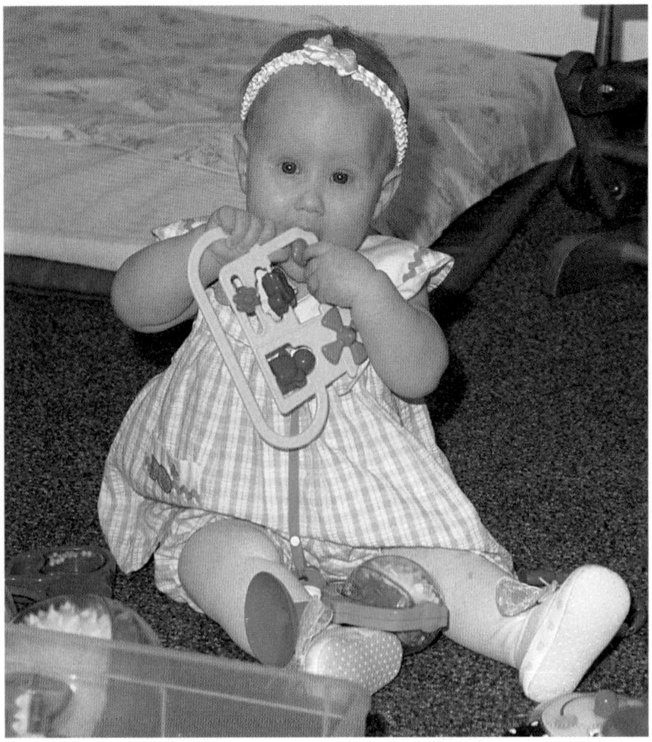

Figure 8-4 Seven-month-old infant sits alone well without support.

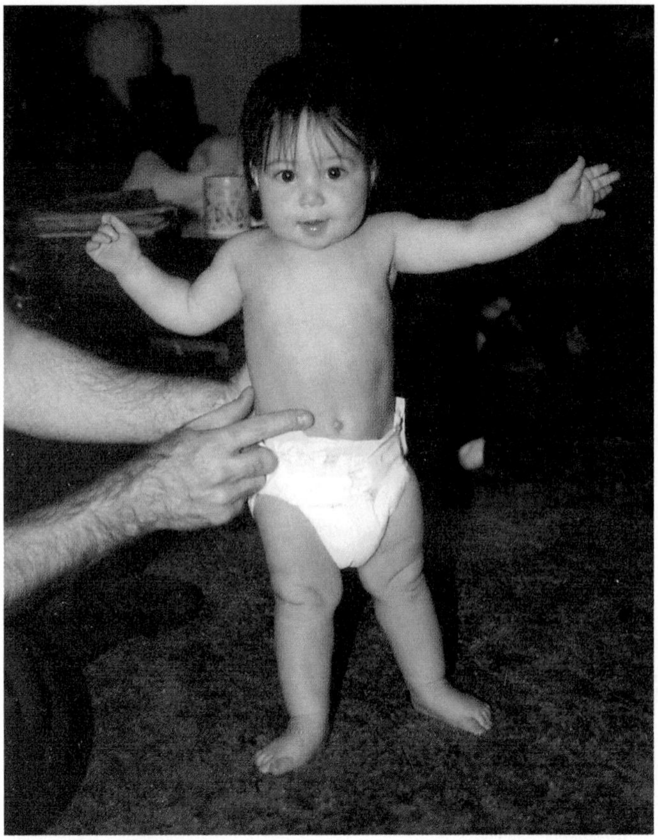

Figure 8-5 Infant Bearing Weight with Support

the infant will be able to move forward (walk), first with assistance, then alone.

By 6 months, the infant can bear most of the body's weight on legs when held in a standing position, and by 8 months can bear weight. From 8 to 10 months of age, the infant demonstrates increasing mobility first by **crawling** (pulling self forward with abdomen touching the floor) and then by **creeping** (moving on hands and knees with abdomen off the floor). By the time infants are creeping, they are able to pull themselves to a standing position.

From 10 to 12 months, infant locomotion progresses rapidly. During this time, deliberate steps will be taken while holding onto something (**cruising**). The infant will start to walk sideways while holding onto furniture, before walking or standing alone (Figure 8-6). Once infants can stand alone, they will attempt to take a few steps alone. A summary of gross motor skills can be found in Table 8-1.

Fine Motor

As development progresses, the infant begins to utilize the hands and eyes to explore and manipulate the environment. Fine motor development is the ability to coordinate hand–eye movement in an orderly and progressive manner.

During the first month of life, a primitive grasp reflex enables the infant to hold objects with a tightly clenched fist. By the end of 2 months, this primitive reflex fades and the infant begins to actively grasp and momentarily hold an object before dropping it.

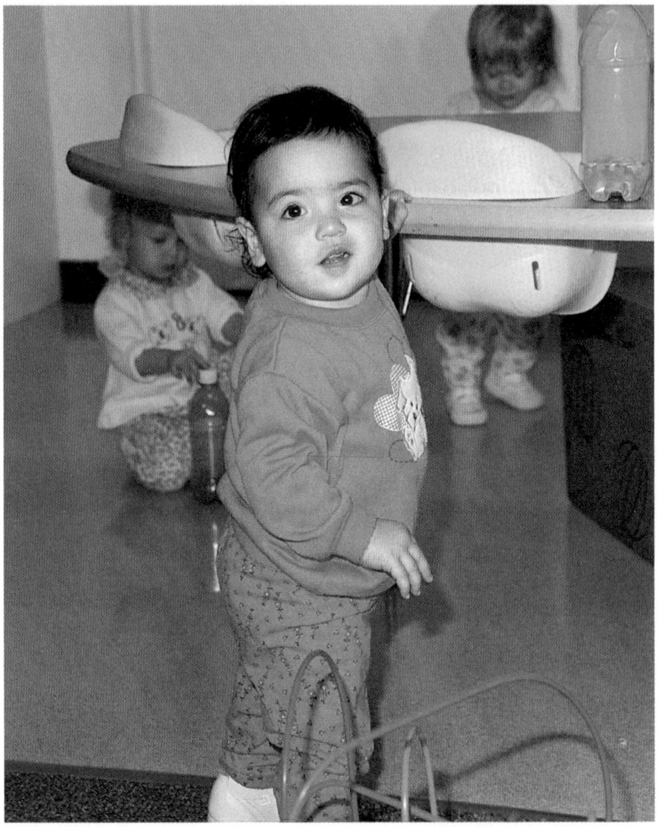

Figure 8-6 Infant Cruising by Holding onto Table

TABLE 8-1 Summary of Gross Motor Development

Age	Motor Skill
2–3 Months	Some head lag when pulled to sitting position
	Holds head up and supports weight on forearms when prone
	Some head bobbing while supported in sitting position
	Rolls from abdomen to back
	Tonic neck and Moro reflexes disappearing
4–6 Months	Good head control with no head lag, holds chest and abdomen up with weight supported by hands while prone
	Sits with support
	Rolls from back to abdomen
	Bears weight in standing position with support
7–8 Months	Sits alone without support
	Bears weight with some support
9–12 Months	Moves from prone to sitting to standing position without assistance
	Stands alone without support
	Goes from crawling to creeping to cruising
	Attempts to walk alone

Kids Want To Know

Sibling Rivalry: I want my mommy all to myself.

- This is a very difficult statement for a mother to handle. It is important to assure the child that his or her mommy loves him very much.
- Encourage the child to help with an infant sibling's care.
- Most importantly, counsel the mother to find special "big kid" time just for the older sibling. "Big kid" activities could be playing with toys that have little pieces, which are normally off limits when the infant is around, painting, reading a book, or going for a walk.

At 3 months of age, the infant has the ability to hold the hand open, look at the fingers, and place them in the mouth, and by 4 months, the infant can look from hand to hand. By 5 months of age, the infant can voluntarily grasp an object with the whole hand (palmar grasp), can actively manipulate all grasped objects and place them in the mouth. Between 6 and 7 months of age, the infant can hold a bottle securely, and readily grasp the feet and pull them to the mouth. In addition, the infant can willingly drop any grasped object.

As the infant's fine motor development progresses, the palmar grasp is replaced with a thumb and finger pincer grasp at approximately 8 months of age (Figure 8-7). At first, the infant can only crudely grasp objects in a pincer fashion with the thumb and index finger. As the infant practices the grasp, a dominant hand begins to emerge. During this developmental time, the infant continues to test the new abilities by reaching for objects, banging them together, and transferring them from hand to hand.

By 10 months of age, the infant's pincer grasp is more refined and reflected in the ability to grasp small finger foods such as Cheerios. Between 10 and 12 months of age, the infant's hand movements become very deliberate, as they purposefully drop or place small objects into a container and remove them. The infant can even hold and mark paper with a crayon. By 12 months of age, the infant will be able to turn multiple pages in a book. A summary of fine motor development can be found in Table 8-2. See Figure 8-7 for development of grasp during the first year.

PSYCHOSEXUAL DEVELOPMENT

Psychosexual development is based on the individual's need to seek pleasure. The individual must be able to balance pleasure seeking with societal expectations. According to Freud's theory, the infant is in the oral stage of development (birth to 1 year), during which the need for pleasure dominates life. Oral stimulation or sucking is the central focus of this stage (Dixon & Stein, 2000). According to Freud, feeding or nutritive sucking becomes the most important source of pleasure and satisfaction. See Chapter 6 for more information on Freud's theory.

As development progresses, the infant learns to connect actions with end results. For example, the infant learns that cries of hunger result in being fed, and eventually the caregiver's touch will be associated with feeding needs being met as infants learn to delay the need for immediate gratification in anticipation of being fed. If the infant is not fed within a few minutes of being held, the infant will start to cry as a signal that the need for the pleasure or comfort from the feeding has not been met.

In addition to feeding, another source of pleasure and satisfaction for the infant is obtained through nonnutritive

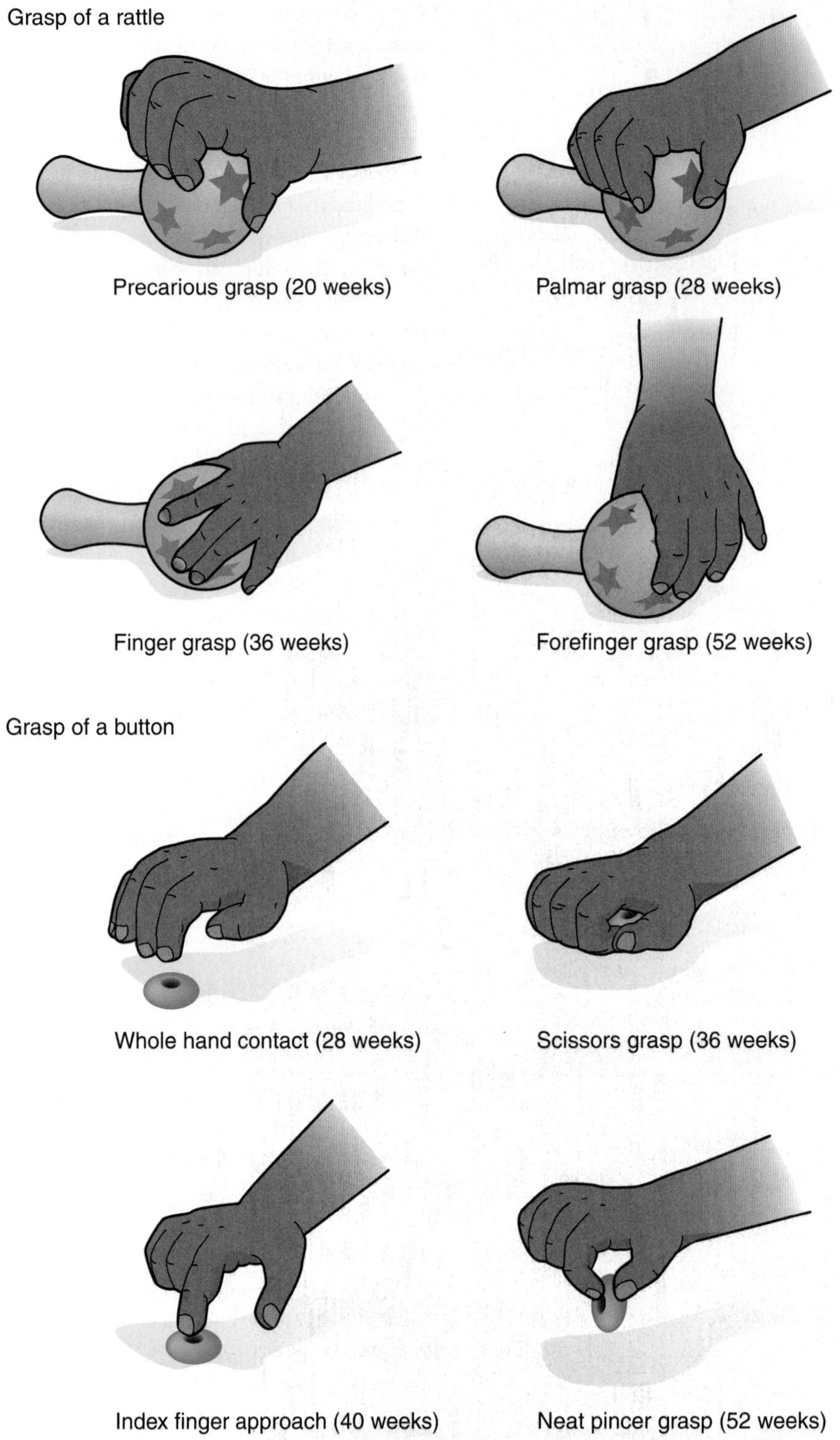

Figure 8-7 Development of Prehension

sucking (Figure 8-8). With the infant's natural tendency to suck, nonnutritive sucking occurs first by accident through the reflex of rooting and then purposefully by actively placing objects, such as toys, fingers, or a pacifier, in the mouth.

COGNITIVE DEVELOPMENT

According to Piaget (1952), an infant is in the sensorimotor stage (birth to 24 months) of cognitive development when knowledge is acquired about an object through interaction

TABLE 8-2 Summary of Fine Motor Development

Age	Motor Skill
2–3 Months	Follows object past midline Holds hands open Regards own hands and fingers when held in front of face Places hand in mouth Briefly reaches at a dangling object
4–5 Months	Reaches for object beyond grasp Looks from object to hand and back again Places object in mouth Uses whole hand to grasp object Plays actively with hands and feet
6–7 Months	Holds objects securely and bangs them together Actively drops objects Transfers object between hands
8–9 Months	Pincer grasp beginning Releases object at will Dominant hand preference emerging
10–12 Months	True pincer grasp present Can self-feed finger foods Can place small objects into a container Can remove small objects from a container Can hold and mark with a crayon Can turn multiple pages in a book

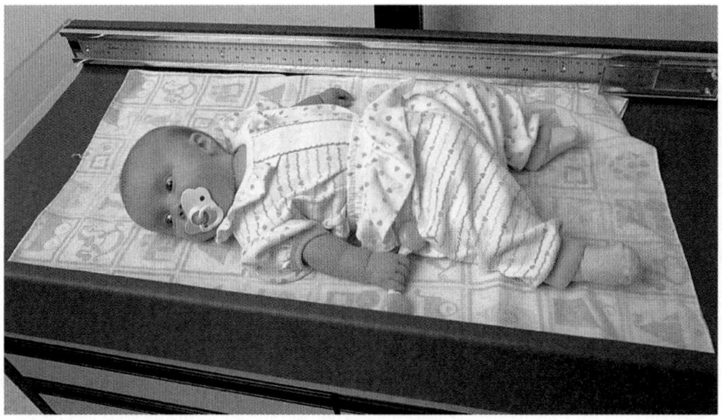

Figure 8-8 Nonnutritive sucking is a source of pleasure and satisfaction for infants.

with that object and use of the senses. The major task for the infant, according to Piaget, is **object permanence,** in which the infant learns that an object is not an extension of the self and that it continues to exist even when it cannot be seen.

Piaget's sensorimotor stage consist of six substages. During the first year of life, the infant will pass through the first four of these substages. In the first substage, the newborn (birth to 1 month) learns about the world through repetitive use of involuntary reflexes. These repetitive acts, such as rooting, sucking, or crying, provide the infant with cause-and-effect experiences. For example, when an infant is hungry, crying will signal the infant has a need. The caregiver understands this cry is due to hunger and will provide the needed nourishment. When the nipple is provided, the infant will stop crying and begin to suck to obtain nourishment. Through these actions, the infant learns crying will result in the appearance of a nipple, followed by sucking, which results in satisfaction and contentment.

The second substage—primary circular reactions—occurs between 1 and 4 months of age; the infant's random movements become voluntary actions. Here, the infant becomes an active observer of the world but continues to be dominated by the need for pleasure. For example, an infant who cries when the diaper is wet will stop when touched by the caregiver in anticipation of the diaper being changed. The infant has learned crying in response to a wet diaper results in a clean, dry diaper.

In addition, up to 4 months of age, the infant begins to develop hand–eye coordination and becomes more interested in the immediate environment. Sounds, such as cooing and smiling, and gestures made by the caregiver are imitated. As objects become familiar, the infant will look and grasp at objects such as a toy rattle placed in the infant's visual field. However, object permanence has not yet developed, since the infant will not search for the familiar object when it is removed from the visual field. To infants this age, the object is "out of sight, out of mind."

Between 4 and 8 months of age, the infant progresses through the third substage—secondary circular reaction—which is characterized by becoming more aware of the surrounding environment and mastery of voluntary actions. The concept of play becomes evident during this period as well. Here, the infant's actions are more intentional and not solely directed by pleasure as the infant learns through repetitive actions to create interesting sights and sounds and begins to focus on the effects of the actions (Figure 8-9). For instance, the infant may repeatedly bang a toy just to produce a different sound.

The beginning of object permanence is evident during this substage, as an object is no longer seen as an extension of the infant but rather as a separate entity. While interacting with a familiar object, the infant will now search for the object if it is removed from the visual field. Although infants will look for the object, they quickly lose interest if it is not readily found. Another example of object permanence is the infant's development of stranger anxiety when left with a new babysitter. Here, the infant actively searches for the caregiver after the caregiver has left and may begin crying when the caregiver is not found.

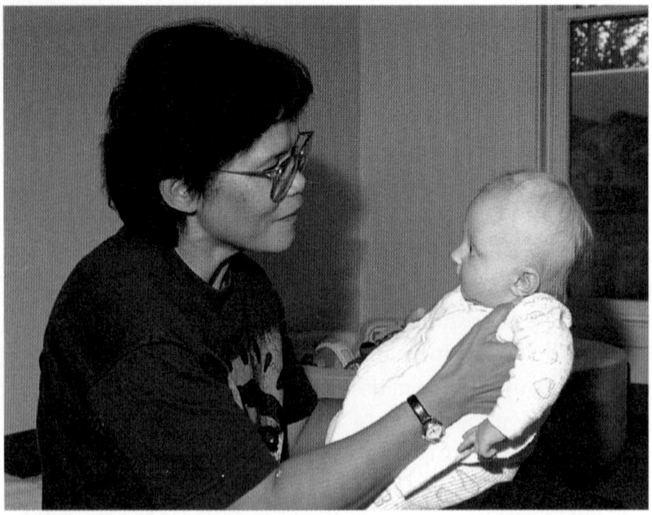

Figure 8-9 Infants like to examine faces.

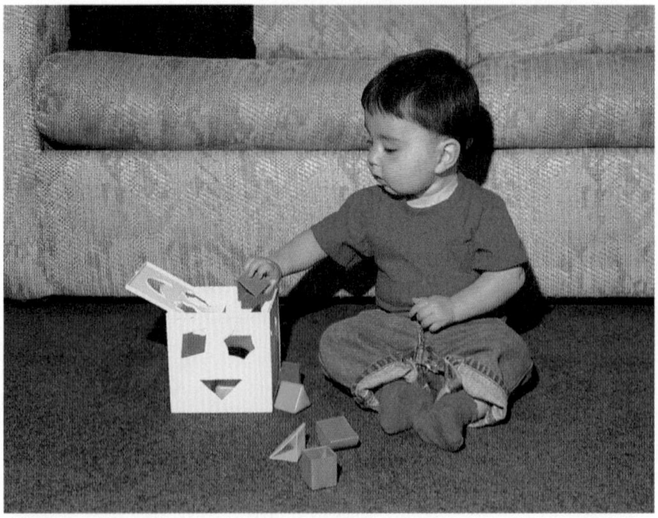

Figure 8-10 Older infants enjoy putting blocks in containers.

The infant applies newly mastered skills to new experiences in the fourth substage (8 to 12 months), called coordination of secondary schema, and is able to put several events together to accomplish an end result. For example, the infant is able to put blocks into a container with various shaped holes, and understand simple words and commands—e.g., no-no, bye-bye, cracker.

Object permanence is apparent and demonstrated when the infant actively seeks a hidden object. The beginning of reasoning is evident when the infant moves any obstacle to uncover a hidden object (Figure 8-10).

PSYCHOSOCIAL DEVELOPMENT

The psychosocial development of an infant, as defined by Erikson (1963), is centered around the concept of trust versus mistrust. According to Erikson, trust is developed when the basic needs of feeding, clothing, and comforting are met by caretakers. If these needs are not met, the infant will develop a mistrust of others.

However, trust development involves more than just meeting basic needs. The quality of the caregiver–infant interaction while providing care also plays a major role. If the caregiver consistently demonstrates nurturing behaviors such as talking, playing, smiling, clothing, and comforting, the infant will develop a strong sense of trust. If these behaviors are absent, trust development may be delayed. Furthermore, the caregiver and infant must learn together ways to achieve satisfaction and decrease frustration during daily routines (Figure 8-11).

Should the infant be in an alternative child care situation (child care workers or sitters), the trust development is continued by the child care provider, who needs to know the infant's:

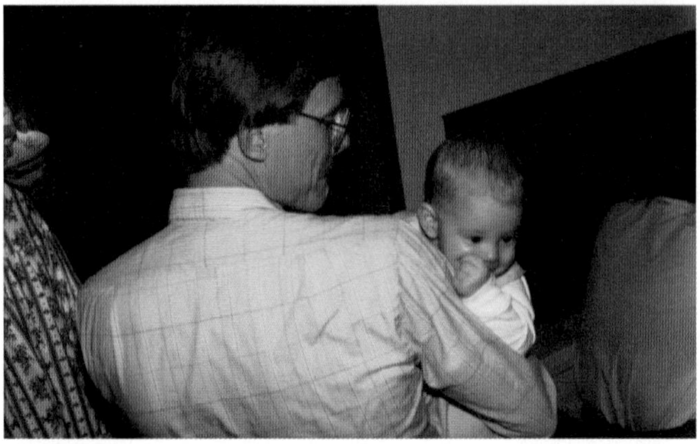

Figure 8-11 Fathers are important caregivers for infants.

- Usual home routines
- Sleep patterns
- Eating habits
- Cues given when frustrated
- Response to comforting methods
- Favorite toys, games, songs, music

Confidence in the child care provider's ability to provide a trusting environment is very important. The caregiver should inquire about:

- The child care provider's experience with infants
- How the child care provider comforts a fussy infant
- Whether there are other children in their care
- The number of children in their care at any given time

Nursing Tip:

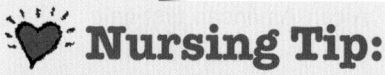

Understanding psychosocial development

To improve your understanding of the infant's psychosocial development and the caregiver's knowledge of psychosocial development, ask yourself:

- Does the infant demonstrate trust in the environment?
- What does the caregiver know about developing the infant's sense of trust?
- Does the caregiver have other factors, i.e., divorce, financial problems, and health problems, that might interfere with the infant's development of a sense of trust?
- Are there any environmental and/or cultural biases that might impede the caregiver's ability to assist the infant in developing a trusting relationship?

If the infant's needs are met in a consistent manner by the caregiver or alternative child care provider, trust in the self as well as trust in others and the surrounding environment will develop. If not, the infant will eventually develop a sense of mistrust.

HEALTH PROMOTION

The health status of the infant, a major concern for caregivers, is based on the ability to adapt to rapid changes.

Nursing Tip:

Family database

To be more effective in health promotion, it is important to be familiar with family circumstances, including the following (Schor, 1995):

- Composition of the household
- Language spoken in the household
- Identity of the primary caregiver
- Caregivers' health status
- Caregivers' employment status
- Caregivers' educational level
- Caregivers' financial status
- Caregivers' use of alcohol, tobacco, and other substances
- Adequacy of the house
- Cultural influences
- Religious affiliation
- Social support and/or conflict

Therefore, the caregiver needs to know the expected physical, emotional, and developmental growth patterns of the infant. As health care providers, nurses are able to assist the caregiver in understanding these patterns. The Nursing Tip and Research Highlight boxes will assist in understanding the family's makeup and particular circumstances. Through education, counseling, anticipatory guidance, and understanding the family's cultural needs, the nurse can assist the caregiver and family and ensure that the infant maintains an optimal level of health and development.

Health Screening

Health promotion and maintenance are important since health status is a good indicator of the infant's ability to adapt to the rapid changes of growth and development. Optimal health enables the infant to adjust to these changes without placing undue stress on the body.

Health screening provides the opportunity to assess for and detect any problems the infant may have and includes tests to detect phenylketonuria (PKU), iron deficiency anemia, lead poisoning, and hypothyroidism. The infant's health screening actually begins immediately after birth with the first Apgar scoring and physical examination. Once discharged home, the infant's health promotion and maintenance becomes the responsibility of the caregiver, who should be encouraged to contact the health care provider for any health concerns.

In the first year, health screening or well-child visits are usually scheduled when the infant is 2 weeks, and 2, 4, 6, 9, and 12 months old. The screening visit typically includes

Family Teaching

When to Call Your Health Care Provider

The following signs and symptoms may indicate the need to contact the health care provider:

- Fever: under 2 months 100.2°F (37.9°C); 3 to 6 months 101°F (38.3°C); over 6 months 103°F (39.4°C)
- Feeding poorly: Lack of interest, poor sucking effort, failure to awaken for feeding
- Vomiting
- Decreased activity or alertness: appears listless
- Inconsolable crying
- Abnormal movement: unusual jerking of body
- Unusual skin color: pale or mottled skin color; bluish around the lips

(Reisser, 1998; Shelov, 1998)

Research Highlight

Parental Concerns of Mexican American First-Time Mothers and Fathers

Study Purpose

To identify the concerns of first-time Mexican American parents during the first 6 months.

Methods

A convenience sample of Mexican American parents (n = 26) living in a rural 170-square-mile area of Hidalgo County of southern Texas were identified by network sampling methods. A majority of the families (62%) had an annual family income of less than $5,000. Families were visited at differing times for the infants' first 6 months and asked about parental concerns. Responses were recorded, transcribed, and translated if necessary. Responses were analyzed and divided into categories of parental concerns.

Findings

Eight areas of parental concerns were identified. These concerns, in decreasing order of importance, are (1) illness of a family member, (2) providing for the material needs of the infant, (3) threatened job loss or the need to find employment, (4) breastfeeding issues and the infant's diet, (5) uncertainty regarding how to rear an infant, (6) threats infants face in the future, (7) lack of assistance in parenting, and (8) other concerns, including changing social involvement, infant crying, and safety of the infant once the infant is mobile. Both parents were equally concerned about most matters, except breastfeeding issues.

Implications

Mexican American parents are very concerned with the health of their infants. Teaching specific skills to recognize illness and how to manage illness and emergencies to parents in clinics and other nurse–client interactions is highly recommended. Basic concepts of infant care and development are also important to new parents and can be taught and emphasized in many areas, including parent education classes.

Citation

Niska, K. J., Lia-Hoagberg, B., & Snyder, M. (1997). Parental concerns of Mexican American first-time mothers and fathers. *Public Health Nursing, 14*(2), 111–117.

health assessment, physical examination, growth indicators (weight, height, head circumference), anticipatory guidance, parental concerns, and administration of scheduled immunizations. Table 8-3 provides an outline of typical health screening visits.

During the visit, the caregiver will probably have questions and concerns regarding the infant's ongoing needs and care. The nurse can be instrumental in providing information related to physical development, nutrition, safety, immunizations, and play. With guidance, the caregiver will be better able to understand the infant's needs and the care required to meet those needs.

Immunizations

The recommended childhood immunization schedule can be found in Appendix C (Advisory Committee on Immunization Practices [ACIP], 2000).

Prior to administering any immunization, the nurse assesses for contraindications to administration. Immunizations are usually not contraindicated when a mild illness such as allergic rhinitis, mild diarrhea, or mild respiratory infection is present (see Chapter 15 for an extensive discussion on contraindication to immunizations). The nurse also provides the caregiver with information about the benefits

TABLE 8-3 Health Screening Visits

Emphasis of Visit	1 Month	2 Months	4 Months	6 Months	9 Months	12 Months
Assessments: Developmental milestones, hearing and vision, nutritional	✔	✔	✔	✔	✔	✔
Physical examination	✔	✔	✔	✔	✔	✔
Growth measurements: Height, weight, head circumference	✔	✔	✔	✔	✔	✔
Immunizations*						
Anticipatory guidance: Infant care, expected growth, and developmental milestones, safety, dental health	✔	✔	✔	✔	✔	✔
Screenings:						
PKU	✔					
Thyroid	✔					
Hematocrit, Hemoglobin	✔				✔	
Lead					✔ or	✔
Parental concerns	✔	✔	✔	✔	✔	✔

Adapted from: Shelov, S. P. (Ed.), (1998). Caring for your baby and young child. New York: Bantam.
** Refer to Appendix C for latest immunization schedule.*

Family Teaching

Home Care with Immunizations

- Most common reactions usually last 1–2 days:
  - Irritability
  - Mild loss of appetite
  - Low-grade fever (<102°F)
  - Redness, swelling, and tenderness at the injection site
- General treatment of reaction:
  - Give acetaminophen at the time of the immunization
  - Administer acetaminophen every 4–6 hours for a total of three doses
- Immunization-specific reaction:
  - Diphtheria, Tetanus, Pertussis (DTaP)—low-grade fever with redness, swelling, and tenderness at injection site
  - Inactivated polio vaccine (IPV)—tenderness at injection site
  - Hepatitis B (hep B)—irritability and redness, swelling, and tenderness at injection site
  - Measles, mumps, rubella (MMR)—mild rash, low-grade fever, and drowsiness beginning 7–10 days after immunization
- Contact the health care provider immediately if the infant develops any symptoms other than the common reactions or if the mild reactions persist longer than 2 days.

(Vaccine Information, 1994; Shelov, 1998)

and risks of the immunizations and answers questions about the immunizations. In addition, the caregiver should receive information about possible reactions the infant might experience after receiving the immunizations (Vaccine Information, 1994).

Vision

Research has shown that even newborns have full visual array with acuity of 20/100 to 20/200 (Behrman, 1996). Therefore, it is important that problems with vision be detected early to prevent significant delays in motor development since visual and auditory abilities have an impact on perception and understanding of the surrounding environment. To enhance visual development, a variety of stimuli should be introduced into the infant's life.

Visual development is demonstrated by the infant's ability to follow a light or object placed within the visual field and the cessation of body movements after fixating on the object (Figure 8-12). Infants prefer the human face, demonstrated by visual attentiveness when interacting with the caregiver. By 6 months, the infant can recognize familiar faces and may experience stranger anxiety. As visual acuity improves and motor skills develop, the infant begins to respond to the variety of colors and shapes in the environment. Of particular interest to the infant is any object with a black–white contrast (Slusher & McClure, 1992). Any caregiver concern regarding visual responsiveness and/or lack of eye contact in their infant may indicate visual problems.

Once the skills of reaching and picking up objects have developed, play behavior can be observed to evaluate vision, since the ability to easily find and pick up small toys is a good indicator of vision in children under 3 years of age. If milestones in visual development are not consistently demonstrated, the infant should be referred for further evaluation (Behrman, 1996).

Nursing Alert

Infant Behaviors Related to Visual Problems

- *Absence of blink*
- *Absence of doll's eye reflex (movement of head to the right or left, in which eyes lag behind and do not immediately adjust to the new position; disappears as infant is able to focus)*
- *Does not fixate on objects*
- *Does not follow objects by 1 month of age*
- *Does not watch own hands and feet by 4 months of age*
- *Does not reach for objects by 5 months of age*
- *Absent or poor hand–eye coordination by 7 months of age*
- *Does not watch objects fall when dropped*

Hearing

The intensity of the infant's response to auditory stimuli may vary depending on the state of alertness. The human voice is an important and readily available sound stimulus, and infants prefer the sound of a human voice to other sounds in their environment. The infant also responds well to musical toys and those making different sounds (Figure 8-13).

Hearing problems should be detected early in life to prevent significant delays in speech development. A hearing problem is when an infant does not consistently achieve hearing milestones in development (Capute & Accardo, 1978).

An infant's development can be profoundly affected by the inability to see and/or hear. Therefore, it is important infant's vision and hearing be assessed regularly (see Chapter 14 for further information).

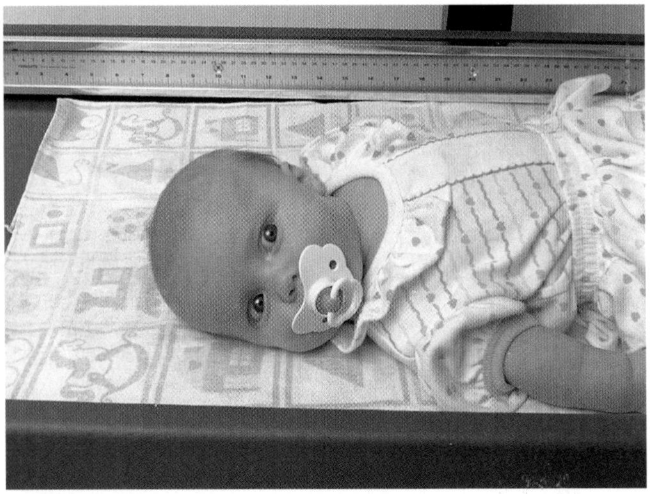

Figure 8-12 At 2 months of age infants can track objects in their visual field.

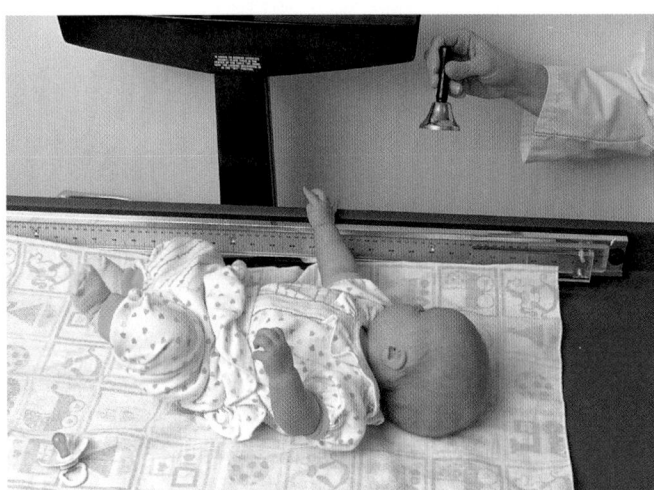

Figure 8-13 At 2 months of age infants can localize sounds.

Nursing Alert

Infant Behaviors Related to Hearing Problems

- *Lack of startle reflex or blink with a loud sound*
- *Failure to be awakened by loud noises in the environment*
- *Failure to turn head toward a sound by 6 months of age*
- *Absent babble or voice inflection by 7 months of age*
- *General indifference to sound*
- *Lack of response to the spoken word*
- *Failure to follow verbal direction*
- *Failure to respond to a human voice*

Nursing Tip:

Parental concerns about infant hearing and vision

Caregivers are in constant interaction with their infant and are usually the first to notice something is wrong with vision and/or hearing. Be alert to any concerns expressed by the caregiver regarding the infant's lack of response or inability to achieve milestones associated with vision and/or hearing.

REFLECTIONS FROM FAMILIES

How could he be deaf? We could not believe what was being said about our baby. But in reality, we had known for some time that something was wrong. By the time Chad was 2 months old, we became increasingly concerned that he might have a hearing problem. We decided to get him checked since Chad did not seem to respond to loud noises or to turn his head to the sound of our voices. Now, we have been told that he is deaf. What will happen now?

Dental Care

Tooth development and eruption are affected by genetics, gender, race, and growth patterns. **Deciduous teeth,** also referred to as primary or baby teeth, are the first teeth to develop and erupt. The eruption of teeth varies among children, but the teething process typically begins around 3–4 months of age. The first teeth to erupt are usually the lower central incisors, followed by the upper central incisors after approximately 4–8 weeks (Shelov, 1998) (Figure 8-14).

Dental hygiene should begin with the eruption of the deciduous teeth, by gently cleaning the infant's teeth and gums with a clean wet cloth using a circular movement or with a small, soft-bristled toothbrush (Jaques, 1993). It is important to establish a routine of dental hygiene early in life to prevent future dental problems.

Fluoride helps to prevent dental caries, and may be given as a supplement if drinking water does not contain enough fluoride. The caregiver should be encouraged to investigate the fluoride content of the drinking water system by contacting their local water board or company.

An infant who is exclusively breastfed or whose formula is prepared with water that is not fluoridated should receive a daily supplement of sodium fluoride (Jaques, 1993) (Table 8-4). According to the American Academy of Pediatrics (AAP) (1995), fluoride supplements should be started at 6 months of life. However, when fluoridation is available in the water and exceeds 0.3 ppm concentration, the infant does not need fluoride supplements. The level that protects tooth enamel without causing tooth staining from an excessive amount of fluoride is 0.6 ppm.

Dental caries can also occur in infants who have frequent and/or prolonged exposure to sugars found in milk, formula, or juice. The longer the sugar stays on the tooth enamel, the more opportunity there is for bacteria in the mouth to combine with sugar to form dental caries (Jaques, 1993; Oppenheim, 1996). This type of dental caries, known as **nursing** or **bottle-mouth caries,** is commonly seen in infants who receive a bottle filled with formula or juice at nap or bedtime. The problem also occurs in infants who breastfeed for prolonged times or on demand after tooth eruption (Oppenheim, 1996) (Figure 8-15).

Nursing Tip:

Estimation of deciduous teeth related to child's age

Caregivers are usually concerned about the number of teeth their child should have at a certain age. While each child gets teeth at a different rate, the following formula is used by many clinicians as a guide to determine the expected number of teeth a child should have at a certain age: Subtract 6 from the child's age in months to equal the total number teeth expected. For example: 18 months old – 6 = 12 teeth expected at 18 months.

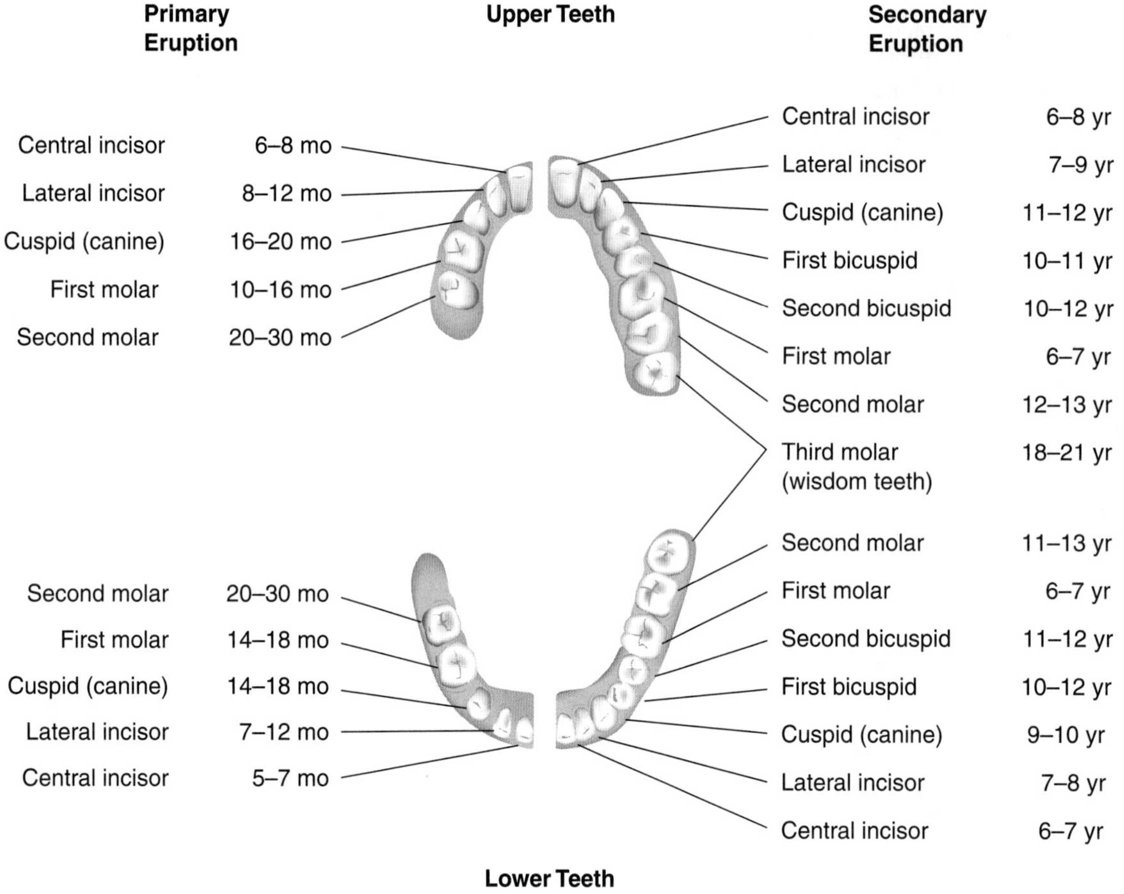

Figure 8-14 Sequence of Tooth Errution

TABLE 8-4 Daily Fluoride Supplementation*

	Fluoride Content of Water		
Child's Age	**< 0.3 ppm**	**0.3–0.6 ppm**	**> 0.6 ppm**
Birth–6 Months	0	0	0
6 Months–3 Years	0.25	0	0
3–6 Years	0.50	0.25	0
6–12 Years	1.00	0.50	0

** Fluoride dose given in milligrams.*
Adapted from the 1995 recommendations of the AAP.

Dental hygiene also includes routine visits to the dentist. The first dental visit usually occurs after several teeth have erupted. Most dentists suggest that this first visit occur before the child is 2 years of age (Jaques, 1993; Oppenheim, 1996). The frequency of dental visits is usually based on the child's state of health, family history of dental problems, and the need for fluoride supplements (McDonald & Avery, 1994).

Teething

During infancy, the period of eruption of deciduous teeth is called **teething** and occurs over several months. During eruption, the periodontal membrane becomes slightly swollen, red, and tender. The infant may have increased drooling and fussiness, mild anorexia, and an increased desire to bite. Other symptoms such as low-grade fever, vomiting, and diarrhea have also been attributed to teething

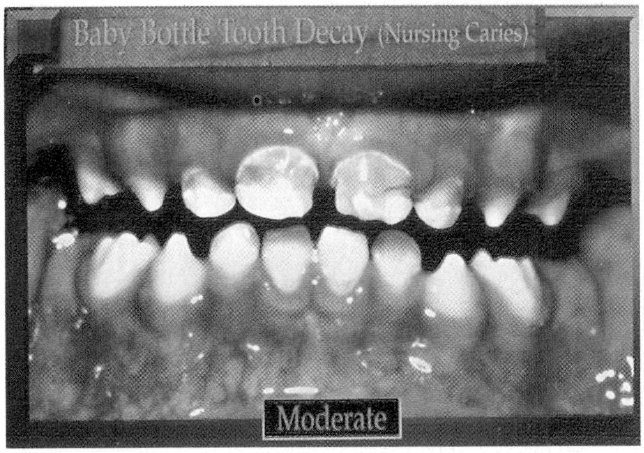

Figure 8-15 Moderate Baby Bottle Tooth Decay. Courtesy of American Academy of Pediatric Dentistry.

Family Teaching

Soothing Swollen, Tender Gums

To soothe swollen, red gums, try:
- Frozen teething ring
- Ice cube in a washcloth
- Zwieback
- Hard rubber toy
- Topical application of an oral anesthetic such as Ora-Gel

For irritability and/or a low-grade temperature, give:
- Acetaminophen according to recommended dosage

(Shelov, 1998). The accompanying Family Teaching box contains several measures that can be used to soothe the infant during the teething process.

Nutrition

Since the infant experiences rapid changes in growth and development over a relatively short time, a good nutritional foundation is necessary. The responsibility for meeting the infant's nutritional needs falls on the caregiver; needs are normally evaluated during a routine assessment or when the caregiver expresses a concern over the infant's pattern of growth and development. During the assessment, the nurse should also take the opportunity to discuss the infant's developmental skills and feeding milestones.

For the first few months of the child's life, the infant will be either breastfed, formula-fed, or a combination of the two. Both breast and formula feedings are nutritionally sound, easy to digest, and provide the infant with the needed nutrients to grow. They also provide approximately 20 kcal/oz. (See Chapter 7 for a discussion of formulas.) The infant's nutritional requirements are based on the physical activity and rate of growth needed to support life. At birth, energy requirements are 120 kcal/kg/day. They gradually decrease to 100 kcal/kg/day by 1 year of age (Whitley, Cataldo, DeBruyne, & Rolfes, 1996), because of the gradual decline in metabolic needs as the infant's growth slows. In addition to energy requirements, the infant must have adequate fluid intake, which is based on daily energy expenditure. Infant fluid requirements are 1–1.5 mL/kcal expended per day (Whitley et al., 1996) (Figure 8-16).

Solid Foods

The American Academy of Pediatrics recommends introducing semisolid foods, i.e., single-grain infant cereal and applesauce, when the infant can sit well with support, the tongue

Nursing Tip:

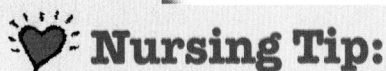

Calculation of infant's caloric and fluid needs

Infant's weight = 4.5 kg; formula = 20 kcal/oz (30 mL)

1. Caloric need: 120 kcal/kg/day

   120 kcal × 4.5 kg = 540 kcal/day

   Amount of formula needed per day:

   540 kcal ÷ 20 kcal/oz = 27 oz of formula

2. Fluid need: 1 to 1.5 mL/kcal/day

   540 kcal × 1 mL = 540 mL/day

   540 kcal × 1.5 mL = 810 mL/day

   Amount of formula needed per day (in ounces):

   540 mL ÷ 30 mL/oz = 18 oz of formula

   810 mL ÷ 30 mL/oz = 27 oz of formula

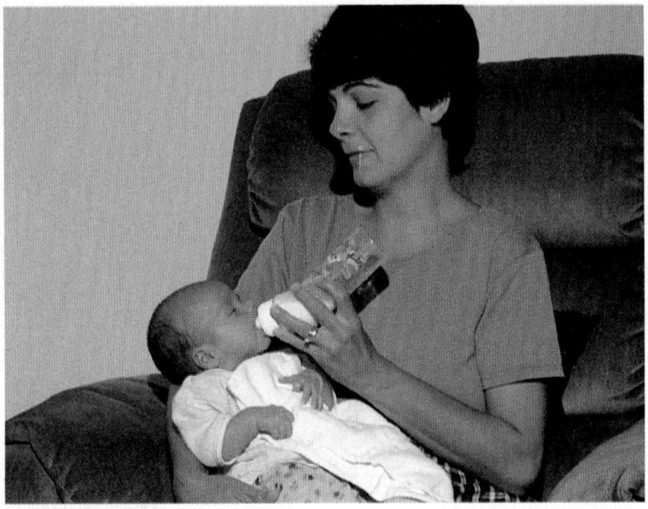

Figure 8-16 Infant being bottle-fed, one method of providing appropriate nutritional requirements.

Nursing Tip:

Salt and sugar content of strained foods

The caregiver should be cautioned about the salt and sugar content of strained foods. Extra sugar intake can contribute to excessive calorie intake. Salt contributes to an increase in extracellular fluid and a slight rise in blood pressure. Over the past few years, companies that commercially prepare strained foods have made an effort to decrease the salt and sugar content in their baby foods (Dietary Guidelines for Infants, 1997).

TABLE 8-5 Developmental Behaviors Related to Feeding

Age	Skill
Newborn–2 Months	Primitive reflexes facilitate feeding Hunger cry initiates feeding interaction
2–4 Months	More alert and interactive during feeding Beginning ability to wait for food Associates caregiver's smell, voice, and cradling with feeding Hand-to-mouth behavior quiets infant
4–6 Months	Readiness for solids Excellent head and trunk control Reaching for objects Loss of extrusion reflex of tongue
6–8 Months	Sits alone with steady head during feedings Chewing mechanism developed Holds bottle Vocal eagerness during meal preparation Much more motor activity during feeding
8–10 Months	Readiness finger foods Grasps spoon but cannot use it effectively Enjoys new textures, tastes Emerging independence
10–12 Months	Increasing determination to feed self Neat pincer grasp Holds cup but frequently spills it More verbal and motor behavior during feeding

Family Teaching

Feeding Infant Solid Foods

Stress the importance of the infant's need to practice the new skill of eating solids (chewing and swallowing) instead of sucking.

- Introducing one new food at a time at 4–7-day intervals allows for identifying food allergies and gives the infant the chance to become accustomed to the new food.
- Feed solids with a spoon. Put a small amount of food (1 teaspoon) on the spoon and place toward the back of the infant's mouth. This enables the infant to overcome the diminishing extrusion reflex and facilitates the newly acquired skills of chewing and swallowing.
- Give solid foods when the infant is hungry then follow with formula or breast milk. This encourages the infant to eat the solids instead of becoming satiated with fluids.
- Gradually increase solid foods to approximately 4 oz per feeding. As solid food intake advances, the infant's daily intake of milk will decrease to approximately 24 oz at 12 months of age.

(Reisser, 1998; Shelov, 1998)

Family Teaching

Common Food Allergies

- Foods to avoid: chocolate, strawberries, citrus fruits, peanut butter, shellfish, egg whites, tomatoes, corn, wheat, nuts
- Common reaction: diarrhea, abdominal pain, nasal congestion, rashes, vomiting

(Reisser, 1998; Shelov, 1998)

thrust (extrusion reflex) has decreased, and the infant's hunger seems unsatisfied after nursing or bottle feeding (Arrigo, 1994; Pipes, & Trahms, 1993); this usually occurs between 4 and 6 months of age. Introduction of solids before this time can contribute to food allergies because food is not completely digested; increased calorie intake, resulting in an overweight infant; and the danger of choking. The decision to introduce solid foods should be individualized. Developmental behaviors related to feeding can be found in Table 8-5 (Arrigo, 1994; Dixon & Stein, 2000).

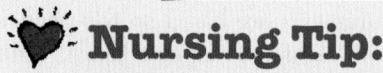

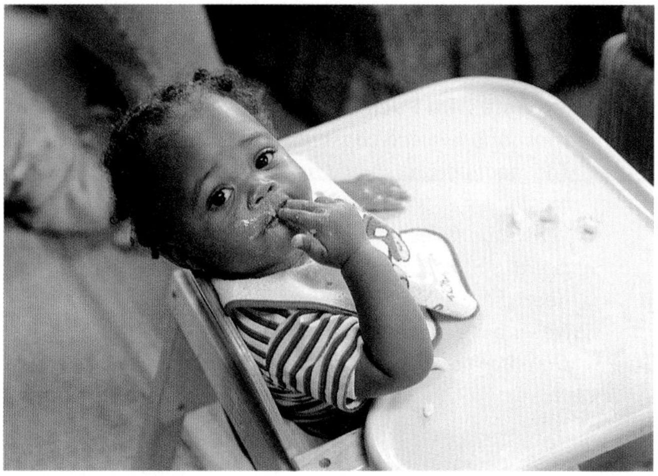

Figure 8-17 Feeding solid foods to infants can sometimes be messy.

Family Teaching

Helpful Hints for Infant Self-Feeding

- Place high chair in an area that can be easily cleaned.
- Place infant in a high chair and fasten safety belt.
- Use a large plastic bib.
- Dress infant in easily removable and washable clothes.

The caregiver may express concern about the sequence of adding solid foods to the diet. Usually, the first food introduced is iron-fortified rice cereal, since it is the easiest to digest and the least likely to cause allergies. The cereal can be mixed with formula or expressed breast milk and, later, fruit or juice. Because of the infant's need for iron, the nurse should stress the benefit of continuing iron-fortified cereal until 18 months of age. Fruits or vegetables are usually the next foods tried. Encourage the caregiver to introduce vegetables before fruits since the infant could become accustomed to the sweet taste of fruits. By 8–10 months of age, most fruits and vegetables should have been introduced and strained meats can be added to the infant's diet. Fruit juices, a good source of vitamin C, which enhances absorption of iron in the cereal, are usually offered the same time as fruits. Because of cultural variations, it is important for the nurse to ask what the infant is eating and support good nutritional habits that are culturally appropriate.

Due to the potential for an allergic reaction during the infant's first year, the Family Teaching box identifies foods that need to avoided until the second half of the first year.

When infants can sit steadily, they are usually allowed to drink from a cup. Finger foods are introduced during the second half of the first year as the finger grasp develops, teeth begin to erupt, and hand–eye coordination improves. Table 8-6 is a guide for introducing solid foods.

TABLE 8-6 Guide for Introduction of Solid Foods

Age	Food	Frequency
4–6 months	Cereal	Twice a day
6–8 months	Vegetables	Once a day
	Fruits	Twice a day
	Juices	Between meals (small amounts)
8–10 months	Meats	Once a day
10 months	Egg yolks	Once a day
9–12 months	Finger foods	At least daily

Family Teaching

Finger Foods

Rule of thumb: Pieces should be the size of the infant's thumb. Food items that are hard and small should be avoided since they can slip easily into the child's throat and may cause choking.

Foods to avoid:

- Nuts, popcorn, kernel corn, chunks of meat (e.g., hot dogs), chips, pretzels, berries, grapes, cherries, raw fruit and vegetables (e.g., apples, carrots, celery)
- Sticky, stringy, and chewy foods (e.g., peanut butter, caramel)
- Small, hard, or round candy (e.g., jelly beans, peppermints, butterscotch)

(Arrigo, 1994; Martin, 1996; Reisser, 1998)

When discussing the infant's developmental readiness for solid foods, the nurse should stress to the caregiver the importance of self-feeding. To encourage autonomy, the infant needs to be given the opportunity to explore the texture, smell, color, and taste of food. The caregiver should expect that self-feeding will be messy. Anticipatory guidance can help this experience become a valuable lesson for the infant.

Weaning

Weaning is a process of giving up one method of feeding for another, such as the transitions from breast to bottle, and from bottle to cup. There is no right way or time to wean an infant. Behaviors consistent with weaning include eating from a spoon, holding the bottle, feeding self with fingers or a spoon, eating foods that require chewing, and the decreasing desire to be held during feeding. If the infant is weaned too soon from breast milk or formula, iron deficiency anemia could occur (Reisser, 1998). Weaning from the breast to a bottle occurs when many nursing mothers return to work or resume activities away from the home (Shelov, 1998). Weaning should be a process in which breastfeeding sessions are gradually replaced by a bottle, and/or the bottle-feeding sessions are gradually replaced by increased amounts of solid foods and drinking from a cup (Reisser, 1998; Shelov, 1998).

Nursing Alert:

Being Safe with Pacifiers

- *Look for one-piece construction.*
- *The mouth guard should be wider than the infant's mouth.*
- *Ventilation holes should be present on the mouth guard.*
- *Keep the pacifier clean.*
- *Never put a pacifier on a string.*
- *Do not leave a pacifier in a sleeping infant's mouth.*

Use of Pacifiers

Oral stimulation or sucking is one of most important sources of pleasure and satisfaction for the infant, and one of the first coordinated muscular activities. There are two forms of sucking, nutritive and nonnutritive (Turgeon-O'Brien, Lachapelle, Gagnon, Larocque, & Maheu-Robert, 1996). Nutritive sucking enables the infant to obtain essential nutrients necessary for life through either bottle- or breastfeeding. Nonnutritive sucking is used as a source of pleasure and satisfaction, which provides the infant the opportunity to

Research Highlight

Breastfeeding and the Use of Pacifiers

Study Purpose

To determine the effects of the use of pacifiers on breastfeeding.

Methods

Breastfeeding was observed in the hospital 4 to 5 days after birth in 82 healthy infant–mother pairs in Sweden with uncomplicated, term births. All mother–infant pairs left the hospital exclusively breastfeeding; 57 pairs had a correct sucking technique and 25 had an incorrect sucking technique. Mothers were contacted by phone at 2 weeks and at 1, 2, 3, and 4 months after delivery and interviewed about breastfeeding habits, problems, and amount of pacifier use.

Findings

Breastfeeding among the pacifier-user group was 44% at 4 months, as compared with 91% in the nonuser group. Pacifier use over 2 hours a day was associated with more breastfeeding problems than with limited or no use of pacifiers. Infants with a correct sucking technique at discharge who did not use pacifiers had a 96% rate of breastfeeding at 4 months. The correct sucking infants who used a pacifier had only a 59% rate of breastfeeding at 4 months. Of the infants with an incorrect sucking technique, 82% of nonusers were still breastfeeding at 4 months and only 7% (one mother) of the pacifier-users were still breastfeeding.

Implications

You should realize that pacifier use is associated with lower levels of breastfeeding success and can educate mothers about the possibility of breastfeeding problems associated with using a pacifier.

Citation

Righard, L., & Alade, M. (1997). Breastfeeding and the use of pacifiers. *Birth, 24,*(2), 112–120.

learn self-gratification. Nonnutritive sucking provides the infant with a means of gaining self-control and as a transition from the stages of waking and sleeping (Wagner, 1997).

Since sucking provides the infant with pleasure and satisfaction, caregivers need to understand the difference between nutritive and nonnutritive sucking. If the infant is fussy and crying, the caregiver may offer a pacifier as a soothing method without understanding the infant's true need. If the infant is hungry, however, offering a pacifier will not calm the infant.

In an attempt to understand infant needs, caregivers are encouraged to note the time and circumstances around their infant's distress. Distress may be due to a need for sleep/food, to be held, or simply to suck (Wagner, 1997). If the infant simply wants to suck, the caregiver may select a pacifier to meet this need, or infants may start sucking on their fingers. As time goes on the infant will decide which method of nonnutritive sucking is the favorite.

If a pacifier is selected, it is important that the caregiver receive appropriate information about pacifier use and safety considerations (see Nursing Alert Box). It should be stressed that the pacifier should not be used as a substitute for general caregiving, nor as an attempt to meet needs other than for nonnutritive sucking. When the caregiver selects a pacifier, the shape should correspond with the shape of the nipple used for infant feeding. Many lactation consultants stress caution in introducing a pacifier if the infant is being breast fed. In fact, according to the La Leche League International, nipple confusion and even refusal to breastfeed can occur if a pacifier is introduced before the nursing relationship has been established (Wagner, 1997) (see Research Highlight).

Communication

Communication enables the infant to express needs, emotions, and attitudes, and involves central nervous system maturation, cognitive abilities, and social interaction. The infant's initial means of communication—crying and smiling—elicit different responses from the caregiver. When the infant cries, the caregiver responds with soothing behaviors such as speaking softly, holding, and establishing eye contact. Caregiver's reactions to an infant's smile include talking, cooing, smiling, and playing. Even though the infant begins smiling as a reflex, by 2 months the infant has a "social" smile used to gain attention and amazement from the caregiver.

The infant's ability to communicate through language follows a predictable course. As maturation progresses so do language abilities. During infancy, **receptive language** (the ability to understand words) is greater than **expressive language** (the ability to speak words). By the end of the first year, the infant can say several words such as "dada" and "mama" as well as understand simple commands such as "bye-bye," "point to your belly," and "no-no." A summary of language development during infancy can be found in Table 8-7.

The nurse's awareness of the expected pattern of language development is important during the infant's routine health screening visits. Assessing the infant's language development

TABLE 8-7 Summary of Language Development in Infancy

Age	Expressive Skills	Receptive Skills
Birth–2 Months	Crying Comfort sound with feeding Coos Vocalizes to familiar voice	Sounds elicit startle reflex Turns and looks for sounds Prefers human voice
3–6 Months	Vocalizes during play and pleasure Squeals Laughs aloud Less crying Uses vowels and consonant sounds that resemble syllables (ma, mu, ba, ga, ah, da)	Watches speaking mouth Shifts gaze between sounds Understands own name Uses sound to get attention
7–9 Months	Increases vowel and consonant sounds Uses two-syllable sounds (baba, dada) Talks along with others	Associates words with activity Responds to simple commands ("no-no") Understands familiar words
10–12 Months	Says "mama" and "dada" to identify caregivers Repeats sounds made by others Makes intentional gestures Learns three to five words	Recognizes family members' names Recognizes objects by name Understands simple commands (say "bye-bye")

by using the Denver II screening tool enables the health care provider to detect any potential problems (Frankenberg, 1990) (see Appendix E).

Language patterns can provide anticipatory guidance to the caregiver to enhance language development as well. Therefore, the caregiver should be encouraged to talk to the infant, make eye contact, and smile during feeding and diaper changes. Once the infant starts to vocalize, the caregiver should repeat these sounds in response to the infant's vocalizations. The names of objects or people should be emphasized when talking to the infant, and the caregiver should always be observant of the infant's response to adult vocalization.

Temperament

Temperament is the way a child interacts with the surrounding environment. Children are thought to be genetically endowed with specific temperamental characteristics, which, when combined with the caregiver's personality, produce a characteristic pattern of social interaction between the child and the environment.

Temperamental characteristics are behavioral tendencies, not implications of a good or bad child, and can be categorized into nine attributes (Thomas, Chess, & Birch, 1968):

1. *Activity*—intensity and frequency of physical activity
2. *Rhythmicity*—regularity of repetitive physiological functions, i.e., sleep cycle, eating patterns, elimination patterns
3. *Approach–withdrawal*—initial reaction to a given stimulus, i.e., people, situations
4. *Adaptability*—ease or difficulty with which the child reacts or adapts to a given stimulus
5. *Intensity of response*—degree of energy used by the child to react to the stimulus
6. *Threshold of responsiveness*—amount of stimulation needed to evoke a child's response
7. *Mood*—amount of happiness versus unhappiness or pleasant/friendly behavior versus unpleasant/unfriendly behavior exhibited in various situations
8. *Distractibility*—effectiveness of the stimulus to alter the direction of the ongoing behavior
9. *Attention span and persistence*—length of time the child pursues an activity and the continuation of an activity despite the obstacles

The attributes provide a framework for three distinct personality types, as described in Table 8-8. Not all children can be placed into these categories easily; children often exhibit a variety of personality types.

The knowledge of temperament can be very useful in achieving a goodness-of-fit in the caregiver–infant relationship (Medoff-Cooper, 1995) (see Research Highlight). The nurse can be instrumental in helping the caregiver understand the uniqueness of the child's personality and provide a guide in child-rearing techniques (Medoff-Cooper, 1995). For exam-

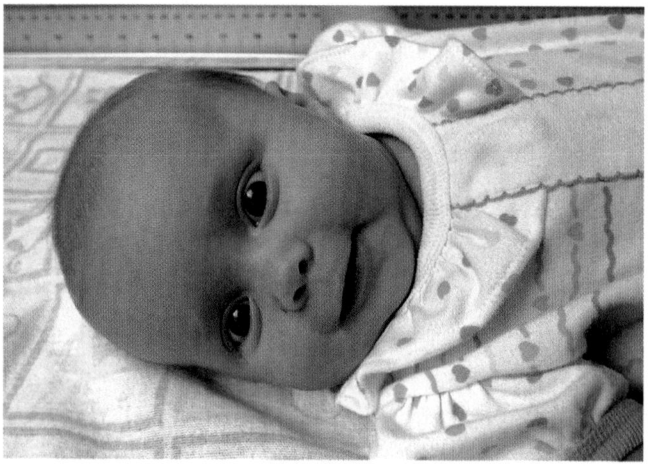

Figure 8-18 A child's temperament is considered to be a combination of genetics and caregivers' personalities.

TABLE 8-8 Summary of Personality Types

Personality Type	Characteristics
Easy	Easygoing and adapts rapidly to stimuli Has an overall positive mood Likes to be around people Sleeps and eats well Has regular and predictable behaviors
Difficult	Adapts slowly to stimuli Has an overall negative mood Requires a structured environment Likes people but can do well alone Seems to be in constant motion Has irregular patterns of behavior
Slow-to-warm-up	Adapts slowly to stimuli but is watchful Quietly withdraws and usually moody Primarily a loner and socially shy Oversensitive and slow to mature Primarily inactive Reacts passively to changes in routine

Adapted from Thomas, A., Chess, S., and Birch, H. (1970). The origin of personality. Scientific American 223*(2), 106–107.*

Research Highlight

Mothers' Parenting Self-Appraisals—The Contribution of Perceived Infant Temperament

Study Purpose

To investigate the relationship of mothers' parenting self-appraisals and their perception of infant temperament while considering maternal attributes (amount of education and child care experience), infant gender, and the personal and social context of parenting (centrality of infant to the mother, and life and relationship changes due to the infant).

Methods

A total of 117 mothers who participated in a family medicine residency program and had delivered healthy, term infants completed questionnaires at 1 and 3 months about their child's temperament and their own parenting experience and problem-solving abilities (mothering self-appraisal). Forms were given to mothers before leaving the hospital postpartum unit and were returned to the clinic receptionist at the infant's next well-child visit.

Findings

At 1 and 3 months, infant temperaments contributed to maternal self-appraisal when infant gender, maternal attributes, and parenting context were controlled. The specific temperament variable of amenability was the most consistent predictor of maternal self-appraisals.

Implications

It is important to recognize that temperament of an infant can affect maternal self-appraisal. When assessing a mother's point of view of her own parenting skills, understanding the infant's temperament may provide insight to nurses about the mother's self-assessment.

Citation

Pridam, K., Chang, A., & Chiu, Y. (1994). Mothers' parenting self-appraisal: The contribution of perceived infant temperament. *Research in Nursing & Health, 17,* 381–392.

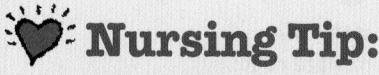

Reflective Thinking

Your Temperament

Recall when you were a child. How would you classify your temperament? Is it similar to how you would classify yourself today? Do others see you the same way?

ple, a consistent routine is important for the child who is easily overwhelmed by changes. If the child has problems falling asleep, it may be helpful to provide a calm and quiet environment during the bedtime ritual. For the child who is easily

Nursing Tip:

Goodness of fit

The nurse can assist the caregiver by:

- Being aware of the cultural norms of the caregiver
- Taking time to ask about the infant's general behavior characteristics
- Asking how the caregiver interprets the infant's behavior
- Asking questions about areas that may be problematic
- Encouraging the expression of feelings about infant–caregiver interactions

distracted while eating, the caregiver should minimize all distractions by providing a quiet setting during the meal.

By increasing the caregiver's understanding of the child's personality, a more effective plan of care can be developed to meet infant needs. Thus, needs are met, a trusting relationship develops, and the caregiver's frustrations associated with child rearing may be diminished.

Colic

Colic, one of the most common health problems seen in infants younger than 3 months of age, describes recurrent episodes of unexplained crying and the inability to be consoled. The onset varies, but it usually occurs around 1–2 weeks of age and subsides spontaneously by approximately 16 weeks of age.

Excessive air swallowing, improper feeding techniques, food allergies, infant behaviors, and parental factors have been implicated as causes of colic, but none of these has been supported through research (Keefe, 1996; Taubman, 1984). The colicky episode is characterized by loud, persistent cry and flexing of the hips toward the abdomen. These physical characteristics are thought to be a result of paroxysmal abdominal cramping. The "rule of 3" has also been used to define colic (Schmitt, 1986). The "rule of 3" states that colic is present if crying occurs during the first 3 months of life, lasts longer than 3 hours per day, occurs more than 3 days in any 1 week, and continues for at least 3 weeks.

Even though colic usually resolves spontaneously, the episodes are very stressful. The family is usually fatigued, frustrated, and expresses feelings of helplessness; caregivers often blame themselves for not being able to console the infant.

Colic management begins by recognizing a problem exists. First and foremost, it is important for the health care provider to eliminate an infectious or organic cause for the infant's discomfort. Once no underlying medical condition has been identified, colic should be approached in terms of managing the infant's episodes as well as the emotional turmoil experienced by the family.

In managing the infant's episodes, the nurse should assess the infant's daily routine and discuss the infant's normal patterns. Refer to Figure 8-19 for some carrying techniques that may soothe a colicky infant. Some suggestions for easing the discomfort of colic include (Dixon & Stein, 2000; Keefe, 1996):

1. Feed the infant slowly, burp frequently, and keep in upright position during feeding to decrease the amount of air swallowed. Do not overfeed the infant, which can be determined by calculating the infant's required calorie needs by body weight.
2. When breastfeeding, avoid eating foods that may contribute to gas formation. Typically these include foods such as onions, cabbage, collards, and dry beans, which cause gas in the caregiver. This is a trial-and-error approach and may take a week before results are seen.
3. Swaddle the infant to decrease self-stimulation by jerky or sudden movements. A front carrier for body contact, swaddling, or gentle movement may be useful.
4. Take the infant for a car ride. Almost all colicky children respond favorably to vibration and movement.
5. Use a swing for at least 20 minutes. This provides movement and allows the family time for a rest period between interactions with the infant.
6. Walk or rock the infant while applying gentle pressure to the infant's abdomen.
7. Gently massage the infant's back while the infant is lying down.
8. Supply background or "white" noise (hair dryer, vacuum cleaner, fan) or play a womb sound tape (known as a "souffle" toy) or some soft music.

Nursing Tip:

Care of the infant with colic

To help the caregiver manage colic:

- Stress that no one is to blame!
- Explain the possible reasons for colic.
- Give suggestions for relieving colicky episodes.
- Explain that colic usually disappears by 16 weeks of age.
- Be supportive, and encourage expression of concerns.
- Encourage talking with others who have experienced a colicky infant.
- Encourage brief periods away from the crying infant.

Reflective Thinking

Caring for the Child with Colic

To improve your understanding of colic and the caregiver's situation, ask yourself:

1. How would you personally feel if your infant cried constantly while you provided the care? Would you feel that people thought you were not a good caregiver?
2. What coping techniques would you use?
3. Who would you call when reaching the point of exasperation?

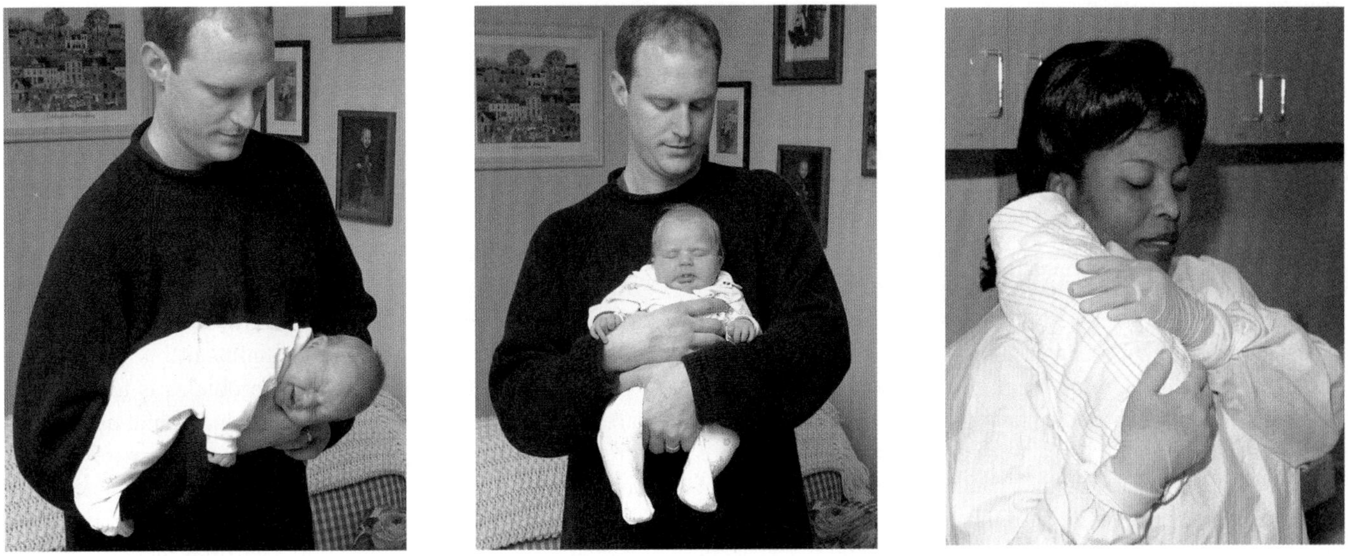

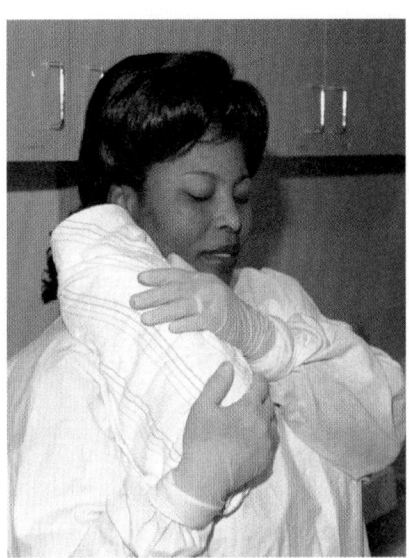

Figure 8-19 Different Types of Infant Carries That May Alleviate Infant Colic Distress

9. Place the infant in a quiet, darkened room to reduce environmental stimuli.
10. Let the infant cry it out in the crib when other measures do not work. Sometimes only fatigue will make the infant fall asleep.

The nurse should encourage the caregiver to avoid the tendency to take the episode personally, to keep a positive attitude, and to remain calm. The caregiver may be encouraged to try breathing techniques to relax, taking some time away from the care of the infant, doing something special when away from the ongoing care of the infant, and/or ask a relative to help in the infant's care.

Sleep

Infants have variable sleep patterns that are influenced by temperament, satisfaction with feedings, caregivers' responses to periodic awakenings, and environmental conditions (Mackin, Medendorp, & Maier, 1989). There is a transition from neonatal sleeping, which is shorter with multiple sleep periods, to the more organized central nervous system maturation after the third month (Table 8-9). As the child matures, the sleep–wake cycle evolves into a pattern of being awake during the day and asleep at night (Dixon & Stein, 2000).

During the first months of life, infants sleep approximately 16 hours a day and experience more rapid eye movement (REM) sleep than at any other time in life (Herzog, 1997). Sleep provides the time needed to rebuild reserves necessary for rapid physical growth and development. In addition, the central nervous system and neurons undergo a great deal of development during REM sleep (Herzog, 1997).

As the infant matures, the amount of REM sleep diminishes, the required hours for sleep gradually decrease, and sleep–wake periods develop into a day/night cycle. These changes develop over time and are termed **sleep consolidation** (fewer periods of sleep with longer durations) and **diurnal cycle** (sleeping through the night alternating with daytime wakefulness) (Weissbluth, 1991). By the time the infant is 3 to 4 months of age, the diurnal cycle is well established and a pattern of 9–11 hours of nocturnal sleep has

TABLE 8-9 Infant Sleep Time

Age	Awake	Day Sleep	Night Sleep
Newborn	7.5 hours	8 hours	8.5 hours
1 Month	8.5 hours	6.75 hours	8.75 hours
4 Months	9 hours	4.5 hours	10.5 hours
6 Months	9.25–9.75 hours	3.25–4 hours	11 hours
1 Year	10.25 hours	2.25 hours	11.5 hours

Adapted from Wright (1994, May). Sleep, little baby. American Baby, *56(5), 75–81.*

developed. This developmental milestone of "sleeping through the night" or "settling-in" is a time the caregiver has been anxiously awaiting. Napping also occurs during this time. The number of naps per day varies with each infant, but generally the infant will take one or two naps by the age of 1 year (Weissbluth, 1991).

After regular sleep patterns develop, the infant may begin to experience periods of awakening during the night, referred to as night wakings. These night wakings seem to coincide with the development of separation anxiety. Even though this is a transient phase, night waking can result in a strained caregiver–infant relationship. During this time, it is not uncommon for the infant to have difficulty falling asleep at night and nap times as well as falling back to sleep if awakened. Methods such as rocking and providing a pacifier and a dim light (night light) may assist the infant in returning to sleep. Usually, the infant can settle back to sleep if left alone during the awakenings that occur every 2–4 hours during the sleep times.

The infant's sleep state can also be influenced by sleeping arrangements. Sleeping arrangements for an infant vary widely from family to family. For the first few months of the child's life or when the infant is ill, the sleeping arrangement known as co-sleeping is a relatively common practice used by many cultures, especially among African-American, Hispanic, and Asian families (Brazelton, 1990; Wright, 1994). According to Tonnessen (1996), approximately 25%–30% of caregivers co-sleep, or share the family bed, with children. Co-sleeping has both advocates and critics, but no evidence has been presented indicating that this practice is dangerous, psychologically harmful, or even habit forming (Tonnessen, 1996; Wright, 1994).

Family Teaching

Family Bed Concerns

- *Once you share the family bed, you will always share the family bed:* No, but you should be prepared for it to take several months to ease the infant out of your bed.
- *Sharing the family bed will encourage your infant to be overly dependent on you:* There is no evidence to support this idea.
- *Sleeping with your infant increases the risk of suffocation:* Rarely. The risk of suffocation can be minimized by not placing pillows, blankets, and/or comforters under the infant, not sleeping on a waterbed, sheepskin, or featherbed, and not overdressing or overbundling the infant for sleep.
- *Sharing the family bed can cause marital problems:* Maybe, if both caregivers do not agree on the sleeping arrangements.

(American Academy of Pediatrics, 1997, 2000; Tonnessen, 1996)

Part of the nurse's developmental assessment of the infant is the evaluation of sleep patterns. The nurse should also keep in mind that the infant's sleep pattern is a common concern for the caregiver. When concern is expressed, the nurse should elicit information related to the history of the problem, daily sleep routine, sleeping position, sleeping arrangements, changes in feeding, environmental problems, and occurrence of stressors in the family unit.

The best way to prevent sleep problems is to assist the caregiver in understanding the infant's individual needs. The caregiver should be given information relevant to healthy sleep patterns and signs of maturation in the infant. When providing this information, the nurse should take the caregiver's cultural practices and personal preferences into consideration. In addition, the nurse should suggest measures that will foster healthy sleep patterns (Anders, Halpern, & Hua, 1992) including (Wright, 1995):

- Establish a bedtime routine such as giving a bath, reading a book, telling a story, singing, holding, and/or rocking.
- Provide a quiet, relaxed environment in a cozy, safe crib.
- Maintain a comfortable room temperature.
- Use low-level lighting in the room.
- Do not use the crib as a playpen.
- Place infant in the bed when drowsy but not asleep.
- Place supine or side-lying for sleep.
- Do not feed during the night; if feeding is necessary, make it brief.
- Do not awaken infant to feed or change a diaper.

The sleeping position of the infant is also important. Even though some infants may seem to sleep better or more soundly on their stomachs (prone), sudden infant death syndrome has been associated with this sleeping position, and the American Academy of Pediatrics recommends that infants be placed on their back (supine) while sleeping (American Academy of Pediatrics [AAP], 2000; Graeber, 1997) (Figure 8-20).

Sudden infant death syndrome (SIDS) is the sudden, unexplained death of an infant under the age of 1 year (most SIDS cases [95%] occur by 6 months of age) (Hunt, 1996), after all known causes have been ruled out through autopsy, death scene investigation, and review of history (AAP, 2000). In statistical data reported prior to 1992, an association between the prone sleeping position (stomach lying) and the incidence of SIDS was identified, resulting in the American Academy of Pediatrics recommending the supine or side-lying position for sleeping infants. Since the 1994 recommendation, the supine sleeping position has statistically been shown to contribute to lower incidence of SIDS (AAP, 2000). In fact, as

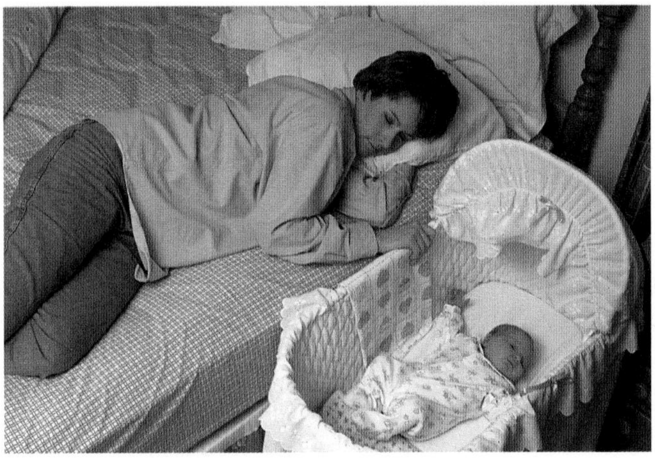

Figure 8-20 Infants should be placed on back to sleep.

of 1996, the rate of SIDS in the United States had fallen to 0.74 per 1,000 live births, a 38% decrease since the American Academy of Pediatrics recommended a supine sleeping position for healthy infants (AAP, 2000). Other risk factors associated with SIDS can be found in the Nursing Tip box. Generally, it is not known what causes SIDS, but the AAP (2000) proposes the following mechanisms:

- A delayed development of arousal or cardiorespiratory control
- Maldevelopment or malnutrition in the brain region, involved with hypercapnic ventilatory response, chemosensitivity, and blood pressure

Nursing Tip:

Risk factors associated with SIDS

Infant

- Prematurity
- Low birth weight
- Male gender
- Asphyxia
- Multiple birth
- SIDS in a sibling
- Age under 6 months

Environmental

- Exposure to cigarette smoke
- Prone sleeping position
- Bottle-feeding in the crib
- Overbundling for sleep
- Overheating
- Soft sleep surfaces
- Loose bedding

(AAP, 2000; Tonnessen, 1996)

Family Teaching

Recommendations to Reduce the Risk of SIDS

Remember SIDS is not:
- Contagious
- Caused by immunization or child abuse
- Anyone's fault

Risk-reduction strategies:
- Place infant in the supine position to sleep.
- Cribs should conform to the safety standards of the Consumer Product Safety Commission.
- Do not let infant sleep on a waterbed, sofa, soft mattress, or other soft surfaces.
- Avoid soft material in the infant's sleeping environment (i.e., pillows, quilts, comforters, stuffed toys).
- Stop smoking around your infant.
- Avoid overheating your infant.
- Avoid bed sharing or co-sleeping.

(AAP, 2000)

- Rebreathing, with associated hypoxia and hypercabia providing noxious stimuli
- Arousal responses to laryngeal chemoreflex diminished, leading to apnea and bradycardia

The incidence of SIDS in the United States is highest in American Indians and African Americans, with a rate of two to three times that of the national average. Due to these factors and incidence, it is important caregivers are given information about SIDS and strategies to reduce the risk of SIDS. Strategies to reduce the risk can be found in the Family Teaching box.

Bathing

Infants do not need much bathing during the first year of life. During the bath, caregivers should never leave the infant unattended to answer the telephone or doorbell. Even though sponge baths are used until the cord falls off, it is always important to keep the diaper area clean to avoid diaper rash. Before bathing, caregivers should gather all supplies, including a basin of lukewarm water, a washcloth, towels, baby shampoo, mild soap, and cotton balls. While giving a sponge bath, the caregiver should expose only those areas on the infant being washed to avoid chilling the infant. A cotton ball can be used to clean the eyes first, moving from the inner to outer areas, before using a washcloth for the remainder of the face. The perineal area is always washed last. It is important to clean all body creases thoroughly, especially the neck folds and perineal area, and wash and dry each body part before moving on to the next area. To prevent **cradle**

Research Highlight

Prevalence and Predictors of the Prone Sleep Position among Inner-City Infants

Study Purpose

To describe infant sleep position in a cohort of infants born to predominantly low-income, inner-city mothers and to identify predictors of the prone sleep position in this population.

Methods

A total of 394 mothers were interviewed shortly after delivery and again at 3 to 7 months postpartum to identify determinants of preventive health care practices. Bivariate associations were assessed using a Fisher exact test for categorical variables and Student's *t* test for continuous variables.

Findings

At 3–7 months of age, 157 infants (40%) were placed in the prone position for sleep. Independent predictors of prone sleep position included poverty (95% confidence interval [CI]), African American race (95% CI), presence of grandmother in the home (95% CI), and intent, as measured shortly after delivery, to place the infant in the prone position (95% CI). Importantly, of the 43 mothers who observed their infants in the prone sleep position while in the hospital, 40 (93%) intended to place their infants prone at home.

Implications

Educational efforts should address both initial intentions and reinforcement of the correct sleep position, once initiated. Hospital health care providers should ensure healthy infants are placed in the supine position for sleep during the postpartum hospital stay.

Citation

Brenner, R., Simons-Morton, B. G., Bhasker, B., Mehta, N., Melnick, V. L., Revenis, M., Berendes, H. W., & Clemens, J. D. (1998). Prevalence and predictors of the prone sleep position among inner-city infants. *JAMA, 280,* 341–346.

cap (seborrhea), a dry, scaly scalp condition, hair should be washed every other day using a mild baby shampoo. If cradle cap does develop, a soft-bristle toothbrush can be used to remove the crusts and mineral oil or petroleum jelly can be used to soften the patches. After the cord falls off, the infant can be bathed in a sink or plastic tub in about 2 inches of warm water. A towel can be placed on the bottom to prevent the infant from slipping. While bathing infants, caregivers should always hold or use a tub ring to stabilize the infant even though the child may be able to sit upright without much support. Since bathing can be an important time for bonding and play, it should be unhurried and nonstressful.

Skin and Nail Care

Generally, infants do not need lotions or baby powder. If lotions are used, they should be hypoallergenic and initially placed on the hands for warming before being rubbed on the skin. Baby powder, typically a mixture of hydrous magnesium silicate (talc) and other silicates can cause a severe aspiration pneumonia, which can often be fatal. Therefore, parents should be told of its danger and discouraged from using it or encouraged to use a corn starch preparation in its place. If a powder is used it should be placed on the hand before being applied to the skin, to avoid creating a cloud of talc dust that is easily inhaled. A nail clippers can be used to keep fingernails and toenails short to prevent infants from scratching themselves. The best time to clip the nails is right after the bath because nails are softer.

Stranger and Separation Anxiety

Stranger and separation anxiety emerge at approximately 8–12 months of age, when the infant develops a sense of object permanence. Stranger and separation anxiety usually peak at 15–18 months and disappear by 2 years of age. **Separation anxiety** behaviors are demonstrated when an infant is separated from the caregiver. **Stranger anxiety** behaviors are demonstrated by an infant when a stranger appears.

When these anxieties emerge, developmentally, the infant can produce a mental image of the caregiver and recall that image even after a separation. Separation anxiety occurs because the infant does not understand that the caregiver will return. However, as time goes on and with repeated episodes of separation, the infant will be able to cognitively cope with the separation and no longer demonstrate the behaviors (Dixon & Stein, 2000).

The infant's ability to produce a mental image of the caregiver enables the infant to also detect a difference in the appearance of an unfamiliar person. For the 8-month-old infant, the ability to recognize a discrepancy occurs rapidly when the stranger and familiar caregiver are seen together. As the child becomes older, the caregiver will not need to be present for the infant to identify a stranger (Mussen, Conger, Kagan, & Huston, 1990) (Figure 8-21).

Typically, the infant who is experiencing stranger and/or separation anxiety will demonstrate overt distress by withdrawing, frowning, whimpering, crying, and clinging. Separation anxiety is more likely to occur if the infant is left in an unfamiliar place or with an unfamiliar person (Mussen et al., 1990). With stranger anxiety, the stranger's approach influences the infant's reaction to the stranger. The infant will usually become anxious if the stranger immediately tries to reach out and touch or pick the child up. When time is provided for adjustment or adaptation to the unknown person, the infant usually reacts with less distress. The caregiver's reaction to the infant's behavior can also either reassure the infant or increase the infant's anxiety (Hoffman, Paris, & Hall, 1994).

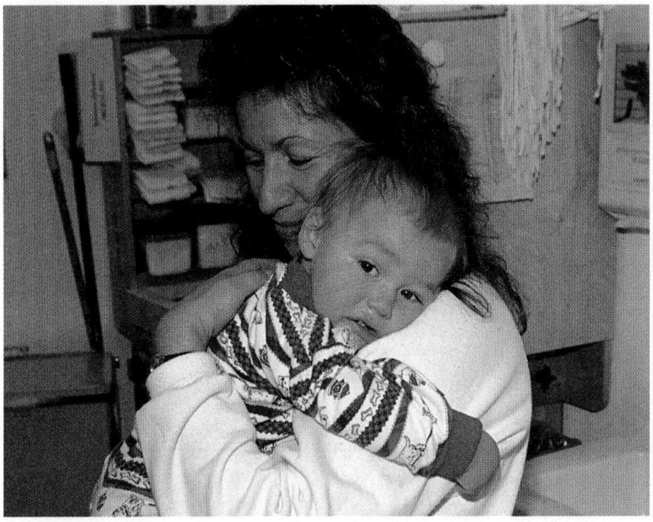

Figure 8-21 With ample time, an infant will warm-up to a "stranger."

Family Teaching

Relieving Stranger and Separation Anxiety

Stranger anxiety:

- Encourage friends and relatives to visit often.
- Let the child see the caregiver's expression when a stranger approaches.
- Have the caregiver talk to the stranger first.
- Encourage the stranger to avoid intrusive movements or expressions.
- Have the caregiver maintain a safe distance from the stranger.
- Allow the child to warm up to the stranger.
- Encourage the stranger to approach on the child's level and use a soothing tone of voice.

Separation anxiety:

- Leave the child in a familiar place or with a familiar person.
- Encourage the caregiver to talk to the child before leaving.
- Do not leave the child without saying good-bye.
- Leave a security object with the child, i.e., a familiar toy or an object belonging to the caregiver.
- Encourage the child to explore at own pace.

REFLECTIONS FROM FAMILIES

Separation anxiety—what a concept. I can remember the first time I experienced this with Carl. He was about 10 months old and I had taken him to the day care he had been attending since he was 6 weeks old. We were in his room when he started crying and clinging to my neck when I said good-bye. I was shocked! What had happened? He didn't do this yesterday!

When Carl started crying, his care provider came over and talked to him in a calm and soothing voice. Eventually he went to her but continued to cry. She encouraged me to continue my "good-bye" routine. As I left him crying I had such a feeling of guilt. Even though I knew what had happened I couldn't help but think, "What do I do?" "Why did he react that way?" "Should I really leave him crying?" When I called after I got to work, his care provider said he had stopped crying within minutes of my leaving, was fine, and playing like he always had.

Stranger and separation anxieties can be disturbing for the caregiver, especially the caregiver who works away from the home. Therefore, it is important to help the caregiver understand that these anxieties are a normal part of infant development. In addition, information related to the time of occurrence, the rationale for the occurrence, the characteristic behaviors to be expected, and when these anxieties usually disappear should be provided. The nurse should also give suggestions to ease the infant's discomfort. Some helpful hints for the relief of stranger and separation anxiety can be found in the accompanying Family Teaching box.

Alternative Child Care

Whether a single parent, a dual-income family, or a family with one working parent, when faced with having to leave their infant with another person, caregivers are challenged to find quality child care (care that is responsive and developmentally appropriate for young children and provides an environment where the child is safe, nurtured, and challenged to learn [DeBord, 1996]). The caregiver must become an informed consumer when searching for quality child care, and the nurse should keep caregivers informed on alternative child care issues such as availability, affordability, and quality. Prior to any investigation into alternative child care, the nurse should stress it is important for the caregiver to:

- Be realistic about challenges.
- Think carefully about the situation.
- Learn to adapt.
- Set priorities based on family values.
- Keep communications open.
- Identify any financial concerns (Duncan, 2000; Sprain, 2000).

Table 8-10 provides information on the various types of child care providers available, with advantages and disadvan-

TABLE 8-10 Types of Alternative Child Care

Types	Advantages	Disadvantages
Center-based care	• Group care for two or more children • Located usually in a home, school, church, or building designed for group care • Include nursery school, preschool, parent cooperative • Licensed by local or state agencies • Staff usually trained in child care and development • Structured program of activities for children usually available • Reliable hours of operation	• Regulations vary from area to area • May be placed on a waiting list for admission • Greater adult:child ratio • Care may not be individualized
Family child care	• Small group care • Good adult:child ratio • Located in provider's home • Special arrangements are easier to make	• Usually includes provider's children • Licensing by local or state agencies usually not required or if required not always licensed • Provider(s) may not be trained in child care and development • Hours of operation may not be reliable
In-home care	• Home care provided by sitter or nanny • Individualized care • Easier to meet special needs (i.e., physical, mental, emotional problem) • Provider may do light home tasks • Do not have to transport child	• Provider may not be trained in child care and development • May infringe on family privacy • Dependent on provider's reliability

Adapted from DeBord, K. (1996). Quality child care: What does it really mean? *[On-line]. Available: www.carefinder.com/parents/choose.html; Scarr, S. (1998). American child care today.* American Psychologist, *53(2), 95–108; and Shelov, S. P. (Ed.) (1998).* Caring for your baby and young child. *New York: Bantam.*

tages of each, and Table 8-11 provides guidelines for choosing quality child care.

While searching for quality child care, the caregiver may inquire about the long-term effects of child care on infant development. Even though this area needs further study, research has shown that quality child care does not seem to have any persistent effect on child development (Scarr, 1998). In fact, most studies report better school achievement, greater social competence, and fewer behavior problems in children who experience quality child care (Bolger & Scarr, 1995). The child who benefits the most from quality child care comes from a socioeconomically disadvantaged environment. Quality care may in fact provide learning opportunities and social and emotional experiences not available for these children at home (Scarr, 1998).

Once equipped with information on quality care, the next step for the caregiver is finding good child care (Figure 8-22). The Family Teaching box provides some suggestions for locating such a setting.

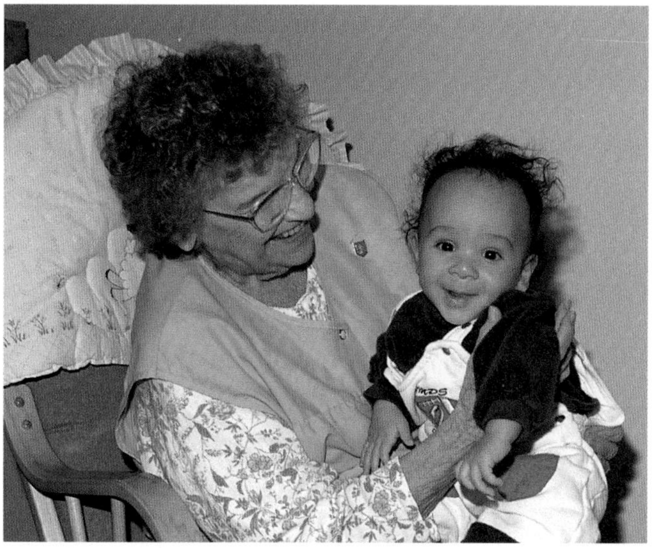

Figure 8-22 Finding quality child care takes effort, time, and patience.

TABLE 8-11 Choosing Child Care

Does Child Care Provider	
Appear warm and friendly?	Accept and respect your family's cultural values?
Seem calm and gentle?	Seem to enjoy cuddling infants?
Seem easy to talk with?	Meet infant physical needs?
Seem to like themselves and the job?	Provide infant stimulation?
Treat each child as special?	Provide dependable and consistent care?
Understand children's stages of development?	Provide consistency between home and child care?
Encourage good health habits?	Seem to have time for all infants?
Have previous experience and trained staff?	
Does the Child Care Setting Have	
Up-to-date license or registration certificate?	Smoke detectors?
A clean and comfortable look?	Covered radiators and protected heaters?
Enough room to allow children to move freely and safely?	Strong screens or bars on windows above first floor?
Appropriate staff:child ratio?	Nutritious meals and snacks?
Late pick-up policy?	A separate place to care for sick children?
Child-proofed environment?	A first-aid kit?
Enough heat, light?	Safe gates at top and bottom of stairs?
Enough furnishings for all children?	A clean, safe place to change diapers, sanitized after each use?
Furnishings that are safe and in good repair?	Cribs with firm mattresses?
Adequate number of clean bathrooms?	Separate linen for each crib?
Fire safety plan and adequate exits?	
Fire extinguishers?	
Are There Opportunities for the Child to	
Play quietly and actively?	Learn to get along, share, and respect themselves and others?
Play alone?	Learn about their own and others' cultures?
Follow a schedule that meets young children's needs?	Crawl and explore safely?
Learn new developmental skills?	

Adapted from Labensohn, D. (2000). Parent checklist for child care *[On-line]. Available: at www.carefinder.com/parents/choose/html.*

Family Teaching

Ways to Find Quality Child Care

- Ask friends and neighbors how they found child care.
- Look in the Yellow Pages of the telephone directory under "Child Care Centers."
- Check classified ads in the local newspaper.
- Place an ad in local newspaper.
- Put up notices on community bulletin boards.
- Talk with family child care associations or provider support groups.
- Ask the local affiliate of the National Association for the Education of Young Children.
- Contact the local Human Development Extension agent (usually a person with a college degree in human development or child psychology who works for the county or state).

(DeBord, 1996)

Reflective Thinking

Alternative Child Care

What are your feelings about alternative child care? Provide statements for and against both parents working outside the home and requiring alternative child care.

Lastly, only the caregiver can make the final decision regarding child care. As an informed consumer, it is most important for the caregiver to do the following (Four Steps, 2000):

- Interview the child care provider by calling first and then visiting.
- Check references.
- Make the decision on what is heard and seen.
- Always stay involved.

Play

Play enhances the infant's maturation and provides an opportunity to practice newly acquired motor skills as well as learn about the environment and the people around them. Active interaction with toys and people also helps develop a sense of predictability, mastery, and control (Hughes, 1991).

Kids Want To Know

Disappointed Sibling

I waited for so long for this baby to come, and she is not fun. She doesn't play or laugh. What is wrong with her?

- First of all assure the child that there is nothing wrong with the baby–this is what newborn babies do. Explain that babies eat and sleep all the time so that they can get enough energy to grow and be able to play.
- Encourage the child to keep talking and singing to the infant, that the baby loves the sibling's voice.
- Explain that in a month or two the baby will watch the older child run around, dance, and sing, and before you know it the baby will be old enough to join in.

Play for the infant moves rapidly from accidental pleasure-producing activities to purposeful, repetitive activities with an increasing awareness of the surrounding environment. By 6 months to 1 year, the infant engages in repetitive activities involving voices, sounds, music, and a variety of toys, which enhance the development of language and sensorimotor skills.

The caregiver's involvement and responsiveness influence the quality of play; interpersonal contact is essential. The infant needs to be played with, not just allowed to play, because the richest play occurs when the caregiver takes an active role.

Caregiver play nurtures the relationship through shared activities, accomplishments, and joys. If the caregiver is uncomfortable playing with the infant, the nurse can be instrumental in assisting the caregiver to become involved. Suggestions to aid the caregiver in being involved in infant play include (Dixon & Stein, 2000):

- Safety first—be sure toys are developmentally appropriate.
- The infant learns by using all five senses—provide toys accordingly.
- Place the infant in a variety of positions throughout the day, i.e., stomach, side, back.
- Encourage the use of hands and feet in play.
- Offer a few new experiences each day.
- Encourage banging toys together.
- Praise often.

During routine infant assessment, the nurse should ask the caregiver about the nature of the infant's play. With the emergence of voluntary reach and grasp, it is important to investigate the infant's motor competency, visual–motor coordination, and the appropriateness of the environment in exploring the object world. To facilitate the infant's continued development, the caregiver should be given information relevant to the toys and activities appropriate for the infant (Dixon & Stein, 2000). Table 8-12 provides a list of developmentally appropriate toys and activities for the infant.

When inquiring about the nature of the infant's play, the nurse should also listen for details about the quality and complexity of play to determine if it is age-appropriate. The caregiver's description of play behavior can be beneficial in screening for problems such as developmental delays, neurologic problems, delayed social skills, autism, learning disabilities, and emotional disturbances (Dixon & Stein, 2000).

TABLE 8-12 Toys and Activities Appropriate for the Infant

Age	Toys/Activity
Birth–3 Months	Black-and-white pattern cards Soft, cuddle toys Nonbreakable mirror Rattles Mobiles Music boxes Talking and singing Rocking and holding Gentle massage Interaction with other people
3–6 Months	Crib gyms Squeaky toys Teething rings Different textured toys Noise-making toys Talking and singing Play pat-a-cake, play peek-a-boo Social interaction with other people
6–9 Months	Safe place to creep/crawl Bath tub toys Jack-in-the-box Nested toys Big, soft blocks Drinking cup Toys to bang together Talking and singing Playing hide-n-seek Social interaction with other people
9–12 Months	Continue with toys for 6–9 months Safe place for exploration Push-pull and motion toys Colorful cloth books Paper for tearing Building blocks Metal pots and pans Different shaped and colored toys Social interaction with other people

Nursing Tip:

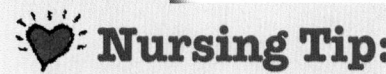

Motor skills and coordination

To have a clearer understanding of the infant's motor competency and visual–motor coordination, ask yourself:

- What motor skills does the infant demonstrate?
- Are these motor skills appropriate for the age of the infant?
- How does the infant use hand and mouth in exploration?
- What toy does the infant choose?
- Does the infant use both hands and arms equally?
- Are the infant's movements smooth?
- How does the caregiver facilitate the infant's play?

Safety Promotion and Injury Prevention

Infants are in a state of perpetual development and refinement of motor skills. In addition, infants have an insatiable curiosity about the environment. When this perpetual change and curiosity are combined, the infant is at risk for accidental injury, the leading cause of infant deaths, especially between 6 and 12 months of age. To ensure a safe environment for the infant, the caregiver must be aware of the safety concerns most associated with each stage of motor development.

The nurse and caregiver should discuss the environmental hazards associated with specific motor development. Anticipatory guidance, provided prior to the skill development, should include:

- The reason why infants are prone to injury
- The importance of injury prevention
- The importance of setting age appropriate limits
- The importance of always anticipating danger and removing the child from the danger

One way to prevent accidental injury is to child-proof the home. A general safety checklist can be found in the Box 8-1.

Of all the places in the home, the infant's bedroom should be monitored most closely because it harbors many hazards for the curious child. First and foremost, the bedroom furniture should meet Consumer Product Safety Commission standards. The crib should be located away from windows and electrical outlets. If there are posts on the crib, they should not protrude more than a half inch (Potter, 1995). The head or footboard should have no cut outs where

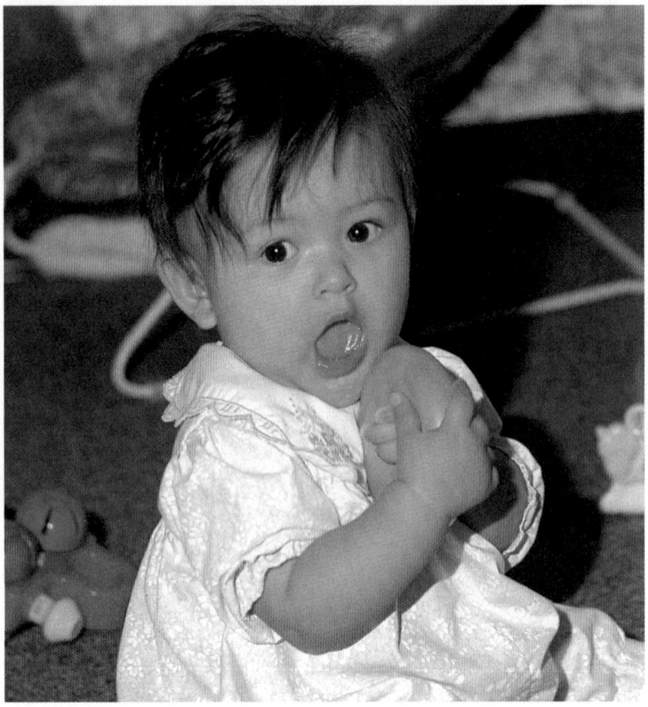

Figure 8-23 For safety reasons, make sure all toys in reach of an infant are age-appropriate.

the infant's head could be trapped, and the spaces between the bed rail slats should be no more than $2^3/_8$ inches. The bed rails should be locked in the highest position when the infant is in the crib to prevent falling. The mattress should fit snugly against the frame so the infant cannot slip between the mattress and frame. Bumper pads should fit snugly and be used until the infant begins to pull to a standing or kneeling position. A pillow should not be used, nor should any object be hung on the crib (Keeping your child safe, 1994). When the infant begins to stand, the mattress should be placed in the lowest setting and the bumper pads removed.

As the infant's ability to explore the environment increases daily, so do the hazards encountered. The caregiver needs to be reminded that the ability to roll and turn makes the infant susceptible to falling if left unattended on the bed, changing table, or counter top. When the infant can reach for and grasp items and bring them to the mouth, the caregiver must be cautious in leaving objects within the infant's reach. With the ability to creep and crawl, the infant can move farther and faster than the caregiver might expect, so the floor should be kept free of small objects and childproof latches used in cupboards. As locomotion improves, the infant will soon be able to stand and walk (cruise) around objects. Once this occurs, the caregiver must constantly be vigilant since the infant is now susceptible to falling, suffocating, and drowning. Table 8-13 provides information related to the appropriate infant safety measures associated with specific developmental achievements and type of injury.

BOX 8-1 General safety checklist

House
- All cleaning supplies, medicines, and cosmetics locked up or out of reach
- All knives or sharp edge objects out of reach
- Poisonous plants in the home removed
- All firearms removed or locked up
- Ammunition stored separately from firearms
- Fans and heaters out of reach
- Carbon monoxide detectors working (Replace batteries every 6 months.)
- All small objects picked up and out of sight
- No removable small parts on toys
- Plastic bags and latex balloons stored out of reach
- Unused large appliances kept locked
- Pool area gated/fenced

Falls
- All unused electrical outlets covered with safety caps
- All electrical wires out of reach or hidden
- Furniture sturdy and in good repair
- Walkways clear of any obstacles
- Stairway gated
- Sturdy handrails on all stairs/steps
- Window screens in good repair
- Nonskid rugs used

Burns
- No smoking around children and all cigarettes and matches out of reach
- Guards on front of heating appliances, furnace, fireplace
- Hot water heater thermostat set at <120°F
- All cooking utensil handles to the back of stove
- No drinking or handling hot liquids around children
- Smoke detectors working correctly (Replace batteries every 6 months.)
- Fire extinguishers easily accessible for adults

Emergency Needs
- Post all emergency numbers by telephones
- House address and phone number by each telephone
- First-aid kit up to date
- Syrup of ipecac in home
- Have and practice an emergency exit plan in case of a fire
- Caregivers know CPR

Adapted from Dixon, S., & Stein, M. (2000). *Encounters with children: Pediatric behaviors and development* (3rd ed.). St. Louis: Mosby.

TABLE 8-13 Infant Safety

Birth to 4 Months

Places objects in mouth
Reaches for objects
Rolls from side to back

Type of Injury	Safety Checklist
Falls	Keep crib rails up. Never leave infant unattended on a high surface.
Drowning	Never leave infant unattended in bathtub.
Burns	Keep hot water heater temperature <120°F. Always check bath water temperature. Do not hold or drink hot liquids when holding infant. Install smoke and carbon monoxide detectors in home. Avoid sun exposure. Do not use microwave oven for warming formula or food. Always check temperature of formula prior to feeding.
Strangulation	Be sure crib slats are $<2^3/_8$ inches apart. Be sure mattress fits tightly against slats. Do not tie anything to crib. Keep infant's crib away from curtain or blind cords. Never tie any string around infant's neck.
Motor vehicle accident	Use only an approved infant-restraint system in the car. Do not leave infant unsecured in car seat. Always put car seat in the back seat facing rear. Never place car seat in front if airbag present or activated.
Choking	Keep small objects out of reach. Never leave infant unattended on the floor.
Suffocation	Do not use pillows in the infant's bed. Keep plastic bags/wrap out of reach.
Ingestion	Do not smoke around infant.

4 to 7 Months

Sits with support
Rolls from back to side
Bears weight in standing position with support
Reaches for object beyond grasp
Actively drops objects

Type of Injury	Safety Checklist (in addition to those listed for birth to 4 months)
Choking and strangulation	Keep floor free of small objects. Never leave infant unattended on the floor. Do not tie toys on infant's crib. Keep infant's crib away from curtain or blind cords.
Burns	Cover all unused electrical outlets with safety caps. Put manufacturer-approved protective covering over heaters, furnaces. Never leave infant unattended on the floor.

continues

TABLE 8-13 *Continued*

Type of Injury	Safety Checklist (in addition to those listed for birth to 4 months)
Falls	Restrain infant in high chair. Do not use walkers. Never leave infant unattended on the floor Gate all stairways.
Ingestion	Use child-proof latches on cupboards/drawers. Never leave infant unattended on the floor. Keep toxic substances/plants out of reach in locked cabinet. Post poison control number by telephone. Keep ipecac syrup handy Do not smoke around infant.

8 to 12 Months

Drops object at will.
Uses pincer grasp.
Can self-feed finger foods.
Places and removes small objects in a container.
Sits alone without support.
Can move from prone to sitting to standing.
Stands alone without support.
Progresses from crawling to creeping to cruising.
Attempts to walk alone.

Type of Injury	Safety Checklist (in addition to those listed for 1–7 months)
Burns	Turn cooking handles toward back of stove. Do not use a dangling tablecloth. Never leave unattended in bathroom. Keep electrical wires or cords out of reach.
Drowning	Never leave unattended in bathroom. Never leave unattended in the yard, pool, or playground.
Falls	Fence all stairways. Be sure furniture is sturdy. Never leave unattended in the yard or playground. Put infant's bed in lowest position.
Ingestion	Keep medicines, cosmetics, toxic substances/plants out of reach. Never leave unattended in the yard or playground. Post poison control number by telephone. Keep ipecac syrup handy. Do not smoke around infant.
Choking	Use caution with finger foods (i.e., berries, grapes, cherries, carrots, popcorn, hot dogs) and coins. Never leave unattended in the yard or playground.
Motor vehicle	Leave infant in the back seat and switch to forward-facing car seat at 20 lb and at least 1 year.

Adapted from American Academy of Pediatrics (1996). Selecting and using the most appropriate care safety seats for growing children: Guidelines for counseling parents. Pediatrics, 97, *761–762; CDC (1995). Air-bag associated fatal injuries to infants and children riding in front passenger seats—United States.* Morbidity and Mortality Weekly Report, 44*[45], 845–847; and Keeping your child safe. (1994).* The parent's almanac. *[On-line.] Available: family.starwave.com/resource/pra/bonus27.html.*

Family Teaching

Check for Hidden Dangers

To ensure the infant's safety, the caregiver is encouraged to crouch down at what is the child's eye level, close to the floor, to survey the environment for hazards that the infant might encounter. It may even be necessary to crawl around to find any hidden dangers. Infants should also be placed in appropriate child safety restraints in the back seat whenever riding in automobiles. See Chapter 7 for further information about child-restraint seats.

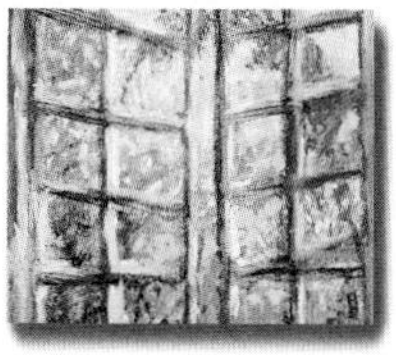

In the Real World

Infancy is nothing short of a miracle; the infant begins life as a completely dependent being and ends as an independent individual in perpetual motion. As a nurse, I watch this period of life with such awe and fascination and count myself lucky to be called a caregiver. Infants deserve only the best from caregivers, who will influence their outlook on this wonderful thing called life. As a child health nurse, my responsibility is to provide necessary information and guidance and to answer any question asked by caregivers so the infant will have the potential to achieve optimal growth and development.

Key Concepts

- It is essential for the nurse to have an understanding of infant growth and development to ensure the infant and family maintain an optimal level of health.
- Motor skill development progresses in an orderly fashion. Gross motor development occurs before fine motor development, and the infant must be able to reach before being able to grasp an object.
- An infant is in the sensorimotor stage of cognitive development. Knowledge is acquired about an object through interaction with that object. The major task for the infant is object permanence.
- Trust can be developed by promptly meeting the infant's basic needs of feeding, clothing, and comforting.
- Health screening includes health assessment, physical examination, and administration of scheduled immunizations and provides the health care provider with the opportunity to detect and evaluate any problems.
- Nutritional requirements are based on physical activity and rate of growth. Energy requirements range from 120 kcal/kg/day at birth to 100 kcal/kg/day by 1 year of age. Fluid requirement is 1–1.5 mL/kcal expended per day.
- Anticipatory guidance provides information on expected milestones and methods to encourage optimal development.
- During infancy, receptive language is greater than expressive language.
- Temperamental characteristics and the caregiver's personality produce a characteristic pattern of social interaction between the child and the environment.
- Infants have variable sleep patterns that are influenced by temperament, satisfaction with feedings, caregiver's response to periodic awakenings, and environmental conditions.
- Play provides the infant the opportunity to practice newly acquired motor skills and to learn about the environment and the people around them.
- The infant's inherent curiosity coupled with limited cognitive ability places them at risk for accidental injuries.

Review Questions

1. What are the physiological growth and developmental milestones of infants, and why are they important?
2. What are the fine and gross motor developmental milestones of infancy? Why are the principles associated with them important?
3. Why are infant psychosexual, cognitive, and psychosocial development important, and how do they interrelate?
4. What health promotion and maintenance activities for infants do nurses need to know about and why?
5. What information would you provide for a parent of an infant related to calorie and fluid requirements?
6. How does infant play change during the first year of life? What activities would you suggest parents provide for their infant to facilitate development?
7. What are the important anticipatory guidance interventions caregivers of infants need to know related to nutritional needs, growth and development patterns, stranger and separation anxiety, and safety?

References

Advisory Committee on Immunization Practices. (2000, January 21). Recommended childhood immunization schedule, United States, January–December 2000. *Morbidity and Mortality Weekly Report, 49*[2], 35- 38).

American Academy of Pediatrics. (1995). Fluoride supplementation for children: Interim policy recommendations. *Pediatrics, 95,* 777.

American Academy of Pediatrics. (1996). Selecting and using the most appropriate car safety seats for growing children: Guidelines for counseling parents. *Pediatrics, 97,* 761–762.

American Academy of Pediatrics. (1997). Does bed sharing affect the risks of SIDS? *Pediatrics, 100,* 272.

American Academy of Pediatrics. (2000). Changing concepts of sudden infant death syndrome: Implications for infant sleeping environment and sleep position. *Pediatrics 105,* 650–656.

Anders, T., Halpern, L., & Hua, J. (1992). Sleeping through the night: A developmental prospective. *Pediatrics, 90,* 554–560.

Arrigo, M. (1994, September). Starting solids. *American Baby, 56*(9), 68–72.

Behrman, R. E. (1996). *Nelson's textbook of pediatrics* (15th ed.). Philadelphia: Saunders.

Bolger, K. E., & Scarr, S. (1995). Not so far from home: How family characteristics predict child care quality. *Early Development and Parenting, 4*(3), 103–112.

Brazelton, T. B. (1990). Parent-infant co-sleeping revisited. *Ab Initio 2*(1), 1–7.

Brenner, R., Simons-Morton, B. G., Bhasker, B., Mehta, N., Melnick, V. L., Revenis, M., Berendes, H. W., & Clemens, J. D. (1998). Prevalence and predictors of the prone sleep position among inner-city infants. *JAMA, 280,* 341–346.

Capute, A., & Accardo, P. (1978). Linguistic and auditory milestones during the first two years of life. *Clinical Pediatrics, 17,* 847–853.

Centers for Disease Control and Prevention. (1995). Airbag associated fatal injuries to infants and children riding in front passengers seats—United States. *Morbidity and Mortality Weekly Report,* 44[45], 845–847.

DeBord, K. (1996). *Quality child care: What does it really mean?* [On-line]. Available: www.carefinder.com/parents/choose.html.

Dietary guidelines for infants. (1997). *Current practices in infant feeding.* [On-line]. Available: www.gerber.com/dietguide.html.

Dixon, S., & Stein, M. (2000). *Encounters with children: Pediatric behaviors and development* (3rd ed.). St. Louis: Mosby.

Duncan, S. F. (2000). *Building family strengths series: balancing work and family.* [On-line]. Available: www.montana.edu/wwwpb/pubs/mt9506.html.

Erikson, E. E. (1963). *Childhood and society* (2nd ed.). New York: Norton.

Four steps to selecting a child care provider. (2000). [On-line]. Available: www.carefinder.com/parents/choose.html.

Frankenberg, W. (1990). *Denver II manual.* Denver: Denver Developmental Materials.

Graeber, L. (1997). Simple steps to sleep. *Parents, 72*(5), 72–74.

Herzog, J. M. (1997). Birth to two. *Sleep.* [On-line]. Available: www.ctw.org.

Hoffman, L., Paris, S., & Hall, E. (1994). *Developmental psychology* (6th ed.). New York: McGraw-Hill.

Hughes, F. P. (1991). *Children, play, and development.* Boston: Allyn & Bacon.

Hunt, C. E. (1996). Sudden infant death syndrome. In R. E. Behrman, R. M. Kliegman, & A. M. Arvin (Eds.), *Nelson's textbook of pediatrics* (15th ed., pp. 1991–1995). Philadelphia: Saunders.

Jaques, S. (1993, October). All about your baby's teeth. *American Baby, 55*(10), 92–95.

Keefe, M. R. (1996). Ask the expert. *The Journal of the Society of Pediatric Nurses, 1*(1), 41–42.

Keeping your child safe. (1994). *The parent's almanac.* [On-line]. Available: family.starwave.com/resource/pra/bonus27.html.

Labensohn, D. (2000). *Parent checklist for child care.* [On-line]. Available: www.carefinder.com/parents/choose.html.

Mackin, M. L., Medendorp, S. V., & Maier, M. C. (1989). Infant sleep and bedtime cereal. *American Journal of Diseases of Children, 143,* 1066–1068.

Martin, D. (1996, April). Introducing solid foods to babies. *Foods and Nutrition* [On-line]. Available: ianrwww.unl.edu/ianr/pubs/extnpubs/foods/g962.html.

McDonald, R. E., & Avery, D. R. (1994). *Dentistry for the child and adolescent* (6th ed.). St. Louis: Mosby.

Medoff-Cooper, B. (1995). Infant temperament: Implications for parenting from birth through 1 year. *Journal of Pediatric Nursing, 3,* 141–145.

Mussen, P. H., Conger, J. J., Kagan, J., & Huston, A. C. (1990). *Child development and personality* (7th ed.). New York: Harper & Row.

Niska, K. J., Lia-Hoagberg, B., & Snyder, M. (1997). Parental concerns of Mexican American first-time mothers and fathers. *Public Health Nursing, 14*(2), 111–117.

Oppenheim, M. N. (1996, February). Early infancy oral health care. *New York State Dental Journal, 62*(2), 22–24.

Piaget, J. (1952). *The origins of intelligence in children.* New York: International Universities Press.

Pipes, P., & Trahms, C. (1993). *Nutrition in infancy and childhood* (5th ed.). St. Louis: Mosby.

Potter, K. (1995). Safety checklist. *Childproofing your home.* [On-line]. Available: www.neosoft.com/~jrpotter/safety.html.

Pridam, K. F., Chang, A. S., & Chiu, Y. (1994). Mothers' parenting self-appraisal: The contribution of perceived infant temperament. *Research in Nursing & Health, 17,* 381–392.

Reisser, P. C. (1998). *Baby and child care.* Wheaton, IL: Tyndale.

Righard, L., & Alade, M. (1997). Breastfeeding and the use of pacifiers. *Birth, 24*(2), 112–120.

Scarr, S. (1998). American child care today. *American Psychologist, 53*(2), 95–108.

Secker, D. (1999). Interpreting growth and growth standards. *HINS Articles.* [On-line]. Available: www.hins.org/growth.

Shelov, S. P. (Ed.) (1998). *Caring for your baby and young child.* New York: Bantam.

Slusher, I. L., & McClure, M. J. (1992). Infant stimulation during hospitalization. *Journal of Pediatric Nursing, 7,* 276–279.

Sprain, J. K. (1998). *Employed parenthood: Do I have a choice?* [On-line]. Available: www.nncc.org/Choose.Quality.Care/qual.employ.html.

Taubman, B. (1984). Clinical trials of the treatment of colic by modification of parent–infant interaction. *Pediatrics, 74,* 998.

Thomas, A., Chess, S., & Birch, H. (1968). *Temperament and behavior disorders in children.* New York: New York University Press.

Thomas, A., Chess, S., & Birch, H. (1970). The origin of personality. *Scientific American, 223*(2), 106–107.
Tonnessen, D. (1996, July). The family bed. *Parents, 71(7),* 47–48.
Turgeon-O'Brien, H., Lachapelle, D., Gagnon, P. F., Larocque, I., & Maheu-Robert, L. (1996). Nutritive and nonnutritive sucking habits: A review. *Journal of Dentistry for Children, 63,* 321–327.
Vaccine Information Materials Instruction Sheet. (1994). In W. Atkinson, L. Furphy, J. Gantt, & M. Mayfield (Eds.), *Epidemiology and prevention of vaccine-preventable diseases* (Appendix G). Washington, DC: U.S. Department of Health & Human Services.
Wagner, H. (1997, February). Pacifier dilemma. *Parents, 72*(2), 80–82.
Weissbluth, M. (1991). Sleep learning: The first four months. *Pediatrics Annuals, 20,* 228–238.
Whitley, E. N., Cataldo, C. B., DeBruyne, L. K., & Rolfes, A. R. (1996). *Nutrition for health and health care.* St. Paul: West.
Wright, J. (1994, May). Sleep, little baby. *American Baby, 56*(5), 75–81.
Wright, J. (1995, May). American baby basics: All about baby's sleep. *American Baby* [On-line]. Available: www.enews.com/da.

Suggested Readings

Bhavnagri, N. P., & Gonzalez-Mena, J. (1997, Fall). The cultural context of infant caregiving. *Childhood Education, 74*(1), 2–8.
Briggs, S. (1998). Little steps for new parents: A week-by-week guide and journal for baby's first year. Washington, DC: National Association for the Education of Young Children.
Brooks-Gun, J. (1995). The learning, physical, and emotional environment of the home in the context of poverty: The infant health and development program. *Children & Youth Services Review, 17,* 251–276.
Caulfield, R. (1996). Physical and cognitive development in the first two years. *Early Childhood Education Journal, 23,* 239–242.
Denham, S. A. (1995). Continuity and change in emotional components of infant temperament. *Child Study Journal, 25,* 289–308.
Elkind, D. (1994). *A sympathetic understanding of child: Birth to sixteen* (2nd ed.). Needham Heights, MA: Allyn & Bacon.
Fields, T. (1996, July). Carrying position influences infant behavior. *Early Child Development & Care, 121,* 49–54.
Gardner, J. M., & Karmel, B. Z. (1995). Development of arousal-modulated visual preferences in early infancy. *Developmental Psychology, 31,* 473–482.
Glass, J. (1998). Gender liberation, economic squeeze, or fear of strangers: Why fathers provide infant care in dual-earner families. *Journal of Marriage & Family, 60,* 821–834.
Halpern, L. F. (1995). Infant sleep–wake characteristics: Relationship to neurological status and the prediction of developmental outcomes. *Developmental Review, 15,* 255–291.
Heet, L. M. (1999, January). SIDS a killer for native infants: Aberdeen study points the way to prevention. *American Indian Report, 15*(1), 24–25.
Honig, A. S. (1997). Infant temperament and personality: What do we need to know? *Montessori Life, 9*(3), 18–21.
Hueston, W. J., Mainous, A. G., & Clarkson, P. (1994). Delays in childhood immunizations in public and private setting. *Archives of Pediatric & Adolescent Medicine, 148,* 1470.
Infant nutrition: Drinking from a cup, eating from a spoon. (1994, Fall). *Texas Child Care, 18*(2), 8–14.
Izard, C. E. (1995). The ortogeny and significance of infant's facial expressions in the first nine months of life. *Developmental Psychology, 31,* 997–1013.
Lew, A. R. (1995). The effects of hunger on hand–mouth coordination in the newborn infant. *Developmental Psychology, 31,* 456–463.
Miller, K. (1997). Play of infants and toddlers: caring for the little ones. *Child Care Information Exchange, 118,* 41–43
New, R. S. (1999, March). Here, we call it "drop off and pick up": transition to child care, American-style. *Young Children, 54*(2), 34–35.
Orcutt, B. (1997). Are there drawbacks to pacifiers? *The Washington Nurse, 27*(5), 14.
Proctor, A. (1995, April). Assessing communication, cognition, and vocalization in the prelinguistic period. *Infant & Young Child, 7*(4), 39–54.
Ramey, C. T., & Ramey, S. L. (1999). Right from birth: your child's foundation for life: Birth to 18 months. Goddard parenting guides. Beltsville, MD: Gryphon.
Recommendations for reducing the risks for SIDS. (2000). [On-line]. Available: www/sidsallaiance.org/facts/.
Rock-a-bye baby . . . on their backs. (1998). *JAMA, 280,* 396.
Rome-Flanders, T., & Crunk, C. (1995). A longitudinal study of infant vocalizations during mother–infant games. *Journal of Child Language, 22,* 259–274.
Rovee-Collier, C., & Boller, K. (1995, January). Current theory and research on infant learning and memory: Application to early intervention. *Infant & Young Child, 7*(3), 1–12.
Rucher, A. S. (1995). Infant and toddler play: Assessment of exploratory style and developmental level. *Early Childhood Research Quarterly, 10,* 297–315.
Schmitt, B. C. (1986). The prevention of sleep problems and colic. *Pediatric Clinics of North America, 33,* 763–774.
Schor, E. L. (1995). The influence of families on child health. *Pediatric Clinics of North America, 42,* 89–99.
Seifer, R. (1996). Attachment, maternal sensitivity, and infant temperament during the first year of life. *Developmental Psychology, 32*(1), 12–25.
Shrivastava, A., Davis, P., & Davis, D. P. (1997). SIDS: parental awareness and infant care practices in contrasting socioeconomic areas in Cardiff. *Archives of Disease in Childhood, 77*(7), 52–53.
Tigges, B. B. (1997). Infant formulas: practical answers for common questions. *The Nurse Practitioner, 22*(8), 70–87.
Vehicle restraints for children: Current recommendations for use. (1993). *Family & Community Health, 15*(4), 26–27.
Weinberger, N. (1998). Making a place for infants in family day care. *Early Education & Development, 9*(1), 79–96.
Wieland, D. (1998). Soothing strategies: successful calming techniques to suit your baby's temperament. *Parents, 73*(7), 28–29.

Resources

Organizations and Websites

American Academy of Pediatrics
141 Northwest Point Blvd.
Elk Grove Village, IL 60009-0927
(847) 434-4000
www.aap.org

Consumer Product Safety Commission
4330 East-West Highway
Bethesda, MD 20814-4408
(301) 504-0990
(800) 638-2772 (toll free)
www.cpsc.gov

I Am Your Child
www.iamyourchild.org
(The I Am Your Child campaign stresses the importance of a child's first years and is sponsored by Rob Reiner's Families and Work Institute.)

National Maternal and Child Health Clearinghouse (NMCHC)
2070 Chain Bridge Rd., Suite 450
Vienna, VA 22182
(703) 356-1964
(888) 434-4624 (toll-free)
(703) 821-2098 (fax)
www.nmchc.org

National Network for Child Care
www.nncc.org

National Sudden Infant Death Syndrome Resource Center
2070 Chain Bridge Rd., Suite 450
Vienna, VA 22182
(703) 821-8955
(703) 821-2098 (fax)
sids@circsol.com
www.sidscenter.org

CHAPTER 9

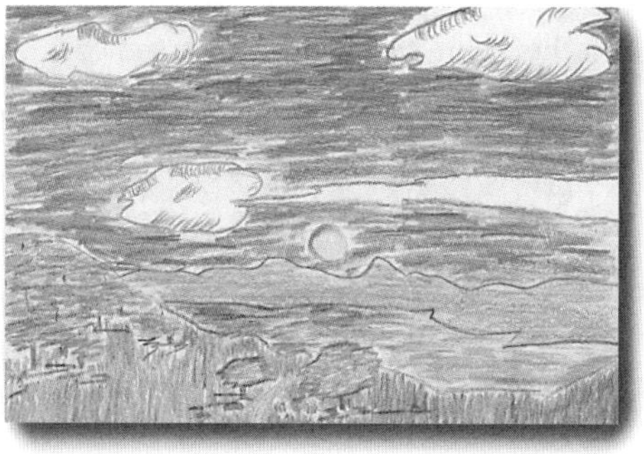

I always thought infants were wonderful, but since Emily became a toddler, I can't believe the magic that has entered our lives. It's hard to believe how Emily's changed since turning 2. She's gone from a dependent infant, needing me for everything, to a rambunctious, flirtatious explorer. She moves continuously, from one toy to another, climbing on the furniture, trying to do and be everything. I can hardly keep up with her! She's independent and wanting to do things her way one minute, clinging to me the next.

GROWTH AND DEVELOPMENT OF THE TODDLER

Barbara C. Woodring, RN, EdD
Debra Ann Mills, RN, MS

COMPETENCIES

Upon the completion of this chapter, the reader will be able to:

- *Describe the toddler's physiological, psychosexual, psychosocial, cognitive, and moral development.*
- *Discuss appropriate nursing interventions affecting the toddler's physiological, psychosexual, psychosocial, cognitive, and moral development.*
- *Describe interventions for temper tantrums, negativism, regression, and ritualism.*
- *Discuss strategies that caregivers can use when developing a disciplinary plan.*
- *Discuss sibling rivalry and appropriate interventions.*
- *Describe the physiological and psychosocial signs of readiness for toilet training and appropriate interventions.*
- *Discuss anticipatory guidance strategies for health promotion, including play, nutrition, sleep, safety, development, and dental hygiene.*

Toddlerhood is a difficult, exciting, and interesting period of life. Fundamental learning processes develop as the child begins to seek autonomy, explores the world, learns how things work, begins to tolerate limitations, expresses desires, and develops relationships. However, the toddler's excitement and frustration make this a period of incredible challenge for caregivers and health care providers alike.

Toddlerhood is the magical time of childhood encompassing the tumultuous twos and the terrific threes. This 24-month-span (12–36 months of age) reflects periods of rapid, unprecedented maturation, and change in the life of the child and family. The toddler evolves from a dependent infant with limited mobility and communication skills, into a more independent, very mobile, verbal, and inquisitive member of the family.

Promoting toddler health and maintaining wellness involves knowledge of normal growth and developmental processes, an understanding of common significant milestones, and the ability to anticipate deviations that may occur within the individual child. Knowledge of concepts and theories that support toddler development is very important. Refer to Chapter 6 for a review of developmental theories related to the toddler years.

As the toddler develops autonomy and a sense of identity, increased motor skills combined with a lack of experience and judgment can present innumerable dangers. Nurses and caregivers, therefore, need to utilize strategies to promote and assist the toddler's mastery of major developmental skills, while at the same time protecting the child from environmental dangers, provide structured guidelines and loving discipline (needed, but seldom desired), and promote a sense of independence and inquisitiveness (Figure 9-1).

Toddler physiological, psychosexual, psychosocial, cognitive, and moral development will be discussed in the following pages. It is always important to remember, however, that development in each area significantly impacts overall growth, development, and maturation, and no area of development can be viewed in isolation. Information about issues commonly arising during the toddler stage will also be presented.

PHYSIOLOGICAL DEVELOPMENT

The physical changes of toddlerhood occur in a fairly predictable manner; however, no child can be held to a rigid time frame of when those milestones will be reached. While some children initially direct their energy toward accomplishing motor activities first, others initially concentrate on verbal mastery. Generally, this does not mean one toddler is advanced and another delayed, but rather it means both will accomplish desired developmental tasks within a normal range of time, but at their own pace. It is important to provide caregivers with information to help them understand and anticipate developmental sequences. It is essential, however, that they also realize the information provides flexible guidelines rather than hard and fast rules.

Physical growth, so rapid in infancy, slows during toddlerhood, but the toddler should show a steady increase in growth, with an average weight gain of about 5 pounds per year and an increase in height averaging 3 inches per year. This slowed growth rate is evidenced by the toddler's decline in appetite and erratic eating habits. Physical appearance also changes markedly. The head gains a more proportional dimension to the rest of the body, reflecting slower brain growth, as the extremities lengthen. Chest circumference increases and soon exceeds the abdominal girth, and the top-heavy, wide base (feet spread) pot-bellied stance and toddling gait of young toddlers eventually gives way to a well-balanced appearance and gait as bones lengthen and strengthen, and abdominal muscle replaces adipose tissue. Children learn to walk at various ages, with some beginning as early as 12 months; however, most toddlers are walking by 15 months and climbing stairs by 18 months—and spending a great deal of time perfecting their efforts, compelled to repeat the process over and over again until the skill is mastered (Figure 9-2).

Neurological System

The toddler engages in many behaviors reflecting central and peripheral nervous system maturation. Brain growth continues slowly, corresponding to advancing intellectual skills and fine motor development. Improved coordination and equilibrium parallels the almost complete (by 2 years) myelinization of the spinal cord as evidenced by the toddler's refined skill in walking, jumping, and climbing.

Increasing eye–hand coordination, manual dexterity, and walking/running skills contribute significantly to the toddler's locomotion and socialization. These skills promote throwing and retrieving a variety of objects, opening and closing containers with lids, and building objects with blocks before knocking them down (Gemelli, 1996) (Figures 9-3, 9-4, and 9-5). The neurophysiologic changes that have the

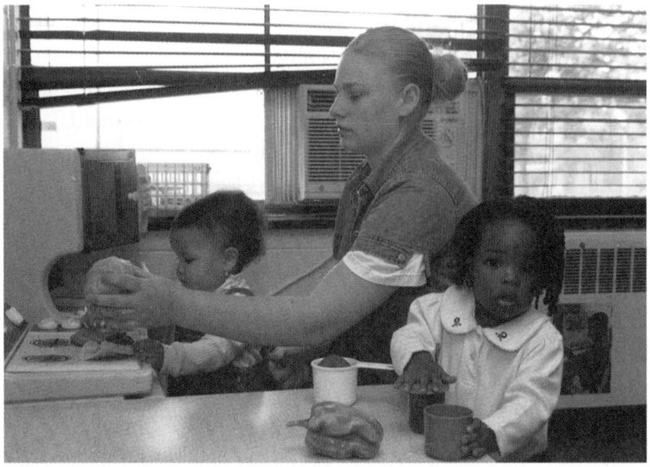

Figure 9-1 Toddlers are usually happy and love to be around others.

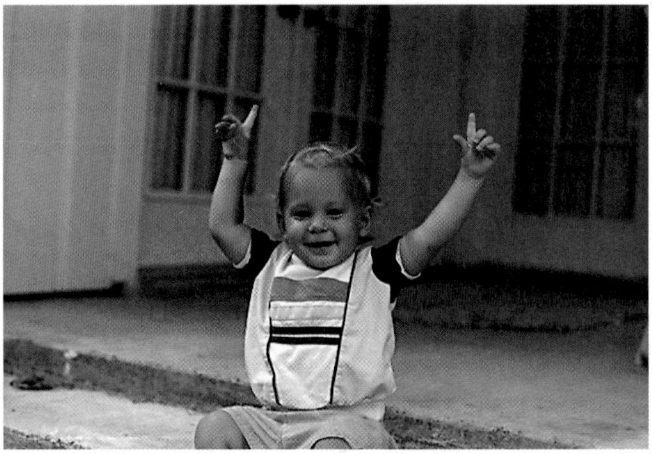

Figure 9-2 Toddlers have an engaging social smile, reach out to others for interaction, and like to be independent.

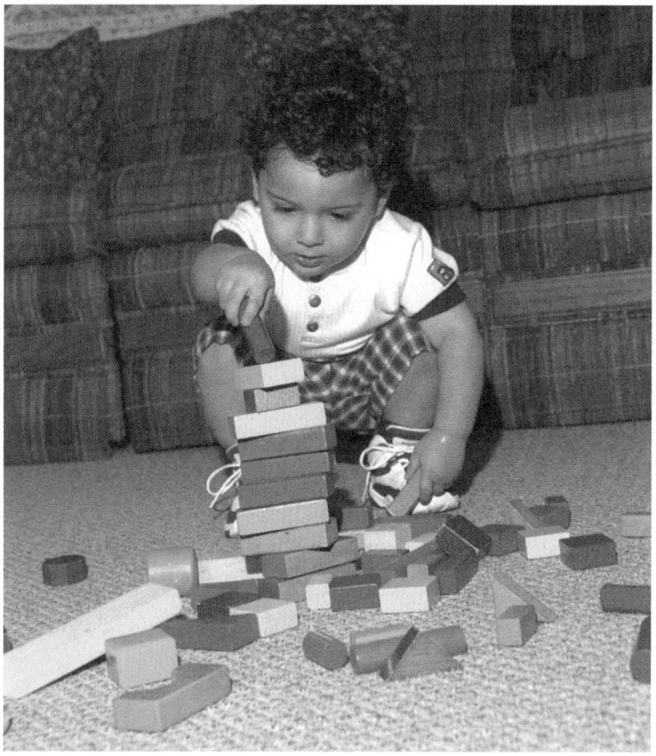

Figure 9-3 Toddlers' fine motor development is enhanced by a variety of learning activities.

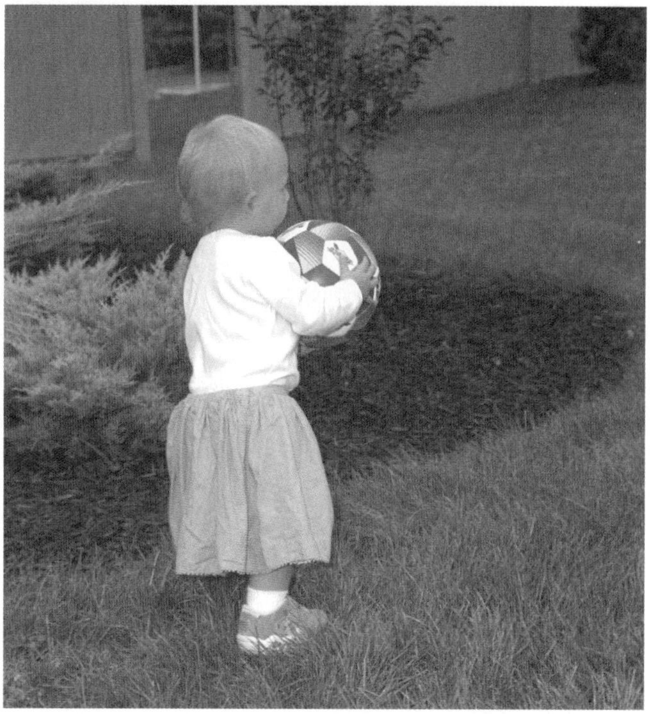

Figure 9-5 A sense of balance and coordination develops as the toddler grows and gains more control over her body.

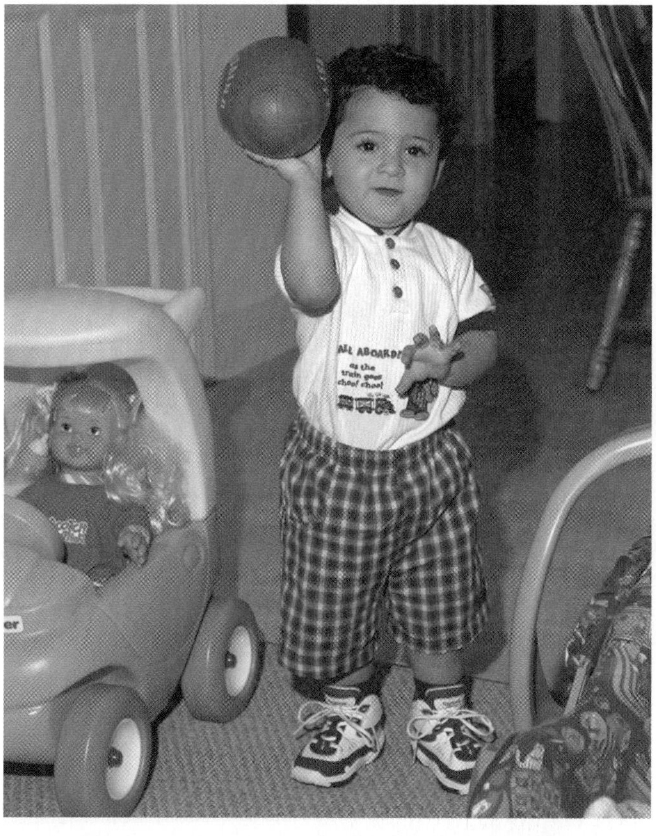

Figure 9-4 Toddlers are developing their gross motor abilities, so they need opportunities to practice these new skills.

greatest impact upon family/child education and suggested nursing interventions are listed in Table 9-1.

Musculoskeletal System

Increased bone length, muscle maturation, and increased muscle strength enable toddlers to develop autonomy. Major advances occurring in the musculoskeletal system during toddlerhood are reflected in Table 9-2.

Gastrointestinal/Genitourinary System

The gastrointestinal/genitourinary system continues to mature during these years. The stomach enlarges in size, allowing consumption of the traditional three meals per day, all deciduous teeth generally erupt by 30 months of age, and improved eye–hand coordination enables self-feeding. This would seem to set the perfect scenario for a toddler growth spurt, however, this does not generally occur. Instead, the toddler enjoys a gradual increase in size, accompanied by a decreased appetite and a ritualistic interest in limited types of food. Toddlers also vary in their energy requirements, eating large amounts of food one day and very little food the next. The food likes and dislikes also differ from day to day. This period of decreased appetite as a result of decreased caloric need is often referred to as a time of **physiologic anorexia.**

TABLE 9-1 Overview of Neurological Changes of Toddlerhood

Significant Changes	Nursing/Caregiver Implications
Anterior cranial fontanel closes at approximately the time of cord myelinization (12–18 months).	Be alert for premature closure as it can impinge on brain growth/function. Prior to closure, a bulging fontanel indicates increased intracranial pressure; sunken fontanel indicates dehydration.
Brain growth continues, reaching 80%–90% of adult size by 3 years.	Increasing head circumference is stimulated by brain growth; small circumference may suggest growth abnormalities, which place child at risk for developmental delay; enlarged size may indicated genetic syndromes or circumference hydrocephalus.
Cognitive development is demonstrated by rapidly expanding vocabulary.	The child begins toddlerhood with a vocabulary of a few words and, by 3 years, uses 300–900 words and 2–3-word phrases.
Control gained over most reflex activity.	Persistence of primitive reflexes may suggest defective cortical development.
Head circumference should approximate chest, with chest enlarging more rapidly after 24 months.	Head circumference should increase 1 inch (2.5 cm) or less per year until school age. Always measure head using a paper tape measure placed 1 inch above top of the ears.
Myelinization completed around 24 months of age.	The child is not able to walk well until myelinization has occurred. Walking well is an indication that myelinization has occurred and the child is physiologically capable of bladder/bowel control.
Spinal cord and vertebral column grow at variable rates; cord ends at L3-4 (in adult cord ends L1).	Be alert for positioning of the toddler for lumbar punctures.

TABLE 9-2 Overview of Musculoskeletal Changes of Toddlerhood

Specific Changes	Nursing/Caregiver Intervention
Bone length increases due to ossification and long bone growth; by 36 months, the child should be 41 inches (104 cm) in height. Pot belly appearance is due to lack of abdominal development. Between 13–18 months: • Walks a few steps without support • Walks upstairs with help, creeps downstairs • Turns book pages • Walks and pulls toys • Able to remove shoes and socks, tries to put on shoes • Unzips zippers • Stacks up to four cubes	Birth length doubles by 2 years. Gains 4–6 inches (10–12 cm) in height per year until school age. Deviations may indicate endocrine and/or growth hormone abnormalities. Consider safety issues with advancing mobility (stairs, running). Toys encouraging use of fine/gross motor skills should be provided. Play activities should encourage physical activity.

continues

TABLE 9-2 *Continued*

Specific Changes	Nursing/Caregiver Intervention
Between 19–30 months: • Goes up and down stairs alone (places both feet on one step before going to next) • Kicks ball forward without losing balance • Turns doorknobs • Rides tricycle (by 2 years) • Builds towers of eight cubes • Moves fingers independently, holds crayons with fingers not fist • Brushes teeth • Dresses self with supervision (buttons, snaps, etc.) but cannot tie shoes • Inserts squares into square holes • Binocular vision well developed By 36 months, large and small muscle groups enlarge, and physically observable actions are refined.	Encourage use of bike helmet and teach basic safety rules (stop/look before crossing street, etc). Child is interested in pictures and drawing, and is able to copy horizontal/vertical lines and circles.

Even though caloric needs diminish during this time, protein requirements, though less, remain higher than for other age groups. Vitamin and mineral requirements—particularly calcium, phosphorous, and iron (essential for bone and muscle growth)—increase slightly. This can create concern since toddlers often go through food fads and have a decreased food intake. Measures should be taken to help reduce the amount of fat in the toddler's diet by providing low-fat or skim milk, lean meats, and low-fat products (cheese).

Bladder and bowel control is typically achieved during this time period, and children are able to retain urine up to 4 hours before needing to void. Specific gastrointestinal and genitourinary changes that can be expected and accompanying nursing interventions can be found in Table 9-3.

TABLE 9-3 Overview of Gastrointestinal/Genitourinary Changes of Toddlerhood

Specific Changes	Nursing/Caregiver Intervention
Increased eye coordination: grasps spoon (15 months), drinks from cup without spilling (18 months)	Encourage self-feeding. Finger foods and appropriately shaped cups/utensils are important to foster independence and dexterity.
Gains 4–6 lbs (1.8–2.5 kg) per year, average weight by 3 years = 30–32 lbs (14–15 kg)	Need for protein and calorie intake remains high; toddler needs 1,000–1,500 kcal/day to support growth and 115 mL/kg of liquids per day to maintain fluid balance; weight should reveal a consistent incline on growth chart.
Slowed growth needs produce physiologic anorexia at 18 months; stomach capacity increases to allow for less frequent, larger meals.	Toddlers become "picky" eaters. Do not use food as a disciplinary tool, or cookies and sweets as behavioral rewards.
Poor eating habits and prolonged use of a bottle can create nutritional anemia and tooth decay.	Obtain an accurate food history; teach caregivers alternatives for bottle feeding, especially at bedtime (e.g., sipper cups, finger foods); expand food options; encourage child to make selections as appropriate; add one new food at a time to avoid overlooking food allergies.

continues

TABLE 9-3 *Continued*

Specific Changes	Nursing/Caregiver Intervention
Primary dentition (20 deciduous teeth) is completed by 30 months.	Poor nutritional intake and/or constipation can also create a pot-bellied appearance; assess carefully to ascertain cause; encourage tooth brushing after meals. Assess need for adding dietary fluoride to assure dental health if the fluoride level in the water is low.
Sphincter control enables bladder and bowel training.	Encourage caregivers to develop realistic expectations related to potty training based on child's developmental abilities and physiologic capabilities; encourage food with high-fiber content (such as whole grain cereals, fruits, and vegetables) and adequate fruit juices and fluids to prevent constipation; large quantities of fruit juices, especially apple juice, can produce diarrhea.
Bladder capacity increases, to allow the retention of urine for 2–4 hours; bladder and kidneys reach near-adult functional levels at about 16–24 months, which normally coincides with the ability to walk.	Urinary output should equal or exceed 1 mL/kg/hr.
Urinary bladder is positioned higher in the abdominal cavity than in adults.	Palpate bladder between umbilicus and symphysis pubis.
Urethral structures are short (1–3 inches, versus 4 inches in adult female and 8 inches in adult male). Toddlers are susceptible to urinary tract infections.	Keep perineal area clean, especially during toilet training. Begin teaching child to cleanse self from front to back; encourage child to take breaks while playing to empty bladder, which prevents incontinence and infections from urinary retention.

Cardiorespiratory System

During toddlerhood, the cardiorespiratory system continues to mature; vital signs become more stable and move closer to adult norms. Respiratory and cardiac rates slow, while blood pressure rises. Other significant factors related to cardiopulmonary assessment can be found in Table 9-4.

Sensory System

In addition to the physiologic changes noted in Tables 9-1 to 9-4, the senses of hearing, smell, taste, touch, and vision develop and begin to connect, since toddlers utilize all five senses to explore the world and exert autonomy and independence. Caregivers and health care providers need to be

TABLE 9-4 Overview of Cardiorespiratory Changes of Toddlerhood

Significant Changes	Nursing/Caregiver Implications
Vessels are easily compressed, obliterating the pulse.	Take pulse apically for 1 full minute. Awake = 70–110; asleep = 60–100 beats/min.; respirations = 25–30 breathes/min.; blood pressure = 90/50 mm Hg.
Circulating blood volume is less than in adult.	Small blood loss, including multiple blood tests, can compromise circulating volume; hypotension is a late sign of circulatory compromise; child may remain normotensive until 25% of blood volume is lost; assess capillary refill as indicator of peripheral circulation status (should refill in 2 seconds).
Lengthening body and decreasing adipose tissues produce thinner chest wall.	Breath sounds are easily heard.
Airway is small and easily compromised.	Asthma and acute allergic reactions may rapidly escalate into respiratory distress; observe for nasal flaring, retractions, and dyspnea.

continues

TABLE 9-4 *Continued*

Significant Changes	Nursing/Caregiver Implications
Cough reflex remains.	Avoid suppressing cough through the use of antitussive medications.
Tracheal diameter approximates size of adult's small finger.	Toddler rapidly reacts with signs of respiratory distress with even small amounts of mucus or obstruction.
Tongue is large in proportion to the size of the mouth.	Airway may become obstructed by tongue if child seizes or loses consciousness.
Larynx cartilage is softer than in adults and is positioned more anteriorly.	Hyperextension of neck may occlude airway, increasing the risk of aspiration/obstruction.
Alveoli are not fully functional.	Watch for rapid onset of respiratory distress due to the tendency for small airways to collapse.
Ear and throat internal structures remain relatively short and straight, tonsils and adenoids are large.	Otitis media, tonsilitis, and upper respiratory infections are common.

aware of behaviors reflecting hearing and vision difficulties such as failure to develop language, unusual responses to loud sounds, or increased falls. Baseline hearing and vision screening should be performed during toddlerhood and appropriate strategies, if necessary, immediately begun. Refer to Chapter 31 for more information.

Toddler vision should be 20/20 to 20/40, with full binocular capabilities reached shortly after 12 months of age. Depth perception continues to develop throughout the toddler years. Developing depth perception, combined with inquisitiveness, poor judgment, and occasional lack of coordination, puts the toddler at risk for frequent falls when learning to walk, run, and climb stairs.

PSYCHOSEXUAL DEVELOPMENT

Attitudes related to gender identity, sex roles, and sexuality are mostly determined by the values and morals of the caregiver and the environment. Toddlers are generally able to recognize gender differences by 2 years of age and begin to explore and recognize body parts, most often during toilet training.

According to Freud (1957), toddlers are in the anal stage of development. (Refer to Chapter 6 for more information on Freud.) Freud also first pointed out the tension revolving around toddler bowel/bladder training, and viewed toilet training as a possible way of resolving conflict and handling stress. He believed improperly managed toilet training could lead to life-long psychological trauma with accompanying physical bowel/bladder responses (Freud, 1957).

Many thoughts and activities of both the caregiver and the toddler tend to be focused on toilet training, and, because of the close proximity of the genitalia to the urinary and anal orifices, toddlers tend to manually manipulate and inspect these areas. Masturbation is common and should be handled in a matter-of-fact-manner, thereby lessening the child's anxiety and feelings of shame. The inquisitive nature of toddlers, combined with their need to explore, the concept of object permanence, and the desire to know about their bodies influences toddlers to behaviors related to toileting.

Domestic mimicry, or imitation of domestic/role activity, is one way toddlers express their understanding of gender roles. For example, in imaginative play, the child takes the role of "mommy," "daddy," or "baby," and develops lifelong attitudes related to gender-specific behavior. Caregiver responses to boys playing with dolls or cooking in the play kitchen, and girls taking a truck a part or building houses in the mud can have a profound influence on later role-related thinking patterns and experiences (Figure 9-6).

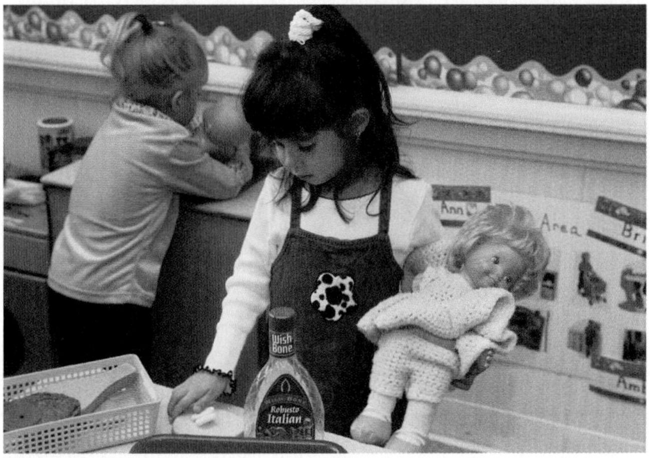

Figure 9-6 Toddlers engage in domestic mimicry when they repeat actions seen in caregivers.

Critical Thinking

Maria's "Brite" Idea

The Lite-Brite board and pieces were among 34-month-old Maria's favorite toys. One afternoon, Maria told her mother that she had hidden her favorite yellow bright-light and now was unable to get it. Her mother accompanied Maria to her bedroom, where she had been playing and began the search. They looked high and low for the yellow bright-light, but did not find it. Maria was very upset and crying—she wanted that particular piece of her toy and could not be consoled. Maria's mother began questioning her more carefully about where she had last been playing with the missing toy. Did she remember laying it down or putting it somewhere for safe keeping? Then Maria, pouting, pointed to her vulva. She had "hidden" the lite-brite in her vagina to see if it would light up in the dark.

Maria was taken to the local emergency department (ED). A pediatric surgeon was able to manually remove the yellow Brite Lite intact (and in working order) from her vagina with only minimal trauma. When asked why she had put the toy into this part of her body, Maria very matter-of-factly answered "it's dark in there, and I wanted to see the yellow light."

Maria's mother was advised not to punish Maria but to firmly reinforce that hiding things in any body opening might make her sick. All seemed well until Maria returned to the ED, about 4 weeks later, to have dried beans removed from her nose!

1. How would you explain this behavior to her caregivers? Does she need psychological help to overcome this problem?
2. Maria's father thinks she should be disciplined for disobeying, since they had to make another trip to the ED for a very similar problem (inserting a dried bean into her nose) after only 4 weeks. How would you help this family determine the best way to deal with the situation?

In a similar fashion, the caregiver's response to the toddler's sexually related actions and questions can influence future sexual attitudes. Therefore, the caregiver needs to clarify what the child really wants to know before beginning detailed explanations. For example, when the $2^1/_2$-year-old asks, "Where does baby come from?" the child may really want to know that the baby *doll* came from the toy box in the bedroom, not the physiological process of reproduction (Brazelton, 1992).

Since the child's gender identity is formulated during toddlerhood, continual rewards for responding in a manner consistent with a specific gender internalizes that identity.

Family Teaching

Accomplishing Positive Psychosexual Outcomes with Toddlers

- Avoid using slang, baby talk, or confusing terms. Teach the child correct anatomical names.
- Provide positive reinforcement as the toddler experiments with various gender-related behaviors. Do not confuse the child with statements such as "big boys don't cry" or "only boys play with trucks."
- Accept manipulation of genitalia and masturbation as a natural, private behavior of toddlerhood.
- Respond to questions with age-appropriate language.
- Do not make toilet training a major confrontational issue for the household; try to tie in educational aspects when possible (e.g., always wash hands, wipe front-to-back, etc).

Gender identity is reinforced by observing same and opposite sex caregivers enact their gender roles, attitudes, and values, and by experiencing the way adults treat children of different genders differently. Refer to the Family Teaching display for guidelines to use in assisting caregivers to encourage appropriate psychological development.

PSYCHOSOCIAL DEVELOPMENT

The three major psychosocial tasks of toddlerhood are gaining self-control, developing autonomy, and increasing independence. Progress toward mastery can be judged through observing specific behaviors such as:

- Tolerating separation from caregiver (stays with sitter or in day care without prolonged crying/distress)
- Withstanding delayed gratification (waits, without a temper tantrum, until toy is removed from box to play)
- Increasing control over bowel/bladder function (maintains dryness for more than 2 hours)
- Utilizing socially acceptable behavior/language (controls temper tantrums/biting behaviors)
- Walking well and seeking new experiences in the environment
- Interacting with others in a less id-centric/ego-centric manner (shares toys more willingly)

In the process of mastering self-control, autonomy, and independence, the toddler must also grapple with new, confusing, and frightening situations (Figure 9-7). The way the child responds to these situations culminates in what Erikson

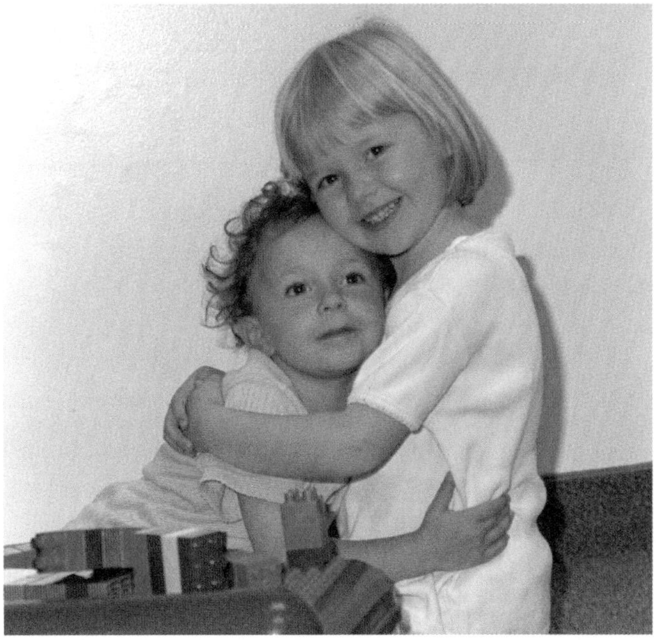

Figure 9-7 Toddlers often find comfort in the familiar such as an older sibling.

refers to as autonomy versus shame and doubt (Erikson, 1963). Either the child masters the situation and autonomy and self-concept are strengthened, or he is unsuccessful and doubts his abilities to succeed in such situations in the future (Figure 9-8). For more information on Erikson's theory, refer to Chapter 6 as well as Table 9-5.

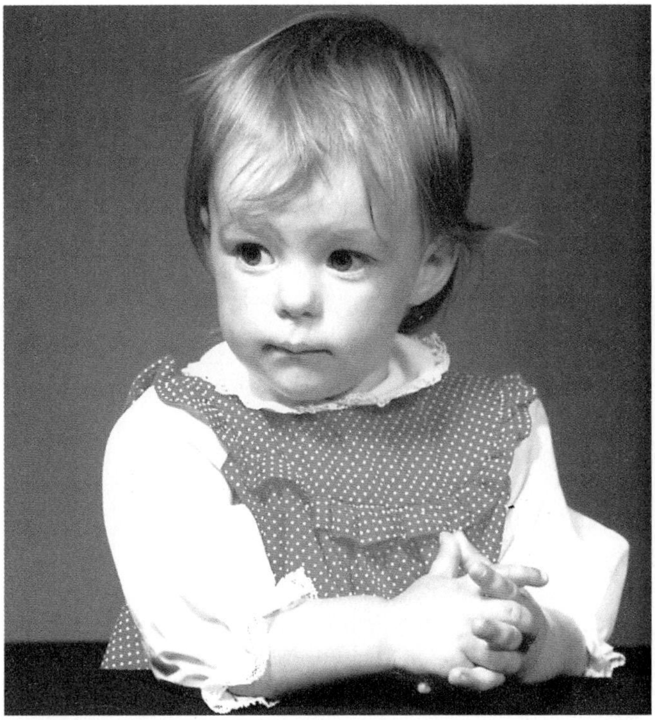

Figure 9-8 Some toddlers are serious and remain that way for much of their life.

TABLE 9-5 Psychosocial Milestones

Age	Description
15 Months	Fears being alone, being abandoned, strangers, objects, and places. Expresses independence by trying to feed/undress self.
18 Months	Negativism predominates; fears water. Temper tantrums and awareness of own gender begins.
24 Months	May resist bedtime and naps, fear the dark and animals; temper tantrums, negativism, and dawdling continue. Bedtime rituals important. Explores genitalia. Shows readiness for bowel/bladder control.
36 Months	Temper tantrums, negativism, and dawdling behaviors subside; self-esteem increases due to increased independence in eating, elimination, and dressing. Explores many emotions in pretend play. Separation fears generally subside; may develop a fear of monsters.

COGNITIVE DEVELOPMENT

The social smile and babbling language of infancy give way to meaningful hand/arm gestures punctuated with rapidly increasing development of speech skills during the toddler years. Language ability develops rapidly. However, it is dependent upon physical maturity as well as environmental influences (parental encouragement and participation). Although most toddlers' comprehension of words is greater than their ability to verbalize, by 36 months of age children are able to converse and begin to acknowledge different points of view. Vocabulary expands from a few words to over 900 words in 2 short years. Speaking in short sentences, using pronouns, and understanding directional commands (Table 9-6) also occur during this time. These advancements suggest the toddler is more mature than their thinking processes since the meanings of all verbalizations are not always understood. Reasoning skills also remain undeveloped during this time, although an understanding of causal relationships is emerging. Guidelines to enhance communication are found in Nursing Tips: How to Communicate with Toddlers. Refer to Chapter 31 for more information on language development.

Cognitively, toddlers are able to recognize and distinguish between shapes of objects, but they are only beginning to classify objects into categories of use. In the mind of a toddler, all objects that look alike have the same function and

Research Hightlight

Emotional Continuity

Study Purpose

To determine (1) if emotions present at 3 years of age continued, intensified, or diminished by 6 years, (2) if associations existed between emotional responses and gender, and (3) if, over time, the child developed an understanding of conflicting emotions.

Methods

Forty-seven children were followed for 3 years, starting when the child was 3 years of age. A variety of psychological tests were administered at 36 months and again at 6 years of age.

Findings

(1) There was significant stability in individual differences over the 3-year period. Emotional understanding at age 3 continued to be significantly related to the child's understanding at age 6, including language ability and participation in discussions about causality. (2) Girls were better at handling and explaining emotions than boys. (3) By 6 years of age, almost all children were able to explain the presence of two emotions occurring simultaneously.

Implications

Everyone dealing with children should be educated about the lasting impact of early emotional development, and the importance of fostering and encouraging frequent and consistent emotional interactions between toddlers and their caregivers, their siblings, and their environment. Caregivers need to understand that the exchanges of toddlers set the pattern for emotional responses used during the rest of the child's life. Children of both genders should be encouraged to express their emotions (e.g., it is appropriate for little boys to cry).

Citation

Brown, J., & Dunn, J. (1996). Continuities in emotional understanding from three to six years. *Child Development, 67*, 789–802.

TABLE 9-6 Toddler Cognitive Milestones

Age	Description
12–15 months	Expresses self by refining hand/arm gestures. Speaks at least three to four understandable words and develops own language often not understood by others. Learns by repetitive experiences (e.g., repeatedly tossing items off tray of high-chair) and by trial and error.
18 months	Concept of object permanence developed. Speaks 10 or more understandable words, frequently uses jargon learned in home environment (e.g., nicknames or cultural terms).
24 months	Engages in symbolic play and domestic mimicry. Egocentric thinking evident in speech and play. Uses pronouns, refers to self by name. Speaks in two- to three-word sentences.
36 months	Is able to name body parts, gives full name. Uses about 900 different words, most are understandable; speaks in three- to five-word sentences.

Nursing Tip:

How to communicate with toddlers

- Acknowledge use of culturally specific terms/actions/rituals.
- Relate time to familiar activities (after lunch).
- Speak at the child's eye level.
- Respect the child's personal space; speak before violating this space.
- Touch the child gently on the shoulder to gain attention.
- Use terms that the child understands and that are acceptable to family when adults are introduced (for instance, the family may prefer that all adults be addressed as Mr/Ms, not by a first name).
- Use child's nickname or most familiar name (not necessarily his legal name).
- Use positive reinforcement often ("You've been very helpful").
- Use short, concrete descriptions ("Put the ball into the toy box, please").
- Avoid using literal phrases ("don't cough your head off," or "this will just be a little stick in your arm").
- Use play to project feelings and gain information ("what if you could . . .", "if you had a wish . . .).
- Answer questions simply.
- Set limits firmly, but gently. Reward acceptable behavior (avoid using food as a reward).
- A child's attention span is approximately equal to his age in years (e.g., 3 years old, attention span of 3 minutes).

are therefore treated equally. For example, a pail is used to collect sand from the sandbox, hold water to scrub the floor, and hold paint. So, in the child's mind, if the toddler is allowed to overturn the pail of sand, then he or she is also allowed to overturn the water pail and the paint pail (Figure 9-9).

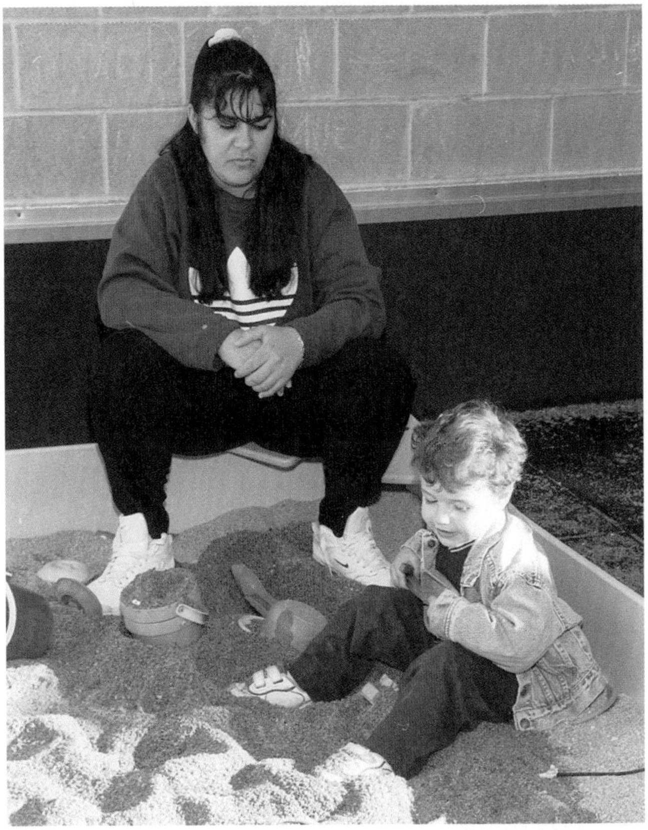

Figure 9-9 Toddlers need a variety of experiences to develop their cognitive abilities.

Piaget (1952) was concerned primarily with how knowledge is acquired and learning takes place; he systematically explained how children processed experiences and situations that touched their lives (culture, neighbors, other children, etc). According to Piaget (1952), toddler cognitive development encompasses three major stages divided into two phases: sensorimotor and preoperational. A summary of Piaget's sensorimotor and preconceptual phase of thinking is found in Table 9-7.

TABLE 9-7 Sensorimotor and Preconceptual Phases of Toddler Development (Piaget)

Stage/Age	Cognitive Changes	Behavioral Changes
Sensorimotor Tertiary circular reactions, 15–18 months	Experiences as many new situations as possible to achieve new skills/abilities. Combines new and old knowledge to experiment and begin early reasoning. Understanding of object permanence is enhanced.	Inquisitive and curious about "world." Uses all senses to explore and test environment. Increases use of physical skills to increase abilities (e.g., transitions from walking to climbing to reach a higher shelf).

continues

TABLE 9-7 *Continued*

Stage/Age	Cognitive Changes	Behavioral Changes
Sensorimotor Tertiary circular reactions, 15–18 months	Learns to differentiate self from objects. Develops awareness of spatial and causal concepts.	Places items in and out of containers; recognizes that items out of sight exist (box of crackers in cupboard). Is comforted by parents' voices, even if they are unseen. Extends separation time from caretakers.
Mental combinations, 18–24 months	Can infer a cause even if only experiencing the effect (threw a toy, child disciplined, and toy put out of reach). Beginning to think before acting. Imitation becomes more symbolic. Beginning sense of memory in early problem solving. Better sense of time relationships. Egocentric in actions and thinking.	Follows directions and understands requests (don't run, you will fall; put your toy here). Imitates role model's speaking (words and animal sounds). Demonstrates domestic mimicry. Uses simple words with meaning (sit, go, up, down). Engages in parallel play and senses ownership (my truck). Refers to self by name. Comfort level requires routine schedule and rituals.
Preconceptual, 2–4 years	Thoughts, play, and actions continue to be egocentric. Sense of time, space, and causality improves. Use of language as mental representation increases. Develops cognitive connection between new experience and things that occurred in the past (refuses to eat food because something before didn't taste good, "icky"). Begins trial and error learning.	Increased vocabulary with phrases of 2–3-words. Has difficulty sharing and is possessive of toys, family members, and other items (mine or my). Uses vocabulary terms that are future oriented (tomorrow). Can follow more complex directions (put this toy in the box behind you). Can put shoes on even if on wrong foot, repeats procedure again and again.

Kids Want To Know

Cognitive Development

I babysit two little boys every Saturday. Jared is 2 years old, and his cousin Jesse is 2 1/2 years old. Most of the time, they are pretty good, but they can't seem to play together very well. I give them each a toy and say, "have fun"! The next thing I know, Jesse has Jared's toy. Jared is crying and sometimes has a red mark from being hit by Jesse. I try to make them share, but it just doesn't work. If Jesse isn't taking Jared's toys, Jared's taking Jesse's. I feel frustrated when this happens, and I don't know what to do!

Your feelings of frustration are not uncommon, but it might help if you know why they act this way. Toddlers live in a world of their own. They only see their side of things and don't see another person's perspective, such as sharing. Each toddler is concerned only with playing with the toy. Jared doesn't realize that taking it way from Jesse will make him unhappy, and vice versa.

MORAL DEVELOPMENT

Toddlers have little concept of right and wrong even though Kohlberg's (1976) theory of moral development could be applied to toddlers because of their willful desires to make independent decisions and their increasing cognitive capacities. (Refer to Chapter 6 for more information on Kohlberg.) However, a child's ability to actually make moral decisions is based upon multiple cognitive and social interactions that exceed the abilities of a toddler.

On the other hand, Fowler (1974) does make a strong case for the consideration of early stages of faith development in this age group. Fowler defined faith as a relational phenomenon, an active relationship with another, a commitment, belief, love, and/or hope, which may be directed toward family, religion, God, or friends. As such, undifferentiated faith, as a foundation for other faith development, may occur as early as 2 years of age. Although religious rituals and symbols may not be understood at this time, the child does enjoy interacting with adults and children around simple religious stories.

HEALTH PROMOTION

As nurses who focus their efforts on meeting the needs of children and their families, we must provide informational and educational supports to equip caregivers to be as well prepared as possible to meet the mounting challenges presented by growing children. When caregivers are informed of expected growth patterns and developmental changes, they can anticipate what should come next, plan for the changes, and note quickly when the expected changes do not occur.

Parenting is a process that one is never totally prepared to begin. Therefore, parents/caregivers of toddlers need preparation and patience to deal with the emotional periods their child will experience during these volatile 24 months of excitement and frustration. Gemelli (1996) has identified three essential roles for parents of toddlers:

- Protecting the toddler from experiencing too many episodes of distressful, over- or understimulation such as violent television shows or long periods without interaction
- Teaching the toddler how to gratify innate needs while keeping within the limits and rules set by the family and society, such as eating off of their own plate at mealtimes
- Providing empathy, encouragement, support, and love, while teaching their toddler that autonomy has limits and restrictions, such as praising the child for trying a new food item or disciplining when a disliked food item in thrown

Nurses need to provide assistance and guidance to caretakers for common issues such as nutrition, sleep, dental hygiene, safety and injury prevention, health screening, negativism, ritualism, regression, discipline, sibling rivalry, temper tantrums, toilet training, child (day) care, and play. Each of these topics will be addressed briefly.

Nutrition

The toddler's ability to chew and swallow as well as use utensils also improves during this time. Caretakers who understand these changes will be better able to introduce new foods reflecting the child's abilities. It is also, however, important to avoid foods that may be major choking hazards (pieces of hot dogs, popcorn, nuts, hard candy); (Forgac, 1995; Feeding the Toddler, 2001).

Caregivers should consider the toddler's abilities by cutting food into small bits, offering dipping sauces, and serving small portions. Most adult food can be provided with some modifications; however, toddlers rarely like new food the first time it is introduced. Juice should be limited to 4 ounces per day, because it is a nutrient-dense food that often replaces calories that should come from more nutritious foods. Since there is an increased incidence of severe peanut allergy in young children, caretakers should be instructed to withhold any food item containing peanuts until 3 years of age.

Mealtimes continue to be messy during this age. Toddlers are still in the process of becoming proficient with a spoon and often spill. Caregivers should be encouraged to provide praise and positive reinforcement since scolding causes tension and stress. Eating habits are established in the first 2–3 years, and forcing food or creating periods of extended tension at mealtime are not healthy. Food issues tend to occur about the same time that the toddler is being encouraged to sit with the family during mealtime, often leading to explosive verbal exchanges, especially during the evening meal.

Caregivers tend to become concerned about the child's decreased food intake and/or the fact that, for weeks, the toddler may eat only cereal (or go on other food jags). Caregivers need to be assured the child will not starve and generally will eat when hungry. A general rule of thumb to use in determining adequacy in the meal is to offer 1 tablespoon of each food group for each year. For example, a 3-year-old would need 3 tablespoons of meat, 3 tablespoons of carbohydrate (rice or potato), 3 tablespoons of vegetable, and 3 tablespoons of fruit.

Different strategies may also be used. Offering smaller amounts of food may encourage the toddler to ask for more. For others, frequent nutritious snacks throughout the day may be more enjoyable. Nurses should also remind caretakers to acknowledge the toddler's ritualistic needs (e.g., same plate, same cup). Encouraging the toddler to explore the world of food should be accompanied by clear limits. The Family Teaching box on picky eaters provides some helpful guidelines in coping with these stressors.

Family Teaching

The Picky Eater

1. Provide healthy snacks every 1–2 hours; place them where the toddler can independently reach them.
2. Plan snacks for the day; regulate their timing with meals.
3. Allow an occasional junk-food snack.
4. Carry crackers and/or vegetable stick snacks while traveling in the car.
5. Be patient, food jags will pass; the child may eat only grilled cheese sandwiches for a month, but will move on to another favorite food in time.
6. Keep distractions to a minimum; turn off the television during mealtimes.
7. Respect the child's speed of eating.
8. Encourage the child to participate in meal preparation.
9. Use snack time to introduce essential nutrients (a good snack contains two of the five food groups):

If the child . . .	**Offer . . .**
Isn't a big milk drinker and needs calcium	Yogurt, frozen yogurt, hot cocoa, pudding
Doesn't eat meat and needs iron	Fortified breakfast cereal (*not* presweetened), raisins, fortified breakfast bars
Eats only white bread and needs more fiber	Fresh fruit and vegetables, bran muffins, bean or pea soup
Doesn't eat vegetables and needs vitamin A	Veggie juice, apricots, sweet potato wedges

REFLECTIONS FROM FAMILIES

My 2-year-old daughter Elena has changed a lot in the past few months. She used to be such a good eater, and now she either doesn't eat or will only eat certain kinds of food. I worry about her almost every day, fearing that she won't develop properly or that I am doing something wrong. The worse thing is that my husband or I fight with her often, and we all leave the dinner table feeling stressed and miserable.

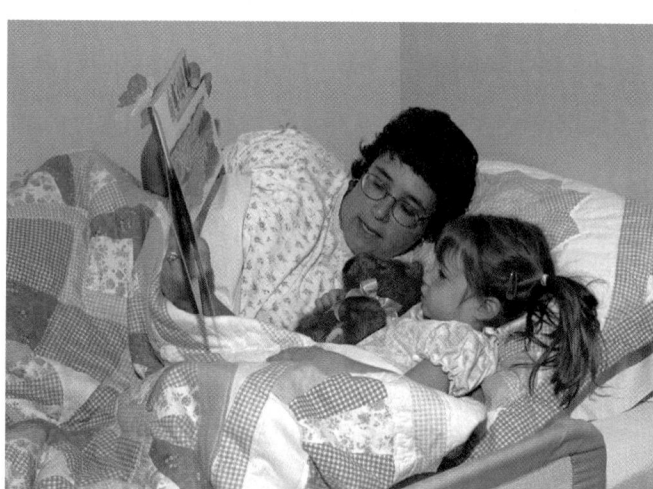

Figure 9-10 Nighttime rituals are especially important to toddlers.

Sleep

Most 2-year-olds require 12–14 hours of sleep each day with a nap generally in the afternoon (some toddlers require a morning nap as well). Sleep is important to reenergize the toddler and promote growth and development. Lack of sleep makes the toddler feel tired, cranky, and irritable. To help the toddler obtain adequate sleep and rest, caretakers can develop naptime and bedtime routines (Figure 9-10). Bedtime protests can be reduced by beginning a winding down period when toddlers are bathed, cuddled, and/or read to prior to being put to bed for the night. Firm consistent limits are needed when the child resists going to bed and dawdles or stalls (asking for water).

Some toddlers wake in the middle of the night and may have trouble returning to sleep. It is important to let the child cry for a short time since this assists the child to learn self-calming and comforting measures. If crying continues, caregivers can offer a hug, backrub, or drink before leaving the room again. A favorite blanket or toy coupled with a calm reassurance can also help facilitate the child's return to sleep. Nightmares are also common in toddlerhood since their dreams seem very real (Grover, 2001a). The toddler will generally respond to gentle reassurances and most often will return to sleep and will not remember the dream the next day.

Dental Health

In addition to routine health care visits, toddlers should also see a dentist. The child's first visit should be soon after the first teeth erupt at about 1 year of age. An important aspect of the visit is assessment of oral health, education of caretakers regarding correct methods of dental hygiene, and counseling on strategies to prevent caries (Grover, 2001c).

Young children are unable to brush all areas of the mouth, and as a result, caretakers will need to assume some responsibility for effective teeth cleaning (Figure 9-11). Toddlers may use only water, disliking the taste and foam of toothpaste. There is, however, some danger if fluoridated toothpaste is swallowed, so caregivers should be cautioned that, if toothpaste is used, it be used sparingly. Caregivers should select small toothbrushes that are soft with short, rounded bristles. After cleansing the teeth, flossing is recommended to remove debris below the gum line and prevent gingivitis (Grover, 2001c). A disclosing agent may help identify areas where plaque exists. Teeth should continue to be brushed until the dye (generally red) is gone.

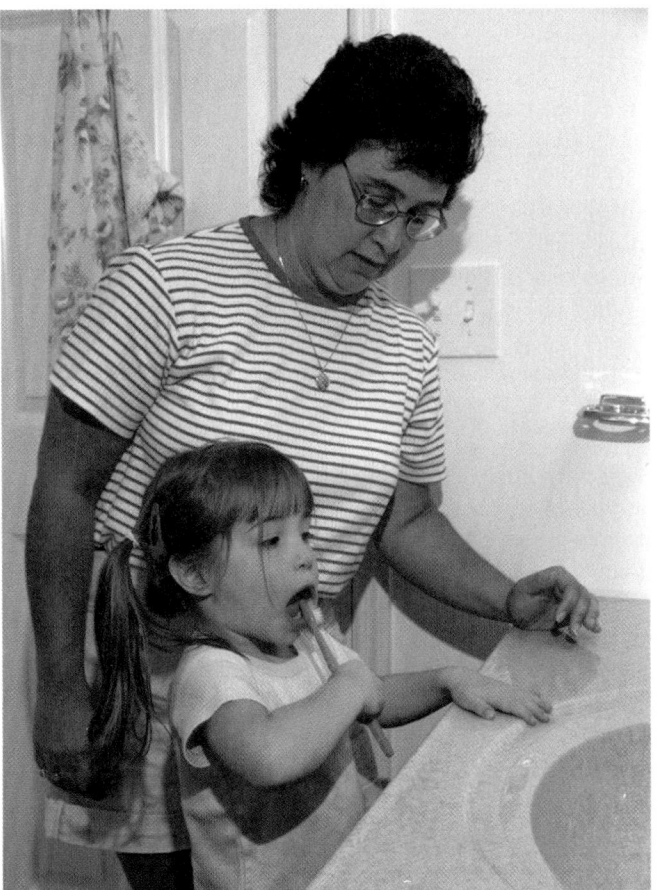

Figure 9-11 Toddlers will need to be supervised when learning to brush their teeth.

The use of fluoride is an effective method to lessen the extent of tooth decay and promote tooth health (American Academy of Pediatrics Committee on Nutrition, 1986). Tooth enamel resists developing caries when adequate amounts of fluoride are consumed before the teeth erupt. The nurse should educate caregivers regarding correct administration of fluoride supplements if it has been determined that fluoridation of water does not exist in the community (American Academy of Pediatric Dentistry, 1996).

Safety Promotion and Injury Prevention

The coupling of an inquisitive mind and a tottering, but mobile body places toddlers at increased risk for injury through accidents. The types of accidents and injuries experienced are directly related to the child's developmental progression (Table 9-8). Most injuries and deaths to toddlers are due to airway obstruction, poisonings, drowning, falls, burns, and automobiles (Online Safety Project, 2001).

Auto Safety

State and federal laws related to child safety seats and seat belt use have produced a marked decrease in injuries and deaths among children; however, the laws are of little value unless caregivers follow them. Toddlers should *always* be strapped into a child-safety seat, appropriate for weight and size (Henson, Hadfield, & Cooper, 1999; Thompson & Emslie, 2000). The safety seat should be placed in the *back seat* of the vehicle. Toddlers should *not* ride in the front seat of a vehicle that has an *air bag,* unless they have specific medical conditions (i.e., tracheotomies, uncontrolled seizures, severe respiratory problems) that require constant observation. In these limited cases, the child should be placed in an appropriate front seat car seat and the air bag mechanically disabled (Flaherty & Snyder, 1998). A booster seat (one without side arms) is not appropriate until a child weighs at least 30 pounds. Transition of a child from a booster seat to lap-shoulder belts should not occur until the child reaches at least 4 years of age, 40 pounds, and/or 40 inches in height.

Nurses should review child passenger safety information with caregivers at every opportunity. The Child-Occupant Safety Checklist (Table 9-9) could become a routine part of your teaching approach.

Keeping toddlers from darting into streets in front of vehicles requires constant attention and repeated teaching. By 3 years of age, the child should begin to understand the concept of stopping and looking both ways before moving into a street. Even if toddlers do not understand the concept of oncoming danger, repetition of the stop–look sequence helps build the concept of safety.

TABLE 9-8 Developmental Specific Injury Prevention

Developmental Characteristics of Toddler (1–3 years)	Prevention Strategies
Walks, runs, may dart into street More independent and developing autonomy Not aware of dangers but is intent on exploring Will stray from caregiver Walks with unsteady gait Explores with mouth Can reach, climb, open lids, turn doorknobs Uses all senses to explore environment	Prevent injuries from motor vehicle accidents (as passenger, cyclist, or pedestrian): • Begin teaching stop–look both ways at curbside; stay off streets with riding toys and tricycle. • Use appropriate car seat. • Do not allow child in front seat of vehicle with air bags. • Supervise—toddler acts impulsively! • Provide fenced play area. • Teach toddler not to enter the car of strangers. Prevent fall-related injury: • Don't run with anything protruding from mouth (e.g., popsicle or lollipop sticks). • Use gates in stairways until child is very stable in walking and climbing stairs. • Remove scatter rugs, which may slide with child. • Remove electrical cords from walkway. • Keep child away from machinery and lawn mowers. • Teach child to wear bike helmets when on tricycle or on back of adult bicycle. • Secure screens in all open windows; use secure window guards. • Keep door to stairwells closed or gates in place. • Remove objects from crib that could be used to climb out of crib or window. • If child climbs out of crib, place in different bed. Prevent aspiration: • Check all toys for small, removable parts (buttons, eyes). • Use Mylar balloons only. • Avoid popcorn, nuts, hard candy, and other small, hard foods or large chunks of meat or hard vegetables. Prevent suffocation: • Keep all plastic bags and similar objects out of reach. • Do not use a plastic bag as liner for trash can in child's room. Prevent burns: • Set water heater at less than 49°C (120°F). • Keep curling iron and cords out of reach. • Turn handles of pans toward center/back of stove. • Do not place containers of hot liquid on table cloth or scarf, which can be pulled. • Use safety covers on electrical outlets. • Keep child away from fireplaces and space heaters. • Keep cigarettes, lighters, and matches out of sight and reach. Prevent ingestion/poisoning: • Store poisonous substances in original containers. • Lock or remove medications and poisonous substances out of reach. • Never refer to medication as candy. • Do not keep medication, including vitamins, on counter, on table top, or in purse or diaper bag. • Discuss meaning of poison with child. • Use Mr. Yuck or similar designation for items that are off limits for child. • Keep syrup of ipecac in home to be used *only* when directed by Poison Control Center. • Post phone number of Poison Control Center by each telephone in house. Promote gun safety; if gun in house: • Keep gun locked up and unloaded. • Store bullets away from the gun. Prevent drowning: • Supervise child while in bathtub. • Instruct child to never go near water alone.

continues

TABLE 9-8 *Continued*

Prevent drowning (*cont.*):
- Provide close supervision around water.
- Instruct child never to run around pool or other bodies of water.
- Standing water should not be left in small wading pools unless a cover is applied.
- A child-approved life vest should be on child whenever on a boat or near water.
- Surround pools with locked fences.
- Teach child to swim but supervise—*closely*.

Miscellaneous:
- Teach child caution when approaching unknown animals (dogs, cats, raccoons).
- Do not expect young children to supervise toddlers.
- Use sun screen.
- Eliminate passive smoke in environment.
- Keep alcohol out of sight and reach.

TABLE 9-9 Child-Occupant Safety Checklist

Criteria	Yes	No
Child in restraint device	❑	❑
In the back seat (middle preferable)*	❑	❑
If more than 20 pounds, child faces forward in auto; if less than 20 pounds, child faces rear.*	❑	❑
Proper position (less than 20 pounds, at approximately a 45 degree recline; more than 20 pounds, upright)	❑	❑
Infant's or child's back firmly against back of safety seat	❑	❑
Head contained within the seat or, if in booster, within automobile seat back	❑	❑
Child car seat intact (no cracks in shell, no frays in straps, straps not torn, no exposed foam, no bent frames)	❑	❑
Car seat straps straight (not twisted)	❑	❑
Shoulder harness on shoulders	❑	❑
Shoulder harness taut (not more than 2 inches from shoulders)	❑	❑
Harness in slots below shoulders for rear-facing position, above shoulders for facing front	❑	❑
Infant/child not wearing bulky clothing or blanket under harness	❑	❑
Auto seat belt across chest (not across face, neck, or under arm)	❑	❑
Auto seat belt used with child car seat	❑	❑
Auto seat belt routed correctly through child car seat	❑	❑
Auto seat belt tight (doesn't slide and has locking clip if sliding type)	❑	❑
Restraint latch releases without difficulty (but doesn't pull out without pressing latch release)	❑	❑
Child car seat stable (can't be pulled forward away from auto seat or side to side)	❑	❑
Child car seat within edges of auto seat (doesn't extend over)	❑	❑
Child car seat made after 1981	❑	❑
Child car seat not on recall list	❑	❑
One infant/child in a restraint device (no sharing a restraint device)	❑	❑
In proper restraint for age and size	❑	❑
Booster seat used with shield/lap belt or lap/shoulder belt	❑	❑

** If there are no adults other than the driver in the car, the child can be placed in the front seat facing the rear, which is safer than back seat facing front. However, if car is equipped with air bags, young children must ride in the rear seat.*

Data from Gaines, S., Benjamin, H., & Deforest, M. (1998). Promoting automobile safety for young children. MCN, *23(3), 148–151.*

Home and Environmental Safety

Homes and surrounding play areas need to be childproofed to prevent drowning, falls, and accidental poisonings (Figures 9-12 and 9-13). Even when caregivers make a conscious effort to protect toddlers, toddlers needs to learn which things they may and may not play with in a home. All medications and toxic substances (e.g., gasoline, pesticides, household cleaning products) must be kept out of the child's reach and preferably locked away. These items should *never* be stored in familiar containers (such as soft drink bottles) and should have a "Mr. Yuck" or similar poison alert symbol affixed. Never tell a child that medication is candy to encourage taking it, and never leave medications (including vitamins) sitting on tables, or in the diaper bag or purse. Homes where toddlers live or frequently visit should have a bottle of syrup of ipecac in case a child accidentally ingests a toxic substance. However, caregivers should be instructed to administer syrup of ipecac *only after* consulting a Poison Control Center.

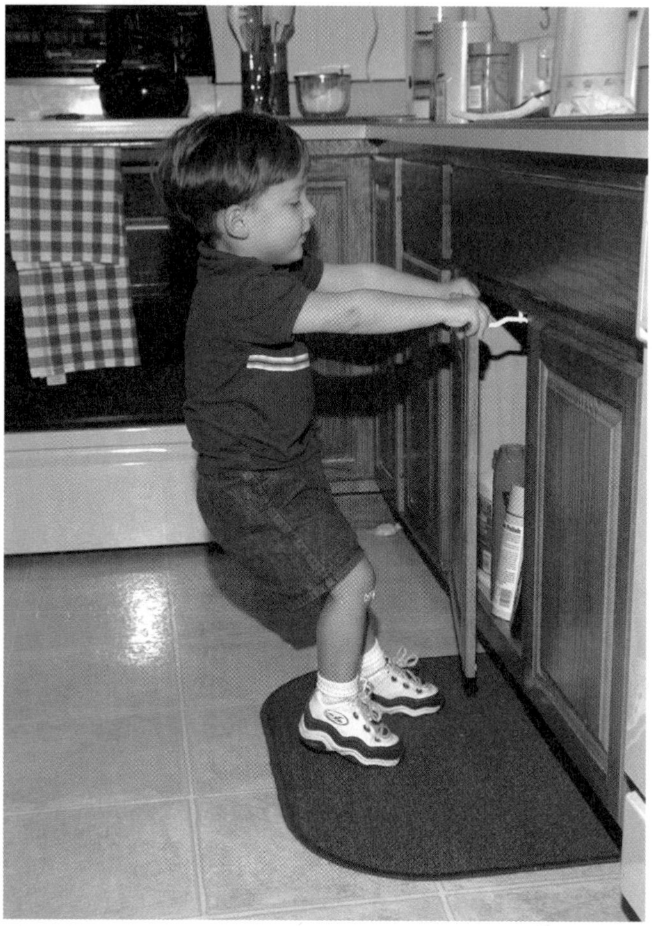

Figure 9-12 A toddler's curiosity may require caregivers to be sure low cabinets have a child safety lock.

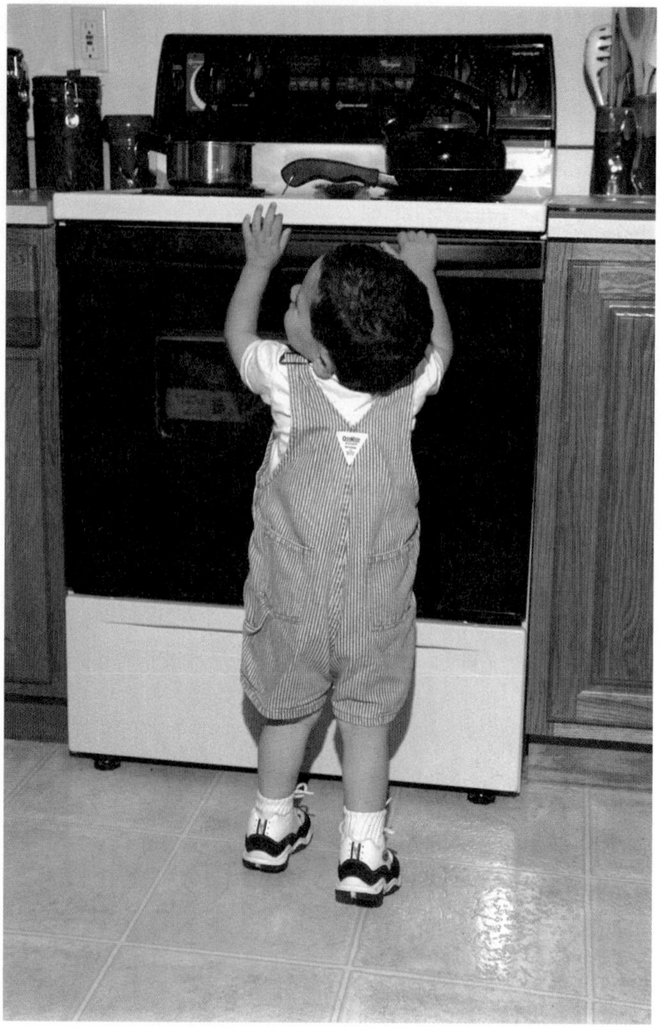

Figure 9-13 All homes where toddlers live or visit need to be childproofed. Be sure all pot handles are always turned away from the front of the stove.

Water Safety

Alertness to water safety issues continues from infancy. The toddler's anatomical configuration (larger head/shorter lower extremities) creates a higher center of gravity and, when combined with an unsteady gait and insatiable curiosity, increases the risk of injury near bodies of water. The fact that a child may drown in 1 inch of water makes every bathtub and mud puddle a potential hazard. Therefore, a toddler should *never* be left alone in a bathtub or pool since the child's attempts to stand may result in a fall. The fall could injure bones, fracture skulls, cause unconsciousness, and/or precipitate drowning. Being alone in the tub may also encourage the inquisitive toddler to turn on the hot water faucet, producing scalding water burns. Standing water should never be left in uncovered kiddie pools, and a locked fence should surround larger outdoor pools. Toddlers should not be allowed to go near any standing water without adult

Research Highlight

Home Use of Syrup of Ipecac

Study Purpose

To analyze if the use of ipecac in the home had an impact upon the outcome and treatment of accidental ingestion of pharmaceutical products by young children.

Methods

Data from 55,436 calls at seven regional Poison Centers were collected, with consideration given to substance ingested, treatment site, use of syrup of ipecac, age of child, outcome, and the experience and work load of employees in center.

Findings

Of the 55,436 calls, 22% related to children under the age of 6 years. The drugs most frequently ingested were analgesics, cold medications, and topical preparations. Referrals from the centers to hospitals varied widely; one center referred as few as 8.6% of the children and another as many as 20%. Lower rates of referral were correlated with increased use of ipecac in the home, with greater staff experience and with risk level of the drug ingested. The outcomes for children treated at home with syrup of ipecac were generally excellent, no deaths occurred and only two children had major adverse reactions.

Implications

The relative consistency among the seven regional Poison Control Centers should reassure professionals and caregivers alike. This system, and the advice provided, has saved many lives and has proven cost effective by reducing the number of emergency department visits required. As in many of life's situations, advice given by more experienced individuals tends to be more accurate and dependable. The use of syrup of ipecac was also validated to be a safe, cost-effective home treatment when administered in consultation with appropriately trained center personnel.

Citation

Bond, G. (1995). Home use of syrup of ipecac is associated with a reduction in pediatric emergency department visits. *Annals of Emergency Medicine, 25*, 338–343.

supervision; life jackets are recommended at poolside and required whenever the toddler is on any boat.

Toy Injuries/Gun Safety

Injuries related to the toys that children play with are central to toddler safety (Figure 9-14). Toys must be strong, safe, and large enough to prevent swallowing. Popped balloons are a major culprit, and for this reason, the use of latex balloons should be discouraged. Mylar, foil-type balloons are the only ones recommended as safe for young children.

Another category of concern to toddler safety is gun safety. It is impossible to teach toddlers the differences between toy guns and real guns since their cognitive abilities are not well enough developed to comprehend gun safety. Therefore, if guns are in the house, they must always be kept locked away from the inquisitive toddler (Society of Pediatric Nurses, 1998).

Routine Health Screenings

Routine health visits to a primary health care provider begun in infancy should continue through toddlerhood. Caregivers should be encouraged to schedule well-child visits at 15, 18, 24, and 36 months of age; additional visits should be made if illness occurs. The routine visits are needed for health monitoring and updating or beginning immunizations if not initiated during infancy. The American Academy of Pediatrics

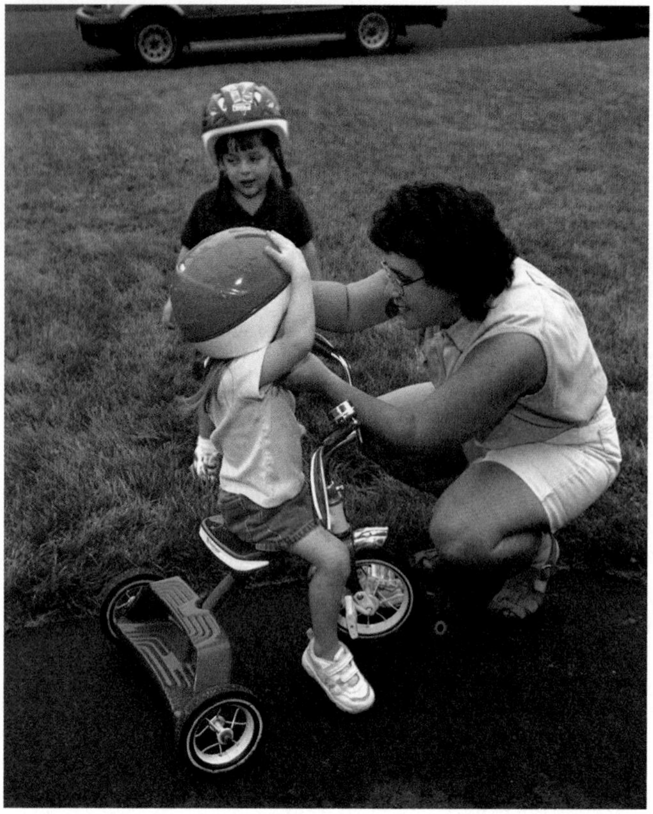

Figure 9-14 Even children as young as toddlers need to learn to wear helmets while riding their tricycles.

(2000) has recently published a revised immunization schedule, which indicates toddlers need boosters of diphtheria, tetanus, and pertussis (DTP, or DtaP), H. influenza (HIB), polio, and hepatitis B (if not received at 6 months of age) by 18 months of age. They also need initial doses of measles, mumps, rubella (MMR) and varicella/chicken pox (Var) vaccines. See Appendix C for the schedule of recommendations for all childhood immunizations. Caregivers should be encouraged to complete the initial immunization series in a timely manner to protect their child and to prevent delayed school entry.

Health screening should always include a complete physical examination (including blood pressure, height, and weight), evaluation of hemoglobin (for iron-deficiency anemia), dental evaluation, and vision and hearing assessment. Before the anterior fontanel closes, the head circumference should be measured. The American Academy of Pediatrics recommends that screening serum lead levels be obtained in children exhibiting poor growth patterns or neurological irritability, or in those living in high-risk areas (AAP, 1998).

Eye On:

Health care providers also need to be sensitive to cultural and ethnic variations when comparing children to preestablished norms. For instance, attention should be given to the height/weight assessment of Asian children. A single evaluation of a child of Asian ancestry, compared to standard U.S. Caucasian norms, may lead to an inaccurate judgment that the child is short in stature or malnourished for age, when actually this should be attributed to genetic makeup.

Negativism

Negativism is an expression of the toddler's constant search for autonomy. The toddler resents being given directions and/or not being allowed to explore what is desired in an expanding environment. Characteristically, the toddler seems to delight in doing the opposite of what is asked and responding "no" to all requests. Caregivers are frequently frustrated when trying to deal with toddler negativism and are delighted to learn that this period typically passes by about 30 months of age.

Caregivers, however, will have to select their own method of dealing with their child's negativism. As with any attention-seeking behavior, it is best to ignore the action as much as future behavior-related issues.

Family Teaching

Handling "No!"

- Reduce the opportunity to say "no." Don't give the child an option if one doesn't really exist. **Don't ask:** "Do you want lunch now?" **Ask:** "Do you want peanut butter or bologna for lunch?"
- Avoid complex requests or overstimulating situations (such as trips to the grocery store) when the toddler is tired or hungry.
- Don't draw attention to negative behaviors, but if you are going to deal with them, do it immediately; otherwise, the child will have forgotten why reprimanding occurred.
- Do not threaten the child, especially as a reaction of frustration or anger. State disciplinary guidelines briefly, in simple terms. Be sure the child understands the consequence. The toddler may not remember both the terms and the consequence with a lengthy explanation. Example: "You need to brush your teeth so we can read your bedtime story," ***not*** "If you don't hurry up and brush your teeth there will be no story tonight."

Ritualism and Regression

As disrupting as negativism can be, another characteristic developing simultaneously is **ritualism,** or the need to maintain sameness (same cup, same spoon). The toddler needs stability within the expanding environment and to know, when off in a new play area, familiar people and places will still be available (Figure 9-15). Rituals, such as mealtime and bedtime routines, provide repetition where the child may gain comfort and security. When rituals are disrupted, as when a child is ill or hospitalized, the child experiences stress, responds by exerting autonomy, and frequently **regresses** (returns to a earlier, safer, more familiar behavior) to dependence and negativism (Erikson's concept of autonomy versus shame and doubt) to cope with the situation.

Many caregivers feel they become slaves to the schedules of their 2-year-old. When a toddler demands things be done in the same way at the same time, the child is not acting out of stubbornness, but asking for needs to be met. Routines provide a sense of security and give a framework to master new skills while providing a sense of control over the environment.

The best initial approach is to ignore regression while complimenting the child on positive attributes and behaviors. When caregivers assess the toddler's behavior, they often assume regression is an act of defiance or willful disobedience. Since the loss of a newly acquired skill is frightening to the toddler, regression should be disciplined cautiously.

It not uncommon for toddlers to demonstrate a variety of behaviors when stressed. These behaviors include aggression, avoidance, distraction, isolation, seeking information, self-consoling activities, and emotional expressions (Figure 9-16). That is why toddlers may use a security blanket, have a favorite teddy bear, ask many questions, argue, cry, or have temper tantrums (Ryan-Wenger, 1992).

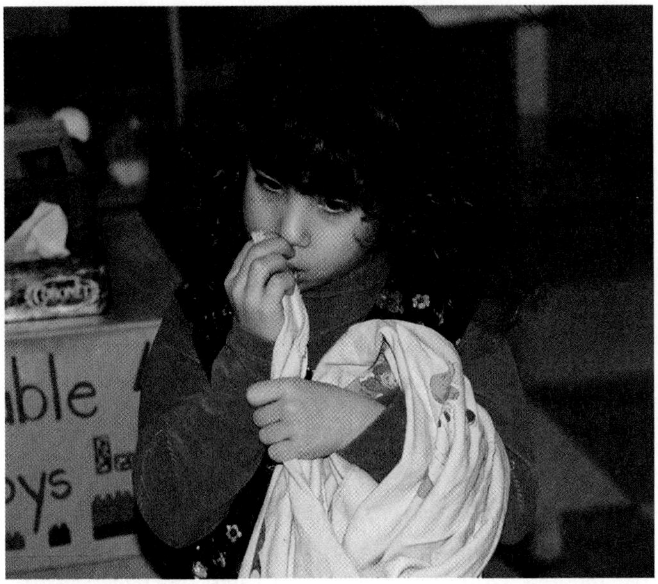

Figure 9-15 Toddlers often have a special object of affections such as a blanket, special toy, doll, or stuffed animal that they receive comfort from.

Family Teaching

Routines That Work

1. Set a schedule that fits both the caregiver's lifestyle and the child's personality whenever possible. For example, if the caregiver works the night shift and the child is an early riser, plan enjoyable activities early in the day (e.g., playing outside, going shopping, doing the bath time routine), so that both can rest in the early afternoon.
2. Stick to a schedule, since routines provide security for toddlers. Establish a bedtime and bedtime routine (e.g., change clothes, brush teeth, read story). Adhere to these unless exceptional circumstances arise.
3. Use a consistent alternate caregiver. It is much easier to develop trust and separate from the primary caregiver if the same person cares for the toddler in the caregivers' absence.

Discipline

In light of their evolving concept of ritualism and the need for familiar routines, toddlers are assisted in developing self-control by consistently applied discipline. Regardless of the methods used, teaching the reasons for the discipline is essential (Blum & Williams, 1995).

Family Teaching

Avoiding or Managing Regression

- Do *not* introduce new foods, activities, and/or expectations.
- Attempt to identify the overwhelming stressor, and consider various options to help the toddler manage the situation.
- Alternating activities and providing more caregiver attention and interaction may help the child develop behavioral stability.
- Remind that regression is a normal expression and generally does not have long-lasting effects.

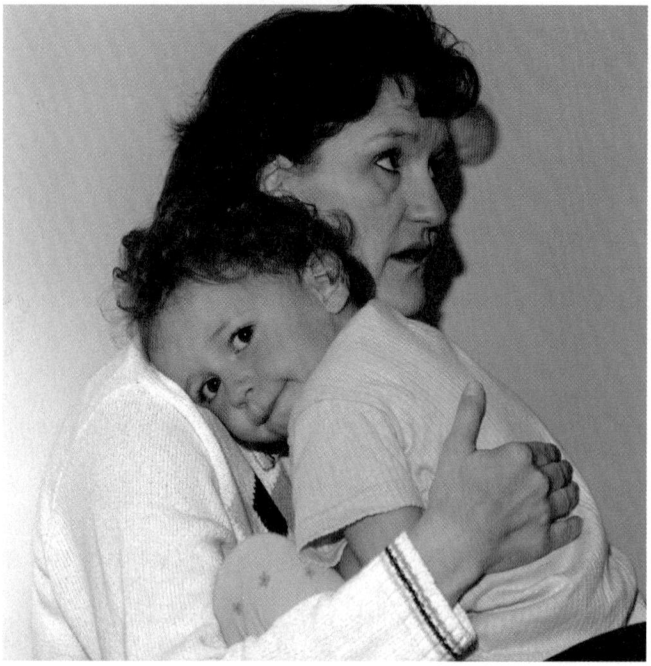

Figure 9-16 Toddlers need extra care and attention in order to cope with stress.

Limit setting (letting the child know what they are able to do and not do in a situation) is an important part of toddler discipline since we all tend to function better when both the expectations and limits defining actions are known. These limits may be established by the child, adult caregivers, or the external environment. Caregivers who provide the toddler with clear and concise limits facilitate autonomy development and help the child gain a sense of order, control, and security (Gottesman, 2000).

Caregivers should agree upon both the limits not to be exceeded and the type of discipline used when established boundaries are pushed. The American Academy of Pediatrics (1998) identifies three essential components of successful and effective discipline: (1) a supportive and loving relationship between parent(s) and child, (2) use of positive reinforcement to promote desired behaviors, and (3) removing reinforcement to reduce and eliminate undesired behaviors.

Family Teaching

Appropriate Toddler Discipline

- Predetermine and communicate limits to the child.
- Allow limit testing.
- Assist in achieving mastery of socially acceptable behavior.
- Provide ways for channeling undesirable feelings into constructive activities.
- Provide assurance child is loved even when certain behaviors are inappropriate.

Reflective Thinking

Corporal Punishment

You see a parent physically punishing a child in public. How do you feel about corporal punishment? What would you do?

Nursing Alert

Toddler Discipline

1. Nurses should never physically discipline a child. (Physical punishment may legally be administered only by a parent or legal guardian and the type and degrees of such punishment are currently under scrutiny.) The American Academy of Pediatrics' (1998) statements related to spanking, discipline, and punishment are accepted as the professional standard and can be found on their website.
2. If the child is hospitalized, discuss with caregivers how you may support their methods of discipline. Explain that hospitalized children frequently display regressive behavioral patterns, and carefully think before implementing any disciplinary measures related to regressive behavior.
3. If you observe inappropriate verbal or physical discipline, as a professional you are mandated to report it. The reporting mechanism will differ from state to state, but your responsibility does not change.

To support and facilitate consistency, all caregivers, including grandparents and babysitters, should be told about established limits and disciplinary actions. Providing *consistent* discipline is critical for understanding, gaining responsibility, and experiencing positive behavioral outcomes. Refer to the Family Teaching box for more information.

The type of discipline utilized will vary from family to family and culture to culture; however, approximately 90% of parents in the United States use **corporal punishment** (physical punishment) in disciplining their children (APA, 1998). Corporal punishment may bring about an immediate change in behavior, but the long-term effect is questionable for toddlers. Use of caregiver role modeling (Bandura, 1986) has been successful in disciplining toddlers, but requires the child to (1) see the correct behavior enacted, (2) remember what the role model did, (3) be physically able to repeat the role model's action and (4) be motivated to engage in the modeled behavior. This works especially well where a strong trust relationship exists with the role model. Role modeling, use of the teaching process, scolding, ignoring, and/or **time out** (placing the child in a nonstimulating environment) seem to be among the most widely used methods of achieving behavioral change with toddlers (Berkowitz, 2001a)

Sibling Rivalry

Sibling rivalry, defined as intense feelings of jealousy between siblings, often is seen when an infant is born into a family with a toddler. The arrival of this new baby can be devastating to toddlers since now they must compete for a caregiver's attention and fear loss of love or abandonment (Berkowitz, 2001b; O'Brien, 1996; Steelsmith, 1997) (Figure 9-17).

See the Family Teaching box for some suggestions for handling this common problem.

Family Teaching

Discipline

1. The sooner discipline is incorporated into the child's life, the easier it is.
2. Discuss discipline philosophies behind closed doors, but when disciplining a child, be unified and supportive of each other.
3. Avoid disciplining in the wrong place, with the wrong motives, or with wrong timing; the child will rebel every time.
4. Avoid threatening to discipline and then not following through.
5. If a rule is broken, corrective actions should follow.
6. Expect respect in all interactions.
7. Follow discipline with love and positive encouragement.
8. Allow crying, but not screaming.

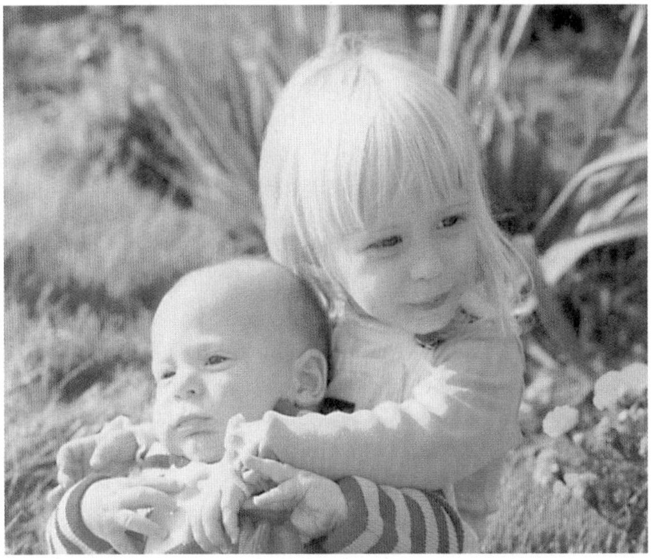

Figure 9-17 The arrival of a new sibling can be less traumatic for the toddler who is involved in the baby's care and made to feel an important member of the family.

Family Teaching

Tips for Dealing with Sibling Rivalry

- Establish a time frame when attention is focused exclusively on the toddler.
- Maintain the toddler's rituals as long as needed.
- Do not introduce new developmental tasks (e.g., toilet training or weaning from nighttime bottle) near the time when a new baby is expected.
- Have the toddler "sleep over" in the home of grandparent or individual who will be caring for him/her when the mother is in the hospital several times before the birth occurs. Reassure the child that his or her mother will return.
- If the toddler will be moved out of a nursery or crib to make room for a new baby, make the move several months in advance, and do not announce the real purpose of the move. Emphasize positive aspects: "you're getting to be so big."
- Do not tell the toddler that the new brother or sister is a playmate. This encourages the toddler to have unrealistic expectations of the neonate and can intensify negative behaviors.
- Be alert for subtle responses (not all sibling rivalry is overt) of sibling jealousy, such as taking the baby's bottle, pacifier, toys.
- After the new baby arrives, encourage visitors to spend time talking to the toddler. Keep small "gifts," which can be given to the toddler when presents are given to the neonate.
- When toddlers demonstrate rivalry, set limits and consistently administer discipline with love.
- Plan joint time with children, equalizing attention as much as possible.
- Encourage participation in the play-time and care of the new sibling; praise positive interactions.

Temper Tantrums

Temper tantrums are outward explosive reactions to inward stressful or frustrating situations that are a normal part of toddler life. Between 2 and 3 years of age, the child is faced with new environments, new rules, and new fears. Toddlers need to express their feelings, wishes, and frustrations, but lack the language skills to do this. All of these new experiences, coupled with the child's quest for autonomy, may create tension and erupt into a tantrum. Tantrums are ways toddlers say, "I have needs, I am important, I need to have some control." A typical temper tantrum—occurring when the toddler can't control his or her emotions, feels overwhelmed, or does not get what is wanted when it is wanted—may involve crying, screaming, falling onto the floor, kicking the feet, flailing the arms, banging the head, and breath holding (Grover, 2001b). Head banging requires intervention if it is continuous and/or unsafe, and to prevent injury, the caregiver should hold the child's head, make few comments (to prevent reinforcement of the negative behavior), and/or provide a protective mat or pillow. Beyond this, as with any attention-seeking behavior, the tantrum should be ignored. Speaking softly and calmly, recognizing the child's feelings, and holding can help.

When breath holding occurs and the child appears to faint or stop breathing, caregivers frequently become frightened and rush into frenzied action, which only reinforces the tantrum behavior. Therefore, caregivers must be taught that breath holding is usually harmless. The child may "faint," but will automatically begin breathing again as soon as carbon dioxide builds up and stimulates the respiratory center. Although caregivers are not encouraged to intervene during a tantrum, they should remain close by to prevent traumatic injuries. It is also helpful to remove the child from public attention.

At the conclusion of the tantrum, the caregiver should offer a toy or option not related to the incident-producing difficulty. ("Why don't we play with your new tea set?") This will redirect the toddler's attention. Disciplining a child after a tantrum usually is of little value. However, if the caregivers have told the child there would be a consequence to this behavior, they should follow through as promised.

Tantrums cannot always be controlled, but caretakers can take measures to lessen their frequency and/or intensity, including developing a regular schedule for the toddler, reducing the need to say "no," allowing choices, rewarding good behavior, and staying calm. Tantrums can sometimes be avoided by using time-outs or by placing a child in a bedroom before the behavior escalates. Temper tantrums are considered a normal developmental response of toddlerhood but should disappear by 4 years of age.

Toilet Training

A major factor contributing to the toddler's goals of independence and autonomy is accomplishing bowel and bladder control. Success, however, depends on the readiness of both the child and the caregiver. Caregivers who understand normal child growth and development will have more realistic expectations and less frustration during toilet training.

Myelinization of the spinal cord and development of sphincter muscle control occur at approximately 12–18 months of age, and must be complete prior to beginning bowel and bladder training since the average toddler is ready to begin toilet training at approximately 18–24 months. The time to begin toilet training, however, varies from culture to culture and family to family. Nurses should educate parents about the signs of readiness for toilet training, which include

Nursing Tip:

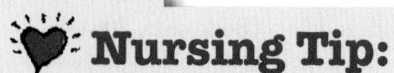

Atraumatic toilet training

- The child needs to achieve this level of independence at her or his own speed.
- Caregivers must reach agreement as to how the toilet training will be handled and determine acceptable words used to describe the activities; a consistent approach and vocabulary must be maintained.
- The child must be physiologically (able to walk well, can pull pants up/down, usually 24–30 months of age) and psychologically (dislikes feeling of wet diapers, wants to go to preschool but can't in a diaper) ready to be potty trained.
- Caretakers should ignore helpful advice from grandparents, aunts, neighbors, and day care workers: focus on the unique characteristics of *this* child.
- Avoid scolding, punishing, or overreacting to accidental soiling.
- Have a child-sized potty available.
- Praise child for each attempt, either verbally or with favorite stickers, whether successful or not.

Reflective Thinking

Toilet Training

Connie, the mother of a 20-month-old daughter (Tasha), is returning to work in a week and is concerned about placing her daughter in child care. Connie feels that Tasha should be potty trained prior to entering child care, and she wants to know if this can be accomplished during the next week. Considering your understanding of growth and development and the signs of toilet training readiness, what is your response?

the ability to demonstrate cognitive awareness of elimination (diaper is wet), follow directions and communicate understanding of elimination needs to the caregiver (pulls on diaper, asks for diaper change), remain dry for longer periods of time (more than 2 hours), independently dress and undress, and sit, squat, and walk well (Berkowitz, 2001c; Vessey, 2000).

Bladder control is often more difficult to attain than bowel control. The toddler usually has only one to two bowel movements per day, but urinates much more frequently. Often, accidental urinary incontinence occurs because the toddler becomes so involved in play activities that the urge to urinate is ignored until it is too late to reach the bathroom. When the toddler is attempting to remain dry and learn bowel control, an emotional tug-of-war often develops between the child and the caregivers, leaving both frustrated and angry. Punishment and coercion can lead to shame and feelings of inferiority. A strategy that is often helpful is giving the child control over the process. Telling the child how the body makes "pee" and "poop" daily and helping the toddler succeed can encourage participation and responsibility. A relaxed approach, with positive reinforcement and praise, will aid in toilet training, as will avoiding constant reminders and providing incentives for using the toilet correctly. Recording the child's progress and not punishing accidents are also important. Consistent day and night dryness should be achieved by 5 years of age, or further evaluation for physical and/or psychological problems is warranted (Berkowitz, 2001c).

Stress may either interfere with toilet training or precipitate regressive bowel/bladder continence. Caregivers need to be informed that such regressions are usually temporary and understanding, gentle support, reinforcement, and encouragement will assist the toddler regain a sense of independence and success.

Child Care

Placing the toddler in a child care setting if both parents are employed outside the home may be necessary in some situations. The child care setting may pose additional threats to the toddler's health and well being. Caregivers might seek support from professionals that use of such facilities is perfectly acceptable in today's society. Refer to Chapter 7 for more information on the use of child care.

Play

Play has been described as "the work of childhood." Certainly, this is an appropriate description since it is through active play and manipulation that toddlers learn about the environment. Object exploration also enhances fine and gross muscle development and coordination. According to Gemelli (1996), play is the primary way toddlers teach themselves; they do not necessarily view their play as play, but a natural aspect of life. As one 2 1/2-year-old replied when asked why he liked to play: "I don't play. This is what I do!" Toddlers most often play alongside, but not with, other children (**parallel play**). The toddler demonstrates little attention to the feelings of play partners, and frequently grabs desired toys or hits others to keep a favorite toy.

Play fulfills three functions for toddlers, including facilitating cognitive development by permitting exploration of the environment, learning about objects, and solving problems. It also advances social development particularly through fantasy play when acting out roles. Finally, it permits problem solving, vents frustrations, uses excess energy, and assists in coping with inner conflicts/anxieties in nonthreatening ways.

Each time a new toy is introduced into the toddler's world, the teaching–learning process should occur: introduce the toy, instruct the child how to use the toy, allow the child to play/practice with the item, and provide feedback and reinforcement on how well they have done (Barnard, 1995). Caregivers may need some instruction about this process, but once established, it provides the basis for a lifelong educational process. The initiation of "why?" and "why not?" questions, which accompany play, especially with a new toy or game, enhances the child's ability to gather data and make decisions (Figure 9-18).

Age-appropriate play does not require expensive, shiny, developmentally approved toys. It does, however, require a patient and innovative caregiver who views play activities as major educational and socializing events in the child's life. Table 9-10 presents toddler play activities.

A portion of the play experience involves make-believe, pretending, or fantasy. Fantasy and make believe help conceptualize what and how a child wishes the world to be. Fantasy helps the toddler cope with parental expectations and aids in denying aspects of reality they prefer to ignore

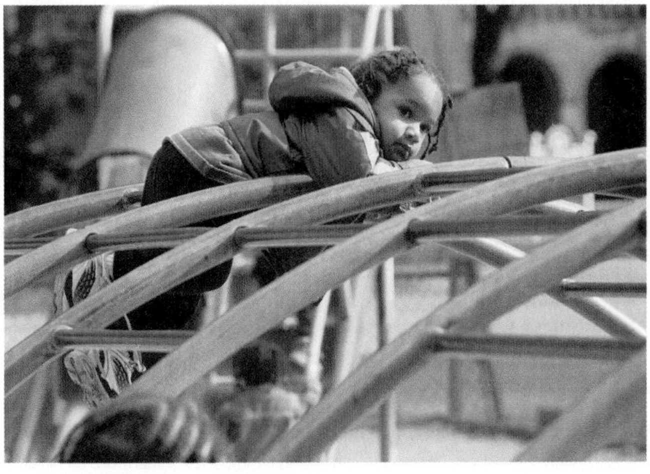

Figure 9-18 This child is exploring her world and demonstrating mastery of both the physiological and cognitive dimensions of development in her play.

TABLE 9-10 Toys and Play Activities for Toddlers

Toy or Play Activity	Development Promoted	Selection Criteria
• Pull toys	• Stimulates gross motor skill and strengths (P) • Stimulates awareness of object when not seen (C)	• Wooden with pull cords • Makes noise indicating their presence (noise may be offensive)
• Picture books	• Teaches page manipulation (P) • Stimulates guided language development (C) • Teaches remembered properties of objects (forms and objects) (C) • Provides social experiences when assisted (S) • Stimulates knowledge and aids in school activities (C)	• Cloth or washable • Nontearable • Facilitates creativity and development of language
• Book of rhymes	• Provides fine distinctions in hearing (P & C) • Social experience and humor (E & S) • Stimulates language development (C & S)	
• Toys as symbols of adult activities • Dress-up kits • Nurse/doctor kits	• Symbols represent actions (e.g., lunch pail equals going to work) (C & S)	• Durable • Nonbreakable
• Scribbling on paper	• Stimulates creativity (C) • Aids in school activities (C) • Stimulates fine motor development (P) • Fosters artistic development (E & C)	• Large nontoxic crayons/markers
• Small push-pull toys • Cars and trucks	• Stimulates gross motor skills and strength (P) • Provides active experimentation with toys, objects, and movements (C & P) • Stimulates self-expression (E) • Aids in creative expression (C)	• Large • No sharp edges • Durable
• Large, crawl-in box • Trapeze set • Slides • Jungle gym • Teeter-totter	• Teaches gross motor skills (P) • Stimulates creativity (C) • Creates own environment (P & C) • Fosters social development (S)	• Durable • Adult supervision with trapeze, jungle gym equipment, and slides
• Stuffed animals • Dolls • Blanket • Blanket surrogate	• Comforts and provides security through familiarity (C, E, & S) • Promotes creativity (C) • Promotes imitative behaviors (C & S)	• No pieces that can be removed and swallowed
• Filling and emptying toys • Take-apart toys • Large size Legos • Loc-blocks • Block set • Hammer and nail sets	• Provides self satisfaction with repetition (P, C, & E) • Provides outlet for emotional expression (E) • Promotes gross motor skill and strength (P) • Promotes creativity (C)	• Durable • Nonbreakable
• Puzzles • Tinker Toys	• Provides awareness of simple shapes (C)	
• Balls • Sandbox • Wagons • Hobbyhorse	• Provides awareness of shapes/textures (C) • Promotes gross/fine motor development (P) • Promotes social development (S)	
• Finger paints • Drums • Modeling clay	• Promotes awareness of textures, colors, shapes (C) • Promotes artistic development (E & C)	• Nontoxic substances • No sharp edges

Key: C, cognitive development; P, physical development; E, emotional development; S, social development.

Adapted from Lee, J., & Fowler, M. (1986). Merely child's play and developmental work and playthings. Journal of Pediatric Nursing, *1(4), 260-269; Florey, L. (1971). An approach to play and play development.* American Journal of Occupational Therapy, *25(6), 275-280; Betz, C. (1983). Teaching children through play therapy.* Journal of Association of Operating Room Nurses, *88(4), 709, 712-713, 716-717; and Betz, C., & Poster, E. (1984). Incorporating play into the care of the hospitalized child.* Issues in Comprehensive Pediatric Nursing, *7(6), 343-355.*

Research Highlight

Pretend Play—A Learning Process

Study Purpose

To determine the age when children knowingly begin to engage in pretend (fantasy) play.

Methods

One hundred and twelve children between 8 and 24 months of age were given a large basket of toys that could be used any way the child wanted. The child's play was videotaped and the tapes analyzed.

Findings

Infants (9–12 months) selected toys and carried out actions indicating they knew the meaning/function of the real object (e.g., touching a small brush to the head), but did not exaggerate the action, suggesting the infants were not consciously pretending at play. At 12–24 months, most children began demonstrating pretend play by adding sound effects and dramatic gestures when they acted out everyday activities (e.g., put cup to lips, throw head back, and pretend to gulp).

Implications

Caregivers need to encourage children to play by showing interest in make-believe play and adding opportunities for pretend play as often as possible (e.g., feed doll pretend cereal at breakfast time, keep miniature dishes in kitchen to encourage mimicry).

Citation

Heller, L. (1996, June). The magic of make-believe. *Parents,* 76–78.

(Figures 9-19, 9-20, 9-21, and 9-22). Toddlers who trust their caregiver's ability to protect them from danger will eventually use these experiences to reconstruct their fantasies into reality-based beliefs (Gemelli, 1996).

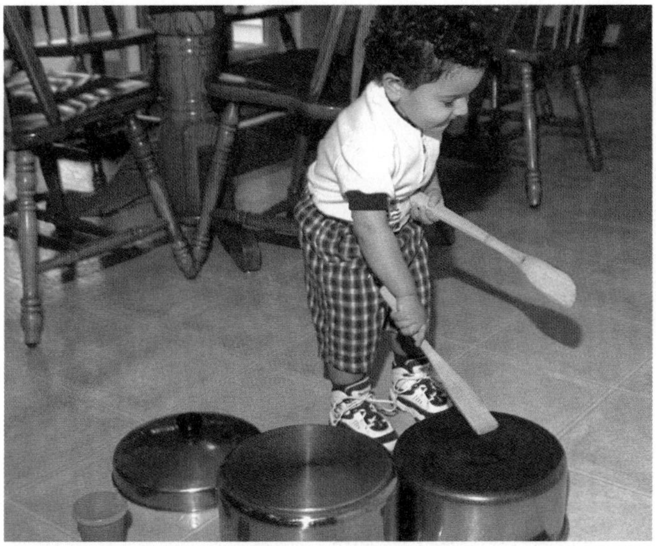

Figure 9-19 Toddlers have very active imaginations and can make toys out of just about anything.

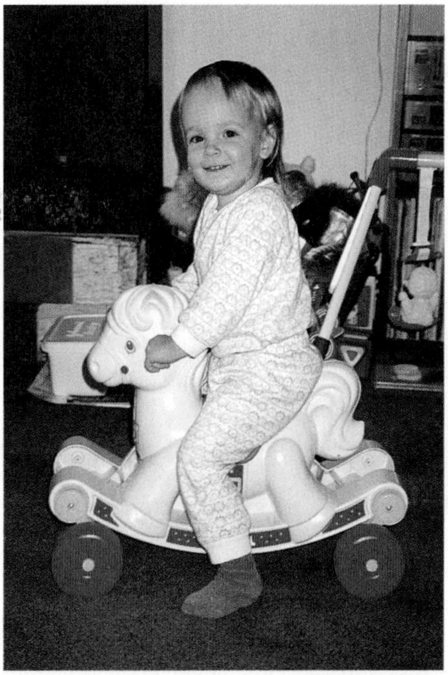

Figure 9-20 Toddler play allows refinement of skills as well as language development and a growing sense of independence.

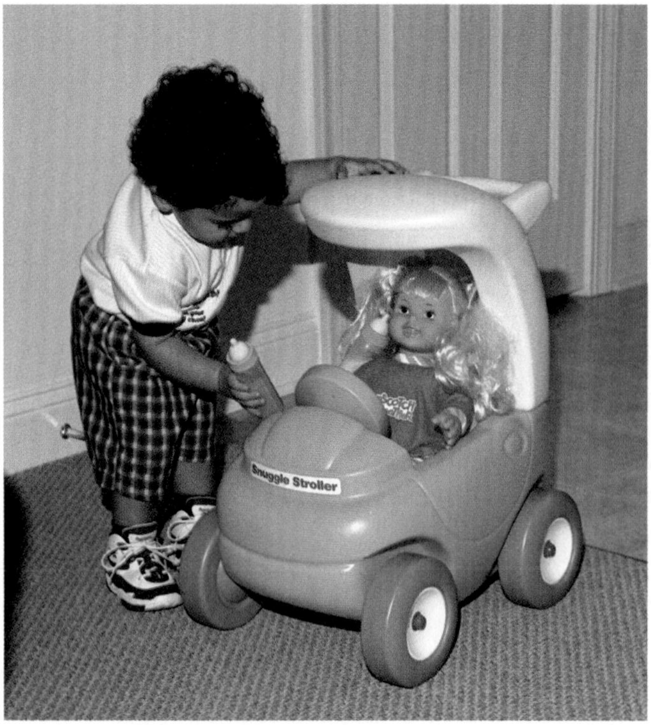

Figure 9-21 Caregivers need to be sensitive to a toddler's abilities and provide play and learning opportunities in line with the child's developmental level.

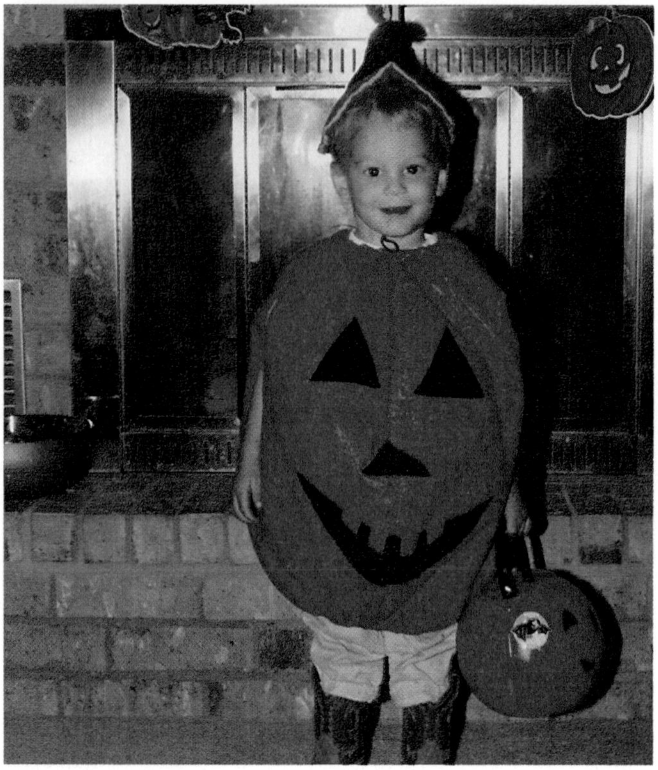

Figure 9-22 Toddlers often wear Halloween costumes throughout the year just to pretend and play dress-up.

NURSING MANAGEMENT

The nurse's role in toddler health promotion is critical. Education should provide ideas, suggestions, and concepts surrounding growth, development, and parenting skills. This knowledge will allow caregivers to become independent in promoting health with respect to nutrition, sleep, dental needs, safety, elimination, and growth and development. Ideally, the toddler should be seen consistently by the same health care provider since the most accurate clinical judgments are made not on one observation alone, but rather based on trends over time.

In the Real World

I hadn't cared for a toddler before and when I did, boy did I learn a lot! Jerry, age $2^1/_2$ years, was admitted for a cleanup for cystic fibrosis. I needed to draw blood, start oxygen, begin medications, and call respiratory therapy. The first thing I did was try to explain about the blood collection: "Jerry, it will only be a little stick in your arm, it won't hurt for very long." The screaming began: "I don't want a stick in my arm, the leaves will look funny!" I'd forgotten about toddler's thinking. I began again using simple terms and getting help from one of the nurses. Although it was a challenge to take care of him, I loved his energy, his sweetness, and his durability.

Key Concepts

- Toddlerhood is a period characterized by Erikson's task of autonomy versus shame and doubt. The toddler struggles to separate from caretakers and develop a sense of self.
- Major developmental tasks surround the toddler's developing locomotion, language, and cognitive development.
- Toddler physical growth slows, resulting in decreased appetite and relatively less demand for calories (physiologic anorexia). Nutritional needs continue, particularly for protein, calcium, magnesium, and iron, to support growth. Caregivers should be educated to facilitate this period of time.
- The combination of increased motor skills (fine and gross), desire to explore, lack of experience (judgment), and immaturity places the toddler at risk for accidental injury. Caretakers should be provided education and guidance in creating a safe home environment.

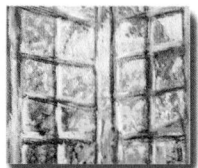

- The provision of structure, guidance, and limit setting is critical for the toddler's development of autonomy, self-control, and mastery of skills. Effective discipline techniques are consistent and firm, and may include time outs, diversion, and positive reinforcement.
- Sibling rivalry reflects the toddler's fear, anxiety, and lack of understanding when a new infant enters the family. It can be minimized with methods such as including the toddler in preparations for the baby, affirming that the toddler is loved and is very special, and setting appropriate limits.
- Nurses can assist caretakers to understand their toddler's readiness for toilet training (recognizing physical and psychological signs) and provide guidance for strategies for success.
- Nurses need to educate caretakers on health promotion such as nutrition, sleep, needed immunizations, hygiene, and safety.

Review Questions

1. Jamie is wearing mom's sweater and her eyeglasses while pouring make-believe tea for her playmate. Which of the following best describes this toddler's behavior?

A. Autism
B. Negativism
C. Parallel play
D. Domestic mimicry

2. Of the physiologic changes that occur during toddlerhood, which of these is *essential* before a child is capable of walking?

A. Calcification of long bones
B. Myelinization of spinal cord
C. Readiness for separation (from caregiver)
D. Stabilization of muscles of the legs

3. There are several major developmental milestones of toddlerhood; which of these should *not* be included in the list?

A. Seeks independence
B. Walks well
C. Plays well with friends
D. Uses over 300 words

4. When a toddler is not able to accomplish a task (such as tying his shoe), he may go quietly into a corner and pout. This behavior demonstrates which of the following theories?

A. Erickson's industry versus inferiority
B. Piaget's sensory-motor stage
C. Erickson's autonomy versus shame
D. Piaget's preconceptual stage

5. A 2-year-old child has been crying ever since his mother left his hospital room. The nurse begins playing an audiotape of his mother's voice, and he quiets down immediately. This response is evidence of:

A. An increased concept of object permanence
B. Differentiation of self from others
C. Symbolic imitation
D. Egocentrism

6. A $2\frac{1}{2}$-year-old boy is having a temper tantrum in the middle of a large family gathering. Which response would you recommend to the caregiver as being *most appropriate* in this situation?

A. Immediately pick him up and carry him from the middle of activities.
B. Toss water in his face when he begins holding his breath.
C. Ignore his behavior completely as long as he is not injuring himself.
D. Threaten to spank him if he doesn't stop his kicking immediately.

7. In assessing a toddler's physical growth, which of these factors would suggest intervention was needed?

A. His weight at 3 years is 15 pounds.
B. She has all of her deciduous teeth by 27 months.
C. His anterior fontanel has not closed by 13 months.
D. She is 28 months old and still not potty trained.

8. The *primary* reason for discontinuing a bedtime bottle of milk is to:

A. Prevent tooth decay
B. Assist in maintaining nighttime dryness
C. Encourage more mature eating habits
D. Prevent dental deformity

9. When planning to meet a toddler's nutritional needs, one should include which of the following?

A. 500 kcal/kg, high fiber
B. 1,000 kcal/day, high protein
C. 2,000 kcal/day, low fat
D. 150 kcal/kg, wide variety of components

10. A 20-month-old boy is running through the church screaming. His father catches him, sits the boy down beside him, and says "I want you to sit here quietly, like Daddy." This is an example of which type of discipline?

A. Scolding
B. Ignoring the problem
C. Guiding behavior
D. Time out

11. From the factors listed below, select the primary purpose for disciplining a child:

A. To identify who is in control
B. To display evidence of good parenting skills
C. To teach punishment/reward system
D. To protect child and others

12. In general, potty training a child can best be accomplished by which of these means?

A. Same-sex parental role modeling
B. Setting specific behavioral limits and adhering to them
C. Describing socially acceptable behaviors to toddler
D. Threatening to withhold items of pleasure (e.g., favorite toy, dessert)

References

American Academy of Pediatric Dentistry. (1996). Reference manual 1996–97. *Pediatric Dentistry 18*(6), 24–77.

American Academy of Pediatrics. (1998). Screening for elevated blood lead levels (RE 9815). *Pediatrics, 101*, 1072–1078.

American Academy of Pediatrics Committee on Infectious Diseases. (2000). *Recommended childhood immunization schedule—United States, January–December, 2000* [On-line]. Available: http://www.aap.org/family/parents/immunize.htm

American Academy of Pediatrics Committee on Nutrition. (1986). Fluoride supplements. *Pediatrics, 77*: 58–761.

American Academy of Pediatrics Committee on Psychosocial Aspects of Child and Family Health. (1998). Guidance for effective discipline: A policy statement. *Pediatrics, 101*(4), 723–728.

Bandura, A. (1986). *Social foundation of thought and actions: A social cognitive theory.* Englewood Cliffs, NJ: Prentice Hall.

Barnard, K. E. (1995). *NCAST II teaching manual.* Seattle: University of Washington.

Berkowitz, C. (2001a). Discipline. In C. Berkowitz (Ed.), *Pediatrics: A primary care approach* (pp. 114–118). Philadelphia: Saunders.

Berkowitz, C. (2001b). Sibling rivalry. In C. Berkowitz (Ed.), *Pediatrics: A primary care approach* (pp. 105–107). Philadelphia: Saunders.

Berkowitz, C. (2001c). Toilet training. In C. Berkowitz (Ed.), *Pediatrics: A primary care approach* (pp. 108–111). Philadelphia: Saunders.

Betz, C. (1983). Teaching children through play therapy. *Journal of Association of Operating Room Nurses, 88*(4), 709, 712-713, 716-717.

Betz, C., & Poster, E. (1984). Incorporating play into the care of the hospitalized child. *Issues in Comprehensive Pediatric Nursing, 7*(6), 343-355.

Blum, N. J., & Williams, G. E. (1995), Disciplining young children: The role of verbal instructions and reasoning. *Pediatrics, 96*(2), 336.

Bond, G. (1995). Home use of syrup of ipecac is associated with a reduction in pediatric emergency department visits. *Annals of Emergency Medicine, 25*, 338–343.

Brazelton, T. B. (1992). *Touchpoints, the essential reference: Your child's emotional and behavioral development*. Reading, MA: Addison-Wesley.

Brown, J., & Dunn, J. (1996). Continuities in emotional understanding from three to six years. *Child Development, 67*, 789–802.

Erikson, E. (1963). *Childhood and society*. New York: Norton.

Feeding the toddler [On-line]. (2001). Available: www.uri.edu/coopext/efnep/toddlers/toddler.p2.html.

Flaherty, L., & Snyder, J. (1998). National Highway Safety Administration: final air bag ruling. *Journal of Emergency Nursing, 24*(3), 260–261.

Florey, L. (1971). An approach to play and play development. *American Journal of Occupational Therapy, 25*(6), 275-280.

Forgac, M. T. (1995). Timely statement of the American Dietetic Association: dietary guidance for healthy children. *Journal of American Dietetic Association, 95*(3), 370.

Fowler, J. (1974).Toward a developmental perspective of faith. *Religious Education, 69*, 207–219.

Freud, S. (1957). In J. Strachey (Ed.), *The standard edition of the complete psychological works of Sigmund Freud* (Vol. 18). London: Hogarth.

Gains, S., Benjamin, H., & DeForest, M. (1996). Promoting automobile safety for young children. *MCN, 21*, 148–151.

Gemelli, R. (1996). *Normal child and adolescent development.* Washington, DC: American Psychiatric Press.

Gottesman, M. M. (2000). Patient education review. Nurturing the social and emotional development of children, a.k.a. discipline. *Journal of Pediatric Health Care, 14*(2), 81–84.

Grover, G. (2001a). Sleep: Normal patterns and common disorders. In C. Berkowitz (Ed.), *Pediatrics: A primary care approach* (pp. 39–44). Philadelphia: Saunders.

Grover, G. (2001b). Temper tantrums. In C. Berkowitz (Ed.), *Pediatrics: A primary care approach* (pp. 118–121). Philadelphia: Saunders.

Grover, G. (2001c). Dental care. In C. Berkowitz (Ed.), *Pediatrics: A primary care approach* (pp. 44–48). Philadelphia: Saunders.

Heller, L. (1996, June). The magic of make-believe. *Parents*, 76–78.

Henson, R., Hadfield, J. M., & Cooper, S. (1999). Injury control strategies: Extending the quality and quantity of data relted to road traffic accidents in children. *Journal of Accident & Emergency Medicine, 16*(2), 87–90.

Kohlberg, L. (1976). Moral stages and moralization: The cognitive-developmental approach. In Likona, T. (Ed.), *Moral development and behavior.* New York: Holt, Rinehart, & Winston.

Lee, J., & Fowler, M. (1986). Merely child's play and developmental work and playthings. *Journal of Pediatric Nursing, 1*(4), 260-269.

O'Brien, M. (1996), Child-rearing difficulties reported by parents of infants and toddlers, *Journal of Pediatric Psychology, 21*(3), 443–446.

Online Safety Project [On-line]. (2001). Available: http://www.safekids.com

Piaget, J. (1952). *The origin of intelligence in children.* New York: International University Press.

Ryan-Wenger, N. (1992). A taxonomy of children's coping strategies: a step toward theory development. *American Journal of Orthopsychiatry, 62*(2), 256–263.

Society of Pediatric Nurses. (1998). Policy statement for prevention of pediatric firearm injuries. In *SPN policy manual.* Denver: Author.

Steelsmith, S. (1997). *Helping young children adjust to a new baby* [On-line]. Available: www.parentingpress.com/t_970705.html.

Thompson, R., & Emslie, A. (2000). Young children and the risk of accidental injury: running an audit at nine months. *Community Practitioner, 73*(10), 799–800.

Vessey, J. A. (2000). Toilet training methods, clinical interventions, and recommendations. *Journal of Child and Family Nursing, 3*(1), 33.

Suggested Readings

American Academy of Pediatrics, Committee on Injury and Poison Prevention (1996). Selecting and using the most appropriate car safety seats for growing children: Guidelines for counseling parents. *Pediatrics, 97*(5), 761–763.

Benasich, A., & Brooks-Gunn, J. (1996). Maternal attitudes and knowledge of child-rearing: Associations with family and child outcomes. *Child Development, 67,* 1186–1205.

Bennetts, L. (1996). Raising intelligent kids: Part 2—Emotional savvy. *Child, March,* 56–64.

Berkowitz, C. (2001). Thumbsucking and other habits. In C. Berkowitz (Ed.), *Pediatrics: A primary care approach* (pp. 127–130). Philadelphia: Saunders.

Berkowitz, C. (Ed.). (2001). *Pediatrics: A primary care approach.* Philadelphia: Saunders.

Blum, N. J. (1995). Developmental assessment. In M. W. Schwarts (Ed.), *Clinical handbook of pediatrics* (p. 30–38). Baltimore: Williams & Wilkins.

Brayden, R. M., & Poole, S. R. (1995). Common behavioral problems in infants and children. *Primary Care, 22*(1), 81–97.

Cassidy, A. (1996). Routines that work. *Parents, June,* 80–82.

Christoffel, K. K., & Naureckas, S. M. (1994). Firearm injuries in children and adolescents: Epidemiology and preventive approaches. *Current Opinions in Pediatrics, 6*(5), 519–524.

Faber, A., & Mazlish, E. (1997). *Siblings without rivalry: How to help your children live together so you can live too.* New York: Norton.

Garling, A., & Garling, M. (1995). Mother's anticipation and prevention of unintentional injury to young children in the home. *Journal of Pediatric Psychology, 20*(1), 23–36.

Gellin, B. G. (2000). Do parents understand immunizations? A national telephone survey. *Pediatrics, 106*(5), 1097–1102.

Green, M. (Ed.). (1994) *Bright futures: Guidelines for health supervision of infants, children and adolescents.* Arlington, VA: National Center for Education in Maternal and Child Health.

Gronlick, W., Bridges, L., & Connell, J. (1996). Emotion regulation in two-year olds: Strategies and emotional expression in four contexts. *Child Development, 67,* 928–941.

Herman, M. (1996). Let them eat snacks. *Child, March,* 83.

Johnston, C., Rivara, F., & Soderberg, R. (1994). Children in car crashes: Analysis of data for injury and use of restraints. *Pediatrics, 93,* 960–965.

Levy, S. M., Kirtsy, M. C., & Warren, J. J. (1995). Sources of fluoride intake in children. *Journal of Public Health Dentistry, 55*(1), 39-52.

Lueg, A. K., Robson, W. L., & Lane, M. (1994). The toddler who does not eat. *American Family Physician, 49*(8), 1789–1792.

Luxem, M., & Christophersen, E. (1994). Behavioral toilet training in early childhood: Research, practice and implications. *Journal of Behavioral Pediatrics, 15,* 370–378.

Nachmias, M., & Gunnar, M. (1996). Behavioral inhibition and stress reactivity: The moderating role of attachment security. *Child Development, 67*(2), 508–522.

National Association of Children's Hospitals and Related Institutions. (1996). *Pediatric excellence in health delivery systems.* Alexandria,VA: Author.

Needleman, R., Howard, B., & Zuckerman, B. (1989). Temper tantrums—when to worry. *Contemporary Pediatrics, 6*(8), 12–14.

Occupant protection law across the nation. (1997). Washington, DC: National Safe Kids Campaign.

O'Flaherty, J. E., & Pirie, P. L. (1997). Prevention of pediatric drowning and near-drowning: A survey of members of the American Academy of Pediatrics. *Pediatrics, 99*(2), 169–174.

Pendrys, D. G. (1995). Risk of fluorosis in a fluoridated population: Implications for the dentist and hygienist. *Journal of the American Dental Association, 126*(12), 1617–1624.

Reau, N. R., Senturia, Y. D., Lebailly, S. A., & Christoffel, K. K. (1996). Infant and toddler feeding patterns and problems: Normative data and a new direction. *Journal of Developmental and Behavioral Pediatrics, 17*(3), 149–153.

Reid, M. J. (1999). Treatment of young children's bedtime refusal and nighttime wakings: A comparison of "standard" and graduated ignoring procedures. *Journal of Abnormal Child Psychology,* February 1999.

Reyes, M., Routh, D., Jean-Gilles, M., Sanfilippo, M., & Fawcett, N. (1991). Ethnic differences in parenting children in fearful situations. *Journal of Pediatric Psychology, 16*(6), 717–726.

Satter, E. (1995). Feeding dynamics: Helping children to eat well. *Journal of Pediatric Health Care, 9*(4), 178–218.

Senturia, Y., Christoffel, K., & Donovan, M. (1994). Children's household exposure to guns: A pediatric practice-based survey. *Pediatrics, 93,* 469–475.

Thorpe, T. (1995). Care of the hospitalized neonate, infant, toddler, preschooler, school age child & adolescent patient. In L. Baker, B. Anderson, & K. Gettrust (Eds.), *Inpatient pediatric nursing* (p. 545–553). Albany, NY: Delmar.

Woodring, B. (1998). The child with a medical-surgical condition. In M.E. Broome (Ed.), *Comprehensive care of the pediatric patient: Prehospitalization through rehabilitation.* Park Ridge, IL: Emergency Nurses Association.

Youngblut, J. M., Singer, L. T., Boyer, C., & Wheatley, M. A. (2000). Effects of pediatric trauma for children, parents, and families. *Critical Care Nursing Clinics of North America, 12*(2), 227–235.

Resources

Organizations and Websites

The American Academy of Pediatrics
141 Northwest Point Blvd.
Elk Grove Village, IL 60007-1098
www.aap.org

The American Academy of Family Physicians
11400 Tomahawk Creek Parkway
Leawood, KS 66211-2672
(800) 274-2237
www.aafp.org

Centers for Disease Control and Prevention
(800) 311-3435
www.cdc.gov

Kid Source Online
This is a group of parents who want to make a positive and lasting difference in the lives of parents and children. Their goal is to provide that knowledge and advice to help you better raise and educate your children.
www.kidsource.com

National Center for Infants, Toddlers and Families
2000 M Street, NW, Suite 200
Washington, DC 20036
(202) 638-1144
A national nonprofit charitable organization whose aim is to strengthen and support families, practitioners and communities to promote the healthy development of babies and toddlers.

National Institute of Child Health & Human Development
Bldg 31 Rm 2A32, MSC 2425
31 Center Dr.
Bethesda, MD 20892-2425
www.nichd.nih.gov

National Network for Child Care
An Internet source of over 1000 publications and resources related to childcare. Publications are research-based and reviewed.
www.nncc.org

The Online Safety Project
www.safekids.com

Your Amazing Baby
This site was designed for those of you looking for information on typical infant and toddler development.
www.amazingbaby.com

Zero to Three
Zero to Three is the nation's leading resource on the first three years of life.
www.zerotothree.org

CHAPTER 10

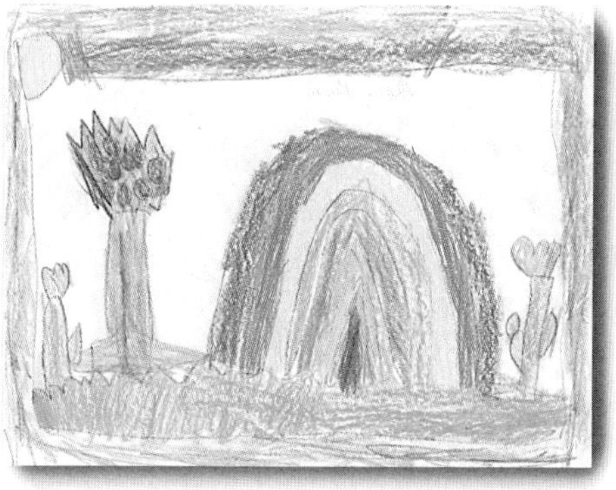

GROWTH AND DEVELOPMENT OF THE PRESCHOOLER

Carolyn C. Reynolds, APRN, MS

I remember when my children were preschoolers. Those were such fun years! The children were always doing something . . . playing in the sandbox or with their trucks or dolls. It seemed like they were busy from morning to night! I remember giving them a paint brush and a pail of water. They "painted" the garage several times over. They were delightful, happy children who rarely needed discipline, and always wanted to learn more about bugs, plants, flowers, and trees.

COMPETENCIES

Upon completion of this chapter, the reader should be able to:

- *Describe normal physiological changes that occur during the preschool years.*
- *Discuss changes in gross and fine motor movement, and identify appropriate activities to help develop these skills.*
- *Provide examples of Piaget's preoperational phase of cognitive development.*
- *Describe the skills obtained during Erikson's phase of developing a sense of initiative versus guilt.*
- *Identify activities of daily living (ADLs) that the preschool child is capable of independently performing.*
- *Describe how a preschooler determines right from wrong.*
- *Encourage ways to maintain optimal health through nutrition, activity, and sleep/rest.*
- *Describe activities and toys that a preschooler would enjoy.*
- *Discuss methods for injury prevention for a family with a preschool-aged child.*
- *Describe ways to evaluate readiness and preparation for school.*
- *Identify appropriate methods of discipline and limit-setting.*

The preschool years directly follow toddlerhood and span ages 3 to 6. Although physical growth and changes slow, this is a time characterized by refinement of the cognitive and social skills begun during the toddler years. The preschooler establishes control of body systems as indicated by the ability to toilet, dress, and feed self, and is also able to tolerate longer periods of separation from caregivers, and interact cooperatively with adults and other children. In addition, the preschooler can use language in a sophisticated manner and has an increased attention span and memory. The refinement of these skills prepares the child for entrance into school (Figure 10-1).

The changes typically occurring in the physiological, psychosexual, cognitive, psychosocial, and moral realms of development during the preschool years are described in the following pages. Health promotion, safety, and common concerns related to normal growth and development during the preschool years are also presented.

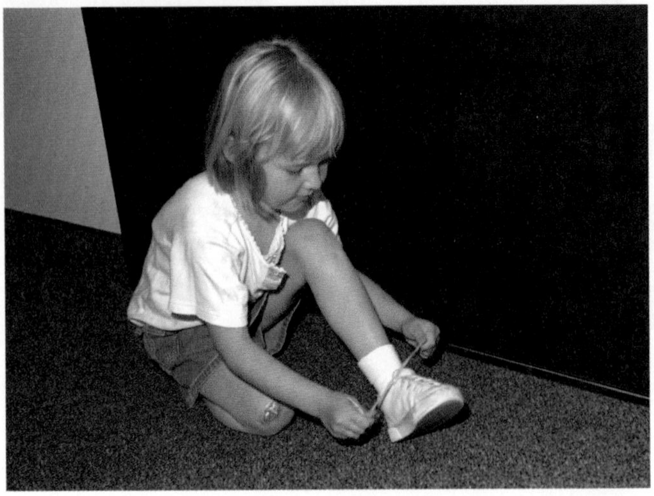

Figure 10-1 During the preschool years, as fine motor skills refine, the child learns how to tie her own shoes.

PHYSIOLOGICAL DEVELOPMENT

Physical Growth

During the preschool years, the rate of physical growth and change slows as compared to the rate experienced during the infant and toddler years. Generally, children will gain an average of 2 pounds per year in weight and 3 inches per year in height. By 5 years of age, half the adult height will be reached (Brazelton, 1994).

The preschooler's body contour also changes. The prominent abdomen, **lordosis,** and wide-legged gait characteristic of the toddler years gives way to a slimmer, taller, more posturally erect contour.

Body systems also continue to mature and stabilize. All the senses mature, and visual acuity reaches 20/20 with intact color vision. (Berry, Simons, Siatkowski, Schiffman, Flynn, & Duthie, 2001). Tonsils may grow and levels of antibodies may increase to assist the preschooler in better fighting infection. Children generally have all 20 of their deciduous teeth by 3 years of age. By the end of the preschool years, the eruption of permanent teeth may begin.

Handedness is established by the end of the preschool years. Muscle and bone growth continues, but maturity is not reached yet. Excessive activity and overexertion can damage growing tissue. Care should be taken to ensure that the preschooler receives adequate rest, nutrition, and exercise to promote optimum development of the musculoskeletal system (Brazelton, 1994).

Bowel and bladder control, including nighttime control, is generally achieved during this period of development as well. However, accidents may still occur if the child becomes absorbed in an activity. Sleep patterns also become more organized with longer periods of sleep and wake.

Gross and Fine Motor Skills

The preschool period is a time of refinement of eye–hand coordination and muscle coordination. Walking, running, and jumping are well established by the preschool years, and by 3 the child is able to ride a tricycle, balance on one foot for a few seconds, jump off the bottom step, and use alternate feet when going up the stairs. At age 4, the child can skip and hop on one foot, walk forward heel-to-toe, catch a ball with both arms, and use alternate feet when going down the stairs. Then, by age 5, the child is able to skip on alternate feet, jump from a height of 12 inches and land on toes, throw and catch a ball well, walk backward heel-to-toe, and begin to learn many other motor skills, including skating, swimming, dancing, and tumbling (Dixon & Stein, 2000) (Figures 10-2 and 10-3).

Fine motor skills also develop at an advanced rate. These skills can be tested through the use of the Denver Developmental Screening Test (DDST), a standardized development test in wide use throughout the United States. The child who is 3 years old builds a tower of nine to 10 cubes, builds a bridge with blocks, copies a circle and may add facial features, and dresses and undresses self. The 4-year-old child can use scissors successfully, draw a stick figure with three parts, lace shoes, do up simple buttons, copy a square or trace a cross/diamond, and show hand preference.

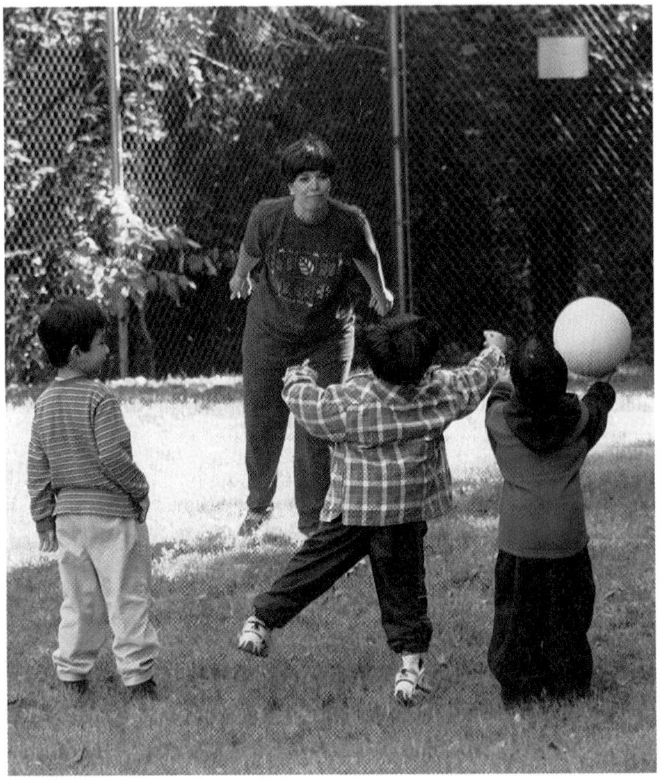

Figure 10-2 As the child progresses through the preschool years, he becomes more proficient in catching a ball.

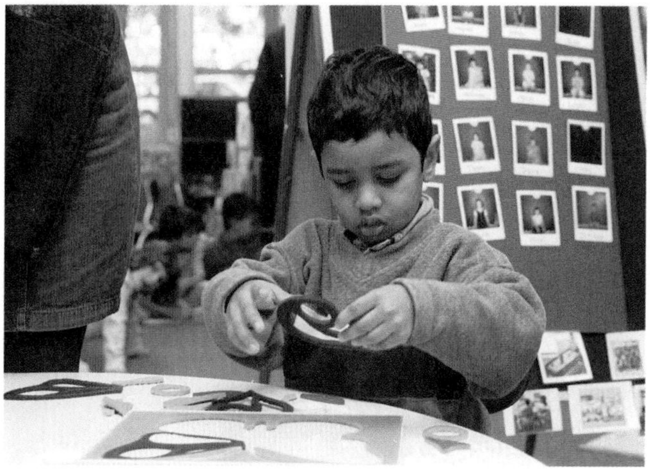

Figure 10-3 Preschoolers enjoy doing puzzles.

The 5-year-old child can begin to tie shoelaces, copy a square and triangle, and draw a person with at least six parts. The 5-year-old also becomes increasingly skilled with the use of a pencil and scissors. Refer to Appendix E for the DDST II.

The refinement and mastery of gross and fine motor skills encourage expression and independence, which leads to a greater sense of self-achievement and success as the child gets ready to enter school. Table 10-1 summarizes the preschooler's physiological development.

PSYCHOSEXUAL DEVELOPMENT

During the preschool years, the child is curious about his or her body, and learns about the physical differences between boys and girls. Freud described this period of time as the **Oedipal,** or **phallic,** stage of psychosexual development (Freud, 1959), when the child experiences subconscious conflicts and an intense attraction and love for the parent of the opposite sex. In turn, the child feels competition with the parent of the same sex for the attraction/affection of the other parent. This is termed the **Oedipus** (preschool boy to his mother) or **Electra** (preschool girl to her father) complex. Caregivers can be reassured that this phenomenon of

TABLE 10-1 Preschool Developmental Milestones (3–6 years)

Physiological Development

	3rd Year	4th Year	5th Year
Growth	Weight increases 4–6 lb (1.8–2.7 kg) per year. Average weight is 32 lb (14.6 kg). Height increases 3 in (7.5 cm) per year. Average height is $37^1/_2$ inches (95 cm). Visual acuity is 20/20. Color vision is fully intact. May have achieved nighttime control of bowel and bladder.	Weight increases at a rate similar to the prior year. Average weight is 37 lb (16.7 kg) Height increases at same rate. Average height is $40^1/_2$ inches (103 cm). Birth length is doubled. Maximum potential for development of amblyopia. Cooperates with Snellen test.	Weight increases at a similar rate. Pulse and respiration rates decrease slightly. Average weight is $41^1/_2$ lb (18.7 kg). Height increases at same rate. Average height is $43^1/_4$ inches (110 cm). Half of adult height. Handedness is established. Eruption of permanent teeth may begin. Pulse and respiration rates decrease slightly.
Gross motor	Walking, running, and jumping are well established. Rides tricycle. Jumps off bottom step. Balances on one foot for a few seconds. Alternates feet going up stairs.	Skips and hops on one foot. Alternates feet going up and down stairs. Able to walk forward heel-to-toe, climbs jungle gym, and catches ball with both arms.	Skips on alternate feet and jumps rope. Jumps from height of 12 inches and lands on toes. Begins to skate and swim. Throws and catches ball well. Rides bike with training wheels. Able to walk backwards heel-to-toe and run on toes. Arms are coordinated with legs when running. Proficient climber.

continues

TABLE 10-1 *Continued*

	3rd Year	4th Year	5th Year
Fine motor	Builds towers of 9–10 cubes. Cannot draw a stick figure but may make a circle with facial features. Copies circle and can build a bridge. Dresses and undresses self.	Uses scissors successfully. Draws stick figures with 3 parts. Can lace shoes but may not be able to tie shoes. Copies a square and traces a cross or diamond. Shows hand preference.	Begins to tie shoelaces. Improved cutting with scissors. Uses a pencil very well. Copies square and triangle. Draws person with at least 6 parts.
Psychosexual Development			
Sexuality	Knows own and others' gender. Begins to adopt culturally prescribed behavior, and roles.	Masturbation may increase. Displays sexual curiosity and interest in bodily differences between girls and boys. May explore differences in gender through play ("doctor" and "nurse"). May have own ideas to explain sexual differences and reproduction.	Displays gender stereotypic roles. Curiosity and sexual exploration continues. Able to understand potential for sexual abuse.
Cognitive Development			
Cognition	Preoperational thinking characterized by egocentrism, concrete/tangible thinking, transductive reasoning, magical thinking, and the inability to distiguish between one's own perception and that of someone else. This is a period of magical thinking and the inability to reason logically. Concepts of time, space, and causality are primitive.		
	Attention span is still short but is increasing. Learns through observing and imitating. Continues to be very self-centered. Believes that objects have human qualities (animism). Begins to learn concepts of time. Asks questions about environment. Fears are more specific, including fear of bodily harm. Active imagination! Color and number recognition begins.	Less self-centered and developing social awareness. Comprehends some simple analogies such as "if fire is hot, ice is cold." Better understanding of time. Understands concepts of long/short, light/heavy, etc. Can sort objects into like categories. Usually separates from family easily. Starts, but may not complete projects.	Questions parents' thinking and principles by comparing to peers and other adults. Learns the "rules" of the culture (values and acceptable behavior). Beginning to see other perspectives but tolerates differences rather than understanding them. Very curious about factual information about the world. Shows more realistic sense of causality. Classifies objects according to similarities. Personality qualities are noticeable.
Language	Knows name and age. Forms sentences of 3–4 words. Asks many questions. Uses mainly "telegraphic" speech. Correct use of plurals and pronouns. May use personal, made-up words and may carry on conversation with self. Vocabulary of about 900 words.	Use of longer sentences (4–5 words). Tells exaggerated stories. Questioning is at peak. Correct use of some prepositions. Names one or more colors. Vocabulary of about 1,500 words.	Use of longer sentences (6–8 words) and uses prepositions, past verb tenses, adjectives, etc. correctly. Vocabulary of about 2,100 words by the end of the 5th year of age. Names four or more colors. Knows names of days of week, months, and other time-associated words. Follows three commands in succession.

continues

TABLE 10-1 *Continued*

Psychosocial Development

	3rd Year	4th Year	5th Year
Psychosocial	Developing a sense of Initiative vs. Guilt (Erikson). This is a period of very energetic play and the child can develop a sense of accomplishment and satisfaction in his/her activities. As the child oversteps his/her limits he/she experiences a feeling of guilt for not having behaved appropriately. This is the beginning of the development of a conscience (superego). The child has mostly overcome stranger anxiety and separation anxiety. More sociable and willing to please. Likes being a helper.		
Family relations	Likes to please parents and conform with their wishes. Is less jealous of younger siblings (may be an opportune time for birth of additional sibling). Is aware of family relationships and sex-role functions.	Takes aggression and frustrations out on parents or siblings. "Do's" and "Don'ts" become important. Rivalry with older and younger siblings increases. May "run away" from home. Is able to run simple errands outside the home.	Gets along well with parents. May seek out parent for reassurance and security, especially when starting school. Begins to question parent's thinking and principles. Enjoys activities such as sports, cooking, shopping, or working.
Social	Feeds self completely and dresses with minimal help. Has increased attention span. Can help to set the table and/or do the dishes.	Very independent in dressing and feeding. Tends to be selfish, impatient, and physically aggressive. Has mood swings. Shows off dramatically to entertain others. Tells family stories to others without restraint.	Less rebellious and quarrelsome. More settled and eager to please. Tries to live by the rules. Trustworthy and can take on responsibilities. Has fewer fears. Has better manners.
Coping	Temper tantrums, negativism, ritualism begin to decrease. Coping behaviors may include regression, denial, projection, displacement, attack, rationalization, and sublimation. Active imagination (may have an imaginary friend).	Begins to verbalize fears about body integrity, animals, or the dark. Uses play and fantasy.	Verbalizes feelings in later preschool years, may temporarily regress. May display independence through noncompliance or express confusion over inconsistent limits.
Play	Learns through play and imitation of adult behaviors. Will play cooperatively with other children and share toys. Plays group games with simple rules. Also likes dramatic play and is very imaginative and creative.		

Moral Development

Moral	Kohlberg Stage 3 (Conventional Level): Child desires to please others or seeks approval through behaviors. Shows concern for others.		
Spiritual	Learns to imitate the religious affect and behavior of parents. Mimics religious gestures although does not comprehend the meaning. Cannot separate feeling from thoughts. Formulates imagined descriptions of God, in other words, God is a friend child can communicate with.		

Every child is unique and has an individual personality. While these descriptions are generally applicable, each child must be assessed as an individual.

competition and romance is normal, but may need help handling feelings of anger and jealousy that may arise. The resolution of the Oedipus or Electra complex comes as the child identifies with the parent of the same sex (Freud, 1959). (See Chapter 6 for more information.)

During this stage, the child becomes aware of himself or herself as a male and female, and begins to take on the behavior of the same sex caregiver (Charlesworth, 2000). For example, a young girl sees her mother putting make-up on and wants to do the same. Or a young boy sees his father vacuuming and wants to help.

Children will display sexual curiosity and interest in bodily differences according to gender. They may explore these differences through play such as "doctor" and "nurse," or ask many questions. If these questions are not answered by an adult, the children might come up with their own answers, which often are inaccurate (Brazelton, 1994). Therefore, caregivers should answer questions simply, by using correct terms for all body parts, including genitalia. Caregivers should be cautioned to only answer questions asked, since often the child is curious only about one aspect of sexuality and not interested in hearing a complete description. This is also an optimum time to teach children that certain body parts are private and should not be touched by "strangers." Table 10-1 summarizes the preschooler's psychosexual development.

COGNITIVE DEVELOPMENT

During the preschool years, many changes in the child's cognitive abilities are also occurring. **Cognitive ability,** or the capacity to understand and use phenomena in the world around us, is best explained by Piaget (Piaget, 1969), who saw the child as an active participant in life, constantly **assimilating,** incorporating experiences into mental and physical structures of action (**schema**). These schema change over time as the child confronts new experiences and seeks to modify behavior and mental structures to handle the change. This change is called **accommodation.** (See Chapter 6 for more information.)

Preoperational Phase

Piaget's **preoperational stage** occurs between the ages of 2 and 6 years (Piaget, 1969). During this period, the child develops the ability to perform mental operations governed by personal perceptions and linkage to events previously experienced. The preschool child can understand experiences only from his or her own point of view, and cannot imagine that another person would have a different perspective (**egocentrism**). There is no separation of internal and external reality. The preschooler uses a personal system for organizing objects and events in his or her mind (**idiosyncratic**) and reasons from one particular to another, often by unrelated events (**transductive reasoning**), when in reality the particulars are not linked at all. **Animism** (belief that objects have human qualities) is also a part of the preschooler's thinking (Dixon & Stein, 2000). See Table 10-2 for examples.

The 3-year-old child's attention span is increasing, but it lasts for a short time. Learning occurs through observation and imitation, as the 3-year-old asks many questions about the world around them, has a beginning concept of time, and begins to recognize colors and numbers (Figure 10-4). Due to the 3-year-old's active imagination, fears, including fears of bodily harm, may be experienced at this time (Charlesworth, 2000).

TABLE 10-2 Preoperational Thinking

Question	Conclusion
Egocentrism	
Why do cars go?	Cars go to take me to the park.
Why does the sun shine?	The sun shines to see me when I play outside.
Why did I get sick?	I hit my sister.
Animism	
How did you get hurt?	The bike threw me off.
Why did you hit the door?	The door hit me in the head.
Transductive Reasoning	
Daddy is home.	It must be time for dinner.
The doctor put that thing in my ear.	I have an earache.
I ate cookies right before dinner.	The cookies made me get sick.

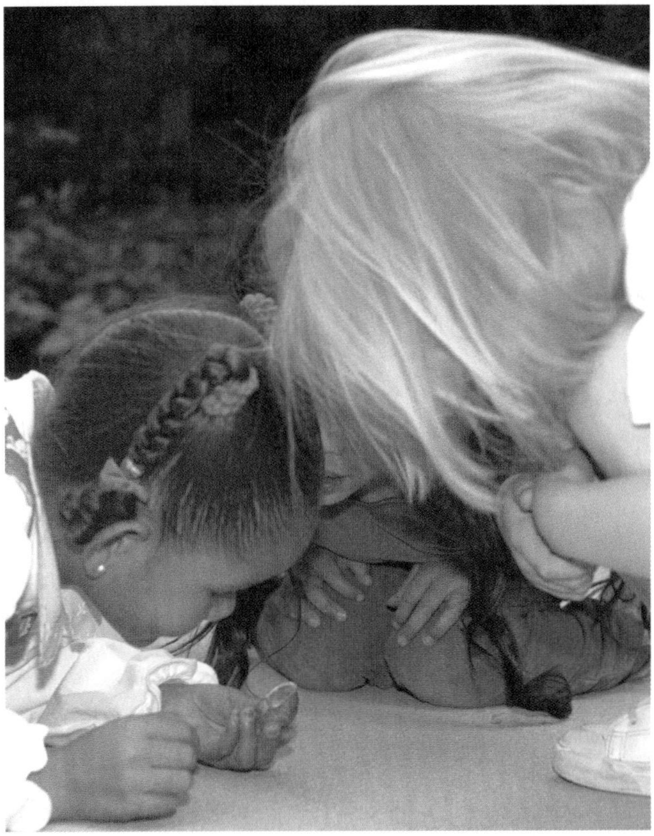

Figure 10-4 As they look at an empty snail shell, these preschoolers wonder where the snail is.

Fear

Preschoolers can become fearful of real or imagined things (bugs, the dark, animals). It is best to counsel the caregiver to tackle the problem directly. Instruct caregivers to find realistic ways to overcome or deal with the fear. For instance, keep a night light on at night. In some cases, continuous exposure to the fear stimulus may diminish the fear. However, it is important to not force a child. For example, if a child has a fear of swimming, the caregiver should encourage the child to put on a swimsuit and life-saving gear, and sit by the edge of the pool. As the child witnesses the safe fun that other children and caregivers are experiencing, they may realize that there is nothing to be afraid of.

The 4-year-old child is less self-centered and has an increasing awareness of others and can comprehend simple analogies, for example, "if fire is hot, ice is cold." The child can also understand time better as well as the concept of opposites, for example, heavy/light and long/short. Finally, the 4-year-old can sort objects into like piles (Charlesworth, 2000).

The 5-year-old is busy learning the values and acceptable behavior of the culture, will question parent's thinking by comparing with peers and other adults, and has a fairly good estimate of time. In addition, the 5-year-old begins to see other perspectives but only *tolerates* differences, rather than understanding them. The 5-year-old also demonstrates a more realistic understanding of cause and effect (Charlesworth, 2000).

Another method of assessing cognition is through the child's use of language. The 3-year-old child has a vocabulary of about 500 words, forms sentences that are three to four words in length (**telegraphic speech**), uses plurals and pronouns correctly, and may make up words or carry on a conversation with himself or herself (Dixon & Stein, 2000).

The 4-year-old has a vocabulary of about 1,500 words, and uses longer sentences (about four to five words long) and some prepositions correctly. This is the age when questioning is at a peak; the child may tell exaggerated stories at this time too (Dixon & Stein, 2000).

The 5-year-old has a vocabulary of about 2,100 words, speaks in longer sentences (six to eight words long), and uses prepositions, adjectives, and past verb tenses correctly. In addition, the 5-year-old can name four or more colors, and recognize time-associated words, such as the days of week and the months of the year (Dixon & Stein, 2000).

PSYCHOSOCIAL DEVELOPMENT

The development of a sense of initiative versus guilt is the chief psychosocial task described by Erikson (1963). (See Chapter 6 for more information.) This is a time of very energetic learning, as the child participates in play and work with energy and enthusiasm, and develops a sense of accomplishment and satisfaction in activities. This increases the child's ability to use initiative, but as established limits are overstepped, feelings of guilt for not behaving appropriately may appear. A feeling of conflict may also arise as the child realizes actions were not appropriate. Feelings of guilt may also arise from thoughts the child has that are different from expected behaviors.

As the child learns to distinguish between the feelings of initiative and guilt, the child also begins to develop a conscience (**superego**). Learning right from wrong and good from bad is the beginning of moral development (Figure 10-5). However, preschoolers generally do not understand the reasons that something is acceptable or unacceptable; rather, preschoolers become aware of appropriate behavior through punishments and rewards handed out by caregivers or other adults. Reliance on caregivers and adults assists the preschooler in developing moral judgment.

In this age group, verbal reminders of established limits are effective, and the preschooler will understand the danger of running out into the road without looking. A reminder of what to do when crossing the street will be sufficient. The preschooler may disagree and question limits, which allows them to develop independence in thought and action as well as socially acceptable behaviors.

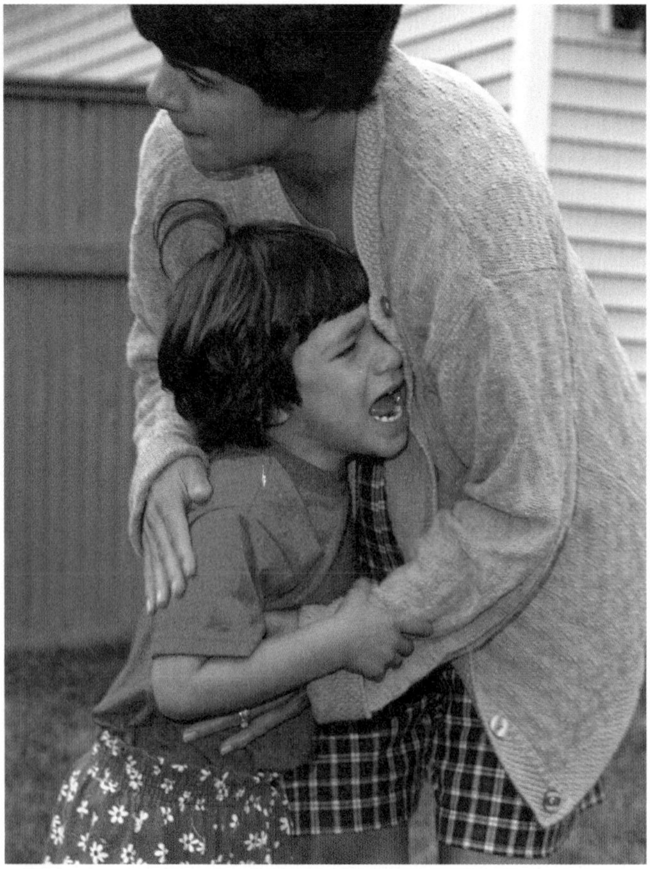

Figure 10-5 Distinguihing right from wrong is a concept learned in the preschool years.

Reflective Thinking

Differences between Boys and Girls

A mother comes to you with concerns about her preschool son Peter's inquisitiveness related to physiological differences between boys and girls. How would you respond? Would you feel awkward in responding? Why?

Socialization

The preschool years are also critical years for the development of social skills—both the skills to care for self (dressing, bathing, eating, acting appropriately in social settings/manners) and the skills to get along with others. The preschool-aged child is less egocentric, more capable of sharing, and able to enjoy play groups, since playing with other children helps teach relating to others, and encourages imitation of adults. Preschool play is also dramatic, imaginative, and creative (Figure 10-6).

As the preschool-aged child matures, arguing with others appears and may progress to the point where the child uses physical aggression to make a point. Although this may appear to be regressive behavior, this is actually normal behavior needed to identify and test roles in the social group and family. The child will gradually become less rebellious and quarrelsome and, by the end of the preschool years, will be more eager to please and take on more responsibilities. The child will also try to live by established rules and enjoys playing group games with simple rules (Brazelton, 1994).

Family Relations

The 3-year-old child likes to please caregivers and conform to their wishes. At this age, the child is also less jealous of a younger sibling, so this may be an opportune time for the birth of an additional sibling. The 3-year-old is also aware of his or her place in the family and understands sex-role functions well.

As the child turns 4, there is a dramatic increase in aggressive behavior, and frustrations may be shown through physical aggression. Rivalry with older and younger siblings increases. The 4-year-old may act out if she doesn't get her way. However, the 4-year-old child is also becoming increasingly able to run simple errands, such as getting a diaper for an infant the mother is changing or a book from another room, and complete assigned tasks.

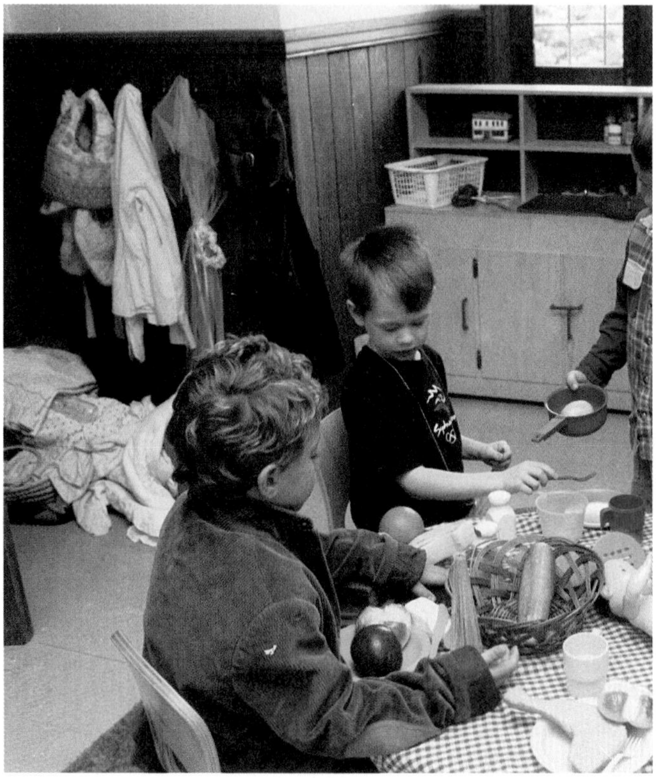

Figure 10-6 Imaginative play is demonstrated by this group of boys.

As the child turns 5, behavior within the family stabilizes and the child gets along well with family members. Parents are looked to for reassurance and a sense of security as the time for attending school nears. The 5-year-old also enjoys helping with cooking, shopping, chores, or other family activities.

MORAL AND SPIRITUAL DEVELOPMENT

Children of preschool age are in the **preconventional** or **premoral** stage of moral development as described by Kohlberg (Kohlberg, 1981). (See Chapter 6 for more information.) The child's moral judgment is at the most basic level, and right and wrong are determined from rules parents have established. Additionally, right and wrong are determined through rewards or punishments the child receives in response to an action. However, the preschool child has little understanding of why something is right or wrong, and if questioned, will often say "because my mother says so." Young preschoolers may have difficulty applying known rules to a different situation. For example, if a parent says "there is no jumping on the couch in our house," the preschooler may jump on the couch in a friend's house. Later, the child is able to direct actions toward satisfying personal needs rather than the needs of others, and develops a concrete sense of justice and fairness.

The preschooler's knowledge of faith or religion is learned from parents and other important adults in their lives. The preschooler may have a concrete concept of a Supreme Being with physical characteristics that are often like an imaginary friend. The child understands simple religious stories and memorizes short prayers. However, understanding the meaning of these rituals is limited, and participation in religious rituals occurs out of self-interest rather than out of a strong spiritual motivation.

HEALTH PROMOTION

As with any age group, it is important to look at the ways that normal growth and development impact daily activities and the health of the child. In the preschool period, families play a major role in ensuring health and preventing injury and illness. The following sections explore the unique issues a preschooler may encounter related to health promotion and injury prevention.

Nutrition

Nutritional health is important in the preschool years as in other ages because of the impact good nutrition has on growth and also for the value of establishing good health habits for the rest of the one's life. By 3 years of age, a child should be eating table foods. The diet of a preschool child should revolve around the principles of the U.S. Department of Agriculture's food pyramid, which suggests six to 11 servings of breads and cereals; three to five servings of vegetables; two to four servings of fruit; three servings of milk products; two to three servings of meat; and sparse use of fats and sweets every day. In addition, this is a good time to switch the preschooler to low-fat or skim milk to decrease the amount of fat intake, since total fat intake should be no more than 30% of total caloric intake per day (American Academy of Pediatrics [AAP], 1999).

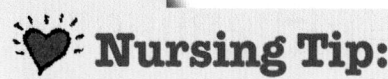

> **Nursing Tip:**
>
> **Vitamins**
>
> Children's vitamins look fun and taste good, so children may be tempted to take more than the one per day. Be sure all vitamins are stored with other medications in a locked cupboard so the preschooler cannot "get into" the vitamins and take too many.

Planning meals and snacks around the pyramid will give the child a well-balanced diet providing all the nutrients necessary to maintain health. If the child is eating a well-balanced diet, it shouldn't be necessary to supplement the diet with vitamins or minerals. If the child does not get a balanced diet, it may be necessary to start vitamins.

It is overwhelming to a preschooler to be served too much of any one food. Because of the decreased rate of growth during the preschool years, the appetite will also be decreased and the child may not be able to eat a large serving at one time. A helpful rule to follow is to serve 1 tablespoon of food per every year of age. It is also a good idea to vary the types of foods offered (Brazelton, 1994). Some children may be labeled "picky eaters," but this is an age of exploration, and something the child refuses one day may be eaten another day. Experimenting with various ways of preparing foods, as well as letting the child help prepare the foods may also increase intake (Green, 1994).

Some preschoolers will go on a "feeding strike" where they will refuse to eat much for a few days. This is normal, since children will often self-regulate their needs and eat when hungry. Other children may have "food jags" or go through a period of time when they will only eat one food or only foods of one color. Once again it is all right for children to make these choices. Caregivers should not fall into the trap of making eating and mealtimes a power struggle. Instead, they should be happy and enjoyable times for the family.

Childhood Obesity

Today, there is an increasing incidence of childhood obesity. This might relate to the growing number of obese adults since

Research Highlight

Parental Perceptions of the Preschool Obese Child

Study Purpose

To determine parents' perceptions of their child's obesity.

Methods

Two hundred parents, identified when they visited WIC or Child Health Services, completed a questionnaire on their child's weight/obesity. Clinic staff then added their perceptions of the child's weight/obesity to the bottom of the questionnaire.

Findings

Thirty-five percent of parents did not believe their obese child was overweight, and 53% had no problem controlling what their child eats. Seventy-eight percent of parents expressed concern about heart disease as a consequence of childhood obesity.

Implications

Parents do acknowledge some health risks associated with obesity, but a large percentage do not perceive their child as obese. Interventions in childhood obesity need to begin with understanding the parents' perception of obesity and then working to alter that perception when necessary.

Citation

Myers, S., & Vargas, Z. (2000). Parental perceptions of the preschool obese child. *Pediatric Nursing, 26*(1), 23–30.

studies have shown, prior to 3 years of age, that parental obesity is the biggest predictor of a child's risk of developing obesity in adulthood (Buiten & Metzger, 2000). Childhood obesity has both immediate and long-term physical and psychosocial effects. The physical effects may be hyperlipidemia, obstructive apnea, pancreatitis, gallbladder disease, non–insulin-dependent diabetes, and hypertension, which often lead to long-term cardiovasular diseases. The obese child also often has lower self-esteem and may find it hard to "fit in" with a group of peers (Buiten & Metzger, 2000).

The prevention and treatment of childhood obesity includes three components: (1) nutritional diets—with a decreased amount of foods with poor nutritional value, for example, candy, chips, and soda pop, and an appropriate serving size for age; (2) increased amounts of physical activity/exercise; and (3) behavior modification to teach the child appropriate ways to lead a healthy life (Roberts, 2000).

Family Teaching

Establishing a Bedtime Routine

The bedtime routine should include various components:

- Establishing a bedtime and sticking to it
- Establishing a wake-up time and sticking to it
- Avoiding stimulants such as sugar or caffeine, or roughhousing near bedtime
- Making the bedroom cozy and inviting
- Avoiding nonsleep activities in bed, for example, watching television
- Maintaining quiet in and near the bedroom
- Making bedtime a fun time to be with the child
- Providing a quiet activity (reading a story) prior to going to bed

Sleep/Rest

Sleep patterns begin to change during the preschool years, and may vary from child to child. Generally, the preschooler will sleep a total of 12 hours every day. Some children sleep 10.5 hours a night and another 1.5 hours during an afternoon nap. Others will sleep for 12 hours every night. If children

REFLECTIONS FROM FAMILIES

It was always hard to get Joshua and Emily to bed when they were preschoolers, especially in the late spring and summer when it was daylight savings time and they could hear their friends playing outside. While this time of year brought the bellyaching of wanting to play with friends, I had established a routine when they were toddlers. I would give them a bath, have them brush their teeth, read them a favorite story, have them say their prayers, and then tuck them in. I also made sure their room was dark by pulling the blinds. While not every day was easy, sticking with a routine was definitely a plus.

participate in preschool or day care centers, they will generally have a nap time. Even though many preschoolers will not sleep during this nap time, it is important to have the children at least rest (Stanford Sleep Center, 2000).

It is critical to establish a bedtime routine for the child, and hopefully, those rituals started during the infant and toddler years can be continued. If bedtime rituals have not been started earlier, this is the time to establish routines that prepare the child for sleep. By participating in the routine consistently, the child will enjoy bedtime and the household will not be disturbed as much (Stanford Sleep Center, 2000).

It is also important to help the child relax and prepare for sleep. Some children like to take a bath, play a quiet game, read a bedtime story, have a chat, say "goodnight moon," listen to soothing music, or have a light left on. All of these can help the child relax, learn how to be calm, and fall asleep.

Sleep Disturbances

An increase in the number and kind of sleep problems are common and normal during the preschool years. They should resolve and diminish, however, as the child gets older, since many are related to irregular sleep habits and/or anxiety about going to bed and falling asleep. By following a bedtime routine and teaching the child ways to become calm and relaxed before bed, the caregiver can minimize the incidence of these problems. Other children suffer from bedtime fears, which may be helped by using a night light and by having an open discussion to resolve those fears (Stanford Sleep Center, 2000).

Nightmares, which are also fairly common, often involve a major threat to the child who wakes up crying because of being scared. If nightmares awaken a child, the parent should comfort and reassure the child that the nightmares are not real, and help the child remain in bed and fall back to sleep (Brazelton, 1994).

Sleep terrors, talking in the sleep, and sleepwalking are other sleep disturbances occurring during the preschool years. In these situations, the child may appear to be awake but in actuality is confused and can't communicate clearly. Most often, children will just experience a single or an occasional episode of sleep disturbance. If the episodes occur several times a night or nightly, the child should be seen by a health care provider. Fortunately, as children mature, these sleep problems should diminish (Stanford Sleep Center, 2000).

Activity

As detailed previously, the preschool child is refining both gross and fine motor coordination and skill. This allows the child to participate in more physical games and sports where motor activity is used (Figure 10-7). An emphasis on physical fitness has emerged in the last few years, and regular physical activity can benefit a child in many ways—for example, improved ability to perform motor skills; enhanced self-confidence and body image; development of lifetime habits; and prevention of disease processes associated with inactivity (Roberts, 2000). Physical activity can also help get rid of tension and excess energy.

By introducing the preschooler to sports, physical fitness can improve. Therefore, the main goal of sports for this age

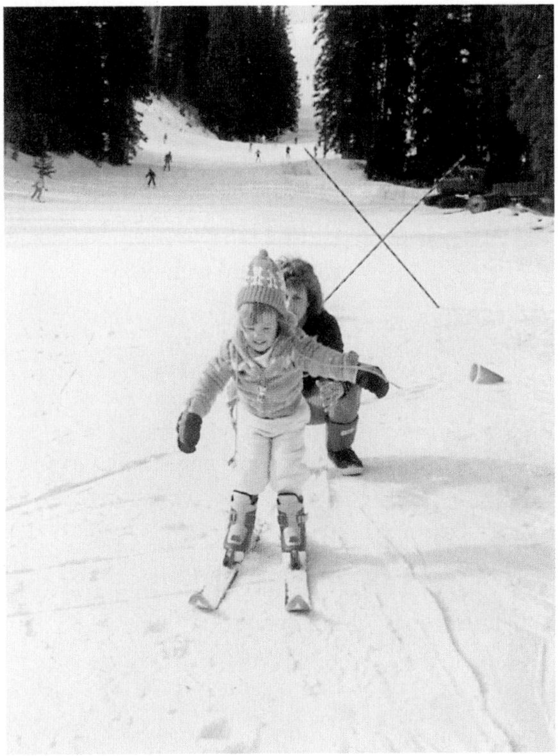

Figure 10-7 Learning to ski not only promotes physical fitness but can enhance a child's self-esteem.

is to have fun, get exercise, and learn to enjoy the activity. However, since not all children will enjoy every sport, it is important to find the right sport for each child in order to make it a positive experience. The American Academy of Pediatrics suggests that caregivers encourage a variety of physical activities in a noncompetitive environment, with an emphasis on fun and safety. Some sports meeting this criteria are T-ball, karate, gymnastics, bicycling, or dance.

Play

Preschoolers enjoy group play. They engage in imitative, dramatic, and imaginative play.

TABLE 10-3 Toys and Activities That Stimulate Development

Skill	Toy/Activity
Hand–eye–mouth coordination	Bubbles Coloring books Scissors Video games Large beads to string Stickers Markers or paint Large building set
Small motor	Crayons Sewing cards Art projects Play dough
Gross motor	Playing catch Kicking a ball Riding a tricycle Building blocks
Dramatic play	Play tools Kitchenette with dishes Dolls Magic wand Dress-up supplies Action figures Cars, trucks, trains Play people and animals
Cognitive	Books Puzzles Educational videos
Problem-solving	Puzzles Shape sorter Board games
Socialization	Group games such as London Bridge and Red Rover Board games Pretend play

A 3-year-old still plays in an egocentric manner but is developing more tolerance of playmates. Appropriate toys and activities for this age may include a tricycle, pounding bench, big blocks, musical/rhythm toys, show and tell, guessing games, and puzzles.

A 4-year-old's play is interactive. The child can also obey limits and often has an imaginary friend. This imaginary friend is often given up by the time the child enters school. Toys and activities may include construction toys, puzzles, memory games, fantasy play, books, and music.

A 5-year-old has achieved impulse control and plays well in groups, so this is an optimal time to introduce the child to group sports and games. The 5-year-old child enjoys pretend play, puppets, dress-up, books, and art activities (Lytle & Lytle, 2000) (Table 10-3).

Literacy

The child's love of reading and interest in obtaining the skill is established during this time period when caregivers spend time reading to young children. The child will show early literacy skills by reciting the name of the books they want to read; retelling the stories in the book; asking questions about the story; pretending to read a favorite book; correcting the reader if a page is skipped; and paying attention through the entire story (USOE Family Literacy Program, 2000).

Preschoolers will also enjoy books with more words that tell stories, especially if the book has lots of pictures. Books about children with similar experiences, including going to the doctor, going to the park, and going to school, or books about friends and families are also appropriate for children this age. Lastly, books with a predictable story line and repeated phrases help keep the child's attention (Figure 10-8).

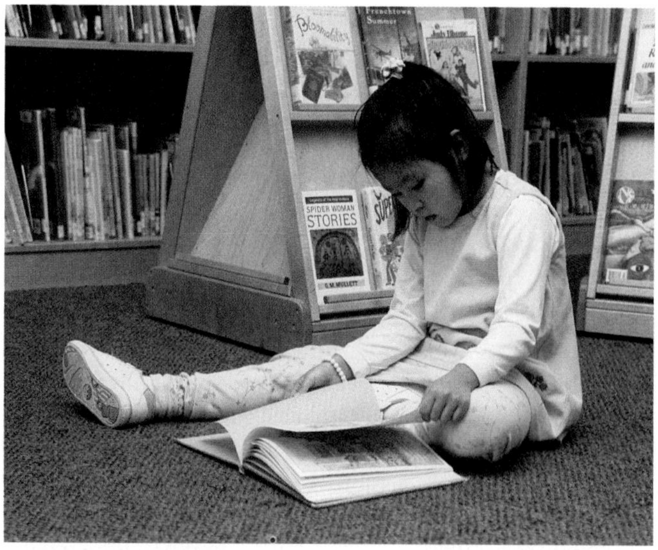

Figure 10-8 Regular visits to the library for story hours and borrowing books encourage a love of reading.

Eye On:

Toys that Teach

Through advertisements, some toys are promoted as "toys that teach," meaning they teach, for example, "cause and effect" and "manual dexterity." While these toys are safe and attractive, the nurse must caution caregivers to be cognizant of deceptive advertising. For instance, an advertisement may imply that, if children do not have this toy, they will be developmentally delayed or that this toy is an adequate substitute for caregiver–child interaction. These claims are not true.

Television/Media

The influence of television and other media on children has become controversial since both can be constructive and positive. Television, however, is not a substitute for education and play, but some programs can reinforce learning, promote creativity, and encourage cognitive growth by teaching colors, numbers, the alphabet, and social skills in a creative and stimulating manner. On the other hand, some programs are inappropriate for young children (Leland, 1999). Since preschoolers often believe that what they see is real, they cannot differentiate between reality and fantasy in television programs. Inappropriate programs give children a distorted view of how to deal with problems, which often is with violence (AAP, 1999).

While the television should not be used as a babysitter, it is virtually impossible to "ban" television viewing. Instead, caregivers should closely monitor and control what a child watches. The AAP recommends a preschooler only watch 1–2 hours of television per day. See Box 10-1.

BOX 10-1 Guidelines for television and video viewing

- Limit child's viewing time to no more than 1–2 hours per day.
- Control what the child watches.
- Watch television with children, especially if the child is viewing a new show or a new video.
- If the child is allowed to watch a program while the parent is occupied with another activity and cannot supervise appropriately, encourage the child to select a video with known content.
- Provide feedback to the networks regarding the quality of children's programming.

Adapted from AAP, Committee on Public Education. (1999). Media Education. *Pediatrics, 104*(2), 341–343.

DENTAL HEALTH

By the beginning of the preschool period, the eruption of the deciduous (primary) teeth is complete. It is essential to preserve these primary/temporary teeth so the permanent teeth will have room to form correctly and the dental arch will not be narrowed. Since the preschooler is also very willing to be involved in brushing his or her teeth, this is an appropriate time to establish good dental habits that will last a lifetime.

The number one dental problem in the preschool years is dental caries or tooth decay, which may cause the premature loss of teeth and a consequent alteration of the dental arch, compromising development of the permanent teeth. Prevention of dental caries is accomplished through daily brushing and flossing of teeth, and preschoolers enjoy imitating parents and older siblings brush their own teeth. Parents or other adults should assist the child to ensure that even the back teeth are brushed thoroughly. If toothpaste containing fluoride is used, only a pea-sized amount of toothpaste should be used (AAP, 1988; Centers for Disease Control and Prevention [CDC], 1991). The preschool-aged child will also need assistance flossing because motor skills are lacking.

The preschool child should visit a dentist at least every 6 months. The first time the child visits the dentist, the child should not be told there will be no pain because, if pain is felt, trust will be lost and the child will become frightened (Hauck, 1991). Most dentists prepare children according to their developmental level before any work begins. The dentist will determine if the child needs to take fluoride supplements depending on the amount of fluoride in the drinking water.

Lastly, children should avoid sugary snacks that may predispose them to dental caries. Instead, parents should provide healthy snacks such as fruit, vegetables, or cheese. When the child is ready to chew gum, it should be sugar-free. When the child does have a sugary treat, the child should brush or at least rinse the mouth out with plain water (Green, 1994).

Night Grinding

Some children grind their teeth at night. This is common during the preschool years and may be a way to release tension and calm oneself in order to fall asleep. Generally, tooth grinding lasts for a short time as the child slips into sleep. Children with cerebral palsy, however, often grind their teeth due to jaw muscle spasticity. If tooth grinding is excessive, the child should be referred to a health care provider.

SAFETY AND INJURY PREVENTION

With the increase in motor skills and coordination, the preschool-aged child is less prone to falls common during the toddler years. However, due to their increased mobility

Critical Thinking

Nighttime Fears

The parents of 3-year-old Tatiana tell you she keeps the whole family awake at night because she is afraid of the dark. How would you help this family?

Kids Want To Know

Why do I have to wear my helmet?

It is safer to wear your helmet when riding your bike because it will protect your head from getting hurt if you fall. Everyone should wear a helmet when riding their bike.

and skills, there are now other dangers. One of the greatest areas of concern is playing near the street or driveway since preschool children still need close, constant supervision by adults to remain safe (Figure 10-9).

It is also important to remember that the preschool-aged child is less reckless, will listen more to rules, and is aware of potential dangers such as hot objects, sharp instruments, or dangerous heights. This makes it easier for the adults who are supervising preschoolers to set limits and expect obedience. However, as this is a time when the child likes to imitate whatever adults do, it is critical that adults also abide by the same rules, for example, putting on a seat belt before the car moves (Murphy, 1999).

Box 10-2 gives guidelines for injury prevention.

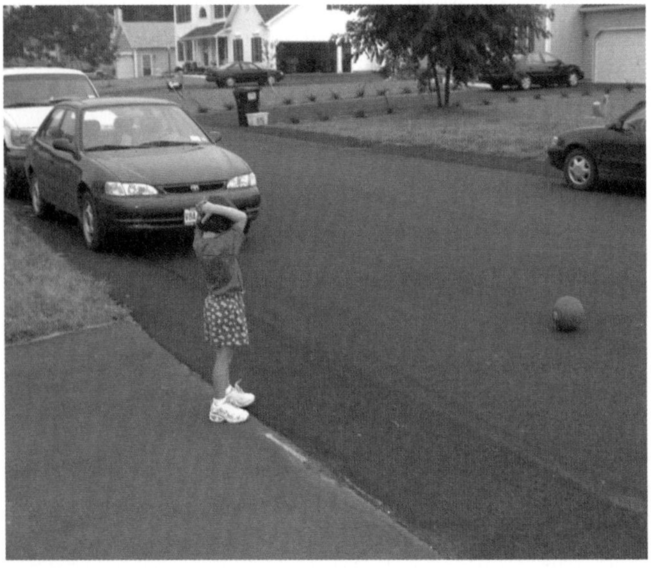

Figure 10-9 Injury prevention includes teaching the preschooler how to cross the street and not to run after a ball that has rolled into the street.

HEALTH SCREENINGS

Health supervision and screenings are important in ensuring the ongoing health of the preschool-aged child. Healthy habits are built through regular screenings that help avert issues that may turn into problems later. A preschooler should see a health care provider yearly, including a physical examination with care taken to assess growth parameters, and vision, hearing, and blood pressure screening. If the young child is uncooperative with the vision screening, another appointment should be scheduled 6 months later (Green, 1994).

The preschooler will also need to be kept current on immunizations, especially prior to starting school. If the child has received all the recommended vaccines/doses as an infant and toddler, then only booster doses of diphtheria, tetanus, and acellular pertussis (DTaP), inactivated polio vaccine (IPV), and measles, mumps, and rubella (MMR) will be needed. Refer to Appendix C for the current schedule of immunizations.

The health screening should also include an assessment for the risk for hyperlipidemia, high-dose exposure to lead, and a tuberculin (TB) test. The TB test is required only once prior to school entrance unless there are risk factors present; then the test can be done annually with the health screening (Green, 1994; Dixon & Stein, 2000).

One of the most common and preventable health problems in the United States is lead poisoning. Common sites of exposure include older homes/apartments that may have peeling lead-based paint, older lead water pipes, or lead dust from renovation of older homes. Extremely high blood lead levels can cause mental retardation, coma, or seizures. However, chronic low-level lead exposure is more common and leads to learning disabilities, impaired growth, anemia, and hearing loss. During the health screening, it is important

Nursing Alert:

Antibiotic Resistance

Not every minor illness should be treated with antibiotics. Evidence is showing that resistance to antibiotics is increasing due to the indiscriminate use of antibiotics during childhood. Antibiotics should only be used for confirmed cases of bacterial infection, for example, strep throat.

BOX 10-2 Injury prevention guidelines

Home safety

- Establish and enforce consistent, explicit, and firm rules for safe behavior.
- Test smoke detectors to ensure that they work properly. Change batteries yearly.
- Keep all poisonous substances, cleaning agents, health and beauty supplies, medicines, and home improvement materials in a locked, safe place. Have safety caps on all medications.
- Keep cigarettes, lighters, matches, and alcohol out of the child's sight and reach.
- Ensure that guns, if in the home, are locked up and that the ammunition is stored separately.

Play safety

- Ensure that playgrounds are safe. Check for impact- or energy-absorbing surfaces under playground equipment.
- Teach the child about playground safety.
- Teach the child about sports safety, including the need to wear protective sports gear.

Water safety

- Ensure that home and neighborhood swimming pools are enclosed by a four-sided fence with a self-closing, self-latching gate. Children should be supervised by an adult whenever they are in or around water.
- Ensure that the child wears a life vest if boating.
- Teach the child how to swim.
- Teach the child safety rules for swimming pools.

Car safety

- Continue to use a car seat or a properly secured booster seat until the child's head is higher than the back of the seat. When the child moves out of a booster seat, ensure that the seat belt is always fastened when the car is moving.
- The child should always ride in the back seat.
- Never leave the child alone in the car or in the house.

Safety with others

- Keep the child away from cigarette smoke. Do not allow smoking in the home.
- Choose sitters carefully. Discuss with them their attitudes about behavior in relation to discipline.
- Teach the child safety rules regarding interacting with strangers.
- Ensure that the child is supervised before and after school in a safe environment.
- Teach the child his phone number and address in case he/she becomes lost.

Outdoor safety

- Put sunscreen on before going outside to play.
- Supervise all play near streets or driveways.
- Teach the child pedestrian and neighborhood safety skills.
- Teach the child about safety rules for getting to and from school.
- Teach the child about safety rules for bicycles. Teach the correct signals for traffic safety.
- Ensure that the child wears a bicycle helmet when riding a bicycle, tricycle, or scooter.

Emergency preparedness

- Keep your address and phone number posted near the phone.
- Keep your list of emergency numbers (doctor, hospital, nearest neighbor, poison control center, etc.) near the phone.
- Keep a 1-oz. bottle of syrup of ipecac in the home and use as directed by the poison control center or health care provider.

Adapted from Green, M. (Ed.) (1994). *Bright futures: Guidelines for health supervision of infants, children, and adolescents.* Arlington, VA: National Center of Education in Maternal and Child Health.

to determine whether or not the child is at risk for exposure to lead. If there is a risk, a venous blood lead level should be drawn as well as a complete blood cell count. If the blood lead level is >20 mcg/dL, medical treatment is necessary (Cohen, 2001).

The common health problems of the preschool years include mostly minor illnesses such as otitis media, colds, or gastrointestinal disturbances. In fact, during the preschool years, minor illnesses are more common than at any other age. This is probably because this is when most children start playing together more frequently, attend child care, or start preschool/school activities resulting in more exposure to illness. Therefore, teaching children hand washing principles (after using the bathroom and before eating) may decrease the incidence of illnesses.

PREPARATION FOR SCHOOL

During the preschool years, many children attend some type of early childhood program, either child care or preschool, which provides an excellent opportunity to encourage development. The experience can bring increased time for interaction with other children of the same age, teach group cooperation skills, stimulate language, physical, and social development, and help them cope with frustration and dissatisfaction (Brazelton, 1994; Dixon & Stein, 2000) (Figure 10-10).

Most early childhood programs include quiet play; active, outdoor activities; group activities and games; art projects; creative or free play; snack time; and rest time. All activities are tailored to provide mastery of skills and to give the child an increased sense of achievement, confidence, and success.

Caregivers often ask health care providers for advice on knowing when the child is ready to attend preschool or school. Even though there are no absolute indicators of school success, the child's social maturity (age, physical abilities, and ability to play with other children) and potential to participate in learning (can follow instructions and has an attention span that is long enough to be able to participate in activities) can provide an indication of readiness (Dixon & Stein, 2000).

Preparation for attending preschool/school can help the transition. Since there will be separation issues when the child initially starts school, this can be lessened by helping the child understand what will happen at school if the experience is presented as fun and exciting. If the child thinks school is an adventure and learning can be fun, the change will be embraced quicker.

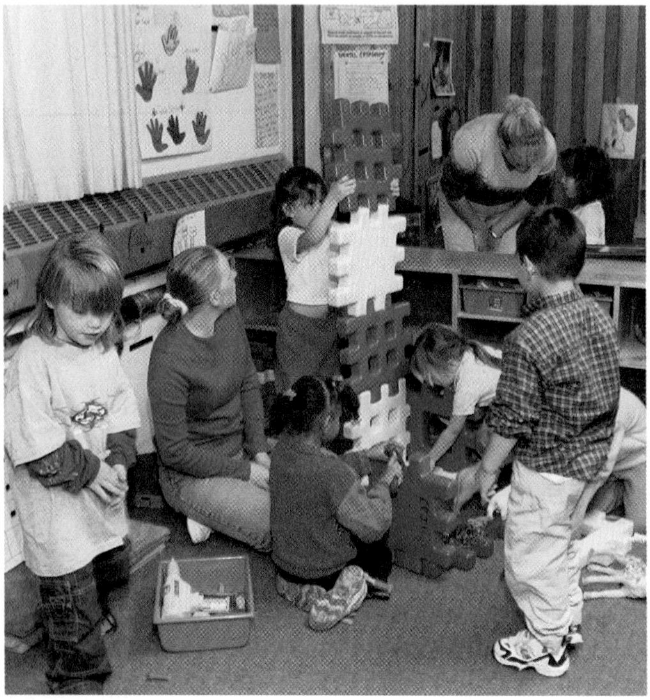

Figure 10-10 Group Cooperation Skills

Family Teaching

Preparation for the First Day of School

- Send detailed information about the child to the school, including familiar routines, favorite activities, food preferences, and names of siblings and parents.
- Put the child on a "school" schedule a few weeks before school actually starts. This will assist the child to feel comfortable with the routine before school actually begins.
- Practice school-type activities: ride the bus, have school lunch at home (play cafeteria), sit in chair at table to color, practice printing name, tie shoes, and have rest.
- Introduce child to the school, surroundings, and the teacher.
- Stay with the child on the first day if possible. Be available but not conspicuous.

DISCIPLINE AND LIMIT SETTING

Poor behavior is normal for all children. As a toddler, the child has learned to throw temper tantrums to get what is wanted. As the child becomes a preschooler, the same kind of tactics may be used. Limits are needed to help the child learn acceptable behavior. Initially, the child will test limits, but in the end, the child will welcome the limits because they define expected behaviors. If the child crosses over these boundaries, disciplinary action must be taken, and the child's behavior redirected in as positive a manner as possible (Green, 1994).

Time-outs can also be an effective method of discipline. No longer than 1 minute per each year of age, time-outs teach the child how to calm down and will give the child enough time to calm down but not too much time to become resentful (Brazelton, 1994).

One of the challenges of working with preschoolers is diverting aggressive behavior. Preschoolers tend to engage in instrumental aggression, that is, aggression designed to unblock a blocked goal such as a getting back an object, territory, or privilege. The caregiver needs to encourage sharing and nonaggressive ways of resolving conflict. Preschoolers engage in modeling, which is imitating behavior that they witness. It is important for caregivers to not only model positive behavior but reward for positive behavior (Charlesworth, 2000).

An effective tool for teaching appropriate behavior is **reverse attention.** Our society tends to give attention to bad behavior and ignores good behavior. The news is filled with reports of robberies, murders, and other bad behavior. Rarely does the news highlight a person who never causes any trouble, pays their bills on time, and takes good care of their families. This trend toward focusing on negative behavior is also seen within the family. The child who is quietly coloring is left alone, but when the child colors on the walls, parents discipline the behavior. Caregivers need to be taught to reward good behavior in addition to disciplining negative behavior (Brazelton, 1994).

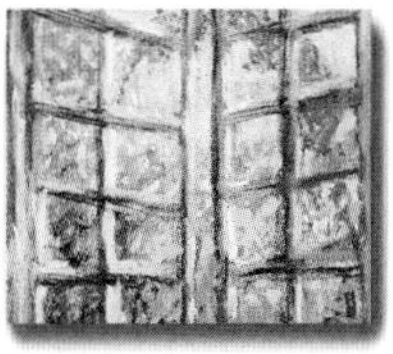

In the Real World

I never thought I would get used to the questions my preschool clients asked. But now, that age is my favorite age to take care of. They are so honest, inquisitive, interested in learning all they can about what is going on around them, and willing to help. I love reading them stories. Many times they know the story by heart and will tell me if I forget to read a paragraph or talk about one of the pictures. Isn't it too bad that, as children get older, they lose the inhibitions they had as preschoolers?

Key Concepts

- The preschool years are characterized by the refinement of physical, motor, cognitive, and social skills.
- The preschooler is in the preoperational stage of cognitive development where he learns to perform mental operations that are governed by his own perception and understanding of events.
- During the preschool years, the child develops a sense of initiative versus guilt.
- The preschooler learns ADLs, including how to dress self, tie shoes, and brush teeth.
- The preschool child learns to cooperate with other children, and enjoys associative and cooperative play.
- The beginning of moral judgment is obtained as the child learns what is right and wrong based on the punishments and rewards established by caregivers.
- Health promotion is directed toward proper nutrition, sleep/rest, activity, and dental health.
- Preschoolers need close supervision in the home, by water, outdoors, or on the playground in order to prevent injury.
- The preschool child should visit a health care provider on a yearly basis for a routine assessment of health and development.
- A child's readiness for participation in school is determined by the child's social maturity and readiness to learn.
- Give attention for good behavior, and ignore negative behavior.

Review Questions

1. Describe physical growth during the preschool years.
2. List several tests of motor function for a 3-year-old that is included on the DDST.
3. Give an example of animism and transductive reasoning.
4. Explain the language development skills of the preschooler.
5. Describe how a child who has achieved a sense of initiative may react to a new situation.
6. Is it normal for the preschooler to have an imaginary friend? When would you be concerned about this imaginary friend?
7. What is a rule to follow when serving food to a preschooler?
8. List some common sleep disturbances that may occur during the preschool years.
9. Why would a preschooler grind his or her teeth at night?
10. When can a preschooler stop riding in a car safety seat?

References

American Academy of Pediatrics, Committee on Public Education. (1999). Media education. *Pediatrics, 104*(2), 341–343.

Berry, B. E., Simons, B. D., Siatkowski, R. M., Schiffman, J. C., Flynn, J. T., & Duthie, M. J. (2001). Preschool vision screening using the MTI-photoscreener™. *Pediatric Nursing, 27*(1), 27–34.

Brazelton, T. B. (1994). *Touchpoints*. New York: Perseus Press.

Buiten, C., & Metzger, B. (2000). Childhood obesity and risk of cardiovascular disease: A review of the science. *Pediatric Nursing, 26*(1), 13–18.

Centers for Disease Control and Prevention. (1991). Public Health Service report on fluoride benefits and risks. *Morbidity and Mortality Weekly Report, 40*(RR-7): 1–8.

Charlesworth, R. (2000). *Understanding child development.* (5th ed.). Albany, NY: Delmar.

Cohen, S. M. (2001). Lead poisoning: A summary of treatment and prevention. *Pediatric Nursing, 27*(3), 125–130.

Dixon, S. D., & Stein, M. T. (2000). *Encounters with children: Pediatric behavior and development* (3rd ed.). St. Louis, MO: Mosby.

Erikson, E. H. (1963). *Childhood and society*. New York: Norton.

Freud, S. (1959). *Collected papers.* New York: Basic Books.

Green, M. (Ed.) (1994). *Bright futures: Guidelines for health supervision of infants, children, and adolescents.* Arlington, VA: National Center of Education in Maternal and Child Health.

Kohlberg, L. (1981). *The philosophy of moral development, moral states, and the idea of justice.* New York: Harper & Row.

Leland, J. (1999, June 19). The magnetic tube. *Newsweek, Special Issue*, 89–90.

Lytle, R., & Lytle, D. (2000, December). Play, playfulness, and expressive activities. *Exceptional Parent Magazine*, pp. 64–70.

Murphy, J. M. (1999). Pediatric occupant car safety: Clinical implications based on recent literature. *Pediatric Nursing, 25*(2), 137–148.

Myers, S., & Vargas, Z. (2000). Parental perceptions of the preschool obese child. *Pediatric Nursing, 26*(1), 23–30.

Piaget, J. (1969). *The theory of stages in cognitive development.* New York: McGraw-Hill.

Roberts, S. (2000). The role of physical activity in the prevention and treatment of childhood obesity. *Pediatric Nursing, 26*(1), 33–41.

Stanford Sleep Center. (2000). *Children's sleep problems* [On-line]. Available: www.stanford.edu/~dement

USOE Family Literacy Program. (2000, October). *Early literacy development.* Paper presented at Seminar, Salt Lake City, UT.

Suggested Readings

American Academy of Pediatrics, Committee on Nutrition. (1988). Fluoride supplementation for children. *Pediatrics, 95*(5), 800.

American Academy of Pediatrics, Committee on Nutrition. (1993). *Pediatric nutrition handbook.* (3rd ed.). Elk Grove Village, IL: Author.

Bibace, R., & Walsh, M. E. (1980). Development of children's concepts of illness. *Pediatrics, 66*, 912–917.

Chen, J., & Kennedy, C. M. (2001). Ask the expert: Television viewing and children's health. *Journal of the Society of Pediatric Nurses, 6*(1), 35–38.

Curry, D. M., & Duby, J. C. (1994). Developmental surveillance by pediatric nurses. *Pediatric Nursing, 20*(1), 40–44.

Davidhizar, R., Havens, R., & Bechtel, G. A. (1999). Assessing culturally diverse pediatric clients. *Pediatric Nursing, 25*(4), 371–375.

Dokken, D., & Sydnor-Greenberg, N. (2000). Exploring complementary and alternative medicine in pediatrics: Parents and professionals working together for new understanding. *Pediatric Nursing, 26*(4), 383–390.

Hall-Long, B. A., Schell, K., & Corrigan, V. (2001). Youth safety education and injury prevention program. *Pediatric Nursing, 27*(3), 141–146.

Hauck, M. R. (1991). Cognitive abilities of preschool children: Implications for nurses working with young children. *Journal of Pediatric Nursing, 6*(4), 230–235.

Henry, J., & Giordano, B. (1992). Introduction-assessment of growth in infants and children: Normal and abnormal patterns. *Journal of Pediatric Health Care*, 5, 289–290.

Kennedy, C. M. (2000). Television and young Hispanic children's health behaviors. *Pediatric Nursing, 26*(3), 283–291.

Knestrick, J., & Milstead, J. A. (1998). Public policy and child lead poisoning: Implementation of title X. *Pediatric Nursing, 24*(1), 37–41.

Manworren, R. C. B., & Woodring, B. (1998). Evaluating children's literature as a source for patient education. *Pediatric Nursing, 24*(6), 548–553.

Sawicki, J. A. (1997). Sibling rivalry and the new baby: Anticipatory guidance and management strategies. *Pediatric Nursing, 23*(3), 298–302.

Schonfeld, D. J. (1993). Talking with children about death. *Journal of Pediatric Health Care, 7*, 269–274.

Selekman, J. (1998). Infectious diseases and the immunizations of today and tomorrow. *Pediatric Nursing, 24*(4), 309–315.

Strasburger, V. C., & Donnerstein, E. (1999). Children, adolescents and the media: Issues and solutions. *Pediatrics, 103*(1), 129–139.

Vessey, J. A. (1995). Developmental approaches to examining young children. *Pediatric Nursing, 21*(1), 53–56.

Resources

Organizations and Websites

The American Academy of Pediatrics
141 Northwest Point Blvd.
Elk Grove Village, IL 60007-1098
(847) 434-4000
www.aap.org

The American Academy of Family Physicians
11400 Tomahawk Creek Parkway
Leawood, KS 66211-2672
(800) 274-2237
www.aafp.org

Centers for Disease Control and Prevention
(800) 311-3435
www.cdc.gov

Kid Source Online
www.kidsource.com

National Institute of Child Health & Human Development
Bldg 31 RM 2A32, MSC 2425
31 Center Dr.
Bethesda, MD 20892-2425

National Safe Kids Campaign
www.safekids.com

CHAPTER 11

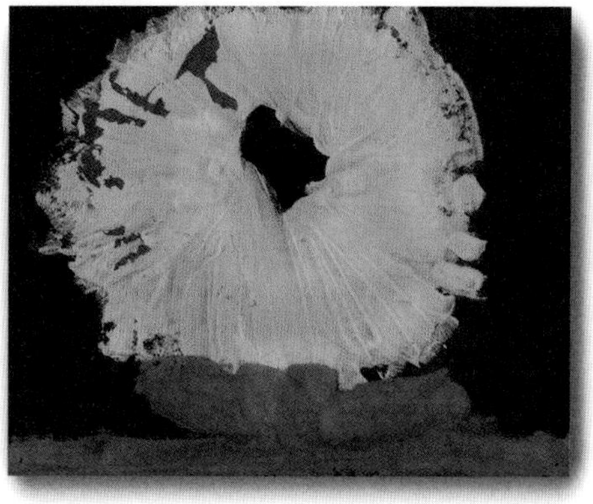

GROWTH AND DEVELOPMENT OF THE SCHOOL-AGED CHILD

Susan O'Conner-Von, DNSc, RNC

I can't believe the differences between Eshawn (6) and Tonjia (12). When Eshawn comes home from school, he jumps up on my lap, hugs me, and eagerly tells me all about his day. Tonjia, on the other hand, quickly greets me, grabs a cookie and soda, immediately goes to her room, turns on her CD player and calls her girlfriends to talk. They also are "into" different things. Eshawn enjoys puttering around the house on Saturdays with his dad, but Tonjia would rather spend the day at the mall with her friends. What a difference 6 years make in children!

COMPETENCIES

Upon completion of this chapter, the reader will be able to:

- *Describe the normal physical growth pattern for the school-aged child.*
- *Discuss Freud's latency phase of psychosexual development.*
- *Offer examples of concrete operations of the school-aged child.*
- *Explain Erikson's major task of school-age psychosocial development.*
- *Describe the characteristics of moral development during school-age.*
- *Explain the nurse's role in caring for school-aged children.*
- *Discuss the significance of school and peers for the school-aged child.*
- *Identify common stressors of the school-aged child and coping strategies to help them manage.*

The phase of development from 6 to 12 years, the **school-age years,** is crucial to establishing positive self-esteem, a sense of belonging, and feelings of competence. It is during this time that the child moves from egocentric thought to experiencing the world through peers and the school environment. Today's child entering school, like never before, can experience the world beyond the classroom with the help of the Internet, electronic mail, educational videotapes and cable television.

This chapter begins with a description of the normal growth and development parameters of the school-aged child, including physiological, psychosexual, cognitive, psychosocial, and moral development and concludes with health promotion and the role of the nurse in safety promotion and injury prevention.

PHYSIOLOGICAL DEVELOPMENT

The school-age years are marked by a steady rate of physical growth. However, caregivers and nurses need to keep in mind that each child is unique and growth is affected by genetics, gender, the presence of acute or chronic illness, and the environment (Rudolph & Kamei, 1998). A vital mechanism influencing physical development during the school-age years is growth hormones. These hormones are carried in the bloodstream and stimulate cells to grow throughout the body. The pituitary gland and hypothalamus, located at the base of the brain, are believed to play key roles in stimulating physical growth. The brain and skull growth slows down during the school-age years, and will increase little from that point.

Musculoskeletal

During the school-age years, the child's weight increases by 5 to 6 pounds per year and height increases by 2 inches per year (Schor, 1999). At 6 years, the average boy weighs 45 pounds and is 46 inches tall; the average girl weighs 43 pounds and is 45 inches tall. At 12 years, the average male weighs 88 pounds and is 59 inches tall; the average female weighs 91 pounds and is 60 inches tall. Skeletal growth is particularly noticeable in the long bones of the extremities. Growing pains, which occur because the long bones grow faster than the attached muscles, affect up to 15% of school-aged children (Rudolph & Kamei, 1998).

Muscle strength and size also increase at a gradual rate during school-age years (Figure 11-1) and six basic gross motor skills (balancing, catching, throwing, running, jumping, climbing) continue to be refined. At the same time, improved balance and coordination enable the school-aged child to explore new physical activities, such as bike riding and rollerblading. These newly found activities are often met with enthusiasm. However, muscles can be easily injured so physical activities should be selected according to the abilities of the child.

Boys have a greater number of muscle cells than females, so it is common to find they do well with gross motor activities, such as throwing and running. In contrast, girls tend to have better dexterity of fingers and hands, so they are more adept at fine motor (small muscle) skills during the school-age years. As eye–hand coordination and motor skills improve, the school-aged child is able to write, tie shoes, and become autonomous in dressing. Motor development progresses in a cephalocaudal and proximal to distal direction, with refinement of both gross motor and fine motor skills occurring as the central nervous system matures (Rudolph & Kamei, 1998).

To meet the increased activity levels during the school-age years, the cardiovascular and respiratory systems

Critical Thinking

Physiological Development

Eight-year-old Ryan and ten-year-old Wally have come to the office for a physical. Ryan weighs 43 pounds and is 45 inches tall. Wally weighs 68 pounds and is 50 inches tall. The boys are accompanied by their mother; she is worried about their weight and height. Why is she showing concern? What does the nurse need to consider when answering the mother?

Kids Want To Know

Why do I wake up at night with cramps in my legs?

Growing pains are temporary and caused by bones growing faster than muscles. The discomfort is usually located in the knees, calves, and thighs. Comfort measures that can be used at home include analgesics, gentle massage, and a warm bath. Shoes that are sturdy and supportive are also helpful.

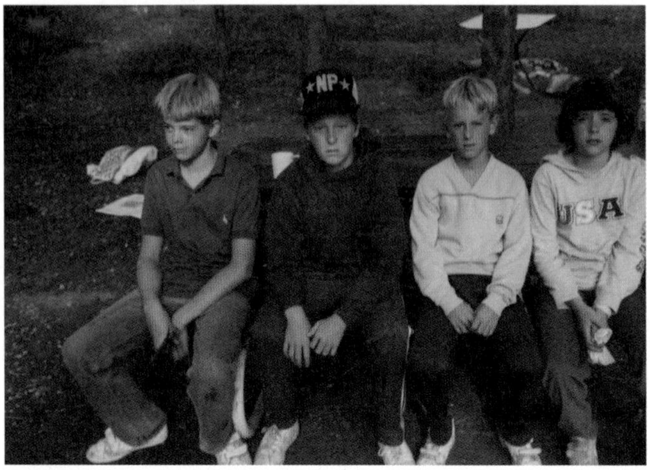

Figure 11-1 School-age children mature at different rates.

Kids Want To Know

Will I have to undress during my check-up? What is happening to my body?

By the time a child reaches 9 years of age, honest discussion by caregivers is warranted about upcoming physical examinations and changes. Caregivers are encouraged to use correct terms when discussing these changes, be aware of the importance of modesty, and stay with their child during an exam to offer support.

Nursing Alert:

Innocent Heart Murmur

As many as 50% of all school-aged children have an "innocent" heart murmur between 6 and 10 years of age. These murmurs are not clinically significant, but may be a concern to the caregiver if found during a routine physical exam.

Family Teaching

Heart Murmur

- Explain to caregivers that an "innocent" murmur is created from the sound of the blood flowing through the heart and can be heard because of the child's thin chest wall.
- Reassure the child and caregiver that the murmur is not associated with heart disease and will no longer be heard when the child reaches adolescence.
- Provide the school nurse with medical documentation confirming the presence of an innocent heart murmur.
- Provide coaches with medical documentation confirming the presence of an innocent heart murmur.

develop in size and capacity. The heart growth slows and the heart assumes a more vertical position in the chest and the diaphragm descends to allow for lung expansion. As the cardiac and respiratory systems become more efficient, the pulse and respiratory rates slow down. The average apical pulse rate for the school-aged child is 90 to 95 beats per minute while at rest. The average respiratory rate for the school-aged child is 20 breaths per minute while at rest. In addition, the **tidal volume** (amount of air inhaled or exhaled with each breath) doubles (Stedman's Medical Dictionary, 2000).

Dental

It is during the school-age years that the 20 **deciduous** or baby **teeth** are shed and the permanent teeth appear. This process usually starts at age 5 years and is complete before adolescence, except for the third molars (wisdom teeth). The first permanent teeth appear by age 6 years and are called the central incisors and first molars. Over the next five years, the deciduous teeth are replaced at a rate of 4 teeth per year. When children start to lose their teeth, the rate of loss is determined by genetics and gender. It is common for girls to lose their teeth earlier than boys. However, for both boys and girls, by the end of the school-age years, the 20 deciduous teeth are replaced by 28 of the 32 permanent teeth (Stedman's Medical Dictionary, 2000). Often the permanent front teeth seem too large for the face giving the child an odd look. This look is also attributed to the face growing faster than the skull (Figure 11-2).

Family Teaching

Dental Health

To maintain proper dental health, regular teeth brushing and flossing are important during the school-age years.

Assess the school-aged child for correct teeth brushing and flossing technique. Advise caregivers to monitor the school-aged child at home, encourage brushing at least twice a day, and schedule regular visits to the dentist (Schor, 1999). Also advise caregivers to purchase a toothbrush with a small brush head with soft bristles for their school-aged child and replace every 2 to 3 months.

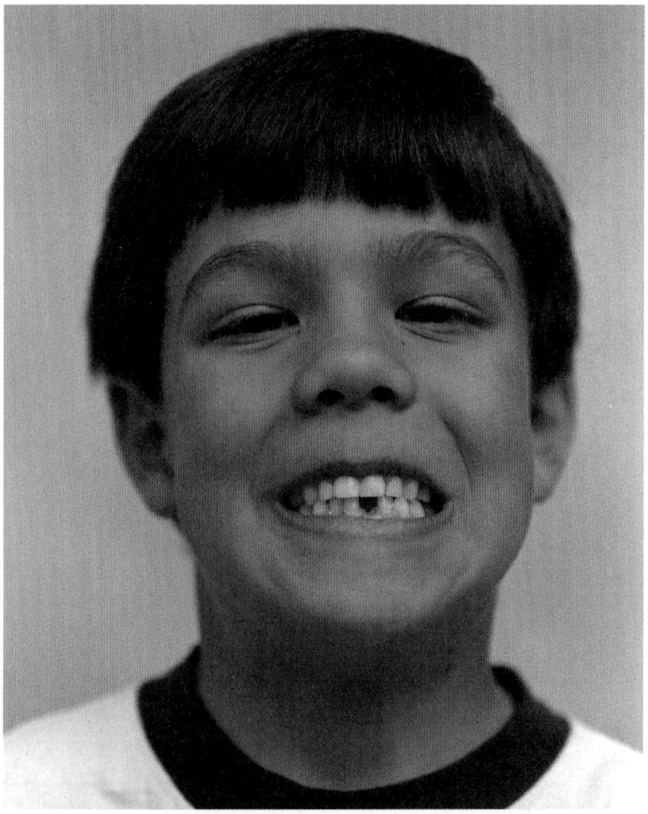

Figure 11-2 During ages 6–11, a child loses his or her deciduous teeth.

During the preschool years, children are exposed to and develop immunity to a variety of microorganisms. Therefore, the school-age years are often one of the healthiest phases of life. Antibodies are produced by the lymphatic system and reach their peak by age 7 years. For example, IgA, which protects the respiratory and gastrointestinal tracts from pathogens, and IgG, which activates destruction of bacteria, are found at adult levels during this time. Because of the increase in body size and maturity of the immune system, school-aged children are able to respond to illnesses similar to adults.

REFLECTIONS FROM FAMILIES

My father never told me about sex, instead I learned about it from the other guys on my little league baseball team. At that point in my life, the thought of sex was repulsive and I thought there is no way I could even think about it. Now that I am a father, I plan to be honest with my son and tell him about sex within the context of a loving relationship.

PSYCHOSEXUAL DEVELOPMENT

Freud (1923) believed that the first five years of life were the most critical to psychosexual development. Starting at age 6 years and throughout school-age, the child enters a calm period in the development of their sexuality, called **latency.** Freud theorized that the school-aged child identifies with the same-sex parent by modeling the behaviors and emotions of this parent (see Chapter 6 for more information on Freud's theory). The child also learns about sex-role behavior and identity by observing caregiver interactions, the media, and friendships with children of the same gender.

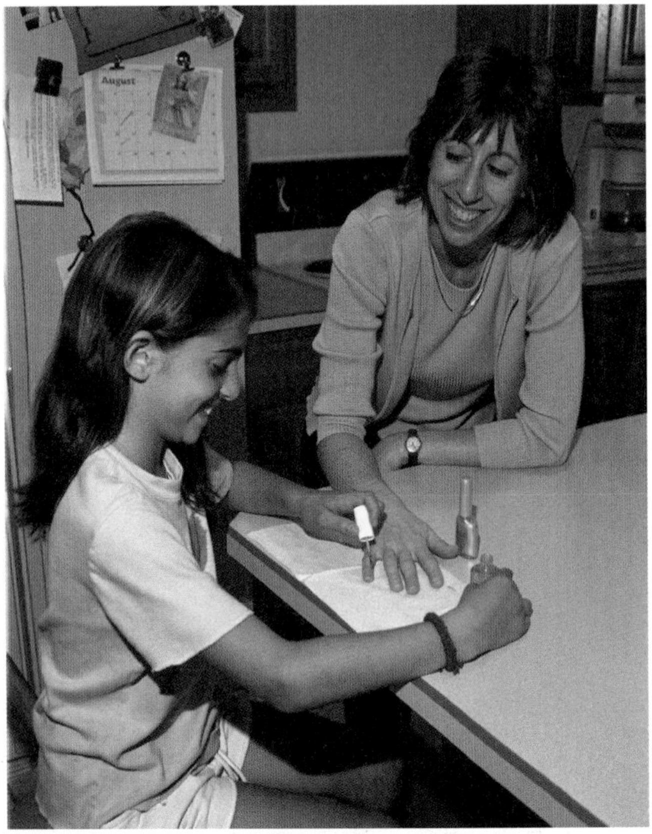

Figure 11-3 Prepubescence starts between the ages of 9 and 12 years of age in females.

Sexual Development

The last years of the school-age period are called prepubescence, meaning the two years before **puberty** (Figure 11-3). Puberty comes from the Latin word *pubertas*, meaning adult (Steinberg, 1999) and is considered the stage of human maturation when secondary sex characteristics begin to develop and females start **menarche** (see Chapter 12). The first physiological signs of prepubescence, such as breast tissue development, can appear as early as 9 years of age in females. However, in the United States, the average age of puberty is 12 years for females and 14 years for males (Santrock, 1998).

COGNITIVE DEVELOPMENT

Piaget (1962) suggested that around 6 years of age, children start to move from the egocentric view of the preschool age to the more open and flexible thought of the school-aged child. As children learn about the ideas of their peers and adults, they are able to see things from another's point of view.

The expanded cognitive abilities enable the child to imagine the world without having to experience it. However, because abstract thought has not been developed, the child is limited to thinking concretely and in the present time frame. During these **concrete operations,** the child gains the skills of **classification** (the ability to group items according to common characteristics), **conservation** (the ability to acknowledge that a change in shape does not mean a change in amount), and **reversibility** (the ability to recognize that actions can move in reverse order). For example, the child who has mastered classification can group animals according to the dog, cat, or horse family, and often collects baseball cards, coins, and rocks. Conservation emerges as the child's

Nursing Tip:

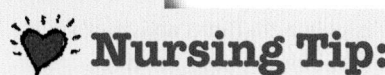

Understanding the concepts of time, height, weight, and volume

Because of the child's skill in concrete operations, more detail can be included when preparing the child for new health care experiences. For example, in preparing a child for an upper gastrointestinal series, the nurse can explain the scheduled date and time of the procedure, how the procedure will be performed, and show the child the amount of barium to be used. This detailed explanation, as well as the child's increased participation in self-care and treatment are important when caring for the school-aged child.

egocentric thinking is replaced by cognitive reasoning, develops over time, and begins with the conservation of numbers, followed by mass, weight, and volume. Reversibility is important when learning addition and subtraction, and is seen when a child can reassemble a toy or play a game in reverse order (Figure 11-4 and Figure 11-5).

Language and Reading

During the school-age years, the child's ability to use language is enhanced and vocabulary expands from 2,000 to 50,000 words (Click, 1998). By six, the school-aged child uses six-word sentences and can follow a story without the use of pictures. By seven, the school-aged child understands time and the difference between right and left and by eight, the child can use language as a tool for reasoning (Dixon & Stein,

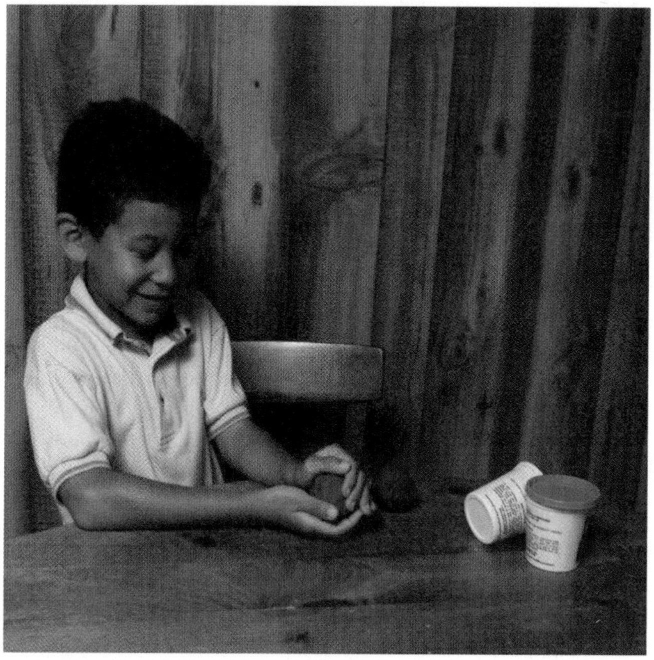

Figure 11-5 This young boy will master the concepts of conservation, reversibility, and classification before moving on to adolescence.

Original	Physical Change	Question	Nonconserving Response	Conserving Response
Child agrees that the same amount of drink is contained in each glass. 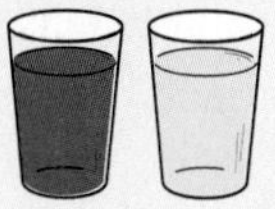	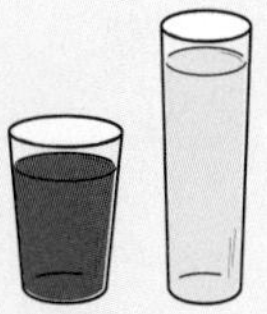	Is there still the same amount of drink in each glass, or does one glass have more?	No, they are not the same; there is more in the tall glass.	Yes, they have the same amount; you just put the drink in a different size glass. It is taller, but it is also thinner.
Child agrees each ball contains the same amount of clay. 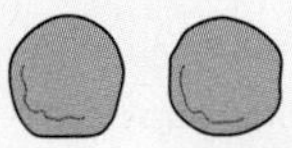	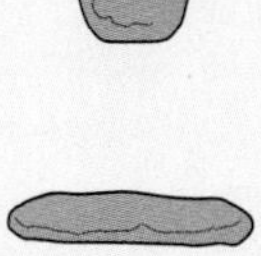	Is there still the same amount of clay in the ball and the snake, ordoes one have more?	No, there is more clay in the snake because it is longer (or more in the ball because it is fatter).	Yes, they have the same amount. You just rolled one ball out in a different shape.

Figure 11-4 Physical Changes in Conservation Tasks. *Source:* Charlesworth, R. (2000). *Understanding child development* (5th ed.). Albany, NY: Delmar.

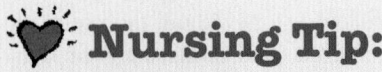

> **Nursing Tip:**
>
> **Explain medical terms**
>
> Language unites groups and cultures. Medicine has a distinct language from mainstream society. Therefore, when caring for school-aged children, it is important to use correct terminology they will understand. Since children of this age may interpret each word literally, avoid using terms such as "taking a CAT scan" or "being put to sleep." Instead, explain the sequence of events the child will experience and exactly what will happen.

2000). School-aged children also can learn the literal meaning of words and are beginning to understand a word's nonliteral meaning. By 11 years of age, metaphors are understood and used in conversation, such as when describing a headache as "drums pounding in my head." However, temperament, social and cultural factors, and verbal and language environment affect language acquisition. This is especially true of expressive verbal skills (Rudolph & Kamei, 1998).

Besides a tool for communication, language becomes a tool for socialization as the school-aged child's language becomes less egocentric. However, because their mental capacity and control of language is not fully developed, nurses need to use words school-aged children can understand and carefully assess their comprehension.

During the school-age years children begin to acquire the ability to read, through letter identification, telling a story from looking at the pictures, and being read to. Reading should be encouraged by choosing books the child enjoys, being read to by an adult, and reading alone.

PSYCHOSOCIAL DEVELOPMENT

The school-age years introduce the child to the world of peers and school. As each child interacts within this new context, a more realistic sense of self and place in this world evolves. A newfound independence from caregivers is discovered and peers become a major socializing agent. Because they are the major socializing agents at this time, children behave according to what they deem is acceptable to their friends. Although school-aged children need the love and support provided by caregivers, peers provide the support needed to gain independence from family as increased amounts of time are spent with peers of the same gender.

The developmental theory of Erik Erikson (1963) identified the major task of the school-age period as **industry** (the ability to be useful or productive) **versus inferiority** (see Chapter 6 for more information on Erikson's theory). During this time, energy is channeled into activities such as school projects, sports, and hobbies. These concrete endeavors become the child's work and bring a sense of accomplishment and worth (Figure 11-6). It is during this stage that the school-aged child also develops the ability to work with others on school projects and athletic teams in preparation for becoming a citizen of the world.

Erikson (1963) believed development is a continual process based on prior success, and if children are not able to realize a sense of industry, feelings of inferiority may develop. This occurs when children feel they cannot live up to the expectations of caregivers or teachers, or when they feel different from peers. In order for school-aged children to feel a sense of competence, it is imperative that they have a positive relationship with an affirming adult (Figure 11-7). If unable to receive the support needed from caregivers or teachers, a school nurse, club leader, or coach may be instrumental in instilling this positive sense of competence.

Self-Concept

The development of a positive self-concept and self-esteem are critical at this time. Self-concept is influenced by physical appearance, athletic ability, academic achievement, approval from caregivers, and is shaped by comparisons with peers (Overbay & Purath, 1997). Caregivers and peers also play a role in determing self-esteem, a global evaluation of self also known as self-image or self-worth. The closer the

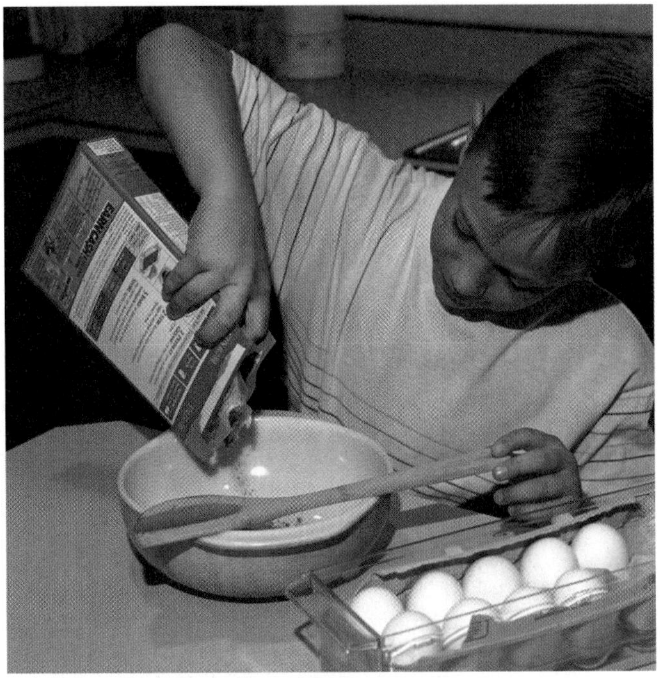

Figure 11-6 Making brownies brings a sense of accomplishment to this young man.

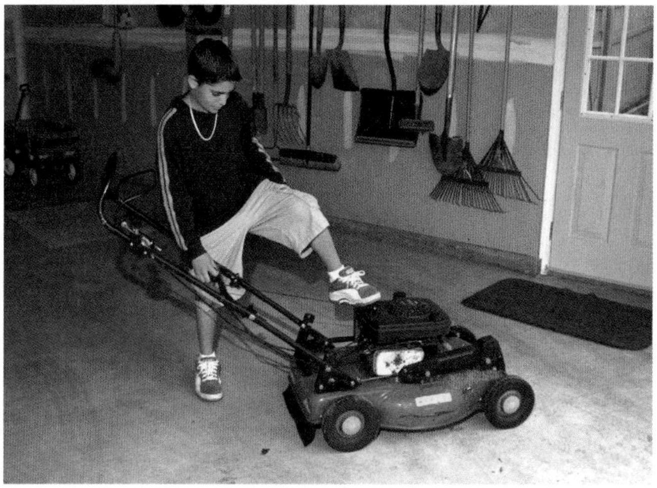

Figure 11-7 School-aged boys can learn role behavior by watching caregivers as they work around the house.

perceived self is to the ideal self (how the child would like to be) the higher the child's self-esteem. Acceptance by peers also influences a child's sense of self-worth and healthy body image. Examples of positive self-esteem include the ability to express an opinion, work cooperatively with others, and initiate a conversation. A child with poor self-esteem may feel shame, inadequacy, and the inability to gain respect from others (Schor, 1999).

MORAL DEVELOPMENT

Kohlberg (1969) proposed eight stages of moral development (see Chapter 6 for more information on Kohlberg's theory). The school-aged child is at the **conventional level** (Stages 3 and 4) of moral development, when the conscience develops an internal set of "rules" that must be followed in order to "be good." During Stage 3 (ages 6 to 10 years), the child's morality is based on avoiding the disapproval of others, and maintaining a positive relationship with friends, family, and teachers (Figure 11-8). Accidents can be viewed as punishment for disobeying. For instance, a toy breaking may be punishment for spilling milk in the family room where drinking is prohibited. During Stage 4 (ages 11 and 12 years), the child is concerned with doing the "right" thing and showing respect for authority figures. Children at this level can also demonstrate rigid behavior in an effort to obey the law. These children can take into account circumstances surrounding an incident rather than just looking at the result. Older school-aged children understand the need to treat others as they would like to be treated.

Table 11-1 describes key milestones for school-aged children.

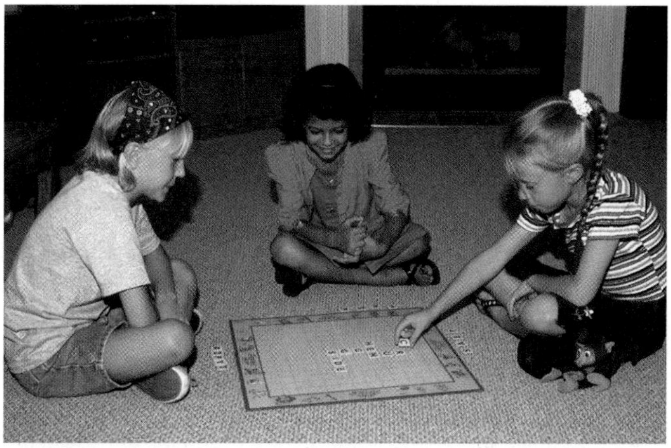

Figure 11-8 School-aged children learn how to abide by rules, making board games a popular choice.

TABLE 11-1 School-age Milestones

6 to 7 Years

Gross and Fine Motor Skill	Cognitive Development	Social Development
Legibly prints letters.	Learning to tell time.	Able to bathe and dress self.
Uses knife, fork, and spoon.	Learning to read. Can read from memory.	Able to fix own hair.
Rides 2-wheel bike.	Understands right and left.	Enjoys games with peers of same gender.
Masters all skills on the DDST.	Knows value of currency.	Shares and cooperates.
Improved dexterity.	Interested in magic and fantasy.	May be jealous of younger siblings.
Cuts, pastes, folds paper.	Defines common objects according to their use.	Needs praise and recognition.
Ties shoe laces.		Fewer mood swings.
Throws overhand.		

continues

TABLE 11-1 *Continued*

6 to 7 Years *(continued)*

Gross and Fine Motor Skill	Cognitive Development	Social Development
Copies a diamond. Walks a straight line.	Understands concept of numbers. Attention span increasing. Enjoys word and spelling games. Obeys three commands. Likes to help. Knows right and left hand. Concrete, animistic thinking Attends first and second grades. Reflective.	Enjoys helping around the house. Participates in school and community activities. Attentive listener. Demonstrates independence. Spends time in quiet play.

8 to 9 Years

Gross and Fine Motor Skill	Cognitive Development	Social Development
Developing eye-hand coordination. More fluid movement. Plays team sports. Body becomes flexible. Able to use household tools. Writes using cursive. Dresses self completely. Jumps, skips, draws three-dimensional figures.	Understands concept of time. Knows the date and month. Collects and classifies objects. Increased ability to read. Learning fractions. Understands space, cause, effect, conservation. Knows similarities and differences of objects. Counts backward from 20. Shows interest in music lessons. Can make change (small currency). Helps around the house. Can be critical of accomplishment and failure. Learns from experiences. Punctual. Improvises simple activities. Less animistic in thinking. Attends third and fourth grades.	Likes competitive games and sports. Runs errands. Social, well behaved. Modest. Demanding and critical of others. Compares self with others. Looks up to adults. Dependable, responsible. Rules are important. Able to do household chores. Best friends are important. Tolerant and accepting of others.

10 to 12 Years

Gross and Fine Motor Skill	Cognitive Development	Social Development
Eye-hand coordination well developed. Fine motor skills well developed.	Developing ability for abstract thought. Able to write stories.	Rules are important. Interest in opposite sex. Quarrelsome with siblings.

continues

TABLE 11-1 *Continued*

10 to 12 Years *(continued)*

Gross and Fine Motor Skill	Cognitive Development	Social Development
Gross motor skills may become awkward with growth spurt. Balances on one foot for 15 seconds. Catches a fly ball. Cooks and sews.	Drawings are detailed. Easily distracted. Knows death is irreversible. More realistic than idealistic. Truthful. Reads for enjoyment; reads well. Knows limits. Interested in the future. Likes to memorize and identify facts. Likes to discuss and debate. Unaware of effect on others. Beginning formal operations.	Developing social competence. Self-disciplined. Easy to please. Obedient. May have best friend. Becoming diplomatic. Affectionate, sensitive. Respects parents. Self-directed and independent. Can stay at home alone for short. periods of time. Increased interest in family.

Nursing Tip:

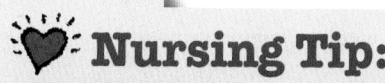

Modeling moral behavior

It is imperative that nurses model moral behavior and use sound moral judgment in caring for school-aged children and families. Nurses need to assist these youngsters in making decisions regarding their health care, keeping in mind they may agree with suggestions in order to do the "right thing." Nurses also need to present good health care options and encourage school-agers to choose the option that works best for them.

HEALTH PROMOTION AND MAINTENANCE

Nutrition

During the school-age years, the child becomes aware of how the body works and can more fully understand physical development and how to remain healthy because a steady rate of physical development is also occurring at this time. The nutritional needs of the school-aged child should remain relatively steady and children should be encouraged to make independent food choices. Eating a healthy breakfast before school is encouraged as a means to provide the essential nutrients needed for academic and physical performance. While at school, it is imperative that nutrition education be a part of the curriculum so the school-aged child will have the knowledge to select the most nutritious and appropriate quantities of food (Figure 11-9).

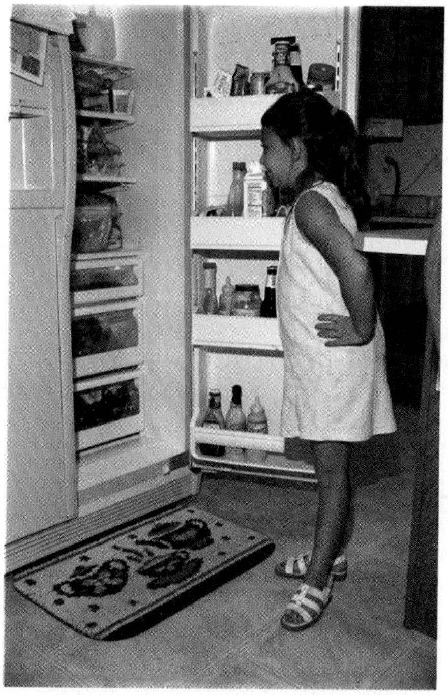

Figure 11-9 School-aged children are able to choose nutritious foods when they are available and should be encouraged to do so.

Eye On:

Dietary Differences

The diet of children raised in a traditional Native American household is usually high (35–50%) in fat and carbohydrates. The diet of children raised in traditional Hispanic American households usually consists of beans, salsa, tortillas, and rice with hot spices, and there is a tendency for these children to be heavier than their counterparts. Nurses need to be cognizant of family and ethnic traditions when counseling on nutrition and try to work these traditions into dietary planning.

Although school-aged children are more independent in making food choices, the influences of culture and caregivers cannot be ignored as eating habits established during childhood may be difficult to alter later in life. Leading a fast-paced life is common for many families today, so nutritious foods like fruits and vegetables must be readily available in order to avoid the temptation to live on fast-foods, which are often high in calories, fat, and sodium, and low in vitamins and minerals. If consumed on a regular basis, fast-foods can lead to obesity, a fact that probably contributes to the increase in obesity in children during the past three decades (Luder & Bonforte, 1996). Statistics collected over 10 years for the National Growth and Health Study revealed 30–32% of African-American girls and 21% of Caucasian girls, ages 9 to 10 years, were considered obese (Evers, 1997). Childhood obesity is a problem because it is associated with social isolation, lowered self-esteem, impaired potential for athletics, health problems, and long-range proclivity for heart disease, cancer, and diabetes (Covington, 1996). See Family Teaching box for steps in preventing childhood obesity.

Caregivers may be hesitant to limit the dietary intake of their school-aged child because of their concern regarding the nutrients needed for physical growth. However, careful meal planning, setting a schedule for snacks and meals, and physical activity are crucial for the physical and emotional health of the school-aged child. Table 11-2 includes the nutritional needs of the school-aged child.

Family Teaching

Steps in Preventing Childhood Obesity

1. Offer a variety of foods that are healthy.
2. Encourage your school-aged child to help with meal preparation.
3. Respect your child's ability to decide how much to eat.
4. Consult your physician if you are concerned about your child's weight.
5. Encourage physical activity and discourage sedentary activities such as watching television (Figure 11-10).

(Evers, 1997)

Sleep and Rest

By the time children reach school-age, most do not need to nap. Although nighttime sleep habits may vary, at 6 years children require at least 10 hours of sleep, and at 12 years children require 8 to 9 hours of sleep. Sleep is essential during the school-age years to foster physical growth and academic performance, and failure to receive adequate rest can lead to irritability and lack of attention span at school, which may lead to falling asleep and the potential of failing grades.

Nightmares and night terrors are less common during the school-age years. However, it is estimated that **somnambulism** or sleep walking, occurs in 15% of all school-aged children and is not uncommon between 4 and 8 years of age (Rudolph & Kamei, 1998). The sleepwalking event is usually not remembered in the morning, occurs more frequently in

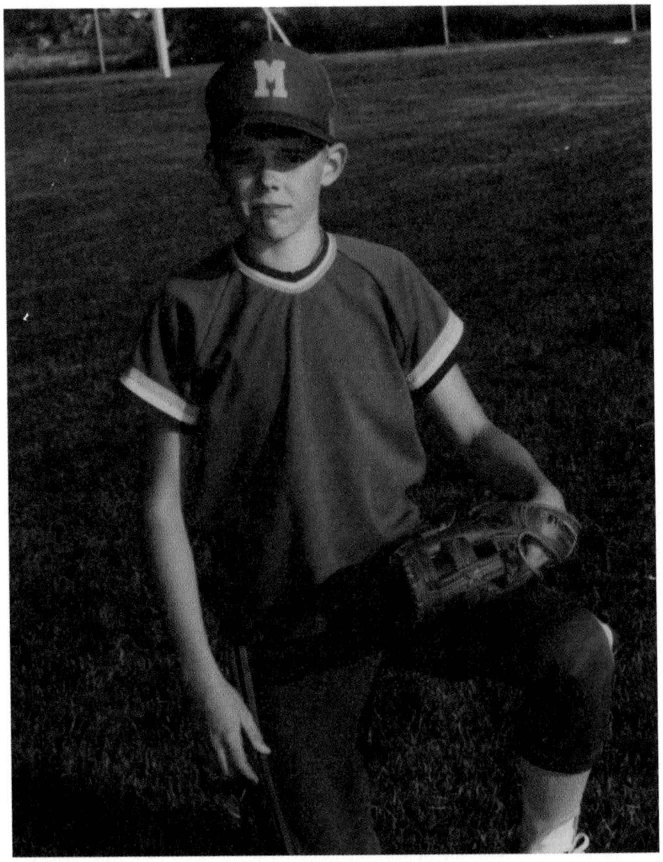

Figure 11-10 Outside activities help prevent obesity in childhood and promote self-esteem.

Research Highlight

Food Choices of Healthy School-aged Children

Study Purpose

To assess the school-aged child's knowledge base of healthy food choices so school nurses and teachers can develop dietary education programs.

Methods

One hundred and twenty-seven school-aged children, between 10 and 12 years or age were questioned regarding their knowledge of healthy food choices. The children attended public and private schools, and represented lower to middle socioeconomic levels. The Children's Nutritional Flash Cards, 23 flash cards with two food items on each, were used to gather data. The investigator showed the child each flash card and then asked the child to choose the healthier food item on each card.

Findings

Results showed most children knew the healthy foods, but were not able to consistently select the healthier food item. Only one child answered all questions correctly.

Implications

Because children become more independent in their food choices during the school years, school nurses and teachers can influence and increase their knowledge of proper nutrition through dietary assessment and education.

Citation

Colizza, D., & Colvin, S. (1995). Food choices of healthy school-age children. *Journal of School Nursing, 11* (4), 17–20.

Table 11-2 Nutritional Needs of the School-aged Child

Food	Daily Servings
Milk (Milk, cheese, yogurt)	2–3
Meat (Lean meat, chicken, fish, beans, eggs, peanut butter)	3 or more
Bread (Bread, cereal, rice, pasta)	6–9
Vegetables	3–5
Fruit	3–5

boys, and can be associated with nocturnal enuresis. Most children outgrow sleepwalking by adolescence. **Somniloquy** or sleep talking can occur at any age across the life span and does not indicate a health concern or need for intervention (Rudolph & Kamei, 1998).

Dental Health

School-aged children should be encouraged to brush at least twice a day and to floss before bedtime, to help prevent cavities. Because of the lack of manual dexterity, it is important to monitor and assist the younger school-aged child with tooth brushing and flossing. Caregivers need to be advised to provide fluoride toothpaste and keep regular dental check-ups in order to ensure healthy teeth. The child's first visits to the dentist can greatly influence future visits, so it is important to seek a pediatric dentist.

During the school-age period, **malocclusion** or an abnormality of the coming together of the teeth can occur when the permanent upper and lower teeth do not approximate, leaving them crowded or uneven and requiring a referral to an orthodontist. If braces are needed, frequent brushing and flossing are critical in preventing dental caries. An **evulsed tooth** (tooth that is knocked out) should be picked up, rinsed gently under water, and placed back in its socket. The child should hold the tooth in place. A dentist should be contacted immediately. If the tooth cannot be held in place, it should be put in cold milk or held in the mouth, under child's or caregiver's tongue until seen by a dentist.

Safety and Injury Prevention

The leading cause of death in this age group is accidents, so health care should be focused on accident prevention (Prescott, 1999). Factors contributing to the high incidence of accidents for this group are their increased independence, desire to have peer approval, and increased involvement in physically challenging activities. Most accidents are related to motor vehicles, but firearm injuries continue to increase in incidence (Children's Defense Fund, 2000). During the 1980s, violent crime for children ages 10 to 14 continued to steadily increase and by 1990, 1 of 8 deaths among children ages 10 to 14 years was caused by a firearm (Fingerhut, 1993). Currently, 12 children die each day from gunfire in the United States, which is one child every two hours. (Children's Defense Fund, 2000).

Because school-aged children may understand but resist rules established by adults in an effort to gain independence and peer approval, safety rules must be clearly defined through education and enforced with discipline. Critical are rules related to motor vehicle, bike, skateboard, and swimming safety, and avoidance of firearms and strangers. The Family Teaching box offers examples of important rules that need to be established and enforced by caregivers, nurses, and teachers.

Nursing Alert:

Children, Pickup Trucks, and Automobiles

- *Children riding in the cargo area of pickup trucks are at risk for death or injury if the vehicle is involved in an accident. Caregivers should be reminded not to allow their children to ride in that area.*
- *Children seated in the front seats of vehicles are at increased risk of death and injury in crashes. This holds especially true in vehicles with passenger-side airbags. Almost all children killed by airbags were either unrestrained or improperly restrained at the time of the crash. Children under 12 years of age should sit in the back seat.*
- *Seat belts fit correctly when the lap portion of the belt rides low over the hips. The well-fit shoulder belt crosses the sternum and shoulder. Correct seat belt fit is usually not achieved until the child is 9 years old.*

Health Screening

When compared to traditional standards, school-aged children enjoy excellent health (Prescott, 1999); when school-

Family Teaching

Safety Rules for School-aged Children

Motor vehicle	Always wear a seat belt, sit in backseat, especially in car with airbags.
Bike/skateboard/Rollerblades	Wear helmet, elbow and knee pads.
Pedestrian	Use caution when crossing streets, obey traffic lights.
Trampolines	Use should be discouraged.
Swimming	Learn how to swim, never swim alone.
	Wear a life jacket while in a boat.
	Do not dive in shallow water.
Firearms	Avoid guns, do not assume a gun is not loaded.
Strangers	Do not talk to strangers or accept rides from strangers.
	Learn home address and telephone number.
	Use 911 if needed and know how to call a safe neighbor.
Medicines	Should be kept out of reach; explain consequences of taking the drugs.
Drug use/Smoking	Teach about illicit drugs; counsel on why and how to avoid their use.
Burns	Teach escape route; cook/bake under supervision of adult.

aged children are sick, it is typically for a minor illness. School-aged children average two health care visits each year, with dental problems being the most frequent reason to visit a health care provider (Schor, 1998). The American Academy of Pediatrics (AAP) recommends routine medical exams for the school-aged child at least every 2 years, and suggests they occur at ages 5, 6, 8, 10, 11, and 12 years. These exams should include height, weight, vital signs, physical exam, vision and hearing screening, and assessment of dietary intake and use of tobacco/alcohol/ drugs (Schor, 1999). Scoliosis screening is also recommended (see Chapter 34 for more information). In addition, annual TB testing is recommended for any high-risk children.

Immunizations

By the time they enter kindergarten, most children have received all the recommended immunizations. For the school-aged child, booster shots of diphtheria, tetanus, and pertussis (DTP), and measles, mumps, and rubella vaccine (MMR) are recommended between the ages of 4 and 6 years. If the MMR booster is not given at this time, it is given at ages 11 to 12 years, as is the Td (tetanus and diphtheria) booster. Td is then repeated every 10 years as well. Refer to Appendix C for the current Immunization schedule.

School

School is an exciting new world because it provides the arena for physical, intellectual, and social development. Schools do affect the evolving character of the school-aged child and every school has the potential to actively encourage prosocial behavior. The teacher can guide and provide a structured environment where learning can take place, regulate what is being learned, how it is being learned, with whom it is being learned, and in what context the learning occurs.

Teachers serve as role models: they strive to stimulate intellectual development; are in a position to influence the child's attitudes and values; and can be an important factor in determining school success. The child facing extreme difficulties of poverty, abuse, and violence may find safe haven at school and learn to cope with life stressors because of a teacher's positive influence. Dedicated teachers must be credited with keeping students' performance at a steady pace when considering the conditions many children and families have faced over the past decades (Children's Defense Fund, 2000).

As social interaction and communication develop between school-aged children, so does their role in facilitating the transmission of knowledge. Vygotsky (1962) suggested that when a child of one stage of development helps another child of the same level of development, both benefit. Nurses can also use cooperative learning as an effective method of teaching the school-aged child in the health care setting.

Homework

School-aged children may occassonally have homework assignments, although many teachers try to allow time within the school day to complete assignments. If children do have school work that needs to be completed at home, the AAP (2001) suggests that caregivers:

1. Provide a positive atmosphere where children can work without being distracted. This means no television and an area that is free of clutter.
2. Show interest in the child's work. Check to see that the homework is complete and be prepared to explain the assignment if the child does not understand what the teacher has asked the child to do.
3. Be prepared to help the child in a particular subject that is difficult, or consider using a tutor.
4. Re-evaluate the after-school activities the child is involved in, especially if these activities leave little time to complete the homework assignment.

Play

Piaget (1962) described play during the school-age years as games with rules as the child is able to think more objectively, thus making group activities a possibility. Socially, school-aged children are beginning to understand the concept of cooperation and reflect this in their play as they work together for the good of their team. Strict adherence to rules provides the framework for playing the game and creating a sense of security. Children of this age enjoy video games and watching television. These activities should be limited as they are sedentary activities (Figure 11-11).

Play also provides the opportunity to learn what the body is physically capable of as gross and fine motor development are stimulated. By the time the school-aged child is

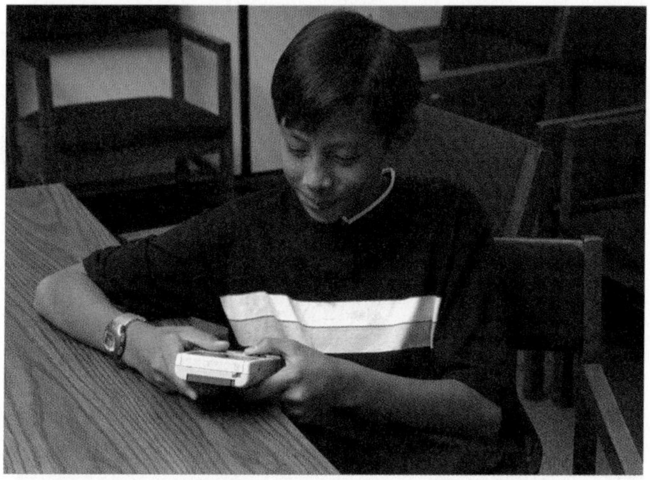

Figure 11-11 Hand-held computer games are popular with school-aged children. Their use should be limited as it is a sedentary activity.

Nursing Tip:

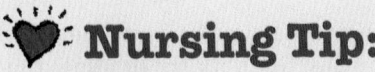

Encouraging play
During play children enact that which they cannot verbalize or physically demonstrate. As nurses, we can incorporate play into health care experiences as a way of helping children express needs and actively cope with experiences. Scribbling, finger painting, coloring, and drawing are useful tension-reducing methods, which are inexpensive and can foster a child's creativity (Ryan-Wenger, 1998).

6 years old, the physical strength and stamina for team sports have developed, contributing to physical health and release of frustrations (Figure 11-12). Children enjoy playing board games, starting collections, participating in, listening to, or playing music.

Physical Activity

Physical activity is important in maintaining a healthy lifestyle (Long & Williams, 1998). Although most school-aged children are physically active, a concern remains related to their decreased physical activity and increased sedentary activities, such as watching television or playing computer games. Biddle and Goudas (1996) found that caregivers' support and encouragement were directly related to their child's level of physical activity, so careful attention must be paid to teaching children and their caregivers about the importance of physical activity. Physical activity for school-aged children can take many forms and includes hiking, spontaneous sports activities, or being a member of an organized community team. It is important for the child to find something enjoyable. This will foster future participation.

Even children with physical limitations should be encouraged to participate in an activity that uses their abilities.

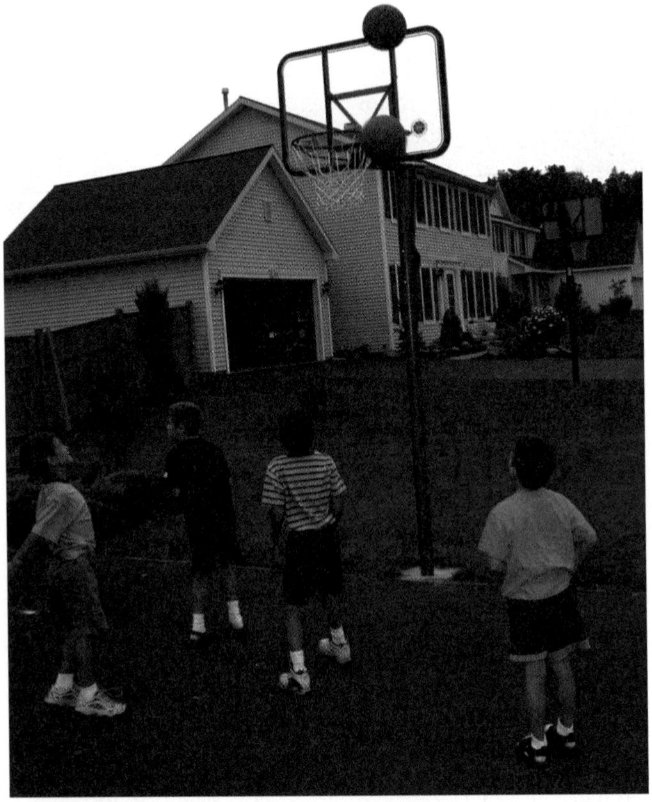

Figure 11-12 Play for school-agers can take a variety of paths and include pick-up basketball.

Sports

As the child's skeleton and muscle size continue to grow at a gradual rate, the gross motor skills of jumping, running, throwing, and catching continue to be refined. However, the child's muscles and bones are easily injured because of immaturity so athletic activities must be carefully selected according to the child's physical development and not the caregiver's wishes. Careful attention must also be paid to limiting activities that stress the child's physical development and endurance, such a contact sports and long distance running.

As the child seeks cooperative play with rules, team sports become interesting. Team play can contribute to not only physical, but also social development as the youngsters learn to play as team members and work for common goals. Sports should encourage everyone to participate and recognize all team members for their contributions, not just a select few. However, during the school-age years, the child is also exposed to the high value placed on winning and competing, and should learn a healthy balance between playing for the sake of playing and always winning or competing.

Peers

During the school-age years, children transition from the central focus of their home and caregivers, to a world of school and peers. As school-aged children become older, gain more independence, and spend more time with peers of the same gender, friendships develop that may influence them for the rest of their life. Peers help each other learn about the world and all its possibilities, influence self-esteem and self-confidence, and are important sounding boards for issues needing to be discussed. Child–child interactions provide opportunities to learn a wide variety of social behaviors and how to cope in situations such as cooperation, competition, aggression, disagreement, and negotiation (Charlesworth, 2000).

Research Highlight

Self-Concept and Health Status

Study Purpose

To examine the relationship between self-concept, physical fitness, and health habits in school-aged children.

Methods

Participants included sixty-one children (38 female and 23 male) enrolled in first through eighth grade. To measure self-concept, each child completed the Martinek-Zaichowsky Self-Concept Scale for Children. To measure physical fitness, each child completed a one-mile walk–run, shuttle run, and curl-ups. Health indicators such as height, weight, and body mass index were also examined. In addition, caregivers completed a questionnaire about their own health habits, their child's health habits, and family history of disease.

Findings

Findings showed school-aged children who exercised on a regular basis had a more positive self-concept than children who led a more sedentary life. No gender differences were found between self-concept and physical prowess.

Implications

This study underscores the importance of regular physical exercise to enhance not only the development of physical strength and coordination, but also improve the school-aged child's self-concept. Nurses need to encourage physical activity as part of the daily lives of school-aged children; incorporating exercise into the child's daily routine can foster a positive self-concept and life-long commitment to physical fitness.

Citation

Overbay, J., & Purath, J. (1997). Self-concept and health status in elementary school-age children. *Issues in Comprehensive Pediatric Nursing, 20*, 89–101.

Body Image

School-aged children are knowledgeable about their bodies and often will compare how they look to how their peers or adults look. Children also are acutely aware of physical differences related to height or weight, and know if they are not as coordinated as their friends. School-aged children who are especially sensitive about these differences may be uncomfortable in a swimming suit or shorts, and not participate in activities where their "differences" may become apparent. If the child has a physical disability, it is not uncommon for other children to call attention to the disabililty, exclude them from activities and, at the same time, worry that they themselves have a similar disability. Caregivers and nurses need to be sure children know each child is different in a special way, yet at the same time, identical to their friends in many other ways. Children who call attention to physical disabilities in others need to realize such comments may have lasting effects and should be discouraged from making hurtful comments.

Bullying

Developing social skills is one of the primary tasks of the school-age years (Schor, 1998). For children who lack such skills, one of the ways to express their anger is the act of bullying, that is, inflicting verbal or physical harm on another. Usually, boys are more likely to engage in bullying than girls, and reasons given for bullying include: to get even; others do it; for fun; because the other child annoys me; to show how tough the child is; because the other child was a wimp; and for money (Rigby, 1998). Reactions to bullying can include

Critical Thinking

Dealing With Bullying Behavior

Consider the following situation: You are a school nurse in a large urban school. Over the past month, 11-year-old Spencer, who is new to your school, has been stopping in your office on a weekly basis with complaints of headache and stomachache. You noticed at this visit that he has a number of bruises on his face. Spencer reluctantly responds to your question about the bruises and admits that a group of bullies have been "beating him up" because he would not steal for them. He tells you he is scared to tell his mother, as she can not afford to send him to another school.

1. Determine the approach you should use with Spencer.
2. Discuss ways you could intervene to prevent future harm.
3. Describe how would you address Spencer's concern about notifying of his mother.
4. Would you notify school administrators? Is so, how would you do this?
5. Identify school and community resources that could help this family.

Nursing Tip:

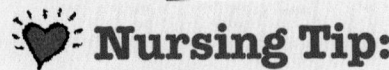

Stress reduction strategies
Nurses need to work in partnership with the child and family to determine effective methods of stress reduction. Since school-aged children often enjoy writing, they can be encouraged to write about their experiences in order to cope. Additional stress reducing techniques such as relaxation, guided imagery, or distraction may also help some children.

Kids Want To Know

My friends tell me that surgery is gross and will hurt a lot. Can I put it off?

Ronnie, age 10 years, is scheduled for outpatient surgery next week. This is his first surgery. Ronnie has not verbalized any concerns about the surgery until today. Upon arriving home from school, Ronnie says his friends warned him about the horrible pain he would have and told him he would be naked during surgery. Ronnie asked that the surgery be postponed.

Without knowing the accuracy of his friends' statements, his caregivers decided to seek the answers. They contacted his surgeon and found their hospital offered a presurgery preparation program for children and caregivers. At the program they were told about the surgery and assured their child's safety and welfare was the primary goal. Ronnie and his caregivers were also told pain management was an important intervention and medication would be available throughout the stay. The caregivers also received information about postoperative pain management at home. Ronnie was relieved to know he would be covered during surgery and his caregivers could visit before surgery, attend the anesthesia induction, and stay with him after the surgery. Attending the presurgery preparation program greatly reduced the stress and allowed Ronnie and his caregivers to be more fully informed about the surgical experience.

sadness, reduced self-esteem, having fewer friends, being less popular or absent from school, as well as complaining of headache, sleep disturbances, and stomachache (Rigby, 1998). School nurses can play a vital role in identifying both the victims and perpetrators of bullying behavior and must take action for the safety and well-being of all involved as some of the recent incidences of school violence and shootings were carried out by students who were bullied by peers.

Stress

Consider the following situations:

a) Twelve-year-old Karl is admitted to the emergency room with an exacerbation of his asthma.

b) Ten-year-old Mary brings home a report card with all A's and one B.

c) Six-year-old Chad is admitted to the hospital for same-day surgery.

d) Eight-year-old Christine's father is diagnosed with cancer and is scheduled for a bone marrow transplant.

Without knowing the children in these situations we cannot know if they experienced stress. We do know, however, that stress is a part of life for everyone, including school-aged children. The school-aged child in today's world is constantly exposed to stress. Like never before, children are subjected to the effects of a high divorce rate, peer pressure, and use of illicit drugs and alcohol. A situation is considered stressful for a child when there is a discrepancy between demands placed on the child and the child's perceived ability to meet these demands (Menke, 1981). In addition, what is stressful for one school-aged child may not be stressful for another; if the child feels resources and supports are available it may be viewed as a positive challenge instead of a negative threat. If stress is viewed as a negative threat and beyond their ability to handle, children may exhibit some of the signs listed in Table 11-3 and need assistance in working through the experience.

Health care experiences can be potential stressors for children as they deal with separation from friends and family, interruption of school, and the threat of injury or pain.

TABLE 11-3 Signs of Stress

1. Frequent fatigue
2. Irritability
3. Change in sleep or eating pattern
4. Complaints of headaches or stomachaches
5. Substance abuse
6. Drop in academic performance

Surgery is an example of a health care stressor that results from the potential loss of control, fear of pain, concern for modesty, and separation from caregivers and friends. Therefore, school-aged children need to be prepared at least a week in advance of a stressful event such as surgery, so they can have their questions answered and formulate coping strategies. Caregivers also need to be prepared because, if prepared, they will be less anxious and better able to provide positive support for their child.

Latchkey Children

Today, in both single- and two-caregiver families, more caregivers are working outside the home. As a result, many children come home after school to an empty house and are home alone for a period of time without adult supervision (**latchkey children**) (Figure 11-13). The current number of latchkey children in this country is difficult to estimate, but

Research Highlight

Worries of School-aged Children

Study Purpose

To discover how worried school-aged children are during particular situations and to determine if caregivers can identify how worried their child is during these particular situations.

Methods

Forty-eight school-aged children, (24 boys and 24 girls) ages 7 to 12, forty mothers, and eight fathers participated. Each child and parent was interviewed in their home and asked to complete a questionnaire with twenty-seven potentially worrisome experiences. The children were asked to rate each item and then rank the five most worrisome items.

Findings

Children ranked the following as the five most worrisome items: (1) being in a war; (2) being lost and not being able to see; (3) being in a fire; (4) having a parent die; and (5) being asked to take drugs. The investigators found parents were readily able to determine what worried their children the most. However, the study revealed parents were not aware of their child's concerns about war, hearing parents quarrel, moving to a new school, or failing an exam.

Implications

Nurses need to encourage caregivers of school-aged children to discuss concerns their child may have related to self, family, or school. By taking a direct approach with open discussion and problem solving, the child's worries can decrease.

Citation

Neff, E., & Dale, J. (1996). Worries of school-age children. *Journal of the Society of Pediatric Nurses, 1* (1), 27–32.

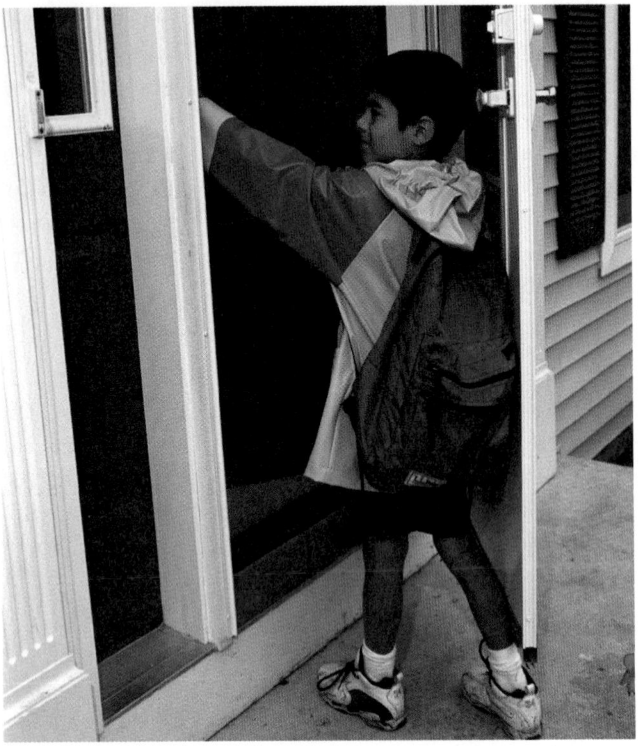

Figure 11-13 Latchkey children usually spend a few hours home alone after school.

Family Teaching

Tips for Latchkey Children

Nurses must take a proactive role in promoting quality after-school programs in their communities. School nurses can encourage students who go home to an empty house to discuss with their caregivers safe rules to abide by while they are alone. The following tips for latchkey children can be reinforced by the school nurse:

1. Do not open the door to anyone you do not know.
2. Do not tell a telephone caller you are home without a caregiver.
3. Make a list of emergency phone numbers and the phone number for a neighbor who can be trusted. Keep this list in a safe place near the phone.
4. Create an after-school routine such as homework, household chores, or caring for pets.

may be as high as 10 million. An even greater number of children whose caregivers work are cared for by an older sibling. Because of this lack of adult supervision, latchkey children are at risk for developing physical and social problems, and anxiety (Schor, 1999).

Reflective Thinking

Caring for a Latchkey Child

1. How would you feel if a 7-year-old boy you are caring for in a health care setting told you that he was left alone for many hours every day without adult supervision?
2. How would you feel about his caregivers and what actions would be appropriate?

Dishonesty

It is not uncommon for school-aged children to steal, cheat, or lie. Although these behaviors may be upsetting for caregivers, they are often just a phase the child goes through, and may be related to immature cognitive development, or on the other hand, indicate a more serious problem. Young children may steal because they want something another person has, feel they were treated unfairly and want revenge, or want to be able to bribe other children. Other children may observe family members take things from one another (money out of a purse, clothes from a drawer) and see nothing wrong in doing the same thing. Children may cheat because they want to win a game they are playing, or do well on an examination. If winning or being the best is important to their caregivers, or if they see caregivers cheat, children are more likely to model that same behavior. Finally, young school-aged children may lie to cover up misbehavior or avoid being punished, whereas older children lie because they may not meet expectations of teachers or caregivers.

Limit Setting and Discipline

Nurturant caregivers place discipline in a warm, supportive, and empathetic relationship with their school-aged child. By providing clear limits of behavior and positive reinforcement for good behavior, the caregiver is better able to help the child develop self-confidence. In effect, caregivers who model responsible behavior can easily be examples of effective values.

Implicit in discipline approaches is a fundamental attitude toward the child. Taking the child seriously and treating the child as a person whose feelings and questions matter is critical. The child's preference, however, cannot always be accommodated but should be considered and never dismissed. The school-aged child is someone with a distinctive point of view and a unique set of needs. The caregiver needs to be not only warm and empathetic but also needs to model for the school-aged child the values of honesty and prosocial behavior (helping, sharing, and caring). Reasoning capabilities of the school-aged child are being developed, so talking about and explaining a negative behavior or act should be encouraged. Withdrawing privileges is often a satisfying method of discipline.

Sexuality

School-aged children may engage in some form of sex play during the late school-age years. This is normal behavior. Caregivers should avoid drawing attention to it or laying on guilt. At a very early age, children are exposed to sexually explicit information through the media. Unless caregivers are honest and open about sexual issues, children will seek answers to their questions from peers. All too often the information from peers is inaccurate; therefore, it is imperative nurses are available to provide education regarding sexuality to children and caregivers. In providing education, it is important to use the appropriate anatomical terms and encourage open discussion between children and caregivers. Caregivers should use truthful information and not shy away from the discussion.

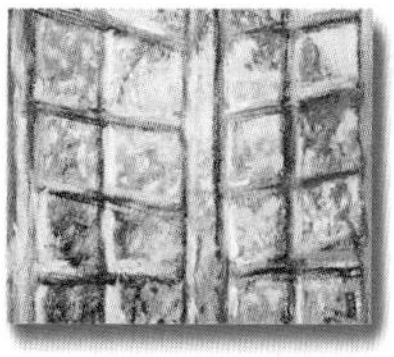

In the Real World

I love caring for school-aged children! They are always so inquisitive and want to learn everything they can about their disease or illness. Most recuperate quite quickly from surgery unless there are complications, and, once their pain is under control, are out in the halls talking to nurses, parents, and other clients. They are also so willing to help the nurses in any way they can. It is not unusual to see a school-aged child sitting at the desk talking to the nurses, especially during the evening hours when things are beginning to wind down on the units. Of course, there are those children who are not like this, but I have not seen too many and when I do, all it takes on my part is a little extra time and attention as they are usually just scared.

NURSE'S ROLE IN FOSTERING HEALTHY SCHOOL-AGED CHILDREN

The school-age years are an exciting time because it is during this time the child learns how to master skills and relate to others. How successful the child feels during this period can shape his or her future success in work and relationships. Although their world revolves around school and relationships with peers, children's caregivers still play a critical role in their lives. The nurse caring for a school-aged child is in an ideal position to serve as a positive role model and teacher for both child and caregiver. Nurses should encourage caregivers to foster independence within their child by promoting acceptable limit-setting and allowing choices. Education about nutrition, exercise, rest, sexuality, and safety can foster healthy habits for life. The rewards are many when a school-aged child is able to realize his or her full potential as a healthy, self-assured individual.

Key Concepts

- During school-age, the child's weight increases by 5 to 6 pounds per year, height increases by 2 inches per year, 20 deciduous teeth are shed, and 28 of the 32 permanent teeth appear.
- During latency, the child ignores his/her own sexuality and instead, identifies with the same-sex caregiver.
- Concrete operations, where thoughts are less egocentric and become more open and flexible, allow the child to gain the skills of classification, conservation, and reversibility.
- According to Erikson's theory of psychosocial development, the major task of the school-age period is industry versus inferiority where the child's work brings a sense of accomplishment and worth.
- Kohlberg proposed the school-aged child is at the conventional level of moral development when the conscience develops an internal set of "rules" that must be followed in order to be "good."
- Schools, teachers, and peers play important roles in the school-aged child's development.
- Play for school-aged children includes quiet time, board games, and sports.
- Latchkey children are at risk for problems associated with poor adult supervision.
- Factors contributing to the high incidence of accidents involving school-aged children are increased independence from caregiver supervision, desire to meet the approval of peers, and increased involvement in physically challenging activities.
- Nursing care of school-aged children involves teaching caregivers and children about nutrition, immunizations, health and safety issues, activity, rest and sleep, and expected developmental changes.

Review Questions

1. Describe the physiological changes occurring during the school-age period.
2. What developmental milestones are associated with the school-aged child?
3. Define the cognitive skills of classification, conservation, and reversibility. Offer examples of each. Explain the importance of gaining these skills in terms of the nurse's plan of care in a health care setting.
4. What are the major influences on moral development of the school-aged child?
5. Why are peers, teachers, and schools so important for the school-aged child?
6. Explain the risks associated with latchkey children.
7. List several safety promotion and injury prevention techniques for school-aged children and their caregivers.
8. Put together a response for a child who asks "how a baby gets in his mother's tummy?".

References

American Acadamy of Pediatrics. (2001). *Back to school tips* [Online]. Available: www.aap.org/advocacy/release/augschool.htm.

Biddle, S., & Goudas, M. (1996). Analysis of children's physical activity and its association with adult encouragement and social cognitive variables. *Journal of School Health, 66*, 75–78.

Charlesworth, R. (2000). *Understanding child development* (5th ed.). Albany, NY: Delmar.

Children's Defense Fund. (2000). *The state of America's children yearbook*. Washington, DC: Author.

Click, P. (1998). *Caring for school-age children* (2nd ed.). Albany, NY: Delmar.

Colizza, D., & Colvin, S. (1995). Food choices of healthy school-age children. *Journal of School Nursing 11*(4), 17–20.

Covington, C. (1996). Childhood obesity: Too much, too little, too late. *Issues in Comprehensive Pediatric Nursing. 19*(4), iii–v.

Dixon, S., & Stein, M. (2000). *Encounters with children: Pediatric behavior and development*. St. Louis, MO: Mosby.

Erikson, E. (1963). *Childhood and society*. New York: Norton.

Evers, C. (1997). Empower children to develop healthful eating habits. *Journal of the American Dietetic Association* 97(10), S116.

Fingerhut, L. (1993). *Firearm mortality among children, youth, and young adults 1–34 years of age: Trends and current status*. United States Department of Health and Human Services. CDC, No. 231.

Freud, S. (1923). *The ego and the id*. London: Hogarth Press.

Kohlberg, L. (1969). *Stages in development of moral thought and action*. New York: Holt, Rinehart, & Winston.

Long, K., & Williams, D. (1998). Health care for the school-age child. In *Annual review of nursing research* (pp. 39–61). New York: Springer.

Luder, E., & Bonforte, R. (1996). Health and nutrition issues during childhood years. *Topics in Clinical Nutrition, 11*(3), 47–55.

Menke, E. (1981). School-aged children's perception of stress in the hospital. *Journal of the Association for the Care of Children's Health, 9*(3), 80–86.

Neff, E., & Dale, J. (1996). Worries of school-age children. *Journal of the Society of Pediatric Nurses, 1* (1), 27–32.

Overbay, J., & Purath, J. (1997). Self-concept and health status in elementary school-age children. *Issues in Comprehensive Pediatric Nursing, 20*, 89–101.

Piaget, J. (1962). *Play, dreams and imitation in childhood*. New York: Norton.

Prescott, B. (1999). Health care of the school age child. *Montana Nurses Association Pulse, 36*(1), 18.

Rigby, K. (1998). Gender and bullying in schools. In P. Slee & K. Rigby (Eds.), *Children's peer relations* (pp. 47–59). London: Routledge.

Rudolph, A., & Kamei, R. (1998). *Rudolph's fundamentals of pediatrics* (2nd ed.). Stamford, CT: Appleton & Lange.

Ryan-Wenger, N. (1998). Children's drawings: An invaluable source of information for nurses. *Journal of Pediatric Health Care, 12*(3), 109–110.

Santrock, J. (1998). *Adolescence* (7th ed.). New York: McGraw-Hill.

Schor, E. (1998). Guiding the family of the school-age child. *Contemporary pediatrics, 15*(3), 75–84.

Schor, E. (Ed.). (1999). *The complete and authoritative guide: Caring for your school-age child*. New York: Bantam Books.

Stedman's Medical Dictionary (27th ed.). (2000). Philadelphia: Lippincott, Williams, & Wilkins.

Steinberg, L. (1999). *Adolescence*. (5th ed.). New York: McGraw-Hill.

Vygotsky, L. (1962). *Thought and language*. New York: Wiley.

Suggested Readings

Biddle, S., & Armstrong, N. (1992). Children's physical activity: An exploratory study of psychological correlates. *Social Science and Medicine, 34*(3), 325–331.

Bossert, E. (1994). Factors influencing the coping of hospitalized school-age children. *Journal of Pediatric Nursing, 9*(5), 299–306.

Brooks, R. (1992). Self-esteem during the school years. *Pediatric Clinics of North America, 39*(3), 537–549.

Cowell, J., Warren, J., & Montgomery, A. (1999). Cardiovascular risk prevalence among diverse school-age children. *Journal of School Nursing, 15*(2), 8–12.

Cutler, B., Smith, K., & Kilmon, C. (1995). Characteristics of fifth-grade children in relation to the type of after-school care. *Journal of Pediatric Health Care, 9*(4), 167–171.

Davidson, L. (1999). School age prostitution: An issue for children's nurses. *Journal of Child Health Care, 3*(2), 5–10.

Finan, S. (1997). Promoting healthy sexuality: Guidelines for the school-age child and adolescent. *The Nurse Practitioner, 22*(11), 62–72.

Garvey, C. (1990). *Play*. Cambridge, MA: Harvard University Press.

Ginsburg, H., & Opper, S. (1988). *Piaget's theory of intellectual development*. Englewood Cliffs, NJ: Prentice Hall.

Hart, D., & Bossert, E. (1994). Self-reported fears of hospitalized school-age children. *Journal of Pediatric Nursing, 9*(2), 83–90.

Hoffert, M. (1997). Weaving the fabric of a life: A phenomenological inquiry of solitude experienced by school age children. *Prairie Rose, 66*(1), 4–6.

Jones, F., & Selder, F. (1996). Psychoeducational groups to promote effective coping in school-age children living in violent communities. *Issues in Mental Health, 17*, 559–571.

Kohlberg, L. (1981). *The philosophy of moral development*. San Francisco: Harper & Row.

Konner, M. (1991). *Childhood: A multicultural view*. Boston: Little & Brown.

Leonard, K. (1999). Firearm safety courses for elementary school-age children. *Canadian Journal of Public Health, 90*(1), 35–36.

Lightfoot, J., & Bines, W. (1997). Meeting the health needs of the school-age child. *Health Visitor, 70*(2), 58–61.

MacBriar, B., Burgess, M., Kottke, S., & Maddox, K. (1995). Development of a health concerns inventory for school-age children. *Journal of School Health, 11*(3), 25–29.

Mattey, E. (1996). Teach us body sense (TUBS): A health education program for primary students. *Pediatric Nursing, 22*(6), 545–551.

McClowry, S. (1995). The influence of temperament on development during middle childhood. *Journal of Pediatric Nursing, 10*, 160–165.

McClowry, S., & McLeod, S. (1990). The psychosocial responses of school-age children to hospitalization. *Children's Health Care, 19*(3), 155–161.

McEvoy, M. (1996). Increasing bicycle helmet use among school-age children. *Nurse Practitioner, 21*(4), 14–16, 150.

Menke, E. (1998). The mental health of homeless school-age children. *Journal of Child and Adolescent Psychiatric Nursing, 11* (3), 87–98.

Rodgers, G. (1996). Bicycle helmet use patterns among children. *Pediatrics, 97*, 166–173.

Schmalz, K., & Larwa, L. (1997). Problems encountered by parents and guardians of elementary school-age children in obtaining immunizations. *The Journal of School Nursing, 13*(1), 10–16.

Schonfeld, D. (1996). Talking with elementary school-age children about AIDS and death. *The Journal of School Nursing, 12*(1), 26–32.

Schwartz, D., Dodge, K., Pettit, G., & Bates, J. (1997). The early socialization of aggressive victims of bullying. *Child Development, 68*(4), 665–675.

Seligson, M., & Allenson, M. (1993). Continuity of supervised care for school-age children. *Pediatrics, 91*(1), S206–208.

Sharrer, V., & Ryan-Wenger, N. (1995). A longitudinal study of age and gender differences of stressors and coping: Strategies in school-age children. *Journal of Pediatric Health Care, 9*, 123–130.

Smith, M. (1993). Pediatric sexuality: Promoting normal sexual development in children. *Nurse Practitioner, 18*(8), 37–44.

Wilson, A., & Yorker, B. (1997). Fears of medical events among school-age children with emotional disorder, parents, and health care providers. *Issues in Mental Health Nursing, 18*(1), 57–71.

Wood, L., & Masterson, J. (1999). Use of technology to facilitate language skills in school-age children. *Seminars in Speech and Language, 20*(3), 219–232.

Resources

Organizations and Websites

After School: School Age Resources
School-Age NOTES
P.O. Box 40205
Nashville, TN 37204-0205
(615) 279-0700
Fax: (615) 279-0800
www.afterschoolalliance.com

The American Academy of Pediatrics
141 Northwest Point Boulevard
Elk Grove Village, IL 60007-1098
(847) 434-4000
Fax: (847) 434-8000
www.aap.org

American School Health Association
7263 State Route 43
P.O. Box 708
Kent, OH 44240
(330) 678-1601
Fax: (330) 678-4526
www.ashaweb.org

Bright Futures Project
NCEMCH
2000 15th Street, North, Suite 701
Arlington, VA 22201-2617
(703) 524-7802
Fax: (703) 524-9335
www.brightfutures.org

The Children's Defense Fund
25 E Street, NW
Washington, DC 20001
(202) 628-8787
www.childrensdefense.org

Children's Health Information Network
1561 Clark Drive
Yardley, PA 19067
(215) 493-3068
www.tchin.org

Kidlink
www.kidlink.org

Kids Health Organization
www.kidshealth.org

Kid Source: On Line
www.kidsource.com

Maternal and Child Health Bureau
Parklawn Building
5600 Fishers Lane
Rockville, MD 20857
www.mchb.hrsa.gov

National Association of School Nurses
Eastern Office
P.O. Box 1300
Scarborough, ME 04070-1300
(877) 627-6476 (1-877-NASN4SN)
Fax: 207-883-2683

Western Office
1416 Park Street, Suite A
Castle Rock, CO 80104
(866) 627-6767 (866-NASN-SNS)
Fax: 303-663-0403
www.nasn.org

National Institute of Child Health and Human Development
Bldg 31, Room 2A32, MSC 2425
31 Center Drive
Bethesda, MD 20892-2425
(800) 370-2943
www.nichd.nih.gov

National Runaway Switchboard
3080 North Lincoln Ave.
Chicago, IL 60657
(800) 621-4000
www.nrscrisisline.org/

Ped info
www.pedinfo.org

U.S. Consumer Product Safety Commission
Washington, DC 20207-0001
(301) 504-0990
Fax: (301) 504-0124 and (301) 504-0025
www.cpsc.gov

CHAPTER 12

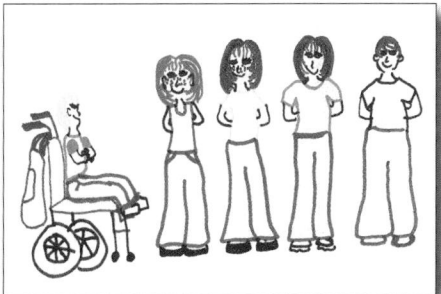

I don't know what I can do about my boys. They are so different! Ryan (age 13) daydreams a lot, is so sensitive, and gets his feelings hurt easily. He also has wide mood swings and spends a lot of time with his friend Luke, who lives on the same street. He never studies and isn't interested in girls at all. On the other hand, Ron, my 16-year-old, is so cooperative. He does anything his dad or I ask him to do, and his room is so neat! He has started to date Sarah, a girl in his Spanish class at school, works part time at his dad's office, and plans to major in accounting when he attends college.

GROWTH AND DEVELOPMENT OF THE ADOLESCENT

Barbara Mandleco, RN, PhD
J. Kelly McCoy, PhD

COMPETENCIES

Upon completion of this chapter, the reader will be able to:

- *Explain the importance and timing of physiological development in adolescence.*
- *Discuss the importance of psychosexual, psychosocial, cognitive, and moral development in adolescence.*
- *Discuss the impact that school, peers, work, and leisure time have on adolescent development.*
- *Describe the major developmental tasks of adolescence, and discuss why they are important for the transition to adulthood.*
- *Discuss several nursing interventions for effectively working with adolescents.*
- *Discuss several health promotion and screening activities related to adolescence and the appropriate nursing interventions.*
- *Discuss several issues or problems facing adolescents today and the appropriate nursing interventions.*

Between childhood and adulthood, individuals experience the unique developmental period known as adolescence (ages 12–21), when young people begin to focus on who they are, how they are similar to or different from those around them, and what they want to become when they reach adulthood. It is a time of exploration, excitement and discovery, and sometimes confusion and despair (Figure 12-1).

Adolescence is second only to infancy in the amount of change individuals encounter physiologically and psychosocially. In order to effectively identify issues and problems commonly seen in adolescence, and consequently deliver appropriate and individualized nursing care, it is important to consider the physiological, psychosexual, psychosocial, cognitive, and moral transformations occurring during this time, as well as changes in adolescents' rapidly expanding social context, including the family, school, and peers.

The concept of an adolescent stage of development is actually a relatively recent phenomenon. During the late 19th century our economy began to change from agricultural to industrialized; as a result, an unskilled workforce made up largely of children and adolescents became much less important to the labor market. This shift created a new and increasingly distinct segment of the population, which was not considered to be made up of either children or adults. In 1904, G. Stanley Hall

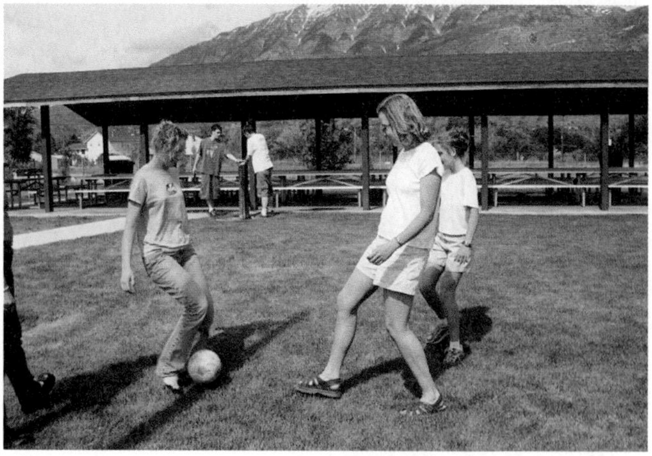

Figure 12-1 Adolescence can be a time of excitement, discovery, and despair.

became the first person recognized for studying this newly created segment of the population when he published a two-volume set of books titled *Adolescence,* earning him the title of "father of adolescence." Hall saw adolescence as a necessary precursor to adulthood, a time likely to be filled with storm and stress (Santrock, 2000). Compared to these early perceptions, adolescence is now considered much less traumatic, but remains an important time in development.

Adolescence consists of early, middle, and late periods. Each is distinguished by several different aspects of adolescents' lives and constitute the ages of 12–14, 15–17, and 18–21 years. Another way to differentiate these periods relates to physiological development: **prepubertal** (early), **pubertal** (middle), and **postpubertal** (late adolescence). A third way relates to the level of education—early, middle, and late adolescence are associated with middle school, high school, and post–high school.

PHYSIOLOGICAL DEVELOPMENT

The physiological changes occurring during adolescence are extensive, do not occur in isolation, and have an impact on the adolescent's psychosexual, psychosocial, and cognitive development. These changes also affect the experiences adolescents have with family members, peers, and others in their social world, as well as their own body image and self-esteem.

Clarification of two terms, commonly associated with this period is needed, however, before discussing the actual physiological changes occurring. **Puberty** is the state of physical development (between ages 12 and 16 for males and ages 10 and 14 for females) when secondary sex characteristics begin to appear, sexual organs mature, reproduction first becomes possible, and the adolescent growth spurt starts (Steinberg, 2001). **Adolescence** begins with puberty and ends when the individual is physically and psychologically mature and able to assume adult responsibilities. The age when puberty begins and how long adolescence lasts varies individually and cross-culturally (Jolley & Mitchell, 1996; Turner & Helms, 1995). In the past, these terms have been used interchangeably even though their meanings are different.

Before puberty, the primary hormone regulating growth is somatotropin, also called growth hormone. However during puberty, the gonadal hormones are responsible for many of the significant physiological changes seen in various body systems (Katchadourian, 1977).

Musculoskeletal System

During the **adolescent growth spurt (AGS),** which lasts about 4.5 years (Gallahue & Ozmun, 1995), the body assumes an adult appearance. Girls may begin their spurt as early as 7.5 or as late as 12 years of age, whereas boys typically begin their growth spurt by age 13. During the AGS, there is rapid acceleration in weight and height gain: boys gain 12–14 lb and grow 3–6 inches; girls gain 8–10 lb and grow 2.5–5 inches.

The AGS is not uniform; weight begins to increase first, followed in 4–6 months by a rapid increase in height (Tanner, 1990). The age of onset, intensity, and duration of the AGS varies from individual to individual, and differs for boys and girls (Figure 12-2).

Typically, height begins increasing in early adolescence for females and in midadolescence for males. Females achieve **peak height velocity (PHV),** the maximum annual rate of growth in height during the AGS, at about 11 years of age, or 6–12 months before menarche. Very few females grow more than 2 inches after menarche. Males reach PHV at about age 13, after axillary and mature pubic hair appears, and growth of the penis and testes begins (Malina &

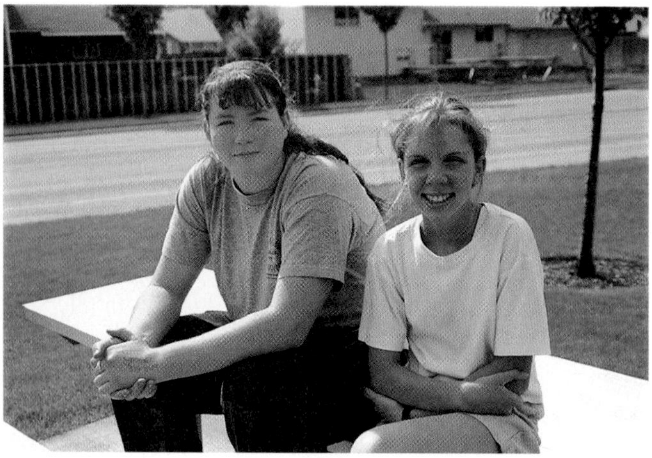

Figure 12-2 Adolescents develop at very different rates. What is considered normal varies greatly.

Bouchard, 1991). Most males do not grow in height after 18 or 20 years of age. See Figures 12-3 and 12-4 for linear growth curves during childhood and adolescence.

Weight increases for adolescents tend to follow the same growth curve as height. **Peak weight velocity (PWV),** the period when weight gain is the most rapid, is greater for males than females, and occurs simultaneously with PHV (Malina & Bouchard, 1991). PWV for females occurs about 6 months after PHV. Females frequently are heavier than their male counterparts during the AGS and tend to weigh more than males until about age 14, when their weight gain begins to level off. Weight gain in adolescent males is due primarily to increases in muscle mass and height, whereas in females, it is due primarily to increases in fat and height (Gallahue & Ozmun, 1995). Males continue gaining weight until about 22 years of age (Dacey & Travers, 1996; Turner & Helms, 1995). Diet, gastric motility, exercise, socioeconomic status, lifestyle, and hereditary factors affect adolescent weight gain.

Significant changes also occur in skeletal size, muscle mass, skin, and adipose tissue. Full bone length is first reached in the extremities and moves inward. Trunk growth begins with lengthening and widening of the hips, especially in females, then involves broadening of the chest and shoulders, especially in males. Males have greater arm and leg length relative to trunk size and delayed skeletal ossification as compared with females. Supporting muscles grow more slowly than the skeletal system, and large muscles develop faster than small muscles, resulting in the characteristic lanky or awkward look of some adolescents. Feet and hands grow out of proportion to the body, resulting in decreased coordination (Katchadourian, 1977). However, fine motor coordination improves as adolescence progresses.

The period of greatest muscular development does not occur until a year after the PHV, and in males it continues into late adolescence. Muscle mass doubles and strength increases for males during this period (Katchadourian, 1977). Endurance increases for both genders, especially with fitness training. Subcutaneous fat decreases in males and increases in females. In males, fat is deposited more commonly on the trunk, whereas in females, it is deposited over the thighs, buttocks, and breasts.

Sebaceous glands increase in size as they become active for both genders (Murray & Zentner, 2001; Steinberg, 2001). Eccrine and apocrine glands mature as well, leading to increased amounts of and a distinct odor to perspiration. Perspiration is also now secreted in response to emotional stimuli. The skin becomes darker, and the texture thickens and toughens in males. Females, on the other hand, develop soft, smooth-textured skin, with fine hair growing on the cheeks and upper lip (Katchadourian, 1977).

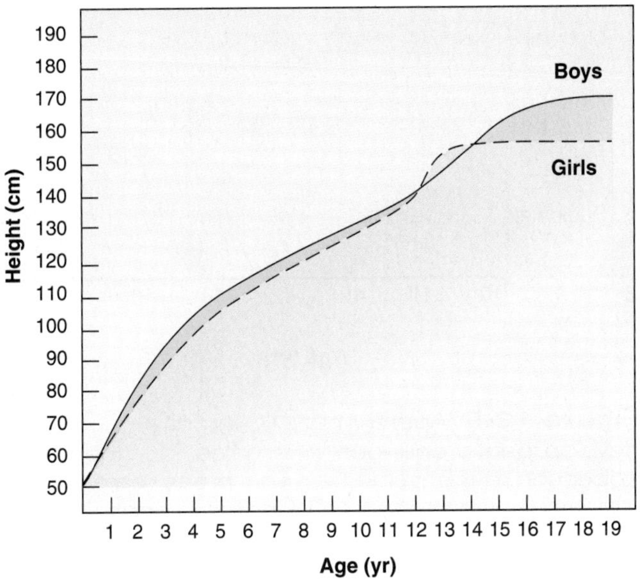

Figure 12-3 Linear Growth Throughout Childhood. From Tanner, J., Whitehouse, R. H., & Takaishi, M. (1966). Standards from birth to maturity for height, weight, height velocity, and weight velocity: British Children, 1965. *Archives of Diseases of Children 41*, 454–471.

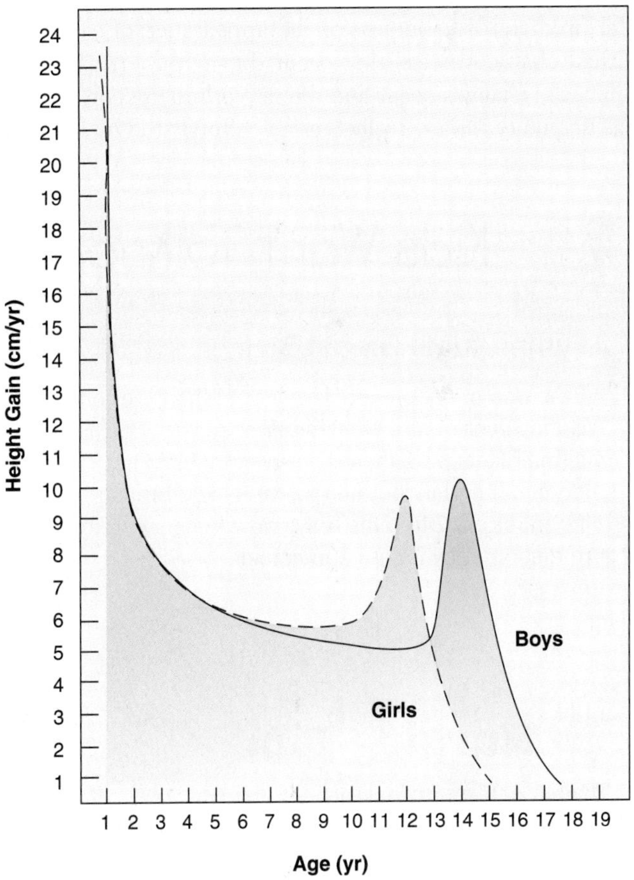

Figure 12-4 Linear Growth in Centimeters per Year. From Tanner, J., Whitehouse, R. H., & Takaishi, M. (1966). Standards from birth to maturity for height, weight, height velocity, and weight velocity: British Children, 1965. *Archives of Diseases of Children 41*, 454–471.

Genitourinary System

Secretion of neurohormonal releasing factors by the hypothalamus stimulate the anterior pituitary gland to release follicle-stimulating hormone (FSH) and luteinizing hormone (LH). In females, FSH stimulates ovarian follicle growth and estrogen production. Estrogen causes breast changes, including enlargement and darkening of the nipple, growth and development of the reproductive organs (vagina, uterus, ovaries), and growth and darkening of pubic and axillary hair. Estrogen also promotes epiphyseal maturation, which in turn inhibits long bone growth. LH initiates ovulation and formation of the corpus luteum, which then produces progesterone. Progesterone prepares the uterus to accept a fetus and maintain a pregnancy (Katchadourian, 1977).

In males, FSH is responsible for sperm production and maturation of the seminiferous tubules. LH promotes testicular maturation and testosterone production. Testosterone causes the musculoskeletal system changes discussed earlier and promotes growth and development of the male reproductive system. It also stimulates epiphyseal maturation, which then inhibits long bone growth (Katchadourian, 1977).

These reproductive hormones are also responsible for the predictable sequence of the appearance of secondary sexual characteristics, that occur during puberty. The age when the changes occur and the rate of progression through the sequence varies. In fact, cross-cultural studies show the onset of these secondary sexual changes varies with environmental conditions, race and ethnicity, geographical location, and nutrition (Eveleth & Tanner, 1990).

This sequence of secondary sexual characteristics has been divided into five stages, called the **Tanner stages.** For females, the stages describe breast and pubic hair growth. For males, the stages describe growth of the testes, penis, scrotum, and pubic hair.

The first visible sign of female sexual maturation is breast development, which may not be symmetrical. This is followed by growth of pubic hair, which begins on average between 11 and 12 years of age, and is complete by about age 14 (Katchadourian, 1977; Marshall & Tanner, 1969). Breast development and pubic hair growth for females is described in Appendix F. Figure 12-5 illustrates the approximate timing of development changes in females.

In females, **menarche** (first menstrual period) indicates puberty and sexual maturity. Most adolescent females are ambivalent about menarche; they are happy for the proof they are women, yet view it as a burden since they are unable to control their bodies. Often, the response reflects

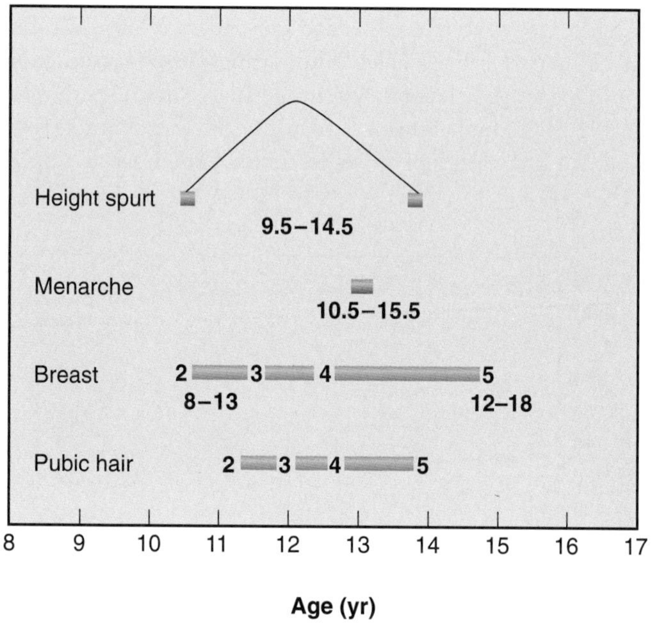

Figure 12-5 Approximate timing of developmental changes in females. Numbers appearing in the pubic hair and breast category indicate the Tanner stage of development. Ranges of ages during which the height spurt, menarche and breast development may begin or end are indicated by inclusive numbers below the categories. The PHV is illustrated by the apex of the line indicating the timing when the height spurt occurs. From Marshall, W. A., & Tanner, J. M. (1970). Variations in the pattern of pubertal changes in boys. *Archives of Diseases in Children, 45*, 22.

Kids Want To Know

Asymmetrical Breast Size

Why is one of my breasts larger than the other one? Will they ever be the same size? Is something wrong with me? Reassure the adolescent that it is not uncommon and in fact normal for female breasts to be different sizes. Often the only one who is aware of the size discrepancy is the teen herself.

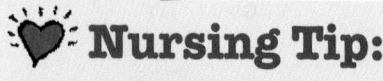

Nursing Tip:

Breast self-examination

Adolescence is a good time to begin teaching breast self-examination (BSE). It is important to remind the adolescent to perform BSE once per month, 8 days following menses or on a given fixed date each month. BSE should be avoided when breasts are tender due to menstruation or ovulation.

REFLECTIONS FROM FAMILIES

First of all, I think one of the biggest ways that I felt I was growing up and becoming a woman was when I got my first period. I thought this was a huge deal. My friends and I would talk about it and saw it as a sign that we were growing up. I also thought that getting my first bra was such a big deal. I wanted to wear a bra because it meant that I was growing up and becoming an adult. There were many other things that I looked forward to too, like shaving my legs, wearing nylons and high heels. I have a sister who is 4 years older than me and she was doing all those things. I wanted to be like her. I felt that these were signs that I was an adult.

Kids Want To Know

Why do I seem to be developing more slowly than my friends?

Sexual maturation and physical development vary considerably from adolescent to adolescent. Assure the adolescent that if development of his secondary sexual characteristics has begun, maturity will soon follow.

feelings about growing up and femininity, and can be influenced by messages and attitudes of peers and parents.

Even though regular menstrual cycles and ovulation typically begin 6–14 months after menarche, adolescent females can become pregnant after their first menstrual period. Menarche occurs about 2 years after breast development starts and after the AGS peaks. The exact time menarche begins, however, varies among populations and is influenced by nutrition, exercise, weight, breast development, health, metabolism, heredity, stress, depressive affect, family relations, and other environmental influences (Brooks-Gunn, 1988; Gallahue & Ozmun, 1995; Graber, Brooks-Gunn, & Warren, 1995; Moffitt, Caspi, Belsky, & Silva, 1992; Warren, Brooks-Gunn, Fox, Lancelot, Newman, & Hamilton, 1991). The average age of menarche in North America (12.88 years in Caucasian girls, and 12.16 in African American girls) has remained stable over the past 45 years (Herman-Giddens et al., 1997). However, in developed countries throughout the world during the past 150 years, the average age of menarche had decreased about 3 months per decade until the 1980s; this was probably due to better nutrition and overall health (Tanner, 1991).

For males, puberty and sexual maturity are initially indicated by growth of the penis and testes, spermatogenesis, and seminal emissions. The first ejaculate, however, usually does not contain mature sperm, and occurs about 1 year after the penis begins its adolescent growth. Testicular enlargement begins between 10 and 13 years of age and is usually complete by age 18 (Katchadourian, 1977; Marshall & Tanner, 1970). A description of male external genitalia development and pubic hair growth is found in Appendix F.

Figure 12-6 illustrates the approximate time developmental changes occur for males according to Tanner staging and age ranges.

During this time, it is not uncommon for one side of the scrotum to grow faster than the other; 60% of males experience transient breast enlargement (gynecomastia), and many after the age of 14 experience nocturnal emissions (loss of seminal fluid during sleep). These situations can be disturbing, and adolescent males may have uncomfortable and embarrassing feelings related to the changes their body undergoes during this period. They are sensitive to suspected deviance and constantly compare their body and appearance to their peers. Teens can also be reassured that as they get older, their body will slim down and fat will be redistributed.

Kids Want To Know

Gynecomastia and Nocturnal Emissions

Why does it look like I'm growing breasts? Will it ever go away? How long will it last? Why are my pajamas damp in the morning when I get up? What causes it? Is it normal? Reassure the teen that many adolescents experience temporary breast enlargement and nocturnal emissions. These situations are normal and will disappear as they progress through puberty.

Cardiorespiratory System

The heart almost doubles in weight and increases in size by about one half during adolescence (Malina & Bouchard, 1991). Although the heart continues to enlarge until age 17 or 18, the rate of growth is slower in comparison with other body systems and the pumping mechanism is somewhat inefficient. This may be one cause of fatigue and symptoms

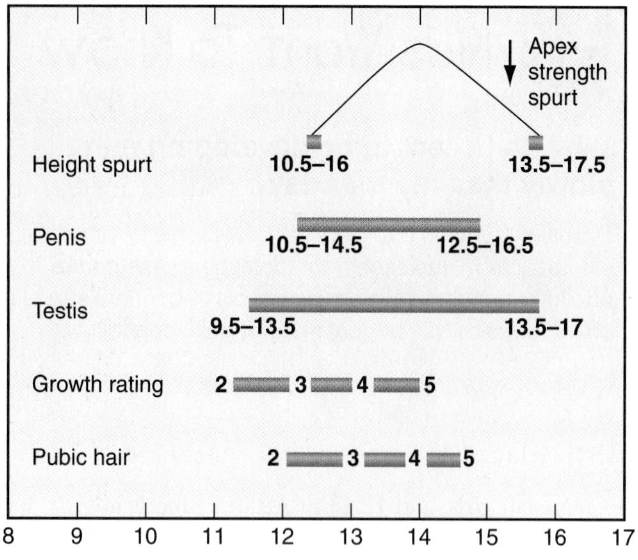

Figure 12-6 Approximate timing of developmental changes in males. Numbers appearing in the pubic hair and growth rating indicate the Tanner stage of development. Ranges of ages during which the height spurt and penis and testis development may begin or end are indicated by inclusive numbers below the categories. The PHV is illustrated by the apex of the line indicating the timing when the height spurt occurs. From Marshall, W. A., & Tanner, J. M. (1970). Variations in the pattern of pubertal changes in boys. *Archives of Diseases in Children, 45*, 22.

of inadequate oxygenation that some adolescents complain about (Murray & Zentner, 2001). Systolic blood pressure accelerates during puberty, before achieving adult values by the end of adolescence. Average blood pressure is 100–120/50–70 mm Hg. The pulse drops from childhood rates to average 60–70 beats per minute. Females have a slightly lower systolic blood pressure and a slightly higher pulse and body temperature than males (French, Perry, Leon, & Fulkerson, 1994; Katchadourian, 1977). Red blood cell mass and hemoglobin concentrations increase and the white blood cell count is decreased in both genders during adolescence. Platelet count and sedimentation rates are increased in females, whereas hematocrit levels and blood volume are increased in males (Katchadourian, 1977).

The lungs increase in length and diameter during adolescence, and the respiratory rate averages 16–20 breaths per minute. Males have greater vital capacity, volume, and rate because of their greater shoulder width and chest size. Their lung capacity, however, matures later than in females, probably due to their general later maturation. The slowness of respiratory system growth relative to the growth of other body systems may be another cause of the inadequate oxygenation and fatigue sometimes experienced by adolescents (Murray & Zentner, 2001).

Critical Thinking

Physiological Development

How can nurses help adolescents struggling with the physiological changes their body undergoes when they have not received correct information from their parents or peers or when they are slower than their age-mates? How can nurses help parents explain correct physiological development to their teenagers?

Family Teaching

Physiological Development

Physiological development can be worrisome and embarrassing to adolescents, especially if they are maturing earlier or later than their peers. You need to discuss maturation of the apocrine and eccrine glands, the importance of frequent showering, and using deodorant and body powders.

Home

Teach caregivers and teens that physiological development may vary among individuals, and even though development may be early or late, these are "normal" and temporary situations. However, if females do not begin breast development by age 13 and males do not demonstrate testicular enlargement of 2.5 cm by age 14, referral may be warranted.

Avoid ridiculing and blaming adolescents about their hygiene; they are trying to gain acceptance from peers and control over their changing body at a time in life when self-esteem is fragile.

School

Teachers need to be aware of different maturity levels of their students and realize late maturers may not feel comfortable showering in front of their early maturing peers. Allow ample opportunity for showering after physical education classes.

Community

Coaches need to be aware of physiological development of their athletes, especially if the adolescents are late maturers.

Neurological System

Brain growth continues during adolescence. The cells that support and nourish the neurons proliferate, even though the number of neurons does not increase. Continued growth of the myelin sheath allows faster neural processing (Graber & Peterson, 1991), and is reflected in the adolescent's increasing ability to think abstractly and to hypothesize.

Gastrointestinal System

Rapid maturation of the gastrointestinal system occurs during adolescence, and by the 21st birthday, all 32 teeth have erupted. Gastric acidity and capacity increase (up to 1,500 mL) to accommodate and facilitate digestion of the increased food intake that occurs in response to rapid growth. Adult size, function, and location of the liver is attained, as are adult elimination patterns (Katchadourian, 1977).

A summary of physiological milestones appears in Table 12-1.

PSYCHOSEXUAL DEVELOPMENT

The basic assertion of Freud's psychosexual theory (see Chapter 6) is that we are motivated by two competing forces; one compels us to appease our inherent biologic drives while the other fosters the desire to live in a social community. Freud contended that virtually all psychological development is an adaptive response to the upsurge in our physiologically based "drives" and our attempts to satisfy these drives while coexisting with others. While these instinctive drives are motivated by several biologic needs (hunger, fatigue, etc.), the sexual instinct, or id, is the most important in establishing individuals' psychological makeup or personality. For Freud, the physical changes of puberty reawaken the sexual and aggressive energies felt toward parents during early childhood, but that were repressed during latency or late childhood. To effectively cope, adolescents need to redirect these newly reemerging energies from

TABLE 12-1 Physiological Milestones in Adolescence

Stage	Boys	Girls	Both
Early (11–14)	Testes, scrotum, penis growing Pubic hair curly, abundant Facial hair fine, downy Axillary hair present PHV 9.4 cm/yr Gynecomastia	Breast development occurs Menarche Ovulation Pubic hair curly, thick, triangular distribution PHV 8.3 cm/yr Heavier than males	Appetite increases PWV achieved Immature cardiovascular pumping mechanism Muscle mass increases Gangly, awkward Fine motor coordination increases Permanent teeth present
Middle (15–17)	Adult genitalia Mature sperm production Facial/body hair present Muscle mass and strength greater than females Increased appetite Gynecomastia decreases Voice changes	Skeletal growth ends Sexual maturation achieved % of body fat decreases Appetite decreases Height gain 6–10.4 cm/yr	Increased fine motor coordination Physical endurance increases Sweat glands function Increased capacity of cardiovascular system Acne
Late (18–21)	Skeletal growth ends		Cardiovascular/respiratory/gastrointestinal/hematopoietic/sexual maturity achieved Stable appetite Motor activity increases Endurance increases Dentition complete

parental relationships to nonfamilial relationships (friendships, love interests) and career endeavors. For this to occur, a separation or detachment from parents is necessary, sometimes resulting in conflict between adolescents and their parents. As adolescents struggle with the inner tension brought on by pubertal change, Freud believed anxiety, heightened distress over how to act out their inner conflict, and a likely demonstration of psychologically regressive or immature behavior occurred.

Thus, Freud argued, many psychological issues adolescents face are attributable to physiological changes. Most researchers now contend the implications of these physiological changes are much more complex than Freud or the psychosexual perspective originally indicated, and in fact, are more a result of how the individual and others respond to the adolescent's physiological changes than to the changes themselves.

Body Image

A primary example of interaction between the psychological and physiological attributes of adolescents is evident in their evolving sense of body image or mental conception of their physical appearance. **Body image** encompasses positive or negative feelings, and the self-perception of physical attractiveness. Implicit in the definition is the assumption that one's body image varies with maturation, and changes across time, situations, and experiences one has with others (Figure 12-7). Constant changes in appearance—including increases in weight and height, appearance of body hair, oversized hands and feet, developing sex organs, and facial blemishes—present the adolescent with new challenges, both real and imagined, that affect their body image.

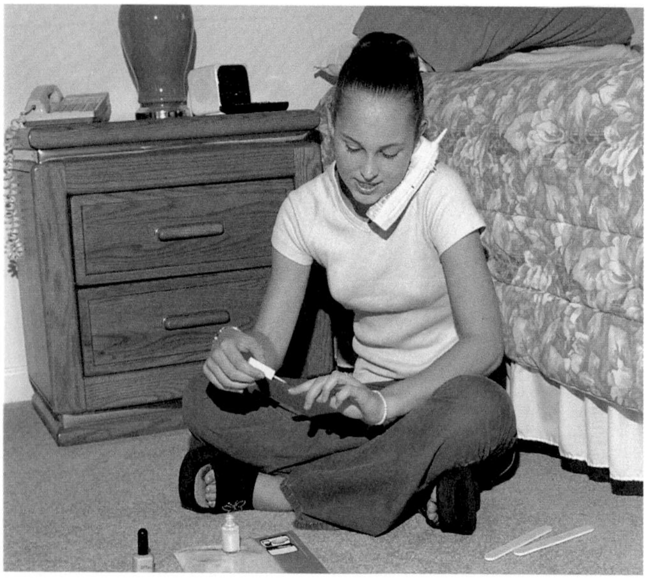

Figure 12-7 As adolescents begin to take on adult features during puberty, their interests and activities begin to change.

This is particularly significant during adolescence because the adjustment required by rapid physiological changes affect self-esteem; few adolescents are satisfied with their physical appearance (Guinn, Semper, Jorgensen, & Skaggs, 1997). Adolescent females tend to be more dissatisfied with their appearance and more likely to be concerned about particular parts of their bodies than their male counterparts (Berger, 1994; Blyth, Simmons, & Zakin, 1985; Rozin & Gross, 1987). Often, they perceive themselves as weighing more than they actually do (Feldman, Feldman, & Goodman, 1988). In fact, in a 1999 survey of American high school students (CDC, 2000), 30% of students nationwide believed they were overweight, and 42.7% reported they were trying to lose weight. This distortion of body image is not only a potentially significant emotional problem for adolescents, but also may motivate the adolescent female to engage in potentially dangerous and life-threatening weight-reducing behaviors such as anorexia, bulimia, vigorous aerobic exercise, or special diets (Whitaker, Davies, Shaffer, Abrams, Walsh, & Kalikow, 1989). In fact, 7.6% of high school students report trying to lose weight by taking diet pills, and 4.8% of high school students had vomited or taken laxatives to lose or avoid gaining weight (CDC, 2000).

While developing a sense of body image, most adolescents look to the cultural ideal valued by their society. In Western culture, this traditionally has been the shapely, thin woman and the muscular, tall man. However, few adolescents, or any individual for that matter, can successfully measure up to these standards. More than vanity, the adolescent's preoccupation with appearance is a recognition of the role physical attractiveness plays in gaining the attention and admiration of the opposite sex. The fact that physique is valued by both genders is understandable. There is a strong relationship between how adolescents feel about themselves and how they feel about their bodies. Looking "awful" or believing others view them as looking "awful" is the same as being "awful." These feelings may be reinforced by the fact that physically unattractive teens tend to have fewer friends than attractive teens (Berger, 1994; Sprinthall & Collins, 1995).

Many factors influence body image, including present and past experiences, level of cognitive development, and identity formation. Other factors are one's degree of attractiveness, size and physique appropriate to gender (including weight and body type), name/nickname, cultural ideals and values, degree of identification with same-sexed parent, peer and sibling relationships, level of aspiration, and ability to reach societal or individual ideals (Berger, 1994; Duke-Duncan, 1991; Murray & Zentner, 2001; Sprinthall & Collins, 1995; Wright & Whitehead, 1987). The rate and timing of maturation can also be an important factor in an adolescent's self-image. In fact, some research suggests that pubertal timing has a greater influence on behavioral and emotional problems than the actual transition to puberty itself (Buchanan, Eccles, & Becker, 1992). The young people who have the most difficult time adjusting to their physical development and body image are those whose body is on a different schedule from their peers. For example, late maturing adolescents may feel a sense of failure about their body if they are not as fully developed as their friends, which affects self-esteem and causes them to feel uncomfortable and insecure. Since, on average, early maturing males and females are shorter than their later maturing counterparts, they too may have difficulties with body image as their later maturing peers catch up and overtake them in height.

Social experiences are different for early and late maturing males and females. For boys, early maturation (appearance of secondary sexual characteristics during early adolescence) is associated with favorable social adjustment, whereas for females the picture is more complex. Some findings suggest that early maturation is associated with high social status and prestige in the peer group, whereas other findings indicate greater vulnerability to social pressures, leading to problems in social adjustment (Magnussen, Stattin, & Allen, 1988). For example, some studies indicate that about 20% of early maturing males are more attractive to peers and adults, given responsibility earlier, often excel in athletics, commonly receive honors, hold offices in student government, and have a positive self-image. They also are more poised and confident in social settings and report more frequent feelings of positive affect, attention, strength, and being in love (Steinberg, 1999). Finally, since for boys, physical ability is most valued, those who develop early have the edge in all realms.

Early maturing females on the other hand, may be socially disadvantaged because they are out of step with their peer group. They may become lonely and experience pressure to become involved in sexual relationships beyond the level of their maturity and coping ability (Simmons & Blyth, 1987). This can result in damaged self-esteem or unwanted sexual activities. Often, those who are taller and more developed early on than their classmates discover there are few peers who share common interests or problems. They may be teased about their developing body; called "boy crazy" by peers; scrutinized by parents; criticized by girlfriends for not spending time with them; be more introspective, unsure, submissive, and withdrawn; and be less poised and expressive. Early maturing females are also less satisfied with their weight and less positive about their bodies than late maturers (Koff & Rierdan, 1991). Often, they violate norms more frequently than their late maturing peers (Magnussen, Stattin, & Allen, 1988; Silbereisen & Kracke, 1993). They are also at heightened risk for engaging in delinquent behavior (Caspi & Moffitt, 1991; Simmons & Blyth, 1987) and are more vulnerable to eating disorders, depression, and deviant peer pressures (Brooks-Gunn & Paikoff, 1993; Ge, Conger, & Elder, 1996; Stattin & Magnussen, 1990) as compared with their late maturing or on-time peers.

About 20% of late maturing adolescents feel a sense of failure about their body because their development lags behind that of their friends. This also influences self-esteem and causes them to feel shy, uncomfortable, and insecure. Later maturing males tend to be less relaxed, poised, and popular with peers; feel more restless and talkative and feel socially inadequate and inferior. As adults they tend to hold fewer leadership positions in their jobs or organizations, and are less responsible, dominant, and controlling. They also have lower educational aspirations; often express a need for sympathy, encouragement, and understanding; and may feel rejected or inferior (Berger, 1994; Steinberg, 1999). Later maturing females on the other hand, are higher on scales of activity, sociability, leadership, prestige, popularity, and expressivity during their early adolescence (Sprinthall &

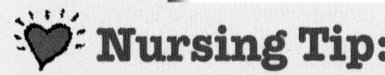

Reflective Thinking

Your Own Adolescence

Were you an early or late maturer? How did puberty affect you as a young adolescent? Has puberty had any long-term effects on you? What advice would you give an adolescent about the rate and timing of maturation?

Nursing Tip:

Concerns about body image

Nurses need to be aware of the importance physical appearance has to adolescents, and offer reassurance and encouragement to late maturing adolescents that they will catch up with their counterparts. Suggestions for becoming involved in activities they may enjoy or do well in can help maintain self-esteem and perhaps make up for slower physiologic development or unhappiness with body type, height, or weight. Early maturing adolescents can be directed to activities in which they will succeed and encouraged to be understanding of their later maturing peers who are not as capable. Parents need to understand the importance of body image to adolescents and refrain from commenting negatively about weight and general appearance. If comments are necessary, they should be couched with tact, understanding, and nurturance.

Collins, 1995). They also are twice as likely as early maturing girls to continue their education beyond the compulsory number of years of high school (Steinberg, 2001).

COGNITIVE DEVELOPMENT

Although the physiological changes associated with puberty are the most apparent indicators of development, equally important to young people's movement toward adulthood are the cognitive changes that occur during this time. As young people's thought processes become more sophisticated, their ability to think about themselves and the world around them changes radically. Piaget, Vygotsky, Selman, and Elkind describe the cognitive changes occurring during adolescence from a variety of perspectives. By far, the majority of research about the changes in young people's thought processes is the result of Jean Piaget's (1972) theoretical ideas (see Chapter 6). During adolescence (Piaget's stage of formal operations), the most distinct feature of young people's thinking is that they can now consider what is possible rather than just what is real. Thinking is no longer constrained by the concrete, physical world of their existence; rather, they are now capable of considering abstract possibilities. No longer are potential solutions based only on previous experiences; young people are able to consider all possible solutions to a problem, both real and abstract, and they can assess options and determine the best solution. Young people can now consider their own thoughts as real objects to be studied and analyzed—they can think about their own thoughts.

One outcome of adolescents' ability to consider abstract possibilities is that they begin to recognize the distinction between how things are and how things could be (the difference between the "real" and the "ideal"). During earlier stages of development, the "real" and the "ideal" are largely the same. However, as adolescents' thinking ability moves beyond the limitations of reality, they begin to conceive of the possible. Out of this ability comes a new sense of idealism and a new set of standards with which they begin comparing themselves to the world around them. Adolescents' critical assessment of their world is most likely to be seen in their interactions with their parents and in the emergence of their social, political, and religious identities.

Another significant cognitive change is language development. Adolescents generally become more sophisticated in their ability to understand words and their related abstract concepts (Figure 12-8). Because of this increased sophistication, adolescents experience a whole new world regarding the meaning of words, including metaphors and satire. Children can generally identify the obvious story that exists in a book or movie, but it is often not until adolescence that they begin to understand more abstract metaphorical meanings. During adolescence, young people also begin to find great joy in the double meaning of puns, satire, and parodies. An example of this new-found appreciation can be seen in the popularity among adolescents of *MAD* magazine, which pokes fun at all aspects of our culture.

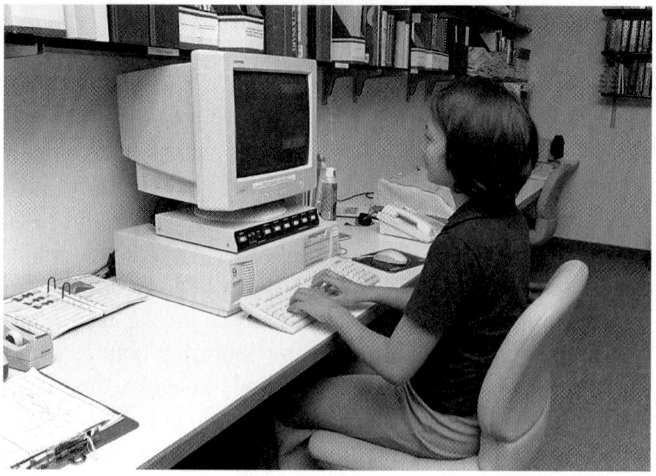

Figure 12-8 As adolescents' ability to think abstractly begins to emerge, their understanding and use of language becomes more sophisticated.

The shift to formal operational thought occurs gradually and varies individually. Formal operational thought consists of two subperiods: early and late (Broughton, 1983). When adolescents first acquire the abilities associated with formal operational thought, their new-found skill to think in hypothetical ways produces unconstrained thoughts with unlimited possibilities. This early stage of thinking results in an inordinate attempt to fit newly available abstract information into their existing immature understanding of how the world works, resulting in a subjective and idealist perception of the world (Santrock, 2001), which can be observed in the almost zealous, simplistic way they frequently embrace political or social causes. As adolescents become more cognitively mature, they are better able to adjust their thinking strategies to fit the new information now available to them. However, although researchers have suggested that a link exists between the timing of pubertal and cognitive development (Newcombe & Dubas, 1987), there are still no conclusive data (Linn & Petersen, 1985).

Cognitive Socialization

Lev Vygotsky, a Soviet cognitive theorist who did not base his work on Piaget's, considered the differences among adolescents' cognitive abilities to be a function of identifiable features of their cognitive environment (Santrock, 2001), and emphasized the way society promotes cognitive growth. For example, Vygotsky believed cognitive development was the result of social relationships with important others (e.g., parents, teachers and peers), rich in cognitively challenging interactions (Figure 12-9). One of Vygotsky's most important concepts is the **zone of proximal development (ZPD)**—tasks that are too difficult for individuals to master alone but

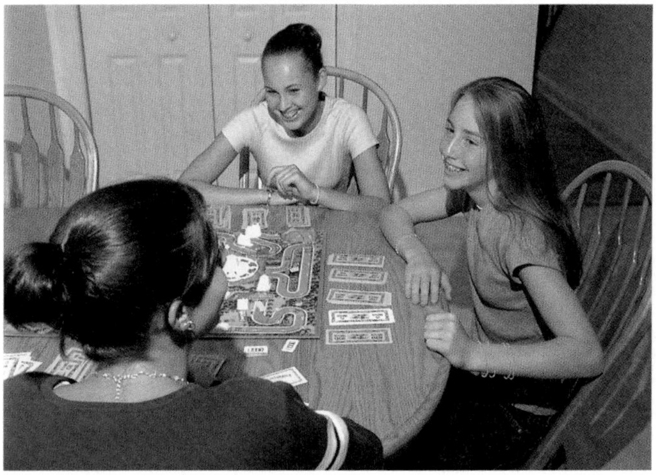

Figure 12-9 One aspect of cognitive development important to adolescents' acceptance among peers is their ability to recognize and correctly interpret the thoughts and emotions of those around them.

Family Teaching

Cognitive Development

- Adolescent is likely to begin questioning many things previously learned and is capable of reasoning problems out for themselves.
- Adolescent will often begin reexamining many parental rules, values, and explanations.
- Provide opportunities to explore the reasons for different religious and political values, attitudes about sexuality and social responsibility, or explanations about injustices they see.
- Clearly explain values and the reasoning behind them.
- Demonstrate greater willingness to listen to and understand adolescents' evolving opinions.

REFLECTIONS FROM FAMILIES

I can remember how my thinking changed. I was able to solve problems more easily. I felt like all of a sudden, I have problem solving skills. I was not only able to work out some of my own problems, but I was able to help out my peers with their problems. I also remember spending a lot of time thinking about things. It always seemed as if there was something to think about or something to wonder about. I even sometimes would ask myself why I was thinking about what I was thinking. I found myself looking at other people's perspectives. I also thought about hypothetical situations, wondering what I'd do and planning what to do ahead of time before those situations could come up. I remember comparing myself to others, wanting to acquire others' ideal characteristics. I remember asking myself really thought-provoking questions and pondering deep subjects such as "What am I? Why am I here? Who do I want to become? What is important in life?"

that can be mastered with the guidance and assistance of adults or more skilled adolescents (Santrock, 2001). The lower limit of this zone is the level of problem solving reached by the adolescent working independently; the upper limit is the level of additional responsibility the adolescent can accept with the assistance of an able instructor. According to Vygotsky, the greatest growth occurs when adolescents are stretched to perform at the upper limit of their ZPD. Cognitive development, therefore, is a function of the social relationships adolescents experience and the extent to which they are challenged within these relationships to think at a level beyond their independent capability. For example, most seventh-grade students would be overwhelmed if they were placed in a college-level calculus course. However, these same students are capable of understanding far more complex ideas (i.e., math operations) if they are coached by an adult or peer who is sensitive to their potential upper limit of understanding and can push them to think at that higher level. Once introduced to new skills, young people then internalize and make use of them on their own (Sprinthall & Collins, 1995).

Social Perspective Taking

Another important aspect of adolescents' cognitive development is their broadening ability to assume another person's perspective. Based on Piaget's work and the symbolic interaction theory of George Herbert Mead, Selman (1980) proposed that an individual's interactions are in large part due to their **social perspective taking ability.** For Selman, an adolescent interacts or communicates with others according to the social–cognitive understanding they have about who they are in relation to those around them. Maturation and social experience changes this over time. Selman argues that between early and late childhood the distinction between self and others moves from one that is behaviorally based to one that is capable of distinguishing between the actions and motives of others or the reasoning behind others' behavior. Young children have difficulty understanding that others' intentions are not always consistent with their resulting behavior; for example, a caregiver's attempt to remove a sliver from the child's hand is meant to be helpful, but it hurts. During adolescence, cognitive reasoning continues to become more complex, where simultaneous, mutual (third-person) perspective taking becomes possible. This allows young people to think not about what is best for each individual in an interaction, but rather what would be best for the relationship between them. Early adolescents' initial attempts to focus on the relationship between self and others is particularly evident in their best friendships, in which there is a high expectation regarding uniformity in dress, interests, and activities in which individual differences are considered threats to friendship. According to Selman, as this mutual perspective taking ability matures, young people come to recognize that relationship needs can be fulfilled through more than one or two relationships and individual differences can be an asset rather than a threat.

Adolescent Egocentrism

Formal operational thought enables adolescents to think about their own thoughts, and also permits them to realize that other people's thoughts are separate and distinct from their own. According to Elkind (1967), this capacity to consider other people's thoughts is the crux of adolescent **egocentrism,** when one is unable to appropriately differentiate between oneself and the objects of one's attention. Although some egocentrism is present at each developmental stage, it is most commonly associated with adolescents' thinking. With the onset of formal operational thought, adolescents are now able to consider the thoughts of others. However, their cognitive immaturity presents difficulties in differentiating their own thoughts and others' thoughts. Although adolescents realize others' thoughts are not the same as their own, they have the mistaken notion that others know what they are thinking, and assume that others are as obsessed with the adolescents' behavior and appearance as they are themselves, resulting in an even greater sense of self-consciousness (Figure 12-10).

As a function of this egocentrism, Elkind identified two types of social thinking particularly evident during adolescence—imaginary audience and personal fable. **Imaginary audience** refers to the adolescents' beliefs of always being on stage. Because adolescents confuse their ability to focus on their own thoughts with others' ability to know what they are thinking, they believe others are just as concerned about their appearance and behavior as they are. This is most evident in concerns about dress or appearance. For example, numerous adolescents have dreaded going to school on a particular day because they were sure that everyone else at school would be as conscious as they are of the unusually large zit on their nose.

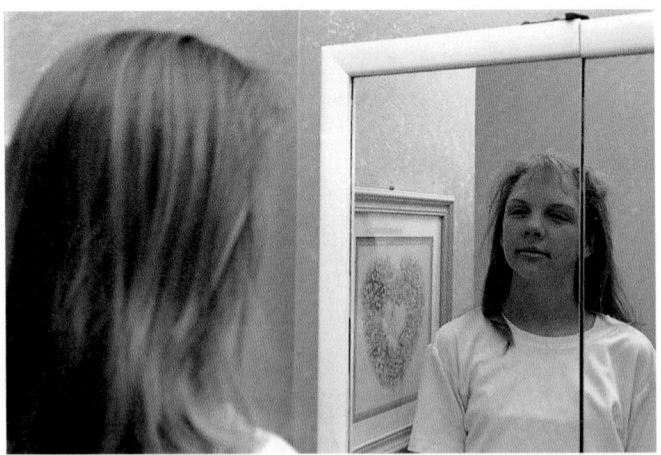

Figure 12-10 Appearance is important for adolescent females, and illustrates their egocentrism.

Connected to the adolescents' imaginary audience is their belief in what Elkind calls their own **personal fable,** in which adolescents have an exaggerated notion of their own uniqueness. Because adolescents frequently believe they are important to so many people (i.e., the imaginary audience), they regard themselves, and particularly their feelings, as special and unique. This personal uniqueness is expressed in two ways—an extreme sense of isolation, believing no one has ever had to endure the feelings or difficult situations they are experiencing (thus the phrase, "You just don't understand"), or they believe they are immortal and thus immune to the bad things that happen to others, including death (Figure 12-11). This sense of immortality is frequently evidenced in adolescents' behaviors relating to driving, drugs, alcohol, and sexuality.

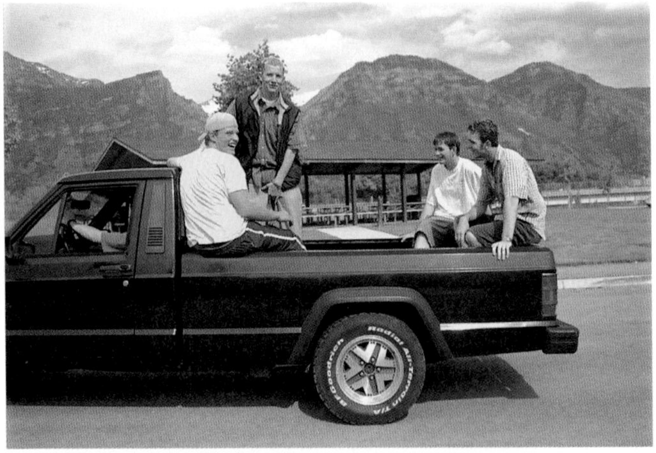

Figure 12-11 The sense of immortality that accompanies adolescents' formation of a personal fable is evidenced by their increased likelihood of engaging in risky behavior.

Reflective Thinking

Personal Fable

Can you recall any friends you had as a teenager who clearly demonstrated a personal fable, thinking they could engage in risky behavior (i.e., drinking and driving, unprotected sexual intercourse, daredevil stunts) without any concern that the existing dangers might happen to them? Did you have a personal fable? What was it?

PSYCHOSOCIAL DEVELOPMENT

Two major tasks for adolescents are answering the question "Who am I?" and attempting to understand the unique place they have in their world. In reality, these two cannot be separated; adolescents, like all of us, cannot understand who they are without understanding how they fit into their home, community, or society (Figure 12-12). This notion, generally referred to as adolescents' psychosocial orientation, has numerous explanations. In addition, adolescents' formation of a psychosocial orientation is based on several primary social contexts, including family, peers, and school.

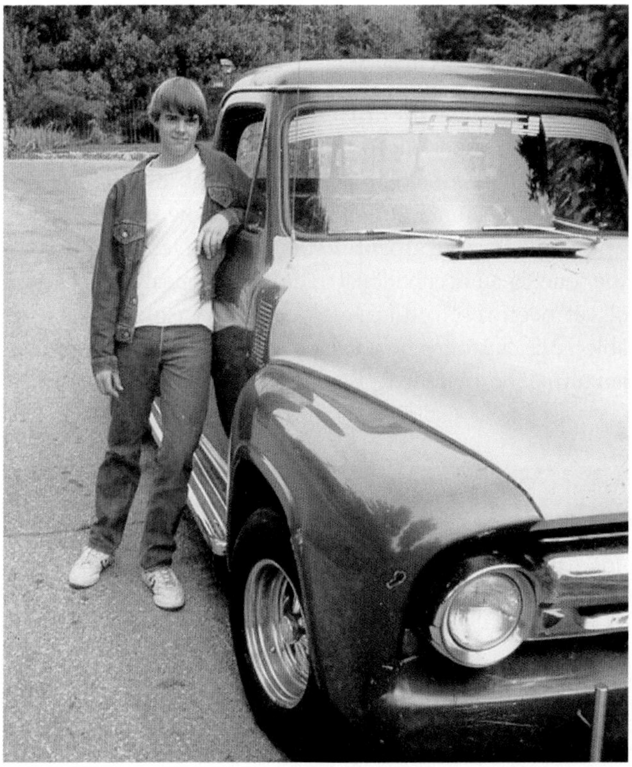

Figure 12-12 There are many aspects of adolescents' lives that contribute to their sense of identity, including relationships, talents, beliefs, and material possessions.

Psychosocial Identity

Adolescents' understanding of who they are is based on a global sense of their own identity, the value they place on that identity, and a sense of what they are able to do (their sense of self-competency). How adolescents define themselves depends on several distinct physiological, psychological, and social changes, including (1) their own pubertal development and the biologic changes of their agemates; (2) the shift to formal operational thought, the resulting changes in their interpersonal behavior, and the moral explanations for that behavior; (3) the increasing level of responsibility they assume at home, at school, and in the workplace; (4) the need to begin thinking about their career; and to a lesser extent (5) the need to begin considering their religious beliefs and political ideology. Based on these events, adolescent establish a unique sense of individual identity. To understand the formation and nature of adolescent identity, it is important to explore the concept of self and self-understanding, followed by an exploration of identity development, its establishment, and some specific dimensions making up an adolescents' broader sense of who they are.

Self, Self-Worth, and Self-Competency

No one knows when children become self-aware. Early on, children begin to distinguish themselves as separate from the world around them (Lewis & Brooks-Gunn, 1979), and this sense of separateness increases as children develop. However, it is not until formal operational thinking develops that young people are able to consider who they are in relation to their abstract roles and characteristics. For example, when asked to describe themselves, early adolescents are likely to identify themselves using roles that define them, such as being a boy or girl, a football player, a dancer, a student, or a computer user. Older adolescents are more likely to use descriptions of the more abstract characteristics that make up their personalities. For example, they might respond with statements about themselves as being a happy person, a lonely person, a quiet person, or a very outgoing person. In either case, young people develop the ability to recognize they are a complex collection of different roles and characteristics. This cognitive representation of the self is referred to as adolescents' **self-understanding.** With this self-understanding, adolescents develop the ability to recognize that who they are is not always consistent and may even present contradictions (Santrock, 2001). During early adolescence, young people begin recognizing that they possess different characteristics in different situations. At first these inconsistencies may create within adolescents a sense of contradiction about who they are. However, as they move through middle and late adolescence they eventually recognize that inconsistencies are part of the differentiated roles that define their overall sense of self (Harter, 1999).

An important part of adolescents' self-understanding is the value they place on their definition of who they are, which involves self-competency and self-worth. **Self-competency** is adolescents' sense of how well they can function within a particular realm, as for example in scholastic activities, sports, with friends, or in other activities defined as important by adolescents or those around them. In contrast, **self-worth** indicates the extent to which adolescents perceive themselves as individuals of worth, either as defined by themselves or those around them. While these two definitions are related, it is possible for young people to feel they are not very competent in many areas, but still believe they have worth; or they may recognize their competence in many areas, but have little sense of personal worth.

Identity

According to Erikson (1968), the major crisis of adolescence is establishing an **identity.** Marcia (1980) suggests:

> Identity is adolescents' definition of who they are based on their cumulative understanding of their inherent motivations, personal belief systems, and previous experiences. When adolescents have a strong sense of identity, their actions will be more self-determined and they will have a more secure sense of who they are and how they are similar to, and different from, those around them.

Adolescents' sense of identity is based on three primary factors: (1) individual identifications (parents, peers, teachers, folk heroes) as well as group ones ("my group of friends," "our generation," other blacks, other Americans) established during childhood; (2) their ability to master each developmental task (i.e., trust versus mistrust, autonomy versus shame and doubt, etc.) presented to them by society; and (3) the establishment of their own ideology, based on the social, political, and religious attitudes and values they adopt (Conger & Petersen, 1984).

Identity Statuses

Although most individuals are approaching a sense of who they are by young adulthood (Meilman, 1979), not all will arrive at a definitive answer. Many will spend much of their lives either avoiding or failing to see a need for establishing a sense of identity. Although many young people won't establish a sense of identity until young adulthood, the process generally begins during adolescence. Marcia (1980) recognized that there are different paths young people take to establish their sense of identity, resulting in one of four identity statuses: identity achievement, foreclosure, identity diffusion, and moratorium. He saw these as four distinct modes for dealing with the identity issues characteristic of late adolescence, and based them on Erikson's belief that young people must experience a period of crisis as they move from childhood to adulthood. While the eventual goal is identity achievement, young people will not necessarily pass through each of the other three statuses en route to achieving an identity. As adolescents resolve the crises they face, they establish a commitment to their choices. **Identity achievement** indicates individuals experienced a crisis period and achieved a sense of commitment to their resulting decisions. These individuals are generally well-adjusted, stable, and mature. **Foreclosed** individuals demonstrate a strong sense of commitment, but have not experienced the crisis or exploratory period necessary for arriving at their sense of commitment. These individuals have typically "borrowed" or been given their ideology or career aspirations by their parents or other authority figures, and appear very mature in their belief systems. On further inspection, however, generally have difficulty explaining why they believe as they do. **Identity diffusion** refers to individuals who have not experienced an identity crisis or made a commitment to any ideologic or occupational direction. These individuals are immature and tend to follow popular fads or trends. Finally, **moratorium** status indicates individuals are experiencing an occupational and/or ideological crisis that has not yet been resolved and delays socially expected actions. Table 12-2 illustrates how each status has different crisis and commitment experiences (Baumeister, 1991; Marcia, 1980).

Table 12-2 Adolescent Identity Status

Position on Occupation and Ideology	Identity Diffusion	Foreclosure	Moratorium	Identity Achievement
Has experienced a period of crisis or exploration	No	No	Currently	Yes
Has come to a sense of commitment	No	Yes	Emerging	Yes

Adapted from Marcia, J. E. (1980). Identity in adolescence. In J. Adelson (Ed.), Handbook of adolescent psychology *(pp. 159–187). New York: Wiley. Reprinted with permission of John Wiley & Sons, Inc.*

Psychosocial moratorium, Erikson's term referring to the period of exploration many people engage in as they attempt to determine their life course, is particularly evident among young people who attend college, an experience that allows them time to explore career options before making a final decision. Adolescents entering the workforce directly after high school are therefore often more likely to have identity achievement as compared with their college-bound peers.

An important determinant of adolescents' identity status appears to be the parenting to which they are exposed. Of particular importance is the extent to which parents promote a strong sense of connectedness among family members while providing their adolescents appropriate opportunities for developing a sense of individuality (Grotevant, 1998). Individuality includes the ability to present one's own point of view and verbally define who one is. Identity achieved adolescents are more likely to come from homes that promote a strong sense of connectedness and individuality (Santrock, 2001). In contrast, adolescents whose homes were high in connectedness, but weak in individuality are more likely to promote a foreclosed identity style, while homes that were weak in connectedness, irrespective of individuality, are likely to promote a diffused identity status.

Gender Identity

Gender identity refers to the way we think about ourselves as either male or female, and is a culmination of biological makeup, personal, and social expectations and recommendations about how males and females should think and behave. From the moment children are born, the world will respond to them differently depending on whether they are male or female. As young children first come to understand the differences between boys and girls they are likely to demonstrate very strong preferences toward gender-appropriate behavior. During late childhood, children continue to recognize the need to engage in gender-appropriate behavior, but become more accepting of themselves and others engaging in behaviors normally identified with the opposite sex. However, as young people approach adolescence there is a reorientation regarding what is considered acceptable behavior for those of each gender. Adolescents are much more traditional in their gender attitudes and behavior as compared with children or adults (Sigelman, Carr, & Bagley, 1986). The greater attitudinal and behavioral differences that emerge between early adolescent boys and girls are likely due to the adolescents' and others' (i.e., caregivers, teachers, peers) responses to the pubertal changes experienced by the adolescents themselves that cause them to look increasingly different as they take on adult male and female physiological characteristics (Lynch, 1991).

Erikson (1968) considered gender to be an important part of establishing young people's individual identity. In fact, one explanation for adolescents' more intolerant attitudes about certain cross-sex behaviors is that this more rigid perspective may help adolescents as they attempt to make sense of who they are (Shaffer, 2000). Gilligan, Lyons, and Hanmer (1990) contend that males and females experience different developmental paths and suggest that gender is particularly important in early adolescent girls' sense of identity formation—girls have a greater relationship orientation

Family Teaching

Psychosocial Development

- Provide positive role models.
- Encourage efforts to establish a sense of hope about the world around them and a purpose and determination about themselves.
- Create a secure environment where adolescents can grow.
- Assist adolescents in finding and developing unique strengths.
- Allow adolescents to participate in family decision making while providing guidance and structure regarding the decisions they make about themselves.
- Create a learning and social environment where young people are encouraged to think and solve problems for themselves.
- Provide opportunities to begin exploring various career options.

REFLECTIONS FROM FAMILIES

I felt a great responsibility to not openly trouble my parents or cause them to worry. I felt that I needed to prove to them and to everyone else that they were still good parents despite my brother's problems. Inwardly there was a constant struggle going on between who I thought people wanted me to be and who I really was. I constantly thought about it—struggling between my feelings of responsibility and the pressure to just once quit being me and be the irresponsible, bad child. It became vital to me that I do things for the right reason. Was I doing it because it was right or because my parents wanted me to? Was I pushing myself to succeed because that was what I wanted or because that would help my parents believe that they hadn't failed?

regarding their interactions with others. During the onset of adolescence, girls become aware that their innate relational orientation is not valued by the male-dominated culture, in which a rules-based orientation is dominant. As a result, many girls silence their unique perspective or "different voice," becoming less willing to assert themselves and their opinions. Others (Archer, 1992; Waterman, 1992) have found that males and females are becoming increasingly similar in their patterns of identity formation.

Intimacy

Erikson (1968) contends that once young people have achieved a sense of who they are, they are better able to commit themselves intimately to another person (Figure 12-13). Marcia (1980) however, states that the paradox of intimacy is that "it is a strength that can be acquired only through vulnerability; and vulnerability is possible only with the internal assurance of a firm identity" (p. 160). According to Erikson (1968), the youth who is not sure of his identity "shies away from interpersonal intimacy or throws himself into acts of intimacy which are 'promiscuous'" (p. 135). Such an individual may be involved in intimate relationships, but is likely to settle for highly stereotyped interpersonal relations, resulting in a lack of fulfillment and "a deep sense of isolation." It is interesting that while we often think of elderly people as the loneliest individuals, surveys have found that the highest level of loneliness often appears in youths and late adolescents (Cutrona, 1982).

MORAL DEVELOPMENT

An important aspect of young people's cognitive maturation is their ever-increasing ability to consider the complexity of their own and others' moral and ethical reasoning. As a result of their gradual movement away from the solitary influence of the home and toward the diverse influence of society and the adult world, and because of their psychosocial development, the concern for moral values and standards is likely never to be more relevant than during adolescence. From a psychoanalytic perspective, moral development arises during childhood out of fear of rejection as a result of an individual's inability to control unconscious sexual and aggressive impulses (Shaffer, 2000). Thus, to keep these impulses in check, young people adopt as their own the rules and prohibitions defined by society generally, and their caregivers specifically. From a social learning perspective, moral development is a result of early experiences and the reinforcement children and adolescents receive for their different behaviors. Hoffman (1980) contends that parental discipline, and more specifically, the discipline techniques applied, are crucial factors in determining whether a response to a moral situation will be internalized. For example, children whose caregivers give explanations or reasons for desired behavioral changes, rather than demanding change based on their authority, are much more likely to internalize the reasoning behind the behavior rather than merely conforming temporarily to the desired changes in behavior.

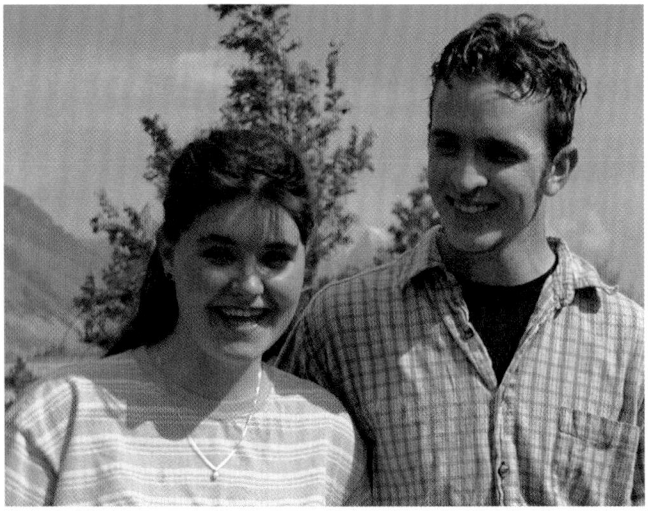

Figure 12-13 Learning about intimacy becomes a significant part of many late adolescents' lives.

While these perspectives are insightful, the major contributor to current thinking regarding moral development is Kohlberg (1976), based largely on the work of Piaget. Kohlberg's conventional level of moral reasoning, which has been shown to emerge during adolescence (Rest, Davison, & Robbins, 1978) and to persist as the predominant stage of moral functioning throughout adulthood, focuses on the acceptance by individuals of those norms and rules defined either by their close social network or by the more formal governmental systems of their culture/society (i.e., local, state, or federal laws). (Refer to Chapter 6.) This level of moral thinking is occupied by two stages or primary orientations; stage 3, or the "good-boy" morality, where the focus is on maintaining good relationships; and stage 4, or the authority-maintaining morality, where the focus is on upholding the law. Gilligan (Gilligan, 1982; Gilligan, Lyons, & Hanmer, 1990) has argued that Kohlberg's stages of moral development are biased toward the rule-oriented reasoning she contends is more evident among males, and more valued by society. As a result, Gilligan believed adolescent males would more likely reflect judgement-based reasoning of the fourth stage of moral thinking, whereas female adolescents would more likely reflect the relationship-based reasoning of the third stage. Most recent research on this issue, however, has failed to support Gilligan's contentions, generally finding no gender differences, or moderate differences favoring females, when using measures of Kohlberg's stages. The ability to consider the moral implications of their own and others' thoughts and actions is crucial to adolescents' developing a personal belief system, which largely defines their social, political, and religious identities.

ADOLESCENTS IN CONTEXT

Families

The family is the first and, in general, the most important socializing agent in one's life. Successful socialization is the process by which children acquire the beliefs, values, and behavior deemed significant by older members of their society (Shaffer, 2000), and is to a large degree, a function of the parenting and other familial interactions experienced while growing up. But do familial experiences change as young people pass through the adolescent period? In particular, do caregiver–child relationships differ as youths move through the second decade of life?

Several changes are likely to have an impact on the type of interactions and quality of relationships adolescents and their caregivers have with one another. First, adolescents experience physiological changes associated with puberty that cause both they and their caregivers to think and respond differently to one another; caregivers begin to expect adolescents to act more like adults. And while they may not always act more mature, adolescents begin to believe they should be treated more like adults. These changes in adolescents' interpersonal interactions with caregivers do appear to be linked to the onset of puberty and the hormonal changes that occur during this period, resulting in greater conflict (Steinberg, 1981).

The cognitive shift to formal operational thinking has an impact on young people's relationships with caregivers as well. Abstract thinking allows adolescents to better distinguish their real and ideal worlds, resulting in caregivers no longer defining adolescents' ideal standard, which is now measured according to what ideal caregivers should be like. In addition, as adolescents' are better able to articulate their own concerns when caregivers make requests they disagree with, they are less likely to comply. If caregivers are not sensitive to adolescents' desires to test their newly found cognitive skills, adolescents are likely to be perceived as defiant.

Adolescents also begin answering the question "Who am I?" and exploring attitudes and values they have been taught. This often increases the level of tension between adolescents and caregivers, since caregivers are also likely to reexperience their own identity issues during this period, often confronting their own mortality and the notion that they are approaching a new stage in their own lives (Steinberg & Steinberg, 1994).

Attachment and Autonomy

As young people approach adulthood, they want more autonomy and need to have a sense of self-direction and independence. Caregivers, however, are often unsure of how to provide their children with opportunities for establishing autonomy. They may even feel threatened by their child's desire for more independence, therefore responding by exerting ever greater control.

Reflective Thinking

Caregiver–Adolescent Relationships

Think back to your adolescence. Do you recall ever feeling embarrassed that your parents were with you when you were at the mall or at a dance, even though you may have enjoyed doing things with them when you were around the house? Why do you think you felt uncomfortable? What suggestions would you give an adolescent who is embarrassed to be seen with their parents?

The interesting dilemma for adolescents is that although they are attempting to establish a sense of autonomy and, as a result often act as if they would rather die than be seen with their parents, the unsureness of this period makes the safety found in the caregiver–child relationship no less important (Figure 12-14). The task for caregivers is to recognize the normalcy of their adolescents' needs to push away and begin to explore the world around them, while at the same time recognizing their need to know there is a secure

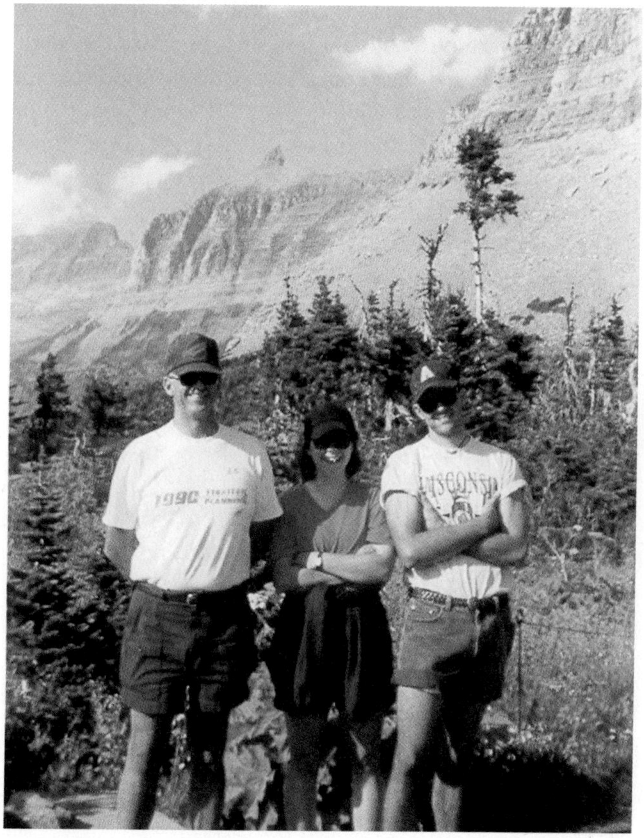

Figure 12-14 Contrary to what many caregivers would guess, they generally continue to be an important part of adolescents' lives.

base to return to if their world becomes too unfamiliar or frightening. Indeed, adolescents' attachment to caregivers is important and has been linked to characteristics such as self-esteem and emotional adjustment (Armsden & Greenberg, 1987; Paterson, Pryor, & Field, 1994; Raja, McGee, & Stanton, 1992).

Caregiver–Adolescent Conflict

As a result of their desire for greater autonomy, and their increased level of reasoning and the associated questioning, adolescents are likely to experience conflict in their relationships with their caregivers (Figure 12-15). Most arguments are the "normal, everyday, mundane family matters such as school work, social life and friends, home chores, disobedience, disagreements with siblings, and personal hygiene" (Montemayor, 1983, p. 91). Rarely do they argue about the hot topics that are typically identified with adolescence, such as sex, drugs, religion, or politics. This is surprising considering the differences in adult and youth attitudes about these topics. Caregivers may indirectly attempt to influence their children's behavior regarding these "hotter" issues through rules and interactions over the more mundane matters families are willing to discuss. For example, caregivers may be uncomfortable discussing their attitudes and beliefs about adolescent sexuality, but will evidence those beliefs through the rules they establish about acceptable clothing, curfews, and dating. Montemayor also found most caregiver–adolescent interactions were peaceful and free of stress. More recently, Barber (1994) found that Caucasian, African-American, and Hispanic caregivers and adolescents all disagree about similar issues (e.g., chores and dress). While there were similar proportions of each group reporting chronic (i.e., daily) conflict, substantially lower levels of conflict were reported by both minority groups as compared with Caucasian families. Barber speculated that this may be a function of Caucasians' greater use of an authoritative parenting style, which encourages adolescents to have a greater say in issues relevant to themselves.

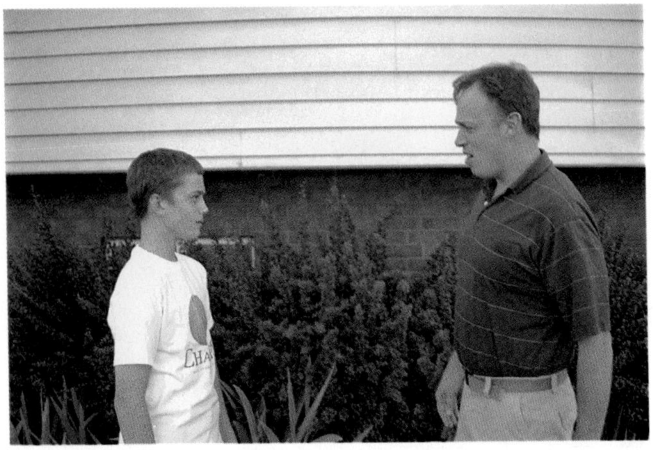

Figure 12-15 Changes in both teens and their caregivers during the adolescent period often result in more conflict between them.

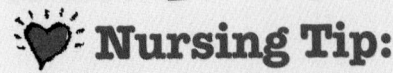

Nursing Tip:

Caregiver–adolescent conflict

Adolescents' attempts for greater autonomy can often result in an escalation in the amount of conflict they have with their caregivers. Discuss with caregivers why adolescents may disagree with rules and expectations. Suggest that caregivers "choose their battles" with adolescents. That is, keeping a bedroom neat and clean may not need to be as important as who their adolescent chooses as peers or what time they need to be home at night. Sometimes allowing adolescents to "win" may be all it takes for them to realize they are "in control" over some parts of their life.

Sibling Relationships

Siblings provide a unique relationship for adolescents because they are generally close in age and are likely to spend a great deal of time with one another. Interestingly, their relationship is one in which there is no choice about membership. Thus, while conflict in friendships may be avoided in order to preserve the relationship, sibling relationships have more warmth and conflict since they do not operate under the same threat of termination (Brody, Stoneman, & McCoy, 1994; Furman & Buhrmester, 1992).

Siblings can have an impact on one another for both good or ill. For example, older adolescents' involvement in illicit drugs and alcohol (Brook, Whiteman, Gordon, & Brenden, 1986; Clayton & Lacy, 1982; Rowe & Gulley, 1992), as well as deviant and sexual behavior (Rowe & Britt, 1991; Rogers & Rowe, 1990), are predictive of their younger siblings' involvement in similar behavior. In contrast, siblings also provide a buffering effect against challenging experiences such as parental divorce (Kempton, Armistead, Wierson, & Forehand, 1991) or poor peer relationships (East & Rook, 1992). For example, East and Rook (1992) found that children who received relatively little support from their school friends often reported receiving support from their favorite siblings.

As youths approach adolescence, several changes occur in their relationships with their siblings. Furman and Buhrmester (1992) found that progression through adolescence was associated with a reduction in perceived sibling support and a corresponding increase in perceived sibling conflict, which apexed between the ages of 12 and 13 years old, followed by an increase in support and a decrease in conflict when youths reached the age of 15 or 16 years old.

Siblings appear to be important socializing agents for adolescents as they transition into the world outside their family since they may provide young people with an environment where they can learn appropriate interpersonal skills in preparation for their nonfamilial interactions, particularly with peers (McCoy, Brody, & Stoneman, 1994; Stocker & Dunn, 1990) (Figure 12-16).

For adolescents who are "only" children—about 20% of all adolescents in the United States—there appears to be little research indicating they are at a loss because of the absence of a brother or sister. Only children have been found to have a fairly high sense of self-esteem and achievement motivation as compared with those with siblings (Falbo, 1992). This may be a result of their increased level of interaction with parents and other adults.

Peers

Friends have long been considered to be of central importance to adolescents. Erikson (1968) believed that the peer group provides a sanctuary of group identity while a young person is passing between the dependency of childhood and the independence of adulthood. Piaget considered peer relationships crucial to youths' understanding of rules and moral behavior and argued that while young children's interactions with adults and siblings tended to emphasize the divine structure of rules, the informal and unsupervised play among peers during childhood and adolescence fosters the kind of spontaneous, flexible rule making and rule enforcing that is necessary in developing a mature moral orientation (Hoffman, 1980).

Because of the developmental importance of peers during early to middle adolescence, friendships experienced during this period are unlike those encountered at any other stage of life (Douvan & Adelson, 1966; Elkind, 1984; Selman, 1980). Friendships during this period demonstrate higher levels of mutuality, interaction, and interdependency. Thus, during childhood, peers are more appropriately characterized as playmates rather than as friends, and their coming together is based more on proximity and common activities than on relationship issues (Douvan & Adelson, 1966; Elkind, 1984). Conversely, the friendships of adulthood are much less intense than those experienced during adolescence as a result of adults' greater sense of individuality and the consequent reduction in their need to "examine and share the internal world with others" (Douvan & Adelson, 1966, p. 178).

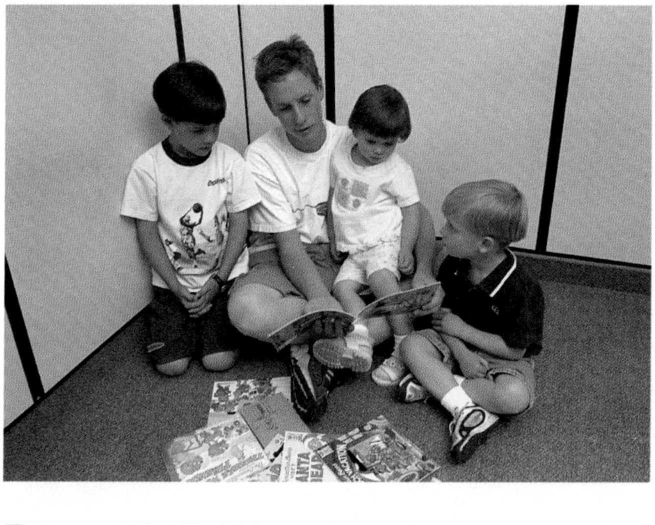

Figure 12-16 Sibling relationships can provide adolescents with significant opportunities for learning how to teach, help, and care about others.

Peer relationships generally exist at one of three levels; the friendship dyad, the clique, and the crowd. The **friendship dyad,** or coming together of two friends, is the most fundamental peer relation and the one most likely to be based on similar interests and emotional support in comparison to friendships that exist largely as part of a larger association of peers. **Cliques,** three to nine "buddies" or "mates" who exhibit a strong sense of cohesion, have been described as constituting an alternative family structure for its members as they acclimate to the world outside the home (Dunphy, 1963). During early adolescence, cliques typically constitute several same-sex friends. The **crowd** is an association of two to four cliques in which relations are less intimate than in the smaller groups (Dunphy, 1963). Formation of the crowd is usually based on a common distinguishing characteristic, evidenced by the labels often associated with different adolescent crowds (e.g., "preppies," "brains," "jocks," "normals," "druggies") (Brown, Mounts, Lamborn, & Steinberg, 1993). For example, an adolescent will have an especially close friendship with someone whom they trust, and are particularly comfortable sharing personal feelings with them; these friends will in turn likely belong to a clique or small group of friends with whom they share similar interests and enjoy "hanging out"; this group of friends is likely to have a larger crowd of individuals with whom they will not necessarily do things outside of large gatherings, but whom they are likely to seek out at the mall or at school events and with whom they identify because of some common characteristic (e.g., athletics, musical interest, deviant behavior, drama). The importance of the peer group at each level varies across adolescence as a function of individual development (Selman, 1980) and the peer groups' developmental stage (Dunphy, 1963) (Figure 12-17).

As youths develop, the structure of their peer relationships changes as it passes through five stages of development (Dunphy, 1963) (Figure 12-18). Beginning with the isolated, unisexual cliques established during childhood, early adolescents begin to explore, as unisexual cliques, interactions with cliques of the opposite sex. During this early period, interaction with the opposite sex is considered daring and only approached in the security of a group setting. Unisexual cliques eventually begin to merge to form heterosexual crowds, where dating begins. In late adolescence, crowds no

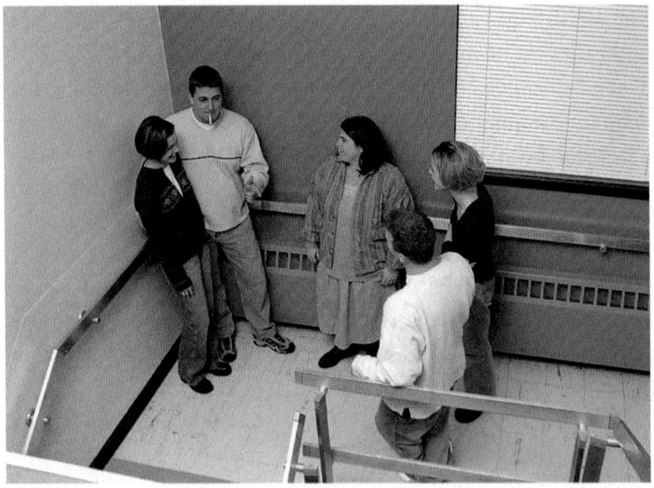

Figure 12-17 Male and female friend groups are often found among adolescents.

longer serve a purpose and are replaced by loosely associated groups of heterosexual couples.

Research concerning same-sex identity formation of adolescents (Cass, 1979; Troiden, 1989) suggests that their peer group experiences will be either similar to or different from heterosexual peer group development based on the timing of their transition toward a homosexual identity; a shift to the gay community as a source of close relationships is the pivotal step.

The number of friends young people have has also been linked to later social well-being. For example, Roff, Sells, & Golden (1972) found in all but the very lowest socioeconomic group, that the least popular sixth- through eighth-grade students were far more likely to have delinquency records 3 to 4 years after they were assessed, as compared with their moderately and highly popular classmates. Other researchers found that children who were less popular or more rejected

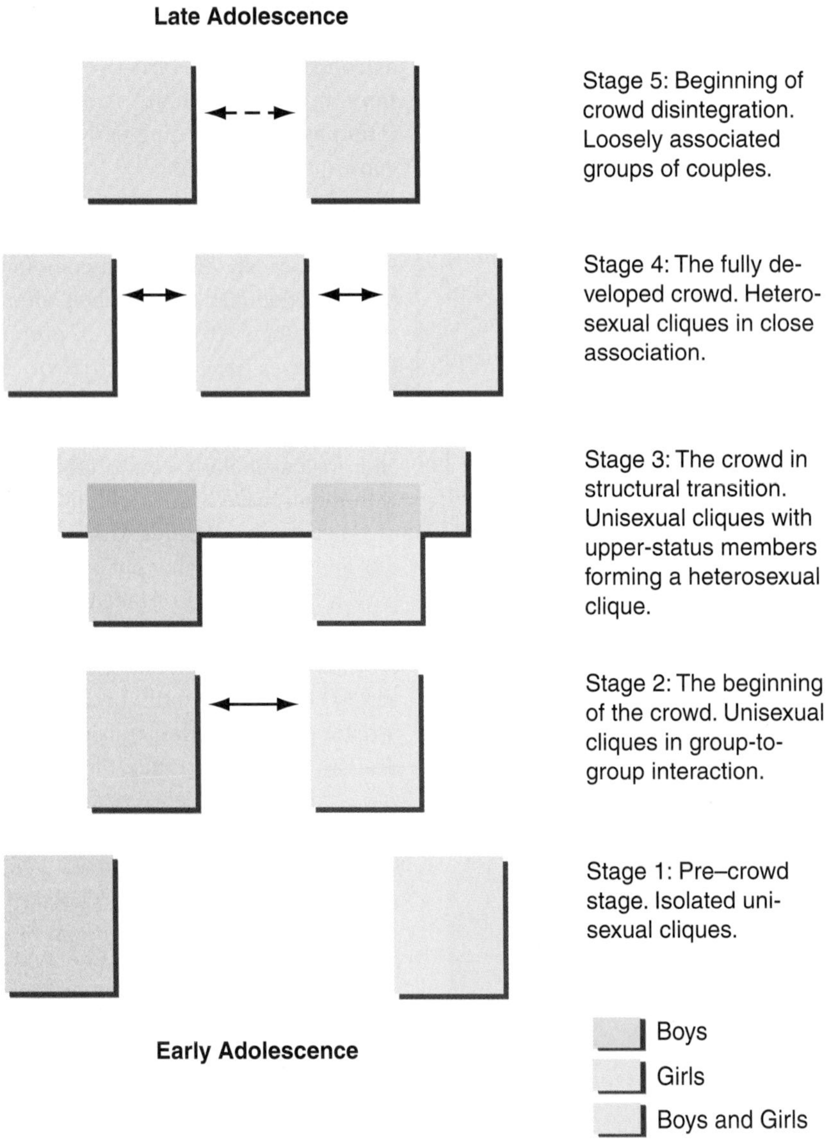
Late Adolescence
Stage 5: Beginning of crowd disintegration. Loosely associated groups of couples.
Stage 4: The fully developed crowd. Heterosexual cliques in close association.
Stage 3: The crowd in structural transition. Unisexual cliques with upper-status members forming a heterosexual clique.
Stage 2: The beginning of the crowd. Unisexual cliques in group-to-group interaction.
Stage 1: Pre–crowd stage. Isolated unisexual cliques.
Early Adolescence
Boys
Girls
Boys and Girls

Figure 12-18 Stages of Group Development in Adolescence

by their peers were more likely to drop out of school and to become involved in juvenile and adult criminal activity (Janes, Hesselbrock, Myers, & Penniman, 1979; Kupersmidt & Coie, 1990; Parker & Asher, 1987; Parker, Rubin, Price, & DeRosier, 1995; Roff, Sells, and Golden, 1972).

Another important aspect of adolescents' peer relationships is the *quality* of the friendships. Quality friendships are characterized by high levels of mutual caring, respect, and trust, in a context of balanced give and take (Youniss & Smollar, 1985). Adolescents who experience these types of close friendships generally report more intimate self-disclosure, more prosocial behavior, and more emotional support or encouragement from their friends, while also reporting less conflictual, domineering, or rivalrous behavior (Berndt & Savin-Williams, 1989; Furman & Robbins, 1985). Although present in childhood friendships, these characteristics become much more pronounced during preadolescence and adolescence (Berndt & Perry, 1986; Sharabany, Gershoni, & Hofman, 1981). Sullivan (1953) proposed that preadolescents develop greater sensitivity toward others through close friendships, and Mannarino (1976) and McGuire and Weisz (1982) found that when preadolescents report having close friendships, they are more likely to be altruistic.

For most adolescents, ethnicity or culture appear to be very important in determining who they select as friends. For example, in one study of an ethnically integrated school (DuBois & Hirsch, 1990) while most students reported having an other-ethnic school friend, only about a quarter of the students reported having contact with those friends outside of school. For many ethnic minority youths, especially immigrants, peer relations formed from their own ethnic group can provide an adaptive support against the sense of isolation that can often exist among their peers of the majority population (Santrock, 2001).

Peer Influence

A major concern for many parents is whether their adolescents are being adversely influenced by their friends. The extent to which adolescents influence friends or are influenced by them varies according to their ability to establish and maintain supportive peer relationships as well as the type of group they belong to. Teevan (1972) contends compliance with peers is often based on the expectation that "such conformity will be rewarded with eventual acceptance into the group" (p. 283). Whether responding to actual peer pressure or merely to perceived expectations, young people who are less secure in their relations with friends are more likely to engage in behavior they would otherwise avoid. The importance of peer influence may be evaluated according to how closely associated the individual is to their friendship group or clique (Figure 12-19). Most adolescents would be expected to fit into the *core* of a particular peer circle, where

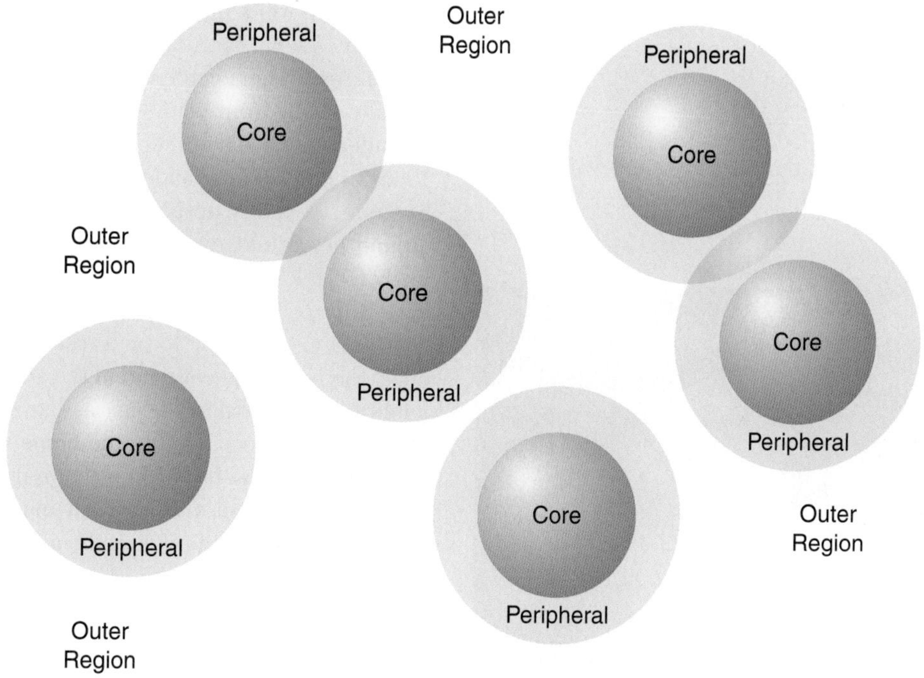

Figure 12-19 Theoretical Conception of Peer Group Structure. Because of peers' increased significance during adolescence, experiences with peers can either increase adolescents' sense of belonging or their sense of isolation. Reprinted with permission of J. Kelly McCoy.

Reflective Thinking

Friendship

Were the friendships you had during early adolescence different from the friendships you have now? How were they different? What advice would you give an adolescent worried about their friends?

there is a strong sense of commitment and collegiality. However, many adolescents instead fit into the *peripheral* region of one or more groups, where there is a sense of tentative belonging and a desire to become a part of the core group (Figure 12-20). Finally, others float unattached, *outside* any particular peer group. Adolescents who exist at the periphery of their identified peer group would be most vulnerable to peer influence as a result of their insecure position in the group. Out of a desire to become a core member of the peer group they identify with, peripheral group members would be most likely to allow peer expectations, or at least perceived peer expectations, to dictate their behaviors. In addition to group placements, the type of group one belongs to is also an important predictor of participation in antisocial or self-destructive behavior. Adolescents identified as being in the "druggies" or "toughs" peer groups are much more likely to report participating in groups encouraging antisocial or self-destructive behaviors as compared with those identified as being "populars," "brains," or "normals" (Stone & Brown, 1998).

Parents and Peers

A major parental concern is that family values will be displaced by peer values. Although there is some justification for this concern, several factors influence whom adolescents are likely to select as peers (Conger & Petersen, 1984). First, there is usually considerable overlap between parental and peer values because of common backgrounds; many adolescents select friends whose values are congruent with their parents'. Second, parents often are unsure of appropriate expectations for certain areas of adolescents' lives, and are thus willing to defer to the expectations of their adolescents' friends. This is especially apparent in current fashions, music, and leisure activities. Third, parents and peers have an impact on different aspects of adolescents' lives; peers are more likely to be influential in matters of short-term importance (i.e., tastes in music and entertainment, fashions in clothing and language, dating and friendship behavior), whereas parents are more likely to be influential in matters of greater and longer-term permanence (i.e., moral and social values, educational aspirations, and occupational choice) (Kandel & Lesser, 1972). Fourth, when adolescents do turn to peers for support, frequently it is not a displacement of parental influence but rather an attempt to fill a void left by their parents' lack of support and involvement. Finally, adolescents' orientations toward parents as compared with peers varies as a function of individual differences within adolescents and their social contexts (Conger & Petersen, 1984). As a result, Conger and Petersen conclude that the degree of conflict between parental and peer influence is less than assumed.

While numerous studies have found that adolescents' behavior is strongly predicted by peers' behavior (Brook, Whiteman, Gordon, Nomura, & Brook, 1986; Needle, McCubbin, Wilson, Reineck, Lazar, & Mederer, 1986; Sussman, Dent, McAdams, Stacy, Burton, & Flay, 1994), several researchers contend that much of this similarity may actually result from young people seeking out friends with attitudes and behavior similar to their own (Billy & Udry, 1985; Cohen, 1977; Kandel, 1978). For example, a girl who becomes sexually active may cease to feel comfortable around her friends who are not sexually active, thus, she is likely to seek out new friends who have a similar sexual status (Billy & Udry, 1985). Because the similarity among friends is just as likely to be a result of selection as is influence, the resemblance found in the attitudes and behavior of adolescent friendships is just as likely to be a function of characteristics developed in the home and in other nonpeer contexts as it is the friendships themselves.

Caregivers can also have an impact on the quality of adolescents' friendships directly, according to four mechanisms: (1) their expectations about the positive and negative implications of peer relations; (2) their monitoring of adolescents' peer activity; (3) their direct interactions with adolescents' friends; and (4) their perceptions of their own roles in their adolescent's friendships (McCoy, 1992). In another study McCoy, Corey, and Owen (1999) found that while many adolescents do seem to determine whether their parents are involved in their friendships, the involvement level

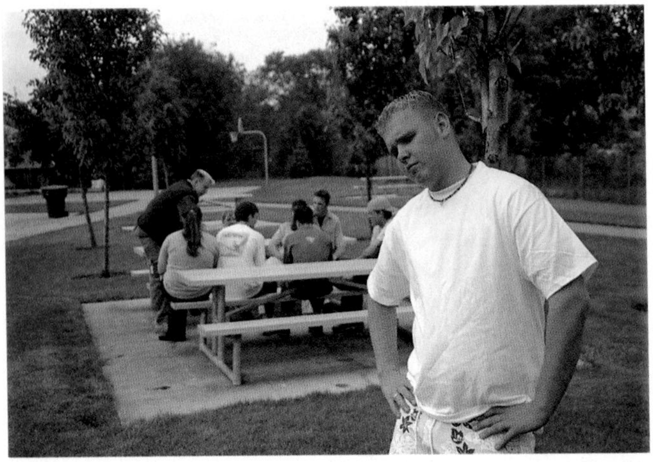

Figure 12-20 Adolescents typically want to be a member of the group.

of many more parents seemed to be determined by the parents' own desire or availability to be involved. Finally, parents' involvement in adolescents' peer relations can be both positive and negative (Ladd & Golter, 1988; Parke et al., 1989) and depends on whether parents act as facilitators, spectators, or controllers of their children's peer relations.

Dating

As previously mentioned, youths' passage through adolescence is marked by the increased significance of peer relationships. This process begins with same-sex friendships. However, during middle and late adolescence, young people begin to explore opposite-sex relationships—frequently through dating. Up until the early part of the past century, dating was a courtship experience used largely to identify an appropriate mate and overseen by parents. Since World War II, we have seen a dramatic shift in the purpose and events that define adolescent dating. Although some adolescents still view early dating experiences as a means of sorting and selecting an appropriate mate, for most, dating has taken on much more of a recreational role. In addition, dating is seen as providing other functions, including a source of status and achievement; a unique socializing experience in which to learn about intimacy, sexuality, and a sense of identity; and an opportunity to develop new and deeper forms of companionship (Paul & White, 1990).

A major shift in the dating experience has been the age when it is likely to begin. Dating now typically begins around age 12 and 13 years for most girls, and between ages 13 and 14 years for boys (McCabe, 1984). By age 16, 90% of all adolescents report having had at least one date (Dickinson, 1975). Although the onset of dating would seem most likely to be triggered by adolescents' individual pubertal development, Dornbusch and his colleagues (1981) concluded that socially defined factors, as measured by chronological age, were much better predictors of dating onset than was individual adolescents' pubertal status. Does this mean pubertal status is unimportant to adolescents' dating experience? Petersen's (1985) notion of the "cohort pubertal effect" may help explain the interaction between social context and pubertal status. Petersen argued that the average pubertal status of a particular age group of adolescents, not individual adolescents' pubertal status, is likely to best predict when certain adolescent behaviors (i.e., talking on the phone at length, conflict with parents, and interest in the other sex) are likely to occur. If this is correct, while the onset of dating is socially defined, those social definitions may coincide with the average age of pubertal onset.

So, as dating becomes more important to adolescents, how do they decide who to consider as potential dating partners? According to one study (Roscoe, Dian, & Brooks, 1987), adolescents' focus about a dating partner shifts with age; early adolescents tend to be more egocentric, focusing on issues of immediate gratification (e.g., recreation and status) regarding who and why they dated, whereas older adolescents focus more on long-term aspects of the dating experience (i.e., companionship and mate selection issues). There are also several gender differences regarding dating choices. Males more frequently listed "sexual activity" as a reason for dating while females were more likely to list "intimacy." When 15-year-old males and females were asked what they liked about their girlfriend or boyfriend, boys were more likely to mention physical attractiveness, whereas girls were more likely to mention support and intimacy (Feiring, 1996).

A process of selection referred to as the **matching hypothesis** (Santrock, 2001), proposes that although individuals may prefer a more attractive person in the ideal or abstract, they will generally end up choosing someone who is close to their level of attractiveness. In other words, although many people dream of dating someone they view as extremely attractive, they will generally select as a dating partner or permanent mate someone who would be considered equal in attractiveness to themselves.

Another important part of the dating process are the **dating scripts** adolescents learn and internalize regarding what is expected of them and what they should expect from their dating partners. Dating scripts will vary based on regional location, community size, socioeconomic status, religious affiliation, and peer group, but they are most differentiated by gender. Dating scripts for males and females differ, with males being responsible for initiating, planning, and paying for the date and for initiating the level of sexual interaction; females are generally responsible for appropriately responding to males' attempts to initiate and carry out the date as well as their initiation of sexual gestures (Rose & Frieze, 1993). Although these gender-defined scripts have changed somewhat over the past several decades—giving males and females more flexibility in what is considered appropriate—they appear to have remained largely unchanged.

The extent to which adolescents' dating experiences have an impact on individual development remains largely unknown. Although this area has received limited exploration, there are some ways in which dating has been found to be important. First, because boys are not encouraged to develop the capacity to be emotionally expressive in their same-sex peer relationships, opposite sex relationships may provide boys with an opportunity to explore intimacy development in a context that is much more socially acceptable (Steinberg, 2001). Second, becoming seriously involved in a steady dating relationship before age 15 can have a somewhat stunting effect on adolescents' psychosocial development, particularly for girls (Neemann, Hubbard, & Masten, 1995). Girls who begin early to date seriously have been found to be less mature, less imaginative, less oriented toward achievement, less happy with who they are, and more superficial. In contrast, adolescent girls who have not dated at all by the time they reach late adolescence have been

Critical Thinking

Dating Scripts

Dating scripts are an important determinant of what is likely to happen during adolescents' dating experiences. But where do adolescents learn the expectations that define their dating scripts? To what extent do you think adolescents learn about dating scripts in their homes from parents and siblings? To what extent are these scripts learned from the media? How important are peers in determining the dating scripts adolescents establish?

identified as having a more retarded social development, excessive dependency on their parents, and greater feelings of insecurity (McDonald & McKinney, 1994; Neemann, Hubbard, & Masten, 1995).

If adolescents postpone dating, and dating behavior remains light to moderate, it can provide a positive opportunity for social development. What has been difficult to determine is whether adolescents' dating experiences are themselves an important positive factor for social development or whether more socially advanced adolescents are simply more likely to date.

Schools

Schools and academic achievement are important in shaping the developing adolescents' sense of autonomy and identity. This is because almost 90% of adolescents attend public secondary school (grades 9 to 12), and they spend an average of 180 days per year in school. In fact, during most of the year, typical adolescents spend more than one-third of their waking hours every week in school or school-related activities. In addition, adolescents remain in school for more years now than they did in the past (Sprinthall & Collins, 1995; Steinberg, 2001). This is due to not having to drop out to support their families. Academic achievement during adolescence is important because it often reflects not only how well the individual accomplishes long- and short-term goals, but also the feelings of success one has in one's own as well as society's eyes. To be effective, schools and curricula for adolescents should be based on principles of learning and development and provide a climate that encourages exploring future directions and goals (Figure 12-21).

Schools can have a positive or negative effect on adolescents. Often, a student's experience varies according to parent and family context, peer group, size of the school, extracurricular activities, and academic track. Berndt and Keefe (1995) also found an adolescent's adjustment to school was influenced not only by the behavior of their friends, but also by the characteristics of the friendship. Students whose friends described themselves as disruptive in the fall of the academic year described themselves as increasing their disruptive behavior during the year. Students whose friendships had positive features increased their involvement in activities during the year; students whose friendships had more negative features were less involved in activities and became more disruptive as the year progressed (Figure 12-22).

For some adolescents, school is a stabilizing, friendly force in their lives. It can encourage cognitive development, establish a climate for social interaction, and provide an

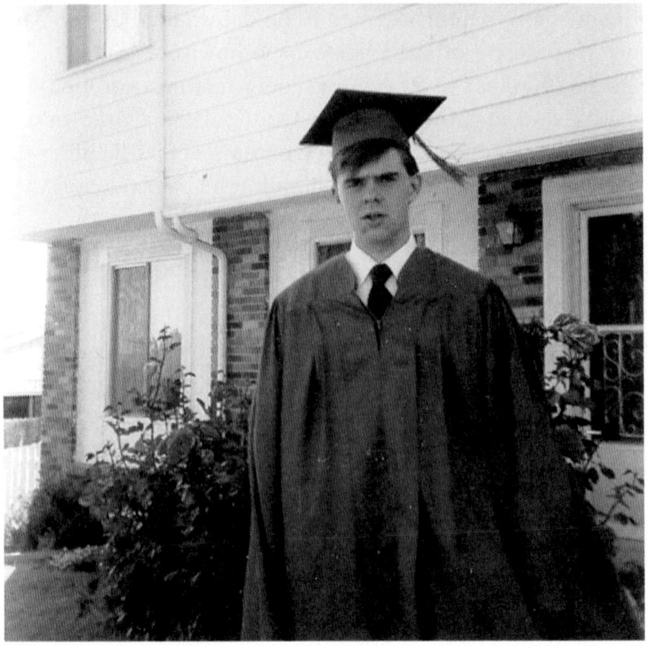

Figure 12-21 High school graduation is an important milestone and accomplishment for teens.

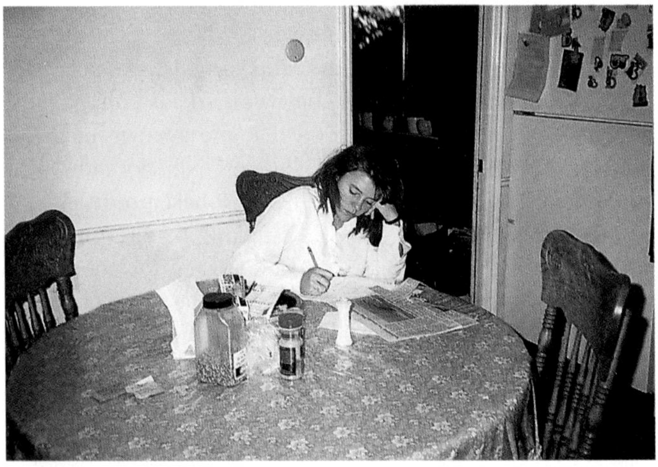

Figure 12-22 Studying and keeping up with homework assignments help adolescents succeed in school.

environment that encourages task completion. School also allows adolescents to have contact with peers and teachers, test new ideas, and validate their thoughts (Figure 12-23). Activities and opportunities at school can provide safe, acceptable outlets for their energy and foster development. Groups such as the honor society, musical and dance groups, student council, athletic teams, school yearbook and newspaper staff, debate teams, special interest clubs, pep squads, cheerleading, and ethnic-identity groups give adolescents a chance to participate in activities with young people who have similar interests, provide experiences in organizations working toward common goals, and allow development of cohesiveness and group loyalty. Schools also can help break barriers related to ethnicity, social class, race, and gender.

School is more likely to have a positive effect on adolescents if they have close friends before, during, and after the transition to secondary school. Academically talented and economically advantaged students also tend to have a more positive experience as compared with their less-affluent or less capable counterparts. These adolescents are more likely to hold positions of leadership, experience classes that are challenging and enjoyable, and have teachers who pay more attention to them (Steinberg, 2001).

For other adolescents, however, school can be a source of stress, where threats to safety and self-esteem and constant change occur (Freiberg, 1992). Some adolescents may experience depression, decreases in perceptions of their athletic and academic abilities or actual academic and athletic performance, or dissatisfaction with school (Sprinthall & Collins, 1995). Moving from an elementary school, where they were the oldest and tallest to a middle school or high school where they are now the youngest and shortest may also cause stress. This "top-dog" phenomenon, where they move from the top position in elementary school to the lowest position in middle school can be difficult and may result in less commitment and satisfaction with school as well as liking their teachers less than they did in earlier years. There are also shifts from the personal to the impersonal; from smaller to larger classes and buildings; from the same class with the same peers and teachers to different classes, different peers, and different teachers; from simple to complex classroom organization; and from slower paced to faster paced curricula.

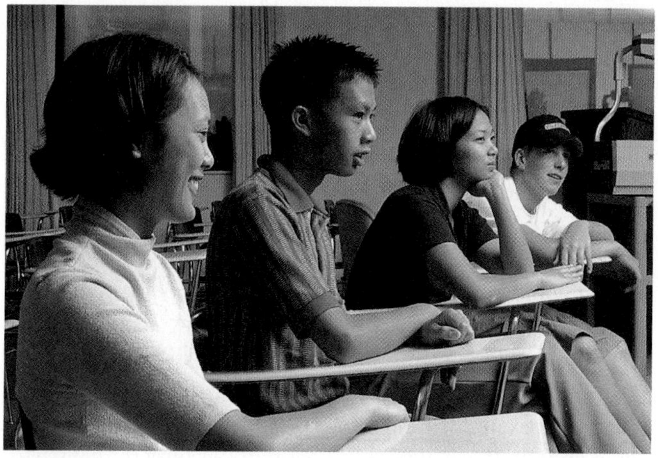

Figure 12-23 Classroom interactions allow for varying points of views and new experiences with teens of different cultures.

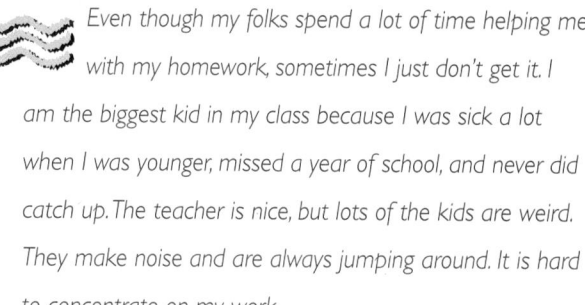

REFLECTIONS FROM FAMILIES

Even though my folks spend a lot of time helping me with my homework, sometimes I just don't get it. I am the biggest kid in my class because I was sick a lot when I was younger, missed a year of school, and never did catch up. The teacher is nice, but lots of the kids are weird. They make noise and are always jumping around. It is hard to concentrate on my work.

In addition, adolescents are dealing with physiological, psychosocial, and cognitive changes that affect their adjustment; junior and senior high schools often have a more open, frightening, combative, and academically taxing environment than elementary school. Teachers provide fewer opportunities for decision making and choices, student–teacher relationships tend to be less positive and personal than in elementary school (Sprinthall & Collins, 1995), and control and discipline are emphasized. Learning activities may often emphasize individual achievement and competition rather than learning for learning's sake. As a result, students may be alienated from the subject matter since these experiences and approaches are not well matched to their developmental needs of greater autonomy and independence. Perhaps that is why levels of unexcused absenteeism, dropout rates, grade failure, and suspensions are higher during this time. Indeed, it is no wonder adolescents with more psychological and academic problems before the transition to secondary school cope less well with the transition to this new environment (Steinberg, 2001).

It is difficult to generalize about the role school plays in adolescent development, however, since different adolescents have different experiences within the same school. Many schools do not promote psychosocial development and have higher dropout rates because of their focus on obedience and conformity and their lack of encouragement for self-reliance, creativity, and independence. However, there are also many good schools that emphasize these qualities and intellectual activities, have classrooms where students actively participate in their own learning, employ committed

Reflective Thinking

School Experiences

What do you remember about the high school you attended? Was the experience primarily negative or positive? Why? What suggestions would you give an adolescent concerned about school experiences?

and autonomous teachers who continually evaluate their programs, and invite parent involvement. They also encourage adolescents to learn about themselves, their relationships with others, the academic material, and society so the students are better able to experience the challenges of adulthood.

Nurses can work closely with parents and school officials to provide accurate, objective information related to health-promotion activities and issues adolescents are concerned about and see as important. School-based health centers (SBHCs) afford unique opportunities for nurses to provide accurate information and nonjudgmental counseling about adolescent issues. Located in or adjacent to schools, these centers provide physical examinations; health education programs; screenings; counseling related to substance abuse, mental health, and sexuality; dental care; and treatment of minor injuries (Anglin, Naylor, & Kaplan, 1996). Often set up to serve poor young people, who are less likely to receive health care than more affluent students, these local centers are in a position to address important adolescent health issues, such as confidentiality, underused services, and preventable diseases (Steinberg, 2001). Adolescents who use SBHCs are more likely to use them for mental health, medical, and substance abuse counseling (Anglin, Naylor, & Kaplan, 1996). See Chapter 5 for a more thorough discussion on school-based health clinics.

Work and Career Development

Part-Time Employment

Adolescents' direct experience with the workplace through part-time employment and their preparation for entering the adult workplace through their exploration of potential career opportunities are important. Greenberger and Steinberg (1986) have identified three important issues to consider: the amount of time adolescents work, the type of work in which they are likely to be involved, and the implication of the work experience on adolescents' lives.

First, nearly two-thirds of all 16-year-olds in the United States will have some kind of part-time work while attending school. Although there is a general conception that adolescents today are lazier than they were a few generations ago, it is interesting to note that adolescents today are twice as likely to have some kind of part-time employment as compared with adolescents in 1960, when only one-third of all adolescents worked part-time while attending school. As compared with other countries, the number of 16-year-olds working in the United States is vastly different. Whereas about 67% of 16-year-olds in the United States work part-time while going to school, only about 37% of the adolescents in Canada combine school and part-time work, about 20% in Sweden, and less than 2% of the 16-year-olds in Japan work part-time while attending school (Greenberger & Steinberg, 1986). Thus, whether adolescents are likely to be employed appears to be very much socially defined.

Secondly, approximately half of all adolescent work opportunities fall into one of two areas; fast food and retail sales. Greenberger and Steinberg (1986) expressed concern over the number of useful skills adolescents are likely to develop as a function of their work experience. In the past young people were likely to receive training to prepare them for the jobs they would take on as adults; however, most of the work available to adolescents today is dull and repetitious. Because adolescents were found to spend only about 5 minutes per hour using skills they were likely to have learned in school, the authors expressed concern that little opportunity was offered adolescents for gaining skills with long-term benefits. A second possible benefit of adolescents' part-time work experience is their potential exposure to the adult workplace and the opportunity to better prepare for full-time entry into the adult world. Again, Greenberger and Steinberg (1986) found that most adolescents worked in age-segregated workplaces, where teens are generally supervised by other teens, and have little opportunity for adult contact or to learn how to interact more effectively in the adult world. The authors concluded the workplace was just as likely as schools to segregate adolescents from adults and the adult world.

A final important issue addressed by Greenberger and Steinberg and others (Mortimer, Finch, Ryu, Shanahan, & Call, 1996; Steinberg & Dornbusch, 1991) has to do with the potential risks and benefits to adolescents' development that may result from part-time work experiences. While a number of benefits do appear to be related to adolescents working (e.g., learning about the business world, learning how to manage money, a greater sense of control over one's own life, and the opportunity to develop a sense of pride in one's abilities and accomplishments), these benefits are most evident among adolescents who work a limited number of hours per week and when adolescents see their work experiences as stimulating and good preparation for later life (Mortimer, et al., 1996). However, when adolescents work more hours per week or are employed in jobs that seem to provide little personal growth, there appear to be a number of potentially negative outcomes. For example, when adolescents who work an average of 20 hours per week were compared with those who did not work, the adolescents who worked had a lower investment in schooling, higher rates of school tardiness and absences, a greater likelihood of lying about incomplete homework, more propensity to engage in deviant acts—including higher rates of alcohol and marijuana use—greater cynicism and tolerance for cheating, less investment in schoolwork, and fewer extracurricular activities (Greenberger & Steinberg, 1986; Mortimer et al., 1996; Steinberg & Dornbusch, 1991; Steinberg & Cauffman, 1995).

Career Development

Another important aspect of adolescents' interactions with the workplace is their exploration of a career or occupation. But, how do adolescents go about choosing a career? First, adolescents are generally very unsettled regarding career plans. For example, in one study only about 26% of students maintained their choice of careers after 1 year and only 17% retained their original career choice after 3 years (Sprinthall & Collins, 1995).

Several researchers have developed theories about the process adolescents go through in their selection of a career (refer to Santrock, 2001, for a more thorough review). Of particular interest is the developmental theory of career selection proposed by Ginzberg (1972), who believed there are three stages of career exploration young people are likely to experience as they move toward a final career choice: fantasy, tentative, and realistic. During the **fantasy stage** (until about age 11), career opportunities are likely to be limited only by children's imagination. When asked what they would like to be when they grow up, children in this stage will likely select careers they are currently the most impassioned about, without considering possible constraints. Between the ages of 11 and 16 years, young people move into the **tentative stage** during which they begin to consider how they might fit in with the various career options they are interested in. They first evaluate what really interests them (11 to 12 years), then evaluate how careers of interest match their own capabilities (13 to 14 years), and then finally determine what types of work are most congruent with the principles they most value (15 to 16 years). Ginzberg identified late adolescence through young adulthood as the **realistic stage,** or the stage when young people begin to extensively explore available careers and then focus on a particular career and job within that career that most realistically matches what they would like to do (Santrock, 2001).

Factors that appear to be important to adolescents' career selection include their own personalities, the attitudes and expectations of their parents and peers, and their broader social context (Steinberg, 1999). Holland (1973, 1987), most identified with exploring the importance of personality for young people's career choices, believes that career selection is a reflection of adolescents' basic personality style, and that once individuals have found a career that fits their personality, they are more likely to enjoy their work and stay with it. Adolescents are also very much influenced by the attitudes and values of their parents and peers.

Reflective Thinking

Career Selection

Do you recall when you first began thinking about what you wanted to do for a living once you had grown up? What did you first want to be? Do you recall the process of selection that you went through to get to the point of career preparation that you are at currently?

Although peer educational and occupational plans are important predictors of adolescents' career aspirations, it is parents who appear to have a greater influence on the types of career paths adolescents are likely to choose (Kandel & Lesser, 1972). Kohn (1977) found that adolescents raised in homes with values more characteristic of middle-class jobs (i.e., autonomy, self-direction, and independence) are more likely to seek those types of jobs irrespective of whether their family situations are more middle class or working class in nature. Also, while gender is an important factor in adolescents' decisions about the type of career they will select (Marini, Fan, Finley, & Beutel, 1996), parents' modeling gender-related career choices was important to adolescents' sex-stereotyped attitudes about work (Barber & Eccles, 1992; Leslie, 1986).

HEALTH PROMOTION

General Nursing Interactions

Any adolescent health promotion effort needs to incorporate the adolescents' perspective of what health means and consider their priorities and concerns relative to health and health care services, as well as the level of their cognitive development. Often, developmental tasks and crises in the physiological, psychosexual, psychosocial, or cognitive domains have an impact on adolescent concerns related to health since the concerns usually have something to do with their own point of view or context.

Many adolescents are reluctant to seek health care because of financial concerns, geographical access, characteristics of the health care provider, or the perceived notion of unavailability of confidential services. Therefore, it is critical that providers be respectful, demonstrate openness, competence, honesty, warmth, compassion, and understanding, and have the ability to communicate effectively with adolescents and their families (Figure 12-24).

Several guidelines are also important for nurses to remember when interacting with adolescents. First, the environment should be caring—positive relationships are

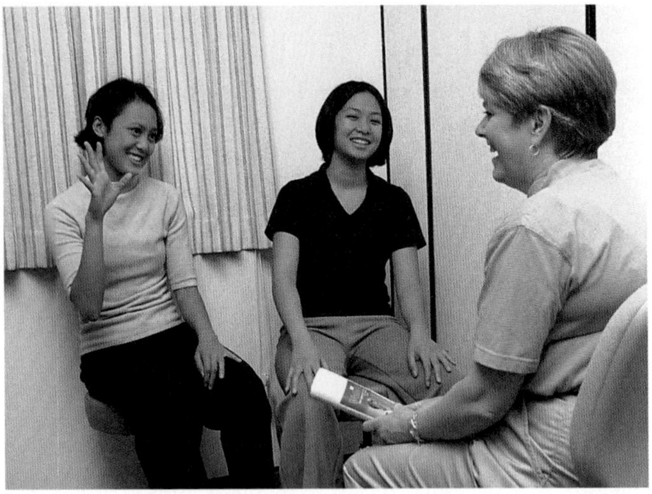

Figure 12-24 Nurse–adolescent interactions need to be relaxed, warm, and accepting.

encouraged, individual differences are valued, and strengths and weaknesses acknowledged. Second, nurses need to treat adolescents with dignity and make it a priority to know them as individuals. Third, assessment with the purpose of improving health, describing health promoting behaviors, and understanding is crucial. Fourth, relationships with families are important to develop and maintain. This means frequent communication between nurses, adolescents, and families and encouraging family participation in many health and other issues.

Effective nurses also need to know and understand age and maturational level, physiological changes have an impact on development, and the specific psychosocial needs and developmental changes expected during adolescence. Interactions should always be individualized, and communications need to convey honesty, general concern, and acceptance. Confidentiality and trust can be important issues for adolescents, which nurses must acknowledge. The physiological, psychosexual, psychosocial, and cognitive changes that normally occur during this period and the many issues and concerns adolescents face today need discussion and explanation. Any program developed for adolescents and/or their caregivers should present information objectively and accurately, and adolescents themselves should be allowed and encouraged to identify and discuss issues and problems they consider important and to provide input into planning.

To work effectively with adolescents, nurses should demonstrate poise, tolerance, warmth, and empathy. They should encourage independence and be aware of hidden adolescent fears or concerns that may be subtly expressed. Nurses also need to be aware of their own biases, which may have an impact on interactions or care delivered. Adolescents should be allowed and encouraged to be responsible for as much of their own personal health care as possible, and helped as needed. Finally, adolescents should be assisted in making appropriate decisions that have an impact on their lives. If they do not know how to make wise decisions and careful choices, nurses should teach them principles of effective decision making and problem solving.

Nursing care should be provided in settings, sometimes away from caregivers, where the self-conscious adolescent feels welcome and comfortable. Allowing sufficient time and privacy for all interactions is essential, so sensitive topics related to physiological growth, sexuality, personal goals, and behaviors (drug abuse, gang membership, promiscuity) can be discussed in an unhurried and nonjudgemental atmosphere. It is not uncommon for successful interactions to resemble conversations between persons with common interests. The interviewer applies developmental principles, so concrete-thinking early adolescents understand answers to their specific questions and older adolescents understand answers to their open-ended and more abstract questions. Confidentiality issues should be discussed early in interactions, since adolescents may confide information to nurses that they prefer their caregivers not know about. It is important to make clear early on, however, that some issues may need to be shared with caregivers, especially when they are younger adolescents still living at home.

Even though adolescence is generally a time of wellness, these young people will seek health care for skin conditions, minor illnesses, school/sports physicals, management of chronic illness, high-risk behaviors, and conditions related to sexuality.

The *Healthy People 2010* (U.S. Department of Health and Human Services, 2000) goals for adolescent health promotion include immunizations, nutrition, oral health, fitness, physical activity, unintentional injury, violence, substance abuse, sexual behavior, and mental health. These areas are particularly relevant to adolescents because they are the major sources of morbidity and mortality for the adolescent age group. Each will be discussed with appropriate nursing interventions.

Immunizations

Until recently, immunization or vaccination programs have not focused on improving coverage for adolescents. Since adolescents continue to be adversely affected by preventable diseases such as measles, rubella, hepatitis B, and varicella, it is important to improve the delivery of immunization services to this age group by implementing the recommended childhood immunization schedule (see Appendix C).

Nutrition

Adolescence is a time of rapid growth in muscle mass, weight, and height. These physical changes mean increased nutritional needs, especially calories, proteins, and minerals (calcium, zinc, and iron). Calcium is needed to meet skeletal growth requirements, prevent fractures, and help prevent osteoporosis later in life (Committee on Nutrition, 1999). Zinc is necessary for final body growth and sexual maturation. Iron intake should be increased to meet normally expanding blood volume needs, the increase in lean body mass, and to replace iron lost through menstruation. Iron requirements increase to as much as 2.2 mg/day and are associated with the size and timing of the growth spurt, sexual maturation, and menses (Beard, 2000). Males will need more calories than females, especially if they are involved in athletics. Typically, female requirements are around 2,000 calories per day; males will need from 2,500 to 3,000 calories per day. Protein needs also increase. Recommended allowances for females range from 44–46 grams per day and for males, from 45–59 g/day (Committee on Dietary Allowances, 1989).

Adolescents always seem hungry but often do not eat appropriate, well-balanced meals. Instead, they prefer snack foods that are easy to prepare, faddish, and often full of empty calories. Adolescent food habits are influenced by concerns of their body image, peer pressure, emotional problems, their busy schedules, or unsupervised meal preparation/purchase. It is also not unusual for teenagers to skip meals (breakfast most commonly), eat fast foods, or snack frequently. Therefore, nurses can help caregivers and adolescents improve their nutrition by explaining the importance of a good diet and encouraging adolescents to be involved in meal planning. Caregivers also need to realize that the adolescents' need for freedom, independence, and peer acceptance may be reflected in their eating habits. If nutritious foods and snacks are available (milk, cheese, yogurt, fruits, vegetables, juices), adolescents are regularly allowed to be responsible for preparing family meals, and food preferences (hamburgers, pizza, burritos) are integrated into meal plans, conflicts about nutritional concerns may decrease. Adolescents and their caregivers also need to be aware of the recommended dietary allowances, and know which foods are high in calcium (milk and milk products), iron (green vegetables, meats), and zinc (milk, meat, fish, eggs). Adolescents should also receive information about nutritious snacks and fast foods available in restaurants (salads, pasta, grilled meats, vegetables, fruits).

All health screening visits for adolescents need to include height and weight measurements as well as questions about eating habits, including dieting, changes in weight, meal patterns, and consumption of empty-calorie, high-fat, high-salt foods. Nutritional evaluations should also include information about family cultural preferences related to food, whether psychological or psychosocial problems affect eating, and whether nutritional requirements are understood or being met.

At least three issues related to nutrition may surface during the nutritional assessment: obesity, anorexia nervosa, and bulimia nervosa. Obesity is one of the most serious health problems facing today's children and adolescents. At least 11% of U.S. children and adolescents are obese, and as many as 22% are overweight (Strauss & Knight, 1999). In some ethnic groups these numbers may even be higher (Hill & Trowbridge, 1998). The rate is increasing (Birch & Fisher, 1998), and children and adolescents of obese parents are at greater risk of being obese than children and adolescents whose parents are thin.

Children today are more sedentary as compared with a generation ago. In fact today, about 25% of children do not participate in any regular physical activity, girls participate less than boys, and as one gets older, physical activity actually decreases (U.S. Department of Health and Human Services, 1997). One reason for this decline in physical activity may be that mandatory physical education classes are decreasing in schools as children get older, and television, computer games and use, and video games are popular with young people (Berkey et al., 2000).

Second, today's children's diets (high in fat, low in fruits and vegetables and complex carbohydrates) promote obesity. High-fat foods tend to be palatable, less satiating, higher in total energy, and of smaller volume, leading to overconsumption (Berkey et al., 2000; Birch & Fisher, 1998; Troiano & Flegal, 1998). In addition, fruits, vegetables, and complex carbohydrates may not be popular with children and adolescents.

Finally, factors related to the home environment—parental obesity (more often maternal than paternal), low family income, lower levels of cognitive stimulation in the home, and parental occupation—promote obesity in children and adolescents. Parental obesity is an important risk factor because of child–parent modeling and genetics. In fact, children from families in which one parent is obese have a 40% risk of being obese as an adult. They have an 80% risk of being obese as an adult if both parents are obese (Behrman & Kleigman, 1998). Low family income may be related to obesity because of less healthy eating patterns, decreased activity, and an environment that provides high-fat foods and few fruits and vegetables (Kennedy & Powell, 1997). Lower levels of cognitive development may be related to obesity in children and adolescents because children raised in stimulating and interactive home environments may engage in fewer sedentary activities (television, video games) and more regular physical activity. Parental occupation is a factor if a parent's education is not used in the occupation or if the occupation is nonprofessional. All these factors are important independently of other socioeconomic factors, including race and caregiver marital status or education (Strauss & Knight, 1999).

Obesity in adolescence may also be connected to not being able or wanting to master the psychosocial and psychosexual tasks of adolescence. Overeating compensates as a regression tactic for self-satisfaction or as a coping mechanism for stress. The resulting obesity becomes yet another obstacle to overcome in achieving developmental milestones. Obesity can ward off the pressures associated with puberty and societal expectations and, as long as an adolescent is obese, can repress emotional maturation. For some, obesity can be the reason for their disappointments and eating a method of coping that keeps them connected to their family. This dependence on food/family also interferes with the developmental tasks of separation and individuation. In addition, obesity can interfere with sexuality issues; excess weight protects the adolescent from unwanted sexual advances or attention. Obesity may also represent a way to bring embarrassment and shame to others (caregiver, family), a way of becoming larger than a person not liked (peer), or aggression directed at the self. It is not unusual for obese adolescents to dislike their own physical appearance, express admiration for thin people, and judge others in terms of their own weight. Psychological counseling as well as nutritional and activity counseling may help adolescents develop more mature methods of coping if their obesity is connected to psychosocial or psychosexual issues.

The obese adolescent's sense of identity can also be affected by derogatory comments made by others, leading to guilt, shame, and consequent overeating, which results in more weight gain, more derogatory comments, and even more poor self-esteem. Box 12-1 provides suggestions on ways to help overweight/obese adolescents lose weight.

Mechanical methods of weight loss frequently advertised in popular magazines are another option that can be used alone or in combination with diet and exercise programs. These methods include steam baths, sauna suits, spot reducers, and special exercise outfits. However, they offer only short-term weight loss. Use of appetite-suppressant drugs, a final treatment option, are typically reserved for adolescents who are severely obese. This option should be managed by a physician or nurse practitioner. On a final note, it is uncommon for weight-reduction plans to be successful with adolescents, even though many are used. A more realistic alternative goal for those who have difficulty losing weight and keeping if off may be just to not gain any additional weight.

Two other issues related to nutrition in adolescence are anorexia nervosa and bulimia nervosa. Although related, they may have different causes and long-term complications. Both, more commonly seen in females (Green, 1994), are characterized by having a distorted self-image and are psychological illnesses with accompanying physical symptoms. People with anorexia severely limit their food intake; those with bulimia have repeated episodes of binge eating followed by the use of laxatives or vomiting. The diagnosis of either should be considered when the adolescent appears underweight, has not achieved normal reproductive milestones for gender, follows a poor diet, or has not achieved anticipated height (Rees, 1996; Sifuentes, 2000). It is important to refer these clients to professionals who specialize in treating eating disorders. See Chapter 35 for a more detailed discussion of adolescent eating disorders.

BOX 12-1 Helping adolescents with their weight

Instruct obese adolescents to:

1. Avoid purchasing empty-calorie foods; remove empty-calorie snack foods from home.
2. Ask self before eating, "Am I hungry?"
3. Make dining pleasurable.
4. Eat only at mealtimes and at the table; avoid empty-calorie snacks, reduce dietary intake by at least 500 calories daily to lose 1 lb a week.
5. Serve individual portions on smaller plates; avoid second helpings.
6. Eat slowly by cutting food into small mouthfuls and putting eating utensils down between bites.
7. Keep a food diary; examine for empty calories and to see if you are eating traditional food groups.
8. Participate in regular exercise (walking, bicycle riding, swimming, etc.)
9. Maintain attractive appearance and proper posture.
10. Avoid using food as a reward.
11. Praise and feel proud of small weight losses.

Dental Health

During adolescence dental visits occur twice a year, good oral hygiene habits have been established, the majority of orthodontic work has begun, and most permanent teeth have erupted. Third molars, however, may erupt in later adolescence (Grover, 1996) or may become impacted, requiring surgical removal. Although the incidence of dental caries decreases during this time, fluoride supplements (or the need for fluoridated water) should continue until age 16 (Committee on Nutrition, 1995).

During adolescence, malocclusion, gingivitis, and dental trauma may occur. Malocclusion occurs due to dental crowding or mandibular/facial bone growth changes. Usually, braces are needed to redirect facial/mandibular growth and correct tooth positioning (Figure 12-25). Gingivitis, the inflammation and consequent breakdown of the gingival epithelium, may be seen during adolescence because of ineffective cleaning, high sugar/simple carbohydrate diets, or increased hormonal activity. The gums may bleed easily and appear swollen and pale. Treatment involves brushing the teeth at least twice a day using a soft-bristled brush and fluoride toothpaste, flossing daily, eating a well-balanced diet, and regular dental visits (American Dental Association, 1998).

Dental trauma, more common in males, often accompanies sports injuries and involves fractured or avulsed teeth, lacerations of the oral mucosa or gums, or jaw fracture. If tooth avulsion (tooth knocked out of socket) occurs, it may be reimplanted successfully if treatment is begun within 30 minutes (Krasner, 1990). If the tooth cannot be repositioned in

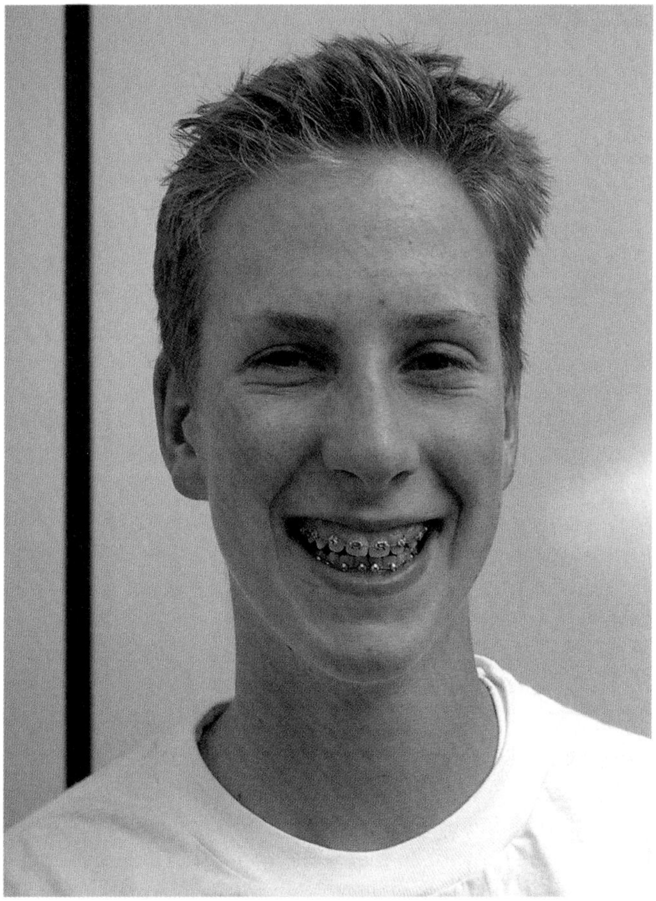

Figure 12-25 It is not uncommon to see adolescents wearing braces to treat malocclusions.

the socket, it should be placed in a container of milk rather than being cleaned, and the adolescent taken immediately to the dentist. All cases of dental trauma should be treated as an emergency and a dentist seen as soon as possible.

Sleep, Rest, and Activity

Adolescents need approximately 8 hours of sleep per night. Because of their busy schedules (social activities, obligations at school, employment commitments) and rapid physical growth, adolescents often do not receive enough sleep. Many appear fatigued, their schoolwork may suffer, and parents may complain that their teens rarely have time to help around the house. Nurses need to educate both parents and adolescents on the importance of adequate rest and sleep and encourage teens to have realistic activity schedules that do not overextend them. An adolescent's excessive anxiety and fatigue may also result in sleep disturbances, which can continue into adulthood since adult sleep cycles and habits are formed during adolescence.

Many adolescents are not as physically active as they should be, even though they are very busy (see discussion of nutrition above). Others exercise regularly and develop physically fit bodies. Often, fitness behaviors adopted during adolescence are predictors of fitness habits later in life (Green, 1994). Adolescents need daily exercise to provide an outlet for tension and anxiety and to maintain muscle tone and development. Regular exercise will also promote healthy sleep patterns and enhance emotional development. Physical activity and fitness may also reduce cardiovascular disease risk factors such as hyperlipidemia, hypertension, and obesity.

The Physical Activity Guidelines for Adolescents (1994) suggest that adolescents should be involved in moderate to vigorous physical activity three or more times a week for at least 30 minutes per session, and be active daily, or nearly every day. *Healthy People 2010* (U.S. Department of Health and Human Services, 2000) goals for adolescents validate these recommendations by encouraging adolescents to increase vigorous activity to at least 20 minutes or more a day for 3 days a week in at least 75% of children and adolescents. However, strength training (a form of physical activity) in adolescence can occasionally lead to significant musculoskeletal injury, such as ruptured intervertebral disks, epiphyseal fractures, and low back bony disruptions (AAP Committee on Sports Medicine, 1990). Injuries can be lessened or prevented if the program followed is based on the physical maturity of the individual. The AAP Committee on Sports Medicine (1990) recommends that if adolescent athletes have reached Tanner stage 5 development, they will have experienced their period of maximal height velocity and be less vulnerable to injury.

Because of rapid musculoskeletal growth, adolescents are also prone to ligament tears and damage to the growth plates of the long bones (Pendergrast & Strong, 1992). Adolescents should be cautioned about involvement in contact sports and encouraged to participate in sports according to their size rather than according to their chronologic age. Weight-lifting is especially dangerous if the body is not physiologically ready. Sports injuries to late maturing boys are more likely to occur if they participate in contact sports with early maturing, muscular agemates. It is better to direct adolescents into activities in which they will succeed rather than those at which they will experience physical and psychological failure. Tennis, swimming, and horsemanship may be some suggestions for alternative, more appropriate activities for adolescents who develop more slowly.

Even though being involved in sports is advantageous for adolescents and participation is increasing, injuries account for substantial cost and morbidity (Cheng, et al., 2000). Most injuries involve falls or being struck by or against objects. Injury rates are higher for males than females, and even noncontact sports (soccer, basketball, baseball, bicycling) may result in head injuries and collisions with other persons (Cheng, et al., 2000).

Nurses can help adolescents increase their physical activity as appropriate to meet the physical activity guidelines for adolescents and avoid injury by considering the

Family Teaching

Activity

- Initiate exercise programs that are enjoyable, realistic, and consider physical limitations and capabilities. 30 to 60 minutes per day three to four times per week will enhance fitness and set the stage for a lifetime of health. However, sports involving physical contact are not recommended until after PHV.
- Seek out physical education courses at times and places conducive to adolescent participation
- Evaluate physical development regarding PHV before allowing participation in contact sports.

Family Teaching

Health Promotion

- Adopt a flexible approach to meals.
- Provide healthy snacks.
- Set realistic sleeping schedules that provide an average of 8 hours of sleep per night.
- Participate in sports according to size rather than according to chronologic age.
- Encourage schools to offer nutritious options that appeal to adolescents.
- Search for a variety of activities (tennis, basketball, baseball, softball, hockey, skateboarding, etc.).

adolescent's physical development and capabilities. Therefore, nurses need to inquire about an adolescent's activity program, including frequency, vigor, and preferences, before making any recommendations, as well as to determine Tanner staging. Adolescents can also be encouraged to develop interests in sports, recreation, active play, or exercise at home, school, or in the community (Figure 12-26).

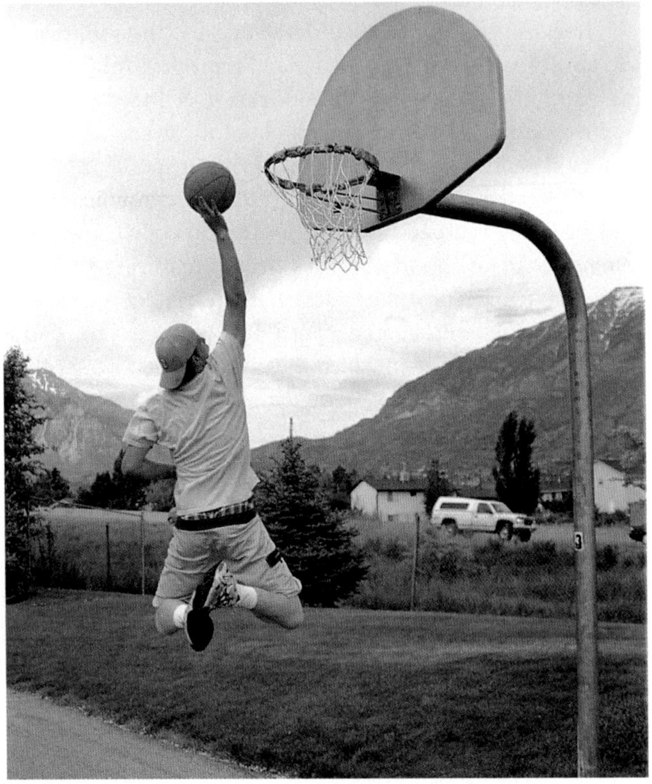

Figure 12-26 Physical acitivity is a popular activity for adolescents, either alone or with others.

In fact, data from the 1996 National Longitudinal Study of Adolescent Health (Gordon-Larsen, McMurray, & Popkin, 2000) suggest that use of a community recreational center and participation in daily school physical education programs were associated with an increased likelihood of engaging in a high level of moderate to vigorous physical activity. Youngsters who participated in physical education classes five times a week were more than twice as likely to be highly active, and those who participated four times a week were 44% more likely to be highly active. Any prescribed programs, however, should allow for warm-up and cool-down periods and develop fitness gradually instead of overnight. Adolescents involved in sports need to wear appropriate protective gear, including helmets, pads, and guards, and be aware of safety rules and regulations.

Safety and Injury Prevention

Unintentional injury is the leading cause of death in adolescents. Nearly half the deaths occurring to individuals between ages 16 and 19 are caused by motor vehicle accidents, and these are more common with teenage drivers who use marijuana, alcohol, or other drugs (Clemen-Stone, Eigsti, & McGuire, 1998; Escobedo, Chorba, & Waxweiler, 1995). Automobiles, motorcycles, motor scooters, mopeds, snowmobiles, minibikes, and all-terrain vehicles cause many adolescent skeletal, head, and spinal cord injuries and abrasions and burns. Approximately 16% of teens report they rarely or never wear seat belts; of those who ride motorcycles, 38% rarely or never wear helmets; 85.3% rarely or never wear helmets when riding their bicycles (CDC, 2000). Adolescents are also more at risk for sports-related injuries and accidents. Therefore, accident prevention and safety promotion programs are extremely important for the adolescent. Nurses can initiate such programs or become involved in them through clinics, schools, or community agencies serving adolescents. In addition, nurses need to educate adolescents and their caregivers about safety issues and accident prevention (seat belts, helmets while riding bicycles, motorcycles, skateboards, and the use of protective equipment while participating in baseball, football, and soccer), and remind them they are not immortal or immune from being injured (personal fable) if they take unnecessary chances. Table 12-3 presents various hazards and developmental characteristics of adolescents as well as appropriate intervention strategies.

Violence

The second leading cause of death for individuals ages 15–19 and the third leading cause of death for adolescents ages 10–14 is homicide, most due to handgun use (American Academy of Pediatrics Committee on Injury and Poison Prevention, 2000; Webster, Gainer, & Champion, 1995). Six percent of high school students reported that they had carried a gun during the past year; 18% reported that they had carried any weapon at least once during the past year (CDC, 2000). The homicide rate for black teens is eight times higher than that for whites of the same age (Danielson, 1998). The World Health Organization reports that the homicide rate for males aged 15 to 24 in the United States is 10 times higher than in Canada, 15 times higher than in Australia, and 28 times higher than in Germany or France (World Health Statistics Annual, 1995). During 1999, comparing schoolgrounds with violent neighborhoods, there was an increasing likelihood of violence having an impact on adolescents. Over 5% of students felt too unsafe to go to school, and 6.9% said they had carried a gun, knife, or club onto school property at least once in the month preceding the survey. More than 7% claimed they had been injured or threatened with a weapon on school property during the year before being surveyed (CDC, 2000). Delinquency rates have increased faster among girls than among boys, and adolescent-related violence in rural areas is rising (Danielson, 1998). Even though most gang-related problems occur in large cities, gang conflict is also seen in smaller cities. Gangs in schools almost doubled between 1989 and

TABLE 12-3 Injury Prevention in Adolescents

Hazard	Developmental Characteristics	Nursing Implications
Firearms	Independent, believe they are invulnerable	Do not carry or use a weapon to deal with conflict resolution Follow firearm safety rules
Motor vehicles	Take unnecessary risks	Enroll in drivers' education courses Wear seat belts (driver/passengers) Follow traffic rules/speed limit Do not drink and drive
Poisoning	Need peer approval	Be aware of dangers of drug/alcohol use
Sports		
Contact sports	Physically active	Wear protective gear, including padding/helmets/clothing when participating in contact sports or riding bicycles, all-terrain vehicles, motorcycles, skateboards Proper use of sports equipment
Exercise programs	Responsible for self/others	Assess exercise/fitness programs for safety and ability
Outdoor activities	Curious	Integrate safety information about outdoor activities (hiking, camping, fishing, backpacking, etc.) into behavior
Water Craft Swimming	Overestimate abilities, stamina, physical development	Avoid drinking alcohol when boating or swimming Learn how to swim Follow rules regarding water safety

Critical Thinking

Violence in the Home

How do you help a child who lives in a home that puts them at risk for violence?

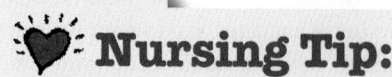

Nursing Tip:

Violence

When working with youths who are victims of violence, ask about the victim's relationship to the perpetrator, circumstances surrounding the event, use of alcohol/drugs, predisposing risk factors (violence in the family, unemployment, truancy), and intentions regarding seeking revenge (Danielson, 1998).

1995, with a simultaneous 25% increase in the number of students victimized by violent crime.

The cause of violent crime committed by young people today has been traced to individual, family, community, and social circumstances. Violent delinquency tends to be more common in working-class than in middle-class teens, and a relationship exists between money-making crimes, unemployment, and poverty. It is not uncommon for violent youth to associate with delinquent peer groups and experience vio-

Research Highlight

Risky Behaviors

Study Purpose

To investigate the relationship between risky behaviors (tobacco use, alcohol use, sexual intercourse, poor school performance), and three components of the current and future-oriented self-concept (popular [well liked], deviant [engaging in problem behaviors], conventional [engaging in culturally sanctioned behavior]).

Methods

One-hundred sixty adolescents from a working-class suburban junior high school completed questionnaires measuring their involvement in the identified risky behaviors (tobacco use, alcohol use, sexual intercourse), their current self-concept, and their future-oriented self-concept during the winter of eighth and ninth grades. Grade point averages were obtained from school records.

Findings

There were high correlations between the four risky behaviors, and the prevalence of these risky behaviors increased from eighth grade to ninth grade. Involvement in risky behaviors during eighth grade predicted current and future-oriented deviant self-concept scores in ninth grade. Current popular self-concept scores in eighth grade predicted risky behaviors in ninth grade.

Implications

It is important to realize that how adolescents feel about themselves (self-concept) may be part of the reason they engage in risky behaviors. In addition, when adolescents engage in these risky behaviors early, they have a greater chance of becoming enduring parts of their later behavior. Intervention efforts should be directed toward not only changing one's self-concept so it is more positive, but also limiting engagement in risky behaviors.

Citation

Stein, K., Roeser, R., & Markus, H. (1998). Self-schemas and possible selves as predictors and outcomes of risky behaviors in adolescents. *Nursing Research, 47*(2), 96–106.

lence at home where there is access to illicit drugs, alcohol, and guns. Violent behaviors in adolescence are also associated with depression, drug abuse, lower church attendance, and hopelessness (DuRant, Treiber, Goodman, & Woods, 1996).

Prevention programs targeted to stem the tide of teen violence are essential, and need to involve health care providers, including nurses, caregivers, schools, and other community agencies. Adolescents need connectedness (feelings of warmth, love, caring) with caregivers and schools so they feel a sense of belonging, concern, and true interest in their welfare. This will help them become directly involved and begin to feel some ownership in programs beneficial to their health and well-being. Intervention efforts directed toward creating prosocial environments in the home and school may help prevent and reduce aggressive and violent behavior as well. Affection, involvement, cohesiveness, effective supervision, and acceptance can assist in preventing delinquency and subsequent violent behavior.

Sexual Activity

Sexual decision making and behaviors are traditionally controlled by family and societal values. In the past, these values were rather conservative and congruent. Today, however, teenagers have more options than in the past, and are faced with family and/or societal values that are more liberal and may not be as congruous as they once were. Today, 49.9% of high school students have engaged in sexual intercourse, and 8.3% experience intercourse before they turn 13 years of age (CDC, 2000). In fact, 56% of female and 73% of male adolescents report having had sexual intercourse before turning 18. First intercourse occurs at an average age of 17 years for females and at an average age of 16 for males. One-fourth of adolescents report having had their first intercourse experience by 15. Nineteen percent of sexually active high school students report having had four or more partners (American Academy of Pediatrics Committee on Adolescence, 2000).

Adolescents' reasons for becoming sexually active include but are not limited to feeling grown-up; to enhance self-esteem; to experiment; to be accepted by friends; to have someone to care about, love, and be close to; for pleasure; to gain control over one's life; to seek revenge; and to prove they are "normal" (American Academy of Pediatrics Committee on Adolescence, 2000; Murray & Zentner, 2001). Since few adolescents have the ego strength or decision-making skills to counter peer pressure from sexually active friends, they may become sexually active against the wishes of their families and some health care providers.

Predictors of early sexual activity include lack of attentive or nurturing parents, early pubertal development, poverty, history of sexual abuse, cultural and family patterns of early sexual experience, poor school performance, lack of school or career goals, and dropping out of school. Factors associated with delay in initiating intercourse include regular attendance at worship services, stable home environment, and higher family income (AAP Committee on Adolescence, 2000).

Sexually active young people participate in behaviors that put them at risk for sexually transmitted diseases and pregnancy because they frequently have multiple partners or do not use condoms or other forms of contraception. Sexually transmitted diseases (STDs), defined as any disease spread from person to person during sexual contact, are highly communicable, currently considered a public health epidemic, and affect an increasing number of persons (Murray & Zentner, 2001). Reasons for the increased incidence of sexually transmitted diseases include lack of understanding about transmission; breakdown of the family unit; increased use of contraceptives; changing sexual patterns, attitudes, and mores; the feeling "it can't happen to me"; and increased societal mobility. Common STDs include chlamydia papilloma infections, genital herpes, gonorrhea, trichomonas, and acquired immunodeficiency syndrome (AIDS).

Most teen pregnancies occur in those 18–19 years old—51% end in a live birth, 35% are aborted, and 14% are miscarriages or still births (AAP Committee on Adolescence, 2000). Although birth rates to women under 20 have declined since the 1970s, the United States continues to have one of the highest teenage pregnancy rates among developed countries (Hewell & Andrews, 1996; Ventura, Peters, Martin, & Mauer, 1997). African-American teen pregnancy rates are higher than rates in Caucasians, and continue to increase (Murray & Zentner, 2001). Most teenage mothers are unmarried. The resulting unplanned pregnancy affects not only the mother and child, but also the child's father and the respective families because adolescents are often not socially, emotionally, educationally, economically, or physically ready for pregnancy and parenthood.

Several factors related to individual, family/friend, and society influence the incidence of adolescent pregnancy. Individual factors include self-destructive or self-hate feelings and behaviors, egocentrism, low self-esteem, loneliness, recent loss, early maturation, independence from family, lack of responsibility, plea for attention, personal fable, self-punishment, and need to prove one's womanhood. Family/friend factors include having a close relative who has experienced an adolescent pregnancy, conflictual mother–daughter or father–daughter relationships, sexually permissive peer group, inadequate communication, history of sexual abuse or incest, few girlfriends, an older boyfriend, lack of religious affiliation, substance abuse by family/friends, and fulfilling caregiver prophecy when parents suggest their daughter will become pregnant if she does not change her behavior. Societal factors include implied acceptance of intercourse outside marriage, a variety of adult behavioral values, media pressure, inadequate access to contraception, and the availability of public assistance/welfare for single young mothers (AAP Committee on Adolescence, 2000; Clemen-Stone, Eigsti, & McGuire, 1998; Dworetzky,1995).

Reflective Thinking

Adolescent Pregnancy

Imagine yourself as a pregnant adolescent. What would you feel? How would your future have been affected?

Nursing Tip:

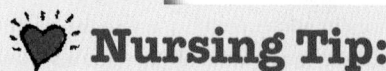

Sexual activity

Assess adolescent's knowledge, feelings, and concerns about sexual preference and activity. Provide accurate information using correct terminology. Refer to appropriate agencies, resources, or caregivers. Ensure that adolescents understand that what they are experiencing is a normal part of moving into adulthood.

There are risks associated with adolescent pregnancies—medical and psychological. Medical risks include low birth weight (more than double the rate for adults) and neonatal death (almost three times as high as in adults). The mortality rate for the teenaged pregnant woman is twice as high as for adult pregnant women. Other problems include poor maternal weight gain, pregnancy-induced hypertension, STDs, anemia, and prematurity. Psychological complications include persistent poverty, separation from the child's father, repeat pregnancy, divorce, school interruption, and limited vocational opportunities (AAP Committee on Adolescence, 2000).

Improved methods of contraception and the increased number of sex education courses in the schools reach only a small percentage of adolescents. Not all those students who are sexually active attend such courses or have them readily available, and those adolescents who do participate in the courses may not integrate this information into their behavior because they do not see pregnancy as a concern for themselves or their partners. Therefore, during routine interactions and/or health assessments, nurses should determine an adolescent's understanding about intercourse, contraception, and reproduction before screening or providing necessary information and support. This includes assessing their understanding and accurate interpretation of risks of being sexually active and then discussing sexual responsibility, including abstinence, how STDs are transmitted, and possible consequences of infection and pregnancy. Adolescents who are sexually active should also receive information about the potential outcomes of their behavior, including ways to reduce their risk of becoming pregnant or infected with STDs or AIDS by limiting the number of sexual partners, using appropriate birth control methods, and consistently using condoms. When adolescents with STDs are identified, they should receive appropriate counseling and medical care. When pregnant adolescents are identified, comprehensive prenatal care is essential to reduce maternal and neonatal complications. Pregnant adolescents should also receive information about available options. Teens who keep their infants need help becoming effective, secure, and comfortable parents. Information about normal infant growth, development, and care should be provided in an accepting, nurturing environment.

Homosexuality

Adolescence is also an important time for developing one's sexual orientation. In fact, in a sample of over 34,000 Minnesota junior and high school students, 10.7% were "unsure" of their sexual orientation, 88.2% described themselves as predominantly heterosexual, and 1.1% described themselves as bisexual or predominantly homosexual. As the age of the subjects increased, uncertainty about their sexual orientation diminished (Remafedi, Resnick, Blum, & Harris, 1992).

Most gay adolescents felt different from other boys as children. The average age they realized they were gay was 12.5 years and the average age of their first crush was 12.7 years. Almost half say they initially tried to deny their identity as a gay person and many were confused when they first became aware of their preferences.

In contrast, development of a same-sex orientation for young females is likely to occur much later and more abruptly (Diamond, 1998). Although development of a same-sex identity for many adolescent females will be similar to the developmental trajectory of adolescent males, most females' progression toward a same-sex orientation is likely to be more subject to nonsexual influences (emotions, personal experience, ideological or political beliefs), less associated with childhood indicators (early and pervasive sense of feeling different and gender-atypical behavior or ideation during childhood), and less stable as compared with adolescent males' development of a same-sex orientation (Diamond, 1998).

Parents with traditional family beliefs (importance of family, having children, religion) tended to be less accepting of their gay sons than parents with less traditional values (Santrock, 2001). In addition, adolescent males, but not females, whose parents have more traditional political ideologies and demonstrate greater religiosity are less comfortable exhibiting behaviors consistent with their gay or lesbian identities (Waldner-Haugrud & Magruder, 1996). When acknowledging their sexual orientation, adolescent reactions ranged from being happy and relieved to depressed, anxious and having suicidal thoughts (Santrock, 2001).

Remafedi (1987a) reported that most subjects in his qualitative study of gay adolescents experienced substance abuse, school problems, and emotional difficulties, and

Research Highlight

Sexual Decision-Making

Study Purpose

To identify reasons adolescents give for engaging in unprotected sexual intercourse, using condoms if they do engage in sexual intercourse, or remaining abstinent.

Methods

Sixty-two male and 53 female adolescents between 16 and 18 years of age, from primarily two-parent, Caucasian, rural homes completed a demographic questionnaire and a study questionnaire. The study questionnaire asked them to respond to a vignette by choosing one of three likely endings (condom use, unprotected sex, abstinence). They then were asked to explain the reason for choosing the story ending they did, and determine how sure they were about their choice on a scale of 1 (not sure at all) to 7 (very sure). Finally, the adolescents were asked what the reason would be for each of the three possible story endings from the perspective of the main characters, and the thoughts and feelings associated with each story ending from the perspective of the main characters. Responses were categorized according to themes.

Findings

Most students chose the story ending where the main characters had either protected or unprotected intercourse; in general, the adolescents were very sure of this decision. Those believing the characters would abstain said the couple did not know each other well enough to have sexual intercourse. The students who believed the story would end with the couple using a condom said it was the responsible and safe thing to do and what was expected. Those thinking the couple would engage in unprotected intercourse said a condom was not available, there was loss of control, or that is what often happens today. Adolescents' perceptions of reasons for being abstinent were relationship issues, moral issues, anxiety or fear, situational constraints, readiness, or fear of a pregnancy or STD. Perceptions of reasons for using a condom were relationship issues, fear of a pregnancy or STD, desire, and responsibility. Perceptions of reasons for engaging in unprotected intercourse were wanting to become pregnant, emotional immaturity, relationship issues, desire, situational constraints, or use of other birth control methods.

Implications

Develop intervention programs for adolescents that encourage abstinence, help adolescents think about positive consequences of using condoms (feeling mature and responsible, freedom from worry), and carefully use fear-inducing strategies, acknowledging and reinforcing the legitimacy of concerns related to pregnancy and STDs.

Citation

Keller, M., Duerst, B., & Zimmerman, J. (1996). Adolescents' view of sexual decision-making. *Image: Journal of Nursing Scholarship, 28*(2), 125–130.

almost half reported conflict with the law or running away from home. In another study by Remafedi (1987b), 43% of the gay adolescents reported strong negative attitudes from parents; 41% reported strong negative attitudes from friends. Fifty-five percent experienced verbal abuse from peers, 37% felt they were discriminated against, and 30% had been physically assaulted.

Nurses need to recognize that even though many young people explore their own sexual orientation or homosexual attractions, few who engage in homosexual behavior during adolescence continue the practice into adulthood (Santrock, 2001). Thus, nurses and caregivers need to help young people recognize that homosexual experimentation is not the same as establishing a homosexual orientation, acknowledge same and bisexual relationships and attractions, and phrase questions about sexuality and sexual activity carefully.

Effect of Television and Other Media on Adolescents

Media in America contribute to more adverse health outcomes than to prosocial or positive outcomes. This is especially true with regard to violence, guns, sex, and drugs. For example, cross-sectional, naturalistic, and longitudinal studies as well as several meta-analyses suggest that there is a relationship between media violence, real-life aggression, and acceptance of aggressive attitudes. Those exposed to violence on television and the media tend to be more likely to commit violent acts. In addition, guns are glamorized in the media; 26% of violent acts committed on the media use guns. Research also suggests that adolescents exposed to greater amounts of alcohol or tobacco advertising are more likely to use or intend to use those products as compared with those adolescents who are not exposed to those products. One-third of teens who smoke could link their smoking to tobacco promotional activities. Alcohol advertising in the media stimulates favorable predispositions, greater problem drinking, and higher consumption by young people (Strasburger & Donnerstein, 1999.) Box 12-2 lists the effects of television and other media on adolescents.

Caregivers need to control or monitor the media programming their teens watch, and remove television sets from teens' bedrooms. Specifically, this means to limit all media use to no more than 1 to 2 hours per day, view television with their adolescents, and monitor their child or adolescent's use of the media (Strasburger & Donnerstein, 1999).

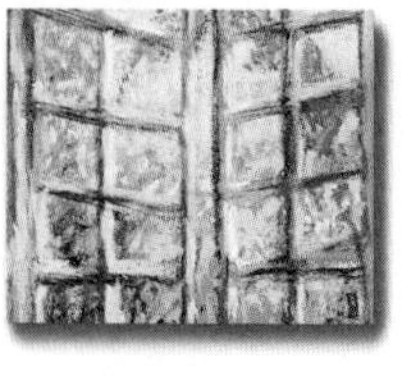

In the Real World

This past week I cared for 16-year-old Morgan, who had had a ureteral resection. Rebecca (the other nurse) and I and spoke with him frankly about procedures, care plans, and equipment. At one point I explained how a pulse oximeter worked to measure oxygen-carrying productivity. This 6-foot, 90-kg young man did not need to be babied, but he did need to be respected and supported in his recovery. Recognizing adolescents' general desire for privacy and sensitivity about anatomy, I tried to keep him well-covered and work as professionally as possible. Morgan was appreciative, polite, and cooperative.

BOX 12-2 Effect of television and other media on adolescents

1. 2–3 hours/day mean less physical activity, reading, and interaction with friends.
2. 10,000 acts of violence viewed/year; 26% involve use of guns.
3. 15,000 sexual references, innuendoes, jokes per year; <170 deal with abstinence, birth control, pregnancy, STDs.
4. 70% of content from prime-time dramatic programs contains references to alcohol, tobacco, illicit drugs; over 50% of movies contain references to tobacco/smoking; for every "just say no" public service announcement, 25–50 beer and wine advertisements will be viewed.

Key Concepts

- In order to effectively identify issues/problems commonly seen in adolescence and consequently deliver appropriate and individualized nursing care, the physiological, psychosexual, psychosocial, cognitive, and moral transformations occurring during this time, as well as changes in adolescents' rapidly expanding social context, including the family, school, and peers should be considered.
- The physiological changes that occur during adolescence are extensive, do not occur in isolation, and have an impact on the adolescent's psychosexual, psychosocial, and cognitive development. These changes also affect the experiences adolescents have with family members, peers, and others in their social world, as well as their own body image and self-esteem.
- Young people are able to consider all possible solutions to a problem, both real and abstract, and can assess options and determine the best solution.
- Elkind identified two types of social thinking particularly evident during adolescence—imaginary audience and personal fable.
- Adolescent psychosocial orientation is affected by their family, peers, and school experiences.
- Adolescent identity is based on individual and group identifications established during childhood; their ability to master each developmental task presented to them by society; and establishing their own ideology, based on the social, political, and religious attitudes, and values.
- Nurses working with adolescents need to be respectful and demonstrate openness, competence, honesty, warmth, compassion, and understanding and have the ability to communicate effectively with adolescents and their families.
- Adolescent health promotion topics include immunizations, nutrition, oral health, fitness, physical activity, unintentional injury, violence, substance abuse, sexual behavior, and mental health.

Review Questions

1. Why is adolescence such an important period of life?
2. What are the Tanner stages and why are they important?
3. How do thinking processes change during adolescence? How are adolescents helped to learn?
4. What factors are important in adolescent identity development?
5. What identity statuses do adolescents experience as they attempt to answer the question, "Who am I?"
6. How do parents, siblings, and peers influence adolescent development?
7. Why does school have such a profound influence on adolescents? What are the positive and negative effects of schools on adolescents?
8. How do work experiences influence adolescents?
9. What are at least five issues adolescents face that have an impact on their health and well-being?
10. How might a nurse interact effectively with adolescents?
11. What are the health promotion/screening activities nurses need to be concerned about with adolescents?

References

American Academy of Pediatrics Committee on Adolescence (2000). Adolescent pregnancy—Current trends and issues: 1998. *Pediatrics, 103*(2), 516–520.

American Academy of Pediatrics Committee on Injury and Poison Prevention (2000, April). *Pediatrics, 105*(5), 888–895.

American Academy of Pediatrics Committee on Sports Medicine (1990, November). Strength training, weight and power lifting, and body building by children and adolescents. *Pediatrics, 86*(5) 801–803.

American Dental Association. (1998). Cleaning your teeth and gums (oral hygiene) [On-line]. Available: www.ada.org/public/faq/cleaning.html#daily

Anglin, T., Naylor, K., & Kaplan, D. (1996). Comprehensive school-based health care: high school students' use of medical, mental health, and substance abuse services. *Pediatrics, 97*(3), 318–330.

Archer, S. L. (1992). A feminist's approach to identity research. In G. R. Adams, T. P. Gullotta, & R. Montemayor (Eds.), *Adolescent identity formation*. Newbury Park, CA: Sage.

Armsden, G., & Greenberg, M. T. (1987). The inventory of parent and peer attachment: Individual differences and their relationship to psychological well-being in adolescence. *Journal of Youth and Adolescence, 16*, 427–454.

Barber, B. (1994). Cultural, family, and personal contexts of parent-adolescent conflict. *Journal of Marriage and the Family, 56*, 375–386.

Barber, B., & Eccles, J. (1992). Long-term influence of divorce and single parenting on adolescent family- and work-related values, behaviors, and aspirations. *Psychological Bulletin, 111*, 108–126.

Baumeister, R. F. (1991). Identity crisis. In R.M. Lerner, A.C. Petersen, & J. Brooks-Gunn (Eds.), *Encyclopedia of adolescence* (vol. 1). New York: Garland.

Beard, J. (2000). Iron requirements in adolescent females. *Journal of Nutrition, 130*, 440S–442S.

Behrman, R., & Kleigman, B. (1998). *Nelson's essentials of pediatrics* (3rd ed.). Philadelphia: Saunders.

Berger, K. (1994). *The developing person through the life span* (3rd ed.). New York: Worth.

Berkey, C. S., Rockett, H. R. H., Field, A. E., Gillman, M. W., Frazier, A. L., Camargo, C. A., Jr., & Colditz, G. A. (2000). Activity, dietary intake, and weight changes in a longitudinal study of preadolescent and adolescent boys and girls. *Pediatrics. 105*(4), 56.

Berndt, T., & Keefe, K. (1995). Friends' influence on adolescents' adjustment to school. *Child Development, 66*, 1312–1329.

Berndt, T. J., & Perry, T. B. (1986). Children's perceptions of friendships as supportive relationships. *Developmental Psychology, 22*, 640–648.

Berndt, T. J., & Savin-Williams, R. C. (1989). Peer relations and friendships. In P. Tolan & B. Cohler (Eds.), *Handbook of clinical research and practice with adolescents* (pp. 203–219). New York: Wiley.

Billy, J. O. G., & Udry, J. R. (1985). Patterns of adolescent friendship and effects on sexual behavior. *Social Psychology Quarterly, 48*, 27–41.

Birch, L. L., & Fisher, J. O. (1998). Development of eating behaviors among children and adolescents. *Pediatrics, 101*(3), 539–549.

Blyth, D. A., Simmons, G. G., Zakin, D. F. (1985). Satisfaction with body image for adolescents. *Journal of Youth and Adolescence, 14*, 207–225.

Brody, G. H., Stoneman, Z., & McCoy, J. K. (1994). Contributions of family relationships and child temperaments to longitudinal variations in sibling relationship quality and sibling relationship styles. *Journal of Family Psychology, 8*, 274–286.

Brook J. S., Whiteman M., Gordon A. S., & Brenden C. (1986). Older brother's influence on younger sibling's drug use. *Journal of Psychology, 114*, 83–90.

Brook, J. S., Whiteman, M. Gordon, A. S., Nomura, C., & Brook, D. W. (1986). Onset of adolescent drinking: A longitudinal study of intrapersonal and interpersonal antecedents. *Alcohol and Substance Abuse in Women and Children* (pp. 91–110). Binghamton, NY: Hawthorn.

Brooks-Gunn, J. (1988). Antecedents and consequences of variations in girls' maturational timing. *Journal of Adolescent Health Care, 9*, 365–373.

Brooks-Gunn, J., & Paikoff, R. (1993). Sex is a gamble, kissing is a game: Adolescent sexuality and health promotion. In S. G. Millstein, A. C. Petersen, & E. O. Nightengale (Eds.).

Promoting the health of adolescents. New York: Oxford University Press.
Broughton, J. (1983). The cognitive developmental theory of adolescent self and identity. In B. Lee & G. Noam (Eds.), *Developmental approaches to self*. New York: Plenum.
Brown, B., Mounts, N., Lamborn, S., & Steinberg, L. (1993). Parenting practices and peer group affiliations in adolescence. *Child Development, 64*, 467–482.
Buchanan, C., Eccles, J., & Becker, J. (1992). Are adolescents the victims of raging hormones: Evidence for activational effects of hormones on moods and behavior at adolescence. *Psychological Bulletin, 111*, 62–107.
Caspi, A., & Moffitt, T. (1991). Individual differences are accentuated during periods of social change: The sample case of girls at puberty. *Journal of Personality and Social Psychology, 61*, 157–168.
Cass, V. C. (1979). Homosexuality identity formation: A theoretical model. *Journal of Homosexuality, 4*, 219-235.
Center for Disease Control and Prevention. (2000). *Youth risk behavior surveillance—United States, 1999*. June 20, 2000/49(5505); 1–96. Atlanta, GA: Author.
Cheng, T., Fields, C., Brenner, R., Wright, J., Lomax, T., Scheidt, P., & DC Child/Adolescent Injury Research Network (2000). Sports injuries: An important cause of morbidity in urban youth. *Pediatrics, 105*(3), e32.
Clayton R. R., & Lacy W. B., (1982). Interpersonal influences on male drug use and drug use intentions. *International Journal of the Addictions, 17*(4), 655–666.
Clemen-Stone, S., Eigsti, D., & McGuire, S. (1998). *Comprehensive family and community health nursing* (5th ed.). St. Louis: Mosby-Year Book.
Cohen, J. M. (1977). Sources of peer group homogeneity. *Sociology of Education, 50*, 227–241.
Coleman, E. (1982). Developmental stages of the coming out process. *Journal of Homosexuality, 7*, 31–43.
Committee on Dietary Allowances, Food and Nutrition Board, National Research Council. (1989). *Recommended dietary allowances* (10th ed.). Washington, DC: National Academy Press.
Committee on Nutrition. (1995). Fluoride supplementation for children: Interim policy recommendations. *Pediatrics, 95*, 777.
Committee on Nutrition. (1999). Calcium requirements of infants, children, and adolescents. *American Academy of Pediatrics, 104*(5), 1152–1157.
Conger, J. J., & Petersen, A. C. (1984). *Adolescence and youth*. New York: Harper & Row.
Cutrona, C. E. (1982). Transition to college: Loneliness and the process of social adjustment. In L.A. Peplau & D. Perlman (Eds.), *Loneliness: A sourcebook of current theory, research, and therapy*. New York: Wiley.
Dacey, J., & Travers, J. (1996). *Human development across the lifespan* (3rd ed.). Madison, WI: Brown & Benchmark.
Danielson, R. (1998). Adolescent violence in America. *Clinician Reviews, 8*(5), 167–184.
Demo, D. H., & Acock, A. C. (1988). The impact of divorce on children. *Journal of Marriage and the Family, 50*, 619–648.
Diamond, L. M. (1998). Development of sexual orientation among adolescent and young adult women. *Developmental Psychology, 34*, 1085–1095.
Dickinson, G. E., (1975). Dating behavior of black and white adolescents before and after desegregation. *Journal of Marriage and the Family, 37*, 602–608.
Dornbusch, S., Carlsmith, J., Gross, R., Martin, J., Jennings, D., Rosenberg, A., & Duke, P. (1981). Sexual development, age and dating: A comparison of biological and social influences upon one set of behaviors. *Child Development, 52*, 179–185.
Douvan, E., & Adelson, J. (1966). *The adolescent experience*. New York: Wiley.
DuBois, D. L., & Hirsch, B. J. (1990). School and neighborhood friendship patterns of blacks and whites in early adolescence. *Child Development, 61*, 524–536.
Duke-Duncan, P. (1991). Body Image. In R.M. Lerner, A.C,. Petersen, & J. Brooks-Gunn (Eds.). *Encyclopedia of adolescence* (pp. 90–94). New York: Garland.
Dunphy, D. C. (1963). The social structure of urban adolescent peer groups. *Sociometry, 26*, 230- 246.
DuRant, R., Treiber, F., Goodman, E., & Woods, E. (1996). Intentions to use violence among young adolescents. *Pediatrics, 98*(6), 1104–1108.
Dworetzky, J. (1995). *Human development: A lifespan approach* (6th ed.). St. Paul: West.
East, P. L., & Rook, K. S. (1992). Compensatory patterns of support among children's peer relationships: A test using school friends, non-school friends, and siblings. *Developmental Psychology, 28*, 163–172.
Elkind, D. (1967). *Egocentrism in adolescence. Child Development, 38*, 1025–1034.
Elkind, D. (1984). *All Grown up and no place to go: Teenagers in crisis*. Reading, MA: Addison-Wesley.
Erikson, E. H. (1968). *Identity: Youth and crisis*. New York: Norton.
Escobedo, L., Chorba, J., & Waxweiler, R. (1995). Patterns of alcohol use and the risk of drinking and driving among U.S. high school students. *American Journal of Public Health, 85*, 976–978.
Eveleth, P.B., & Tanner, J.M. (1990). *Worldwide variation in human growth* (2nd ed.). Cambridge, UK: Cambridge University Press.
Falbo, T. (1992). Social norms and the one-child family: Clinical and policy implications. In F. Boer & J. Dunn (Eds.), *Children's sibling relationships* (pp. 71–82). Hillsdale, NJ: Erlbaum.
Feiring, C. (1996). Concepts of romance in 15-year-old adolescents. *Journal of Research on Adolescence, 6*, 181–200.
Feldman, W. R., Feldman, E., & Goodman, J. (1988). Culture versus biology: Children's attitudes toward thinness and fatness. *Pediatrics, 81*, 190–194.
Freiberg, K. (1992). *Human development: A life-span approach*. Boston: Jones and Bartlett.
French, S., Perry, C., Leon, G., & Fulkerson, J. (1994). Weight concerns, dieting behavior, and smoking initiation among adolescents: A prospective study. *American Journal of Public Health, 84*, 1818–1820.
Furman, W., & Buhrmester, D. (1992). Age and sex differences in perceptions of networks of personal relationships. *Child Development, 63*, 103–115.
Furman, W., & Robbins, P. (1985). What's the point? Issues in the selection of treatment objectives. In B. Schneider, K. Rubin, & J. Leddingham (Eds.), *Children's relations: Issues in assessment and intervention* (pp. 41–54). New York: Springer-Verlag.
Gallahue, D., & Ozmun, J. (1995). *Understanding motor development* (3rd ed.). Madison, WI: Brown & Benchmark.
Ge, X., Conger, R., & Elder, G. (1996). Coming of age too early: Pubertal influences on girl's vulnerability to psychological distress. *Child Development, 67*, 3386–3400.

Gilligan, C. (1982). *In a different voice*. Cambridge, MA: Harvard University Press.

Gilligan, C., Lyons, N., and Hanmer, T. (Eds.). (1990). *Making connections: The relational worlds of adolescent girls at Emma Willard School*. Cambridge, MA: Harvard University Press.

Ginzberg, E. (1972). Toward a theory of occupational choice: A restatement. *Vocational Guidance Quarterly, 20*, 169–176.

Gordon-Larsen, P., McMurray, R., & Popkin, B. (2000, June). Determinants of adolescent physical activity and inactivity patterns. *Pediatrics, 105*(6), e83 ff.

Graber, J., & Peterson, A. (1991). Cognitive changes at adolescence: Biological perspectives. In K. Gibson & A. Peterson (Eds.). *Brain, maturation and cognitive development*. New York: Aldine de Gruyter.

Graber, J., Brooks-Gunn, J., & Warren, M., (1995). The antecedents of menarchial age: Heredity, family environment, and stressful life events. *Child Development, 66*, 346–359.

Green, E. W. (Ed.). (1994). *Bright futures: Guidelines for health supervision of infants, children, and adolescents*. Arlington, VA: National Center for Education in Maternal and Child Health.

Greenberger E. & Steinberg, L. (1986) *When teenagers work*. New York: Basic Books.

Grotevant, H. D. (1998). Adolescent development in family contexts. In W. Damon (Ed) & N. Eisenberg (Vol. Ed.), *Handbook of child psychology* (5th ed.) (Vol. xx, *Social, emotional, and personality development*. New York: Wiley.

Grover, G. (1996) Dental care. In C. Berkowitz, (Ed.). *Pediatrics: A primary care approach* (pp. 45–49). Philadelphia: Saunders.

Guinn, B., Semper, T., Jorgensen, L., & Skaggs. (1997, March). Body image perception in female Mexican-American adolescents. *Journal of School Health, 67*(3), 112–116.

Hall, G. S. (1981). *Adolescence*. Norwood: USA Telegraph Books.

Harter, S. (1999). *The construction of the self: A developmental perspective*. New York: Guilford.

Herman-Giddens, M., Slora, E., Wasserman, R., Bourdony, C., Bhapkar, M., Koch, G., & Hasemeier, C. (1997). Secondary sexual characteristics and menses in young girls seen in office practice: A study from the pediatric research in office settings network. *Pediatrics, 99*(4), 505–512.

Hewell, S., & Andrews, J. (1996). Contraceptive use among female adolescents. *Clinical Nursing Research, 5*(3), 356–363.

Hill, J. O., & Trowbridge, F. L. (1998). Childhood obesity: future directions and research priorities. *Pediatrics, 101*(3), 570–574.

Hoffman M. L. (1980). Moral development in adolescence. In J. Adelson (Ed.), *Handbook of adolescent psychology* (pp. xx–xx). New York: Wiley.

Holland, J. L. (1973). *Making vocational choices: A theory of careers*. Englewood Cliffs, NJ: Prentice Hall.

Holland, J. L. (1987). Current status of Holland's theory of careers: Another perspective. *Career Development Quarterly, 36*, 24–30.

Janes, C. L., Hesselbrock, V. M., Myers, D. G., & Penniman, J. H. (1979). Problem boys in young adulthood: Teachers' ratings and twelve-year follow-up. *Journal of Youth and Adolescence, 8*, 453–472.

Jolley, J., & Mitchell, M. (1996). *Lifespan development: A topical approach*. Madison, WI: Brown & Benchmark.

Kafka, R., & London, P. (1991, Fall). Communication in relationships and adolescent substance use: The influence of parents and friends. *Adolescence, 26*(103), 587–597.

Kandel, D. B. (1978). Homophily, selection, and socialization in adolescent friendships. *American Journal of Sociology, 84*, 427–436.

Kandel, D. B., & Lesser, G. S. (1972). Parental and peer influences on educational plans of adolescents. *American Sociological Review, 34*, 213–223.

Katchadourian, H. (1977). *The biology of adolescence*. San Francisco: Freeman.

Keller, M., Duerst, B., & Zimmerman, J. (1996). Adolescents' view of sexual decision-making. *Image: Journal of Nursing Scholarship, 28*(2), 125–130.

Kempton, T., Armistead, L., Wierson, M., & Forehand, R. (1991). Presence of a sibling as a buffer following parental divorce: An examination of young adolescents. *Journal of Clinical Child Psychology, 20*, 434–438.

Kennedy, E., & Powell, R. (1997). Changing eating patterns of American children: a view from 1996. *Journal of the American College of Nutrition, 16*, 524–529.

Koff, E., & Rierdan, J. (1991). Menarche and body image. In R.M. Lerner, A. C,. Petersen, & J. Brooks-Gunn (Eds.), *Encyclopedia of adolescence* (pp. 631–636). New York: Garland.

Kohn, M. (1977). *Class and conformity* (2nd ed.). Chicago: University of Chicago Press.

Kohlberg, L. (1976). Moral stages and moralization: The cognitive-development approach. In T. Lickona (Ed.), *Moral development and behavior*. New York: Holt, Rinehart and Winston.

Krasner, P. (1990). The treatment of avulsed teeth. *Journal of Pediatric Health Care, 4*(2), 86–90.

Kupersmidt, J. B., & Coie, J. D. (1990). Pre-adolescent peer status, aggression, and school adjustment as predictors of externalizing problems in adolescence. *Child Development, 61*, 1350–1362.

Ladd, G. W., & Golter, B. S. (1988). Parents' management of preschooler's peer relations: Is it related to children's social competence? *Developmental Psychology, 24*, 109–117.

Leslie, L. (1986). The impact of adolescent females' assessments of parenthood and employment on plans for the future. *Journal of Youth and Adolescence, 15*, 29–49.

Lewis, M., & Brooks-Gunn, J. (1979) The development of self-knowledge. In C. B. Kopp & J. B. Krakow (Eds.), *The child: Development in a social context*. Reading, MA: Addison-Wesley.

Linn, M. C., & Petersen, A. C. (1985). Emergence and characterization of sex differences in spatial ability. *Child Development, 56*, 1479–1498.

Lloyd, B., & Lucas, K. (1997). *Smoking in adolescence: Images and identities*. London: Routledge.

Lynch, M. E. (1991). Gender intensification. In R. M. Lerner, A. C. Petersen, & J. Brooks-Gunn (Eds.), *Encyclopedia of adolescence* (Vol. 1). New York: Garland.

Magnussen, D., Stattin, H., & Allen, V. (1988). Differential maturation among girls and its relations to social adjustment: A longitudinal perspective. In E. M. Hetherington, & R. Parke, (Eds.), *Contemporary readings in child psychology* (3rd ed.; pp. 97–116). New York: McGraw-Hill.

Malina, R., & Bouchard, C. (1991). *Growth maturation and physical activity*. Champaign, IL: Human Kinetics.

Mannarino, A. P. (1976). Friendship patterns and altruistic behavior in preadolescent males. *Developmental Psychology, 12*, 555–556.

Marcia, J. E. (1980). Identity in adolescence. In J. Adelson (Ed.), *Handbook of Adolescent Psychology* (pp. 159–187). New York: Wiley.

Marini, M., Fan, P., Finley, E., & Beutel, A. (1996). Gender and job values. *Sociology of Education, 69*, 49–65.

Marshall, W.A., & Tanner, J.M. (1969). Variations in the pattern of pubertal changes in girls. *Archives of Disease in Childhood, 44*, 291–303.

Marshall, W.A., & Tanner, J.M. (1970). Variations in the pattern of pubertal changes in boys. *Archives of Disease in Childhood, 45*, 13–23.

McCabe, M. (1984). Toward a theory of adolescent dating. *Adolescence, 19*, 159–169.

McCoy, J. K. (1992). *The importance of individual and family characteristics in predicting adolescent friendship quality*. Unpublished doctoral dissertation, University of Georgia, Athens, GA.

McCoy, J. K., Brody, G. H., & Stoneman, Z. (1994). A longitudinal analysis of sibling relationships as mediators of the link between family processes and youths' best friendships. *Family Relations, 43*, 400–408.

McCoy, J. K., Corey, A. M., & Owen, C. L. (1999, April). *Early adolescents' relationship patterns with parents and peers and parents' involvement in their children's friendships*. Paper presented at the Biennial Conference of the Society for Research in Child Development, Albuquerque, NM.

McDonald, D., & McKinney, J. (1994). Steady dating and self-esteem in high school students. Journal of *Adolescence, 17*, 557–564

McGuire, K. D., & Weisz, J. R. (1982). Social cognition and behavior correlates of preadolescent chumship. *Child Development, 53*, 1478–1484.

Meilman, P. W. (1979). Cross-sectional age changes in ego identity status during adolescence. *Developmental Psychology, 15*, 230–231.

Moffitt, T., Caspi, A., Belsky, J., & Silva, P. (1992). Childhood experience and the onset of menarche: A test of a sociobiological model. *Child Development, 63*, 47–58.

Montemayor, R. (1983). Parents and adolescents in conflict: All families some of the time and some families most of the time. *Journal of Early Adolescence, 3*, 83–103.

Mortimer, J., Finch, M., Ryu, S., Shanahan, M., & Call, K. (1996). The effects of work intensity on adolescent mental health, achievement, and behavioral adjustment: New evidence from a prospective study. *Child Development, 67*, 1243–1261.

Murray, R., & Zentner, J. (2001). *Health assessment and promotion strategies throughout the lifespan*. (7th ed.). Stamford,CT: Appleton & Lange.

Needle, R., McCubbin, H., Wilson, M., Reineck, R., Lazar, A., & Mederer, H. (1986). Interpersonal influences in adolescent drug use—the role of older siblings, parents, and peers. *International Journal of the Addictions, 21*, 739–766.

Neemann, J., Hubbard, J., & Masten, A. (1995). The changing importance of romantic relationship involvement to competence from late childhood to late adolescence. *Development and Psychopathology, 7*, 727–750

Newcombe, N., & Dubas, J. (1987). Individual differences in cognitive ability: Are they related to timing of puberty? In R. Lerner & T. Foch (Eds.), *Biological-psychosocial interactions in early adolescence* (pp. 249–302). Hillsdale, NJ: Erlbaum.

Parke, R. D., MacDonald, K. B., Burks, V. M., Carson, J., Bhavnagri, N., Barth, J. M., & Beitel, A. (1989). Family and peer systems: In search of the linkages. In K. Kreppner & R. M. Lerner (Eds.), *Family systems and life-span development*. Hillsdale, NJ: Erlbaum.

Parker, J. G., & Asher, S. R. (1987). Peer relations and later personal adjustment: Are low-accepted children at risk? *Psychological Bulletin, 102*, 357–359.

Parker, J. G., Rubin, K. H., Price, J. M., & DeRosier, M. (1995). Peer relationships, child development, and adjustment: A developmental psychopathology perspective. In D. Cicchetti & D. J. Cohen (Eds.), *Developmental psychopathology, Vol 2. Risk, disorder, and adaptation* (pp. 96–161). New York: Wiley.

Paterson, J., Pryor, J., & Field, J. (1994). Adolescent attachment to parents and friends in relation to aspects of self-esteem. *Journal of Youth and Adolescence, 24*, 365–376.

Paul, E. L., & White, K. M. (1990). The development of intimate relationships in late adolescence. *Adolescence, 25*, 375–400.

Pendergrast, R., & Strong, W. (1992). Sports medicine. In W. McAnarney, R. Kreipe, D. Orr, & G. Comerci (Eds.). *Textbook of adolescent medicine*. Philadelphia: Saunders.

Peterson, A. C. (1985). Pubertal development as a cause of disturbance: Myths, reactions, and unanswered questions. *Genetic, Social, and General Psychological Monographs, 111*, 205–232.

Physical Activity Guidelines for Adolescents. (1994). *Pediatric Exercise Science, 6*, 299–463.

Piaget, J. (1972). Intellectual evolution from adolescence to adulthood. *Human Development, 15*, 1–12.

Raja, S. N., McGee, R., & Stanton, W. R. (1992). Perceived attachments to parents and peers and psychological well-being in adolescence. *Journal of Youth and Adolescence, 21*, 471–485.

Rees, J. (1996). Eating disorders in adolescence: A model for broadening our perspective. *Journal of the American Dietetic Association, 96*(1), 22–24.

Remafedi, G. (1987a). Adolescent homosexuality: Psychosocial and medical implications. *Pediatrics, 79*(3), 331–337.

Remafedi, G., (1987b). Male homosexuality: The adolescent's perspective. *Pediatrics, 79*(3), 326–330.

Remafedi, G., Resnick, M., Blum, R., & Harris, L. (1992). Demography of sexual orientation in adolescents. *Pediatrics, 89*(4), 714–721.

Rest, J., Davison, M., & Robbins, S. (1978). Age trends in judging moral issues: A review of cross-sectional, longitudinal, and sequential studies of the Defining Issues Test. *Child Development, 49*, 263–279.

Roff, M., Sells, S. B., & Golden, M. M. (1972). *Social adjustment and personality development in children*. Minneapolis: University of Minnesota.

Rogers, J. L., & Rowe, D. C. (1990). Influence of siblings on adolescent sexual behavior. *Developmental Psychology, 24*(5), 722–728.

Roscoe, B., Dian, M. S., & Brooks, R. H. (1987). Early, middle, and late adolescents' views on dating and factors influencing partner's selection. *Adolescence, 22*, 59–68.

Rose, S., & Frieze, I. R. (1993). Young singles' contemporary dating scripts. *Sex Roles, 28*, 499–509.

Rowe, D. C., & Britt, C. L. (1991). Developmental explanation of delinquent behavior: Common vs. transmitted effects. *Journal of Quantitative Criminology, 7*, 315–322.

Rowe, D. C., & Gulley, B. L. (1992). Sibling effects on substance use and delinquency. *Criminology, 30*, 217–233.

Rozin, J. C., & Gross, J. (1987). Prevalence of weight reducing and weight gaining in adolescent boys and girls. *Health Psychology, 6*, 131–147.

Santrock, J. W. (2001). *Adolescence* (8th ed.). Dubuque, IA: Brown & Benchmark.

Selman, R. L. (1980). *The growth of interpersonal understanding*. New York: Academic.

Shaffer, D. R. (2000). *Social and personality development*, (4th ed.). Pacific Grove, CA: Brooks/Cole.

Sharabany, R., Gershoni, R., & Hofman, J. E. (1981). Girlfriend, boyfriend: Age and sex differences in intimate friendship. *Developmental Psychology, 17*, 800–808.

Sifuentes, M. (2000). Eating disorders. In C. Berkowitz, (Ed.). *Pediatrics: A primary care approach* (2nd ed., pp. 429–433). Philadelphia: Saunders.

Sigelman, C. K., Carr, M. B., & Bagley, N. L. (1986). Developmental changes in the influence of sex-role stereotypes on person perception. *Child Study Journal, 16*, 191–205.

Silbereisen, R., & Kracke, B. (1993). Variation in maturational timing and adjustment in adolescence. In S. Jackson & H., Rodriguez-Tome (Eds.), *Adolescence and its social worlds* (pp. 67–94). Hillsdale, NJ: Erlbaum.

Simmons, R., & Blyth, D. (1987). *Moving into adolescence: The impact of pubertal change and school context*. New York: Aldine de Gruyter.

Sprinthall, N. A., & Collins, W. A. (1995). *Adolescent psychology: A developmental view*. New York: McGraw-Hill.

Stattin, H., & Magnussen, D. (1990). *Pubertal maturation in female development: Paths through life* (Vol. 2). Hillsdale, NJ: Erlbaum.

Stein, K., Roeser, R., & Markus, H. (1998). Self-schemas and possible selves as predictors and outcomes of risky behaviors in adolescents. *Nursing Research, 47*(2), 96–106.

Steinberg, L. (2001). *Adolescence* (5th ed.). New York: McGraw-Hill.

Steinberg, L., & Cauffman, E. (1995). The impact of employment on adolescent development. In R. Vasta (Ed.), *Annals of Child Development* (Vol. 11). London: Kingsley.

Steinberg, L., & Dornbusch, S. (1991). Negative correlates of part-time work in adolescence: Replication and elaboration. *Developmental Psychology, 17*, 304–313.

Steinberg, L., & Steinberg, W. (1994). *Crossing paths: How your child's adolescence triggers your own crisis*. New York: Simon & Schuster.

Steinberg, L. D. (1981). Transformations in family relations at puberty. *Developmental Psychology, 17*, 833–840.

Stocker, C., & Dunn, J. (1990). Sibling relationships in childhood: Links with friendships and peer relationships. *Journal of Developmental Psychology, 8*, 227–244.

Stone, M. R., & Brown, B. B. (1998). In the eye of the beholder: Adolescents' perceptions of peer crowd stereotypes. In R. E. Muuss & H. D. Porton (Eds.) *Adolescent behavior and society: A book of readings* (pp. 158–169). Boston: McGraw-Hill College.

Strasburger, V., & Donnerstein, E. (1999, January). Children, adolescents, and the media: Issues and solutions. *Pediatrics, 103*(1), 129–139.

Strauss, R. S., & Knight, J. (1999). Influence of the home environment on the development of obesity in children. *Pediatrics, 106*(6), 85.

Sullivan, H. S. (1953). *The interpersonal theory of psychiatry*. New York: Norton.

Sussman, S., Dent, C., McAdams, L., Stacy, A., Burton, D., & Flay, B. (1994). Group self-identification and adolescent cigarette smoking: A 1-year prospective study. *Journal of Abnormal Psychology, 103*, 576–580.

Tanner, J. M., (1990). *Fetus into man: Physical growth from conception to maturity* (2nd ed.). Cambridge, MA: Harvard University Press.

Tanner, J. M. (1991). Menarche, secular trend in age of. In R.M. Lerner, A. C., Petersen, & J. Brooks-Gunn (Eds.), *Encyclopedia of adolescence* (pp. 637–641). New York: Garland.

Tanner, J. M., Whitehouse, R. H., & Takaishi, M. (1966). Standards from birth to maturity for height, weight, height velocity, and weight velocity: British children, 1965. *Archives of Diseases of Children, 41*, 454–471.

Teevan, J. J., Jr. (1972). Reference groups and premarital sexual behavior. *Journal of Marriage and the Family, 34*, 283–291.

Troiano, R. P., & Flegal, K. M. (1998). Overweight children and adolescents: Description, epidemiology, and demographics. *Pediatrics, 101*(3), 497–504.

Troiden, D. (1989). The formation of homosexual identities. *Journal of Homosexuality, 17*, 43–73.

Turner, J., & Helms, D. (1995). *Lifespan development* (5th ed.). New York: Holt, Rinehart & Winston.

U.S. Department of Health and Human Services. (1997). Guidelines for school and community programs to promote lifelong physical activity among young people. *MMWR 46*, 1–36.

U.S. Department of Health and Human Services. (2000). *Healthy People 2010: National health promotion and disease prevention objectives*. Washington DC: Author.

Ventura, S. J., Peters, K. D., Martin, J. A., & Maurer, J. D. (1997). Births and deaths: United States 1996. *Monthly Vital Statistics Report, 46*(1), Supplement 2.

Waldner-Haugrud, L. K., & Magruder, B. (1996). Homosexuality identity expression among lesbian and gay adolescents: An analysis of perceived structural associations. *Youth & Society, 27*, 313–333.

Warren, M., Brooks-Gunn, J., Fox, R., Lancelot, C., Newman, D., & Hamilton, W. (1991). Lack of bone accretion and amenorrhea in young dancers: Evidence for a relative osteopenia in weight bearing bones. *Journal of Clinical Endocrinology and Metabolism, 72*, 847–853.

Waterman, A. S. (1992). Identity as an aspect of optimal psychological functioning. *Adolescent identity formation*. Newbury Park, CA: Sage.

Webster, D., Gainer, P., & Champion, H. (1995). Weapon carrying among inner-city junior high students: Defensive behavior vs. aggressive delinquency. *American Journal of Public Health, 85*, 1604–1608.

Whitaker, A., Davies, S., Shaffer, D., Abrams, S., Walsh, B., & Kalikow, K. (1989). The struggle to be thin: A survey on anorexic and bulimic symptoms in a non-referred adolescent population. *Psychological Medicine, 19*, 143–163.

Wright, E., & Whitehead, T. (1987). Perceptions of body size and obesity: A selected review of the literature. *Journal of Community Health, 12*, 117–129.

World Health Statistics Annual, 1994 (1995). Geneva, Switzerland: World Health Organization.

Youniss, J., & Smollar, J. (1985). *Adolescent relations with mothers, fathers, and friends*. Chicago: University of Chicago Press.

Suggested Readings

Adler, E., & Clark, R. (1991). Adolescence: A literary passage. *Adolescence, 26*(104), 757–768.

Amato, P. R. (1993). Children's adjustment to divorce: Theories, hypotheses, and empirical support. *Journal of Marriage and the Family, 55*, 23–38.

Amato, P. R., & Keith, B. (1991). Parental divorce and adult well-being: A meta-analysis. *Journal of Marriage and the Family, 53*, 43–58.

American Academy of Pediatrics Committee on Adolescence (2000, April). Suicide and suicide attempts in adolescents. *Pediatrics, 104*(4), 871–874.

American Academy of Pediatrics Committee on Infectious Diseases (1997, March). Immunization of adolescents: Recommendations of the Advisory Committee on Immunization Practices, the American Academy of Pediatrics, the American Academy of Family Physicians, and the American Medical Association (RE9711). *Pediatrics, 99*(3), 479–488,

American Medical Association (1996). Guidelines for adolescent preventable services (GAPS): Recommendations for physicians and other health professionals. Available: www.ama-assn.org

Anderson, R., Crespo, C., Bartlett, S., Cheskin, L, & Pratt, M. (1998, March). Relationship of physical activity and television with body weight and level of fatness among children. *Journal of the American Medical Association, 279*(12): 938–942.

Barber, B. (1992).Family, personality, and adolescent problem behavior. *Journal of Marriage and the Family, 54*, 69–79.

Bradford, M. (1996). Health concerns and prevalence of abuse and sexual activity in adolescents at a runaway shelter. *Applied Nursing Research, 8*(4), 187–190.

Cole, T. J. (1991). Weight-stature indices to measure underweight, overweight, and obesity. In J. H. Himes, (Ed.), *Anthropometric assessment of nutritional status* (pp. 83–111). New York: Wiley Liss.

Connelly, C. (1998). Hopefulness, self-esteem, and perceived social support among pregnant and nonpregnant adolescents. *Western Journal of Nursing Research, 20*(2), 195–209.

Conrad, N. (1991). Where do they turn? Social support systems of suicidal high school adolescents. *Journal of Psychosocial Nursing, 29*(3), 14–20.

Dietz, W. H. (1998). Health consequences of obesity in youth: Childhood predictors of adult disease. *Pediatrics, 101*(3), 518–525.

Domel, S. B., Thomson, W. O., Davis, H. C., Baranowski, T., Leonard, S. B., & Baranowski, J. (1996). Psychosocial predictors of fruit and vegetable consumption among elementary school children. *Health Education Research, 11*, 299–308.

Dryfoos, J. (1998). *Safe passage: Making it through adolescence in a risky society*. New York: Oxford University Press.

Estes, M. E. (2002). *Health assessment and physical examination* (2nd ed.). Albany, NY: Delmar.

Fine, M. A., & Kurdek, L. A. (1992). The adjustment of adolescents in stepfather and stepmother families. *Journal of Marriage and the Family, 54*, 725–736.

Flegal, K. M. (1993). Defining obesity in children and adolescents: epidemiologic approaches. *Critical Review Food Science Nutrition, 33*, 307–312.

Grossman, M., & Rowat, K. M. (1995). Parental relationships, coping strategies, received support, and well-being in adolescents of separated or divorced and married parents. *Research in Nursing and Health, 18*, 249–261.

Hetherington, E. M. (1972). Effects of father-absence on personality development in adolescent daughters. *Developmental Psychology, 7*, 313–326.

Hetherington, E. M. (1989). Coping with family transitions: Winners, losers, and survivors. *Child Development, 60*, 1–14.

Hetherington, E. M., Anderson, E. R., & Hagan, M. S. (1991). Divorce: Effects on adolescents. In R. M. Lerner, A. D. Petersen, & J. Brooks-Gunn (Eds.), *Encyclopedia of adolescence* (Vol. 1). New York: Garland.

Hetherington, E. M., Bridges, M., & Insabella, G. M. (1998). What matters? What does not? Five perspectives on the association between marital transitions and children's adjustment. *American Psychologist, 53*(2), 167–184.

Hetherington, E. M., Stanley-Hagan, M., & Anderson, E. (1989). Marital transitions: A child's perspective. *American Psychologist, 44*, 303–312.

Himes, J. H., & Dietz, W. H. (1994). Guidelines for overweight in adolescent preventive services: recommendations from an expert committee. The Expert Committee on Clinical Guidelines for Overweight in Adolescent Preventive Services. *American Journal of Clinical Nutrition, 32*, 607–629.

Holland, W., & Fitzsimons, B. (1991) Smoking in children. *Archives of Diseases in Childhood, 66*, 1269–1274.

Igoe, J. (1991). Empowerment of children and youth for consumer self-care. *American Journal of Health Promotion, 6*, 55–65.

Irwin, C., (1993). Topical areas of interest for promoting health: From the perspective of the physician. In S. Millstein, A. Petersen, & E. Nightengale, (Eds.). *Promoting the health of adolescents: New directions for the twenty-first century* (pp. 328–332). New York: Oxford University Press.

Jacobson, L., & Wilkenson, C. (1994). Review of teenage health: Time for a new direction. *British Journal of General Practice, 44*, 313–424

Johnson, S. L., & Birch, L. L. (1994). Parent's and children's adiposity and eating style. *Pediatrics, 94*, 653–661.

Kurdek, L., & Fine, M. (1994). Family acceptance and family control as predictors of adjustment in young adolescents: Linear, curvilinear, or interactive effects. *Child Development, 65*, 1137–1146.

Kurdek, L., & Sinclair, R. (1988). Relation of eighth graders' family structure, gender, and family environment with academic performance and school behavior. *Journal of Educational Psychology, 80*, 90–94.

Lamborn, S., Mounts, N., Steinberg, L., and Dornbusch, S. (1991). Patterns of competence and adjustment among adolescents from authoritative, authoritarian, indulgent, and neglectful families. *Child Development, 62*, 1049–1065.

Lee, S., & Gruggs, L. (1995). Pregnant teenagers' reasons for seeking or delaying prenatal care. *Clinical Nursing Research, 4*(1), 38–49.

Maccoby, E. E., & Martin, J. A. (1983). Socialization in the context of the family: Parent–child interaction. In P. H. Mussen (Ed.), *Handbook of child psychology* (4th ed., Vol. 4, pp. 37–56). New York: Wiley.

Mahon, N. (1994). Positive health practices and perceived health status in adolescents. *Clinical Nursing Research, 3*(2), 86–103.

Mahon, N., Yarcheski, A., & Yarcheski, T. (1993). Health consequences of loneliness in adolescents. *Research in Nursing and Health, 12*, 23–31.

Mechanic, D., & Hansell, S. (1989). Divorce, family conflict, and adolescent well-being. *Journal of Health and Social Behavior, 30*, 105-116.

Millstein, S., Petersen, A., & Nightengale, E. (Eds.). (1993). *Promoting the health of adolescents: New directions for the twenty-first century*. New York: Oxford University Press.

Needle, R. H., Su, S. S., & Doherty, W. J. (1990). Divorce, remarriage, and adolescent substance use: A prospective study. *Journal of Marriage and the Family, 52*, 157–169.

Riesch, S., Jacobson, G., & Tosi, C. (1994). Young adolescents' identification of difficult life events. *Clinical Nursing Research, 3*(4), 393–413.

Riesch, S., Tosi, C., Thurston, C., Forsyth, D., Kuenning, T., & Kestly, J. (1993). Effects of communication training on parents and young adolescents. *Nursing Research, 42*(1), 10–16.

Rosenbaum, M., & Leibel, R. L. (1998). The physiology of body weight regulation: relevance to the etiology of obesity in children. *Pediatrics, 101*, 525–539.

Steinberg L. D. (1990). Autonomy, conflict, and harmony in the family relationship. In S. Feldman & G. Elliott (Eds.), *At the threshold: The developing adolescent* (pp. 255–276). Cambridge, MA: Harvard University Press.

Steinberg, L., Lamborn, S., Darling, N., Mounts, N., and Dornbusch, S. (1994). Over-time changes in adjustment and competence among adolescents from authoritative, authoritarian, indulgent, and neglectful families. *Child Development, 65*, 754–770.

Stevens-Simon, C. (1993). Clinical applications of adolescent female sexual development. *Nurse Practitioner, 18*(12), 18–29.

Troiano, R. P., Flegal, K. M., Kuczmarski, R. J., Campbell, S. M., & Johnson, C. L. (1995). Overweight prevalence and trends for children and adolescents: The National Health and Nutrition Examination Surveys, 1963 to 1991. *Archives of Pediatric Adolescent Medicine, 149*, 1085–1091.

Wagner, W. (1996). Optimal development in adolescence: What is it and how can it be encouraged? *The Counseling Psychologist, 24*(3), 360–399.

Williams, J. O., Achterberg, C., & Sylvester, G. P. (1995). Targeting marketing of food products to ethnic minority youths. In C. L. Willams & S. Y. Kim (Eds.), *Prevention and treatment of childhood obesity. Annals of the New York Academy of Sciences, 699*, 107–114.

Yarcheski, A., Mahon, N., & Yarcheski, T. (1997). Alternate models of positive health practices in adolescents. *Nursing Research, 46*(3), 85–92.

Yarcheski, A., Mahon, N., & Yarcheski, T. (1998). A study of introspectiveness in adolescents and young adults. *Western Journal of Nursing Research, 20*(3), 312–324.

Resources

Organizations and Websites

Adolescence Directory On-Line (ADOL)
www.education.indiana.edu/cas/adol/adol.html
(an electronic guide to information on adolescent issues)

AMA Archives of Pediatrics and Adolescent Medicine
www.ama-assn.org/public/journals/ajdc/ajdchome.htm
(a vehicle for increased attention to adolescent health, the education of pediatric health care professionals, and disease prevention and health promotion)

American Academy of Child and Adolescent Psychiatry (AACAP)
3615 Wisconsin Ave. NW
Washington, DC 20016
(202) 966-7300
www.aacap.org

American Academy of Pediatrics (AAP)
141 Northwest Point Blvd.
Elk Grove Village, IL 60009-0927
(847) 981-5005
www.aap.org

Consumer Product Safety Commission
(800) 638-2772
www.cpsc.gov

National Highway Traffic Safety Administration
400 7th St. SW, Rm. 5319
Washington, DC 20005
(800) 424-9393

National Runaway Switchboard
3080 North Lincoln Ave.
Chicago, IL 60657
(800) 621-4000

Planned Parenthood Federation of America, Inc.
810 Seventh Ave.
New York, NY 10019

Public Health Service AIDS Information Hotline
(800) 342-AIDS

Sex Information and Education Council of the U.S. (SIECUS)
32 Washington Pl.
New York, NY 10003
(212) 673-3850

STD Hotline
(800) 227-8922

Tough Love
P.O. Box 1069
Doylestown, PA 18901

Youth Indicators 1993: Trends in the Well-Being of American Youth
National Center for Education Statistics, U.S. Department of Education
www.ed.gov/pubs/YouthIndicators/

UNIT III

Unique Considerations in Children

CHAPTER 13

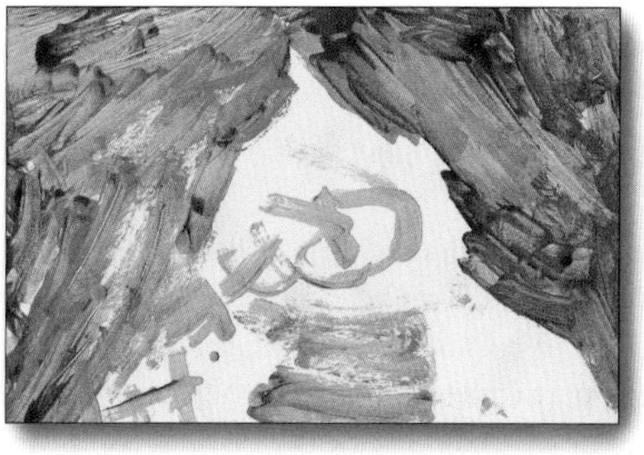

CHILD AND FAMILY COMMUNICATION

Frances J. Dotton, RN, PhD
Barbara Mandleco, RN, PhD

My 4-year-old and only child, Tatiani, was running a high temperature and complaining of an earache. We were up most of the night. It really hurts a parent to see their child who is normally very happy and active, listless and laying on the couch crying in pain. Instead of being comforting and giving me the answers to my questions about what I could do for Tatiani, the doctor's receptionist gave me information about their office rules and told me to bring her into the office. Since that was impossible for me to do at the time, I was only frustrated and angry after my call, in addition to having a child in pain. When I saw the impact of a child's suffering on their parents in my own practice, I made it a priority to reserve time in any interaction to deal with the parent's feelings. My care of the parent may be simply answering questions and saying something reflecting empathy with their present situation such as "Who said raising a child was easy?"

COMPETENCIES

Upon completion of this chapter, the reader will be able to:

- *Explain what communication is and its importance in developing positive relationships with children and their families.*
- *Discuss barriers encountered in communication.*
- *Describe verbal and nonverbal communication.*
- *Discuss the elements of communication, including rapport and trust, respect, empathy, listening, providing feedback, and conflict management.*
- *Describe the impact and challenges that a child's developmental level has on communication.*
- *Describe effective communication strategies that assist nurses' work with infants, children, and adolescents.*
- *Discuss the impact that a person's cultural background may have on their communication patterns.*
- *Explain the concept of communicating with children who have special needs.*

Enhancing understanding of a child's condition can reduce fear and pain, as well as encourage active participation in care decisions (Rushforth, 1999). This understanding is especially enhanced when effective communication occurs among nursing staff, children, and their caregivers and families. In fact, the ability to communicate effectively is recognized as a basic and central component in delivering care to children and their caregivers (Riesch, 1997; Stuart & Sundeen, 1995). Therefore, it is essential that nurses practice and integrate effective communication skills into every facet of interaction. Effective communication expressed in an authentic, nonjudgmental, empathetic manner improves not only the quality of care but also determines the success of relationships established in delivering care. Since one cannot *not* communicate, learning effective communication skills is essential to delivering effective care and can be compared to learning aseptic skills; once one understands the principles behind effective communication, one can integrate these principles into practice.

THE COMMUNICATION PROCESS

Communication is defined as the exchange of meanings between and among individuals through a shared system of symbols. The sender, message, channel, receiver, and feedback are major components of the communication process. The **sender** generates a message in response to a need to relate to others, to create meaning, or to understand various situations. The **message** is a verbal or nonverbal stimulus produced by a sender and responded to by a receiver. The **channel** is the medium through which a message is transmitted. It may be visual, auditory, or kinesthetic. Visual channels include sight, observation, and perception. Auditory channels include the spoken word and cues. Kinesthetic channels include sensations experienced, as in touch. The **receiver** is the person intercepting the sender's message. **Feedback** provides the sender with information from the receiver about the message. The sender can then adjust the message so that it is understood more effectively by the receiver the next time it is sent (Estes, 2002).

Communication is both talking and listening. Nurses must be able to not only use words to explain information to caregivers and children, but also to listen to what caregivers and children say. The ability to prepare and present ideas, feelings, and thoughts accurately (by talking) and to respond to messages accurately (by listening) reduces distortion and results in effective communication.

BARRIERS TO COMMUNICATION

Barriers to communication include physical factors and psychological factors. Physical or environmental factors include the physical space or distance between the receiver and sender, the temperature or ventilation in the environment, and distracting noises such as the radio or television. They can also include health status, especially if the child (or family) is disoriented or has a hearing or visual handicap. Since effective communication will not occur when children and families do not understand the medical terminology used, explanations should include common words and simple terms. Finally, hearing or speech difficulties, including accents and speech impediments, may become barriers for some (Estes, 2002; Marquis & Huston, 1992).

Psychosocial barriers include one's personal judgments, past experience, emotions, developmental level, or social values. Preconceived ideas and allowing feelings to influence behavior, opinions, or beliefs may also be problematic. Expressions of personal opinions need to be carefully shared with children and their caregivers since nurses represent authority figures. Finally, facial expressions that convey disapproval may become a psychosocial barrier if the child or family suspects disapproval (Estes, 2002; Marquis & Huston, 1992).

MODES OF COMMUNICATION

Communication can be examined and described according to whether it is formal/informal or verbal/nonverbal. **Formal communication** refers to communication that occurs in an organized way, with a particular agenda, as when teaching a child's care to the caregiver upon discharge. Formal communication needs to be clear and understandable. **Informal communication** occurs when individuals talk using no particular agenda or protocol. Often, informal communication occurs sporadically when caring for children and their caregivers in day-to-day interactions.

VERBAL COMMUNICATION

Verbal communication refers to messages that are communicated through words and language (Estes, 2002). Verbal communication is most effective if it is brief, clear, effectively toned, paced appropriately, relevant, and well timed. The receiver will be confused if more words than necessary are used or if the speaker does not speak slowly and clearly. Important points should be repeated and medical jargon avoided, especially when talking to children and their caregivers and families. Messages also need appropriate pacing; they should not be too slow or fast, and there should be few pauses and periods of silence. Only important and relevant information should be conveyed, and the tone should be pleasant. Messages should also be sent at the appropriate time. For example, teaching will not be effective if delivered when children are in pain or have visitors, or when caregivers are preoccupied with personal thoughts. When interacting with families, it is also essential to convey interest and warmth; to avoid distractions, yes/no questions, and personal bias; and not to monopolize the conversation. **Paraverbal cues,** also part of verbal communication, include the tone and pitch of the voice; volume, inflection, and speed; and grunts or other vocalizations not considered language (Luckman, 1999). These cues add meaning to the words spoken, and can and often do influence the listener more than the actual words themselves (Estes, 2002). Confusion results when verbal messages are inaccurate or unreliable.

NONVERBAL COMMUNICATION

Nonverbal communication conveys feelings, attitudes, and intentions (Luckman, 1999). It enables one to decode

Research Highlight

The Effect of Human Touch on Preterm Infants

Study Purpose

To evaluate the effects of gentle human touch (GHT) on preterm infants.

Methods

An experimental design followed 30 preterm (26–32 weeks at birth) infants hospitalized in a level III neonatal intensive care unit (NICU). The infants had no congenital anomalies, no surgery, no administration of pancuronium bromide, no medical orders prohibiting GHT, and no known substance-abusing mother. Infants were randomly assigned to a control group, which received no GHT, or an experimental group, which received 15 minutes of GHT each day for 5 days beginning between 6 and 9 days of age. Effects measured included (a) oxygen saturation or heart rate levels before, during, and after GHT, (b) amount of quiet sleep and active sleep during GHT compared to before and after GHT, (c) motor activity and behavior signs of distress during GHT compared to before and after GHT, (d) morbidity scores, (e) number of days receiving supplemental oxygen, (f) number of days receiving phototherapy, (g) average daily weight gain, and (h) patterns of behavioral organization.

Findings

GHT significantly lowered the amount of active sleep for the experimental group and decreased motor activity. No difference was seen in oxygen saturation or heart rate, amount of quiet sleep, morbidity scores, numbers of days on supplemental oxygen, or weight gain.

Implications

Nurses caring for preterm infants should be encouraged to use GHT since no adverse effects were found on oxygenation or heart rate. In fact, GHT, which decreases active sleep, motor activity, and behavioral stress, may serve to calm these infants. NICU nurses can encourage the caregivers of preterm infants to use GHT in the early weeks of life while monitoring each infant's individual responses.

Citation

Harrison, L., Olivet, L., Cunningham, K., Bodin, M. B., & Hicks, C. (1996). Effects of gentle human touch on preterm infants: Pilot study results. *Neonatal Network: Journal of Neonatal Nursing, 15*(2), 35–42.

verbal communication and transcend the literal content of the message. Nonverbal communication is especially apparent when emotions cause observable body changes, and comes through more powerfully and effectively when there is incongruence between the verbal and the nonverbal message. In fact, most communication is nonverbal, and most verbal communication contradicts nonverbal messages. Nonverbal communication is important because the listener will believe the nonverbal message rather than the verbal message if they contradict each other. Therefore, it is critical to always consider nonverbal communication in any interaction since it contributes to what others "hear."

Nonverbal communication also includes spatial relationships (the distance between participants); appearance (clothing, grooming, hair style); eye contact; body posture (slouching, standing erect with the head leaning to receiver); gestures (which sometimes add emphasis to words); facial expressions (which need to agree with the message); timing (hesitation may imply untruthfulness or diminish the effect of the message); and, with children especially, touch (Luckman, 1999) (Figure 13-1). In fact, touch may be one of the most important communicative behaviors nurses use since it conveys warmth, understanding, affection, willingness to become involved, nurturance, and caring (Fredriksson, 1999). Touch, however, may have special meanings to children and their families depending on their gender or ethnic background. Therefore, nurses always need to be sensitive to the message transmitted when touching,

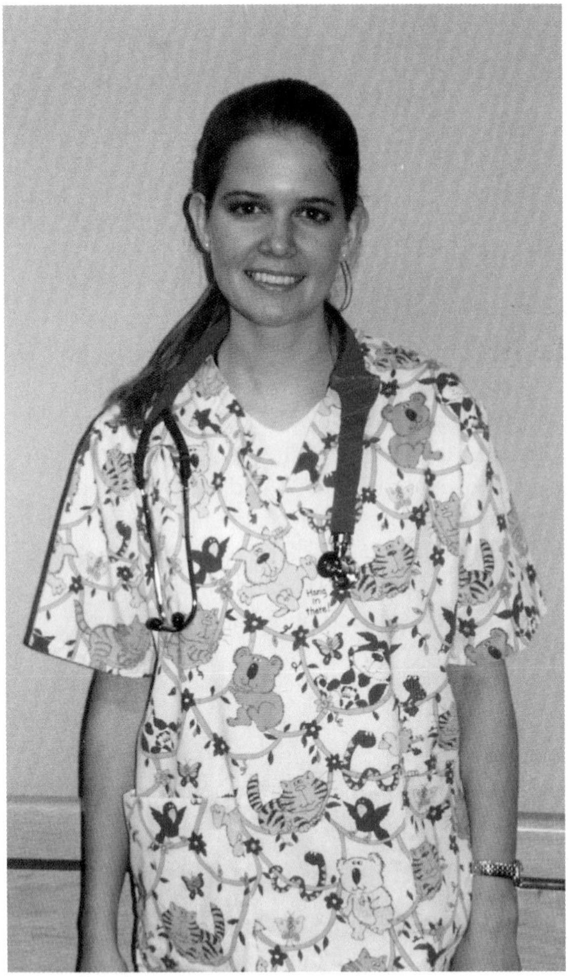

Figure 13-1 In the pediatric setting, nurses' demeanor and uniform are a nonverbal method of communicating.

since, for some, touch may mean concern and empathy, whereas, for others, it may mean dominance, interpreted as the nurse overstepping her bounds, or a desire for intimacy, resulting in uncomfortableness.

NURSE, CHILD, AND FAMILY COMMUNICATION

Effective communication requires sensitivity to the child and family's needs and a well-developed and carefully thought-out plan. In fact, the nurse's ability to establish a therapeutic relationship with children and their caregivers is strongly tied to communication abilities and must be a high priority for all nurses as they interact with clients and families. Nurses always need to be aware of client and family needs for education and use communicative interactions as an entree into providing new or reinforcing old information. Increasing knowledge and providing information regarding a child's illness, symptoms, care needed, or developmental level can empower families and ultimately increase well-being. Before communication can be effective, several key elements must be addressed, including establishing rapport, building trust, showing respect, conveying empathy, listening actively, providing appropriate feedback, managing conflict, and establishing professional boundaries (Figure 13-2).

Rapport and Trust

Nurses must develop trust and rapport with clients, and clients must be willing to talk, listen, and provide honest answers. Nurses may also need to be available and open to questions that caregivers and children may have. To build rapport with the child and the caregivers, the nurse must be accepted by them and be willing to discuss non-health-related issues to convey warmth and friendliness. To establish trust, a nurse must follow through on promises, keep appointments, respect patient confidentiality, and carefully explain procedures in a way that is acceptable to the family (Luckman, 1999).

Respect

To establish respect, the nurse should address the child by first name (the formal name unless given permission to use a nickname) and the caregivers by Mr., Ms., or Mrs. and then the last name. Before addressing the caregivers by first name, it is imperative that the caregivers give their consent. Respect is also conveyed by considering the family's feelings, cultural views, and values. Nurses need to convey that they have time to spend with the child and the family. This will allow the family to share their thoughts and concerns and ask questions. If nurses communicate they do not have time, for example, by standing near the doorway, frequently looking at the clock while talking, or confiding to the child and family how busy they are, caregivers and children will soon believe that the nurse is too busy or doesn't really care. These messages interfere with establishing trust and respect, and should be avoided. Interference in establishing respect also occurs when a child is in isolation and nurses are required to wear gloves and masks. Indeed, children in these situations may feel isolated since they are not visited frequently and verbal communication is muffled or difficult to understand. Therefore, the nurse should make a concerted effort to speak more clearly without appearing as if yelling. Smiling is also important; although the child cannot see a smile from the nurse's mouth, since it will be covered by a mask, the child will see it in the nurse's eyes.

Empathy

Empathy forms the basis of a helping relationship and is an important element in communication. **Empathy** refers to

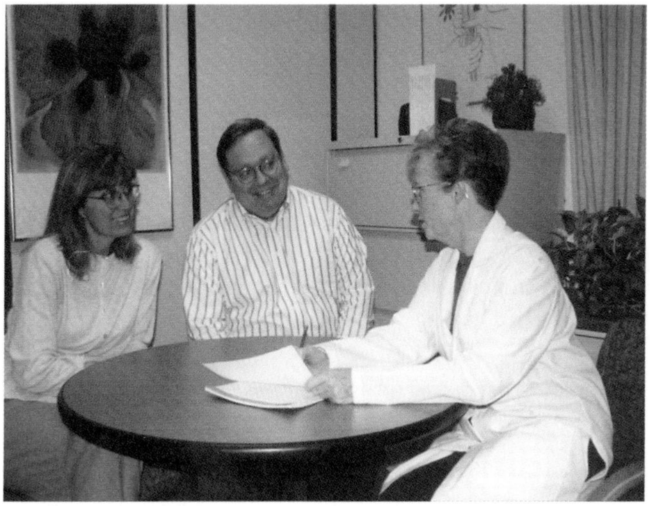

Figure 13-2 When interacting with parents, nurses need to be sure the environment is conducive to effective communication.

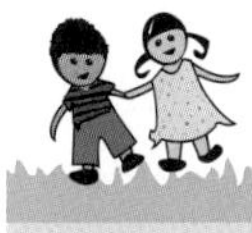

Taking Medication

Child: "I don't want to take that. It tastes yucky."
Nurse: "I feel so proud of you when you take your medicine. I understand it doesn't taste good and you don't like to do it. I am pleased you want to help yourself feel better by taking your medicine." Feelings are emphasized, and the "I" statements express ownership of the feelings. Empathy is illustrated when the child understands what the nurse is thinking.

the ability to put one's self in the other person's shoes—to feel as well as to intellectually know what the other person is experiencing (Luckman, 1999). Empathetic nurses are able to appreciate and understand children and caregivers as unique individuals, and allow them to feel cared about and accepted. For this to happen, the nurse's empathy needs to be integrated with verbal and nonverbal behavior. Empathy, however, is not to be confused with sympathy. The empathetic nurse maintains a sense of objectivity, and is supportive, understanding, and able to plan and implement helpful behaviors by teaching and giving examples that facilitate the ability of the child and the caregivers to function in difficult and sad situations. The sympathetic nurse, on the other hand, offers condolence and pity, and is not able to develop or carry out behaviors that engage the child or parent in activities that help them to maintain their relationship and ability to function in difficult situations. For example, Shawn, an 11-year-old boy with an inoperable brain tumor, is being cared for at home by his parents. The nurse sympathizer feels sorry for Shawn and is often near tears when she looks at him and tries to talk to his parents. She assumes all of Shawn's care. The nurse empathizer would teach the parents how to participate in Shawn's care, make suggestions on how to conserve Shawn's energy, and outline diversional activities that all might enjoy together given Shawn's condition. The nurse empathizer would direct energy toward finding ways to enable the parents to have quality time and experiences with Shawn and might even "share tears with" parents as they talk about what to expect in the end. The nurse empathizer is able to establish an accurate understanding of the child and the caregivers from their perspective, build rapport, and relate to the child and caregivers in such a way as to allow them to express their feelings and concerns.

Listening

Listening consists of providing verbal and nonverbal cues that communicate interest (Luckman, 1999). It is an activity that requires attention and effort as one not only listens to the words of the child and the caregivers, but one also listens to how words are used and decides whether or not what is said is what is meant. Accurate listening does not happen without effort. It requires actively attending to what is verbalized, observed, and created by the entire communication context (Fredriksson, 1999). It is important not to allow one's mind to wonder, daydream, prejudge what is being said, or think about what will be said as a response; one must listen attentively and wait for others to finish what they are saying. Attentive listening goes beyond hearing and includes what is not said or what is conveyed through gestures. Active listening also includes maintaining eye contact, taking an open and relaxed posture, and facing the child or caregivers (Luckman, 1999). See Box 13-1 for more information on effective listening.

When working with children and caregivers, the nurse should encourage and allow each to give input, discuss concerns, express feelings, and acknowledge problems. Respecting other's feelings and views, and appreciating each other's understandings and fears even though they are different than one's own are also important. While listening to children, the nurse must consider their developmental level, cognition, and emotional behavior. Children who are social and verbal may seem to be more in control and able to understand, and think more logically and rationally than children who engage in shy, clinging, and dependent behaviors. Nurses should use developmentally appropriate language and behavior with children and attend to their behavioral cues for clues as to their concerns and fears (Figure 13-3). For example, a child may continue talking and asking questions in order to avoid beginning a treatment.

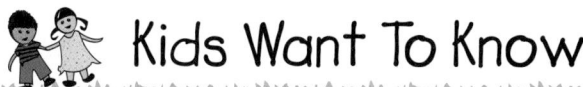

Reflective Thinking

Jumping the Gun

Active listening takes conscious effort, time, and practice. When nurses listen, they are able to convey in their own words what children and their caregivers have said and the feelings that were expressed. If nurses construct responses before children or caregivers finish speaking, or answer questions while they are being asked, listening isn't occurring. Can you in your own words express the thoughts and feelings of the children and caregivers? If you cannot, you are not listening. Evaluate yourself. How well do you listen?

BOX 13-1 Four *B*s of effective listening

Be attentive; eliminate distractions.

Be clear about the message; clarify if necessary.

Be empathetic; convey concern and caring.

Be open minded; avoid prejudices.

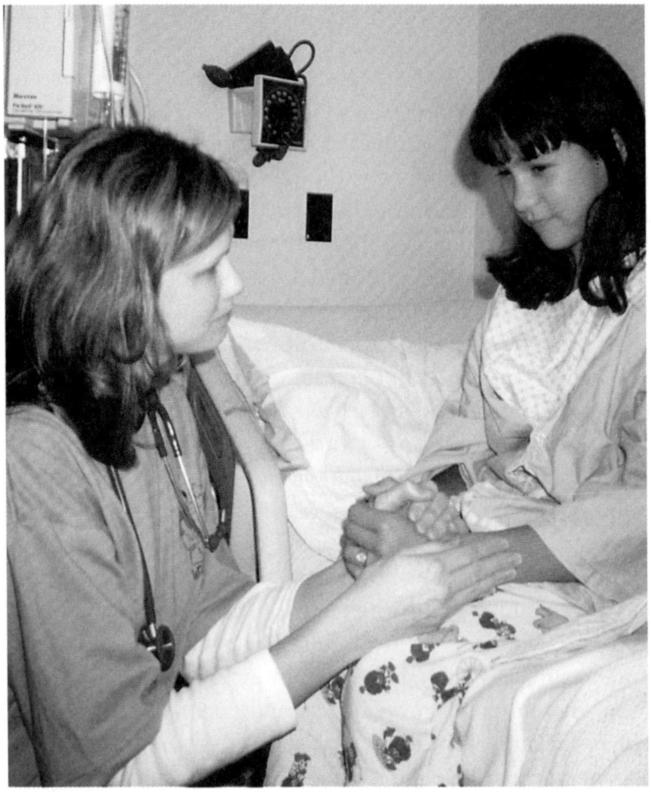

Figure 13-3 Adolescents often need reassurance when they are to undergo treatments or procedures. Used with permission of Baystate Medical Center Children's Hospital.

Nursing Tip:

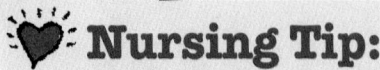

Healing chitchats

Provide a quiet, private time to talk without interruption about troubles that a child or the caregivers may be experiencing. No feedback should be offered or judgments made. An opportunity to verbalize hurt feelings and discuss problems without reproach is a step toward healing.

Providing Feedback

Providing feedback can include nodding of the head, reflecting back to the client what was said, asking questions to clarify, seeking validation from the client to ensure one is talking about the same thing, and focusing on a single idea and exploring it further. Focusing means to direct the conversation based on a statement made by the client. For instance, during a conversation with a child regarding her broken leg, the child mentions that another child on the playground has been pushing her around. The nurse may want to direct the conversation and delve more deeply into the fear the child may be experiencing due to the playground incident, other violent interactions the child may have had in the past, and what may occur during interactions in the future.

Conflict Management

There are three ways to approach conflict resolution: win-win, lose-win, and win-lose. The win-win approach occurs when both parties are committed to solving the conflict. They work together toward a resolution, searching for a variety of ways to resolve the problem so that they are able to finally arrive at a solution acceptable to all parties. The lose-win situation occurs when one person allows a resolution at their own expense; the win-lose approach occurs when one person resolves the conflict by having their needs and wants satisfied, but forces others to agree with their solution. It is important for the nurse to strive for the win-win approach. This allows the child and caregivers to feel in control, and there is more likelihood of adherence to whatever decisions are made.

Professional Boundaries

The nurse should create and maintain professional boundaries in relationships with children and their caregivers. Therapeutic relationships should be caring and empathetic, but should avoid emotional overinvolvement and overprotectiveness. It is always helpful to explain to children and families the type of care that will be provided, when the care will be provided, and how both parents and children can assist in the care. Identifying needs and establishing expectations will enhance and facilitate interactions. The nurse should never interfere with the relationship between the child and the caregivers. Rather, the nurse best serves the child by assisting the caregivers in caring for and nurturing the child, and by recognizing the need of the caregivers to feel accepted by the professionals and to be recognized as important to the child's well-being. Finally, nurses should avoid personal behaviors that signal overinvolvement such as socializing with the child or their family, sharing personal information such as home addresses or telephone numbers, and giving or accepting gifts. See Box 13-2 for more information about how to avoid becoming overinvolved.

Additional Skills Useful in Communicating

Several additional skills have been found especially useful when communicating with children and their caregivers. These include observation, silence, being aware of the environment, humor, play, writing, drawing, and using third parties.

Observation

Observational skills enable the nurse to validate and interpret what children and caregivers do not say. Nonverbal behavior provides meaningful information about what the child and caregivers are communicating to each other and to the nurse. How words are delivered is as important as what words are used. Congruence between the meaning of the words and all other behaviors validates the message. Observing the eyes (position, movement, gaze, and expression), mouth, furrowing of the brow and nasolabial area, general emotional mood, bodily movements, and posture is important. Cues also need to be interpreted from within the child's cultural perspective to avoid erroneous interpretations. For example, in some cultures, eye contact and directness are signs of paying attention. However, in other cultures, looking someone directly in the eye is considered rude. The nurse should also observe the ways children and caregivers respond to each other's request for attention, and behave and interact in disciplinary or nurturing situations. These observations can help the nurse assess the effectiveness of the communication patterns between children and caregivers and allow development of health-related strategies that are respectful of the relationship.

BOX 13-2 To avoid overinvolvement

Do not have contact with children and families after discharge.

Do not purchase gifts for children and families.

Do not share personal information with children and families.

Silence

Silence may be another method used to communicate. Silence should be interpreted in relation to the environment where communication occurs and the normal behavior of those interacting. A child who is shy and hesitant with strangers may be silent when the nurse approaches for care. A caregiver who is silent after being told of a child's terminal diagnosis is likely to be experiencing shock and disbelief and to be trying to come to grips with the reality of what was just heard. Children may be silent out of separation anxiety and fear, as in the case of a 4-year-old child who is hospitalized and must spend time in a strange environment without caregivers nearby. Silence also may demonstrate comfort, respect, and concern as when a nurse sits with parents after upsetting news is heard or when the child is falling asleep after an upsetting procedure.

Environment

The environment can affect communication events among the nurse, the child, and the caregivers even more than the spoken words. The way in which nurses exist in the environment and use space to make people more or less comfortable as they seek care is important. Nurses who are effective in nurse–client communication develop and demonstrate a respect for the client's sense of physical and personal space. For example, when sensitive issues or feelings of anxiety need to be discussed and the environment is in a four-bed unit where roommates can overhear the conversation, sharing fears and anxieties and asking questions may be difficult. A quiet, private environment should be provided before discussion begins. Nursing behaviors such as knocking before entering a child's room, calling the child and caregivers by name, addressing each directly, and asking permission to examine demonstrate respect and engender a sense of ownership over physical and personal space. Clients in caregiving settings such as hospitals and clinics will experience less stress, irritability, and fatigue when they remain in relative control of their physical and personal space. Environments that facilitate therapeutic communication reduce psychological distress so that children can attend to their health care situation. When children are relaxed or not experiencing fear, they are able to cope with people and the environment, and more willingly converse. However, children may vary in their communication levels based on their personality, temperament, experiences, and developmental abilities. The nurse should use concern, care, and knowledge of child development, and be willing to use a variety of communication approaches with the same child during different interactions or with different children in similar interactions.

Humor

Humor is healing and can bridge communicative gaps even when the direct communication is feared and/or offensive (Andrews & Boyle, 1999); it is recognized as an effective method of helping children and adolescents to cope with illness, pain, and hospitalization (May, 1999). For example, nurses who are able to laugh at themselves may be forgiven, and nurses who can make others laugh can't be all bad (or frightening). The nurse should use tasteful humor in dealing with pediatric patients and their caregivers to promote therapeutic interactions.

Play

Play, a natural childhood behavior, should be encouraged in health care environments and employed as a method of communicating (May, 1999). Using puppets, dolls, or stuffed animals, drawing pictures with crayons and paints, or employing a storytelling approach to give information engages the child. Because play is familiar and a daily form of natural behavior, children do not associate it with stress, anxiety, or fear. Play helps the child to relax and shed inhibitions, however temporarily, brought about by health care environments. The nurse who engages in play is likely to be legitimized as someone who can be trusted in communication. For more information about children's play, see Chapter 16.

Writing and Drawing

An especially effective method of communicating with older, school-aged children and adolescents, writing can include keeping a journal or diary, or writing a letter that is not delivered. Other examples include encouraging the child or adolescent to write down thoughts or feelings that are not easy to express verbally to keep track in written form of experiences related to a health care situation, or to write a story or essay about an experience (May, 1999). Sometimes just being able to articulate thoughts and feelings in writing can serve as a springboard for later discussions or concerns.

Drawing can be helpful for younger children since it provides clues to a child's emotional state and feelings (May, 1999). Evaluating the drawings or having a child tell a story about the drawing allows the nurse a window into the child's inner self. One needs to be cautious, however, since the evaluation of drawings should take place in conjunction with the evaluation of other information such as observation of behavior and communication with the child directly. Examination of drawings should include the evaluation of the gender of figures, the order in which the figures are drawn and the position of each in relation to other figures in the drawing, the exclusion of certain individuals, the accentuation or absence of particular body parts, the placement and size of the drawing on the page, whether or not the drawing is made with bold or light strokes, and the colors used (Sorensen, 1993).

Third-Party Communication

The nurse can promote dialogue with children by using indirect methods such as employing a third party. Here, the nurse directs her attention to the child through a trusted friend (e.g., a stuffed toy). By doing this, the nurse is taking an interest in the child's normal activity, is employing a stress-reducing communication method to create a therapeutic environment, and is helping the child to focus on the content of the message rather than on anxieties and fears. See Box 13-3.

Another third-party approach used with older children and adolescents is to attribute feelings or thoughts to other children. This method can be a safe form of interaction that uses the thoughts and feeling of the group rather than of the child or adolescent directly. Using group feelings helps a child or adolescent to feel comfortable talking to an adult because someone else is talking; the adult is told what the third person thinks without the child or adolescent being held responsible for the statement since the statement is made by the third person. For example, when explaining how one learns how to give oneself insulin injections, monitor blood glucose, or manage the diet during daytime hours while at school, the nurse could state that Christine, one of her 16-year-old patients, often will excuse herself from her friends, go to the restroom to check her sugar levels, and give herself insulin if needed. The nurse could also mention that Christine has told her friends that she is diabetic, wears a med alert bracelet, and always carries hard candy in her purse.

Storytelling

Storytelling is another effective communication strategy that nurses may use to promote therapeutic environments with children. Storytelling techniques can be used to establish rapport, to assess and help resolve children's anxieties and fears, to explain treatments and procedures, to teach health, and to prepare for painful or emotional events. The nurse

BOX 13-3 Using a toy to communicate

A 4-year-old boy is sitting in bed holding a stuffed bear. Instead of directly addressing the child, the nurse approaches and uses the toy as a medium for introduction

Nurse: Hi Mr. Teddy Bear! How are you? My name is ____________. What is your name? (wait for an answer). Oh, I guess I'll have to call you Mr. "no name" bear. Mr. "no name" bear, who is your friend?

Child: His name is Billy Bear! (in clinical practice, it has been found that even shy children will not let their friend be called Mr. "No Name" and will quickly provide their teddy bear friend's name.)

Nurse: Billy Bear! What a nice name. I bet he is fun to play with.

can devise or use stories so that the child can adopt either of the two storytelling roles: teller and listener. For example, a child can be read or told a story about a boy who had surgery, or be asked to tell a story about a boy who has had surgery. The former might be used to explain what will happen when going to surgery. The latter might be used to elicit information about the child's experience when the nurse devises a story and takes turns with the child to fill in the content. Called "mutual storytelling" (Gardner, 1986), the nurse might say, "I'll start the story, and when I nod, you fill in the next part of the story." The nurse begins with, "Once upon a time a boy broke his leg and had to have surgery. He . . ." The nurse nods to the child to fill in the blank. The nurse then uses the child's response to extend the story a bit, followed by nodding to the child to elicit another response. The nurse then analyzes the themes presented by the child, which may reveal important feelings.

Children begin to experience storytelling as infants and toddlers. It is a natural part of their early lives, and the use of story plots helps a child to make the transition from preoperational to concrete operational thinking (Arnold & Boggs, 1995). For nurses, however, storytelling is a skill, and confidence and competence are gained through use and practice. Storytelling may be carried out in a variety of ways, for example, by telling stories from books related to the subject at hand, telling stories based on previous experiences with children or told to you by other children, and telling stories adapted from articles printed in nursing journals. Composing a story specific to the child and content area can be useful as well. Using drawings, dances, mime, poetry, or cut-outs from newspapers, comics, or magazines for illustration may also encourage communication between children and nurses. Refer to Box 13-4 for further information.

REFLECTIONS FROM FAMILIES

When Helen was first born, I was so frightened. You see, I was a single mother in my early thirties with little to no experience taking care of children. While I am an outgoing, personable person who is verbally adept and observant, this whole experience of becoming a mother threw me for a loop. Even with supportive people around me, the highs and lows of raising a child alone was staggering.

Helen is five years old now. I am much more relaxed, even though I sometimes find myself at wit's end with the constant chatter and questions, and relentless energy of my soon to be kindergarten student. As I think back on some of the nurses I have interacted with these last several years, only a few stand out "softly and brightly" in my mind. There are the few who asked me how I was getting along and actually waited for an answer. They're the few who were not too busy to listen, and then suggested alternatives as to how I might want to handle Helen's health problems. I wish all nurses, and doctors for that matter, could learn to empower a parent as I know these few nurses did for me. After all, it is the parent who raises a child; nurses and doctors only help.

BOX 13-4 Principles of effective communication in pediatric settings

1. Talk to caregivers initially if child is shy or appears hesitant.
2. Use objects (toys, dolls, stuffed animals) instead of questioning child directly.
3. Provide opportunities for older children and adolescents to talk privately with the nurse or other care provider.
4. Use clear, specific, simple phrases in confident, quiet, unhurried speech.
5. Position yourself so that communication is at eye level.
6. Allow expression of thoughts and feelings.
7. Provide honest answers.
8. Offer choices only if they exist.
9. Use a variety of age-appropriate methods and techniques.

Family Teaching

Communicating with Caregivers

1. Explain equipment and procedures thoroughly.
2. Address the questions and concerns of caregivers honestly.
3. Teach caregivers what to expect the child will look like and feel like during treatment.
4. Help caregivers to understand the bigger picture—that is, the long-range as well as the short-range effect of treatment.
5. Teach and allow the caregiver to carry out as many aspects of the child's care as feasible.
6. Make reassurance a part of family interactions; ask caregivers how they are doing as time passes.

DEVELOPMENTAL FACTORS AFFECTING COMMUNICATION

Effective communication will enhance the preparation of a child and the caregivers for their experiences related to health and illness (Rushforth, 1999). However, the nurse must incorporate knowledge of human growth and development when communicating with children. Children should be encouraged to become active contributors to their health as soon as they are developmentally able to understand and carry out health-promoting behaviors. Until then, the nurse works directly with caregivers and reinforces their self-confidence in caring for and teaching the child. Refer to Chapter 31 for additional information on language development, which is critical when communicating with children, and to Table 13-1 for general principles for communicating with children of various ages.

Infants

Infancy is a time when communication is achieved through nonverbal means. Even though the adult may use language to relate to an infant, the tone, pitch, and speed of words as well as touch and the bodily movements accompanying the words generate meaning to the infant rather than the words used. However, loud, sudden noises may cause startle reactions and crying, while soft, song-like tones delivered in an upbeat tempo may soothe and comfort. Gentle rubbing or patting while securely holding an infant is also a method to communicate pleasure and security. Infant responses are nonverbal, such as vocal cues, including crying, cooing, and whining, and body language, such as stiffness or relaxation, arm or leg movement, pushing away with hands and feet against the adult, opening or closing the mouth, and gripping or pushing objects such as rattles and blankets. Infant expressions of comfort and discomfort become more direct and overtly explicit with age. That is, a 2-week-old infant will cry and flail

TABLE 13-1 Communication Principles Based on Developmental Level

Developmental Level	Communication Principles
Infants	Allow the infant time to warm up to strangers. Respond to the infant's cries in a timely manner. Use motherese*, and a soothing and calm voice. Talk to the infant directly
Toddlers	Approach the toddler carefully; the child may be fearful. Integrate the toddler's words for familiar objects or activities into care. Prepare for procedures right before they are to be carried out. Integrate dolls, storytelling, and picture books into conversations.
Preschoolers	Allow choices as appropriate. Use play, storytelling, puppets, and third parties. Speak honestly, use simple language, and be concise. Prepare for procedures 1–3 hours before they are to be experienced.
School-aged children	Use books, diagrams, and videos in preparing for procedures. Prepare for procedures several days in advance. Allow for honest expression of feelings and adequate time for questions to be answered.
Adolescents	Prepare for up to 1 week prior to experiences. Respect the adolescent's need for privacy. Use appropriate medical terminology. Use creative methods to explain experiences and procedures.

* *Motherese is child-directed speech that adults use when talking to young children. It uses simple, short sentences, spoken slowly in a high-pitched voice. There is also repetition and exaggerated emphasis on key words, which are usually words for activities and objects.*

arms and legs when hungry, while a 6-month-old infant may kick the legs and arm-wave, or suck on toys, fingers, or blankets when hungry. Caregivers soon learn to distinguish their infant's cries and will differentiate the cry of hunger from the cry of pain or anger. As the caregiver understands the meaning of infant behavior, satisfaction and attachment increase. As the caregiver learns how to turn the infant's tears into satiation, contented sleep, or cooing wakefulness, interactions and communication are positively reinforced.

Prior to developing stranger anxiety, infants will respond positively to the nurse and other strangers who provide comforting behaviors through feeding, diapering, rocking, and other forms of nonverbal communication. After the onset of stranger anxiety, incorporating the caregiver into the health care procedures reduces the infant's discomfort. Whenever the nurse needs to hold or give an infant care, caregivers should be involved. If this is not possible, the nurse should hold the infant so that the caregiver is in view. The nurse's movement should be firm and gentle, allowing time for the infant to get to know the nurse; abrupt movements will only increase the infant's distress. Using calm, soft, and soothing vocalizations and purposeful, slow movements enhances therapeutic communication with infants (Figure 13-4). For more information, refer to Chapter 8.

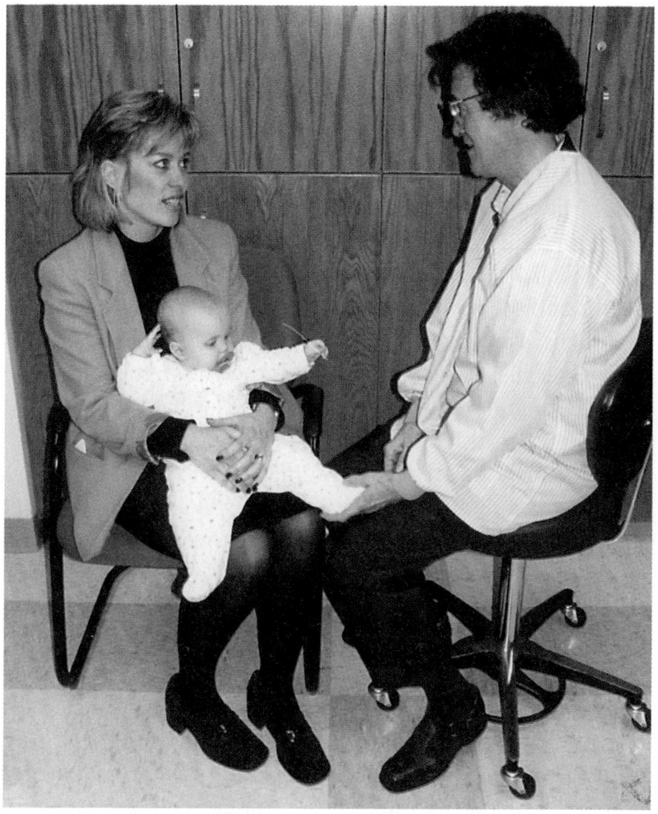

Figure 13-4 When communicating with infants, nurses often need to move slowly, and interact with parents initially.

Critical Thinking

Communicating with Infants

Ronnie, a 6-month-old infant diagnosed with meningitis, is fussy whenever you enter his room. How could you communicate with him when providing care?

Toddlers

The toddler continues to experience the world through hearing, seeing, smelling, tasting, and touching, and remains dependent on caregivers. Independence emerges, and satisfaction is derived from repetition and routine as the environment is explored. Language in the form of two-word combinations emerges as well as the ability to participate in turn-taking rules of social communication, such as the fact that an answer follows a question and that someone listens when someone speaks. Gestures and simple language are used to convey wants and needs. One-word sentences that are part babble with "bye-bye" may be used to express whole ideas, aided by accompanying gestures that provide clues to the meaning. "Bye-bye" with hat in hand may mean "I want to go out and play," while "bye-bye" after being kissed by dad prior to walking out the door, may mean "I want to go bye-bye with Dad." Two-word utterances become common at about 2 years of age. The two-word sentence consists of a noun and verb such as "me do." By the age of 3 years, complete sentences are constructed using all parts of speech, and the child's vocabulary has progressed to approximately 900–1,000 words. Toddlers also engage in monologues as a way of practicing speech, and as they mature, egocentric thought and monologue speech become more socialized. Increasingly, they engage in more conversation with others (Berkowitz, 2000).

Nurses interacting with toddlers should be observant of the situation surrounding one-word utterances and gestures. Learning the words that toddlers use for common items or behaviors, and using them in conversation is recommended. For instance, instead of saying it is "time for bed," the nurse may want to use an expression that for the child means bedtime, such as "it is time to hear the night-night angel sing." Using the expression that indicates bed- or naptime, while following the child's ritual of falling asleep while a music box plays is a comforting, familiar way of interacting that brings safe and familiar experiences to the child's mind. Using play or books to demonstrate or describe activities or procedures immediately before they are to occur is a good way to prepare toddlers for experiences. Refraining from wordy explanations and preparing for procedures well in advance are not toddler friendly. Being aware of the child's response and approaching the child calmly and positively are important. For more information, see Chapter 9.

Preschoolers

During the preschool years, a child's articulation becomes clearer, there are improvements in correct grammatical usage, and an expansion of word combining occurs. The child's vocabulary rapidly expands, and the child is able to use words appropriately even when the meaning is not fully appreciated. Since the preschooler is striving for independence, but still needs adult encouragement and support, it is important to allow the child to initiate activities and make choices if possible. For example, let the child decide whether to have "water or a mouthful of Jell-O after your medicine." Nurses may need to remind the children how to cooperate in an activity or to wait for their turn. Asking the child's cooperation by giving them something to do or hold may engage them cooperatively and allow the procedure to be performed. Using picture books, stuffed toys, and puppets to prepare a child for a procedure will allow the child to experience the procedure in a nonthreatening way (Figure 13-5). A child may also answer the nurse's question through a teddy bear: "Hi, Mr. Teddy bear, do you think your friend, Johnny, would like some Jell-O after his medicine or would a mouthful of chocolate pudding be better?"

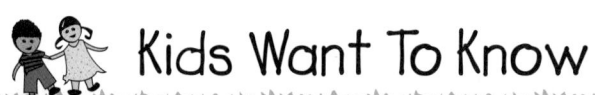

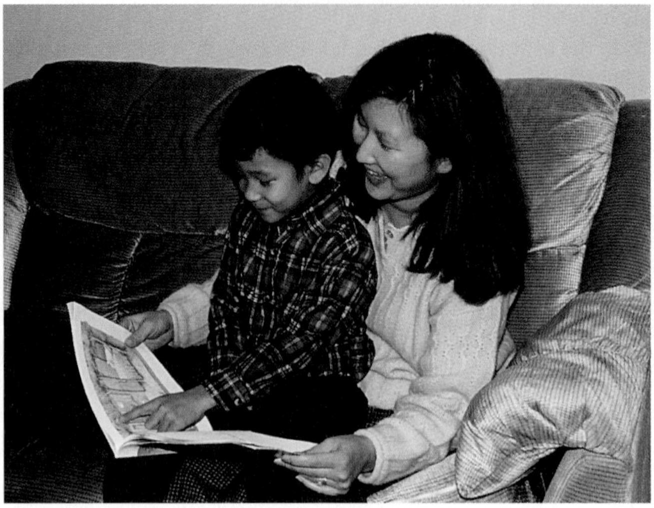

Figure 13-5 Establishing rapport with preschoolers often can be done by reading a story.

Preschoolers are egocentric, and magical thinking predominates during the preschool years; these children see things only from their perspective. When they lack information or do not understand something, they fill in the gaps with their imagination. Since an avid imagination can be far worse than any reality, it is better to communicate with honesty, in simple sentences using concrete language. The nurse should never smile or laugh when giving an injection, say something won't hurt when it will, or use words with double or literal meanings such as a "shot" or a "stick in the arm." It is also not helpful to tell the child about others or what "good boys or girls" do. Allowing the preschooler to touch and manipulate equipment they will see and experience is essential. Telling preschoolers how it will feel when they come in contact with the equipment (cold, warm, pressure, tickles, etc.) and how they can behave is also important. For example, tell them that it is okay to squeeze the teddy bear, cry, or bang on the bed with their hand, etc. For more information, see Chapter 10.

Kids Want To Know

Why do they have to do that test? Will it hurt?

Whenever talking to preschoolers, use simple words that answer the questions asked; avoid detailed answers. "You will go to the X-ray department so that they can take a picture of your tummy. They want to find out why you have a tummy ache. The bed you lie on will be cool, but they will put a blanket on you to keep you warm. The test should not hurt."

School-Aged Children

A school-aged child's relational experiences expand to include people and environments outside the family and home. They are taught rhymes, chants, and rituals by other children, which can serve as a means of emotional-social control in frightening and confusing contexts. We all remember examples, such as "cross your heart and hope to die," "star light, star bright, first star I see tonight," and "knock on wood," which we used to minimize the bad that could befall us. Humor and riddles are tension releasers and assist a child with their social identity, i.e., "knock, knock, who's there?" During early school years, interaction with other children increases and close friendships are developed. Children of this age group may be verbally aggressive, bossy, opinionated, and argumentative.

School-aged children learn to accept responsibility for their actions, they understand rules, and they become oriented to rules and sanctions. They are interested in learning and have increased attention spans. They learn to master classification, serialization, and spatial, temporal, and numerical concepts. Concrete thinking emerges and predominates. They learn to focus on more than one aspect of an experience and to explore and consider many alternatives to a problem. They are increasingly able to understand their body and their environment and to use language as a means of control and appreciate it as a method used by others to control them. School-aged children also have expanding vocabularies that enable them to describe feelings, thoughts, and concepts. They are able to carry on conversations with others and to appreciate their viewpoints. However, words with multiple meanings and words that describe things they have not experienced are still not thoroughly understood.

When working with the school-aged child, the nurse should spend time with the child to explain treatments and procedures well in advance of the scheduled time (Figure 13-6). Photographs, books, drawings, and videos may be used to aid understanding and assist in answering questions that may follow. Immediate and subsequent opportunities should be allowed for questions, and repetition of explanations and enhanced details of what will happen to them should be provided. Fears and concerns about body integrity should be assessed and truthfully answered. Conversation that encourages critical thinking should be promoted. For more information, see Chapter 11.

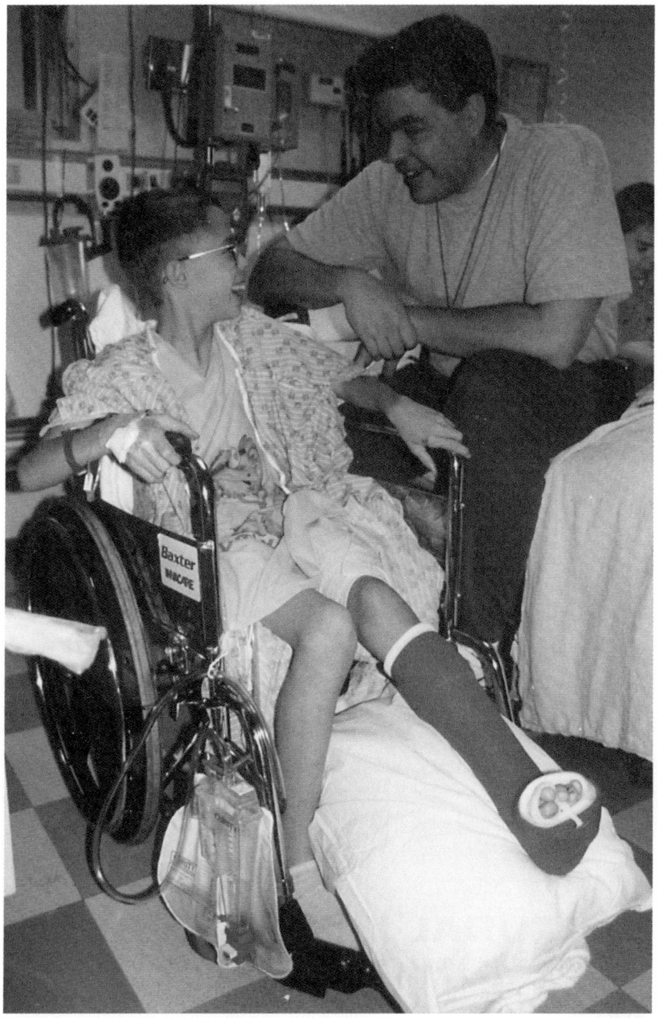

Figure 13-6 When communicating with school-aged children, nurses need to assume a relaxed demeanor and convey interest.

Adolescents

Adolescents are able to think logically and abstractly, and are able to verbalize and comprehend most adult concepts. They are able to create hypothetical situations and generate explanations for and about situations they encounter. Privacy and independence are sought in activities and relationships. The adolescent makes personal discoveries about their relationships and events, and will discuss these discoveries with peers and trusted adults in an effort to construct ideals.

An adolescent's preoccupation with what should or could be produces conflict in relationships with people who are unwilling to listen to them express their thoughts. They need to verbalize what the world should be like in order to analyze their own ideas and come to their position short of the ideal. The *ideal* world they construct must be merged with the *real* world by listening to themselves and others.

Attentiveness and acceptance are necessary. Caregivers and other adults need to be patient and actively listen to matters that the adolescent considers significant, even if trivial to adults (Figure 13-7). The adolescent should be allowed the freedom to work through issues and should be provided the guidance necessary to develop and decide on a positive course of action. Since adolescents may be moody and argumentative, interactions between adolescents and caregivers or other adults will be more cooperative when the adolescent participates in working toward a solution and is permitted to participate in the selection of the final decision and subsequent course of action.

The nurse should communicate support during interactions with adolescents by actively listening, without

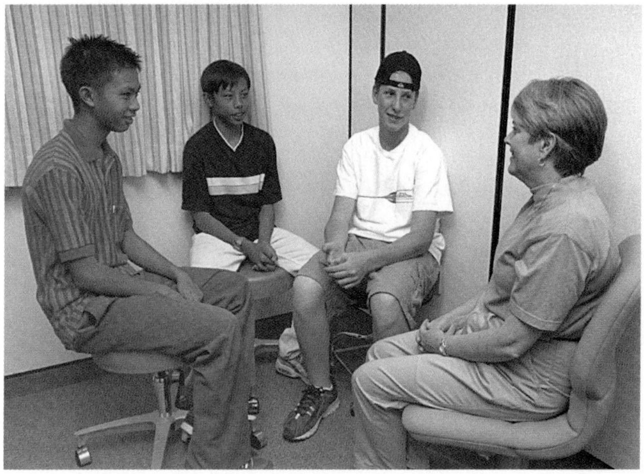

Figure 13-7 Listening is especially important when interacting with children and adolescents.

Research Highlight

Adolescent–Parent Communication

Study Purpose

To examine the relationship between adolescents' views of communication with their caregivers and decision making, conflict and conflict resolution, family satisfaction, self-esteem, well-being (physical health, psychosocial health, experience of positive and negative affect, general life satisfaction), and coping. The effects of age, gender, and level of intellectual ability/education goals were also examined.

Methods

Two studies were carried out. One focused on areas of life at home (decision making, conflict and conflict resolution, family satisfaction). The other focused on the adolescents' personal development. Study I included 413 adolescents living in The Netherlands ages 13–15 from three different levels of education based on the Dutch secondary school system. Adolescents completed several self-report measures and scales. Study II included 660 adolescents ages 13–15. The adolescents were again divided by education level. These adolescents completed several scales measuring health perception, self-esteem, and life satisfaction.

Findings

Study I and II agreed that adolescents are generally satisfied with communication with their parents. However, study I showed that communication with the mother was more favorable than with the father. Children in early adolescence were more positive about communication with parents than those in mid-adolescence in both studies. Adolescents with a higher level of education had a more positive level of communication with caregivers than those with a lower level of education. Study I differed from study II in that it showed a more positive communication between sons and fathers than daughters and fathers. Well-being, self-esteem, and aspects of coping correlated with positive communication patterns.

Implications

Nurses need to recognize that communication between caregivers and adolescents is important and may affect adolescents' overall well-being. Interventions should be directed toward improving parent–adolescent communication, especially between fathers and daughters. Caregivers of adolescents should be supported in their communication efforts.

Citation

Jackson, S., Bigstra, J., Oostra, L., & Bosma, H. (1998). Adolescents' perceptions of communication with caregivers relative to specific aspects of relationships with caregivers and personal development. *Journal of Adolescence, 21*, 305–322.

demonstrating surprise, disapproval, or trivialization. The nurse should avoid questioning, giving personal advice, or taking sides. It may be necessary for the nurse to initiate multiple interactions before an adolescent feels safe and secure enough to ask questions or discuss concerns. Short, nonthreatening contacts may serve as icebreakers, which may lead to involved conversations. For more information, see Chapter 12.

CULTURAL IMPACT ON COMMUNICATION

The nurse's relationship with children and their families should be caring, supportive, and respectful and, just as important, congruent with their acceptable cultural perspective. This is important so that the nurse's intentions and behavior are not perceived as culturally insensitive. This requires that the nurse know and understand how personal cultural values and beliefs affect behavior in providing nursing care, and learn about and be nonjudgmental of the cultural values and beliefs of those cared for. Nurses also need to know how to respond to gestures or questions, how to listen to concerns, how and when to be sensitive to child/family reactions, when to use an interpreter, and how to consider illness- and health-related beliefs when delivering care (Luckman, 1999). Refer to Table 13-2 for information related to specific cultures and their communication patterns and Box 13-5 for information about using an interpreter. Remember that what is most important is to treat and understand each person as an individual who may or may not incorporate the communication patterns of their ethnic group into their value system.

The care that is planned and implemented with a child and/or caregiver should be congruent with their values and consistent with their understanding of health care. During contact, the nurse needs to incorporate questions and make observations that elicit information about family practices that

TABLE 13-2 Traditional Communication Patterns of Various Cultures

Cultural Group	Communication Styles
Chinese	• Self-expression is repressed. • Silence is valued. • Hesitant to ask questions. • Nonverbal and contextual cues are important. • An individual may smile even if the individual does not understand. • Touching is limited.
Japanese	• Listen empathetically. • Are stoic. • Value politeness, personal restraint, and self-control. • Attitudes, actions, and feelings are more important than words. • Direct eye contact is considered a lack of respect. • Touching is limited.
Vietnamese	• Disrespectful to question authority figures. • Value harmony and modesty of speech and action. • Avoid direct eye contact. • There is a relaxed concept of time. • Respect titles, family, and generational relationships.
Filipino	• Respect personal dignity, nonverbal communication, and preserving self-esteem. • Avoid direct eye contact, expressions of disagreement, especially with authority figures, and discussion of personal topics. • Small talk is important before serious discussions.
African Americans	• Cautious around and distrustful of the majority. • Value direct eye contact. • Use nonverbal expressions.

continues

TABLE 13-2 *Continued*

Cultural Group	Communication Styles
African Americans *(continued)*	• Sensitive to incongruence between verbal and nonverbal messages. • Tend to test those in the majority before submitting to their suggestions and care. • May use Ebonics, an English dialect.
Hispanic Americans (Mexican)	• Use direct eye contact. • Use gestures and voice tone changes in speech. • Unassertive if others appear busy or rushed. • May smile and nod even if do not understand. • Perceive touch as reassuring, comforting, and sympathetic • Many are bilingual, but may use nonstandard English. • Small talk is important before serious discussion. • Appreciate open ended questions and a nondirective approach. • It is important for the father to be present when speaking with a male child. • Discussions of personal topics are easier if the nurse is of the same gender as the client.
Puerto Ricans	• Value personal and family privacy; questions regarding family are considered presumptuous and disrespectful. • A relaxed concept of time. • May not use standard English. • Many are bilingual. • New immigrants and older individuals may speak Spanish.
Cubans	• Most new immigrants are bilingual. • Small talk is important before serious discussion.
Native Americans	• Value nonverbal communication. • Silence is essential to understanding and respecting another. • Direct eye contact is considered insulting. • May be reticent in forming opinions of health care providers. • Pauses after being questioned are common; they signify thoughtful consideration. • Hesitant to discuss personal affairs unless trust has developed and prefer that these discussions occur with a person of the same gender. • Sensitive about having their behaviors and words written down. • Believe it is ethically wrong to speak for another.
Middle Eastern	• Use silence to show respect. • Men and women do not touch each other unless they are in the immediate family or are married. • Touching or embracing is common among those of the same gender.

continues

TABLE 13-2 ***Continued***

Cultural Group	Communication Styles
European Americans	• Hugs/embraces are tolerated among intimates and close friends only. • Understanding or agreement is noted by nods. • Use neutral facial expressions in public. • Individuals separate into gender-specific groups at social events, unless the activity is for couples. • Prefer personal space. • Speak warmly and pleasantly and smile to put others at ease. • A firm handshake symbolizes goodwill; a pat on shoulder/back denotes camaraderie.

Adapted from Estes, M. E. Z. (2002). Health assessment and physical examination. *Albany, NY: Delmar.*

BOX 13-5 Surmounting language barriers between health care providers and children/families

A. With an interpreter

1. Determine language(s) and dialect (if relevant) a client is familiar with and speaks at home; the language may not be identical to the one commonly used in their country of origin. Some clients may be multilingual, and a language other than their mother tongue can be used.
2. Avoid using interpreters from groups (countries, regions, religions, tribes) where there may be past or present conflicts.
3. Be sensitive to and make allowances for differences with regard to age, culture, gender, and socioeconomic status between the client and interpreter.
4. Request as verbatim a translation as possible.
5. Be aware that an interpreter not related to the client may request compensation.
6. Maintain a list of potential interpreters.
7. Contact institutions (hospitals, universities, etc.), organizations, and translation services, including telephone companies, that may be able to provide interpreters, emergency translations, and other relevant information.

B. Without an interpreter

8. Always be polite, formal, patient, and attentive to the client's (or client's family) attempts to communicate.
9. When greeting the client, smile, use the client's complete or last name, indicate your name by saying it while gesturing to oneself, and offer a handshake or nod.
10. Speak in a low and moderate tone.
11. If possible, use words from the client's language.
12. Use simple words–no idiom, no jargon (medical or otherwise), no slang. Avoid the use of contractions and pronouns, which may be unclear to the client.
13. Give instructions clearly, in simple language (with a minimum of words), and in the correct order.
14. Talk about one topic at a time.
15. Use hand signs freely and act out actions while talking.
16. Check the client's understanding by requesting that he or she describe/illustrate the procedure, pantomime the meaning, or repeat the instructions.
17. Try using Latin phrases or phrases from other languages that have become universal.
18. Write simple sentences in English or another language, since some people understand the written, but not spoken languages, and some accents may be confusing.
19. See if a family member or friend can act as an interpreter for the client. If not, and if the health provider cannot find one, enlist the family in networking to find one.
20. Use phrase books and flash cards.

Adapted from Luckman, J. (1999). *Transcultural communication in nursing.* Albany, NY: Delmar.

may impact care. These include questions about their communication and decision-making strategies, child rearing, and health and illness practices. Once this information is obtained, it can be used to determine priorities and develop an individualized treatment plan that is culturally consistent with the family's values and beliefs and that will engender their commitment and compliance See Box 13-6 for more information.

For caregivers who would normally depend on their extended family for support and find themselves without them in their present environment, extra time or assistance may be necessary to help them make critical health care decisions (Figure 13-8). Anticipating the arrival of members who must travel to reach a child and family, or providing a quiet place for the family to telephone distant extended family members is an appropriate nursing intervention.

BOX 13-6 Questions to elicit pertinent information about health care practices/beliefs

Who do you discuss your child's health/illness problems with?

Who assists you in making decisions about your child's health/illness problems?

Who assists you or your family when you need help related to health care?

Nursing Tip:

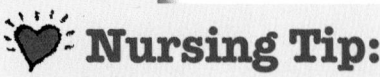

Be proactive for children or caregivers who speak English as a second language

Enunciate clearly, and speak slowly.

Avoid situations that prevent the listener from seeing lip movements, facial expressions, or gestures.

Speak in the active voice.

Avoid using contractions, slang, and idiom.

Eye On:

Touch

Avoid touching a Cambodian, Vietnamese, Thai, or Hmong child on the head during an initial assessment or conversation, since the head has traditionally been considered the site of the soul for these cultures. On the other hand, Hispanics view touch as a gesture of sincerity and are used to gentle embraces. Therefore, when caring for Hispanic children and families, shaking hands and sitting/standing closer are important, as is gentle touch on the hand or head.

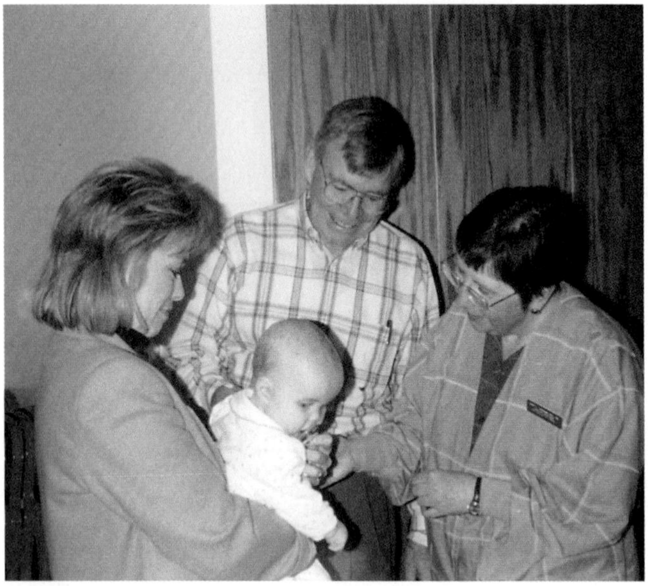

Figure 13-8 It is important to interact with all family members when caring for infants, children and adolescents.

COMMUNICATING WITH CHILDREN WITH SPECIAL NEEDS

Communicating with children who have special needs can be particularly challenging and may require adopting alternative methods of interacting. Whenever communicating with children with special needs, it is imperative to involve families and to carefully assess the child's skills and abilities. Principles of communicating with children with special needs and their families are the same as those discussed in this chapter. However, refer to Chapter 31 for specific information on communicating with children who have a visual or hearing impairment and to Chapter 33 for specific information on communicating with children who have a significant cognitive impairment.

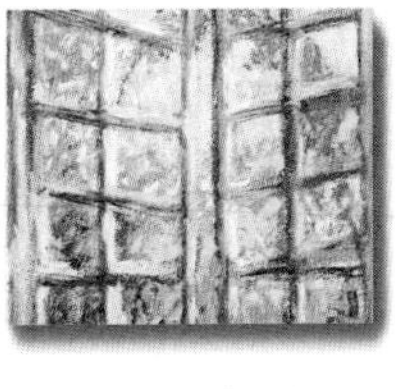

In the Real World

Because of his age (12), I tried to allow Luke (admitted for incision and drainage of an abscess on his leg) to be as modest and independent as possible. As I helped him with his bed bath, he began to open up about his interests, friends, and hospital stay. Although I only spent 20–30 minutes performing these simple activities, the time allowed for trust to develop and communication lasted throughout the day. Furthermore, he was more relaxed and cheerful. When I changed him from a PCA to oral pain meds, I explained the importance of staying on top of the pain and he indicated he understood. Later on that day, when his IV line was heplocked, I let him help me. By letting Luke become more involved in the procedure, I think it became less scary for him and I communicated my trust.

The definition of communication includes transferring knowledge and information. Besides discussing pain control and heplocks with Luke, I do not feel I did a lot of patient teaching. However, I did transfer knowledge about feelings and trust, and I believe that this is especially important since often pediatric patients may not understand why procedures need to be done. Communicating information has an empowering effect on patients and allows them to assume more control of their environment and care. With empowerment comes an increased effort to improve and a better attitude about treatment. Communication is that aspect of therapeutic nursing interventions which helps standards of practice be effective.

Key Concepts

- The ability to communicate effectively is recognized as a basic and central component in delivering care to children and their caregivers.
- The sender, message, channel, receiver, and feedback are major components of the communication process.
- Barriers to successful communication will impede the message, and include physical factors and psychological factors.
- Communication can be formal/informal and verbal/nonverbal.
- Empathy, listening effectively, observing accurately, using silence appropriately, being aware of the environment, humor, play, writing, drawing, and using third parties are effective methods of communicating with children and adolescents.
- Effective communication requires sensitivity to the child's developmental level, and to the needs of the child and family's, and a well-developed and carefully thought-out plan.
- Cultural background can play a role in the determination of an individual's communication pattern.
- Communication with children with special needs requires knowledge of their skill and ability level, and may require adopting alternative methods of interacting.

Review Questions

1. Describe a developmentally appropriate communication approach for each of the following age groups: infant (0–12 months), toddler (1–2 years), preschooler (3–5 years), school-aged child (6–11 years), adolescent (12 years plus).
2. Describe two behaviors that negatively affect communication between nurse and child, or nurse and caregiver, and discuss each.
3. Describe two behaviors that positively affect the relationship between nurse and child, or nurse and caregiver, and discuss each.

References

Andrews, M. M., & Boyle, J. S. (1999). *Transcultural concepts in nursing care* (3rd ed.). Philadelphia: Lippincott.

Arnold, E., & Boggs, K. (1995). *Interpersonal relationships: Professional communication skills for nurses* (2nd ed.). Philadelphia: Saunders.

Berkowitz, C. (2000). *Pediatrics: A primary care approach*. Philadelphia: Saunders.

Estes, M. E. Z. (2002). *Health assessment and physical examination* (2nd ed.). Albany, NY: Delmar.

Fredriksson, L. (1999). Modes of relating in a caring conversation: A research synthesis on presence, touch, and listening. *Journal of Advanced Nursing, 30*, 1167–1176.

Gardner, R. (1986). *Therapeutic communication with children* (2nd ed.). New York: Science Books.

Harrison, L., Olivet, L., Cunningham, K., Bodin, M. B., & Hicks, C. (1996). Effects of gentle human touch on preterm infants: Pilot study results. *Neonatal Network: Journal of Neonatal Nursing, 15*(2), 35–42.

Jackson, S., Bigstra, J., Oostra, L., & Bosma, H. (1998). Adolescents' perceptions of communication with parents relative to specific aspects of relationships with parents and personal development. *Journal of Adolescence, 21*, 305–322

Luckman, J. (1999). *Transcultural communication in nursing*. Albany, NY: Delmar.

Marquis, B. L., & Huston, C. J. (1992). *Leadership roles and management functions in nursing: Theory and application*. Philadelphia: Lippincott.

May, L. (1999). "I've got tummy ache in my head": Communicating with sick children. *Pediatric Nursing, 11*(2), 21–23.

Riesch, S. (1997). Parent–adolescent communication in non-distressed families. *Annual Review of Nursing Research, 15*, 123–152.

Rushforth, H. (1999). Practitioner review. Communicating with hospitalized children: Review and application of research pertaining to children's understanding of health and illness. *Journal of Child Psychology and Psychiatry, 40*, 683–691.

Sigelman, C. (1999). *Lifespan human development* (3rd ed.). Albany, NY: Brooks/Cole.

Sorensen, E. (1993). *Children's stress and coping*. New York: Guilford Press.

Stuart, G., & Sundeen, S. (1995). *Principles and practice of psychiatric nursing* (5th ed.). St. Louis, MO: Mosby.

Suggested Readings

Bradley, J. C., & Edinberg, M. A. (1990). *Communication in the nursing context* (3rd ed.). East Norwalk, CT: Appleton & Lange.

Edelman, L., Greenland, B., & Mills, B. L. (1993). *Family-centered communication skills*. St. Paul, MN: Pathfinder Resources.

Hawks, J. (1992). Empowerment in nursing education: Concept analysis and application of philosophy, learning and instruction. *Journal of Advanced Nursing, 17*, 609–618.

Haynes, W. O., & Shulman, B. B. (l994). *Communication development: Foundations, processes, and clinical applications*. Englewood Cliffs, NJ: Prentice Hall.

Jeppson, E. S., & Thomas, J. (l995). *Essential allies: Families as advisors*. Bethesda, MD: Institute for Family-Centered Care.

LaMontagne, L. L. (1993). Bolstering personal control in child patients through coping interventions. *Pediatric Nursing, 19*, 235–237.

LeReche, L., & Dworkin, S. F. (1984). Facial expression accompanying pain. *Social Science in Medicine, 19*, 1325–1330.

Marta, E. (1997). Parent–adolescent interactions and psychosocial risk in adolescents: An analysis of communication, support, and gender. *Journal of Adolescence, 20*, 473–487.

McClowry, S. G. (1993). Pediatric nursing psychosocial care: A vision beyond hospitalization. *Pediatric Nursing, 19*, 146–148.

Ricchini, W. (1997). Kid stuff tips for communicating with children. *Advances for Nurse Practitioners*, 5(2), 83–85.

Roehlkepartain, E. C. (l999). *You can make a difference for kids*. Minneapolis, MN: Search Institute.

Smith, D. R. & Williamson, L. K. (1987). *Interpersonal communication roles, rules, strategies, and games* (3rd ed.). Dubuque, IA: Wm. C. Brown.

Spector, R. E. (1996). *Cultural diversity in health and illness* (4th ed.). East Norwalk, CT: Appleton & Lange.

Watzlawick, P., Beavin, J. M., & Jackson, D. (1967). *Pragmatics of human communication*. New York: W. W. Norton.

Resources

Organizations and Websites

National Institute of Health
www.nih.gov

National Center for Health Statistics
www.cdc.gov/nchs

Minority Health Network (MHNet)
www.pitt.edu/~ejb4/min/desc.html

Child Development Institute
www.childdevelopmentinfo.com/parenting

Talking with Kids
www.talkingwithkids.org

CHAPTER 14

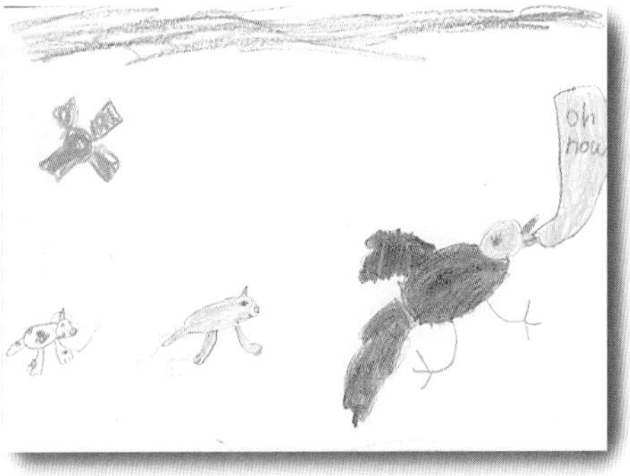

Although we always try to look at our situation with an optimistic outlook, there is great trepidation when our son's cardiologist appointment is approaching. As we cherish and live each day to the fullest, far back in our minds there is a voice that quietly asks: What if something is wrong this time? What if we need to look into another surgery? What if it looks like his heart has done as much as it can on its own? What if we need to put him on the transplant list? This one appointment could change our future dramatically. Ironically, the same appointment usually confirms that all is well, but this can never ease the nervousness. What is termed a simple appointment is actually a significant life-changing event for us every time.

PEDIATRIC ASSESSMENT

Kathy Murphy, MSN, RN, CS

COMPETENCIES

Upon completion of this chapter, the reader will be able to:

- *Elicit a complete health history from a child and caregiver using standard components of a pediatric health history.*
- *Discuss the purpose of a nutritional assessment and its components.*
- *Explain the purpose of developmental assessment.*
- *Identify various techniques of approaching children at different developmental levels before initiating the physical assessment.*
- *Perform inspection, palpation, percussion, and auscultation in a head-to-toe assessment of a child.*
- *Identify normal and abnormal findings obtained during the physical assessment.*

Children are unique individuals who undergo rapid changes from birth through adolescence. Physical growth, motor skills, and cognitive and social development are evidence of the numerous changes that family members, friends, and health care professionals observe throughout a child's maturing years. In an assessment of the child, the nurse must be aware of these changes while continually reassessing what is considered within normal limits.

PHYSICAL GROWTH

One important set of parameters required for pediatric health assessment is physical growth. The parameters of weight, length, or height, and head circumference (dependent on age) are essential in serial physical growth measurements. (Chest circumference is of less importance.) For example, by plotting a child's growth on a chart (see Appendix B), the nurse is able to determine normal or abnormal growth curves according to the child's age. Refer to Chapters 7–12 for specific weight and height parameters for age groups.

HEALTH HISTORY

Because the historian in a pediatric history is less often the child and most likely the caregiver, it is very important to document the historian's relationship to the child. The child should be included in the history taking as is appropriate for her or his age and development.

Nursing Tip:

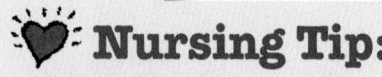

Adjusting chronological age

For the infant born prematurely, you will need to adjust the chronological age on the growth chart. For instance, the corrected age for a 6-month-old infant who was born 2 months prematurely would be 4 months. Plot the obtained weight and length on the growth chart under the child's corrected age, and mark above the weight "corrected." The corrected age rule applies until the child is 18 months old.

Biographical Data

Child's Name

In addition to the child's name, obtain the full name of the legal guardian. Occasionally, the caregiver is not the legal guardian, for example, when the child is a ward of the court or state.

Address and Phone Number

Obtain the address and phone number of the caregiver if different from those of the child.

Source of Information

Other than the child or caregiver, information can be obtained from medical and school records, diaries, clinic notes, and agencies such as crippled children's services, public health departments, and home health agencies.

Chief Complaint: The caregiver is often the individual who seeks health care for the child and provides a description of the perceived problems, especially for infants, toddlers, and young preschoolers whose age and mental status prevent them from offering genuine descriptions of their problem. You must frequently rely on the caregiver's intuition in such cases. The caregiver is usually acutely aware of cues to the child's illness. For instance, changes in sleeping patterns (difficulty falling asleep, reversion to night waking), regression to outgrown behaviors (bedwetting, finicky eating, thumb sucking), and unusual physical complaints in an otherwise healthy child (headaches, stomachaches) are important signs that the child may be experiencing stress or illness, and warrant further investigation. The older preschooler, school-aged child, and adolescent are able to provide verbal descriptions of their complaints.

Past Health History

Pertinent information should be elicited regarding the birth history, including prenatal, labor and delivery, and postnatal history.

Birth History

Obtaining the birth history may be one of the more sensitive topics of the past health history. You must feel comfortable and show sensitivity when inquiring about whether the pregnancy was planned, the date prenatal care was first sought, and birth order of pregnancy, taking into account miscarriages and abortions.

Prenatal:

1. Did you plan your pregnancy for ______ (insert month)?
2. How many weeks after thinking that you were pregnant did you go to a health care provider for a check-up?
3. How many children have you carried to full term?
4. Were there any pregnancies that you were not able to carry to full term? What happened?
5. Did you take any prescribed or over-the-counter medications?
6. Did you drink alcohol or caffeine, or smoke cigarettes during pregnancy?
7. Did you take any drugs during pregnancy, such as marijuana, crack cocaine, amphetamines, or hallucinogens such as LSD and mescaline? If so, what were the amounts and frequency of use?
8. Were there any problems or illnesses that either you or your health care provider were worried about during pregnancy (pregnancy-induced hypertension, preterm labor, gestational diabetes, TORCH infection [toxoplasmosis, rubella, cytomegalovirus, and herpes])?

Labor and Delivery:

1. How many weeks did you carry the baby before delivering?
2. Was the labor spontaneous or induced?
3. How many hours long was the labor?
4. Was the baby delivered vaginally or by cesarean section? If by cesarean section, why?
5. Was any analgesia or anesthetic used?
6. Did you hold your baby immediately after delivery? (This question will provide information about the neonate's condition at delivery.)
7. Immediately following delivery, what was the baby's color?
8. What were the baby's Apgar scores at 1 and 5 minutes?
9. What were the birth weight and length of the baby?
10. Was the baby's father at the birth with you?
11. Where was the baby born (home, hospital, automobile, or other location)?

Postnatal:

1. Did you and your baby go home together? (If answered no, inquire as to the reason for separate discharges.)

2. If hospital delivery, how long was the hospitalization for you and the baby?
3. Did the baby have any breathing or feeding problems during the first week?
4. To your knowledge, did your baby receive any medications during the first week?
5. How would you describe the baby's color at 1 week? (For the light-skinned baby, ask if the skin was pale, pale pink, blue, or yellow. For the dark-skinned baby, inquire about the color of the sclera, oral mucosa, and nailbeds.)
6. Was the baby circumcised?
7. Did you start breast- or bottle-feeding your baby?
8. Were there any problems with your choice of feeding?
9. Did you or the baby have a fever after delivery?
10. Did you have anyone to help you take care of the baby in the first few weeks after delivery?

Medical

Inquire about the circumstances and outcomes of any hospitalizations or emergency department visits. Keep in mind that some children's caregivers may use the emergency department for episodic health care and may not have regular health care providers.

Injuries/Accidents

Determine if the child has a pattern of frequent injuries or accidents. Repeat trauma may indicate abuse.

Childhood Illnesses

Document past and current exposure to measles, mumps, rubella, pertussis, and chickenpox.

Immunizations

Immunizations provide protection against many contagious diseases of childhood. Maternal antibodies pass through the placenta and breast milk, offering the baby limited protection from disease. A schedule of recommended childhood immunizations is located in Appendix C. Many health care providers follow the immunization schedule as a guide for well-child check-ups. A record of immunizations is often important for school admission and to avoid repeat vaccinations.

Family Health History

Inquire about age and health status (if deceased, age and cause of death) of the child's mother, father, siblings, grandparents, aunts, and uncles. Ask about diseases in the family that could affect the child's health, including heart disease, diabetes, mental retardation, seizures, allergies, asthma, congenital disorders, alcoholism, and attention deficit hyperactivity disorder (ADHD). Also ask about sudden infant death syndrome (SIDS).

Social History

Work Environment

Day care facilities and schools are the child's equivalent of a work environment. Inquire about the number of hours the child attends a day care facility per week. Inquire about the child's academic performance. In addition, ask if the child is home alone before or after school.

Home Environment

Ask about potential exposure to lead in chipping paint because lead is harmful to the developing brain and nervous system of fetuses and young children. This group is four to five times more likely to absorb lead by ingestion than are older children (Fisher & Vessey, 1998).

Child's Personal Habits

1. Determine what activities the child enjoys.
2. Ask how the child copes with stress and if a security object (blanket, stuffed toy) helps calm the child.
3. Determine if the child is prone to temper tantrums and what type of discipline is used.

Health Maintenance Activities

Sleep

Determine if the child takes naps and if the child shares a bedroom, because children's different sleep habits may lead to interrupted sleep.

Diet

Questions concerning diet need to be tailored to the child's developmental level. Refer to *Nutritional Assessment, Dietary History* for questions appropriate to each developmental level.

Safety

Childproofing the environment, especially for young children, is an essential practice. Box 14-1 lists questions to include in your interview.

NUTRITIONAL ASSESSMENT

Good nutrition is essential for optimal health and disease prevention. Educating a child early in life about the importance of healthy eating habits can play a role in safeguarding the child against future disease. Never has there been a time in our history where so much emphasis is being placed on health promotion and preventing diet-related diseases or

BOX 14-1 Questions about childproofing the environment

1. Would you tell me how you have childproofed your home?
2. Do you have gates on the top and bottom of the stairs?
3. Are the slats on the crib less than $2^3/_8$ inches apart?
4. Have you taken the crib mobile down and taken out the bumper pads (applies to infants who are trying to pull up)?
5. Is all sleepwear flame retardant?
6. Is the hot water thermostat turned down to 120° Fahrenheit?
7. Have you installed potty locks to keep the toilet lid down?
8. Do you keep curtain and blind strings out of reach?
9. Have you placed all sharp items such as razors and knives out of reach of the child?
10. Do you monitor your child in the bathtub?
11. Do you always drain the water in the tub after getting out?
12. Have you placed cushioned covering on the tub's water faucet and drain lever?
13. Do you use a nonskid bath mat in the tub?
14. Are there outlet covers on every outlet in the house?
15. When you are cooking, do you keep the pot or pan handles turned in?
16. Have you taken tablecloths off all tables?
17. Do you keep the phone cord out of reach?
18. Is the slack taken up on all electrical appliance and lamp cords?
19. If you have a raised hearth, have you covered it with bumpers, pads, or towels?
20. Are all of your plants out of reach?
21. Are slip protectors under all rugs?
22. If you have a pool in the yard, is it fenced in, or is there a protective cover on top?
23. Do you empty pails that contain liquid after using them?
24. Are medications, cosmetics, pesticides, gasoline, cleaning solutions, paint thinner, and all other poisonous materials out of the child's reach?
25. Do you have your local poison control telephone number next to each phone?
26. Do you have syrup of ipecac in the house? Do you know why it is used and its expiration date?
27. Do you have smoke detectors close to or in the child's bedroom, and on each floor of the house?
28. Do you have a fire extinguisher on each floor?
29. Have you devised and practiced an escape route plan in case of fire?
30. Are you CPR trained?
31. What would you do in case of an emergency?
32. Where do you place your child's car seat–in the front or back seat, facing front or rear? Do you place your child in the car where an air bag is supplied?
33. Does your child use protective gear such as a helmet or knee and elbow pads if participating in an activity in which injuries may occur?
34. Do you keep plastic dry cleaner overwraps, latex balloons (unattended by a caregiver), plastic trash bags, and grocery bags out of the child's reach?

deficiencies. Nutritional assessment enables the nurse to provide anticipatory guidance, identify at-risk individuals, and collaborate with the health care team for early referral of the child as needed. A variety of methods are employed to assess the child's nutritional status, including history of dietary intake, analysis of laboratory data, anthropometric data, and physical examination.

Dietary Intake

There are numerous ways to determine if a child is receiving adequate nutrition. One vehicle for doing so is through a record of dietary intake. Dietary intake is elicited through a 24-hour recall, food diary, or food frequency questionnaire. As with all open-ended questions, an accurate response is variable. Accuracy is hard to obtain if the child has multiple caregivers. Involving the primary caregiver and extended caregivers will be an important task. When obtaining the 24-hour food recall, inquire about the previous 24 hours. Involve any family members present during your interview. Ask the individual to recall the amount and types of food eaten by the child, including the amount and type of liquids consumed during the past 24 hours. A food diary is quite similar to the 24-hour recall in that you are requesting the family to keep track of the same information for a 3–7-day time span. Instruct the caregiver to allow others such as day care providers to record the time, type, and amount of foods and liquids consumed directly on the diary. A food frequency questionnaire can be used during the interview to collect information about consumption of foods from all the food groups. Information collected includes what type, and the amount and frequency of consumed liquids and foods.

Dietary History

Another important tool for assessing dietary risk factors is a diet history. Dietary histories can identify a host of nutritional and behavioral problems, and anticipatory guidance can be provided for deficient areas of nutritional health. The following questions concerning diet are divided into age groups:

A. Infants (0–12 months)

1. Are you breast- or bottle-feeding? (Breastfeeding provides superior immunologic properties.)
2. How many wet diapers does your baby have in a 24-hour period? (Infants should have at least six very wet diapers every 24 hours.)
3. If bottle-feeding, is the formula iron-fortified?
4. How much formula does your baby drink per day, or how often does your baby breastfeed and how long are the feedings? (Newborns to 1 month of age drink up to 32 ounces per day, 1–3-month-olds drink up to 42 ounces a day, 3–6-month-olds drink up to 40 ounces day, 6–12-month-olds drink up to 32 ounces per day; breastfed babies may want to feed every 2 hours, and should take at least one breast and suck for 10 minutes to completely empty the breast.)
5. How long does it take for your baby to finish a bottle? (Generally, an infant should complete their bottle within 15–20 minutes. An oral/motor dysfunction or congenital heart disease could be suspected if the infant is unable to complete a bottle within the normal time frame.)
6. Does your baby go to bed with the bottle in the crib? (Allowing the baby to fall asleep or keep the bottle in the crib may lead to dental caries.)
7. Have you introduced iron-fortified cereal? (Iron-fortified cereal can be introduced between 4 and 6 months of age and should be continued until the second birthday. Often, the child's hematocrit will fall about 1 year of age as a result of being a "picky eater.")
8. Do you give your baby honey? (Honey should not be given to children younger than 1 year of age because of the risk of botulism.)
9. Have you started solid foods? (Readiness cues include sitting without support, extrusion reflex present, being able to lean forward indicating desire for more, and turning away to indicate refusal of food.)
10. If solid foods have been started, how often do you introduce a new food? (Introduce one new food every 3–5 days in order to differentiate food allergies. Many pediatricians recommend starting vegetables first to avoid a "sweet tooth" phenomenon, then following with fruits, and starting meats at about 8–9 months of age.)
11. Do you give your baby fruit juices? (Excessive use of fruit juices can leave the baby feeling full and not wanting to take adequate amounts of formula.)

B. Toddlers (1–3 years old)

1. Have you started your child on whole milk? (Whole milk can now be safely substituted for formula. The caregiver is encouraged to switch from whole to 2% milk at 2 years of age.)
2. How much milk does your child drink? (The recommended amount of milk per day is 16 ounces, with a maximum of 1 quart.)
3. Is your child drinking from a cup? (Transitioning the child from bottle to cup occurs at or before 1 year of age. An early transition helps prevent dental caries. If the child is filling up on milk via a bottle, a variety of foods are not being taken in.)
4. Have you transitioned your child to soft table foods? (Generally, at about 12 months of age, a child is able to chew soft food.)
5. Are you present in the room while your child is eating? (Supervising the child is important to prevent choking.)
6. Does your family include the child during mealtimes? (Starting family meals at an early age has many positive benefits such as establishing routines and communication between family members.)
7. Is your child starting to feed him- or herself? (During the later phase of infancy and early toddlerhood, the child will begin to take an interest in self-feeding.)
8. Do you let your child eat any of the following foods: nuts, popcorn, whole hot dogs, grapes, raw vegetables, or hard candy? (These foods/snacks may present a choking hazard.)
9. Do you offer your child at least two healthy snacks per day? (Offering small nutritious snacks throughout the day will help provide the toddler with adequate nutrition not achieved at mealtimes.)
10. Is your child eating foods from all food groups? (A good rule of thumb for determining the right amount of food for a child is ensuring they eat 1 tablespoon

of each food group per age in years; thus, a 2-year-old would need to eat 2 tablespoons of vegetables.)

C. Preschooler (3–5 years)

1. How much milk does your child drink per day? (The preschooler needs to drink at least 20 ounces of milk per day.)
2. How much juice does your child drink? (Limiting juice to no more than 8–12 ounces per day will help the child take more food at meals and snacks.)
3. Does your child eat a variety of foods from all food groups? (Utilize the same rule of thumb for adequate food intake as described for toddlers.)
4. Many of the same questions for the toddler group apply to the preschooler (questions 5, 6, and 9).

D. School-aged child (6–12 years)

1. How many servings of milk does your child drink per day? (School-aged children should receive 800 mg of calcium per day, which is equivalent to about 21 ounces of milk.)
2. Has your child switched from 2% to skim milk? (At the age of 6, children should switch to skim milk.)
3. Is your child eating three meals per day? (Children often skip breakfast because of early morning time constraints.)
4. Does your family sit down together for at least one meal per day? (Meals at this age tend to occur on the run because of extracurricular activities planned for dinnertime.)
5. Does your child eat a hot lunch at school? (A school lunch will provide approximately one-third of the total recommended daily allowance.)
6. Does your child brush their teeth at least two times per day? (Caregivers are encouraged to brush their child's teeth at least once a day until the child has mastered cursive writing. You can foster autonomy by allowing your child to brush his or her teeth in the morning.)
7. Does your child eat sugary snacks? (Limit sugar intake to prevent dental caries and avoid empty calories.)
8. Do you allow your child to sit in front of the television and eat a meal? (Obesity is on the rise, and spending excessive time watching television seems to contribute to decreased physical activity.)
9. How often does your child eat fast food per week? (Incidence of obesity increases with frequent consumption of fast food.)

E. Adolescent (13–18 years): The same questions asked during the school-aged child's interview can be used, but answers to the questions of the adolescent directly may yield important information.

Laboratory Evaluation

Data gathered during a nutritional assessment will give the interviewer an indication of at-risk factors. Inadequate caloric intake is a nutritional problem. Two commonly ordered laboratory tests are serum albumin and prealbumin. Both tests reflect adequate calorie and protein intake. A serum albumin reflects the previous month's food intake. The prealbumin reflects a shorter period of time, which is the previous 1 week of intake. A complete blood cell count, which includes hemoglobin, hematocrit, and red cell indices, provides an indication of adequate iron status. Cholesterol screenings have become more frequently ordered in children whose family history predisposes them to elevated cholesterol levels.

Anthropometric Data

Anthropometric measurements refer to the science of measuring the human body as to height, weight, and size of component parts, including skinfolds. Anthropometric data provides information about growth patterns and the nutritional status of children. The physical growth parameters of weight and length/height are found in Appendix B. Measurements of skinfold thickness and arm circumference are important indicators of body fat stores, nutritional status, and skeletal muscle mass.

Skinfold thickness is a more reliable indicator of body fat than is weight. The most common measurement site is over the tricep muscle in the child. This measurement may be threatening for the child. To alleviate anxiety let the child sit in the caregiver's lap. While the child's arm is dangling at her or his side in a fully relaxed position, lift the fold of subcutaneous tissue and skin away from the triceps muscle. Place the calipers on the skin next to the fingers, while lifting the fold of skin. Hold the skinfold in place while measuring the triceps skinfold. Repeat this step twice and average the three readings to obtain the skinfold thickness value.

Arm circumference is measured at the midpoint of the upper arm. To locate the midpoint of the upper arm, have the child flex the arm at a 90° angle. Measure from the **acromion process** (the lateral extension of the spine of the scapula, forming the highest point of the shoulder) to the **olecranon process** (a proximal projection of the ulna that forms the point of the elbow) and mark the midpoint with a washable ink pen or marker. Ask the child to hold their arm in a relaxed position at their side. Using a tape measure, measure the circumference.

Physical Examination

The physical examination of nearly all body systems can identify nutritional deficiencies. Examination techniques are described throughout this chapter. Table 14-1 summarizes physical signs and symptoms of poor nutritional status.

TABLE 14-1 Physical Signs and Symptoms of Poor Nutritional Status

	Subjective	Objective
General appearance	Fatigue, poor sleep, change in weight, frequent infections	Dull affect, apathetic, increased/ decreased weight
Skin	Pruritis, swelling, delayed wound healing	Dry, rough, scaling, flaking, edema, lesions, decreased turgor, changes in color (pallor, jaundice), petechiae, ecchymoses, xanthomas (slightly elevated yellow nodules)
Nails	Brittle	Dry, splinter hemorrhages, spoon-shaped, pale
Hair	Easily falls out, brittle	Less shiny, dry, changes in color pigment
Eyes	Vision changes, night blindness, eye discharge	Hardening and scaling of cornea, conjunctiva pale or red
Mouth	Mouth sores	Lips: cracked, dry, swollen, fissures around corners Gums: recessed, swollen, bleeding, spongy Tongue: smooth, beefy red, magenta, pale, fissures, sores, increased or decreased in size, increased or decreased papillae Teeth: missing, caries
Head and neck	Headaches, decreased hearing	Xanthelasma (creamy, yellow plaque on eyelid due to hypercholesterolemia), irritation and crusting of nares, swollen cheeks (parotid gland enlargement), goiter
Heart and peripheral vasculature	Palpitations, swelling	Cardiac enlargement, changes in blood pressure, tachycardia, heart murmur, edema
Abdomen	Tender, changes in appetite, nausea, changes in bowel habits	Edema, hepatosplenomegaly
Musculoskeletal system	Weakness, pain, cramping, frequent fractures	Muscle tone is decreased, flabby muscles, bowing of lower extremities
Neurological system	Irritable, changes in mood, numbness, paresthesia	Slurred speech, unsteady gait,tremors, decreased deep tendon reflexes, loss of position and vibratory sense, paresthesia, decreased coordination
Female genitalia	Changes in menstrual pattern	None

Courtesy of Estes, M. E. (2002). Health assessment and physical examination *(2nd ed.). Albany, NY: Delmar.*

Evaluation of Data

Utilizing the diet history, compare and contrast this information with the Food Guide Pyramid (Figure 14-1). Determine if the child is receiving the recommended amount/variety of food per day. The evaluation involves piecing together data obtained from the dietary history and physical examination, and extrapolating information to define the child's nutritional status. A referral to a specialist is made if suspected nutritional inadequacy exists.

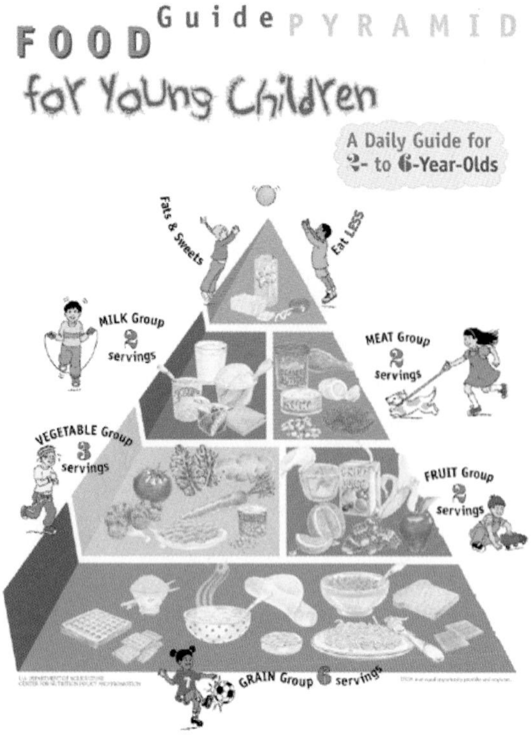
FOOD Guide PYRAMID
for Young Children
A Daily Guide for 2- to 6-Year-Olds
Fats & Sweets
Eat LESS
MILK Group
2 servings
MEAT Group
2 servings
VEGETABLE Group
3 servings
FRUIT Group
2 servings
GRAIN Group 6 servings

Figure 14-1 Food Guide Pyramid for Young Children. Courtesy of U.S. Department of Agriculture.

DEVELOPMENTAL ASSESSMENT

Evaluation of developmental functioning is an essential component of any health assessment. A developmental assessment has several purposes: (1) validation that a child is developing normally, (2) early detection of problems, (3) identification of concerns of caregivers and child, and (4) provision of an opportunity for anticipatory guidance and teaching about age-appropriate expected behaviors. Several screening tests are currently available for developmental assessment (Table 14-2). These tests evaluate a variety of aspects, including fine and gross motor skills, social and language skills, behavior, temperament, cognition, memory, and the child's home environment. Screening procedures using these measures quickly and reliably identify children whose development is below normal and may also be used to monitor developmental progress. Some developmental assessments instruments can be administered in a variety of settings with a minimal amount of preparation, whereas others require proper training and supervision. Caution should always be taken to guarantee that administration is accurate; directions and explanations to caregivers and children need to be clear and concise. Following administration, it would be helpful to ask caregivers if the child's performance was typical, since

TABLE 14-2 Developmental Assessment Measures for Infants and Children

Test Name	Ages	Features Evaluated
Carey–Revised Infant	4 to 8 months	Temperament, patterns of feeding, sleeping, elimination, responses to different situations
Denver Articulation Screening Exam	2.5 to 6 years	Intelligibility; articulation of 30 sound elements
Denver II	Birth to 6 years	Personal-social, fine motor-adaptive, language, gross motor
Developmental Profile II	Birth to 9 years	Physical, self-help, social, academic, communication skills
Early Language	Birth to 3 years	Auditory expressive and receptive, visual components of speech
Goodenough–Harris Drawing Test	5 to 17 years	Child's drawing of a person; analyzed for body parts, clothing, proportion, perspective
HOME (Home Observation for Measurement of the Environment)	Birth to 6 years	Organization, play materials, parental control, stimulation, punishment or restriction
McCarthy Scales of Children's Abilities	2.5 to 8.5 years	Intellectual and motor development, memory, quantitative, perceptual-performance, general cognition

retesting may be necessary if the behavior was atypical. All results should carefully be communicated to caregivers so that misunderstandings and misinterpretations are kept to a minimum. Before administering any measure, it is essential to read and follow instructions carefully.

A commonly used tool for assessing neuromuscular development of the child from birth through 6 years of age is the Denver Developmental Screening Test II (Denver II; Frankenburg, 1994; see Appendix E). The test is composed of four sections: personal-social, fine motor-adaptive, language, and gross motor. There are a total of 125 items described on the test. Some items can be accomplished easily by observing the child without commands from the observer. For instance, the child may be smiling spontaneously, saying words other than "mama" or "dada," or sitting with the head held steady. Certain items can be given an automatic pass mark if the caregiver indicates that the child is able to accomplish the corresponding item, such as drinking from a cup, washing and drying hands, or dressing without help.

Documentation is reflected by using a "P" for pass, "F" for fail, "R" for refuses, and "no" for no opportunity. Give up to three trials before documenting the particular item's score on the Denver II. At the end, complete the five Test Behavior questions. A normal test consists of no delays and a maximum of one caution. A caution is failure of the client to perform an item that has been achieved by 75–90% of children the same age. A delay is a failure of any item to the left of the age line. A suspect test is one with one or more delays and/or two or more cautions; in these instances, retest the child in 1–2 weeks.

Keep in mind that current illness, lack of sleep, fear and anxiety, deafness, or blindness can affect a child's performance. If these or other logical rationale can explain a child's failure to successfully complete a series of Denver II items during a session, readminister the test in 1 month, providing resolution of the preexisting condition is accomplished, where appropriate. If the child does in fact have a developmental disability, early detection can lead to appropriate intervention and assistance.

Physical Assessment

Techniques for approaching children vary from one age group to the next. A basic principle during any physical assessment is building a trusting relationship; this can be done in a variety of ways. First, always explain what will be done prior to each portion of the assessment and answer questions honestly. Second, praise the child for positive behaviors, e.g., cooperating during assessment of the middle ear. Portraying a caring attitude will greatly influence both the child's and the caregiver's sense of trust. Show respect for the child as an individual and allow expression of feelings (whimpering, crying). Refer to Box 14-2 for information about approaches to pediatric physical assessment.

Nursing Tip:

Facilitating the pediatric assessment

- Use game playing and distraction to increase child cooperativeness. It is important to have available different items of distraction that can be used when a child is uncooperative or focusing on what will be done next. Distractions include small toys that easily hook onto a stethoscope, wind-up musical toys, and humming or whistling.
- Demonstrate procedures on a doll, stuffed toy, or even the caregiver prior to performing them on the child.

All needed equipment should be assembled and readily available. The following items are recommended for a physical examination on a child:

- Clean gloves
- Scale (infant or stand-up)
- Appropriately sized blood pressure cuff
- Disposable centimeter tape measure
- Snellen E eye chart
- Allen cards
- Otoscope and speculum (2.5 or 4.0 mm) with pneumatic attachment
- Opthalmoscope
- Pediatric stethoscope
- Growth charts
- Skinfold calipers
- Marking pen
- Peanut butter or chocolate
- Small bell
- Brightly colored object
- Denver II materials

Vital Signs

The act of measuring vital signs is often disturbing to a young child. Past experiences influence the degree of cooperation you will encounter. Vital signs may be obtained at the beginning of the assessment or during the assessment of a certain system.

If the child is particularly anxious, it is best to integrate the assessment of vital signs into the overall assessment. Vital signs include temperature, respiration, pulse, and blood pressure, which are compared to normal ranges for the child's age. These measurements provide information about the child's basic physiological status.

BOX 14-2 General approaches to pediatric physical assessment

1. Assess the child in a warm, quiet room. To prevent hypothermia, always keep infants under the age of 6 months warm during the examination.
2. Use natural lighting, if available, during the assessment. Fluorescent lighting makes assessing varying degrees of cyanosis and jaundice difficult.
3. To help reduce anxiety and uncooperativeness (especially when assessing young children), have a familiar caregiver present during the assessment.
4. Talk to the child in a soothing voice; even an infant who cannot understand your words will take comfort in a calm and supportive approach.
5. Explain all procedures and allow older infants, toddlers, preschoolers, and younger school-aged children to manipulate medical equipment.
6. To promote the child's feeling of security, allow the infant who cannot sit up and the younger child to sit on the caregiver's lap for as much of the examination as possible.
7. Until the infant or toddler is comfortable, maintain eye contact with the caregiver while the assessment is taking place. Maintaining eye contact with the child who experiences anxiety in the presence of strangers can interfere with completing the examination. Maintain eye contact with the caregiver if other means of alleviating the fears are not successful.
8. Interview the older school-aged child or adolescent separately, without the caregiver. Talking to the individual without the caregiver present may yield important information not gained during a group interview (e.g., that the child is using drugs).
9. Respect the child's modesty.
10. Warm your equipment (e.g., stethoscope).
11. Avoid making abrupt movements because these may startle a child.
12. If the child is sleeping, take advantage of the situation by performing simple procedures (length, head circumference) and system assessments that require a quiet room (such as the cardiac and respiratory assessments) first.
13. Perform all invasive or uncomfortable procedures (ear inspection, hip palpation) last because they may cause discomfort, crying, fear, and increased heart rate.
14. Always provide comfort measures following pain. It is especially helpful to allow the caregiver the opportunity to provide supportive measures. This shows the child that you are genuinely concerned about his or her feelings.
15. To prevent falls, always keep one hand on any infant who is placed on the examination table.
16. Prior to completing the examination, ask the caregiver and child what questions they have.

Nursing Tip:

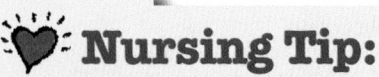

Integrating vital signs into the pediatric examination

1. An apical heart rate can be obtained during the cardiac assessment.
2. The respiratory rate can be obtained when auscultating the lungs.
3. Blood pressure and rectal temperature measurements are more threatening and should be performed toward the end of the assessment, preferably before using the otoscope.

Temperature

There are four basic routes by which temperature can be measured: oral, rectal, axillary, and tympanic. The site is based on the child's age, development, and condition. The oral route is convenient and accessible, but an accurate measurement is difficult to obtain in most toddlers and preschoolers because the child must be cognitively capable of following instructions for safe use. Therefore, the oral route is usually reserved for children ages 5–6 years and older. A rectal temperature is considered the most accurate and can be taken in children of all ages. However, it is not appropriate in all instances, for example, in the child who presents with a history of diarrhea.

An axillary temperature is safe, noninvasive, and can be taken in all age groups. This route may be contraindicated when accuracy is especially critical or in the initial stages of fever, when the axilla may not be sensitive to early temperature changes. When taking an axillary temperature, have the child sit or lie on the caregiver's lap to free your hands for other observation or to prepare for the next area of assessment. Explain to the child that this type of temperature measurement does not hurt. To pass the time, ask the caregiver to read the child a story. A tympanic temperature is convenient, safe, and noninvasive; yet, research is inconclusive as to the accuracy of reading and correlations with other body temperature measurements.

Children dislike having a rectal temperature taken, so your approach to explanation should be matter of fact: "I need to measure your temperature in your bottom. You need to hold very still while I do this. Your mommy [or other appropriate person] will be right here with you." Caution is required in children less than 2 years of age due to risk of rectal perforation or breakage, especially with a mercury thermometer. Place the child in either a side-lying or a prone position on the caregiver's lap or place the child on the back on the examination table and firmly grasp the feet with your nondominant hand. After lubricating the stub-tipped thermometer, insert it gently into the child's rectum: 1/2 inch for newborns, 3/4 inch for infants, and 1 inch for preschoolers and older children. Hold the thermometer firmly between your fingers to avoid accidentally inserting it too far (Figure 14-2).

Normal body temperature (afebrile) varies with the age of the child (Table 14-3). A temperature above 38.5°C or 101.5°F is interpreted as hyperthermia. An elevated body temperature can be related to severe illnesses such as meningitis, or common childhood illnesses such as otitis media and streptococcus pharyngitis, or heat exposure. In contrast, hypothermia is a body temperature below 34.0°C or 93.2°F. A low body temperature can be related to sepsis, ambient cold exposure, or submersion cold injury.

Respiratory Rate

Try to obtain the respiratory rate early in the assessment, when the child is most cooperative and not crying. If the child is crying, the measurement will not be accurate and should be retaken. Refer to the Pediatric Nursing Skills CD-ROM for information about obtaining respiratory rate. Remember to observe the expansion of the abdomen in infants and toddlers. Table 14-4 lists the normal respiratory rates for children.

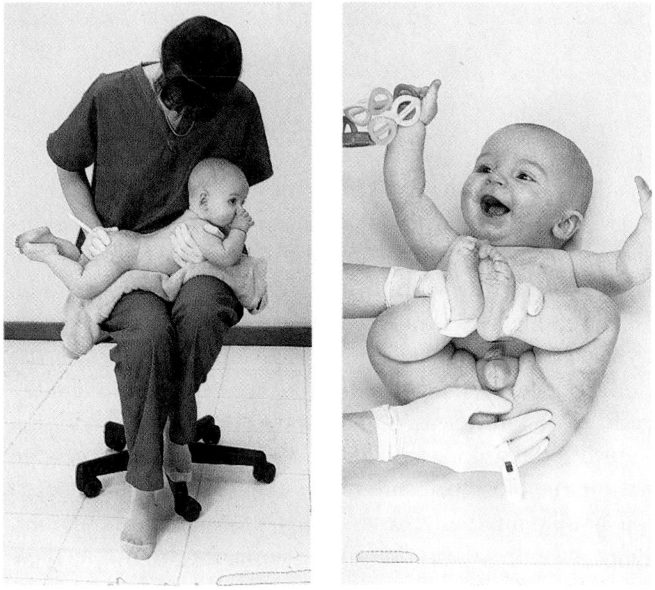

(A) (B)

Figure 14-2 Rectal Temperature. (A) Infant in Prone Position (B) Infant in Supine Position

TABLE 14-3 Body Temperature: Normal Range According to Age

Age	Centigrade	Fahrenheit
Newborn to 1 year	37.5–37.7°	99.4–99.7°
3 to 5 years	37.0–37.2°	98.6–99.0°
7 to 9 years	36.7–36.8°	98.1–98.3°
10 years and older	36.6°	97.8°

Pulse

An apical pulse should be taken on neonates, infants, and young children (under 2 years of age) and on all children with cardiac problems or on digitalis preparations. To determine the pulse, place your stethoscope over the child's **precordium,** which is the part of the front of the chest wall that overlays the heart, great vessels, pericardium, and some pulmonary tissue. A radial pulse can be obtained on children over 2 years of age. Refer to the Pediatric Nursing Skills CD-ROM for information about obtaining an apical and radial pulse rates. An elevated heart rate or tachycardia is indicative of fever, anxiety, dysrhythmia, congestive heart failure, or medications. A slow heart rate or bradycardia would suggest a surgically induced or congenital heart block, digoxin toxicity, or cold submersion injury. Table 14-5 depicts ranges for normal pulse rates by age.

Blood Pressure

The most important aspect of obtaining a blood pressure is choosing the correct cuff size. The bladder of the cuff width

TABLE 14-4 Respiratory Rate

Age	Resting Respiratory Rate	Average
Newborn	30–50	40
1 year	20–40	30
3 years	20–30	25
6 years	16–22	19
10 years	16–20	18
14 years	14–20	17
18 years	16–20	18

Courtesy of Estes, M. E. (2002). Health assessment and physical examination. *Albany, NY: Delmar.*

Research Highlight

Compare Methods of Newborn Temperature Measurement

Study Purpose

The purpose of this study was to (a) compare newborn temperature measurements obtained by digital disposable, electronic, and tympanic thermometers with glass mercury thermometers, and (b) compare the financial implications of each method.

Methods

In this correlational study, 12 perinatal and neonatal nurses obtained temperature measurements of 184 newborns between 1 and 168 hours of age. The sample–stratified and convenience–was selected using medical records numbers. Instruments for measuring temperature included glass, tympanic, electronic, and digital thermometers. Data were analyzed by Pearson *r* coefficients, mean, standard deviation, and range using an SPSS statistical package.

Findings

The glass, electronic, and digital thermometer temperature readings were highly correlated (0.748–1.0). The tympainc thermometer had a low correlation coefficient (0.35). Use of the glass thermometer was the most costly, whereas the tympanic thermometer was the most cost effective.

Implications

In healthy newborns, the use of electronic and digital thermometers is appropriate if there is a concern about using glass thermometers. However, these results cannot be extrapolated to sick infants. Although tympanic thermometers had the lowest cost, their lack of correlation with the gold standard glass thermometers makes them a poor choice for healthy newborns.

Citation

Sganga, A., Wallace, R., Kiehl, E., Irving, T., & Witter, L. (2000). A comparison of four methods of normal newborn temperature measurement. *Journal of Maternal Clinical Nursing, 25*(2), 76.

Table 14-5 Pulse Rate: Normal Range According to Age

Age	Resting Pulse Rate (Beats/Minute)	Average
Newborn	100–170	140
1 year	80–170	120
3 years	80–130	110
6 years	70–115	100
10 years	70–110	90
14 years	60–110	85–90
18 years	60–100	72

Courtesy of Estes, M. E. Z. (2002). Health assessment & physical examination (2nd ed.). *Albany, NY: Delmar.*

should be 40% of the arm's circumference measured midway between the olecranon and acromion. The cuff bladder should cover 80–100% of the arm circumference (National High Blood Pressure Education Program Working Group, 1986; see Figure 14-3). Place the cuff on the upper extremity. Locate the brachial pulse with your finger. Place the stethoscope over the antecubital fossae. Manually inflate the cuff. As you are releasing the air, observe the dial and listen to record the systolic and diastolic numbers. You will need to palpate the blood pressure in the infant and toddler. Record the systolic number. Causes of hypertension are numerous. Renal disease, coarctation of the aorta, stress, and medications can result in hypertension. Causes of hypotension include hemorrhage, sepsis, septic shock, and medications. Tables 14-6 and 14-7 present general ranges for normal blood pressure at different ages.

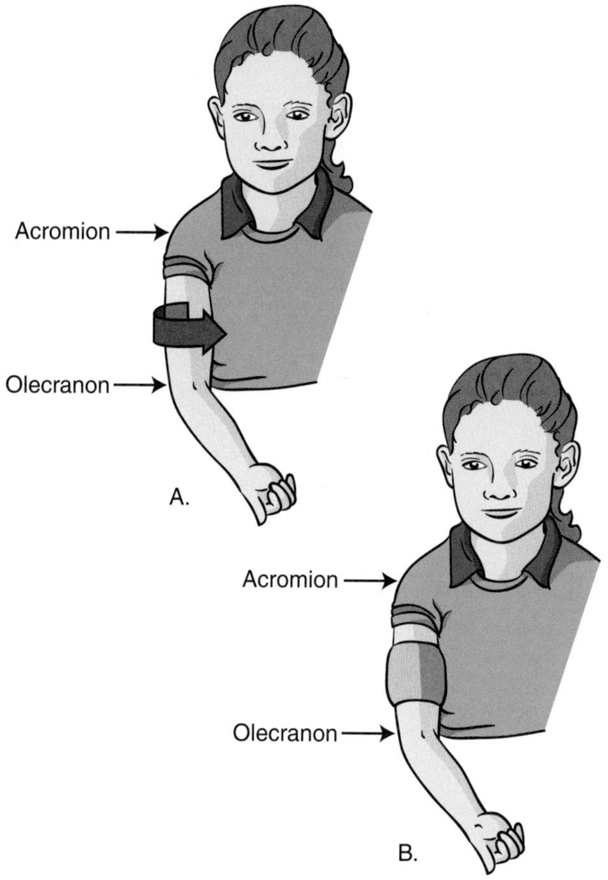

Figure 14-3 Determination of Proper Blood Pressure Cuff Size. (A) The cuff bladder width should be 40% of the circumference of the arm measured midway between the olecranon and acromion. (B) The cuff bladder covers 80–100% of the arm's circumference.

Nursing Tip:

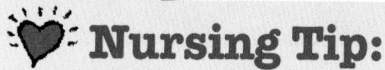

Determining normal systolic blood pressure
In children 1 year of age and older, an easy rule of thumb for determining normal systolic blood pressure is: normal systolic BP (mm Hg) = 80 + (2 × age in years). Normal diastolic blood pressure is generally two-thirds of systolic blood pressure.

Physical Growth

Weight

The type of scale and method for obtaining weight vary depending on the age. Use the same scale at each visit, if possible, to prevent variations in serial weight checks. The scale should be balanced before weighing. If using an infant scale, cover it with paper. Place infants and young toddlers nude on the scale (Figure 14-4). Always keep one hand on the child to prevent falls and lift your hand slightly when obtaining the actual weight reading. Children who can stand without support can be weighed on a standard platform scale, wearing underpants. Weight should be noted and recorded and plotted on a standardized growth chart (see Appendix B). Usually, neonates lose approximately 10% of birth weight by the third or fourth day after birth, then regain it by 2 weeks of age. This expected change in weight is called physiological weight loss, and it is due to a loss of extracellular fluid and **meconium.**

Table 14-6 Blood Pressure Levels for the 90th and 95th Percentiles of Blood Pressure for Boys Aged 1 to 17 Years by Percentiles of Height

Age, years	Blood Pressure Percentile*	Systolic Blood Pressure by Percentile of Height, mm Hg†							Diastolic Blood Pressure by Percentile of Height, mm Hg†						
		5%	10%	25%	50%	75%	90%	95%	5%	10%	25%	50%	75%	90%	95%
1	90th	94	95	97	98	100	102	102	50	51	52	53	54	54	55
	95th	98	99	101	102	104	106	106	55	55	56	57	58	59	59
2	90th	98	99	100	102	104	105	106	55	55	56	57	58	59	59
	95th	101	102	104	106	108	109	110	59	59	60	61	62	63	63
3	90th	100	101	103	105	107	108	109	59	59	60	61	62	63	63
	95th	104	105	107	109	111	112	113	63	63	64	65	66	67	67
4	90th	102	103	105	107	109	110	111	62	62	63	64	65	66	66
	95th	106	107	109	111	113	114	115	66	67	67	68	69	70	71
5	90th	104	105	106	108	110	112	112	65	65	66	67	68	69	69
	95th	108	109	110	112	114	115	116	69	70	70	71	72	73	74

continues

Table 14-6 *Continued*

Age, years	Blood Pressure Percentile*	Systolic Blood Pressure by Percentile of Height, mm Hg†							Diastolic Blood Pressure by Percentile of Height, mm Hg†						
		5%	10%	25%	50%	75%	90%	95%	5%	10%	25%	50%	75%	90%	95%
6	90th	105	106	108	110	111	113	114	67	68	69	70	70	71	72
	95th	109	110	112	114	115	117	117	72	72	73	74	75	76	76
7	90th	106	107	109	111	113	114	115	69	70	71	72	72	73	74
	95th	110	111	113	115	116	118	119	74	74	75	76	77	78	78
8	90th	107	108	110	112	114	115	116	71	71	72	73	74	75	75
	95th	111	112	114	116	118	119	120	75	76	76	77	78	79	80
9	90th	109	110	112	113	115	117	117	72	73	73	74	75	76	77
	95th	113	114	116	117	119	121	121	76	77	78	79	80	80	81
10	90th	110	112	113	115	117	118	119	73	74	74	75	76	77	78
	95th	114	115	117	119	121	122	123	77	78	79	80	80	81	82
11	90th	112	113	115	117	119	120	121	74	74	75	76	77	78	78
	95th	116	117	119	121	123	124	125	78	79	79	80	81	82	83
12	90th	115	116	117	119	121	123	123	75	75	76	77	78	78	79
	95th	119	120	121	123	125	126	127	79	79	80	81	82	83	83
13	90th	117	118	120	122	124	125	126	75	76	76	77	78	79	80
	95th	121	122	124	126	128	129	130	79	80	81	82	83	83	84
14	90th	120	121	123	125	126	128	128	76	76	77	78	79	80	80
	95th	124	125	127	128	130	132	132	80	81	81	82	83	84	85
15	90th	123	124	125	127	129	131	131	77	77	78	79	80	81	81
	95th	127	128	129	131	133	134	135	81	82	83	83	84	85	86
16	90th	125	126	128	130	132	133	134	79	79	80	81	82	82	83
	95th	129	130	132	134	136	137	138	83	83	84	85	86	87	87
17	90th	128	129	131	133	134	136	136	81	81	82	83	84	85	85
	95th	132	133	135	136	138	140	140	85	85	86	87	88	89	89

** Blood pressure percentile was determined by a single measurement.*
† Height percentile was determined by standard growth curves.
Reproduced with permission from Pediatrics, *98, 653–654, 1996.*

Table 14-7 Blood Pressure Levels for the 90th and 95th Percentile of Blood Pressure for Girls Aged 1 to 17 Years by Percentiles of Height

Age, years	Blood Pressure Percentile*	Systolic Blood Pressure by Percentile of Height, mm Hg†							Diastolic Blood Pressure by Percentile of Height, mm Hg†						
		5%	10%	25%	50%	75%	90%	95%	5%	10%	25%	50%	75%	90%	95%
1	90th	97	98	99	100	102	103	104	53	53	53	54	55	56	56
	95th	101	102	103	104	105	107	107	57	57	57	58	59	60	60
2	90th	99	99	100	102	103	104	105	57	57	58	58	59	60	61
	95th	102	103	104	105	107	108	109	61	61	62	62	63	64	65
3	90th	100	100	102	103	104	105	106	61	61	61	62	63	63	64
	95th	104	104	105	107	108	109	110	65	65	65	66	67	67	68
4	90th	101	102	103	104	106	107	108	63	63	64	65	65	66	67
	95th	105	106	107	108	109	111	111	67	67	68	69	69	70	71

continues

Table 14-7 *Continued*

Age, years	Blood Pressure Percentile*	Systolic Blood Pressure by Percentile of Height, mm Hg†							Diastolic Blood Pressure by Percentile of Height, mm Hg†						
		5%	10%	25%	50%	75%	90%	95%	5%	10%	25%	50%	75%	90%	95%
5	90th	103	103	104	106	107	108	109	65	66	66	67	68	68	69
	95th	107	107	108	110	111	112	113	69	70	70	71	72	72	73
6	90th	104	105	106	107	109	110	111	67	67	68	69	69	70	71
	95th	108	109	110	111	112	114	114	71	71	72	73	73	74	75
7	90th	106	107	108	109	110	112	112	69	69	69	70	71	72	72
	95th	110	110	112	113	114	115	116	73	73	73	74	75	76	76
8	90th	108	109	110	111	112	113	114	70	70	71	71	72	73	74
	95th	112	112	113	115	116	117	118	74	74	75	75	76	77	78
9	90th	110	110	112	113	114	115	116	71	72	72	73	74	74	75
	95th	114	114	115	117	118	119	120	75	76	76	77	78	78	79
10	90th	112	112	114	115	116	117	118	73	73	73	74	75	76	76
	95th	116	116	117	119	120	121	122	77	77	77	78	79	80	80
11	90th	114	114	116	117	118	119	120	74	74	75	75	76	77	77
	95th	118	118	119	121	122	123	124	78	78	79	79	80	81	81
12	90th	116	116	118	119	120	121	122	75	75	76	76	77	78	78
	95th	120	120	121	123	124	125	126	79	79	80	80	81	82	82
13	90th	118	118	119	121	122	123	124	76	76	77	78	78	79	80
	95th	121	122	123	125	126	127	128	80	80	81	82	82	83	84
14	90th	119	120	121	122	124	125	126	77	77	78	79	79	80	81
	95th	123	124	125	126	128	129	130	81	81	82	83	83	84	85
15	90th	121	121	122	124	125	126	127	78	78	79	79	80	81	82
	95th	124	125	126	128	129	130	131	82	82	83	83	84	85	86
16	90th	122	122	123	125	126	127	128	79	79	79	80	81	82	82
	95th	125	126	127	128	130	131	132	83	83	83	84	85	86	86
17	90th	122	123	124	125	126	128	128	79	79	79	80	81	82	82
	95th	126	126	127	129	130	131	132	83	83	83	84	85	86	86

** Blood pressure percentile was determined by a single reading.*
† Height percentile was determined by standard growth curves.
Reproduced with permission from Pediatrics, *98, 653–654, 1996.*

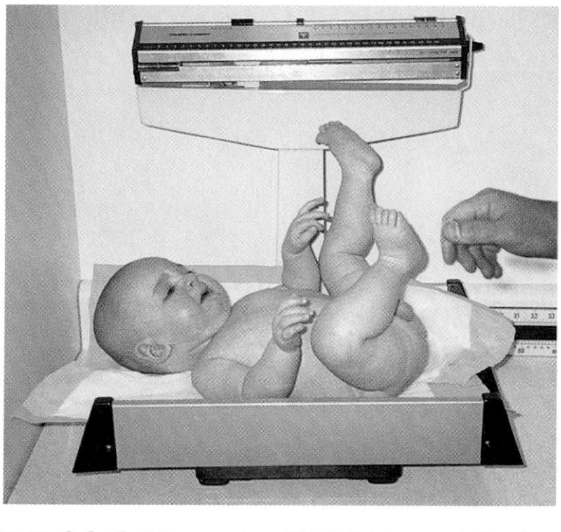

Figure 14-4 Measuring Weight in an Infant

Critical Thinking

A Child Below the 3rd Percentile

You obtain the weight and height on a 2-year-old girl and plot these measurements on the appropriate growth chart. She is in the 2nd percentile. What would you do about this?

Length/Height

Recumbent length is measured for children younger than 2 years old. Position the measuring board flat on the examination table. Place the child's head at the top of the board and the child's heels at the foot of the board, making sure the legs are fully extended. If a board is not available, place the child in a supine position and mark lines on the paper at the tip of the head and at the heel (Figure 14-5A), making sure the legs are fully extended. Measure between the lines and record. Height for all other age groups can be measured in the same fashion as for an adult. Figure 14-5B shows a preschooler's height being measured. Length/height should be plotted on a standardized growth chart (see Appendix B). A height below the 5th or above the 95th percentiles warrants investigation, as does the child who falls two standard deviations below his or her own established curve. Any such finding is abnormal.

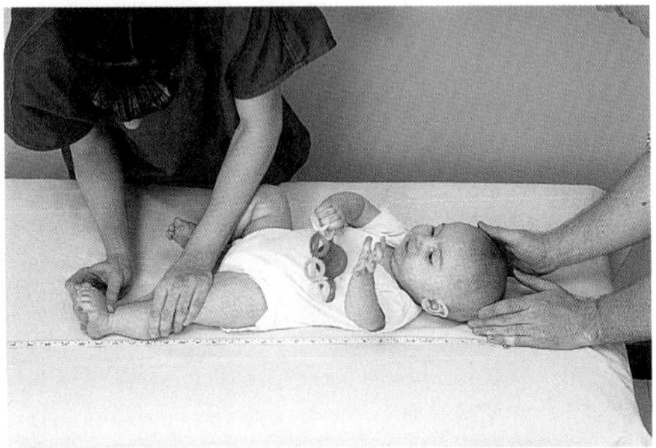

(A)

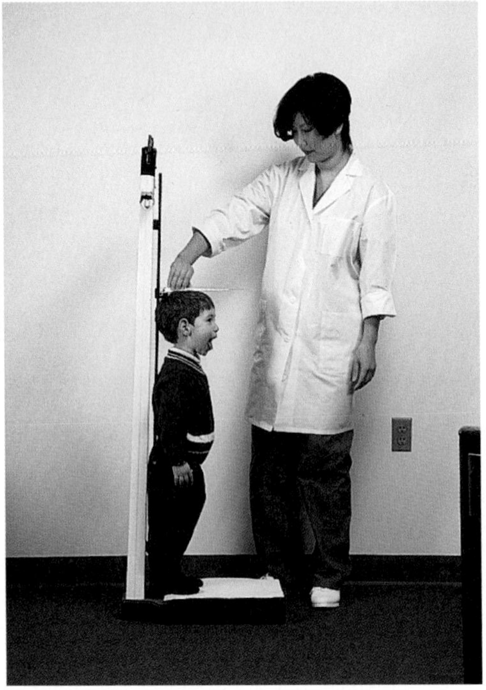

(B)

Figure 14-5 Measuring Length and Height in Children. (A) Recumbent Length in Infant (B) Height in Preschooler

Eye On:

Variations in Height

Children of different races vary in height. African American and Caucasian children are the tallest, followed by Native American children, who are similar or a little shorter. Next in height are Mexican American children, followed by the shortest group–Asian American. Within the same racial group, children from families with higher socioeconomic status are taller than those from lower socioeconomic status families. Obese children are taller than lean children (Seidel, Ball, Dains, & Benedict, 1995).

Nursing Tip:

Obtaining length/height in children under 2 years of age

1. If measuring a recumbent length, always plot on the birth-to-36-month chart.
2. If measuring height, plot the measurement on a birth-to-36-month growth chart and subtract 1 centimeter, or plot on a 2-to-18-year chart.

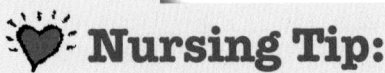

Head Circumference

Head circumference is measured in all children less than 2 years of age or in children with known or suspected hydrocephalus. Place the child in a sitting or supine position. Using a tape measure, measure anteriorly from just above the eyebrows and around posteriorly to the occipital protuberance (refer to Figure 14-6; also see Appendix B, head circumference for girls and boys birth to 36 months. Normal average head growth is 1.0–1.5 cm per month during the

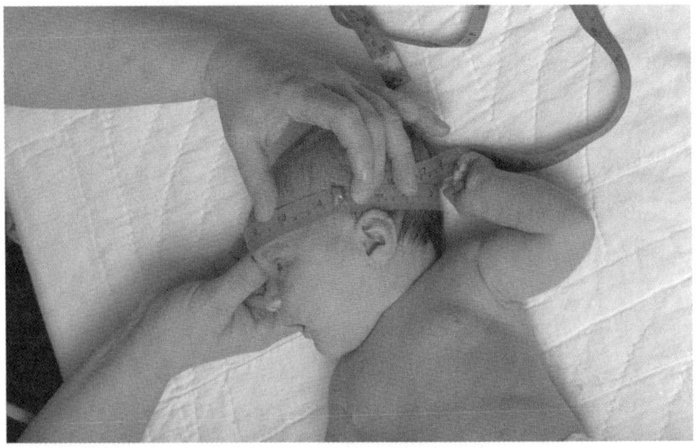

Figure 14-6 Measuring Infant Head Circumference

first year. Premature infants often have small head circumferences.

Microcephaly, a congenital anomaly characterized by a small brain with a resultant small head and a mental deficit, is an abnormal finding. Another abnormality, **hydrocephalus,** is an enlargement of the head without enlargement of the facial structures. For more information about microcephaly and hydrocephalus refer to Chapter 32.

Chest Circumference

Chest circumference is measured up to 1 year of age. It is a measurement that, by itself, provides little information but is compared to head circumference to evaluate the child's overall growth. Measure the chest circumference by placing the tape measure around the chest at the nipple line (Figure 14-7). Measure at the end of exhalation. From birth to about 1 year, the head circumference is greater than the chest circumference. After age 1, the chest circumference is greater than the head circumference. A measured chest circumference below normal limits is abnormal. A below-normal chest circumference for age can be attributed to prematurity.

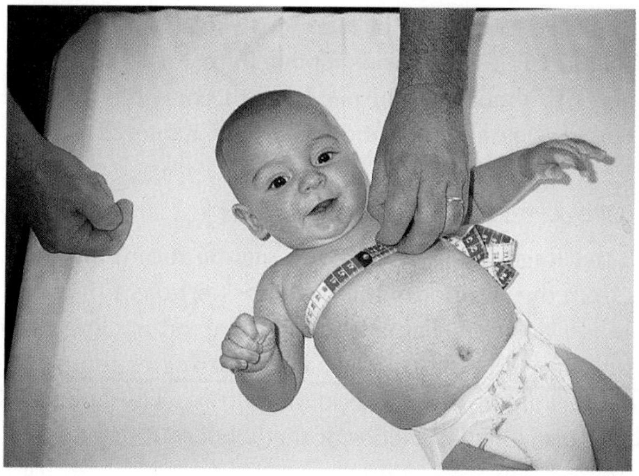

Figure 14-7 Measuring Chest Circumference

> **Reflective Thinking**
>
> **Suspecting Child Abuse**
>
> A young mother of five children brings her 2-year-old child, who is wheezing and having difficulty breathing, into the emergency department. The mother tells you she was up all night with the child. On auscultation of the posterior lung fields, you note three 4-mm rounded areas on the upper back that appear to be second-degree burns. There is erythema and tissue destruction surrounding the borders of each area.
>
> 1. What would be your first reaction?
> 2. How would you proceed with the assessment? What questions would you ask the mother?
> 3. Do you know your institution's policy and your state's laws on reporting suspected child abuse?
> 4. Are you, as a nurse, a mandated reporter?

Skin

Inspection

Color

Observe the color of the body, especially at the tip of the nose, the external ear, the lips, the hands, and the feet. These areas are prominent locations for detecting cyanosis or jaundice.

Lesions

Inspect the skin for lesions, noting the anatomic location, distribution, shape, color, size, and exudate. No skin lesions should be present except for freckles, birthmarks, or moles (nevi), which may be flat or elevated. Several abnormal skin conditions are associated with lesions. Eczema or atopic dermatitis (AD) is a common skin disorder involving inflammation of the epidermis and superficial dermis. The lesions of AD are usually symmetrical, scaly, erythematous patches or plaques with possible exudation and crusting. Inhaled allergens such as pollens, molds, or dust mites, or food allergens are thought to induce mast-cell responses that cause AD. Erythema toxicum, a benign rash whose cause is unknown, appears as small, erythematous, maculopapular lesions that erupt on the newborn. Another lesion is **telangiectatic nevi,** commonly known as stork bites. Refer to Chapter 7 for specific information. Diaper dermatitis is characterized by diffuse redness, papules, vesicles, edema, scaling, and ulcerations on the area covered by a baby's diaper. It is the result of a bacteria and urea reaction on the skin. A dark-black tuft of hair or a dimple over the lumbosacral area is abnormal and may indicate that the neonate has a vertebral defect known as spina bifida occulta.

Palpation

Temperature

Temperature is assessed by palpating the skin with the back of the hand. Skin surface temperature should be warm and equal bilaterally. Hands and feet may be slightly cooler than the rest of the body. Generalized hyperthermia may be indicative of a febrile state, hyperthyroidism, or increased metabolic function caused by exercise. Generalized hypothermia may be indicative of shock or some other type of central circulatory dysfunction.

Texture

Use the finger pads to palpate the skin. The technique of palpating the skin of a younger child can be accomplished by playing games. For example, use the finger pads to walk up the abdomen and touch the nose. The skin of a child normally is smooth and soft. A common variation occurring in the infant is **milia,** which are small, white papules on the cheeks, forehead, nose, and chin due to sebum that occludes the opening of the follicles. Milia resolve spontaneously within a few weeks. Newborns may also have **vernix caseosa,** a thick, cheesy, protective, integumentary deposit that consists of sebum and shed epithelial cells.

Turgor

Skin turgor or elasticity reflects the child's state of hydration. It is assessed by pinching a small section of the child's skin between your thumb and forefinger and quickly releasing it. The upper arm and abdomen are optimal areas to assess. Good turgor and adequate hydration is evidenced when the skin rapidly returns to its original contour after it is released. Decreased skin turgor, a sign of dehydration, is present when it slowly returns to its original contour or remains pinched or "tented" after it is released.

Edema

Edema, an accumulation of fluid in the interstitial spaces, is assessed by pressing the thumb into an area of the body that appears puffy or swollen. Edema is most evident in dependent parts of the body (arms, hands, legs, ankles, feet, sacrum). Periorbital edema may be observed in children on the eyelids. Normally the skin surface stays smooth. If pressure leaves an indentation, pitting edema is present.

Hair

To evaluate the scalp for lesions or signs of infestations, don gloves and lift the scalp hair by segments. Note the scalp's color, which should be similar to the child's skin. There should be no signs of lesions or infestations. Seborrheic dermatitis (cradle cap), caused by increased production of sebum, looks like yellow, greasy-appearing scales and crusts on the scalp of a light-skinned infant. In dark-skinned infants, the scaling is light gray. Head lice (pediculosis capitis) may be seen crawling within the hair. Refer to Chapter 30 for more information about seborrheic dermatitis and head lice.

Head

Inspection

Shape and Symmetry

With the child sitting upright either in the caregiver's arms or on the examination table, observe the symmetry of the frontal, parietal, and occipital prominences. Normally, the shape of a child's head is symmetrical without depressions or protrusions. The anterior fontanel may pulsate with every heart beat. The infant of Asian descent generally has a flattened occiput, more so than infants of other races. A flattened occipital bone with resultant hair loss over the same area is abnormal and is usually caused by the infant being in the supine position for prolonged periods of time.

Head Control

Head control is assessed when the infant is in a sitting position. With the head unsupported, observe the infant's ability to hold the head erect. At 4 months of age, most infants are able to hold the head erect and in midline. To evaluate for head lag, pull the infant by the hands from a supine to a sitting position. Again by 4 months of age, the head should stay in line with the body when being pulled forward. Documented prematurity, hydrocephalus, and illnesses causing developmental delays are possible causes of head lag. Significant head lag after 6 months of age may indicate brain injury and should be further investigated.

Palpation

Fontanel

Place the child in an upright position. Using the second or third finger pad, palpate the anterior fontanel at the junction of the sagittal, coronal, and frontal sutures. Palpate the posterior fontanel at the junction of the sagittal and lambdoidal sutures. Assess for bulging, pulsations, and size. Crying will produce a distorted, full, bulging appearance. The anterior fontanel is soft and flat. Size ranges from 4 to 6 centimeters at birth. The fontanel gradually closes between 9 and 19 months of age. The posterior fontanel is also soft and flat. The size ranges from 0.5 to 1.5 centimeters at birth. The posterior fontanel gradually closes between 1 and 3 months of age. It is normal to feel pulsations related to the peripheral pulse.

If palpation reveals a bulging, tense fontanel, this is abnormal and indicates increased intracranial pressure. A sunken, depressed fontanel occurs with dehydration. A wide anterior fontanel in a child older than $2^1/_2$ years is an abnormal finding. An anterior fontanel that remains open after $2^1/_2$ years of age may indicate disease such as rickets. In rickets, there is a low level of vitamin D relative to decreased phosphate level. A posterior fontanel greater than 1.5 cm in diameter is abnormal and occurs with congenital hypothyroidism. For more information, refer to Chapter 28.

Suture Lines

With the finger pads, palpate the sagittal suture line, which runs from the anterior to the posterior portion of the skull in a midline position. Palpate the coronal suture line, which runs along both sides of the head, starting at the anterior fontanel. Palpate the lambdoidal suture. The lambdoidal suture runs along both sides of the head, starting at the posterior fontanel. Ascertain if these suture lines are open, united, or overlapping. Grooves or ridges between sections of the skull are normally palpated up to 6 months of age. Suture lines that overlap or override one another, giving the head an unusual shape, warrant further investigation. **Craniosynostosis** is premature ossification of suture lines, whereby there is early formation and fusion of skull bones. Craniosynostosis may be caused by metabolic disorders or may be a secondary consequence of microcephaly. Figure 14-8 illustrates a superior and lateral view of an infant head.

Surface Characteristics

With the finger pads, palpate the skull in the same manner as the fontanels and suture lines. Note surface edema and contour of the cranium. Normally, the skin covering the cranium is flush against the skull and without edema. A softening of the outer layer of the cranial bones behind and above the ears combined with a ping-pong ball sensation as the area is pressed in gently with the fingers is indicative of **craniotabes,** an abnormal finding. Craniotabes is associated with rickets, syphilis, hydrocephaly, or hypervitaminosis.

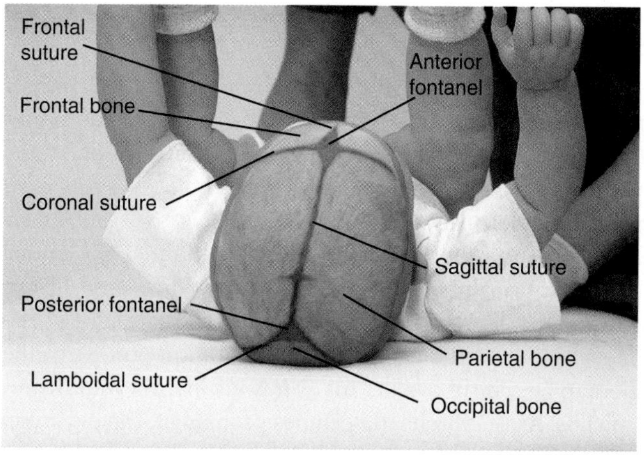

(A)

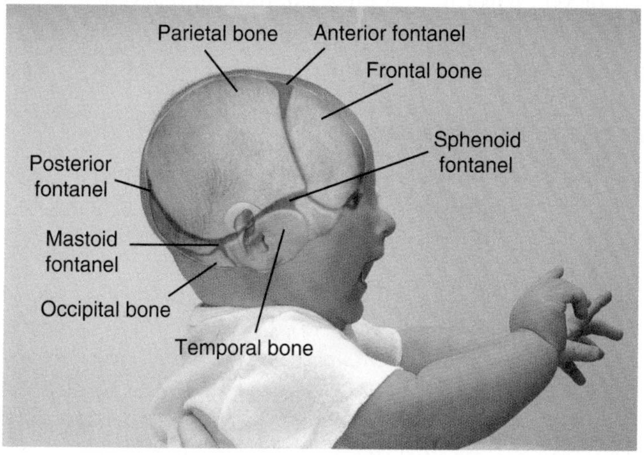

(B)

Figure 14-8 Infant Head Structures. (A) Superior View (B) Lateral View

Another abnormal finding in a newborn is a **cephalhematoma,** or a localized, subcutaneous swelling over one of the cranial bones. Refer to Chapter 7 for additional information about a cephalhematoma.

Another variation in the newborn that causes the shape of the skull to look markedly asymmetric is known as **caput succedaneum** or swelling over the occipitoparietal region of the skull. A newborn's head may also feel asymmetric due to **molding** of the cranial bones as a result of induced pressure during delivery. For more specific information on caput succedaneum and molding, refer to Chapter 7.

Eyes

General Approach

From infancy through about 8–10 years, you should assess the eyes toward the end of the assessment, with the exception of testing vision, which should be done first. Remember that the child's attention span is short, and attentiveness decreases the longer you evaluate. Young children generally are not cooperative for eye, ear, and throat assessments. Place the young infant, preschooler, or school-aged or adolescent child on the examination table. The older infant or the toddler can be held by the caregiver.

Vision Screening

General Approach

Several screening tests are available to evaluate visual acuity in children including the adult Snellen, Snellen E, and Allen. The child's age and developmental level determine the measures used. The adult Snellen chart can be used on children as young as 6 years, provided they are able to read the alphabet. The Snellen E chart, which shows the letter "E" facing in different directions, is used for a child over 3 years of age or any child who cannot read the alphabet. Test every 1–2 years through adolescence. If the child resists wearing a cover patch over the eye, make a game out of wearing the patch. For example, the young child could pretend to be a pirate exploring new territory. Use your imagination to think of a fantasy situation. The Allen test (a series of seven pictures on different cards) can be used with children as young as 3 years of age (American Academy of Pediatrics Committee on Practice and Ambulatory Medicine, Section on Opthalmology, 1996).

Snellen E Chart

Ask the child to point an arm in the direction the E is pointing. Observe for squinting. Vision is 20/40 from 2 to approximately 6 years of age, when it approaches the normal 20/20 acuity. The test is abnormal if results are 20/40 or greater in a child 3 years of age or 20/30 or greater in a child 6 years or older, or if results are different in each eye.

Nearsightedness or myopia is the result of congenital cataracts, retinal trauma, or a tumor.

Allen Test

With the child's eyes both open, show each card to the child and elicit a name for each picture. Do not use any pictures with which the child is not familiar. Place the 2–3-year-old child 15 feet from where you will be standing. Place the 3–4-year-old child 20 feet from you. Ask the caregiver to help cover one of the child's eyes. Show the pictures one at a time, eliciting a response after each showing. Show the same pictures in different sequence for the other eye. To record findings, the denominator is always constant at 30, because a child with normal vision should see the picture on the card (target) at 30 feet. To document the numerator, determine the greatest distance at which three of the pictures are recognized by each eye, for example, right eye = 15/30, left eye = 20/30. The child should correctly identify three of the cards in three trials. Two- to three-year-old children should have 15/30 vision. Three- to four-year-old children should be able to achieve a score of 15/30 to 20/30. Each eye should have the same score. If the scores for the child's right and left eyes differ by 5 feet or more or either or both eyes score less than 15/30, refer the child to an ophthalmologist.

Strabismus Screening

The Hirschberg test (corneal light reflex) and the cover-uncover test screen for strabismus. The latter is the more definitive test.

Hirschberg Test

Hold a pen light by the side of your head with one hand so the light is facing straight ahead. The pen light should be approximately 12 inches from the child's head. Using your other hand turn the child's head so the light is in the midline position toward the child's eyes. Make a general observation of the light reflection relative to both cornea noting symmetry and central location. The reflected light should be seen symmetrically in the center of both corneas.

Esotropia, thought to be congenital, occurs when the light reflection is displaced to the outer margin of the cornea as the eye deviates inward. Some theories suggest that neurological factors contribute to its development. **Exotropia** occurs when the light reflection is displaced to the inner margin of the cornea as the eye deviates outward. This abnormality can result from eye muscle fatigue or can be congenital. More information on eye abnormalities can be found in Chapter 31.

Cover-Uncover Test

This test is performed on infants greater than 6 months of age through school-age. Stand 2 feet in front of the child. Place the child in a seated position on the examining table or caregiver's lap. Ask the child to focus attention on the pen light by the side of your head. Place a cover card or your hand over one eye. Wait until the uncovered eye focuses then remove the occluder and evaluate the eye just uncovered for focusing movement.

The normal finding is neither eye moves when the occluder is being removed. Infants younger than 6 months of age display strabismus due to poor neuromuscular control of eye muscles. It is abnormal for one or both eyes to move to focus on the penlight during assessment. Assume strabismus is present. Strabismus after 6 months of age is abnormal and indicates eye muscle weakness.

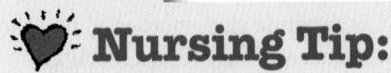

> **Nursing Tip:**
>
> **Pseudostrabismus**
>
> Some infants have an epicanthal fold that gives the false appearance of strabismus. This situation is termed **pseudostrabismus.** However, in these infants the corneal light reflex is normal.

Inspection

Eyelids

Sit at the child's eye level. Observe for symmetrical **palpebral fissures** (opening between the margins of the upper and lower eyelids) and position of eyelids in relation to the iris. Normally, the palpebral fissures of both eyes are positioned symmetrically. The upper eyelid covers a small portion of the iris, and the lower lid meets the iris. Epicanthal folds are normally present in children of Asian descent. An epicanthal fold is an excess skinfold over the angle of the inner canthus of the eye. It is abnormal for a portion of the sclera to be seen above the iris as it is in children with hydrocephalus. As the forehead becomes prominent, the eyebrows and eyelids are drawn up, creating a setting sun appearance of the child's eyes. Children with Down syndrome have a fold of skin covering the inner canthus and lacrimal caruncle. During embryonic development, the fold of skin slants in a downward direction toward the nose.

Lacrimal Apparatus

If lacrimal duct obstruction is suspected, use the index finger to lightly palpate the lacrimal sac area while bracing the

> **Nursing Tip:**
>
> **Lid eversion in children**
>
> Lid eversion is not performed in children unless you are assessing for an infection or foreign body. If performed, the technique is the same as for an adult.

child's head with the other hand. Note drainage from the lacrimal duct orifice. The child's caregiver reports that the child is unable to produce tears, an abnormal finding. The lacrimal ducts should be open by 3 months of age. **Dacryocystitis** is an infection of the lacrimal sac caused by obstruction of the lacrimal duct. It is characterized by tearing and discharge from the eye.

Anterior Segment Structures

Sclera

The sclera is observed mainly to determine its color. Normally, the newborn exhibits a bluish-tinged sclera related to thinness of the fibrous tissue. The sclera is white in light-skinned children and a slightly darker color in some dark-skinned children. A yellowish color to the sclera indicates jaundice, which is due to hemolysis of red blood cells, non-functioning liver cells, or obstruction of bile in the common or hepatic duct.

Iris

Using the light source on the opthalmoscope, observe the iris for lesions and color. Up to about 6 months of age, the color of the iris is blue or slate gray in light-skinned infants and brownish in dark-skinned infants. By 12 months of age, complete transition of iris color has occurred. Small white flecks, called Brushfield's spots, noted around the perimeter of the iris are abnormal. Brushfield's spots are found on the iris of the child with Down syndrome. The spots develop during embryonic maturation.

Pupils

The pupils should be inspected for size, shape, equality, and response to light. Pupils should be equal in size; however, a small number of individuals (5%) normally have pupils of different sizes (Jarvis, 1996). To test for pupillary light reflex, dim the room lights. Position the child according to age. Move the lighted instrument in from the side and observe the change in the size of the pupils. The pupils should react equally and accommodate to light. An abnormality is suspected if one or both pupils are nonreactive. Any central nervous system insult (e.g., head injury, meningitis, seizures) may cause an abnormal response.

Utilize the pupillary reflex to elicit an optical blink reflex in the newborn. When the pupils' reaction to light is assessed, a newborn will normally blink and flex the head closer to the body. This is called the optical blink reflex.

> **Nursing Tip:**
>
> **Recording pupillary response**
>
> The normal response of the pupils is recorded as PERRLA, which means the **P**upils are **E**qual in size, **R**ound in shape, and **R**eact to **L**ight and **A**ccommodate.

Posterior Segment Structures

General Approach

Observe the red reflex, retina, and optic disc. The assessment is easier to accomplish if the infant or toddler is lying supine on an examination table. The assistance of another individual, such as the caregiver, to hold the child in position is essential. The older child may be allowed to sit, if cooperative.

Inspection

Red Reflex

Turn the opthalmoscope to 0 diopters. Stand 10–12 inches from the client and observe the pupil through the opthalmoscope's window. Note the color of the reflex within the eye. In children, the red reflex appears as a brilliant, uniform red glow. In newborns and infants, the red reflex will appear lighter. In many darker-skinned individuals, the reflex will appear darker. Black spots or opacities within the red reflex are abnormal and may indicate a cataract. Chromosomal disorders, intrauterine infections, and ocular trauma are possible causes of cataracts in newborns. A yellowish or white light reflex (cat's eye reflex) is also abnormal and may indicate retinoblastoma, a malignant glioma located in the posterior chamber of the eye.

Retina

Assess the retinal background for color. Divide the retina into four quadrants and follow the retinal arteries and veins from the disc to periphery. Note the size and distribution of retinal arteries and veins. The retina's background is generally pink but may be lighter in some Caucasians and darker in African American individuals. There is no difference in normal vasculature among children and adults. A red to dark-red color is abnormal. Some areas may be rounded or flame shaped. Hemorrhage is seen in trauma. Bleeding into the optic nerve sheath is found in children who have been physically shaken.

Optic Disc

At a 15° lateral position to the eye, move in closer to the eye approximately 1 inch from the child. Move the diopter to –5 to 0. Locate a vessel and move medially (nasal side) to locate the disc. Observe the color of the disc along with margin definition. The disc is creamy yellow to salmon in color. The disc is lighter in an infant. It measures about 1.5 mm in diameter and is round in shape. The margins of the disc are regular and clearly defined. If abnormal, the margins are blurred. In papilledema, the optic disc margins are abnormal. The margins are poorly defined (blurred) related to increased intracranial pressure.

Ears

Auditory Testing

General Approach

Perform auditory testing at about 3–4 years of age or when the child can follow directions. Prior to 3 years of age, the following are a few parameters for evaluating hearing:

1. Does the child react to a loud noise?
2. Does the child react to the caregiver's voice by cooing, smiling, or turning eyes and head toward the voice?
3. Does the child try to imitate sounds?
4. Can the child imitate words and sounds?
5. Can the child follow directions?
6. Does the child respond to sounds not directed at him or her?

External Ear

Inspection of Pinna Position

Position the child on the caregiver's lap or examining table. Draw an imaginary line from the outer canthus to the top of the ear. The top of the ear should be at or a little above the imaginary line. An abnormal finding occurs when the top of the ear is below the imaginary line drawn from the outer canthus to the top of the ear. Kidneys and ears are formed at the same time in embryonic development. If a child's ears are low set, renal anomalies must be ruled out. Low-set ears can also occur in Down syndrome. Additional information on Down syndrome can be found in Chapter 33.

Internal Ear Inspection

A cooperative child may be allowed to sit for the assessment. A young child may be held as shown in Figure 14-9A. Restrain the uncooperative young child by placing him or her supine on a firm surface (Figure 14-9B). Instruct the caregiver or assistant to hold the child's arms up near the head, embracing the elbow joints on both sides of either arm. Restrain the infant by having the caregiver hold the infant's hands down (Figure 14-9C).

With your thumb and forefinger grasping the otoscope, use the lateral side of the hand to prevent the head from jerking. Your other hand can also be used to stabilize the child's head. Pull the lower auricle down and out to straighten the canal. This technique is used in children up to about 3 years of age. Use the adult technique after age 3. Insert the speculum about $\frac{1}{4}$ to $\frac{1}{2}$ inch, depending on the child's age. Suspected otitis media must be evaluated with a pneumatic bulb attached to the side of the otoscope's light source. Select a larger speculum to make a tight seal and prevent air from escaping from the canal. If a light reflex is present, focus on the light reflection. Gently squeeze the bulb attachment to introduce air into the canal. Some nurses prefer to gently blow air through the tubing rather than squeezing air into the canal. Observe the tympanic membrane for movement.

The tympanic membrane is transparent and pearly gray to light pink in color. The membrane is smooth and continuous. Light from the otoscope is reflected off the membrane. The tympanic membrane moves when air is introduced into the canal.

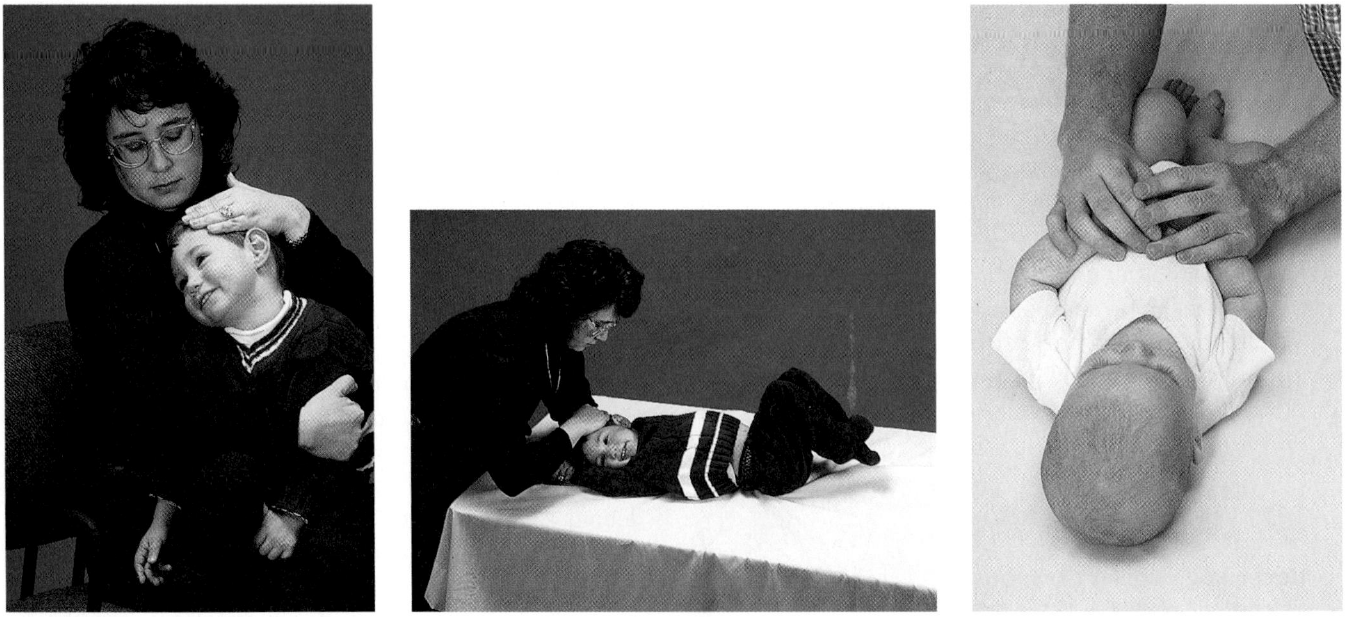

(A) (B) (C)

Figure 14-9 Restraining the Child for the Otoscopic Examination. (A) Preschooler in a Sitting Position (B) Preschooler in a Supine Position (C) Infant

Nursing Tip:

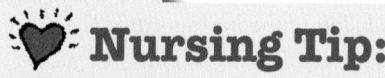

False impression of otitis media

If the child is screaming and crying, a flush or erythema on the tympanic membrane will be present. After allowing the caregiver to comfort the child, attempt to reassess. The flush or erythema can give false impressions of otitis media.

More information about otitis media can be found in Chapter 24.

Nose

Observe the size and shape of the external nose, which should be symmetric and positioned in the center of the face. A short and small, large, or flattened nose may indicate congenital anomalies. Observe the external nose for flaring, discharge, or odor. Nasal flaring indicates respiratory distress. Purulent yellow or green discharge accompanies an infection. Clear, watery secretions may indicate allergic rhinitis, the common cold, or a foreign body. A foul odor may indicate a foreign body lodged in the nasal cavity. In an infant and young child, the nasal cavity can be visualized by tilting the head back and pushing the tip of the nose upward. The nasal mucosa should be firm and pink.

Nursing Tip:

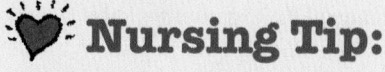

Assessing for choanal atresia

1. Select an appropriately sized catheter (10–12 French).
2. Place the newborn in a supine position on the examination table.
3. Stand at the newborn's side, and use the nondominant hand to hold the newborn's head in a midline position.
4. Use the dominant hand to insert the catheter through the nasal passage and into the nasopharynx.
5. Remove the catheter.
6. Perform the test through the opposite nare to evaluate patency.

Normally, the catheter does not meet resistance and is able to pass freely to the nasopharynx. Inability to insert the catheter into the nasopharynx coupled with symptoms of snorting respirations, feeding problems, and cyanosis are indicators of choanal atresia.

Patency of the nares must be determined at birth because newborns are obligatory nose breathers. With the infant's mouth closed, block one nostril and then the other. Observe the respiratory pattern. If total obstruction exists, the infant will not be able to inspire or expire through the uncompressed nostril. If obstruction is suspected, an assessment for choanal atresia should be performed. Information about the assessment can be found in Chapter 7. In **choanal atresia,** there is a unilateral or bilateral bony or membranous septum between the nose and the pharynx.

Mouth and Throat

Inspection

Lips

Observe if the lip edges meet, which is normal. Cleft lip is seen as a separated area of lip tissue. It involves the upper lip and sometimes extends into the nostril. A cleft lip is an obvious finding during a newborn assessment. It occurs mainly on the left side and is more frequently found in males. A cleft lip develops during the fifth to sixth week after fertilization. Genetics plays a small role in etiology. Refer to Chapter 23 for a full discussion of cleft lip.

Buccal Mucosa

If the child is unable to open the mouth on command, use the edge of a tongue blade to lift the upper lip and move the lower lip down. The buccal membranes are pink, moist, and smooth. Thrush, a thick, curdlike coating on the buccal mucosa or tongue, is abnormal. It can be acquired when a newborn passes through the vagina during delivery.

Teeth

Count the number of teeth present on the gum line. Observe the condition of teeth surface for caries or chips. Infants cut their first tooth between 5 and 8 months. By one year of age there are normally eight teeth. Between 5 and 6 years of age, a child will shed the lower central incisors. About 1 year after deciduous shedding, the first permanent teeth erupt. A lack of visible teeth coupled with roentgenographic findings revealing absence of tooth buds is abnormal. Absence of deciduous teeth beyond 16 months of age signifies an abnormality most commonly related to genetic causes. It is abnormal for the teeth to turn brownish black, possibly with indentations along the surfaces of the teeth. These brownish black spots may be caries (cavities), which can be caused when a child falls asleep with a bottle in the mouth (Jones, Berg, & Coody, 1994).

Hard/Soft Palate

Observe the palate for continuity and shape. For infants, you will need to use a tongue depressor to push the tongue down. Infants usually cry in response to this action, which allows visualization of the palates. The roof of the mouth is continuous and has a slight arch. It is abnormal if the roof of the mouth is not continuous. This anomaly is called cleft palate. Cleft palates vary greatly in size and extent of malformation. The degree of malformation is classified into two groups. A midline malformation may involve the uvula or extend through the soft or hard palates or both. If associated with cleft lip, the malformation may extend through the palates and into the nasal cavity. Cleft palates form between the sixth and tenth week of embryonic development, during fusion of the maxillary and premaxillary processes. Genetics plays a small role in etiology. Chapter 23 includes more information on cleft palate.

Epstein's pearls in the newborn appear on the hard palate and gum margins and are abnormal. The pearls are small, white cysts that feel hard when palpated. These cysts result from fragments of epithelial tissue trapped during palate formation.

Oropharynx

Observe the position and color of the uvula. Observe the color and size of tonsillar tissue in the oropharynx. The tonsils are part of the lymphatic system and normally are hypertrophied in early childhood. Beginning at age 10 years, they gradually shrink in size. Tonsillar size ranges from +1 to +4 (Figure 14-10). Up to the age of 10 years, a tonsil grade of 2+ is considered normal. Tonsils should not interfere with the act of breathing. Excessive salivation is an early sign of a tracheoesophageal fistula (TEF). Drooling is accompanied by choking and coughing during the child's feeding. The esophagus failed to develop as a continuous passage during embryonic formation. Refer to Chapter 23 for additional information on TEF.

Neck

Inspection

General Appearance

Observe the neck in a midline position while the child is sitting upright. Note shortening or thickness of the neck on both right and left sides. Note any swelling. Normally, there is a reasonable amount of skin tissue on the sides of the neck and no swelling. Unilateral or bilateral swelling of the neck below the angle of the jaw is abnormal (Figure 14-11). Enlargement of the parotid gland occurs in parotitis or mumps, an inflammation of the parotid gland. There is pain and tenderness in the affected area.

Palpation

Thyroid

Use the first two finger pads to palpate the thyroid gland and its lobes. Have the younger child who is unable to swallow on command take a drink from a bottle. Upon palpation, note any tenderness, enlargement, or masses. An enlarged thyroid gland can be indicative of hyperthyroidism. For additional information about hyperthyroidism, refer to Chapter 28.

Lymph Nodes

Because of the infant's short neck, you must extend the chin upward with your hand before proceeding with palpation. With the finger pads, palpate the submental, submandibular, tonsillar, anterior cervical chain, posterior cervical chain, supraclavicular, preauricular, posterior auricular, and occipital lymph nodes (Figure 14-12). Use a circular motion. Note location, size, shape, tenderness, mobility, and associated skin inflammation of any swollen nodes palpated. Lymph nodes are generally not palpable. Children often have small, movable, cool, nontender nodes referred to as "shotty" nodes. These benign nodes are related to environmental antigen exposure or residual effects of a prior illness and have no clinical significance. Enlargement of the anterior cervical chain, which is abnormal, occurs in bacterial infections of the pharynx, such as strep throat. Enlargement of the occipital nodes or posterior cervical chain nodes is abnormal. This can occur in tinea capitis and acute otitis externa.

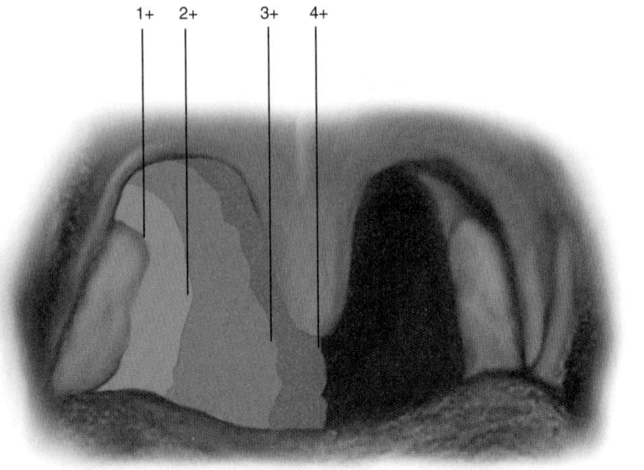

Figure 14-10 Grading of Tonsils

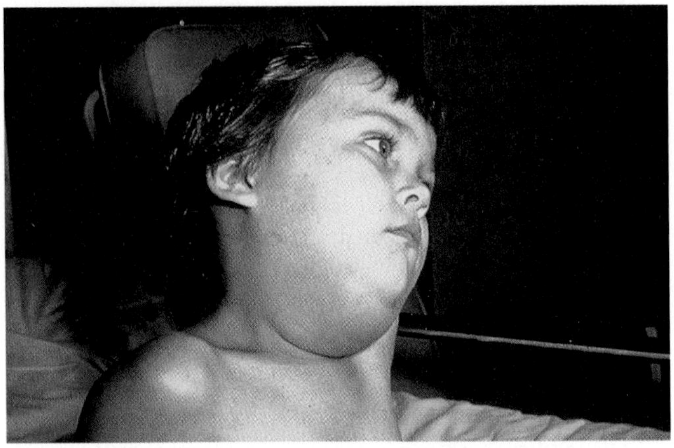

Figure 14-11 Parotitis (Mumps) (Courtesy of the Centers for Disease Control and Prevention.)

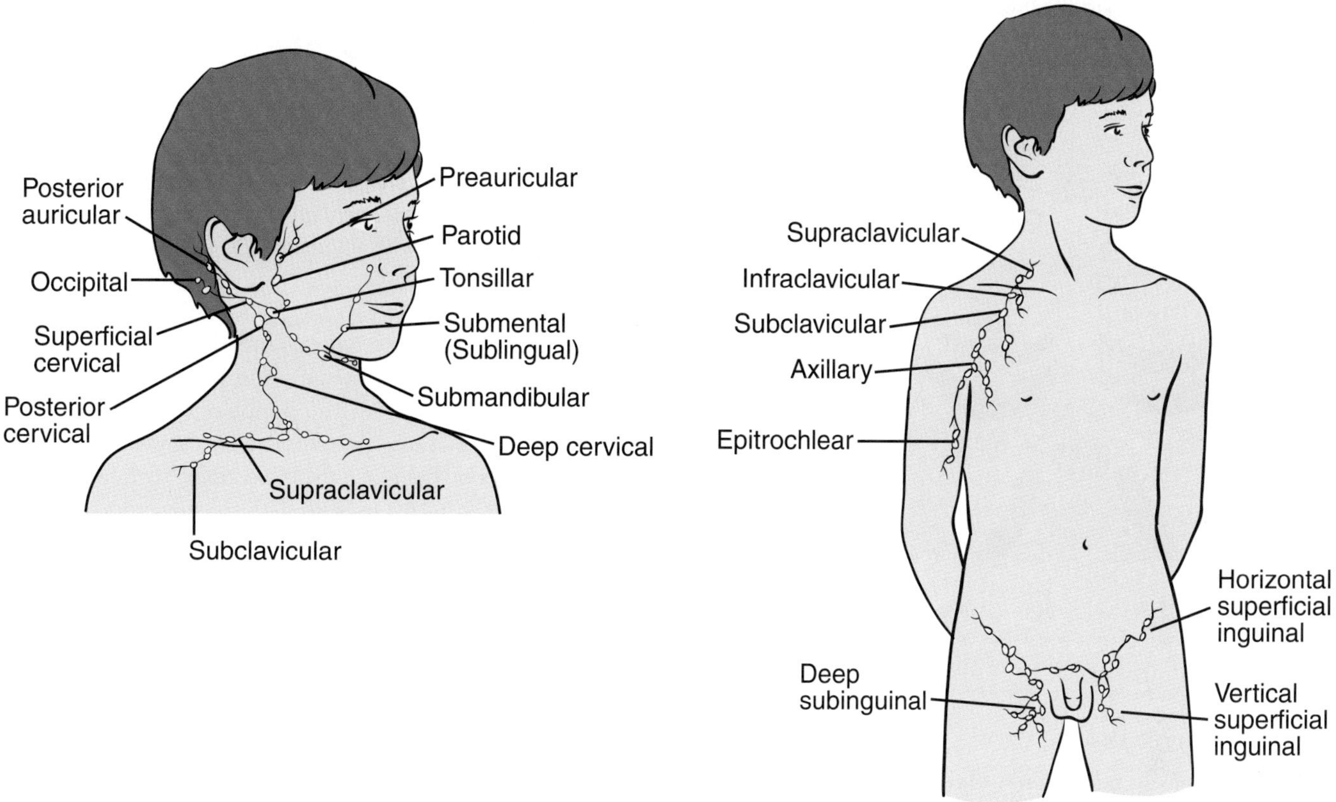

Figure 14-12 Lymph Nodes

Breasts

Inspection of the breasts is performed throughout childhood. Palpation is not usually performed on the child until puberty, unless otherwise indicated.

Thorax and Lungs

Inspection

Shape of Thorax

Observe the configuration of the thorax noting bony structures and musculature. Note the anterior-posterior to lateral diameter and shape of the sternum. The infant has a rounded thorax with the anterior-posterior and transverse diameters approximately equal. By age 6, the chest attains the adult configuration of a lateral diameter greater than the anterior-posterior diameter. If a school-aged child has an abnormal chest configuration, suspect pathology such as cystic fibrosis (CF), which can lead to an altered anteroposterior-transverse diameter. Refer to Chapter 24 for information about CF. Pectus excavatum or funnel chest is a depression in the lower body of the sternum. In severe cases, the sternum can press against the right ventricle, thus interfering with cardiac function. The deformity tends to be progressive from birth. In pectus carinatum, or pigeon chest, the sternum projects forward. This is usually detected when the child is a preschooler or at early school age. This deformity can result from a congenital anomaly.

Retractions

In children, it is important to evaluate intercostal muscles for signs of increased work of breathing. If at all possible, perform this examination when the child is quiet because forceful crying will mimic retractions. Retractions can occur in a variety of locations including the suprasternal (above the sternum), substernal (below the sternum), supraclavicular (above the clavicles), intercostal (between the ribs), and subcostal (below the ribs) regions (Figure 14-13). The trapezus, scalenus, and sternocleidomastoid muscles can also be affected. Acute phases of pneumonia and asthma can produce a condition known as respiratory distress. Clinical features of respiratory distress include retractions of varying severity. Chapter 24 has additional information about pneumonia and asthma. With upper airway obstruction, an increase in respiratory effort ensues creating an increase in negative intrathoracic pressure. The net result is retractions.

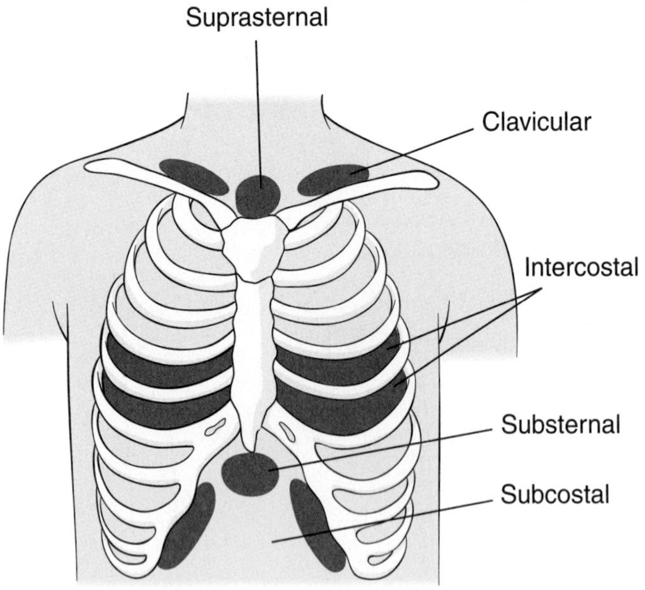

Figure 14-13 Location of Retractions

Palpation

Tactile Fremitus

Fremitus is easily felt when a child cries. If the infant or young child is not crying, it is advisable to defer this procedure until later in the assessment, perhaps after the throat and ear examinations, which usually produce crying. With the child in the same position as inspection, instruct the older child to repeat "99." As the child is crying or repeating "99," use both hands to palpate the chest simultaneously. Repeat the procedure until the anterior, posterior, and lateral sides are assessed, comparing the contralateral side. A soft vibration over the chest wall is normal. Increased sound production is caused by consolidation, as in pneumonia. Decreased sound production is caused by conditions such as pulmonary edema or pleural effusions.

Percussion

Percussion is performed to further assess the underlying structures of the thorax. The chest is percussed to determine dullness or hyperresonance caused by consolidation, fluid, or air trapping. However, in the newborn it is usually unreliable because an adult's fingers are too large in relation to the small chest (Seidel, Ball, Dains, & Benedict, 1995). Normal diaphragmatic excursion in infants and young toddlers is one to two intercostal spaces.

Auscultation

Breath Sounds

Use the same assessment techniques as for an adult. Sometimes, it is difficult to differentiate the various adventitious sounds because a child's respiratory rate is rapid; for example, differentiating expiratory wheezing from inspiratory wheezing can be difficult. Mastering the technique takes time and practice. Of the three types of breath sounds—bronchial, bronchovesicular, and vesicular—the bronchovesicular are normally heard throughout the peripheral lung fields up to 5–6 years of age, because the chest wall is thin with decreased musculature. Lung fields are clear and equal bilaterally.

The common terms used to describe adventitious breath sounds are crackles (formerly called rales), rhonci, and wheezes. Crackles may be caused by conditions such as bronchiolitis, CF, and bronchopulmonary dysplasia. Wheezing during infancy and early childhood may be common. Children with asthma and bronchiolitis may present with wheezing. Stridor is a high-pitched inspiratory crowing sound occurring with croup and acute epiglottitis. Additional information about these respiratory disorders can be found in Chapter 24.

> **Nursing Alert:**
>
> **Stridor in Children**
>
> *Stridor is indicative of upper airway obstruction, particularly edema in children. Inspiration accentuates stridorous sounds. To prevent medical emergencies such as epiglottitis, prompt attention must be sought for children who present with stridor.*

Heart and Peripheral Vasculature

General Approach

The cardiovascular physical assessment has two major components: (1) assessment of the precordium and (2) assessment of the periphery. It is best to perform the cardiac assessment near the beginning of the examination, when the infant or young child is relatively calm. Do not get discouraged during the assessment. The novice nurse is not expected to identify a murmur and location within the cardiac cycle. Be patient because skill will come only with practice. Cardiac landmarks change when a child has **dextrocardia.** In this condition, the apex of the heart points

> **Kids Want To Know**
>
> **Why does the nurse have to listen to my heart in so many places?**
>
> Meredith is 8 years old and is curious about why the nurse puts the stethoscope in different locations on her chest. The nurse replies "your heart has valves that open to allow blood to flow and close to stop the flow. I am listening for specific sounds that indicate the valves are working correctly."

toward the right thoracic cavity, thus heart sounds are auscultated primarily on the right side of the chest.

Inspection

Apical Impulse

With the child's entire chest exposed, look diagonally across the chest for the apical impulse. In infants and young children, the heart lies more horizontally in the chest than in an adult; therefore, the apical impulse is located at the fourth intercostal space and just left of the midclavicular line. The apical impulse of a child 7 years or older is at the fifth intercostal space and to the right of the midclavicular line. The impulse may not be visible in all children, especially in those who have increased adipose tissue or muscle. If the apical impulse is shifted toward the left side or downward expect pathology. Cardiac enlargement or a pneumothorax can cause the location of the apical impulse to deviate. The apical pulse moves laterally with cardiac enlargement. A pneumothorax shifts the apical impulse away from the area of the pneumothorax, which occurs when air enters the pleural cavity from a perforation, commonly as a result of injury to the chest wall.

Precordium

Observe the precordium for any movements other than the apical impulse, which is normally visible. Movements other than the apical impulse are abnormal, and if noticed, they should be described in terms of type, location, and timing in relation to the cardiac cycle. Another abnormality is a **heave,** or a lifting of the cardiac area secondary to an increased workload and force of the left ventricular contraction. A child with congenital heart disease is at risk for developing congestive heart failure (CHF) with associated volume overload and may have heaves. Large left-to-right shunt defects, such as a VSD, cause right ventricular volume overload. More information about cardiac alterations can be found in Chapter 25.

Palpation

Thrill

A **thrill** is a vibration that is similar to what one feels when a hand is placed on a purring cat. It is most commonly produced by blood flowing through a narrow opening from one chamber to another such as in a septal defect. Palpate as for an adult or use the proximal one-third of each finger and the areas over the metacarpophalangeal joints. Place the hand vertically along the heart's apex and move the hand toward the sternum.

Place the hand horizontally along the sternum, moving up the sternal border about $1/2$ to 1 inch each time. When at the clavicular level, place the hand vertically and assess for a thrill at the heart's base. Use the finger pads to palpate a thrill at the suprasternal notch and along the carotid arteries. A thrill is not found in the healthy child. A thrill's anatomic location corresponds to a particular structural abnormality within the heart. For example, a thrill in the pulmonic area is felt at the second and third intercostal space on the upper left sternal border. A thrill at the second intercostal space on the right upper sternal border is attributed to pathology in the aorta.

Peripheral Pulses

Use the same finger to assess each peripheral pulse. The sensation of one finger pad versus another can be different. Use the finger pads to palpate each pair of peripheral pulses simultaneously, except for the carotid pulses. The carotid pulses should not be palpated together because excessive stimulation can elicit a vagal response and slow down the heart. Palpating both carotid pulses at the same time could also cut off circulation to the child's head. Palpate the brachial and femoral pulses simultaneously. Pulse qualities are the same in the adult and the child. A brachial-femoral lag, when femoral pulses are weaker than brachial pulses when palpated simultaneously, is abnormal and occurs in a cardiac defect know as coarctation of the aorta (COA). COA is due to a narrowing of the aorta before, at, or just beyond the entrance of the ductus arteriosus, which causes reduced blood flow to the lower body.

If coarctation of the aorta is suspected (as when a brachial-femoral lag is present), obtain all four extremity blood pressures and compare the upper and lower extremity readings on each side. Remember to use an appropriately sized cuff. Refer to the section *Vital Signs: Blood Pressure* for information about determination of proper cuff size. Take the upper extremity blood pressure in the right arm. Because weak or absent leg pulses accompany coarctation, measurements are difficult to obtain. Use a Doppler transducer to intensify the sound of the pulse. Until you feel proficient, the Doppler technique requires two people for accurate measurement; have the caregiver hold the child's leg still while you assess the pulse. Locate the posterior tibial pulse with the Doppler transducer and make an "X" with a pen where the pulse is felt or heard. Place an appropriately sized cuff on the lower right leg. The lower edge of the cuff should be $1/2$ inch to 1 inch above the presumed posterior tibial pulse location. Apply a small amount of ultrasound gel to the area surrounding the presumed pulse. Turn the Doppler transducer on and adjust the volume control while the attached probe is locating the pulse. When a pulse is identified, proceed with the blood pressure measurement. Only the systolic number is obtained with this technique. Repeat the steps on the left side of body.

Normally, upper and lower extremity blood pressures are equal. If the systolic blood pressure in the leg is lower than that in the arm and femoral, popliteal, posterior tibial, or dorsalis pedis pulses are weak or absent, you can assume coarctation of the aorta is present. If undiagnosed, as the child becomes older, the upper extremity pulses are bounding.

REFLECTIONS FROM FAMILIES

My 2-year-old son is always so frightened and upset when he goes in for his well-child checkup. I was so relieved during his last visit because the nurse practitioner knew exactly how to help him calm down. She kneeled down so she was on his level and talked with him before the exam. She allowed him to handle some of the equipment, like the stethoscope, before using it on him. At no time was he completely undressed. He was so cooperative and never cried. The whole experience was better than it had ever been.

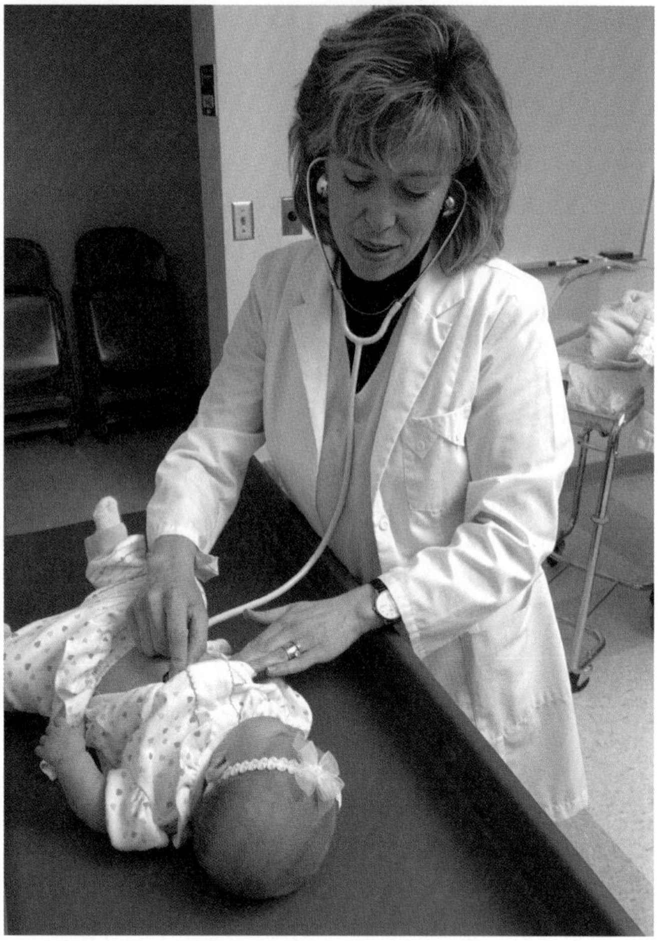

Figure 14-14 Auscultation of the heart requires a quiet infant.

Auscultation

Heart Sounds

Auscultating the infant's or the young pediatric child's heart is difficult because the heart rate is rapid and breath sounds are easily transmitted through the chest wall. Have the child lie down. If this position is not possible, the child should be held at a 45° angle in the caregiver's arms. A quiet environment and child is optimum in order to properly listen to the heart (Figure 14-14). Use the Z pattern to auscultate the heart. Place the stethoscope in the apical area and gradually move it toward the right lower sternal border and up the sternal border in a right diagonal line. Move gradually from the child's left to the right upper sternal borders (Figure 14-15). Perform a second evaluation with the child in a sitting position.

Fifty percent of all children develop an innocent murmur at some time in their lives. Innocent murmurs are not associated with pathology and are accentuated in high cardiac output states such as fever. When the child is sitting, they are heard early in systole at the second or third intercostal space along the left sternal border and are softly musical in quality; they disappear when the child lies down. Refer to Chapter 25 for specific information about types of murmurs. Be aware of sinus arrhythmias during auscultation of the heart's rhythm. Sinus arrhythmia is normal in many children. On inspiration, the pulse rate speeds up, the pulse rate slows with expiration. To determine if the rhythm is normal, ask the child to hold his or her breath while you auscultate the heart. If the heart rate variability stops, then a sinus arrhythmia is present.

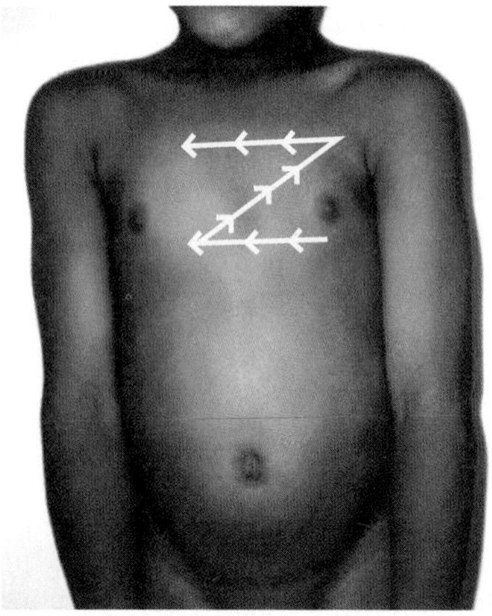

Figure 14-15 Z Auscultation Pattern for Young Children

S_1 is best heard at the apex of the heart, left lower sternal border. S_2 is best heard at the heart base. A fixed split S_2 that does not vary with respiration is abnormal, and you can suspect an atrial septal defect (ASD). In children, S_2 physiologically splits with inspiration and becomes single with expiration. This phenomenon is due to a greater negative pressure in the thoracic cavity. In children, S_3 often sounds like the three syllables of the word "Kentucky," especially when accompanied by tachycardia. A loud third heart sound may be present in children with CHF or VSD.

Nursing Tip:

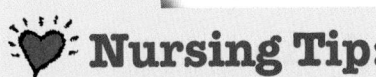

Assessing for umbilical hernias in children

If the child is upset and crying, assess the umbilicus for an outward projection, which is indicative of an umbilical hernia. If an umbilical hernia is present, palpate the area to determine if the hernia reduces easily. Approximate the size of the inner ring (the diameter of the hernia).

Abdomen

General Approach

If possible, ask the caregiver to refrain from feeding the infant prior to the assessment because palpation of a full stomach may induce vomiting. Children who are physically able should be encouraged to empty the bladder prior to the assessment. The young infant, school-aged child, or adolescent should lie on the examination table. For the toddler or preschooler, have the caregiver hold the child supine on the lap, with the lower extremities bent at the knees. If the child is crying, encourage the caregiver to help calm the child before you proceed with the assessment. Observe nonverbal communication in children who are not able to verbally express feelings. The order of abdominal assessment is inspection, auscultation, and palpation. Auscultation is performed second because palpation can alter bowel sounds. During palpation, listen for a high-pitched cry and look for a change in facial expression or for sudden protective movements that may indicate a painful or tender area.

Inspection

Observe the abdomen for a distinct separation of the rectus muscles with a visible bulge along the midline known as **diastasis recti.** Normally the abdominal musculature is continuous. A separated abdominal muscle that lies vertically is abnormal. The gap between the two edges may range from 1 to 5 centimeters. Diastasis recti is more common in African-American infants and usually disappears by early childhood.

Nursing Tip:

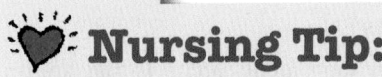

Measuring the abdomen in children

If abdominal distension is seen during inspection, evaluate its circumference. Place the tape measure around the abdomen at the level of the umbilicus. If serial abdominal circumference measurements are to be taken, use a marking pen to indicate the location where the tape measure was placed.

Peristaltic Wave

Observe the abdominal wall below the xiphoid process and above the symphysis pubis for wave-like movements. Peristalsis is not normally visible. Visible peristaltic waves seen moving across the epigastrium from left to right are abnormal and may occur in the gastrointestinal disorder pyloric stenosis. In this condition, the pyloric muscle hypertrophies, resulting in obstruction at the pyloric sphincter. Refer to Chapter 23 for more information about pyloric stenosis.

Auscultation

After performing auscultation of the lungs, it is helpful to proceed to auscultating the abdomen because doing so allows you to complete a good portion of auscultation all at once. If the child is not cooperating, a simple distracting phrase such as "I can hear your breakfast in there" is helpful during auscultation.

Palpation

General Palpation

Perform the exact same technique and sequence of light and deep palpation as done with the adult. On palpation, an olive-shaped mass felt in the epigastric area and to the upper right of the umbilicus is abnormal and is indicative of pyloric stenosis. Abdominal distension coupled with palpable stool over the abdomen and the absence of stool in the rectum is abnormal. An aganglionic segment of the colon is responsible for Hirschsprung's disease, which produces these abnormal gastrointestinal (GI) findings. A sausage-shaped mass that produces intermittent pain when palpated in the upper abdomen is abnormal. This is a manifestation of another GI disorder called intussusception. Bowel sounds heard in the thoracic cavity, a scaphoid abdomen, an upward displaced apical impulse, and signs of respiratory distress are abnormal findings in the newborn and suggest a diaphragmatic hernia. More information on gastrointestinal alterations are found in Chapter 23.

Liver Palpation

For infants and toddlers, use the outer edge of your right thumb to press down and scoop up at the right upper quadrant. For the remaining age groups, use the same technique as for an adult. The liver is not normally palpated, although the liver edge can be found 1–2 cm below the right costal margin in a normal, healthy child. The liver edge is soft and regular. It is abnormal for the liver edge to be palpated more than 2 cm below the right costal margin and be full with a firm, sharp border. Hepatomegaly occurs in several disease states such as viral or bacterial illnesses, tumors, congestive heart failure, and fat and glycogen storage diseases. Viral and bacterial illnesses and tumors cause liver cells to multiply in number, creating an enlarged liver. In heart failure, the hepatic veins and sinusoids enlarge from congestion, resulting in hemorrhage and fibrosis of the liver. In fat and glycogen storage diseases, fat and glycogen accumulate within the liver, and fibrosis ensues.

Musculoskeletal System

General Approach

The extent or degree of assessment depends greatly on the child's or caregiver's complaints of musculoskeletal problems. Be aware that, during periods of rapid growth, children complain of normal muscle aches. Try to incorporate musculoskeletal assessment techniques into other system assessments. For instance, while inspecting the integument, inspect the muscles and joints. Inspecting the musculoskeletal system in the ambulatory child is accomplished by allowing the child to move freely about and play in the examination room while you inquire about the health history. Your observations of the child enable you to assess posture, muscle symmetry, and range of motion of muscles and joints. Do not rush through the assessment. Throughout the assessment, incorporate game playing that facilitates evaluation of the musculoskeletal system. Observe range of motion and joint flexibility as the child undresses.

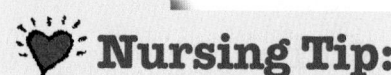

> **Nursing Tip:**
>
> **Palpating muscle strength in children**
> Playing games will assist you if the child is resistant to formal examination. For example, you can test plantar flexion by asking the child to pretend that the feet are pushing the brake on a car while you bear the force with your hands.

Inspection

Muscles

Assessment of the muscles includes examination of muscle mass (size), muscle tone, muscle strength, gross and fine motor ability, and involuntary movements.

Muscle Mass (Size)

Note the symmetry and alignment of muscle mass by comparing one side of the body with the other. Muscles should have a firmness when palpated. In most instances muscle size and firmness will be equal. Muscles should be measured if hypertrophy or atrophy is suspected.

Muscle Tone

Muscle tone is best evaluated by observation of active range of motion. Note any resistance, rigidity, spasticity, hypotonia, flaccidity, or paralysis as the child performs range of motion of the neck, spine, and extremities. Increased muscle tone (spasticity) is abnormal and may indicate cerebral palsy (CP), which results from a nonprogressive abnormality in the pyramidal motor tract. One of the more common contributing factors, perinatal asphyxia, causes abnormal posture and gross motor development and varying degrees of abnormal muscle tone. Refer to Chapter 32 for more information about CP.

Muscle Strength

To evaluate the strength of the infant's shoulder muscles, place your hands under the axillae and pull the infant into a standing position. The infant should not slip through your hands. Be prepared to catch the infant if needed. Evaluate the infant's leg strength in a semi-standing position. Lower the infant to the examination table so the infant's legs touch the table. Place the infant older than 4 months in a prone position. Observe the infant's ability to lift the upper body off the examination table using the upper extremities.

In children beyond infancy note the symmetry of strength by testing muscles with and without your resistance. To test hand strength, ask the child to squeeze your fingers hard. To test upper extremity strength, have the child flex each of her/his arms while you attempt to pull the forearm into extension. To test lower extremity strength, ask the child to keep the legs extended straight while you attempt to push each into flexion. Another method of testing the legs involves asking the child to stand, rising from a supine position. The child with good muscle strength is able to rise to a standing position without using the arms for leverage. The inability to rise from a sitting to a standing position is abnormal and occurs in the child with Duchenne's muscular dystrophy (MD) due to generalized muscle weakness. A further discussion of MD can be found in Chapter 34.

Gross and Fine Motor Ability

Assessment of gross motor function determines the child's ability to move large muscles in a coordinated and integrative manner. The status of gross motor function may be noted through observation of the coordination of the body in walking, sitting, and other activities that require the use of large muscles and joints. Fine motor function is assessed by determining the child's ability to coordinate small muscles. These types of movements require more precision and refinement in execution and in the visual-perceptual integration. Examples of these skills include grasping, holding, manipulating, and releasing objects. Use the Denver II to screen gross and fine motor skills that are appropriate for the child's specific age.

Involuntary Movements

Normally, no involuntary movements occur. If they are present, note their location, frequency, rate, and amplitude. Note if the movements can be controlled at will. Abnormalities include tremors, tics, twisting, and jerking and irregular movements.

Joints and Spine

Observe the medial, lateral, toe, and heel aspects of both shoes for signs of abnormal wear. Compare one shoe to the other for signs of excessive wear. Ask the ambulatory child to walk at least 10 feet. Note the scapula's position and symmetry. Note the flexibility of the radiocarpal, elbow, shoulder, hip, tibiofemoral, and tibiotalar joints while the child is walking. Inspect the joints from head to toe. The infant's spine is C-shaped. Head control and standing create the normal S-shaped spine of the adult. Lordosis, an exaggerated lumbar curvature of the spine, is normal as the child begins to walk. A toddler's protruding abdomen is counterbalanced by an inward deviation of the lumbar spine. Lordosis is abnormal after 6 years of age. Lordosis can be attributed to bilateral developmental dislocation of the hip or postural factors such as progression of congenital kyphosis, or can occur secondary to contractures of hip flexors. The spine should also be assessed for scoliosis. Refer to Chapter 34 for the procedure and further information.

Count the fingers and toes. **Polydactyly,** extra fingers or toes, may be found in certain congenital syndromes. A fusion between two or more digits, called **syndactylism,** is abnormal. It is also associated with certain congenital syndromes. It is abnormal for a young male (usually 2–12 years old) to present with a painless limp from the affected hip. The limp is accompanied by limited abduction and internal rotation, muscle spasm, and proximal thigh atrophy. These are manifestations of Legg-Calvé-Perthes disease, also called coxa plana. It is caused by an interruption in the blood supply to the capital femoral epiphysis with avascular necrosis of the femoral head resulting. More information can be found in Chapter 34.

Tibiofemoral Bones

Instruct the child to stand on the examination table and with the medial condyles together. Measure the distance between the two medial malleoli. Measure the distance between the two medial condyles. Normally, the distance between the medial malleoli is less than 2 inches (5 cm). The distance between the medial condyles is less than 1 inch (2.5 cm). If the distance between the medial condyles is less than 1 inch (2.5 cm) and the distance between the medial malleoli is more than 2 inches (5 cm), the child has knock-knee, or genu valgum. This is common between 2 and 4 years of age. Genu valgum persisting after 6 years of age is abnormal. If the measured distance between the two medial condyles is greater than 1–2 inches, bowleg or genu varum is present. Genu varum is a common finding in infants and toddlers until walking has been firmly established. Genu varum persisting after 2 years of age is abnormal and may be caused by rickets.

Palpation

Joints

Palpate the joints for heat, tenderness, and swelling. Joint flexibilty values are within the same range as an adult. Findings are the same as the adult. Swollen, inflamed, painful joints, seen in juvenile rheumatoid arthritis (JRA), are abnormal. JRA causes synovial inflammation and degeneration of the joint. Its cause is unknown.

Feet

Stand in front of the child. Hold the right heel immobile with one hand while pushing the forefoot (medial base of great toe) toward a midline position with the other hand. Observe for toe and forefoot adduction and inversion. Repeat on the left foot.

Normal findings are that the toes and forefoot are not deviated. Metatarsus varus (club foot) is characterized by medially adducted and inverted toes and forefoot. Clubfoot usually results from an abnormal intrauterine position of the fetal foot. Heredity also plays a role in the etiology.

Hip and Femur

The hips should be evaluated to detect developmental dysplasia of the hip (DDH) (see Chapter 34). One method, the Ortolani maneuver, should be performed by a trained individual at the very end of the assessment because it may produce crying. The test is performed on one hip at a time. Evaluate the hips up until 12 months of age. Place the infant supine on an examination table with the feet facing you. Stand directly in front of the infant. With the thumb, hold the lesser trochanter of the femur and with the middle and third fingers, hold the greater trochanter (Figure 14-16A). These two fingers should rest over the hip joint. Slowly press outward and abduct until the lateral aspects of the knees nearly touch the table (Figure 14-16B). The tips of the fingers should palpate each femoral head as it rotates outward. Listen for an audible clunk, which indicates a positive Ortolani's sign. With the fingers in the same locations, adduct the hips to elicit a palpable clunk (Ortolani's sign). As each hip is adducted, it is lifted anteriorly into the acetabulum. Abnormal findings indicating DDH include a positive Ortolani's sign; a sudden, painful cry during the test; asymmetrical thigh skin folds; uneven knee level; and limited hip abduction. Epidemiology of DDH is related to familial factors, maternal hormones associated with pelvic laxity, first-born children, and breech presentations.

Neurological System

The neurological examination includes evaluation of function within six major areas: (1) the cerebrum, (2) cranial nerves, (3) the cerebellum, (4) the motor system, (5) the sensory system, and (6) reflex status.

Cerebral Function

Cerebral function is tested through an evaluation of behavior and mental status and includes appearance, judgment, memory, thought processes, language and speech, mood and affect, and orientation. An infant functions mainly at the subcortical

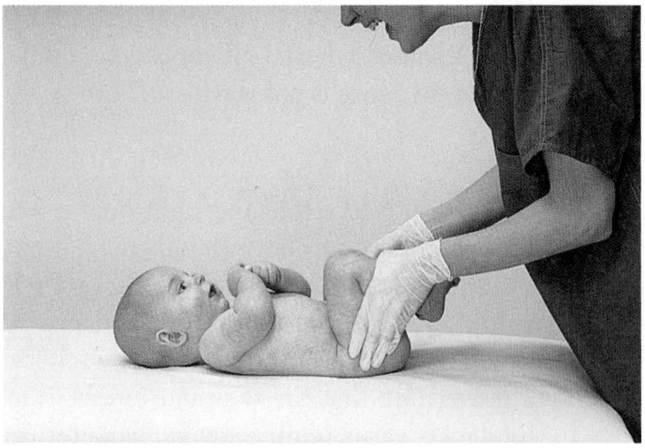

(A)

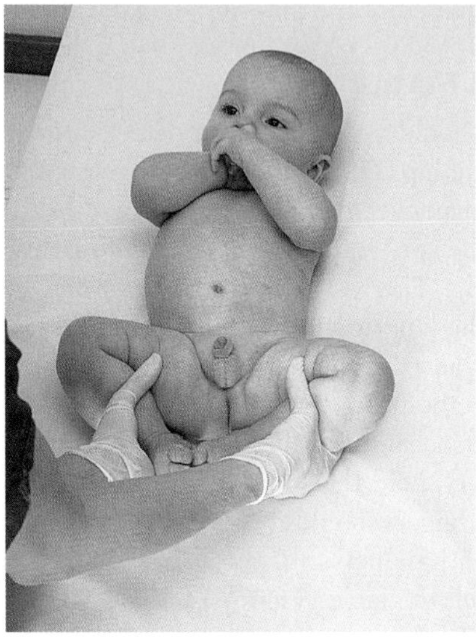

(B)

Figure 14-16 Ortolani Maneuver. (A) Hand Placement (B) Hip Abduction

level. Memory is about three-fourths developed by 2 years of age, when cortical functioning is acquiring dominance. Level of consciousness is also assessed as a function of the central nervous system. Because the infant cannot verbally express level of consciousness, instead assess the newborn's ability to cry, level of activity, positioning, and general appearance.

Cranial Nerves

A thorough assessment of cranial nerve function is difficult to perform on the infant less than 1 year old. Difficulty is also encountered with toddlers and preschoolers because they often cannot follow directions or are not willing to cooperate. Testing for the school-aged child or the adolescent is carried out in the same manner as for an adult.

Infant (Birth to 12 Months)

To test cranial nerves (CNs) III (oculomotor), IV (trochlear), and VI (abducens), move a brightly colored toy along the infant's line of vision. An infant older than 1 month responds by following the object. Also evaluate the pupillary response to a bright light in each eye. CN V (trigeminal) is tested by assessing the rooting or sucking reflexes. CN VII (facial) is tested up until 2 months by assessng the sucking reflex and by observing symmetrical sucking movements. After 2 months of age, an infant will smile, allowing assessment of symmetry of facial expressions. A positive Moro reflex in an infant less than 6 months old is evidence of normal functioning of CN VIII (acoustic). CNs IX (glossopharyngeal) and X (vagus) are examined by using a tongue blade to produce a gag reflex. Do not test if a positive response was already elicited by using a tongue blade to view the posterior pharynx. To test Cranial Nerve XI (accessory), evaluate the infant's ability to lift the head up while in a prone position. CN XII (hypoglossal) is assessed by allowing the infant to suck on a pacifier or a bottle, abruptly removing the pacifier or bottle from the infant's mouth, and observing for lingering sucking movements.

Toddler and Preschooler (1 to 6 Years)

The older preschooler is able to identify familiar odors. Most children readily identify the smell of peanut butter and chocolate. Test CN I (olfactory) one side at a time by asking the child to close the eyes and to identify the smell of peanut butter and chocolate. Test each nostril with different substances while occluding the other nostril with your finger. Test vision (CN II [optic]) using Allen cards. CNs III, IV, and VI are tested in the same fashion as for the infant. CN V is tested by giving the child something to eat and evaluating chewing movements. Sensory responses to light and sharp touch are still not easily interpreted in these age groups. Observe facial weakness or paralysis (CN VII) by making the child smile or laugh. An older preschooler may cooperate by raising the eyebrows, frowning, puffing the cheeks out, and closing the eyes tightly on command. To evaluate CN VIII, ring a small bell out of the child's vision and observe the response to unseen sounds. Test CNs IX and X in the same manner as for the infant. CN XII is difficult to assess in this particular age group.

Cerebellar Function

Tests for cerebellar function mainly involve evaluation of posture, balance, and coordination. General evaluation of

Nursing Alert:

Allergic Reaction to Inhaled Substances

Be aware of the child's allergies prior to testing CN I. For example, even the smell of peanut butter can cause a severe allergic reaction in some children. In such cases, use a different aromatic source when testing CN I.

function includes observation of the child's body posture, stance, and gait; watching the child walk heel-to-toe, jump, skip, hop, and throw. The Romberg test is administered to evaluate balance by having the child stand with feet together, arms at side, and eyes open and then closed. If the child falls, loses balance, or leans to one side, the result is positive and indicates cerebellar dysfunction.

Motor System

Motor system function usually is evaluated as part of the musculoskeletal system examination and was discussed in that section.

Sensory System

Sensory function involves the body's response to various types of stimulation and usually is assessed during testing of cranial nerve function.

Reflex Status

Assessment of reflex status includes deep tendon reflexes (DTR), superficial, and newborn (often referred to as infant) reflexes.

Deep Tendon Reflexes

Measurement of the DTRs reveals the intactness of the reflex arc at specific spinal levels and are tested in the same manner as with an adult. The following reflexes are routinely tested: upper extremities—biceps, triceps, and brachioradialis; lower extremities—patellar and Achilles. DTRs are evaluated for strength and symmetry of right and left sides, which should be equal. The tendon is slightly stretched and tapped with a reflex hammer. The expected response is contraction of the muscle.

Superficial Reflexes

With superficial reflexes the receptors are in the skin rather than the muscles as in the DTRs. Superficial reflexes that are tested include the abdominal, cremasteric (testes), gluteal (buttocks), and plantar. They are elicited by stimulating the skin.

Newborn (Infant) Reflexes

During infancy, examination includes identification of the presence or absence of newborn reflexes, which must be lost before motor development can proceed. See Chapter 7 for discussion of these reflexes.

Female Genitalia

General Approach

Place the up-to-preschool-aged child on the caregiver's lap or examination table. Ask the caregiver to assist by holding the legs in a froglike position. Place the child older than 4 years on the examination table in a semilithotomy position, without the feet in stirrups. Reserve the lithotomy position with the feet in stirrups for the older adolescent. Explain the procedure prior to the assessment. Never ask the caregiver of the infant or young school-aged child to leave the room during this portion of the examination because the caregiver is a source of comfort to the child. Drape the older-than-preschool-aged child.

A vaginal/pelvic exam is not routinely performed on young females; however, it is warranted when signs of possible sexual abuse are present. Refer to Chapter 36 for information regarding sexual abuse. The assessment is undertaken by a health care provider who is trained to perform pediatric vaginal examinations and can evaluate these problems. Any female who has reached menarche needs to be evaluated for a pregnant uterus.

Inspection

Perineal Area

Stand directly in front of the child. Assess Tanner's stage (Appendix F). Use the thumb and forefinger to separate the labia. Identify the labia majora and minora, clitoris, urethral meatus, hymen, and vaginal orifice. Observe color, size, and discharge from structures. Observe intactness and scarring of the hymen and vaginal orifice. The infant's labia minora are sometimes larger than the labia majora. The hymen is sometimes intact up until the point of sexual activity. It is abnormal for the female infant to display a rudimentary penis in the clitoral area, which is a finding in ambiguous genitalia. Genital ambiguity occurs during embryonic development as a consequence of genetic causes or androgens or androgen inhibitors that reverse genital characteristics. A bloody discharge noted at the vaginal opening or on the diaper is abnormal. It is not uncommon to note pseudomenstruation in an infant under 2 weeks of age. Maternal hormones such as estrogen are the cause.

Male Genitalia

General Approach

Female nurses may encounter difficulty assessing a reluctant adolescent. Be firm when explaining that this portion of the assessment is a required part of his examination. Infants and toddlers do not object to the assessment. In case the infant or toddler urinates during the examination, have a diaper or disposable cloth available to catch the stream of urine. The older school-aged child and the adolescent should be draped in order to maintain modesty. Assess Tanner's stages during inspection.

Penis

Note the position of the urethral meatus. Note the size of the penis. If you are not able to determine circumcision status, ask the caregiver if the child was circumcised. The meatus is normally found on the tip of the penis. A disappearing penis phenomenon occurs normally in infants with increased adipose tissue in the area surrounding the penis. Reassure the caregiver that this is normal and will resolve after adipose tissue is lost. It is abnormal for the urethral meatus to be located behind or along the ventral side of the penis, a condition known as hypospadias. During the third month of fetal development, the urethral meatus fails to move toward the glans penis. Mothers who take phenytoin (Dilantin) for epilepsy are at greater risk for having children with hypospadias. Another abnormality is epispadius in which the meatal opening is on the dorsal surface of the penis. During the third month of fetal development, the urethral meatus fails to move toward the glans penis.

Scrotum

Evaluate scrotal size and color. Note if the testes are seen in the scrotal sac. The scrotum appears proportionately large in size when compared to the penis. The sac color is brown or black in dark-skinned children and pink in light-skinned children. Two testes should be present, but, in infants, they may retract into the inguinal canal or abdomen due to various stimuli, including cold and palpation.

Palpation

Scrotum

Place the infant in a supine position on the examination table. Instruct the young child to sit cross-legged to inhibit the **cremasteric reflex** (retraction of the testes from the scrotum) from occurring. Locate each testis within the scrotal sac by using the fingers of one hand in a milking motion to descend the testes. Palpate and note the size, shape, and mobility of each testis. Both testicles are palpated in the scrotum. They are smooth, round, or oval shaped and freely movable. It is abnormal to be unable to palpate the testes. **Cryptorchidism** is a failure of the testis to descend into the scrotal sac. One or both testes failing to descend within the inguinal canal occurs during embryonic development. An enlargement of the scrotum is abnormal and is seen in a congenital hydrocele, which results from failure of the fetal male reproductive tract to develop properly. This mass will transilluminate. Refer to Chapter 22 for additional information about genitourinary disorders.

Hernia

Place the infant supine on the examination table. All other children should stand during the examination. Use your little finger for the infant's exam and the index finger for the younger child's. Follow the inguinal canal as is done on an adult male. If possible, perform the assessment on a crying infant. Have preschoolers and early school-aged children attempt to blow up a balloon while you palpate the inguinal areas. Palpate the inguinal areas while the older school-aged child or adolescent coughs. No swelling or masses are palpated. A hernia palpated above the inguinal ligament is an abnormal finding. Indirect inguinal hernias occur during embryologic development as a result of persistent patency of the processus vaginalis testis.

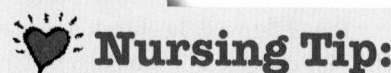

> **Nursing Tip:**
>
> **Anal reflex and sexual abuse**
>
> Anal trauma, such as occurs in sexual assault, manifests as poor anal sphincter control. Consider sexual abuse if a child exhibits an absent or slow anal reflex.

Anus

As a rule, rectal assessments are not performed on children unless you detect a problem or suspect abuse. In these cases, refer the child for further evaluation if you are not trained specifically for this procedure and follow your institution's guidelines.

Inspection

Ask the child to lie on the abdomen. Gently separate the buttocks to allow direct visualization of the anal opening. Observe for bleeding, fissures, prolapse, skin tags, hemorrhoids, lesions, and pinworms. During separation of the buttocks, observe any movement of the anus. Stroke the perianal area with your finger, and note any movement. This is called the anal reflex or anal wink. No bleeding, fissures, prolapse, skin tags, hemorrhoids, lesions, or pinworms should be present. An anal reflex normally is observed. An absent anal reflex is abnormal. Conditions such as a spinal cord lesion, trauma, and tumors that interrupt nervous innervation to the anal sphincter cause this finding.

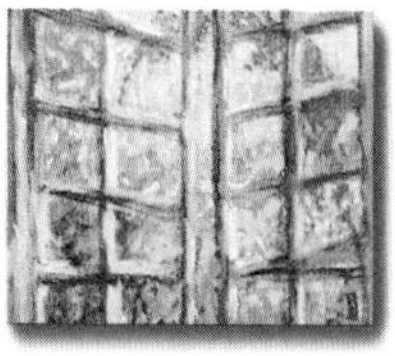

In the Real World

As a nursing student I was completely overwhelmed by the numerous sounds that the heart made. I could not always tell if I was listening to an infant's second or third heart sound because their heart was beating so rapidly. How was I going to describe the murmur? One of the pediatricians I worked with told me not to worry. He further said it had taken him at least a thousand settings of auscultating hearts before he could differentiate various sounds in pediatrics.

Case Study/Care Plan

The Client with Congenital Heart Disease

Lisa is a 6-month-old infant born with a complete atrioventricular canal (CAVC) defect and Down syndrome. Mrs. Mitchell, Lisa's mother, took her for a routine 6-month check-up.

Health History

Legal Guardian

Rose Mitchell (biological mother and caregiver)

Source of Information

Caregiver

Patient Profile

6-month-old BF

Chief Complaint

(Per caregiver): "I have noticed Lisa taking a lot more time to eat & she is always working hard to breathe."

History of Present Illness

2 d PTA, Mrs. Mitchell noticed pt was taking 45 min to feed in contrast to her nl 20–30 min. During the feed, pt diaphoretic. Mrs. Mitchell feels pt's respirations are more labored; changing 4 wet diapers/d (had been 7–8).

Past Health History

Birth History

Prenatal

2 prior spontaneous miscarriages; denies drug, ETOH, tobacco, or caffeine use during pregnancy; viral illness in 1st trimester; sought prenatal care at 2 mo p̄ missed period; unplanned pregnancy for caregivers

Labor and Delivery

38-wk gestation delivered via C-section (failure to progress) p̄ a 24-hr labor, not able to hold baby p̄ birth in delivery room, baby's mucous membranes pale pink, does not remember Apgar scores, birth wt 8 lb, length 22 in.

Postnatal

Pt transported to another facility at 2 d for cardiac catheterization, d/c at 2 wk of age, caregivers visited infant qd in hospital, poor feeding, d/c on NGT (q other feeding), afebrile during hospitalization

Medical

CAVC defect, Down syndrome

Surgical

None

Medications

Digoxin 0.02 mg po bid (q 12°), Lasix 3 mg po bid (q 12°), Aldactone 6.25 mg po qd am

continues

continued

Communicable Diseases

Mother denies exposure to TB, HIV

Allergies

NKDA, Enfamil c̄ Fe produces diarrhea & wt loss

Injuries/Accidents

None

Disabilities/Handicaps

Developmentally delayed

Blood Transfusions

None

Childhood Illnesses

0 recent exposure to MMR, pertussis, chickenpox

Immunizations

Has had 2 DTP (2 mo, 4 mo), 2 OPVs (2 mo, 4 mo), 2 hepatitis B vaccines (2 mo, 4 mo), 2 Hib (2 mo, 4 mo)

Family Health History

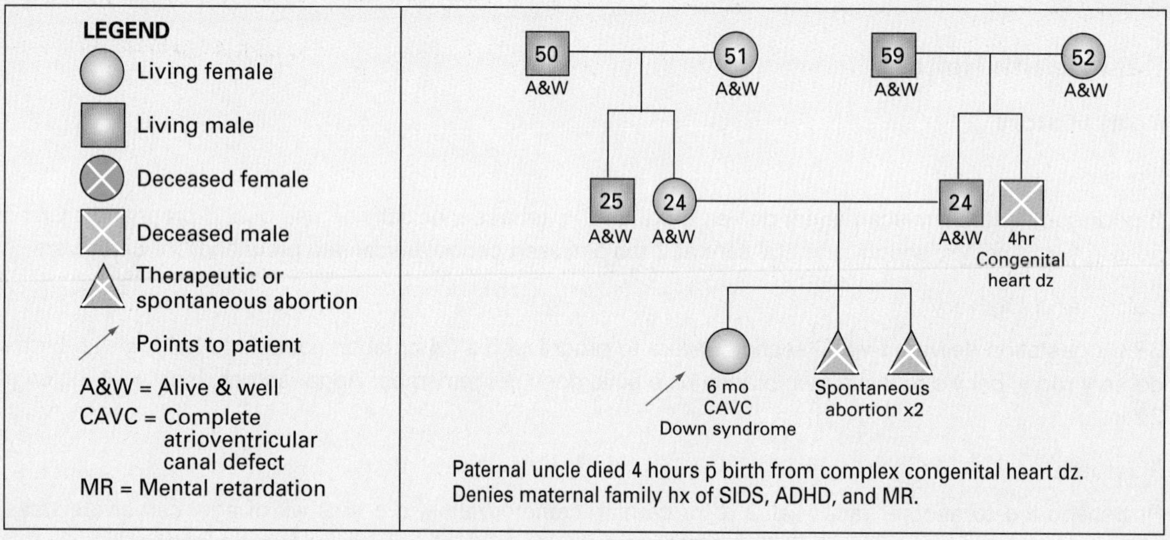

Social History

Alcohol, Tobacco, Drug Use, Sexual Practice

N/A

Travel History

Never left her home town

School Performance

Enrolled in county's early intervention program, has PT & OT 2 ×/wk, mom does PT exercises on remaining days

continues

continued

Home Environment

Family lives in 3 BR home built in 1978; 0 guns in home; neither caregiver drinks ETOH or takes illicit drugs; 0 pets

Hobbies, Leisure Activities, Stress, Education

N/A

Economic Status

Lisa's parents have hl care insurance that covers most expenses

Military Service

N/A

Religion

Baptist

Ethnic Background

African American

Roles/Relationships

Caregivers married; mom stays at home c̄ infant; FOB assists when home; 0 recent life changes; both caregivers collaborate on hl care decisions

Child's Personal Habits

Does best c̄ mom holding her during stressful periods

Characteristic Patterns of Daily Living

Wakes at 7 AM, takes meds then formula; lies on mat c̄ toys while mother fixes breakfast; 5 ×/wk mother does PT for 30 min, then pt takes formula, naps 45 min, sits in bouncer seat while mother fixes lunch; mother plays c̄ pt until next feed, when pt takes formula; mother sings & reads stories; pt naps 45 min; outdoor walk in stroller; pt takes formula, then sits in swing while mother makes supper; FOB comes home from work & plays c̄ pt; pt sits in bouncer seat c̄ parents at dinner; FOB gives bath, administers meds & gives formula; pt goes to bed at 8 PM.

Health Maintenance Activities

Sleep

11 hr at night, 2 naps (45 min each)

Diet

Bottle-fed c̄ Isomil plus Moducal added to formula to yield 30 calories/oz; was taking 28 oz qd; in past 2 d, has ↓ to 23 oz qd; no solids have been introduced, no MVI given

Exercise

PT

Stress Management

N/A

continues

continued

Use of Safety Devices

Car seat in rear-facing position in back seat only

Safety

House has been childproofed c̄ outlet covers, gates on stairs, poisons & cleaning supplies in locked cabinet, meds in shoe box on highest shelf in closet, table edge protectors, bumpers over hearth's edge, poison control # posted next to phone, smoke detectors upstairs & downstairs, fire extinguisher in kitchen; have not devised escape route for fires; parents both CPR trained ā pt d/c from hospital, would dial 911 for an emergency

Health Check-Ups

At 2 & 4 mo; sees cardiologist q month

Development

Motor

Able to roll from side to back, follows moving object c̄ eyes, attempts to hold objects & attempts to hold head up while in prone position

Cognitive

Gurgles & coos

Social

Smiles, pays attention to familiar voices, & recognizes caregiver

Physical Assessment

Vital Signs

T: 99.6°F Ⓡ; apical HR: 140; RR: 60; BP: 88/42 mm Hg (RUE, supine)

Physical Growth

Wt: 10 lb 8 oz; length: 25 in; head circumference: 40.0 cm; chest circumference: 39.5 cm

Skin

Inspection

No erythema, papules, vesicles, edema, scaling, or ulcerations; Mongolian spot 4 × 5 cm noted over lumbar-sacral area

Palpation

Soft, smooth s̄ roughness, dryness, scaliness, or keratic areas; turgor WNL, diaphoretic along hairline & forehead; arms & legs warm & clammy bilaterally

Hair and Nails

Inspection and Palpation

s̄ alopecia, infestations; cap refill 4 sec UE & LE

Head

Inspection

Symmetrical, round, no bulges or prominence of forehead or involuntary mvt, face symmetrical, unsteady head control

continues

continued

Palpation

Anterior fontanel soft & flat (1.5 cm × 1.0 cm), posterior fontanel closed, suture lines not overriding, no edema

Eyes

Vision Screening

Bilateral symmetrical light reflex c̄ Hirschberg test, no malalignment of eyes c̄ cover-uncover test

Inspection

No ptosis, inner epicanthal folds present, producing tears, sclera light & muddy, conjunctiva pale pink, cornea smooth & transparent, iris brown, Brushfield's spots around perimeter of iris (OU), PERRL, ⊕ red reflex, optic discs creamy pink, round, borders regular s̄ hemorrhages

Ears

Auditory Testing

Reacts to loud noises

Inspection (External Ear)

Top of pinna positioned $^{1}/_{8}$" below outer canthus, pinna s̄ lesions or masses

Palpation (External Ear)

No pain c̄ mvt

Inspection (Internal Ear)

No erythema; sm amt cerumen in EAC; bilateral TMs pearly s̄ retraction, bulging, perforation, fluid, or air bubbles; mobility c̄ pneumatic bulb; landmarks intact; ⊕ light reflex

Nose

Inspection

Patent nares c̄ flaring, mucosa pale pink, septum midline, no edema of turbinates

Mouth and Throat

Inspection

Lips pale pink, no fissures/cracking, edges meet; buccal mucosa pale pink s̄ lesions; Ø teeth; tongue pale pink, thick, & midline, protrudes slightly, s̄ fasciculations; high, arched palate; both hard/soft palates intact s̄ lesions; tonsils 1+, no erythema or exudate; uvula midline; oropharynx pink s̄ exudate

Neck

Inspection

Symmetrical, short & thin, s̄ edema; active ROM

Palpation

Thyroid nonpalpable, trachea midline, s̄ lymphadenopathy

Breasts and Regional Lymphatics

Inspection

Tanner stage I; no retractions, erythema, venous distention, edema, ulcerations; areolas circular & even bilaterally, neg masses & ulcerations; nipples circular s̄ retractions/inversions, erythema, d/c, ulcerations or supranumerary nipples

continues

continued

Palpation

Breasts neg for nodes glands, masses, or tenderness; axillary area: nonpalpable nodes, neg tenderness or masses

Thorax and Lungs

Inspection

Thorax rounded, moderate intercostal retractions

Palpation

↓ Tactile fremitus RLL

Percussion

Diaphragmatic excursion 1 ICS on Ⓛ (hyperresonant), unable to obtain on Ⓡ (dull)

Auscultation

Breath sounds = bilaterally, bronchial sounds over trachea, bronchovesicular breath sounds throughout peripheral lung fields, coarse crackles throughout

Heart and Peripheral Vasculature

Inspection

Apical impulse at 4th ICS to Ⓛ of MCL; 0 heaves, lifts of precordium; 0 clubbing of fingers or toes; neg JVD

Palpation

Neg thrills on precordium, suprasternal notch & carotids; 0 brachial-femoral lag using Ⓡ brachial, Ⓡ femoral artery; pulses 2+/4+ bilaterally

Auscultation

Apical HR even & regular, nl S_1, narrowly split S_2, ⊕ S_3, 0 S_4, III/VI systolic ejection murmur along LSB

Abdomen

Inspection

Rounded & symmetrical c̄ inverted umbilicus, abd musculature continuous, 0 visible peristalsis

Auscultation

Hyperactive BS in 4 quadrants; 0 venous hums, 0 bruits @ femoral, iliac, renal, and aortic areas; 0 peritoneal friction rub

Percussion

Tympanic; neg fluid shift

Palpation

0 pain or tenderness, 0 masses, liver edge down 3.0 cm from RCM, spleen tip 1.0 cm from LCM, kidneys not palpable

continues

continued

Musculoskeletal

Inspection

AROM & hyperextensibility of all 4 extremities, attempts to hold head up in prone position, unable to lift chest off table in prone position, C-shaped spine

Palpation

Strength: $^{2}/_{5}$ of all muscle groups; toes & forefoot not deviated; neg for hip pain & limitation of mvt; neg Ortolani's maneuver

Neurological

Inspection

Alert, smiling, reaching for objects; ⊕ Babinski, ⊕ suck; CN III–XII grossly intact; DTR 2+/4+

Female Genitalia

Inspection

Tanner stage I, labia dark pink s̄ hypertrophy, excoriation, ulcerations; no vaginal d/c; perineum smooth s̄ lacerations; hymen intact

Anus

Inspection

Anal area darker pink in color than perineum; s̄ lesions, bleeding, fissures, prolapse, hemorrhoids

Laboratory Data

Chemistry

	Pt's Values	Normal Range
Sodium	139 mEq/L	135–145 mEq/L
Potassium	5.4 mEq/L	3.5–5.0 mEq/L
Chloride	89 mEq/L	95–105 mEq/L
Carbon Dioxide	37.0 mEq/L	18–27 mEq/L
Calcium	11.1 mg/dl	8.0-11.0 mg/dl
Glucose	98 mg/dl	60-100 mg/dl
BUN	14 mg/dl	6.0-23.0 mg/dl
Creatinine	0.5 mg/dl	0.2–0.5 mg/dl

Diagnostic Data

Radiological Report

AP and Lateral Chest X-Ray

The overall heart size is enlarged, with the right heart border being unusually rounded, suggesting right atrial prominence. The lungs are grossly hyperinflated, with uneven aeration and patchy infiltrate in the right upper lobe. The pulmonary vascularity is increased and slightly congested. The aortic arch is left-sided.

Key Concepts

- The parameters of weight, length, or height, and head circumference (dependent on age) are essential for assessing physical growth. Using standardized growth charts, these measurements are used in determining normal and abnormal patterns.
- A pediatric health history includes biographical data, past health history, family health history, social history, and health maintenance activities.
- A nutritional assessment enables the nurse to provide anticipatory guidance, identify at-risk individuals, and collaborate with the health care team for early referral of the child as needed.
- A developmental assessment has several purposes: (1) validation that a child is developing normally or detects problems early, (2) identification of concerns of caregivers and child, and (3) provision of an opportunity for anticipatory guidance and teaching about age-appropriate expectations.
- In performing the physical assessment, techniques for approaching children vary from one age group to the next. However, a basic principle during any physical assessment is building a trusting relationship.
- Vital signs include temperature, respiration, pulse, and blood pressure, which are compared to normal ranges for the child's age. These measurements provide information about the child's basic physiological status.
- The skin is observed for color and lesions and palpated to determine temperature, texture, turgor, and edema.
- The head is inspected for shape, symmetry, and control, and the fontanels, suture lines, and surface characteristics are palpated.
- Examination of the eyes includes vision and strabismus screening, and assessment of the anterior and posterior segment structures.
- The thorax and lungs are examined using inspection, palpation, percussion, and auscultation.
- Assessment of the heart and peripheral vasculature consists of inspection (apical impulse, precordium), palpation (thrills, peripheral pulses), and auscultation of heart sounds.
- The order of abdominal assessment is inspection, auscultation, and palpation.
- The extent or degree of musculoskeletal assessment depends on the caregiver's and child's complaints of problems.
- A neurological examination includes assessment of infant reflexes (depends on age) and cranial nerves.

Review Questions

1. Describe the components of a health history for a child. What information is gathered in the following areas: (a) past health history, (b) social history, and (c) health maintenance activities?
2. List two environmental problems that put a child at risk for illness or death.
3. What is the purpose of a nutritional assessment?
4. What information is included in a nutritional assessment?
5. Describe factors that could lead to invalid results from a developmental screening test?
6. State an easy rule of thumb for determining normal systolic blood pressure in children older than 1 year.
7. How would the nurse obtain a height and weight for a 12-month-old child?
8. Describe the sequence for assessing the abdomen.
9. Describe the cranial nerve assessment of an infant and a toddler.

References

American Academy of Pediatrics Committee on Practice and Ambulatory Medicine, Section on Opthalmology. (1996). Eye examination and vision screening in infants, children, and young adults. *Pediatrics, 98*(1), 153–157.

Estes, M. E. (2002). *Health assessment and physical examination* (2nd ed.). Albany, NY: Delmar.

Fisher, A. M., & Vessey, J. A. (1998). Preventing lead poisoning and its consequences. *Pediatric Nursing, 24*(4), 348–350.

Frankenburg, W. K. (1994). Preventing developmental delays: Is developmental screening sufficient? *Pediatrics, 93*(4), 586–593.

Jarvis, C. (1996). *Physical examination and health assessment* (2nd ed.). Philadelphia: Saunders.

Jones, K. F., Berg, J. H., & Coody, D. (1994). Update in pediatric dentistry. *Journal of Pediatric Health Care, 8*(4), 160–167.

National High Blood Pressure Education Program Working Group. (1996). Update on the 1987 task force on high blood pressure in children and adolescents. A working group report from the national high blood pressure education program. *Pediatrics, 98*, 649–657.

Seidel, H., Ball, J., Dains, J., & Benedict, G. (1995). *Mosby's guide to physical examination* (3rd ed.). St. Louis, MO: Mosby.

Sganga, A., Wallace, R., Kiehl, E., Irving, T., & Witter, L. (2000). A comparison of four methods of normal newborn temperature measurement. *MCN, 25*(2), 76.

U.S. Department of Agriculture. (1999). T*he food guide pyramid for young children*. Washington, DC: U.S. Government Printing Office.

Suggested Readings

Coats, K., & Jenkins, R. (1997). Vision assessment of the pediatric patient: Refinements. *American Academy of Opthalmology, 1*(1), 1–12.

Erikson, R., Meyer, L., & Woo, T. (1996). Accuracy of chemical dot thermometers in critically ill adults and children. *Image Journal of Nursing Scholarship, 28*(1), 23–28.

Gessner, I. H., & Victoria, B. E. (1993). *Pediatric cardiology*. Philadelphia: Saunders.

Giger, J. N., & Davidhizar, R. E. (1995). *Transcultural nursing*. St. Louis: Mosby.

Hay, W. W., Hayward, A., Levin, M., & Sondheimer, J. (2000). *Current pediatric diagnosis and treatment*. Stamford, CT: Appleton & Lange.

Hennigen, L., Kollar, L., & Rosenthal, S. (2000). Methods for managing pelvic examination anxiety: Individual differences and relaxing techniques. *Pediatric Health Care, 14*(1), 9–12.

McCance, K. L., & Huether, S. E. (1994). *Pathophysiology: The biologic basis for disease in adults and children* (2nd. ed.). St. Louis: Mosby.

Prazer, G. (1998). The aural infrared thermometer: A practitioner's perspective. *Journal of Pediatrics, 133*, 471–472.

Resources

Organizations and Websites

American Academy of Pediatrics
141 Northwest Point Blvd.
P.O. Box 747
Elk Grove Village, IL 60009-0747
(847) 434-4000

Denver Developmental Materials, Inc.
P.O. Box 6919
Denver, CO 80206-9019
(303) 355-4729
(800) 419-4729

National Association of Pediatric Nurse Associates and Practitioners
1101 Kings Highway North, Suite 206
Cherry Hill, NJ 08034-1912
(856) 667-1773
(877) 662-7627

CHAPTER 15

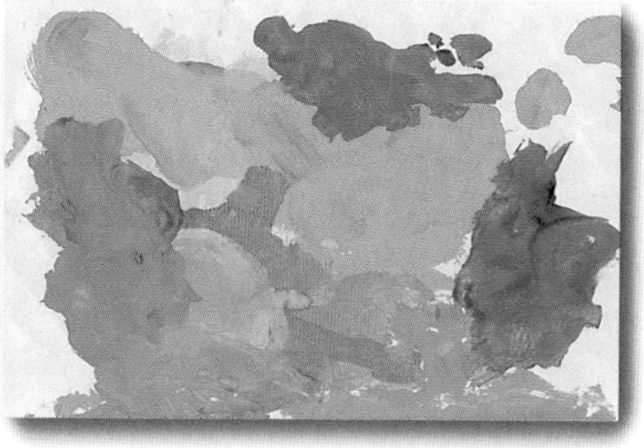

INFECTIOUS DISEASES

Barbara S. Kiernan, PhD, RN, CS, PNP

"Grandma, could you go with me to the health clinic today? Mom's at work and the baby needs to get her first set of shots?" my 25-year-old granddaughter asks as I hear her plaintive voice over the telephone. "I'm scared and not sure she needs to get this done. I hate to see her be hurt. I just need to have some moral support." As a retired nurse and doting grandmother, I am usually consulted when health crises arise.

However, I can understand why my granddaughter is thinking the way she is. Immunizations are not without controversy, but I can reflect as well about the progress that has been made in this country in preventing the incidence of childhood diseases through planned immunization practices. I remember my mother's stories of growing up in the early 20th century. Of the eight children born to her parents, only three survived into adulthood. Infectious diseases took their toll in her family by causing the deaths of five children, each one under the age of four. As a child in the early 1930s, I suffered through the throes of several infectious diseases without any consequences other than the inconvenience of being ill and feeling miserable. Immunizations came into practice as I was having children of my own, yet at the time of their childhood there was no protection against measles, mumps, rubella, or chickenpox. Polio was the scourge when my children were young. My children and grandchildren benefited from the research and development of vaccines. Now my baby great-granddaughter is ready to begin that process. With the history of how my family has been affected by infectious diseases, I prepare to stand by my granddaughter and her baby as they keep their appointment.

COMPETENCIES

Upon completion of this chapter, the reader will be able to:

- *Describe the mode of infectious disease transmission.*
- *Discuss how a child's developmental level affects the transmission of infectious disease.*
- *Discuss the impact of day care and school settings on the incidence of infectious diseases.*
- *Describe the etiology, clinical manifestations, treatment, and nursing management of common infectious diseases.*
- *Identify measures used to prevent common infectious childhood diseases, including immunizations.*
- *Identify the educational needs of families whose child has an infectious disease.*
- *Discuss the importance of adhering to the laws and policies related to infectious diseases, including immunizations.*

In the early part of the 20th century, infectious illnesses were responsible for the high incidence of infant and childhood mortality in the United States. The discovery of antibiotics and the development of specific immunizations has decreased the morbidity and mortality rates associated with most communicable and infectious diseases particularly in industrialized countries. Yet, resistance to antibiotics and the emergence of new infections continues to plague the global community. The prevention of disease, disability, and death from infectious diseases, including those prevented by vaccines, is a major goal for ensuring the health care of all people (U.S. Department of Health and Human Services, 2000).

Throughout the years from infancy to adolescence, children will be exposed to a number of infectious diseases. An **infectious disease** is any disease caused by invasion and multiplication of microorganisms in the body. It may or may not be communicable. A **communicable disease** is a disease caused by an infectious agent that is transmitted to a person by direct or indirect contact, vehicle or vector, or airborne route. Infectious diseases are common occurrences during infancy, childhood, and adolescence. For purposes of this chapter, the term infectious disease will be used. Before the age of 3, children typically experience six to 10 infectious illnesses for each year of life (Grover, 1996). These include both respiratory and gastrointestinal infections. Although the majority of infectious illnesses are not life-threatening, some illnesses may cause serious lifelong disabilities or even death.

Many of these illnesses are preventable by receiving immunizations or by health promotion practices that avoid exposure to certain pathogens. Nurses play an important role in health promotion and education by intervening with children and their caregivers at all levels and in many environments. Awareness about developmental stages and anticipated behavior plus knowledge of disease processes enable nurses to be more effective in promoting children's health and wellness. This chapter provides an overview of the common infectious diseases that are prevalent during childhood and adolescence, including specific risk factors based on developmental age. Guidelines for current immunizations recommended are discussed. Risk reduction measures are provided to decrease the incidence of illnesses for which no vaccinations are available.

ANATOMY AND PHYSIOLOGY

Children experience higher incidences of infectious diseases than adults because of an immature immune system and developmental and biological variances. Maternally acquired antibodies decrease as the infant grows and develops. Children gradually develop immunity after exposure to diseases or through immunizations. Because young children are unable to verbalize that they do not feel well, a disease may be advanced before it is detected. Thus, a contagious child may inadvertently expose others in day care or school settings even before symptoms occur. In these settings, infectious diseases may readily be transmitted from child to child because of handling common objects.

Infectious diseases are caused by **pathogens** (disease-producing microorganisms) that invade the body. Once established, they reproduce and multiply, creating a wide variety of symptoms and disease states. The seriousness of the disease is dependent upon several factors, including the microorganism, the method of transmission, the concentration of pathogens, and the environment. Infectious microorganisms or pathogens include bacteria, viruses, fungi, and parasites. Illness may be manifested by local cellular injury, secretion of toxins, or antigen–antibody reaction.

The transmission of disease is dependent upon six factors, which are referred to as the chain of infection (Figure 15-1). They include infectious agent, reservoir, portal of exit, mode of transmission, portal of entry, and susceptible host.

1. Infectious agent—The specific pathogen must be present in sufficient numbers to cause disease. Some organisms have a greater **virulence** (the degree or power of microorganisms to cause disease) than others and can be more devastating, depending on the age of the child and the development of the immune system.
2. Reservoir—A place where pathogens can survive without multiplication. Reservoirs can be animate (living), such as humans, animals, and insects, or inanimate (not living), such as soil, water, other environmental sources, and medical equipment (intravenous [IV] solutions and urine collection devices).
3. Portal of exit from reservoir—Pathogens can leave the reservoir through the blood or body secretions such as urine, feces, respiratory secretions, and saliva.
4. Mode of transmission—Pathogenic organisms are spread by direct contact from person to person through saliva, droplets from the respiratory tract, body contact,

Family Teaching

The Spread of Infection

Home:

- Instruct caregivers about ways in which infections are spread as well as simple preventive measures.
- Emphasize careful handwashing before and after eating, after using the bathroom, prior to and after having bodily contact with another, and after coughing or sneezing.
- Discuss the importance of cleanliness and sanitation especially if their children attend institutional settings such as day care or preschool.
- Have caregivers explore the sanitary practices of day care and school staff.

Day care or school:

- Instruct personnel in these settings to wipe surface areas used for diaper changing with a disinfectant after each use.
- Avoid changing diapers on rugs, upholstered furniture, and bed coverings.
- Supervise children in handwashing before and after eating, after using the bathroom, prior to and after having bodily contact with another, and after coughing or sneezing.

Community:

- Educate community groups about methods to decrease the spread of infection.
- Act in a consultant role to groups in the community and offer education about the spread of illness to the following: church groups, senior citizens groups, parent–teacher groups, and youth groups.
- Discuss the importance of keeping immunizations up to date for children as well as adults and senior citizens.
- Promote yearly immunizations against influenza for groups that are susceptible to be exposed.

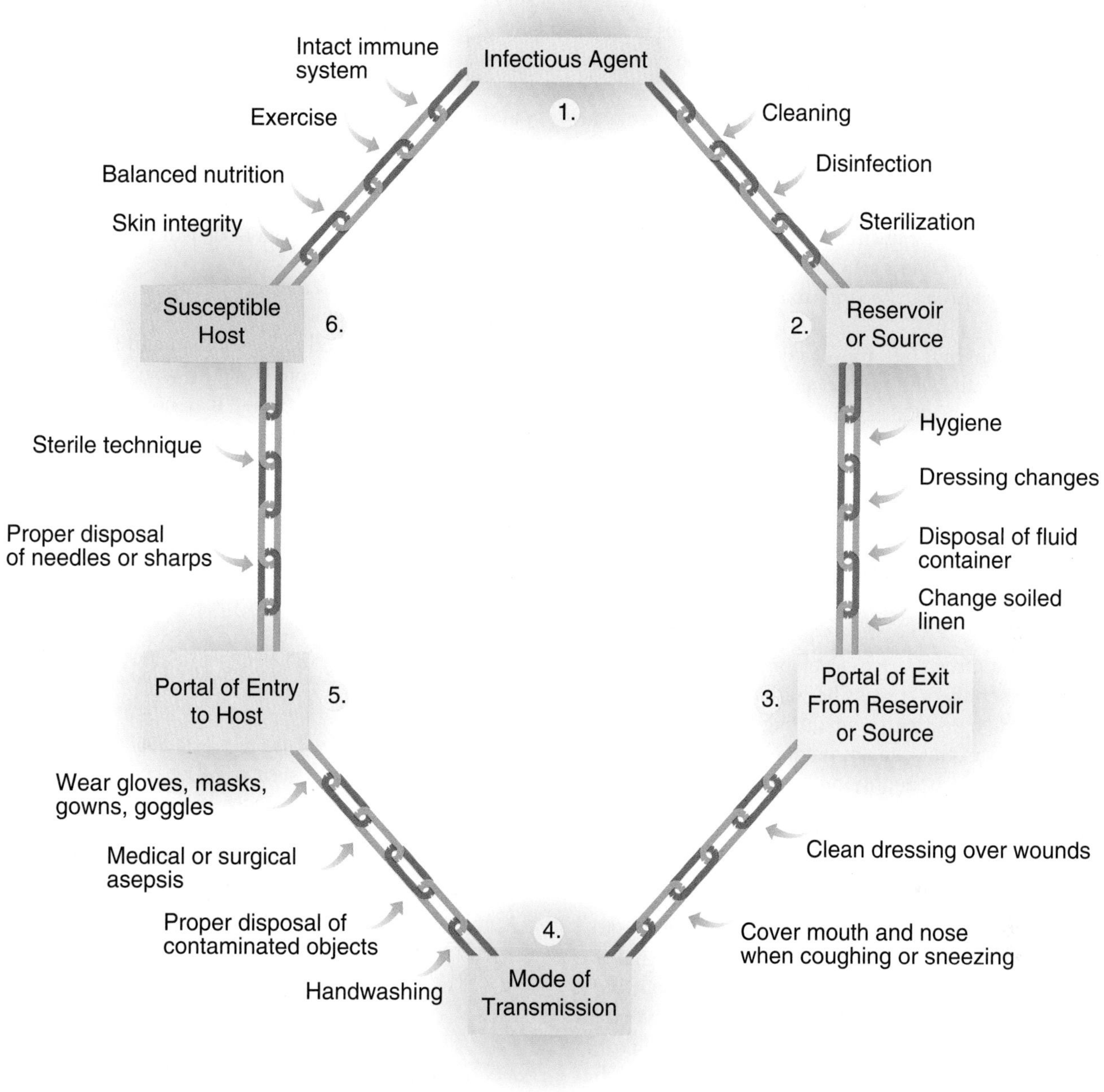

Figure 15-1 Chain of infection is the process by which organisms are transmitted from the environment to a host, invade the host, and cause an infection. Preventive measures for breaking the chain follow each link.

blood, and body fluids in the urinary, gastrointestinal, and reproductive systems. Pathogens can also be transmitted on objects, in contaminated water or food, or by **vectors** (animals or insects that carry the infectious organism from one host to another).

5. Portal of entry to the host—Pathogens can enter the body through the respiratory tract, the gastrointestinal tract, the urinary tract, and the skin and mucous membranes, and across the placenta.

6. Susceptible host—Pathogens cause illness when the individual lacks immunity to specific organisms or when the immune system is dysfunctional.

Other factors that support the development of disease include (1) the ability of the pathogens to survive in the environment, (2) the asymptomatic or carrier state, and (3) the dose of the pathogen. Regarding the first factor, many organisms remain viable from hours up to several weeks on environmental surfaces such as toys or changing tables in a day care center. Children put fingers and toys in their mouths during play time, thus increasing the possibility of infection if the environment is not cleaned properly. Examples include hepatitis A, rotavirus, and *Giardia* cysts (American Academy of Pediatrics [AAP], 2000).

Regarding the second factor, many children may remain asymptomatic but are able to transmit pathogens before they become ill. For example, children exposed to the varicella virus, which causes chickenpox, are contagious the day prior to becoming ill but may exhibit none of the characteristic lesions at that time. Others may be **carriers** (persons who can harbor and spread the organism to others without becoming ill).

Regarding the third factor involved in developing disease (the dose of the pathogen), the concentration of pathogens in a particular sample of fluid or blood determines whether or not infection occurs after a single exposure.

DEVELOPMENTAL STAGES AND THE RISK OF INFECTION

As children pass through each developmental stage they are susceptible to certain organisms because of psychosocial and physiological changes that occur during specific periods of life. At every stage, children are uniquely at risk of developing certain infections beginning *in utero* and extending through adolescence.

Infancy

During prenatal life, the developing fetus is susceptible to a number of illnesses through maternal infection that are potentially life threatening. The process of transmitting a disease from one generation to another is known as **vertical transmission.** It can occur through the placenta while the infant is *in utero*, during delivery, or through breast milk following delivery. Among the infections transmitted in this way are rubella, herpes, and human immunodeficiency virus (HIV). Newborns are susceptible to invasive infection by bacterial organisms such as staphylococci or *Escherichia coli*, which in older children or adults are considered part of the normal flora.

As infants begin to grow, develop, and become more mobile, they come in contact with a variety of persons, objects, and surfaces that have the potential for causing illnesses and diseases. Potentially pathogenic organisms are spread through the respiratory tract as droplets through sneezing, coughing, and talking. If caregivers neglect to wash their hands frequently, they can introduce organisms from their hands into the infant's nose or mouth while changing diapers via the fecal–oral route. Hand-to-mouth behavior on the part of the infant is another source of infection. The common adult habit of kissing an infant's fingers and hands can be a potential source of infection to the infant who then puts the fingers in his or her mouth. Additionally, infants who place unclean objects in their mouths can become ill. These objects, in turn, become a potential source of infection for other infants in that same environment (Figure 15-2). Infants are more susceptible to respiratory and enteral viruses. Therefore, they are at greater risk for metabolic problems as a result of fever, decrease in appetite and fluid intake, diarrhea, and subsequent dehydration.

Toddlers and Preschoolers

Toddlerhood is a period of exploration and further development. Most toddlers become toilet trained during this phase. Because they are learning, they may not always be diligent about washing their hands, so they are still at risk for developing diseases transmitted through the fecal–oral route. Day care and encounters with other toddlers in diapers add to the risk. Toddlers and some preschoolers still put objects in their mouth. It may be difficult to break the cycle of infection if sanitary conditions in these situations are lax.

Nursing Alert:

Use of Aspirin

Caregivers should not use aspirin to treat the pain and fever of viral illnesses such as influenza and varicella (chickenpox) in children under 13 years of age. The use of acetylsalicylic acid has been linked to the subsequent development of Reye's syndrome, which is a disorder combining both encephalopathy and fatty degeneration of the liver (see Chapter 32). Acetaminophen is the drug of choice for febrile illness in infants and children.

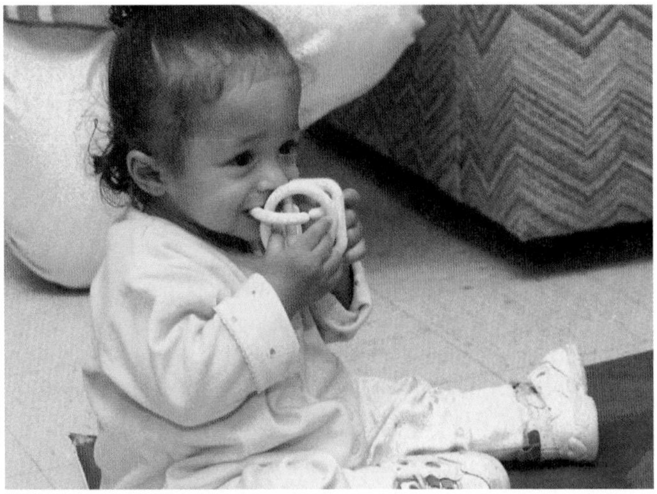

Figure 15-2 Infants learn through hand and mouth exploration.

Some toddlers and preschoolers enjoy encounters with small animals such as dogs or cats; however, their inquisitiveness places them at risk for being scratched or bitten. Organisms present in animal saliva or on their bodies can cause illness in any child who is scratched or bitten. Playing with infected animals may cause tinea corporis (ringworm of the body; see Chapter 30).

The school-aged section next contains some information that is true of toddlers and preschoolers in day care centers.

School-Aged Children

Schools are a perfect breeding ground for the spread of infection. Many children are lax in hygienic practices such as washing hands before eating and after using the bathroom. Some schools may operate on strict schedules; therefore, children are not given the opportunity to wash up when they should. Same-sex friendships are common in school-aged children and frequently result in the mutual sharing of items of clothing, grooming devices, food, and toys. Children may spend the night together at each others' homes or on camping trips. Sharing beds and linens as well as personal items such as combs can result in outbreaks of head lice, scabies, pinworms, tinea corporis, and tinea capitis.

The leading cause of pneumonia for this age group is *Mycoplasma pneumoniae* and can be found where children are grouped together. This infection is highly contagious and can result in illness ranging from inflammation of the trachea and bronchioles to pneumonia. Behaviors exhibited among some schoolchildren such as not covering one's mouth while coughing or sneezing and not washing hands afterwards are contributing factors. Another common illness, erythema infectiosum or Fifth's disease, has a characteristic rash and is highly contagious. The illness is caused by parvovirus B19. By the time the rash erupts, children are no longer contagious, but the epidemic nature of this disease and the uniqueness of the rash (intensely red with a slapped-cheek appearance) can give caregivers cause for concern.

Adolescents

Adolescents present unique challenges regarding the spread of infectious diseases. Adolescents are basically well individuals and do not seek care unless they are ill. For this reason, they are less likely to have continuity of preventative health care such as immunizations (Gordon, Zook, Averhoff, & Williams, 1997). Adolescents need to receive booster doses of vaccines to maintain high levels of immunity (see Nursing Tip: Adolescent Immunizations). When they do not, they are susceptible to developing the illness. A decrease in the protective levels of childhood immunity for measles, mumps, rubella, tetanus, and diphtheria has been reported in the adolescent age group (Averhoff, Williams, & Hadler, 1997). In addition, adolescents generally lack immunity against hepatitis B, a viral infection that could be acquired during this period or early adulthood through sexual contact.

The prevalence of sexual intercourse as well as the rate of sexually transmitted diseases (STDs) has increased among adolescents. Factors associated with the increase in STDs in this age group include frequent unprotected sex, biological

Nursing Tip:

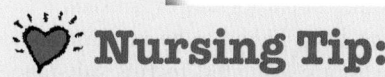

Family teaching about disease transmission

Each encounter with children and their caregivers is an opportunity for nurses to review the principles of disease transmission. It is important to assess basic knowledge about disease transmission. Nurses may find that caregivers as well as children have misconceptions about the cause of illness such as going out in cold weather without a coat. Education should focus on personal hygiene, ways of staying healthy, and the basics of nutrition that support the immune system. Children's literature that reviews germ theory and illness prevention can be used by nurses to illustrate important concepts. As caregivers are encouraged to take responsibility for the sex education of their children, nurses need to remind them to include open and frank discussion about sexually transmitted diseases.

Nursing Tip:

Adolescent immunizations

Assess for immunization status each time an adolescent is seen for a health encounter. Adolescents need booster doses of tetanus and diphtheria vaccine (Td) about 10 years after their last dose received prior to starting kindergarten. They may not have received the measles–mumps–rubella vaccine (MMR) as a booster prior to entering elementary school. If they have not received the hepatitis B series in early infancy or childhood, it should be started in adolescence. Some states may allow adolescents to consent for their own immunizations. Nurses need to be familiar with the laws of the state in which they work.

College-bound adolescents and their families should receive information about the importance of vaccination against meningococcal disease. This group of adolescents is at particular risk for the development of meningitis, especially if they plan to live in dormitories or residence halls. The vaccine is effective for approximately 3–5 years (American College Health Association [ACHA], 1999).

REFLECTIONS FROM FAMILIES

I have just been diagnosed with chlamydia and am taking some medication to treat it. I have had sex with both of my girlfriends during the past year and am too embarrassed to tell them so they can get tested. I didn't use condoms because they're too inconvenient. I guess I really don't need to tell them because we didn't have sex often enough for them to be infected.

susceptibility to disease, and difficulty in accessing and utilizing confidential health care. Those at high risk for disease include intravenous drug users, sexually active heterosexuals, and male homosexuals (Centers for Disease Control and Prevention [CDC], 1998a).

Many adolescents do not believe that they are at risk for becoming infected or pregnant. The majority of adolescents who are having sexual intercourse are doing so without protection against pregnancy or sexually transmitted diseases. Thus, the early introduction to sexual activity, with an increase in the frequency of activity with multiple partners, places them at higher risk (Sieving, Resnick, Bearinger, Remafedi, Taylor, & Harmon, 1997). Intercourse can cause microscopic tears in both the vaginal and anal mucosa, thus creating a portal for the entry of pathogenic organisms.

Crack cocaine use has been linked to an increased rate of STDs. Adolescents who are addicted to this substance report a greater number of sexual partners, exchanging sex for drugs, or having sex with those who inject drugs, which increases their risk not only for STDs but also HIV (Word & Bowser, 1997). Currently, the rate of adolescents who become newly infected with the HIV virus is rising.

Preadolescents and adolescents should be seen alone, apart from their caregivers, during a portion of the interview to assess their knowledge about disease transmission, especially STDs. Adolescents may be concerned about changes in their body, which may or may not be significant as they relate to infectious diseases. Nurses can assess whether adolescents are sexually active and if their behaviors are placing them at risk for sexually transmitted diseases. The majority of states have provisions that allow adolescents to consent to the confidential diagnosis and treatment of STDs without parental knowledge and consent. Other states may allow adolescents to obtain HIV counseling and testing without consent. Still other states permit adolescents to obtain necessary vaccinations without parental consent (CDC, 1998a). Nurses need to be familiar with the laws and regulations in their own states to provide the correct information to families.

Reflective Thinking

Caring for Adolescents with Sexually Transmitted Diseases

To increase self-awareness and comfort level in discussing the care and treatment of STDs with adolescents, ask yourself:

1. How comfortable do I feel about asking adolescents personal questions about their sexual practices?
2. How knowledgeable am I about the extent and types of STDs affecting adolescents?
3. Can I be nonjudgmental when discussing health promotion practices that decrease the risk of illness?
4. Am I comfortable enough about my own sexuality and sexual behavior to be able to deliver care in a positive manner?

INFECTIOUS DISEASES IN DAY CARE AND SCHOOL SETTINGS

It is estimated that more than 15 million children under the age of 5 spend all or part of their day outside of the home in day care facilities (Donowitz, 1999). There are several factors that can influence the incidence of infection as young infants and children are cared for in out-of-home settings such as day care and school, including the following (AAP, 2000; Holmes, Morrow, & Pickering, 1996):

- Personal hygiene and immunization status of the caregiver
- Sanitation of the environment
- Procedures for the handling and preparation of food
- Immunization status and age of the children
- Caregiver-to-child ratio
- Quality and physical space of the facility

Family Teaching

Nurses can make an impact in the decision-making process by acting as resources to caregivers who are considering the placement of their children in day care or preschool. Caregivers need to know about the characteristics of optimal day care as it relates to the health of the children. One topic concerns the facility policies related to illness. Will they allow a child with a temperature of 101°F to attend? How many days after a fever subsides can the child return?

Research Highlight

Handwashing Promotes Wellness

Study Purpose

Many caregivers of young children lack information on the transmission of infectious diseases, while young children often do not have the skills and knowledge to maintain proper hygiene. The purpose of this study was to determine if an instructional program on germs and handwashing could reduce the prevalence of infectious disease in day care participants.

Methods

A longitudinal study on handwashing practices was conducted involving preschool children (ages 3–5) and their teachers at two similar child care programs. The test group comprised eight teachers and 26 children, while the control group had eight teachers and 12 children. The teachers in the test group received training on infectious diseases and proper handwashing. The children were given developmentally appropriate instruction on handwashing and infection control. The control group did not receive any instruction. An assessment checklist was filled out by both caregivers and teachers in both groups to monitor any infectious illness or symptomatology occurring the previous week. Over the 21-week period of the study, over 700 checklists were collected from the test group and more than 400 from the control group.

Findings

Chi-square analysis showed that, during the weeks of the peak cold and flu season, the test group reported significantly fewer colds than the control group.

Implications

The results suggest that, when proper handwashing practices as well as developmentally appropriate germ theory is incorporated into the preschool curriculum for both children and teachers, the spread of infectious disease can be decreased.

Citation

Niffenegger, J. P. (1997). Proper handwashing promotes wellness in child care. *Journal of Pediatric Health Care, 11*, 26–31.

If the child appears with a red, watery eye, what is the center protocol? Many centers will provide caregivers with a written illness policy. Some programs may have facilities to care for children with minor illnesses. Another topic concerns sanitation. Caregivers need to ask about changing facilities if the children are still in diapers. Are children who are toilet trained separated from those who are not? Does the staff use frequent handwashing? When staffing is less than adequate, practices regarding handwashing may be relaxed. What about food preparation? Is it performed in an area separate from areas where diapers are changed? Nurses can help caregivers prepare a list of questions to ask when evaluating prospective child care facilities.

In addition to teaching the family, nurses who work in a day care or school setting should be resources to staff and students about the prevention of common illnesses as well as managing outbreaks of illness as they occur during the school year. Providing materials and references to teachers and caregivers may help reduce the anxiety that sometimes accompanies episodic illness.

The majority of illnesses occurring in children who spend the better part of their day in out-of-home settings are caused by respiratory tract and enteric pathogens (Churchill & Pickering, 1997). Early introduction to child care outside of the home may have some benefit. When children enter elementary school, they may be less at risk for respiratory illness because of prior exposure (McCutcheon & Woodward, 1996). Enforcing hygienic measures and ensuring current immunizations are important factors in infection control that should be instituted in all child care facilities.

Many out-of-home facilities, whether they are private homes, licensed centers, or schools, have policies regarding the admission of ill children. Children who have fever, diarrhea, irritability, open mouth sores, rashes, and purulent conjunctivitis are excluded until the illness is treated appropriately or resolves. Other diseases, including tuberculosis, scabies, head lice, hepatitis A, streptococcal pharyngitis, impetigo, varicella, mumps, measles, and pertussis, require specific treatments and time periods during which the disorder becomes noninfectious. Most of these children need physician proof of no longer being contagious in order to return to school or day care (AAP, 2000).

IMMUNIZATIONS

Immunizations are an important part of health promotion and disease prevention for all children. The vaccines used for immunizing against diseases are prepared from microorganisms or genetically engineered antigens, and introduced into the body to evoke an immune response. The term immunization often is used interchangeably with vaccine. The majority of vaccines are administered by injection, though some vaccines are given by the oral route, and others are given by aerosol.

Schedule of Immunizations

The periodic scheduling of immunizations reinforces and ensures regular health supervision visits with a primary care provider (Green & Palfrey, 2000) as well as providing optimal intervals to facilitate the development of the immune response. Immunization schedules change periodically based on knowledge about the safety and efficacy of current as well as newly developed vaccines. In general, recommendations for childhood immunizations are based on the consensus of the Advisory Committee on Immunization Practices (ACIP) of the Centers for Disease Control and Prevention (CDC), the American Academy of Pediatrics (AAP), and the American Academy of Family Physicians (AAFP). The current recommended childhood immunization schedule is updated annually (Figure 15-3). It is important that nurses who work with families of growing children keep abreast of the latest immunization schedules so they can address questions and concerns that caregivers may have. Nurses should assess for immunization status at every opportunity when children enter any part of the health care system so that immunizations can be kept current. Caregivers often are aware of the importance of immunizations but find that long waiting times to get services or difficult access to the health care setting are barriers to care (Evers, 2000). Clinic staff who remind families of keeping immunization appointments can facilitate adherence to immunization guidelines.

While adhering to the recommended schedule is ideal, many children for one reason or another fall behind in receiving the routine vaccinations. Factors such as illness, caregiver mobility, inconvenience, lack of caregiver knowledge about the importance of immunizations, and difficulty in accessing health care may contribute to incomplete immunizations (Pruit, Kline, & Kovaz, 1995; Strobino, Keane, Holt, Hughart, & Guyer, 1996). When a child receives only one or two doses of vaccine and does not receive the remaining vaccines according to the recommended schedule, the series does not need to be restarted. Instead, only the missed doses need to be given according to the recommended immunization schedule for children not immunized during the first year in Table 15-1. Nurses can help plan the remaining schedule with the family according to what the child has already received. Those who administer vaccines routinely should have the most up-to-date copy of the vaccine schedule on hand for reference.

Many practitioners recommend a variety of methods to determine children's immunization status to avoid missed opportunities. The combination of caregiver-linked and provider-validated methods is the gold standard for measuring immunization status. Caregivers are asked to identify all those who provided immunizations to their children and contact them for validation. All immunization records are combined into one record. A copy can be given to the caregivers for reference. The ultimate goal is for the implementation of computer-based immunization registries for all children.

Reflective Thinking

How Many Injections Will an Infant Receive?

The average infant who is immunized by the age of two according to current national guidelines will receive a total of 15–16 injections if each vaccine is given separately. This is based on using inactivated polio vaccine (IPV) as recommended for the series. Using combination vaccines such as DTP and Hib together may reduce the number to 11. In addition, many practitioners are now immunizing against pneumococcal disease. This could increase the number of vaccines by four injections depending on the infant's age when the vaccine is initiated. How do you feel when caregivers ask about the necessity for so many injections? What do you tell them? What can you do to alleviate the discomfort of the caregivers and especially the child? How can you prepare children and caregivers to decrease the discomfort from immunizations?

Vaccines[1] are listed under routinely recommended ages. [Bars] indicate range of recommended ages for immunization. Any dose not given at the recommended age should be given as a "catch-up" immunization at any subsequent visit when indicated and feasible. (Ovals) indicate vaccines to be given if previously recommended doses were missed or were given earlier than the recommended minimum age.

Age ► / Vaccine ▼	Birth	1 mo	2 mo	4 mo	6 mo	12 mo	15 mo	18 mo	24 mo	4–6 yrs	11–12 yrs	14–18 yrs
Hepatitis B[2]		[Hep B #1]										
			[Hep B #2]			[Hep B #3]					(Hep B[2])	
Diphtheria, tetanus toxoids, and pertussis[3]			DTaP	DTaP	DTaP			[DTaP[3]]		DTaP	[Td]	
H. influenzae type b[4]			Hib	Hib	Hib	[Hib]						
Inactivated polio[5]			IPV	IPV		[IPV[5]]				IPV[5]		
Pneumococcal conjugate[6]			PCV	PCV	PCV	[PCV]						
Measles, Mumps, Rubella[7]						[MMR]				MMR[7]	(MMR[7])	
Varicella[8]							[Var]				(Var[8])	
Hepatitis A[9]											[Hep A–in selected area[9]]	

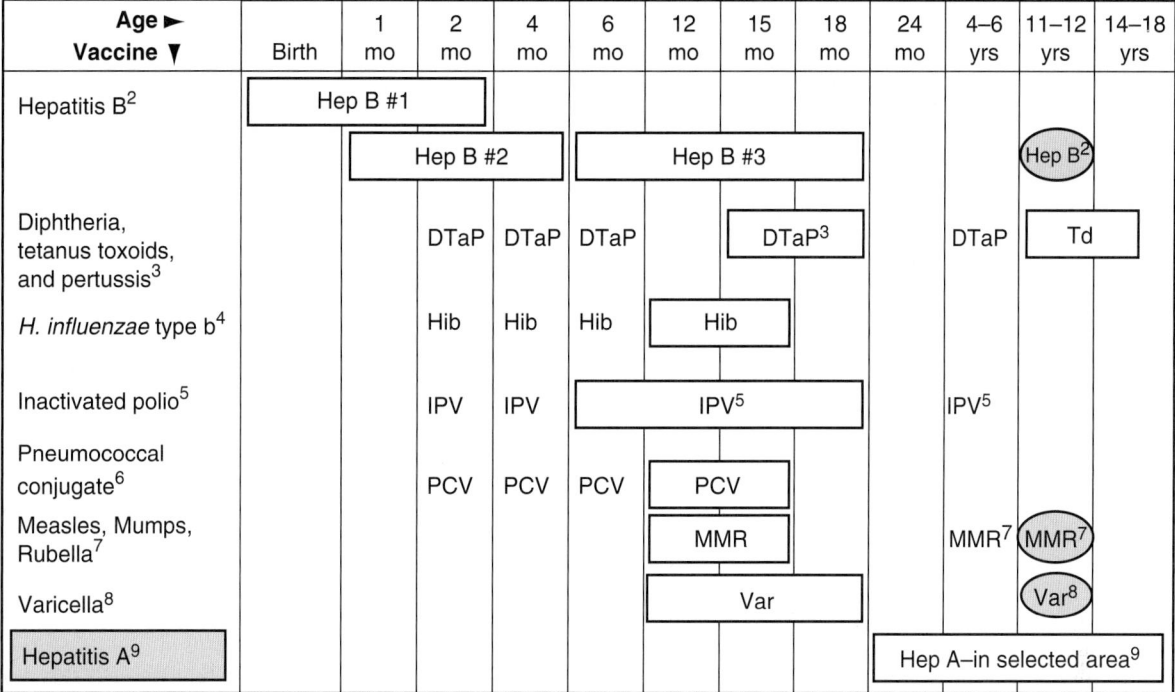

Approved by the Advisory Committee on Immunization Practices (ACIP), the American Academy of Pediatrics (AAP), and the American Academy of Family Physicians (AAFP).

1. This schedule indicates the recommended ages for routine administration of currently licensed childhood vaccines, as of 11/1/00, for children through 18 years of age. Additional vaccines may be licensed and recommended during the year. Licensed combination vaccines may be used whenever any components of the combination are indicated and its other components are not contraindicated. Providers should consult the manufacturers' package inserts for detailed recommendations.

2. *Infants born to HbsAg-negative mothers* should receive the 1st dose of hepatitis B (Hep B) vaccine by age 2 months. The 2nd dose should be at least one month after the 1st dose. The 3rd dose should be administered at least 4 months after the 1st dose and at least 2 months after the 2nd dose, but not before 6 months of age for infants.
Infants born to HbsAg-positive mothers should receive hepatitis B vaccine and 0.5 mL hepatitis B immune globulin (HBIG) within 12 hours of birth at separate sites. The 2nd dose is recommended at 1–2 months of age and the 3rd dose at 6 months of age.
Infants born to mothers whose HbsAg status is unknown should receive hepatitis B vaccine within 12 hours of birth. Maternal blood should be drawn at the time of delivery to determine the mother's HbsAg status; if the HbsAg test is positive, the infant should receive HBIG as soon as possible (no later than 1 week of age).
All children and adolescents who have not been immunized against hepatitis B should begin the series during any visit. Special efforts should be made to immunize children who were born in or whose parents were born in areas of the world with moderate or high endemicity of hepatitis B virus infection.

3. The 4th dose of DTaP (diphtheria and tetanus toxoids and acellular pertussis vaccine) may be administered as early as 12 months of age, provided 6 months have elapsed since the 3rd dose and the child is unlikely to return at age 15–18 months. Td (tetanus and diphtheria toxoids) is recommended at 11–12 years of age if at least 5 years have elapsed since the last dose of DTP, DTaP or DT. Subsequent routine Td boosters are recommended every 10 years.

4. Three *Haemophilus influenzae* type b (Hib) conjugate vaccines are licensed for infant use. If PRP-OMP (PedvaxHIB® or ComVax® [Merck]) is administered at 2 and 4 months of age, a dose at 6 months is not required. Because clinical studies in infants have demonstrated that using some combination products may induce a lower immune response to the Hib vaccine component, DTaP/Hib combination products should not be used for primary immunization in infants at 2, 4 or 6 months of age, unless FDA-approved for these ages.

5. An all-IPV schedule is recommended for routine childhood polio vaccination in the United States. All children should receive four does of IPV at 2 months, 4 months, 6–18 months, and 4–6 years of age. Oral polio vaccine (OPV) should be used only in selected circumstances.

6. The heptavalent conjugate pneumococcal vaccine (PCV) is recommended for all children 2–23 months of age. It also is recommended for certain children 24–59 months of age.

7. The 2nd dose of measles, mumps, and rubella (MMR) vaccine is recommended routinely at 4–6 years of age but may be administered during any visit, provided at least 4 weeks have elapsed since receipt of the 1st dose and that both doses are administered beginning at or after 12 months of age. Those who have not previously received the second dose should complete the schedule by the 11–12 year old visit.

8. Varicella (Var) vaccine is recommended at any visit on or after the first birthday for susceptible children, i.e. those who lack a reliable history of chickenpox (as judged by a health care provider) and who have not been immunized. Susceptible persons 13 years of age or older should receive 2 doses, given at least 4 weeks apart.

9. Hepatitis A (Hep A) is shaded to indicate its recommended use in selected states and/or regions, and for certain high risk groups; consult your local public health authority.

For additional information about the vaccines listed above, please visit the National Immunization Program Home Page at http://www.cdc.gov/nip/ or call the National Immunization Hotline at 800-232-2522 (English) or 800-232-0233 (Spanish).

Figure 15-3 Recommended Childhood Immunization Schedule, United States, January–December 2001. *Source:* Committee on Infectious Diseases, American Academy of Pediatrics. (2000). *2000 Red Book: Report of the Committee on Infectious Diseases* (25th ed.). Elk Grove Village, IL: American Academy of Pediatrics.

TABLE 15-1 Recommended Immunization Schedules for Children Not Immunized in the First Year of Life*

Recommended Time/Age	Immunization(s)†	Comments
Younger Than 7 Years		
First visit	DTaP, Hib,‡ HBV, MMR	If indicated, tuberculin testing may be done at same visit. If child is 5 y of age or older, Hib is not indicated in most circumstances.
Interval after first visit		
1 mo (4 wk)	DTaP, IPV, HBV, Var§	The second dose of IPV may be given if accelerated poliomyelitis immunization is necessary, such as for travelers to areas where polio is endemic.
2 mo	DTaP, Hib,‡ IPV	Second dose of Hib is indicated only if the first dose was received when younger than 15 mo.
≥8 mo	DTaP, HBV, IPV	IPV and HBV are not given if the third doses were given earlier.
Age 4-6 y (at or the before school entry)	DTaP, IPV, MMR‖	DTaP is not necessary if the fourth dose was given after fourth birthday; IPV is not necessary if the third dose was given after the fourth birthday.
7–12 Years		
First visit	HBV, MMR, dT, IPV	
Interval after first visit		
2 mo (8wk)	HBV, MMR,‖ Var,§ dT, IPV	IPV also may be given 1 mo after the first visit if accelerated poliomyelitis immunization is necessary.
8–14 mo	HBV,¶ dT, IPV	IPV is not given if the third dose was given earlier.

** Table is not completely consistent with all package inserts. For products used, also consult manufacturer's package insert for instructions on storage, handling, dosage, and administration. Biologics prepared by different manufacturers may vary, and package inserts of the same manufacturer may change. Therefore, the physician should be aware of the contents of the current package insert. Vaccine abbreviations: HBV indicates hepatitis B virus; Var, varicella; DTaP, diphtheria and tetanus toxoids and acellular pertussis; Hib,* Haemophilus influenzae *type b conjugate; IPV, inactivated poliovirus; MMR, live measles-mumps-rubella; dT, adult tetanus toxoid (full dose) and diphtheria toxoid (reduced dose), for children 7 years of age or older and adults.*

† If all needed vaccines cannot be administered simultaneously, priority should be given to protecting the child against diseases that pose the greatest immediate risk. In the United States, these diseases for children younger than 2 years usually are measles and Haemophilus influenzae *type b infection; for children older than 7 years, they are measles, mumps, and rubella. Before 13 years of age, immunity against hepatitis B and varicella should be ensured. DtaP, HBV, Hib, MMR, and Var can be given simultaneously at separate sites if failure of the patient to return for future immunizations is a concern.*

‡ See Haemophilus influenzae *Infections.*

§ Varicella vaccine can be administered to susceptible children any time after 12 months of age. Unimmunized children who lack a reliable history of varicella should be immunized before their 13th birthday.

‖ Minimal interval between doses of MMR is 1 month (4 wk).

¶ HBV may be given earlier in a 0-, 2-, and 4-month schedule.

Adapted from Committee on Infectious Diseases, American Academy of Pediatrics. (2000). 2000 Red Book: Report of the Committee on Infectious Diseases *(25th ed.). Elk Grove Village, IL: American Academy of Pediatrics.*

All states require children to be immunized prior to entry into licensed child care or school. Many states also have regulations requiring immunization of children in upper grades and those entering college. State immunization requirements may be obtained from state and local health departments. Since specific requirements for entry level programs vary, it is important that nurses become familiar with the immunization requirements of the state in which they practice.

Combination Vaccines

Because of the number of injections that some infants and children may be receiving at one appointment, vaccine manufacturers have been researching ways to combine vaccines into a single dose. The diptheria–tetanus–pertussis injection is an example of a combination vaccine. The present vaccine (DTap) now contains acellular pertussis, which prevents many of the side effects of the whole-cell pertussis vaccine (DTwP). Other examples include measles–mumps–rubella vaccine (MMR) and trivalent (three strains) inactivated polio vaccine (IPV). Hepatitis B and hemophilis influenza B have also been combined. Combination vaccines currently under study include (1) DTap, IPV, and HepB; (2) DTap, IPV, and Hib; and (3) MMR and varicella (AAP, 1999).

Combining vaccines is subject to the U.S. Food and Drug Administration (FDA) approval. Combination vaccines have some drawbacks. Some of the difficulties encountered with combination vaccines include immunological problems that arise when certain antigens are combined, as well as chemical incompatibility (ACIP, 1999). Additionally, vaccine combinations that require different schedules may result in confusion when they are administered by several providers who use different products (AAP, 1999). However, combination vaccines might improve current immunization coverage as well as provide catch up for children who are delayed in their immunizations. Reducing fear of needles and pain plus ensuring safety and efficacy should be a prime concern of all personnel involved with providing immunizations. As these new vaccine debut, nurses need to update their knowledge base about these preparations.

Nurses are the primary administrators of vaccines in health care settings. In addition to immunization requirements, nurses must be familiar with the appropriate site for injectable vaccines, the appropriate storage of vaccines, the specifications of the National Childhood Vaccine Injury Act of 1986, expected reactions to various vaccines, reportable vaccine-related events, and contraindications to specific vaccine use.

Vaccine Handling and Storage

Inappropriate handling or storage of vaccines can result in a decrease in vaccine potency and ineffective immunization. Some vaccines are sensitive to heat while others are affected by freezing. The most current recommendations for the handling and storage of vaccines can be obtained from the package insert. With the rapid development of new immunizations, it is imperative that package inserts be reviewed.

The National Childhood Vaccine Injury Act

The National Childhood Vaccine Injury Act of 1986 was established in response to concerns about serious vaccine-related injuries and deaths. It is a system in which persons who have suffered an injury or death as a result of vaccines may seek compensation. No negligence must be proven, and the program provides an alternative to civil litigation. The act requires every child to have a personal immunization record that is maintained in a permanent medical record. It mandates that the following information be recorded at the time of each immunization:

- Month, day, and year of administration
- Vaccine administered
- Manufacturer
- Lot number and expiration date
- Site and route of administration
- Name, address, and title of the health care provider administering the vaccine

Caregivers are asked to read and sign consent forms granting permission before any immunization is administered. Information regarding immunizations is presented to caregivers verbally and in writing. Most health care settings where immunizations are administered require written

Nursing Tip:

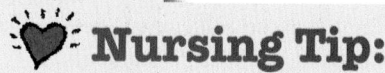

Importance of immunization records

Caregivers should be given a copy of their child's immunization record. Nurses need to stress the importance of keeping this record in a safe place and bringing it with them to each visit to the health provider. Telling caregivers that this record is "the child's passport to day care or school" places importance on the value of knowing their child's immunization status.

Nursing Alert:

Vaccines with Thimerosal

Thimerosal, an organic compound containing mercury, is a preservative found in most vaccines. It is used to reduce the risk of bacterial contamination in opened vaccine vials. While there has been no evidence of harm caused by the trace amounts of thimerosal in vaccines, some infants may be exposed to cumulative levels of mercury during the first 6 months of life that exceed the Environmental Protection Agency (EPA) recommendations. At very high doses, thimerosal has been associated with neurotoxity and nephrotoxity. Therefore in 1999, the American Academy of Pediatrics and the U.S. Public Health Service issued a joint statement calling for the removal of the preservative from vaccines (Ball, Ball, & Pratt, 2001). To date, many manufacturers are planning to remove thimerosal from vaccines. Some have already removed the preservative from certain vaccines.

consent. Nurses must ensure that caregivers understand the information provided. Some may be reluctant to reveal that they cannot read or understand the written handouts. If the nurse assesses that the caregiver cannot read, then the contents of the consent form must be explained in terms that are understood. When working with non–English-speaking populations, nurses need to be aware of and use consent forms written in that particular language as well as seeking the assistance of an interpreter as indicated.

Precautions and Contraindications

Although immunization is generally considered safe and effective, some children will have reactions ranging from minor to life-threatening, while others will not receive the level of protection from disease that is expected. Nurses must be aware of the relatively few contraindications to immunizations (Table 15-2) so that children are not pre-

TABLE 15-2 Guide to Contraindications and Precautions to Immunizations, January 2000[a]

Vaccine	Contraindications	Precautions[b]	Not Contraindications (Vaccines May Be Given)
General for all vaccines (DTaP/DTP,[c] IPV, OPV, MMR, Hib, HBV, Var)	Anaphylactic reaction to a vaccine contraindicates further doses of that vaccine Anaphylactic reaction to a vaccine constituent contraindicates the use of vaccines containing that substance	Moderate or severe illnesses with or without a fever	Mild to moderate local reaction (soreness, redness, swelling) following a dose of an injectable antigen Low-grade or moderate fever following a prior vaccine dose Mild accute illness with or without low-grade fever Current antimicrobial therapy Convalescent phase of illness Prematurity (same dosage and indications as for healthy, full-term infants) Recent exposure to an infectious disease History of penicillin or other nonspecific allergies or fact that relatives have such allergies Pregnancy of mother or household contact Unimmunized household contact
DTaP/DTP[c]	Encephalopathy within 7 days of administration of previous dose of DTaP/DTP	Temperature of 40.5°C (104.8°F) within 48 hours after vaccination with a prior dose of DTaP/DTP Collapse or shock-like state (hypotonic-hyporesponsive episode) within 48 hours of receiving a prior dose of DTaP/DTP Seizures within 3 days of receiving a prior dose of DTaP/DTP[d] Persistent inconsolable crying lasting 3 hours, within 48 hours of receiving a prior dose of DTaP/DTP GBS within 6 weeks after a dose[e]	Family history of seizures[d] Family history of sudden infant death syndrome Family history of an adverse event after DTaP/DTP administration

continues

TABLE 15-2 *Continued*

Vaccine	Contraindications	Precautions[b]	Not Contraindications (Vaccines May Be Given)
IPV	Anaphylactic reactions to neomycin or streptomycin	Pregnancy	—
OPV[f,g]	Infection with HIV or a household contact with HIV Known altered immunodeficiency (hematologic and solid tumors, congenital immunodeficiency, and long-term immunosuppressive therapy) Immunodeficient household contact	Pregnancy	Breastfeeding Current antimicrobial therapy Mild diarrhea
MMR	Pregnancy Anaphylactic reaction to neomycin Anaphylactic reaction to gelatin Known altered immunodeficiency (hematologic and solid tumors, congenital immunodeficiency, severe HIV infection, and long-term immunosuppressive therapy)	Recent (within 3 to 11 months, depending on product and dose) immune globulin administration[h] Thrombocytopenia or history of thrombocytopenic purpura[h,i]	Tuberculosis or positive PPD Simultaneous tuberculin skin testing[j] Breastfeeding Pregnancy of mother of recipient Immunodeficient family member or household contact Infection with HIV Nonanaphylactic reactions to eggs or neomycin
Hib	None	—	—
Hepatitis B	Anaphylactic reaction to baker's yeast	—	Pregnancy
Varicella	Pregnancy Anaphylactic reaction to neomycin Anaphylactic reaction to gelatin Infection with HIV Known altered immunodeficiency (hematologic and solid tumors, congenital immunodeficiency, and long-term immunosuppressive therapy)	Recent immune globulin administration Family history of immunodeficiency[k]	Pregnancy in the mother of the recipient Immunodeficiency in a household contact Household contact with HIV

[a] *DTaP indicates diphtheria and tetanus toxoids and acellular pertussis; DTP, diphtheria and tetanus toxoids and pertussis; IPV, inactivated poliovirus; OPV, oral poliovirus; MMR, measles-mumps-rubella; Hib,* Haemophilus influenzae *type b; HBV, hepatitis B virus; Var, varicella; GBS, Guillain-Barré syndrome; HIV, human immunodeficiency virus; and PPD, purified protein derivative (tuberculin).*

continues

TABLE 15-2 *Continued*

[b] *The events or conditions listed as precautions, although not contraindications, should be reviewed carefully. The benefits and risks of administering a specific vaccine to a person under the circumstances should be considered. If the risks are believed to outweigh the benefits, the immunization should be withheld; if the benefits are believed to outweigh the risks (for example, during an outbreak or foreign travel), the immunization should be given. Whether and when to administer DTaP (or DTP) to children with proven or suspected underlying neurologic disorders should be decided on an individual basis.*

[c] *DTP is no longer recommended in the United States.*

[d] *Acetaminophen given before administering DTaP (or DTP) and thereafter every 4 hours for 24 hours should be considered for children with a personal or with a family (ie, siblings or parents) history or seizures.*

[e] *The decision to give additional doses of DTaP (or DTP) should be based on consideration of the benefit of further vaccination vs the risk of recurrence of GBS. For example, completion of the primary series in children is justified.*

[f] *A theoretical risk exists that the administration of multiple live virus vaccines within 30 days (4 weeks) of one another if not given on the same day will result in suboptimal immune response. No data substantiate this risk, however.*

[g] *OPV is no longer recommended for routine use in the United States.*

[h] *An anaphylactic reaction to egg ingestion previously was considered a contraindication unless skin testing and, if indicated, desensitization had been performed. However, skin testing no longer is recommended as of 1997.*

[i] *The decision to vaccinate should be based on consideration of the benefits of immunity to measles, mumps, and rubella vs the risk of recurrence or exacerbation of thrombocytopenia after vaccination, or from natural infections of measles or rubella. In most instances, the benefits of vaccination will be much greater than the potential risks and justify giving MMR, particularly in view of the even greater risk of thrombocytopenia after measles or rubella disease. However, if a prior episode of thrombocytopenia occurred in temporal proximity to vaccination, not giving a subsequent dose may be prudent.*

[j] *Measles vaccination may temporarily suppress tuberculin reactivity. MMR vaccine may be given after, or on the same day as, tuberculin testing. If MMR has been given recently, postpone the tuberculin test until 4 to 6 weeks after administration of MMR. If giving MMR simultaneously with the tuberculin skin test, use the Mantoux test and not multiple puncture tests, because the latter require confirmation if positive, which would have to be postponed for 4 to 6 weeks.*

[k] *Varicella vaccine should not be given to a member of a household with a family history of immunodeficiency until the immune status of the recipient and other children in the family is documented.*

This information is based on the recommendations of the Advisory Committee on Immunization Practices (ACIP) and of the Committee on Infectious Diseases of the American Academy of Pediatrics (AAP). Sometimes these recommendations vary from those in the manufacturers' product label. For more detailed information, providers should consult the published recommendations of the ACIP, AAP, and the manufacturers' package inserts. These guidelines, originally issued in 1993, have been updated to give current recommendations as of 2000 (based on information available as of December 1999).

Adapted from Committee on Infectious Diseases, American Academy of Pediatrics. (2000). 2000 Red Book: Report of the Committee on Infectious Diseases *(25th ed.). Elk Grove Village, IL: American Academy of Pediatrics.*

Nursing Tip:

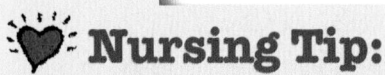

Immunization history

Before giving vaccines, ask the caregivers about the child's response to the last dose. Ask them to recall what vaccine was given and where. That way, you will be able to assess if the reactions were normal or not. You can choose an alternate site for the present vaccine. Make sure that all immunizations are recorded on the child's record. Document both the amount of vaccine used and the sites of the injections.

vented from receiving protection against possible life-threatening, preventable diseases. There are only two true, permanent contraindications to vaccination: (1) a history of severe anaphylactic reaction to a vaccine or its component and (2) encephalopathy within 7 days of administration of DTP/DTaP. Mild common illnesses such as otitis media, upper respiratory infections, colds, and diarrhea are *not* contraindications to immunizations.

Despite the availability of vaccines to prevent the majority of communicable diseases, some children and adolescents may be exposed to certain viruses or bacteria and may not be fully immunized or may have inadequate levels of immunity to these organisms. Epidemics of certain illnesses such as pertussis continue to occur despite the availability of immunization (Christie, Marx, Marchant, & Reising, 1994).

NURSING MANAGEMENT

Caregivers often look to nurses for guidance and counseling regarding the care of their children when an infectious dis-

Eye On:

What happened to polio drops?

Most families who have young children receiving immunizations have been immunized themselves when they were infants and children. Many caregivers recall receiving oral polio vaccine either on sugar cubes or as drops. When told by health care providers that their children will be immunized with a polio vaccine given as an injection, they may wonder and ask "I thought polio has been eradicated, why does my child need this immunization?" Health care providers must be prepared to answer their questions. It is important to let caregivers know that, although polio has been eliminated in the United States, there is still a need for immunization against polio. The infection still exists in many parts of the world, and there is a possibility that the virus could be introduced accidentally, thus leading to an epidemic (Wadsworth, 1999).

The first type of polio vaccine developed by Jonas Salk was licensed in 1955. It was a killed, inactivated vaccine, or IPV, that induced immunity through the blood system but was incapable of causing paralytic polio. The oral form of polio vaccine developed by Albert Sabin soon followed and was licensed in 1961. The oral preparation of polio vaccine (OPV) contained live but weakened virus, which acts in the intestines to produce immunity. It is capable of producing paralytic polio. Infants who receive their first dose orally (live virus) are susceptible to developing paralytic polio, although the chance is small. Weighing all of the variables, it remains imperative to continue vaccination against polio but with the killed virus, which is only available by injection.

Nursing Alert:

MMR Vaccine in Adolescent Females

When administering MMR vaccine to adolescent females, it is important to assess for the possibility of pregnancy. The vaccine is a ***teratogen*** *(any substance or process that interferes with normal prenatal development) and can cause developmental abnormalities in the fetus when given during the first trimester. If the vaccine is given, nurses need to caution the adolescents against pregnancy for at least 3 months.*

Critical Thinking

Implementing a Plan for Lapsed Immunizations

As the nurse in a pediatric clinic, you interview Ms. Cooper, the parent of 2-year-old Leslie. According to Leslie's immunization record, she has had the first and second hepatitis B vaccines plus the first diptheria–tetanus–pertussis and polio vaccines. Ms. Cooper relates that "This is all she has ever received," and asks "Will she have to start over again?" What will you tell Ms. Cooper about Leslie's current immunization status? What vaccines need to be administered today? How will you plan the remainder of Leslie's immunizations so that her mother knows when to return to the clinic?

ease occurs. Nurses are often asked questions such as "My child has been exposed to chickenpox. What are her chances of getting it? When will that happen?" or "Several children at school have Fifth's disease. Should I worry about my child catching it?" Nurses need to be knowledgeable about the clinical manifestations, etiology, incidence, and incubation period, as well as the therapeutic management of each disease. Table 15-3 presents some of the more common infectious diseases seen in children, with recommendations for treatment and prevention.

Several excellent resources are available for information about immunizations and vaccine recommendations. The main sources are publications and the Internet, which include the following:

- *Red Book: Report of the Committee on Infectious Diseases* of the AAP. This text is updated every 3 years and may be purchased from the AAP's website at www.aap.org/.
- *Morbidity and Mortality Weekly Report (MMWR)* of the CDC. This is a weekly newsletter and is available from the CDC's website at www.cdc.gov/.
- Statements and recommendations of the ACIP of the CDC.

Nurses can refer to these resources when giving anticipatory guidance and instructing caregivers on the care and management of children with infectious diseases. Nurses must seize the opportunity to educate caregivers about routine immunizations and the potential consequences of nonadherence to recommended schedules.

The majority of children who experience infectious or communicable diseases are managed at home. Home is the ideal environment because the spread of the infection is limited to those in the immediate environment. A small percentage of children may need to be hospitalized because of complications or secondary infection. Still other children may require respiratory or nutritional support. When these

TABLE 15-3 Infectious Diseases in Children

Disease	Clinical Manifestations	Etiology	Incidence/Incubation/Control	Therapeutic Management
Cytomegalovirus (CMV)	Most CMV infections are asymptomatic; most infants with congenital CMV infection are asymptomatic; however, 5% have significant manifestations of fetal damage (intrauterine growth retardation, jaundice, hepatitis, hepatosplenomegaly; brain damage, petechial rash, retinitis) **Diagnosis:** viral culture specimens from urine, pharynx, cervical secretions, human milk, semen, peripheral blood leukocytes; presence of IgM CMV antibodies in cord blood identifies congenitally infected infants; polymerase chain reaction detects CMV DNA in tissues **Complications:** psychomotor retardation, microcephaly, hearing loss, seizures, learning disabilities	Cytomegalovirus, a member of the herpes family of viruses **Transmission:** direct person-to-person contact with virus-containing secretions and from mother to infant before, during, or after birth	**Incidence:** CMV infection is distributed worldwide; most humans have become infected by the time they reach adulthood; CMV causes congenital infection in 1–2% of all live births **Incubation:** unknown for person-to-person transmission **Control:** at greatest risk are susceptible pregnant women exposed to urine and saliva of CMV-infected children who attend day care centers; handwashing and simple hygienic measures should be reinforced in this population	Administer ganciclovir, an antiviral drug, to treat life-threatening CMV infections in immunocompromised hosts (individuals with AIDS and recipients of bone marrow, heart, and kidney transplants) and to treat retinitis.
Diphtheria	Low-grade fever; gradual onset of membranous nasopharyngitis, obstructive laryngotracheitis **Diagnosis:** nose and throat cultures **Complications:** thrombocytopenia, myocarditis, vocal cord paralysis, ascending paralysis	*Corynebacterium diphtheriae* bacillus **Transmission:** intimate contact with discharges from the nose, throat, eye, and skin lesions	**Incidence:** more frequent in fall and winter; most common and most severe in unimmunized or inadequately immunized individuals **Incubation:** usually 2–5 days **Control:** universal immunization with diphtheria toxoid; prophylactic treatment of frequent close contacts with erythromycin or benzathine penicillin; notification of public health officials	Administer single dose of equine antitoxin IV after sensitivity testing. Administer erythromycin or penicillin. Initiate strict isolation of hospitalized individuals until two sequential nose and throat cultures are negative. Monitor respiratory status. Assess for signs of complications. Offer comfort measures such as rest, fluids, and fever management.

TABLE 15-3 *Continued*

Erythema Infectiosum (Fifth Disease) 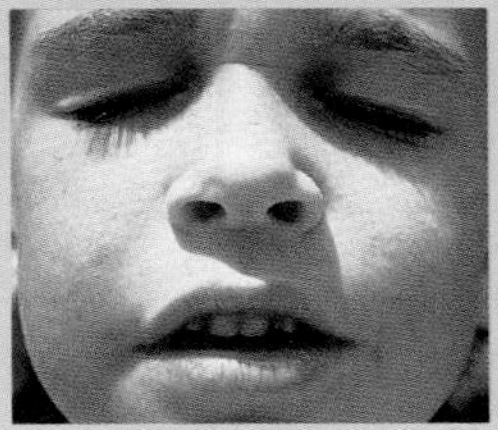 *Courtesy of the Centers for Disease Control and Prevention (CDC)*	Mild systemic symptoms, occasional fever, red facial rash giving a "slapped cheek" appearance, circumoral pallor, and symmetric lacy rash on trunk and limbs. Rarely seen in dark skinned individuals. Rash can recur for weeks with exposure to heat or sun **Diagnosis:** by clinical findings **Complications:** arthralgia, arthritis	Human parvovirus B19 **Transmission:** contact with respiratory secretions; contagious before onset of illness	**Incidence:** often has outbreaks in elementary or junior high schools during the spring **Incubation:** 4–14 days; can be as long as 20 days **Control:** good hygiene practices including handwashing and disposal of tissues contaminated with respiratory secretions	Manage fever and offer comfort measures if needed. Allow children to attend school since they are not contagious after appearance of the rash.
Infectious Mononucleosis	Fever, fatigue, exudative pharyngitis, lymphadenopathy, hepatosplenomegaly, atypical lymphocytosis; occasional rash **Diagnosis:** Usually confirmed by monospot and/or heterophile antibody blood tests **Complications:** aseptic meningitis, encephalitis, Guillain-Barré syndrome; rare: splenic rupture, thrombocytopenia, agranulocytosis, hemolytic anemia, orchitis, myocarditis	Epstein-Barr virus, a herpesvirus **Transmission:** contact with respiratory tract excretions and close personal contact	**Incidence:** common in group settings of adolescents, also found in children, no seasonal pattern **Incubation:** estimated to be 30–50 days **Control:** good hygiene practices including handwashing and disposal of tissues contaminated with respiratory secretions	Steroids may be considered when complications are present. Encourage rest. Manage fever. Maintain fluid intake with cool, nonacidic fluids, jello, popcicles. Suggest saline gargles for older children. Strongly advise avoidance of contact sports until splenomegaly resolves.

continues

TABLE 15-3 *Continued*

Disease	Clinical Manifestations	Etiology	Incidence/Incubation/Control	Therapeutic Management
Lyme disease 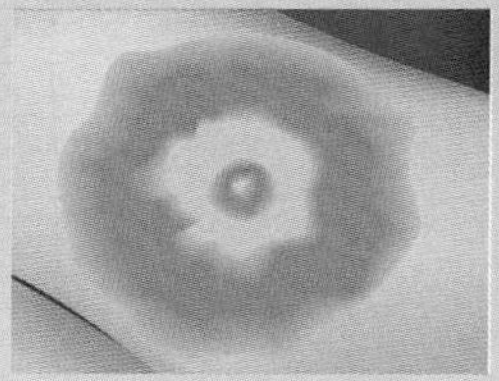 *Courtesy of the Centers for Disease Control and Prevention (CDC)*	Early stage: rash (erythema migrans), begins as a small papule and spreads peripherally; characterized by raised, red margin and clearning in the center at the site of the tick bite; fever; malaise; fatigue; headache; stiff neck; arthralgia. Late stage: arthritis of large joints, especially the knee, beginning months after the initial infection. **Diagnosis:** based on history and serologic testing **Complications:** rare in children: involvement of neurological and cardiac systems	*Borrelia burgdorferi*, a spirochete **Transmission:** to humans through the bite of infected tick, especially deer or black-legged tick; person-to-person is not possible	**Incidence:** localized to three regions of the United States—northeast (Maryland to Massachusetts), midwest (Wisconsin and Minnesota), west (northwest California); incidence is highest in children 5–10 years of age **Incubation:** 7–14 days (range 3–30 days) **Control:** avoid tick infested areas; use tick repellent with DEET; wear light-colored long-sleeve top and pants (light color makes tick identification easier); inspect clothing and body daily after possible tick exposure; remove ticks from body immediately; immunize persons over 15 years of age who reside or recreate in geographical areas of high risk	Antibiotics—doxycycline (Vibramycin) or amoxicillin (Augmentin)
Mumps	Mild systemic symptoms, swelling of the salivary glands, meningeal signs in 10–30% of cases **Diagnosis:** complement–fixation test **Complications:** encephalitis, orchitis rare: arthritis, renal involvement, thyroiditis, mastitis, pancreatitis, hearing impairment	Paramyxovirus **Transmission:** direct contact with respiratory secretions	**Incidence:** late winter and spring; peak incidence in 10–14 year olds **Incubation:** usually 16–18 days; may be as long as 25 days **Control:** universal immunization of children; good hygiene practices including handwashing and disposal of tissues contaminated with respiratory secretions	Manage fever and comfort measures. Exclude from school until 9 days after onset of parotid swelling.

TABLE 15-3 *Continued*

Pertussis (whooping cough)	Begins with mild upper respiratory symptoms known as the catarrahal stage; progresses to severe paroxysms of cough, often with a characteristic inspiratory whoop followed by vomiting. Apnea is common in infants under 6 months **Diagnosis:** nasopharyngeal culture **Complications:** seizures, pneumonia, encephalopathy, death	*Bordetella pertussis* bacillus **Transmission:** close contact with respiratory secretions; most contagious during mild respiratory symptoms	**Incidence:** occurs in unimmunized or partially immunized infants and children; adolescents and adults are a major source; no seasonal pattern **Incubation:** 6–20 days **Control:** Universal immunization; erythromycin prophylaxis for household and other close contacts; good hygiene practices including handwashing and disposal of tissues contaminated with respiratory secretions	Infants under 6 months and other clients with severe disease are usually hospitalized. Administer erythromycin orally for 14 days. Observe respiratory isolation for 5 days after initiation of antibiotic treatment. Maintain airway. Maintain fluid intake. Provide a restful environment. Offer supportive care for respiratory distress and feeding difficulties. Support anxious parents by explaining about the illness and the nature of the cough.
Polio	Nonspecific illness with low-grade fever and sore throat **Diagnosis:** stool culture **Complications:** Aseptic meningitis; rapid onset of asymmetric acute flaccid paralysis and residual paralytic disease involving the motor neurons; paralysis of respiratory muscles	Enterovirus **Transmission:** fecal–oral and possibly respiratory	**Incidence:** more common in infants and young children; most common in summer and fall; all endemic cases since 1979 have been associated with oral poliovirus vaccine **Incubation:** 3–6 days **Control:** universal immunization; good hygiene practices including handwashing and handling of diapers	Offer comfort measures and supportive treatment depending on extent of complications present. Refer for physical therapy if required.

continues

TABLE 15-3 *Continued*

Disease	Clinical Manifestations	Etiology	Incidence/Incubation/Control	Therapeutic Management
Rocky Mountain Spotted Fever 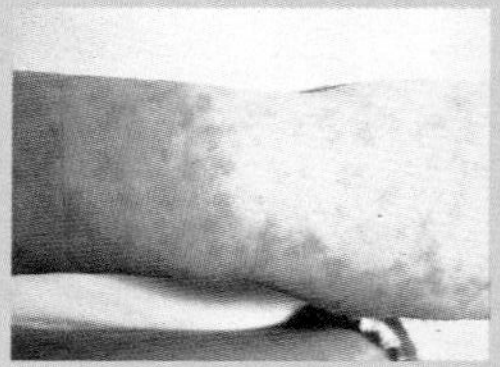 *Courtesy of the Centers for Disease Control and Prevention (CDC)*	Fever, headache, myalgia, nausea, vomiting, anorexia, confusion, erthematous and macular rash on ankles and wrists (may spread to rest of body) **Diagnosis:** history and serologic tests **Complications:** CNS disease; multisystem organ failure; disseminated intravascular coagulation (DIC); shock, and death	*Rickettsia rickettsii* **Transmission:** to humans through the bite of infected tick; reservoir—dogs, wild rodents	**Incidence:** occurs in spring and summer; disease is widespread in United States; most cases reported in south Atlantic, southeastern, and south central states **Incubation:** 1 week (range of 2–14 days) **Control:** same as Lyme disease	Chloramphenicol (Chloromycetin) or doxycycline (Vibramycin)
Roseola (Human herpesvirus 6) 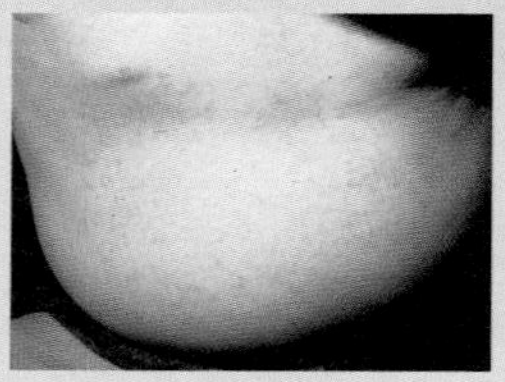 *Courtesy of Robert A. Silverman, M.D., Clinical Associate Professor, Department of Pediatrics, Georgetown University*	High fever for 3–5 days followed by a red maculopapular rash lasting up to several days **Diagnosis:** by clinical presentation **Complications:** seizures, encephalitis	Human herpesvirus 6 **Transmission:** contact with respiratory secretions	**Incidence:** highest in children between 6 and 24 months of age; rare before 3 months and after 4 years of age; no seasonal pattern **Incubation:** estimated to be about 9 days **Control:** good hygiene practices including handwashing	Manage fever. Manage fluid intake. Offer comfort measures.
Rotavirus	Diarrhea, usually preceded or accompanied by vomiting and low-grade fever; in severe cases, isotonic dehydration, electrolyte imbalances; and acidosis **Diagnosis:** history and clinical presentation; immuno-assays **Complications:** death	*Rotaviruses* **Transmission:** fecal–oral route; possibly respiratory	**Incidence:** most common in infants and children under 2 years of age and day care centers **Incubation:** 48 hours **Control:** good hygiene; children in whom diarrhea cannot be contained by diapers or toilet use should be excluded from day care centers until diarrhea ceases	Prevention and treatment of dehydration; no antiviral therapy is available.

TABLE 15-3 *Continued*

Rubella (German measles) 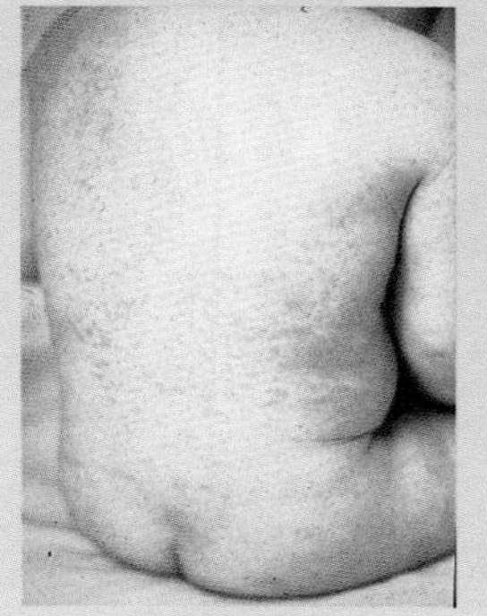 *Courtesy of the Centers for Disease Control and Prevention (CDC)*	Slight fever, red maculopapular discrete rash, lymphadenopathy; 25–50% of cases are asymptomatic. First day of rash: head and upper torso heavily covered with rash. By third day lower half is heavily covered with rash with upper part lessening in rash severity. **Diagnosis:** nasal secretion culture; acute and convalescent antibody titers **Complications:** transient polyarthralgia and polyarthritis. rare: encephalitis, thrombocytopenia teratogenic effect on fetus if client is pregnant.	Rubella virus **Transmission:** direct or droplet contact with nasopharyngeal secretions	**Incidence:** peaks in late winter and early spring **Incubation:** 14–21 days **Control:** universal immunization; good hygiene practices including handwashing and disposal of tissues contaminated with respiratory secretions	Initiate isolation and school exclusion for 7 days after onset of the rash. Offer supportive care and comfort measures.
Rubeola (measles) 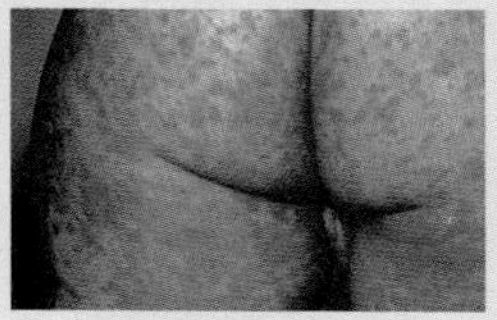 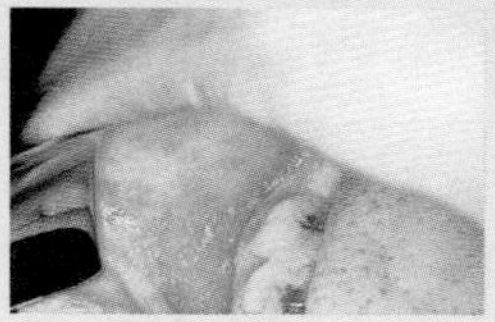 Koplik's spots appearing on the lingual and buccal mucosa in Rubeola. They are small red spots with bluish-white centers. *Courtesy of the Centers for Disease Control and Prevention (CDC)*	Acutely ill with fever, cough, coryza, conjunctivitis, Koplik spots. Rash begins light on upper body and head on first day. By third day the upper body rash has increased and progressed to lower body. **Diagnosis:** viral tissue culture from nasopharyngeal secretions; acute and convalescent antibody titers **Complications:** otitis media, bronchopneumonia, croup, diarrhea, encephalitis resulting in permanent brain damage, death	Morbillivirus **Transmission:** direct contact with infectious droplets; occasionally by airborne spread	**Incidence:** peaks in winter and spring, primarily in unimmunized individuals **Incubation:** 8–12 days **Control:** universal immunization; good hygiene practices including handwashing and disposal of tissues contaminated with respiratory secretions	Initiate respiratory isolation for 4 days after onset of rash. Consider administration of vitamin A if deficiency is suspected. Encourage hospitalization of infants and children with severe cases or complications. Observe fever control measures. Offer comfort measures, including dimming the lights in the presence of photophobia.

continues

TABLE 15-3 *Continued*

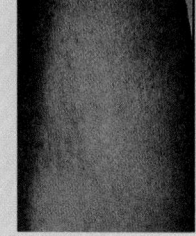

Disease	Clinical Manifestations	Etiology	Incidence/Incubation/Control	Therapeutic Management
Scarlet Fever  *Courtesy of the Centers for Disease Control and Prevention (CDC)*	Acute fever, sore throat, rhinitis, headache, red sandpaper-like rash prominent in creases, white strawberry tongue (day 1), flush cheeks, red strawberry tongue (day 2) **Diagnosis:** throat culture **Complications:** otitis media, sinusitis, peritonsillar and retropharyngeal abscesses, cervical adenitis, rheumatic fever, acute glomerulonephritis	Group A beta-hemolytic streptococci (GAS) **Transmission:** contact with respiratory secretions	**Incidence:** most frequent among school-aged children in late fall, winter, and spring **Incubation:** 2–5 days **Control:** prompt treatment; good hygiene practices including handwashing and disposal of tissues contaminated with respiratory secretions	Administer antibiotics for 10 days (penicillin, erythromycin, amoxicillin, cephalosporins). Encourage school exclusion for at least 24 hours after initiation of treatment and until afebrile. Manage fever. Maintain fluid intake with cool, nonacidic fluids, jello, popcicles. Suggest saline gargles for older children. Offer comfort measures.
Tetanus	Early signs—headache, restlessness, followed by spasms of masticatory (chewing) muscles, difficulty opening mouth (**trismus**), dysphagia; eventually, **opisthotonos** (severe spasm of back muscles causing back to arch acutely, head to bend back on neck); seizures; dysuria and urinary retention; bowel incontinence; and fever **Diagnosis:** based on clinical presentation **Complications:** airway obstruction and asphyxiation due to laryngeal and respiratory muscle spasms; death	*Clostridium tetani*–spore-forming bacillus produces a neurotoxin that affects the central nervous system (spinal cord and brain stem) **Transmission:** to humans through wound in skin from contact with soil contaminated with animal feces	**Incidence:** worldwide; prevalent in nonimmunized populations. Mortality rate is high. Spores, found in soil, dust, and intestinal tracts of humans and animals, especially horse and cattle. **Incubation:** 4–14 days (average 8 days) **Control:** active immunization with tetanus toxoid; tetanus prophylaxis should be followed as part of wound management; prompt surgical cleansing and debridement of wounds	Administer human tetanus immune globulin (TIG) to neutralize the neurotoxin in the child's system in order to stop continuation of the infectious process. Administer Penicillin G, IV initially, for 10–14 days. Surgically cleanse and debride wound. Administer diazepam (Valium) to reduce muscle spasms and control seizures. Respiratory support and intervention as needed. Provide quiet environment since muscle spasms are aggravated by external stimuli.

TABLE 15-3 *Continued*

Varicella (chicken pox) 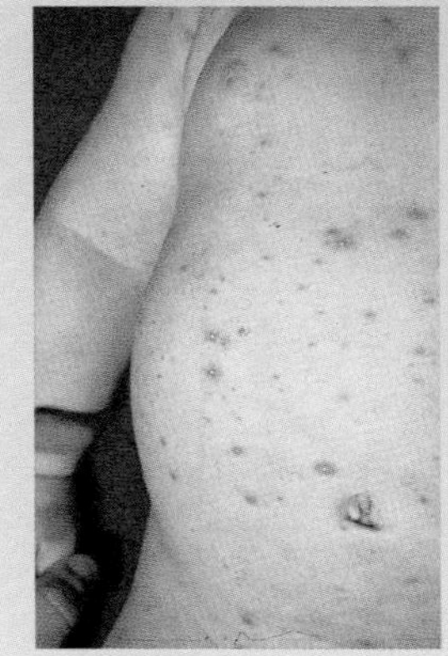 *Courtesy of Robert A. Silverman, M.D., Clinical Associate Professor, Department of Pediatrics, Georgetown University*	Mild fever and systemic symptoms; generalized pruritic, vesicular rash **Diagnosis:** usually by clinical findings **Complications:** bacterial superinfection of lesions, thrombocytopenia, arthritis, hepatitis, encephalitis, meningitis, glomerulonephritis, Reye's syndrome	Varicella-zoster virus, a herpesvirus **Transmission:** highly contagious; direct contact and airborne spread from respiratory secretions	**Incidence:** most often in children under 10 years of age; most common in late winter and early spring **Incubation:** 10–21 days **Control:** universal immunization; good hygiene practices including handwashing and disposal of tissues contaminated with respiratory secretions	Oral acyclovir may be given in some cases, but is not recommended for routine treatment of uncomplicated cases in otherwise healthy children. Manage fever (aspirin is contraindicated since it increases risk of Reye's syndrome). Observe strict isolation for at least 5 days in hospitalized clients. Manage pruritus with oral antihistamine (benadryl), baking soda or oatmeal baths, and calamine lotion to keep child cool. Maintain fluid intake with cool, non-acidic fluids, jello, popcicles. Prevent secondary infection by controlling pruritus and keeping child's fingernails clean and short. School exclusion until all lesions are dry and crusted over.

Adapted from Committee on Infectious Diseases, American Academy of Pediatrics. (2000). 2000 Red Book: Report of the Committee on Infectious Diseases *(25th ed.). Elk Grove Village, IL: American Academy of Pediatrics; and Centers for Disease Control. (2000).* Epidemiology and prevention of vaccine-preventable diseases *(6th ed.). Atlanta, GA: U.S. Department of Health and Human Services.*

Kids Want To Know

Can my classmates get chickenpox from me?

Martina, a 10-year-old, has chickenpox and has not been at school for the past 7 days. She returned 8 days after the onset of the rash. Her classmates are afraid to get near her because of all the lesions on her face, arms, and legs. The nurse explains that the infectious period is 1–2 days before the eruption of the rash to 6 days after the onset of the lesions, when crusts have formed. Although she has many lesions, they have all crusted over. Therefore, Martina can tell the other kids that they cannot get chickenpox from her.

children are hospitalized, isolation procedures may need to be instituted depending on the etiologic agent and the method of transmission. The hospital's infection control department is the best resource in directing the parameters of the isolation and precautions associated with the particular illness. Even at home, caregivers may want to isolate the ill child from well siblings to prevent the spread of infection.

Caregivers who treat their children at home need teaching regarding supportive care and comfort measures. Many caregivers may be unfamiliar with the types of treatment that will promote their children's comfort while restoring them back to health. Others may rely on home remedies, some of which may be harmful to children. For example, the use of alcohol sponging to reduce fever is still promoted by some family members but can be dangerous to small infants and children.

Fever is often present during the earliest stage of the illness, also known as the **prodrome** (the earliest phase or sign of a developing condition or disease). Fever management may include the use of tepid sponges, dressing in cool clothing, and antipyretic medications such as acetaminophen or ibuprofen. These medications are analgesic as well as antipyretic and may be used to relieve the discomfort of other accompanying symptoms such as headache, malaise, sore throat, or muscular aches and pains.

Some illnesses may be accompanied by vomiting or diarrhea. Caregivers will need to know the signs and symptoms of dehydration, as well as how to prevent dehydration and manage fluid intake (see Chapter 21). Some viral diseases that cause mouth lesions, such as varicella (chickenpox) may make oral intake difficult. Fluids that are soothing such as gelatins or popsicles should be offered. Once children begin to recover, they gradually may progress to their normal diets.

Children who manifest pruritic lesions may be treated with antihistamines such as diphenhydramine hydrochloride (Benadryl) or hydroxyzine hydrochloride (Atarax). Baking soda, oatmeal, or colloid preparations in bath water may assist in relieving discomfort. Topical drying agents such as calamine can be used to decrease itching. Fingernails should be cut short and kept clean to prevent secondary infections. Covering an infant's hands with cotton mittens or socks may inhibit the tendency to scratch, especially during periods of sleep.

Many respiratory illnesses may be accompanied by coughing, which may be **paroxysmal,** or severe, in character. Children may need extra humidification; this can be accomplished by room humidifiers or by placing the child in the bathroom with the mist from a shower. A mist tent can be constructed by draping a sheet over the crib or bed and directing the humidifier at the head of the bed. Sick children may need quiet activities to occupy their time during the convalescent period. Soft music, reading to children, and age-appropriate games and videos may provide some comfort and diversion to children and their families.

Caregivers will need to know approximately how long the illness will last, the period of communicability, plus the appropriate time for children to return to school or day care. All of the these factors are specific to the etiology of the illness. Although the incidence of complications from childhood infectious diseases is rare, caregivers will need to know what signs and symptoms indicate problems. Neurological signs such as severe headache, irritability, stiff neck, altered levels of consciousness, and seizures may indicate viral encephalitis, an inflammation of the brain, which is a rare sequella of chickenpox, measles, mumps, or rubella infection. A disease that affects the respiratory system such as pertussis may cause respiratory distress and apnea. Part of the educational process should be directed to an under-

Nursing Alert:

Use of Acetaminophen

Acetaminophen (Tylenol) is available in liquid, tablet, and suppository form in a variety of strengths. Nurses will need to discuss the variation in concentration with caregivers to ascertain which particular form will be used. This will prevent either underdosing or overdosing of the medication. Regardless of the form of the acetaminophen, the recommended dose for infants and children is 10–15 mg/kg/dose every 4 hours, but not more than five times a day. The major toxicity from overdose is liver damage. Many over-the-counter cold remedies contain acetaminophen. Caregivers may not be aware of this and want to use a combination product in addition to acetaminophen. Instruct caregivers to read labels carefully to prevent overdosing, and keep this and all medications out of reach of children in the household.

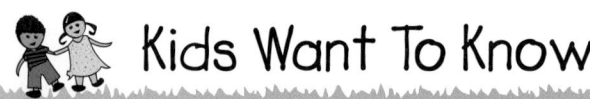

standing of the pathophysiology of the disease, the rationale for the therapy, and monitoring for signs of complications.

The infectious diseases that adolescents experience are most frequently related to their sexual activity. Adolescent behavior regarding sexuality has been discussed here and in Chapter 12. Table 15-4 lists some of the common sexually transmitted diseases experienced by adolescents. Nurses need to be aware that diseases thought of as being sexually transmitted may be seen in younger children. Some of these such as chlamydia, gonorrhea, syphilis, and HIV (other than perinatally transmitted) can be suggestive of sexual abuse. If sexual abuse is suspected, it must be reported (see Chapter 36).

Intestinal parasites including parasitic worms and protozoa are described in Table 15-5.

Many infectious diseases are reportable by law to local and state health departments who, in turn, must report them to the CDC. At the CDC, information about the occurrence and nature of such diseases is collected. With this data, the CDC monitors trends of disease, evaluates the effectiveness of disease-focused interventions, and makes recommendations to health care agencies for infection control and prevention. Some of the diseases discussed in this chapter are among those required to be reported (Box 15-1). The list of reportable infectious diseases may change based on suspected prevalence of particular diseases. It is important that the pediatric nurse be familiar with the current list of reportable infectious diseases.

BOX 15-1 Selected infectious diseases that must be reported to the Centers for Disease Control and Prevention

Acquired immunodeficiency syndrome (AIDS)
Chancroid
Congenital rubella syndrome
Diphtheria
Encephalitis, post chickenpox and mumps
Gonorrhea
Hepatitis B
Measles
Mumps
Pertussis
Paralytic polio
Rubella
Syphilis, all stages
Varicella

Adapted from American Academy of Pediatrics. (2000). *2000 red book: Report of the Committee on Infectious Diseases* (25th ed.). Elk Grove Village, IL: Author.

FUTURE DIRECTIONS

Since the introduction of immunization practices for children, which began in the 1940s, the recommendations and requirements for vaccines continue to evolve. Researchers continuously engage in the practice of seeking treatments and cures for disease, with a primary goal of prevention through vaccine development. As newer vaccines are developed, they must undergo strict research and FDA approval before their release. A vaccine for rotavirus was developed and placed on the recommended schedule of immunizations for 1999 (CDC, 1999). Within the year, the vaccine was withdrawn voluntarily from the market because of an association with intussusception.

A new vaccine, pneumococcal conjugate (Prevnar), has been developed for pneumococcus (*Streptococcus pneumoniae*), the most common cause of sepsis, sinusitis, pneumonia, otitis media, and menigitis in children under the age of 2 (ACIP, 2000). Previously, a form of vaccine, pnuemococcal polysaccharide (Pneumovax, Pnu-Imune), was shown to be effective for children over 2 years of age and given to those who had chronic illnesses such as HIV infection and sickle cell anemia. It was not recommended for younger children (younger than 2 years of age) and infants because of poor antibody response. However, the new vaccine, Prevnar, has proven to be highly effective at inducing the desired response and preventing infection in children under 2 years old and infants. Therefore, it is recommended that all children receive it at the 2, 4, 6, and 12–15 months visits (Overturf & the Committee on Infectious Diseases, 2000).

Although deaths from infectious diseases decreased markedly during the past century, there has been an increase in mortality over the past two decades, attributable in part to the emergence of new pathogens, specifically HIV (CDC, 1998b). Influenza continues to reemerge periodically and cause epidemics. *Mycobacterium tuberculosis*, which includes new drug-resistant strains, has made a comeback and is especially devastating to those infected with the HIV virus. Drug resistance due to the overuse of antibiotics has presented some distinct challenges, as noted by the growing incidence of penicillin-resistant *Streptococcal pneumoniae*, vancomycin-resistant enterococci, and methicillin-resistant *Staphylococcus aureus*. There are several factors that have contributed to this phenomenon, including population growth and crowding; increased use of day care and community living centers; destruction of natural habitats; increasing numbers of persons who are immunosuppressed; aging of the population; use of antimicrobial drugs; and globalization of food distribution, commerce, and travel. It is now known that the bacterium *Helicobacter pylori* is responsible for the majority of peptic ulcers thought to be due to stress and diet. Once diagnosed, the infection is easily treated by a drug combination, which includes antibiotics and H_2 receptor antagonists (text continues on page 450).

TABLE 15-4 Sexually Transmitted Diseases in Adolescents

Disease	Clinical Manifestations	Etiology	Incidence/Incubation/Control	Therapeutic Management
Gonorrhea	**Female:** purulent discharge, urethritis, endocervicitis, pelvic inflammatory disease (PID) **Male:** purulent discharge, urethritis **Both sexes:** pharyngitis, conjunctivitis, proctitis **Neonates:** infection of the eyes; scalp abcess related to fetal monitor probe **Diagnosis:** Gram stain **Complications:** acute epididymitis, acute PID, arthritis, dermatitis, meningitis, disseminated gonococcal infection, infertility	*Neisseria gonorrhoeae* a gram-negative diplococcus **Transmission:** intimate contact, sexual intercourse, sexual abuse (sexual abuse should be considered when a diagnosis of gonorrhea is made in any child who is not sexually active), perinatal	**Incidence:** 132/100,000 in U.S. Highest rate reported in adolescents 15–19 years of age **Incubation:** 2–7 days **Control:** Obtain an endocervical culture as part of prenatal care; evaluation for other sexually transmitted diseases; treatment of contacts; notification of public health officials	Administer ceftriaxone IM or cefixime PO in a single dose plus doxycycline twice a day for 7 days or azithromycin PO in a single dose. Evaluate for other STDs including syphilis, HIV, chlamydia, hepatitis B. Chlamydia occurs in 45% of cases of gonorrhea and should be treated. Encourage abstinence until treated and symptom free. Offer education regarding medication administration and importance of adherence to treatment regimen. Avoid sexual contact until cured. No need to return for test of cure one week after completing therapy unless symptoms persist.
Syphilis 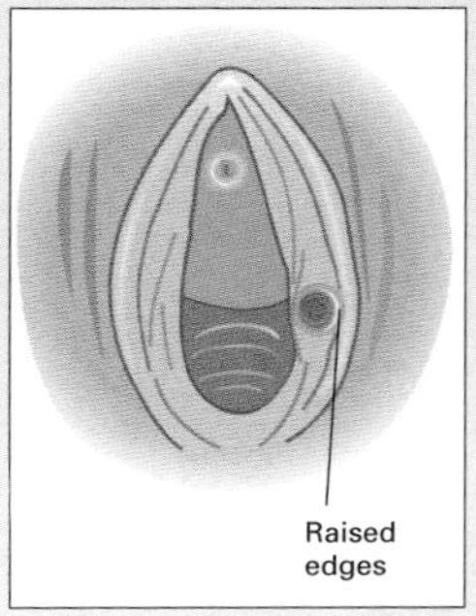 	**Congenital:** Stillbirth, prematurity, hydrops fetalis, multisystem sequelae including hepatosplenomegaly, mucocutaneous lesions, lymphadenopathy, thrombocytopenia. **Acquired:** **Primary stage:** one or more painless ulcers of mucous membranes and skin usually on genitalia.	*Treponema pallidum* spirochete **Transmission:** Congenital: Transplacental during pregnancy or at time of delivery: **Acquired:** intimate contact, sexual intercourse, sexual abuse (sexual abuse should be considered when a diagnosis of acquired syphilis is made in any child who is not sexually active)	**Incidence:** 2.6 per 100,000 **Incubation:** 3 weeks with a range of 10–90 days **Control:** Screen women early in pregnancy and at delivery; education and treatment of sexual contacts with reporting to public health authorities	**Congenital:** Administer aqueous crystalline penicillin G IV q12h for 7 days then q8h for 3 additional days for a total of 10 days or single dose of procaine penicillin G IM daily for 10 days. **Early acquired syphilis:** Primary, secondary, or tertiary of < 1 year's duration Administer single dose of benzathine penicillin G IM once

TABLE 15-4 *Continued*

	Secondary stage: maculopapular rash on palms and soles, fever, enlarged lymph glands, sore throat, headache, splenomegaly, arthralgia. **Tertiary stage:** neurosyphilis, skin, bone or visceral changes, aortitis. **Diagnosis:** Serologic testing: VDRL, RPR **Complications:** If left untreated, client can experience manifestations of secondary and tertiary syphilis.			**Pregnancy:** Benzathine penicillin G IM two doses one week apart **Penicillin allergy:** Administer tetracycline qid for 14 days or erythromycin bid for 14 days (this does not apply to clients who are pregnant) Offer education regarding the importance of adherence to medication administration. Advise client to refer sexual contacts for evaluation and treatment. Advise to avoid sexual activity until cured. Encourage follow-up to monitor serology as recommended. Instruct to use latex condoms to prevent further reinfection.
Chlamydia	Symptomatic or asymptomatic **Female:** Mucopurulent cervicitis, urethritis, salpingitis, and proctitis **Male:** Nongonococcal urethritis **Diagnosis:** Chlamydia culture Enzyme immunoassay for screening **Complications:** Pelvic inflammatory disease, infertility, ectopic pregnancy **Neonates:** ophthalmia neonatorum, chlamydial pneumonia	*Chlamydia trachomatis* bacterial agent **Transmission:** Sexual transmission In neonates, contact with infected genital tract during delivery	**Incidence:** 236/100,000 Most common STD in adults less than 25 years old Rate in pregnancy: 6–12% Rate during adolescence: as high as 37% **Incubation:** About a week **Control:** Refer sexual contacts for evaluation and treatment. Screen for infection during routine gynecological and prenatal exams.	Administer doxycycline BID for 7 days or azithromycin 1 gram in a single dose or erythromycin QID for 7 days. Encourage abstinence until treated and symptom free. Offer education regarding medication administration and importance of adherence to the treatment regimen. Advise to avoid sexual contact until cured. Instruct in the use of latex condoms to prevent further reinfection.

continues

TABLE 15-4 *Continued*

Disease	Clinical Manifestations	Etiology	Incidence/Incubation/Control	Therapeutic Management
Herpes genitalis (HSV-2) 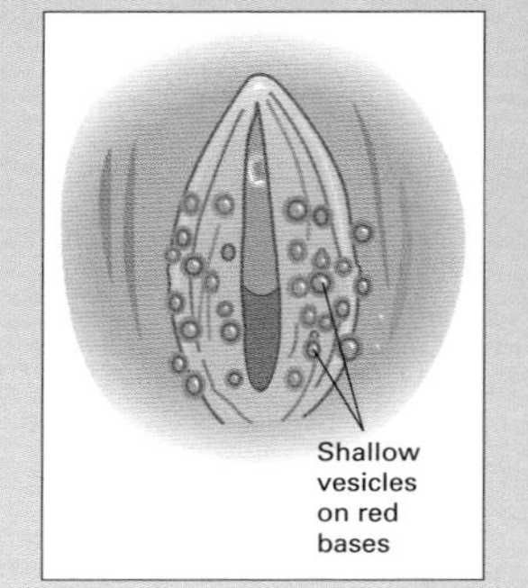	Characterized by periods of latency between initial outbreak and recurrence. **Primary infection:** Itching or intense burning at site of outbreak; may be accompanied by flu-like symptoms. Inguinal lymphadenopathy Initial lesions are painful raised vesicles. Recurrent lesions are less painful and resolve more quickly. Virus can be shed when client is asymptomatic and is contagious. **Diagnosis:** Viral culture **Complications:** In newborns, generalized systemic infection including CNS and liver involvement; infections of skin, eyes, and mouth. High mortality rate in neonatal herpes infection.	*Herpes Simplex type 2* virus **Transmission:** In neonates, acquired during pregnancy through the placenta or contact with infected genital tract during delivery. Sexual intercourse.	**Incidence:** 1 out of 5 adults over age 12 30,000,000 cases annually **Incubation:** About 6 days **Control:** Abstinence during outbreak Use of condoms at other times since transmission has been noted without evidence of lesions	No effective cure **Primary lesions:** Administer oral acyclovir within 6 days of onset to shorten median duration of viral shedding from primary lesion and signs and symptoms by 3–5 days. **Recurrent lesions:** Administer oral acyclovir within 2 days of symptom onset to shorten clinical course. Oral acyclovir decreases frequency of recurrence (6 or more episodes per year) Valacyclovir and famciclovir can also be used. Counsel about asymptomatic viral shedding and potential for recurrent outbreaks. Keep lesions clean and dry. Encourage abstinence during active stage when lesions are present. Advise use of latex condoms to prevent infection in sexual partners.
Human Papillomavirus (HPV) 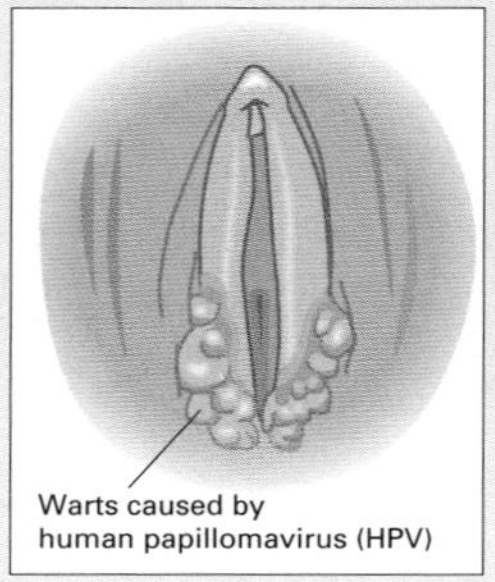	Soft, fleshy, single or multiple papules which occur in the anogenital area and are known as genital warts. Pain, pruritus Can be asymptomatic or subclinical **Female:** Warts located on perineum, vulva, cervix, vagina, urethra, anus, oral cavity	*Human papillomavirus* over 20 types; most common types 6 or 11 **Transmission:** Direct sexual contact Perinatal contact during delivery	**Incidence:** 50 per 100,000 population—3,000,000 cases annually **Incubation:** 3 months to several months **Control:** Encourage sexual partner to be examined.	Treatment depends on the location of the lesions: **Client application:** Instruct client in self application of Podofilox 0.5% solution or gel BID for 3 days, or Imiquimod 5% cream for 16 weeks.

TABLE 15-4 *Continued*

	Male: Warts located on penis, perineum, anus, oral cavity **Diagnosis:** Clinical presentation; biopsy **Complications:** Cervical, anal, or vaginal dysplasia Can lead to cervical cancer Reoccurrence Laryngeal papilloma in newborn		Counseling sex partner of client with HPV. Cervical cancer screening for female partner of client with HPV	**Provider application:** Administer cryotherapy with liquid nitrogen every 1–2 weeks. Apply odophyllin resin 10–25% application to lesions every week. Apply trichloroacetic acid to lesions weekly. Assist in surgical removal by excision or laser surgery. Provide client with patient education regarding need for periodic screening for cervical cancer as well as examination of sexual partners for presence of warts
Hepatitis B (HBV)	General fatigue, muscle and joint pain, loss of appetite **Diagnosis:** History of illness including sexual history, IV drug use, hepatitis panel **Complications:** Chronic carrier state Chronic persistent hepatitis Progressive liver disease with cirrhosis or hepatocellular carcinoma	*Hepadnavirus* **Transmission:** Contact with infected blood or body fluids; sexual contact, perinatal transmission	**Incidence:** 10,258 new cases 5–10% become chronic carriers **Incubation:** Average 120 days with a range of 45–160 days Infected person can infect others approximately 4–6 weeks before symptoms appear **Control:** Prenatal screening: universal precautions; immunoprophylaxis with hepatitis B vaccine Condom use for sexual activity	No specific treatment Symptomatic management Administer interferon alpha-2b antiviral medication, which is 40% effective in eliminating chronic HBV infection. Administer Hepatitis B Immune Globulin when exposed to HBV. Offer counseling for clients who are chronic carriers of Hepatitis B.

continues

TABLE 15-4 *Continued*

Disease	Clinical Manifestations	Etiology	Incidence/Incubation/Control	Therapeutic Management
Human immunodeficiency virus (HIV type 1, more common in U.S.; HIV type 2, more common in West Africa)	Symptomatology of acute retroviral syndrome including fever, sore throat, skin rash, lymphadenopathy, malaise, arthralgia, myalgia, headache, nausea, and vomiting. **Diagnosis:** HIV RNA PCR test in infants less that 18 months of age. HIV antibody test in infants and children greater than 18 months of age and Western blot. HIV culture **Complications:** Progression to AIDS as late manifestation (in 85% of cases within 17 years after infection) Opportunistic infections such as *Pneumocystis carinii pneumonia* (PCP), Kaposi's sarcoma (KS), *Mycobacterium avium complex* (MAC) AIDS	*Retrovirus, RNA virus* **Transmission:** Contact with infected blood or body fluids; sexual contact, perinatal transmission	**Incidence:** 40,000–80,000 new infections annually **Incubation:** Signs and symptoms may appear 2–12 weeks after infection. Seroconversion (the ability of antibodies to HIV to be detected in the blood) may not occur until 4–12 weeks or longer after infection. The period when antibodies remain undetected is known as the "window period" **Control:** Avoid sex with individuals having multiple partner use; consistent use of latex condoms; avoid needle sharing; offer testing to HIV positive women during pregnancy	No known cure Informed consent necessary to obtain HIV testing. Pre and post test counseling by trained professionals is essential to discuss the options for treatment if a test is positive. Treatment assists to slow the decline of the immune system. Current treatment includes highly active antiretroviral therapy (HAART) consisting of three classifications of medications: nucleoside reverse transcriptase inhibitors; non-nucleoside reverse transcriptase inhibitors; and protease inhibitors. Treatment is individualized based the client's immune status and sensitivity to the specific drug. Treatment goals include maintaining high CD4 counts and decreased viral loads. Counseling, social support, behavioral change, referral for care.

Adapted from American Academy of Pediatrics. (2000). 2000 Red Book: Report of the Committee on Infectious Diseases *(25th Ed.). Elk Grove Village, IL: Author; and Centers for Disease Control and Prevention. (1997). 1998 guidelines for treatment of sexually transmitted diseases. Morbidity and* Mortality Weekly Report, *47(RR1), 1–111.*

TABLE 15-5 Intestinal Parasites (including Helminths [Parasitic worms] and Protozoa)

Disease	Clinical Manifestations	Etiology	Incidence/Incubation/Control	Therapeutic Management
Giardia	May be asymptomatic; chronic or relapsing diarrhea (may be watery or greasy, foul-smelling); crampy abdominal pain; anorexia leading to weight loss and failure to thrive; flatulence **Diagnosis:** identification of cysts in fecal sample or enzyme immunoassay to detect *G. lamblia* antigens **Complications:** lactose intolerance	*Giardia lamblia*, a protozoan **Transmission:** humans are main reservoir, but the organisms can infect dogs, cats, beavers, and other animals; animals can contaminate water with feces containing cysts; direct transmission: hand-to-mouth transfer of cysts from feces of infected person; indirect: ingestion of cyst contaminated water or food	**Incidence:** more common in children than adults; endemic in areas of world with poor sanitation; associated with day care centers and residential institutions for the mentally retarded **Incubation:** 1–4 weeks (average 8 days) **Control:** improved sanitation and personal hygiene in day care centers; good handwashing, especially after diapering infants and toileting; exclude infected child from day care centers until diarrhea resolves; educate families who camp and hike to avoid drinking water from streams	Drug of choice furazolidone (Furoxone); other drugs available: quinacrine hydrochloride (Atabrine) and metronidazole (Flagyl)
Pinworms (enterobius)	Nocturnal anal itching, sleeplessness **Diagnosis:** direct visualization of worms or microscopy; eggs detected on transparent tape pressed against perianal region in morning before child has a bowel movement **Complications:** movement of worm to appendix, female genital tract, and peritoneal cavity	*Enterobius vermicularis* **Transmission:** fecal-oral; ingestion or inhalation of eggs of worm; eggs are transmitted by fingers and hands from scratching anal area; eggs remain infective in indoor environment for 2-3 weeks and contaminate anything they contact such as shared toys; bedding, clothing, toilet seats, baths, and food	**Incidence:** most common helminth infection in United States; occurs frequently in preschoolers and school-aged children, crowded conditions, institutions, and families **Incubation:** 1-2 months **Control:** good handwashing after contact with infected child, bed linens, clothes, after toileting and before eating; keep child's fingernails short to minimize chance of eggs collecting under nails from scratching	Drug of choice: mebedazole (Vermox) or pyrantel pamoate (Antiminth); all household members are treated simultaneously

continues

TABLE 15-5 *Continued*

Disease	Clinical Manifestations	Etiology	Incidence/Incubation/Control	Therapeutic Management
Ascariasis	Mild infection: asymptomatic; moderate infection: abdominal pain, distention, enlarged abdomen, anorexia, weight loss, fever **Diagnosis:** eggs can be detected by microscopic stool examination **Complications:** intestinal obstruction, pulmonary involvement (pneumonitis) with cough and blood-stained sputum, perforation of intestines by migration of worms resulting in peritonitis, obstruction of common bile duct by migration of worms	*Ascaris lumbricoides*, a roundworm **Transmission:** ingestion of eggs via contact with contaminated soil, food, fingers, and toys; food can be contaminated wherever human feces are used as fertilizer	**Incidence:** most common in warm climates, in areas of poor sanitation; most prevalent in young children aged 1–4 years **Incubation:** prolonged, as the life cycle of the worm is 4–8 weeks, and feces contain eggs about 2 months after ingestion of embryonated eggs **Control:** sanitary disposal of feces; treatment of human feces before use as a fertilizer; vegetables cultivated in areas where human feces fertilizer is used must be thoroughly cooked or soaked in a dilute iodine solution before eating	Mebedazole (Vermox) or pyrantel pamoate (Antiminth); reexamination of stools 3 weeks after therapy to determine if worms have been eliminated; if partial or complete intestinal obstruction due to large number of worms, administer piperazine citrate (Piperazine) via NG tube which paralyzes worms and allows them to be passed easier.

Adapted from American Academy of Pediatrics. (2000). 2000 Red Book: Report of the Committee on Infectious Diseases *(25th ed.). Elk Grove Village, IL: Author.*

Case Study/Care Plan

A CHILD WITH VARICELLA

Susan is a 7-year-old girl who lives with her mother and father and two siblings, 10-year-old Jennifer and 9-month-old Michael. She is sent home from school complaining of being achy and "feeling yucky." Being concerned, her mother takes her temperature and finds it registers 100.6°F. She is worried that Susan may have an infection and gives her some acetaminophen to make her comfortable. During the course of the evening, she begins to develop a rash. The lesions begin as red bumps on her chest and back and soon become filled with fluid. She soon complains of itching at the site of the lesions. Her mother calls the Pediatric Hotline for guidance. The nurse takes a careful history and notes that chickenpox has been reported in the community. She shares this information with the mother and asks about other children in the household and what the immune status of the family is. Both of Susan's parents had chickenpox (varicella) as children; however, Michael and Jennifer have not had the disease nor the immunization for the disease. Since infection usually confers lifelong immunity, Susan's parents should be immune. Jennifer is at high risk for developing varicella since she has never had the disease. Michael may be at risk but should still be protected by maternal antibody to varicella. Susan's mother asks about what to expect regarding Susan's illness and the implications for the rest of her family. Susan is most contagious within the two days prior to the onset of the rash and until 6 days after the rash appears or sooner providing all the lesions have dried and crusted over. Since Jennifer has been exposed and is at highest risk, she should receive a dose of varicella vaccine within 72 hours and possibly up to 120 hours after exposure (AAP, 2000). Michael is too young to receive the vaccine.

Assessment The nurse should obtain a history of Susan's exposure to varicella (chickenpox). Susan's immunization status needs to be determined, in other words, if and when was she given the varicella vaccine. Ask about her current symptoms. During the physical examination, note the lesions: their appearance, configuration, and distribution. Obtain her vital signs, especially noting if her temperature is elevated. Assess for associated manifestations such as malaise, loss of appetite, and pruritus.

Nursing Diagnosis #1

Impaired skin integrity related to inflammation, scratching from pruritus, and/or infection of lesions

Expected Outcomes

1. Susan will have improved skin integrity.
2. Susan will experience minimal discomfort from pruritus.
3. Susan will not experience any signs of secondary infection during the course of her illness.

Interventions/*Rationales*

1. Keep skin clean with mild soap and warm water. *Good hygiene prevents the occurrence of secondary bacterial infections caused by streptococcus or staphylococcus.*

2. Keep fingernails short to prevent and/or minimize excoriation or scarring by scratching. *Since the lesions are pruritic, Susan is prone to scratching.*

3. Use antipruritic measures such as baking soda baths, drying lotions such as calamine, and medications such as diphenhydramine hydrochloride (Benadryl), or hydroxyzine HCL (Atarax or Vistaril). *If pruritus is controlled, Susan will be more comfortable, scratch less, and reduce her chances of causing secondary infection.*

4. Teach caregivers about the signs and symptoms of secondary infection such as increased redness, warmth, presence of pus in the lesions, prolonged fever, and pain. *Caring for the skin using the above measures will decrease the incidence of secondary infection, but caregivers need to be vigilant of the signs of secondary infection and be able to report them to the health care provider.*

continues

continued

Evaluation

Susan's skin is intact, and lesions are healing. She experiences minimal discomfort and pruritus. She scratches the lesions infrequently or not at all.. The lesions remain free of secondary infection.

Nursing Diagnosis #2

Deficient knowledge related to the transmission of varicella as evidenced by caregiver questions

Expected Outcomes

1. The caregivers will voice understanding of the transmission of the virus.
2. The caregivers will notify their health care provider at the onset of the virus in the siblings to be able to use acyclovir in symptom reduction.
3. The caregivers will be able to manage the care and treatment of the illness without undue stress.

Interventions/*Rationales*

1. Discuss the etiology, clinical manifestations, and treatment of varicella with caregivers. *Anticipatory guidance is helpful to reduce anxiety and to increase the caregivers' abilities in coping with the illness.*
2. Prepare the caregivers about the probability of infection in Susan's siblings. The incubation period is 10–21 days after contact with the infected person. *Knowing the parameters of varicella infection and the measures available to ameliorate the effects of the disease will assist the caregivers in preparing to manage potential problems.*
3. Discuss the probable administration of acyclovir for Michael and Jennifer if either should develop varicella. Acyclovir is an antiviral drug that inhibits the activity of herpes viruses including varicella. It does not cure but lessens the effects of the virus. It has been shown to decrease the number of lesions, the amount of fever, and shorten the healing time while still producing an effective antibody response. It should be given orally within 24 hours after the onset of varicella lesions. The dose is 20 mg/kg/dose four times a day for five days. *If used in this manner, acyclovir can decrease the duration and extent of the fever as well as the number and duration of skin lesions.*

Evaluation

Susan's mother and father state how the virus is transmitted, and the signs and symptoms of the prodrome. They are vigilant in observing their other two children for the signs and symptoms of varicella. They verbalize appropriate home care.

The interplay of infectious diseases and the normal course of growth and development in humans is evident. Nurses have a unique opportunity to intervene at many levels and in many ways. The broad-based education of professional nurses gives them the foundation for assessment, planning, intervention, and education. The information regarding infectious diseases is constantly changing as new vaccines and drug therapy are developed. Health professionals have a better understanding of the distinctive properties of infectious agents and can better inform the public as to ways of prevention and treatment so that these illnesses may be kept to a minimum and eventually eradicated.

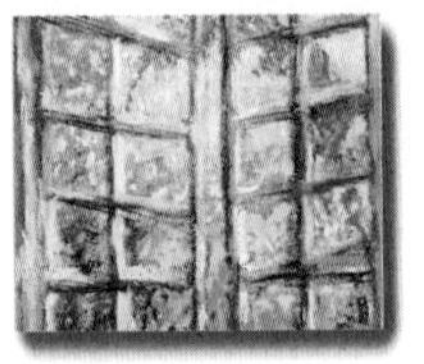

In the Real World

Quote from a veteran nurse with over 15 years of working in ambulatory pediatrics: "When I first became a nurse, the recommendations for immunizations were relatively simple. Now, if it weren't for the continued updates, I would be lost. As newer vaccines are developed, I have to keep abreast of all of the latest requirements. It keeps you on your toes and alert to assessing every child at every instance in order to keep up the level of protection."

Key Concepts

- The transmission of disease is dependent upon six factors, which are referred to as the chain of infection.
- The development of children's immune systems begins early in fetal life. The intrauterine environment does not always protect children from contracting infectious illnesses.
- Handwashing is the best defense against the spread of infectious disease.
- The transmission of many infectious diseases can be traced to the developmental stage of children. Certain behaviors make children more vulnerable to infectious illnesses at different ages.
- Immunizations play a major role in the prevention of illness, and in reducing morbidity and mortality. Caregivers need to be instructed in the importance of this preventative health care measure.
- Health care personnel who administer immunizations must be knowledgeable about the rationale, care and handling, administration, and effects of each specific vaccine.
- Treatment of infectious disease is aimed at the reduction of symptomatology. Pharmacological therapy such as antibacterial, antiviral, and antifungal medications may be prescribed depending upon the etiology of the illness.
- The prevalence of sexual intercourse as well as the rate of sexually transmitted diseases (STDs) has increased among adolescents.
- Adolescents need to be assessed for the possibility of STDs.
- Caregivers can adequately care for children with infectious diseases at home. Most caregivers can be taught how to provide supportive care for their children.
- It is important for the nurse to understand the laws and policies related to communicable disease including reporting the incidence of certain diseases.

Review Questions

1. Explain why infants and children are more prone to infection than adults.
2. When should caregivers be instructed about immunizations?
3. Identify strategies to facilitate adherence to immunization schedules from infancy through adolescence.
4. Identify the common ways in which infants and children facilitate the spread of infectious disease.
5. Explain why acetaminophen is the drug of choice when treating viral illnesses.
6. What should be included in a plan to teach the staff of a day care center how to prevent the spread of illness?
7. What factors are associated with the spread of STDs in adolescents?
8. Explain why adolescents with herpetic lesions may be at risk for developing HIV infection.
9. Discuss the rationale for reporting certain infectious diseases to the proper health authorities.

References

Advisory Committee on Immunization Practice (ACIP). (1999). Combination vaccines for childhood immunizations. *Morbidity and Mortality Weekly Report, 48*(RR05), 1–15.

Advisory Committee on Immunization Practice (ACIP). (2000). Preventing pneumococcal disease among infants and children. *Morbidity and Mortality Weekly Report, 49*(RR09), 1–38.

American Academy of Pediatrics (AAP). (1999). Combination vaccines for childhood immunization: Recommendations of the Advisory Committee on Immunization Practices, the American Academy of Pediatrics, and the American Academy of Family Physicians. *Pediatrics, 103*(5), 1064–1077.

American Academy of Pediatrics (AAP). (2000). *2000 Red Book: Report of the Committee on Infectious Diseases* (25th ed.). Elk Grove Village, IL: Author.

American College Health Association (ACHA). (1999). *Frequently asked questions* [On-line]. Available: http://www.acha.org./special-prj/men/faq.htm

Averhoff, F. M., Williams, W. W., & Hadler, S. C. (1997). Immunization of adolescents: Recommendations of the Advisory Committee on Immunization Practices, the American Academy of Family Physicians, and the American Medical Association. *Journal of School Health, 67,* 298–303.

Ball, L., Ball, R., & Pratt, D. (2001). An assessment of thimersal use in childhood vaccines. *Pediatrics, 107*(5), 1147–1154.

Centers for Disease Control and Prevention (CDC). (1998a). 1998 Guidelines for treatment of sexually transmitted diseases. *Morbidity and Mortality Weekly Report, 47*(RR1), 1–127.

Centers for Disease Control and Prevention (CDC). (1998b). *Preventing emerging infectious diseases: A strategy for the 21st century.* Atlanta, GA: U.S. Department of Health and Human Services.

Centers for Disease Control and Prevention (CDC). (1999). Withdrawal of rotavirus vaccine recommendation. *Morbidity and Mortality Weekly Report, 48*(43), 1007.

Christie, C. D., Marx, M. L., Marchant, C. D., & Reising, S. F. (1994). The 1993 epidemic of pertussis in Cincinnati: Resurgence of disease in a highly immunized population of children. *New England Journal of Medicine, 331,* 16–21.

Churchill, R. B., & Pickering, L. K. (1997). Infection control challenges in child-care centers. *Infectious Disease Clinics of North America, 11,* 347–365.

Donowitz, L. G. (Ed.). (1999). *Infection control in the child care center and preschool* (4th ed.). Baltimore: Williams & Wilkins.

Evers, D. B. (2000). Insights on immunizations from caregivers of children receiving Medicaid-funded services. *Journal of the Society of Pediatric Nurses, 5,* 157–166, 182.

Gordon, T. E., Zook, E. G., Averhoff, F. M., & Williams, W. W. (1997). Consent for adolescent vaccination: Issues and current practices. *Journal of School Health, 67,* 259–264.

Green, M., & Palfrey, J. S. (Ed.). (2000). *Bright futures: Guidelines for health supervision of infants, children, and adolescents* (2nd ed.). Arlington, VA: National Center for Education in Maternal and Child Health.

Grover, G. (1996). Fever and bacteremia. In C. D. Berkowitz (Ed.), *Pediatrics: A primary care approach* (pp. 127–132). Philadelphia: Saunders.

Holmes, S. J., Morrow, A. L., & Pickering, L. K. (1996). Child-care practices: Effects of social change on the epidemiology of infectious diseases and antibiotic resistance. *Epidemiological Reviews, 18*(10), 10–28.

McCutcheon, H., & Woodward, A. (1996). Acute respiratory illness in the first year of primary school related to previous attendance at child care. *Australian & New Zealand Journal of Public Health, 20*(1), 49–53.

Niffenegger, J. P. (1997). Proper handwashing promotes wellness in child care. *Journal of Pediatric Health Care, 11,* 26–31.

Overturf, G., & Committee on Infectious Diseases. (2000). Prevention of pneumococcal infections, including the use of pneumococcal conjugate and polysaccharide vaccines and antibiotic prophylaxis. *Pediatrics, 106*(2), 367–376.

Pruitt, R., Kline, P., & Kovaz, R. (1995). Perceived barriers to childhood immunziations among rural populations. *Journal of Community Health Nursing, 12*(2) 65–72.

Sieving, R., Resnick, M. D., Bearinger, L., Remafedi, G., Taylor, B. A., & Harmon, B. (1997). Cognitive and behavioral predictors of sexually transmitted disease risk behaviour among sexually active adolescents. *Archives of Pediatrics & Adolescent Medicine, 151,* 243–251.

Strobino, D., Keane, V., Holt, E., Hughart, N., & Guyer, B. (1996). Parental attitudes do not explain underimmunization. *Pediatrics, 98,* 1076–1083.

U.S. Department of Health and Human Services. (2000). *Healthy People 2010: Understanding and improving health.* Washington, DC: U.S. Dept of Health and Human Services.

Wadsworth, L. (1999). Polio immunization: Dealing with new recommendations and helping parents understand the changes. *Journal of Pediatric Health Care, 13*(Supplement, Part 2), S21–S29.

Word, C. O., & Bowser, B. (1997). Background to crack cocaine addiction and HIV high-risk behavior: The next epidemic. *American Journal of Drug and Alcohol Abuse, 23,* 67–77.

Suggested Readings

Bob, P., & Famolare, N. (1998). Teaching and communication strategies: Working with the hospitalized adolescent with pelvic inflammatory disease. *Pediatric Nursing, 24*(1), 17–20.

Diggle, L., & Deeks, J. (2000). Effect of needle length on incidence of local reactions to routine immunizations in infants aged 4 months: Randomized controlled trial. *British Medical Journal, 32*(7266), 931–933.

Grabenstein, J. (1999). How to interpret immunization schedules and records. *Hospital Pharmacy, 34*(4), 482–491.

Horner, S., & Murphy, L. (1999). Creating alternative immunization clinics to maintain and improve community immunization rates. *Journal of Community Health Nursing, 16*(2), 121–132.

Selekman, J. (1998). Infectious diseases and the immunizations of today and tomorrow. *Pediatric Nursing, 24*(4), 309–315.

Twomey, J. (1998). Varicella exposure in a child at risk of being immunosuppressed. *Pediatric Nursing, 23*(5), 459–464.

Watson, B., & Rothstein, E. (1999). Varicella vaccine: Progress 4 years after licensure. *Pediatric Annals, 28,* 516–529.

For children:

Berger, M. (1985). *Germs make me sick!* New York: HarperCollins.

Resources

Organizations and Websites

Association for Professionals in Infection Control and Epidemiology
1275 K Street, NW, Suite 1000
Washington, DC 20005-4006
(202) 789-1890
www.apic.org

Centers for Disease Control and Prevention
Includes all of the essential information on both global and national disease trends, prevention, and treatment with specific guidelines for immunizations, including international travel. Services include Advisory Committee on Immunization Practices (ACIP)
1600 Clifton Road, NE
Atlanta, GA 30333
(404) 639-3311
(800) 232-2522 (Immunization Hotline)
www.cdc.gov

Immunization Action Coalition
1573 Selby Avenue, Suite 234
Saint Paul, MN 55104
(651) 647-9009
www.immunize.org

National Immunization Program
The Pink Book—Epidemiology and Prevention of Vaccine-Preventable Diseases can be downloaded from the CDC website at www.cdc.gov/nip.
Centers for Disease Control and Prevention
1600 Clifton Road, NE
Atlanta, GA 30333
(800) CDC-SHOT
www.cdc.gov/nip/default.htm

National Vaccine Injury Compensation Program
U.S. Department of Health and Human Services
Health Resources and Services Administration
Parklawn Building, Room 8A-35
5600 Fishers Lane
Rockville, MD 20857
(800) 338-2382
www.hrsa.dhhs.gov

CHAPTER 16

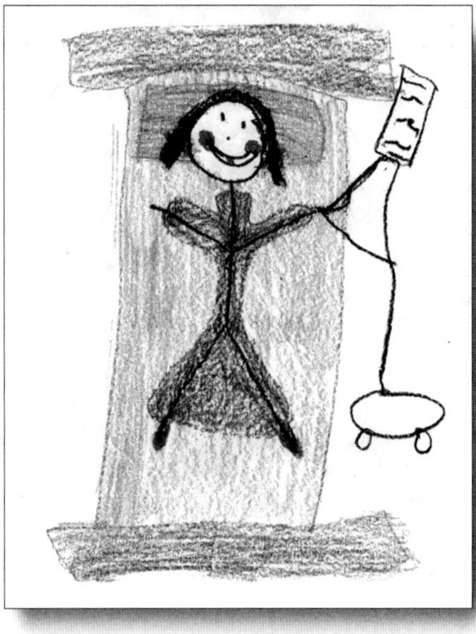

CARE OF CHILDREN WHO ARE HOSPITALIZED

E. Ann Sheridan, RN, MS, EdD

That experience of being in the hospital was so scary for Helen! She was only six when she had to spend a week in the hospital. She was riding her bicycle and was hit by a car. Not only did she have surgery because of abdominal injuries, but she also had to be in traction because her upper leg was broken. She had a hard time adjusting when she got to come home too. Helen was so independent before the accident, but afterwards had trouble sleeping, would awaken frequently during the night, and didn't want me to leave her even if it was just to go to the store.

COMPETENCIES

Upon completion of this chapter, the reader will be able to:

- *Describe the effects of illness and/or hospitalization on children, their caregivers, and their families.*
- *Discuss the contributions of theorists and nurse researchers in understanding phenomena and intervention efforts related to the experiences of children and families during illness and/or hospitalization.*
- *Describe the major factors that help children cope with illness and hospitalization.*
- *Describe a participative nursing model designed to maximize establishing and maintaining helping relationships with children and caregivers.*
- *Describe how caregiver attitudes and coping skills affect children's responses and abilities in learning ways of mastering fears and concerns related to illness and hospitalization.*
- *Describe the needs of hospitalized children and their families according to their developmental level with appropriate nursing interventions that can reduce stress and promote coping.*
- *Discuss the importance of delineating clear clinical outcomes related to the psychosocial health of children and evaluating these outcomes in determining the effectiveness of nursing interventions.*

It is vitally important that nurses carefully learn the art and science of caring for ill and hospitalized children and their families in order to assuage their fears and promote well-being. Developing the skills of the expert pediatric nurse begins with an understanding of the nature and culture of childhood and parenthood, the influence of the stages of growth and development on the life of the child, and the experiences of families in contemporary society. The art of identifying the needs of children and families is highly complex, and requires astute observation of nonverbal and verbal behavior, validation of information, accurate interpretation, and appropriate responses and interventions. The care of children is rooted in science and research as the continuous expansion of knowledge informs nursing practice.

Perhaps the most complex skill to learn is selecting relevant concepts and principles from nursing, the physical and social sciences, and the arts and humanities, and then applying this knowledge while delivering care to children and their families. The importance of this approach has evolved over many years as nursing and child health leaders studied the experiences of ill children and pursued ways of improving their health and welfare. Understanding historical dimensions provides the context for recognizing the critical contributions of these early leaders and for assessing new trends and practices.

TRADITION OF CARING FOR ILL AND HOSPITALIZED CHILDREN

Traditionally, the medical care of children was referred to as pediatrics, or the science of the child, with the primary focus on applying medical knowledge and techniques to diagnosing and curing disease. Children were regarded as small adults with limited recognition of physiological or psychosocial differences, individuality, or other attributes that directly affected care, treatment, and outcomes. With advances in medical science, increased attention to the uniqueness of childhood, and the desirability of having separate facilities, children's hospitals were constructed toward the end of the 19th century. For many years, it was believed that limited caregiver visits were in the best interest of hospitalized children because of the intense physical and emotional reactions to separation at the time of leave-taking. It was thought, at the time, that this kind of desperate response was detrimental to recovery. Other reasons for restricting visits included fears of infection, disrupting the work of the staff, interfering with the child's rest, and confidentiality issues (Giganti, 1998).

After an extensive study of the care of children in hospitals in Britain and the issuance of the Platt Report in 1959, changes occurred (Shields & Nixon, 1998). This historic document described policies and practices in the care of hospitalized children, how these practices adversely affected child development and recovery, and the kind of changes necessary for child-centered pediatric care and education. As knowledge about the psychology of childhood, the detrimental effects of separation, and the impact of hospitalization on the emotional life of the child expanded, hospital policies and practices gradually changed. In the late 1950s, liberal visiting policies, rooming-in practices, and a focus on family-oriented care began to be implemented in many hospitals throughout the United States. One of the most significant changes was liberalizing caregiver visiting from weekly or a few hours each day to 24 hours a day with rooming-in accommodations. Although the benefits of changes have been well documented, restricted visiting practices in pediatric intensive care units continued to exist as recently as 1994 (Giganti, 1998).

Pioneers in pediatric nursing generated new knowledge and deeper understanding of children during periods of illness through their astute observations and extensive study of individual children and their responses. These theorists proposed that the unique experiences of children and families, their growth and developmental stages, and their talents and strengths were critical factors in coping with illness and hospital stays (Figure 16-1). Through their research, writing, and teaching, they clearly documented the significant contributions of nursing to the health and welfare of children and families and to the community of health professionals who work together to implement policies beneficial to these children and families. Their work was the impetus for creating the knowledge base in the field and the emergence of sophisticated research designs that have revolutionized the care of ill and hospitalized children. Refer to Box 16-1 for a summary of the contributions of the leaders in the development of pediatric nursing.

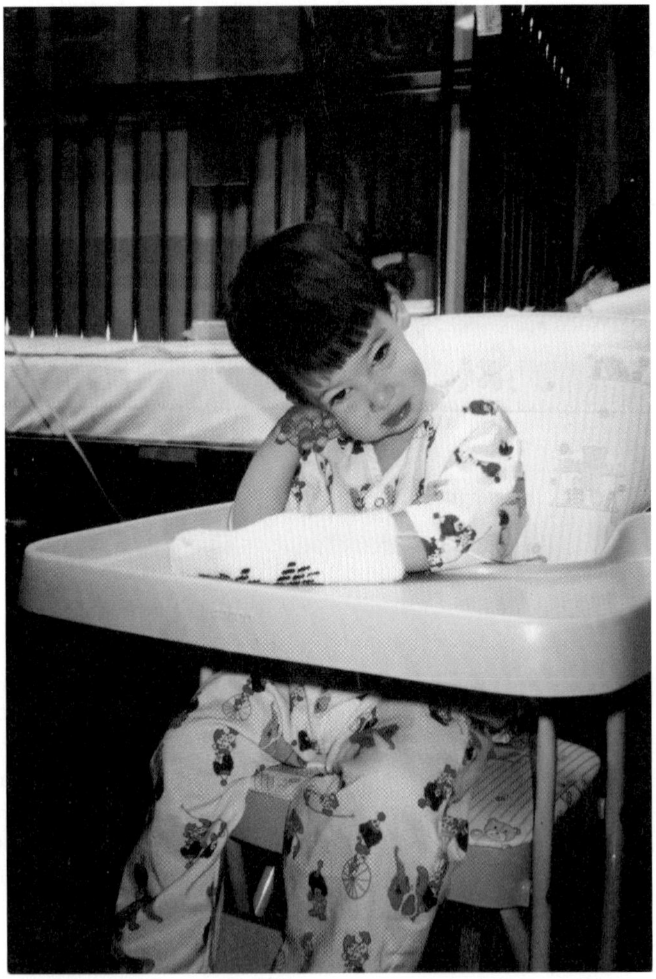

Figure 16-1 The Sentiments of a Child in the Hospital. Published with permission of Baystate Medical Center Children's Hospital.

BOX 16-1 Leaders in pediatric nursing

- **Gladys Sellew** (1887–1977) was a nurse, nurse educator, sociologist, and humanitarian. Her work in the tenements, ghettoes, and settlements of Cincinnati, Cleveland, Chicago, and Washington D.C. brought richness, reality, and a community dimension to the field of pediatric nursing. Her thesis on black families was the first research in nursing to be based on an original investigation that used as its methodology participant observation (Hawkins, 1988). Early in her career as a nurse, she conducted a study of the time required for nursing care in a pediatric ward, and in 1926, she wrote a text, *Pediatric Nursing*, which was translated into several languages.
- **Florence G. Blake** (1907–1982) was the first nurse to systematically study how children and parents cope with hospitalization and document the effectiveness of nursing in allaying and managing the fears and concerns of hospitalized children. She published extensive case studies in national and international journals, an early textbook entitled *The Child, His Parents and the Nurse* (1954) and at least nine editions of the textbook *Nursing of Children*. She was the first to identify the importance of understanding the experience of illness and hospitalization from the child's perspective, applying knowledge of growth and developmental theory, using play in caring for hospitalized children, and involving family in pediatric care. Her belief that children can "grow" by managing crises successfully was a revolutionary idea in the field of child care in hospitals. She is also credited with designing and implementing two of the earliest graduate programs in Pediatric Nursing in the United States at the University of Chicago (1946) and the University of Wisconsin–Madison (1963).
- **Florence H. Erickson** (b. 1914) was a professor and researcher in the field of nursing and child development. She started the masters program in the Nursing of Children in the late 1950's and the first Ph.D. program in Nursing in the 1970s, both at the University of Pittsburgh. She published an important monograph, *Play Interviews for Four Year Old Hospitalized Children* (1958), which was the impetus for extensive study on the benefits of using hospital equipment during play sessions with children to help them express feelings and understand their experience. This was influential in initiating the therapeutic advantages of using play in hospitals, a practice that evolved into the current Child Life Programs. Dr. Erickson cofounded the *Maternal-Child Nursing Journal* (now MCN) and *The American Journal of Maternal-Child Nursing*.
- **Dorothy Marlow** (1921–1992) was a nurse educator, administrator, author, and director of the Maternal-Child Health Master's Program at the University of Pennsylvania who wrote *Textbook in Pediatric Nursing*, which paralleled the major medical text *Textbook of Pediatrics* (originally authored by Waldo E. Nelson). Her unique contribution was to arrange the content of child care by age groups with concurrent concepts and theories of growth and development, and the most common short- and long-term conditions of that age group, followed by children's responses to illness and ways to assist children during these developmental periods.
- **Eugenia Waechter** (1925–1982) was a pioneer in both pediatric nursing and nursing research. She conducted the first controlled study done directly with children, published as "Death Anxiety in Children with Fatal Illness." Her writings about the care available to children and families guided the development of a theoretical base in pediatric nursing. With Blake, she authored two later editions of the text *Nursing Care of Children*.

With the change in orientation from child-centered to family-centered care, parents and significant others in the life of the child have become essential partners in the health care team. Changes in health care, health care systems, and methods of financing have also affected patterns of child care and hospitalization. The length of hospitalization has been shortened considerably, and alternatives to inpatient care, such as same-day surgery, have replaced many hospital admissions (Dougherty, 1998). The reduced number of hospital admissions has been beneficial because children recover best in their own surroundings. A concomitant result, however, has been a higher level of illness acuity in pediatric inpatient units and an urgent need for nurses with advanced education, and highly developed skills and expertise in the care of infants, children, adolescents, and their families.

Changes in health care financing threaten both the quality and quantity of care for children who are ill and hospitalized. Increased numbers of unlicensed personnel and decreased numbers of experienced nurses and nurses with advanced preparation in the care of children limits the possibilities for preventing the untoward effects of severe illness, surgery, or life-threatening conditions. With additional changes in staffing patterns to increased numbers of part-time nurses and contract nurses, the continuity of care so essential to the developmental needs of infants and young children, may be seriously compromised. Both qualitative and quantitative research needs to be conducted in light of these changes to reexamine the experiences of children who are ill and hospitalized, particularly those who are most vulnerable to emotional trauma.

PREPARATION FOR CLINICAL NURSING IN THE CARE OF CHILDREN AND THEIR FAMILIES

To begin learning about the care of ill children, it is important to reflect on one's own experiences and strengths, review theories about child growth and development, and realize that, even through the trauma and stress of illness and hospitalization, children continue to grow physically, emotionally, socially, and spiritually. The predominant goal is to identify and preserve the strengths of children while trying to enhance their growth in the midst of stress and intrusions into their bodies, their space, and their very being. To do this successfully takes an understanding of the lives of individual children and their families, and the courage and commitment to accurately discern and meet their emerging needs. Introspection, reflection, and understanding of personal styles and journeys in learning make it possible for nurses to mature in the transition from novice to expert.

While preparing for the care of children and their caregivers, several assumptions and questions may arise. The questions in Box 16-2 are designed to direct the kind of inquiry that will lead to accuracy and effectiveness in providing sensitive nursing care. These are in addition to those ques-

Reflective Thinking

Viewing a Pediatric Unit from Different Perspectives

First, from the perspective of a child:

Enter the pediatric unit as if you were a young child being admitted to the hospital for the first time. Be aware of the sights, smells, sounds that are detectable, and the conversations of others. Use your imagination to identify thoughts, feelings, and anxieties that come to mind as you experience this process. Make a few notes as you proceed. For 10–15 minutes, walk around the unit and into a child's room as if this were to be your room. Be aware of the questions you would ask and the fears you may have. Continue to "look around the unit" absorbing the general atmosphere and responses to you from children or staff. Take another 15 minutes to reflect on this experience and to record your reflections to share with colleagues.

Second, from one's own perspective:

Tour the unit again, and take this opportunity to introduce yourself to members of the staff, a caregiver, and a child. Be aware of your own thoughts and feelings as you spend about 20 minutes becoming acquainted with personnel and the general environment. Then, reflect on this experience, writing about your impressions and your thoughts about how you feel as you begin to assume responsibility for learning about the care of children and caregivers. Discuss these reflections with colleagues.

BOX 16-2 Guiding questions to address while learning the role and responsibilities of a nurse caring for a child who is hospitalized

What child characteristics will have a bearing on the plan of care? (e.g., body dimensions for determining the appropriateness of dosages of medications, level of cognitive development)?

What is the nature of the caregiver–nurse partnership during the hospital experience? What is the pattern of the caregiver's role in providing direct care, e.g., bathing, feeding?

What is the history of the illness, sequence of symptoms, or conditions of the injury? Are there other existing health problems or recent stressful experiences?

What emergency measures or remedies have been used? How recent were treatments and medications given?

What is the current status of the illness; e.g., is the condition improving or worsening? Examine the progress and sequence of events during the past 24 hours.

What have been the most helpful interventions to date?

What is the child's and caregivers' perceptions and understanding of the nature of the health problem, therapeutic measures, and plans for care?

What are the strengths of the child and family in coping with stressful situations (e.g., ways of comforting one's self and being comforted by others)? Does the child have a transitional object or favorite toy that provides comfort?

What are the usual routines at home, e.g., daily activities, caregiving patterns, play/school, sleeping, eating, and elimination routines?

What are the most significant relationships in the child's life?

What are the expectations of the child, family, and nurse during this experience?

With the implementation of the plan of care/clinical pathways, what are the predictions regarding outcomes?

tions directly related to the ongoing plan of care and clinical pathways. Thorough assessment and understanding the rationale for plans are included in the initial phase of preparation.

THE NATURE OF ILLNESS IN CHILDHOOD

Illness in infants, children, and adolescents is characterized by acute or traumatic episodes, chronic conditions, or situations requiring surgical intervention or for which surgery is the elective treatment. Some health problems require medical or surgical treatment before birth; others are incompatible with life but amenable to surgical correction (e.g., some forms of congenital heart disease, tracheoesophageal atresias, gastrointestinal atresias). Genetic and environmental factors and general vulnerability, particularly in situations of poverty and stressful living conditions, also influence the incidence of disease and injury in childhood and adolesence.

REACTIONS AND RESPONSES OF CHILDREN TO THE STRESSORS OF ILLNESS AND HOSPITALIZATION

High levels of anxiety in children are created by the rapid onset of illness and injury, particularly when there have been limited experiences with childhood disease. Even children who have been previously hospitalized fear repeating those events that caused pain and stress. Many factors contribute to the distress of young children during hospitalization; existing fears and fantasies may be intensified. Their logic may be illogical; many have not developed a concept of time; and others may have fantasies that are real to them as they try to explain the unknown. Normal fears are exacerbated, and children become anxious when they think they may be in pain, separated from caregivers, harmed, or mutilated in some way (Algren & Algren, 1997). They often perceive a threat to basic needs for love and protection, control and independence, and fulfillment of basic physiological needs when in reality none exist. Some fear they may die (Lamontagne, Hepworth, Byington, & Chang, 1997). To allay these fears, children need the constant support of caregivers and nurses directly responsible for care and guidance.

The developmental level of the child and their perceptions and interpretations of experiences are more important than the actual events. Their limited life encounters and immature intellectual capacities contribute to difficulty in comprehending what is happening. This is particularly true when there are physical intrusions into the bodies of toddlers and preschoolers. For them, the intactness of their bodies is important; they feel the distress of exposure and intrusion acutely. The impact of hospitalization is also affected by the nature and severity of the health problem, the condition, and the degree to which activities and routines differ from those of everyday life.

Children's anxieties are also due to separation from caregivers and familiar persons and environments; the presence of strangers; equipment that looks ominous; the distress of other children; and the pain and discomfort of intrusions and interventions. Although age, maturity, vulnerability to anxiety, and previous experiences make a difference in the intensity of stress responses, there are many stressors pervading the hospital experience for children of all ages. The primary fears producing stress are lack of control, fear of intrusions and "hurt," and separations from the significant persons in their lives.

The cultural variations of families, their values and practices related to illness, general responses to stress, and attitudes regarding child rearing also have a significant influence on the child's behavior and responses. The potentially negative impact of illness and hospitalization may be modified by a variety of factors, including age, developmental level, anxiety level of caregivers, individual characteristics/temperament of the child, child and caregiver coping skills, caregiver–family–child relationships, religion, previous hospital/surgery experiences, ethnic and cultural beliefs, and the type and quality of preparation for hospitalization and/or surgery (Fox, 1997).

Children, like persons of all ages, share fears of the unknown, unfamiliar environments, and situations where control is difficult to maintain. It is also distressing when language is heard but not understood. Children notice and become anxious when they see ominous-looking apparatus and strangers in unusual attire (surgical caps, masks, and garb), when they hear unfamiliar noises, or smell strange odors. They become distressed when they hear or see other children crying and wonder what may happen to make them cry also. They are also uncertain about how they will fulfill their essential needs if no one is nearby.

REFLECTIONS FROM FAMILIES

Most of the time, someone was within calling distance, but when our 5-year-old, Karl, was first brought from the emergency room in a cast, he had to "go to the bathroom," so he put on his light as instructed to do when he "needed anything." Over the intercom, he heard a voice ask, "What do you want?" Perplexed, Karl looked all around, wondering where the person was, and then he said, "what do you say to a wall?" I went for the nurse directly. Karl then did not want us to leave because he was afraid of having an "accident" if someone doesn't come right away.

ALLEVIATING THE ANXIETIES OF CHILDREN

To lessen the anxieties of children, it is helpful to understand the common situations creating distress and then intervene in such a way so stressors are minimized or eliminated. Those procedures involving any bodily intrusion are most feared, as are those involving equipment and technology (Figure 16-2). It is particularly stressful when darkness is involved as often happens in radiological examinations. Stress-point nursing, which includes thoughtful preparation for situations anticipated to be stressful by using both procedural (description of the treatment and sequence of steps) and sensory information (how this might feel) according to the cognitive level of the child, identification of the child's role during the event, and rehearsal with the same nurse who provides supportive care throughout can help children manage stressful events (Wolfer & Visintainer, 1975). The principles embedded in stress-point intervention are most effective when occurring during difficult stressors, e.g., new tasks, and when interventions are focused on the issues of greatest concern to the family (Burke et al., 1999).

Even those situations that may appear minor to an adult are frightening to a young child. An example is when children are being transported to another area of the hospital for tests and become anxious and resist because of fears that caregivers may not be able to find them. Anticipating this would prompt the nurse to put a sign on the door, so the child could be "found." In a similar situation, children may not want to leave their room with anyone other than their caregiver because they fear getting lost. Reassurance of always being with someone and having a picture of an animal or cartoon character (different for each room) on the wall inside and outside the room helps children feel more confident about their place. To strengthen children's sense of feeling secure, it is important for nurses to let them know when they are leaving for the day, say good-bye, and tell them about their new nurse and when they will return.

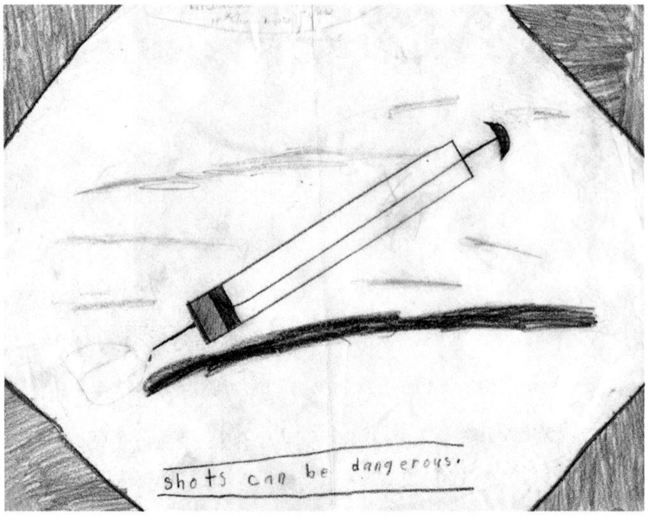

Figure 16-2 Injections are a cause of anxiety for most children.

Nursing Alert:

Psychological First-Aid in Times of Stress

Although many stressful situations are foreseeable and untoward reactions preventable, children may exhibit acute responses even when the cause is not clear, e.g., crying, outbursts of emotion, covers over head. Whenever there are signs or symptoms of obvious emotional distress, psychological "first aid" should be applied immediately. The specific interventions are situation-specific and most effective when nurses know and understand the individual child, and his/her unique circumstances and developmental level. Effective interventions may include holding, explanation/reassurance related to fears/concerns, and/or play activities. The child with an outburst of anger could be helped by carefully listening, clarifying misconceptions, playing out, or using hand puppets to express feelings.

MAJOR FACTORS THAT SUPPORT COPING DURING ILLNESS AND HOSPITALIZATION

During illness, there are several dominant factors influencing the child's ability to cope and learn to use coping methods. These include the inner strengths, talents, and attributes of the child and several external determinants including the expertise of the nurse, the support of families, the quality of the partnership between the nurse and the family, the supportiveness of the environment on the children's unit, and the effectiveness of support through play.

Inner Strengths, Talents, and Attributes of the Child

Each child is a unique individual with different temperaments and capacities for managing adverse situations. Inner strengths include the ability to cope because of past episodes of getting through difficult situations with the assistance of adults in their world. Some children however, may appear to be more resilient than they are because they want to appear strong or stoic. Other inner strengths include the abilities to express thoughts and fears, seek information in order to understand situations and expectations, and then feel the success of mastery.

Children's talents also help in coping. For example, through drawing, writing prose or poetry, and other creative activities, children not only express their thoughts and feelings, but also use these media to cope. Others may have a curiosity about how things work and seek information and opportunities to discuss their condition and experiences, or use computers. Some have the kind of personality, charm, and ability to interact and communicate in a way that attracts others. Although it is difficult to contemplate, physical attractiveness or the nature of a child's illness or situation may also facilitate coping because staff members may prefer to care for and support children with certain characteristics or health problems. For example, children who are cute or highly responsive to others, or those with oncologic problems, cardiac diseases, unusual conditions, or complex technological care may be more appealing or challenging to staff. Although this is an area for future research, relationships between physical attractiveness and nurses' perceptions and interpretation of behavior has been demonstrated (Bordieri, Solodky, & Mikow, 1985).

Expertise of the Nurse

With extensive study and experience, nurses become experts in understanding the verbal and nonverbal behavior of ill children, discerning the meaning intended, and responding skillfully and accurately (Figure 16-3). The expert nurse knows nursing practice is a discipline where one must be constantly attentive to changes and unpredictable signs and symptom. Depth of knowledge about nursing as an art and science, growth, development, and family theory is the source of wise and effective clinical judgments and interventions for both the child and caregiver. It is important to recognize that in any given situation, one nurse may succeed where another may not, giving rise to the need for appreciating the contributions of many nurses and the need for consultation and collaboration.

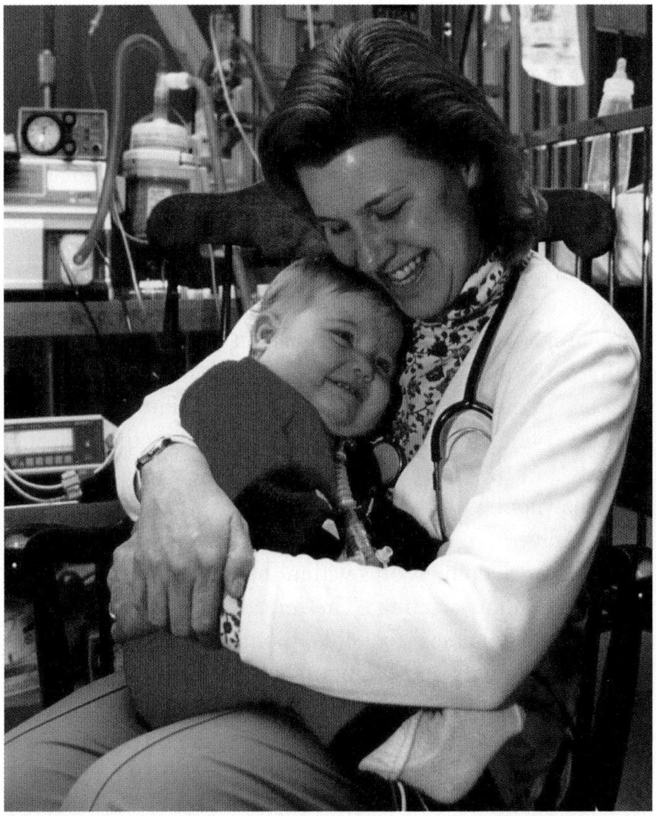

Figure 16-3 Nurse Comforting a Child during Hospitalization. Used with permission of Alfred I. duPont Hospital for Children, Wilmington, Delaware. Photographer: Cynthia Brodoway.

The expert nurse sees the strengths of each child and uses these to design, implement, and evaluate nursing care. They lend their own strengths to children and caregivers, who rely on them to learn and use coping skills, and to understand and manage the exigencies of illness successfully. These nurses also understand the emotional and physical comfort of the child is most important, rather than personal satisfactions gained when children or caregivers like them or express appreciation for their care and concern.

All the nurse's physiological and psychological senses are critical in identifying and meeting children's needs. Children are often so acutely ill that they are unable to communicate their needs. It is important not only to look, but to see; not only to listen, but to hear; not only to touch, but to feel; and not only to smell and to taste, but to discriminate. The nurse's senses and the ability to read and interpret verbal and nonverbal behavior are the best means of assessing children's needs. The nurse can see the subtle changes of a child indicating early signs of dehydration, and facial or body indicators of fear or sadness; can hear the sounds of distress, both physiologically and psychologically including changes in breathing, or cries of pain or misery; and can feel the tension of anxiety. Nurses have diagnosed acute illness through the odor of the acetone breath of a child not previously known to have diabetes, the unique cry of an infant with cri du chat syndrome, or through the salty taste a grandmother described on the face of an infant with cystic fibrosis. The highest level of skill is attained when the nurse accurately identifies the child and/or family needs for help, validates the need, uses knowledge and all resources available to meet this need, and then evaluates the effectiveness of interventions. This is in essence, the classic, dynamic nurse–patient relationship first iterated by Orlando (1961).

The experienced nurse may also be described as a nurse-artist because of the sensitivity exemplified in grasping the meaning of behavior in light of past and evolving events and the creative, skillful actions that reflect depth of understanding, and commitment to attending to each child and family in unique ways. This nurse is thoroughly familiar with current knowledge and research in the field and is highly successful in working with colleagues to provide holistic care and guidance to children and families. Such a nurse has an expanded repertoire of advanced assessment methods including the use of drawings to assess emotional health (Clatworthy, Simon, & Tiedeman, 1999); as well as skill in a wide variety of interventions such as therapeutic play and the use of the arts and humanities, e.g., music, art, drama, and movement therapy.

Support of Children by Caregivers

The support of families is a critical factor in the way that children respond to and cope with illness (Wolfer & Visintainer, 1975; Melnyk, 1995; Lamontagne et al., 1997) (Figure 16-4). With the turn of the century, the differences and complexities of family life become more evident, and many caregivers have difficulty in being physically or emotionally available to children. Stress may be intensified by existing problems or recent changes, e.g., moving, divorce, newly blended families, families with adopted and foster children, and those with other members experiencing serious physical and mental health problems. Depending on the situation surrounding an illness or trauma, caregivers themselves may find coping to be an arduous task while trying to support their child.

REFLECTIONS FROM FAMILIES

When my daughter, Mary, was 2 1/2 years old, there was a serious accident, and she suffered severe burns on her face. She was hospitalized for several days, and I will never forget her dear face, covered with bandages and tears, and how my feelings of guilt, anxiety, and sadness felt so overwhelming. Each day in the hospital, Mary clung and said over and over, "Me go home," and it was heart wrenching for me to leave her. The doctor consented to her discharge if I would do the dressings at home, and this was one of the hardest things I have ever had to do.

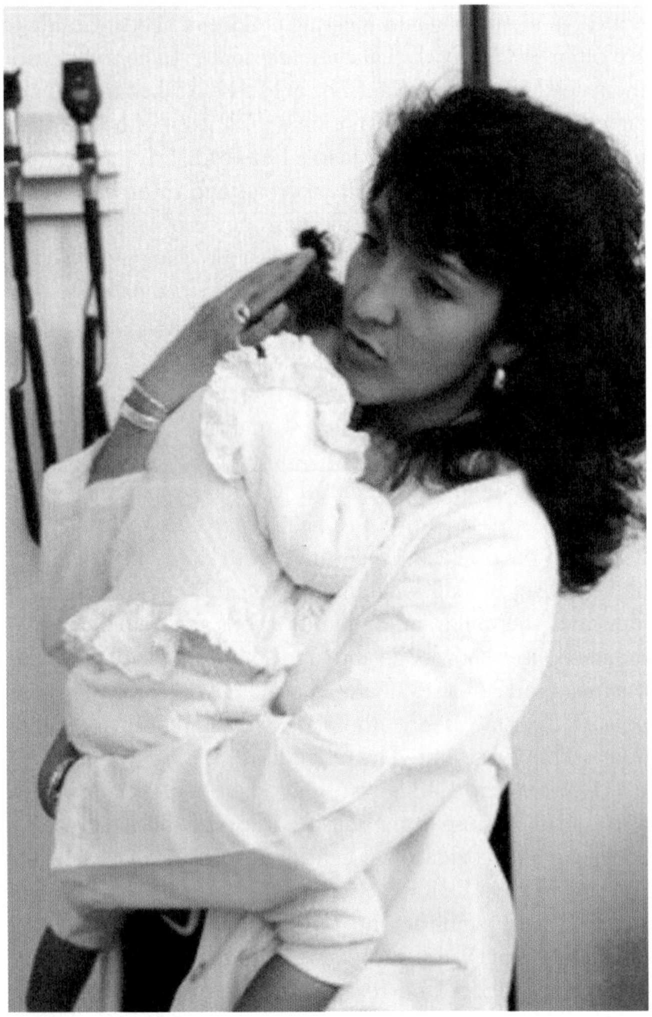

Figure 16-4 Support of caregivers is essential in helping children to cope while hospitalized. Published with permission of Baystate Medical Center Children's Hospital.

In many situations, caregivers may find it difficult to be psychologically or emotionally ready to manage. At these times, it is beneficial to have a network of friends and family able to offer their strengths, time, and assistance. The support of caregivers is dependent upon the empathic responses, assistance, and cooperation rendered by nurses, physicians, and other family members, as well as their own strengths in managing stressful situations.

The presence of caregivers is of paramount importance particularly for young children, yet the issues surrounding the ability to stay with children and facilities to accommodate caregivers are considered in light of the needs of the family and the child. The critical importance of caregiver presence in the hospital may need to be explained to families because young children are often cared for by others during the day, and the impact of separation in a strange environment may not be fully understood.

Usually, there are choices of accommodations: rooming-in; caregiver sleeping rooms within the pediatric unit; or day-visiting and home-sleeping. The selection of arrangements is complex, but, whenever possible, rooming-in is of the highest priority for infants and young children. Whatever arrangements are chosen, caregivers need assurance that children will receive support and comfort, particularly during times of discomfort and discontent. They also need to know that if they are unable to be present other supportive adults (e.g., grandparents, other significant adults) could stand in their stead. Many hospitals also enlist the skills of volunteer grandmothers and grandfathers for rocking, cuddling, reading, and providing comfort and companionship for children.

Relationship Between Nurses and Families

The quality of collaborative relationship and interactions between nurses and caregivers is fundamental to facilitating a child's coping ability. A highly successful design based on this philosophy is the **nursing mutual participation model of care** (NMPMC) used by Brody (1980) in outpatient pediatric settings and Curley (1988, 1997) in children's hospitals. This model was designed to alleviate stress and to empower caregivers to maintain their role during their child's acute illness and recovery. Using this approach, caregivers are equal partners in planning, implementing, and evaluating care. In order for this model to be effective, however, it is essential for the nurse to believe the presence and support of families is essential for optimal healing, recovery, and prevention of additional trauma. Rather than a hierarchical relationship, where the nurse and other health professionals assume an authoritarian role, caregivers and nurses form a partnership, where each lends their talent and expertise to benefit the child and the family (Figure 16-5).

Nurses who use this interactive, participative model of practice engage in a deliberative method of establishing and maintaining helping relationships with caregivers by creating a caring, trusting atmosphere for discussion, and exploring needs and issues of concern. This is best accomplished by consistently identifying and validating immediate needs for help and exploring how these can best be met. Mutuality in the relationship is nurtured by honesty, openness, sensitivity, and commitment to fostering a healing environment for the child. Refer to Box 16-3 for ways of implementing the NMPMC.

This model assumes understanding the changes occurring in families when children are hospitalized and recognizing the needs of caregivers as well as children. Working successfully and cooperatively minimizes the detrimental effects of illness experiences and requires considerable skill on the part of the nurse.

As one gains skill and competence in these participative models, it is helpful to understand that a maturational process occurs in reaching a level of confidence in relating to children and their caregivers. There is also a gradual transition from the role of novice to the expert who has developed the skills and insights necessary for sensitive, evidence-based nursing practice. It is a continuous process of learning by consistently and critically reflecting on actions and reactions, routinely examining the literature, and being aware of one's own process of learning.

Climate of the Pediatric Unit as a Supportive Environment

As a place of healing, the environment of the pediatric unit should be conducive to feelings of safety and security (Figure 16-6). This is often difficult when sights and sounds are strange and unfamiliar. Although it is important to have aesthetically pleasing surroundings, sensitivity to the decor and child-centered accouterments is secondary to the expertise, morale, satisfaction, and quality of the working relationships between and among the staff. Most critical is the conscious attention to the philosophy of family-centered care, where all involved in caring for children meld their talents and expertise on behalf of the health and welfare of those entrusted to their care. Because children sense the anxieties of adults, attending to the needs of adults, including health professionals, in the environment is important. The mental and physical health of nurses is vital to creating an environment where children and caregivers experience the comfort, knowledge, and strength that prevails when nurses use themselves as instruments for healing.

Each child should have a place for their own possessions and mementos, including their favorite things, regardless of

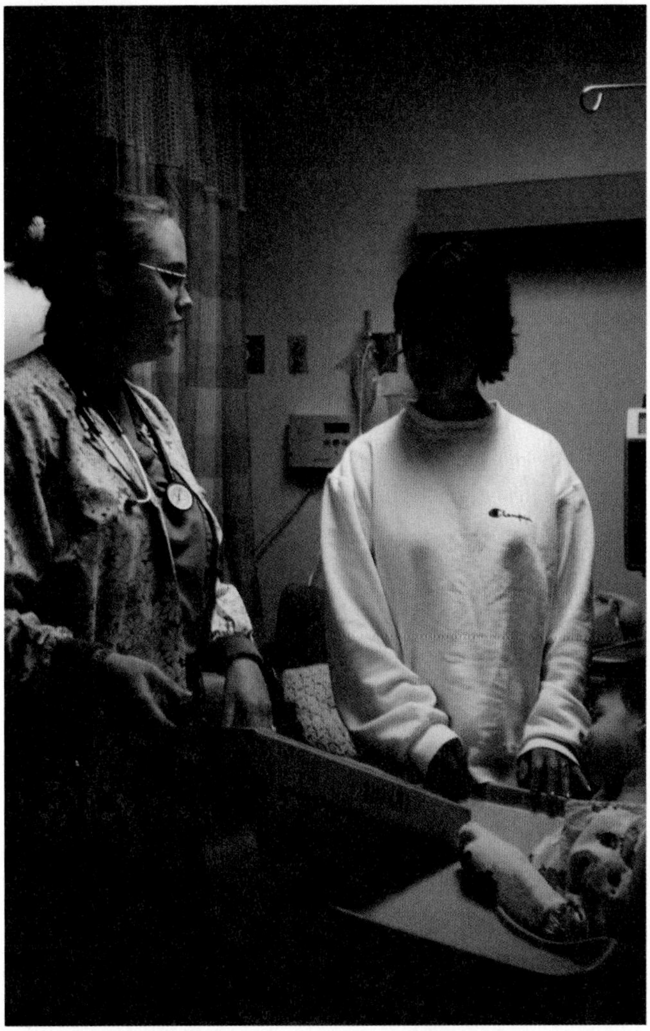

Figure 16-5 Nurse and Parent Engaged in Discussion of Child's Care. Published with permission of Baystate Medical Center Children's Hospital.

BOX 16-3 The nursing mutual participation model of care: A brief description

1. Establish a caring atmosphere by the use of open-ended questions such as "How is it going for you?"
2. Elicit and focus on parental goals and expectations through direct questions such as "How did you hope I could help you (parent your child) today?"
3. Ascertain the parent's perception of the child's condition through questions such as "How does your child look to you today? How do you think you child is doing? . . . What problems do you anticipate in the future?" Information and support can then be targeted to the parent's needs through steps such as validating observations, clarifying misconceptions, explaining nursing actions, and, if necessary, arranging a meeting with the physician.
4. Encourage the parent in the caregiving role by eliciting suggestions and preferences and negotiating any disagreements about the plan of care: "Do you have any questions or suggestions about your child's care? Is there anything you personally wish to do for or with your child?"

Adapted from Curley, M. A. (1988). Effects of the nursing mutual participation model of care on parental stress in the pediatric intensive care unit. *Heart and Lung, 17*(6), 682–688. Used with permission.

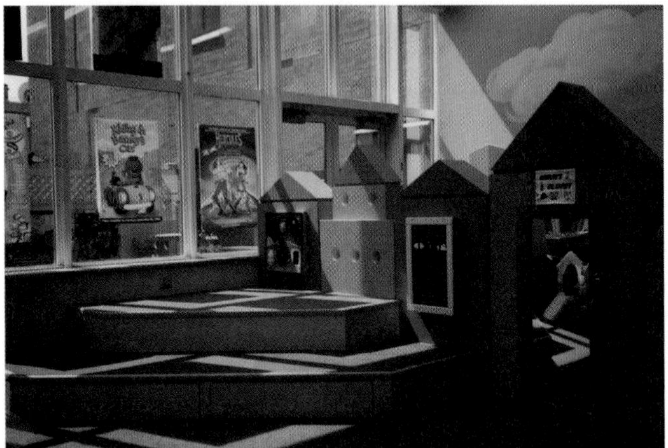

Figure 16-6 The environment of the pediatric unit should be pleasant and conducive to feelings of security. Published with permission of Baystate Medical Center Children's Hospital.

the often well-worn appearance, even though parents may be reluctant to bring the skinned, well-loved, stuffed animal or the remains of other transitional objects such as blankets and items of clothing to the hospital. Shoes should be in sight because these are symbols of mobility and reminders of going home; these are to the child what a hat may be to an elderly gentleman in a similar situation—a symbol of life outside of the hospital. The demeanor, attitude, and kindliness of those caring for children is thought to be far more influential in children's responses than what is worn. Although the attire of those who care for children has been the subject of much controversy, colored or patterned clothing is often worn in pediatric units because many believe children may associate white clothing with fear of being hurt. However, there are some aspects related to attire that may be of consequence, e.g., fingernails or rings, which can harbor harmful organisms or cause injury; hoop earrings, which small fingers might pull on; or designs on clothing that may be frightening (large animal prints). Conversely, a small, fuzzy, animal figure attached to a stethoscope and other equipment or pleasant distractions help reduce children's fears.

Every pediatric unit needs a playroom as a safe haven where no painful treatments or scenes are encountered; a place where children are empowered to cope with stressful events on a day-to-day basis. This area is highly significant to children as evidenced by a 5-year-old child who was discharged from the hospital after extensive abdominal surgery. Just as she was about to leave, she took her mother by the hand, led her to the playroom and then kissed all the toys that were so important to her . . . including the little bear to which she "gave an operation." The inclusion of play is so important that children should be brought to the playroom by any means possible (carts, wheelchairs, beds) and when not feasible, play activities should be brought to the bedside. Play is the work of children, their source of learning and, as such, is an integral component of the plan of care for each child.

The environment needs to be flexible enough to accommodate the needs of family both for visiting and staying through the night; one that provides the amenities needed for families' rest, comfort, and nourishment. Consideration of visits from siblings, grandparents, and significant others may be critically important to some children.

Sibling visitation has become a well-established practice in pediatric and newborn care units. There are considerable benefits to the child, sibling, and family with minimal risks such as infections (Andrade, 1998). Siblings have fears and fantasies about what is happening to their sister or brother, and seeing them helps alleviate concerns, since siblings may fear they may have caused illness or injury by something they did or didn't do. They also may think they might get sick too (Figure 16-7).

Child-siblings who may find it most difficult when their sister or brother is hospitalized are those who are emotionally close to their sibling or feel distanced from caregivers. Helping caregivers understand the reactions of siblings and implementing ways to help them manage the crisis of illness

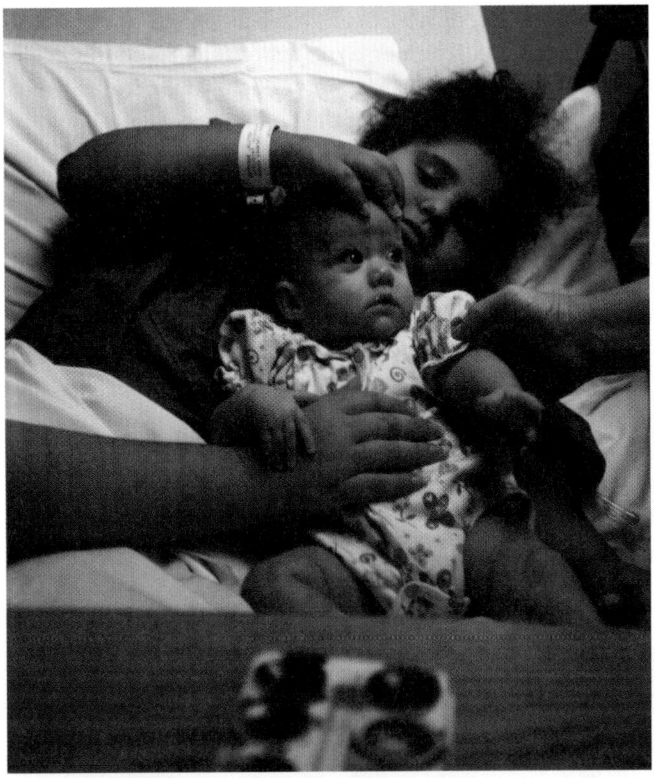

Figure 16-7 Child clients benefit when siblings visit. Published with permission of Baystate Medical Center Children's Hospital.

is also within the purview of family-centered care. In fact, many hospitals have sibling programs to respond to questions and help them understand the hospital experience. Books for siblings of children having illness or disability are also recommended (Ahmann, 1997) (Figure 16-8).

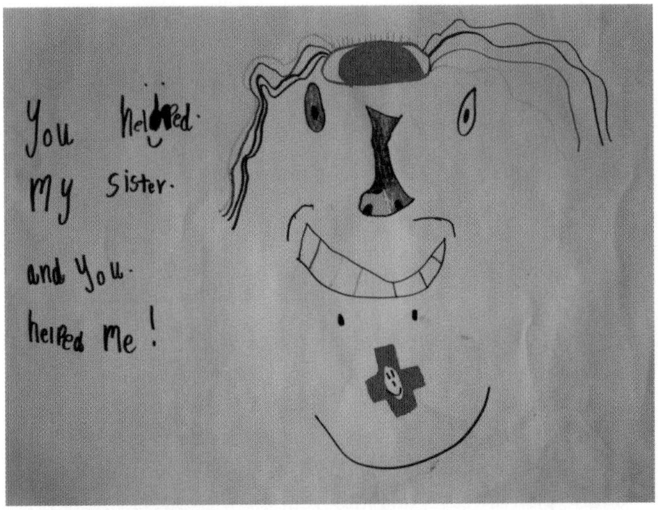
You helped
my sister.
and you
helped me!

Figure 16-8 Drawing of a Sibling while Younger Sister Is Hospitalized. Published with permission of Baystate Medical Center Children's Hospital.

Play as Therapeutic in Facilitating Coping

Hurlock (1978) defined play as any voluntary activity engaged in for the purpose of enjoyment. Play fosters the development of cognitive, psychomotor, language, and psychosocial skills. Blake (1954) proposed the child gains mastery of fears and relief from the tension within through play.

Therapeutic play is an intervention used by nurses and **child life staff** prepared in this technique, to aid ill and hospitalized children express thoughts and feelings. This kind of play also helps nurses better understand the thoughts, feelings, and experiences of children (Kuntz, Adams, Zahr, Kellen, Cameron, & Wassen, 1996). Play moderates reactions to stress and has beneficial physiological benefits as well (Zahr, 1998). For example, anger and pent-up energy can be released through physical activities such as pounding boards and punching bags/balls and games like throwing beanbags in holes for points. Play situations are created, but the child chooses the items and decides on the way to use these according to their level of comfort and readiness.

Art supplies and materials, including paper, crayons, pencils, paint, brushes, finger-paints, water, and clay encourage creative expression thoughts and feelings. A miniature house that contains hospital clothing, child and adult doll figures, hospital equipment, and supplies fosters the inclination of children to don the roles of hospital personnel and treat "their patients" in a safe, simulated setting. This kind of play dramatizes perceptions of their experiences and gives children the opportunity to act out and talk through situations, particularly those difficult to understand or accept. The use of play, including clothing and hospital equipment, is also highly effective in teaching and preparing children for situations related to their specific hospital experience as well as playing out events after they have occurred.

It is highly advantageous for a pediatric unit to have an organized **Child Life Program,** a well-equipped playroom with toys, games, and facilities for the use of hospital equipment, and a schoolroom for children with prolonged hospitalizations. The availability of a variety of dolls facilitates play and acting out thoughts and feelings, e.g., figure dolls of adults, nurses, and doctors, anatomically correct dolls, crying dolls, and those representing many different ages and cultures. Many hospitals provide plain stuffed dolls shortly after admission, and children are encouraged to draw faces and clothes on these to make them special (Gaynard, Goldberger, & Laidley, 1991). Children then have the option of using their doll when procedures and treatments are being demonstrated and in therapeutic play (Figure 16-9).

When children are admitted for same-day surgery, there are fewer negative behavior changes at home after surgery when play with hospital equipment is part of their care (Schmidt, 1990). It is also advantageous for each nurse to

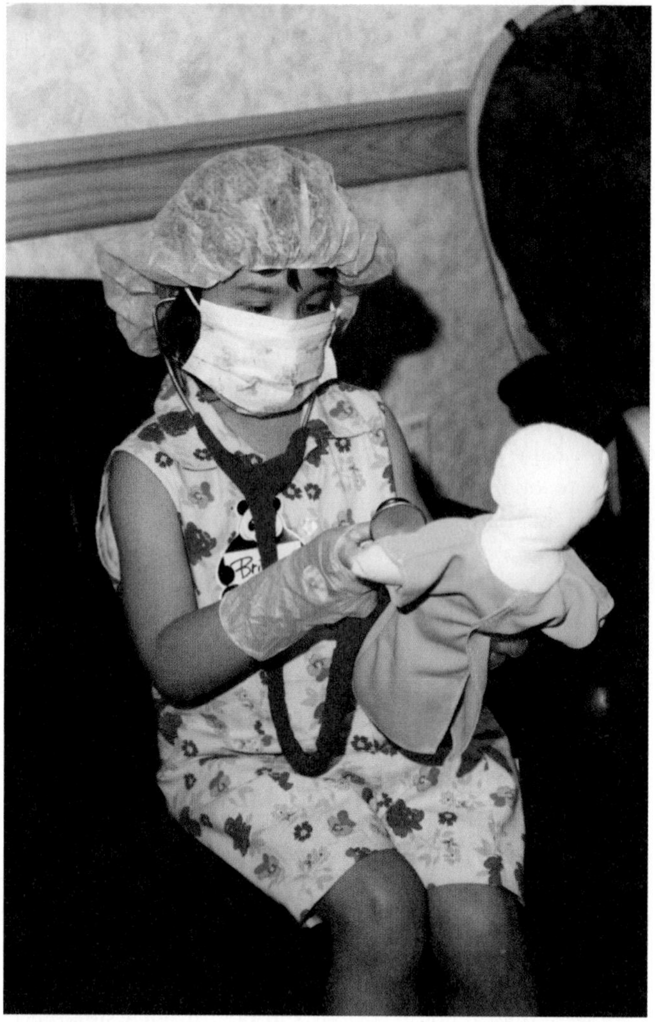

Figure 16-9 Hospitalized Child during Doll Play

create their own small, readily available small suitcase or basket that contains nurse, doctor, adult, and child dolls; frequently used hospital equipment; and a few hand-puppet figures. It is difficult for children to resist play but for those who have difficulty in engaging in active play due to fatigue, immobility, diminished readiness, or other problems, there are ways of providing vicarious involvement, e.g., observing the play of other children, nurses simulating play, conversations between hand held puppets, puppet shows, etc.

Nurses have the responsibility of determining the needs of children for therapeutic play and incorporating these skills in the plan of care for individual children. One example not often considered is when children are distressed about being restrained. When intravenous materials are also involved, it is advisable to provide restraint materials along with those related to the intravenous, e.g., armboard and tape, when providing play materials. Each nurse also needs to develop a basic understanding and skill in using play figures to explain concepts and events. For example, if a toddler needs to have a cast applied, one can be applied to a doll first, and when the removal takes place it can be done first to the doll, and then to the child. The nurse can act out the responses of the child in play situations, by saying, "ouch, you're hurting me," and observe the response of the child, asking what could be done so it won't hurt or help it to be better. Children often have creative and unique solutions to problems that are related to taking medications or having painful treatments revealed through play activities.

Sufficient time each day needs to be allocated for play experiences, particularly for immobilized children who are often in a "state of waiting and increased vigilance" (Gillis, 1989) (Figure 16-10). In expanding their focus beyond their illness, children are better able to manage their perceptions of the slowness of the passage of time and engender positive feelings toward themselves and others. All children in hospitals need opportunities to express their thoughts and feelings about experiences, particularly those that are difficult and

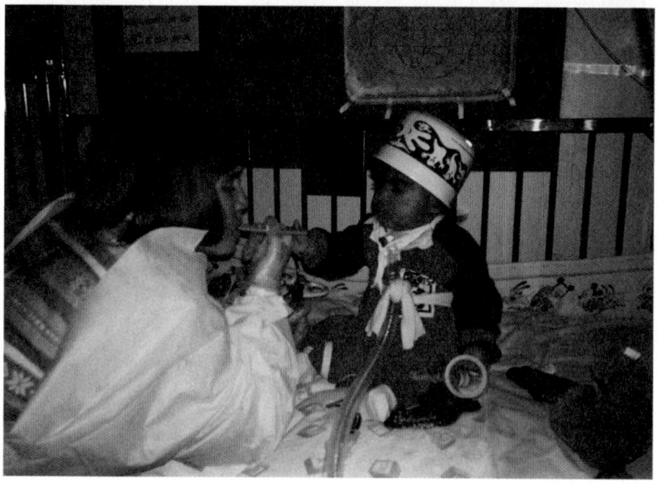

Figure 16-10 Play Activities when a Child Is Unable to Go to the Playroom. Published with permission of Baystate Medical Center Children's Hospital.

Nursing Tip:

Play interviews/sessions with young children in hospitals

Conducting therapeutic play interviews and play sessions with young children requires depth of understanding and skill in this technique. It is wise for novices to read extensively about therapeutic play as an intervention, plan opportunities to observe therapeutic play, practice this intervention with supervision on several occasions, and receive feedback on this practice.

perplexing. Creating environments and situations where children laugh and have fun while hospitalized is an important consideration in the recovery process.

PREPARATION OF CHILDREN AND FAMILIES FOR HOSPITALIZATION

To reduce the potentially adverse effects of hospitalization, preparation for this experience should take place prior to admission whenever possible. The primary purposes of teaching at this time are to provide information, encourage emotional expression, establish trusting relationships, and teach coping strategies. These goals are met most effectively when the age and experiences of the child and honesty and responsiveness to concerns and questions characterize the preparation process. Most childrens' hospitals have programs and learning activities designed to prepare children for hospital experiences, day-stay surgery, and diagnostic procedures. Preparation materials and presentations are most helpful when these reflect the learning needs of children of different ages and stages of development, and accurately depict the sights, smells, sounds, policies, and procedures of the actual setting (Figure 16-11).

With cognitive development and language skills as key factors, both the content and timing of preparation are important considerations. For infants, the best approach is to prepare caregivers. By allaying their fears and concerns they will be better able to communicate a sense of calmness and well being to their infants. For planned admissions, the age of the child should be a guide to timing for preparation for hospitalization or surgery: 1–2-year-olds, the day or evening before or day of admission or surgery; 2–3-year-olds, 2–3 days before; 4–7-year-olds, 4–7 days; and over 7 years, a few weeks before admission or surgery (Fox, 1997). Through tours, use of puppets, medical play, children's literature, and audiovisual media, children learn about the experience and their role in the recovery process. Whenever possible, children should have the opportunity to actively participate, e.g., handling equipment such as blood pressure apparatus, stethoscope, and IV fluid tubing.

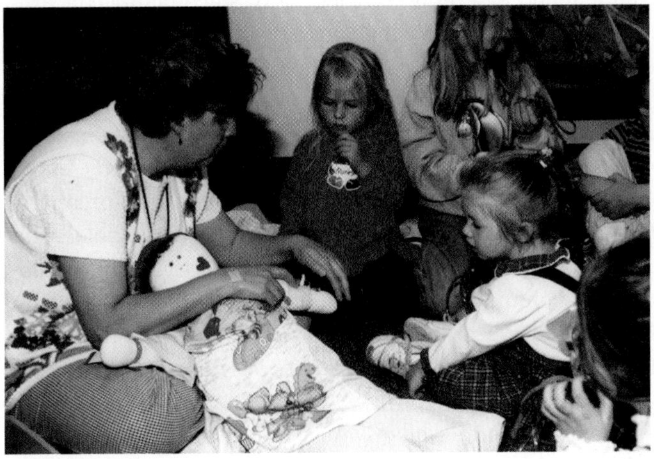

Figure 16-11 Preparing a Child for Hospitalization By Using Dolls

Group preparation is often effective for school-aged children. Adolescents need opportunities to explore the meaning and consequences of the experience in addition to explanations relevant to preparation for surgery and/or hospitalization. Additionally, they need time to discuss fears, concerns, options, and alternatives. Although it is important for children and adolescents to understand as much as possible about the experience, it is equally important for parents to have information that will help them maintain their parental role. When caregivers have accurate information and feel confident, they can transmit a sense of security to their children.

Unexpected hospitalizations of young children under the age of six constitute most admissions to pediatric units. When parents and children are not prepared for the sudden changes and stresses, this results in higher anxiety levels and a higher risk for negative outcomes both during and after hospitalization (Melnyk, 1994). Because of the urgency of admission or when attending a preadmission program is not possible, an orientation is initiated at the time of admission. The child needs to know about their new environment, routines, and expectations, and also needs ongoing, simultaneous explanations about what is occurring and the rationale. The family needs to know essential information to cope with the immediacy of the situation. This is best accomplished by anticipating needs and responding to questions and concerns as they arise.

CARE OF CHILDREN DURING ADMISSION TO A HOSPITAL

The process of admission begins with establishing a helping, trusting relationship with the child and caregivers. The first greeting of welcome should include a smile with the message of expecting their arrival followed by introductions. Shaking hands with caregivers and children (when age-appropriate) is a symbolic gesture of beginning the relationship. At this time the formal name and title of the nurse is followed by a brief discussion of the name each person prefers to be called. When young children are admitted to the hospital, the nurse should first establish a relationship with caregivers. As the child sees their caregivers trust the nurse, it is easier for the children to engage in a relationship with the nurse. Being at eye level and having eye contact while talking to children facilitates positive responses.

During this time, it is also advisable to explain the pattern of staffing and names of other nurses who may be involved in the child's care. Knowing the role, responsibilities, and length of time the nurse will be caring for the child is helpful information, as are the names of health care practitioners, other nurses, and personnel who will be involved during the first day (a process that should be repeated each day). This is followed by a brief description of the general policies. Preferably, the nurse during the initial orientation phase will be the primary nurse or at least one who will provide care during hospitalization.

The admission routines (which may vary according to organization policies) continue with detailed history taking and complete assessment. In addition to obtaining precise information about the child's routines, reactions to stress, and understanding about the reason for hospitalization, information about prior experiences with illness and hospitalization should be ascertained, including the significant experiences of others in the child's home/school environment. Some children may have had recent experiences with the hospital as a place of birth or death. The association may be quite direct as for example when a child has a "heart problem" and experienced the hospitalization and death of someone who had a "heart attack." There also needs to be explicit clarification of the reason for hospitalization so perceptions can be clarified. One female child of about 5 asked, "where is my baby?" when she was leaving the hospital. Her older sister had recently gone to the hospital to have her baby. The importance of accuracy in communication and careful interpretation of verbal and nonverbal behavior cannot be overemphasized.

When children with chronic illnesses are admitted to the hospital, they need to know how this hospitalization is different than other experiences. For younger children, it is helpful to ask parents to write down the home routine for feeding, exercises, and elimination. One mother of a toddler with cystic fibrosis had a plan that she entitled, "the care and feeding of one Nicholas Francis," a detailed account of his daily activities, routines, treatments, and medications. This kind of written plan provides an excellent source of information for consistency of routines and rituals, so reassuring to young children.

Depending on the age of the child and the acuity of illness at the time of admission, it is helpful to have an orientation to the unit stressing those areas of greatest relevance, e.g., play room and toilet facilities. The time of admission is also the time to explore the needs and desires of caregivers regarding their comfort, their involvement in the direct care of their child, and how the nurse, health care practitioners, and staff will work together during the child's hospitalization. It is a unique opportunity to explain the philosophy of family-centered care and the participative model of practice where caregivers are integral partners in providing the best care possible, understanding that the level of direct involvement may vary depending on a variety of circumstances. Establishing helping, supportive relationships at this time influences the way nurses and caregivers work harmoniously in caring and healing.

An initial **nursing interview** with caregivers provides nurses with an opportunity to establish helping relationships while learning essential information about the child and family, and discovering ways of working together for the benefit of the child. Many hospitals have forms for this interview and there may be sections for the child's growth and development and for the medical history and immunizations, which caregivers can complete separately. These data can be used as a source for follow-up questions. It is also helpful to have a separate interview with the child or adolescent in order to understand their perceptions related to their illness and hospitalization. In addition to interview and data collection forms, most pediatric units have written guides for patients and families that contain answers to frequently asked questions and helpful information. Usually included are explanations about philosophy of family-centered care, hospital procedures and resources, policies and practices of the pediatric unit, suggestions for helping children and siblings cope, and safety measures. Informational booklets are prepared by individual hospitals, e.g., Baystate Medical Center (see Resources).

PREPARATION OF CHILDREN FOR SURGERY

When children are admitted for surgical procedures or examinations requiring anesthesia, both the timing and the content of the child's and family's preparation should be considered. Generally, children should be prepared close to the time of the surgical procedure and the dialogue, audio, and visual materials should be age appropriate and relevant to the child's cognitive development (Figure 16-12). Prior to instruction, it is helpful to ascertain what they know and how they feel (Lamontagne, et al., 1997).

Preparing parents also helps improve the child's understanding and ease in asking questions, since family concerns and anxieties strongly influence the child's reaction to preoperative experience (Noble, Micheli, Hensley, & McKay, 1997). Children's fears focus mainly on the unfamiliar environment, pain, mutilation, and separation from parents, and with parental presence these fears may be alleviated (Algren & Algren, 1997). For example, in uncomplicated preoperative situations where caregivers are prepared and able, their presence during induction of anesthesia is reassuring to children and minimizes the stress of separation. The need for heavy sedation decreases with parent-present induction (PPI), promoting more rapid recovery from anesthesia (LaRosa-Nash & Murphy, 1997).

Most hospitals have well-established protocols and resources to prepare children and caregivers for different kinds of surgery. These include tours of the facility and the

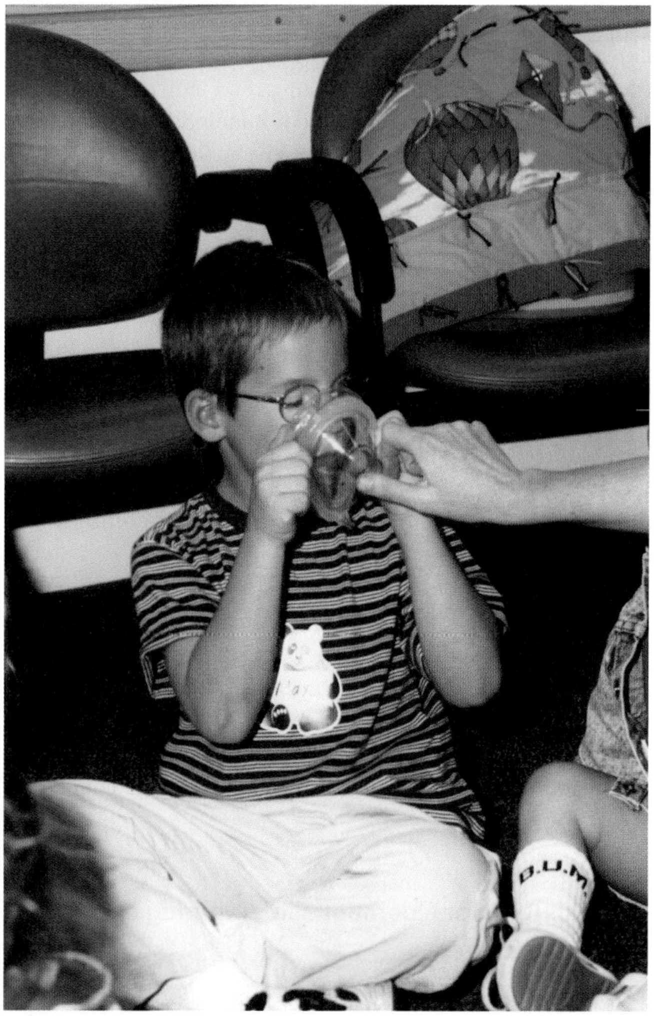

Figure 16-12 Preparing a School-aged Child for Surgery

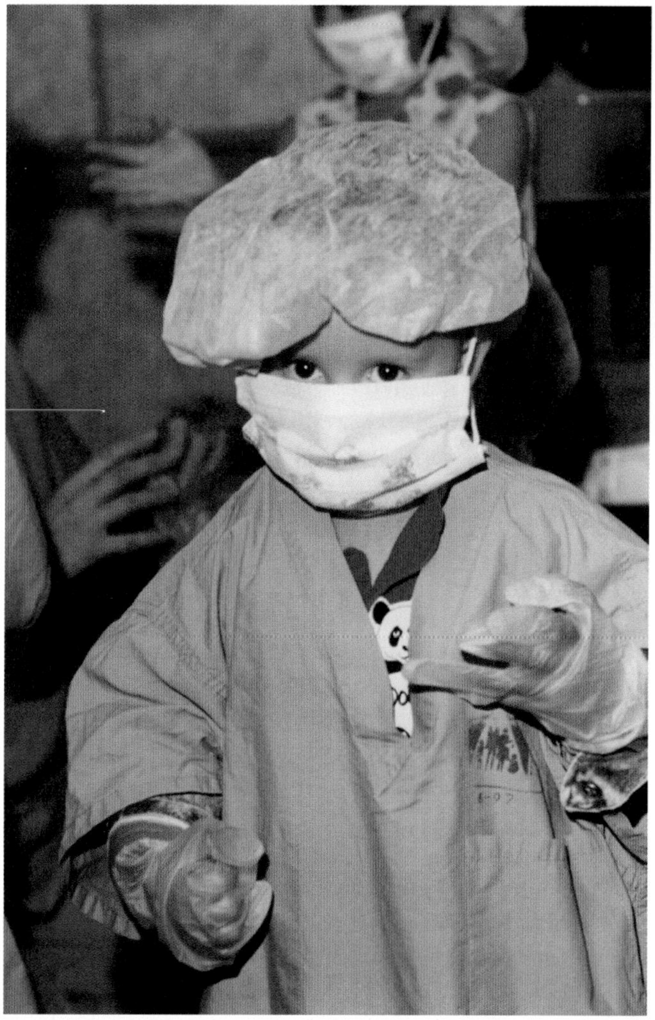

Figure 16-13 A Toddler Becoming Familiar with Surgical Garb

use of films, puppets, and discussions (Figure 16-13). Books are also helpful, and a list of children's literature to prepare children for surgery is in the resource section at the end of this chapter.

Most children want to know if it will hurt and may be afraid something will go wrong or they will wake up during the operation. It is reassuring to know that the "anesthesia doctor" is always there during the surgery and that this will not occur. Explanations regarding anesthesia need to be carefully considered. For example, the phrase "put to sleep" may be frightening, particularly when this has been used in reference to a euthanized pet. Among alternatives to reduce this kind of fear may be a phrase like, "a special kind of sleep" and adding, "you will be awakened when it's over and come back here where (person in family) will be waiting for you."

During a child's immediate preparation for surgery, every effort should be made to minimize stress. Young children who do not understand the rationale for withholding food and fluids need to be carefully observed so they do not take food or fluids inadvertently. When children of young ages have same-day surgery, it is advisable for caregivers to snack-proof the house on the evening before and not eat in the presence of the child on the day of surgery. Using a matter of fact approach rather than emphatic denials of food requests avoids an association of food deprivation and disapproval. Saying, "remember that the nurse said that all children having surgery (or this test) are allowed to eat and drink only after their operation (test) but not before, so you will feel better faster," is more encouraging during the waiting period.

To prevent fear associated with preoperative injections, noninjectable medications should be used whenever possible. In transporting young children to the surgical suite, it is unwise to use their crib, because doing so may precipitate postoperative fears related to sleep; e.g., the young child may reason that if you fall asleep, you may be taken away again. For example, for several days after surgery, 3½-year-old Danny was "awake all night" and only fell asleep when

Critical Thinking

Preparation of a Child/Family for Surgery

Think of a preschooler you know. Imagine that he or she is to be admitted to the hospital for repair of a ventricular septal defect in a week.

- What are the strengths of this child and the strengths of the family that will be influential in preparing this child for hospitalization and surgery, and for coping with these experiences?
- Using all resources available, what would you include in a teaching plan for this child and parents?

If you were the nurse at the time the child was going to surgery, what is the sequence of activities during the immediate preparation to the time that anesthesia is given?

If this child were to be hospitalized for 5 days, describe the nursing interventions that would most likely be effective in helping this preschooler and caregivers cope with this experience. What behaviors would indicate difficulty in coping?

he was on the sofa in the playroom or sitting on his mother's lap. In play, he took several dolls and aggressively put them in and then took them out of their "hurt beds"—he then used buses and trucks to take them outside the room so no one could find them. In subsequent play sessions, his fears were expressed and misconceptions explained, following which he gradually returned the dolls to their beds and resumed more restful nighttime sleep several days later.

The goal for optimal preoperative preparation is to provide and reinforce information for children and parents, encourage emotional expression and fears, and teach coping strategies while minimizing intrusive, distressing, and painful procedures.

FACILITATING COPING WITH EXPERIENCES OF DIAGNOSTIC/THERAPEUTIC PROCEDURES

When children know what to expect, there is greater potential for maintaining control and mastering fears during uncomfortable and frightening procedures. Although time may be limited, as often happens in acute illnesses, an explanation should always come first. When caregivers understand the procedure, they are better able to enhance the explanation by making comparisons to previous experiences or using terms most familiar to the child. The presence of supportive caregivers during treatments and procedures cannot be overemphasized. However, there may be circumstances where they are unable or prefer not to participate, and caregiver involvement should not include restraining.

Because infants and toddlers are in the formative stage of developing language and cognitive skills, the presence of caregivers with their gentle handling and soothing words decreases the pain and anxiety of procedures. The role of adults during and after is also critical in alleviating the emotional and physical discomforts experienced. Preschoolers benefit most from the use of demonstrations and role-play using play equipment, e.g., using a doll or animal to apply a cast, change a dressing, or start intravenous fluids. The child should choose the subject of the procedure as many do not like to use their favorite doll or toy animal. Box 16-4 describes various components of preparing children and caregivers for treatments and procedures.

During procedures, the nurse should continue to guide and coach the child, using soft, reassuring words and giving praise intermittently for cooperation and following directions (e.g., "it's real hard to stay still, but you're doing this very well") (Figure 16-14). It is inadvisable to use words like "you're good girl," particularly for young children who may associate this experience with punishment. At the conclusion

BOX 16-4 Considerations in preparing children for procedures

- Assess the cognitive level, previous experiences with the particular procedure, and readiness for learning.
- Explain honestly and simply, using terms understandable to the child–include what will happen and associated sensations.
- Use the least aggressive language, e.g., "fixing the bandage or making it better" rather than "taking it off or taking it out."
- Include brief rationale and ways the child can safely participate, e.g., holding the adhesive tape.
- Offer opportunities to manipulate the equipment in advance of the procedure when possible (rehearsal is helpful).
- Practice alternate ways of maintaining control during the procedure, e.g., guided imagery, holding/squeezing a hand or a favorite toy, or counting.
- At the conclusion of the initial preparation, ask the child to explain what is going to happen during the procedure and clarify areas of misunderstanding.
- Decide on an activity or comforting measure for after the treatment/procedure, e.g., read a story, glass of juice, going to the playroom, or play activity.

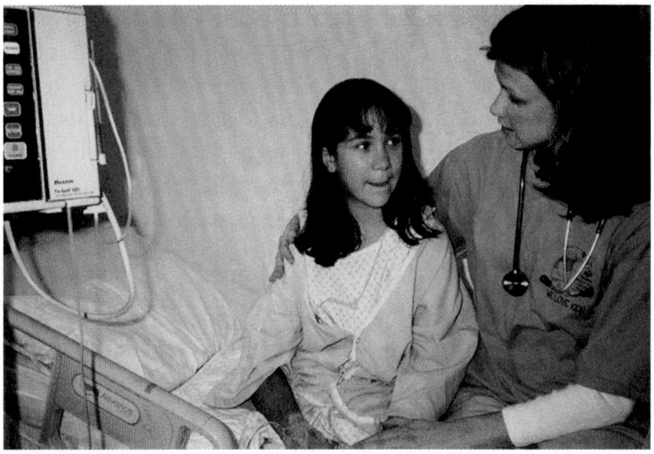

Figure 16-14 Nurses comfort children in many ways. Published with permission of Baystate Medical Center Children's Hospital.

of treatments, offer a simple apology if the child experienced discomfort or pain, e.g., "I'm sorry if I hurt you." Follow-up includes the fun activity or comfort measure agreed on in advance, encouraging expression/description of how the child experienced the procedure through conversations, and/or play. Considerable insight can be gained by asking children and caregivers what could have been done to make the experience easier to manage. Questions like "now that this is over, what helped you the most in getting ready [or during the procedure]?" or, "what should I be sure to tell other children about what it is like and how it feels when they have their bandages changed?" may help with future explanations.

CONSIDERATIONS FOR COMMUNICATING WITH CHILDREN

Sometimes words are confusing and cause distress. For example, a child was in her room crying and stopped long enough to ask "is this tomorrow?," to which the nurse replied "no, it's today." Her crying escalated and the nurse discovered that, the day before, the doctor said that she could go home tomorrow. When the nurse assured her that this was "tomorrow," the child was much relieved and could prepare for going home.

Children often do not understand the different language of the hospital setting or may misinterpret what is said to them or to others. To be effective, communication should be clear, honest, and understandable to the child. A prime example is when children are told they are to have "a shot," and even though this is commonly used to describe an injection, the child may conjure up visions of being maimed or harmed beyond the pain of the injection (Figure 16-15). They may think that they will be shot. Often, children hear, "this won't hurt," or "it will only hurt a little," when something is known to be painful. What is needed more is the truth and the support of another in coping with and managing hurtful experiences. Sometimes words used are frightening and evoke fantasies of doom. One example is the shriek response of a child when the technician said that she would put in dye for a test. The child reacted so vehemently because he thought, "I might die."

Nurses also need to know the words children commonly use for toileting and other vital needs and ways of communicating when they are unable to express themselves verbally (Figure 16-16). Some children have difficulty understanding because of hearing, cognitive, or neurological impairments, and others may not understand or have the ability to express their needs because of language and cultural differences. In a situation of a 4-year-old girl who understood only her native language, her mother left three cards with her when she had to leave, each one of a different color. On the yellow, it was written "I have to go to the bathroom," on the blue, "I want a drink of water," and on the red (only to be used in an emergency), " I want to call my mother."

In communicating with children, the use of their preferred name is important. A 6-year-old whose name was Charles Brown was admitted to the hospital for a spinal cord injury following an automobile accident in which he had been hit by a car. (When asked, "what happened?" he said, "I didn't run fast enough.") The staff nurses amusingly called him "Charlie Brown" from the time he was admitted until one nurse asked him, "what do your parents call you?," to which he answered, "Chuckie." When his own nickname was

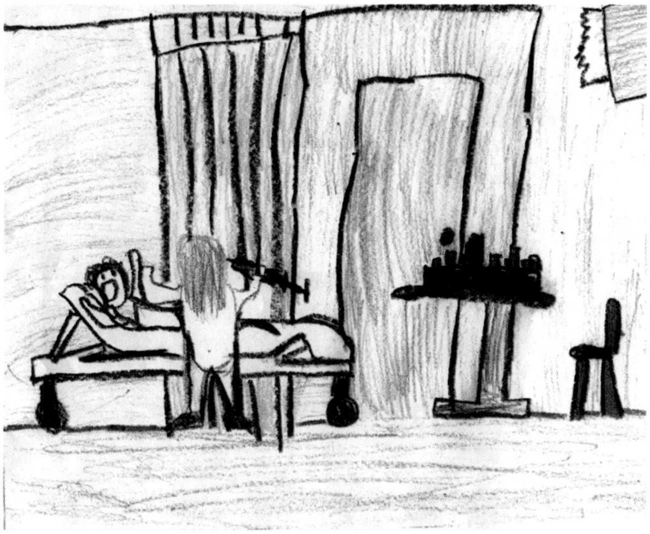

Figure 16-15 Drawing of a 10-Year-Old Male Child Indicating Perception of What It Is Like To Have an Injection

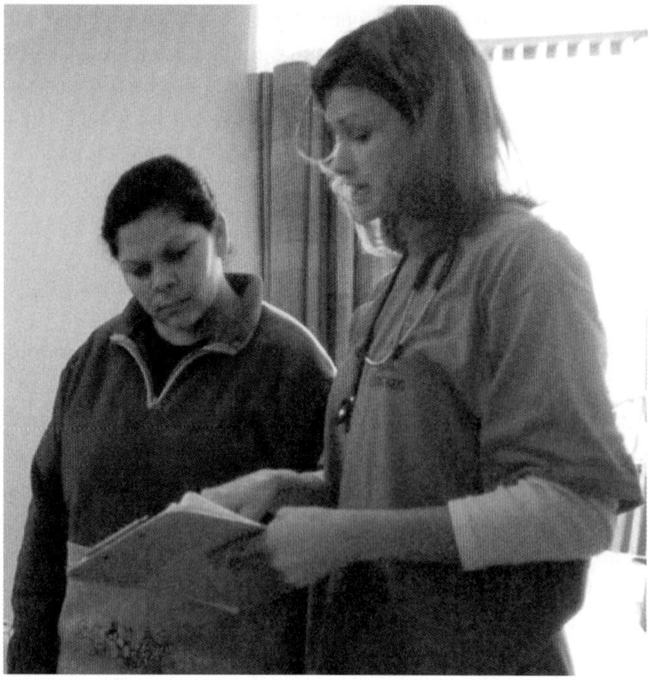

Figure 16-16 Careful listening and responding is important in helping children to cope during hospitalization. Published with permission of Baystate Medical Center Children's Hospital.

used, there were notable changes in the way that he engaged in rehabilitation therapy, and he talked more openly about his family and school.

The language used in reference to children is also important. To refer to children as "kids" or to an individual child as "this kid" minimizes the dignity of children. Even though these terms are commonly used in everyday conversation to refer to children as a group or to a child as an individual, the appropriateness in professional nursing practice is highly questionable. Similarly, one should be aware of the detrimental effects of labeling or stereotyping children and/or caregivers. Instead of saying "he's a diabetic," the phrase "he is a child with diabetes" emphasizes that he is a child with a health problem and not one who is identified by a disease.

Honesty in explanations, responses to questions, and general information demonstrates understanding that children need to be trustful of others. This should be considered in minor situations as well, so when nurses say, "I'll be right back," they should return promptly because situations like this are symbolic of trusting relationships.

NURSING CARE AND GUIDANCE OF INFANTS

Newborns and infants during the first year of life may be hospitalized at a time of rapid growth and development. Some are hospitalized for long periods after birth, with transitions from newborn intensive care units to pediatric units, home, and return to hospital for surgery, diagnostic tests, etc. Others are admitted for congenital and adventitious conditions requiring short- or long-term care. Their healthy attachment to caregivers and their progress toward optimal development are of paramount concern during these times.

Special Needs of Infants

From the time of birth, infants depend on others for nurturance and protection. Gaining a sense of trust is facilitated when needs for bonding, contact comfort, and nutritional sustenance are fulfilled, and as rhythmical, reciprocal patterns develop. Infants need the kind of security predisposing them to restful sleep, satisfaction of oral and nutritional needs, relaxation of the body and body systems, and to spontaneous respond to communication and gentle environmental stimuli.

Caregiver–infant attachment is critical to psychological health and infants need their primary caregiver during illness. Infants beyond the age of 5–6 months are acutely aware of the absence of their mothers and, within a few months, develop stranger anxiety and become fearful of unfamiliar persons. For hospitalized infants, it is essential not only to support caregivers in their role, but to also assure consistency in sensitive, responsive, and interactive nursing care.

The basic source of infant satisfaction is through satiation of oral needs. During illness, there is often disruption in the consistency of feeding patterns, contact comfort, sleeping, elimination, and stimulation. Nurses should be particularly aware of the effects of situations that interfere with the gratification of oral needs, e.g., oral surgery, vomiting, distasteful medications, withholding food and fluids as well as periods of nonoral feedings. When oral satisfaction is threatened, it is difficult for infants to maintain pleasure through sucking, swallowing, digesting, and eliminating. An example of this is when tube feeding is required; the use of a pacifier during the time of the feeding helps the infant develop the relationship between oral pleasure and the feeling of fullness and satiation when hunger is relieved.

Direct Care of Infants

Nurses have many responsibilities in securing optimal health for infants both in teaching caregivers and families and in providing direct care. For consistency, the patterns of care at home are a helpful guide to planning care in the hospital. For first-time mothers of young infants, the nurse is often a model for baby care.

Infants learn through sensorimotor experiences. Talking to infants slowly, singing lullabies, moving them gently and carefully, and rocking and cuddling are ways to help infants reduce tension. Smooth, continuous movements, gentle stroking, and holding confidently are additional methods to reduce stress responses. In some hospitals, grandmothers and other volunteers often provide contact comfort by rocking and cuddling, particularly those with prolonged hospitalizations (Figure 16-17). External stimuli, such as pictures, mirrors, music, and mobiles provide the kind of visual stimulation needed for growth.

Infant massage is an intervention used by nurses who are prepared to use this technique to soothe infants and provide physical stimulation (Field, 1995; Lindrea & Stainton, 2000). Swaddling, by wrapping the infant snugly in a soft blanket, is a practice used by many cultural groups to promote infant comfort and security. See Box 16-5 for more suggestions on caring for infants.

BOX 16-5 Points of emphasis in caring for infants

Safety:

- Always have at least one hand on the infant when the crib sides are down.
- Place the child on the opposite side of the crib when lowering the crib sides.
- Put crib sides up all the way when infant is in a crib, and push against the crib side when it is up to be sure that it is held securely in place.
- Avoid leaving objects small enough to be swallowed or harmful objects in the crib or within reach.
- Examine toys for safety and washability.

Other:

- Be aware of both obvious and subtle signs of discomfort and discontent (crying, furrowed brow, body tension, wringing hands), and respond to needs.
- Assume en face position while feeding and holding infants—encourage eye contact by smiling and talking to infants during bathing.
- Decrease the number of painful or uncomfortable procedures to minimize negative situations that may affect trust development.
- After painful or distressing experiences, comfort infant by holding and using soothing tones and movement.
- Supporting caregivers is the primary way to support infants coping with tension.
- When it is difficult for parents to be present during procedures, their wishes should be respected and supported with reassurance.

NURSING CARE AND GUIDANCE OF TODDLERS

From babyhood to toddlerhood, children develop remarkable skills in all aspects of growth and development. They are now their own person as demonstrated by their awareness of self as a being with the power to use words and actions to express their will. They learn how their behavior affects others as they become individuals, while at the same time being conscious of the need for care and protection by others. When toddlers are hospitalized, preservation of the protective relationships of caregivers continues to be critical to their healthy development and healing.

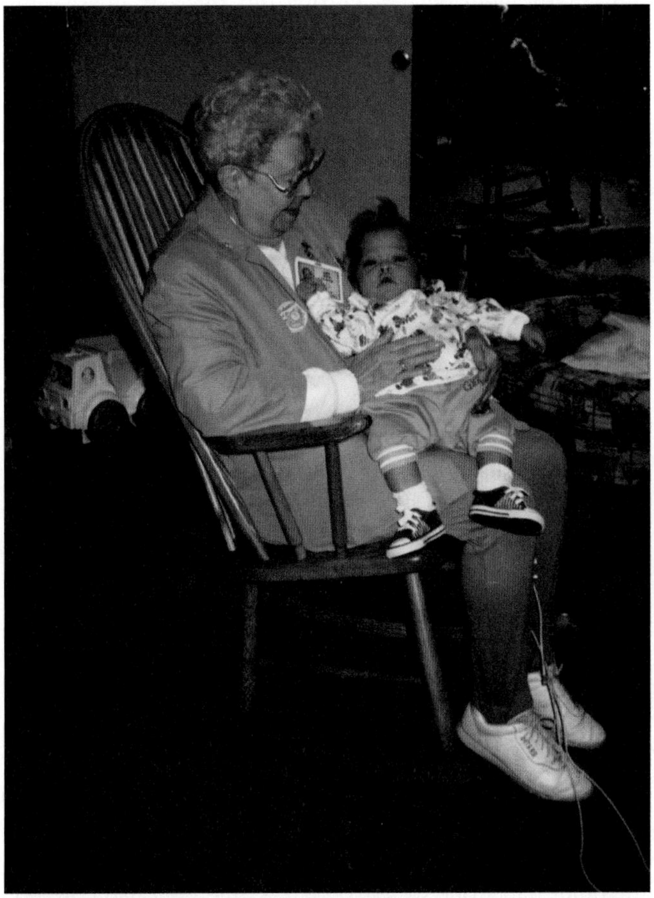

Figure 16-17 Volunteer grandmother comforts a toddler. Published with permission of Baystate Medical Center Children's Hospital.

Special Needs of Toddlers

Hospitalization and/or surgery impose movement restrictions and changes that undermine beginning confidence in skill development. While in the midst of learning to feed themselves or learning sphincter control with all the praise and affirmation usually accorded these efforts, there may be little attention paid to these accomplishments in the hospital. Putting diapers on a child who has mastered toileting diminishes their sense of competence and control. To preserve developing autonomy and minimize shame and doubt in themselves, it is important to know the accomplishments of individual toddlers and maintain mastery insofar as possible. With different routines, separations from caregivers, misinterpretations of language and behavior, and being prevented from moving, enjoying, and controlling their bodies, toddlers become perplexed and may respond with regression, aggression, or withdrawal. Of great concern is the actual separation from caregivers in an unfamiliar environment when family members are not able to stay. When there are short separations, and toddlers have become familiar with a primary nurse, adaptation is facilitated.

However, in the hospital, everything is different and unpredictable. The presence of caregivers, especially during critical times of procedures, treatments, and before and after surgery is essential. It is advisable for each child to have a family member present throughout the hospital stay. The primary goals in planning care for a toddler who is hospitalized are to sustain child-family bonds, to preserve their sense of autonomy by assuring opportunities to exercise their will, and to strengthen their ability to mature in the development of cognitive and psychomotor skills. Effective nurse–caregiver relationships and consistency of care provide the kind of secure environment toddlers need to cope with the changes of illness and hospitalization (Figure 16-18).

Effects of Prolonged Separation on Toddlers

One of the most serious consequences of hospitalization is the response that occurs when prolonged hospital stays are combined with the inability of caregivers to spend extended time with their toddler. If caregivers leave and consistently return after short periods, toddlers can regain security, but if they do not reappear for long periods and children need them desperately, separation anxiety poses a serious threat to healthy development. The literature is replete with the progressive and potentially long-term effects of this kind of crisis. Bowlby (1965) was one of the first to study the psychological distress of children separated from their families during World War II. Spitz (1954) documented the effects of prolonged separation on infants in foundling homes, observing that many infants succumbed even though adequate physical care was provided.

Robertson (1958) studied the effect of separations of young children from their parents due to hospitalization and described three phases of response: protest, despair, and denial. In the initial stage of **protest,** the toddler cries loudly and desperately, making every effort to bring them back. They are inconsolable and constantly look in the direction of where their parent departed. This way of communicating their displeasure is often misinterpreted by caregivers and nurses. Caregivers may think they should stay away so the child will not become so upset, and nurses may try to encourage the child to be "good and not cry," instead of understanding this as a healthy and appropriate expression of emotion.

If separations continue, withdrawal, refusals of food, diminished communication, and general loss of interest in the environment occurs. During this **despair** phase, children may lie quietly and come to others, yet their internal distress is such that they do not express their feelings easily. When caregivers return, the toddler may look away or focus on toys or objects as if to ignore caregivers who disappointed them by going away. If separation is further extended, the child enters a phase of **denial,** or detachment, having lost hope for permanent reunion. There is an outward appearance of indifference and the toddler appears to be settled in, compliant, "adjusted," and indiscriminate in relationships with others and to the situation. This denial of emotion is often misinterpreted as coping well with their plight. Although these developments are now rare because of comparatively short hospitalizations, constant vigilance is necessary to prevent these severe responses (Figure 16-19). In the eyes of a child, even short separations during times of stress can be perceived as much longer than they really are.

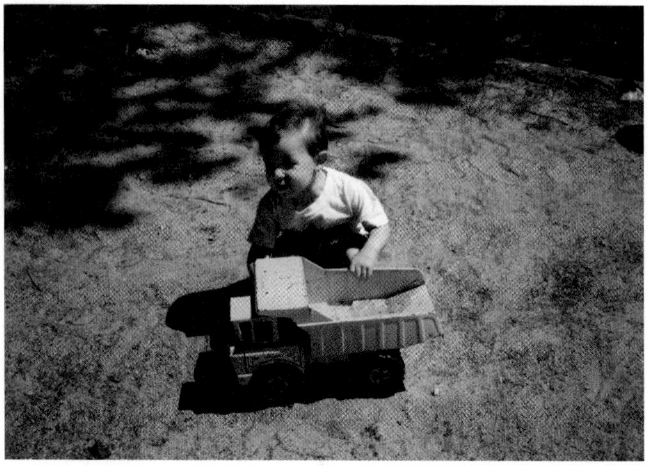

Figure 16-18 A Toddler at Play, Developing a Sense of Autonomy

Direct Care of Toddlers

There are many constructive ways of applying knowledge of growth and development during hospitalization. For example, understanding the concept of the task of autonomy in toddlers and the negativism that is part of this task is evident with choices for a toddler. If the nurse asks, "do you want to take a nap now?", this implies a choice that is not age-appropriate and often precipitates a negative response. If, on the other hand, one were to say, "it's time for a nap now—do you want Pooh Bear or Barney to come with you?" the toddler has the opportunity to exert autonomous behavior and cooperation is more likely.

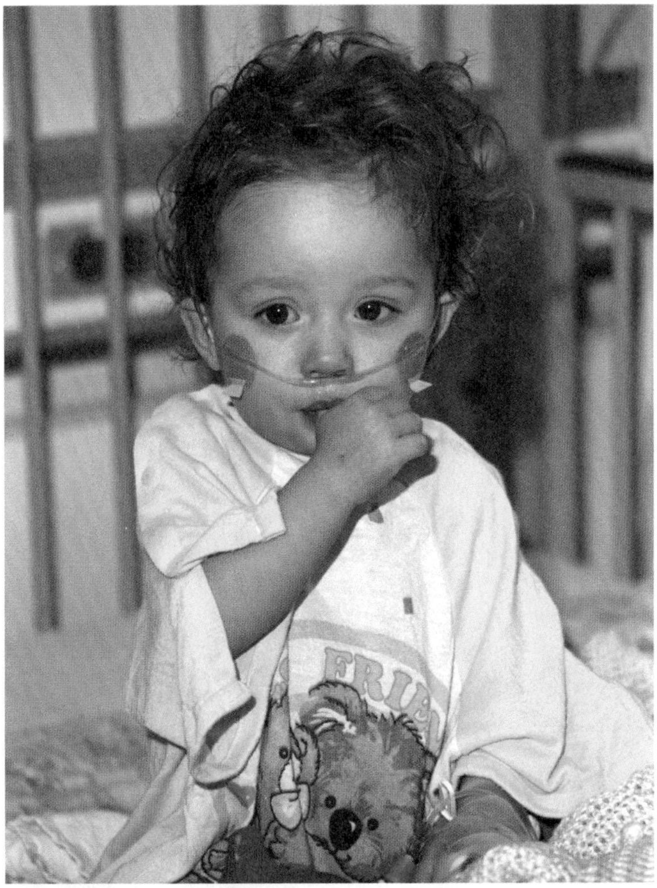

Figure 16-19 It is important to monitor toddlers constantly to prevent severe responses to hospital stay.

Critical Thinking

A Toddler Who Is Immobilized

Andrew, a healthy, active child of 20 months, has been admitted to the hospital and is placed in traction for treatment of a fractured femur. A hip spica cast will be applied within a few days, and a clinical pathway has been determined regarding care in traction, care after the cast is applied, and discharge instructions. He is the youngest of four children and is rarely cared for by adults other than parents. His mother plans to stay with him throughout the hospital stay except for brief periods of a few hours each day.

What kind of assessment data at the time of admission would assist the nurse in understanding the effects of this child's experience on the child and family? What strengths of a child of this age would facilitate coping? What strengths of the family would facilitate coping?

What are ways of helping this child to manage immobility, diminished control, and brief separations?

To maintain areas of comfort, the child's bed and the playroom should not be used for painful procedures. A treatment room, with supportive persons (caregiver and nurse) present to provide comforting during and after the procedure, is a better place. Each day, time should be allocated to provide comfort measures for each child, like rocking or reading to, to balance the stressors of being hospitalized (Figure 16-20). Those measures that are comforting to individual children are most effective in alleviating stress. See Box 16-6 for more information on caring for toddlers.

NURSING CARE AND GUIDANCE OF PRESCHOOL CHILDREN

Preschool children are hospitalized for a variety of reasons, including injuries, infectious or inflammatory processes, surgical procedures, and long-term illnesses. Although they are naturally curious, have facility with language and other skills, and enjoy the beginning independence that comes during

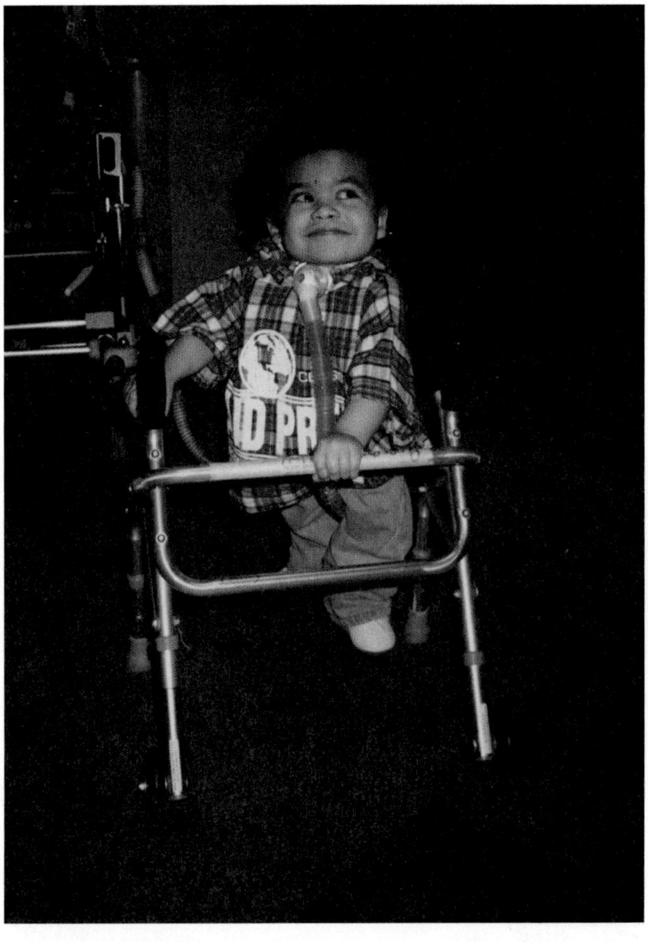

Figure 16-20 Encouragement of mobility is important for toddlers. Published with permission of Baystate Medical Center Children's Hospital.

BOX 16-6 Points of emphasis in caring for toddlers

Safety:

- Assess crib safety and minimize the possibility of climbing out and possible injury (hospital cribs, e.g., Springfield model, have been designed to prevent injuries from climbing out of the crib).
- Never leave child unattended.
- Be aware of any hazardous objects or situations, e.g., sharp objects, materials, toxic substances, and electrical outlets.
- Avoid hard candies, balloons, plastic bags, or foods that may cause accidents.

Other:

- Observe verbal and nonverbal behavior for signs of grief or discontent.
- Explain the response of protest when caregivers must leave for short periods, and encourage them to leave an article of clothing such as a scarf, cap, or small purse so the child will have an object belonging to the person as a symbol of returning. Also explain that it is not wise to leave when child is sleeping, but at a time when their nurse is present. Then, even though it may be hard, encourage the child to wave and say good-bye.
- Play games of peek-a-boo or a variation of hide and seek with dolls to reinforce going away and coming back.
- Provide home routines and as much independence as possible in eating and mobility.
- Ascertain the way the toddler likes to be comforted when in distress.
- Provide for as much mobility/activity as possible.
- Take care of special toys or transitional objects.
- Keep a picture of the toddler and members of family close by and talk about family.
- Observe behavior closely for regression and aggression.
- Maintain locomotion even when walking is limited, e.g., stroller, cart, or moving the bed to the playroom.
- Provide simple directions and appropriate choices.

these years, preschoolers are also acutely aware of their need for the presence and support of the adults in their lives.

Special Needs of Preschool Children

Preschoolers learn best through observation and manipulation of objects (Figure 16-21). Abstractions or things not seen are difficult to understand. Many have not yet learned correct anatomical terms and most have had limited experience in learning about the body. They may think the skin holds them together and any disruption in integrity threatens their sense of being. They often think that, with intrusive procedures, their "insides may come out" or "they will lose all their blood and die." They are often distressed when urine or stool samples are obtained because this is a private matter, and vomiting or diarrhea is perplexing and disturbing because of their perceived loss of control.

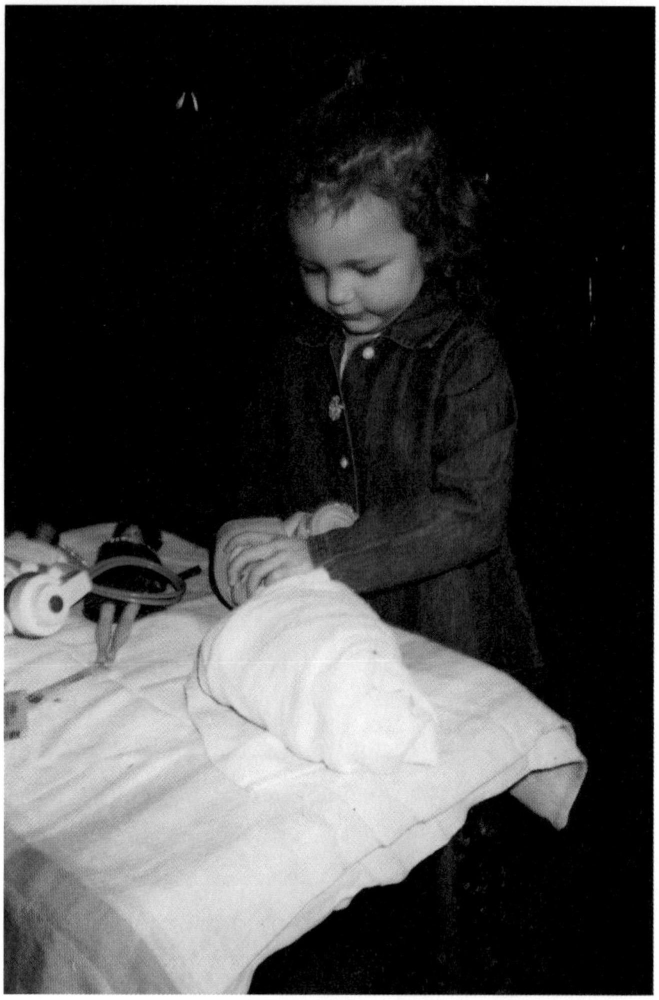

Figure 16-21 Intensity of Play of a 3-Year-Old

Seeing blood or "taking blood" is frightening because of its symbolic nature because to many children "red is the color of hurting" (Shore, 1965). Children need explanations about their body organs and functions, and bandaids to cover any wounds, either by accident or by others, both physical and psychological.

Children of this age also need caregivers present to protect them from their fears and fantasies, and to explain events in terms they understand. They also need to know the sequence of what is to be done in tests or procedures and carefully prepared using play equipment followed by therapeutic play after stressful events. Even though they explore their environment through intrusion, their greatest fears are related to intrusion into their bodies.

Direct Care of Preschool Children

To foster a sense of initiative, preschool children need to be as involved as possible in all aspects of their care and have opportunities for choices. They often experience illness and hospitalization as a consequence for misdeeds and it is essential they understand painful procedures are not punishment. Additionally, they may fear if they are not good or if they cry, further harm will ensue. It is helpful to tell preschoolers it is all right to cry, and to say "I'm sorry" when pain is incurred. Young children also benefit from learning active methods of coping such as guided imagery (Ott, 1996). Providing opportunities for playing out stressful events helps avoid feelings of being victimized.

Teaching is also a primary intervention in the care of preschoolers. This is most likely to be successful when children have adequate time to learn, but not too much time to worry. Continued teaching throughout procedures with opportunities for involvement when possible (e.g., hand the tape for a dressing) and an explanation after the procedure to clarify any misconceptions is important. Follow-up opportunities for play completes a cycle for learning.

Preschoolers are usually sociable, and group play and activities are often successful. Sometimes when children are having difficulty taking fluids, a tea party, or playing restaurant when "drinks" are ordered is more helpful than frequent encouragement to take fluids. It is advisable for children to have meals at a table or in an area with other children whenever possible. Children need praise for cooperation, regardless of their coping ability. Building on strengths is a key concept in fostering the ability to cope. See Box 16-7 for more information on caring for preschoolers.

Kids Want To Know

Frequent questions:

- How long do I have to be here?
- What are you going to do to me?
- How long will it take?
- How much will it hurt?
- When will it be over?

Answer: The test will take until lunch time. They will take a picture of your leg by using a machine called an X ray machine. It won't hurt to take the picture. It will be over when the picture has been checked by the lady taking the picture.

NURSING CARE AND GUIDANCE OF SCHOOL-AGED CHILDREN

The school years are perhaps the healthiest of all ages; however, children are hospitalized during this time for many reasons, e.g., accidents, infections, autoimmune, and oncological conditions. Their developing confidence and self-esteem brought about by success in meeting challenges, competence in learning, and skill in relating to adults and peers are often strengths. During hospitalization, every effort needs to be put forth to help those whose primary focus is school-related to continue to learn and maintain their individual strengths.

BOX 16-7 Points of emphasis in caring for preschool children

Safety:

- Anticipate stressful situations, and observe for behavior indicating signs of distress.
- Encourage adults to accompany preschool children.
- Keep environment free of harmful objects/equipment.
- Wear shoes instead of slippers when ambulating.

Other:

- Understand fears of unfamiliar environment, abandonment, and punishment, and fears related to body integrity and deprivation.
- Have the picture of an animal or object outside and inside the door of each hospital room, so that the child can easily identify their place.
- Encourage involvement in learning to maintain a sense of initiative.
- Provide play activities and reactive materials. They are essential to learning how to cope with stressful situations.
- Tell child who is caring for them and who to call for help.
- Being familiar with common television shows and movies for children facilitates conversation.
- Explore child's perceptions and understanding of their illness and treatments.
- Emphasize treatments are not punishment by explaining reason why these are necessary.

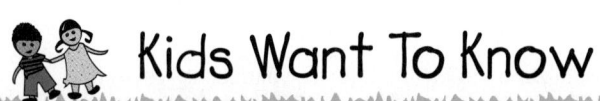

Special Needs of School-Aged Children

The anxiety of illness, diagnostic tests, and therapeutic interventions is expressed in many ways and there are many factors involved in the success of school-aged children in managing the stressors of hospitalization. Some children do not express distress openly, and an outwardly calm child may not be coping successfully. In fact, hospitalized children who were admitted for acute illnesses were more likely to perceive their coping as effective than those with chronic illnesses, and children with low anxiety as a trait were more likely to describe their coping behaviors as effective than those with high trait anxiety (Bossert, 1994).

There is an additional stressor when illness or surgery produces changes in appearance or threatens success in developing or maintaining friendships. For some, there is fear that other children "will make fun of me," "tease," or "not like me anymore." Especially when children have overt changes in appearance due to medications such as corticosteroid therapy, loss of hair or limbs, or scarring. In some situations, it is advisable to seek consultation with psychologists and/or clinical nurse specialists in psychiatric-mental health for ongoing counseling.

Direct Care of School-Aged Children

For some school-aged children, the ability to master the stress of hospitalization may be a source of accomplishment that increases their confidence in coping and mastering other difficult situations. Continuous, deliberative support, positive relationships, and coaching during stressful times are some measures leading to success in mastery and learning coping skills.

A brief description of some methods used effectively are in Table 16-1. Other alternative methods are aromatherapy, biofeedback, self-hypnosis, dance therapy, prayer, medita-

TABLE 16-1 Alternative Ways of Helping Children Cope during Hospitalization

Therapy	Definition
Art therapy	A variety of art forms to encourage children to express thoughts and feelings, e.g., drawings of self and hospital experiences. Use of clay, finger-painting, etc. Also used as adjunctive mental health treatment (*Mosby's Medical Nursing and Allied Health Dictionary*, 5th ed., 1998).
Creative art and crafts	Paper, crayons, paint, pencils, and other materials, etc. for release of creative potential. Through conscious interaction promotes expression of imagination, development of self-esteem, and contributes to sense of accomplishment (Ward, 1998).
Focused breathing	Rhythmic breathing to manage or reduce stress by attending to the process of inhaling and exhaling.
Guided imagery	Guiding imagination and visualization to facilitate (creative imagery) relaxed, focused concentration on images and scenes of pleasurable activity during tests and treatments as a way of empowering children and promoting coping abilities (Ott, 1996; Ward, 1998).
Massage	Effleurage (stroking), petressage (kneading), rubbing, or tapping soft tissues of the body to increase circulation, improve muscle tone, and promote relaxation (Field, 1995; Ward, 1998).
Music therapy	Use of music as background or active child involvement (e.g., singing, sing-along) during play or during invasive procedures as a calming or distracting influence (Berlin, 1998; Kouretas,1999).
Progressive muscle relaxation	Alternately tensing and relaxing muscle groups sequentially.
Written expression	Poetry, journals, diaries, composing songs/lyrics, letters to friends (or imaginary friends or pets) to reflect and express thoughts, feelings, and/or responses to illness experiences.

tion, therapeutic touch, humor, and pet therapy (Figure 16-22). To extend the repertoire of alternative methods, nurses need to study each adjunctive technique thoroughly and feel confident in using these to help children and parents learn new ways of coping. Assessment of the appropriateness of using any particular method and evaluating the effectiveness of the method are essential components of these interventions.

When children are hospitalized, the important events in their lives and ongoing problems should be understood, particularly at times of prolonged hospitalization. If children are isolated because of communicable disease or for low immunity, every effort should be made to help them manage this confinement by minimizing the potential for sensory deprivation and the experience of being separated from others. They also need to clearly understand the reason and length of time (Figures 16-23 and 16-24).

School-aged children who have developed reading skills benefit from books as well as Internet sources to understand their experiences. Most children's units have literature and instructions available to access these resources. Because their writing skills have been developed, there are several creative ways to express thoughts and feelings (described in Table 16-1). If hospitalized for an extended period, contact with schoolmates, teachers, and resuming schoolwork is recommended as soon as possible. To preserve their sense of industry, children should be complimented for learning during hospitalization. See Box 16-8 for more information on the care of school-aged children.

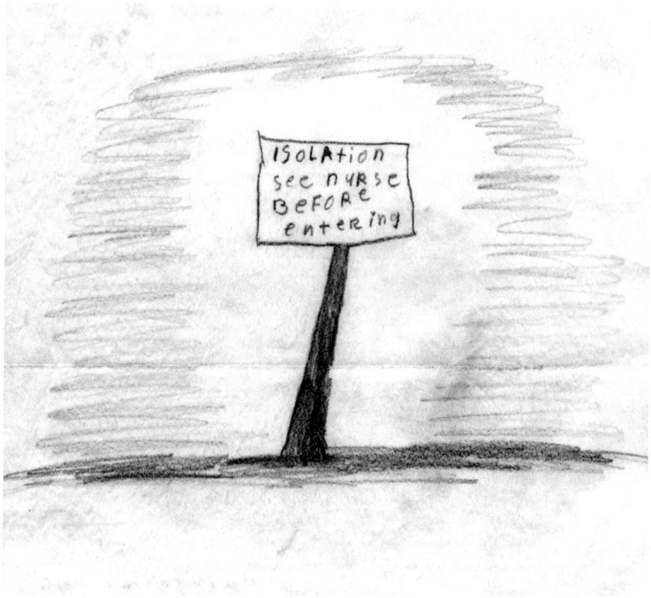
ISOLAtion
see nuRse
BeFORe
enteRing

Figure 16-23 Drawing of a 12-Year-Old Girl in a Single Room

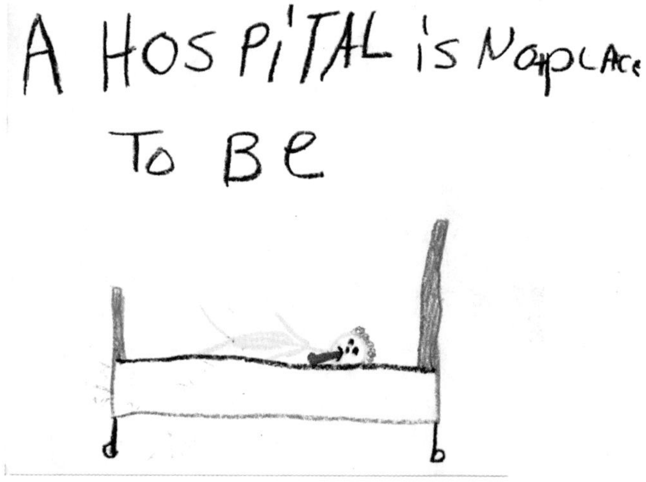
A HOSPiTAL is NoPLACe
TO Be

Figure 16-24 Art of an 11-Year-Old Expressing Sentiments about Being Hospitalized

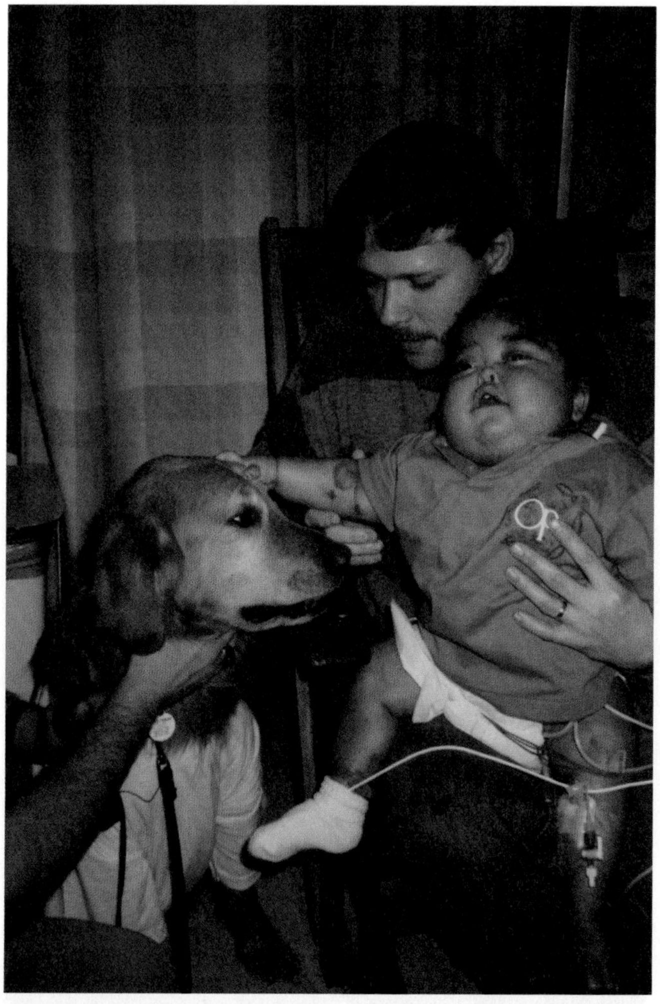

Figure 16-22 Pet therapy helps children cope while hospitalized. Published with permission of Baystate Medical Center Children's Hospital.

BOX 16-8 Points of emphasis in caring for school-aged children

Safety:

- Be cognizant of responses to stress and methods of coping.
- Explain rules to prevent injury; e.g., hospital is not a place for running.

Other:

- Reduce fear of the unknown through explanations and teaching.
- Use a variety of teaching-learning methods in preparing children–visual aids and stories are helpful.
- Help children to understand the nature of their illness and or surgery.
- Encourage creative expression of responses to their experiences, including drawing pictures of themselves in the hospital and writing in journals.
- Use humor and jokes to help in coping and reducing anxiety.
- Be explicit in helping children see what they are learning in the hospital.
- Encourage contact with friends, and introduce other children on the unit who are of similar ages.
- Encourage schoolwork as soon as possible.

Critical Thinking

A School-aged Child Being Discharged

At the time of discharge, Wally, a 12-year-old boy with advanced cystic fibrosis, hospitalized for 7 days for treatment of bilateral lung infection, said, "I wish I didn't have to go back to school" and then hesitatingly said, "it's so embarrassing." As his nurse, you responded with encouragement: "all your friends will be glad to see you . . . so will your teachers, and besides there are only a few months left." His father soon arrived to drive him home, and said, "you look great, let's go." Later, you recalled these interactions and reflected about the response of the nurse in this situation. What assumptions were made that prompted the nurse's response to his comment about school, that is, what might have been the thoughts of the nurse or the feelings of the nurse about his comment? In recapturing and analyzing this situation, construct alternative responses by the nurse and the rationale for any changes.

NURSING CARE AND GUIDANCE OF ADOLESCENTS

The concerns and anxieties of adolescents are often masked by the appearance of sophistication, maturity, and what may be described as bravado. Their confidence and insecurities are often juxtaposed in such a way that hospitalization experiences are often perplexing and difficult. Their need for communication, understanding, and being understood by adults and peers are important in meeting the challenges of their experiences and decisions related to illness and hospitalization.

Special Needs of Adolescents

Adolescents who become ill are often in the midst of conflicts and struggles to establish a sense of identity as social and sexual beings (Figure 16-25). Many adolescents who are admitted to hospitals have sustained severe body injury or are experiencing an acute phase of a long-term illness. Regardless of the kind of health problem, adolescents fear disfigurement, changes in body image, and loss of control of their bodies. Having gained some measure of mental, physical, and social competence, they may be threatened by the stress of illness, treatments, and surgery. At a time when they have become more independent, there may be needs for dependence that lead to feelings of frustration, anger, and ambivalence about the situation and about those who provide assistance.

Adolescents who are hospitalized adapt best when they are with other adolescents in a separate unit where they have privacy and the opportunity to participate in the governance of their space. The environment should reflect their needs for such accouterments as mirrors, refrigerators, telephones, computers, areas of privacy, and a place for valuable possessions, including their own clothes.

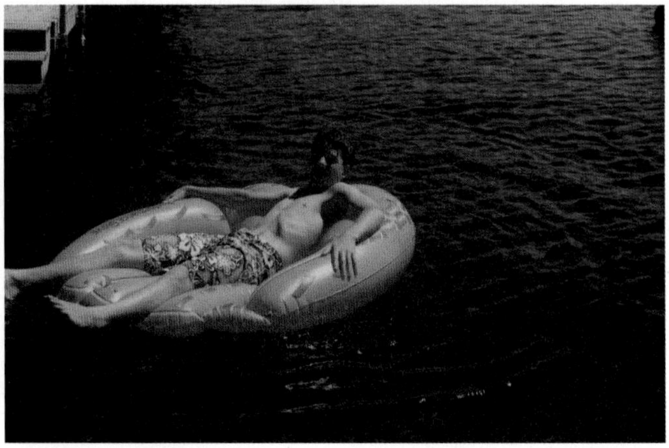

Figure 16-25 Early adolescence is a time to develop a sense of identity.

Direct Care of Adolescents

Nurses with special preparation and interest in caring for adolescents are most successful in helping them cope with the exigencies of illness at a time when self-esteem and self-control are major aspects of development. Even though there may be ambivalent feelings toward adults, it is helpful when caregivers understand adolescents' need for coaches and opportunities to talk through situations of concern, e.g., impending surgery, diagnostic tests. Viewing the nurse and other health care professionals as high-status friends rather than persons in authoritarian roles facilitates their ability to engage in open, trusting relationships.

Nothing is more important than talking to adolescents and listening carefully to what they say and how they say it. Their need for uninterrupted time is very important to the process of developing coping skills. Adolescents are quick to identify those who have a genuine interest in them, and are equally sensitive when interest is feigned or when a person doesn't have time. Adolescents respond positively to those who have a sense of humor and are spontaneous and honest in their responses to questions and concerns. Attention to symptoms or explanations about treatments is not enough for adolescents to feel understood and cared for.

Establishing a helping relationship with adolescents may be difficult because they are seeking independence. However, it is within this kind of relationship that adolescents feel free to express their thoughts and feelings about situations they confront, and are more inclined to discuss personal issues not discussed with parents. They are also better able to cope with the problems they face during illness and hospitalization (Figure 16-26). When the nurse senses there are difficult questions, statements like, "other teens with this problem wondered about/asked about . . . and this is how I usually answer these questions" may help.

Adolescents may also develop crushes on nurses as a part of the process of developing a sense of identity and testing one's self in the formation of sexual identity. This often occurs with young nursing staff and students, who need to understand that this kind of response is related to developmental issues. Sometimes adolescents are openly curious about the personal lives of others as they seek to clarify their own lives and activities. In these situations, it is helpful to be direct and honest in setting boundaries, while understanding the need for working out relationships with others. See Box 16-9 for more information on caring for adolescents.

EXPECTATIONS AND NEEDS OF CAREGIVERS DURING HOSPITALIZATION OF CHILDREN

From the time of admission, caregivers expect collegial relationships with health care professionals. What they need and what they need to know may be different than the health care professionals' assumptions. When difficulties arise, usually due to discrepant expectations, they may cause significant difficulties for caregivers relative to therapeutic goals, expectations about hospitalization and the child's relations, and perspectives about family involvement. There may also be misunderstandings about expectations regarding the amount of time spent with their child and the degree of participation in care.

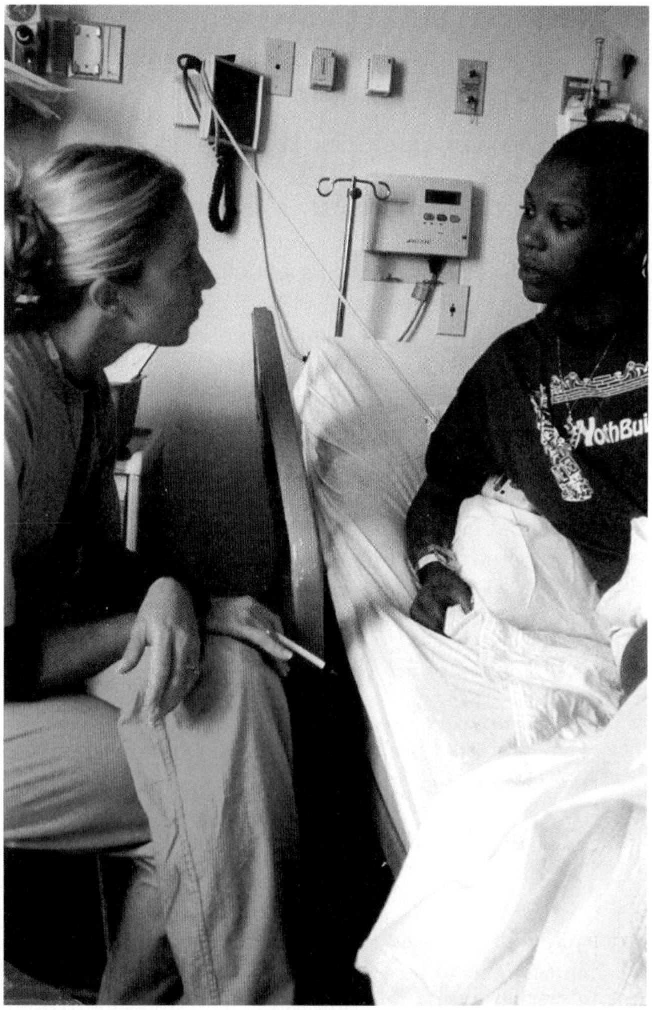

Figure 16-26 Development of helping relationships with adolescents facilitates coping.

The needs of caregivers during the crisis of hospitalization include the need to have accurate and timely information; to trust the competence of physicians and nurses; and to know their child is comfortable and free from pain. They also need health professionals to trust them (Graves & Hayes, 1996; Kristsjinsdottir, 1995). Scott (1998) proposed that, although the priorities of caregivers' needs may vary, common needs are for information, assurance, and proximity to children when critically ill. Through developing a helping relationship with caregivers, these needs and concerns can be prioritized and incorporated into the plan of care. Caregivers also need to feel cared for in the social sense in

BOX 16-9 Points of emphasis in caring for adolescents

- Plan uninterrupted time to teach and discuss responses.
- Encourage communication and involvement in decision-making.
- Do not assume coping is effective if adolescent appears indifferent or full of bravado.
- Encourage reflective journals and creative means of expression, e.g., drawing, poetry.
- Use correct language and explain unfamiliar terms; a discussion rather than lecture format is usually more effective.
- Review recommended reading materials in advance; emphasize areas of greatest relevance–encourage writing questions and reflections each day as a basis for discussion.
- Refer to others who have had similar problems, and say, "other teens in a situation like yours asked about . . . is this something that you wondered about?"
- Use the Internet to converse with others about similar conditions.

order to feel more positive about their experiences and better able to cope. Future studies related to caregiver needs should focus on different ethnic and cultural groups as well as the needs of the family.

The complexity of relationships between children, caregivers, and nurses requires extensive understanding. In addition, there is potential for difficulties in communication and the development of adversarial relationships. Sometimes, nurses may not realize they subtly compete for the child's positive responses and must be cautious that their need for approval and self-satisfaction does not supercede their responsibilities.

In situations where children are hospitalized for extended periods of time, support groups for caregivers are an effective way of creating an environment to express concerns and strengthening coping abilities. Support groups in the community are also available for caregivers of children with special needs and for those whose children have succumbed to illness or injury. Each hospital has information about these resources.

CHILDREN WITH CHRONIC ILLNESS

Children with long-term health problems are well acquainted with health care settings, and each new experience is framed within the context of previous experiences. Caregivers of these children are often experts about disease processes and treatments on a day-to-day basis and the children themselves become increasingly competent in self-care as they get older. Nurses also become highly skilled as coordinators of family-centered care and assume roles of coordinator, leader, teacher, team member, and primary care provider. Care conferences to promote caregiver–professional collaboration are an excellent medium for planning when children have been hospitalized for long periods of time (McClain & Bury, 1998).

The field of pediatric rehabilitation nursing has evolved over the past 25 years to become a specialty committed to the care of families and children with disabilities and other chronic conditions (Edwards, Hertzberg, Hays, & Youngblood, 1999). Pediatric rehabilitation facilities as well as clinics and community agencies are sites for offering extensive services by interdisciplinary teams of health care providers to meet the needs associated with these children's complex, long-term health problems, including developmental, educational, economic, mobility, psychosocial, and vocational services. As children grow and develop over time, individual and family needs change, requiring many adaptations and transitions to different health care facilities or health care personnel.

EMERGENCY CARE

Many children and adolescents with acute and life-threatening illness and injuries are first diagnosed and treated in an emergency room. The caregiver and child's stress and anxiety is often overwhelming because of the uncertainties, acuity, and decisions integral to these situations. Painful, invasive, and perplexing tests and treatments are performed quickly, with minimal opportunities for optimal preparation and support. However, most caregivers want to be present when invasive procedures are performed and nearly all want to participate in the decision about their presence (Boie, Moore, Brummett, & Nelson, 1999)

PEDIATRIC INTENSIVE CARE UNITS

The pediatric intensive care unit (PICU) is a special environment because of the crisis orientation of care. There is also a potential for sensory overload and sensory deprivation.

HOME CARE

With technological innovations and changes in health care system financing and administration, children today are usu-

Research Highlight

School-aged Children Coping with Repeated Hospitalization

Study Purpose

It is often difficult for nurses and other members of the health professions to fully understand the way that children with chronic illness experience the stressors of repeated hospitalizations. The perceptions of these children are important to explore in order to gain insight and skill in reducing and managing the stressor of repeated hospitalization. The purpose of this study was to describe the stressors of these children, their coping mechanisms, and how they believed others can help them cope.

Methods

Using a qualitative design and grounded-theory methodology, the researchers studied six hospitalized school-aged children with chronic illness who experienced repeated hospitalizations. In-depth interviews were conducted, and artwork and journals were reviewed in the process of obtaining thorough, accurate, and relevant perspectives for analysis and interpretation.

Findings

The researchers concluded that the major stressors were invasive procedures, fear of death, loss of control, and isolation. Their coping strategies were described as behavioral distraction, social support, avoidance, submission, and emotional expression. Family and friends were identified as most important in helping them cope physically and emotionally, vividly described as "the mere presence of family and friends as vital." Health care professionals were identified as facilitating coping if they explained procedures, afforded privacy, were patient and gentle, and had a sense of humor. Further, these school-aged children affirmed that health care professionals who did not exhibit these qualities hindered coping.

Implications

- Children who are hospitalized should be encouraged to identify their own stressors and coping mechanisms.
- Family and friends are very important in assisting children to cope.
- Pediatric nurses should stress in word and deed the importance of family presence and incorporate the family into each aspect of care.
- Nurse behavior can assist or hinder a child's coping.
- Regardless of professional stressors, nurses must explain procedures, offer privacy, and be patient and gentle with hospitalized children.

Citation

Boyd, J. R., & Hunsberger, M. (1998). Chronically ill children coping with repeated hospitalizations: their perceptions and suggested interventions. *Journal of Pediatric Nursing, 13*, 330–341.

ally hospitalized for very short periods of time and return to their home with complex, multi-system health problems. Examples of children previously cared for in hospitals or long-term care facilities, who are now cared for at home include those who are respirator-dependent; require parenteral nutrition; or have severe physical and cognitive impairment. Extensive coordination is required to provide respite care, day care, and schooling. There are many community resources available to create environments most conducive to the health and welfare of these children and their families.

DISCHARGE AND THE AFTER EFFECTS OF HOSPITALIZATION

Throughout hospitalization, children and caregivers need to be prepared for discharge, post-hospital and/or post-surgical care, and the effects of this experience. This often involves extensive teaching and preparation for the transition especially when there has been prolonged hospitalization, painful treatments and procedures, or changes in body image. For these children, adolescents, and families, it is important to prepare them, teachers, and other significant persons to reenter home, school, and community.

The kind of preparation is dependent on the continued needs of the child and caregivers for care and support in coping with fears and anxieties. In those situations where there is a change in appearance or mobility, the transition from hospital to home may be difficult. Some may benefit from spending brief periods with family and friends outside the hospital during the rehabilitation process to adapt gradually, e.g., those who have had an amputation or neurological changes. Peers may also need to be prepared by using discussions and films.

Changes in behavior post hospitalization are most evident in children between 6 months and 6 years of age. These include changes in eating, sleeping, and elimination, and in psychosocial behavior such as regression or becoming more aggressive, withdrawn, or fearful. The intensity and duration of these responses are dependent on many factors including the impact of the illness and hospitalization, frequency of intrusive procedures, level of cognitive development and maturity, previous experiences, and perceptions about being comforted in the process of coping with stressful events. When caregivers of children younger than 5 who spent a day in ICU were interviewed about their child's behavior, they reported changes related to regressive behaviors and withdrawal, aggression and demanding behavior and fears and anxieties about sleeping and separation (Youngblut & Shiao, 1993).

Most changes in behavior may occur after 2–3 days of hospitalization because children encounter multiple tests, treatments, and separations from those who provide support. This is also a time when caregivers are anxious and may be less able to give psychological support (Thompson & Vernon, 1993). In fact, moderate lengths of stay that involve more than minimal separation from home, yet insufficient time for accommodation may place children at greater risk for post hospital distress than longer or shorter stays.

There are many considerations in teaching caregivers about the potential changes in behavior after hospitalization. In addition to responding to illness and hospitalization, children may react to previous home sleeping arrangements, particularly when the caregiver has slept closely adjacent to the child while in the hospital. Therefore, for some children, it may be helpful for the caregiver to sleep in a separate room from the child for a few nights prior to discharge.

As the time for discharge approaches, caregivers may feel relief about resuming their family life, yet also feel apprehensive about caring for the child at home. In addition to preparing the family for physical aspects of care, it is also important to know of the potential for the child's behavioral changes in response to the hospital experience. Therefore, it is advantageous to first ask caregivers how they think their child will respond to this experience of illness/hospitalization at home. Their responses are helpful as a basis for an indi-

Family Teaching

Preparing Caregivers for Potential Behavior Changes of Infants and Young Children Post Hospitalization

- Infants and young children may continue to react to hospitalization for a few weeks after discharge and gradually resume their developmental patterns and routines.
- Young children whose caregivers have roomed-in may have difficulty in adapting to sleeping in a room alone or with siblings.
- Changes in behavior may include clinging behaviors and crying even if going to another room, whining, tearfulness at bedtime and wakefulness during the night, intensified protest when leaving child in care of another person, resistance to changing clothes or diapers, outbursts of anger, frustration or aggression in the form of temper tantrums or aggressive play, regression to earlier behaviors (thumb-sucking, changes in use of language), or withdrawal.
- Understanding guidance and consistency in response while giving complimentary responses for positive behaviors is helpful during the transition from hospital to home.
- Siblings need to understand behavioral changes (their own and their sibling's) and be helped and helpful in reestablishing family routines and relationships.
- Telling a story about a child who was in the hospital who learned a lot about hospitals, nurses, and doctors may also be helpful. Tips on helping alleviate fear and how children learn to help themselves when they need to do things that are necessary, but feel afraid are also beneficial.

In the Real World

In pediatric nursing, one of the greatest challenges is to reach out beyond the physical and emotional strengths that exist and build on all the cultural assets a child, his family, and his social group may possess. There is so much to be learned from respectful observation and conversation.

Nursing Alert:

Identification of Children at Risk Following Hospitalization or Surgery

Nurses studying the outcomes of children following hospitalization and surgery are able to identify several situations where children are at greatest risk for less than positive outcomes. They include (Eldridge, 1997):

- *Young children between the ages of 6 months and 6 years or children with developmental delays*
- *Moderate hospital stay of 4–8 days or prolonged hospital stay (longer than 8 days)*
- *More serious illnesses or trauma, especially those resulting in pain or painful procedures*
- *Hospitalizations that necessitate isolation of the child from the family*
- *Caregivers who exhibit high anxiety and/or limited skills in coping*
- *Insufficient preparation of the child and caregivers for hospitalization/surgery*
- *Children who have had multiple hospital or surgical experiences or who have had previous, unresolved negative experiences*

vidualized teaching plan using the considerations in the Family Teaching box.

Implementing a parent-focused program (COPE—Creating Opportunities for Parent Empowerment) has also been used to improve young children's outcomes during and after hospitalization by effectively reducing anxiety and enhancing involvement in their child's care (Melnyk & Alpert-Gillis, 1998). In fact, in posthospital experiences, children of mothers who received child behavioral information through the COPE program (potential changes in behavior and ways to manage in the hospital and at home) had fewer negative behavioral changes than mothers who did not receive the information (Melnyk, 1994). This suggests it is helpful for caregivers to know children may act differently after discharge particularly in sleeping, eating, and separations.

When children become ill, injured, or hospitalized, both they and their caregivers feel vulnerable as they seek to maintain some level of control and mastery in delicate and difficult situations. Because children have not yet reached maturity, they have greater difficulty in coping with the uncertainties, fears, and emotions that surround them. Simultaneously, caregivers struggle to regain their confidence and trust in themselves and others as they too experience the anxieties of the unknown. Nurses are the health professionals who engage most consistently in helping relationships during these times of stress and are well prepared to minimize the potentially adverse effects of unmet needs and iatrogenic stressors. Their role in maintaining the psychological well-being of children and their caregivers, and helping them grow during the crisis of illness is critical. In using themselves as instruments of healing, nurses accurately and wisely use their expertise to protect the mental health of children and caregivers from stress encountered during illness and hospitalization. Developing this level of expertise is a continuous process of learning and applying knowledge and research to evidence-based practice that demonstrates a commitment to excellence.

Critical Thinking

A 4-Year-Old's Hospital Visit

Johnny is a 4-year-old boy who has been ill since birth with respiratory and feeding difficulties; including coughing during or after oral feedings, wheezing, and pneumonias. He had been seen and evaluated by many physicians and treated with antibiotics, positional feeding, and postural drainage, and was hospitalized many times. Based on his symptoms, several conditions like cystic fibrosis, asthma, and allergies were considered and ruled out. Nutrition has been maintained through oral, thickened feedings, nasogastric feeding tubes, and intermittent parenteral feeding. Several weeks ago, he was examined by a resident, who immediately, after hearing the history and sequence of his health problem and observing his delayed physical growth (3rd percentile for height and weight), said, "I think I know his problem . . . I think he has a small tracheoesophageal fistula." With further radiological examination, the diagnosis was confirmed and surgery

continues

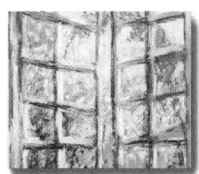

continued

was planned. The nurse explained the procedure briefly, and after the arrangements were made for surgery in 2 weeks, she gave his caregivers a booklet about the hospital and a map. His father was a nurse, so it was assumed that he would prepare him for hospitalization and surgery.

Johnny was quite advanced in speech and cognitive ability and was the star mascot for his sister's softball team. As he reluctantly packed his bag for getting "his tracks fixed," he said he really didn't want to go, but wanted to "eat regular" and "be like the other kids." He brought his ragged, skinless "Velvie" (named for his favorite story of the Velveteen Rabbit), his old pajamas and underpants to wear for the surgery, and his softball hat. He was admitted on the morning of surgery, identification bands were placed on him and "Velvie," and he was prepared verbally for what would happen before the surgery. Mom waved good-bye, and Dad accompanied him to the preinduction room.

Following successful surgery, he returned to the postanesthesia unit, where his parents were waiting. When he was extubated and awoke, tears spilled down his face as he softly said, "they hurt me . . . you said they wouldn't" . . . then dozed off. When he awakened more fully, he found his rabbit and then noticed his pajamas and underpants were gone. "Where are they" he said, then lifted the sheet, looked, and said, "how come they took off 'em off?" The nurse said she would find them, and he was then returned to a room on the pediatric unit in a crib. When he entered, he saw that the other child in the room was a "baby" (15-month-old) who was to have surgery the following day.

Johnny's parents gradually gained confidence in caring for him and became more comfortable in their relationship with others. After 5 days, nutritional IVs were discontinued when it was ascertained that he was able to take and retain fluids and pureed foods. During the first few days postoperatively, he was wheeled to the playroom in a go-cart and play materials were offered. His play sessions were initially restrained as he carefully arranged the doll figures, beds, and stretchers in a long line. He then played with a few matchbox cars and put them in line; then a baby doll went into the parade. When he saw that the baby was anatomically correct, he took the stethoscope and examined the genital area and said, "OK." The next day, he played primarily with clay and finger-paints and went back to the doll figures; he poked the throat and chest of the doctor doll very hard and said, "that hurts, doesn't it . . . well doesn't it?, then took the mommy doll and said "don't talk . . . it's not true . . . you better grow up."

Johnny's mother and father alternated staying at the hospital with him; his brother (age 6) and sister (age 9) visited after school almost every day. He was discharged after 8 days in the hospital. When his mother was contacted several days later, she said he was eating but just "picking at his food" and didn't want to go back to preschool. She thought he was more aggressive than usual, shouted at his brother for just looking at him, and said emphatically, "Don't look at me." But, she added, "It's OK" . . . he's better and that's all that's important. Now I hope he will grow."

1. In considering Johnny's past history, what do you surmise were his parent's initial reaction to the diagnosis of tracheoesophageal fistula? What of the child's response to going to the hospital to have surgery?
2. Reflecting on the role of the nurse in the initial preparation for hospitalization, what was done that may have been effective? What could have been done at this time?
3. As a 4-year-old with previous hospital experiences, what would be the most effective way of preparing Johnny and his parents for a hospital admission within 2 weeks?
4. As he prepared himself by packing his suitcase and expressing he didn't want to go, but would, then bringing his rabbit, old pajamas, and underpants, what do you think about his assuming he would wear these clothes to surgery and that his rabbit would go with him—is this an advisable practice?
5. Johnny seemed upset with his mother when he awakened from anesthesia because he didn't think there would be any "hurting." What could have been said if this had been overheard? What might have been his concern when he saw he didn't have his own clothes on?
6. When Johnny returned to his room he was sleeping, and when he awoke, he saw the baby in the crib next to his. What do you think of this environment for him at this time?
7. Johnny spent considerable time in the playroom, and when he was walking again, engaged in play and the use of hospital equipment. Although there was no indication of an adult to respond to his play and dialogue, his words and actions had meaning. What are some of the feelings that he seemed to convey through play?
8. Sibling involvement is an important dimension of the care of children. In this situation, what may have been the responses to this situation? How could they be best prepared for this experience?
9. Johnny's parents were able to stay in the hospital with him (bedside lounge-chair, rooming-in), but also needed to do occasional errands and transport the older children to activities and the hospital. Considering his age and stage of development, how could Johnny best be prepared for brief separations?
10. In planning for discharge, what would be most helpful for this family in helping Johnny make the transition to home?
11. From the information available, how would the strengths of this family be described? What are Johnny's strengths?
12. Formulate two or three questions that you think are important to ask about the care and guidance of Johnny and his family.

Key Concepts

- Advanced education, leadership, and research in nursing has had a significant impact on the quality of health care delivered to ill and hospitalized children and families.
- The history of caring for children in hospitals, and research related to the effects of hospitalization on children have influenced the development of current philosophies, policies, and practices in pediatric units and children's hospitals.
- Learning the role and responsibilities of the nurse in minimizing stressful experiences of children and caregivers, and maximizing the use of successful coping is a complex process enhanced by applying knowledge from the arts, sciences, and humanities, astute observations of the behavior of children and caregivers, and reflective nursing practice.
- Stressors and responses of infants, children, adolescents, and caregivers to hospitalization are influenced by their perceptions of events, development and cognitive levels, previous experiences, and facility in using coping methods.
- The physical and psychosocial environments of pediatric units have a profound influence on the effectiveness of the care and comfort of children and caregivers.
- A primary goal in the care of children is to help them and their families grow during experiences of adversity and stress, and learn meaningful ways of coping.
- Play is the work of children and integral to their development as recreation, creativity, and as a means of expressing and exploring thoughts and feelings about events and experiences in their lives.
- Collaboration and communication with other health care professionals is essential to the care and well-being of children and caregivers before, during, and after hospital experiences.
- Family-centered care embraces the concerns and care of siblings in order to minimize their stressors in response to the illness experiences of their sister or brother.
- When caregivers' stress is reduced, they are better able to assist their children in coping with the stressors of hospitalization.
- The transition from being a patient/caregiver in a pediatric hospital to home or other facilities requires preparation.

Review Questions

1. Compare and contrast how hospitalization affects infants, children, preschoolers, school-aged children, and adolescents.
2. Discuss the various factors affecting a child's reaction to a hospital experience.
3. Describe how the relationship between nurses and families of hospitalized children can be strengthened.
4. Describe how play can be used in helping hospitalized children cope with their experiences.
5. Discuss appropriate nursing interventions for hospitalized children of various developmental ages.
6. Discuss the behaviors caregivers might see in a child after the child is discharged from the hospital.

References

Ahmann, E. (1997). Family matters: books for siblings of children having illness or disability. *Pediatric Nursing, 23*(5), 500–502.

Algren, C. L., & Algren, J. T. (1997). Pediatric sedation: essentials for the perioperative nurse. *Nursing Clinics of North America, 32*(1), 17–30.

Andrade, T. M. (1998). Sibling visitation: Research implications for pediatric and neonatal patients. *On-line Journal of Knowledge Synthesis*, 5(6).

Blake, F. G. (1954). *The child, his parents and the nurse.* Philadelphia: Lippincott.

Boie, E. T., Moore, G. P., Brummett, C., & Nelson, D. (1999). Do parents want to be present during invasive procedures performed on their children in the emergency department? A survey of 400 parents. *Annals of Emergency Medicine, 34*(1), 70–74.

Bordieri, J. E., Solodky, M. S., & Mikow, K. A. (1985). Physical attractiveness and nurses perceptions of pediatric patients. *Nursing Research, 34*(1), 24–26.

Bossert, E. (1994). Factors influencing the coping of hospitalized school-age children. *Journal of Pediatric Nursing, 9*(5): 299–306.

Bowlby, J. (1965). *Child care and the growth of love.* Baltimore, MD: Penguin Books.

Boyd, J. R., & Hunsberger, M. (1998). Chronically ill children coping with repeated hospitalizations, their perceptions and suggested interventions. *Journal of Pediatric Nursing: Nursing Care of Children and Families, 13*, 330–341.

Brody, D. S. (1980). The patient's role in clinical decision making. *Annals Internal Medicine, 93*, 718–722.

Bruno, L. C. (1999). Stress reduction. In *Gale Encyclopedia of Medicine*. Gale Research Inc., 2738.

Burke, S. O., Kauffmann, E., Harrison, M.B., & Wiskin, N. (1999). Assessment of stressors in families with a child who has a chronic condition. *MCN American Journal of Maternal Child Nursing, 24*(2), 98–106.

Clatworthy S., Simon, K., & Tiedeman M. E. (1999). Child drawing: Hospital—an instrument designed to measure the emotional status of hospitalized school-aged children. *Journal of Pediatric Nursing, 14*(1), 2–9.

Curley, M. A. Q. (1988). Effects of the nursing mutual participation model of care on parental stress in the pediatric intensive care unit. *Heart & Lung, 17*(6), 682–688.

Curley, M. A. Q. (1997). Mutuality—An expression of nursing presence. *Journal of Pediatric Nursing: Nursing Care of Children and Families, 12*(4), 208–213.

Dougherty, G. (1998). When should a child be in the hospital? *Pediatrics, 101*(1), 6.

Edwards, P. A., Hertzberg, D. L., Hays, S. R., & Youngblood, N.M. (1999). *Pediatric rehabilitation nursing*. Philadelphia: Saunders.

Field, T. (1995). Massage therapy for infants and children. *Developmental and Behavioral Pediatrics, 16*(2), 105–111.

Fox, J. A. (1997). *Primary health care of children*. St. Louis: Mosby-Year Book.

Gaynard, L., Goldberger, J., & Laidley, L.N. (1991). The use of stuffed body-outline dolls with hospitalized children and adolescents. *Childrens Health Care, 20*(4), 216–224.

Giganti, A. W. (1998). Families in pediatric critical care: the best option. *Pediatric Nursing, 24*(3), 261–265.

Gillis, A. J. (1989). The effect of play on immobilized children in hospital. *International Journal of Nursing Studies, 26*(3), 261–269.

Graves, C., & Hayes, B. E. (1996). Do nurses and parents of children with chronic conditions agree on parental needs? *Journal of Pediatric Nursing: Nursing Care of Children and Families, ll*(5), 288–299.

Hurlock, E. B. (1978). *Child development* (6th ed.). New York: McGraw-Hill.

Kristjansdottir, G. (1995). Perceived importance of needs expressed by parents of hospitalized two to six year-olds. *Scandinavian Journal of Caring Sciences*, 9(2), 95–103.

Kuntz, N., Adams, J. A., Zahr, L., Kellen, R., Cameron, K., & Wassen, H. (1996). Therapeutic play and bone marrow transportation. *Journal of Pediatric Nursing, 11*(6), 359–367.

Lamontagne, L. L., Hepworth, J. T., Byington, K. C., & Chang, C. Y. (1997). Child and parent emotional responses during hospitalization for orthopaedic surgery. *MCN: American Journal of Maternal Child Nursing, 22*(6), 299–303.

LaRosa-Nash, P., & Murphy, J. M. (1997). An approach to pediatric perioperative care. *Nursing Clinics of North America, 32*(1), 183–199.

Lindrea, D. B., & Stainton, M. B. (2000). A case study of infant massage outcomes. *MCN: The American Journal of Maternal-Child Nursing, 25*(2), 95–99.

McClain, C., & Bury, J. (1998). Family matters: the heart of the matter: Care conferences to promote parent-professional collaboration. *Pediatric Nursing, 24*(2), 151–154.

Melnyk, B. M. (1994). Coping with unplanned childhood hospitalization; effect of informational interventions on mothers and children. *Nursing Research, 43*(1), 50–55.

Melnyk, B. M. (1995). Parental coping with childhood hospitalization: a theoretical framework to guide research and clinical intervention. *Maternal-Child Nursing Journal, 23*(4), 123–131.

Melnyk, B. M., & Alpert-Gillis, L. J. (1998). The COPE Program: A strategy to improve outcomes of critically ill young children and their parents. *Pediatric Nursing, 24*(6), 521–539.

Mosby's medical, nursing and allied health dictionary (5th ed.). St. Louis: C.V. Mosby.

Noble, R., Micheli, A. J., Hensley, M. A., & McKay, N. (1997). Perioperative considerations for the pediatric patient: a developmental approach. *Nursing Clinics of North America, 32*(1), 1–16.

Orlando, I. J. (1961). *The dynamic nurse-patient relationship: Function, process and principles*. Philadelphia: J.P. Putnam's Sons.

Ott, M. J. (1996). Imagine the possibilities! Guided imagery with toddlers and preschoolers. *Pediatric Nursing, 22*, 34-38.

Robertson, J. (1958). *Young children in hospitals*. New York: Basic Books.

Schmidt, C. K. (1990). Pre-operative preparation: effects on immediate pre-operative behavior, post-operative behavior and recovery in children having-day surgery. *Maternal-Child Nursing Journal, 19*(4), 321–330.

Scott, L. D. (1998). Perceived needs of parents of critically ill children. *Journal of the Society of Pediatric Nurses, 3*(1), 4–12.

Shields, L., & Nixon, J. (1998). "I want my mummy": Changes in the care of children in hospital. *Collegian, 5*(2), 16–23.

Shore, M. F. (Ed.). (1965). *Red is the color of hurting*. Rockville, MD: U.S. Department of Health and Human Services, Public Health Service, National Institute of Mental Health.

Spitz, R. A. (1954). Hospitalism: An inquiry into the genesis of psychiatric conditions in early childhood *Psychoanalytic Study of the Child, 1*, 53.

Thompson, R. M., & Vernon, D. T. (1993). Research on childrens' behavior after hospitalization: A review and synthesis. *Journal of Developmental and Behavioral Pediatrics, 14*(3), 28–35.

Wolfer, J., & Visintainer, M. A. (1975). Pediatric patients' and parents' stress responses and adjustment. *Nursing Research, 24*, 244–255.

Youngblut, J. M., & Shiao, S. P. (1993). Child and family reactions during and after pediatric ICU hospitalization: A pilot study. *Heart & Lung: Journal of Critical Care, 22*(1), 46–54.

Zahr, L. K. (1998). Therapeutic play for hospitalized preschoolers in Lebanon. *Pediatric Nursing, 23*(5), 449–454.

Suggested Readings

Ahmann, E. (1994). Family-centered care: shifting orientation. *Pediatric Nursing, 20*(2), 113–117.

Ahmann, E. (1995). Family matters: resources for family-centered care, an annotated bibliography. *Pediatric Nursing, 21*(3), 300–302.

Alfaro-LeFevre, R. (1995). *Critical thinking in nursing: A practical approach*. Philadelphia: Saunders.

Baker, L. D., & Anderson, B. (1995). *Inpatient pediatric nursing: plans of care for specialty practice*. Albany, NY: Delmar Publishers.

Bar Mor, G. (1997). International pediatric nursing. Preparation of children for surgery and invasive procedures: Milestones on the way to success. *Journal of Pediatric Nursing, 12*(4), 252–255.

Baystate Medical Center Children's Hospital. (2001). *Welcome to Baystate Medical Center Children's Hospital: A guide for patients and their parents*. Springfield, MA: Author.

Berlin B. K. (1998). Music therapy with children during invasive procedures: Our emergency department's experience. *Journal of Emergency Nursing, 24*(6): 607–608.

Blake, F. G. (1965). A search for Kathy's problem. *International Journal Nursing Studies, 2*, 125–136.

Bricher, G. (2000). Children in the hospital: Issues of power and vulnerability. *Pediatric Nursing, 20*(3), 277–282.

Chambers, M. A. (1993). Play as therapy for the hospitalized child. *Journal of Clinical Nursing, 2*(6), 349–353.

Child Life Council. (1995). *Child Life Position Statement*. Rockville, MD: Author.

Cleary, J. (1992). *Caring for children in hospital: Parents and nurses in partnership*. London: Scutari Press.

Coyne, I. T. (1996). Parent-participation: A concept analysis. *Journal of Advanced Nursing, 23*(4), 733–740.

Curley, M. A. Q., & Wallace, J. (1992). Effects of the nursing mutual participation model of care on parental stress in the pediatric intensive care unit—A replication. *Journal of Pediatric Nursing, 7*(6), 377–385.

Curry, J. (1993). Pediatric nursing: preserving a national treasure. *American Journal of Nursing, 3*, 83–92.

Dunst, C. J., & Trivette, C. M. (1996). Empowerment, effective helpgiving practices, and family-centered care. *Pediatric Nursing, 24*, 283–290.

Durham, E. S., & Frost-Hartzer, P. (1994). Relaxation therapy for children and families. *MCN American Journal of Maternal Child Nursing, 19*(4), 222–225.

Eldridge, T. M. (1997). Preparation for painful procedures, hospitalization, and surgery. In J. A. Fox (Ed.), *Primary health care of children* (982–991) St. Louis, MO: Mosby-Year Book.

Ellerton, M., Ritchie, J. A., & Caty, S. (1994). Factors influencing young children's coping behaviors during stressful healthcare encounters. *Maternal-Child Nursing Journal, 22*(3), 74–82.

Endacott, R. (1998). Needs of the critically ill child: A review of the literature and report of a modified Delphi study. *Intensive Critical Care Nursing, 14*(2), 66–73.

Erickson, E. H. (1958). *Play interviews for four year old hospitalized children. Monograph, 23(3)*. Lafayette, IN: Society for Research in Child Development.

Erikson, E. H. (1963). *Childhood and society*. New York: Norton.

Fischer, M. D. (1994). Identified needs of parents in a pediatric intensive care unit. *Critical Care Nurse, 6*, 82–90.

Freitas, J. D. (1997). To tell you the truth: Children reflect on hospital care. *Issues in Comprehensive Pediatric Nursing, 20*(4), 195–206.

Gravelle, A. M. (1997). Caring for a child with progressive illness during the complex phase: parents' experience of facing adversity. *Journal of Advanced Nursing, 25*, 738–745.

Hart, D., & Bossert, E. (1994). Self-reported fears of hospitalized school-age children. *Journal of Pediatric Nursing, 9*(2), 83–89.

Hawkins, M. E. (1988). In M. Kaufman (Ed.). *Dictionary of American Nursing Biography*. New York: Greenwood Press.

Huckabay, L. M. D., & Tilem-Kessler, D. (1999). Patterns of parental stress in PICU emergency admission. *DCCN—Dimensions of Critical Care Nursing, 18*(2), 36–42.

Jones, D. (1994). Effect of parental participation on hospitalized child behavior. *Issues in Comprehensive Pediatric Nursing, 17*(2), 81–92.

Kaufman, E., Harrison, M. B., Burke, S. O., & Wong, C. (1998). Family matters: stress point intervention for parents of children hospitalized with chronic conditions. *Pediatric Nursing, 24*(4), 362–366.

Kaufman, M. (Ed.). (1988). *Dictionary of American Nursing Biography*. New York: Greenwood Press.

Koplewicz, H. S., & Goodman, R. F. (1999). *Childhood revealed: Art expressing pain, discovery & hope*. New York: Harry N. Abrams. Inc.

Kouretas, D. (1999). More on music therapy with children during invasive procedures (letter). *Journal of Emergency Nursing, 25*(3), 167.

Kristensson-Hollstrom, I., & Elander, G. (1997). Parents' experience of hospitalization: different strategies for feeling secure. *Pediatric Nursing, 23*(1), 361–367.

Kristjansdottir, G. (1991). A study of the needs of parents of hospitalized 2-to-6-year old children. *Issues in Comprehensive Pediatric Nursing, 14*, 49–64.

Kuntz, K. R. (1998). Pediatric nursing resources in cyberspace. *Journal of the Society of Pediatric Nurses, 3*(9), 155–160.

Lamontagne, L. L. (1993). Bolstering personal control in children and parents through coping interventions. *Pediatric Nursing, 19*, 235–237.

Langley, P. (1999). Guided imagery: a review of effectiveness in the care of children. *Pediatric Nursing, 11*(3), 18–21.

Lynch, M. (1994). Preparing children for day surgery. *Childrens Health Care, 23*(2), 75–85.

Manworren, R. C. B., & Woodring, B. (1988). Children's literature as a source for patient education. *Pediatric Nursing, 24*(6), 548–551.

Melnyk, B. M., Alpert-Gillis, L. J., Hensel, P. B., Cable-Beiling, R. C., & Rubenstein, J. S. (1997). Helping mothers cope with a critically ill child: A pilot test of the COPE intervention. *Research in Nursing & Health, 20*(1), 3–14.

Nash, P., & Murphy, J. M. (1997). An approach to pediatric perioperative care: parent-present induction. *Nursing Clinics of North America, 32*(1), 183–199.

Newton, M. S. (2000). Family-centered care: Current realities in parent-participation. *Pediatric Nursing, 26*(2), 164–168.

Orr, M. J., & Allen, S. S. (1986). Optimal oral experiences for infants on long-term total parenteral nutrition. *Nutrition in Clinical Practice, 9*, 288–295.

Orsuto, J., & Corbo, B. H. (1987). Approaches of health caregivers to young children in a pediatric intensive care unit. *Maternal-Child Nursing Journal, 16*(2), 157–175.

Patterson, E. T., & Lipman, T. H.(1999). Toward evidence-based practice. *MCN: The Journal of Maternal-Child Nursing, 24*(3), 159.

Peterson, A. C. (1985). Pubertal development as a cause of disturbance: Myths, realities, and unanswered questions. *Genetic, Social, and General Psychological Monographs, 111*, 205–232.

Petrillo, M., & Sanger, S. (1980). *Emotional care of hospitalized children: An environmental approach*. Philadelphia: Lippincott.

Platt, H. (1959). *The welfare of children in hospital*. London: Ministry of Central Health Services Council.

Pollillio, A. M., & Kiley, J. (1997). Does a needleless injection system reduce anxiety in children receiving intramuscular injections. *Pediatric Nursing, 23*(1), 46–49.

Powers, K. S., & Rubenstein, J. S. (1999). Family presence during invasive procedures in the pediatric intensive care unit: A prospective study. *Archives of Pediatrics & Adolescent Medicine, 153*(9), 955–958.

Prugh, D. G., Staub, E., Sands, H., Kirschbaum, R., & Lenihan, E. (1953). A study of the emotional responses of children and families to hospitalization and illness. *American Journal of Orthopsychiatry, 23*, 70.

Robinson, C. A. (1987). Roadblocks to family centered care when a chronically ill child is hospitalized. *Maternal-Child Nursing Journal, 16*(3), 181–193.

Rossen, B. E., & McKeever, P. D. (1996). The behavior of preschoolers during and after brief surgical hospitalizations. *Issues in Comprehensive Pediatric Nursing, 19*(2), 121–133.

Safier, G. (1977). *Contemporary American leaders in nursing: An oral history*. New York: McGraw-Hill.

Sheldon, L. (1997). Hospitalising children: A review of the effects. *Nursing Standard, 12*(1), 44–47.

Smart, G. (1997). Helping children relax during magnetic resonance imaging. *MCN: The Journal of Maternal-Child Nursing, 22*(5), 237–241.

Spitz, R., & Wolf, K. M. (1945). Hospitalism: an inquiry into the genesis of psychiatric conditions in early childhood. In *Psychoanalytic Study of the Child, Vol. 1*. New York: Basic Books.

Standley, J. M., & Hanser, S. B. (1995). Music therapy research and applications in pediatric oncology treatment. *Journal Pediatric Oncology Nursing, 12*(1), 3–10.

Taylor, J., & Miller, D. (1995). *Nursing adolescents: research & psychological perspectives*. Cambridge: Oxford Press.

Tiedeman M. E. (1997). Anxiety responses of parents during and after the hospitalization of their 5- to 11-year old children. *Journal of Pediatric Nursing, 12*(2), 110–119.

Turner, G. (1998). Parents' experiences of ambulatory care. *Pediatric Nursing, 1099*, 12–13.

Vessey, J., & Mahon, M. (1990). Therapeutic play and the hospitalized child. *Journal of Pediatric Nursing, 5*(5), 328–333.

Ward, S. L. (1998). Caring and healing in the 21st century. *Journal of Maternal Clinical Nursing, 23*(4), 210–215.

Wells, P. W., DeBoard-Burns, M. B., Cook, R. C., & Mitchell, J. (1994). Growing up in the hospital: Nurturing the philosophy of family-centered care. Part 2. *Journal of Pediatric Nursing, 9*(3), 141–149.

Wright, M. C. (1995). Behavioral effects of hospitalization in children. *Journal of Pediatric Child Health, 31*, 165–167.

Young, J. (1992). Changing attitudes towards families of hospitalized children from 1935 to 1975: A case study. *Journal of Advanced Nursing, 17*(12), 1422–1429.

For caregivers:

Foltz-Gray, D. (1999). *When your child goes to the hospital*. Parenting, *13*(9).

Manczak, D. W. (1999). *Hospitalization: Helping a child cope*. Clinical Reference Systems, July 1, 1999, 731. (helpful suggestions for families before, during, and after a child is hospitalized)

Oakes-Brin, J., Berkowitz, C. M., & Cunningham, N. (1997) *Caring for the seriously ill child*. Mothering, 82, 22-6. (ways for parents to cope in order to help in the care and recovery of their child)

Rivlin, F. (1999). *Books for children with chronic illnesses*. Contemporary Pediatrics. 16(4), 185. (appropriate ages included)

For children:

Books to prepare children for surgery (adapted from Manworren & Woodring, 1998)

Brown, E., W. (1996) *A sick 'kid's' journey into cyberspace*. Medical Update 19(8), 3-4. A description of Steven Spielberg's Starbright World designed to lessen the isolation, anxieties and the pain of seriously and chronically ill children by using cyberspace. (Speilberg explains, "Starbright engages children and allows them to meet new friends, talk candidly about why they're in the hospital, and compare notes with each other...that's pretty cool" (Brown, 1996, 3). www.starbright.org

Ciliotta, C., & Livingston, C. (1981). *Why am I going to the hospital?* Secaucus, N.J. Lyle Stuart Inc. (middle school age)

Coleman, W. L. (1981). *My hospital book*. Minneapolis MN: Bethany House Pub. (middle school age)

Elliot, I. G. (1981). *Hospital roadmap*. Cambridge MA: Resources for Children in Hospitals. (early school age)

Hautzig, D., & Mathieu, J. (1985). *A visit to the Sesame Street Hospital*. New York: Random House. Inc. (pre-school)

Howe, J. (1985) *A night without stars*. New York: Athaneum Publishers. (ages 11-13 years)

Karu, T., & Karu, T (1999). *Henry & the white wolf*. New York: Workman Publishing. (An outstanding book creatively and sensitively written by a young sister and brother to help children understand the experience of illness and treatments.)

Rogers, F. (1997). *Going to the hospital: A Mister Rogers first experience book*. (A Paperstar Book) New York: The Putnam & Grosset Group. (Describes what happens during a stay at the hospital, including some of the most common forms of medical treatment.)

Shimke, A. (1999). *Kids Health Concerns*. A world wide website that provides information for children about diseases and other health problems.

Resources

Organizations and Websites

American Academy of Pediatrics
(information and guidelines for child health)
www.aap.org

Child Life Council
(resources and information about Child Life Programs)
Parklawn Drive Suite 202
Rockville, MD 20852

Institute for Family-Centered Care
(resources and information)
Wisconsin Avenue, Suite 405
Bethesda, MD 20814
www.familycenteredcare.org

National Information Center on Children and Youth with Disabilities
(information regarding care and resources)
Box 1492
Washington, DC 20013-1492
www.nichcy.org

Net Wellness
(a children and adolescent health care information resource that includes "Ask an Expert")
www.netwellness.org

The author acknowledges the help of members of the staff at the Children's Hospital at Baystate Medical Center, Springfield, Massachusetts: Sheila Rucki, Ed.D., RN, Clinical Nurse Specialist, and Jacque Bell, Director of the Child Life Program who assisted with the resources for this chapter.

CHAPTER 17

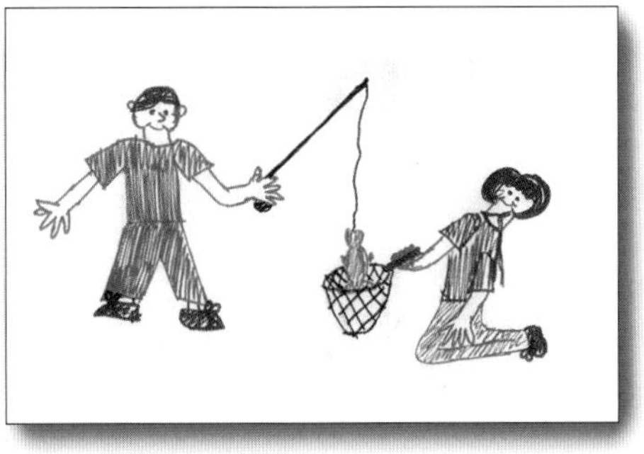

My daughter was born with Treacher-Collins syndrome, which is a craniofacial abnormality. It is characterized by absent cheekbones, downward slanting eyes, a small chin, and malformed or absent external ears. She has had several major surgeries and will require more in the future to build the bones in her face and repair her external ears. She has a trach and wears hearing aids. We met a lot of resistance when I tried to enroll her in school. The trach scared the teacher, principal, and staff. I finally took Lisa to a meeting with the school personnel, and she showed them how to suction. They couldn't fight much once they saw this child could do that by herself. Sometimes I get so tired of having to fight for everything for Lisa. She's not really different from other kids. She even wants to get her ears pierced—as soon as the ears are done.

CHRONIC CONDITIONS

Joan Schmitke, DSN, RN, CS, FNP
Pam Schlomann, PhD, RN

COMPETENCIES

Upon completion of this chapter, the reader will be able to:

- *Identify dimensions of childhood chronic conditions.*
- *Discuss the major focus of the deficit-orientation, health-orientation, and ordinary models used to understand childhood chronic conditions.*
- *Describe aspects of living with childhood chronic conditions from the perspective of the child, caregiver, and siblings.*
- *Explore the impact of cultural values on the child with a chronic condition and on those who interact with the child.*
- *Discuss the nursing management of children with chronic conditions.*

While there is no one accepted definition of the phrase "chronic condition," the term typically refers to a medical state or degree of health that exists for a minimum of three months. All would agree that spina bifida is a chronic condition. But what about hay fever? Or recurrent ear infections? Or chronic constipation? A **chronic condition** has been viewed as a physical, psychological, or cognitive condition that places limitations on day-to-day functioning or requires reliance on special treatments and is expected to last for at least several months (Stein & Westbrook, 1997). Other authors have used a more restrictive definition of the phrase "chronic condition," and therefore, research about childhood chronic conditions has tended to focus on the more severe conditions, while ignoring the mild ones.

Disability and handicap are two words that are frequently mentioned with chronic health conditions. **Disability** refers to a functional limitation that prevents or interferes with a person's ability to perform age-expected activities. In contrast, a **handicap** is a barrier imposed by society, the environment, or one's self in response to perceived differences. For example, lower extremity paralysis from spina bifida results in a disability when the child is unable to walk. By itself, this is not a handicap. However, a handicap would exist if the child is excluded from playing basketball, if a park is not wheelchair accessible, or if the child does not participate in activities because of the erroneous belief that the disability prevents participation. Figure 17-1 illustrates steps that are inaccessible for the girl in the wheelchair. Is this a disability or a handicap?

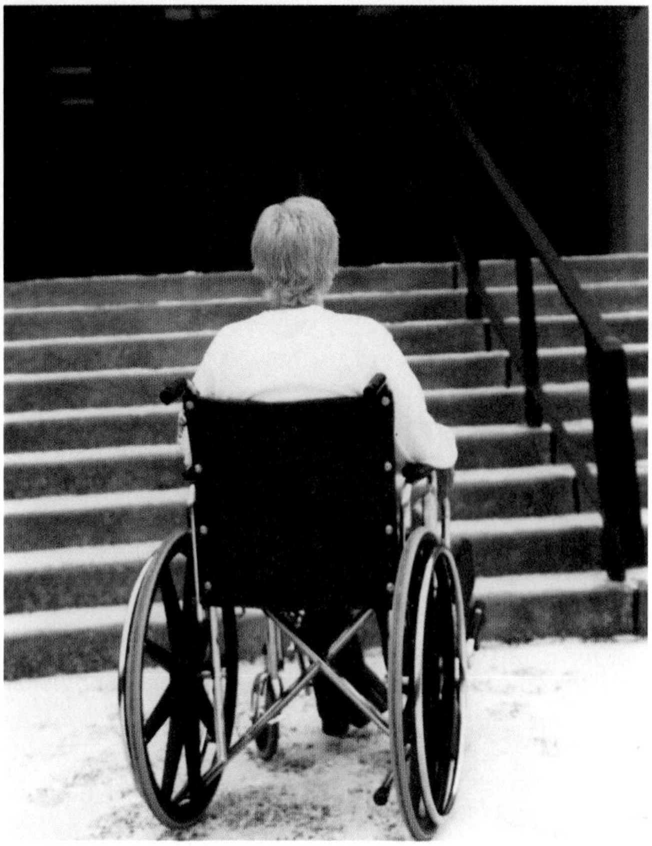

Figure 17-1 These steps are inaccessible for the girl in the wheelchair. Is this a disability or a handicap? Copyright 2001 PhotoDisc, Inc.

Critical Thinking

Is it a Chronic Condition?

A 16-year-old youth was caught smoking pot outside of his school. The counselor referred the adolescent to a local facility for evaluation for substance abuse. The evaluator decided that the incident had been a one-time event and that no further treatment was needed. However, 3 months later, the adolescent was again caught smoking pot and was enrolled in an outpatient treatment program. Does this adolescent have a chronic condition? Why or why not?

As with other age groups, the significance of chronic conditions during childhood appears to be growing. Technological advances have enabled children with serious illnesses to live longer, at times with a newly acquired chronic condition. In addition, occasionally, technology has resulted in iatrogenic (treatment-induced) chronic conditions. However, the actual incidence of childhood chronic conditions has been difficult to estimate. Classic studies estimated that 10–15% of all children in the United States have chronic health conditions and that 10% of those children have conditions that are classified as serious (Hobbs, Perrin, & Ireys, 1985). More recent studies have found that 18% of all children have a chronic condition (Newacheck, Strickland, Shonkoff, Perrin, McPherson, McManus, Lauver, Fox, & Arango, 1998) and that 6.5% of children experience some degree of disability (Newacheck & Halfon, 1998). Clearly, millions of children and their families live with chronic conditions, and nurses need to develop skills to effectively manage the care of these clients. This chapter discusses the dimensions of childhood chronic conditions and appropriate nursing management.

DIMENSIONS OF CHILDHOOD CHRONIC CONDITIONS

For more than two decades, there has been a growing awareness that a disease-specific approach to childhood chronic conditions might not be the most helpful way of understanding them. As an alternative, clinicians have attempted to identify dimensions of chronic conditions and to understand how these affect the child's and the family's adjustment to the condition. For instance, knowing that a child has cerebral palsy might not be as important as knowing whether the condition affects mobility and the ability to care for one's self, and that the condition is not life-threatening or progressive. Important dimensions of chronic conditions include:

1. Nature of onset: Was it a congenital condition or did it begin after a period of relative health? How do the child and family explain the cause of the condition?
2. **Trajectory** or progression of the condition: Will it get better, worse, or stay the same? Does it have episodic exacerbations or crises or is it stable? Is it terminal?
3. Effects on appearance: How visible is the condition? If visible, what is affected—the face, limbs, behavior?
4. Effects on daily functioning: Is the child able to do age-appropriate tasks? Is life-long dependence anticipated?
5. Effects on behavior and ability to relate to others: Is the child's behavior and/or ability to relate age-appropriate and socially appropriate?
6. Care required: Does it require special procedures or equipment? Constant vigilance? Frequent hospitalizations or surgeries? Frequent visits to medical facilities?

As researchers have attempted to uncover the significance of these dimensions, some unexpected, and many conflicting, findings have emerged. One unexpected finding in a number of studies is that the less visible the condition, the

Reflective Thinking

Viewing Chronic Illness

If you were to be diagnosed with a chronic condition, which would you least like to have and why? A condition like diabetes for which you would be required to do frequent monitoring and needle sticks? A condition like cerebral palsy for which you would have to use a walker in order to be mobile? A seizure disorder for which you would have to take daily medications? A condition that would not allow you to be independent, such as quadriplegia from a spinal cord injury? A condition like sickle cell anemia in which you would experience severe bouts of pain?

greater the difficulties the child, caregivers, and siblings often have in adjusting to it. In an early study, this phenomenon was explained with the concept of **marginality,** a situation in which a condition is less visible to others resulting in ambiguity about whether an individual is different from or like others (McAnarney, Pless, Satterwhite, & Friedman, 1974). This leads to a conflict between "normal" (age-appropriate and socially appropriate expectations) and "different," which affects how others relate to the child and the expectations that are placed on the child. For example, a child with a non-visible condition, such as diabetes, may be treated as if no condition existed, and therefore, be subjected to unrealistic expectations.

This visibility has been conceptualized as entailing both functional status and appearance. Unexpectedly, research suggests that these dimensions are inversely related to the impact of a condition on the family. That is, the family and

Research Highlight

Triggers of Parental Uncertainty

Study Purpose

To discover the sources, characteristics, and management of the sense of uncertainty that accompanies life-threatening childhood chronic conditions.

Methods

In a qualitative design, a total of 31 families of children with life-threatening chronic conditions were interviewed. Data were analyzed using the procedures of grounded theory.

Findings

Seven triggers were found to increase the sense of uncertainty for parents. These, along with an example of each, were routine medical appointments (results of laboratory tests), body variability (decrease in appetite), keywords and provocative questions (high risk), changes in therapeutic regimen (discontinuing a treatment), evidence of negative outcomes (someone who dies of the condition the child has), new developmental demands (allowing an adolescent to manage the condition), and nighttime (anxiety, fear).

Implications

Professionals should provide explanations of test results and reasons for changes in therapeutic regimens in a timely manner. Anticipatory guidance can be used to prepare caregivers for normal developmental changes. Ideally, the health care professional should maintain "an ongoing connection with the family" (p. 77) in order to be sensitive to their needs, questions, interpretations of statements, and the child's condition.

Citation

Cohen, M. H. (1995). The triggers of heightened parental uncertainty in chronic, life-threatening childhood illness. *Qualitative Health Research, 5*(1), 63–77.

Reflective Thinking

Dimensions of Chronic Conditions

What dimensions of chronic conditions might be important to a child's or family's everyday life? Why? Check the literature to see if there is support for your opinion.

child experience more negative responses when the child is less functionally impaired and when the condition is less visible. This phenomenon can be explained with the concept of **uncertainty.** Uncertainty exists as to whether the child is "normal" or has a limiting condition. Uncertainty, or ambiguity about what can be expected, creates a sense of limited control, which is stressful and has negative consequences for those involved (Jessop & Stein, 1985). More recently, others have found that uncertainty, regardless of its cause, has many ramifications and is an important dimension of chronic conditions (Ray & Ritchie, 1993; Sharkey, 1995).

While early studies suggested that the need to do special procedures in the care of a child with a chronic condition had no bearing on the child's and family's adjustment, more recent findings have challenged this. Over time, the degree of care that is provided by family members has increased. Family members may be responsible for 24-hour per day care of children who require constant observation and are dependent on sophisticated equipment such as ventilators. Some caregivers have reported that the constancy of care contributes to the burden of that care and can be overwhelming (Ray & Ritchie, 1993).

For some of the proposed dimensions of chronic conditions, there is a lack of adequate knowledge to ascertain how and if the dimensions affect the child and family. Professionals have often assumed that certain dimensions would have a negative impact. For example, contrary to expectations, the severity of the child's condition has little relationship to the stability of the parents' marriage (Eddy & Walker, 1999). Such findings do not mean that the child's health status has no effect on the parents' relationship, but rather suggest that we still have a lot to learn about people's responses to chronic conditions.

LIVING WITH CHRONIC CONDITIONS

A variety of models have been used to understand childhood chronic conditions and their influence on other's perceptions of and interactions with people living with chronic conditions. These models are helpful in framing the child's, caregiver's, and sibling's perspectives on living with the chronic condition. The effects of cultural and societal backgrounds are also considered.

Models of Chronic Conditions

Historically, chronic conditions were thought of as pathological states with major negative consequences in all aspects of life. This approach is an example of a **deficit-orientation model,** which assumes that people with chronic conditions are lacking important aspects of life, and thus, clinicians look for abnormalities and problems in these individuals. Recently, **health-orientation models** have emerged that portray chronic conditions as variations in life. However, the deficit-orientation models continue to be influential, and perhaps, to even dominate thinking about chronic conditions. According to this model if a child indicates that a major disability does not affect self-esteem, the child is considered maladjusted or in denial. According to health-orientation models, the same child is considered well-adjusted, having accepted the disability and chosen to focus on other aspects of life. The **ordinary model** is an example of a research-based health-orientation model in which the child's awareness of the chronic condition changes as the child goes through the developmental sequence. However, the chronic condition does not assume a central or relevant role in the development of identity or in activities of daily life. Those with chronic conditions view themselves as leading ordinary lifestyles (Admi, 1996) (Figure 17-2).

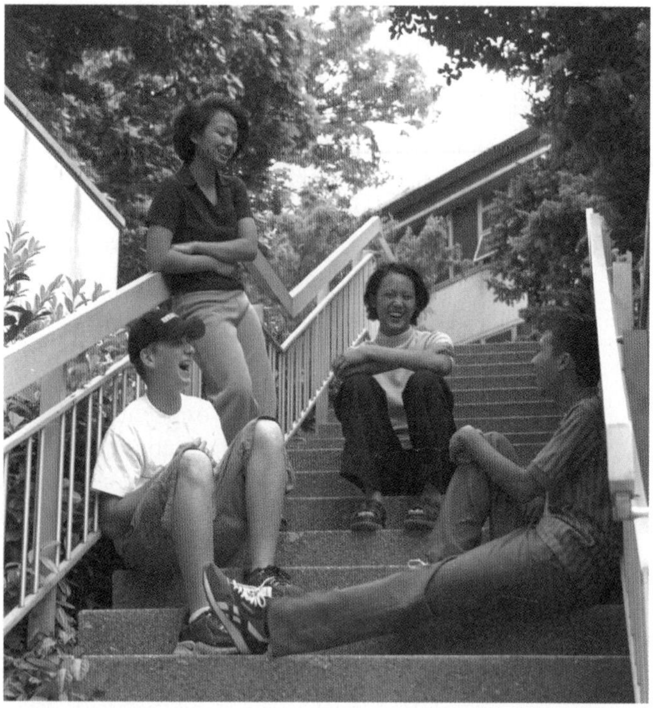

Figure 17-2 Some chronic conditions are not readily apparent. As you look at this group of adolescents, would you be able to discern which adolescent has a chronic condition?

In addition, health-orientation models tend to be critical of professionals who make negative appraisals of those with chronic conditions, such as saying the individual is in denial. These negative appraisals are viewed as misplaced projections of the health care professional's discomfort with disabilities. Health-orientation model proponents do not deny that children with chronic conditions and their families may be maladjusted, but instead focus on positive aspects of the individual's life rather than assuming maladjustment (Admi, 1996).

In addition to determining how professionals view individuals with chronic conditions, the model that one uses has implications for how the individual interacts with and what role she/he assumes with clients with chronic conditions. The deficit-orientation models tend to establish the professional as "the expert" who has the authority to diagnose and treat the client's illness. Some believe that this approach results in dehumanizing and paternalistic modes of interactions. In contrast, health-orientation models portray the relationship between client and professional as a partnership, with each individual bringing a different type of expertise to the situation. Families are central in the relationship and decision making. Focus shifts from treatment to prevention. The professional's role is to empower and enable clients to achieve their self-selected goals for self-identified concerns (Hulme, 1999). Health-orientation models encourage approaches to the management of chronic conditions that are more holistic and consistent with nursing values. Nurses need models that keep the "interests, the experience, and the voice of the person with chronic illness in the center" (Chinn, 1996, p. vi).

Six major themes, representing 20 conceptual categories, have been identified from an extensive review of the literature on chronic illness (Dluhy, 1995). These six themes will provide the framework for a discussion of living with chronic conditions in the remainder of this chapter (Table 17-1).

The Child's Perspective

> "I just went out and played like every other kid, you know, sports, and got my share of trouble. Breaking windows and doing all that fun stuff."—Youth with cystic fibrosis (Admi, 1996, p. 170)

Discussions about living with chronic conditions can focus so much attention on the condition that the essence of the individual is lost. Children with chronic conditions are first and foremost children. While chronic conditions may affect many aspects of life, they do not define the children.

Demands and Challenges

Very little is known about the child's perspective in managing a chronic condition. One study looked at children with cystic fibrosis as an example of children growing up with any chronic health condition. The children talked about two important aspects of living with cystic fibrosis: (a) managing symptoms and (b) managing treatments. The primary symptoms that were of concern to these youth were slim physical appearance, frequent coughing, and bowel movement problems (odor, pain, and flatus). Fatigue and respiratory difficulties were of concern to some (Admi, 1996). One could imagine that health care professionals might not generate the same list of concerns as would children, or would prioritize entries differently. By listening to the children's perspectives professionals can learn from them and provide more effective care.

Management of symptoms is often condition specific. For spina bifida, the child may be concerned about incontinence.

TABLE 17-1 Themes and Concepts in Chronic Illness

Themes	Conceptual Areas
Demands and challenges	Fatigue; dyspnea; pain; uncertainty; stress/adaptation
Emotional and cognitive responses	Defense mechanisms; control/mastery; coping/adaptation; attributions
Day-to-day tasks of living with illness	Life management/normalizing symptoms
Being chronically ill in the culture of a "healthy" society	Role transitions; disability; stigma; social definitions of illness
Changing interactional patterns with family and health care providers	Social support; relationship with health care providers
Potential life outcomes	Quality of life; meaning in illness; redefining the illness situation

Used with permission from Dluhy, N. (1995). Mapping knowledge in chronic illness. Journal of Advanced Nursing, *21, 1055.*

For asthma, the child may be concerned about limitations in sporting activities. Developmental issues are also a factor that affects the child's concerns. At one developmental stage, children with a given condition may tend to be concerned with one set of symptoms, while at a different age they may identify other symptoms. For example, younger children tend to identify pain more than adolescents who tend to be more concerned with other disease-related problems (Spirito, Stark, Gil, & Tyc, 1995).

Children with a chronic condition must learn to manage the treatments associated with the condition as well as its symptoms. Again, developmental issues affect how children deal with this. For example, one study found that treatments that were difficult, time-consuming, or visible and interfered with daily activities were problematic to school-aged children (Admi, 1996). This view is partially due to the children's concrete thought processes and limited ability to understand disease processes. The school-aged child may not understand why treatments are necessary during symptom-free periods or when the benefits are not immediately apparent. In addition, school-aged children often responded to treatments with manipulative behavior or testing of boundaries. For example, a child may refuse to do physical therapy activities or do them in such a way as to minimize their effectiveness.

Research suggests that early adolescence is another difficult period for children with chronic conditions (Admi, 1996). The growing understanding of the disease process often resulted in extreme responses, from preoccupation with the disease and very strict adherence to treatments all the way to disregarding the condition, nonadherence, and risk-taking behaviors. In late adolescence, the youth developed a more balanced, responsible position with more flexible approaches to treatment management. The goal was to manage the disease without having either symptoms or treatment assume a central and controlling role in their life.

Nurses need to be cognizant of developmental issues and the child's perspective as they are involved in managing chronic conditions and as they facilitate movement of the child toward assuming increasing responsibility. Rather than making assumptions about what is of concern to the child, professionals should ask open ended, age-appropriate questions to elicit this information. Additionally, nurses may need to reframe flexible approaches to treatments as adaptive rather than noncompliant.

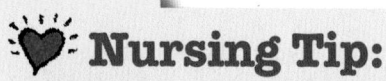

> **Nursing Tip:**
>
> **Child's perspective**
>
> Use open-ended, nonjudgmental questions to explore how the child is managing the condition and its treatment. For example, "What kind of things have you tried? Has that worked? Were there problems with it?" Based on your knowledge of potential problem areas at different developmental stages, use statements that give the child permission to talk about these issues. For example, "Some children your age who have asthma don't like to use their inhalers in front of other kids. How has it been for you?"

Emotional and Cognitive Responses

Most of the research on living with chronic conditions from the child's perspective has dealt with emotional and cognitive responses. Children with and without chronic conditions have been compared based on various psychosocial measures of adjustment, such as measures of self-esteem, anxiety, and depression. While there is some indication that children with chronic conditions are at-risk for maladjustment, results have been inconsistent and often dependent on the model of chronic conditions that was used.

Children use various coping strategies to deal with their chronic conditions. Some have a positive and optimistic attitude about their disorder, and focus more on how their lives are similar to rather than different from their peers. They concentrate on what they are able to do and what they have. Involvement in their own care and being as independent as possible are important to them. They use an adaptive coping style, have high self-esteem, and few behavior problems. On the other hand, some children with chronic conditions view themselves as different from other children. Their coping strategies include withdrawal, blaming themselves or others for their condition, negativity, and irritability. They tend to exhibit low self-esteem and feelings of unworthiness (Austin, Patterson, & Huberty, 1991). Although the choice of coping strategies is for the most part dependent on the situation, age and gender are also factors (Spirito, et al. 1995). Asking the child about coping strategies that are utilized and about their effectiveness is an important aspect of assessment. If those strategies are inadequate, the child should be assisted to develop different ones.

Day-to-day Tasks of Living with a Chronic Condition

Two important factors of day-to-day living for children are developmental issues and school issues. These factors are also important for children with chronic conditions.

Developmental Issues

While the development pattern of children with chronic health conditions may be somewhat complicated by their condition, these children have the same developmental tasks as any other child. Additionally, they experience the same common childhood illnesses and demonstrate similar age-dependent behaviors, such as the "terrible two's." Little is known about how various symptoms or treatments of chronic conditions affect development. Based on developmental theories, one might speculate that various aspects of conditions affect a child's ability to master different developmental tasks. For example, conditions that affect sensations (such as sight or hearing impairment) or mobility would decrease a toddler's ability to explore the environment. According to Piaget's theory, one might expect that this would hamper the child's cognitive development. Similarly, a complicated medical regime may complicate an adolescent's attempts at establishing independence; or differences in physical appearance or function may affect the youth's ability to develop a positive body image. According to Erikson's theory, both of these could be problematic for the psychosocial development of the adolescent. These speculations obviously reflect a deficit model of chronic conditions. Rather than focusing on this aspect, one might consider creative ways in which children with chronic conditions and their caregivers can maximize development. For example, a child who uses a wheelchair may not achieve a sense of athletic accomplishment from playing football, but may do so from doing wheelies or playing wheelchair basketball (Figure 17-3).

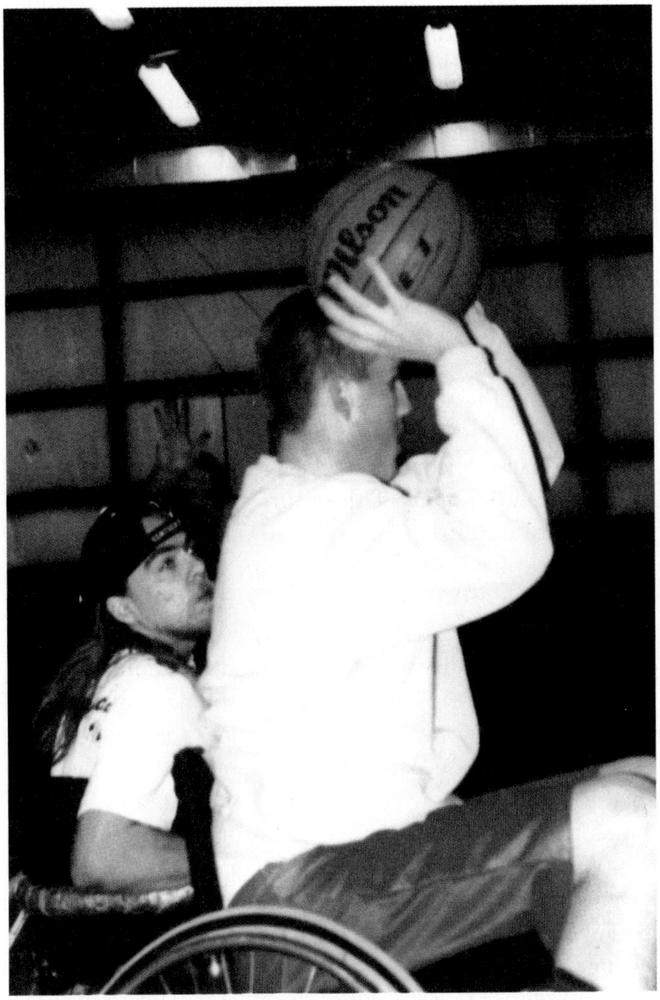

Figure 17-3 Wheelchair Basketball

School Issues

One critical aspect of day-to-day living for children with chronic conditions is school, including attendance and performance. School attendance and accomplishment are typically viewed as essential aspects of normalizing life and promoting healthy development. Nevertheless, school attendance may be negatively affected by illness exacerbations, protective caregivers, the response of the child to the condition, and by the school's response to the child and medical appointments (Figure 17-4). Children with chronic conditions tend to experience more academic problems than their healthy peers (Spirito, et al. 1995; Thies, 1999; Williams & McCarthy, 1995).

By law, there is a mandate to provide appropriate education to all children. Public Law 94-142, Education for All Handicapped Children Act of 1975, requires a free, appropriate public education for all children ages 5–18 years regardless of the severity of the disability. This education must be provided in the least restrictive environment that is appropriate for the child, which can range from a regular classroom placement to the child's home. This stipulation has led to the placement of children with chronic conditions in settings that permit more interactions with others without chronic conditions. This concept has been referred to as **mainstreaming.** The benefits of the inclusive classroom for both groups of students have been well documented (Figure 17-5). In young children, however, interactions are limited unless teachers plan specific activities to facilitate social integration.

This law also requires schools, at no cost to the family, to provide related services that would facilitate the child's development and capacity to benefit from the educational experience. Related services include a variety of offerings

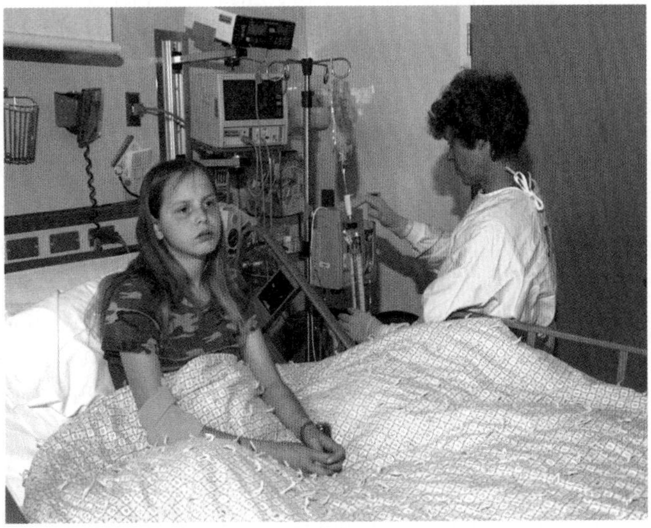

Figure 17-4 When a child with a chronic condition has to return to the hospital, it often raises questions from peers as to why their friend is not in school, when will she be back?

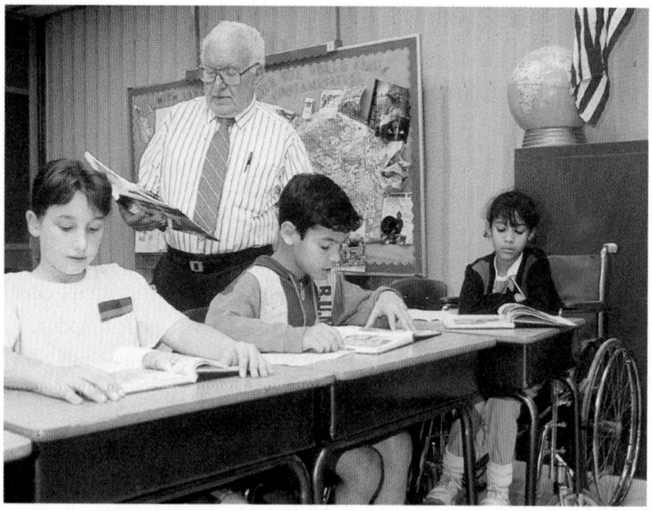

Figure 17-5 Teachers report that when children with special needs are included in regular classes, they become part of the class, without their disability being their most important characteristic.

Reflective Thinking

Education for All Handicapped Children Act

A child with multiple disabilities is in the first grade in a small rural community. The caregivers have requested that the school purchase an expensive computer system that will facilitate the child's communication. The school's very limited budget would be significantly affected by this purchase. This would affect the education of all children in the school. What are the requirements of P.L. 94-142 in relation to this situation? Is it appropriate that this child's needs be placed above the educational needs of other children? Explain your answer.

such as special transportation; speech, occupational, and physical therapy; counseling; and certain health-related services. This has been a contested issue; cases have gone through the court systems all the way to the Supreme Court to define the responsibilities of the schools (American Academy of Pediatrics, 2000).

Part H of Public Law 102-119, Individuals with Disabilities Education Act (formerly P.L. 99-457, Education for the Handicapped Amendments of 1986) first extended the components of Public Law 94-142 to children age 3–5 who are handicapped or at risk for later delay, and then to the age period from newborn to 3 years. It later extended the coverage to 21 years of age. Early identification of at-risk children is critical. At risk includes not only children with identified health problems, but also those who have environmental factors (such as poverty or homelessness) that may negatively affect their development. Additional aspects of this law that are of interest to nurses are that it (a) focuses on community-based, early intervention with the hope of maximizing development and preventing problems; (b) has family-centered care as an integral component, and (c) dictates a coordinated, interdisciplinary approach.

Reflective Thinking

Family Day Care Decisions

You are the parent of a 3-year-old child who attends a family day care. Your day care provider has informed you that she has been mandated to accept a 2-year-old child, who is HIV positive. How would you feel about your child attending the same family day care as the 2-year-old HIV positive child? How would you feel if you were the family day care provider? Explain your answer.

Another law, the Americans with Disabilities Act of 1990, is having an impact on the educational experience of children with chronic health conditions. The law prohibits discrimination based on disability and requires institutions to make reasonable accommodations for individuals with disabilities. Accessibility and accommodations can be denied only if they would create an undue financial burden on the institution or would create a public health or safety risk (e.g., a contagious disease). One application of this law has been to require educational facilities, including family day care, day care centers, and preschool programs, to accept children who have chronic conditions, including those who are HIV positive. While many of these programs have been very resistant to enrolling children with chronic conditions in general, they have often been adamant about restricting children who are HIV positive (Craig & Haggart, 1994; Child Care Law Center, 1994).

The 1997 Individuals with Disabilities Education Act (IDEA) continues to expand upon these previous laws. The purpose of this law is to raise expectations for children with disabilities, increase parental involvement in the education of these children, improve teacher training, and increase funding for schools and for early intervention programs.

While these laws have made major changes in the lives of children with chronic health conditions, they are not a panacea; attitudes cannot be mandated but take time to change. Additionally, laws do not necessarily supply adequate resources to carry out the mandates. Therefore, compliance with the laws may be difficult, and sometimes impossible. Finally, the effort that families often have to exert to require institutions to comply with the law may be overwhelming. Professionals need to be knowledgeable about laws affecting children with chronic conditions and, when appropriate, to act as child and family advocates.

Having a Chronic Condition in the Culture of a Healthy Society

Two aspects of having a chronic condition in the culture of a healthy society have emerged in the literature. The first is an outcome issue. What are the effects of living with a chronic condition in a healthy society on the development of the child's self-concept and self-esteem? While a deficit-orientation model would suggest that this situation would have a negative impact, the research is actually mixed and, overall, refutes that notion. In fact, there is some indication that children with chronic conditions are as popular and have as many friendships as other children (Graetz & Shute, 1995).

The second aspect is a process issue. How does the child mediate negative responses such as stares, comments, misinformation, and stereotypic expectations? Based on deficit-orientation models, one might expect children with chronic conditions to experience stigmatizing responses and discrimination. Interestingly, this phenomena has not been systematically assessed. Mothers have reported that discrimination of their children exists in the form of exclusion from certain school activities, mockery by peers, and inaccessible public places (Turner-Henson, Holaday, Corser, Ogletree, & Swan, 1994). Children have reported both rejection and acceptance (Admi, 1996). They also have experienced difficulties with others being wrongly concerned that their conditions are contagious or fatal. How children respond to these situations is a very complex process. Children and their families must learn how to manage condition-related information and be able to determine what and how much to tell, to whom, when, and where (Admi, 1996). While caregivers have a major role in coaching children about managing questions about their condition, nurses can also help by listening and by providing age-appropriate information.

Kids Want To Know

What should I do when people stare at me?

Stares and stigmatizing responses are common problems for individuals with chronic conditions. Stares, fears about touching, assumptions about abilities, etc. are common things to which they must respond. Following are tips for the nurse in responding to the child:

- Anticipate occurrences (when a child is going into a new situation or has experienced a change in appearance or function).
- Listen to and explore the child's concerns. Give the child an opportunity to talk about negative responses of others.
- Coach children about how to react to negative responses; role play situations with the child:
  1. Frontal approach: When other children are staring at you, ask them if they have a question.
  2. Indirect approach: Underscore own strengths without directly addressing stigmatizing responses. For example, you said the kids on the baseball team tease you and say you can't play because of your asthma. They said you have to stop too often to use your inhaler. You can reply with a statement that emphasizes your strengths such as, "Although I can't play this time, I know all the rules of baseball and can be the scorekeeper."
  3. Ignore: Affirm right to choose what to tell to whom.
- Facilitate the interaction of children with chronic conditions so they can support one another.
- At all times (not just in response to a negative situation), counter the stigmatizing message with one that affirms the child's value, appearance, and abilities.

Reflective Thinking

Age-Related Responses to Chronic Conditions

Visualize a child with cerebral palsy walking with an unsteady gait through a shopping mall. What responses to stranger's stares would you anticipate from a child who is 4 years old and a child who is 14 years old? Using the same ages, what differences would you anticipate in their responses to questions about their chronic conditions?

Changing Interactional Patterns

Very little is known about the interactional patterns of children with chronic conditions with the health care system and with peers. What is known, though, gives important insight for health care professionals and identifies interactional patterns as an area for further study. When adults encounter the health care system, they frequently feel objectified and frustrated by the experience. While children's views about health care have not been studied as much as adults', their reactions indicate similar responses. For example, adolescents report that they do not tell their health care providers when they deviate from a planned course of treatment, even when they believe these modifications are beneficial (Admi, 1996). This suggests that they do not perceive their relationship with the health care provider as a partnership. One might speculate that the reason for the concealment relates to the adolescents' beliefs that their perspectives would not be valued and that knowledge of deviation from the planned care regimen might have negative consequences.

Peer relationships are considered a vital aspect to the healthy development of children with chronic conditions, just as it is with other children. While there is some indication that chronic conditions negatively affect peer relationships and create a greater sense of isolation, there is growing evidence that relationships are not significantly strained. The process of living with and managing others' responses to a chronic condition may in fact improve the child's understanding of complex social situations (Rubovits & Siegel, 1994). One more aspect of peer relations for children with chronic conditions is that older children have indicated that talking with another child with the same condition is one of the best coping strategies available (Novakovic, Fears, Wexler, McClure, Wilson, McCalla, & Tucker, 1996; Wildrick, Parker-Fisher, & Morales, 1996).

Potential Life Outcomes

As emphasized earlier, children with chronic conditions are children *with* a chronic condition. The condition, while a part of the child's identity, is not typically focal. In fact, these children exert some degree of effort to maintain the boundaries of the condition to prevent it from becoming central in their lives. Interestingly, and contrary to expectations, this is true even when the condition is a terminal illness (Admi, 1996). Adolescents with terminal illnesses acknowledge the terminal nature of the illness and plan optimistically for the future. They need permission both to acknowledge the illness and to maintain an optimistic outlook. Quality of life and finding meaning in the chronic illness situation are dependent on maintaining a balance that puts boundaries on risk-taking behaviors while not allowing the reality and treatment routine of the condition to encroach on all aspects of life. For example, an adolescent with diabetes may occasionally choose to go to a fast food restaurant with his peers, even though this will interfere with control of his blood sugar.

Understanding and defining a chronic condition follows a developmental path for children. As expected, with increasing age, children are able to understand more complex and abstract descriptions of the disease process and treatment. Because of their experiences, children with chronic conditions may have more sophisticated explanations than expected for their developmental stage (Rubovits & Siegel, 1994). Health care providers must learn the child's particular perspective.

Chronic conditions are often conceptualized as requiring dependence. This may affect not only immediate but also long-term expectations, hopes, and dreams for the child. A growing emphasis is to develop a mindset and resources that enable individuals with chronic conditions to be contributing members of society as adults.

Reflective Thinking

Dependence or Independence?

In the video, "My Body Is Not Who I Am" (1995), a lady with quadriplegia explains that she is not dependent on an aide who dresses, feeds, and positions her. Rather, she explains, she directs the aide, an employee, to do the tasks she needs done. Is this any different than having an auto technician repair one's car, a hair dresser to style one's hair, a dentist to do a root canal? What does it mean to be independent? Dependent? Interdependent? What does it mean to be a "contributing member of society"?

The Caregiver's Perspective

The caregivers of children with chronic conditions also face demands and challenges, emotional and cognitive responses, and changing roles within the family and society. They must learn to access and eventually coordinate professionals and services as they work for the best interest of the child. Eight adaptive tasks have been identified for them: (1) accepting the condition, (2) managing the condition, (3) meeting the child's developmental needs, (4) meeting the developmental needs of other family members, (5) coping with stress and crisis, (6) assisting family members to manage feelings, (7) educating others about the condition, and (8) establishing a support system (Canam, 1993).

Demands and Challenges

The initial challenge of parenting a child with a chronic condition often revolves around finding out what is ailing the child. Some disorders are immediately obvious, while others have subtle symptoms that may be uncovered only after multiple visits to health care providers (Knafl, Ayres, Gallo, Zoeller, & Breitmayer, 1995). In addition to the variation in the amount of time between the onset of symptoms and learning about the diagnosis, chronic conditions vary in severity and in the amount of care required. Caring for a child with a chronic condition that is mild or does not have significant limitations is quite different than caring for a child whose condition requires the constant presence of a caregiver. Whatever the condition, however, one of the caregiver's challenges is to learn the skills required to care for the child. For example, the caregiver of a child with diabetes must learn how to test the blood for the presence of glucose and how to calculate and inject the appropriate amount of

REFLECTIONS FROM FAMILIES

Whole

I said he was not whole
But I wonder what I meant.
He cannot walk
or talk
or perform any life skill
unassisted,
But he can giggle
and cry
and flirt;
He expresses—and attracts—
love,
His body and mind, though constrained,
"Successfully shelter his human soul
And will do so throughout his entire life."
This—
most human
most godlike—
I can affirm
He is greater than his parts.
He is not disabled in his soul.

—Cherry Winkle Moore, February 6, 1993
(Used with permission of the author.)

insulin. The caregiver of a child with short gut syndrome may have to learn how to give parenteral or tube feedings. If a child is dependent on a ventilator, the caregiver will learn how to suction the child and when the machine is malfunctioning, how to identify the problem. For all skills, in addition to learning to handle the technology, the caregiver must learn to look at the child and ascertain impending difficulties such as signs of hypoglycemia or signs of respiratory distress.

Another challenge for the caregiver is time management. Providing the care needed by the child and taking her or him to various appointments while working outside the home may produce stress or be impossible. The decision for the caregiver to stop employment may not be financially feasible. Suitable day care for children with chronic conditions is extremely limited and often very expensive (Craig & Haggart, 1994; Gabor & Farnham, 1996). Finding time for other family members, particularly siblings of the child with a chronic condition, may also present a challenge to time management. The caregiver's efforts to minimize the perceived harmful effects on siblings is an additional challenge.

Some of the challenges of caregiving involve adjustment to a new role, changing roles within the family, and the necessity of regular contact with the health care system. Particularly during the adjustment to caregiving responsibilities, caregivers may become frustrated with themselves because the intensity of their emotional responses to a given incident seems out of proportion. Lack of sleep for the caregiver may decrease coping abilities, heighten emotional responses, and increase conflict within the family. The term **caregiver burden** has been used to describe the effect of the challenges and demands of caring for a child with a chronic condition (Ray & Ritchie, 1993). Most often, mothers assume the primary responsibility of caregiver and are at greatest risk for caregiver burden. However, the assumption should not be made that this is always the situation; others may have this role. Additionally, health care providers have a role in facilitating involvement of others, such as fathers, for whom society does not typically grant this role (May, 1996).

Respite care is often beneficial to families with a child with a chronic condition. To those caring for a child with complex health needs, it may be essential (Gravelle, 1997). **Respite care** involves having a person who relieves the usual caregiver of caregiving responsibilities for a period of time. The substitute may provide care in the home of the child with a chronic condition, or may provide care for the child in another home or institution. Some caregivers have a substitute on a regular basis, for example, the substitute may care for the child two afternoons each week. Other families prefer to have a substitute less frequently, but for a longer time period; for example, a substitute may provide respite care while the rest of the family goes on vacation each year. Respite care facilitates normalization and reduces stress levels for caregivers and siblings (Sherman, 1995). Nevertheless, the lack of competent, affordable respite care continues to be a major problem for many families with children with chronic conditions. Additionally, caregivers frequently have trouble relinquishing control to and trusting respite care providers.

Critical Thinking

Respite Care: What's in a Name?

A caregiver of three small children needs a break from child care responsibilities and hires a babysitter. A caregiver of a child with a chronic condition also needs a break and arranges respite care. What are the implications of calling these services by different names?

Exploring the need for, availability of, and reasons for not using respite care are important aspects of nursing care for the family experiencing a child with a chronic health condition. Additionally, as a profession, nurses need to be active in increasing accessibility to respite care.

Emotional and Cognitive Responses

The literature suggests that families with children with chronic conditions do not typically have more psychosocial problems than families with healthy children. Additionally, the situation of caregivers of children with severe chronic conditions appears to be different. Often, the condition of these children does not improve and the hope that a child will become independent does not exist. These children often require intensive daily care that involves medical technology. Time demands result in isolation and fatigue. Respite care and/or a strong support system are critical to the family's functioning.

When asked about their experiences at the time they learned their child had a chronic condition, caregivers report that they initially felt grief, a sense of being alone, and frustration with themselves, their partners, and health care professionals. In this early time period they searched for information about the condition and its consequences from the professionals. As their knowledge increased, they developed a sense of competence and confidence, which mitigated their sense of frustration. They also learned to see the positive aspects of the situation (Gibson, 1995).

Adjustment to having a child with a chronic condition has been described as similar to the grief process, which includes the stages of shock and denial, anger, guilt, and finally acceptance. An alternative way of viewing the adjustment process is as one of **chronic (cyclic) sorrow,** a concept developed to explain the experience of parents with developmentally delayed children, and later applied to other chronic conditions (Gravelle, 1997; Kraft & Kraft, 1998; Olshansky, 1962). The notion is that the adjustment process and grief experience do not happen just once with a final resolution as suggested by the stage perspective. Instead, they reoccur at predictable times and, perhaps with increasing intensity, during the child's life. Examples of those times include unmet or delayed developmental milestones, such as walking, learning to read, and getting a driver's license. Other problematic times are (a) when younger siblings achieve expected milestones before the older sibling with a chronic condition and (b) at culturally defined celebrations and age-dependent rites-of-passage, such as reaching age 18 or 21 in mainstream U.S. culture or age 13 in the Jewish culture.

Caregivers use many coping strategies to deal with chronic sorrow: maintaining involvement in personal interests, using respite care, seeking information, focusing on positive aspects of life, focusing on the day and not getting bogged down in thoughts about the future, and talking with others (Eakes, Burke, & Hainsworth, 1998; Sterling, Jones, Johnson, & Bowen, 1996). Nurses should assess the effectiveness of coping strategies used by caregivers and suggest additional strategies as necessary. Anticipatory guidance, based on knowledge of trigger events, and acknowledgment of the difficulties involved in caring for their child may also be beneficial to the caregivers.

Reflective Thinking

Caregiver Responsibilities

Imagine that you have just become the caregiver of a child with a severe disability. The child requires constant supervision as she is dependent on a ventilator. How would your life change? How would your plans and dreams for the future change? What supports would you have available? What role might a nurse have in helping you adjust to the situation?

Day-to-day Tasks of Living with a Chronic Condition

As part of adjustment to caring for a child with a chronic condition, the family rearranges life schedules and routines to include long-term care of the child. In this process, there is an emphasis on continuous efforts to facilitate day-to-day normalization of life for the child and the family. **Normalization** is defined as cognitive and behavioral strategies used by a family of a child with a chronic condition in order to view itself as normal. While the caregiver acknowledges the condition and its impact on the child and family, effort is made to define the situation as normal, to maintain important aspects of their preillness lifestyle, and to interact with others based on this perspective (Deatrick, Knafl, & Murphy-Moore, 1999). Therefore, caregivers both adjust their lifestyle to meet treatment regimens and adjust treatment regimens to fit into their lifestyle. Sometimes this can mistakenly be labeled as "noncompliance." As part of normalization, caregivers also may focus on positive aspects of their child and be labeled as "in denial." Another way in which caregivers strive for normalization is to facilitate normal, age-appropriate development for the child and siblings (Frauman & Brandon, 1996; Reichenbach, 1996). Efforts are made to continue usual involvement in family and outside activities for siblings and the child with a chronic condition.

Having a Chronic Condition in the Culture of a Healthy Society

Coming to terms with the realization that the child with a chronic condition is not going to be cured through the efforts of the professional is one of the most difficult aspects of the caregiver's role. In addition, the caregiver must frequently redefine expectations as the child gets older. If the child with the chronic condition is expected to eventually assume responsibility for self-care, the caregiver must negotiate with the child regarding when and how to shift responsibility for care to the child. The child's age, developmental level, and interest are factors that are considered in the negotiation process. For example, a child diagnosed with diabetes as a toddler should assume increasingly greater responsibility for independent management of the condition. Initially, the caregiver will do all insulin adjustments. As the child reaches preschool age, the caregiver will verbalize the need for more insulin or food. During the early school-age time, the caregiver will verbalize specific amounts and rationale for insulin adjustments. Gradually, the child will be expected to verbalize this information with opportunity for correction and affirmation by the caregiver. By the end of elementary school, many children will be independently making these decisions. One way of conceptualizing this process is as a planned and systematic leadership transition, in which the caregiver's role moves from provider to manager to supervisor to consultant. At the same time, the child's role shifts from receiver to coprovider to manager to supervisor and, finally, chief executive officer (CEO) of care (Kieckhefer & Trahms, 2000) (Figure 17-6). The nurse functions as a teacher/coach in supporting this transition.

Changing Interactional Patterns

The relationship of the caregivers of children with chronic conditions has received much attention. While early studies, based on deficit-orientation models, attempted to demonstrate negative consequences on their relationship, research has not supported this (Graves & Hayes, 1996). The caregiver's relationship with health care providers also changes as the individual becomes more competent and confident in the role. The caregiver becomes an advocate for the child and is able to persist in getting what is thought to be best for the child. Ideally, the health care providers and caregivers become partners, combining professional and caregiver expertise in caring for the child (Hulme, 1999). Professionals need to respect the caregiver's right to make decisions about treatment or caregiving options.

Caregivers report that relationships with professionals are both helpful and harmful. Negative comments generally address either professionals' disregard for the family's knowledge and interests, or problems associated with fragmented care. Critical time periods for the formation of the caregiver's perceptions of the partnership with the health care provider occur at the time of initial diagnosis and during hospitalizations. At the initial diagnosis of the child's condition, caregivers report being bombarded with information that is not pertinent to their child or to the present moment. While information helps families and children to cope, inappropriate information is overwhelming and confusing (Edwards-Beckett & Cedargren, 1995). This may be especially true in the situation of a newborn. Focusing too

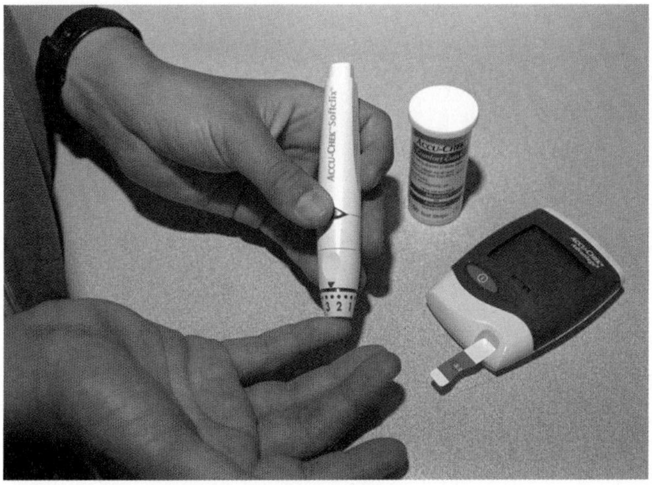

Figure 17-6 As the child becomes older, he will take on responsibilities of managing his condition.

Nursing Tip:

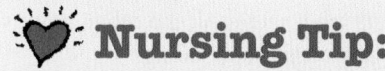

Caregiver–professional partnership

Discuss with caregivers strategies for developing effective partnerships with health care professionals such as:

- Make a list of questions to be asked and information to be provided prior to appointments.
- Ask for immediate clarification of any terminology, information, or technology with which you are unfamiliar.
- Know your rights in any given circumstance. Federal laws protect you and your child.
- Expect your expertise to be respected. As caregiver, you know your child and your family best. You know what has worked, what hasn't worked, and have insight in how new approaches might be integrated into your situation.
- In situations in which you feel uncomfortable or adversarial, take a support person (e.g., nurse, social worker, clergy, friend, representative from Protection and Advocacy). Discuss with the support person, prior to the situation, what your concerns are and what you hope to achieve.
- Directly express frustration and confront discounts of your expertise with statements such as, "When you [professional's problem behavior or communication], I feel like . . . [you are discounting me as caregiver, you are discounting my knowledge]."

intensely or exclusively on a chronic condition and its trajectory can prevent caregivers from seeing all the other aspects of their baby and may negatively affect bonding.

During their child's hospitalizations, caregivers report frustration because their expertise and unique ways of managing their child's care are ignored. While nurses acknowledge the need to collaborate with families and to be responsive to their needs, they report this is very inconsistently done (Bruce & Ritchie, 1997). Besides being frustrating, this can have negative consequences for the child's well-being. Caregivers also express annoyance with home health professionals who expect the family to follow rigid hospital protocols of care. Part of the normalization process is to adapt care so that it maximizes both the child's and entire family's well-being (Sharkey, 1995).

Potential Life Outcomes

In the midst of chronic sorrow, caregivers typically make sense of and find meaning in the situation. They often discover positive outcomes in their experiences of caring for a child with a chronic condition. For example, family relationships may be strengthened as a result of working together. As caregivers come into contact with other caregivers of children with chronic conditions, they become aware of situations that are worse than their own. This process of downward comparison, which assumes that someone else's situation is worse than one's own, enables them to view their own in a more favorable light (Gibson, 1995). Networking with other caregivers also helps them to obtain information and to receive emotional support. Interestingly, many caregivers find networking most effective at an individual, informal level rather than through support groups because caregiving responsibilities make formal support group attendance difficult (Edwards-Beckett & Cedargren, 1995). Internet contacts are also a potentially powerful resource for caregivers.

REFLECTIONS FROM FAMILIES

His Gifts

I have a first-born son
Who is severely disabled
But he brings great gifts to me.

He brings to my life
Sweetness.
He looks at me.
He fully accepts me as I am.
He knows what love is
And because of him
I do, too.

He brings to my life
Focus.
He points my life in new directions.
He opens doors I hadn't seen.
I cannot heal my son
but I can look where he points.
I can go through doors he opens
And I do.

He brings to my life
A new pace.
Because of him I walk more slowly.
I walk more humanly in a fallen world.

My son brings to my life
An abundance of God's grace.
He is a means of grace to me.
He makes me more aware of my blessings.
He will not let me ignore the grief of others.

All of these gifts I would gladly exchange
For a whole son
but that is not mine to choose.
I may choose to thank God
And my son
and I do.

—Cherry Winkle Moore, 1990
(Used with permission of the author.)

Critical Thinking

Caregiver Assessment

Parents are scheduled to visit your clinic with their 2-year-old child who was recently diagnosed with cystic fibrosis. They also have a 4-year-old child. What areas/issues would you explore when assessing the caregivers in this situation? How would you phrase questions to address these assessment areas? Reflect on those questions. Will they empower and affirm the caregivers? Will they help you identify strengths as areas where growth and/or assistance might be needed?

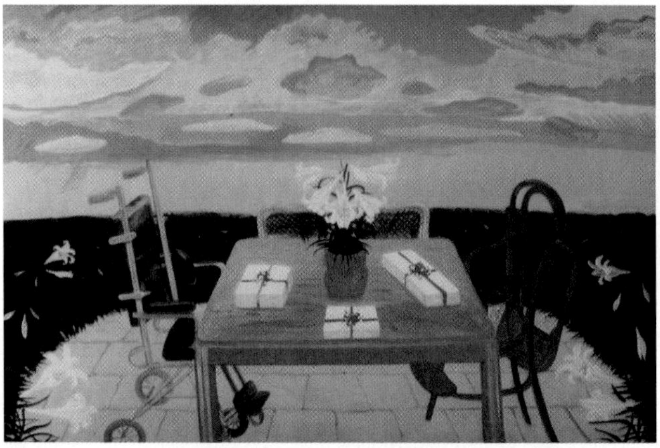

Figure 17-7 "His Gifts," an acrylic. Courtesy: Cherry Moore, mother of chronically ill child. Reprinted with permission.

In addition to identifying the positive outcomes in the process of finding meaning and making sense of their situation, caregivers also identify the strains of caring for a child with a chronic condition. Caregivers of children with severe chronic conditions often ask questions such as "But when do I get on with *my* life?" For some families, the burden (financially, emotionally, physically, socially) is excessive and compromises individual and family integrity.

The Sibling's Perspective

The perspectives of siblings of children with chronic conditions are not often addressed in research or in practice, yet the development of the healthy sibling may be profoundly affected by the experience of living with the child with a chronic condition. An overview of the available literature reveals a lack of consistency of findings on almost every aspect of life for the healthy child (Faux, 1993).

Demands and Challenges

Little information exists about the demands and challenges faced by the healthy siblings; however, it is known that this child must live with the emotional responses of the others in the home and usually receives less attention because of increased demands on the caregiver. There is some evidence that siblings often assume greater responsibilities such as for housework and caring for younger family members (Faux, 1993).

Emotional and Cognitive Responses

Research suggests that siblings of children with chronic conditions have no greater risk of developing psychosocial problems than do siblings of healthy children (Thompson, Curtner, & O'Rear, 1994). Nevertheless, when siblings were asked, they reported feeling worried about the child's illness, feeling jealous about decreased attention, experiencing negative feelings within themselves, noting negative feelings in those around them, and feeling that family events were restricted (Derouin & Jessee, 1996; Sargent, Sahler, Roghmann, Mulhern, Barbarian, Carpenter, Copeland, Dolgin, & Zeltzer, 1995). On the positive side, they reported an increased closeness within the family and an increase in their own ability to care because of their experiences with their brother or sister.

> **Nursing Tip:**
>
> **Helping siblings cope**
>
> Encourage siblings of children with chronic conditions to participate in support groups in which they can gain knowledge, share feelings and emotions, and get help in coping with the sibling's condition.

Day-to-day Tasks of Living with a Chronic Condition

Although schedules for siblings may be tied to the needs of the child with a chronic condition, there is little information on the day-to-day effects. The sibling may be required to accompany the caregiver and the child with a chronic condition to frequent therapy sessions or health care appointments. These visits and other caregiving activities may limit the sibling's participation in sports, school, or church activities. Siblings may be involved in the actual care for the ill child. For example, one of the tasks identified by them was reminding the brother or sister to take medicines (Derouin & Jessee,1996).

Having a Chronic Condition in the Culture of a Healthy Society

Because of close identification between siblings, characteristics of the chronically ill child may be associated with the sibling. Therefore, the sibling may share some of the stigma faced by the ill child. Often, stigmatization results from a lack of knowledge. In an attempt to counteract misconceptions, siblings recommended telling others up front that the condition (cerebral palsy, for example) of the brother or sister is not contagious (Derouin & Jessee, 1996). Like the child with the chronic condition, the sibling may benefit from coaching and role playing to explore ways to respond to peers. For example, the siblings of a child with cystic fibrosis who plays on a baseball team may be asked why their brother has a tube coming out of his nose or why he coughs so much. Coaching the sibling to provide simple explanations that the tube helps him breathe and the coughing is not contagious would be appropriate.

Changing Interactional Patterns

Siblings have identified being able to be involved in the child's care and experiencing an increased sense of closeness with other family members as positive changes, while the lack of attention from caregivers was considered a negative aspect. However, caregivers' opinions of sibling adjustment to the changes involved in living with a child a chronic condition were often based on the caregivers' view of the chronic condition itself. If the caregivers viewed the condition as severe and not amenable to control, they perceived multiple negative changes for the sibling. On the other hand, if the caregivers viewed the condition as not severe and as very amenable to control, they perceived few negative changes for the sibling and viewed the sibling as well-adjusted (Gallo, Breitmayer, Knafl, & Zoeller, 1993).

Potential Life Outcomes

Potential life outcomes for siblings have seldom been researched. Siblings worry about the possible death of the brother or sister. In addition, they may worry about their own future if the brother or sister lives to adulthood but is unable to function independently as an adult. The sibling may be expected and groomed to assume the caregiver role at some point in the future when the present caregivers can no longer meet the needs of the child with the chronic condition. The anticipation and preparation for this role and/or the exploration of alternative options have a significant effect on the well-sibling's life experience.

CULTURAL ISSUES

"The impact of ethnicity and culture on the family's response to illness has not received the attention it deserves" (McCubbin, Thompson, Thompson, McCubbin, & Kaston, 1993, p. 1064). With limited research-based knowledge regarding the interactions between ethnicity, culture, and illness, particularly chronic illness, stereotypes prevail. In addition to inhibiting communication between people of different cultures, stereotypes prevent intra-group differences from being taken into account. The global nature of health care and the multiethnic, multicultural composition of people in the United States requires that sensitivity be embraced in all health care interactions. Caregivers from cultures different from the culture of the health care provider report that professionals do not establish a partnership role with them (Groce & Zola, 1993). In addition, caregivers do not have the power base from which to access available services for their child, and this problem is compounded if the family is part of a minority group.

One of the advantages of health-oriented models is its intercultural applicability. In this model, the child, caregiver, and professional are seen as partners in identifying and proposing solutions to problems. The knowledge and expertise of each partner and an attitude of mutual respect are assumed. This foundation promotes an increased sensitivity to the cultural aspects of care and views the child in context of the family. By combining a partnership approach and sensitivity to the culture, health care professionals and caregivers are able to propose solutions that conform to the value system of the family. If proposed solutions do not conform to the value system/culture of the family, they are not likely to be followed.

One caution must be mentioned in utilizing the health-oriented model interculturally. For some cultures, the professional is viewed as the expert and the client is viewed as the passive recipient. In this situation, caregivers could perceive requests for their input as evidence that the professional lacks knowledge. Culturally sensitive role negotiations are necessary for an ongoing effective relationship.

Eye On:

Differences in Developmental Expectations Across Cultures

In addition to being sensitive to the cultural values of the caregivers, the professional should take into account the differences in normal developmental or age-appropriate expectations between cultures. For example, in some cultures, the child is carried until approximately the age of 1 year. At that point, there is a celebration, a foot-touching-the-ground ceremony. Without considering cultural perspectives, a professional could interpret consistently carrying around an 11-month-old child as "babying" the child. If the child has a chronic condition, such as cystic fibrosis, the caregiver may be labeled as overprotective. However, recommendations to put the child down would not make sense to these caregivers.

Height and weight charts are used in health care settings to provide objective measurements of appropriate physical growth in children. The measurements in these charts are based on "normal" growth parameters for mainstream U.S. children. However, children from other backgrounds may be larger or smaller than the parameters designated on these growth charts. Children with chronic conditions are often smaller than their agemates. When a child with a chronic condition is also part of an ethnic group that is typically of short stature, the child may be deemed ever further outside the "normals." The health care professional may advise the caregivers that the child is extremely small, when in reality, the individual may be only slightly smaller than agemates of the same ethnic heritage. Interpreting growth charts in light of the parents' stature will help minimize this problem.

In order to effectively care for people from other cultures, professionals need to examine their own ethnocentrism, particularly as this relates to health and illness. **Ethnocentrism** is the tendency for all individuals and cultures to believe their values are the best, the most correct. Ethnocentrism prevents professionals from learning from people of other cultures or perhaps even from seeing that other cultures have anything worth learning. In reality, professionals could learn a great deal about ways of conceptualizing illness and identifying and solving problems as they work with people from other cultures. For example, some cultures do not have a word for disability. Instead, everyone is "accepted and valued regardless of their physical condition along the continuum" (McCubbin, et al., 1993, p. 1067). The person's abilities rather than the disability are valued and emphasized. Professionals are now beginning to shift from a deficit orientation to a health orientation. This perspective has been present in some other cultures for a long time. An openness to learn from children with chronic conditions and their caregivers, particularly those from other cultures, will facilitate effective care.

SOCIETAL ISSUES

Children with chronic conditions are often viewed in terms of their cost to society. This is not totally without basis. The cost of caring for these children is high. They are about four times as likely to be hospitalized; spend about eight times as many days in the hospital; and visit a doctor more than two times as often as children without chronic conditions (Newacheck & Halfon, 1998; Newacheck, et al., 1998). This does not include cost of special services at school, cost of special equipment, loss of employment for caregivers, or intangible costs to families. Even in Canada where medical expenses are fully paid by the government, families identified financial impact of a childhood chronic condition as a major stressor (Ray & Ritchie, 1993).

In spite of the many resources used by children with chronic conditions, their level of care and access to health care is often inadequate and frequently distributed unevenly throughout society. Children with chronic conditions are more likely to be behind on immunizations and basic health screenings than other children because of illness, hospitalization, or relative lack of importance. The emergence of managed care has had a further impact on accessibility and quality of care for children with chronic conditions. There is a potential for positive effects—more comprehensive, coordinated, community-based care with an emphasis on prevention. However, there is also a potential for negative effects—reduced access to services and disruption in care arrangements. Monitoring is necessary to validate these potential effects (Perrin, Kuhlthau, Walker, Stein, Newacheck, & Gortmaker, 1997; Newacheck, Stein, Walker, Gortmaker, Kuhlthau, & Perrin, 1996).

While access to health care is a major problem for poor children, it is worse if they have a chronic condition. In fact, 11.2% of children with special health care needs have no public or private insurance coverage. Poor children with chronic conditions were four times as likely to be without insurance coverage than other children (Newacheck, McManus, Fox, Hung, & Halfin, 2000). Compared to Caucasian children, African-American children with chronic conditions have poorer outcomes, including more relapses, more hospitalizations, and more complications (Weekes, 1995). This is partially explained by poverty. There is a higher proportion of children with disabilities living in rural poverty than those in urban areas or those not living in poverty. If the child living in a rural community has a severe disability, the situation is critically complicated (Lishner, Richardson, Levine, & Patrick, 1996). Universal access to comprehensive health care is needed to provide adequate care to children with chronic conditions and to prevent the occurrence of many conditions.

Caring for children with chronic conditions is expensive; for those with severe, chronic conditions, the costs can be staggering. In light of recent trends in health care management, more children with severe, chronic conditions are being cared for at home rather than in institutions. Although this arrangement is less expensive, society must consider the potential harm being done to families if caring for the child at home is the only option available to them. There are few available institutional placements for children with severe disabilities. Besides having a long waiting list or being of questionable quality, the facility may be located at great distance from the family's home. This creates a burden for the family because it becomes difficult for them to remain involved in the child's life. Society must decide if decisions about home versus institutional placement of children with severe, chronic conditions will be exclusively driven by economic issues. As family and child advocates, nurses have a major role in the development of policies that provide for adequate resources for the these families.

NURSING MANAGEMENT OF CHILDREN WITH CHRONIC CONDITIONS

Children with chronic conditions and their caregivers have frequent, ongoing contacts with health care professionals, especially nurses. Nursing care may take place in an acute care setting, a clinic, school, home, or other community facility. Because of the chronic nature of the child's condition, communication between professionals in all settings and with the child and caregiver are crucial to effective nursing care.

Demands and Challenges

Research has suggested that nurses often overidentify caregiver needs and may focus on their deficits rather than strengths (Graves & Hayes, 1996). While knowledge of potential problems a caregiver may encounter is useful, nurses must realize that each family's experience with chronic conditions is unique. Nursing assessment should include strengths and areas for growth from the caregivers' perspectives. Affirming and building on the caregivers' strengths is an effective strategy in providing information and in collaboratively planning for the child's care.

Nurses often teach the child and caregivers about the chronic condition and its potential trajectory. Before beginning to teach the child and caregivers, the nurse needs to thoroughly assess the family's current level of knowledge, skills, and resources. The family may have cared for the child

Family Teaching

Caring for the Family of a Child with a Chronic Condition

Home:
- Supply the family with information about the child's chronic condition, its trajectory, and its therapies.
- Provide educational sessions and materials for caregivers to learn skills needed to provide optimum care.
- Educate the family about the normalcy of feelings of denial, anger, grief, etc. related to having a child with a chronic condition.
- Assist caregivers to talk with siblings about the child's condition and to assess their needs and concerns. Make a referral to groups for siblings with children who have a similar condition.
- Arrange frequent care conferences with the caregivers and the health care team. Encourage caregivers to take an active role in discussions about their child's condition and care.
- Encourage caregivers to identify support systems, i.e., other family members, friends, clergy, and community support groups.
- Encourage interaction with other families who have a child with a similar chronic condition.

School:
- Communicate with school personnel about the child's functional potential and needed modifications in the child's activities.
- Communicate to teachers when homebound or hospital education is needed.
- Promote the child's participation in school and afterschool social activities.
- Reinforce with caregivers the importance of regular communication with the school nurse.
- Teach school personnel about the use and maintenance of medical or adaptive equipment to be used by the child.

Community:
- Involve the family in social and recreational activities sponsored by disease-related organizations.
- Provide a referral to a visiting nurse or a home care nurse for assistance in complex care.
- Make a referral to a community health nurse to provide reinforcement of teaching conducted in acute care settings.

for a number of years and may know more than the nurse about these areas. In this situation, the nurse can acquire valuable information from the family.

If the condition has been recently diagnosed, the family needs information about the condition in order to provide appropriate care, to decrease uncertainty, and to hold realistic expectations for the child. They may also need to acquire complex skills and knowledge about how to access resources. Although the information is needed, it may overwhelm the family. Nurses need to assess the readiness of caregivers to learn and will need to adjust the pace and the amount of information based on that assessment. In addition, nurses should be sensitive to the responses of caregivers to the teaching and to assess their understanding of the information by asking appropriate questions or by having them demonstrate a newly acquired skill. Again, the amount and type of information and the number of sessions may need to be altered in light of caregivers' responses or understanding. The provision of written instructions as a follow-up to teaching sessions enhances learning.

Emotional and Cognitive Responses

In working with families, nurses need to be careful not to assume that (a) emotional or psychosocial problems exist for the child, the caregivers, or the siblings just because a child in the home has a chronic condition, (b) the nurse's and the family's perceptions of what constitutes a problem are the same, and (c) the problems encountered by the child, caregiver, or siblings are fewer or less significant because the condition is less visible or involves fewer functional impairments. By consciously decreasing assumptions and by listening to and understanding the family's perspectives, nurses can facilitate coping for the child and family.

Initially and periodically, nurses need to assess the family's coping. This assessment should include the nurse's observations of coping strategies, family interactions, and attitudes, as well as their responses to direct questions. Nurses should ask specifically about caregiver burden, their perceptions of the efficacy of coping strategies, their sense of control/mastery of the situation, and problems encountered.

Families also need to know that negative emotions are normal and should be expressed in appropriate ways rather than suppressed. Caregivers should be taught to encourage the child with the chronic condition and siblings to express emotions. Support groups provide an avenue for the expres-

Nursing Tip:

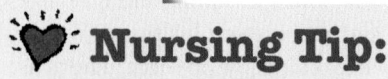

Facilitating mastery/control
Nurses can use the interview time to facilitate an increased sense of control or mastery on the caregiver's part by giving them recognition and praise.

sion of thoughts and feelings and can be helpful for the entire family.

Day-to-Day Tasks of Living with a Chronic Condition

Many of the day-to-day tasks include efforts at normalization in physical and emotional development and in daily activities. Nurses can monitor the child's developmental progress and use anticipatory guidance in making suggestions for facilitating development. For example, the nurse can encourage the caregivers of a toddler to find creative play activities that encourage exploration of the environment, which in turn facilitates independence in the child. For adolescents, the nurse can encourage the development of relationships with peers of both genders. Sexuality develops in children with chronic conditions just as it does in children without those conditions. Nevertheless, children with chronic conditions are often treated as asexual and also know less about sexuality-related topics than other children do. This aspect of development needs to be considered when working with children with chronic conditions. The child and family need information and opportunities to discuss puberty, reproduction capacity, safe sex practices, and intimate relationships. Key times for explaining these topics include after diagnosis, prepubescence, mid-puberty, and prior to transfer to the adult health care system (Kelton, 1999).

Nurses can also play a role in normalizing day-to-day living by working with the family in getting the child into an appropriate school placement. The nurse can educate teachers and other personnel in order to facilitate the child's reentry into school. Depending on the situation, the child's peers may also be prepared for the child's placement or return to school.

The day-to-day tasks of living with a chronic condition most often take place in the child's home where the child and caregivers have developed routines for providing daily care. However, when the child is hospitalized, these routines are frequently interrupted and may cause frustration for everyone. Nurses need to help facilitate the implementation of these day-to-day routines in the acute care setting.

> **Critical Thinking**
>
> **Facilitating School Entry**
>
> You are a school nurse. A first grader with spina bifida is enrolling in the school and will be placed in a regular classroom. The child is ambulatory with a walker, will need intermittent catheterization, and is on medications for seizures and bladder control. What role will you have with the teacher, child, caregivers, and classmates? If the teacher is resistant to having the child in the class, how would you proceed?

Having a Chronic Condition in the Culture of a Healthy Society

One way that nurses can facilitate a positive self-concept in a child with a chronic condition is to promote normalcy by emphasizing what the child can do and encouraging involvement in age and developmentally appropriate tasks. Nurses may be involved in the decisions as to when and how the caregiver can begin to shift the responsibility for care to the child. Observations by the nurse and the caregiver's opinions about the child's readiness to assume responsibility for care are crucial to a successful transition.

As the child and family interact with others, they may be subject to discrimination, stares, and inappropriate questions and advice. The child may encounter mocking from other children. Assessment should periodically include questions about the child's and family's experiences as they interact with others. Not all situations can be prevented; however, the nurse, the child, and the caregiver will need to develop acceptable ways to respond to negative responses from others. Examples of coping strategies include getting involved in support groups of other children with similar conditions, communicating directly and providing information about the condition and its limitations, ignoring responses of others, and emphasizing capabilities of the child.

Changing Interactional Patterns

In the process of caring for a child with a chronic condition, caregivers and sometimes siblings redefine their roles. For the caregiver of a child with a newly diagnosed chronic condition, the nurse may use anticipatory guidance in facilitating role transition. Periodic, ongoing assessment of family interaction patterns will be necessary, particularly as the child and the family go through times of change such as the addition of a family member or the beginning of school. The nurse can listen and suggest ways to reframe role expectations or to make transitions.

Interactions with professionals also change as caregivers become more knowledgeable about the effects of the condition on the child, more competent in working with the child, and more confident in their abilities to serve as an advocate. Ideally, the partnership between the family and the nurse will utilize their complementary areas of expertise to benefit the child and maximize family adjustment. For the nurse, viewing the caregiver as a partner may reemphasize the importance of listening intently to others' perspectives and suggestions, being willing to learn as well as teach, being sensitive to cultural differences, and being flexible and willing to try different approaches. These attitudes are crucial to an effective partnership with the caregiver and the child.

Potential Life Outcomes

Nurses have the privilege of working closely with caregivers and children as they struggle to make sense of their situations, to adjust to the child's illness, to maintain some sort of normalcy for these families. Nurses will be involved with the families in times of encouragement and optimism, in times of discouragement and grief, and in the struggle to make sense of the situation in the context of their lives. This provides opportunities for nurses to create new meanings for themselves as they reflect on their own lives.

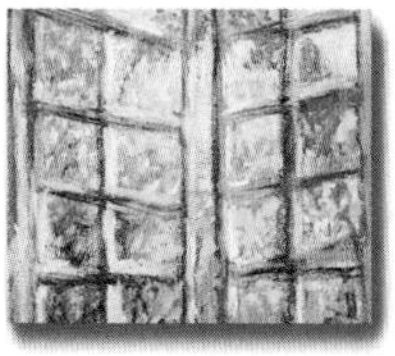

In the Real World

I am a school nurse at an elementary school. We have several students who have chronic conditions. In September, a new child was enrolled in a second grade class. Rory suffers from seizures at least one to two times a day. During the second week of school, Rory had a seizure. The students—some with looks of fear, horror, and puzzlement—watched as the aides quickly took measures so Rory would not injure himself. When the seizure was over and the room settled down, the children had many questions regarding what had happened. It was decided between Rory's parents, Rory, myself, and the second grade teacher to meet with the students and discuss seizures, why they happen, and what to do when they happen.

The discussion took place the very next day. The students were very inquisitive as we provided an explanation. They seemed to have absorbed the information quite quickly. They felt comfortable with information and the events that will take place when Rory has a seizure.

The next time Rory had a seizure the students knew to clear the area of items that he may injure himself with while the teacher and aides placed him on his side. After the seizure was over, the students asked Rory how he was and then resumed their normal activities. Rory felt better emotionally that his classmates knew about his condition and that he was still needed and wanted as a friend without a moment's hesitation.

Key Concepts

- Childhood chronic conditions include a variety of physical, emotional, and cognitive problems that last for at least three months and may prevent the child from accomplishing age-appropriate physical, intellectual, psychological, and sociocultural developmental functions. The conditions may range in severity from mild to severe.
- Dimensions of childhood chronic conditions include nature of onset, trajectory of the condition, effects on appearance, effects on daily functioning, effects on behavior and ability to relate to others, and the kind and amount of care required.
- A chronic condition requires the child, siblings, and caregivers to adjust to the changes in roles and responsibilities, to learn new skills, to deal with the uncertainty regarding the impact of the condition, and to attempt to normalize life.
- The adaptive tasks that have been identified for caregivers include: accepting the condition, managing the condition, meeting the child's developmental needs, meeting the developmental needs of other family members, coping with stress and crisis, assisting family members to manage feelings, educating others about the condition, and establishing a support system.
- Meeting the needs of a child with a chronic condition may lead to caregiver burden, a sense of being overwhelmed with the responsibilities at hand.
- Caregivers of children with chronic conditions may experience chronic sorrow as they repeatedly come to terms with the changes in the life of the child and in their own lives.
- Chronic fatigue, a constant state of vigilance, and the demands of caregiving contribute to caregivers' stress.
- Siblings of children with chronic conditions have no greater risk of developing psychosocial problems than do siblings of healthy children.
- Nurses play a major role in listening, mutual problem identification and solving, and teaching, thereby empowering the caregivers to have a sense of control.

Review Questions

1. Discuss the potential effects of the visibility of a chronic condition on the child, the family, and others who come into contact with the child.
2. Describe the implications of lifelong dependency for a child with a chronic condition on the child, siblings, and caregivers.

3. The caregivers of a child with a newly diagnosed chronic condition meet with a nurse to discuss the care of their child. Describe the approach that would be used if the nurse followed the pathologic or deficit model of chronic conditions. Describe the approach that would be used if the nurse followed a health-oriented model of chronic conditions.
4. Give an example of the way in which the developmental level will affect a child's response to having a chronic condition. How might a chronic condition affect a child's development?
5. How are public law (PL) 94-142, part H of PL 102-119, and the Americans with Disabilities Act applicable to children with chronic conditions?
6. Describe some of the challenges faced by caregivers of children with chronic conditions.
7. Describe the relationship between culture and chronic conditions in children.
8. Describe the impact of poverty on the care received by children with chronic conditions.
9. What would be an appropriate response for the nurse when a caregiver tells a sibling of a child with a chronic condition never to get angry with the child?

References

Admi, H. (1996). Growing up with a chronic health condition: A model of an ordinary lifestyle. *Qualitative Health Research, 6*(2), 163–183.

American Academy of Pediatrics. (2000). Provision of educationally-related services for children and adolescents with chronic disease and disabling conditions. *Pediatrics, 105*(2), 448–451.

Austin, J., Patterson, J., & Huberty, T. (1991). Development of the coping health inventory for children. *Journal of Pediatric Nursing, 6*(3), 166–174.

Bruce, B., & Ritchie, J. (1997). Nurses' practices and perceptions of family-centered care. *Journal of Pediatric Nursing, 12*(4), 214–222.

Canam, C. (1993). Common adaptive tasks facing parents of children with chronic conditions. *Journal of Advanced Nursing, 18,* 46–53.

Child Care Law Center. (1994). *Caring for children with HIV or AIDS in child care.* (PN. 9302). San Francisco: Author.

Chinn, P. L. (1996). From the editor, living with chronic illness. *Advances in Nursing Science, 18*(3), vi.

Cohen, M. H. (1995). The triggers of heightened parental uncertainty in chronic, life threatening childhood illness. *Qualitative Health Research, 5*(1), 63–67.

Craig, S. E., & Haggart, A. G. (1994). Including all children: The ADA's challenge to early intervention. *Infants and Young Children, 7*(2), 15–19.

Deatrick, J. A., Knafl, K. A., & Murphy-Moore, C. (1999). Clarifying the concept of normalization. *Image: Journal of Nursing Scholarship, 31,* 209–214.

Derouin, D., & Jessee, P. O. (1996). Impact of a chronic illness in childhood: Siblings' perceptions. *Issues in Comprehensive Pediatric Nursing, 19,* 135–147.

Dluhy, N. M. (1995). Mapping knowledge in chronic illness. *Journal of Advanced Nursing, 21,* 1051–1058.

Eakes, G., Burke, M., & Hainsworth, M. (1998). Theory: Middle-range theory of chronic sorrow. *Image: Journal of Nursing Scholarship, 30*(2), 179–184.

Eddy, L., & Walker, A. (1999). The impact of children with chronic health problems on marriage. *Journal of Family Nursing, 5*(1), 10–33.

Edwards-Beckett, J., & Cedargren, D. (1995). The sociocultural context of families with a child with myelomeningocele. *Issues in Comprehensive Pediatric Nursing, 18*(1), 27–42.

Faux, S. A. (1993). Siblings of children with chronic physical and cognitive disabilities. *Journal of Pediatric Nursing, 8*(5), 305–317.

Frauman, A. C., & Brandon, D. H. (1996). Toilet training for the child with chronic illness. *Pediatric Nursing, 22*(6), 469–472.

Gabor, L. M., & Farnham, R. (1996). The impact of children with chronic illness and/or developmental disabilities on low-income single-parent families. *The Transdisciplinary Journal, 6*(2), 167–180.

Gallo, A. M., Breitmayer, B. J., Knafl, K. A., & Zoeller, L. H. (1993). Mothers' perceptions of sibling adjustment and family life in childhood chronic illness. *Journal of Pediatric Nursing, 8*(5), 318–324.

Gibson, C. J. (1995). The process of empowerment in mothers of chronically ill children. *Journal of Advanced Nursing, 21*(6), 1201–1210.

Graetz, B., & Shute, R. (1995). Assessment of peer relationships in children with asthma. *Journal of Pediatric Psychology, 20*(2), 205–216.

Gravelle, A. M. (1997). Caring for a child with a progressive illness during the complex chronic phase: Parents' experience of facing adversity. *Journal of Advanced Nursing, 25,* 738–745.

Graves, C., & Hayes, V. E. (1996). Do nurses and parents of children with chronic conditions agree on parental needs? *Journal of Pediatric Nursing, 11*(5), 288–299.

Groce, N. E., & Zola, I. K. (1993). Multiculturalism, chronic illness, and disability. *Pediatrics, 91*(5Pt2), 1048–1055.

Hobbs, N., Perrin, J., & Ireys, H. (1985). *Chronically ill children and their families: Problems, prospects, and proposals from the Vanderbilt Study.* San Francisco: Jose-Bass.

Hulme, P. (1999). Family empowerment: A nursing intervention with suggested outcomes for families of children with a chronic health condition. *Journal of Family Nursing, 5*(1), 33–50.

Jessop, D., & Stein, R. (1985). Uncertainty and its relation to the psychological and social correlates of chronic illness in children. *Social Science and Medicine, 20*(10), 993–999.

Kelton, S. (1999). Sexuality education for youth with chronic conditions. *Pediatric Nursing, 25*(5), 491–496.

Kieckhefer, G., & Trahms, C. (2000). Supporting development of children with chronic conditions: From compliance toward shared management. *Pediatric Nursing, 26*(4), 354–363.

Knafl, K. A., Ayres, L., Gallo, A. M., Zoeller, L. H., & Breitmayer, B. J. (1995). Learning from stories: parents' accounts of the pathway to diagnosis. *Pediatric Nursing, 21*(5), 411–415.

Kraft, S., & Kraft, L. (1998). Chronic sorrow: Parents' lived experience. *Holistic Nursing Practice, 13*(1), 59–67.

Lishner, D., Richardson, M., Levine, P., & Patrick, D. (1996). Access to primary health care among persons with disabilities in rural areas: A summary of the literature. *Journal of Rural Health, 12*(1), 45–53.

May, J. (1996). Fathers: The forgotten parent. *Pediatric Nursing, 22*(3), 243–247.

McAnarney, E., Pless, I., Satterwhite, B., & Friedman, S. (1974). Psychological problems of children with chronic juvenile arthritis. *Pediatrics, 53*(4), 523–527.

McCubbin, H. I., Thompson, E. A., Thompson, A. L., McCubbin, M. A., & Kaston, A. J. (1993). Culture, ethnicity, and the family: Critical factors in childhood chronic illnesses and disabilities. *Pediatrics, 91*(5), 1063–1070.

Newacheck, P., Stein, R., Walker, D., Gortmaker, S., Kuhlthau, K., & Perrin, J. (1996). Monitoring and evaluating managed care for children with chronic illnesses and disabilities. *Pediatrics, 98*(5), 952–959.

Newacheck, P., & Halfon, N. (1998). Prevalence and impact of disabling chronic conditions in childhood. *American Journal of Public Health, 88*(4), 610–617.

Newacheck, P., Strickland, B., Shonkoff, J., Perrin, J., McPherson, M., McManus, M., Lauver, C., Fox, H., & Arango, P. (1998). An epidemiologic profile of children with special health care needs. *Pediatrics, 102*(1), 117–123.

Newacheck, P., McManus, M., Fox, H., Hung, Y., & Halfon, N. (2000). Access to health care for children with special health care needs. *Pediatrics, 105*(4), 760–767.

Novakovic, B., Fears, T. R., Wexler, L. H., McClure, L. L., Wilson, D. L., McCalla, J. L., & Tucker, M. A. (1996). Experiences of cancer in children and adolescents. *Cancer Nursing, 19*(1), 54–59.

Olshansky, S. (1962). Chronic sorrow: A response to having a mentally defective child. *Social Casework, 43*(94), 190–193.

Perrin, J., Kuhlthau, K., Walker, D., Stein, R., Newacheck, P., & Gortmaker, S. (1997). Monitoring health care for children with chronic conditions in a managed care environment. *Maternal and Child Health Journal, 1*(10), 15–23.

Ray, L., & Ritchie, J. (1993). Caring for chronically ill children at home: Factors that influence parents' coping. *Journal of Pediatric Nursing, 8*(4), 217–225.

Reichenbach, M. B. (1996). Promoting normalcy in chronically ill children. *Orthopaedic Nursing, 15*(1), 37–42.

Rubovits, D. S., & Siegel, A. W. (1994). Developing conceptions of chronic disease: A comparison of disease experience. *Children's Health Care, 23*(4), 267–285.

Sargent, J. R., Sahler, O. J., Roghmann, K. J., Mulhern, R. K., Barbarian, O. A., Carpenter, P. J., Copeland, D. R., Dolgin, M. J., & Zeltzer, L. K. (1995). Sibling adaptation to childhood cancer collaborative study: Siblings' perceptions of the cancer experience. *Journal of Pediatric Psychology, 20*(2), 151–164.

Sharkey, T. (1995). The effects of uncertainty in families with children who are chronically ill. *Home Healthcare Nurse, 13*(4), 37–42.

Sherman, B. R. (1995). Impact of home-based respite care on families of children with chronic illness. *Children's Health Care, 24*(1), 33–45.

Spirito, A., Stark, L. J., Gil, K. M., & Tyc, V. L. (1995). Coping with everyday and disease-related stressors by chronically ill children and adolescents. *Journal of the American Academy of Child and Adolescent Psychiatry, 34*(3), 283–290.

Stein, R., & Westbrook, L. (1997). The questionnaire for identifying children with chronic conditions: A measure based on a noncategorical approach. *Pediatrics, 99*(4), 513–522.

Sterling, Y. M., Jones, L. C., Johnson, D. H., & Bowen, M. R. (1996). Parents' resources and home management of the care of chronically ill infants. *Journal of the Society of Pediatric Nurses, 1*(3), 103–112.

Thies, K. (1999). Identifying the educational implications of chronic illness in school children. *Journal of School Health, 69*(10), 392–398.

Thompson, A. B., Curtner, M. E., & O'Rear, M. R. (1994). The psychosocial adjustment of well siblings of chronically ill children. *Children's Health Care, 23*(3), 211–226.

Turner-Henson, A., Holaday, B., Corser, N., Ogletree, F., & Swan, J. H. (1994). The experiences of discrimination: Challenges for chronically ill children. *Pediatric Nurse, 20*(6), 571–577.

Weekes, D. (1995). African American children, adolescents, and chronic illness. In R. Johnson (Ed.), *African American voices: African American health educators speak out* (pp. 95–112). New York: National League for Nursing Press.

Wildrick, D., Parker-Fisher, S., & Morales, A. (1996). Quality of life in children with well-controlled epilepsy. *Journal of Neuroscience Nursing, 28*(3), 192–198.

Williams, J. K., & McCarthy, A. M. (1995). School nurses' experiences with children with chronic conditions. *Journal of School Health, 65*(6), 234–236.

Suggested Readings

Dwight, L. (1997). *We do it!* New York: Star Bright Books.

Gallo, A., & Knafl, K. (1998). Parents' reports of "tricks of the trade" for managing childhood chronic illness. *Journal of the Society of Pediatric Nurses, 3*(3), 93–100.

Huegel, K. (1998). *Young people and chronic illness: True stories, help, and hope.* Minneapolis: Free Spirit Publishing.

Jessop, D., & Stein, R. (1994). Providing comprehensive health care to children with chronic illness. *Pediatrics, 93*(4), 602–607.

Katz, S., & Krulik, T. (1999). Fathers of children with chronic illness: Do they differ from fathers of healthy children? *Journal of Family Nursing, 5*(3), 292–315.

Kriegsman, K. H., Zaslow, E. L., & D'Zmura-Rechsteiner, J. *Taking charge: Teenagers talk about life and physical disabilities.* Bethesda, MD: Woodbine House, Inc.

Lutkenhoff, M., & Oppenheim, S. (1997). *Spinabilities: A young person guide to spina bifida.* Bethesda, MD: Woodbine House, Inc.

Perrin, E., Lewkowicz, C., & Young, M. (2000). Shared vision: Concordance among fathers, mothers, and pediatricians about unmet needs of children with chronic health conditions. *Pediatrics, 105*(1), 277–285.

Sterling, C., & Friedman, A. (1996). Empathic responding in children with a chronic illness. *Children's Health Care, 25*(1), 53–69.

Transition Project Staff. (1966). *Transition tips and tools.* Minneapolis, MN: Pacer Center, Inc.

Wallander, J., & Noojin, A. (1995). Mothers' report of stressful experiences related to having a child with a physical disability. *Children's Health Care, 24*(4), 245–256.

Resources

Organizations and Websites

Access to Respite Care
c/o Chapel Hill Training Outreach Project
800 Eastowne Dr.
Chapel Hill, NC 27514
(919) 490-5577
(800) 473-1727 Ext. 243
www.chtop.com

American Association of People with Disabilities (AAPD)
1819 H Street NW, Suite 330
Washington, DC 20006
(202) 457-0046
(800) 840-8844
www.aapd.com

Family Village: Global Community of Disability-Related Resources
www.familyvillage.wisc.edu
(Provides links to disability-related resources including disease specific information, chat rooms, educational information, recreational opportunities, spiritual resources.)

Federation for Children with Special Needs
95 Berkley St., Suite 104
Boston, MA 02116
(617) 482-2915
(800) 331-0688
www.fcsn.org

Internet Resources for Special Children
www.irsc.org
(Parent developed web site with links to disability-related sites.)

National Early Childhood Technical Assistance System
Frank Porter Graham Child Development Center
500 Nations Bank Plaza
137 E. Franklin St.
Chapel Hill, NC 27514
www.nectas.unc.edu
(Provides information about the legal requirements for educating children with disabilities)

National Father's Network
16120 N.E. 8th St.
Bellevue, WA 980008-3937
(206) 747-4004
www.fathersnetwork.org

National Information Center for Children and Youth with Disabilities
P.O. Box 1492
Washington, DC 20013
(202) 884-8200
(800) 695-0285
www.nichcy.org

Parents Helping Parents: The Family Resource Center
www.php.com
(Provides links to resources about parenting workshops and support groups, equipment exchanges, and other helpful information for parents of children with special needs.)

Videos

Equal Partners: African-American Fathers and Systems of Health Care. (Tells the story of several black fathers of children with special needs. Produced by the National Fathers' Network, 16120 N.E. 8th St., Bellevue, WA 98008-3937)

Families of Young Children with Special Needs (Series)(1996). Irvine, CA: Concept Media.

My Body Is Not Who I Am. (1995). Aquarius Productions, Sherborn, Mass. (People with disabilities discuss the struggles and triumphs they have experienced living in a body that is physically disabled)

Parenting Children with Special Needs, and Parents' Views of Living with a Child with Disabilities. United Learning, Inc.

CHAPTER 18

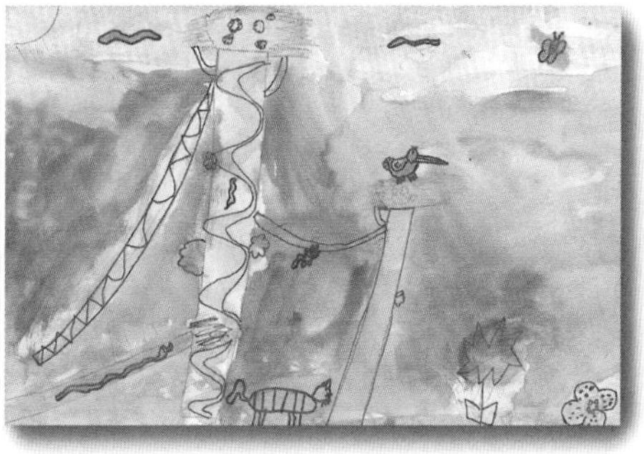

I couldn't believe how quickly Meghana recuperated from her tonsillectomy. She was only 4 years old when she had the surgery and didn't complain of much pain except right after she returned from the operating room. She was enjoying Popsicles and cold drinks within a few hours and, within a few days, had no sore throat at all. That was so different from my husband Carl, when he had his tonsils out when he was 28. I think it took him about two weeks before his throat stopped hurting. He was miserable. Such a different reaction from Meghana.

PAIN MANAGEMENT

Jennifer Obrecht, RN, MS

COMPETENCIES

Upon completion of this chapter, the reader will be able to:

- *Describe the physiology of pain, including the gate control theory.*
- *Discuss common pain misconceptions.*
- *Discuss developmental differences in pain behavior and assessment strategies.*
- *Describe various pediatric pain assessment scales and their application to children of varying developmental/cognitive levels.*
- *Describe nonpharmacologic techniques for pediatric pain management.*
- *Discuss the use, dose, and side effects of opioid and non-opioid pain medications.*
- *Differentiate acute from chronic pain.*
- *Discuss information families need to know when caring for a child experiencing pain at home.*

Pain, an important symptom seen in children, can be caused by pressure, over stretching, injury, or reduced oxygen supply to body tissues. It also can be a unique problem, a symptom of a specific disease or health problem, or the result of disease or treatment. However, since many health care professionals are still under the impression children do not experience pain or are less sensitive to pain than adults, information about pediatric pain management strategies is essential to delivering holistic, effective care.

Appropriate pain relief is important for physiological as well as psychological reasons. For example, babies have improved mortality and morbidity after cardiac surgery when they receive appropriate pain medications (Anand & Hickey, 1987). Proper and effective pain management also promotes wound healing and decreases the length of hospital stay. Therefore, infants and children treated throughout the health care spectrum should be afforded the opportunity for effective **analgesia**—pain control using medications or other interventions.

This chapter discusses the pediatric pain experience. The text provides information about the developmental implications of pediatric pain, especially in infants and toddlers who generally cannot describe their pain. **Acute pain,** pain lasting three to five days, and attributed to a specific cause such as surgery or an injury, is differentiated from **chronic pain,** or pain that lasts for long periods of time or comes and goes frequently over long periods of time. Treatment options for all pain problems are reviewed and appropriate assessment techniques for pediatric clients, including formal assessment scales, a review of physiological pain indicators, and a description of pediatric pain behaviors are included. The importance of nursing care and advocacy for children in pain is stressed throughout the chapter.

PAIN PHYSIOLOGY

The nerve receptors specific to pain, called **nociceptors,** are located throughout the body in many types of tissue. There are two types of nociceptors, the **C-nerve fibers** (slowly conducting unmyelinated axons that transmit diffuse, dull, burning, and chronic pain) and the **A-delta nerve fibers** (mylinated nerves that fire impulses more rapidly and transmit sharp, well localized pain). A pain impulse starts when these receptors are stimulated by noxious stimuli (mechanical, chemical, thermal) provoking an electrical activity, called **transduction** (Annand, 2000). Transduction is followed by **transmission** whereby the pain impulse moves along peripheral sensory nerves to the spinal column and then to the brain (Price & Wilson, 1999) (Figure 18-1).

The intensity and duration of the pain impulses are affected by neural activity and chemical factors, termed **modulation** (Urban & Gebhart, 1999). Specifically, the prolonged firing of the C-fibers causes a chemical cascade that stimulates the **N-methyl-D-asparate (NMDA) receptors,** causing the spinal column receptors to be more responsive (Bennett, 2000). The release of chemical mediators such as **substance P** (McHugh & McHugh, 2000), a neuropeptide, sensitizes the nerve endings and increases the rate of firing (Zubrzycka & Janecka, 2000). Investigating the role of these chemical mediators may lead to new understanding and treatment of pain.

The **perception** of pain completes the transmission cascade. Perception takes place in the cerebral cortex where meaning or recognition of the pain impulse occurs (Woolf & Decosterd, 1999). Until recently, the central role of pain was thought to be passive. However, studies over the past decade have shown that an extensive central pain network including the thalamus and some somatosensory structures exist (Schnitzler & Ploner, 2000). As the mechanism of the pain cascade continues to be studied, new information about treatment and pharmacologic management should improve.

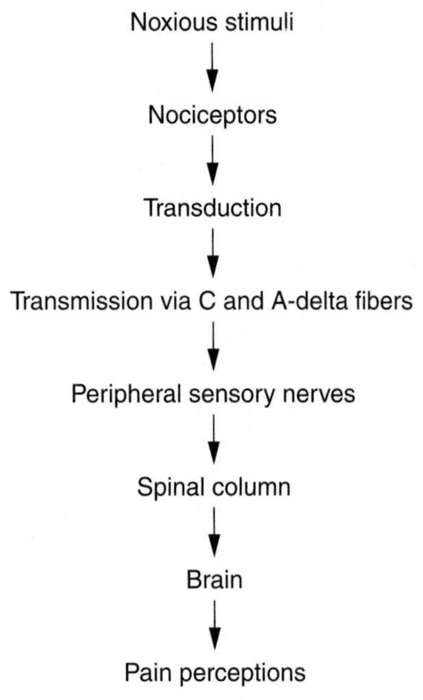

Figure 18-1 Physiology of Pain

GATE CONTROL THEORY

The **gate control theory** explains how pain impulses travel and are interpreted in the body (Melzack & Wall, 1965). At the level of the dorsal horn, a gating mechanism opens and closes to allow pain impulses through. The input of large fiber closes the gate (inhibits pain sensations) and the input of small fibers (allows pain sensations to travel to the brain) opens the gate. However, stimulating the larger afferent nerves that carry the pain impulses, such as rubbing an injured finger or applying cold or heat to an injury, can also blunt pain sensations. The gate's ability to open and close is influenced by stimulation, emotion, anxiety, distraction, sensation, and memory, and supports assessing and treating pain by using both physiological and psychological techniques.

PEDIATRIC PAIN RESEARCH

Early description of pediatric pain focused on under-managing children with acute or postoperative pain. Often, comparisons with adults experiencing pain after similar procedures were described (Eland & Anderson, 1977). The role of the nurse, physician, and parent in treating a child's pain was the focus, and research was conducted generally with hospitalized children.

Anand and Hickey (1987) were two of the first to describe the phenomena of pain in infants. In a double-blind controlled study, these authors compared the effect of pain management in infants to morbidity and mortality. The infants in the control group received no anesthesia or pain medication for thoracotomy, as was the standard of care at the time. The experimental group received general anesthesia and postoperative pain management and demonstrated remarkable improvement in postoperative morbidity and mortality.

Research has also been conducted on assessing pain and developing and testing a variety of assessment scales for use in children (Beyer, Denyes, & Villarruel, 1992; Hunter, McDowell, Hennessy, & Cassey, 2000; Wong & Baker, 2001). In addition, researchers have described the ability of children to quantify and accurately describe their pain response.

Today, a growing body of research examines alternative or adjunct therapies for treating cancer, procedural, and immunization pain in children (Ching, 1999). For example, burn patients listening to music during dressing changes had a decreased pain rating after the procedure and decreased vital sign changes during the procedure than those who did not listen to music (Fratianne, Prensner, Huston, Super, Yowler, & Standley, 2001; Prensner, Yowler, Smith, Steele, & Fratianne, 2001). Similar responses have also occurred when behavioral therapies such as guided imagery, hypnotism, and relaxation techniques were used.

Other researchers have explored the nurse's perceptions of pain (Burokas, 1985; Gonzalez & Gadish, 1990; Pederson, Matthies, & McDonald, 1997). Educational level, personal pain experience, and the number of years in practice play a role in nurses' decision to medicate or not medicate a child for pain. Findings indicate many nurses have let personal pain perceptions influence their treatment modalities for clients in pain. In addition, accurate assessment and improvement in consistent pain treatment correlate with nurses' education about pain and years of nursing experience. A general rule of thumb regarding pain in children is if an intervention would hurt an adult it will also hurt a child. As the nurse caring for a child, it may be effective to consider whether or not the procedure or intervention is painful. If so, it undoubtedly is painful to a child.

COMMON PAIN MISCONCEPTIONS

Over the years, several misconceptions related to children's pain have surfaced.

Misconception 1: Infants do not feel pain. The 30-week human fetus is capable of transmitting pain impulses to the brain, and newborns have been observed withdrawing purposefully from painful stimuli and crying in response to pain. Even though the human fetus and newborn transmit and receive pain impulses, this transmission occurs more slowly than in children or adults because of immature myelination. Therefore, it is inaccurate to assume pain does not affect newborns because they cannot remember the pain. Effective and judicious pain relief for newborns and infants is important.

Misconception 2: Infants and children are more sensitive than adults to opioid pain medication. Infants and children need to receive weight appropriate doses of opioid pain medication. They are no more susceptible to the unwanted side effects of respiratory depression or hypotension than older children or adults, and several authors have documented the safety of opioids for children (Anand, 2001). Risks associated with some medications do not outweigh the analgesic benefit.

Misconception 3: Pain is a character building experience. Some people believe less medication is a good thing and children will have to learn to deal with the pain. However, pain interrupts a child's appetite, sleep, and play. Indeed, pain is traumatic and not character building. It is true the pain from a surgical procedure or childhood illness differs in severity, duration, and cause from the normal bumps and bruises of childhood, but appropriate pain treatment is warranted for ill or hospitalized children.

Misconception 4: Children and adolescents will become addicted to opioids if used to treat pain. The actual risk of addiction is very low in these age groups (Agency for Health Care Policy and Research, 1992). In studies where adolescents are permitted to self-administer pain medication, they generally use less medication for shorter periods of time, and even when used for long periods of time, adolescents do not exhibit sign of dependence on pain medication. Concerns about psychological dependence on controlled substances, however, should be considered when medicating for chronic or long-term pain. Refer to Box 18-1 for definitions related to addiction, tolerance, and physical dependence.

Misconception 5: Children who are playing, sleeping, or can be distracted are not experiencing pain. Toddlers and preschool age children will look for ways to escape their pain and engage in developmentally appropriate tasks (play, make-believe) to relieve themselves from pain. Infants may sleep but still be in pain. A withdrawn adolescent may deny pain and be perceived as exhibiting developmentally appropriate behavior, but actually be experiencing unreported pain.

BOX 18-1 Terminology

Addiction: the psychological and physical need to use a medication for non-prescribed purposes. The desired effect is usually the euphoric feeling or "high" associated with opioid analgesics.

Tolerance: the need to use an increasing dose of a medication over time to achieve the desired effect. The body adapts to the presence of the medication and the analgesic effect can be reduced.

Physical dependence: physical adaptation to the presence of the medication in the blood stream. Patients should be weaned from the medication rather than abruptly stop receiving the medication

CHILD DEVELOPMENT AND PAIN

Children of various ages perceive pain in the context of their development level and their perceptions and understanding of the world around them colors their behaviors and perceptions about pain (Table 18-1).

Infants

A full-term newborn can localize and purposefully withdraw from painful stimuli. Infants have a distinctive cry when

TABLE 18-1 Developmental Stages and Pain Responses

Phase	Developmental Task	Unique Pain Response
Infancy	Trust vs. mistrust Sensorimotor	Cry, withdraw, furrowed brow, taut mouth.
Toddlerhood	Autonomy vs. shame and doubt Sensorimotor; Preoperational thought	Cry, scream, protest, withdraw.
Preschooler	Initiative vs. guilt Preoperational thought	Cry, localize body part, anticipate painful procedures. Body image concerns.
School-aged	Industry vs. inferiority Concrete operations	Body image concerns, may assume pain is punishment.
Adolescent	Identity vs. role confusion Formal operations	Assume pain will be treated, can conceptualize pain relief.

experiencing acute pain, characterized as high-pitched and shrill, followed by a period of apnea, then several short gasps or bursts of crying. This pattern is repeated throughout the painful experience (Frank & Gregory, 1993). Often, this cry is thought to be a response to another noxious stimuli, such as hunger or cold, but the distinct nature of this cry should alert the nurse to the presence of pain. A facial expression of pain may also accompany the cry. Here, the brow is furrowed, the mouth opens in a taut fashion, and the tongue is thrusted during the cry. Nasal flaring is usually present, and the facial expression is of distress, indicating pain.

Toddlers

Hospitalization or a health care experience (i.e., visits to the physician's office) is a new and challenging experience for a toddler, and often exposure to a painful procedure is associated with separation from parents or primary caregivers, heightening the toddler's anxiety and exacerbating the pain. Therefore, the toddler's age-appropriate protest to unpleasant or noxious stimuli may be confused with a response to pain. It is easy to identify when toddlers are in pain, but difficult to assess when the pain worsens as all painful stimuli demonstrate the same degree of intensity.

Preschoolers

The pain response may be subdued or less physical than expected for this age group, and lack of physical activity may indicate the preschooler is experiencing pain, because preschoolers, when healthy, are not capable of sitting or lying for long periods of time. The child of this age who does not readily run, jump, or wiggle may be in pain. Preschoolers also may not be capable of localizing pain, and use a general term like "stomach." However, they usually can not accurately differentiate what part of their "stomach" hurts, that is, chest, torso, back, or abdomen pain.

Preschoolers benefit from medical play prior to a painful procedure as touching and exploring the unfamiliar medical equipment may provoke some familiarity that helps them cope (Figure 18-2). However, the playing preschooler can be deceiving as many youngsters play despite pain, because this is normal and helps distract them from their pain. Play also helps these children cope with pain as some preschoolers use play to exhibit pain. For example, drawing or acting out the situation may help a preschooler explain

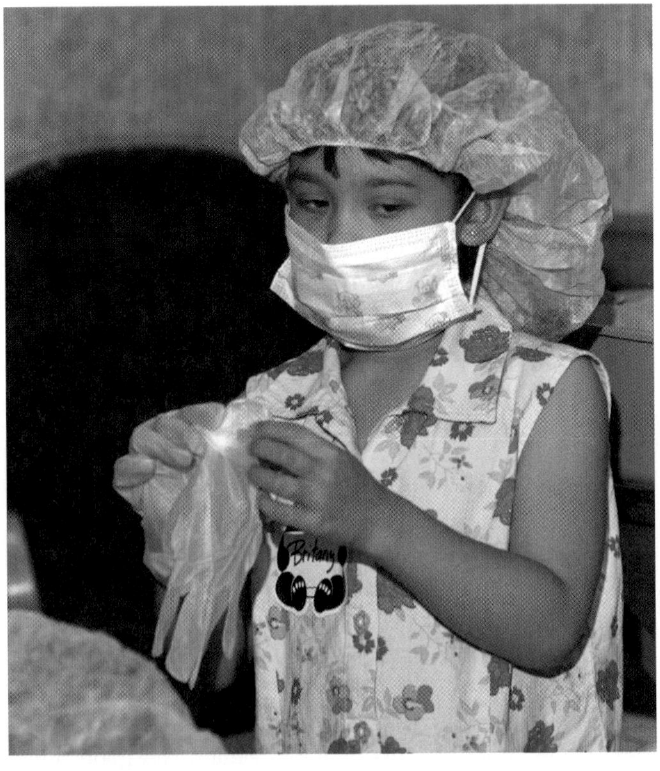

Figure 18-2 Medical play prior to procedures provides familiarity to help children cope with a painful experience.

pain as they describe "bad" or "sick" feelings without specifically saying they hurt or something is painful.

School-Age

School-aged children are concrete thinkers, learning cause and effect, and often experience pain in an "all or nothing" phenomena. When prompted, school-agers can recall today's hurt may be less intense than yesterday, but in response to open ended questions about pain, often maintain it continues until it is completely gone. Some school-aged children may have preconceived ideas about pain and its treatment. School-aged children also have many body image concerns and some fear their insides will leak out after receiving an injection or undergoing surgery. Therefore, covering all wounds can decrease their anxiety and help decrease their pain perception. School-aged children need to gain some control over their environment and should also be given choices whenever possible. Allowing a child to choose the limb for a painful procedure, or breaking down the procedure into as many steps as possible, highlighting that only one small part is painful, may help. In addition, they may view their pain as punishment or something they caused. This anticipation and anxiety may heighten their pain perception. Therefore, discussing treatment options prior to the painful event may help the child cope. However, preparation should be near the time the procedure is carried out and explained in age-appropriate terms.

Adolescents

Adolescents may feel they need to hide their pain ("grin and bear it"), and hesitate to report pain if they think everything is already being done to relieve it. Frequently, they deny pain to prove strength or in hopes of a quicker discharge from the hospital. Adolescents are also eager to demonstrate maturity by coping with significant pain, may be able to conceptualize their pain relative to other situations, and understand when pain has improved or will improve. Some adolescents deny pain because they are concerned about taking medications for pain. In addition, cultural or family values regarding the use of drugs can strongly influence how an adolescent experiences pain and how the pain is treated.

> **Critical Thinking**
>
> **An Adolescent in Pain**
>
> What would you say to Heather, a 16-year-old in obvious pain who refuses medications because she fears addiction? What if her family agreed and supported her decision?

Therefore, in caring for adolescents in pain, the nurse should acknowledge and frequently assess their pain. Although adolescents crave independence, it is important to include parents or family members in discussions regarding effective pain treatment.

Adolescents may also use distraction to relieve their pain by watching videos, listening to audiotapes, playing games, or sleeping. The lack of interest in discussing pain does not mean adolescents do not have pain, but they might need assistance developing assessment strategies to best treat their pain. The adolescent should be included in these discussions and consulted regarding treatment options.

PAIN ASSESSMENT

Accurate and complete assessment of a child's pain can lead to better and more effective intervention. Several areas related to pain assessment follow.

Pain Interview and History

The initial assessment should include comprehensive information about the child's pain experiences, treatments, and successes. The nurse should also query the child and caregiver about interventions and coping strategies that have helped in the past. Questions should be asked about procedural and other types of painful experiences, and the PQRST format used to find out about pain. Following the PQRST system, the child is given the opportunity to describe and rate his or her pain using a self-rating scale (Box 18-2).

Caregivers should also be asked about the child's pain. For children developmentally or cognitively too young to rate or discuss their own pain, parent information should be valued as if the client had responded. Table 18-2 lists questions that the nurse can use in obtaining a pain history.

Assessment Measures

A number of assessment measures have been developed to quantify a child's pain. They are divided into two categories:

> **BOX 18-2 The PQRST pain assessment**
>
> P–presence of pain "Are you hurting today?"
>
> Q–quality "What words describe your pain?" (i.e., sharp, burning, tingling ...)
>
> R–radiation/location "Where is your pain? Does it shoot or radiate anywhere else?"
>
> S–severity "Give me a number between 0–10 for your pain."
>
> T–timing "How long have you had this pain? How long does it last when the pain comes?"

TABLE 18-2 Pain History Questions

Child Questions	Caregiver Questions
Tell me what pain is to you.	What words does your child use to describe pain?
Tell me about times you have hurt before today.	Describe the pain experiences your child has had.
Who do you tell if you hurt?	Who does your child tell when he/she hurts?
What do you do for yourself when you hurt?	How do you know when your child is in pain?
What do you want others to do for you when you hurt?	How does your child usually react when he/she is in pain?
What don't you want others to do for you when you hurt?	What do you do to help your child when he/she is hurting?
What helps the most to take your pain away?	What does your child do to help himself/herself when he/she hurts?
	What works best to decrease or relieve your child's pain?
Is there anything else you want to tell me about when you hurt? (If yes, describe)	Is there any thing special you would like me to know about your child's pain? (If yes, describe)

Adapted from Hester, N.O., & Barcus, C.S. (1986). Assessment and management of children in pain. Pediatrics: Nursing Update, 1, *2–8.*

objective measures used by the nurse or other health care professional to score client behavior or vital sign changes, and self-reporting instruments designed so children may rate their own pain.

Objective Measures

Objective pain measures are ideal for the infant, preverbal child, or developmentally delayed child who is not able to actively participate in pain assessment. Most objective rating measures score behaviors and physiological changes to determine the intensity of pain experienced, and are most useful for acute pain since reliability and validity are less well established for long-term pain. Objective pain assessment measures are most effective when combined with self-reporting tools for children and adolescents because they are able to report or score their own pain. The postoperative pain scale is valid for children over 12 years of age as a measure of acute pain and provides an objective means of assessing the pain. However, instruments like this are best used for acute or short-term pain or when a child is unable to readily communicate pain. Objective measures are also a useful method of documenting improvements in pain intensity over time, especially postoperatively.

Reflective Thinking

Two Boys–Differences in Pain Perception

You are caring for two young boys of approximately the same age who underwent the same operative procedure on the same day. Abraham is walking in the hall three times per day, playing video games, and talking on the phone. Joshua lies in bed moaning, is reluctant to walk, and is not interested in any activities. Both children have the same pain rating by objective or subjective measure. Would you discount one rating based on a comparison of the children's behaviors? Would your perceptions affect the care you deliver or pain medication given to relieve each child's pain?

Eye On:

Perception of Pain

Culture determines the way persons derive meaning from their lives and also determines appropriate behaviors. One's cultural upbringing teaches behaviors, including those that are exhibited when in pain. People from different cultures use different types of words to describe pain (for example, in sensory or emotional terms). These differences should not be ignored, but the nurse also needs to be careful not to prejudge a client based on cultural background or ethnicity. Due to the unique experience of pain, the person will exhibit individualized behaviors even though they are influenced by cultural upbringing.

From White, L. (2001). *Foundations of nursing.* Albany, NY: Delmar.

Subjective (Self-rating) Measures

In all types of pain, the most information can be gained when children measure the pain themselves. Several methods assist children rate their own pain, and the choice of a specific measure should be based on the child's developmental level and preferences, institutional policies, and instrument availability (Figures 18-3, 18-4, and 18-5). A quantifiable measure of pain also adds to validity when discussing pain treatment with members of the health care team because reporting a child's pain by numbers or measures is more credible than saying "she says she hurts."

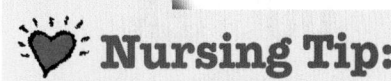

> **Nursing Tip:**
>
> **Pain assessment measures**
>
> Many institutions where children are cared for agree on a consistent pediatric pain assessment measure. Recommend a measure of your choice if there is not one consistently used where you practice.

However, the limitation to all instruments is their availability and consistency of use when accurately assessing pain. Table 18-3 describes several pediatric pain assessment tools.

Research Highlight

Pain Perception/Assessment after Cardiac Surgery

Study Purpose

To examine children's perception of pain after cardiac surgery and review current and previous nursing practice in regards to pain assessment, intervention, and evaluation for children after cardiac surgery.

Methods

A retrospective chart review was used initially to examine the care, pain assessment, and interventions children ages 0–3 and 3–18 received. Children, ages 3–18, were then enrolled in the study to have their pain assessed after cardiac surgery. The child's perception and nurses' assessments of pain were compared to the practices identified in the chart review so that comparisons of the nurses' perceptions of pain with children's perceptions could be made.

Findings

The nurses' assessments of the child's pain and the child's perceptions differed. The interventions the nurse performed did not match the child's pain ratings. Factors affecting the child were the perception of pain including location of the incision and previous cardiac surgery experiences. Factors affecting the amount of analgesic administered included the postoperative day (more medication administered closer to surgery), the child's age, and whether or not the child was intubated (extubated patients received less medication). Several areas of nursing practice, including consistent use of pain assessment, pain assessment at regular intervals, and use of pain rating scales for all children were identified as needing future study.

Implications

Nurses need to develop pain assessment strategies and integrate them on a regular basis into bedside care as the child's overall medical status is not always an indicator of the level of pain. Nursing staff should also receive consistent education about pain assessment and interventions for children with similar medical diagnosis.

Citation

McRae, M., Rourke, D., & Imperia-Perez, F. (1997). Development of a research-based standard for assessment, intervention and evaluation of pain after neonatal and pediatric cardiac surgery. *Pediatric Nursing 23*(3), 263–271.

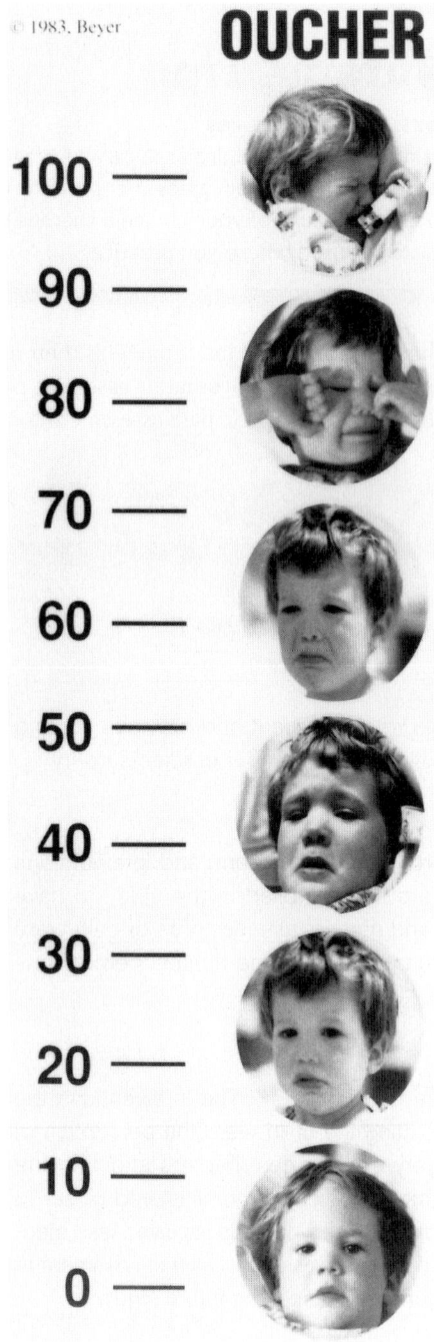

Figure 18-3 The Oucher Pain Assessment Tool: For Use with Children 3–12 Years of Age. Caucasian, Hispanic, and African-American versions are available. The Caucasian version of the Oucher, developed and copyrighted by Judith E. Beyer, RN, PhD, 1983. Used with permission.

For the verbal child, a simple pain assessment scale of 0 to 10 or 0 to 5 may be the most helpful. Here, the nurse asks the child to rate pain on a scale where "zero is no pain at all" and ten is "the worst pain ever you can imagine" (Figure 18-6). The scale points should be documented

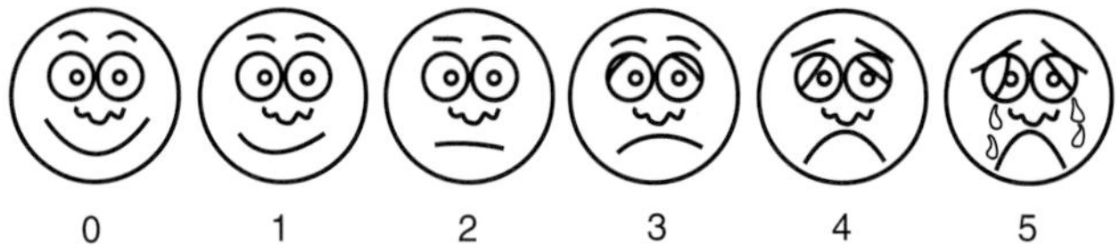

Figure 18-4 Wong/Baker FACES Pain Rating Scale. From Wong, D. L., Hockenberry-Eaton, M., Wilson, D., Winkelstein, M. L., & Schwartz, P. (2001). *Wong's Essentials of Pediatric Nursing*, 6th ed., p. 1301, St. Louis: Mosby. Copyright Mosby. Reprinted with permission.

when recording the child's measure of pain (i.e., "rates pain 5 out of 10" rather than "rates pain a 5"). Drawing a ten centimeter line and asking the child to point to the level of pain on the line may also be effective.

MANAGEMENT OF ACUTE PAIN

Feeling pain is a likely experience for most children when they come in contact with the health care system. With careful planning and consideration, much of this pain can be minimized or eliminated. Therefore, the nurse caring for the child in any situation should advocate for the child and parent or caregiver to help treat the child's pain. Every child has the right to appropriate and safe pain relief and nurses play a major role in assessing, treating, and managing a child's pain.

Goals of Acute Pain Management

Pain associated with a surgical procedure or a specific disease state is described as acute pain. The intensity of acute pain fades predictably over a few days or a week, and most hospitalized children experience a phase of acute pain that is nearly resolved by discharge.

The impact of effective pain treatment for children cannot be underestimated. Pain has serious physical and psychological consequences, such as increased oxygen uptake in the blood and alteration in blood glucose metabolism. The benefits of aggressive pain treatment before, during, and after surgery or invasive procedures, has longer-term benefits. Prevention is better in treating acute pain because pain that has already occurred and is severe is difficult to control. Children and their families should be told that effective pain treatment is available and an expected part of their recovery care.

Goals and expectations of pain management should also be discussed with the child and family as they can be involved in choosing assessment strategies and developing pain management techniques. Whenever possible, the child and family should be prepared for pain associated with a procedure or surgical intervention. Finally, the preparation

CODE ____________

DATE ____________

Adolescent and Pediatric Pain Tool (APPT)

INSTRUCTIONS:

1. Color in the areas on these drawings to show where you have pain. Make the marks as big or small as the place where the pain is.

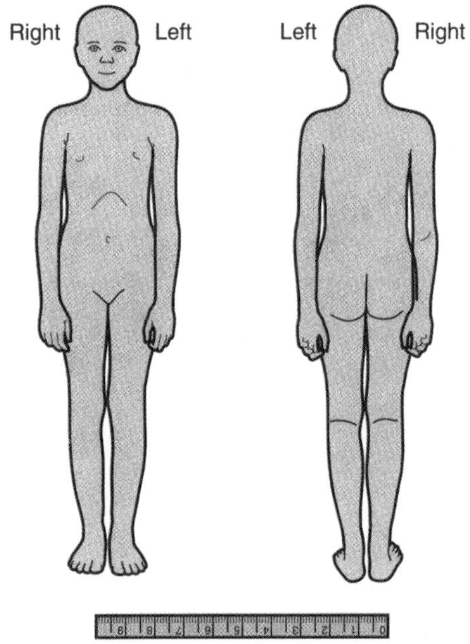

2. Place a straight, up and down mark on this line to show how much pain you have.

No pain — Little pain — Medium pain — Large pain — Worst possible pain

3. Point to or circle as many of these words that describe your pain.

1: annoying, bad, horrible, miserable, terrible, uncomfortable

2: aching, hurting, like an ache, like a hurt, sore

3: beating, hitting, pounding, punching, throbbing

4: biting, cutting, like a pin, like a sharp knife, pin like, sharp, stabbing

5: blistering, burning, hot

6: cramping, crushing, like a pinch, pinching, pressure

7: itching, like a scratch, like a sting, scratching, stinging

8: shocking, shooting, splitting

9: numb, stiff, swollen, tight

10: awful, deadly, dying, killing

11: crying, frightening, screaming, terrifying

12: dizzy, sickening, suffocating

13: never goes away, uncontrollable

14: always, comes and goes, comes on all of a sudden, constant, continuous, forever

15: off and on, once in a while, sneaks up, sometimes, steady

If you like, you may add other words:

____

____

____

For office use only.

BSA: ________
IS: ________

#S (2-9)	____	/37= ____	%
#A (10-12)	____	/11= ____	%
#E (1,13)	____	/8= ____	%
#T (14,15)	____	/11= ____	%
Total	____	/67= ____	%

Figure 18-5 Adolescent and Pediatric Pain Tool. From Savedra, M. C., Tesler, M. D., Holzemer, W. L., & Ward, J. A. (1992). University of California, San Francisco, School of Nursing, San Francisco, CA 94143-0606. Copyright © 1989, 1992. Used with permission.

TABLE 18-3 Pediatric Self-rating Pain Assessment Tools

Description	Resources	Comments
Photos of children in pain	Oucher (Beyer, et al., 1992)	The Oucher pediatric pain intensity scale consists of two scales: a 0 to 100 numeric scale and a 6-point facial scale. If the child can count from 1 to 100 by ones or by tens, the numeric scale can be used; if not, the facial scale can be used. The facial scale has been successfully used in children as young as 3 to 4 years (see Figure 18-3).

continues

TABLE 18-3 *Continued*

Description	Resources	Comments
Drawn faces of children in pain	Faces (Wong & Baker, 2001); the Faces Pain Scale (Bieri, et al., 1990)	The Wong/Baker Faces Pain Rating Scale can be used with children as young as 3 years. It helps children express their level of pain by pointing to a cartoon face that most closely resembles how they are feeling. Directions available in Spanish (see Figure 18-4).
Body image to locate pain	Adolescent and Pediatric Pain Tool (APPT) (Savedra, et al., 1992). Eland Color Tool (Eland, 1993)	Front and back body images used to locate pain; APPT also contains lists of words to describe pain and line to plot pain severity (see Figure 18-5). Eland uses colors to signify varying pain locations of increasing intensity.
Numbers or other quantifiers	Hester Poker Chips (1979); Visual Analogue Scale	The Poker Chip Tool uses of four red poker chips. The chips are aligned horizontally on a hard surface in front of the child, and they are described as "pieces of hurt." The chips are described from left to right as just a little bit of hurt, a little more hurt, more hurt, and the most hurt you could ever have. The child is then asked, "How many pieces of hurt do you have right now?" This tool can be used with children 4 to 13 years old. Visual Analogue Scale has pain descriptor words that correspond with numbers, from 1-10. Hester has instructions in English and Spanish.

From Eland, J. (1993). Children with pain. In O. B. Jackson & R. B. Saunders (Eds.), Child health nursing. *Philadelphia: J.B. Lippincott.*

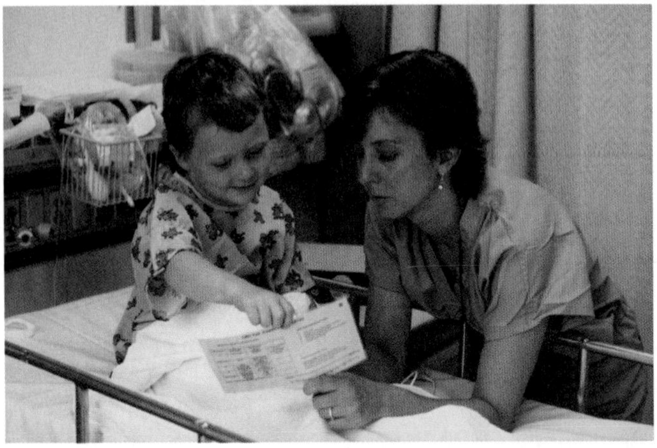

Figure 18-6 Nurse and children review a pain rating scale prior to the child experiencing pain.

and discussion should include treatment options. The main goals of effective pain management are to relieve pain, maximize function, and minimize side effects.

Relieve Pain

The chosen treatment should first and most importantly improve or relieve the pain. However, it may not be practical or possible to relieve all the pain unless the child is unconscious. Children and their families need to understand the limitations of effective pain management.

Maximize Function

Effective pain treatment allows the child the opportunity to walk, eat, and otherwise participate in the recovery process. Adequate pain control may contribute to a shorter hospital stay and promote quicker return to normal function.

Minimize Side Effects

All medications have side effects; some are unpleasant. Most commonly prescribed pain medications also have the potential for unpleasant or harmful side effects, but these drugs are dosed or delivered so side effects are minimized. For example, a patient controlled device may deliver intravenous opioids so the client receives the amount of medication desired with few side effects. If side effects do occur most can be adequately treated with adjunct medication that promotes pain relief without other effects.

Nonpharmacologic Pain Management

A strong nurse-client-family relationship promotes accurate reporting of pain as the client learns to trust pain will be managed. An understanding of methods to comfort the child when caregivers are not available can assist in managing the child's pain. Several specific pain management modalities, which are most effective when taught prior to the anticipated pain, should be discussed with the child and caregivers. Some techniques may be practiced prior to the painful situation or the child may use strategies that worked in the past. However, it may not be practical or effective to use more than one modality at a time. In addition, nonpharmacologic techniques should be used in conjunction with pharmacologic treatments whenever possible because the intent of these strategies is not to replace pharmacologic treatments for pain but rather to enhance the effects of the medications.

Many children and caregivers have developed their own independent strategies to deal with pain. The nurse should always explore these individualized strategies of pain management with the child and family and inform other members of the health care team. All attempts should be made to promote and continue these strategies in the acute care setting. Specific nonpharmacologic pain management strategies are described in Table 18–4.

TABLE 18-4 Non-pharmacologic Pain Management Techniques

Name of Intervention	Step-by-step Description	Uses
Distraction	1. Ask the family/child to identify the child's favorite activities, toys, and so forth. 2. Consider incorporating audio or videotapes, television, music. 3. Promote play as the child would in his or her usual state of health. 4. Encourage interactions with same age children.	All age groups. Strategies are good for ongoing acute pain (i.e., after surgery) or for procedural pain (i.e., burn patients during dressing changes).
Preparation	1. Explain in developmentally appropriate terms what the child can expect to see, feel, hear, smell, or taste. Confirm the child understands the explanation. 2. Give realistic time frames for each sensation. 3. The younger the child, the closer to the time of the procedure preparation should occur. Prepare the child for what to expect and be honest about pain. 4. Encourage the child to safely play with equipment and act out the procedure on a doll or toy.	Most effective for preschool, school-aged, or adolescent patients. Limited use in toddlers, not appropriate for infants. Should occur prior to a procedure expected to cause pain.
Relaxation	1. Position the child in a comfortable position. 2. Ask the child to take a deep breath, relaxing as they breathe in and out. 3. Starting with the toes, instruct the child to progressively relax body parts until the head is reached. 4. Decrease as much outside stimulation as possible	For school–aged or adolescent clients. Ideally, the instructions should be made prior to the pain. Useful for chronic pain. May be used as frequently as desired.
Cutaneous stimulation	1. Rub affected area in a consistent manner. 2. Apply ice or heat as warranted and desired to affected area or contralateral area. 3. Apply consistent gentle pressure to site of pain. 4. Use of a TENS (transcutaneous electrical nerve stimulator) also possible.	Useful for all age groups as tolerated. Combining techniques (i.e., heat and rubbing) is of maximum benefit.
Self exercises	1. Positive Thinking—Gives the child a positive focus "I will get better soon." 2. Thought Stopping—Memorize and repeat a statement focusing on positives of situation. "Short procedure, nice nurse, go home soon."	Most appropriate for older children. Encourage creativity and parent input. Good for children with chronic or cancer pain.

continues

TABLE 18-4 *Continued*

Name of Intervention	Step-by-step Description	Uses
Self exercises *(cont.)*	3. Guided Imagery—Formal exercise to help children through painful situations. Ask the child to envision a pleasant situation (real or imagined). Encourage the child to "go there" whenever the pain occurs. The child may need to develop a script of pleasant places and record it or write it down. When needed, the script may be played or read to the child. Details about the experience (sounds, smells, colors, textures) are included. Encourage the child to concentrate on the pleasant experience whenever pain is felt.	
Hypnosis	Focused attention, altered state of consciousness (Valente, 1991). Specially trained personnel should induce hypnotic state.	Used with painful procedures, especially those with burns, sickle cell disease, cancer, nausea, and vomiting associated with cancer treatment (Valente, 1991).

Other successful nonpharmacologic interventions include biofeedback, caregiver involvement, hypnosis, cutaneous stimulation (rubbing, massaging, holding), and applying heat (promotes muscle relaxation, increases blood circulation) or cold (slows ability of pain fibers to transmit pain, decreases inflammation, decreases edema).

Pharmacologic Pain Management

The nurse is responsible for understanding the expected action, potential side effects, and interactions of medications prescribed for clients. Because nurses may be administering medication, they also need to be able to answer the family's questions and observe for side effects. With appropriate dosing, the medications can be used for children of all ages. A broad understanding of the classifications of analgesics follows.

Opioid Analgesics

Opioid analgesics are a class of medications derived from the opium plant for the specific purpose of relieving pain. Used alone or in combination with other medications, opioids are among the strongest pain medications and the cornerstone of management for moderate to severe pain, including acute pain (postoperative pain) and long-term chronic pain (cancer pain). Research confirms that the use of opioids for pain relief is unlikely to result in addiction even when used for the long term (Paice, 1992).

Opioid analgesics are effective when administered in small, frequent doses. The technique of delivering small doses of the medication until the desired effect (pain relief) is observed is called **titration.** Titrating the dose up or down may be necessary in order to obtain adequate analgesia with minimal side effects. Opioids are unique in that they have no **ceiling dose** (there is no point after which they are no longer effective). In the most severe pain situations, opioid analgesics can be titrated to extremely high doses if needed to achieve adequate analgesia with minimal side effects.

Morphine is the gold standard of opioids, and the effectiveness, cost, and uses of other opioids are compared to morphine. For children, opioids are dosed by weight. Neonatal doses are reduced by one-third to one-quarter to account for their immature liver function and differences in metabolism. (See Table 18-5 for specific dosing recommendations). Larger children (greater than 50 kilograms) may receive adult doses. Appropriate dosing is an important aspect of pain management and care should be taken to appropriately individualize the dose so as to promote adequate analgesia and minimize side effects. Most intravenous opioids can also be converted to oral doses of the same or similar opioids. Side effects of opioids are most commonly nausea, vomiting, and itching.

Rather than discontinue the use of opiods, side effects should be treated. If a child is experiencing severe side effects from an opioid analgesic and not receiving adequate pain relief, a different, non-opioid pain medication should be added to the pain management protocol to augment pain relief while minimizing side effects.

Respiratory depression and hypotension are rare and dangerous side effects of opioid analgesic that can be treated with naroxolone (Narcan) at a dose that reverses respiratory

TABLE 18-5 Selected Opioid Pain Medications for Children

Medication	Initial (starting) dosing guidelines	Comments
Morphine Sulfate	Parenteral: 0.05–0.1 mg/kg q 3–4 hours Oral: 0.3–0.5 mg/kg q 4 hrs	Oral formulation in elixir and tablets. Elixir ideal for younger children who cannot swallow tablets.
Fentanyl	Parenteral: 0.5–2 mcg/kg q 1–2 hours Transmucosal/transdermal: 10–15 mcg/kg	Unique side effect with parenteral dosing is chest wall rigidity. (Reversed with naloxone Narcan). Transmucosal (Fentanyl Oralet) for single dose administration. Transdermal not recommended in children.
Meperidine	Parenteral: 1 mg/kg q 3–4 hours Oral: 1–1.5 mg/kg q 6 hours	Not usually recommended in children as metabolite accumulation (normeperidine) lowers seizure threshold.
Methadone	Parenteral/Oral: 0.1–0.2 mg/kg q 8–12 hours	Parenteral to oral conversion is 1:1. Oral formulation available as elixir or tablets.
Hydromorphone	Parenteral: 0.015 mg/kg q 3–4 hours Oral: 0.02 mg/kg q 3–4 hours	Often associated with less itching, nausea/vomiting side effects than other opioids.
Codeine	Parenteral: not recommended because of poor and painful site absorption and high occurrence of side effects Oral: 1mg/kg q 3–4 hrs	Available as elixir and tablets combined with acetaminophen. This form is less expensive than codeine alone.
Oxycodone	Parenteral: not available Oral: 0.1 mg/kg q 4–6 hours	Available as elixir and tablets combined with acetaminophen (Percocet; Tylox).
Hydrocodone	Parenteral: not available Oral: 0.1–0.2 mg/kg q 4–6 hours	Available as elixir and tablets combined with acetaminophen (Vicodin) or ibuprofen (Viciprofen).

Adapted from Agency for Health Care Policy and Research (1992). Acute pain management in infants, children and adolescents: Operative and medical procedures; *Yaster, M., et al., (Eds.). (1997).* Pediatric pain management and sedation handbook; Children's Memorial Hospital formulary handbook *(1999).*

depression but does not reverse analgesic effects. Dosing of Naroxolone is given in Box 18–3.

Opioids can be dosed at different intervals; commonly, they are on a PRN schedule and administered when pain is assessed or reported. However, this dosing interval is inappropriate for children. First, PRN dosing places the onus to request medication for pain on the child and many children do not report their pain. Second, children may fear the treatment for pain will be an injection. Third, despite repeated instructions, children may forget the pain medication is available upon request. Finally, very young children are not able to request pain medication because of undeveloped language skills. Therefore, an alternative to PRN dosing is "reverse PRN" medication delivery. Here, the nurse asks about or assesses the client's pain at the prescribed time interval the medication may be administered. Medication is

BOX 18-3 Naroxolone (Narcan) dosing

0.1 mg/kg, IV, ETT, q 1–2 minutes to maximum, 2 mg/kg.

Nursing Alert:

Fentanyl

Fentanyl has a unique, additional side effect: chest wall rigidity. Here, the client is unable to breathe because of ineffective movement of the chest wall muscles, and manual ventilation is difficult. Carefully screen clients for this side effect, which is reversible with Naroxolone.

Nursing Tip:

Reverse PRN method

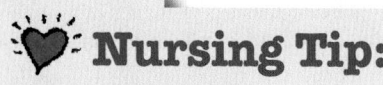

When using the reverse PRN method, prompt children by informing them pain medication is available and will be available again. For example, "It is time for your pain medication. Would you like it now?" The children can make their own decisions regarding accepting or declining the medication. For infants and toddlers, perform a pain assessment when it is time to administer the medication and administer as warranted.

REFLECTIONS FROM FAMILIES

Barbara was really hurting after her appendectomy. I had visions of her being in agony for hours. I was so impressed with the nurses. They gave her pain medication right after she got to the unit from the recovery room and would always check her within a short time to be sure her pain was lessened. They also asked her a few hours later how her pain was since it was probably time for more medication.

then administered if pain is present. Often children respond favorably to this method.

Analgesics may also be administered using an around-the-clock dosing schedule. Here, the child receives pain medications at preset intervals. However, the effects of the medication should be continually reassessed to assure the child is receiving adequate analgesia. The side effects and level of analgesia are also continually monitored, and if side effects appear, the medication may be titrated, discontinued, or a substitute analgesic given.

Nursing Alert:

Opioid-induced Respiratory Depression

Opioids can have a cumulative effect. Monitor clients on an around-the-clock dosing schedule for oversedation leading to respiratory depression.

Nonsteroidal Anti-inflammatory Drugs (NSAIDs)

Nonsteroidal anti-inflammatory drugs (NSAIDs) may be used independently to treat mild to moderate pain or in conjunction with opioids to treat more severe pain. NSAIDS work by inhibiting prostaglandins at the site of the pain. The most common NSAIDS are ibuprofen (Advil), naproxen (Naprosyn), and ketorolac (Toradol). Aspirin is also an NSAID, but rarely used in children because of its association with Reye's syndrome. Table 18-6 reviews dosing for this class of medications.

Other Drugs

Acetaminophen is not an anti-inflammatory drug because it does not inhibit prostaglandins. The drug of choice for fever in children, acetaminophen is also effective for relieving mild to moderate pain, and may be used in conjunction with opioids or NSAIDS for moderate to severe pain.

Patient-Controlled Analgesia

Patient-controlled analgesia (PCA) is a computer operated pump that allows the patient to self-administer pain medication. By pushing a button on the pump, children as young as 5 or 6 years old may self-administer intravenous opioids to relieve pain. Patient-controlled analgesia is available to most children in the acute care setting and may also be administered at home. The PCA dosing regime allows for a steady drug state and more consistent analgesia while avoiding the undesired side effects associated with delivering relatively large doses of bolus analgesics. The delivery of small frequent doses of opioids provides better pain relief without sedation. By maintaining a steady amount of the analgesic, the child receives better pain control at less risk (Figure 18-7).

There are several advantages of PCA pain relief over traditional treatment modalities. Aside from the already mentioned advantages of superior analgesia and safer drug delivery, PCA offers the child the ability to immediately and independently relieve pain. The dose is tailored to the patient's weight and easily titrated for a child's changing pain control needs. A number of medications are now available for delivery via a PCA pump: morphine, meperdine (Demerol), fentanyl, and hydromorphone (Dilaudid).

PCA pumps offer several programming options. The pump may be programmed in "PCA only" mode, where doses of the medication are delivered only when the client demands a dose by pushing the button. In the "PCA plus (+) continuous" mode, the pump delivers a pre-programmed background infusion of the analgesic and administers additional medication according to patient request. The PCA (+) continuous mode is especially effective for young children who are often remiss or do not realize they need to push the button to administer their analgesic. The use of different modalities should be tailored to the child's ability to push the

TABLE 18-6 Selected Nonsteroidal Anti-inflammatory Pain Medications

Medication	Initial Dosing Guidelines	Comments
Ibuprofen	4–10 mg/kg po q 6 hours.	Associated with gastric irritation. Administer with food or milk. Available as solution or chewable or swallowable tablet. Do not administer with other NSAIDs.
Acetylsalicylic acid/ Aspirin	10–15 mg/kg po q 4 hours Maximum daily dose: 75 mg/kg/day up to 4 gm/day	Associated with Reye's syndrome. Do not administer to any child with viral illness within the last 4 weeks.
Ketorolac	Oral dose: 10 mg/dose (Adult) Parenteral: 0.5mg/kg q 6 hours Maximum single dose: 30 mg Maximum daily dose: 120 mg/day	Do not administer for longer than five continuous days because of increased incidence of gastric bleeding, renal insufficiency. Do not administer with other NSAIDs.
Naproxen	5–7 mg/kg po q 8–12 hours Maximum dose: 1.5 gm/day	Available as solution or tablets. Do not administer with other NSAIDs.

Adapted from Agency for Health Care Policy and Research (1992) Acute pain management in infants, children and adolescents: Operative and medical procedures; *Yaster, M., Cote, C., Krane, E., Kaplan, R., & Lappe, D. (Eds.). (1997).* Pediatric pain management and sedation handbook; Children's Memorial Hospital formulary handbook *(1999).*

PCA button, considering developmental level and the anticipated pain management needs.

Local/Regional Anesthesia

Several techniques are now available to relive pain using local or regional anesthesia. Here, the area of the body where the pain is expected to be may be numbed by using a local or regional anesthetic injection with or without an opioid. Procedural pain (lumbar puncture, bone marrow aspirate) may also be reduced by using a euteric mixture of local anesthetics (EMLA) (lidocaine and prilocaine) or TAC (tetracaine, adrenoline, cocaine) two local anesthetic creams (Zempsky & Karasic, 1997). Both are applied to the skin prior to the procedure (EMLA up to 3 hours), covered with an occlusive dressing, and can eliminate the pain of the initial injection for most children (Figure 18-8).

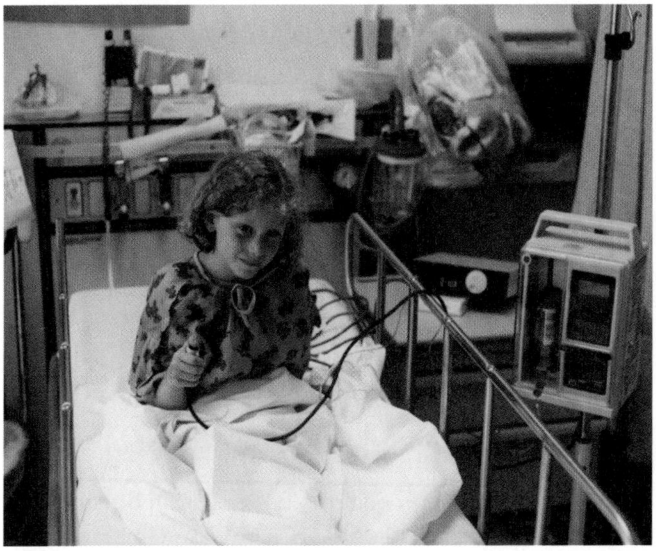

Figure 18-7 This child is using her PCA pump.

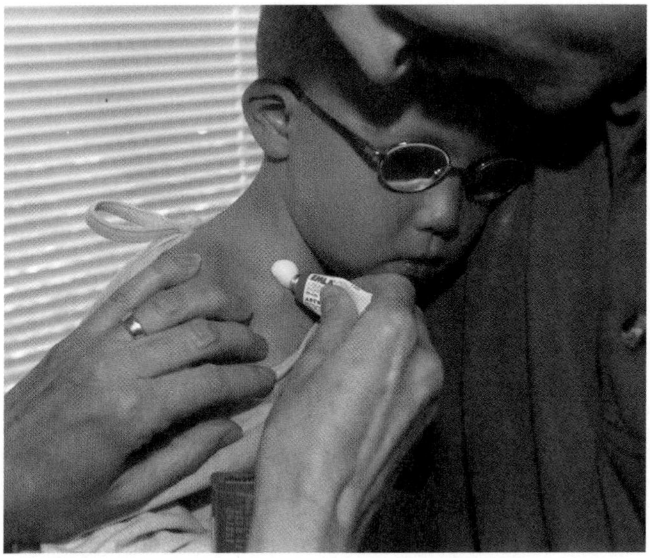

Figure 18-8 EMLA Application

Case Study/Care Plan

Pain Management

Ryan is a 2-year-old boy who had surgery twelve hours ago for a congenital hip problem. He is in a full body cast and constantly cries and grabs at his cast. The night shift nurse is concerned he is not getting adequate pain relief from his current analgesic regime of 2 mg IV morphine every 3 hours PRN and acetaminophen rectally every six hours. Ryan is scheduled to go home in the morning with his grandmother, Mary, his primary caregiver. She, too, is concerned about his current pain and how she will manage his pain at home.

Nursing Care Plan

Assessment

1. Assess and quantify Ryan's pain on a 0–5 or 0–10 point scale.
2. Incorporate feedback from Mary regarding his usual behavior and response to pain.
3. Review vital sign trends since surgery to ascertain changes associated with pain.

Nursing Diagnosis

Pain related to surgical procedure.

Expected Outcomes

1. Ryan will receive relief from his pain.
2. Caregiver will support him during his painful experience.

Interventions/*Rationales*

1. Administer morphine every 3 hours. *A two-year-old child is too young for PRN dosing and unable to consistently request pain medication.*
2. Request oral acetaminophen dosing if he will tolerate it. *The pain medication should be delivered in the least invasive route.*
3. Apply cold packs to painful area by laying them on cast. *The cold will minimize the inflammation at the site of pain.*
4. Ask Ryan's grandmother how he usually sleeps at home and position him accordingly. *Provides Ryan with his usual means of comfort.*
5. Provide age-appropriate distractions. Incorporate familiar or favorite objects from home. *The anxiety from the hospitalization may contribute to his pain.*
6. Involve Ryan's grandmother in all aspects of his care. *As his primary caregiver, she is most familiar with how to comfort him.*

Evaluation

Evaluate Ryan's pain 30 minutes after analgesic administered with the same assessment tool. Document improvements in pain.

Regional anesthesia is applied to a region of the body, usually in association with a surgical procedure by blocking or numbing specific nerves or nerve segments prior to the surgical procedure to prevent the pain sensation. Some surgeries or procedures are performed using only local or regional anesthesia. In such cases, the area may be numb for a period of time (2–12 hours) following the procedure.

Kids Want To Know

Numbness

"I can't feel my foot. Is it still there?" Peter asks after receiving a local anesthetic.

Assure Peter that the feeling of numbness is temporary from medication and will subside.

Show Peter his foot by moving blankets, using a mirror, or repositioning.

Family Teaching

Chronic Pain

Household activities should not revolve around the child's pain. Advise caregivers not to question the child every day regarding the pain, so as not to emphasize the experience or promote secondary gains. The child should be asked to only discuss pain if there is a significant change in the pain experienced.

Epidural or Intraspinal Analgesia

Opioids and/or local anesthetics can also be administered via the epidural or intraspinal route. This method of delivery provides complete analgesia for surgery or postoperatively, when medications are delivered via a single injection that last 2–12 hours or by an indwelling catheter that remains in for 1 to 5 days. The catheter is generally removed after five days, because of the increased risk of infection.

Conscious Sedation

Conscious sedation allows a child to be both pain free and also sedated for a procedure (bone marrow aspirate, wound care, endoscopy, MRI, liver biopsy). Children also have less anxiety and rarely remember the procedure (Litman, 1995). This depressed state of consciousness, obtained by IV analgesia, leaves protective reflexes intact and allows the child to respond to verbal instructions while the procedure is occurring (American Academy of Pediatrics, Committee on Drugs, 1992). Commonly used drugs for this method of pain management include morphine, fentanyl, midazolam (Versed), pentobarbitol (Nembutal), and chloral hydrate.

CHRONIC PAIN

Chronic pain, when compared to acute pain, varies in its presentation, treatment, and expected outcomes. Persisting for long periods of time, generally longer than 3 months, chronic pain hinders daily function and changes a child's opportunity to participate in age-appropriate activities. Chronic pain, difficult and frustrating to treat, can appear as headache or abdominal pain in children.

Headaches

Recurrent and chronic headaches are a common neurologic complaint in children. In fact, 2.5% of 7 year olds suffer from headaches, and when 15 years old, 15.7% of these same children have similar complaints (Johnson & Oski, 1997). Children experience several types of headaches and special attention should be paid to rule out an organic cause of the headache. Headache can be the presenting symptom for several types of brain tumors (see Chapter 29) and major depression in children (Johnson & Oski, 1997). For other children, headache may be the diagnosis rather than a symptom of another disorder. Common headaches seen in children and adolescents include migraine and chronic tension headaches.

Migraine or cluster headaches are intense and often associated with nausea or photophobia (light sensitivity). They tend to involve the frontal or temporal regions of the head or are localized retro-orbitally (Johnson & Oski, 1997). The child can often predict the onset of a migraine headache by an **aura,** or premonition of its beginning. They last from several hours to days and can be very debilitating. Often, there is a positive family history of migraines. Several medications have been effective in treating migraine headaches, including Fiorinal, Midrin, and sumatriptan (Imitrex). Biofeedback and relaxation therapy as well as prophylactic treatment with propanolol (Inderal), phenobarbital, and amitriptyline (Elavil) have also proven successful (Johnson & Oski, 1997).

Chronic tension headaches are most often seen in adolescents or older school-aged children. They tend to involve the temporal or occipital regions bilaterally, are diffuse, extend to the neck, and are continuous during the day (Johnson & Oski, 1997). Stress in the child's life is a contributing factor in this type of headache and steps should be taken to identify the stressors. Often, these children become accustomed to having a headache and can no longer identify the inciting triggers or situations. Children suffering from chronic tension headaches are best treated with a program combining stress management, behavior management, and individual and family therapy (Johnson & Oski, 1997).

Abdominal Pain

Abdominal pain is another common chronic pain complaint in children (Berkowitz, 2000; Kirschner & Black, 1998). It is classified as visceral (dull or crampy and poorly localized), somatic (reflects peritoneal inflammation; is localized to the area of the involved viscera), or referred (caused by local irritation and referral along the organ's innervation pathway) (Kirschner & Black, 1998). An organic cause of a child's abdominal pain should always be explored because it may indicate colic, food allergy, intusussception, appendicitis, Meckel's diverticulum, peritonitis, urinary tract infection, or other pathology (Berkowitz, 2000).

Periumbilical pain is often associated with recurrent abdominal pain syndrome (RAPS), a common childhood disorder affecting children between the ages of 5 and 12 years of age that is severe enough to affect activities (Kirschner & Black, 1998). The pain rarely occurs at night and does not interrupt sleep. Sometimes, constipation is associated with RAPS. Nursing care for the child with chronic abdominal pain consists of support, education about coping techniques, assurance the experience is common and probably will be outgrown, and, if applicable, a bowel program regime (Kirschner & Black, 1998). However, 30–50% of children with RAP will experience abdominal pain as adults as well (Berkowitz, 2000).

HOME CARE OF THE CHILD IN PAIN

Many children with pain conditions are now managed at home. Whether the source of the pain is a chronic condition, a pain syndrome, or following a surgical or invasive procedure, caregivers should be instructed in the home care of the child experiencing pain. Medications, including route, doses, actions, and the administration schedule are taught to the caregivers and child, if appropriate. The family is also encouraged to use specific home remedies or their own nonpharmacologic interventions to relieve the child's pain. Some families may wish to use herbal or folk remedies. However, caregivers should be cautioned that when ingesting herbal remedies, dosing information, safety, and drug interactions might not be known. Families wishing to utilize such remedies should consult their health care provider and every effort made to investigate the safety of such interventions.

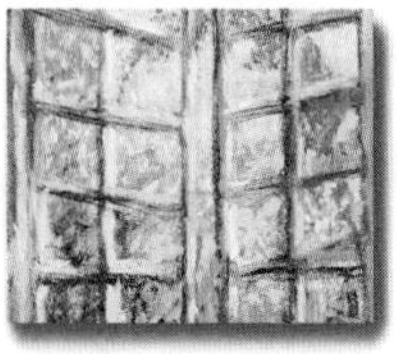

In the Real World

I used to work on an adult med-surg floor before transferring to the peds unit. I really love the children and enjoy caring for them. They rarely complain of pain postoperatively unless they had major surgery, have overvigilant parents, or are anxious. Most cannot wait to have their PCA removed so they can go to the playroom.

Key Concepts

- Pain physiology involves transmission, transduction, modulation, and perception.
- The gate control theory is the most common pain theory.
- Misconceptions of pain in children include infants do not feel pain, infants and children are more sensitive to opioids than adults, pain is character building, children and adolescents will become addicted to opioids if used, and children who are playing, sleeping, or can be distracted are not in pain.
- Children experience pain in the context of their developmental level, social and psychological experiences, and their environment
- Several objective and subjective measures are available to determine a child's pain experience or responses to treatment.
- Non-pharmacologic pain treatment can be used as an alternative to or in conjunction with pharmacologic pain treatment.
- For moderate to severe pain, opioids are the treatment of choice with doses tailored to the child's height, weight, and individual analgesic needs.
- Non-opioid pain medications, such as topical preparations, NSAIDs, and acetaminophen may be used to treat mild to moderate pain or given in conjunction with opioids to treat more severe pain.
- Local or regional anesthesia, used before, during, or after a procedure, is an appropriate method of treating pain in children.
- Chronic pain, including headaches and abdominal pain, is a unique and difficult-to-treat problem with specific treatment regimes for long-term management.
- In caring for the child at home, families can incorporate their own treatments for pain with prescribed pharmacologic and non-pharmacologic interventions. However, home or folk remedies, including herbal treatment, should be carefully reviewed for possible drug interactions or dangerous side effects.

Review Questions

1. Describe the physiology of pain. Chart or diagram the cycle of the pain impulse through the nervous system; include the components of the gate control theory.
2. Describe common pediatric pain misconceptions. Delineate scientific information correcting the misperceptions.
3. How do infants experience pain? What indicates an infant is experiencing pain?
4. What unique pain behaviors do toddlers exhibit? Preschoolers? School-aged children?
5. What differentiates an adolescent's pain experiences from those of adults?
6. Describe the components of a complete pain assessment.
7. Choose three common pediatric pain assessment tools. Describe their implementation. For what age child is each appropriate?
8. How are opioids dosed in children? How is patient-controlled analgesia used in children?
9. How are opioid side effects managed in children? (Specify side effect and management.)
10. Describe regional analgesia.
11. What are the characteristics of chronic pain in children? How is chronic pain treated ?
12. What would you include in a home treatment pain management plan? What treatments would you caution a family to use at home?

References

Agency for Health Care Policy and Research. (1992). *Acute pain management in infants, children and adolescents: Operative and medical procedures. Clinical practice guidelines.* (AHCPR Publication No. 92-0020). Rockville, MD: Author.

American Academy of Pediatrics, Committee on Drugs. (1992). Guidelines for monitoring and management of pediatric patients during and after sedation for diagnostic therapeutic procedures. *Pediatrics, 89*(6) 1110–1115.

Anand, K., & Hickey, P. (1987). Pain and its effects on the human fetus and neonate. *New England Journal of Medicine, 317*, 1321–1329.

Anand, K. J. (2001). International evidence-based group for neonatal pain. Consensus statement for the prevention and management of pain in the newborn. *Archives of Pediatrics & Adolescent Medicine, 155*(2), 173–180.

Annand, F. (2000). The phenomenon of pain: A study guide. *Point of View, 38*, 14–19.

Bennett, G. (2000). Update on the neurophysiology of pain transmission and modulation: Focus on NMDA-receptors. *Journal of Pain and Symptom Management, (19, Suppl.)*, S2–6.

Berkowitz, C. (2000). Abdominal Pain. In C. Berkowitz (Ed.). *Pediatrics: A primary care approach* (2nd ed.) (pp. 425–419). Philadelphia: Saunders.

Beyer, J., Denyes, M., & Villarruel, A. (1992). The creation, validation and continuing development of the Oucher: A measure of pain intensity in children. *Journal of Pediatric Nursing, 7*, 335–346.

Bieri, D., Reeve, R., Champion, G., Addicoat, L., & Ziegler, J. (1990). The Faces pain scale for self-assessment of the severity of pain experienced by children: Initial validation, and preliminary investigation for ratio scale properties. *Pain, 41*, 139–150.

Burokas, L. (1985). Factors affecting nurses' decisions to medicate pediatric patients after surgery. *Heart & Lung, 14*, 373–379.

Children's Memorial Hospital. (1999). *Children's Memorial Hospital formulary handbook*. Chicago: Lexi-Comp.

Ching, C. (1999). Contemparory therapy: Aromatherapy in management of acute pain. *Contemporary Nurse, 8*, 146–151.

Eland, J. (1993). Children with pain. In O. B. Jackson & R. B. Saunders (Eds.), *Child health nursing*. Philadelphia: J.B. Lippincott.

Eland, J., & Anderson, J. (1997). The experience of pain in children. In A. Jacox (Ed.). *Pain: A source book for nurses and other health professionals* (pp. 453–473). Boston: Little, Brown & Co.

Frank, L., & Gregory, G. (1993). Clinical evaluation and treatment of infant pain in the neonatal intensive care unit. In N. Schecter, C. Berde, & M. Yaster (Eds.). *Pain in infants, children and adolescents* (pp. 519–536). Baltimore: Williams & Wilkins.

Fratianne, R. B., Prensner, J. D., Huston, M. J., Super, D. M., Yowler, C. J., & Standley, J. M. (2001). The effect of music-based imagery and musical alternate engagement on the burn debridement process. *Journal of Burn Care & Rehabilitation, 22*(1), 47–53.

Gonzalez, J., & Gadish, H. (1990). Nurses' decision in medicating children postoperatively. In D. C. Tyler & E. J. Krane (Eds.). *Advances in pain research and therapy: Pediatric pain*. New York: Raven Press.

Hester, N. O., & Barcus, C. S. (1986). Assessment and management of children in pain. *Pediatrics: Nursing Update, 1*, 2–8.

Hunter, M., McDowell, L., Hennessy, R., & Cassey, J. (2000). An evaluation of the Faces Pain Scale with young children. *Journal of Pain and Symptom Management, 20*, 122–129.

Johnson, K., & Oski, F. (1997). *Oski's essential pediatrics*. Philadelphia: Lippincott-Raven.

Kirschner, B., & Black, D. (1998). The gastrointestinal tract. In B. Kliegman (Ed.), *Nelson's essentials of pediatrics* (3rd ed.) (pp. 419–458). Philadelphia: Saunders.

Litman, R. (1995). Recent trends in management of pain during medical procedures in children. *Pediatric Annals 24*(3), 158-163.

McHugh, J., & McHugh, W. (2000). Pain: Neuroanatomy, chemical mediators, and clincal implications. *AACN Clinical Issues, 11*, 168–72

McRae, M., Rourke, D., & Imperia-Perez, F. (1997). Development of a research-based standard for assessment, intervention and evaluation of pain after neonatal and pediatric cardiac surgery. *Pediatric Nursing, 23*(3), 263–271.

Melzack, R., & Wall, P. (1965). Pain mechanisms: A new theory. *Science, 150*, 971–979.

Paice, J. (1992). Pharmacologic management. In J. Watt-Watson & M. Donovan (Eds.), *Pain management: Nursing perspective*. St. Louis: Mosby.

Pederson, C., Matthies, D., & McDonald, S. (1997). A survey of pediatric critical care nurses' knowledge of pain management. *American Journal of Critical Care, 6*, 289–295.

Prensner, J. D., Yowler, C. J., Smith, L. F., Steele, A. L., & Fratianne, R. B. (2001). Music therapy for assistance with pain and anxiety management in burn treatment. *Journal of Burn Care & Rehabilitation*, 22(1), 83–88.

Price, S. A., & Wilson, L. M. (1999). *Pathophysiology clinical concepts of disease processes*. St. Louis: Mosby.

Savedra, M., Tesler, M., Holzmer, W., & Ward, J. (1992). *Adolescent pediatric pain tool: User manual*. San Francisco: University of California.

Schnitzler, M., & Ploner, M. (2000). Neurophysiology and functional neuroanatomy of pain perception. *Journal of Clinical Neurophysiology, 17*, 592–603.

Urban, M., & Gebhart, G. (1999). Central mechanisms in pain. *Medical Clinics of North America, 83*, 585–596.

Valente, S. (1991). Using hypnosis with children for pain management. *Oncology Nursing Forum, 18*(4), 699–704.

White, L. (2001). *Foundations of nursing*. Albany, NY: Delmar.

Wong, D., & Baker, C. (2001). Smiling faces as an anchor for pain intensity scales. *Pain, 89*, 294–300.

Wong, D. L., Hockenberry-Eaton, M., Wilson, D., Winkelstein, M. L., & Schwartz, P. (2001). *Wong's Essentials of Pediatric Nursing*, 6th ed., St. Louis: Mosby.

Woolf, C., & Decosterd, I. (1999). Implications of recent advances in the understanding of pain pathophysiology for assessment of pain in patients. *Pain, (Suppl.6)*, S141–7.

Yaster, M, Cote, C., Krane, E., Kaplan, R., & Lappe, D. (Eds.). (1997). *Pediatric pain management and sedation handbook*. St. Louis: Mosby.

Zempsky, W., & Karasic, R. (1997). EMLA versus TAC for topical anesthesia of extremity wounds in children. *Annals of Emergency Medicine*, *30*(2), 163.

Zubrzycka, M., & Janecka, A. (2000). Substance P: Transmitter of nociception. *Endocrine Regulation, 35*, 195–201.

Suggested Readings

Colwell, C., Clark, L., & Perkins, R, (1996). Postoperative use of Pediatric Pain Scales: Children's self-report versus nurse assessment of pain intensity and affect. *Journal of Pediatric Nursing, 11*, 375–382.

Forrest, J. B., Heitlinger, E. L., & Revell, S. (1997). Ketorolac for postoperative pain management in children. *Drug Safety, 16*, 309–329.

Hester, N. (1979). The preoperational child's reaction to immunization. *Nursing Research (4)*, 250–254.

Keuren, K.V., & Eland, J. (1997). Perioperative pain management in children. *Nursing Clinics of North America, 32*, 31–44.

Ko, C., Thompson, J., Alcantra, A., & Hiyama, D. (1997). Preemptive analgesia in patients undegoing appendectomy. *Archives of Surgery, 132*, 874–877.

Manworren, R. (2001). Development and testing of the pediatric nurses' knowledge and attitudes survey regarding pain. *Pediatric Nursing, (27)*, 151–158.

McCarthy, C., Cool, V., & Hanrahan, K. (1998). Cognitive behavioral interventions for children during painful procedures: Research challenges and program development. *Journal of Pediatric Nursing, 13*, 55–63.

McGrath, P. J., Beyer, J., Cleeland, C., Eland, J., McGrath, P. A., & Portenoy, R. (1990). American Academy of Pediatrics Report of the Subcommittee on Assessment and Methodologic Issues in the Management of Pain in Childhood Cancer. *Pediatrics, 86* (5 Pt 2), 814–817.

Vincent, C. (2001). Nurses' analgesic practices with hospitalized children. *Journal of Child and Family Nursing (4)*, 79–89.

World Health Organization (1998). *Cancer pain relief and pallative care in children*. Geneva: WHO.

Resources

Organizations and Websites

American Pain Society
4700 W. Lake Ave.
Glenview, IL 60025
(847) 375-4715
Fax: 877-734-8758
www.ampainsoc.org/

American Society of Pain Management Nurses
7794 Grow Dr.
Pensacola, FL 32514

AstraZeneca, Corp.
www.emla-usa.com/questions/
Includes *Q&A on Pediatric Pain* and *Meet the Experts*.

Center for Research Dissemination and Liaison
AHCPR Publications Clearinghouse
P.O. Box 20907
Silver Springs, MD 20907
Write to obtain free copies of Clinical Practice Guidelines
Acute Pain Management in Infants, Children and Adolescents, Cancer Pain

Children's Hospice International
Guidelines and manuals for families and nurses.
901 North Pitt St. #230
Alexandria, VA 22314
(800) 2-4-Child
Fax: 703-684-0226
www.chionline.org

Pediatric Pain Discussion Group
www.santel.lv/SANTEL/pediat/ped-pain.html

Pediatric Pain: Science helping Children
www.is.dal.ca/pedpain/
Includes an interesting section on the role of patients, children, and health care professionals.

University of Iowa College of Nursing
www.nursing.uiowa.edu/sites/pedspain.
Website for patients, families, and health care professionals.

CHAPTER 19

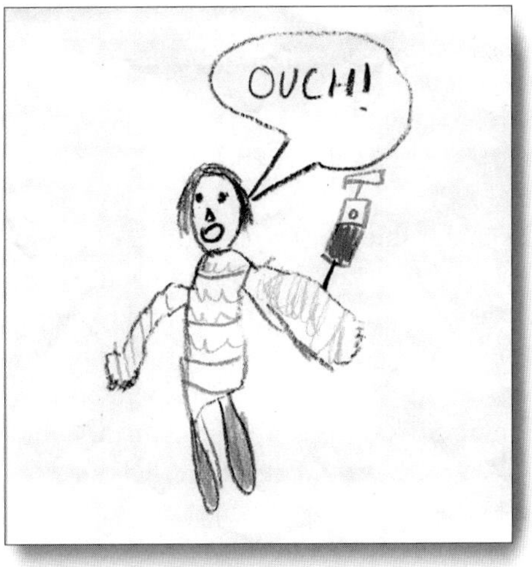

It is so hard to get my children to take their medicines. Helen and Wendy say "it tastes terrible" or "it makes me sick to my stomach." I've tried pleading and cajoling, bribing, threatening, or forcing the medication into their mouth. It distresses me to see Helen and Wendy upset at a time when they are not feeling well. I wish it were easier. I don't envy the nurses who have to give medications to kids every day.

MEDICATION ADMINISTRATION

Mary E. Tiedeman, PhD, RN

COMPETENCIES

Upon completion of this chapter, the reader will be able to:

- *Describe pharmacokinetic and pharmacodynamic processes.*
- *Discuss age-related differences in pharmacokinetic and pharmacodynamic processes.*
- *Discuss the impact of psychosocial and cognitive development on giving medications to infants and children.*
- *Discuss special considerations and approaches for safely administering medications to infants and children.*
- *Discuss appropriate methods for calculating a pediatric medication dose.*
- *Discuss age-appropriate techniques for administering medications to children via the oral/enteral, intravenous, intramuscular, subcutaneous, rectal, ophthalmic, otic, nasal, and topical routes.*
- *Describe the advantages and disadvantages of each route of pediatric medication administration.*

Assuring safe administration of medications to children is an important part of providing appropriate pediatric nursing care. Physiological, psychosocial, and cognitive differences between children and adults have implications for pharmacologic intervention with children. Understanding and applying knowledge of these differences will facilitate safe medication administration to children (Pollard, 1998). This is particularly important since research on pharmacologic intervention with children has been fairly limited due to ethical constraints related to informed consent. Since most drugs have not been adequately tested in the pediatric population, infants and children are at risk for adverse reactions, including age-specific adverse reactions, and ineffective treatment. To alleviate this problem, the Food and Drug Administration (FDA) has just issued new regulations requiring pediatric studies for new drugs and biological products (Clark, Queener, & Karb, 2000; Hood, 1997; Kanneh, 1998a; Regulations Requiring Manufacturers to Assess the Safety and Effectiveness of New Drugs and Biological Products in Pediatric Patients, 1998).

PHYSIOLOGICAL CONSIDERATIONS

In general, physiological differences between children and adults make children more sensitive to drugs and increase the risk of adverse drug reactions. Differences in body size and composition, and the immaturity of various organ systems account for these differences. Of particular significance are body fluid composition and differences in cardiovascular, gastrointestinal, renal, and neurological system functioning. These age-related physiological differences, which change as children grow and develop, are responsible for alterations in pharmacokinetic and pharmacodynamic processes (Brucker & Wallin, 1998; Lehne, 2000; Gutierrez, 1999; Niederhauser, 1997). It is these processes that determine how a drug is administered, how often it is given, and its dose (Clark, et al., 2000).

Pharmacokinetics is concerned with the movement of drugs throughout the body by the processes of absorption, distribution, biotransformation, and excretion. It deals with how drugs enter the body, how they reach their site of action and in what concentration, and how they are eliminated. Thus, pharmacokinetics addresses the body's effects on the drug (Clark, et al., 2000; Hood, 1996a; Kanneh, 1998a: Lehne, 2000; Turley, 1999).

The processes of absorption, distribution, biotransformation, and excretion are different in neonates, infants, and children than in adults. These processes influence drug concentration at the site of action, intensity of effects, and duration of drug action, making it important to understand developmental differences when giving medications to children (Brucker & Wallin, 1998; Carlson & Byington, 1998; Gutierrez, 1999; LeDuc, 1999).

Absorption is the process whereby drugs move from the site of administration into the bloodstream. The rate and extent of absorption determine how soon the effects of the drug start and how intense those effects will be. Absorption is a major determinant of **bioavailability,** i.e., the portion of a drug that reaches general circulation and is available to exert its effect at its site of action (Gutierrez, 1999; Hood, 1996a; Kanneh, 1998a; Lehne, 2000; Turley, 1999). Physiological differences in infants and children also impact this process.

Gastric emptying time and pH are two factors influencing the absorption of orally administered drugs (Hood, 1996a; Kanneh, 1998b; Pollard, 1998). Gastric emptying time is slower in neonates and infants (up to 6–8 hours). It reaches adult values (2 hours) around 6 months of age, although peristalsis is irregular and unpredictable. Delayed gastric emptying will delay the absorption of drugs designed to be absorbed from the intestine. Since most drugs are mainly absorbed from the intestine due to its larger absorptive area, the absorption and, therefore, therapeutic effect of most drugs are delayed. However, there may be more complete absorption than anticipated for drugs absorbed primarily in the stomach (Bindler & Howry, 1997; Blaho, Winbery, & Merigan, 1996; Gutierrez, 1999; Hood, 1996a; Kanneh, 1998b; Koren, 1998; LeDuc, 1999; Lehne, 2000; Niederhauser, 1997; Pollard, 1998).

Gastric pH is higher (more alkaline) in the newborn and gradually decreases (becomes more acidic) to reach adult levels around 2–3 years of age. Acidic drugs are better absorbed from an acidic environment; basic drugs are better absorbed from an alkaline environment. Therefore, in infancy, basic drugs will be more readily absorbed from the stomach, and acidic drugs will be less well absorbed from the stomach compared to older children and adults (Blaho, et al., 1996; Brucker & Wallin, 1998; Carlson & Byington, 1998; Hood, 1996a, 1997; Kanneh, 1998b; LeDuc, 1999; Lehne, 2000; Pollard, 1998)

Additional factors that influence the absorption of orally administered drugs include intestinal transit time and transport substances such as enzymes. With more rapid transit time, less drug will be absorbed; with slower transit time, more drug will be absorbed. Peristalsis is irregular in the neonate and young infant. Therefore, the amount of drug absorbed in the small intestine may be unpredictable. In addition, infants have lower levels of some substances needed for absorption and transport of certain drugs. For example, the activity of α–amylase and other pancreatic enzymes is low in infants up to 4 months of age and neonates have lower concentrations of lipase and bile acids. Overall, variations in the gastrointestinal system result in slower, more erratic absorption of orally administered drugs during the first 6 months of life (Blaho, et al., 1996; Carlson & Byington, 1998; Koren, 1998; LeDuc, 1999; Niederhauser, 1997).

Absorption of drugs administered intramuscularly is affected by muscle mass and perfusion of the area. Neonates and infants have less muscle mass than older children or adults (25% of body weight compared to 40% of body weight in adults). The smaller muscle size results in less volume capacity and less absorptive surface. There is also decreased muscle tone and lower muscle oxygenation in this age group. In addition, neonates and infants have vasomotor instability with diminished and unpredictable peripheral blood flow. Thus, absorption of drugs administered intramuscularly is slower and unreliable in neonates and infants. Perfusion to the area also influences the absorption of drugs administered subcutaneously. When there is diminished blood flow, absorption is delayed. When perfusion is adequate, the subcutaneous route facilitates the rapid absorption of nonirritating, lipid-soluble drugs (Brucker & Wallin, 1998; Hood, 1997; Kanneh, 1998b, Koren, 1998; LeDuc, 1999; Lehne, 2001; Pollard, 1998).

There is more rapid absorption of topical medication in infants and children due to greater body surface area (BSA) to weight ratio. The skin is also thinner and more permeable (Hood, 1997; Kanneh, 1998b; Pollard, 1998). Absorption is further increased if skin integrity is compromised, there is prolonged contact time, or an occlusive dressing is applied. These factors necessitate careful attention to instructions for using topical medication, especially since plastic coated diapers can be considered an occlusive dressing (Kanneh, 1998b; Niederhauser, 1997; Pollard, 1998).

Distribution is concerned with the movement of a drug from blood to interstitial spaces and from there into cells, i.e., the distribution of the drug throughout the body and the amount of drug in body tissues, fluids, and spaces (Hood, 1996a; Lehne, 2000; Turley, 1999). Factors influencing drug distribution in the body include body composition and fluid distribution, protein binding, and blood flow in the tissue (Hood, 1997; Pollard, 1998).

Neonates, infants, and young children have a higher percentage of body water than adults; most of this water is in the extracellular fluid. This difference is most pronounced in children under 2 years of age (adult values are reached around 6–7 years of age) and leads to a dilution of water-soluble drugs and a consequent decreased concentration in the blood. Therefore, higher mg/kg doses of water-soluble drugs may be required, especially in children under 2 years of age (Blaho, et al., 1996; Brucker & Wallin, 1998; Carlson & Byington, 1998; Clark, et al., 2000; Kanneh, 1998b; Hood, 1997; Pollard, 1998).

Body fat percentage varies by age and gender as well as between individual children. Fat comprises 14–15% of body weight of a newborn. For the premature infant, the percent of body weight comprised of fat may be as little as 1%. The percentage of body fat increases up to 6 months of age and then decreases slightly, with body fat comprising 23–24% of body weight of a 1-year-old. For boys, the percentage of body fat continues to decrease through adolescence, except for a slight increase in body fat percentage around 12 years of age. For girls, the percentage of body fat decreases until around 10 years of age, and then increases throughout adolescence. The percentage of body fat influences drug distribution throughout the body and affects the concentration of the drug remaining in the circulatory system and at its site of action. Lipid-soluble drugs have a high affinity for adipose tissue and can be stored in body fat. This can leave less drug available in circulation and at the site of action. Thus, with lipid-soluble drugs, body fat must get saturated before drug blood levels begin to rise, requiring different mg/kg dosages, depending on the amount of body fat, to achieve therapeutic blood levels. An individual with a higher percentage of body fat requires a higher mg/kg dose of a lipid-soluble drug than an individual with a lower percentage of body fat (Carlson & Byington, 1998; Gutierrez, 1999; Koren, 1998; LeDuc, 1999; Lehne, 2000; Walker & Watkins, 1997).

Immaturity of the liver in neonates and infants results in lower serum protein levels and fewer protein binding sites. In addition, the albumin in neonates and infants has a lower binding capacity for certain drugs than in adults. With drugs that tend to bind to protein, decreased protein binding increases the serum level of unbound drug. Since it is the unbound drug that exerts an effect, decreased protein binding intensifies the drug's effect, potentially leading to toxicity. Drugs excreted in their active form (not biotransformed but excreted unchanged) may be more rapidly eliminated from the body since it is the unbound portion of a drug that can be excreted. Due to the increased serum levels and more rapid excretion, some drugs may require a decreased dose but an increased frequency of administration (Blaho, et al., 1996; Brucker & Wallin, 1998; Carlson & Byington, 1998; Clark, et al., 2000; Gutierrez, 1999; Hood, 1996a, 1997; Kanneh, 1998b; LeDuc, 1999; Pollard, 1998; Turley, 1999).

Certain drugs also compete with endogenous substances, such as free fatty acids, bilirubin, or steroids, for protein-binding sites. Since the number of binding sites is already limited in young children, competition for binding sites may lead to higher levels of unbound drug necessitating lower drug doses or higher levels of the endogenous substances. In neonates, competitive drug binding may lead to increased concentrations of unbound, unconjugated bilirubin leading to Kernicterus or bilirubin encephalopathy (Blaho, et al., 1996; Brucker & Wallin, 1998; LeDuc, 1999; Lehne, 2000; Niederhauser, 1997).

The immature blood–brain barrier in children under 2 years of age allows relatively easy access to the central nervous system (CNS), making these children more sensitive to drugs that act on the brain and increasing the risk of CNS toxicity. Therefore, lower doses of certain drugs may be required to protect young children from undesired effects (Blaho, et al., 1996; Hood, 1997; LeDuc, 1999; Lehne, 2000).

Biotransformation, also called metabolism, refers to the transformation or alteration of chemical structures from their original form. This transformation facilitates the eventual excretion of the substance via the renal system. Most biotransformation of drugs occurs in the liver (Blaho, et al., 1996; Clark, et al., 2000; Hood, 1996a; LeDuc, 1999; Niederhauser, 1997; Turley, 1999).

Due to liver immaturity, the drug metabolizing capacity of neonates is low. However, the liver matures rapidly from about 1 month to 23 months of age. Therefore, during this time, drugs metabolized by the liver have a longer **half-life** (time required for 50% of administered dose of a drug to be eliminated from the body) and there is an increased risk of toxicity. This requires reducing dosages of some drugs as well as adjusting the frequency of administration, i.e., less frequent. During early childhood, drugs requiring oxidation are typically metabolized more rapidly, necessitating higher doses and/or more frequent administration. Adult levels of liver maturity are reached at puberty (Blaho, et al., 1996; Brucker & Wallin, 1998; Carlson & Byington, 1998; Gutierrez, 1999; Hood, 1997; Kanneh, 1998b; LeDuc, 1999; Lehne, 2000; Pollard, 1998).

Some metabolism of drugs may occur in the gastrointestinal tract where gut microflora alter their physiochemical property. Since infants have lower levels of gut flora, there is less metabolism of these drugs in the gastrointestinal tract. For example, digoxin-reducing microorganisms do not reach adult levels until approximately 2 years of age (Kanneh, 1998b).

Some biotransformation of orally administered drugs occurs before the drug reaches the general circulation. For example, drugs absorbed from the stomach and small intestine pass through the portal circulation where some biotransformation occurs before the drug reaches the general circulation. This phenomenon, known as **first-pass effect,** decreases the bioavailability of orally administered medications. Therefore, drugs administered orally may require larger mg/kg doses for therapeutic effect than drugs administered by other routes. Drugs that are highly cleared by the liver may undergo considerable biotransformation via first-pass effect. Examples of such drugs are analgesics such as morphine and meperidine, certain tricyclic antidepressants such as amitriptyline, and antiarrhythmics such as propranolol (Clark, et al., 2000; Gutierrez, 1999; Hood, 1996a; Kanneh, 1998a; Turley, 1999).

Excretion refers to the movement of a drug or its metabolite from the tissues back into the circulation and then to the organs of elimination. This process removes the drug or its metabolite from the body (Gutierrez, 1999; Lehne, 2000, Kanneh, 1998a).

The kidneys are the primary route of drug excretion. The kidneys are immature at birth and during infancy, renal blood flow, glomerular filtration, and active tubular secretion are all low, resulting in reduced renal excretion. Adult levels of renal functioning are reached around 1–2 years of age. Reduced renal excretion results in a longer half-life and increases the risk of toxicity to drugs that are excreted primarily by the renal system. Therefore, reduced dosages are required during infancy (Blaho, et al., 1996; Brucker & Wallin, 1998; Carlson & Byington, 1998; Gutierrez, 1999; Hood, 1996a, 1997; Kanneh, 1998b; Lehne, 2000; Pollard, 1998).

Pharmacodynamics is concerned with the biochemical and physiological effects of drugs (drug effect, response resulting from drug action) and their mechanisms of action within the body (drug action). That is, what drugs do to the body and how they do it. Drug action may involve nonspecific modification of the cellular environment, as for example altering the pH of the surrounding body fluid. Drug action also occurs at the cellular level through an interaction of the drug and cellular components. Most drugs are thought to act at the cellular level by attaching to receptors on the cells where they mimic or block the action of endogenous regulatory molecules. For example, propranolol blocks beta-adrenergic receptors thus decreasing heart rate, whereas albuterol stimulates (mimics) beta-adrenergic receptors thus producing bronchodilation (Carlson & Byington; 1998; Clark, et al., 2000; Guiterrez, 1999; Hood, 1996a, 1996b; Kanneh, 1998a; LeDuc, 1999: Lehne, 2000).

Even though the mechanism of action of a drug remains the same in all individuals, infants and children may demonstrate variations in drug effects related to the immaturity of target organs and receptor sensitivity. An infant or child may require a lower or higher dose of a drug than expected. In general, infants and children have heightened sensitivity to drugs (Carlson & Byington, 1998; Hood, 1997; LeDuc, 1999; Lehne, 2000).

> Critical Thinking
>
> **Medication Administration to a Child with Impaired Renal Function**
>
> Three-year-old Denise, with renal failure secondary to trauma, is receiving morphine for pain. What concerns do you have regarding giving morphine? What adjustments might be needed in dose and administration?

DEVELOPMENTAL CONSIDERATIONS

Administering medications to children requires an understanding of all aspects of growth and development and its impact on the approach to giving medications. Of particular importance are the child's psychosocial and cognitive development. Physical and motor development are also important (e.g., ability to swallow tablets and size of muscles) and will be discussed in relation to their impact on the various routes of administering medication.

Infants are developing trust and are helped by consistency, both in caregivers and in approaches to nursing care. In later infancy, stranger anxiety may make the infant less receptive to care by the nurse. Involving parents in medication administration can make this experience less stressful for infants. Parents can administer oral medications and they can hold and comfort the infant when medication is administered by other routes.

Toddlers are developing autonomy and commonly display negativism. Following rituals and routines can give toddlers some sense of control and may enhance cooperation in taking medications. Giving choices and allowing toddlers to handle equipment also foster a sense of control and may enhance cooperation. At this age, choices should be kept simple, that is, a choice between two things. For example, "Do you want mommy or the nurse to give you your medicine?' As with infants, toddlers can benefit from parental participation in medication administration.

A history specific to past experience with taking medication and approaches that were successful is essential. Toddlers should be approached in a positive manner conveying a belief in their ability to accomplish the needed behavior, e.g., successfully taking the medication. When giving medications to toddlers, administer them promptly, restrain as needed, and reward positive behavior. Toddlers should not be told or given the message that they are bad when not able to fully cooperate in taking medications (LeDuc, 1999).

Preschoolers are developing initiative. They benefit from the opportunity to play with equipment and respond positively to explanations and comforting. To help foster a sense of control, choices should be offered when possible. However, the number of choices should be limited—e.g., "Do you want to take the pink medicine or the white medicine first?" or "Do you want water or juice with your medicine?" Care should be taken not to inadvertently offer a choice that does not really exist—e.g., "Will you take your medicine now?" Preschoolers can also benefit from parental involvement in medication administration. Giving suppositories may be upsetting to preschoolers because of their fears of bodily intrusion and mutilation. As with toddlers, preschoolers should not be given the message they are bad when not able to fully cooperate with medication administration (LeDuc, 1999).

School-aged children are developing industry. They benefit from explanations regarding the purpose of medications and can be active participants in their care. School-aged children are generally cooperative in taking medication. However, a reward system may serve as an effective feedback mechanism for school-aged children thus enhancing their cooperation. Play activities also can help with coping. School-aged children also should be given choices; older school-aged children can handle a broader range of choices—e.g., "What do you want to drink for taking your medication?" (LeDuc, 1999).

Adolescents may be approached in the same manner as adults. A more detailed discussion of growth and development of the specific age groups can be found in Chapters 7 through 12.

One situation nurses may encounter with psychosocial implications is when parents or other caregivers use the threat of needles or shots to influence children's behavior. Such a situation can be a challenge for the nurse who needs to assure the child that painful or frightening interventions are not a consequence of behavior, while still fostering trust between the child and caregiver. The nurse needs to tactfully provide the caregivers with factual information regarding growth and development, children's fears and anxiety with regard to hospitalization, and suggest and role model alternative ways of dealing with undesired behavior. At the same time, the nurse must acknowledge and accept the caregivers' feelings and frustrations regarding their child's behavior. In intervening with children, the nurse must use age-appropriate teaching approaches regarding illness and treatment while being careful not to convey negative feelings about caregivers' behaviors.

MEDICATION ADMINISTRATION

Medication administration for the pediatric population requires special considerations and approaches. Techniques used in administering the medication are based on the growth and developmental level of the individual infant or child. General as well as specific considerations such as preparation for safe administration, dosage determination, and considerations related to the various routes of medication administration will be discussed.

General Considerations

Before administering medications to infants and children, it is important to give developmentally appropriate explanations. It is essential that explanations be truthful; however, the language used should be minimally threatening. For example, "the medicine may taste different than anything you have tasted before" rather than "the medicine will taste bad." Explanations should include why the drug is given, what the child will experience, what is expected of the child, and how the parents can participate or help support their child. After any distressing procedure, age-appropriate comfort should be provided. For example, the infant could be held and cuddled (LeDuc, 1999; Pollard, 1998).

Preparation for Safe Administration

As with adults, medication administration to pediatric patients adheres to the five rights—right patient, right drug, right dose, right route, and right time. The nurse should not expect the pediatric client to correctly self-identify. Infants and preverbal children are unable to self-identify; young children may disavow their identity in an attempt to avoid an unpleasant experience. Adolescents may consider it fun to misidentify themselves to authority figures. In addition, children may play in each others' beds (Brucker & Wallin, 1998). Therefore, it is essential client identification bands be applied at the time of admission and checked at the beginning of

Eye On:

Possibility of Herbal/Medication Interactions

It is important to check for herbal supplement use prior to medication administration. There is a possibility of herbal and prescribed drug interaction.

REFLECTIONS FROM FAMILIES

Seven-year-old Holly, who received an injection earlier in the day states, "My mom and nurse told me it wouldn't hurt. It did. I wish they had told me the truth."

each shift and before every medication administration. The nurse should remember client identification bracelets may come off accidentally, be removed by the child, or occasionally be removed by the staff. Care must be taken to replace identification when it is removed or lost. Comparing the client identification to the medication administration record (MAR) will help ensure the right client receives the right medication.

Verification of right drug, right dose, right route, and right time is a basic safety measure. Before administering medications the nurse should check the MAR against the physician orders. This is generally done once every 24 hours (as each new MAR record is begun) and as each new medication order is written. There should be a place on the MAR to indicate that each medication order has been verified.

Determining the right dose in the pediatric population requires more than verifying that the dose to be delivered is the same as ordered by the physician. The nurse must also verify that the ordered dose is within the recommended dosage range for the child as described in the following section. Whenever there is a discrepancy between the ordered dose and the recommended dose, further action is necessary. The nurse may contact the pharmacist for additional reference information and check the client chart for any notations that could explain the ordered dose. For some medications it is appropriate to check laboratory reports for drug peak and trough level results.

Appropriate medication administration includes determining that in addition to having the right drug, one has the appropriate formulation and concentration for the intended route (Lehne, 2000). Certain drugs, e.g., digoxin, insulin, and morphine, which bring about critical responses must be double-checked before administration (Brucker & Wallin, 1998). (Hospital policies and procedures will indicate specific drugs that need to be double-checked and the procedure for doing so.)

Dosage Determination

A number of rules are available for calculating appropriate pediatric drug dosages from the recommended adult dosages. Clark's rule uses the child's weight in the calculation, while Fried's rule and Young's rule use the child's age. The rules based on age inaccurately assume children of the same age have the same height, weight, and physiology. Rules that calculate pediatric doses from adult doses based on the child's weight do not take into consideration that children may require different mg/kg doses than adults. Therefore, these rules are no longer the preferred method for calculating appropriate pediatric drug dosages (Brucker & Wallin, 1998).

Appropriate drug dosages in children are most commonly calculated on the basis of unit of drug per kilogram of body weight or unit of drug per BSA (Hood, 1997; Kanneh, 1998b). BSA can be obtained from the child's height and weight using a West nomogram (Figure 19-1). A number of references that provide recommended pediatric dosages based on weight and/or BSA are listed under suggested readings at the end of the chapter. When calculating appropriate drug dosages for an individual child it is essential that the correct recommended dosage be used in the calculation since recommendations differ based on age, route of administration, and purpose. Most dosage recommendations are for a 24-hour period (mg/kg/24 hours). However, some dosage recommendations are for a single dose (mg/kg/dose). It is essential that the nurse differentiate between these when doing calculations. Whether weight or BSA is used to compute recommended dose, as a general rule, the pediatric dose should not exceed the minimum recommended adult dose. Once the child weighs 40 kg or more, weight is not generally used to compute the recommended dose (Blaho,

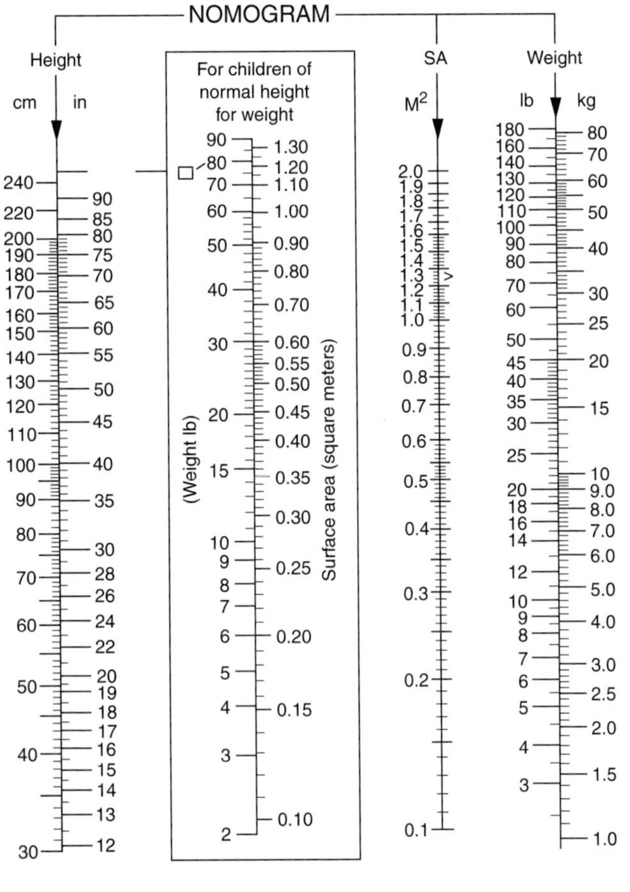

Directions for use: (1) Determine client height. (2) Determine client weight. (3) Draw a straight line to connect the height and weight. Where the line intersects on the SA line is the derived body surface area (M²).

Figure 19-1 Nomogram for Estimating Body Surface Area. Reprinted with permission from Behrman, R.E., Kliegman, R., & Arvin, A (Eds.). (1999). *Nelson's textbook of pediatrics* (16th ed.). Philadelphia, PA: Saunders.

et al., 1996; Kanneh, 1998b). Exceptions to these general rules may occur and should be checked with the hospital/unit policy and/or the pharmacist before calculating and administering the drug.

For drugs that do not have a recommended pediatric dosage, BSA may be used to extrapolate a dosage from the adult dosage. The formula can be found in Box 19-1.

Oral Medication

Preparation

Oral medications come in several forms—liquid, powder, tablets, and capsules. Liquid medications include syrups and elixirs, where the medication is dissolved and distributed throughout the liquid, and suspensions, which contain undissolved particles of drug suspended in the liquid. Suspensions require shaking before administration to distribute the medication evenly throughout the liquid so an appropriate dose is administered each time. Since children under 5 years of age generally are unable to swallow tablets or capsules, it may be necessary to crush tablets or open capsules and remove the powder or liquid if a liquid form of the medication is not available. Before crushing a tablet or opening a capsule it is essential to determine if this will interfere with the pharmacokinetics of the drug, e.g., enteric coated or timed release tablets should not be crushed. Crushed tablets or capsule contents generally have a bitter taste. Therefore, to make the medication more palatable it can be mixed with a pleasant tasting liquid or non-essential food before administering. Common vehicles include flavored syrups provided by the pharmacy, jelly, honey (not for the infant since there is risk of botulism), pudding, ice cream, or applesauce. The medication should not be mixed with formula or other essential foods since the child may associate the medicine taste with the food (Bindler & Howry, 1997; Brucker & Wallin, 1998; Kanneh, 1998b).

BOX 19-1 Calculating recommended pediatric dose from BSA and adult dose

Formula:

$$\frac{\text{BSA} \times \text{adult dose}}{1.73} = \text{recommended pediatric dose}$$

Example: Dosing guidelines for Ketorolac (Tordal) are not established for children 2–16 years

Adult dose recommended is 30 mg IV q 6 hours.

Calculation of the recommended dose for a child with a BSA of 0.6 m^{2}:

$$\frac{0.6 \times 30\text{mg}}{1.73} = 10.4\text{mg q 6 hours}$$

Critical Thinking

Assuring Administration of an Appropriate Medication Dose

Six-year-old Elaine is receiving IV gentamicin for an infection. She weighs 18.5 kg. The recommended dose is 2–2.5 mg/kg /dose every 8 hours. The order is for 30 mg every 8 hours. Consider whether this is an appropriate dose and what actions, if any, you need to take.

Administration

The administration of oral medications in the pediatric population may be a challenge since the appearance, smell, and/or taste of the medication may make children reluctant to accept them. Therefore, a firm, matter-of-fact approach, based on developmental level and ability, usually results in cooperation. For example, ask children to administer the oral drug to themselves or use the syringe to squirt the medicine into their mouth (Brucker & Wallin, 1998; Kanneh, 1998b; Clark, et al., 2000).

Liquid medication can be administered in a medicine cup, a measured medicine spoon, an oral syringe, a dropper, or through a nipple without the bottle attached. A dropper or oral syringe can be used to administer liquid medication to infants and young children. The liquid is directed posterior and to the side of the mouth and given slowly in small quantities (0.2–0.5 cc), allowing the child to swallow before more medication is placed in the mouth. A nipple also may be used for administering liquid medication to infants. The medication is placed directly in the nipple; care should be taken to

Nursing Alert:

Giving Oral Medications When the Child Is Not Cooperative

Never pinch the nose or force a screaming child to swallow medication. This increases the risk of aspiration.

Nursing Alert:

Use of Spoons in Administering Liquid Medication

Do not substitute an ordinary teaspoon or tablespoon or kitchen measuring spoons for a measured medication spoon. Such spoons are not consistently calibrated and may alter the dose of medication that a child receives.

Kids Want To Know

What will the medicine taste like?

Rae Jeanne, a four-year-old, is receiving a liquid antibiotic for an ear infection. She asks "What does it taste like?" and "Does it taste bad?" Be honest in your reply. If you don't know what it tastes like, you can say "some children tell me it tastes like cherry. You can tell me what it tastes like to you." Another response could be "it smells like cherry. You can tell me what it tastes like to you." If you have tasted the medicine, you may say "it tastes like cherry to me." Remember that what one person thinks tastes okay, another person may think tastes bad. You should give descriptions of taste or smell rather than labeling the taste good or bad.

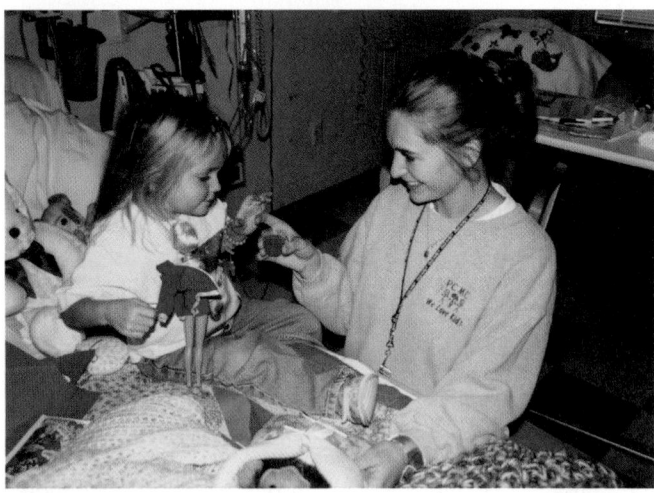

Figure 19-2B Toddlers and preschoolers will often take their oral medications cheerfully if placed in a small cup.

keep the nipple filled with medication so the infant does not suck air while taking the medication. To avoid aspiration, the infant or child should be placed in an upright position, at least at a 45 degree angle, never flat (Bindler & Howry, 1997; Brucker & Wallin, 1998). Older children are able to take liquid from a medicine cup or measured medicine spoon. Toddlers and preschoolers may enjoy using an oral syringe to "squirt" medicine into their mouth. See Figure 19-2A–C.

As children mature, they learn how to swallow tablets or capsules. The nurse can facilitate learning this skill by having children practice by placing the medication in a small amount of food such as ice cream and then having the child swallow the spoonful of food. The child should be told medication is in the food. This helps the child learn a new skill.

For some pediatric clients, oral medications are administered via a nasogastric, a gastrostomy, or a nasojejunal tube.

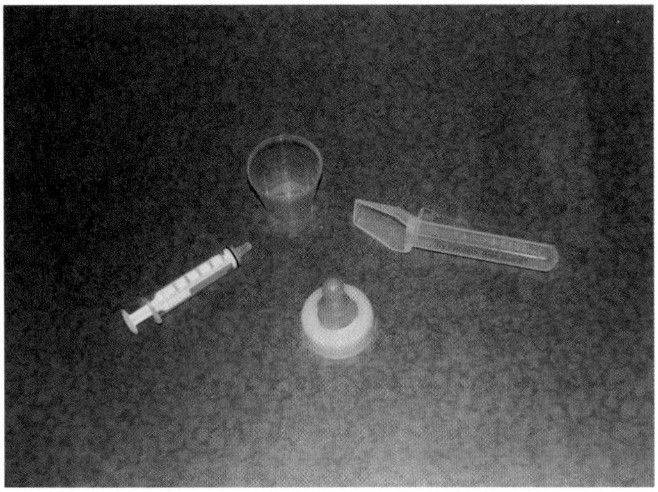

Figure 19-2C Oral medications can be administered to children through a variety of devices: cup, syringe, dropper, nipple, or medicine spoon.

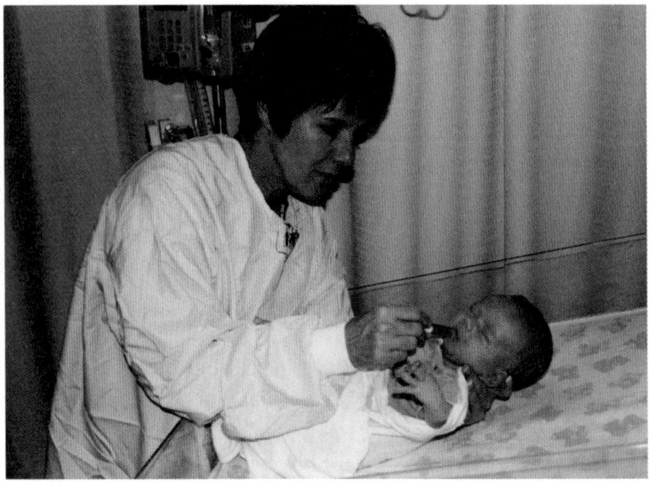

Figure 19-2A Using a syringe to administer oral medications to an infant.

Before administering oral medications in this manner it is essential to determine proper placement of the tube. In addition, medications that act directly on the stomach, e.g., liquid antacids, will be ineffective if given via a nasojejunal tube. A syringe is used to flush the tube before administering the medication. The medication is then put through the tube using a syringe, followed by a sufficient amount of water to ensure the medication enters the gastrointestinal system rather than remaining in the tube.

Intravenous Medication

Intravenous (IV) administration of medication improves the therapeutic blood level of the medication and eliminates the discomfort associated with repeated intramuscular or subcu-

Family Teaching

Safe Administration of Oral Medications

Home:
- Teach caregivers generic and brand name of medication.
- Teach caregivers purpose of medication, why it is necessary, and its expected effects.
- Teach caregivers potential side effects of medication and what to do if they occur.
- Teach caregivers how to give medication, that is, amount to give, frequency of administration, and length of time medication is to be given. Provide a demonstration and allow caregivers to give a return demonstration.
- Teach caregivers about acceptable measuring devices for liquid medications, for example, oral syringes, measured medicine spoons, or medicine droppers calibrated for a specific medication and not to use ordinary table or teaspoons or kitchen measuring spoons for measuring medication.
- Teach caregivers that medication can be mixed with small amounts of nonessential food, such as pudding or ice cream.
- Teach caregivers what to do if child vomits following medication administration or if a dose is forgotten.
- Teach caregivers to inform health care provider of any over-the-counter medications or herbal preparations that are being given.

School:
- Teach caregivers to be aware of and follow local school policy regarding medications taken at school.
- Have caregivers inform appropriate school personnel of the medication the child is taking, the purpose of the medication, how long the child will be taking the medication, and any special precautions or considerations needed while the child is taking the medication.

Community:
- Encourage caregivers to inform other community care takers of needed information for administering the medication safely

taneous injections. Since the medication is placed directly into the bloodstream where it can have an immediate effect, the nurse must follow guidelines related to concentration of medication, rate of delivery, and compatibility of solutions to help ensure the safety of the patient when using this method of administering medications.

Family Teaching

Safe Storage, Use, and Disposal of Medications

Home:
- Teach caregivers to store all medications out of reach of children, in a locked place if possible.
- Teach caregivers not to remove labels from medications or to store medications in other than original container.
- Teach caregivers to dispose of outdated medications or medications which are no longer needed by flushing them down the toilet.
- Teach caregivers not to save medication to give at a later time.
- Teach caregivers not to give medication that has been prescribed for another individual even if the illness is similar.
- Teach caregivers not to refer to medicine as candy.

School:
- Have caregivers check school policy regarding medications at school.
- Teach children not to share their medications with others.
- Teach children not to accept medications from others.

Community:
- Provide caregivers with phone number of local poison control center.
- Have parents educate other care providers, such as grandparents and day care center staff, regarding safe storage, use, and disposal of medications.

Preparation

Before administering IV medications, the nurse should consult pharmacologic references for the recommended time of infusion, maximum concentration of the drug in solution, and compatibility of the drug with IV solutions and other IV medications administered concurrently. The nurse should check the IV site just before giving the medication to ensure the IV is still in the vein and there is no swelling, redness, or tenderness at the site. This will ensure the medication is given intravenously and not into the surrounding tissue, and that it is not given into an inflamed and irritated vein. In addition, the nurse must be sure the drug is completely dissolved and does not contain any particles. If possible, the medication should be ready for administration before entering the child's room to avoid causing unnecessary anxiety. Necessary labels also should be prepared so all care providers are aware an IV medication is being administered (Bindler & Howry, 1997; Lehne, 2000).

Administration

Intravenous medication can be administered in several ways—by syringe infusion pump, buretol (metriset, soluset), piggyback, IV push, or retrograde. Factors to consider when selecting an appropriate method of delivery include (a) volume of solution necessary to dilute the medication, (b) volume of solution tolerated by child, and (c) hospital policies and procedures. Whatever method is used, the amount of fluid used for the medication and flushes must be included in the child's daily fluid intake (Kanneh, 1998b). Figure 19-3A–C offers some examples of equipment and setups.

Syringe infusion pumps, allowing medications to be delivered in a small volume of fluid over a prescribed period of time, are appropriate when larger fluid volumes are contraindicated. Tubing used with syringe infusion pumps is generally low volume (less than 5 cc, some as small as 0.5 cc) so only a small amount of solution is needed to flush the medication through the tubing so the entire dose is received by the patient. The tubing for the syringe infusion pump is primed with IV solution, generally normal saline, and then the syringe containing the medication is attached to the tubing. The syringe is then placed in the infusion pump and the pump is programmed to deliver the medication in the prescribed amount of time. Once the syringe is empty, the tubing is flushed, generally with normal saline. The tubing or syringe should be clearly labeled to indicate the presence of medication or flush.

Medications that can be placed in a larger volume of solution may be administered via a buretol (metriset, soluset). After cleansing the injection port, the medication is placed in the buretol and the IV rate is set to allow infusion

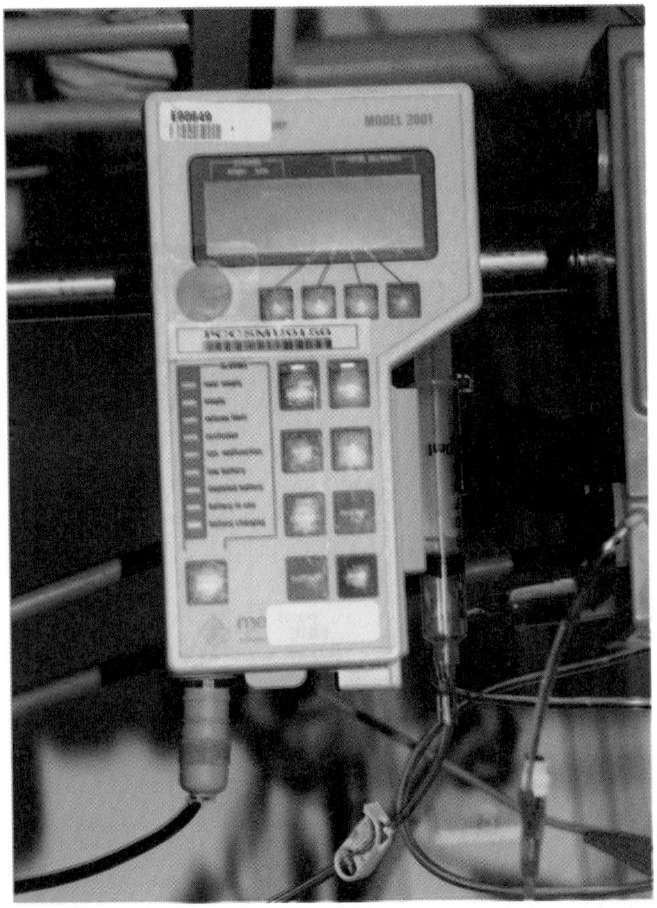

Figure 19-3A A Syringe Pump

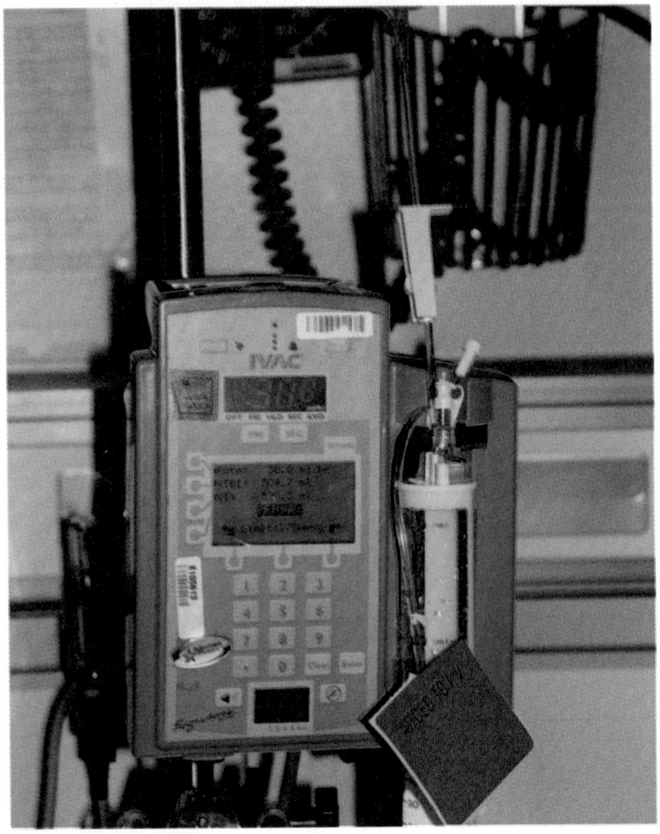

Figure 19-3B An IVAC Pump with a Buretrol Labeled with a Medicine

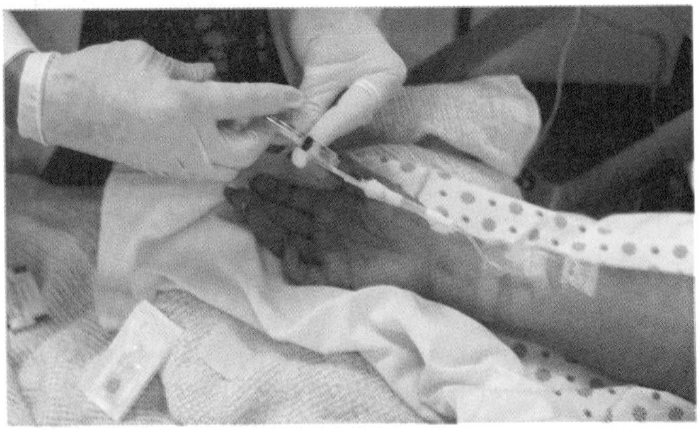

Figure 19-3C Administering an Intravenous Medication

Research Highlights

Saline versus Heparin for Maintaining Peripheral Infusion Devices

Study #1

Study Purpose

To compare the effectiveness of saline and heparin flush solution (10 units/cc) in maintaining peripheral intermittent infusion devices in hospitalized children.

Methods

The study used a randomized, double-blind, quasi-experimental design. The sample included 68 peripheral intermitted infusion devices (PIIDs) in 53 children ages 1 month to 19 years.

Findings

There was significantly more patency and less tenderness in PIIDs flushed with heparin. Those PIIDs flushed with saline had more problems with clotting and infiltration.

Implications

PIID protocols should continue using dilute (10 units/cc) heparin flush solution for hospitalized children.

Citation

Gyr, P., Burrough, T., Smith, K., Mahl, C., Pontious, S., & Swerczek, L. (1995). Double blind comparison of heparin and saline flush solutions in maintenancy of peripheral infusion devices. *Pediatric Nursing, 21*(4), 366, 383–389.

Study #2

Study Purpose

To determine the efficacy of saline versus heparin flush solution (10 units/cc) to maintain patency of peripheral IV locks in a pediatric population.

Methods

The study used a prospective, randomized, double-blind design. The sample included 124 peripheral IVs in 124 children ages 1 month to 22 years.

Findings

There was no significant difference between the heparin and saline groups for total hours duration of the IV and for incidence of complications.

Implications

Saline is as effective as heparin solution in maintaining patency of peripheral IV locks in children over 28 days of age.

Citation

Kleiber, C., Hanrahan, K., Fagan, C. L., & Zittergruen, M. A. (1993). Heparin vs saline for peripheral IV locks in children. *Pediatric Nursing, 19*(4), 376, 405–409.

General Implications

Controversy still exists regarding the use of heparin solution or saline for maintaining IV locks in a pediatric population. The nurse should follow the agency protocol of care of intermittent infusion devices and continue to be alert to research studies that further address this question.

of the medication in the prescribed amount of time. A larger volume of fluid is required to flush the tubing (up to 20 cc) after the administration of the medication. The flush must run at the same rate set for the infusion of the medication. Once the flush is completed, the IV rate is returned to its ordered rate, or the IV may be locked as ordered. When medication is in the buretol it should be clearly labeled or flagged in some way so the IV rate is not changed and no additional fluid is added to the chamber until the medication has completely infused. There also should be a method to indicate the flush is running so the rate of the IV is not changed resulting in the child getting the portion of the medication in the tubing too rapidly or too slowly (Bindler & Howry, 1997).

Larger volumes of medication also can be administered by the piggyback method. Here, the medication is diluted in 50- or 100-cc bags, usually 5% dextrose and water or normal saline. The IV tubing is primed, attached to the bag with the medication, and then connected into the indwelling IV line. These small IV bags can be infused using gravity or they can be incorporated into the IV pump, which will monitor IV rate and volume. Since gravity infusion is subject to the child's movements, which can alter drip rate, the nurse must assess the infusion frequently to maintain appropriate flow rate. Whether the medication is given via the buretrol (metriset, soluset) or piggyback, parents and children should be instructed not to tamper with the IV rate or level of fluid in the buretol.

Some medications may be delivered by direct, slow IV push into the injection port closest to the child. These medications are generally of small volume and can be administered over a period of several minutes, e.g., 3–5 minutes. The nurse must carefully time the administration of the medication to be evenly spaced over the recommended time. For example, when giving 5 cc over a period of 5 minutes, each 1 cc should be administered slowly over a 1-minute period of time.

A final method for administering IV medication is the retrograde method. The IV line to the client is clamped off, and the medication is injected into the injection port that has been cleaned. The medication goes up the tubing toward the IV bag. The line is then opened and the medication flows into the client with the IV solution. Tubing should be labeled to indicate the presence of medication in the IV line. Figure 19-4 illustrates venous access sites in infants.

Nursing Tip:

Giving IV medication through a heparin-locked line

When giving IV medication through a line that has been locked, the acronym SAS or SASH can help the nurse remember the steps of the procedure. S—saline, A—administer medication, S—saline, or S—saline, A—administer medication, S—saline, H—heparin. Which acronym is appropriate depends on the policy of the institution.

Nursing Tip:

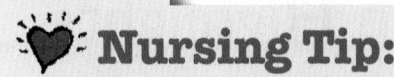

Cleaning IV injection or access ports

The procedure for cleaning injection or access ports on central IV lines may differ from that of peripheral IV lines. Check your hospital/unit procedure manual before injecting medications into a central line.

Intramuscular Medication

Due to the associated discomfort and psychological distress, intramuscular (IM) injections are not recommended for the pediatric population (Kanneh, 1998b). However, at times, it may be necessary to administer medication by this route. Selection of needle size and injection sites as well as techniques of administration are important considerations.

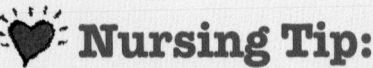

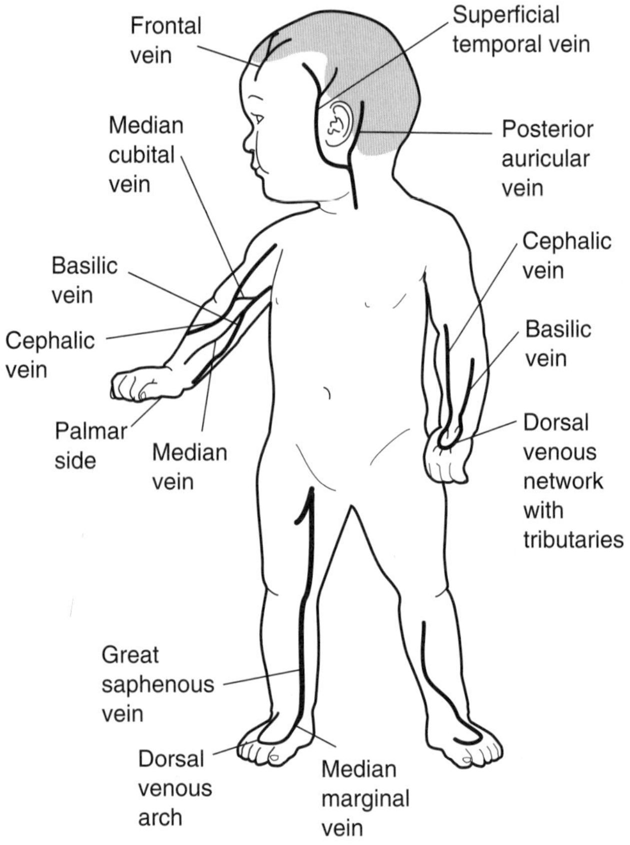

Figure 19-4 Venous Access Sites in Infants

Selecting Needle Size

Needle length and gauge are selected based on the child's size, amount of subcutaneous fat over the injection site, and viscosity of the medication. Age-based guidelines for selecting needle length and gauge can be found in Table 19-1, although each child and situation must be assessed individually. Viscosity of the solution to be injected must be considered when selecting the needle gauge since more viscous solutions require a larger gauge needle (smaller gauge number). The nurse should use the smallest gauge needle that will effectively deposit the medication in the muscle.

Injection sites are determined primarily on muscle development and the amount of fluid to be injected. The preferred injection site for infants is the vastus lateralis. The rectus femoris is also an acceptable site and may be used as an alternative or to rotate injection sites. For the toddler, the vastus lateralis or rectus femoris are still the preferred sites for injection. The dorsogluteal site may be used for the child who has been walking for at least one full year. The ventrogluteal muscle may be used for children older than 3 years of age who have been walking for several years. The deltoid muscle is generally used only in children over 4–5 years of age due to the small muscle mass. The deltoid muscle may be used for immunizations in the child over $1^{1}/_{2}$ years of age since only a small amount of fluid is injected. Figure 19-5 illustrates injection sites.

TABLE 19-1 Age-Based Guidelines for Selecting Needle Length and Gauge

Age Group	Needle Length	Needle Gauge
Infant	$^{5}/_{8}$ inch	25–27
Toddler/Preschool	1 inch	22–23
School-age/ Adolescent	$1–1^{1}/_{2}$ inch	22–23

Reflective Thinking

Getting a "Shot"?

Reflect back to when you were a child and went to the doctor's office for a checkup that required immunizations. Compare your experiences with what you have learned about how to administer subcutaneous and intramuscular injections. Do you recall someone explaining what was going to happen? Imagine you were the nurse responsible for the injection. How would your care differ from what you experienced?

The amount of solution that can be safely injected intramuscularly varies according to the age of the child and the specific muscle. Age-based guidelines for the amount of solution that can be injected can be found in Table 19-2.

Administration

Before administering IM injections, the skin at the injection site should be cleaned with alcohol or an antiseptic solution and allowed to dry. The nurse should insert the needle into the

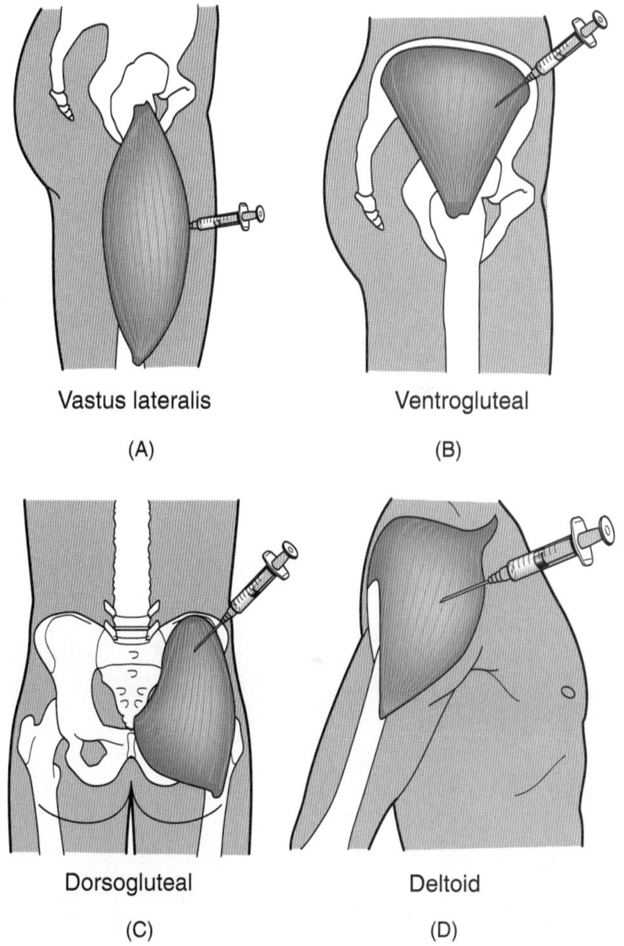

Figure 19-5 Intramuscular Injection Sites. (A) Vastus lateralis: Identify the greater trochanter. Place hand at the lateral femoral condyle. The injection site is in the middle third and anterior to the lateral aspect. (B) Ventrogluteal: Place palm of left hand on right greater trochanter so the index finger points toward the anterosuperior iliac spine. When middle finger is spread to form a V, the injection site is in the middle of the V. (C) Dorsogluteal: Place hand on iliac crest and locate the posterosuperior iliac spine. The injection site is the outer quadrant when an imaginary line is drawn between the trochanter and the iliac spine. (D) Deltoid: Locate the lateral side of the humerus. One finger width below the acromion process is the deltoid.

TABLE 19-2 Age-Based Guidelines for Amount of Solution to be Injected Intramuscularly

	Age group				
Muscle	**Infant**	**Toddler**	**Preschooler**	**School-aged Child**	**Adolescent**
(Age in years)	0–1.5	1.5–3	3–6	6–15	≥ 15
Vastus lateralis/Rectus femoris	0.5–1 cc	1 cc	1.5 cc	1.5–2 cc	2–2.5 cc
Dorsogluteal	**	*1 cc	1.5 cc	1.5–2 cc	2–2.5 cc
Ventrogluteal	**	*1 cc	1. 5 cc	1.5–2 cc	2–2.5 cc
Deltoid	**	*0.5 cc	0.5 cc	0.5 cc	1 cc

***Not recommended; *not recommended unless other sites are not available.*

skin at a 90 degree angle, aspirate (except when contraindicated), and inject the medication. In infants with a smaller muscle mass, the injection may be given at a 45 degree angle toward the knee to keep the needle in the muscle mass. Positioning the infant/child to relax the muscle being used for the injection may lessen the degree of discomfort experienced. For example, flexing the knee may promote relaxation of the vastus lateralis, while lying on the side and flexing the top leg at the knee may relax the ventrogluteal muscle (Bindler & Howry, 1997; Brucker & Wallin, 1998; Pollard, 1998).

When administering the IM injection, the infant and young child should be securely restrained to avoid injury due to a broken needle or giving the injection at the wrong site. It is best to have two adults help hold the child when giving IM medications to toddlers and preschoolers. The school-aged child also may need some help to remain still. It is also necessary to have a firm grip on the lower portion of the syringe to ensure safety should the infant or child move (Bindler & Howry, 1997; Brucker & Wallin, 1998). Figure 19-6a–b illustrates two methods of restraining an infant when giving an IM injection.

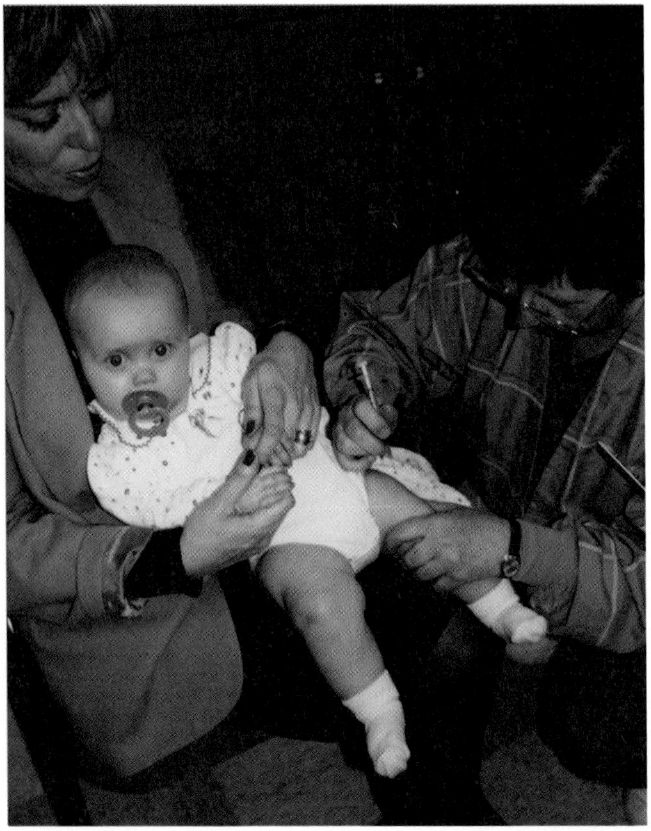

Figure 19-6a Restraining an Infant on the Mother's Lap When Administering an Intramuscular Injection

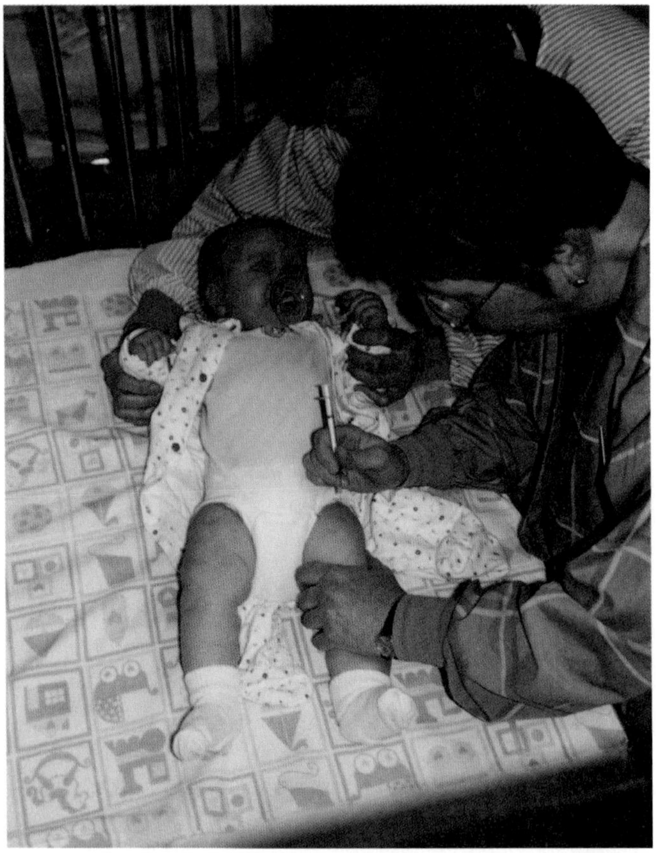

Figure 19-6b Restraining an Infant's Leg for an Intramuscular Injection When the Infant Is on a Bed

Nursing Alert:

Giving IM Medication to a Combative Child

It may require more than two adults to safely restrain a child who is combative. Using a matter-of-fact approach, the child should be gently but firmly restrained and the procedure accomplished as quickly as possible.

Subcutaneous Medication

Medication administered subcutaneously (SC) is placed in the subcutaneous fat layers of the body. Fat deposits differ between infants/children and adults, and must be considered when administering medication by this route. The anterior thigh, buttocks, upper arms, and abdomen are the preferred sites for injection. Pinching up the subcutaneous layer isolates the site and prevents injection into a muscle, especially when the infant or child has little subcutaneous tissue. The infant/child should be restrained as necessary. The technique for injection is the same as for an adult (Bindler & Howry, 1997).

Rectal Medication

Rectally administered drugs may be erratic and unpredictable in their absorption and are not the most desirable route of medication administration for pediatric clients. However, this route of administration may occasionally become the route of choice if the child is vomiting or is NPO. This invasive procedure may be extremely upsetting to toddlers and preschoolers because of age-related fears; school-aged children and adolescents may be embarrassed by this procedure. Therefore, age-appropriate explanation and reassurance are needed, as is proper restraint. The suppository, the most common form of drug used rectally, is lubricated with a water-soluble lubricant and inserted in the rectum beyond the rectal sphincter. The fifth finger is used in infants and children under 3 years of age. The index finger can generally be used in children over 3 years of age. After inserting the suppository, the buttocks should be held together for several minutes or until the child loses the urge to defecate to prevent expulsion of the suppository. If the child has a bowel movement within 10–30 minutes after administration of a suppository, examine the stool for the presence of the suppository. If it is seen, notify the physician/nurse practitioner since the drug may need to be readministered (Bindler & Howry, 1997).

Ophthalmic Medication

Administering ophthalmic medication requires special consideration in the pediatric population. Age-related concerns cause young children to fear having anything placed in their eyes and even infants may close their eyelids so tightly it is difficult for the nurse to open them. Proper restraint is necessary to control the head, keep the child's hands from interfering, and prevent injury to the eye. This may require the help of more than one person especially with infants and toddlers. Children who are old enough to comprehend the procedure should be given an age-appropriate explanation, which may help gain their cooperation. If possible, avoid giving ophthalmic medications when the child is crying since this limits contact of medication with the eye and decreases its therapeutic value (Bindler & Howry, 1997).

To administer eye drops or ointment, the child should be placed in a supine position. Hyperextension of the neck with the head lower than the body may help disperse the medication over the cornea. The hand used to instill the medication should be stabilized by resting the heel of the hand on the child's forehead with the dropper or tube of ointment held with the forefinger and thumb. This is a safety precaution to help prevent injury to the eye, and it also helps ensure the medication goes in the eye and not on the face. The lower eyelid should be retracted and the medication placed in the conjunctival sac using sterile technique. Ointment should be placed in the sac from the inner canthus outward. The dropper or tube of ointment should not touch the eye lashes or the eye, ensuring sterility as well as protecting the eye. Once the medication has been instilled, the child who is old enough to cooperate should be asked to gently close the eyes to allow greater contact of the medication with the conjunctival area (Bindler & Howry, 1997; Brucker & Wallin, 1998) (Figure 19-7).

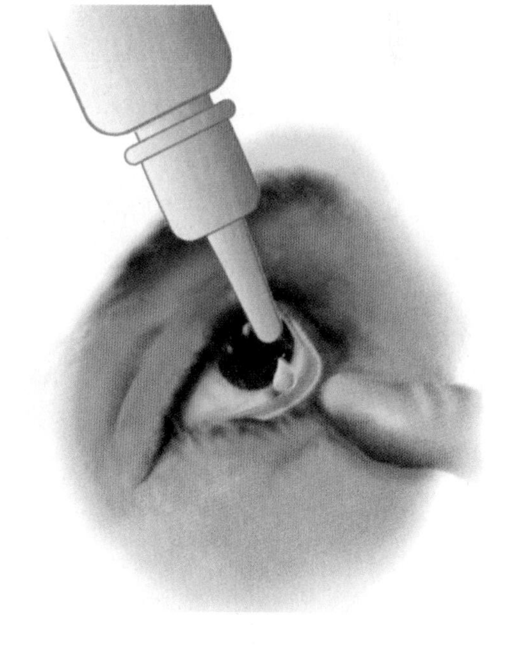

Figure 19-7 When administering an eye medication, gently press the lower lid down and have the child look upward while you instill the drops into the lower conjunctival sac.

Otic Medication

Age-related fears are also a concern when administering otic medications to young children. The younger child may need to be restrained to prevent movement of the head during instillation of the medication. An explanation may help the older child cooperate with the procedure. Unless the tympanic membrane is ruptured, the instillation of otic medication is not a sterile procedure.

The child should be placed in a side-lying position with the affected ear exposed. For children under 3 years of age the pinna is pulled downward and back. For the child older than 3 years of age, the pinna is pulled up and back as with adults. After instillation of the medication, the child should remain in the side-lying position for several minutes. If cotton is placed in the ear canal, it needs to be loose enough to allow discharge of any drainage (Bindler & Howry, 1997; Brucker & Wallin, 1998) (Figure 19-8).

Nasal Medication

The infant and young child may react negatively to nose drop instillation and proper restraint is necessary to safely accomplish the procedure. The infant or child is placed in a position with the head hyperextended. This can be accomplished by extending the head over the parent's lap, the bed, or an examining table. The child should remain in that position for at least 1 minute following the instillation of the nose drops. Nose drop instillation is a clean procedure (Bindler & Howry, 1997; Brucker & Wallin, 1998) (Figure 19-9).

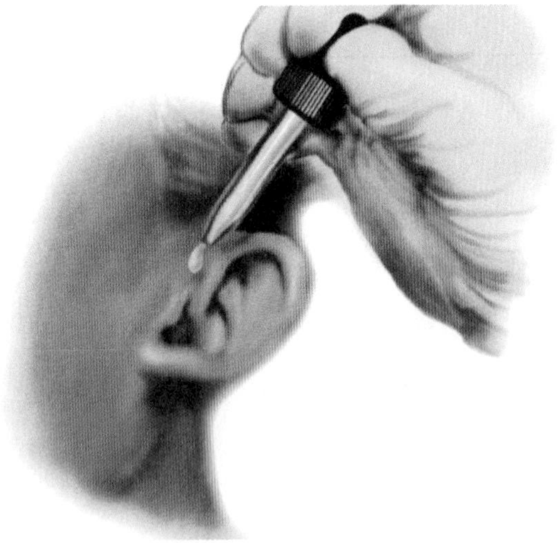

Figure 19-8 When instilling ear drops, hold the dropper 2 inches above the ear canal.

Topical Medication

Administering topical medication to children is the same as for an adult. If the skin is broken, sterile technique is required. The biggest challenge for the nurse administering topical medication to infants and children may be preventing the child from scratching an irritated or infected area. Nails should be kept short and clean, and the child's hands may need to be covered or restrained (Bindler & Howry, 1997).

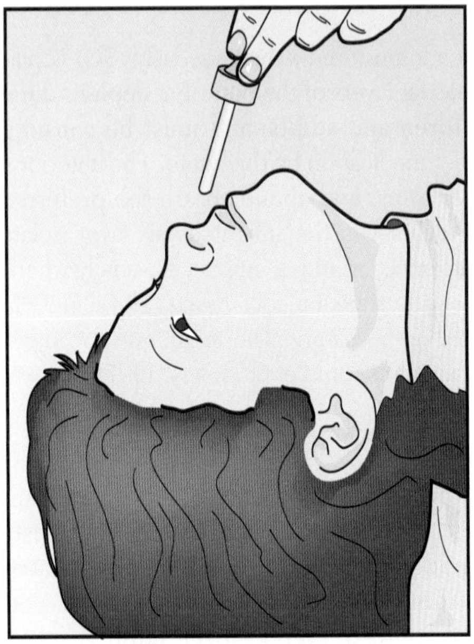

Figure 19-9 When instilling nose drops, the child should be placed on their back with the head tilted down or over the side of the bed. This will allow the medication to reach the back of the nose.

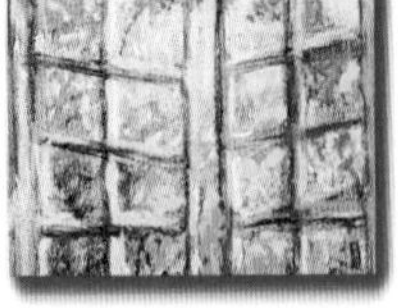

In the Real World

As a student, I felt overwhelmed when I first started administering medications to infants and children. There were all these calculations needed to determine a safe, appropriate dose and the amount (volume, number of pills) of medication to be given. Often the amount given was small and required transferring liquids into smaller syringes or cutting pills in half in contrast with my unit dose experience when caring for adults. In addition, at times I had to crush pills, and it was sometimes challenging to get them dissolved in a medium that the child would accept. As I progressed through my pediatric nursing experience, the supervised practice I received in giving medications to children increased my skills and my confidence in my ability to perform this task safely and efficiently.

Key Concepts

- Most drugs have not been adequately tested in the pediatric population; therefore, standardized doses have not been established, and children may be at risk for adverse reactions and/or ineffective treatment.
- Physiological differences between children and adults make children more sensitive to drugs and increase the risk of adverse drug reactions.
- Age-related physiological differences are responsible for alterations in pharmacokinetic and pharmacodynamic processes and determine the method, dose, and frequency of drug administration.
- Safe drug administration in a pediatric population requires an understanding of physiological differences and their impact on pharmacokinetic and pharmacodynamic processes.
- Approaches to children and techniques of medication administration must be based on growth and development, including physical, psychosocial, and cognitive development.
- Children should be given developmentally appropriate and truthful explanations about medication administration.
- The form of oral medication administered and the method of administration should be developmentally appropriate.
- Intravenous administration of medication improves the therapeutic blood level of medication and eliminates the discomfort associated with repeated injections.
- Injections (IM, subcutaneous) are not the preferred route in children since they are painful and distressing. In addition, physiological factors make this a less effective route in infants.
- When injections are necessary, care should be taken to select the appropriate injection site and size of needle based on the child's size. The needle size selected should be the shortest and smallest gauge possible.
- Administration of rectal, ophthalmic, otic, and nasal medications are invasive procedures that may illicit body integrity fears in toddlers and preschool-aged children.

Review Questions

1. What are the four pharmacokinetic processes?
2. How does gastric emptying time influence the absorption of orally administered drugs? What are the implications for administering medications to infants and children?
3. How does protein binding influence distribution of a drug? What are the implications for administering medications to infants and children?
4. What is the definition of half-life? What physiological factors influence the half-life of drugs administered to infants and children? How is this related to appropriate dose of a drug and the frequency of its administration?
5. What are two psychosocial/cognitive aspects of toddler growth and development that influence the administration of medication to this age group? How would you approach giving medication to this age group based on your knowledge of these aspects of growth and development?
6. What actions should the nurse take before administering a medication when there is a discrepancy between the ordered dose and the recommended dose?
7. A 3-year-old has an order for Cefazolin 300 mg IV every 8 hours. He weights 9.8 kg. The recommended dose for Cefazolin is 50–100 mg/kg/24 hours. Calculate the recommended dosage range for this child and compare it with the ordered dose. Is the ordered dose appropriate? If not why not?
8. What are two methods for administering an oral liquid medication to an infant? How you would administer the medication using each method, including any safety precautions?
9. The nurse is administering an intravenous (IV) medication to a child and has verified the five rights of medication administration, including comparing the ordered dose with the recommended dose. What additional information is needed in order to safely administer the IV medication?

References

Bindler, R. M., & Howry, L. B. (1997). *Pediatric drugs and nursing implications* (2nd ed.). Stamford, CT: Appleton & Lange.

Blaho, K., Winbery, S., & Marigan, K. (1996). Pharmacologic considerations for the pediatric patient. *Optometry Clinics, 5*(2), 61–90.

Brucker, J. M., & Wallin, W. D. (1998). Pharmacotherapeutics for the neonate and pediatric patient. In M. A. Kuhn (Ed.), *Pharmacotherapeutics: A nursing process approach* (4th ed.), (pp. 74–86). Philadelphia: Davis.

Carlson, J. D., & Byington, K. C. (1998). Fundamental principles of pharmacology. In B. P. Williams & C. L. Baer (Eds.), *Essentials of clinical pharmacology in nursing* (3rd ed.), (pp. 11–30). Springhouse, PA: Springhouse.

Clark, J. B., Queener, S. F., & Karb, V. B. (2000). *Pharmacologic basis of nursing practice* (6th ed.). St Louis: Mosby.

Gutierrez, K. (1999). *Pharmacotherapeutics: Clinical decision-making in nursing.* Philadelphia: Saunders.

Gyr, P., Burrough, T., Smith, K., Mahl, C., Pontious, S., & Swerczek, L. (1995). Double blind comparison of heparin and saline flush solutions in maintenancy of peripheral infusion devices. *Pediatric Nursing, 21*(4), 366, 383–389.

Hood, P. (1996a). The principles of pharmacology (1). *British Journal of Theatre Nursing, 6*(5), 21–25.

Hood, P. (1996b). Educational supplement. The principles of pharmacology (2). *British Journal of Theatre Nursing, 6*(9), 21–24.

Hood, P. (1997). Educational supplement. The principles of pharmacology (3). *British Journal of Theatre Nursing, 6*(12), 15–22.

Kanneh, A. (1998a). Pharmacologic principles applied to children. *Paediatric Nursing, 10*(3), 17–20.

Kanneh, A. (1998b). Pharmacologic principles: Part 2. *Paediatric Nursing, 10*(4), 24–27.

Kleiber, C., Hanrahan, K., Fagan, C. L., & Zittergruen, M. A. (1993). Heparin vs saline for peripheral IV locks in children. *Pediatric Nursing, 19*(4), 376, 405–409.

Koren, G. (1998). Special aspects of perinatal & pediatric pharmacology. In B.G. Kutzung (Ed.), *Basic & clinical pharmacology* (3rd ed.), (pp. 979–988). Stamford, CT: Appleton & Lang.

LeDuc, K. (1999). Pediatric pharmacotherapeutics. In K. Guitierrez (Ed.), *Pharmacotherapeutics: Clinical decision-making in nursing* (pp. 93–104). Philadelphia: Saunders.

Lehne, R. A. (2000). *Pharmacology for nursing care* (4th ed.). Philadelphia: Saunders.

Niederhauser, V. P. (1997). Prescribing for children: Issues in pediatric pharmacology. *The Nurse Practitioner, 22*(3), 16–30.

Pollard, R. (1998). Paediatrics and medication administration. Some practical issues. *The Australian Nursing Journal, 6*(5), suppl, 1–4.

Regulations Requiring Manufacturers to Assess the Safety and Effectiveness of New Drugs and Biological Products in Pediatric Patients; Final Rule Fed Reg. Vol. 63, No. 231, pp. 66631–66672 (December 2, 1998) (FR Doc 98-31902 Filed 11-27-98).

Turley, S. M. (1999). *Understanding pharmacology for health professionals* (2nd ed.). Upper Saddle River, NJ: Prentice Hall.

Walker, W. A., & Watkins, J. B. (Eds.). (1997). *Nutrition in pediatrics* (2nd ed.). Hamilton, Ontario, Canada: Decker, Inc.

Suggested Readings

Siberry, G. K., & Iannone, R. (Eds.). (1999). *The Harriet Lane handbook: A manual for pediatric house officers* (15th ed.). St Louis: Mosby.

Taketoma, C. K., Hoddling, J. H., & Krause, D. M. (1999). *Pediatric dosage handbook* (6th ed.). Hudson (Cleveland), OH: Lexi-Comp.

Resources

Organizations and Websites

Medication administration policies

www.familymanagement.com/childcare/policies/medication.administration.html

NASN Position Statement: Medication Administration in the School Setting

www.nasn.org/positions/medication.htm

Preventing Medication Errors in Children—Pediatric Pharmacotherapy A Monthly Review for Health Care Professionals of the Children's Medical Center

www.hsc.virginia.edu/cmc/pedpharm/v5n10.htm

For additional resources on the Internet, search:
www.dogpile.com
This mega-search engine searches from multiple search engines at the same time.

CHAPTER 20

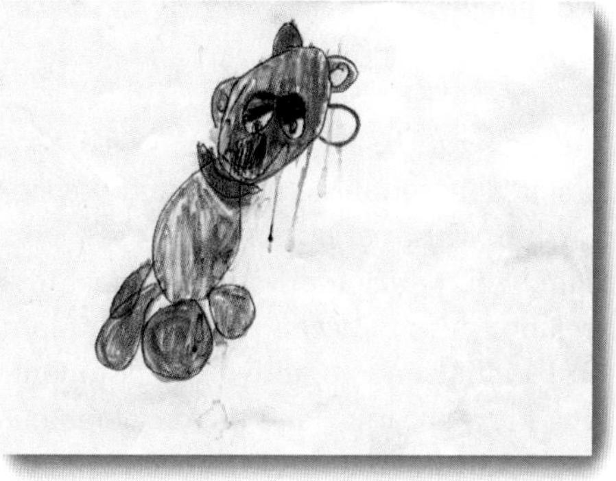

After 19 years as a pediatric nurse, I can still say that assisting children and families cope with separation, loss, and bereavement remains a challenge. My first significant experience with loss and bereavement came at the age of 16 years when my mother died. During that time, I was not able to verbalize my feelings, but looking back some 28 years later, I know that I felt helpless, confused, anger, pain, sadness, and even relief. Some years later I experienced the death of my pet dog Akidu. I experienced some of those same feelings, mainly sadness and anger. These 19 years have also taught me that children experience loss and separation not only related to a person but to pets and objects as well; and as adults grieve, so do children."

When caring for children experiencing loss, I try to incorporate the knowledge gained from my experience. At the same time, I try to remember that many factors influence how an individual copes with loss, and that there is no prescriptive way a person responds to loss. I also teach students that in order to assist clients cope with loss and bereavement, we must recognize and acknowledge the feelings of the individual which may be both verbal and nonverbal.

LOSS AND BEREAVEMENT

Hazel M. Sanderson, EdD, RN

COMPETENCIES

Upon completion of this chapter, the reader will be able to:

- *Describe common situations that can lead to feelings of loss and separation in children.*
- *Explain how children of various ages conceptualize death.*
- *Explain the process of grief and bereavement.*
- *Discuss factors that influence children's reactions to loss.*
- *Discuss the common responses of children to loss.*
- *Explain how children respond to the death of a parent or sibling.*
- *Discuss strategies to help communities cope with loss due to disaster/traumatic events.*
- *Discuss the role of the nurse in providing care to families experiencing a life-threatening illness of a child.*
- *Explain why hospice might be a good alternative to hospital care for the terminally ill child.*
- *Discuss the importance of self-care for nurses caring for the terminally ill child.*

When one thinks of loss, separation, or bereavement, the death of a person comes to mind; yet, on average, children experience loss and bereavement through a myriad of situations that are not related to the death of a person (Box 20-1). These early experiences are important and help shape an individual's ability to cope with loss later in adult life (Butler & Lagoni, 1996).

SITUATIONS LEADING TO LOSS

Relocation

In today's society, the average family will most likely move at least one time in their life. The effects of relocation may initiate feelings of anxiety and loss not only for adults but also for children. Relocation may be a positive or negative experience based on the circumstances. Relocation may mean a new job, better finances, and larger living space, or it may be the result of a need to be close to elderly parents, or it may be the result of a disruption in a family such as divorce. For children, such a move may be seen as a loss of comfortable and familiar things, people, and surroundings; moving to a new school or even starting a new grade may trigger feelings of anxiety and loss.

BOX 20-1 Common situations leading to feelings of loss and separation in children

- Relocation
- Loss of a possession
- Pet loss
- Parental separation/divorce

REFLECTIONS FROM FAMILIES

I don't remember how old I was when we moved to another state. My mother said I was 5 years old. I know I was sad because my aunt and uncles were not moving with us. I remember crying and telling my mother that I did not want to go. My aunt kept saying "I'm going to miss you." I could not sleep in my bed any longer, I did not like being by myself. I slept with my mother or one of my uncles. I know I was afraid, but I don't know what I was afraid of. I am now 18 years old and am preparing to go away to college. I have a small box with three items in it—a trophy, a cap, and a little wooden house. These items were given to me by my uncles and aunt the day my mother and I left. They told me to choose one item from each of them to take with me. Now I am going off to college and my family will not see me as often. I will give everyone an item of mine. My father will get one of my caps, my mother will get a tee-shirt. I don't know what I will give my two little brothers, but I think I will let them choose something from my room.

Loss of a Possession

Children at an early age develop attachments to objects such as toys and items of clothing. Such objects may bring about a sense of relaxation, security, and comfort. A blanket snuggled close to the body during naptime or while crying may be soothing and reassuring. A favorite toy that accompanies the child to the baby sitter, the day care center, or to the health care provider, helps maintain a sense of security and belonging. The loss of the treasured item can cause feelings of anxiety in young children and may be a child's initial experience with loss and separation.

Pet Loss

To understand pet loss, it is important to understand the significance of pet ownership. Most pet owners view their pets as members of the family and attribute human characteristics to them. Many relationships between pets and children are positively related to children's cognitive development, their ability to be empathic and caring, and the development of competence and social adjustment (Butler & Lagoni, 1996). Pets may be the friend who understands the child's feelings when (in the child's perspective) no one else does. A pet may provide unconditional love and acceptance, and may provide children with increased feelings of self-worth when they successfully care for the pet's needs. Hence, the loss of a pet may be of great significance to a child. Because children view pets as friends, the loss of the pet (death, lost from running away, or stolen) may be the child's first real experience with loss, separation, and grieving. Pet loss may be anticipated (old age or terminal illness), or unexpected (lost, stolen, acute illness, or accidental death). Regardless of the reason, children tend to feel much the same way about the loss (Figure 20-1). Therefore, the manner in which adults interact with children after the loss of a pet can greatly impact how children learn to cope with separation and loss later in life.

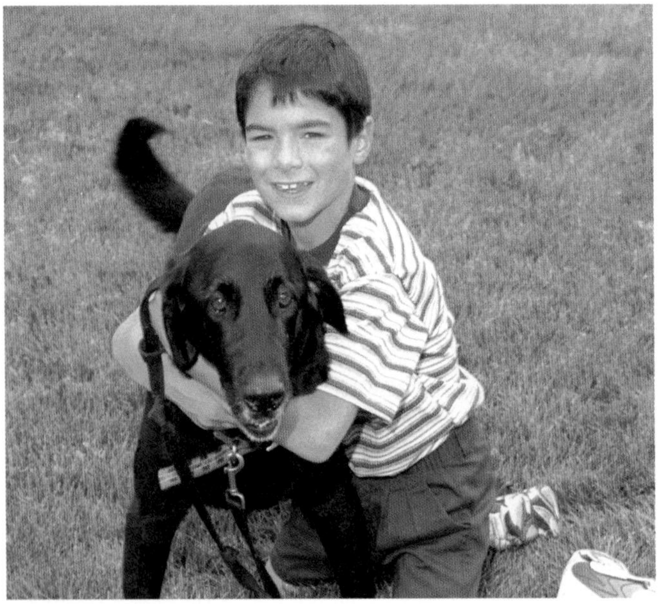

Figure 20-1 Children grieve when their pets become ill or die.

Parental Separation/Divorce

Divorce, an extremely stressful event in the life of a family, is a leading cause of separation experienced by families. It is termed a "taxing multistage process" that continues to affect more than 1 million children annually (Melynck & Alpert-Gillis, 1997). In 1998, approximately 28% of all children under 18 years of age lived with just one parent (*United States of Commerce News*, January 1999), and it is projected that, in this century, approximately 40% of children will experience the divorce of their parents.

Many children adjust well after parental divorce, but others suffer adjustment problems requiring therapeutic interventions (Behrman & Quinn, 1994). Children of divorce are more likely to have academic problems, exhibit externalized behaviors and internalizing disorders, and have lower self-esteem and problems in their relationships with parents, siblings, and peers (Amato 1994; Hetherington, Bridges, & Insabella, 1998). The impact of divorce often causes significant changes in the social, physical, and economic state of the family, but because of increased enforcement of noncustodial fathers' child support payments and changes in the labor force for women, it has been speculated that custodial mothers and their children may no longer experience such drastic economic declines following divorce (Hetherington, Bridges, and Insabella, 1998).

Two major factors in children's reaction to loss is age and cognitive development (Corr & Corr, 1996; Worden, 1996; Grollman, 1995; Mohon & Paige, 1995). In regards to divorce, preschoolers who are able to sense the conflict in the house tend to feel confused and bewildered though they may have a limited understanding about what is taking place. Children at this age perceive divorce as one parent moving away or leaving. The child often assumes that he or she did something wrong. This is turn causes the child to fear abandonment by the custodial parent. Children who are afraid of being abandoned tend to manifest clinging or hanging on behaviors with the custodial parent. These children may temporarily lose any independence recently acquired, and return to bed wetting, thumb sucking, or even bottle feeding. Preschoolers may experience nightmares or sleep disturbances and their play may become aggressive as they attempt to act out their feelings of confusion (Trimm, 1995).

School-aged children may believe that their parents' emotional distress is related to how they have been behaving and can perceive the divorce as a rejection of themselves, resulting in feelings of guilt. Fear of being replaced may exist along with low self-esteem. Children in this age group may have fantasies of reunification of parents and family, and may lie in an attempt to make this fantasy come true (Melnyk & Alpert-Gillis, 1997; Trimm, 1995).

Older school-aged children (9–12 years) may experience conflicts with loyalty and also exhibit outburst of anger toward either or both parents. **Parentification,** the role of assuming the caregiver (parent role), is also common in this age group. These children may also manifest their distress in anger, somatic complaints, and social withdrawal. Parentification is also common in the adolescent group, especially when daily activities of the home are neglected. Adolescents may distance themselves from one or both parents, or may be openly critical or both. Antisocial behaviors such as delinquency, becoming physically violent, smoking, alcohol abuse, or truancy may occur. For some adolescents, school may become a refuge from turmoil at home, and they may spend all their energies in school activities to avoid thinking about the situation at home. An emotional attachment to a member of the opposite sex may provide some form of compensation for family life, whereas others may sever any newly formed relationships (Melnyk & Alpert-Gillis, 1997; Amato, 1994).

CHILDREN'S AWARENESS OF DEATH

The 1990s brought changes in health care management and saw the role of the nurse expand from traditional sites to nontraditional settings such as schools, urgent care centers, HMOs, shelters, and other community organizations. At the same time, our society witnessed an increase in accidental deaths and violent crimes. In addition, we began to enjoy an advancement in technology that brought every new event directly into our living rooms via the Internet and television. Information once shielded from young children, such as death and violence, is now readily discussed in our playgrounds, school yards, and neighborhoods.

Nurses caring for children in any arena are now facing the challenges of caring for children and families affected by death. In order to provide care to children experiencing this loss, it is important nurses understand how children perceive the concept of death at various stages of development.

Concept of Death

The concept of death can be defined as having four distinct components including universality, irreversibility, nonfunctionality, and causality (Corr & Corr, 1996). **Universality** refers to the notion that all things die, death is all inclusive, and it comes to every living thing; death is inevitable. **Irreversibility** means that when the physical body dies it cannot come back to life—death is permanent. **Nonfunctionality** means that when a person or living thing dies, all functions that make the being alive stop. **Causality** refers to the notion that death has an internal and external cause. These causes may be natural, unnatural, good, or evil.

Younger children are more likely than older children to state death is not universal, avoidable, and occurs in the remote future. In essence, it is temporary and reversible. This thinking is reinforced in cartoons and particularly in video games where characters die temporarily. Also, words that adults use to describe death to younger children may reinforce this thinking. For example, oftentimes phrases such as *at rest, is asleep,* and *took a final journey* indicate that the state is reversible. Older children are more apt to grasp the key element of death—that it is permanent.

Understanding Death—A Developmental Process

The literature on children's understanding of death reveals that on average children under the age of 4 years have little to no understanding of the concept of death (Speece & Brent, 1996). Yet, it is quite early in infancy that children develop a sense of cause and effect, learning that when they cry the caregiver provides some form of comfort. It is in these early years that children first experience and react to separation, even though it is temporary. Between infancy and early toddlerhood, children experience separation anxiety, and learn to overcome it. Children also master the concept of object permanence and no longer cry when the caregiver leaves the room, or leaves them at school. It is theorized that these early experiences and losses later in life may be a precursor to an individual's ability to cope with separation. For example, a preschooler in day care cries when he is left by the caregiver. He does not want the parent to leave, and the day is spent crying and sometimes clinging to the teacher. This may continue for a while until the child learns a routine of the day, knowing that at a particular time the caregiver will return.

Piaget's theory of cognitive development provides a theoretical basis for conceptualizing the process of how children perceive and understand death (Table 20-1).

The second stage of cognitive development, according to Piaget occurring between the ages of 2 and 7 years, is the preoperational stage, and incorporates egocentricity and tangible thinking. Children begin to explore the world around them and begin to question, share, and interact with others. Between the ages of 3 and 4 years, children begin to question the sequence of time and events, and develop a limited understanding of death, which often is viewed as a reversible process. The limited understanding of death is illustrated in the preschooler who after being told that a loved one has died, initially feels sad and cries, and then in a short time asks when the deceased will return. By the age of 5 years, children's definition of death is more focused on function. People die when they are unable to breathe, eat, talk, and walk, for example. These two examples of functionality or the cessation of function raises the question on whether young children define nonfunctionality as the cause or the outcome of death.

Concrete operations, Piaget's third stage of cognitive development, occurs between the ages of 7 and 11 years. Here, children begin to develop skills necessary for organizing and sorting information and problem solving. Children of this age are no longer governed by egocentricity and develop the ability to deal with different views of a situation and consider another person's point of view. It is during this

Family Teaching

Talking with Children About Death

In the home:

- Allow the child to grieve.
- Provide child with quiet time (remember age and development).
- Communicate feelings about how this incident affects parents.
- Provide opportunities for all members of the family to share their grief.
- Loss or grief may be exhibited physiologically, socially, and psychologically.

In school:

- Provide opportunities for children to talk about their feelings.
- Offer further supportive counseling.

TABLE 20-1 Theoretical Basis of Understanding Concept of Death

Age	Piaget	Behavioral Manifestation	Understanding of Death
0–2 years	Sensorimotor	Egocentric	None
2–3 years	Preoperational	Egocentric	Reversible temporary
5–6 years	Preoperational	Egocentric	Avoidable
7–11 years	Concrete operations	Completion of task	Causality
12–17 years	Formal operations	Role confusion/intimacy	Selective universality (does not include self)

time that concrete thinking and inductive reasoning develop. Here, children begin to develop a more accurate concept of death with emphasis on its cause (causality), and must be helped to understand the true causes of death (Schonfield, 1993).

Formal operation includes the age group of 12–17 years; here, the individual learns to achieve emotional separation from parents, strives towards mastery, control, and competence, and later establishes intimacy and commitment (Corr & Corr, 1996). Although the adolescent is capable of understanding and conceptualizing death as permanent and universal, often there is an exclusion of the self from this concept. In other words, there is the notion that "it won't happen to me." Adolescents tend to participate in high-risk activities such as driving at high speeds, Rollerblading between traffic, and other activities that may place them at high risk for injury and death.

GRIEF AND BEREAVEMENT

Grief, an individual's response to loss, is viewed as a natural and healthy process. It is a complex range of feelings, cognitions, and behaviors that an individual has in reaction to a loss and includes cognitive, affective, and behavioral changes in the bereaved person after the loss. Worden (1996) views grief as the personal experiences, thoughts, and feelings associated with a loss. **Bereavement** is seen as an adaptation to a loss, and **mourning** is the process one goes through on his or her way to adaptation. To help clarify these terms, one can describe grief as the reaction an individual has to a loss, and bereavement as the behaviors one exhibits after the loss. Mohan and Page (1995) and McGlauflin (1996) explain that each person's response is different, therefore, each person's bereavement will be different.

Grieving and Mourning

Kubler-Ross (1969) identified five distinct stages of the grieving process (Table 20-2). Grieving, an individual's reaction to a loss, is viewed as a passage of time through which an individual may progress at different rates, sometimes moving in and out of the various stages.

Denial is a time of shock and disbelief. Like all phases of the grieving process, it is a healthy reaction to a shock but may become detrimental when individuals are unable to move past the disbelief and accept support to help them with their feelings. When the grieving person experiences feelings of **anger** (feeling of rage, envy, and resentment) over a loss, the anger may be directed toward God—for taking away the loved one, or at the custodial parent or both parents as seen in divorce.

Bargaining is seen at times when there is impending loss. The loss does not have to be limited to death, but may include loss of good health, an appendage, or even a way of life. **Bargaining** is an attempt to postpone the occurrence of the event, as the griever bargains with family and health care provides for one more chance to complete a task, or may wish to make a deal with God. In the event of divorce, children may bargain with parents. For example, the child might begin completing household tasks in the event that the good behavior might keep the family intact. **Depression** is a time when the reality of the situation is subconsciously beginning to take hold. The individual becomes confused, irritable, and sometimes sad. It is a time when a great deal of support is needed to assist the griever make sense of what is happening.

Acceptance is a time when the griever is consciously aware of what has happened or what is most likely to occur. If the griever is the terminally ill individual, he or she may be ready to participate in health care activities prescribed by the health care providers, or may choose palliative care with the aid of a health care proxy or living will. If the child is experiencing the separation of a parent because of divorce, he or she may be concerned with developing avenues whereby contact with the noncustodial parent are maintained.

Worden (1996) views mourning as a process an individual must undergo in order to adapt to a loss. In order to assist an individual adapt to a loss, the four tasks must be facilitated (Table 20-3).

Task I. Accepting the Reality of the Loss

Before children can deal with the loss, they must believe the deceased is dead and will not return to life. To negotiate this

TABLE 20-2 Understanding the Grieving Process According to Kubler-Ross

Stage	Responses to Loss Separation/Divorce	Death
1. Denial	"I don't believe you."	"It is not so."
2. Anger	"I hate you."	"I don't like God anymore."
3. Bargaining	"Will daddy come back if I behave?"	"I'll be a good boy, don't take my mother away."
4. Depression	"Don't leave me."	"Don't leave."
5. Acceptance	"Please call me every day."	"My daddy is living in heaven."

TABLE 20-3 Worden's Tasks of Mourning and Helpful Strategies

Worden's Four Tasks of Mourning	Strategies to Facilitate the Task
Task I—To accept the reality of the loss	• Tell child about the death in appropriate age-related language. • Depending on child's age, repetition may be needed.
Task II—To experience the pain or emotional aspects of the loss	• Allow child to express feelings. • Acknowledge child's feelings or behaviors associated with the loss.
Task III—To adjust to an environment in which the deceased is missing	• Help the child determine the relationship that the deceased person played in the child's life.
Task IV—To relocate the dead person within one's life and find ways to memorialize the person	• Help the child find a place in their heart or mind for the deceased.

Used with permission from Worden, J. W. (1996). Children and grief: When a parent dies. *New York: Guilford Press.*

task, Worden suggests children should be told about the death in appropriate age-related language. Depending on the age of the child, the information may need repeating.

Task II. To Experience the Pain or Emotional Aspects of the Loss

This task requires that behaviors and feelings of children are recognized and acknowledged. A child's ability to process the pain of loss will be influenced by observing an adult's experience of the loss.

Task III. To Adjust to an Environment in Which the Deceased is Missing

Adjustment is closely related to the roles and relationships that the deceased played in the child's life as well as the family. Worden states this adjustment goes on over time, and mourning for a childhood loss can be revived at any point in life. For example, the loss of a parent during childhood may be revived again when the individual has accomplished a significant task. A graduation from college, marriage, or birth of a child may revive the loss, as the individual may wish the parent could be there to share the joy.

Task IV. To Relocate the Dead Person Within One's Life and Find Ways to Memorialize the Person

The author states that this involves finding a new and appropriate place for the deceased in one's emotional life. For example, the deceased might be relocated to a special place in the heart or the mind.

UNDERSTANDING HOW CHILDREN REACT TO LOSS

Children's response to grief is influenced by many factors as listed in Box 20-2.

Children may have long periods when they are overcome with grief which is then followed by an interval when they do not seem to be affected by the loss. For example, within a few weeks after the death of a close relative, the child who was depressed and upset may seem to have forgotten about the loss and resume activities without any mention of the deceased. Nurses must help grieving caregivers understand that the child's behavior is a normal process of grieving since children do not grieve the same as adults (Trimm, 1995; Smith & Boardman, 1995). A major factor influencing how children react to grief is the relationship with the deceased. For example, a child may have little reaction to the death of an older sibling where there has been lit-

BOX 20-2 Factors influencing children's reaction to loss (separation or death)

- Developmental level
- Concept of loss (death)
- Relationship with the deceased/grieved
- Circumstances surrounding the loss
- Caregiver's ability to communicate and provide emotional support
- Emotional reaction to separation
- Support from peers and others
- Prior experience with loss
- Religious and cultural belief systems (Grollman, 1995)

tle contact or interaction, yet may react significantly to the loss of the after-school care provider where there was a close relationship.

Children's reactions to loss whether it be due to separation or death are also related to their personality, family structure, cultural and religious affiliation, age, and cognitive development. Reactions may be manifested in both physical and psychosocial ways (Table 20-4).

Although young children may have little comprehension of death and separation, they manifest behaviors indicative of what they are sensing. Preschool children often manifest sleep disturbances, including nightmares, bed wetting, or fear of falling asleep. They may also demonstrate clinging behaviors such as holding on to caregivers, crying, or not wanting to be left alone or separated from loved ones. Other behaviors in this age group are temper tantrums and regression. School-aged children may experience feelings of guilt about what they thought or said about the deceased person. They may also take on the role of caregiver (parentification), where they assume responsibilities such as looking after siblings, organizing household chores, or taking care of their caregiver. Other behaviors could include psychosomatic symptoms such as headaches, abdominal pain, and overall feelings of not feeling well. (Corr & Corr, 1996; Grollman, 1995; Worden, 1996; Trimm, 1995; Barnard, Morland, & Nagy, 1999).

The adolescent years are usually times of turmoil, finding a direction for self, forging one's own independence, selecting friends (peers), and developing a sense of self-confidence. The bereaved and grieving adolescent may be angry and depressed but may not share their feelings with relatives and keep their feelings hidden inside. Parents and significant others may interpret these behaviors as signs of uncaring, but it is usually the adolescent's way of maintaining individuation. The adolescent may also act out angry feelings in activities such as consuming alcohol, using drugs, dropping or staying out of school, isolating themselves from peers, and severing recently formed relationships (Grollman, 1995; Doka, 1996; Worden, 1996).

CHILDREN'S RESPONSES TO DEATH

Death of a Caregiver

The death of a parent is an extremely traumatic experience and a major crisis in the life of a child. Nearly 5% of American children experience the death of a parent before they are 16 years old, and that translates to approximately 1.5 million children in the United States living in a single-parent home because of the death of one parent.

The death of a parent and its consequences in the home and family change the very core of the child's existence (Worden, 1996). Siegal, Karus, and Ravies (1996) state that few events hold as much potential to disrupt a child's family pattern of life and place (the child) at risk for enduring psychological stress as the death of a parent. Children's reaction to the loss of a parent is often influenced by the manner in which the surviving parent and other adult family members react to the loss. When the surviving parent expresses feelings, openly grieves, and is able to spend time talking to the children about the loss in a positive and loving manner, and when such behaviors are demonstrated by the grieving parent and other significant caregivers, children may openly express their feelings in age-appropriate ways. When a grieving child reaches out to the surviving parent and is scolded or dismissed, but comforted by another adult relative, the child may become confused about how to feel or react to the loss.

The death of the mother may bring about a change in the roles of family members. Routines, schedules, and responsibilities may change. For example, an older sibling might now be responsible for caring for younger siblings.

TABLE 20-4 Common Responses of Children to Loss

Age Group	Physical Responses	Psychosocial Responses
Preschooler	Decreased activity Decreased appetite Regression such as bed wetting	Irritability Fear Anxiety
School age	Physical complaints such as not feeling well, abdominal pains, headaches, body aching, nausea, joint and muscle pains	Depression Fear of being rejected Fantasies of parental reunification
Adolescent	Decreased appetite Decreased or increased activity Increase in smoking, alcohol, drug use	Feelings of betrayal Anger Distancing self from parents/family Increase or decrease in school activities Withdrawal

REFLECTIONS FROM FAMILIES

Don, a 36-year-old male, and his seven siblings talk about the impending death of their father. Don tells his siblings that he must tell his 6-year-old daughter, Grace, that her grandfather will die soon. When questioned about the urgency of his actions, Don states he will not allow Grace to go through what was done to him and his younger siblings when their mother died when he was 10 years old. Don tells his siblings that he can still remember how frightened he felt that morning, sensing something had happened but no one was responding to his request for an answer to what had happened. He still remembers that morning, sitting with his two younger brothers all huddled together in one chair. There seemed to be an eerie silence, followed by a great deal of activity, yet no one informed them that their mother had died, even though they suspected something terrible had happened.

BOX 20-3 Preparing a child for the death of a parent

When planning to discuss with parents and other caregivers about what and how much information should be told about the death of a parent or other significant relative, nurses should base their plan on the knowledge that children should be given accurate information, in a clear manner using age-appropriate language. The information should be given by an individual whom the children trust and whom they feel comforted by. Children should be allowed to express their feelings (verbal, nonverbal, games, role play, letter writing) and provided with bereavement support, nurturing, and continuity. The physical and emotional availability of the surviving grandparent are important to the child's adjustment after the loss, and talking about the deceased is important. Finally, children should be included in activities related to funeral and burial rites when appropriate (Grollman, 1995; Bowden, 1995; Carroll & Griffin, 1997).

Additional caregivers may be introduced into the family such as a baby sitter, grandparent, or aunt, who now carries out activities and chores that were once done by the mother. The death of the mother, the primary caregiver in most families, may leave grieving children with feelings of anxiety as their refuge for comfort and security is gone. The loss of a father, oftentimes the principal financial provider in a two-parent family, may bring concerns about financial issues. Children of single parent families whose parent dies experience additional hardships as the entire home environment changes. Children may be placed with relatives or foster parents. These children lose their parent, their haven, and their home.

Although children grieve differently than adults, they also need support, encouragement, a listening ear, a lap or a shoulder, and arms to hold them. When working with families experiencing the loss or the impending loss of a parent, nurses must be aware of the needs of the children who are sometimes removed from the immediate environment, which more often than not, is their own home. When providing support for the surviving parent, support measures should be considered for the children also. The way in which children are informed of the death of a parent oftentimes remain indelible in their minds forever. See Box 20-3.

Death of a Sibling

Sibling relationships are the most consistent and frequently the longest ongoing relationship one has in life, as it embodies the entire gamet of emotion—love, caring, sharing, protecting, comforting, envy, and blaming (Bowden, 1995). Stahlman (1996) describes a characteristic of sibling relationship as "universal ambivalence," and all of these emotions may be the catalyst for growth, maturity, and the ability of individuals to build relationships with others. To children, siblings are peers, friends, rivals, mentors, protectors, and teachers. To parents, children are the hopes, dreams, and future of a family, so when a child dies, not only is the child lost, but also the hopes tied to that child (De Maso, Meyer, & Beasley, 1997). Sibling loss is becoming a somewhat common phenomenon as the number of children who die yearly increases, since approximately 1.8 million children under 19 years of age experience the death of a brother or sister (Hogan & DeSantis, 1996). These losses are attributed to illness (acute and chronic), and an increase in sudden and traumatic deaths. Regardless of the cause, a child's death can have a profound and lasting effect on surviving siblings (Walker, 1993), and the roles of surviving siblings may change immediately.

Oftentimes following the death of a child, surviving siblings are overlooked, as support is generally provided to grieving parents. For example, when a parent, grandparent, or child dies, support is initially directed toward the adult—the surviving spouse, adult child, or parent. Children are sometimes sent to neighbors or relatives while support is provided to the grieving adult. Regardless of the cause of death or who dies, children should be allowed to grieve and be supported in their grief. Because sibling relationships run the gamet of emotions, a surviving sibling may experience not only sorrow at the loss of a brother or sister, but also guilt about something that was thought or said about the deceased. Guilt or ambivalent feelings can have an impact on how the surviving sibling copes with the loss. Davies (1995) states that the closer the relationship was before death, the more behavior problems the surviving siblings demonstrate afterward. Also, emotional closeness that existed between siblings prior to the death of one tends to be related to the outcome of the surviving child's grieving process.

Walker (1993) states that, when a child dies, the surviving sibling loses not only a brother or a sister but the functional loss of the grieving parent since frequently parents are unable to attend to the needs of the surviving siblings. Oftentimes, grieving children are overlooked as the needs of the grieving parents are being supported. Depending on the circumstances of the death, siblings may feel guilty, angry, or sad. Some of the emotions expressed and experienced by the surviving sibling may be characterized as universal ambivalence. After the death of a sibling, surviving siblings may experience a sense of increased vulnerability, anger at parents for not protecting the deceased, survivor guilt, or protectiveness of parents (Mohan, 1993; Walker, 1993; Worden, 1996). It is important for nurses to understand that because grieving parents may be emotionally unavailable to the surviving children and because support is generally directed toward parents, siblings are often the most neglected family member when a child dies (Davies, 1995; Bowden, 1995; Walker, 1993). Box 20-4 offers some facts to remember when helping children cope with sibling loss.

BOX 20-4 Facts to remember when helping children cope with sibling loss

- Remember that children have a need to grieve.
- Be prepared to answer loaded questions.
- Expect behavioral changes and responses.
- Allow children to express their feelings.
- Be aware that parents might be emotionally unavailable to surviving children.
- Inform the school community of the child's loss.
- Provide peer support groups.

Case Study/Care Plan

A Child Dies

Darren, 12 years old, is in the final stage of a terminal illness. His immediate family keeps vigil at his bedside. Darren is no longer alert.

Nursing Diagnosis #1

Anticipatory grieving by family related to prognosis.

Expected Outcomes

The family will be made aware of steps to facilitate the grieving process and given opportunities to begin the grieving process.

Interventions/*Rationales*

1. Allow family private time to spend with Darren. *Provides privacy and opportunities to gather and grieve as a family.*
2. Provide family with private space to meet and grieve. *Helps family maintain a sense of control and belonging as a family without the interruption and intrusion of others.*
3. Provide opportunities for family to express feelings to each other and to the staff. *Provides support and to clarify feelings and concerns as well as provides psychosocial support where appropriate.*
4. Provide support for family. *Allows family members to grieve and to understand and accept individual style of grieving.*
5. Encourage family to participate in Darren's care. *Promotes dignity, respect, and self-worth of all individuals.*

continues

continued

6. Minimize the number of health care personnel providing information to family. *Decreases the risk of overwhelming and confusing family members. Allows for more accurate identification of family's needs.*
7. Maintain optimum care to Darren. *Helps family maintain a sense of control and belonging.*

Nursing Diagnosis #2

Anticipatory grieving by staff related to prognosis.

Expected Outcomes

The staff will exhibit signs that they have begun the grieving process in a healthy manner.

Interventions/*Rationales*

1. Provide peer support to staff members. *Peer support allows staff members to express feelings, to exchange ideas and experiences, and to teach and learn from each other.*
2. Encourage staff to discuss their feelings. *Discussion of feelings helps minimize fears and clarify issues and misconceptions.*
3. Maintain supportive working environment. *Promotes physical and mental health of the individual and the team.*
4. Maintain optimum care to Darren. *Fosters dignity, respect, and self-worth of individuals.*

Evaluation

Two days later Darren dies, his family was at his bedside. The nurse remained late that day to say her final good-bye to Darren and to provide post-mortem care. Information about the funeral was sent to the nursing unit, a number of nursing staff attended the funeral.

One month later, Samantha, the 7-year-old sister of Darren, is admitted to the hospital with acute abdominal pains. Her parents are extremely nervous, and Samantha is visibly afraid and crying. She clings to her mother and becomes hysterical when left alone. Samantha tells her mother she is afraid that she will die like her brother.

Nursing Diagnosis #3

Anxiety (caregiver) related to hospitalization of child.

Expected Outcomes

Family will exhibit lessened anxiety level related to hospitalization of child.

Interventions/*Rationales*

1. Provide opportunities for caregivers to express their feelings. *Provides support for caregivers to express their feelings.*
2. Provide key personnel to communicate information to caregivers. *Decreases the risk of overwhelming and confusing family members. Allows for more accurate identification of family's needs.*
3. Keep caregivers informed about child's conditions. *Helps family maintain a sense of belonging and control.*
4. Involve caregivers in plan of care. *Helps family maintain a sense of belonging and control.*
5. Provide support services for family. *Helps maintain the physical and psychological health of the family.*

Nursing Diagnosis #4

Increased anxiety and fear related to hospitalization and recent death of sibling.

Expected Outcomes

Child will exhibit lessened anxiety level related to hospitalization and death of sibling.

continues

continued

Interventions/*Rationales*

1. Encourage caregiver to remain with child. *Promotes a sense of safety and belonging for the child and decreases anxiety.*
2. Allow Samantha to express feelings. *Helps to understand child's perceptions, and to provide appropriate interventions.*
3. Minimize the number of staff interacting with Samantha. *Decreases the risk of overwhelming the child.*
4. Explain procedures and treatment in age-appropriate language. *Helps to promote child's understanding of events taking place.*
5. Refrain from using words and terminology that can be misconstrued. *Decreases the chances of misunderstanding, decreases anxiety.*
6. Encourage caregiver involvement in Samantha's care. *Helps child and caregivers maintain a sense of control and normalcy.*
7. Encourage self-care. *Helps promote sense of independence and control.*
8. Provide Samantha with avenues to express self (drawing, painting, writing, puppet play). *Helps staff and family to understand how child feels and to provide appropriate interventions.*

Evaluation

Three days later, Samantha is discharged home. The interdisciplinary team recommend that the family continue to receive counseling to help deal with the two stressful events.

Critical Thinking

When a Child Is Dying

You are in your pediatric clinical rotation in a hospice unit and assigned to a 13-year-old in the terminal stage of an acute illness.

What would you say to the child and family about dying and death?

What would you do or say if the client says the following: "I don't want to die."?

DISASTERS/TRAUMATIC EVENTS

The rise in violent crimes committed by children in generally safe environments such as schools, playgrounds, and homes has propelled this generation of children to a level and kind of unprecedented risk. Children may suffer the effects of a disaster regardless of whether they are directly involved or were witnesses (Barnard & Morland, 1999). The effects of the disaster or traumatic event may have long-term consequences, interfering with the child's ability to engage in productive behavior and function adequately socially, academically, and professionally (Nardar, 1996). See Box 20-5 for the long-term consequences of traumatic loss in children.

In addition to grieving the loss of classmates, friends, peers, or significant others such as teachers or other adults, children have to cope with the experience of the trauma. In other words, not only did someone die, but it is the circumstances under which the individual or individuals died or became injured that is traumatic. Children who experience traumatic losses often experience the same reactions, but in addition, may exhibit rage, sleep disturbances, repeatedly have thoughts about the incident, an increased alertness to dangers, and fear attending school or any other environment similar to the traumatic incident (Barnard & Morland, 1999).

When prioritizing supportive care to children who experienced a violent and traumatic incident, it is important to

BOX 20-5 Long-term consequences of traumatic loss

- Cognitive dysfunction (emotional regression)
- Health disturbances (depression)
- Altered personality trait (may appear uneasy)
- Disruption in moral development
- Attempts at masking emotions

note that such incidents or crimes are crimes against a community and not just individuals. For example, the consequences of a shooting occurring in a school is felt by everyone in the community and beyond, and has ramifications nationwide. When support is provided it must be provided to the community at large. Box 20-6 lists some ideas to help communities cope with traumatic incidents.

REACTIONS OF FAMILY TO A CHILD WITH A LIFE-THREATENING OR TERMINAL ILLNESS

Children are supposed to lead strong and healthy lives, and outlive their parents and other caregivers. However, children may suffer from a variety of life-threatening illnesses, from congenital to acquired—including heart defects or disease, cystic fibrosis, accidents, cancer, and AIDS. The anguish a family experiences from the time of diagnosis to the final outcome can only be described as excruciatingly painful—a time when life instantly becomes chaotic and unpredictable.

The experience of coping with a life-threatening illness presents many challenges to both the family and the health care providers. Doka (1996) suggests the experience of a life-threatening illness can be viewed as a series of phases, each with its own unique issues or tasks. Understanding the various phases and tasks can help nurses and other health team members provide appropriate care to clients and families as the sequence of events from diagnosis to final outcome unfolds (Table 20-5).

BOX 20-6 Helping communities cope with violent traumatic incidents

- Provide counselors from within and outside the community (Red Cross, other agencies). Counselors and other health care providers who live in the community may be dealing with their own sense of loss in regards to the incident.
- Encouraging discussion at community board meetings helps identify the needs of the community.
- Educate the community about how children grieve.
- Allow children to grieve.
- Facilitate grieving of children–allow them to see and hear how adults are dealing with the traumatic loss, which will help them express their feelings.
- Listen to the children, provide opportunities such as plays, writing, drawing, dancing, and music. Listening helps adults understand how children are feeling about the incident. The use of other avenues of expression will provide opportunities for children to express their feelings both verbally and nonverbally.

REFLECTIONS FROM FAMILIES

It's been 15 years since the accident. Whenever I think about the morning they told me she might not survive, I get that numb but tight feeling in my throat. Donna was only 8 years old and was happily riding her bike when she was hit by a car. I was confused and dazed for a very long time. I don't remember events of the hospitalization, probably I don't want to remember. I believe I woke up out of my confusion when Donna was placed in rehab and had to learn to walk and eat again. It's something I pray will not happen to another parent.

Reflective Thinking

Personal Experiences with Death

Have you ever experienced the death of a close family member, friend, or a pet? If yes, how has that shaped your view of dealing with loss? If no, how do you imagine you will deal with a future loss?

Loss of a Newborn

Loss of a newborn remains a stressful and traumatic event for parents, families, nurses, and others regardless of the reason for the loss. When preparing the deceased newborn for viewing by the parents, it is important that the newborn be washed and dressed appropriately. This helps parents see their deceased newborn as their child. Clothing the infant in an outfit and wrapping it in a blanket selected by the parents helps the family to take ownership of the deceased and the loss. The area for viewing the deceased newborn should be clean, quiet, and in an area appropriate for the living. That means it should not be in a utility room or other area not designated for clients. The manner in which nurses prepare the deceased newborn for viewing can have a major impact on how parents and relatives remember the event. A hostile or unwelcome environment may give the parents a feeling of being discarded. Therefore, the deceased newborn can be placed in a basinette, fully clothed and swaddled in a blanket. Chairs should be provided. Parents should be allowed to hold the baby and to stay as long as they can. A nurse should be available to present the baby to the parents just as would be done if the newborn were alive.

TABLE 20-5 Nursing Care of Families Experiencing Life-Threatening Illness of a Child

Phase	Definition	Behaviors/Task	Nursing Care
Prediagnostic	From suspicion to time of medical attention	Guilt. What did I do wrong? Increase in anxiety about the unknown.	• Allow family members to express feelings. • Provide information to family in a timely manner.
Diagnostic/ acute phase	Period when tests and studies to determine the diagnosis occur.	Afraid. Feeling of uncertainty and helplessness. Family life at a standstill. Overwhelmed with information in regards to the diagnosis. May seek second or third opinions.	• Continue to allow family members to express feelings and ask questions. • Assess need for psychological and spiritual support. • Maintain communication among members • Provide information to family in a timely manner.
Chronic phase	Treatment in progress.	• Family's anxiety level may be decreased slightly. • Parents and others may be physically exhausted. • May question therapies and seek opinions or alternate forms of treatment.	• Continue supporting the expression of feelings. • Assess parents' need for rest. • Provide information about therapies. • Encourage other health team members to provide information to family in a timely manner. • Assess siblings need for additional support since parents may be physically and mentally exhausted.
Terminal phase	Recovery is not an option.	• Family must prepare for death of child. • Parents may have difficulty accepting treatment modality that is more palliative.	• Provide support to family. • Assist family in communicating their wishes to the interdisciplinary team. • Minimize the number of personnel providing information to family. • Provide appropriate support for decision making regarding hospice care, hospital care, home care, DNR, and other therapies.
Recovery phase	May include living with long-term consequences of the illness.	• Family must now learn to live with the effects of the death. • May include a change in previous lifestyle for family.	• Provide avenues for discussion of feelings, fears, concerns. • Provide family teaching regarding care of child. • Provide information regarding support services for family and child.

How Much Should the Child Be Told?

A great deal of discussion remains regarding how much information should be provided the terminally ill and dying child. Some parents and caregivers in their desire to protect may not want the child to know many details about their diagnosis. It is imperative that the interdisciplinary team and caregivers discuss what and how much information the child should receive. Also, there should be discussions about the information given siblings. Doka (1996) suggests that attempts to protect children from illness and death are often futile and that, by middle childhood, children are exposed to information about diseases and many have already experienced loss of some kind. Under normal circumstances, children can sense something is wrong by the way adults treat them. Since there is often a tendency to walk away from the child when issues are being discussed, this behavior suggests to the child something is wrong. Therefore, in efforts to protect children from knowing they are ill, nonverbal behaviors may alert the child that something is wrong and cause increased anxiety.

Kids Want To Know

Am I going to die?

One day Ronnie, a 7-year-old with a terminal illness, said to the nurse, "I don't feel better any more, am I going to die? Everyone is acting kind of weird."

- Do not trivialize Ronnie's comments.
- Determine what Ronnie knows about his current status
- Discuss with parents/family/caregivers and health-care team what Ronnie needs to know, who will tell him, and what is being told.

What Should the Child Be Told?

Children as early as preschool age should be told they are ill. Information should be concise, clear, and simple. For example, a young child (5–9 years old) with leukemia can be told blood cells in the body are not strong enough to fight off infection, and the medicines and treatments will help strengthen those cells. An older child (10–12 years old) may need to know more about leukemia and the reasons for specific therapies. Today, children have many avenues to obtain information such as books, television, and the Internet; however, not all the information available is accurate; therefore, it is important that family and the health care team collaborate to provide appropriate and necessary information.

Who Should Tell the Child?

When planning to discuss who will be responsible for informing a child about his or her illness, caregivers and the interdisciplinary team should discuss the matter. No rule exists on who should inform a child about illness, but a small group of individuals who will be primary care providers are the best. The small group may consist of parents or caregiver, a nurse, and the physician/primary health care provider. An older sibling and/or another family member with whom the child has a significant relationship should be included. A cadre of caring and loving individuals with whom the child has a trusting relationship, along with members of the interdisciplinary team with whom a relationship will or has developed would help the child maintain a sense of security, love and trust, and belonging. Nurses can play a pivotal role in maintaining a sense of security and a trusting relationship with the ill child.

DECISIONS ABOUT HOSPICE

Just as caregivers are given options for types of treatment for the ill child, they should also be given options and opportunities to plan where and how the child will spend the final chapter of life. Children's hospice care, a growing alternative to hospital care for the dying child and family, incorporates a holistic approach providing psychosocial, spiritual, and physical support to the child and family. In this setting, the parent and child are the primary decision makers with the interdisciplinary team functioning in a more supportive role. Hospice can be provided at home, the hospital, or in a facility for hospice care. Professional support to the family continues long after the child's death. The support team for the child in hospice includes the family, significant support individuals and the interdisciplinary hospice team. Hospice provides physical, respite, and bereavement care to the child and family. The primary focus of physical care is to maintain a comfortable and pain-free environment for the child, through the implementation of pain management programs. Parents and other caregivers also have the opportunity to provide physical care for the child, and the child is allowed the right and dignity to be a child, and cared for by a parent or other family members.

Hospice service also provides respite care to allow family members to take a break or time off for themselves before resuming the primary care of the child. Hospice personnel are also trained to recognize the signs of anticipatory grieving in the child and/or family, and to support them through this healthy process.

ORGAN AND TISSUE DONATION

The discussion of tissue donation is a very sensitive and uncomfortable topic for many health care providers, since the possible hope for life or living for one person means the death of another. It is an awkward time for the health care providers, whose actions may seem cruelly intrusive on a grieving family. Therefore, the timing for discussion must be planned and well coordinated. Most large hospitals and acute care settings have established programs with well-trained health care personnel who are responsible for discussing tissue and organ donation with families.

Nurses caring for the dying child are aware of the total plan of care for their clients and at a pivotal position to evaluate family concerns about the issue, and provide avenues for family members to openly discuss their concerns with the transplant team. In order to maintain the rights and dignity of a dying child and family, and in order not to be viewed as vultures, specific criteria are established for the procurement of tissue and organs, which may vary according to individual health care agencies.

AUTOPSY

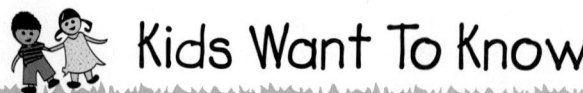

The decision to perform an autopsy is a requirement of law when death is caused by unnatural causes such as murder or suicide, if it occurs within 24 hours of hospitalization, or if death occurs at home or in an institution when a person has not been under the care of a physician. Nurses can only emphasize to the family that the decision to perform the autopsy is not a decision based on hospital policy, but a requirement of state law.

CARE FOR NURSES WORKING WITH TERMINALLY ILL CHILDREN

The idea of dying is not easily discussed in U.S. society, as it represents the end of life as we know it and fear of the unknown. The association between death and children is paradoxic because children represent life and future, whereas death is just the opposite. When children are terminally ill and expected to die, all individuals involved in the care of the child are emotionally affected. Nurses, the primary caregivers to the child and the family, often experience emotional battles within themselves as they attempt to provide the best care to the child and family and put their own feelings aside. Nurses providing physical and emotional care to others often times neglect their own need for support and place themselves at risk both physically and emotionally.

The care of terminally ill children is usually provided in specialty areas, units, or institutions, where the majority of the clients are at high risk of dying. Therefore, the atmosphere of the environment is usually one of urgency, with various levels of anxiety and stress among staff and families. Just as the ill child and family have special needs, so do the nurses; unfortunately needs of the nurses often go unmet. One reason for this is that the nursing staff may not recognize they too are grieving the loss. When nurses do not tend to their need to grieve, they may feel anger, frustration, and depression, manifested by sick calls, breakdown in communication at work and at home, feelings of not being appreciated, and sometimes guilt.

When death involves a child, the acceptance and acknowledgment of the death is more difficult to understand. At times, nurses who are experiencing those feelings begin to question the technology, the profession, and even their faith. During this time, these nurses are not able to appropriately attend to the needs of the dying child or the family, must come to terms with their own feelings about dying and death, and must allow themselves to grieve so they can help others. To do so, nurses must seek assistance.

To maintain the physical, emotional, and psychological integrity of the nursing staff, institutions should provide a caring or health promoting environment with an emphasis on wellness and the promotion of health. Assistance programs for employees or staff are examples of such service. Nurses and other health care providers may be given the opportunity to use mental health days or recharge time when they can seek the assistance of providers such as psychologist and psychiatrist to assist them in dealing with their concerns and feelings. Some institutions have support groups established, others initiate support services when the psychological integrity of the staff is being threatened. Interventions should be ongoing, where nurses can meet individually, privately, or in groups to discuss their needs and concerns.

Nurses caring for terminally ill children and their families must actively focus on promoting their own health. The following questions should be kept in mind and attempts should be made to answer them and to seek help when needed:

1. How do I feel about the concept of dying?
2. Am I comfortable caring for the needs of the dying child?
3. Can I cope with the family's needs also?
4. Am I becoming overwhelmed with caring for this child and family?
5. Who can assist me find ways to deal with my needs and concern?
6. How can I preserve my own health and well-being?

Nurses should be given opportunities to share the answers to their questions with other health care professionals, with the goal being that these feelings and concerns are only human experiences and concerns.

THE NURSE AND TERMINALLY ILL CHILD

The nurse providing care to the terminally child is involved in caring for physical, psychosocial, and spiritual needs. The child may be alert and responsive some times, and at other times may be weak and uncomfortable. The plan of care should not only be individualized and realistic, but also based on the immediate needs of the child. When the terminally ill child is dying, the nurse must cope with the additional needs of the child and the family.

Responding to the Physiological Needs of the Dying Child

A primary goal at this time is keeping the child comfortable and pain free. Maintaining a clean environment, providing hair and oral care, and other aspects of daily hygiene can help maintain the dignity of the human experience and promote the psychological integrity of the family. The administration of therapies to reduce pain, promote comfort, maintain hydration and nutrition, and promote respiratory and circulatory integrity remains important. Nurses must continue to provide care to these clients with the same zeal and enthusiasm even when they question the purpose of their interventions.

Research Highlight

Nurses' Experiences When Caring for Dying Children

Study Purpose

To begin to construct theory about the changes in nurses' behaviors toward children with chronic illness who are in the terminal phase of illness.

Methods

Twenty-five nurses who cared for at least one chronically ill child who died participated in the study. The condition of the children included cancer, renal disease, cystic fibrosis, and premature birth. All nurses were females between 23 and 45 years; six of them had children. The pediatric clients ranged in age from newborn to 18 years. Nurses were interviewed about their feelings about their unique experiences caring for a dying child.

Findings

Nurses experienced distress when caring for dying children. The distress resulted from the final recognition that the child's death was inevitable. A major struggle for nurses was the need to express their sad feelings in an environment that deemed such behavior as unprofessional. Nurses who had difficulty expressing or were not encouraged to express their feelings became withdrawn; others stated that they became task-oriented. Those who acknowledged their feelings and were encouraged to do so were better able to manage their distress. Nurses who acknowledged the need to express feelings and received support from their peers were better able to cope. They later stated that this was a positive learning experience.

Implications

Nurses who work with dying children should find ways to express their concerns and grief and should be provided with professional support. Nurses must be willing to mentor inexperienced nurses involved in the care of a dying child for the first time. This practice should not be limited to pediatric nurses working in hospital settings, but can be applied to nurses working with clients and families experiencing the death of a loved one regardless of the setting.

Citation

Davies, B., O'Loane, M., Clarke, D., Mackenzie, B., Stutzer, C., Connaughty, S., and McCormick, J. (1996). Caring for dying children: Nurses' experiences. *Pediatric Nursing, 22*(6), 500–506.

Responding to the Psychosocial Needs of the Dying Child

Attending to the psychosocial needs are more difficult and taxing for nurses to fulfill particularly when the nurse may be psychologically uncomfortable with personal feelings about dying and death. Many individuals upon hearing of the death of an older adult are more accepting of the outcome since the older person most likely lived a full life. However, when death involves a child, acceptance and acknowledgment is more difficult to understand. When providing care to terminally ill children nurses must:

- Revisit their own thoughts and feelings about dying and death
- Understand the process of grieving
- Talk to children in age-appropriate language

- Help children verbalize their feelings about dying and death
- Be consistent in care provided
- Be honest in discussions

During the time of death, nurses must also uphold and respect the cultural and religious beliefs and rituals of the family.

Eye On:

Cultural Practices Related to Death and Dying

Ragda, a young girl from a Middle Eastern country, is in the process of dying. Her parents ask the nurses to allow Ragda to be prepared for death. To do this, the child must be dressed daily in a specific garment and her head adorned with a specific head dress. Since the parents cannot do this every day, they teach the nurses how to apply the garment and head dress. The nurses respectfully apply the apparel under the watchful eyes of family members. Regardless of the time the family visited, Ragda was properly attired. Although comatose, the parents were relieved to know that when death occurred Ragda was ready.

Attendance of Nursing Staff at Funerals

Questions arise about the attendance of nurses at the funeral of a child cared for. Although there is no hard and fast rule, it may be a venue for nurses to acknowledge their loss and to put closure to the experience. At times, the request for the attendance of nursing staff at the funeral is made by the family through announcement of funeral arrangements sent to the unit. Nurses need to determine for themselves on an individual basis what works best.

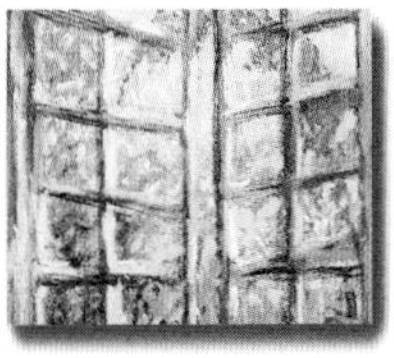

In the Real World

I feel nurses should talk with families about the treatment options and use empathy skills. I have seen that decision making in situations of life and death can be emotionally charged and extremely complicated. I believe it is within nurses' stewardship to help families understand information and access resources necessary for making the wisest choices. I also realize that once decisions are made, nurses have an obligation to respect families' choices and continue providing the best care possible regardless of personal opinions.

Key Concepts

- Children experience loss and separation (divorce, moving to a new neighborhood, changing schools) long before they experience the death of a loved one.
- Four components of the concept of death are universality, irreversibility, nonfunctionality, and causality.
- Understanding the concept of death is a gradual process related to the individual's age, cognitive development, culture, religious belief, and psychological development.
- Children grieve differently than adults; their responses are both physical and psychosocial.
- Children's reaction to the death of a loved one is often influenced by the relationship the child had with the deceased and ways those around them react to the loss.
- After the death of a sibling, children may experience a sense of increased vulnerability, anger, survivor guilt, and parent overprotectiveness.
- Hospice care incorporates a holistic approach providing psychosocial, spiritual, social, and physical support to the terminally ill child and family.
- Nurses must come to terms with their own feelings about dying and death, and allow themselves to grieve in order to help others.

Review Questions

1. What information should the nurse give to parents to assist them explain to their 6-year-old child that a grandfather has died?
2. How can the school nurse assist children cope with the death of a classmate?
3. How are children's reactions to parental separation or divorce similar to that of death?
4 What factors influence a child's response to the death?
5. How can the nurse help a terminally ill child and family prepare for impending death?
6. How can nurses help a community cope with a traumatic event?
7. What are the benefits of hospice care for the terminally ill child and family?
8. Why is caring for self important for nurses caring for the terminally ill child?

References

Amato, P. R. (1994). Life-span adjustment of children to their parents' divorce. *The Future of Children, 4*, 143–164.

Barnard P., & Morland, I. (1999). When children are involved in disasters. In P. Barnard, I. Morland, & J. Nagy (Eds.), *Children, bereavement and trauma: Nurturing resilience* (pp. 21–30). Philadelphia, PA: Jessica Kingsley Publishers.

Barnard, P., Morland, I., & J. Nagy. (1999). *Children, bereavement and trauma: Nurturing resilience*. Philadelphia, PA: Jessica Kingsley Publishers.

Behrman, R., & Quinn, L. (1994). Children and divorce. Overview and analysis. *The Future of Children, 4*(1), 4–14.

Bowden, S. (1995). Young children's experiences of sibling death. *Journal of Pediatric Nursing, 10*(1), 72–79.

Butler, C. L., & Lagoni, L. (1996). Children and pet loss. In C. A. Corr & D. M. Corr (Eds.), *Handbook of childhood death and bereavement* (pp. 179–199). New York: Springer House Company.

Carroll, M. L., & Griffin, R. (1997). Reframing life's puzzle: Support for bereaved children. *The American Journal of Hospice and Palliative Care*, Sept/Oct, 231–235.

Corr, C., & Corr, D. (Eds.). (1996). *Handbook of childhood death and bereavement*. New York: Springer House Company.

Davies, B. (1995). Toward Siblings' Understanding and Perspective of Death. In E. A. Grollman (Ed.), *Bereaved children and teens. A support guide for parents and professionals* (pp. 61–74). Boston: Beacon Press.

Davies, B., O'Loane, M., Clarke, D., Mackenzie, B., Stutzer, C., Connaughty, S., & McCormick, J. (1996). Caring for dying children: Nurses' experiences. *Pediatric Nursing, 22*(6), 500–506.

De Maso, D., Meyer, E., & Beasley, P. (1997). What do I say to my surviving children. *Journal of the American Academy of Child and Adolescent Psychiatry, 36*(9), 1299–1302.

Doka, K. (1996). The cruel paradox: Children who are living with life-threatening illnesses. In C. Corr & D. Corr (Eds.), *Handbook of childhood death and bereavement* (pp. 89–105). New York: Springer Publishing Company.

Grollman, E. A. (Ed.). (1995). *Bereaved children and teens. A support guide for parents and professionals*. Boston: Beacon Press.

Hetherington, E., Bridges, M., & Insabella, G. (1998). What matters? What does not? Five perspectives on the associations between marital transitions and children's adjustment. *American Psychologist, 53*(2), 167–184.

Hogan, N., & DeSantis, L. (1996). Adolescent sibling bereavement: Toward a new theory. In C. A. Corr & D. E. Balk (Eds.), *Handbook of adolescent death and bereavements* (pp. 173–195). New York: Springer Publishing Company.

Kubler-Ross, E. (1969). *On death and dying*. New York: MacMillan.

McGlaufin, H. (1996). Grieving children: Training volunteers and professionals to work with grieving children and their families. *American Journal of Hospice and Palliative Care, 13*(2): 22–26.

Melnyk, B., & Alpert-Gillis, L. (1997). Coping with marital separations: Smoothing the transitions for parents and children. *Journal of Pediatric Health Care, 11*(4), 165–174.

Mohan, M. (1993). Children's concept of death and sibling death from trauma. *Journal of Pediatric Nursing, 895*, 335–344.

Mohan, M., & Page, M. (1995). Childhood bereavement after the death of a sibling. *Holistic Nursing Practice, 9*(3), 15–26.

Nardar, K. (1996). Children's exposure to traumatic experiences. In C. Corr and D. Corr (Eds.), *Handbook of childhood death and bereavement* (pp. 201–220). New York: Springer Publishing Company.

Schonfield, D. (1993). Talking to children about death. *Journal of Pediatric Health Care, 7*, 269–274.

Siegel, K., Karus, D., & Ravies, V. (1996). Adjustment of children facing the death of a parent due to cancer. *Journal of American Academy of Child and Adolescent Psychiatry, 35*(4), 442–450.

Smith, K., & Boardman, K. (1995). Comforting a child when someone close dies. *Nursing, 95*, 58–59.

Speece, M., & Brent, S. (1996). The development of children's understanding of death. In C. Corr & D. Corr (Eds.), *Handbook of childhood death and bereavement* (pp. 29–50). New York: Springer Publishing Company.

Stahlman, D. (1996). Children and the death of a sibling. In C. Corr & D. Corr (Eds.), *Handbook of childhood death and bereavement* (pp. 149–164). New York: Springer Publishing Company.

Trimm, R. F. (1995). Divorce and death: Helping children cope with family loss. *Comprehensive Therapy, 21*(3), 135–138.

United States of Commerce News, January 1999.

Walker, C. (1993). Sibling bereavement and grief responses. *Journal of Pediatric Nursing, 8*(5), 325–334.

Worden, J. W. (1996). *Children and grief: When a parent dies*. New York: Guilford Press.

Suggested Readings

Alderman, L. (1989). *Why Did Daddy Die?* New York: Pocket Books.

Banks, A. (1990). *When Your Parents Get a Divorce—A Kid's Journal*. New York: Penguin Books.

Bonkowski, S. (1990). *A Workbook for Divorced Parents and Their Children*. Chicago: Acta Publications.

Buscaglia, L. (1982). *The Fall of Freddie the Leaf*. New York: Slack.

Gipson, F. (1989). *Old Yeller*. New York: Harper and Row

Grollman, E. (1977). *Talking about Death: A Dialogue between Parent and Child*. Boston: Beacon Press.

Krementz, J. (1988). *How It Feels When a Parent Dies*. New York: Knopf.

Kushner, H. (1982). *When Bad Things Happen to Good People*. New York: Avon Books.

McLendon, G. H. (1982). *My Brother Joey Died*. Julian Messner.

Nagy, J. (1999). The practice of working with bereaved children. In P. Barnard, I. Morland, and J. Nagy (Eds.), *Children, bereavement and trauma: Nurturing resilience* (pp. 13–20). Philadelphia: Jessica Kingsley Publishers.

North American Nursing Diagnosis Association. (2001). *NANDA nursing diagnoses: Definitions and classification 2001–2002*. Philadelphia: Author.

Rofes, E. (Ed). (1982). *The Kids' Book of Divorce—By, for and about Kids.* New York: Vintage Books.

Rogers, F. (1988). *When a Pet Dies.* New York: Putnam

Sesame Street. (1984). *I'll Miss You, Mr. Hooper.* New York: Bantam Books.

White, E. B. (1952). *Charlotte's Web.* New York: Harper Row

Wright, B. R. (1991). *The Cat Next Door.* New York: Holiday House Books.

Resources

Organizations and Websites

Association for Pet Loss and Bereavement
P.O. Box 11230
Brooklyn, NY 11230
(718) 382-0690
www.aplb.org

Bereavement Research Network
www.bereavement.org

Candlelighters Childhood Cancer Foundation
7910 Woodmont Avenue
Bethesda, MD 20814

Children's Hospice International
2202 Mt. Vernon Avenue, Suite 3C
Alexandria, VA 22301

The Compassionate Friends for Bereaved Parents and Siblings
P.O. Box 3696
Oak Brook, IL 60522

UNIT IV

Alterations in Nutrition and Elimination

CHAPTER 21

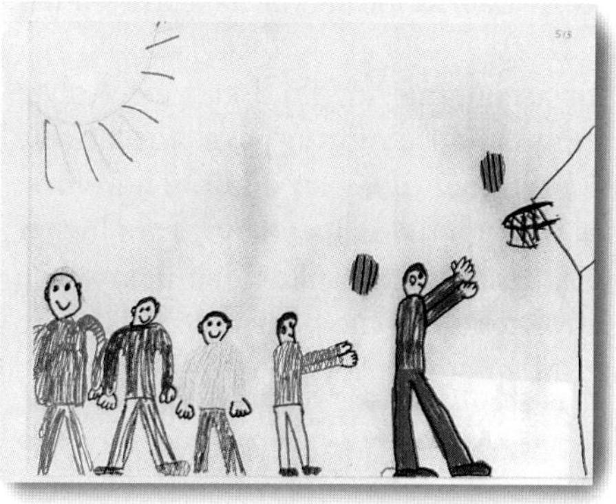

FLUID AND ELECTROLYTE ALTERATIONS

Elaine R. Graf, PhD, PNP, CS

It all happened so quickly. We were all caught off guard. It seemed like the whole family got the flu this year, one after another. How was I to know that the baby would get so much sicker? When the baby started vomiting, I just thought here we go again, another family member with the flu. She would not drink her formula and would not take clear liquids. Everything she did drink she vomited back up within 15 minutes. She was very fussy, so I put her to bed. Four hours later when I went to check on her, I could not wake her up. She was very limp and felt hot. I knew she was in big trouble. We raced her to the emergency room, and the nurses started an IV immediately. As the fluids ran in her arm, she began to wake up and cry. It was amazing how quickly her condition changed for the worst and then got better with fluids. I never would have thought that the baby would have gotten this sick so quickly. Her 5-year-old brother and her father all seemed to do fine, even though they also had the same symptoms. Why did this happen to the baby? How could I have gotten her to drink when she pushed the bottle away? How can I prevent this in the future?

COMPETENCIES

Upon completion of this chapter, the reader will be able to:

- *Identify differences among adults, children, and infants related to fluid requirements, fluid therapy, and electrolytes.*
- *Calculate daily maintenance fluid requirements for children of various ages.*
- *Explain the principles of acid-base imbalances.*
- *Explain the causes and clinical manifestations of the four major types of acid-base imbalances.*
- *Compare mild, moderate, and severe dehydration.*
- *Describe the treatment of the child with gastroenteritis based on the degree of dehydration.*
- *Discuss common types of burn injuries in children and their prevention.*
- *Describe the treatment and nursing management of the child with a major burn injury.*

An understanding of body fluids, electrolytes, and acid-base **buffers** (a substance that either releases or absorbs hydrogen ions to maintain a stable blood pH) is essential in the treatment of many childhood illnesses. Alterations in electrolytes, fluids, and acid-base metabolism can occur quickly in children and, as a result, can be life threatening. Any illness that alters a child's intake, elimination, or need for water and electrolytes has the potential to cause imbalances. The child's survival hinges on the ability of health care providers to accurately assess at-risk situations, diagnose the alteration, initiate the appropriate treatment plan, and implement prevention strategies.

This chapter begins with an introduction of the principles associated with the movement of fluids and electrolytes within a child's body, followed by a discussion of how the body buffers these fluids in order to maintain a stable body pH. Next is a discussion of the common alterations, including dehydration, acute gastroenteritis, edema, and burns, which cause fluid shifts to occur in children. Emphasis is placed on the nurse's ability to quickly recognize these alterations and implement an appropriate plan of care.

ANATOMY AND PHYSIOLOGY

The complex chemical and physiological processes that sustain life depend on the presence of water and the body's ability to maintain **homeostasis,** a dynamic equilibrium of the body that is maintained by processes of feedback and regulation. The most abundant body fluid is water. Four key physiological factors are responsible for the fluid and **electrolyte** (a charged particle found in body fluid) differences between children and adults. These include (1) percentage and distribution of body water, (2) body surface area, (3) rate of basal metabolism, and (4) status of kidney function. Infants and children have a higher proportionate body water content than adults. Water constitutes approximately 50% of the body weight of adults and adolescents, 65% of body weight in children, and 80% of the body weight of infants.

The body's water is found in two main fluid compartments: within the cell (intracellular, or ICF) and outside the cell (extracellular, or ECF). **Intracellular fluid** is body fluid that is located inside the cells and contains large amounts of potassium, phosphate, sulfate, and proteins. **Extracellular fluid** includes **interstitial fluid** (the fluid between the cells and outside the blood and lymph vessels), **intravascular fluid** (within the blood vessels, e.g., plasma), and lymphatic fluid. Extracellular fluid is predominately saline because it contains large amounts of sodium, chloride, and bicarbonate (Figure 21-1).

The distribution of water between these two compartments is also different in infants and children as compared to adults. Forty percent of body water in the newborn is in the extracellular compartment, as compared with 20% in the adult. By the time infants are 1 year of age, 30% of their body water is extracellular. Children reach adult water distribution percentages by the time they are 5 years old (Fann, 1998). During illness states (vomiting, diarrhea, or hemorrhage), fluid that is located in the extracellular compartment is lost first. Therefore, children are more at risk for fluid alterations because a higher percentage of their body weight is water and more of that water is located in the extracellular compartment (Figure 21-2).

The second factor accounting for fluid and electrolyte differences is that infants and children have a relatively greater body surface area than does an adult. Therefore, insensible water losses through the skin and lungs are higher for children, and any situation that results in an increase in loss of water and electrolytes alters the body fluid balance to a greater degree than in an adult. Additionally, infants and young children will lose water more quickly than adults because they have a higher basal metabolic rate (BMR). Due to their higher BMR, the fluid intake per kilogram of body weight per day must exceed the per kilogram fluid requirements of an adult. Further, their bodies cannot regulate homeostatic changes as quickly as adults due to immature kidneys and buffering systems. They need more water to excrete a given amount of solute.

The distribution and movement of body fluids between the ICF and ECF compartments are affected by the amount and type of solutes present, the type of membrane to be crossed, and changes in the permeability of the capillary beds. A **solute** is a substance that is dissolved in a solution (e.g., a teaspoon of salt dissolved in a glass of water is an example of a solute). Solutes found in the human body include electrolytes, such as potassium, sodium, and calcium; nonelectrolytes, such as glucose, urea, and creatinine; and large molecules, such as plasma proteins.

Primarily, fluids move as a result of diffusion, filtration, and osmosis. **Diffusion** is the movement of a solute across a membrane when the pressures on either side of the membrane are equal. In this situation, solutes will flow from an area of higher concentration to an area of lower concentration until an equilibrium is reached. **Filtration** is the move-

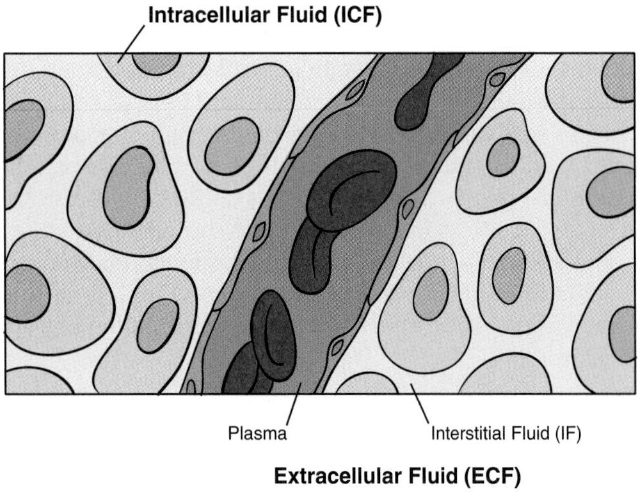

Figure 21-1 Body Fluid Compartments

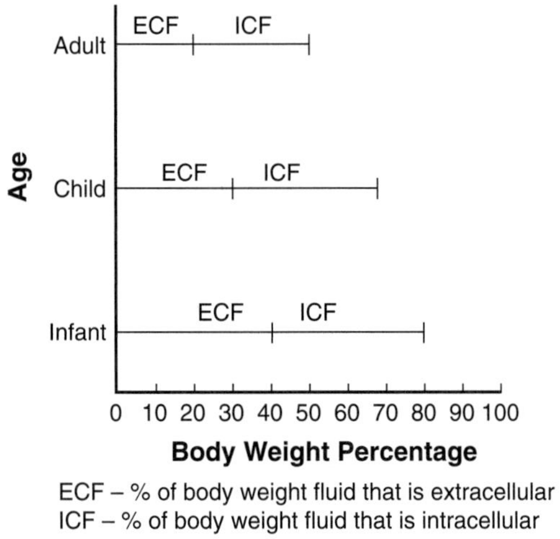

Figure 21-2 Distribution of Total Body Water by Age

ment of a solute based on the force exerted by the weight of the solution. The fluid containing the solute will move from an area of greater pressure to an area of lesser pressure. **Osmosis** is the movement of water across a semipermeable membrane from a solution that has a lower solute concentration to one that has a higher solute concentration. Osmosis accounts for the movement of fluid between intracellular and extracellular spaces. The concentration of a solute in a fluid creates a type of pressure called **osmotic pressure** (a force within the capillary beds that tends to pull water into the capillaries). Osmotic pressure is determined by the type and thickness of the capillary membrane, and the size and concentration of circulating molecules.

Oncotic pressure, which is caused by the amount of plasma proteins present in the vascular system, holds fluids in the capillaries. A decrease in plasma proteins would allow fluid to escape into interstitial spaces. Capillaries are normally impermeable to plasma proteins. However, in certain illnesses, such as sepsis and burns, capillary permeability increases, allowing proteins to move into interstitial spaces along with water, resulting in the formation of edema. Finally, another pressure within the body that is responsible for the movement of fluids is hydrostatic pressure. **Hydrostatic pressure** is the pressure of blood against the capillary walls generated by the contraction of the heart. Hydrostatic pressure within the capillary bed pushes fluid across capillary membranes into the interstitial space and is balanced by osmotic pressures. It is measured by blood pressure and is important in maintaining the fluid balance within the vascular system.

During various illness states (e.g., shock, burns, dehydration), it becomes important to maintain osmotic pressure within the body. This is often accomplished by giving intravenous solutions at a rate sufficient to replace the loss of fluids. If the child is not able to tolerate fluids orally, the rate also needs to include fluids to cover the daily maintenance requirements. While administering intravenous fluids, it is important to decide the type of solution based on the intended need and to determine the appropriate rate. Table 21-1 provides a classification of common intravenous fluids.

Critical Thinking

Examples of Diffusion, Filtration, and Osmosis

Many examples of diffusion, filtration, and osmosis occur in everyday life. Think of two examples of each—one that occurs outside the body and one that occurs inside the body.

ELECTROLYTE IMBALANCES

Serum electrolyte concentrations within the ICF and ECF are the same for adults and children. Although many electrolytes are found in the body, all serving vital functions, sodium, potassium, and chloride are the major electrolytes that influence fluid balance. Normal serum levels of these electrolytes are listed in Table 21-2. Electrolytes influence the formation and retention of water in the ICF and ECF, and can have a dramatic effect on the function of vital organs.

Sodium Imbalance

Sodium, the major extracellular electrolyte, is responsible for establishing and maintaining the **osmolarity** (the concentration of solute within a solution measured by the number of moles per liter of water) and volume of ECF. A decrease in the serum sodium concentration (hyponatremia) produces a decrease in the intravascular **osmolality** (the concentration of solute within a solution measured by the number of moles per kilogram of water). In this situation, free water moves

TABLE 21-1 Intravenous Fluid Classifications

Hypertonic Solutions	Isotonic Solutions	Hypotonic Solutions
10% glucose in water	Ringer's lactate (RL)	Water
Dextrose 5% in 1/2 NS	Normal saline (NS)	
Dextrose 5% in RL	Dextrose 5% in 0.2% NS	
	Dextrose 5% in water	

Adapted from Klotz, R. S. (1998). The effects of intravenous solutions on fluid and electrolyte balance. Journal of Intravenous Nursing, *21(1), 20–26.*

Nursing Tip:

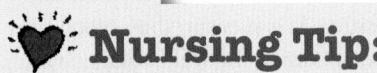

Assessing daily maintenance fluid requirements and minimum urine output

Maintenance of homeostasis requires that the child ingest adequate amounts of fluids and excrete adequate amounts of urine. The following formulas are used to calculate these requirements and also to assess intake and output status.

Maintenance fluid requirements for 24 hours

Weight	*Fluid requirement*	*Examples*
1–10 kg	100 ml/kg	2.5-kg infant = 250 ml 10-kg infant = 1,000 ml
10–20 kg	1,000 ml + 50 ml/kg over 10 kg	11-kg infant = 1,050 ml 13-kg infant = 1,150 ml 20-kg infant = 1,500 ml
>20 kg	1,500 ml + 20 ml/kg over 20 kg	21-kg toddler = 1,520 ml 30-kg child = 1,700 ml

Minimum urine output by age group

Infant and toddler	>2–3 ml/kg/h
Preschoolers and young school-aged child	>1–2 ml/kg/h
Older school-aged child and adolescent	>0.5–1 ml/kg/h

TABLE 21-2 Normal Serum Concentration for Sodium, Potassium, and Chloride

Sodium	136–146 mEq/L (newborns only) 139–146 mEq/L (infant) 135–148 mEq/L (child) 135–146 mEq/L (adult)
Potassium	3.0–6.0 mEq/L (newborns only) 3.5–5.0 mEq/L (infants to adults)
Chloride	97–110 mEq/L (infant) 98–111 mEq/L (child) 95–106 mEq/L (adult)

Critical Thinking

What Does a Measure of Serum Sodium Mean?

Identify what the following serum sodium levels mean. What effect will they have on the fluid compartments of the body?

140 mEq/L from a 6-year-old child
120 mEq/L from an infant
168 mEq/L from a newborn

from the intravascular to the interstitial space until the osmolality of the compartments is equal. Low serum sodium levels (<135 mEq/L) are associated with increased gastrointestinal output such as diarrhea, vomiting, nasogastric suctioning, diuretics, excessive sweating, and renal disease. Signs and symptoms are headache, muscle weakness, abdominal cramps, lethargy, oliguria, and cerebral edema. An excessive intake of sodium or an increased water loss related to sodium loss (e.g., watery diarrhea) causes an increased serum sodium level (hypernatremia). If that level is >145 mEq/L, water will be pulled out of the cells into extracellular spaces (seen as edema) and, if not compensated for, will cause an intracellular fluid deficit. An intracellular fluid deficit can be suspected if a child has flushed skin, dry mucous membranes, an elevated temperature, and intense thirst.

Potassium Imbalance

Potassium is the major electrolyte found in the ICF, and the difference between the intracellular and extracellular potassium determines the excitability of neurons and muscles. The serum potassium concentration (3.5–5.0 mEq/L) represents the minority of total body potassium. The majority of the body's potassium is in ICF (about 140 mEq/L). Potassium is also necessary for the transmission of glucose into cells. Extracellular potassium, measured by a blood sample of plasma serum, is extremely important to monitor because any imbalance will greatly affect heart muscle contraction. An elevated serum potassium can cause cardiac irritability, which can lead to ventricular fibrillation. The cardiac irritability associated with an elevated or decreased serum potassium can be seen by an electrocardiogram (EKG) reading.

Concentration of hydrogen ions also affects the movement of potassium in and out of cells. Hydrogen ions affect the pH of body fluids. An excess serum hydrogen concentration will cause potassium to move from intracellular to intravascular spaces, while a decreased hydrogen concentration will move potassium from the bloodstream into the cells.

Hypokalemia (potassium of <3.5 mEq/L) can occur with a loss of gastric or intestinal fluids or when IV fluids do not adequately replace body fluid losses. Signs and symptoms include lethargy, confusion, dizziness, arrhythmias, diarrhea, a decreased blood pressure, and EKG changes (flattened T wave and ST wave depression). Hyperkalemia (potassium >5.0 mEq/L) can occur with tissue necrosis, hemolysis, renal failure, or a rapid infusion of IV potassium. Signs and symptoms include abdominal cramps, muscle weakness, arrhythmias, and EKG changes (tall peaked T waves and a widened QRS complex), and will lead to cardiac arrest if not treated quickly.

Chloride Imbalance

Chloride is primarily an extracellular electrolyte responsible for maintaining electroneutrality in the ECF. Chloride levels usually parallel sodium levels, meaning, if sodium levels are increasing, chloride levels will increase and vice versa. Hypochloremia (chloride of <98 mEq/L) will occur with diarrhea, vomiting, gastric suctioning, sweating, and excessive use of diuretics. The child will have hypotonic muscles and decreased respirations, and will often be very irritable.

Hormones

Hormones can also affect fluid balance in the body. Two major hormones are the antidiuretic hormone (ADH) and aldosterone. ADH is secreted by the posterior pituitary when serum osmolality increases, causing the renal tubules of the kidneys to reabsorb water. ADH is secreted during times of dehydration, since it causes an immediate increase in vascular volume and a decrease in urine output. Aldosterone is a mineralocorticoid produced by the adrenal cortex, which causes the distal renal tubules of the kidneys to reabsorb sodium and excrete potassium. Aldosterone is excreted when the body wants to retain fluids, since the increased sodium retention leads to water reabsorption. Table 21-3 provides a summary of common disturbances in water, potassium, and sodium balances.

TABLE 21-3 Disturbances in Fluid and Electrolyte Balances

Type/Causes	Signs and Symptoms	Nursing Management Approaches
Water loss		
Failure to intake or absorb water Inappropriate ADH secretion Diabetes (glycosuria) Fluid loss from gastrointestinal tract • Diarrhea • Vomiting • Nasogastric suctioning • Gastrointestinal fistula Excessive perspiration Prolonged fever Impaired skin integrity (burns) Hemorrhage Overuse of diuretics Inadequate fluid management	Thirst Dry skin and mucous membranes Poor skin turgor Weight loss ↓ Pulse pressure, urine output Slow capillary refill Fatigue Tachycardia ↑ Urine specific gravity > 1.020 ↑ Hct, BUN, serum osmolarity	Calculate replacement needs based on losses and maintenance fluid needs Measure intake and output Assess for electrolyte imbalances Assess vital signs Monitor urine specific gravity
Water excess		
Intake > output Excessive water intake Hypotonic fluid overload Use of plain water enemas ↑ Output with normal intake Kidney failure Congestive heart failure	Edema Pulmonary edema, rales Weight gain ↑ Venous pressure ↓ Urine specific gravity ↓ Hct, serum electrolytes	Take full history to determine cause Monitor urine specific gravity Limit fluid intake Administer diuretics and monitor for effects Monitor vital signs Assess for electrolyte imbalances

continues

TABLE 21-3 *Continued*

Type/Causes	Signs and Symptoms	Nursing Management Approaches
↓ Potassium (hypokalemia) Poor food intake Malabsorption Diuresis Fluid loss from gastrointestinal tract Diabetes mellitus Nephritis Corticosteroid use or administration Over use of thiazide diuretics Alkalosis	Muscle cramping, weakness Irritability, fatigue Cardiac arrhythmias Hypotension Ileus ↓ Serum potassium ≤3.5 mEq/L Abnormal EKG findings Flattened T waves ↓ ST segment, ↑ PVCs	Determine cause and treat appropriately Monitor vital signs and EKG Administer potassium IV: give slowly, only after assured of adequate urine output Oral: give high potassium food and fluids If giving oral KCL—mix in juice Assess for acid-base imbalances
↑ Potassium (hyperkalemia) Renal disease and failure Addison's disease Dehydration Burns (cellular destruction) Hemolysis ↑ Intake of potassium foods Improper IV potassium administration Metabolic acidosis	Muscle weakness, twitching ↑ Reflexes Oliguria Ventricular fibrillation/arrest ↑ Serum potassium ≥5.5 mEq/L Abnormal EKG findings Flat P wave, tall peaked T wave Widened QRS complex, ↑ PR interval	Determine cause and treat appropriately Monitor vital signs and EKG Monitor serum potassium levels Administer calcium gluconate, as ordered (used to alter cardiac effects) Administer IV insulin, sodium bicarbonate, or glucose (causes K to move into cells) Assess for acid-base imbalances
↓ Sodium (hyponatremia) ↓ Sodium intake Inappropriate ADH syndrome Loss of gastrointestinal fluids Diuretics DKA Renal disease Excessive sweating Liver failure Low sodium diet	Cerebral edema Muscle weakness Abdominal cramps Weight loss Headaches Lethargy Oliguria Dehydration ↓ Serum sodium <130 mEq/L	Determine cause and treat appropriately Monitor serum electrolyte levels Monitor vital signs Administer IV fluids, as ordered
↑ Sodium (hypernatremia) Excessive intake or retention of sodium Diabetes insipidus Use of mineralocorticoid Hyperglycemia ↑ Insensible water losses Fever	Dry, sticky mucous membranes Thirst Flushed skin Firm skin turgor Disorientation, irritability Convulsions ↑ Serum sodium ≥150 mEq/L ↑ Plasma volume Alkalosis	Determine cause and treat appropriately Measure intake and output Monitor neurologic status Monitor laboratory studies Administer fluids as ordered Monitor vital signs

ACID-BASE BALANCE AND IMBALANCE

Homeostasis in body fluids is also affected by acid-base metabolism. The balance of free acids and bases within the body is regulated by the respiratory and renal systems and must be maintained within a very limited range in order to sustain life. The acidity of body fluids is affected by the concentration of hydrogen ions in the blood, or blood pH. Blood pH is best measured by obtaining an arterial blood gas (ABG). Normal blood pH ranges from 7.35 to 7.45. A blood pH below 6.80 or higher than 7.80 is incompatible with life.

Acidosis is indicated by a blood pH below 7.35, while **alkalosis** is indicated by a blood pH above 7.45.

The respiratory system controls acid-base metabolism by retaining or releasing carbon dioxide (CO_2), thereby causing a shift in the bicarbonate-carbonic acid buffering system. The amount of dissolved carbon dioxide in the blood (pCO_2) is measured by an arterial blood gas, and ranges from 35 to 45 mm Hg. Carbonic acid (H_2CO_3), is a weak, unstable acid, formed when carbon dioxide combines with water (H_2O), that will dissociate into bicarbonate and one hydrogen ion (HCO_3 + H^+). The free hydrogen ions will combine with oxygen to form water. Bicarbonate and water can then be released or retained by the kidneys in order to maintain the necessary balance. Bicarbonate levels are measured by an arterial blood gas and range from 22 to 26 mEq/L. The ability of the kidneys to excrete hydrogen ions and bicarbonate can be inferred from the blood bicarbonate level obtained from an arterial blood gas.

To maintain a stable acid-base balance, the body will try to maintain a 20:1 ratio between bicarbonate and carbonic acid, and an equilibrium of the carbonic acid and dissolved carbon dioxide found in blood. The lungs will compensate for pH changes caused by metabolic disorders (e.g., diabetes, vomiting, diarrhea) by controlling the carbon dioxide level in the blood. Hyperventilation or deep rapid breathing (Kussmaul respirations) will occur in an attempt to blow off carbon dioxide. The kidneys will compensate for pH changes caused by respiratory problems or a buildup of metabolic acids (e.g., lactic acid, hydrochloric acid, pyruvic acid, sulfuric acid) by controlling hydrogen ion and bicarbonate levels in the blood. However, renal compensation is much slower than respiratory compensation and often requires days to restore balance. **Compensation** is a body process used to restore blood pH to normal by changing the partial pressure of carbon dioxide (pCO_2) or the bicarbonic ion concentration. (Figure 21-3 illustrates acid-base balance and imbalance.)

Acid-base imbalances are common in children and fall into four categories: respiratory acidosis, respiratory alkalosis, metabolic acidosis, and metabolic alkalosis. The body will compensate for these disturbances by using a renal or a respiratory buffering mechanism. These responses are monitored by arterial blood gas analysis. Table 21-4 lists the causes, clinical manifestations, and management of the four acid-base disturbances.

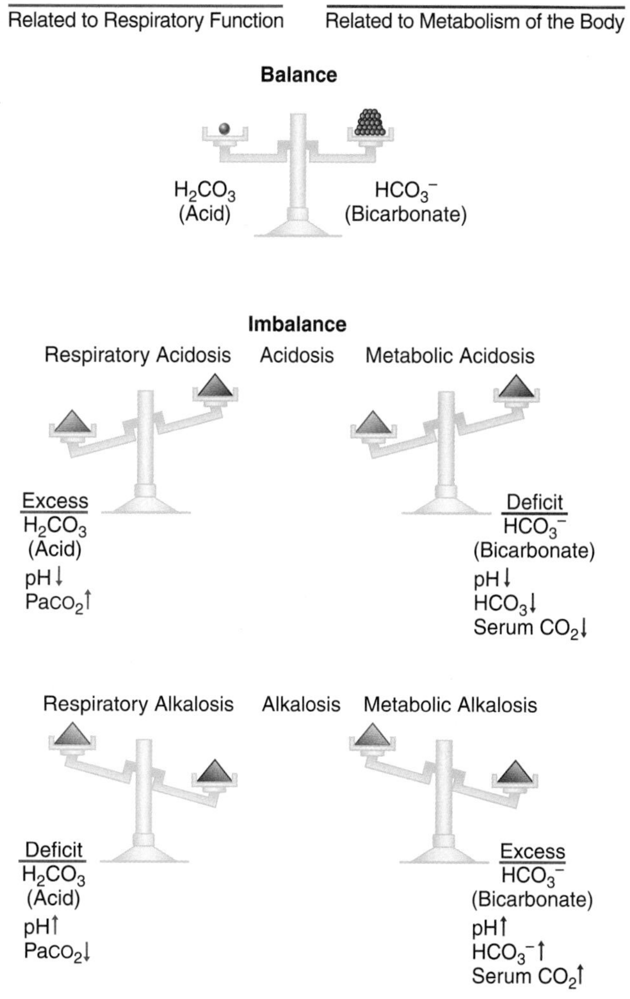

Figure 21-3 Acid-Base Balance and Imbalance

Respiratory Acidosis

Respiratory acidosis can be caused by any condition that decreases a child's respiratory effort. Slowed or shallow respirations will result in a buildup of carbon dioxide, which combined with water forms carbonic acid and leads to acidosis (↓ pH, ↑ pCO_2). Many clinical conditions can cause respiratory acidosis and are listed in Box 21-1.

Acidosis causes central nervous system depression. As a result, the child will be lethargic, confused, and disoriented, may complain of a headache, and, if not treated, may become comatose. Efforts are directed toward correcting the underlying cause by improving ventilation. Without correction, the body, via the kidneys, will attempt to neutralize the increased acid by increasing the retention of bicarbonate. However, the body's attempt at compensation does not correct the underlying problem, and renal compensation is always slow.

Respiratory Alkalosis

Respiratory alkalosis occurs when the carbon dioxide level is too low. This most commonly occurs from conditions that cause the child to hyperventilate (e.g., anxiety, pain, meningitis, gram-negative septicemia, early response to salicylate poisoning, mechanical overventilation). The child will often feel numbness or tingling in toes and fingers, lightheadedness, and confusion, and may faint. Renal compensation for respiratory alkalosis is rarely seen clinically because the underlying condition is often corrected before the kidneys have time to respond. However, if seen, the kidneys would

TABLE 21-4 A Comparative Analysis of Acid-Base Disturbances

Condition/Primary Cause	Clinical Manifestations	Management Approaches
Respiratory acidosis		
Alveolar hypoventilation: ↑ pCO_2 Chronic respiratory disease Depression of CNS Inadequate mechanical ventilation Pneumothorax Neuromuscular disease	Dyspnea ↑ Use of accessory muscles Cyanosis CNS depression ↑ Intracranial pressure Tachycardia	Monitor blood gases Improve ventilation Give oxygen, consider intubation Administer sodium bicarbonate Monitor vital signs
Respiratory alkalosis		
Alveolar hyperventilation: ↓ pCO_2 Anxiety Sepsis Heart failure Hepatic failure Fever/hypermetabolic states Salicylate poisoning Overzealous mechanical ventilation	Tachypnea Numbness, tingling of toes and fingers Lightheaded, dizzy Syncope Diaphoresis	Monitor blood gases Encourage slow ventilation Use rebreathing oxygen masks or bag Administer sedative, if ordered Monitor vital signs
Metabolic acidosis		
↑ Body acids or ↓ HCO_3 Diabetic ketoacidosis (DKA) Alcoholic ketoacidosis ↑ Intake of acids (salicylates) Diarrhea Renal failure Starvation Shock	Confusion Lethargy Deep, rapid respirations Acetone odor to breath Tachycardia Cold, clammy skin (mild acidosis) Warm, dry skin (severe acidosis)	Correct underlying problem Administer sodium bicarbonate Administer oxygen Correct DKA with insulin/glucose Monitor vital signs
Metabolic alkalosis		
↓ Body acids or ↑ HCO_3 Vomiting Prolonged NG suctioning Overuse of antacids Hypokalemia Diuretics	Slow, shallow respirations Tremors, muscle twitching Disorientation Seizures	Correct underlying problem Administer sodium NaCl and KCl Replace loss of fluids Take seizure precautions Monitor intake and output Monitor electrolyte status

BOX 21-1 Clinical conditions associated with respiratory acidosis

Head trauma	Asthma
General anesthesia	Croup/epiglottitis
Drug overdose	Cystic fibrosis
Brain tumor	Atelectasis
Sleep apnea	Muscular dystrophy
Mechanical under ventilation	Pneumothorax

retain free hydrogen ions and excrete bicarbonate. The child's urine pH would increase as a result of the increased bicarbonate excretion.

Metabolic Acidosis

Metabolic acidosis is most commonly caused by a loss of bicarbonate in the stool or an increase in ketone bodies (e.g., acetoacetic acid, acetone, beta-hydroxybutyric acid) in the blood. These conditions most frequently result from diarrhea and diabetic ketoacidosis. Children are often confused, lethargic, and tachycardic. The body compensates by

Nursing Alert:

Electrolyte Shift in Metabolic Acidosis

Metabolic acidosis causes an electrolyte shift: hydrogen and sodium ions move into the cell, and potassium moves into the ECF. Hyperkalemia may cause ventricular fibrillation and death.

Critical Thinking

Respiratory Buffer Response to Metabolic Acidosis

Consider the answers to the following questions related to metabolic acidosis.

1. What effect does metabolic acidosis have on the pH of blood?
2. What is the underlying imbalance (carbon dioxide, bicarbonate, hydrogen ion)?
3. What does the body accomplish by increasing the rate and depth of respiration?

increasing the depth and rate of respirations in order to blow off carbon dioxide.

Metabolic Alkalosis

Metabolic alkalosis occurs as a result of bicarbonate retention or hydrogen ion loss. It is most commonly seen in children with prolonged vomiting, but also occurs with ingestion of large quantities of bicarbonate antacids, massive blood transfusions, loss of nasogastric fluids, and hypokalemia. A child experiencing metabolic alkalosis is often weak and dizzy, and may complain of muscle cramps. The respiratory response would be to increase pCO_2 by decreasing the rate and depth of respirations (hypoventilation).

Critical Thinking

Why Would Vomiting, Hypokalemia, Cystic Fibrosis, Loss of Nasogastric Fluids, or Blood Transfusions Cause Metabolic Alkalosis?

Consider the above alterations. Explain why they can lead to metabolic alkalosis. How can a nurse prevent metabolic alkalosis in the above illness states?

Nursing Tip:

Assessing fluid, electrolyte, and acid-base alterations

Assessing a child who has an alteration in fluid, electrolytes, or acid-base balance requires an understanding of developmental norms for vital signs and behavior, and excellent observation skills. Ask yourself the following questions:

- Has the child been ill recently?
- What are the presenting symptoms?
- Is the child's intake and output balanced?
- How many times has the child voided in the last 24 hours?
- Has the child gained or lost weight recently, or as a result of this illness?
- Are the child's vital signs within normal limits for age?
- Does the child's skin reflect a dehydrated state or an edematous state?
- Are the child's mucous membranes dry?
- Are the fontanelles flat, sunken, or bulging?
- Does the child have tears when crying?
- What is the child's general appearance and behavior?
- What does the child's urine specific gravity reflect?
- What does the child's lab work for electrolytes and blood gases reflect?

The answers to these questions will help in determining if the child has a fluid and electrolyte problem, and in confirming the correct nursing diagnosis.

DEHYDRATION

Dehydration is a critical condition that results from an extracellular fluid loss. Since a large portion of a child's body fluid is located in extracellular spaces, a child is more susceptible to dehydration states than an adult. Dehydration that is not corrected will lead to hypovolemic shock and death.

There are three types of dehydration: hypotonic, isotonic, and hypertonic. **Hypotonic dehydration** occurs when there is a sodium loss that is greater than the water loss, resulting in the serum sodium falling below 130 mEq/L. When this occurs, the intracellular fluid becomes more concentrated and the body responds by moving fluid from extracellular spaces to intracellular spaces. While this response helps to reestablish an osmotic equilibrium within the body, it also increases the extracellular fluid losses and, if untreated, can result in shock. Hypotonic dehydration is commonly caused by inappropriate IV therapy, gastroenteritis, nephrosis, adrenal insufficiency, or not replacing gastric secretions. The child with this type of dehydration will appear sicker than the one with isotonic dehydration.

Isotonic dehydration occurs when the loss of sodium and water are equal so that the serum sodium level remains normal. Fluid loss is from both intracellular and extracellular spaces. Since there is no osmotic variation to cause a redistribution of water, the major loss of fluid comes from the extracellular spaces. This is the most common form of dehydration in children. Isotonic dehydration reduces plasma volume and can result in hypovolemic shock. Losses are usually replaced by intravenous fluids that are high in sodium to prevent a drop in the serum sodium level. It is important that the serum sodium level be maintained between 130 and 150 mEq/L. If sodium drops below 130 mEq/L, the condition then becomes hypotonic dehydration.

Hypertonic dehydration occurs when the loss of water is greater than the loss of sodium. Infants who are treated for diarrhea with fluids containing high concentrations of electrolytes may develop this type of dehydration. In this situation, the serum sodium level will rise >150 mEq/L, and serum osmolarity will increase. The body will compensate by pulling water from intracellular spaces to the intravascular compartment; thus, intravascular volume is maintained, and shock is less apparent. However, it is the most dangerous type of dehydration because the fluid replacement strategy is much more difficult to determine and manage. Hypertonic dehydration can also occur if the child has severe vomiting or diabetes insipidus.

Incidence and Etiology

Although the exact incidence of dehydration is not known, many common illnesses or any hospital procedure that requires a prolonged NPO status can cause a child to become dehydrated. Infants and young children are particularly vulnerable to developing dehydration. Some conditions that cause dehydration are listed in Box 21-2.

BOX 21-2 Conditions causing dehydration

- Vomiting
- Diarrhea
- Burns
- Hemorrhage
- Nasogastric suctioning and drainage loss
- NPO status or inadequate fluid/food intake due to illness
- Overuse of diuretics or enemas
- Adrenal insufficiency

Critical Thinking

Heart and Kidney Responses to Extracellular Fluid Losses

Draw a picture of the body's response to an extracellular fluid loss. Describe the effects of epinephrine, antidiuretic hormone, and the renin-angiotensin system. Why is venous constriction and sodium retention beneficial to a child with an extracellular fluid loss? How could you describe these compensatory mechanisms to a caregiver?

Pathophysiology

The body compensates for extracellular fluid losses in very specific ways. A decrease in the fluid circulating in the vascular system lowers cardiac output and can lead to hypotension (a decrease in blood pressure). Blood pressure sensors in the heart, kidneys, and brain react quickly to increase cardiac output and increase sodium and water retention. Any decrease in blood pressure triggers sensory nerves in the aortic arch to stimulate the sympathetic nervous system, causing the fight or flight response or a release of epinephrine. Epinephrine improves cardiac output by increasing heart rate, cardiac contractility, and venous constriction. This compensatory mechanism helps to circulate the remaining blood faster but does not increase the circulating volume. Compensatory mechanisms within the kidneys activate the renin-angiotensin system, which improves circulating fluid volume by increasing sodium retention. Additionally, blood pressure sensors in the brain respond by releasing ADH, which stimulates thirst and retention of water by the kidneys. These compensatory mechanisms are the body's first line of defense but are only temporary. Without prompt recognition and treatment, cardiac ischemia and arrhythmias will develop.

Clinical Manifestations

The clinical manifestations of dehydration depend on the degree of dehydration; however, in general, they include weight loss, rapid-thready pulse, hypotension, decreased peripheral circulation, decreased urinary output, increased specific gravity, decreased skin turgor, dry mucous membranes, absence of tears, and a sunken fontanel in infants. Clinical dehydration is classified as mild (<5% weight loss), moderate (5–10% weight loss), or severe (>10% weight loss). Table 21-5 lists the clinical manifestations associated with the degree of dehydration.

Diagnosis

A diagnosis of dehydration is determined based on the clinical manifestations that are identified during the history,

TABLE 21-5 Clinical Manifestations Associated with Degree of Dehydration

Assessment	Mild	Moderate	Severe
Loss of body weight	<5%	5–10%	>10%
Skin color	Pale, cool	Dusky, grayish	Mottled*
Skin turgor	Decreased elasticity	Decreased	Markedly decreased
Anterior fontanel	Flat	Depressed	Very sunken
Thirst	Slight	Moderate	Intense
Tears	Present	Decreased	Absent
Mucous membranes	Normal to dry	Dry	Parched, cracked
Pulse	Normal or increased slightly	Increased, weak	Rapid, thready*
Blood pressure	Normal	Decreased	Low*
Urine output	Decreased	Oliguria	Azotemia*

** Classic symptoms of impending shock.*

Nursing Alert:

Fluid Losses Due to Hemorrhage

A hemorrhage that results in external losses of blood and fluid is very easy to assess. On the other hand, an internal hemorrhage causing extracellular fluid (blood) to accumulate in a third-space compartment such as the thoracic or peritoneal cavity is often very difficult to detect because the blood loss is not visible. A nurse must consider if the child is at risk for an internal hemorrhage and then assess for signs and symptoms such as a decreasing blood pressure, hematocrit, and pulse. The child with an internal hemorrhage has the same risk for hypovolemic shock as a child with an external hemorrhage. Signs and symptoms of hypovolemic shock such as hypotension, bradycardia, weak peripheral pulses, and decreased urine output will be the same for both conditions, except that the child with an internal hemorrhage will not lose weight.

physical examination, and laboratory tests. The most reliable method for diagnosing dehydration is measurement of acute weight loss. However, because a child's true pre-illness weight is rarely known in the acute care setting, an estimate of fluid deficit is made based on clinical assessment (Gorelick, Shaw, & Murphy, 1997). Laboratory findings are dependent on the type of dehydration. In hypotonic and isotonic dehydration, hemoglobin, hematocrit, glucose, blood urea nitrogen, creatinine, and protein are elevated due to a loss of circulating plasma fluid (hemoconcentration). Usually the urine is highly concentrated with a specific gravity exceeding 1.030, is dark amber in color, and has a strong odor.

Treatment

How the dehydration state is treated depends upon the degree to which the child is dehydrated. Management focuses on correcting the fluid and electrolyte imbalances, and treating the underlying cause. The section on acute gastroenteritis discusses treatment of mild, moderate, and severe dehydration associated with diarrhea and vomiting. Initially, fluids are replaced by giving an oral rehydration solutions (ORS). Oral rehydration therapy (ORT) has been recommended as the treatment of first choice for children with mild or moderate dehydration (American Academy of Pediatrics [AAP], Subcommittee on Acute Gastroenteritis, Provisional Committee on Quality Improvement, 1996). Rehydration solutions should contain glucose, sodium, potassium, and bicarbonate. Glucose must be present in order for the intestines to absorb sodium chloride. Appropriate oral rehydration solutions such as Pedialyte, Lytren, Infalyte, and Resol are available commercially. Other popular liquids such as soft drinks, fruit juices, broth, and athletic drinks (e.g., Gatorade, Powerade) should not be used for rehydration because they have high-carbohydrate

Nursing Alert:

Rehydration Fluids

The World Health Organization recommends the following electrolyte concentrations for rehydration fluids: 20 g glucose/L, 90 mEq sodium/L, 80 mEq chloride/L, 20 mEq potassium/L, and 30 mEq bicarbonate/L. Encourage caregivers to look at product labels and make sure that the rehydration fluid they are choosing has the above electrolyte concentrations.

content and low-electrolyte concentrations (Hugger, Harkless, & Rentschler, 1998).

For those who cannot afford to purchase commercially available rehydration solutions, a homemade solution can be prepared. The ability of the caregivers to follow formulation instructions should be assessed prior to recommending this alternative in order to assure accurate preparation. The recipes in Box 21-3 are examples for homemade ORS.

Whenever possible, fluids should be replaced by the oral route. However, when dehydration is severe or life-threatening, when vomiting is uncontrollable, and when the child is unable to drink for other reasons, intravenous therapy is initiated. The rate of fluid replacement is dependent on the child's degree of dehydration and the presence of cardiac, pulmonary, or renal problems. The volume of fluid to be given is based on the child's weight and clinical signs and symptoms. The type of solution used varies with the type of dehydration. Generally, isotonic dehydration (most common type in children) is treated with **isotonic fluids** (fluids that have the same concentrations as normal body fluid), hypotonic dehydration with **hypertonic fluids** (fluids that are more concentrated than normal body fluid), and hypertonic dehydration with **hypotonic fluids** (fluids that are less concentrated than normal body fluid). (Refer to Table 21-1.) Common solutions are Ringer's lactate (RL) and normal saline (NS), including one-fourth and one-half strength.

Eye On:

Cost as a Barrier to Use of Oral Rehydration Solution (ORS)

A major barrier to the use of ORS may be the out-of-pocket expense for caregivers.

Pedialyte, which is the most widely used ORS in the United States, costs approximately $5–6 per liter. For a child with dehydration due to moderate diarrhea, the cost per day could be $10–12 to replace excess stool losses. Additionally, ORS is usually not included as a benefit with insurance plans (Duggan, et al., 1998).

BOX 21-3 Recipes for homemade oral rehydration solution

1 tsp	Baking soda
3/4 tsp	Salt
8 tsp	Sugar
1 cup	Orange juice
1 L	Clean water

Combine ingredients and stir until well mixed.

OR

2 cups	Clean water
1/2 cup	Dry, precooked baby rice cereal
1/4 tsp	Salt

Combine ingredients, and stir until well mixed.

With permission from American Academy of Family Practitioners, 8880 Ward Parkway, Kansas City, MO 64114.

Nursing Management

Assessment

The skin is assessed for color, warmth, and turgor. Color indicates the state of perfusion and will turn from pink to pale, dusky, or gray as perfusion decreases. Perfusion is also reflected in the temperature of the skin. The skin will feel cool, and the child may complain of cold fingers and toes with decreased perfusion. Assess for capillary refill time, which will be increased. Additional measures of the quality of systemic perfusion include assessment of heart rate, blood pressure, and peripheral pulses. A postural change in heart rate is a useful cue in assessing fluid status in children over 4 years of age. When the child moves from a lying to a standing position, an increase greater than 20 beats per minute indicates hypovolemia. Changes in postural blood pressure have not been found to be useful in children under 9 years of age (Eliason & Lewan, 1998). Extracellular fluid losses will cause the skin to become dry and loose, referred to as a loss of skin turgor. Decreased skin turgor results in a tenting of the skin when pinched and indicates a decreased fluid state.

Mucous membranes are assessed for the presence of dry, sticky mucus and the absence of tears. Tears should be present if the child is crying. The loss of tears indicates fluid loss of at least 5% of the child's body weight. In a child less than 18 months of age, it is also important to check the anterior fontanel. The fontanel should be even with the contour of the skull. When the child is dehydrated, the fontanel is often depressed or sunken in appearance. Weight is a critical indicator of the child's fluid status and should be compared

Nursing Tip:

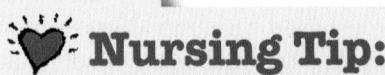

Calculating fluid loss from weight loss

Fluid lost can be calculated according to weight lost. One kilogram of body weight equals 1 L of water. Therefore, each kilogram of weight lost is equal to 1,000 ml of fluid lost.

with a pre-illness weight, if available, or the weight from the previous day.

Intake and output should also be assessed. An assessment of output should include measurements of urine, stools, emesis, wound drainage, and an estimate of insensible fluid loss. The child's urine should be observed for amount, color, and odor. Note the presence of blood or mucus in the stools. Watery stools should also be measured or estimated, and documented as output. If the child has any draining wounds, the dressings should be weighed to estimate fluid loss. Finally, excessive perspiration may require estimating fluid loss by weighing clothing or linens. The use of radiant warmers or warming lights can also increase insensible fluid losses in small infants and should be monitored. Several behavioral changes may also be present in children with dehydration. These include decreased activity levels, loss of interest in their environment, restlessness, irritability, lethargy, and a high-pitched, weak cry. The last assessment should include a review of serum electrolyte results.

Nursing Diagnoses

Nursing diagnoses appropriate for a child with dehydration may include:

1. Deficient fluid volume related to excessive fluid volume loss or inadequate fluid intake.
2. Risk for injury (fall) related to orthostatic (postural) hypotension.
3. Deficient knowledge (caregiver) related to lack of exposure to information about preventing/detecting dehydration.

Outcome Identification

1. The child will receive sufficient fluids to replace losses.
2. The child will exhibit signs of adequate hydration.
3. The child will not fall or sustain other injuries while hypotensive or lethargic.
4. Caregivers will demonstrate understanding of conditions that can lead to dehydration and of the early signs and symptoms.

Planning/Implementation

Nursing interventions include administration of IV fluids, assessment of daily weight, vital signs, and maintenance of accurate intake and output records. Injury due to falls can be prevented by making sure that the side rails of the bed are raised, assessing level of consciousness, and monitoring the serum sodium level. An elevation in serum sodium will cause the brain cells to dehydrate and result in a loss of consciousness if not corrected quickly. An informed nurse will be able to recognize the signs and symptoms of dehydration as they develop and to initiate an appropriate plan of care immediately.

Nursing Alert:

Adding Potassium to Intravenous Solutions

- *Be sure that the child is able to void (1–2 ml/kg/hr) before adding potassium to the IV. Children who are dehydrated are oliguric and can become anuric. An anuric child will not be able to excrete electrolytes that are in the IV solution; therefore, if potassium is added to the IV, it would result in an elevated serum potassium. An elevated serum potassium can cause cardiac irritability and ventricular fibrillation.*
- *Always check the dose and dosage calculations prior to giving. Never give more than 40 mEq/L at a rate not to exceed 1 mEq/kg/hr.*
- *After adding potassium to an IV bag, shake it to make sure the potassium is equally distributed.*
- *Never give potassium by IV push.*

Evaluation

Evaluation is accomplished by assessing for a decrease or absence of the defining characteristics of dehydration or electrolyte imbalance. This is accomplished by continued reassessments. To evaluate the effectiveness of the nursing interventions, explore the answers to the following questions: Is the child able to take in adequate fluids and food? Is the child gaining weight? Are the child's electrolytes within normal limits? Is the child alert and interactive? Does the family understand how to manage the child's care at home?

Family Teaching

Dehydration can be managed at home if the caregivers are well informed and prepared. They need to know the signs of dehydration. They should watch for lethargy or changes in their child's normal behavior. Recommend rehydration fluids, and discuss how to administer them. Caregivers should also be alert to changes in their child's urine output. How often has the child voided? How much with each void? Is the urine dark or concentrated? Help them to be able to make accurate decisions as to when to contact a health care provider (no improvement after 4 hours of rehydration fluid, inability to retain fluids, decreasing urine output, and change in mental alertness).

ACUTE GASTROENTERITIS

Acute gastroenteritis, an inflammation of the mucous membranes of the stomach and intestines, is defined as diarrheal disease of rapid onset with or without accompanying manifestations such as nausea, vomiting, fever, and abdominal pain. Most cases of gastroenteritis are self-limited; however, more severe or prolonged illnesses can result in dehydration with significant morbidity and mortality.

Incidence and Etiology

Acute gastroenteritis accounts for as many as 4.5 million deaths each year worldwide (Gerchufsky, 1995). In the United States, this illness is responsible for 200,000 hospitalizations and 500 deaths in children younger than 5 years of age (AAP, 1996). Children who attend day-care centers, schools, institutions, and other facilities are especially susceptible to episodes of gastroenteritis.

The etiology is due to a variety of organisms such as viruses, bacteria, and parasites. Table 21-6 lists the causes of acute gastroenteritis. In the United States, the majority of cases are of viral origin, specifically Rotavirus and Norwalk virus (Eliason & Lewan, 1998). Rotavirus infection occurs in cooler months, beginning in November in the Southwest and peaking in February or March in the East. It is transmitted via the fecal-oral route, primarily affecting children 6 months to 2 years of age. By age 2 years, most children are immune to severe dehydrating rotaviral diarrhea (Meyers, 1995). Norwalk viruses primarily affect older children and are a major cause of epidemic gastroenteritis worldwide, especially in developing countries. Several pathogens (*Shigella, Salmonella, Campylobacter*) are responsible for bacterial infection. *Shigella* is spread by person-to-person contact or by ingestion of contaminated food. *Salmonella* is transmitted through contact with infected animals, such as pet turtles, hamsters, dogs and cats, and from contaminated food products, such as poultry, eggs, and milk. *Giardia* and *Cryptosporidium* are the most common intestinal parasites that produce disease. *Giardia* is transmitted through ingestion of cysts either from contact with an infected individual or from food or water contaminated with infected feces. It is endemic in some areas, with a very high occurrence rate in day-care centers.

Pathophysiology

The pathophysiological process of viral infection is poorly understood; however, it is hypothesized that the virus destroys or damages the epithelial cells lining the intestines. Viral illness is self-limiting, and recovery involves regeneration of these cells. There are three processes that produce bacterial gastroenteritis (Box 21-4).

TABLE 21-6 Causes of Acute Gastroenteritis

Viruses	Bacteria	Parasites
Rotavirus	*Shigella*	*Giardia lambia*
Norwalk	*Salmonella*	*Cryptosporidium*
Adenovirus	*Campylobacter*	*Entamoeba histolytica*
	Escherichia coli	
	Clostridium difficile	
	Yersinio	

Clinical Manifestations

The clinical manifestations depend on the causative organism; however, in general, signs and symptoms include diarrhea, nausea, vomiting, abdominal pain, weight loss, fever, dehydration, and electrolyte imbalances.

Diagnosis

Diagnosis is based on the history, physical exam, and laboratory studies focused on evaluating the child's hydration status and identifying the causative agent. The history should include the following data:

- Recent exposure to infectious agents
- Travel history, especially if outside the Unites States
- Exposure to contaminated food and water supplies
- Exposure to turtles
- Attendance at a day-care center

The child's hydration status is evaluated, including a history of fluid intake, such as types, amounts, and how tolerated. The stooling pattern, frequency, and volume, as well as urination frequency, amount, and color is also investigated. Current weight compared to pre-illness weight is useful in determining fluid loss.

BOX 21-4 Pathophysiology of bacterial gastroenteritis

- The organism destroys the mucosal cells of the villi in the small intestines, resulting in decreased surface area and less capacity to absorb fluid and electrolytes.
- The organism penetrates the mucosa and submucosa of the intestines causing damage to the cells, necrosis, and ulceration. Eventually, the organism may reach the systemic circulation. Diarrhea ensues and is often mixed with red and white blood cells (e.g., *Shigella, Campylobacter*).
- The organism produces enterotoxins that stimulate secretion of fluid and electrolytes from the primary secretory cells in the small intestines. Action of the enterotoxin also interferes with the absorptive function of the surface area of the upper small intestines. Thus the imbalance between fluid secretion and absorption leads to the loss of water in the stool. Diarrhea associated with this process is profuse and watery, leading to dehydration and acidosis (e.g., *Shigella*, enterotoxigenic *E. coli*).

Generally, if no systemic manifestations are present (fever, lethargy, malaise) and if dehydration is absent, diagnostic laboratory tests are not indicated. Stool cultures should be performed for children with a fever lasting more than 24 hours, blood or mucus in the stool, a family or household member with similar symptoms, or a positive stool white blood cell stain (Galen, 1997). The finding of white blood cells should prompt further investigation to rule out invasive bacterial disease. Rotavirus can be diagnosed by testing the stool using a commercially available kit or electron microscopy. In cases where a parasitic infection is suspected, the stool is examined for ova and parasites.

If dehydration is present, additional tests may be performed to evaluate hydration status such as CBC, urinalysis, blood urea nitrogen (BUN), and electrolyte studies. If the child is dehydrated, the hemoglobin, hematocrit, and BUN will be elevated. The presence of ketones in the urine reflects increased fat metabolism due to caloric deprivation. Metabolic acidosis is common with severe dehydration and diarrhea.

Treatment

Treatment for acute gastroenteritis focuses on fluid replacement and correction of electrolyte disturbances, and is dependent on the degree of dehydration (Table 21-7). Initially management should begin at home since early interventions can reduce complications such as dehydration and poor nutrition. The most important aspect underlying home treatment is the need to administer increased volumes of appropriate fluids as well as to maintain adequate caloric intake.

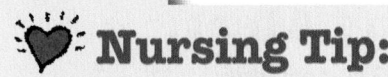

> **Nursing Tip:**
>
> **Refusal to take ORS**
>
> Children who are dehydrated rarely refuse ORS; however, those with vomiting and diarrhea without dehydration may dislike the salty taste. The flavored solutions may be more palatable and can be frozen into an ice-pop or are available in ice-pop form, which may appeal to some children.

Children with no dehydration and mild diarrhea may be treated with 10 ml/kg of ORS to replace fluid lost with each stool. However, since most children who are not dehydrated dislike ORS, they can be offered age-appropriate foods and additional fluids. Breast milk, cow's milk, and full-strength formula can continue to be consumed (Hugger, et al., 1998).

If the child is mildly dehydrated, 50 ml/kg of ORS should be given over 4 to 6 hours. Losses from diarrhea stools and emesis are replaced with an additional 10 ml/kg. Once the dehydration is corrected, the child can resume solid foods. Although there is controversy about which foods are best for refeeding, complex carbohydrates, lean meats, fruits, and vegetables are well tolerated (AAP, 1996).

TABLE 21-7 American Academy of Pediatrics Practice Parameters for Rehydration

Degree of Dehydration	Treatment
Minimal: <3%	Give 10 ml/kg ORS per stool
Mild: 5%	Give 50 ml/kg ORS in 4 hours. Replace each loss from diarrhea and reassess every 2 hours. Resume foods (especially carbohydrates). Avoid foods high in fat or simple sugars.
Moderate: 6–9%	Administer 100 ml/kg ORS and replace losses over 4–6 hrs. Reassess hourly. Treat in a supervised setting.
Severe: >10%	Treat as an emergency. Begin IV therapy (40 ml/kg/hr) until child improves; then offer 50–100 ml/kg ORS. Obtain and monitor electrolyte levels. Reassess frequently. Provide ORS when alert.

Used with permission from Hugger, J., Harkless, G., & Rentschler, D. (1998). Oral rehydration therapy for children with acute diarrhea. The Nurse Practitioner, *23(12), 52–64.*

Nursing Alert:

The BRAT Diet for Gastroenteritis

The traditionally recommended BRAT diet, consisting of bananas, rice, applesauce, and toast or tea, should be avoided for children with acute gastroenteritis because it is low in energy, protein, and fat.

Nursing Tip:

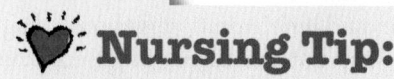

Preventing gastroenteritis

The most effective treatment for gastroenteritis is prevention, specifically good handwashing (after defecation or diapering, and before food preparation and consumption) and proper diaper disposal.

The child with moderate dehydration should be given 100 ml/kg of ORS over 4 to 6 hours, with replacement of losses from diarrhea and vomitus over this same period. When dehydration is corrected, feeding can be resumed as discussed previously. Severe dehydration requires intravenous therapy using isotonic solutions. The fluid is administered in boluses of 15 to 30 ml/kg every 20 minutes until hypovolemia is corrected (Eliason & Lewan, 1998). Electrolyte levels must be determined, and frequent reevaluation of the child's condition is essential. ORT can be instituted when the child's condition stabilizes. When rehydration is completed, the child can be fed according to the AAP guidelines (complex carbohydrates, lean meats, fruits, and vegetables).

Vomiting occurs frequently in children with gastroenteritis; however, most of them with this manifestation and dehydration can be treated with ORT. The guiding principle is to administer small volumes (5 ml) frequently (every 1 to 2 minutes). As vomiting diminishes, larger amounts of ORS can be given at longer intervals.

For most cases of bacterial or viral gastroenteritis, the use of antiemetics, absorbent agents, and gut motility medications is not recommended. The vomiting and diarrhea accompanying this illness are the body's method of eliminating the infecting organism, and these drugs can decrease the speed at which this is accomplished. When *Salmonella* or *Shigella* are the causative organisms, the gastroenteritis is usually self-limiting, and antibiotic therapy is unnecessary. However, antibiotics are recommended for infants under 3 months of age who are at risk for *Salmonella* bacteremia. There are no effective antiviral medications. Parasitic infections are treated with medications such as quinacrine hydrochloride (Atabrine), furazolidone (Furoxone), or metronidazole (Flagyl).

Case Study/Care Plan

The Child with Acute Gastroenteritis

Hannah Torres is a 23-month-old infant brought by her mother to a local emergency room at 8 PM with a history of persistent diarrhea and vomiting for the past 36 hours. Mrs. Torres states that Hannah was seen earlier in the day by their primary doctor who felt she had a viral infection and should be given Pedialyte and allowed to rest. Mrs. Torres became concerned when she continued to have diarrhea and vomit and was difficult to wake up.

Assessment Initial assessment should include the child's hydration status since there is a potential for shock developing with dehydration. The onset, frequency, color, and amount of stools is obtained. If the child is vomiting, assess the frequency, amount, and type of vomitus. The child's intake and tolerance for fluids and solids is assessed. Current weight is compared with last known weight.

Nursing Diagnosis #1

Deficient fluid volume related to losses associated with diarrhea.

Expected Outcomes

1. Child will exhibit signs of rehydration.

continues

continued

2. Child will be free from fluid and electrolyte deficits.
3. Child will maintain weight within normal parameters.

Interventions/*Rationale*

1. Administer oral rehydration solution. *To replace essential fluids and electrolytes.*
2. Administer and monitor IV fluids as prescribed. *IV therapy is based on degree of dehydration.*
3. Monitor and record intake and output. *To evaluate hydration status and effectiveness of fluid replacement.*
4. Check urine specific gravity every 8 hours. *Increasing specific gravity indicates increasing dehydration.*
5. Weigh child daily on same scale at the same time of day. *To assess for dehydration. Weight is an important indicator of fluid status.*
6. Assess for signs of dehydration: decreased or absent tearing, dry mucous membranes, loss of skin turgor. *To evaluate effectiveness of fluid replacement.*

Evaluation

Child has signs of normal hydration such as presence of tears, improved skin turgor, moist mucous membranes, and urine output of at least 1–2 ml/kg/hr.

Nursing Diagnosis #2

Impaired skin integrity related to moisture (irritation) from frequent stools.

Expected Outcomes

1. Child will maintain intact skin in perineal and perianal areas.

Interventions/*Rationale*

1. Change diaper frequently. *To minimize exposure of skin to stool.*
2. Clean diaper area with water and mild soap after each stool. *To remove diarrheal stool, which is acidic and very irritating to the perineum. Commercial baby wipes contain alcohol and may cause further irritation.*
3. Leave diaper area open to air as often as possible. *To promote healing.*
4. Apply creams and ointments (A&D Ointment, zinc oxide, Desitin, petroleum jelly). *To provide a protective barrier from frequent stools.*

Evaluation

The child's skin remains intact and pink.

Family Teaching

Teach the child and other family members that careful handwashing must be practiced, especially after diapering, after using the toilet, and before feeding or eating.

Caregivers should be instructed to change diapers frequently to prevent irritation to the skin. Wash perineal area with mild soap and water after each diarrheal stool. Apply protective ointments to buttocks. Avoid the use of commercial baby wipes.

Teach them the method for monitoring intake and output: record amount of fluids taken; frequency, consistency, and color of stools; frequency and characteristics of vomitus; number of wet diapers per day; weighing wet diapers; and number of voids per day.

Explain signs and symptoms of dehydration, and reinforce the importance of administering ORS and maintaining hydration even in the presence of vomiting. Explain proper food handling techniques (cleaning of cutting boards and food preparation surfaces with hot water and soap; washing hands before and after food preparation; not allowing fresh foods to be contaminated by contact with meat, poultry, or seafood juices).

Tell the caregivers to contact health care provider when (a) the child seems confused or disoriented; (b) vomiting continues for more than 12 hours; (c) blood appears in the diarrhea or diarrhea increases in frequency (bowel movement every hour for more than 8 hours; more than 10 watery bowel movements in one day); (d) there is continuous abdominal pain or intermittent pain that is severe enough to make the child cry or to awaken from sleep; (e) temperature over 100°F for more than 72 hours; (f) child does not urinate for more than 6 hours; (g) crying produces no tears; or (h) infant's anterior fontanel appears sunken.

EDEMA

Edema is an excess accumulation of interstitial fluid that usually results from a disturbance in the fluid exchange between capillaries and interstitial spaces.

Incidence and Etiology

Edema is associated with many illnesses. Heart failure, renal failure, and acute pulmonary edema cause an increase in blood hydrostatic pressure that results in the formation of edema. A loss of blood protein or albumin (often seen with liver disease, nephrotic syndrome, or malnutrition) will cause a shift of fluid into interstitial spaces due to a decrease in blood osmotic pressure. Burns, allergic reactions, and inflammation alter the integrity of the capillary membrane, resulting in the movement of fluid and blood proteins into interstitial spaces. Hypothyroidism and tumors that obstruct the lymphatic system cause an increase in interstitial osmotic pressure that will pull fluid into the interstitial space, resulting in the formation of edema.

Pathophysiology

Edema develops as a result of changes in normal capillary dynamics. Normal capillary dynamics are maintained by balancing hydrostatic and osmotic pressures both within the capillaries and within the surrounding interstitial spaces. Hydrostatic pressures tend to push fluid out of a compartment, and osmotic pressures pull fluid into a compartment. Edema may be caused by four mechanisms: increased blood hydrostatic pressure, decreased blood osmotic pressure, increased interstitial fluid osmotic pressure, and impaired lymphatic drainage.

Increased Blood Hydrostatic Pressure

Blood hydrostatic pressure is the pressure of blood against the capillary walls that tends to push fluid out of the capillaries into the interstitial spaces. When this pressure is increased (as in increased capillary flow), excess fluid may enter the interstitial area, and edema is the result. Venous congestion may also increase the blood hydrostatic pressure by back pressure, as seen in heart failure.

Decreased Blood Osmotic Pressure

Severe and widespread edema may occur when the serum albumin is decreased. Albumin normally contributes to the inward pull of blood osmotic pressure. With decreased numbers of albumin particles, this inward pull diminishes and fluid leaks out into the interstitial area. A decrease in serum albumin may be caused by either albumin loss or diminished albumin synthesis. The most common condition associated with massive albumin loss is nephrotic syndrome. Decreased albumin synthesis accompanies severe protein-calorie malnutrition.

Increased Interstitial Fluid Osmotic Pressure

Normally the interstitial fluid osmotic pressure is small compared to the blood osmotic pressure because of the absence of large amounts of protein in the interstitial fluid. If protein leaks into this fluid, increased interstitial fluid osmotic pressure results, and edema develops. The major cause of this process is increased capillary permeability due to major burns and locally with inflammation (sprained ankle) and hypersensitivity reactions (bee sting).

Impaired Lymphatic Drainage

The lymph vessels normally drain small amounts of fluid and protein from the interstitial spaces and return them to the capillaries. However, if the lymph drainage is impaired through obstruction by a tumor or surgery, fluid and proteins accumulate in the interstitial area, causing edema.

Clinical Manifestations

Edema results in swelling, either localized or general. In most cases, edema in children is manifested initially periorbitally or dependently. If the child is ambulatory, dependent edema will be evident in the ankles. Children on bed rest will have edema in the sacral area. Pitting edema is always a clear sign of an extracellular fluid excess. It is assessed by pushing a finger gently into the edematous tissue and observing for an indentation on the skin. The degree of edema is rated on a four-point scale:

+0 = No persisting indentation
+1 = $^1/_4$" indentation (mild)
+2 = $^1/_4$ – $^1/_2$" indentation (moderate)
+3 = $^1/_2$ – 1" indentation (severe)
+4 = greater than 1" indentation (very severe)

Edematous areas may also appear shiny and full. Additional signs may include a sudden weight gain, an elevation in blood pressure, a bounding pulse, neck vein distention, and dyspnea.

Diagnosis

A diagnosis of edema is determined based on the clinical manifestations that are identified during the history and physical examination. It is important to determine the underlying cause so that appropriate treatment is initiated.

Treatment

Treatment for edema is focused on correcting the underlying condition and often includes the use of diuretics and restriction of sodium and fluid intake. Diuretics are given to promote fluid excretion through the kidneys. Since most diuretics cause potassium losses, it is extremely important to monitor serum potassium levels and provide potassium supplements as necessary. Edema that is due to an inflammatory response, such as an injury or allergic reaction, can be treated by applying cold compresses to reduce blood hydrostatic pressure by decreasing capillary blood flow.

Nursing Management

Nursing management begins with a thorough history and physical assessment. Note the location and extent of the edema. The caregiver may note that the child complains of tight shoes by the end of the day; eyes may appear puffy due to periorbital edema; or the child may complain that his fingers are swollen or feel like sausages. The child may also voice concerns about looking fat. Assess for alterations in body image. Ask if the edema is causing any pain or restriction of movements.

The nurse must maintain accurate measurements of intake and output as well as body weight, which should be measured on the same scale at the same time each day. When diuretics are used, blood electrolytes should be monitored for a potassium depletion. If daily measurements of an edematous limb or abdomen are performed, it should be taken at the exact same location with the same measuring tape. Double check any measurement that shows a dramatic increase or decrease. Edematous limbs should also be checked for circulation integrity by assessing peripheral pulses. Elevating the limb on a pillow will also help the reabsorption of extracellular fluids. Vital signs are important to monitor especially blood pressure and respiratory rate. An increasing blood pressure reflects an increased loss of fluids into extracellular spaces; an increased respiratory rate, along with the presence of rales, often reflects pulmonary edema. Consider elevating the head of the bed if pulmonary edema is suspected.

Family Teaching

Prevention of skin breakdown is paramount. Teach caregivers the importance of good skin care for their child. Edematous tissue is very fragile and, if not kept dry and free from friction, it can easily break down. Special care must be taken to keep the diaper area clean and dry. An infant or child on bed rest should be turned every 2 hours to prevent pressure sores. If the child is on a potassium-depleting diuretic, encourage caregivers to include potassium-rich foods and fluids in the diet such as bananas, apricots, cantaloupe, dates, tomato juice, orange juice, peaches, potatoes, raisins, and figs. Older children may need to be reassured that the edema will be temporary.

BURNS

Significant research-based advances over the past 50 years in fluid therapy, wound care management, respiratory, metabolic, and nutritional support have improved the survival rate for children with burns (Greenfield & Jordan, 1996; Periti & Donati, 1995). The delivery of ideal burn care requires a team of health care providers working together, and carefully assessing and timing the treatments necessary for survival. The team must establish a communication system that includes the child's family so that they can be fully informed of the current care and prepared for future treatments. Although these advances are noteworthy, burns still result from accidents that, for the most part, could have been prevented. Health care providers need to be concerned not only with burn management but also with burn prevention (Forjuoh, 1998).

Incidence and Etiology

Estimates show that 1.25 million people in the United States are burned yearly, 5,500 people die from fire-related burns, 51,000 people are admitted to hospitals for burn care, and 80–90% of the burn injuries are potentially preventable (Brigham & McLoughlin, 1996). Approximately one-third to one-half of the yearly hospitalizations for burns occur in children younger than 18 years of age (Hansbrough & Hansbrough, 1999). At least half of these accidents involve children under 15 years of age, with 1,000 deaths a year in this age group. Deaths from fires and burns are second only to those from motor vehicle accidents in these children (American Academy of Pediatrics, Committee on Injury and Poison Prevention, 2000).

There are four major types of burns: thermal (most common in children), electrical, chemical, and radiation. (1) Thermal burns occur from flames, flash, scalds, or contact with hot objects. Flame injuries are caused by ignition of combustible materials and contact with the fire; household or residential fires are responsible for most flame burns. Flash injuries are caused by explosions, especially of combustible fuels such as gasoline, kerosene, and charcoal lighter. Scald burns occur when hot liquids spill on a child or from hot tap water. Contact burns result from exposure to a hot object such as an oven, hot irons, and radiators. (2) As children become more mobile and curious, they are exposed to additional household burn hazards such as electricity. Chewing on electrical wires or inserting objects into electric sockets can cause electrical burns. (3) Chemical burns are caused when children ingest or are exposed to caustic agents such as household cleaning products. (4) Radiation burns commonly result from overexposure to the ultraviolet rays of the sun.

The majority of burn injuries in children are related to scalds (85%), which are most common in those under 4 years of age (Hansbrough & Hansbrough, 1999). Flame burns predominate in older children and adolescents and account for 13%. The remainder include electrical and chemical.

Since 16% of burns are due to child abuse, it is extremely important to make a determination of cause (Herrin & Antoon, 1996). Was the burn accidental or intentional? Physical findings that are inconsistent with the reported history or incompatible with the child's motor ability, an unclear history of the injury, a delay in seeking treatment, and conflicting stories about how the burn occurred should alert the health care provider to the possibility of an inflicted injury. Additionally, certain types of wounds are noted in child abuse cases: immersion burns (i.e., stocking and glove burns with a clearly demarcated line at the ankle or wrist), doughnut-shaped burns on the buttocks, burns from a cigarette or an iron. This information should be documented thoroughly (Hultman, et al., 1998). If abuse is suspected, a referral should be made to hospital and community resources. Figure 21-4 illustrates an immersion burn of a child's hand. More information on child abuse can be found in Chapter 36.

Pathophysiology

The impact of a burn can range from a minor local injury to a multisystem involvement when a major burn is sustained. All organs and body systems are affected. Table 21-8 lists the alterations of the cardiovascular, renal, respiratory, gastrointestinal, and central nervous systems as well as the changes in metabolism.

Clinical Manifestations

The severity of the burn is determined by the depth of the tissue destroyed and the total body surface area involved. In the past, burns were classified as first, second, third, and fourth degree. However, currently burns are categorized based on the depth of tissue destruction into superficial, partial, and full thickness wounds. First degree burns are categorized as superficial thickness, second degree as partial thickness, and third and fourth degree burns as full thickness. Both classification methods are used in many clinical settings. Figure 21-5 illustrates the tissues involved with different depths of injury.

Superficial (first degree) burns involve only the epidermis, are very painful and red, and heal spontaneously in approximately 5 to 10 days without scarring. Systemic effects are uncommon. An example of a superficial burn is a minor sunburn (Figure 21-6). In a partial thickness burn (second degree), the epidermis and upper layers of the dermis are destroyed. The skin is moist, bright red, extremely painful, and sensitive to cold air. It is common to see blisters form that will blanch with pressure. These wounds will usually heal within 14 to 21 days and may result in some scarring if the burn involves the deep dermal layers of the skin (Figure 21-7). Third degree burns (full thickness) involve the epidermis, dermis, and extend into the subcutaneous tissues. These burns usually will form **eschar,** thick leather-like dead skin (Figure 21-8). Fourth degree burns, also known as full thickness, extend into the tendons, muscles, and bones and are usually caused by electrical burns. Full thickness burns are characterized by a whitish,

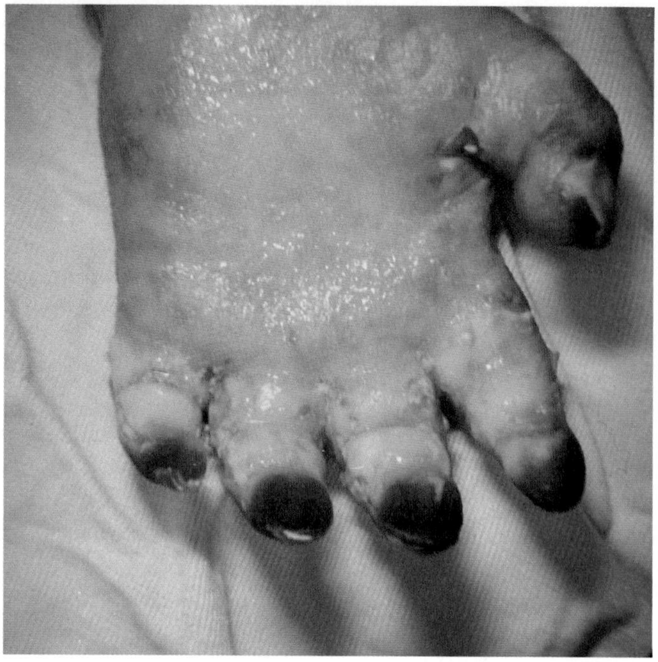

Figure 21-4 Immersion Burns of a Child's Hand. Courtesy of Dr. Robert Arensman, Chief Pediatric Surgery. Children's Memorial Medical Center, Chicago.

Kids Want To Know

When will my burn scars disappear?

Scars from a burn never disappear completely. They can be altered through plastic surgery or camouflaged with creative use of makeup so that they're not so noticeable. The redness appearance of the scars will decrease as the wounds mature.

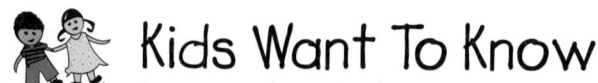

TABLE 21-8 Body System Manifestations after Major Burn

Response	Treatment
Cardiovascular System	
First 24–48 hrs postburn	
↓ Cardiac output resulting from ↑ capillary permeability and vasodilation	Adequate fluid replacement Monitor vital signs, especially BP
↑ Metabolic acidosis hematocrit	Assess blood gases
48–72 hrs postburn	
Capillary permeability is restored	Monitor vital signs
Interstitial fluids move back into bloodstream	Monitor urine output
↓ Hematocrit	↓ IV fluids
↓ Platelet count	Monitor PTT
Renal System	
Reduced blood flow to kidneys leads to ↓ urine output	Monitor I/O
Potential for acute renal failure	Administer IV fluids at a rate that maintains urine output of 1–2 cc/kg/hr
↑ BUN, ↑ Creatinine	
With fluid remobilization, ↑ urine output as interstitial fluid is mobilized and eliminated	Anticipate fluid remobilization Assess BP
Respiratory System	
Upper airway edema and obstruction from inhaling heated gases	Monitor respirations Assess for rales, wheezes
Lower airway obstruction and pneumonia from smoke inhalation	Assess depth of respirations
Carbon monoxide poisoning and hypoxia from inhaling end products of combustion causes mucosal erythema and edema	Monitor blood gases
Atelectasis and respiratory failure	Assess for equal respirations
Pulmonary edema from too vigorous fluid replacement	
Restriction of chest excursion from edema and eschar formation with circumferential burns	Notify health care provider and prepare client for escharotomy
Gastrointestinal System	
↓ Perfusion of GI tract and liver due to ↓ blood flow	Monitor bowel sounds
↓ Gastric acid production for 48–72 hrs followed by ↑ acid production and risk of stress ulcers	Assess liver enzymes Assess NG drainage for evidence of blood
↓ GI motility	Place NG tube for decompression of stomach
Central Nervous System	
Burn-related encephalopathy due to hypoxemia, hypovolemia, and septicemia	Monitor fluids and blood gases Assess signs of infection
Manifestations include:	Assess neurologic status frequently
Hallucinations, personality changes, delirium, seizures, and coma	Initiate seizure precautions
Metabolism	
↑ Metabolic rate from nitrogen losses and stress of injury	Monitor intake of calories Give parenteral nutrition as needed
↑ Heat losses through damaged skin	
Rapid protein breakdown and muscle wasting	Give diet high in proteins
↑ Blood glucose levels due to insulin resistance and breakdown of glycogen stores	
Delayed growth and maturation from need to use energy to repair burned tissues	Give multivitamin, ↑ vitamins C and A

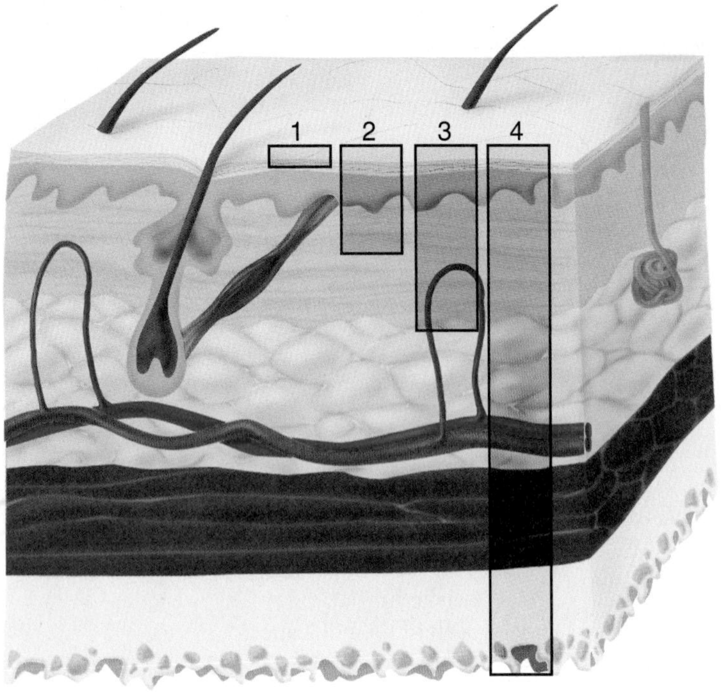

Figure 21-5 Depths of Burns and Corresponding Tissues Involved. Courtesy of Dr. Robert Arensman, Chief Pediatric Surgery. Children's Memorial Medical Center, Chicago.

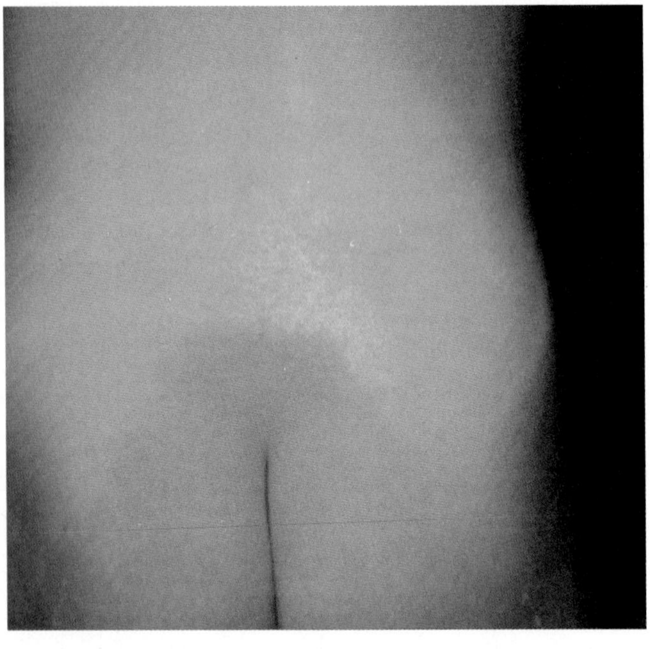

Figure 21-6 Child with a Superficial-Thickness (First Degree) Burn. Courtesy of Dr. Robert Arensman, Chief Pediatric Surgery. Children's Memorial Medical Center, Chicago.

leathery, dry appearance that has a decreased sensation to pain. These burns will result in scarring and contractures and will require skin grafting, skin flaps, or possible amputation to fully heal (Greenfield & Jordan, 1996).

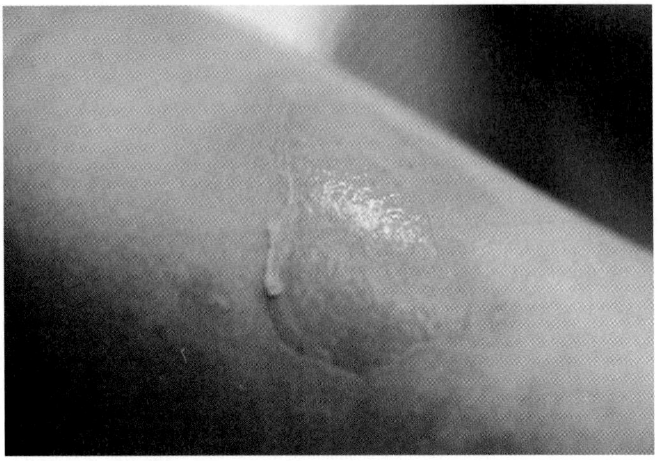

Figure 21-7 Child with a Partial-Thickness (Second Degree) Burn with a Blister. Courtesy of Dr. Robert Arensman, Chief Pediatric Surgery. Children's Memorial Medical Center, Chicago.

The extent of the burn injury is usually expressed as the percentage of the total body surface area (TBSA) affected. In children, the most accurate method of determining the area burned is by mapping the injured areas on a Lund and Browder–like body chart, taking into account the proportional changes that occur during growth. Figure 21-9 is an example of a chart for estimating the extent of burns on a child. If such a chart is not available, the palm of the child's hand, representing 1% of body surface area, can be used to

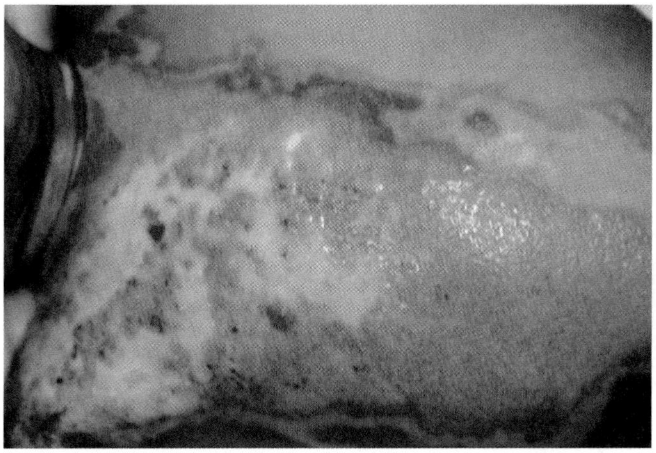

Figure 21-8 Child with a Full-Thickness (Third Degree) Burn. Courtesy of Dr. Robert Arensman, Chief Pediatric Surgery. Children's Memorial Medical Center, Chicago.

estimate the extent of the burn. Calculation of the percent of body surface area burned is important in determining fluid resuscitation needs.

Once the extent and depth of the burn is determined, the burn can be classified as minor, moderate, or major (Table 21-9). Additional variables to consider should include the type of burn, the presence of associated injuries, the age of the child, and the presence of any chronic health conditions and/or social problems. Minor burns can generally be treated on an outpatient basis, while moderate and severe burns require hospitalization. Community hospitals are usually equipped to manage moderate burns. However, a child with major burns or involving the hands, feet, face, eyes, ears, and genitalia should be stabilized and then transferred to a pediatric burn unit, PICU, or pediatric burn care center.

Diagnosis

A diagnosis of burns is determined based on the clinical manifestations that are identified during the history and physical examination.

Treatment

The emphasis of treatment for major burns includes the following: respiratory management, fluid resuscitation, pain management, wound care, prevention of impaired mobility, nutritional support, and psychological support.

Respiratory Management

Initial treatment consists of assessing for patency of the airway and establishing and/or maintaining it. Pulmonary complications remain the leading cause of death in thermal burns. Anticipate respiratory involvement if the burn occurred in an enclosed space or if the child was found unconscious. Oxygen should be administered if hypoxia is present. It is important to assess the child's ability to expand the chest. Full thickness burns that fully extend around the child's trunk may interfere with breathing. An **escharotomy,** an incision made into constricting eschar to restore peripheral blood circulation, may be required to release the chest constriction. Arterial blood gases will also provide evidence of smoke inhalation and the adequacy of gas exchange. A child who has upper body burns, facial burns, or smoke inhalation is at risk for airway obstruction from edema (Figure 21-10). Intubation may be performed if the child exhibits face and neck edema, soot in the nose or mouth, or singed nose hairs.

Fluid Resuscitation

All burn injuries alter capillary permeability and, if severe enough, will require fluid replacement. Fluid resuscitation is a major focus of seriously burned children during the initial treatment period in order to prevent hypovolemic shock. The goal is to infuse intravenous fluids (usually Lactated Ringer's solution) at a sufficient rate and volume to compensate for increased capillary permeability and the loss of intravascular fluids. A large-bore central venous catheter is used in order to administer massive fluid loads. A variety of formulas are available as guidelines for fluid volume and rate of administration; however, each is based on the relationship between body weight and total body surface area burned. The Parkland formula is one that is frequently used (Box 21-5).

The fluid formula requirements are generally 2–4 ml/kg of body weight times the TBSA. Formulas are only guides to resuscitation, and actual fluid administration rates are based on the child's response. Adequacy of the resuscitation is reflected in urine output of 1–2 ml/kg/hr, stable vital signs, and alert and oriented mental status. A Foley catheter is inserted to facilitate urine output measurement. If the urine output falls below this amount, the child is not receiving adequate fluids and may develop renal tubular obstruction if not corrected quickly.

After initial fluid resuscitation, capillary permeability is regained. At this time, the child's urine output will increase dramatically because interstitial fluids are pulled back into the bloodstream. Intravenous fluids should be decreased to maintenance levels to prevent fluid overload and pulmonary edema. The type and amount of fluid used will be based on the results of blood electrolyte tests.

Nursing Alert:

Preventing Hypothermic Shock

Do not apply ice or cold water to any burn. This will cause hypothermia, may intensify a shock condition, and will cause further ischemic injury to the burned area.

Burn Estimate and Diagram
Age vs Area

Initial Evaluation

Cause of burn____________________

Date of Burn____________________

Time of Burn____________________

Age____________________

Sex____________________

Weight____________________

Date of Admission____________________

Signature____________________

Date____________________

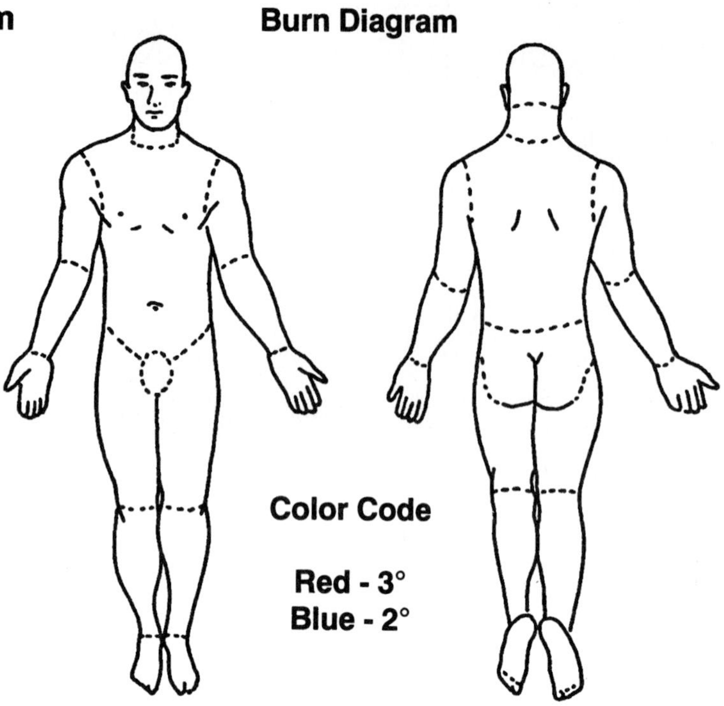

Area	Birth 1 yr.	1-4 yrs.	5-9 yrs.	10-14 yrs.	15 yrs.	Adult	2°	3°	Total	Donor Areas
Head	19	17	13	11	9	7				
Neck	2	2	2	2	2	2				
Ant. Trunk	13	13	13	13	13	13				
Post. Trunk	13	13	13	13	13	13				
R. Buttock	2 1/2	2 1/2	2 1/2	2 1/2	2 1/2	2 1/2				
L. Buttock	2 1/2	2 1/2	2 1/2	2 1/2	2 1/2	2 1/2				
Genitalia	1	1	1	1	1	1				
R.U. Arm	4	4	4	4	4	4				
L.U. Arm	4	4	4	4	4	4				
R.L. Arm	3	3	3	3	3	3				
L.L. Arm	3	3	3	3	3	3				
R. Hand	2 1/2	2 1/2	2 1/2	2 1/2	2 1/2	2 1/2				
L. Hand	2 1/2	2 1/2	2 1/2	2 1/2	2 1/2	2 1/2				
R. Thigh	5 1/2	6 1/2	8	8 1/2	9	9 1/2				
L. Thigh	5 1/2	6 1/2	8	8 1/2	9	9 1/2				
R. Leg	5	5	5 1/2	6	6 1/2	7				
L. Leg	5	5	5 1/2	6	6 1/2	7				
R. Foot	3 1/2	3 1/2	3 1/2	3 1/2	3 1/2	3 1/2				
L. Foot	3 1/2	3 1/2	3 1/2	3 1/2	3 1/2	3 1/2				
						Total				

Figure 21-9 Estimation of the Extent of Burns in Children. Courtesy of The Shriners Burn Hospital; Cincinnati, Ohio.

Pain Management

The pain following a burn is both acute and chronic. Thermal destruction of tissue results in one of the most severe and prolonged types of pain known. Pain from the injury is compounded by performing procedures on the wound, especially dressing changes. It is considerably reduced when the child is at rest. Other factors such as fear and anxiety contribute to the child's perception of pain. For children with major burns, intravenous narcotics such as

TABLE 21-9 Classification of Burn Injuries

Minor	Moderate	Major
Partial thickness burn <10% TBSA	Partial thickness burn 10–15% TBSA	Partial thickness burn >15% TBSA
Full thickness burn <2% TBSA	Full thickness burn 2–10% TBSA	Full thickness burn >10% TBSA
Child older than 2 years of age	Child younger than 2 years with otherwise minor injuries	Child <10 years of age with otherwise moderate injury
Excludes involvement of face, ears, hands, feet, and perineum	Includes small areas of involvement of face, ears, hands, feet, and perineum	Includes large areas of involvement of face, ears, hands, feet, and perineum
Excludes all electrical, chemical, and inhalation burns	Includes small electrical and chemical burns Includes children where smoke inhalation is suspected	Includes electrical and chemical burns, all significant inhalation injuries, burns involving fractures or other major trauma, and all poor-risk individuals
Recommended treatment location: outpatient	Recommended treatment location: community hospital	Recommended treatment location: pediatric burn unit, PICU, or pediatric burn center

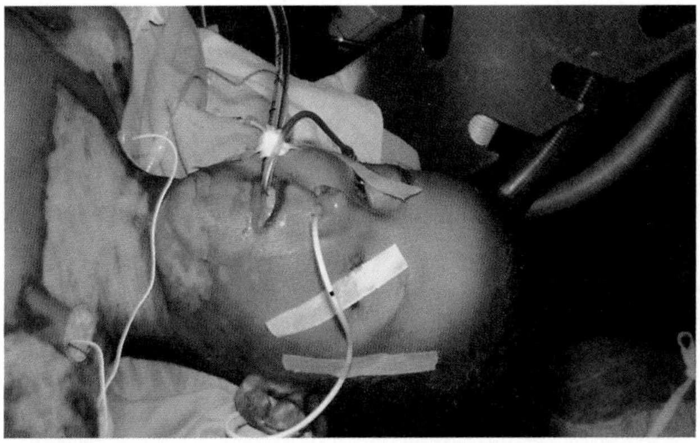

Figure 21-10 A Girl Who was Wearing Flame Retardant Pajamas with Burns from a House Fire. Courtesy of Dr. Robert Arensman, Chief Pediatric Surgery. Children's Memorial Medical Center, Chicago.

BOX 21-5 Parkland formula for fluid resuscitation

4 ml Lactated Ringer's solution × kg of body weight × % total body surface area burned

- One-half of total is given in the first 8 hours postburn.
- One-fourth of total is given in the second 8 hours postburn.
- One-fourth of total is given in the third 8 hours postburn.

Note: Time is calculated from the time of the injury, not the time of admission to the hospital.

Nursing Tip:

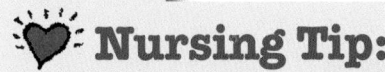

Calculating maintenance IV fluid rate using the 4:2:1 rule

To calculate the hourly IV rate, first determine the child's daily maintenance fluid requirement, then divide that number by 24. In practice, this process can be simplified by using the 4:2:1 rule without sacrificing accuracy. Try it out.

IV rate = 4 ml/kg for each kg of weight up to 10 kg
+ 2 ml/kg/hr for each kg of weight between 10 and 20 kg
+ 1 ml/kg/hr for each kg over 20 kg

Example: Daily IV fluid rate for a 45-kg child who is NPO would be:
40 ml
20 ml
25 ml
85 ml/hr

morphine sulfate are indicated. Initially, these drugs are administered intravenously because the fluid shift limits absorption from the subcutaneous and intramuscular areas, and the pain will not be relieved. Acetaminophen with codeine is usually given to children with minor burns. Children should always be assessed for pain using appropriate assessment tools for the child's age. (Refer to Chapter 18 for a thorough discussion of pain management.) Nurses have a tendency to undermedicate children due to an unrealistic

Eye On:

Effect of Therapeutic Touch on Pain and Anxiety in Burn Patients

The benefits of therapeutic touch have long been debated and are highly controversial. Use in the care of pediatric burn clients has been questioned. However, recent study findings lend support for its use (Turner, Clark, Gauthier, & Williams, 1998). Therapeutic touch is an intervention in which human energies are therapeutically manipulated. The name is really a misnomer because actual touch or physical contact with the skin is not necessary. Therapeutic touch can be implemented by holding the hands 2–5 inches from the patient's body. The therapy is based on the assumption that the human energy field extends beyond the skin. Therefore, not having to touch the child avoids the discomfort associated with direct touch of the burn wounds.

fear of respiratory depression (Ashburn, 1995; Patterson, 1995). Pain medications should be given prior to all painful procedures. Children often do better if they have some control over their pain. Therefore, patient-controlled analgesia is now commonly used with children and has been found to be effective in decreasing pain (Ashburn, 1995). Children also respond well to behavioral interventions such as imagery, relaxation therapies, and hypnosis.

Wound Care

Initial wound care is started after the child has been stabilized. Care should be taken to use aseptic techniques when cleaning the burned areas and to medicate the child prior to the procedure. The wounds are gently cleaned and debrided. **Debridement** is the removal of dead tissue from the burn site and is associated with severe pain. This procedure is performed by soaking the wound for about 10 minutes to soften the tissue. The wound is then washed from the inner to outer edges using a firm, circular motion. Any loose or dead tissue is removed by gently lifting it up with forceps and cutting it away. After the wound and surrounding areas are cleaned, an antimicrobial cream, such as silver sulfadiazine (Silvadene), is applied to minimize bacterial proliferation and prevent infection. Some type of dressing is then applied. Table 21-10 lists several topical agents used in treating burn wounds. Figure 21-11 shows a child having Silvadene applied to a burn wound.

TABLE 21-10 Topical Antimicrobials Used in Burn Care

Antibiotic	Use	Activity	Advantages	Disadvantages
Mafenide acetate (Sulfamylon cream)	Topical applied QD or BID without dressings Apply to depth of $^1/_{16}$"	Gram-positive Gram-negative organisms	Penetrates through full-thickness eschar. Easy application and removal. Able to monitor wound appearance. Allows for movement.	Very painful May cause metabolic acidosis
Silver sulfadiazine (Silvadene)	Topical applied QD or BID Cleanse wound between applications Apply to depth of $^1/_{16}$"	Gram-positive Gram-negative organisms	Painless, soothing Good for outpatient use Easy application and removal Able to monitor wound appearance Allows for movement of burned area	Poor penetration through eschar May cause leukopenia Cross sensitivity with sulfonamides
Silver nitrate 0.5% dressings (soaks)	Used to dampen dressings q2hr Change dressing BID or TID	Wide range of pathogens, including fungal infections	Painless on application No resistant organisms Minimizes heat and water losses	No penetration of eschar Labor intensive Difficult to monitor wound Discoloration of skin and clothes May cause fluid and electrolyte imbalances

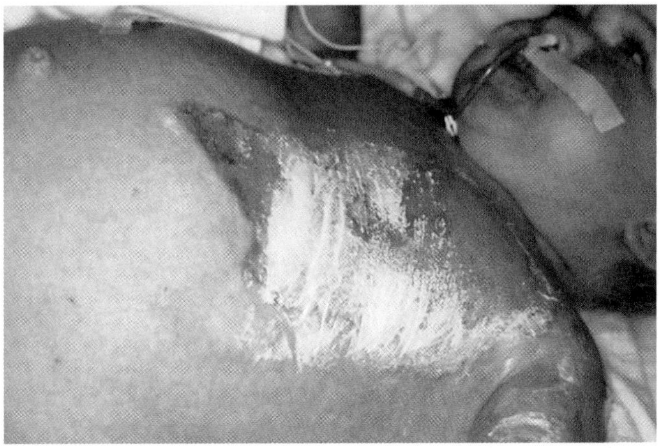

Figure 21-11 A Child Having Silvadene Applied to a Scald Burn of the Chest. Courtesy of Dr. Robert Arensman, Chief Pediatric Surgery. Children's Memorial Medical Center, Chicago.

Hydrotherapy is used to soften dead tissue to help in the debridement process and to improve circulation to the wound. The experience is very painful and scary for all burn clients (Greenfield & Jordan, 1996). Children should be medicated prior to hydrotherapy and dressing changes. It is helpful if caregivers can be present to comfort and distract the child. Figure 21-12 shows a child in a whirlpool bath.

Burn dressings are changed once or twice a day. Sheridan, Petras, Lydon, and Slavo (1998) studied the frequency of burn dressing changes in 50 children with an average burn size of 11% TBSA and found that once daily dressing changes were just as effective as twice daily. Results showed a significant savings of nursing staff time and a decreased need for pain medication with no change in infectious morbidity. Since dressing changes are very frightening, painful, and costly, the researchers recommend changing burn protocols appropriately.

Once the wounds have been debrided and are beginning to heal, various temporary skin grafts can be used to facilitate the healing process. These include **homografts** (cadaver skin), **heterografts** (pig skin), and synthetic skin coverings. (Greenfield & Jordan, 1996; McCain & Sutherland, 1998). Homografts can remain in place until donor site tissues are available. Typically, homografts will begin to slough off around 14 days. Pigskin dressings are replaced daily or every other day. They are often used in children with scald burns of the hands and face because they allow free movement and reduce risk of contracture formation. Temporary grafts accelerate wound healing by creating an environment that promotes epithelial growth in the form of granulation tissue. Adequate granulation tissue must be present before the child can be permanently grafted. Figure 21-13 demonstrates a child's hand with red granulation tissue.

Extensive full thickness burns will require a permanent skin graft, an autograft, to fully heal. The skin for an **autograft** is taken from an unburned area of the child's own skin. Once an autograft is placed on the wound, the area must be immobilized. This is often difficult in children requiring the use of splints or casts (Staley & Serghiou, 1998). Another permanent skin graft is a **cultured epithelial autograft,** which is only used in children with burns covering ≥80% TBSA. They are sheets of skin grown in the lab from a small skin biopsy of the child. Long-term follow-up studies to

Reflective Thinking

Looking at Burns

Burns are often difficult to look at.

How would you feel about working with a child who has been severely burned? Could you move past the way burns look to deliver adequate care?

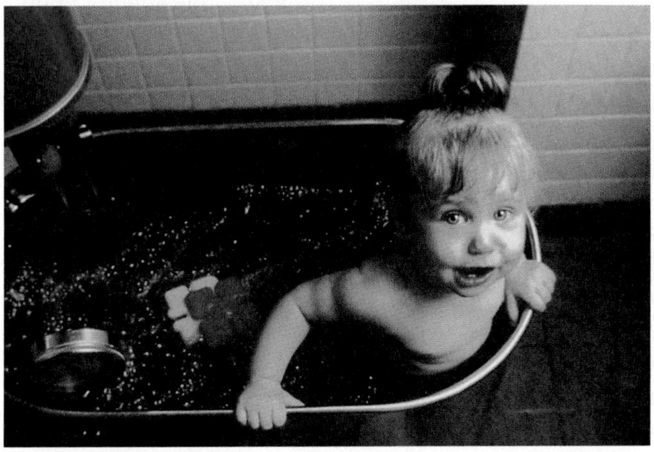

Figure 21-12 A Child with Burns on the Legs in a Whirlpool. Courtesy of Dr. Robert Arensman, Chief Pediatric Surgery. Children's Memorial Medical Center, Chicago.

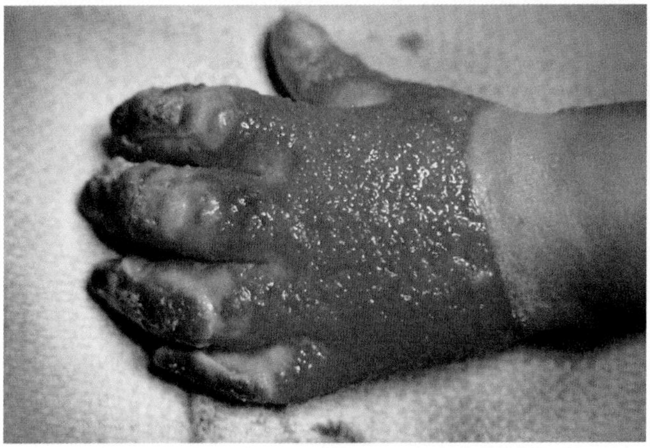

Figure 21-13 A Child's Hands with Red Granulation Tissue. Courtesy of Dr. Robert Arensman, Chief Pediatric Surgery. Children's Memorial Medical Center, Chicago.

REFLECTIONS FROM FAMILIES

At first I was in shock. How could this have happened to my child? Will he be all right? Will he have scars? I worried about the way his face was going to look and I constantly watched all of his machines, looking for signs of improvement. It takes time to put everything in order. I could not remember simple things. I often asked the same questions over and over. I just could not seem to concentrate. The accident disrupted our whole family life. If it wasn't for the compassionate care that the nurses gave to my son and their understanding of my anxieties and stress, I do not know how I would have gotten through this ordeal.

Kids Want To Know

What do I tell people who stare at me?

Sometimes people stare to figure out what it is that looks different, not bad or ugly. Sometimes they stare when they really have questions they want to ask you. When this happens, you can ask them kindly if they have a question you could answer. You can also ask that they please stop staring because it makes you feel uncomfortable. It is also important for you to have someone with whom you can freely discuss your feelings. Many kids find it helpful to talk with another child who has experienced burns and has a similar frustration with people staring. Most communities have support groups for burn survivors.

determine effectiveness are still pending. However, the ability to grow cultured epithelium offers the possibility of an unlimited source of skin for children with extensive burns.

After the grafts heal, pressure dressings are applied to prevent the formation of contractures and to minimize scarring. These dressing may be elastic wraps, pressure splints, or pressurized garments that provide continuous and uniform pressure over the burned areas. The elasticized garments are usually worn for several months, and therefore, need to be altered as the child grows.

Prevention of Impaired Mobility

Children are at risk for impaired mobility and the development of contractures due to prolonged bed rest, muscular atrophy and shortening, and stiffening of burned tissues. It is essential to implement appropriate positioning strategies to prevent deformities and an exercise program to maintain muscle strength and joint mobility. When joints are not being exercised, they should be maintained in maximal extension using splints if needed. Particular attention should be paid to the hands and neck since these are the most prone to rapid contractures. Early exercise is encouraged and compliance can be improved with judicious use of analgesics. Range of motion exercises are performed actively at least three times a day. Active range of motion of muscles is possible in infants and toddlers by using familiar toys; however, most of the joints will require passive range of motion exercises. Caregivers can support and encourage older children to participate in active range of motion.

Nutritional Support

Children have limited glycogen stores to meet the increased energy demands of a burn injury. The burned child will require two to three times the normal amount of calories in order to heal. Children with severe injuries will require some form of caloric supplementation. The diet should be high in protein (23% of total calories) to maintain weight and muscle function (Demling & DeSanti, 1998; Mayes, Gottschlich, & Warden, 1997). Nutrition protocols also call for the addition of a multivitamin with increased amounts of vitamins A and C to help replace the losses from the changes in metabolism and losses from the open burn wounds (Mayes, et al., 1997). Children should be offered a variety of foods and be allowed to choose meals when they feel better. They will often eat more if they have their meals with other children or family members. Most children with major burns are unable to meet their nutritional requirements orally; therefore, it is necessary to use enteral feedings. Changes in stools (increased stooling, diarrhea) may indicate that the child is not tolerating the feedings.

Psychological Support

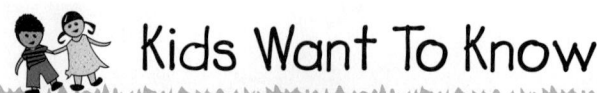

Anxiety for the child and caregivers can be overwhelming. Play therapy is used to help the child deal with the frustrations of burn therapy. It encourages the child to move and actively participate in activities with other children. As recovery continues, counseling with various support services may be implemented to foster the child's self-esteem. Caregivers also need to be supported and encouraged to participate in the care of their child, which is often very reassuring for both of them (Barnum, Snyder, Rapoff, Mani, & Thompson, 1998; Kendall-

Research Highlight

Physical and Psychologic Rehabilitation Outcomes for Pediatric Patients with Severe Burns

Study Purpose

The purpose of this study was to examine the issue of expected quality of life for children who survive massive burn injuries by determining their long-term functional and psychological adaptation. Two research questions were posed: (1) whether children with massive burn injuries achieved age-appropriate developmental milestones and independent self-care skills, and (2) whether they were judged by themselves and significant others to be competent in psychosocial areas.

Methods

Forty-one survivors with 88% (TBSA) burns and 85% mean third degree TBSA burns from a local burn center participated in this longitudinal follow-up study. Behavior, maturation, and emotions were assessed by means of standardized psychological assessments.

Several physical parameters of development and activities of daily living (ADL) skills were used that assessed mobility, self-care, dressing, and feeding. For assessment of functional adaptation, each task of the ADL was scored as independent or dependent. To establish whether massive injuries had an impact on functional independence, they were defined as the presence of any finger amputations, upper or lower extremity amputations, joint fusions, or brain anoxia.

Findings

Thirty-three of the 41 participants (80%) were independent in basic ADL skills. Eighty-six percent of the participants who were ages 10 or older were independent in advanced ADL skills. Patients with amputations were significantly more dependent than those without amputations ($p < 0.05$). Mean psychosocial adjustment scores were within normal limits as compared with standardized scores, and were not significantly related to functional independence in ADL skills.

Implications

The data support previous findings that children who have massive burn injuries adapt well, both physically and psychologically. Only the combination of a major burn with amputations or brain anoxia were associated with physical dependence. The psychosocial adjustment of these children also appears to be normal. However, the borderline scores on the competency scales of the dependent children support previously expressed concerns about diminished social competency. The development of a social skills training program may help to boost self-competence in social situations and thereby enhance the self-sufficiency and self-esteem of burn victims. More studies are needed to assess issues of transition from adolescence to early adulthood.

Citation

Meyers-Paal, R., Blakeney, P., Robert, R., Murphy, L., Chinkes, D., Meyer, W., Desai, M., & Herndon, D. (2000). Physical and psychologic rehabilitation outcomes for pediatric patients who suffer 80% or more TBSA, 70% or more third degree burns. *Journal of Burn Care & Rehabilitation, 21*(1), 43–49.

Case Study/Care Plan

A Child with Major Burns

Jorge Santiago, a 6-year-old boy, sustained 40% partial and full-thickness scald burns to his hands, chest, and both thighs. He was helping his big sister who was cooking macaroni and cheese for lunch. He tried to take the pot of boiling macaroni to the sink, but it was heavier than he thought. It slipped out of his hands, and the boiling water splashed on him. When he arrived at the emergency department, he was alert but crying.

Nursing Care Plan

Assessment During the immediate hours following the injury, nursing assessment focuses on respiratory, cardiac, and renal status and includes monitoring airway, breathing, circulation, vital signs, infusion of fluids, and urine output. The nurse should also assess for additional injuries that may have occurred at the time of the burn. The history should include the following:

- Description of how and where the burn occurred, including the agent of injury and length of time in contact with the skin
- When the injury occurred
- Circumstances surrounding injury
- Initial treatment of the burn

After the initial period (48 hours after the injury), physical assessment findings are directed to maintenance of the cardiovascular and respiratory systems.

Nursing Diagnosis #1

Risk for deficient fluid volume related to increased capillary permeability, extracellular fluid shift, and fluid losses through the burn wounds

Expected Outcomes

1. Jorge will remain hydrated

Interventions/*Rationale*

1. Assess for signs/symptoms of fluid volume deficit: hypotension, tachycardia, pale/cool skin, decreased urine output, change in mental status (restlessness, disorientation). *Decreases the risks associated with hypovolemic shock.*

2. Monitor lab values for abnormal electrolyte values. *To identify fluid and electrolyte disturbances.*

3. Monitor vital signs. *Fluid excess or deficit can cause changes in vital signs.*

4. Monitor intake and output. Measure specific gravity of urine. Report if urine output is < 1–2 ml/kg/hr. *Assures prompt recognition and treatment of hypovolemia. Urine output is the most sensitive indicator of cardiac output and tissue perfusion.*

5. Administer IV fluids as prescribed and maintain patency. *Restores adequate intravascular volume and replaces ongoing fluid losses.*

6. Monitor daily weight to assess for fluid retention or diuresis. *Weight is an indicator of hydration status.*

Evaluation

Jorge remains well hydrated as evidenced by the following:

Electrolyte values remain within normal ranges.

Urine output remains adequate for weight with a specific gravity ranging between 1.005–1.025.

continues

continued

Nursing Diagnosis #2

Ineffective tissue perfusion due to edema or circumferential injuries to extremities.

Expected Outcomes

1. Jorge will maintain adequate tissue perfusion as evidenced by:
   Absence of complaints of numbness or tingling in the extremities
   Presence of peripheral pulses with good capillary refill
2. Jorge will be able to move all extremities and digits.

Interventions/*Rationale*

1. Question Jorge regarding sensation in extremities and fingers. *To ascertain adequacy of circulation.*
2. Assess peripheral pulses and capillary refill frequently. Notify health care provider of any changes in distal pulses. *To assess adequacy of circulation.*
3. Assist with performing escharotomies as needed. *Eschar can constrict peripheral circulation.*
4. Position carefully to prevent compromising the blood flow to the extremities. *Enhances circulation and promotes venous return.*

Evaluation

Jorge maintains adequate sensation, circulation, and movement in all extremities and digits.

Nursing Diagnosis #3

Impaired gas exchange/ineffective airway clearance related to airway obstruction, pulmonary edema, and hypoventilation.

Expected Outcomes

1. Jorge will demonstrate a normal spontaneous respiratory rate, effort, depth, and adequate air movement.
2. Jorge will have normal arterial blood gases
3. Jorge will exhibit an absence of adventitious breath sounds or pulmonary edema.

Interventions/*Rationale*

1. Monitor respiratory rate and effort and assess for hoarseness. *Increased respiratory rate and effort and developing hoarseness are indications of airway obstruction.*
2. Monitor pulse oximetry and arterial blood gases and notify health care provider of hypoxemia or hypercarbia. *To ascertain changes in acid-base balance. Changes in respiratory status can be quickly detected by measuring oxygen saturation.*
3. Provide oxygen therapy as needed and monitor response. *Enhances respiratory effort.*
4. Encourage turning, coughing, and deep breathing. *Promotes lung expansion, facilitates mucus clearing, and prevents development of pneumonia.*
5. Be prepared to assist with intubation and mechanical ventilatory support as needed. Make sure that emergency equipment is close by. *Prophylactic intubation may be performed in children with known facial burns.*

Evaluation

Jorge's respiratory status remains stable as evidenced by normal rate, effort, and ease of breathing.

continues

continued

Nursing Diagnosis #4

Pain related to tissue destruction, debridement, dressing changes, and exercise of burned extremities.

Expected Outcomes

1. Jorge will indicate reduction or elimination of pain.
2. Jorge and family will express satisfaction with pain control measures.
3. Jorge will be able to tolerate activities of daily living and care.

Interventions/*Rationale*

1. Assess level of pain frequently and as needed using an age-appropriate assessment tool. *Provides consistent measurement of pain.*
2. Administer pain medication IV on a scheduled basis rather than p.r.n. *Pain associated with burns is severe.*
3. Assess factors that aggravate or alleviate pain and modify care appropriately. *Individualizes treatment to child's needs.*
4. Ensure adequate analgesia before all painful procedures such as wound care and dressing changes. *Helps ease the pain.*
5. Provide diversional activities as additional method of pain relief. *Techniques such as relaxation, distraction, and therapeutic touch can help alleviate pain.*

Evaluation

Jorge's level of pain is reduced or eliminated as indicated and quantified by decreased scores on pain assessment tools.

Nursing Diagnosis #5

Risk for infection due to tissue destruction and prolonged used of invasive therapies (indwelling catheters, central venous catheters).

Expected Outcomes

1. Jorge's burned skin areas and graft sites will heal within appropriate time intervals.
2. Jorge will demonstrate no signs of systemic sepsis.

Interventions/*Rationale*

1. Monitor for signs of infection (increasing temperature, increasing WBC, purulent foul smelling drainage from wounds, redness or swelling around invasive lines) and of sepsis (fever, ileus, disorientation, tachypnea, tachycardia). *Monitoring allows prompt recognition and treatment.*
2. Monitor lab values as ordered (CBC, wound cultures, blood cultures). *Assesses for potential complications and ascertains any changes in wound flora growth.*
3. Maintain sterile or aseptic techniques, as appropriate, with invasive procedures and dressing changes. *Minimizes exposure to infectious agents.*
4. Administer tetanus toxoid as indicated. *Prevents Jorge from acquiring tetanus.*
5. Administer intravenous/topical antibiotics per order. *Controls bacterial growth.*
6. Ensure good handwashing technique by all members of health care team before and after contact with child. *Minimizes exposure to infections.*

Evaluation

Jorge has no signs of systemic infection as evidenced by stable vital signs and normal wound culture.

continues

continued

Nursing Diagnosis #6

Imbalanced nutrition: less than body requirements, related to increased basal metabolic rate and reduced caloric intake.

Expected Outcomes

1. Jorge will show steady weight gain prior to discharge.
2. Jorge's wounds will heal appropriately.

Interventions/*Rationale*

1. Provide a high calorie, high protein diet. *Avoids protein breakdown and meets additional caloric requirements.*
2. Monitor ability to tolerate oral, tube, or parenteral feedings by assessing for abdominal distention, vomiting, diarrhea, reflux, or increasing gastric residuals. *Avoid feeding intolerances.*
3. Measure and record weight weekly. *Monitors nutritional status.*
4. Provide oral hygiene each shift and as needed. *Encourages appetite.*
5. Involve Jorge in food selection and encourage the family to provide child's favorite foods. *Stimulates the appetite and meets nutritional requirements.*
6. Allow adequate uninterrupted time for meals that encourages socialization with family or other children on the unit. *Meets nutritional requirements by providing a homelike environment.*
7. Monitor and record intake and output. *Allows evaluation of sufficiency of intake.*

Evaluation

Jorge consumes an appropriate amount of nutrients and has restored weight to preburn status.

Nursing Diagnosis #7

Deficient knowledge (caregivers) regarding home management.

Expected Outcomes

1. Caregivers will express and demonstrate confidence regarding home care needs.

Interventions/*Rationale*

1. Plan discharge teaching based on assessment of Jorge and family's level of cognition, psychosocial, and physical needs. *Assures comprehension of knowledge taught.*
2. Record response to all discharge teaching. *To document progress and facilitate further education by other healthcare providers.*
3. Encourage questions and return demonstrations of all procedures that will need to be done at home. *Assures full understanding and ability to do psychomotor skills.*
4. Provide written and verbal home instructions and indications for contacting health care provider. *Written instructions provide family with documents to refer to when questions arise at home.*
5. Arrange for follow-up appointments and referrals. Provide family with phone numbers and office locations. *To provide continuity of care.*

Evaluation

The caregivers demonstrate confidence in Jorge's home care needs and know who, when, and how to contact if questions arise.

Grove, Ehde, Patterson, & Johnson, 1998; Meyers-Paal, et al., 2000; Thompson, Boyle, Tell, Wambach, & Cramer, 1999).

Research on the long-term adjustment of children and families has found that they adjust well to school and their communities with the support of teachers, social workers, and community outreach groups such as burn camps (Kendall-Grove, et al., 1998; Thompson, et al., 1999). Caregivers recover on a slower basis and are often faced with divorce and many financial concerns.

In the Real World

As a student, I wondered if nurses really had to interpret their client's fluid and electrolyte status. Wasn't this what the physician did? I found it very difficult to remember how to differentiate acidosis from alkalosis and memorize lab values. Understanding fluid and electrolyte physiology and pathophysiology is not easy. There is no anatomical model to pull apart and put back together. It just seemed like a set of disjointed facts to memorize and study for the next test. As a practicing nurse, I no longer wonder if this is important information to know. I use it every day on all my patients to assess if their fluids are balanced. Are they dehydrated or fluid overloaded? What do their electrolyte values tell me about their response to treatment? What information is critical that the physician should be notified of immediately? Being able to interpret a child's fluid and electrolyte status is the foundation on which my assessment begins and from which my critical thinking about my client's condition begins.

Family Teaching

The home care needs of the family should be addressed long before the child is ready for discharge. Discharge teaching often includes nutrition and diet requirements, daily dressing changes and skin care, application of elasticized garments (Jobst jacket or pants), application of splints, and daily range of motion exercises. Discharge teaching books are often helpful for families to refer to as they learn. However, these books must take into consideration the educational, ethnic, and language backgrounds of the caregivers (Jenkins, Blank, Miller, Turner, & Stanwick, 1996). Caregivers need support and encouragement to perform these treatments appropriately. Remember, most of these daily routines will be painful for the child. If not done well, the child's wounds will not heal appropriately. Caregivers, who may feel guilt because of the child's burns, often have trouble doing painful procedures without support. Home care should emphasize returning the child to as many independent tasks as possible. Home tutors may be necessary to help the child keep up with school. Support is often needed to help the child and school personnel prepare for the child's return to the classroom. Encourage all involved to explore their feelings and be supportive of the child's return to the community.

Burn Injury Prevention

All burns are preventable by establishing a few safety precautions. Since house fires are responsible for the majority of burn-related deaths in children under five years of age, families should be encouraged to have working smoke detectors in their home and establish a prearranged escape route. Scalds are the most common nonfatal burn, so remembering to turn pot handles inward on the stove and keep young children away from bowls and cups of hot liquid will help prevent burns. Setting the hot water heater thermostat no higher than 120°F will help to prevent scald burns from bath water. Erecting barriers around space heaters and keeping children away from stoves will also help. Electrical burns can be prevented by inserting plastic plugs into light sockets and keeping electrical cords out of sight and reach so that children cannot chew on them. Chemical burns from cleaning solutions can be prevented by storing all cleaning solutions in locked cabinets and by watching children carefully when cleaning solutions are being used. Radiation burns from ultraviolet light are easily prevented by using sunscreens and wearing protective clothing (Forjuoh, 1998). Burn prevention strategies should be discussed openly with caregivers during all health care encounters with the family.

Key Concepts

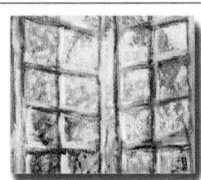

- Forty percent of an infant's body water is located in extracellular spaces. ECF is the first to be lost during illnesses, putting infants at a greater risk for dehydration.
- Body fluids move as a result of the type of membrane to be crossed, changes in the permeability of capillaries, and the amount and type of solutes present.
- The respiratory system compensates for changes in blood pH caused by metabolic conditions by retaining or releasing carbon dioxide.
- The kidneys compensate for changes in blood pH caused by respiratory problems or a buildup of metabolic acids by controlling hydrogen ion and bicarbonate levels in the blood.
- Renal compensation is much slower than respiratory compensation.
- Urine output should be maintained at 1–2 ml/kg of body weight per hour.
- Assessing the specific gravity of the urine is a quick way to assess the hydration status of a child. The higher the specific gravity, the more dehydrated the child.
- Nursing management for the child with acute gastroenteritis includes assessing fluid and electrolyte sta-

tus, administering ORS or IV therapy for severe dehydration, providing an appropriate diet, and giving skin care.

- Burns alter the integrity of the capillary membrane, resulting in the easy movement of fluid and blood proteins into interstitial spaces.
- Immediately following a major burn, body fluids shift from intravascular to interstitial spaces due to increased capillary permeability and cause hypovolemic shock if not corrected quickly.
- Pain management should be integrated into the plan of care based on frequent assessments using an age-appropriate pain scale. Children should not have to experience severe pain after a burn injury. Medicate based on child's need, not the comfort level of the health professional.
- Family involvement is essential for the child to cope with body image and self-esteem issues that arise as a result of a burn.

Review Questions

1. Differentiate between the concepts of diffusion, filtration, and osmosis.
2. What are the normal serum concentrations for sodium, potassium, and chloride?
3. Describe what would happen within the body if there was an excess or a depletion of sodium or potassium?
4. Describe the effects that antidiuretic hormone and aldosterone have on the body. Under what conditions would the body release these hormones?
5. Describe how the body compensates for metabolic acidosis.
6. What signs and symptoms would you expect to see if a child was experiencing respiratory acidosis? What clinical situations might cause respiratory acidosis?
7. What clinical situations might cause metabolic alkalosis?
8. How does the body compensate for acid-base imbalances?
9. Outline the treatment and nursing management for a child with dehydration.
10. What would you include in a discharge teaching plan for caregivers of a child recovering from dehydration?
11. Discuss the treatment of the child with acute gastroenteritis who has diarrhea and vomiting, and moderate dehydration.
12. What nursing interventions will achieve the goal of maintaining skin integrity in an edematous child?
13. Outline the treatment and nursing management for a child during the first 24 hours postburn.
14. Describe how you will determine if the child is receiving adequate IV fluids.
15. What is the most appropriate way to administer pain medication to a burned child? Give the rationale behind your answer.
16. What nursing interventions would you include in a plan of care for a child experiencing a burn dressing change? What role would the caregivers play? How would you facilitate their involvement?
17. Differentiate between the various types of skin grafts.

References

American Academy of Pediatrics, Committee on Injury and Poison Prevention. (2000). Reducing the number of deaths and injuries from residential fires. *Pediatrics, 105*(6), 1355–1357.

American Academy of Pediatrics, Subcommittee on Acute Gastroenteritis, Provisional Committee on Quality Improvement. (1996). Practice parameter: The management of acute gastroenteritis in young children. *Pediatrics, 97*(3), 424–436.

Ashburn, M. A. (1995). Burn pain: The management of procedure-related pain. *Journal of Burn Care & Rehabilitation, 16*(3), 365–371.

Barnum, D. D., Snyder, C. R., Rapoff, M. A., Mani, M. M., & Thompson, R. (1998). Hope and social support in the psychological adjustment of children who have survived burn injuries and their matched controls. *Children's Health Care, 27*(1), 15–30.

Brigham, P. A., & McLoughlin, E. (1996). Burn incidence and medical care use in the United States: Estimates, trends, and data sources. *Journal of Burn Care & Rehabilitation, 17*(2), 95–107.

Demling, R. H., & DeSanti, L. (1998). Increased protein intake during the recovery phase after severe burns increases body weight gain and muscle function. *Journal of Burn Care & Rehabilitation, 19*(2), 161–168.

Duggan, C., Lasche, J., McCarty, M., Mitchell, K., Dershewitz, R., Lerman, S., Higham, M., Radzevich, A., & Kleinman, R. (1998). Oral rehydration solution for acute diarrhea prevents subsequent unscheduled follow-up visits. *Pediatrics, 104*(3), e29.

Eliason, B., & Lewan, R. (1998). Gastroenteritis in children: Principles of diagnosis and treatment. *American Family Physician, 58*(8), 1769–1777.

Fann, B. (1998). Fluid and electrolyte balance in the pediatric patient. *Journal of Intravenous Nursing, 21*(3), 153–159.

Forjuoh, S. (1998). The mechanisms, intensity of treatment, and outcomes of hospitalized burns: Issues for prevention. *Journal of Burn Care & Rehabilitation, 19*(5), 456–460.

Galen, B. (1997). Acute gastroenteritis. *Lippincott's Primary Care Practice, 1*(3), 328–335.

Gerchufsky, M. (1995). Diarrhea in children. *Advances for Nurse Practitioners, 3*(3), 12–16.

Gorelick, M., Shaw, K., & Murphy, K. (1997). Validity and reliability of clinical signs in the diagnosis of dehydration in children. *Pediatrics, 99*(5), e6.

Greenfield, E., & Jordan, B. (1996). Advances in burn wound care. *Critical Care Nursing Clinics of North America, 8*(2), 203–215.

Hansbrough, J., and Hansbrough, W. (1999). Pediatric burns. *Contemporary Pediatrics, 20*, 117–124.

Herrin, J., & Antoon, A. (1996). Pediatric burn injuries. In R. Behrman, R. Kliegman, & A. Arvin (Eds.), *Nelson textbook of pediatrics* (15th ed., pp. 270–277). Philadelphia: Saunders.

Hugger, J., Harkless, G., & Rentschler, D. (1998). Oral rehydration therapy for children with acute diarrhea. *The Nurse Practitioner, 23*(12), 52–64.

Hultman, C. S., Priolo, D, Cairns, B. A., Grant, E. J., Peterson, H. D., & Meyer, A. A. (1998). Return to jeopardy: The fate of pediatric burn patients who are victims of abuse and neglect. *Journal of Burn Care & Rehabilitation, 11*(4), 367–376.

Jenkins, H., Blank, V., Miller, K., Turner, J., & Stanwick, R. (1996). A randomized single-blind evaluation of a discharge teaching book for pediatric patients with burns. *Journal of Burn Care & Rehabilitation, 17*(1), 49–61.

Kendall-Grove, K. J., Ehde, D. M., Patterson, D. R., & Johnson, V. (1998). Rates of dysfunction in parents of pediatric patients with burns. *Journal of Burn Care & Rehabilitation, 19*(4), 312–316.

Klotz, R. S. (1998). The effects of intravenous solutions on fluid and electrolyte balance. *Journal of Intravenous Nursing, 21*(1), 20–26.

Mayes, T., Gottschlich, M. M., & Warden, G. D. (1997). Clinical nutrition protocols for continuous quality improvements in the outcomes of patients with burns. *Journal of Burn Care & Rehabilitation, 18*(4), 365–368.

McCain, D., & Sutherland, S. (1998). Nursing essentials: Skin grafts for patients with burns. *American Journal of Nursing, 98*(7), 34–39.

Meyers, A. (1995). Modern management of acute diarrhea and dehydration in children. *American Family Physician, 51*(5), 1103–1115.

Meyers-Paal, R., Blakeney, P., Robert, R., Murphy, L. Chinkes, D., Meyer, W., Desai, M., & Herndon, D. (2000). Physical and psychologic rehabilitation outcomes for pediatric patients who suffer 80% or more TBSA, 70% or more third degree burns. *Journal of Burn Care & Rehabilitation, 21*(1), 43–49.

Patterson, D. R. (1995). Non–opioid-based approaches to burn pain. *Journal of Burn Care & Rehabilitation, 16*(3), 372–376.

Periti, P., & Donati, L. (1995). Survival and therapy of burn patients at the threshold of the twenty-first century: A review. *Journal of Chemotherapy, 7*(6), 475–502.

Sheridan, R. L., Petras, L., Lydon, M., & Slavo, P. M. (1998). Once-daily wound cleansing and dressing change: Efficacy and cost. *Journal of Burn Care & Rehabilitation, 18*(2), 139–140.

Staley, M. S., & Serghiou, M. (1998). Casting guidelines, tips, and techniques: Proceedings from the 1997 American Burn Association PT/OT casting workshop. *Journal of Burn Care & Rehabilitation, 19*(3), 254–260.

Thompson, R., Boyle, D., Tell, C., Wambach, K., & Cramer, A. (1999). A qualitative analysis of family member needs and concerns in the population of patients with burns. *Journal of Burn Care Rehabilitation, 20*(6), 487–496.

Turner, J. G., Clark, A. J., Gauthier, D. K., & Williams, M. (1998). The effect of therapeutic touch on pain and anxiety in burn patients. *Journal of Advanced Nursing, 28*(1), 10–20.

Suggested Readings

Ahern-Gould, K., & Stark, J. (1998). Quick resource for electrolyte imbalance. *Critical Care Nursing Clinics of North America, 10*(4), 477–490.

Banco, L., Lapidus, G., Zavoski, R., & Braddock, M. (1994). Burn injuries among children in an urban emergency department. *Pediatric Emergency Care, 10*(2), 98–101.

Boorse-Fabius, D. (1998). How to recognize electrolyte imbalances on an ECG. *Nursing98, 98*(2), 32hn1–32hn6.

Hathaway, W., Hay, W., Groothuis, J., & Paisley, J. (1993). *Current pediatric diagnosis and treatment* (11th ed.). Norwalk, CT: Appleton & Lange.

Kee, J. L., & Paulanka, B. J. (2000) *Handbook of fluid, electrolyte, and acid-base imbalances.* Albany, NY: Delmar.

Phipps, A. (1998). Evidence-based management of patients with burns. *Journal of Wound Care, 7*(6), 299–302.

Purvis, R. J., Law, E., Still, J. M., Belcher, K., Kito, N., & Borman, J. B. (1998). Nurses' attitudes toward do-not resuscitate orders. *Journal of Burn Care and Rehabilitation, 19*(6), 538–541.

Rutecki, G. W., & Whittier, F. C. (1997). Acid-base interpretation: Part 1: Applying five rules in everyday cases. *Consultant, 37*(12), 3067–3070, 3073.

Stark, J. (1998). A comprehensive analysis of the fluid and electrolyte system. *Critical Care Nursing Clinics of North America, 10*(4), 471–475.

Tasota, F. J., & Wesmiler, S. W. (1998). Balancing act: Keeping blood pH in equilibrium. *Nursing98, 98*(12), 34–40.

Toedt, M. E. (1996). A short-cut method of determining maintenance fluid rates in children. *Consultant, 36*(9), 1868.

Ulmer, J. F. (1998). Burn pain management: A guideline-based approach. *Journal of Burn Care & Rehabilitation, 19*(2), 151–159.

Resources

Organizations and Websites

American Burn Association
625 N. Michigan Avenue, Suite 1530
Chicago, IL 60611
(312) 642-9260
(800) 548-2876
www.ameriburn.org

American Society for Parenteral and Enteral Nutrition
8630 Fenton Street, Suite 412
Silver Spring, MD 20910-3805
(800) 587-6315
www.clinnutr.org

Burn Prevention Foundation: Prevention Through Education
www.burnprevention.org

Burn Survivors Online
www.alpha-tek.com/burn
Provides information and support for burn survivors and their families.

Cool the Burn
www.cooltheburn.com
Site for children and adults that offers information on burn injuries, grafting, rehabilitation, and wound care.

International Medical Education Foundation
Burnsurgery.org—Educating Burn Wound Professionals Worldwide
www.burnsurgery.org

International Shriners Headquarters
2900 Rocky Point Drive
Tampa, FL 33607-1460
(800) 237-5055
(800) 282-9161 (within Florida)
www.shrinershq.org

National Safety Council
1121 Spring Lake Dr.
Itasca, IL 60142-3201
(800) 621-7615
www.nsc.org

Shriners Burn Care Hospitals
www.shrinershq.org/Hospitals/BurnInst

Boston
51 Blossom Street
Boston, MA 02114
(617) 722-3000

Galveston
815 Market Street
Galveston, TX 77550
(409) 770-6600

Cincinnati
3229 Burnet Avenue
Cincinnati, OH 45229
(513) 872-6000

Sacramento
2425 Stockton Blvd.
Sacramento, CA 95817
(916) 453-2000

CHAPTER 22

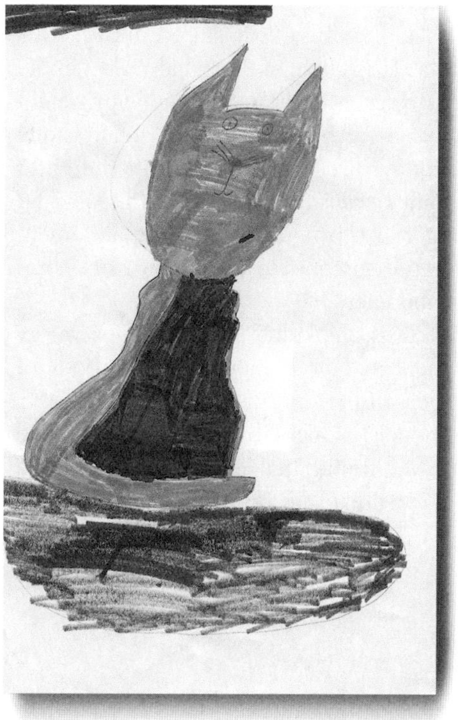

Enuresis. An awful sounding word to a child who suffers from it. My son is six. He had diurnal enuresis. Until we had it under control, going to school or playing with friends could turn out to be traumatic. Was he going to have an accident? Would it be noticeable? Would the children make fun of him?

Observing his personality now, I wonder if perhaps he would not be so shy and withdrawn if things had been different. Would he enjoy going to a friend's house without the fear that he would have a reoccurrence of enuresis? My wife and I support him and offer him encouragement. Is that enough?

GENITOURINARY ALTERATIONS

Stephanie Rockwern Amlung, PhD, RN
Barbara J. Keating, RN, MS
Carole Kenner, RNC, DNS, FAAN
Kerry Fitzgerald Zebold, RN, MSN

COMPETENCIES

Upon completion of this chapter the reader will be able to:

- *Identify the anatomy and physiology of the urinary tract and pediatric variations.*
- *Describe the etiology, clinical manifestations, treatment, and nursing management of urinary tract infections (UTI) in children.*
- *Explain the causes of enuresis and differentiate the disorder from incontinence.*
- *Describe the etiology, treatment, nursing support, and management of common genitourinary alterations.*
- *Describe the etiology, clinical manifestations, treatment, and nursing management of common congenital malformations of the urinary tract and external genitalia in children.*
- *Identify the educational needs of families and children with genitourinary alterations.*
- *Explain the types of renal failure and their treatment.*

The genitourinary system is responsible for the maintenance of homeostasis of the body (water and electrolytes) and for the excretion of waste products. Homeostasis is essential for creating an optimal environment for many other functions of the body. In the male client the urinary system also has a reproductive role and, hence, is critical in a child's development past the phase of toilet training. Because of these essential functions, any alteration in the kidneys and other urinary system organs can pose a major threat to the child's health. Such alterations include infections, structural disorders, and disease processes.

Problems involving the genitourinary system can range from the simple, such as urinary tract infections and enuresis, to the complex, such as renal failure and exstrophy of the bladder. This chapter will discuss infections of the urinary tract, the voiding didorder enuresis, structural defects (vesicoureteral reflux, hypospadias, cryptorchidism, inguinal hernia, hydrocele), glomerular disorders (acute glomerulonephritis, nephrotic syndrome, hemolytic uremic syndrome), and renal failure.

ANATOMY AND PHYSIOLOGY

The genitourinary system is composed of the kidneys, ureters, bladder, and urethra (Figure 22-1). The kidneys are situated posteriorly on the abdominal wall behind the intestines. The medulla and nephrons of the neonatal kidney are functional at birth; however, the peripheral tubules are small and immature. These will slowly mature, so that by adolescence, the kidneys are of mature size and weight. The bladder presents itself in young children close to the anterior abdominal wall, and with growth, lowers into the pelvis. For these reasons it is easy to palpate a full bladder on infants and young children.

Anatomically, the kidneys are a pair of symmetrically shaped organs located in the posterior abdominal cavity adjacent to the lumbar spinal column. The right kidney is slightly lower than the left. The kidneys are partially protected by the ribs and are further protected by a tough outer capsule embedded in adipose tissue and supported by the renal fascia. The kidneys produce urine and transport it via the ureters into the bladder where it is stored until it exits the body via the urethra. The weight of the kidney is less in the child than the adult. However, in the infant and young child the kidney makes up a larger proportion of the child's total body weight. The kidneys are less protected in the child compared with an adult because of unossified ribs, less fat padding, and the larger size proportional to the abdomen. Therefore, they are more susceptible to trauma from compression force to the abdomen.

To control homeostasis, the kidneys have both excretory and nonexcretory functions. The kidneys clear the body of wastes such as urea, creatinine, uric acid, phosphates, sulfates, nitrates, and phenols, along with excreting fluids and electrolytes. It is this fine-tuning that maintains the volume and osmolarity of extracellular and intracellular fluids. The

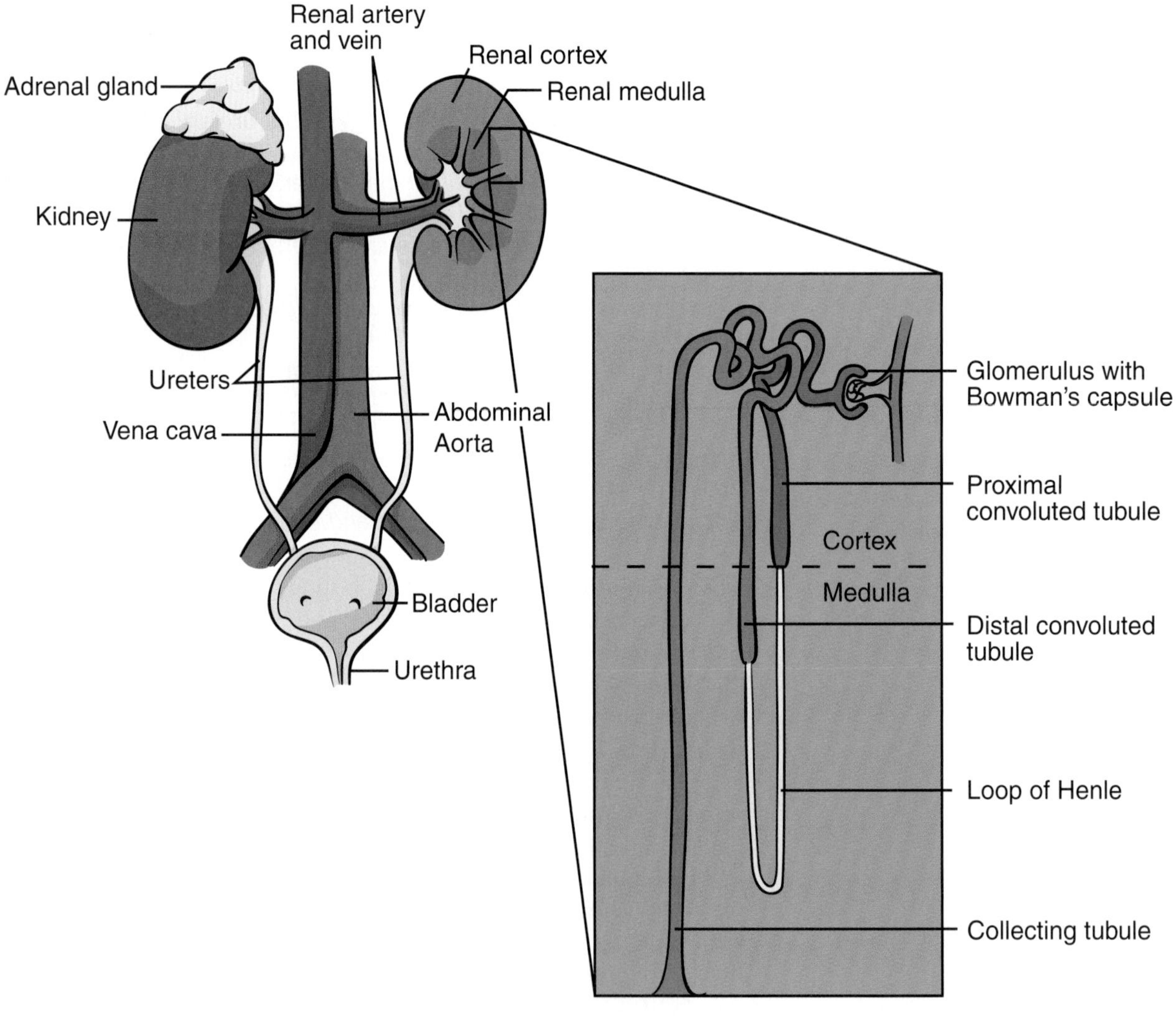

Figure 22-1 Anatomy of the Genitourinary System with Inset of a Nephron

Nursing Tip:

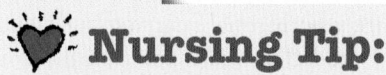

Calculating bladder volume
Bladder capacity in ounces = Age of child + 2
Example: A 3 year-old child has a bladder capacity of approximately 5 oz. (3 + 2 = 5).

kidneys also play a role in the excretion of some drugs and hormones. Nonexcretory functions include the secretion of renin, carbohydrate metabolism, and regulation of vitamin D. Embryologically, the fetal kidney begins to develop before many women realize they are pregnant. Prior to birth, the main function of the kidney is to maintain adequate amniotic fluid levels. In utero, the placenta carries out the functions of blood cleansing and homeostasis for the fetus. By the 7th week of gestation, **nephrogenesis,** or development and growth of the kidney, begins and continues to 32–36 weeks. Urine production begins in the third month, and by the fifth month the collecting tubules and renal pyramids have formed.

At birth the kidney suddenly assumes the role of the placenta, and its response to this change is largely influenced by the gestational age at delivery. Renal blood flow increases dramatically at birth. Urine production is readily established. Ninety-nine percent of newborns void within the first 48 hours post delivery. Serum creatinine levels, which are maternally influenced at birth, decrease by 50% during the first week of life. At birth the amount of fluid that is filtered by the glomeruli (**glomerular filtration rate**) (GFR) is lower than in adults. The GFR reaches adult levels by 2 years of age. The ability to concentrate urine is not well developed in the newborn for several months and even more restricted in the premature infant (specific gravity of 1.001 to 1.015). The neonate's excretory units are underdeveloped and cause disruption in reabsorption of amino acids and bicarbonate, thus causing the infant to be in a state of mild acidosis (plasma pH of 7.11 to 7.36).

URINARY TRACT INFECTION

Urinary tract infection (UTI) is an infection of one or more structures of the urinary tract and can be classified as lower urinary tract (cystitis, urethritis) or upper urinary tract (pyelonephritis). The most common site is the bladder (**cystitis**) with infection confined to the urethra called **urethritis** and to the kidneys (**pyelonephritis**). Pyelonephritis is usually considered more severe and is accompanied by an increase in the severity of symptoms. Identification of the site of infection is important in determining the treatment.

Incidence and Etiology

UTI is the most common disorder of the genitourinary tract. The incidence of UTI in newborns is approximately 1%, with a greater frequency in males. However, after the first year of life, the incidence is more common in girls than boys, with 3% developing UTI during childhood compared with 1% in boys (Rushton, 1997). UTI is more common in Caucasian girls compared with African-Americans. Boys who are uncircumcised are more likely to have UTI than those who are circumcised (Shaw, Gorelick, McGowan, Yakscoe, & Schwartz, 1998).

The most common bacteria that infects the urinary tract is *Escherichia coli*, likely because of its presence in the gastrointestinal tract and perianal skin. Less commonly seen colonization occurs from *Klebsiella pneumonia, Enterobacter, Proteus* species, and *Pseudomonas.* The latter four are usually associated with more complicated UTI often seen in children with chronic conditions that alter the urinary tract, such as neurogenic bladder in individuals with spina bifida. Virus and fungi, particularly *Candida* species, may also cause UTI.

Pathophysiology

In infancy, bacteria frequently enter the urinary tract through the blood and cause infection. After infancy, almost all UTI occur when bacteria enter the urinary tract by ascending through the urethra. Females are especially at risk for infection because of the structure of the lower urinary tract, the short urethra. Males are less susceptible to UTI because of a longer urethra and secretions from the prostate that have antibacterial properties. Structural anomalies and abnormal function of the urinary tract have an important role in the pathogenesis of UTI. Such anomalies include vesicoureteral reflux and neurogenic bladder, which is common in children with spina bifida (see Chapter 32). Other factors that predispose a child to infection include urinary stasis, congenital anomalies of the urinary tract, an obstruction in the urinary tract, and urinary catheters. Urinary stasis increases the risk of UTI. Normally, emptying the bladder frequently completely washes out any organisms. Stasis may be caused by reflux, dysfunction of the voiding mechanism, and infrequent voiding.

Clinical Manifestations

The presenting signs and symptoms of UTI are often vague, especially in young children. Symptoms in the older child generally include malodorous urine, **dysuria,** (difficult or painful urination), urinary frequency, fever, vomiting, diarrhea, irritability, poor feeding, or loss of appetite. Table 22-1 lists the clinical manifestations of UTI in children of various ages. Typically, cystitis is distinguished from pyelonephritis, a syndrome involving fever often greater than 101°F, chills, and back pain. Children with pyelonephritis will also appear to be quite ill.

Diagnosis

A urinalysis (UA) and urine culture with sensitivity (urine C&S) will be performed to diagnose UTI. The means by which a urine sample is obtained has great impact on the interpretation of results. Urine specimens obtained by collection bag methods in non-toilet trained children have been widely utilized for initial evaluation of UTI. This method of collection is not suitable for culture because of its high degree of contamination (Johnson, 1999). However in practice, many health care practitioners will opt for this method of collection because it is the least traumatic. If repeated infections develop, it is prudent to perform either sterile catheterization or suprapubic aspiration of urine to evaluate true infection status. Infants and children less than 3 years of age with fever of unknown origin should be screened for urinary tract infections with a urinalysis and urine culture (Johnson, 1999).

The Pediatric Nursing Skills CD-ROM explains the urine specimen collection procedure. An adequate specimen, usually 5–10 cc of urine (may differ among institutions) must be obtained prior to any antimicrobial therapy to avoid affecting the bacterial count and to ensure an accurate diagnosis. The presence of bacteria (**bacteriuria**) and white blood cells (**pyuria**) in the urine confirm the diagnosis of a UTI. Laboratory confirmation of a positive urine culture indicates the presence of greater than 100,000 colony forming units (CFU)/ml of a urinary tract pathogen. The child with pyelonephritis usually presents with an elevated white blood cell count (WBC), an elevated erythrocyte sedimentation rate (ESR), and an increased C-reactive protein (CRP) (Reynolds & Hoberman, 1995).

The health care provider may recommend renal scanning with dimercaptosuccinic acid or glucoheptonate to identify anatomic abnormalities that may be the cause of UTI. This study identifies both renal scarring and acute pyelonephritis but does not differentiate between the two. However, it is helpful in identifying children who require long-term follow-up and is more sensitive than the traditional intravenous pyelogram (IVP), which is still utilized to rule out urinary tract obstructions. Other testing that may be ordered include a renal ultrasound and a voiding cystourethrogram (VCUG). A renal ultrasound may identify certain abnormalities, such as **hydronephrosis,** an abnormal swelling in the kidney, while the VCUG is utilized to identify urethral and bladder abnormalities, in particular vesicoureteral reflux.

Treatment

Treatment for UTI includes (1) eradicating the infection, (2) preventing reinfections by identifying contributing factors, (3) correcting underlying causes of infection, and (4) preserving renal function. Treatment depends upon a variety of factors, including the child's age, other existing medical conditions, and his or her ability to maintain hydration. Oral antibiotic therapy is used to treat UTI. Antibiotics such as trimethoprim in combination with sulfamethoxazole (Bactrim, Septra), amoxicillin (Amoxil), a cephalosporin, or nitrofurantoin (Furadantin) are given for seven to ten days. Follow-up urine culture should be performed 48 to 72 hours after initiating treatment. For infants or young children 2 months to 2 years of age who are assessed as toxic, dehydrated, or unable to retain oral fluids, initial antibiotic therapy should be given intravenously and hospitalization should be considered (American Academy of Pediatrics Committee on Quality Improvement and Subcommittee on Urinary Tract Infection, 1999). Untreated UTI can lead to a variety of complications including renal scarring. Of those clients who develop scarring, some may develop kidney stones, hypertension, end stage renal disease, and possible compli-

TABLE 22-1 Clinical Manifestations of Urinary Tract Infections in Children of Various Ages

Infants	Preschoolers	School-Age and Adolescents
Malodorous urine	Malodorous urine	Malodorous urine
Malaise	Malaise	Malaise
Irritability/colic	Hematuria	Hematuria
Jaundice in neonates	Fever	Fever and chills
Fever	Dysuria	Dysuria
Poor feeding	Frequency	Frequency
Poor weight gain	Abdominal pain	Abdominal pain
Vomiting and diarrhea	Flank pain	Flank pain
	Costovertebral angle tenderness	Costovertebral angle tenderness
	Vomiting and diarrhea	Avoidance of urination
		Vomiting and diarrhea

cations of pregnancy. It is therefore imperative that urinary tract infections be evaluated and treated carefully. With appropriate management, many of these severe complications can be prevented.

Nursing Management

Assessment

Initial assessment includes interviewing the caregivers and child (if appropriate) regarding changes in urine elimination, in particular, patterns of elimination. Frequency, hesitancy, dysuria, urgency, and bed-wetting in a child who has already established nighttime control are symptoms of UTI. A careful history can assist the health care practitioner in determining the diagnosis of UTI and its possible causes. The nurse also assesses the knowledge level of the caregiver and child.

Hydration is required to maintain renal blood flow and flush out bacteria and debris; therefore, assessment for dehydration is performed. To assess for dehydration the nurse should observe for signs of tachycardia, poor skin turgor, dry mucous membranes, sunken fontanels, hemoconcentration, and decreased peripheral perfusion. Weight checks and urine specific gravity analysis should also be performed. Lastly, assessing the child's level of comfort is important in determining need for analgesics and/or teaching distraction techniques. Without pain management, a caregiver cannot concentrate on learning new concepts if the child remains uncomfortable.

Nursing Diagnoses

Nursing diagnoses for the child experiencing UTI include:

1. Risk for injury related to complications of infection (chronic renal disease and kidney damage).
2. Risk for deficient fluid volume related to decreased fluid intake and fever.
3. Acute pain related to UTI.
4. Deficient knowledge (caregiver) related to lack of information of disease process, diagnostic procedures, management, and prevention of UTI.

Outcome Identification

1. The child will be free of complications and recurrent UTI.
2. The child will maintain adequate fluid intake.
3. The child's pain will be diminished or absent.
4. The caregivers will verbalize an understanding of disease process, diagnostic procedures, management, and prevention of recurrent UTI.

Planning/Implementation

Nursing care focuses on antibiotic therapy, maintaining good hydration, managing fever with antipyretics, providing comfort measures and distraction, and educating the child and caregivers. Antibiotics and antipyretics are administered as ordered. The nurse needs to educate the caregivers regarding alternative techniques to reduce fever, for example, using tepid baths (making certain that water temperature is not so cool that the child may be chilled and start to shiver, which will elevate body temperature); promoting surface cooling by undressing the child; and encouraging oral fluids. The nurse should administer analgesics as ordered and provide and teach alternative comfort measures. If bladder spasms are present, the child may respond to warm moist heat to the abdomen provided it does not increase body temperature. The nurse should offer and assist with distraction techniques. Nurses play a key role in assuring adequate hydration for the child. Accurate documentation of intake and output is essential as the child's ability to concentrate urine may be impaired during the initial phase of renal inflammation (Reynolds & Hoberman, 1995).

Evaluation

Because of the inflammatory response of the bladder, fever may persist in a child for up to 2 to 3 days after antibiotics are begun. However, urine obtained between 24 and 48 hours after initiation of antibiotics should be negative for bacteria because of the high concentration of medication cleared via the bladder. The child should show a decrease in the degree of pyuria and leukocytes in the urine from the initial specimen, although some WBCs may persist for several days depending on the underlying pathology. If fever persists, evaluation of the initial urine culture and sensitivity is needed to assure that appropriate antibiotic therapy is being instituted. Ongoing evaluation of the child's response to fever management, hydration, response to pain, and overall understanding of the plan of care is essential to providing complete care.

Family Teaching

If this is the first episode of UTI, the nurse will need to instruct the family in a wide range of concepts, including anatomy and physiology of the urinary tract, disease process, diagnostic testing, management, prevention of UTI, and follow-up care. The nurse needs to stress the importance of follow-up appointments, radiologic studies, urinalysis, and cultures. Caregivers need to understand the importance of antimicrobial therapy and possible use of prophylactic antibiotics. Furthermore, families must be instructed that although the child may no longer feel ill, the individual must complete a full course of antibiotics and comply with follow-up testing to prevent long-term complications, such as recurrent infection, renal scarring, and subsequent kidney damage and deterioration. Education should also include the need for the child to frequently and completely void and to increase quantities of fluids, especially water. Prevention techniques include instructing caregivers on perineal hygiene and, for girls, wiping from front to back and avoiding the use of bubble baths and perfumed soaps, which tend to be irritating to the urethra. Cotton underwear, because of its breathability, should be worn instead of nylon.

ENURESIS

Enuresis is defined as involuntary voiding of urine beyond the expected age at which voluntary control should be achieved, usually five years of age (Maizels, Rosenbaum, & Keating, 1999). Enuresis differs from incontinence in that incontinence results from a structural abnormality, usually an anatomic malformation (Maizels, et al., 1999). Enuresis can be primary or secondary, diurnal or nocturnal, or both. A child who has never achieved a period of dryness for at least three months is referred to as a primary enuretic. Secondary enuresis occurs when a child has been dry for at least three to six months and then resumes wetting. Diurnal enuresis is wetting that occurs only during the daytime and nocturnal enuresis is wetting that occurs only at night.

Enuresis can have a great impact on a child's life. Children with enuresis may avoid participating in activities with their peers. Social activities such as a sleepover or a camping trip can cause a great deal of stress for these children. Children with daytime wetting often face more problems. Staying dry during the school day can be a challenge and concealing wet clothing can be the largest obstacle of all. These children may also have problems with odor control.

Incidence

Because the age at which urinary continence is achieved covers a wide range of normal, the incidence is difficult to determine. However, it is estimated at 15–20% in 5-year-olds and 5% in 10-year-olds. Most children have nocturnal enuresis, and most are primary enuretics. Primary nocturnal enuresis is more common in boys, whereas primary diurnal enuresis is more common in girls (Riley, 1997). In contrast to enuresis, incontinence is caused by a malformation of the urinary tract and is the least common cause of wetting, affecting about 1–3% of children.

Etiology and Pathophysiology

Enuresis is a symptom, not a disease, and many hypotheses have been proposed to describe its causes (Karlowicz, 1995). Etiologic factors are classified as organic (having a physical basis) and non-organic or functional (exogenous or with no physical disorder or disease). Organic factors should be ruled out before non-organic ones are considered. Organic causes include:

- Neurologic developmental delay in which the child is unable to inhibit bladder contraction
- Urinary tract infections; a child with a urinary tract infection may involuntarily lose urine, however, this is caused by the physiological response of the irritable bladder (Karlowicz, 1995)
- Structural disorders of the urinary tract such as obstructive lesions and small bladder capacity; the child may not be able to hold the large volume of urine produced and therefore may experience urgency and the involuntary loss of urine
- Disorders that affect the concentrating ability of the kidneys such as chronic renal failure
- Diseases associated with an excessive production of urine (**polyuria**), as in diabetes mellitus and diabetes insipidus
- Chronic constipation

Non-organic or functional causes include:

- Sleep arousal pattern problems, that is, sleeping soundly so the child does not awaken in the night to void
- Sleep disorders such as enlarged tonsils and sleep apnea
- Psychological stress and family disruptions such as divorce, death, or birth of a new sibling
- Inappropriate toilet training, that is, early chronologic or developmental age, overly demanding or punitive caregivers

Clinical Manifestations

Most children achieve urinary and bowel control between two and a half and three and a half years of age. The typical sequence for the development of bladder and bowel control is (1) nocturnal bowel control, (2) daytime bowel control,

Eye On:

Enuresis

There are many myths and misconceptions about children with enuresis. If a child is not successfully dry during the day and night by four to five years of age, it may reflect negatively on the child and caregivers. Our society considers nighttime wetting normal behavior for infants and toddlers, but it is not acceptable for school-aged children. Families often view enuresis as a problem when their child is around five years of age.

(3) daytime control of voiding, (4) nighttime control of voiding (Rushton, 1995). It is unclear why some children are not able to accomplish bladder control while other children of the same age have attained control. Any child who continues to experience nighttime wetting after the age of five warrants an evaluation for enuresis. Possible presenting clinical manifestations of a child with enuresis are presented in Box 22-1.

Diagnosis

Physical examination and a careful family history are the hallmarks of determining a diagnosis of enuresis or incontinence. A thorough physical examination to distinguish between organic and nonorganic (functional) enuresis should be performed initially. The examination should include assessing the abdomen and genitals for any abnormalities. A neurologic exam of the peripheral reflexes, perianal sensation, anal sphincter tone, and inspection of the lower back to rule out any spinal defects should also be included.

Results of the history, voiding diary (keeping track of frequency and amount of void), and physical examination may determine which diagnostic tests are required for further evaluation. Some of the more frequently required tests include urinalysis, urine culture, renal ultrasound, and VCUG for children with a history of urinary tract infections. Urine flow rates determine voiding characteristics. One can determine if structural problems are present by measuring the amount of urine voided and the time it takes the child to void, as well as the force of his or her urine stream.

BOX 22-1 Possible clinical manifestations of enuresis

- Dribbling after voiding
- Urgent need to void (child may be seen leg-crossing, dancing, or holding genitals to avoid wetting)
- Constant dribbling with ineffective stream
- Infrequent and painful voiding
- Straining to void
- Incontinence when laughing (Kelleher, 1997)

Treatment

The following treatments can be used separately or in combination to treat children with wetting problems: medication(s), bed-wetting alarms, motivational therapies, elimination diets, and bowel programs for children who are constipated. If the child is experiencing incontinence, the structural cause will need to be determined and treated. Successful treatment requires both the child and caregivers to commit to active involvement in an enuresis program. The most commonly used medications to treat enuresis are oxybutynin chloride (Ditropan), desmopressin (DDAVP), and imipramine hydrochloride (Tofranil) (Table 22-2). Medications are often used in conjunction with other treatments for the most effective outcomes. Medications for enuresis should not be considered a cure but as part of the treatment and solely symptom relief. Children with the best

TABLE 22-2 Common Medications to Treat Enuresis

Name of Medication	Actions	Adverse Reactions
Oxybutynin chloride (Ditropan)	Anticholinergic used for children with small functional bladder capacity. Ditropan affects the bladder muscle by reducing uninhibited bladder contractions, inhibiting voiding, and increasing voluntary control of the urethral sphincter.	Facial flushing Dry mouth Constipation Heat intolerance Drowsiness Insomnia Blurred vision
Imipramine hydrochloride (Tofranil)	Tricyclic antidepressant. Decreases depth of sleep during latter part of night.	Dry mouth Nervousness Insomnia Changes in personality
Desmopressin acetate (DDAVP)	A synthetic analog of vasopressin that works by increasing water retention and urine concentration. By concentrating urine and decreasing the amount of urine produced, the child may not reach bladder capacity and therefore stays dry.	Headaches Nausea Nasal congestion Nose bleeds

Nursing Alert:

Contraindications for DDAVP

DDAVP should not be used for children who are hypersensitive or who have a potential for fluid and electrolyte imbalances (cystic fibrosis, renal disease) because of the potential for water intoxication and hyponatremia.

Nursing Alert:

Warning for Imipramine Overdosage

Fatal accidental overdoses caused by cardiac arrhythmias may occur from imipramine; therefore, labeling should include this information. Nurses should educate families that this medication should be stored in a childproof bottle in a secure place out of the reach of children. Imipramine must only be dispensed by adults.

long-term outcomes for staying dry most often used a combination of treatments in conjunction with medications.

Bed-wetting alarms are in the widely used treatment for enuresis. Some models are meant to be placed under the bottom sheet of the child's bed (Figure 22-2). Most alarms consist of a moisture sensor that is attached to the child's underwear or pajamas (Figures 22-3A and 22-3B). The alarm starts to buzz as the first few drops of urine are detected. The sound of the alarm arouses the child, and the urinary flow is interrupted. The child is instructed to turn off the alarm and go to the bathroom to complete voiding. The alarm teaches the child to recognize bladder fullness and awaken before bed-wetting occurs. When the bed-wetting alarm is used as the only method of treatment, there is a 70% success rate. Although 30% of these children may relapse, overall they respond quickly to a short treatment program where the alarm is reinstated for a brief period of time (Maizels, et al., 1999; Mosier, 1998).

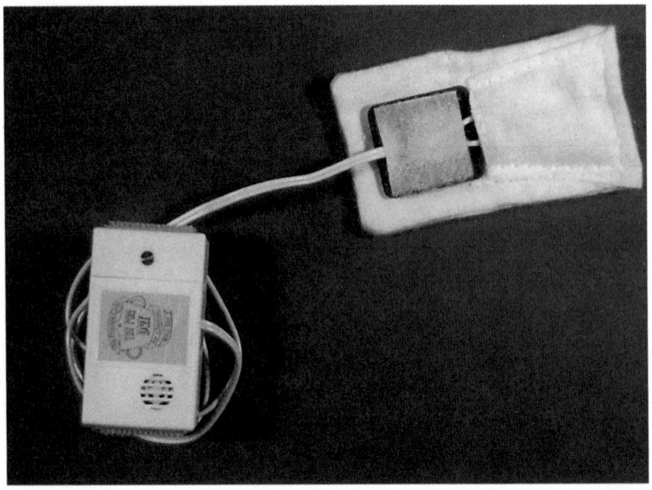

Figure 22-2 A bed-wetting alarm is often used to treat enuresis. Courtesy of Kerry Zebold.

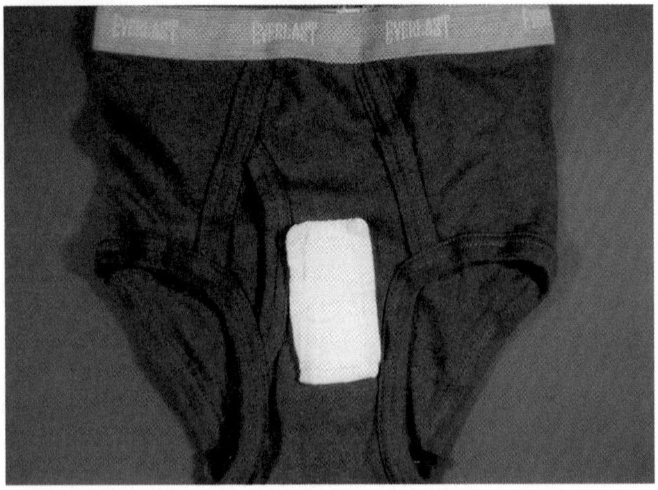

Figure 22-3A Proper Attachment of Bed-Wetting Alarm (male)

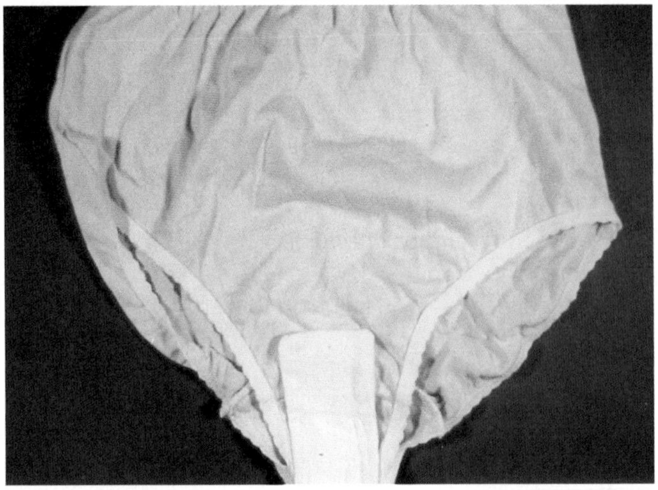

Figure 22-3B Proper Attachment of Bed-Wetting Alarm (female)

Motivational therapies may include using star charts to record the child's progress during the treatment program (Figure 22-4). Rewarding the child for dry nights is effective because over time the behavior may be changed when the child feels proud of his or her accomplishments. The child should be included when designing a reward program. By rewarding a child with special treats (stickers, collectable cards, etc.) or privileges that they value, it increases the chances that the rewarded behavior will occur again. Rewards are most effective if they are given to the child

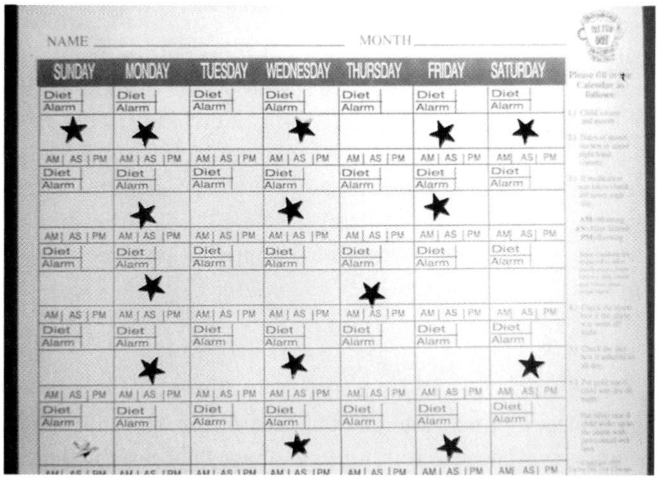

Figure 22-4 Behavior Modification Star Chart is often used to reward desired behavior in children with enuresis.

immediately after the desired behavior. Reward programs should be used with caution. If a child consistently fails to receive rewards, it can decrease self-esteem and motivation to continue the program.

Certain foods may be irritants to the bladder and increase a child's wetting problems. Eliminating foods or beverages that are known irritants may decrease the number of wetting episodes a child has. Foods to eliminate include carbonated beverages, dairy products, beverages with artificial coloring, citric fruit, heavily sugared foods, and beverages with caffeine. Five to 10% of children who wet benefit from the elimination diet (Maizels, et al., 1999).

Many children with wetting problems also experience constipation. The cause of constipation may be one or a combination of several factors such as insufficient fluid intake, low fiber diet, history of painful bowel movements and holding back of stool, changes in daily routine, lack of physical activity, and no routine for daily bowel movements. Stools may be infrequent, hard or large, and may be painful to pass. These children may not completely empty the colon of stool and further perpetuate the cycle of constipation. Treatment for enuresis may not be successful if constipation management is not addressed at the same time. Children may show improvement with wetting once they are on a successful bowel program. To assess for constipation a rectal exam, X ray, or ultrasound of the abdomen can determine if the child has a large mass of stool.

Nursing Management

Assessment

In assessing a child who presents with wetting problems, the history will provide important information for formulating a plan of care. Questions to cover during the assessment of the enuretic child are listed in Box 22-2.

BOX 22-2 Assessment questions—Enuresis

1. Has the child ever been toilet trained by day and/or night and at what age?
2. How frequently does the child have wetting episodes?
3. Does the child have a history of dysuria, polyuria, frequency, or urgency?
4. Has the child ever experienced urinary tract infections?
5. Is there a family history of enuresis or voiding problems?
6. Does the child have any sleep problems, such as deep sleep, snoring, sleep walking?
7. Is there a history of constipation, fecal soiling, large bowel movements, or painful bowel movements?
8. How is the family currently handling the wetting problems?
9. Have they tried any treatments or medications for the wetting?
10. What are the child's and family's feelings or attitudes about enuresis?

Nursing Diagnoses

1. Impaired urinary elimination related to lack of bladder control.
2. Impaired skin integrity related to contact with urine.
3. Disturbed sleep pattern related to bed-wetting and the use of bed-wetting alarms.
4. Low self-esteem related to urinary incontinence or bed-wetting.
5. Impaired social interactions related to urinary incontinence.

Outcome Identification

1. The child will achieve bladder control.
2. The child will be free of skin irritation in the perineal area.
3. The child will have minimal disturbance during sleep.
4. The child will use expressions that indicate positive self-esteem.
5. The child will actively participate in age-appropriate social interactions.

Planning/Implementation

Nursing care of the enuretic child most often includes ongoing family education and support during a long treatment phase. The nurse can provide the child and family with information about the causes of enuresis and the variety of

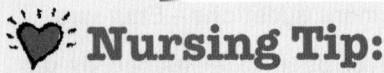

> **Nursing Tip:**
>
> **Feeling comfortable with the alarm system**
> Have younger children practice using the alarm with a doll or stuffed animal to help them feel comfortable with the system.

treatment options. The family should be involved in the decision about the treatment plan. As appropriate to the treatment, the child and family need instruction on the use of bed-wetting alarms, medications, behavior modification, and elimination diets. The family should be encouraged to emphasize the child's strengths and praise attempts at control to increase confidence and self-esteem. The nurse needs to assist the child and family to verbalize feelings of frustration.

Evaluation

Evaluation is based upon the family's report of the child's progress with the program. Families are instructed to follow up with the nurse by telephone one week after starting the program, or sooner if problems develop. Monthly appointments may be necessary until the child achieves 14 consecutive dry nights.

Family Teaching

Nurses can provide children and caregivers with information on hygiene and treatment/prevention of skin breakdown caused by exposure of skin to urine. They will need education about the use of bed-wetting alarms. Explain to the caregivers that the child's sleep will be disrupted during the program, and that it may be beneficial to the child to have an earlier bedtime. Nurses can also educate children and caregivers on the use, schedule, and adverse reactions of medications prescribed as part of the enuresis program. Families and children need support and encouragement during the treatment for enuresis. Nurses should provide children with positive feedback for complying with the prescribed programs. The nurse needs to discuss with the child feelings of embarrassment or guilt as a result of the enuresis. The nurse should encourage keeping an extra set of clothes at school until enuresis is resolved.

STRUCTURAL DEFECTS

Structural defects include vesicoureteral reflux, hypospadias, cryptorchidism, inguinal hernia, and hydrocele.

Vesicoureteral Reflux

Vesicoureteral reflux (VUR) is defined as the backflow of urine from the bladder up the ureter to the kidney. VUR results when the **ureterovesical/vesicoureteral junction** (site where the ureter enters the bladder) fails to maintain a unidirectional flow of urine from the ureter to the bladder. Normally, urine is produced in the kidneys and travels down the ureters into the bladder for storage. In the normal bladder, the junction of the ureter into the bladder forms a one-way valve mechanism or flap valve that allows urine to flow into the bladder while preventing regurgitation back into the ureters and/or kidneys.

Incidence and Etiology

VUR is the most common anatomic disorder affecting the genitourinary tract (Kaefer, et al., 2000). The exact incidence is unknown because routine screening of children without a history of urinary tract infection is not practiced. However, VUR has been consistently found in approximately one-third of children who have at least one UTI (Craig, Irwig, Knight, & Roy, 2000). Often it is diagnosed when the child is between the ages of two and three years. However, in some cases it may be diagnosed in older children or infants depending upon the underlying pathology. For example, children with spina bifida are usually screened for reflux as infants.

It is important to note that reflux has a genetic component. Familial reflux is common. Reflux is present in approximately one-third of siblings who have an affected brother or sister. Of those, 75% do not present with any urinary tract symptoms. Recent studies have also revealed a high incidence of transmission of reflux from parent to child. The incidence of vesicoureteral reflux is also significantly lower in African-American children versus Caucasian when screening is done following a urinary tract infection. Distribution of reflux by gender reveals a possible higher frequency in females than males, although this data is influenced by other factors such as circumcision and age at diagnosis (Belman, 1995).

Pathophysiology

Anatomically, the ureter extends from its respective kidney downward to the top of the bladder **trigone** (a small triangular area at the base of the bladder where the ureters normally join the bladder). It then passes obliquely through the bladder wall for a distance that enables the ureter to act as a sphincter despite not having an anatomic sphincter. The ureter at this point functions as a one-way valve to prevent reflux. When this length is not sufficient, backward flow of urine, hence vesicoureteral reflux, will ensue. With growth, the ureter tunneling through the bladder wall may elongate, and this increase in tunnel length will help promote the resolution of reflux.

Clinical Manifestations

The clinical manifestations of VUR usually are not directly apparent. However, persistent and repeated urinary tract infections are the most common indicator of reflux.

Therefore, the child with repeated UTI should be evaluated. Other manifestations of reflux less commonly seen are enuresis, flank pain, and abdominal pain. However, these symptoms can be vague in children too young to describe and localize their symptoms and may be easily confused with other diagnoses.

Diagnosis

The diagnosis of VUR is made by radiographic evidence of back flow of urine on a **cystogram** (radiograph of bladder, urethra, and ureters), or **voiding cystourethrogram** (VCUG) (radiograph of bladder, urethra, and ureters during voiding). Reflux is graded to determine its severity on a scale of I to V. The degree to which contrast material from the bladder travels up the ureters to the kidneys is graded I to V, with I being the least severe and V the most severe.

Treatment

The medical treatment for vesicoureteral reflux is determined by the severity of the reflux and the fact that some degrees of reflux resolve spontaneously as the child grows. The less severe the reflux (grades I and II), the greater the likelihood of resolution. The goals of medical management for children with reflux include prevention of UTIs, prevention of kidney damage, and prevention of the subsequent complications of reflux and renal scarring. Currently, treatment options include long-term use of antibiotics to prevent UTI, and on occasion the use of anticholinergics. Anticholinergics such as oxybutynin chloride (Ditropan) are used to decrease bladder pressure.

Other treatment options include surveillance of the child over time to observe for signs of deterioration such as increase in incidence and severity of UTIs. Deterioration in a child would necessitate an advance in treatment, such as a change in prophylactic antibiotics and an increase in anticholinergic medication. Lastly, surgery to correct reflux is indicated when medical treatment options have failed. Indications of failure include breakthrough UTIs, particularly pyelonephritis, despite strict compliance to medical management and pharmacotherapy, or increased renal damage, which threatens the survival of the kidney (Tanagho, 1995).

Surgical management may be performed endoscopically or with traditional surgical techniques involving an abdominal incision. When kidney function is impaired and the ureters are massively dilated, a urinary diversion may be recommended to improve renal function and allow the dilated ureters to reestablish tone. This is usually a temporary measure to allow time to consider further reconstruction or reestablishment of the ureters into the bladder (Tanagho, 1995). Surgery involves reimplantation of the ureter into a position on the trigone that allows for sufficient submucosal length to prevent the reflux from recurring.

Nursing Management

Because the non-surgical management for a child with VUR focuses on UTI prevention and management, an important aspect of nursing care focuses on education of the child and caregivers. The child and caregivers should be aware that the treatment may continue for years and compliance with the medication regimen is important. They must also maintain close contact with their health care provider and inform the individual when the goals are not being achieved (i.e., recurrent UTI), hence, necessitating more aggressive management.

If surgery is necessary, the nurse provides the child and caregivers information about the surgical procedure and preoperative and postoperative care. Immediate postoperative care for a child after reimplantation of one or both ureters can be challenging. While managing the acute pain the child may be experiencing it is important to strictly monitor intake and output. The well-organized nurse will label all drainage devices and stents and note where they originate (i.e., ureter, bladder, or peritoneum). The nurse should assess the integrity of all tubes and drainage bags; breaks in tubing can increase risk for infection by introducing bacteria into the drainage system. Noting any kinks or disruptions will assure accurate I & O.

Hypospadias

Hypospadias is a common congenital malformation in which the urethral meatus is on the ventral surface (underside) of the penis (Figure 22-5). The position of the uretheral opening may vary, occurring at any point along the ventral surface of the penis or on the scrotum or perineum.

Incidence and Etiology

Hypospadias occurs in 8.2 per 1,000 live births (Zaontz & Packer, 1997). Rates are highest among Caucasians, lowest among Hispanics, and intermediate among African-Americans. There is some genetic predisposition as evidenced by a family history of another male with hypospadius (Paulozzi, Erickson, & Jackson, 1997). The exact etiology is unknown and may be multifactorial. Some affected boys have defects in testosterone metabolism or testosterone receptors. This suggests that hypospadias can result from an abnormality in endocrine factors that influence the development of the male genitalia.

Pathophysiology

Hypospadias is a congenital birth defect caused by altered embryogenesis or an insult to the developing fetus during the 3rd through 5th months of gestation. In utero, the penile urethra develops from the urogenital sinus. By the 12th week of gestation, the endodermal edges of the secondary urethral groove fuse to form a tube. The urethra fuses in a proximal to distal direction. Failure of this fusion results in the urethral meatus opening other than the tip of the penis, and failure of

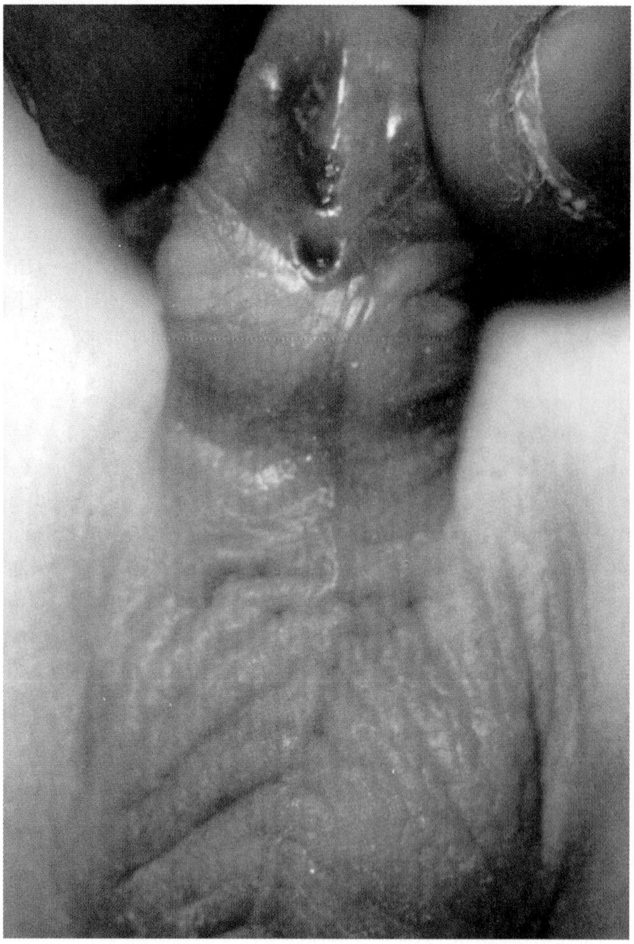

Figure 22-5 Hypospadias is a congenital anomaly in which the urethral meatus is on the ventral surface (underside) of the penis. Photo courtesy of Casimir Firlit, MD, PhD, William E. Kaplan, MD, Max Maizels, MD, and Jeffrey Palmer, MD, Children's Urology Ltd.

the foreskin to develop properly. The foreskin usually appears as a hood in children affected with hypospadias.

Clinical Manifestations

The **prepuce** or skin forming a hood over the glans is abnormally small ventrally and may be redundant dorsally. Many caregivers of infants with hypospadias claim it appears that their newborn son has already been circumcised. Associated conditions may include **chordee** (downward curvature of the penis and an incomplete foreskin), undescended testes, and inguinal hernia. In some cases the urinary stream may be deflected downward secondary to the ventral position of the meatus.

Diagnosis

Diagnosis is based on physical examination. Careful inspection of the external genitalia of all newborn males should be performed at birth.

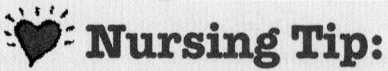

> **Nursing Tip:**
>
> **Testosterone cream side effects**
>
> It is imperative to instruct caregivers about some of the side effects of the testosterone cream. Along with enlargement and growth of the male genitalia, localized acne and pubic hair may appear. Caregivers should be instructed that these side effects will resolve when the cream is discontinued.

Treatment

Treatment for hypospadias involves surgical correction of chordee, placement of the urethral meatus to the tip of the penis. Successful surgery will enable the child to void in a standing position, have a cosmetically normal appearing penis, and have a sexually adequate penis. Historically, surgery to correct hypospadias was performed in stages and involved lengthy hospitalizations and uncomfortable postoperative treatments and drains. Currently, because of advances in surgical technique, the surgery can be performed in one single outpatient procedure. In more severe cases a two-stage repair also may be performed.

Surgery is usually performed before the child is 18 months of age, prior to toilet training and the development of body image or gender identity, thus minimizing psychological trauma (Sugar, Firlit, & Reisman, 1993). Several surgical techniques are available and vary depending on the severity of the anomaly and the surgeon's preference. All techniques involve reconstruction to elongate the urethra, bring it to the tip of the penis, and straighten the chordee. The foreskin is frequently used as a graft whereby it is rolled into a tube and fashioned into a urethra. Hence, no neonatal circumcision should be performed on these infants. On occasion, the size of the penis is augmented preoperatively with testosterone cream or injections to allow for growth of the tissue and hence facilitate surgery.

Several types of dressings may be utilized postoperatively. Some may be as extensive as a compression type dressing, most commonly a penile wrap type dressing, and still some may have no application of a dressing at all. Postoperatively, a urethral stent or foley catheter may be used to facilitate urination and prevent obstruction of urine flow secondary to edema.

Nursing Management

Assessment

Preoperatively, the nurse should assess the infant or child for evidence of other genitourinary defects such as undescended testes, inguinal hernia, or hydrocele. The caregivers' understanding of hypospadias, the surgical procedure, and their expectations of the appearance of the penis after surgery is investigated. The nurse needs to assess their response to having a newborn with a genital defect. Postoperatively, an assessment for adequate urinary output is essential. The nurse observes for signs of wound and urinary tract infection, e.g., penile incision for purulent drainage and excessive erythema, increase in temperature, cloudy urine with a foul odor. The infant or child is assessed for signs and symptoms of pain from incision and bladder spasms.

Nursing Diagnoses

The nursing diagnoses for a child undergoing surgical hypospadias repair are similar to those for many urologic abnormalities. They include:

1. Pain related to surgical incision.
2. Deficient knowledge (caregivers) related to the diagnosis, surgery, postoperative care, and prognosis of hypospadias.
3. Risk for infection related to indwelling catheter and/or stents and surgical incision.

Outcome Identification

1. The child will have minimal to no pain postoperatively.
2. Caregivers will verbalize an understanding of the disorder, the surgical procedure, and prognosis, and will participate in postoperative care.
3. The child will be free of infection of the urinary tract and the incision.

Planning/Implementation

Postoperative pain is usually minimal following repair of hypospadias. A dorsal or caudal nerve block provides adequate pain relief for most children; however, occasionally acetaminophen (Tylenol) may be helpful for a few days to alleviate incisional discomfort. Anticholinergics such as oxybutynin chloride (Ditropan) may be administered if ordered to alleviate bladder spasms while the urethral stent is in place. Caregivers should be informed that anticholinergic medication might cause facial flushing and dry mouth. The child should be encouraged to take in adequate fluids to maintain adequate urinary output and the patency of the stent.

Discharge instructions should include information regarding antibiotic use to prevent infections, timing of dressing and stent or Foley catheter removal, and anticipatory guidance for the caregiver and older child regarding postoperative appearance of the penis. They should understand that the penis will look bruised, wrinkled, and swollen because of the trauma and that it will resolve in a few days to weeks.

These instructions may differ between surgeons. Some may remove the dressing in 4–5 days while others may maintain a larger compression dressing for longer periods depending on the severity of the hypospadias and surgical technique. If a small layered penile dressing is used, the caregiver will be instructed to have the child soak for 20 minutes in a bathtub filled to the child's waist with clear warm water prior to the appointment for removal. This allows the dressing to loosen and often fall off at home.

Complications of hypospadias repair can occur. Urethral fistula, or an opening along the urethra that leaks urine to the skin surface, strictures at the anastomosis site, and retrusion of the urethral meatus to its original position has been reported. If the fistula does not resolve, repeat surgery may be indicated 6 months after the initial repair (Stock, Scherz, & Kaplan, 1995).

Evaluation

The child should be comfortable and participating in age-appropriate activities. The caregivers can explain the surgical intervention and the postoperative course and care involved. They are participating in their child's care. The child should not exhibit signs of UTI or incisional infection.

Cryptorchidism

Cryptorchidism or undescended testis (UDT) is defined as failure of one or both testes to descend through the inguinal canal into the scrotum (Figure 22-6). Further classification is based on whether the testis is retractable or ectopic. A retractile testis is one that has descended normally but readily retracts with physical stimulation and exam, and is often mistakenly diagnosed as UDT. An ectopic testis is one that is found outside the normal path of descent. It may be in the groin, perineum, or abdominal wall.

Incidence and Etiology

UDT is a common urologic problem. The incidence of UDT increases as the degree of prematurity increases. In full-term

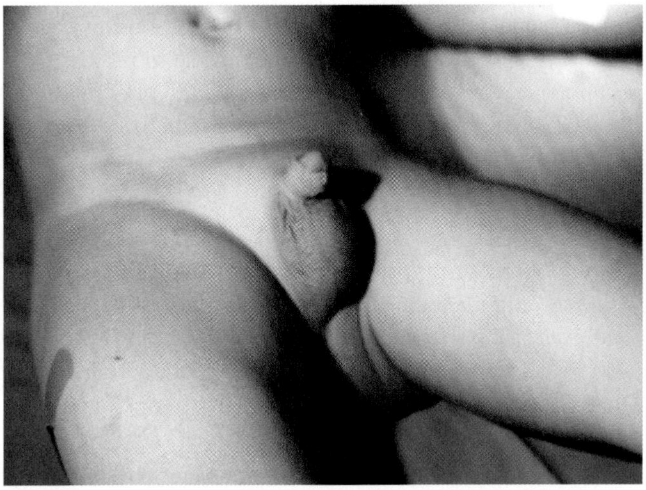

Figure 22-6 Cryptorchidism. Photo courtesy of Casimir Firlit, MD, PhD, William E. Kaplan, MD, Max Maizels, MD, and Jeffrey Palmer, MD, Children's Urology Ltd.

newborns it is between 3% and 5% (Rozanski & Bloom, 1995). Low birth weight and premature infant boys have a higher incidence of UDT. Incidence of cryptorchidism decreases with age so that by 3 months of age the incidence is 1%, and 0.8% at 9 months of age. In many cases the testes descend spontaneously; however, after 1 year of age, spontaneous descent does not usually occur.

Pathophysiology

Sexually indifferent gonads are found at three to five weeks gestation. During the 7th week of gestation the gonads begin to differentiate into a testis or ovary. As the testes increase in size a network of strands form into the seminiferous tubules where spermatozoa are produced. During the third trimester, the testis begins its descent into the scrotum through the inguinal canal. Many theories attempt to explain the failure of the testes to descend into the scrotum including increasing abdominal pressure and hormonal influences (Rozanski & Bloom, 1995). In the undescended testis sperm production is decreased and may cause infertility. The child with UDT also has a 20% to 44% increase in risk for developing a malignant testicular tumor in adulthood (Gonzalez, 1996).

Clinical Manifestations

UDT, which may be unilateral or bilateral, is unilateral in 85% of males and most often affects the right testis. Infants diagnosed at birth with bilateral UDT represent 15% of affected boys (Rozanski & Bloom, 1995). One side of the scrotum (unilateral) or the entire scrotum (bilateral) appears flaccid, non-pendulous, and smaller than normal.

Diagnosis

The diagnosis of cryptorchidism involves primarily the physical examination in which the scrotum is palpated for the testis, a small nodule. It is important to perform the physical examination without stimulating the testicle to retract by the examiner having warm hands and the child being relaxed. If the testis is not palpable, ultrasound may be used to determine its location.

Treatment

Management of cryptorchidism may involve observation while awaiting spontaneous descent of the testis during the first year of life. Human chorionic gonadotropin (HCG) may also be used to stimulate testosterone production to help induce descent of the testis into the scrotum. Limited success with this technique has been reported. However, HCG does increase testicular vasculature and size thereby assisting in locating the testis either before or during surgery (Sugar & Hoyler-Grant, 1995). If the testis fails to descend spontaneously or with the administration of HCG, surgery, orchiopexy, is performed. The optimal timing for surgical correction is when the child is between one and two years of age. The goals of surgical correction are to bring the testis into the scrotum and secure it by scrotal fixation without damaging the testicle.

Nursing Management

Assessment

At birth and the first well-child visit the nurse can evaluate for the presence of both testes. By gently compressing both inguinal canals, a small nodule should be felt on both sides. The nurse should assess the caregivers' understanding of UDT and the importance of timely surgical correction.

Nursing Diagnoses

1. Deficient knowledge (caregiver) related to cryptorchidism and its treatment.
2. Anxiety (caregiver) related to the possible decreased fertility and increased risk of malignancy.

Outcome Identification

1. The caregivers will verbalize an understanding of the disorder and treatment.
2. The caregivers' anxiety will be decreased by explaining that the child should have appropriate referrals for fertility testing when appropriate and should perform testicular self-exam beginning at adolescence.

Planning/Implementation

Education of the caregiver should include clarification and reinforcement of information gleaned from the surgeon, including the use of HCG if ordered. Caregivers need simple explanations regarding how to prepare their child (if age-appropriate) for surgery and what to expect postoperatively. The issue of fertility is of great concern to the caregivers of children with UDT. Biopsies of these testes reveal histologic abnormalities including decreased number of germ cells. Sperm counts in a nondescended testis decrease proportionally with age after the second year of life. The contralateral testis even if normally positioned may also demonstrate abnormal histology. Even after successful orchiopexy, the testes may continue with decreased spermatogenesis (Rozanski & Bloom, 1995).

Family Teaching

Nurses are helpful in teaching and preparing both the child and caregivers for surgery. If HCG therapy is utilized, the caregiver should be aware of the desired effects as well as secondary effects. For example, caregivers may express concern during this treatment when they observe increased penile growth and increased pigmentation of the scrotum as well as growth of pubic hair. Caregivers should be reassured that these side effects will dissipate after therapy is discontinued. They should also be instructed that their child will have discomfort postoperatively. Loose clothing is recommended so as not to apply pressure to the wounds immediately after surgery. Analgesics such as acetaminophen (Tylenol) and acetaminophen with codeine are routinely ordered. The child may appear to have difficulty walking related to tenderness, but this will resolve in a few days. The scrotum will appear quite edematous and ecchymotic. Caregivers need reassurance that all these are expected because of surgery but will resolve in a few days to several weeks.

Sutures and dressings are minimal. Usually dissolving sutures are utilized to close the groin and scrotal wound. Hence, the child does not require suture removal that may induce further fear and trauma. Tegaderm, or other clear plastic type dressings, cover the groin wound and may be removed at home one week after surgery. Nurses must teach the caregiver to observe for signs of infection including increased pain, redness, swelling, and drainage from the incisions, along with fever. Frequent diaper changes and proper hygiene will reduce the risk of infections. Lastly, caregivers should be instructed to help the child avoid strenuous activity, sports, and riding toys that may be straddled until appropriate healing has taken place. The child should be instructed on testicular examination monthly once he reaches puberty to regularly evaluate and assist in early detection of tumors. Nurses are essential in assisting the caregiver to develop a supportive environment in which the child has opportunities to ask questions regarding sexuality and fertility as he becomes an adolescent.

Inguinal Hernia and Hydrocele

Inguinal hernia and hydrocele are similar disorders, both clinically and in their treatment. An inguinal hernia is a scrotal or inguinal swelling, or both, that includes the abdominal contents. A hydrocele is a collection of peritoneal fluid in the scrotal sac.

Incidence

Inguinal hernias occur in children at a rate of approximately 10 to 20 per 1,000 live births (3.5% to 5% of term infants) and occur more frequently in boys than girls (ratio of 4:1) (Figure 22-7A). The incidence increases dramatically with other risk factors including prematurity and low birth weight (Skoog & Conlin, 1995). The majority of infantile inguinal hernias are diagnosed in the first month of life. Hydroceles occur in approximately 6% of full-term infant boys (Figure 22-7B). Children who also present with ventriculo-peritoneal shunts (see Chapter 32) and those receiving **dialysis** (treatment that acts as a filtration system outside the body to rid the body of waste products) are also at increased risk for development of hernias and hydroceles secondary to the persistence of increased intra-abdominal pressure (Skoog & Conlin, 1995).

Etiology and Pathophysiology

An inguinal hernia is caused by abdominal contents exiting the peritoneal cavity and protruding into the **processus vaginalis** (a fold of peritoneum that precedes the testicle as

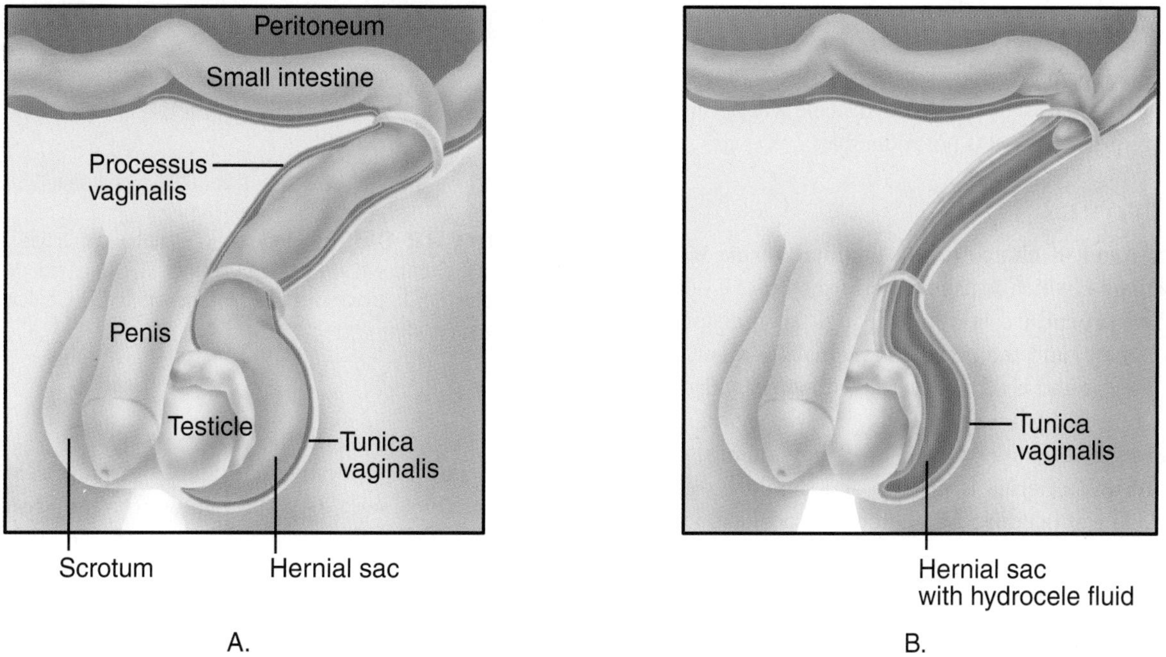

Figure 22-7 (A) An inguinal hernia is a scrotal or inguinal swelling, or both, that includes the abdominal contents. (B) A hydrocele is a collection of peritoneal fluid in the scrotal sac.

it descends through the inguinal canal into the scrotum). An incomplete or abnormal obliteration of the processus vaginalis at birth allows peritoneal fluid or abdominal contents to enter the scrotum, resulting in a hydrocele or inguinal hernia. The processus vaginalis follows the same descending pathway of the testes into the scrotum. Normally fusion of the processus vaginalis occurs spontaneously after the testis is in the scrotum (Skoog & Conlin, 1995).

Clinical Manifestations

An inguinal hernia presents as a bulge or a swelling in the scrotum or groin whose size increases because of increased intra-abdominal pressure from crying or straining (Figure 22-8A). Pain is usually not associated with the hernia unless it becomes strangulated. A hernia can become strangulated when the herniated intestines are trapped within the defect and become edematous and twisted. With strangulation, the blood supply to the herniated segment is cut off. There is ischemia and obstruction of the bowel, which can lead to necrosis and possible perforation. Clinical manifestations include scrotal color changes (redness); pain; intense, inconsolable irritability; vomiting; abdominal distention; and tachycardia.

When a hydrocele is present, the scrotal swelling is painless and does not change in size and shape when the infant cries or coughs (Figure 22-8B). It is not reducible but can be easily transilluminated (Sugar & Hoyler-Grant, 1995).

Diagnosis

The diagnoses of hernia and hydrocele are based on the physical examination of the scrotum and inguinal area. Differentiation between the two may be made on physical exam. Upon palpation a hernia may feel boggy and may be reduced by applying gentle upward pressure on the enlarged area of the hernia. In contrast, a hydrocele will be fluid filled and feel more tense and is not reducible.

Treatment

The treatment of choice for an inguinal hernia is surgery (herniorrhapy), which is usually performed on an outpatient basis. The procedure is done through an incision in the inguinal crease, and the processus vaginalis is identified and ligated. The wound is often covered with a protective sealant after surgery. A hydrocele usually resolves by one year of age. However, if it does not resolve spontaneously by this time, it means a hernia is present and should be surgically repaired. The procedure is called a hydrocelectomy and is the same as for a hernia.

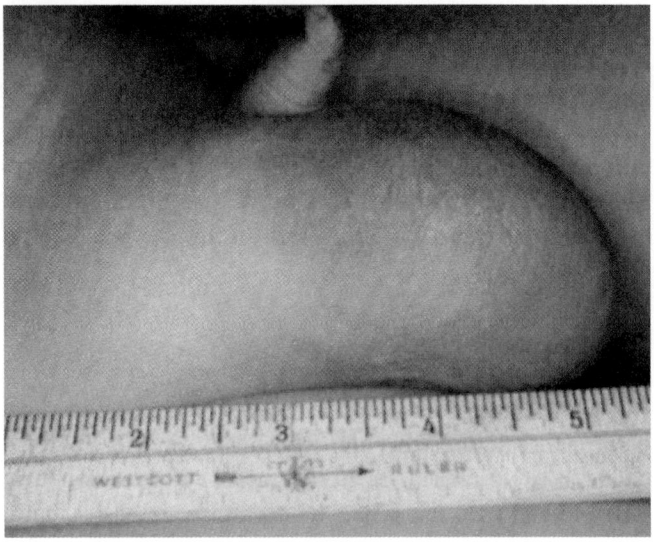

Figure 22-8A An inguinal hernia presents as a bulge in the scrotum. *Source:* Liebert, P. S. (1996). *Color atlas of pediatric surgery* (2nd ed., p.102). Philadelphia: W. B. Saunders. Used with permission.

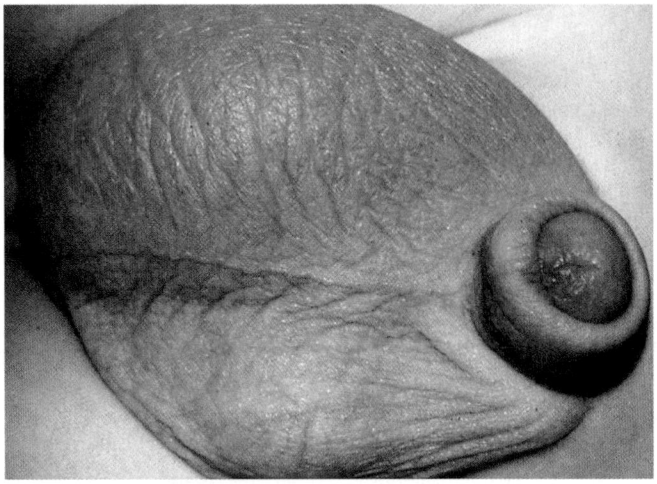

Figure 22-8B Hydrocele. Photo courtesy of Casimir Firlit, MD, PhD, William E. Kaplan, MD, Max Maizels, MD, and Jeffrey Palmer, MD, Children's Urology Ltd.

Nursing Management and Family Teaching

Nursing care for inguinal hernia and hydrocele focuses on teaching the caregivers about the surgical procedure, preoperative and postoperative care, and signs and symptoms of complications such as wound infection and strangulation (preoperatively). Preoperatively the nurse needs to be vigilant for signs of **incarceration** (strangulation of a portion of the bowel leading to circulation impairment and tissue necrosis). After surgery the surgical site is observed for bleeding, drainage, and recurrence of the hernia. The nurse instructs the caregivers that the infant requires frequent diaper changes to prevent infection, and that there are no activity or dietary restrictions. They should be instructed to observe the wound for signs of infection, that is, redness, elevated temperature, and drainage.

ACUTE GLOMERULONEPHRITIS

Acute glomerulonephritis (AGN) is an acute or sudden inflammation of the glomeruli within the kidney. This inflammation results in acute renal failure. Because the inflammation results in damage to the glomeruli within the kidney, it is often referred to as intrarenal acute renal failure. It is classified further according to the exact site of the damage, for example, the glomerular capillaries or the membrane.

Incidence and Etiology

The exact incidence of AGN is not reported. It peaks at seven years of age, is unusual in children younger than three years of age, and occurs more often in males with a ratio of 2:1 (Simckes & Spitzer, 1995). The etiology is usually an infectious agent that has been present in the body for at least 2 to 3 weeks prior to the clinical renal manifestations. There may have been other signs and symptoms that were more systemic prior to the onset of the renal manifestations.

The agents usually involved are bacterial or viral. The most common organism is streptococcus (group A beta). The primary site of infection is typically the throat or the skin. In these cases the disease is referred to as acute poststreptococcal glomerulonephritis (APSGN). Other causes of this condition are systemic or chronic diseases that eventually affect the glomeruli as the disease progresses, such as sickle cell anemia.

Pathophysiology

Either a bacterial or viral agent invades the child's system. The immune system responds by trying to fight the infection and produces antibodies to attack the foreign antigens. This antibody/antigen reaction within the kidney glomeruli forms immune complexes and inflammation occurs. The end result is damaged/scarred glomeruli. Membrane permeability is altered by this immune response, thus allowing protein to leak into the urine. Sodium is retained within the serum and water follows a decrease in the plasma filtration. The accumulation of water and sodium leads to edematous tissues. The glomerular filtration rate is slowed as the passage through the kidney gets narrower.

Clinical Manifestations

The clinical manifestations of AGN are **hematuria** (presence of blood in urine), dependent and periorbital edema, diminished urinary output, proteinuria, hypertension, fatigue, diminished glomerular filtration rate, elevated serum sodium levels, and elevated potassium. Hypertension occurs in 60% to 80% of children with APSGN (Simckes & Spitzer, 1995). All these symptoms are related to the inflammatory process, the changing permeability of the glomerular membrane, and progressive kidney damage. BUN and creatinine levels may also be elevated, and a low-grade fever may be present. Again these symptoms are related to progressive kidney damage and loss of protein. Urine may appear grossly bloody or just blood tinged, smoky or tea colored, and greatly reduced in volume depending on the degree of inflammation. Hematuria is essential for the diagnosis.

Diagnosis

The diagnosis is dependent upon the clinical manifestations listed above. Other diagnostic tests include the WBC with differential. This count may or may not be within normal limits depending on the length of the infection and its severity. Immunologic tests include (1) serum complement (c3) test for complement cascade of the immune system (usually low); (2) streptozyme, which will be positive if the renal condition is caused by a streptococcal infection; and (3) a culture of the primary site of infection such as the throat. If a culture is not possible or is negative, then the diagnosis is made on the renal symptoms, especially the presence of hematuria and the history of a prior streptococcal infection. The complement system is composed of about 20 serum proteins that assist the specific immune system to fight infection. Because there are so many proteins involved, the system responds in a cascade fashion to enhance the immune response. When infection is present, especially bacterial infection, the complement is depleted from the serum as it moves to create an inflammatory effect at the site of infection. Specific renal tests besides the serum chemistries might include a renal biopsy if there is no clear diagnosis from any other source of testing.

Treatment

Treatment depends in part on the degree of kidney damage and is symptomatic. The aims of the treatment are: to identify and treat the source of the inflammatory process; to maintain fluid and electrolyte balance; and to maintain the blood pressure within the normal range. As the primary source of glomerulonephritis is usually not renal, a thorough physical examination must be done. A history of symptoms over the past few weeks must be taken. Areas to focus on include: exposures to other sick children/adults; treatment for any minor infections including over-the-counter medications for fever or aches and pains; the respiratory system, especially the upper respiratory area; the throat for any redness or inflammation; any coughs (productive or non-productive); respiratory difficulties, such as difficulty sleeping in a child who usually does not wake up during the night.

Children with normal blood pressure and urine output can usually be managed at home. However, those with generalized edema, significant oliguria, hypertension, and gross hematuria should be hospitalized because of the possibility of developing acute renal failure. If the edema is generalized, it may be necessary to give diuretics. Antihypertensive agents are given for hypertension. Dietary restrictions are based on the severity of the disorder, especially the extent of edema and hypertension. Sodium, potassium, and fluids may be restricted. The prognosis for children with APSGN is excellent with most recovering completely.

Case Study/Care Plan

Child with Acute Glomerulonephritis

Troy was a 6-year-old male, who had a streptococcal infection two weeks ago. He presented in the emergency room pale, lethargic, with a low-grade fever, dependent and periorbital edema, and, according to the mother, low urine output with a tea color. Vital signs other than the temperature were within normal limits. After a thorough physical examination and diagnostic tests, it was determined he had acute glomerulonephritis.

Nursing Care Plan

Assessment The child needs to be assessed for signs and symptoms of fluid overload. Assess for edema, especially dependent (in the lower extremities) and periorbital. Observe the skin for tautness or redness indicating breakdown. Assess the respiratory system for cough, tachypnea, adventitious lung sounds, and increased work of breathing. Vital signs should be assessed, especially for elevated temperature or blood pressure. Weight should be obtained daily.

Nursing Diagnosis #1

Excess fluid volume related to compromised renal perfusion as evidenced by decreased urine output and edema.

Expected Outcome

The child will exhibit no signs of compromised renal perfusion as evidenced by a normal urinary output and no edema.

Interventions/*Rationale*

1. Measure intake and output every 2 to 4 hours. *Comparisons of the intake and output will help to determine if the renal function is returning.*
2. Measure urine specific gravity every 2 to 4 hours. *The urine specific gravity is an indicator of how well the kidneys are able to concentrate urine. A high specific gravity indicates a poor urine output, dehydration, or other particles in the urine such as blood.*
3. Weigh the child daily on the same scale and with the same clothing on at the time. *An increase in weight can indicate fluid retention. Loss of weight can mean the renal function is returning or the intake is less than body requirements.*
4. Observe for signs of edema. *Presence of edema indicates poor renal function.*
5. Give diuretics as ordered. *Diuretics help rid the body of excess fluid.*

Evaluation

The child exhibited a normal urine output, normal specific gravity, and no signs of edema.

Nursing Diagnosis #2

Imbalanced nutrition: Less than body requirements related to dietary restrictions as evidenced by a decreased oral intake.

continues

continued

Expected Outcome

The child will exhibit no decreased oral intake.

Interventions/*Rationale*

1. Offer small frequent, low sodium and protein meals. *Small frequent meals are more easily tolerated by sick children. The protein and sodium restrictions necessary for children with renal problems often makes food less appealing.*

2. Give the child some choices as to foods he likes. *Giving the child some choices increases the chance he will eat.*

3. Weigh the child on the same scale with the same type of clothing daily. *Daily weights will indicate if the child is losing water weight as well as weight from a decreased intake.*

4. Perform intake and output measurements every 2 to 4 hours. *Comparisons of intake and output will give an indication of how well the child is maintaining his fluid and electrolyte and nutritional balance.*

Evaluation

The child had a normal intake of food and fluids.

Nursing Diagnosis #3

Risk for impaired skin integrity related to the presence of edema as evidenced by reddened or taut skin or actual breaks in the skin.

Expected Outcome

The child will exhibit no signs of impaired skin integrity as evidenced by the lack of redness or tautness or actual skin breaks.

Interventions/*Rationale*

1. Observe the skin for signs of redness or edema at least every 4 hours. *Assessing the skin frequently allows for early signs of impaired skin integrity to be found.*

2. Change the child's position at least every 2 hours. *Changing the position keeps pressure sores from appearing.*

3. Give bath daily and cleanse skin as needed. *Attention to hygiene deters skin breakdown.*

4. Use lotions over areas of dry skin. *Lotions help add moisture to the skin to decrease the chance of skin breakdown.*

5. Use a support pillow under any edematous extremity. *A support pillow will increase circulation and decrease pressure points that might lead to skin breakdown.*

Evaluation

The child's skin remained intact with no signs of redness or tautness or skin breaks.

Nursing Diagnosis #4

Fatigue related to infectious process as evidenced by complaints of tiredness or of not wanting to participate in activities.

Expected Outcome

The child will not experience fatigue as evidenced by no complaints of being tired or not wishing to participate in activities.

continues

continued

Interventions/*Rationale*

1. Assess the child for signs of fatigue such as excessive sleepiness, yawning, or inability to help with activities of daily living. *A child may show signs of fatigue in subtle ways such as sleeping more than usual, yawning, or reluctance to help with bath or feeding activities.*

2. Ask the child what he wants to play with or what activities he wishes to engage in today. *A child of six years usually wants to play no matter how sick he is. If he has some choice he may play more than if he was told what to do.*

3. Observe the child's ability to do activities even if these are bed games. *Observation will indicate the child's tolerance of an activity and level of fatigue.*

Evaluation

The child showed little or no signs of fatigue and was able to participate in activities as desired.

Nursing Diagnosis #5

Pain related to presence of an infection and edema as evidenced by complaints of pain, or wincing on movement.

Expected Outcome

The child experienced no pain as evidenced by no complaints of pain or wincing on movement.

Interventions/*Rationale*

1. Assess the child for signs of pain such as grimacing, crying, staying quiet, verbal complaints of pain, or reluctance to move. *Assessment of the child's pain level allows for early intervention to make the child more comfortable.*

2. Gently move and reposition the child every 2 hours if he is to remain in a bed or chair position. *Moving the child gently promotes circulation of the blood, lessens chance of pain, and helps comfort the child.*

3. Position an edematous extremity on a support pillow. *Supporting a swollen leg or arm will help decrease the pain.*

4. Keep the room quiet and at even temperature. *A calm, moderate temperature room helps comfort the child.*

Evaluation

The child exhibited no signs of pain as evidenced by absence of non-verbal or verbal complaints of discomfort.

Family Teaching

Caregivers need explanations regarding the prognosis for their child. The normal course of this disorder is one to three weeks of therapy without residual effects. They need to be taught:

- Signs of edema or worsening of the renal failure
- Dietary and fluid restrictions such as a low sodium diet, which is essential for the care of this child if urinary output is compromised (low or absent) or edema is present
- Skin integrity and the need for cleanliness. The caregivers are taught to observe for red areas, excessively dry areas, open areas or abrasions, pressure areas that may appear red or bruised.
- Need to reposition the child or encourage the child's moving about at least every two hours.
- Elevation of lower extremities on a pillow when sitting in a chair. This position will decrease the chance of dependent edema and encourage cardiac circulation.

- Rest periods during activities are important because the child will fatigue easily.
- Signs of dehydration and the importance of reporting them immediately to the health care provider
- Signs of a worsening condition, which include grossly bloody urine, increased edema, increased lethargy or activity intolerance, restlessness, or any change in respiratory status. These signs would usually warrant hospitalization.

NEPHROTIC SYNDROME

Nephrotic syndrome (NS) is a clinical entity characterized by massive proteinuria and **hypoalbuminemia** (low levels of albumin in the blood) leading to edema and hyperlipidemia. NS can develop during the course of renal or systemic diseases and can be classified as either primary or secondary. Primary, or idiopathic, NS results from glomerular disease of the kidney. Secondary NS results in renal malfunctioning as a result of a systemic disease, drugs, or toxins such as liver malfunction, hepatitis, systemic lupus erythematosus, lead poisoning, childhood cancer or its therapies, or other diseases that ultimately put a stress on the renal system. The most common type of NS in children is primary.

Incidence and Etiology

The incidence of NS has been reported to be 0.02–0.07 per 1,000 (Bergstein, 1996). It is more common in males than females with a ratio of 2:1 (Constantinescu, Shah, Foote, & Weiss, 2000). It usually affects children between the ages of 2 and 6 years. The etiology of the primary form is believed to be an immune response. The immune response is to glomerular disease or a systemic infection by the body that alters the structure of the glomerulus.

Pathophysiology

Nephrotic syndrome results when there is a threat to the immune system and an inflammatory response is evoked. Figure 22-9 illustrates the pathophysiology of NS. The glomeruli become increasingly permeable to plasma protein resulting in massive urinary protein loss or proteinuria. When protein is lost, fluids shift from the intravascular to the interstitial spaces. The result is tissue edema, ascites or accumulation of fluids in the abdominal cavity, and hypovolemia. Once the volume diminishes in the vascular spaces then renal blood flow declines. Renin production is stimulated to maintain volume and systemic pressure. The result is excretion of aldosterone and tubular reabsorption of sodium. Water follows the sodium leading to edema. Serum cholesterol and triglyceride levels rise from the stimulation of lipoprotein production in the face of hypovolemia and falling serum protein levels. This stimulation is an attempt to make up for the lost proteins and is seen in conditions of starvation. If immunoglobulin levels are monitored, IgG levels are diminished. As blood volume falls, red blood cell and platelet concentrations are increased. The net result is a slowing of the blood flow and ultimately the clumping or clotting of red blood cells and platelets. That coupled with protein losses puts the child at risk for coagulation or clotting problems.

Clinical Manifestations

These children exhibit the same symptoms as any other child with renal failure. Edema is usually the first clinical feature. Initially, it is often mild, being periorbital in the early morning hours and becoming more generalized after the child has been ambulatory (Hogg, et al., 2000). Anorexia, abdominal pain or tenderness caused by the inflammation of the kidney, abdominal swelling, fatigue, history of recent respiratory infection, increased weight or rapid weight gain, and vital signs (initially including blood pressure) within the normal range may also be noted.

Diagnosis

The diagnosis is dependent upon proteinuria. Serum albumin levels are diminished (hypoalbuminemia). Laboratory evaluation includes urinalysis for protein, red blood cell casts, serum albumin (<2.5 g/dl—hypoalbuminemia), serum cholesterol, triglycerides, hemoglobin, hematocrit, platelet count, electrolytes, BUN, creatinine, complement levels, antistreptolysin O (ASO) titer, and streptozyme. The presence of proteinuria, and red blood cells indicates kidney inflammation. The rise in serum cholesterol, triglycerides (in the face of a falling hemoglobin), hematocrit, and platelet count indicates some problem with hypoproteinemia in the serum. The serum electrolytes will be altered as renin and aldosterone levels change and sodium is reabsorbed. The BUN and creatinine rise as kidney function falls. The complement level will fall as the condition worsens as complement (serum proteins) move from the serum to the site of inflammation. The ASO titer and streptozyme are tests to determine if there has been a streptococcal infection.

Treatment

Treatment focuses on reducing proteinuria, controlling edema, and preventing infection. The mainstay of treatment is corticosteroid therapy with prednisone and prednisolone (Prelone) in order to obtain a remission. Corticosteroids decrease the inflammation and the loss of proteins, thus restoring oncotic pressure and promoting diuresis. Oral preparations of prednisolone allow for accurate dosing and increased palatability in young children. A typical protocol is to start with a high dose of either drug (2 mg/kg/day; maximum of 80 mg/day). Treatment is continued until the child becomes free of proteinuria or for a period of four to eight

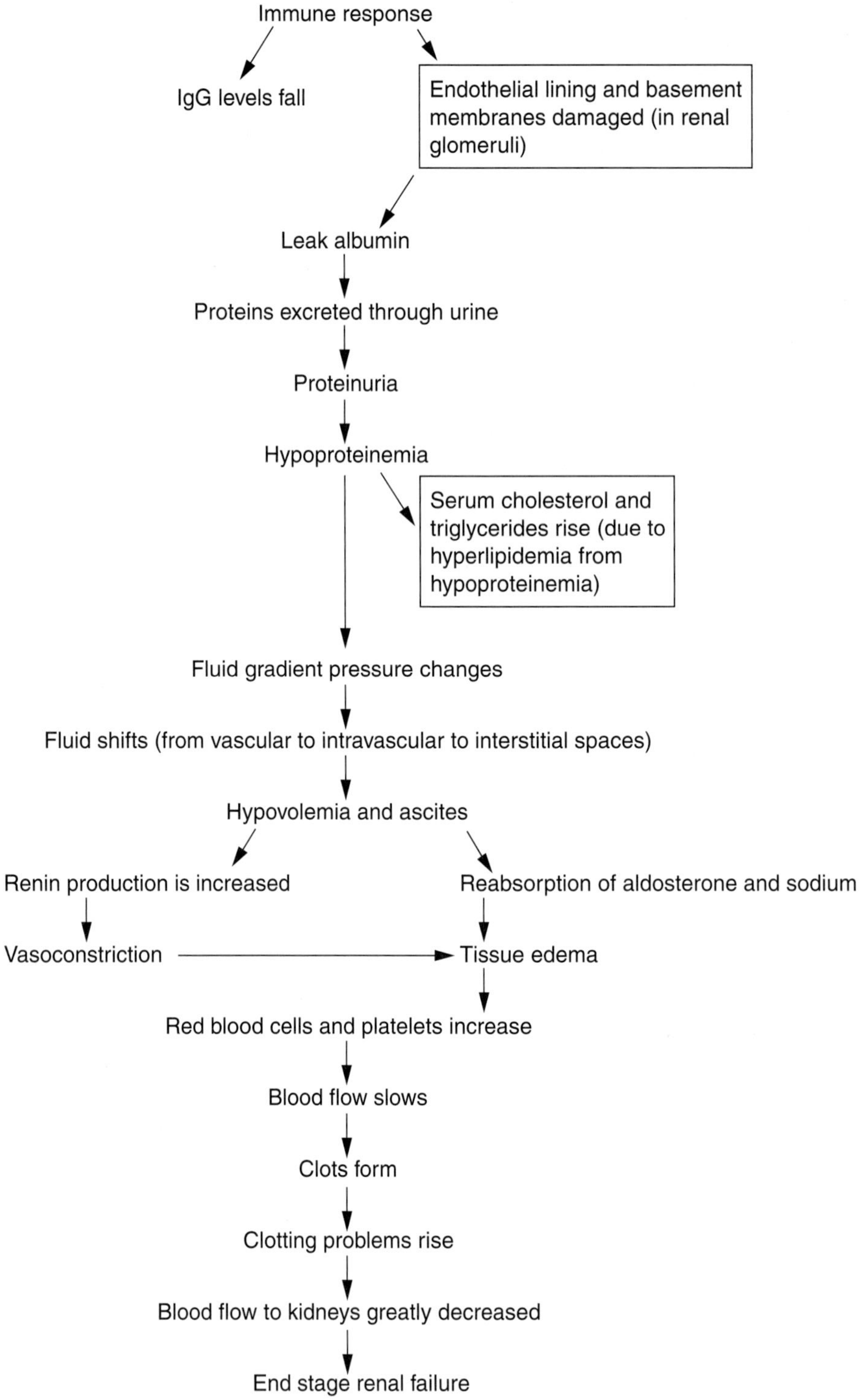

Figure 22-9 Pathophysiology of Nephrotic Syndrome

weeks (Hogg, et al., 2000). The medication is gradually tapered over a period of several weeks and then stopped as long as the child remains asymptomatic. However, the rate of relapses is high, 60–70% (Constantinescu, Shah, Foote, & Weiss, 2000). Relapse is treated with a short course of high-dose daily steroids until the child is free of proteinuria for three days. When there is failure to respond to steroid therapy or when their side effects are troublesome, other immunosuppressant medications are given. These include cyclophosphamide (Cytoxan), chlorambucil (Leukeran), or cyclosporin (Sandimmune). If an infection develops as a result of long-term steroids, an antibiotic is ordered.

Nursing Tip:

Terms used to define response to treatment

Remission is achieved when a urine dipstick measures negative or trace proteinuria for three days or urinary protein excretion is less than 4 $mg/m^2/hr$. Relapse is defined as a urine dipstick measurement of 2+ proteinuria or more for three days or a child found to have 3–4+ proteinuria plus edema.

REFLECTIONS FROM FAMILIES

We were so worried about the use of steroids with our son Adam, who is 4 years old. We had heard all the bad things that can happen with steroids. For example, his health care provider had talked about such things as depression of the immune system, which could put him at risk for infection, growth retardation, and bone demineralization. Will these drugs put Adam at risk for infection? Will they stop his bones from growing? Will his bones become brittle and break easily?

Diuretics, such as furosemide (Lasix), should not be used to treat mild degrees of edema; however, they may be used if the child has severe edema. Because diuretics can precipitate hypovolemia, hyponatremia, and hypokalemia, electrolyte levels should be monitored closely. Albumin may be given if the edema is marked and causes the child to have decreased mobility, poor oral intake, or decreased urine output. Albumin helps to restore normal plasma oncotic pressure and promotes the movement of interstitial fluid back into the intravascular compartments. The albumin is followed by furosemide to reduce potential for fluid volume overload and to enhance diuresis. Salt intake is usually limited to control edema and reduce the risk for hypertension especially when daily glucocorticoids are given.

Nursing Management

Nursing management focuses on maintaining fluid and electrolyte balance, administering medications, preventing infection and skin breakdown, and education. The child's vital signs should be monitored every 4 hours or at least every shift. Low blood pressure and tachycardia are signs of hypovolemia. Intake and output are documented every shift. The nurse should monitor fluid with special attention to sodium restrictions if ordered. Any urine output less than 1–2 ml/kg/hr is to be reported immediately. Serum and urine electrolytes as ordered need to be evaluated. Nurses should assess for signs of edema and dehydration. These include dry skin, or dry mucous membranes, poor skin turgor, slowed capillary refill, pitting edema, sunken eyeballs, or dependent edema. Daily weights should be measured at the same time of day and on the same scale. Assessment of breath sounds for rales or wheezes may indicate pulmonary edema. Medications (diuretics, steroids, or immunosuppressive agents) should be administered as ordered. Signs of infection, including elevated temperature, changing CBC with differential, cough, sore throat, or other systemic complaints are evaluated. The child should be protected from visitors, personnel, or other clients who may have infections. Nurses should use good handwashing while caring for the child, and give antibiotics as ordered to prevent and/or treat infection. The child's skin needs to be protected from breakdown especially if edema is present. The child should be repositioned every two hours. The nurse should place an edematous extremity on a pillow or other support making sure the circulation is not impeded. Skin should be assessed for areas of redness or discoloration. For boys with edematous scrotums, padding and support to this area should be provided.

Family Teaching

Nurses should explain to caregivers what is known about nephrotic syndrome and its expected course. Caregivers should be allowed to ask questions and to express their feelings. Nurses must teach caregivers how to perform urine dipstick protein level measurements and the importance of measuring and recording the readings daily. They should be instructed to obtain daily weights for their child. The nurse needs to explain how important their role is in identifying relapses, the first signs of which are increases in weight and levels of protein in the urine. Caregivers should be taught about steroids and their immunosuppressive action and the need to protect their child against infection. They also need

Nursing Alert:

The Appetite-Stimulating Effect of Steroids

A side effect of steroids in some children is a ravenous appetite, which causes them to gain a significant amount of weight. Nurses should provide explanations to caregivers and the child, if age-appropriate, about the appetite-stimulating effects of these medications. Recommendations should be made for a nutritious, relatively low-fat diet with age-adjusted daily allowances of protein, carbohydrates, and other components.

to know that steroids can increase appetite, and may benefit from having a nutritionist consultation prior to discharge to help with the child's diet.

Caregivers should be instructed to notify the health care provider if the child is exposed to chickenpox if she/he has not had the disease or the vaccine. Live viral vaccines should not be given to children receiving high doses of steroids or other immunosuppressive medications, and caregivers need to be cautioned about this.

HEMOLYTIC UREMIC SYNDROME

Hemolytic uremic syndrome (HUS), an acute renal disease, is the most frequent cause of acute renal failure (ARF) in children.

Incidence and Etiology

Though relatively uncommon, HUS gained attention after children acquired the disorder as a result of an *Escherichia coli* (*E. coli*) infection from eating contaminated beef. It is more prevalent in developing countries where sanitation and the undercooking of meats are a problem. It is most common in children ages 6 months to 3 years. About 80% of all cases of HUS are found in children age 4 and under, occurring equally in both sexes (Neumann & Urizar, 1994). The exact etiology of HUS has not been determined, but it is thought to be associated with bacterial toxins, viruses, and chemicals. The organisms involved include *E. coli*, shigella, rickettsia, coxsackievirus, ECHO virus, adenovirus, pneumococci, and salmonella.

Pathophysiology

The pathophysiology of HUS is complex. The most frequently seen sequence is a bacterial invasion of the gastrointestinal tract leading to vomiting and diarrhea. The bacteria cling to the intestinal mucosa where they quickly multiply. Intestinal peristaltic action is slowed. An endotoxin is produced from the bacteria. An inflammatory response is created that leads to capillary wall damage and occlusion of the surrounding blood vessels. This same reaction occurs within the renal system deep in the glomerular arterioles. The endothelial lining of the affected tissues swell, and platelets move to the injured site. This move results in clot formation and intravascular coagulation. In HUS, the platelet clot or aggregate slows the blood flow through the renal system. Renin production is stimulated resulting in systemic hypertension. The platelet count falls as these platelets are damaged in the same manner as the red blood cells and the result is thrombocytopenia (less than 100,000/µl) which lasts 1 to 2 weeks (Neumann & Urizar, 1994). When the vessels of the glomeruli are affected, the result is a lowered glomerular filtration rate, eventually urine output is lower, and acute renal failure with hypertension follows. These clots and the inflammatory process can occur in any organ of the body, although it is most common in the gastrointestinal, respiratory, and genitourinary systems.

Clinical Manifestations

The clinical manifestations of HUS are a triad of symptoms, which include acute renal failure, thrombocytopenia, and anemia. The prodromal symptoms are gastrointestinal with diarrhea and vomiting or an upper respiratory infection. Once the hemolytic process starts, it may last from a few days to 2 weeks. The child becomes progressively more irritable, lethargic, and anorectic. Soon the child experiences anemia, and as it worsens, pallor increases, the hematocrit falls, and urine output diminishes. As the platelet count falls, there is increased chance of bleeding, bruising, and purpura. As the urinary system becomes more restricted with clot formation, the blood pressure rises leading to hypertension.

Diagnosis

Upon physical examination, hepatosplenomegaly (the enlargement of the liver and spleen) may be present. Edema, hypertension, congestive heart failure, and abdominal tenderness or pain are the common manifestations. The child may be pale, lethargic, dehydrated, and irritable. The history may include bloody diarrhea, vomiting, decreased urinary output, and slight abdominal pain. There may be altered levels of consciousness or seizure activities reported especially if the serum electrolytes, calcium, and phosphorus levels are outside normal limits. The rationale is that if there is an increase in workload on the heart from the edema, the blood pressure rises, and blood flow to the kidneys is diminished. The toxins normally cleared from the kidneys build up and the tubular reabsorption or excretion of ions such as sodium and potassium are altered. The result is an adverse effect on the central nervous system leading to seizures and altered consciousness.

Treatment

Primarily the treatment is symptomatic. If the serum electrolytes are outside normal limits and renal failure is severe, hemo- or peritoneal dialysis and/or fluid restriction may be necessary to raise the serum sodium levels that have fallen because of dilutional or volume overload. Dialysis is most often reserved for those children who are **anuric** (without urine output) for 24 hours or have oliguria and are extremely hypertensive or experiencing seizures. If the serum potassium level is high because of a decreased excretion of this ion by the renal system, a Kayexalate enema or nasogastric solution may be given. Serum glucose levels may also be low because of increased metabolic needs; therefore, dextrose or total parenteral nutrition must be given. If the pancreas has been affected by clot formation, the insulin production may be altered. Some children may develop hyperglycemia and must receive insulin therapy.

Calcium and phosphorous levels are affected with calcium falling and phosphorus rising. Calcium is excreted by the kidney and reabsorbed in the tubules. It is also dependent on intestinal function and transport across the epithelial tissue. In HUS these systems fail resulting in falling calcium with the rebound of phosphorus, which is normally filtered by the kidney. Either calcium gluconate or calcium chloride can be given depending on institutional policy or health care provider's wishes. Aluminum hydroxide gel may be given orally to bind the rising phosphorous. Treatment for hypertension is accomplished with hydralazine (Apresoline) and captopril (Capoten). The child may also be acidotic because of metabolic acidosis from the inability of the kidney to buffer normally produced acids in the body, and may require bicarbonate therapy. If there are central nervous system symptoms, such as altered consciousness or seizures, a central venous line may be placed for central venous pressure (CVP) monitoring. If the bleeding has been severe or the blood counts are low, then blood transfusions with fresh, packed red blood cells are given. Any time that fluids are given, even in the form of packed cells, fluid overload must be considered and prevented, if possible. Some institutions will give plasma products to these children to avoid the increased volume needed with packed red blood cells. Oral feedings may be resumed once the vomiting and diarrhea are controlled. More than 90% of children with HUS recover with normal renal function (Bergstein, 1996). However, there is potential for the development of chronic renal failure.

Nursing Management

Nursing management focuses on maintaining renal function and fluid and electrolyte balance, and providing family support. Nurses should assess the child for signs of dehydration: increased temperature, pulse, respirations, falling blood pressure, decreased peripheral perfusion, dry skin and mucous membranes, decreased urine output with a rising urine specific gravity, and poor skin turgor. Intake and output should be documented at least every 4 hours. If the child is in intensive care, this may be done every 1 to 2 hours. Nurses should check weights daily, and administer fluids and check serum electrolytes, BUN, creatinine, Hct, Hgb, WBC, and arterial blood gases as ordered. If the child experiences any central nervous system symptoms, a central venous catheter may be placed to measure this pressure. A cardiorespiratory monitor should be placed on the child. Attention should be paid to any changes in EKG tracings, such as a peaked T wave (related to potassium rises) and a widened QRS complex, or signs of heart block.

The child is assessed for signs of edema: tachycardia, tachypnea, hypertension, visible edema, and increased pulmonary secretions. Upon auscultation of the lungs, rales or wheezes may be heard. Weights must be monitored at least daily or more frequently as necessary. Urine output will be low and will need close monitoring. A Foley catheter may be placed for strict intake and output measurements. Chest X rays should be done to determine any pulmonary edema or cardiomegaly. Nurses should monitor electrolytes and blood counts as indicated and monitor CVP. If it measures 15 or greater, dialysis may be necessary. Oxygen may be required to support ventilation.

The child is evaluated for signs of bleeding or injury related to thrombocytopenia, and any signs of petechiae, bleeding, excessive bruising, or rashes are documented. Any invasive procedures should be avoided when possible. Nurses should monitor vital signs for changes from baseline, and assess neurologic status, including increasing restlessness, irritability, or lethargy, difficulty in arousal, or decreased sensation to touch or pain.

Nurses should assess the child for signs of possible increased intracranial pressure. These include changes in level of consciousness; inability to respond appropriately to verbal cues, touch, or pain; and changes in movements of the extremities or a decreased muscle tone in one or all four extremities. Pupillary changes or seizure activity should be noted also. The head of the bed should be elevated at least 30 degrees, and the room should be quiet and without excessive lights. If the neurologic status is impaired and the central venous pressure is rising, hypotonic IV solutions should be avoided. Osmotic diuretics should also be avoided as they add to problems of hypervolemia caused by fluid shifts.

Nurses should assess for gastrointestinal disturbances, document any vomitus and stools and describe the characteristics, and auscultate for bowel sounds. If none are present, a nasogastric tube may need to be placed to assist with gastric decompression. Antacids are used if the gastric pH is less than 5. Once feeding can be tolerated, small frequent feedings should be started and increased as tolerated.

Family Teaching

The caregivers may feel guilty that they missed something and did not know their child was so sick. They need reassurance that the symptoms are very subtle. They should be told as much of the pathophysiology as is known and helped to understand the normal course of HUS. They should be encouraged to participate in their child's care (MacPhee, 1995).

RENAL FAILURE

Renal failure refers to a condition that adversely affects the kidney resulting in decreased functioning of this organ system. It may take two main forms: acute or chronic.

Acute Renal Failure

Acute renal failure is a sudden onset of impaired renal function. Most children with ARF regain renal function. ARF is classified according to the part of the renal system that is affected. Three main types exist: prerenal, intrarenal, and postrenal.

Incidence

ARF is uncommon in children, but it can be life-threatening when it does develop.

Etiology and Pathophysiology

Prerenal ARF is characterized by a sudden decrease in renal blood flow or perfusion to the kidneys. This type of renal failure can result from dehydration, hypovolemia or shock, sepsis, renal artery obstruction, or perinatal asphyxia (Stewart & Barnett, 1997). *Intrarenal ARF* is associated with damage to the tissues of the kidney. The causes are iatrogenic secondary to antibiotic therapy (aminoglycosides or other nephrotoxic medications), contrasts dyes, ureterovesical obstruction, glomerulonephritis, pyelonephritis, hemolytic uremic syndrome, or other infections that affect renal tissue. *Postrenal ARF* results from an obstruction of urine at some point between the kidney and the urinary meatus. It is usually an outflow obstruction that causes a "back-up" of urine within the kidney, putting pressure on the endothelial lining and ultimately diminishing renal function. The causes that can occur in utero or during postnatal life are:

- Posterior ureteral valves
- **Ureterovesical obstruction**—an obstruction at the junction of the ureters into the bladder
- **Ureteropelvic obstruction**—an obstruction at the junction of the ureters into the renal pelvis
- Neurogenic bladder, primarily one without innervation
- Wilms tumor—a nephroblastoma or solid mass, which is the most common renal tumor in children (see Chapter 29)
- Renal calculi

Clinical Manifestations

The most common clinical manifestations are fluid and electrolyte imbalance, metabolic acidosis, and signs of dehydration or edema. Pallor, listlessness, lethargy, anorexia, vomiting, and in some cases seizures may also be observed. The child's vitals signs may or may not be within normal limits depending upon the cause and duration of the renal dysfunction.

Diagnosis

The diagnosis is based on history, laboratory evaluation, and physical examination. Anuria or a urine output of <1 ml/kg/hr is a potential finding, although some children will have a normal volume of urinary output. Renal serum panel usually reveals a rising BUN and creatinine; serum electrolytes, especially sodium and potassium, may also be elevated. As the renal blood flow falls, the glomerular filtration rate falls, and the amount of sodium that is filtered by the kidney diminishes. The child may have dependent, pitting, or periorbital edema. There may be hypertension accompanying the edema. This hypertension is caused by changes in blood flow throughout the body and the build up of edema. As the blood flow to the kidneys decreases, renin production increases leading to vasoconstriction. The heart works harder to pump the blood thus raising the blood pressure. Pulmonary edema occurs in some children presenting with increasing respiratory distress.

Treatment

As with nephrotic syndrome, the aims of the treatment for the child with acute renal failure are to increase renal perfusion and to restore and maintain fluid and electrolyte balance. This treatment may be with or without dialysis. The treatment without dialysis is as follows. If the sodium level is too high and edema is present, fluid and sodium restriction are necessary. If the potassium level is too high, then polystyrene sodium sulfonate (Kayexalate) orally or per rectum is given. This resin binds potassium and removes it from the body. If metabolic acidosis is present, treatment is sodium bicarbonate to replace the lacking renal buffer.

If these interventions do not control the fluid and electrolyte balance or pulmonary edema or if congestive heart failure is present, then dialysis must be considered. Other indications for dialysis are severe systemic hypertension, a BUN >120 mg/dl, hyperkalemia, and increasing metabolic acidosis. There are three main types of dialysis: hemodialysis, peritoneal dialysis, and hemofiltration.

Nursing Tip:

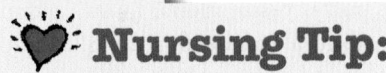

Nephrotoxicity

Many medications such as some forms of antibiotics, aminoglycosides, for example, are detoxified and excreted through the kidneys. These medications, when given in the presence of diminished renal function, can be nephrotoxic (Kenner, 1998). Always question the health care practitioner or nurse practitioner when a medication should be given if renal output is low. Peak and trough levels of these medications must be monitored to determine if the levels are rising indicating that renal clearance is impeded.

Hemodialysis is a hemofiltration system that occurs outside the body. It requires an arteriovenous (AV) fistula or shunt to be placed in a large vessel. This central line provides access to the blood system to pump the blood out from the body to an external extracorporeal circuit and through a filtration system. This serves to remove the body's waste products that can no longer be effectively filtered through the kidneys. This arteriovenous shunt in a large vessel requires surgical placement. The nurse must aseptically maintain it. Hemodialysis can be performed on an intermittent time-cycled basis, either in a hospital, dialysis center, or home setting. It is usually a 3 to 4 hour procedure repeated 3 to 4 times per week. It is more efficient at removing nitrogenous wastes than any other form of dialysis (Madder & Milberger, 1996).

Peritoneal dialysis requires the placement of a catheter into the peritoneal cavity for the purposes of removing excess fluids, solutes, and nitrogenous wastes (Figure 22-10). This placement may or may not require an open surgical procedure. It usually does not require a heparinized line. The treatment or filtration process involves the slow flow of fluid through the catheter into the peritoneal cavity until the desired fluid level has been administered. At that time a clamp is put in place allowing the fluid to dwell for a time in the peritoneal cavity to remove waste products. When the clamp is released, the fluid drains into the dialysis system. This cycle is repeated either automatically or manually four to five times per day. The procedure is usually repeated for several days and is normally done at home. Peritoneal dialysis is problematic for infants requiring dialysis, as the clearance of toxic wastes, solutes, and fluids is slow. Their abdominal areas are small and, if the treatment is not successful, the hypervolemia may be worse, a condition not tolerated well by small infants.

Hemofiltration is a continuous form of dialysis by means of a continuous arteriovenous (CAV) or venovenous (CVV) shunt. These shunts, like hemodialysis, require an extracorporeal circuit through which the blood flows into a filter system. The filter is placed between the arterial and venous lines along with a collecting bag. The blood flows from the child through the circuit continuously to remove nitrogenous wastes, solutes, and fluid. When the arteriovenous shunt is used, movement of the fluid is caused by the body's own pressure gradient (hydrostatic pressure from cardiac output and oncotic pressure from plasma proteins) rather than an external pumping device. If the venovenous shunt is used, a pump is necessary to move the blood through two separate venous cannulas or two ports in multilumen cannula (Madder & Milberger, 1996). Both ports are in veins so blood leaves through a venous route and returns via a vein. Either of these ultrafiltration systems has the advantage of using a very slow process that continuously adjusts as the body's solute load changes. The pressure of the body's own plasma proteins helps regulate the system so there is less stress on it. The circuit is heparinized so there is a danger of bleeding with this type of dialysis. However, this danger is less than with hemodialysis because less volume of blood flows through the circuit

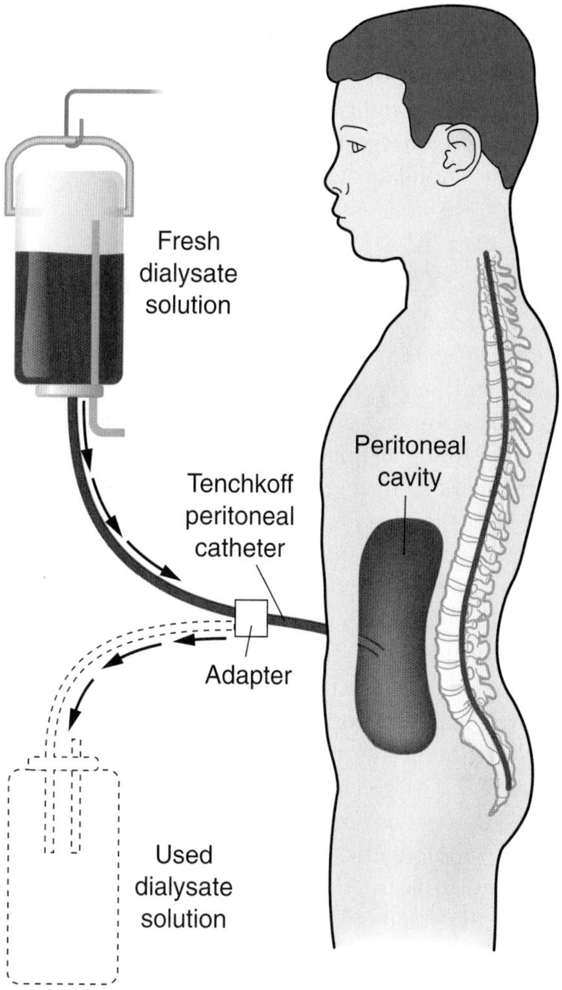

Figure 22-10 Peritoneal Dialysis Setup

Critical Thinking

Dialysis

1. What is the purpose of dialysis?
2. What is the difference between hemodialysis and peritoneal dialysis?
3. Why is intraperitoneal bleeding a potential complication with peritoneal dialysis?

at any one time with hemofiltration. This process is slow and is not as effective at removing large molecules such as urea. When any form of dialysis is used, there are risks. Morbidity and mortality for children on dialysis are most often related to intraperitoneal bleeding, peritonitis, or vessel blockage (Kohli, et al., 1997).

Nursing Management

This section will be divided into two parts. The first will be for the child and family that does not require dialysis but is experiencing acute renal failure. The second part will be for the child and family with acute renal failure who requires dialysis. The nursing care for both groups of children is aimed at restoring and maintaining fluid and electrolyte balance. In addition, for the child and family undergoing dialysis, the focus is also on maintaining the integrity of the circuit, protecting the child from bleeding at the shunt site, and preventing injury or infection. For both groups of children, a thorough history must be taken to elicit the underlying cause of the acute renal failure. Questions should focus on those conditions described as potential etiologies of prerenal, intrarenal, and postrenal acute renal failure, such as, have there been any previous urinary tract infection, episodes of low oxygen levels as with a premature infant, any antibiotic therapy, or renal stones? Physical examination, initially and subsequently, includes vital signs, weight, intake and output, urine specific gravity, and laboratory values, especially BUN and creatinine. The remainder of the nursing management is the same as that described for the child with nephrotic syndrome.

Family Teaching

Fear and anxiety are very real emotions for caregivers of a child with acute renal failure. They need honest and thorough explanations about what is known about the cause and the expected course of the illness. They need time to express their feelings. They may benefit from referrals to clergy or to support groups, especially if the treatment will be prolonged. Encourage them to participate in the child's care as they feel comfortable.

For the child and family undergoing dialysis, teaching regarding medications is necessary. They must be aware that if the urine output diminishes from what they have come to accept as normal, the health care provider should be called prior to medication administration. They need to be taught to maintain the routine schedule or cycling of the dialysis, either at the clinic or in the home, and to maintain meticulous clean care of the catheter site to protect the child from infection. If the dialysis is to be performed in the home, there must be a telephone and running water available. The electric company as well as the police and fire departments need to be notified to make sure that power is restored immediately to this family in case of electrical failure. A backup generator should also be available in the home to be used until power can be restored. It is also necessary for the nurse to assess the child and family for signs of depression or severe anxiety as these are common findings that may require a mental health consultation. This child and family will require a lot of emotional support. If the child is school age, encourage discussion of his or her fears, concerns about peers, and any self-esteem issues he or she may have.

- Instruct the child and family about the need for a low protein diet if this is to be maintained at home.
- Teach the child and family about signs of infection or the worsening of the renal problem. Signs would

Kids Want To Know

What is a renal ultrasound and will it hurt?

A 10-year-old girl with a diagnosis of acute renal failure is scheduled for a renal ultrasound. Before the scan she asks, "What will the scan do to me? Will it hurt?"

The young girl is old enough to probably know what a computer scan is but may not have any concept of what or how a renal scan is done. You can reply by explaining that the scan will not hurt, how the picture is taken, and that the machine will move over her. She may be afraid she has to be sent through a machine for the picture to be taken. Honest answers may calm her fears.

Reflective Thinking

Caring for Children Undergoing Dialysis

To increase self-awareness about children undergoing dialysis, ask yourself:

1. How do I feel about caring for children undergoing dialysis?
2. Is my care affected by the child's appearance? (The child may be edematous with very shiny, taut skin, or have a moon face and be very pale).
3. Do I spend less time interacting with these children because I feel uncomfortable?
4. How do I ensure that these children receive the same quality of care as those children who do not have a chronic illness or life-threatening disease?

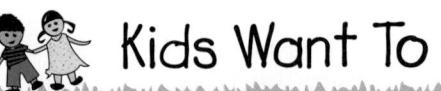

include weight gain caused by edema, headache that could indicate hypertension, flank pain, decreased urine output, fever, sore throat, or flu like symptoms.

- Instruct the family that the child can pursue activities as tolerated each day.
- Encourage the caregivers to teach the child to stay away from other children who have obvious colds, flu, or other infections.
- Encourage the caregivers to teach the child about good handwashing especially at school where there are many other people.
- Allow the child to decide whether the teachers or friends will be told about the renal problem.
- Refer the child and family to resource groups such as the National Kidney Foundation or local support groups.

Chronic Renal Failure and End Stage Renal Failure

Chronic renal failure (CRF) is a progressive disease. The damage that is done to the renal system in some cases is irreversible. This condition is considered chronic when approximately 50% of the renal function remains and the condition has lasted for at least several months. If it is considered to be permanent and irreversible, then it is classified as end stage renal failure (ESRF). All chronic renal failure will first progress to uremia. **Uremia** is a condition where toxic nitrogenous waste products, blood urea, and creatinine build up in the system. If this condition is not reversed, it progresses to ESRF.

Incidence and Etiology

The incidence of CRF is between 1.5 and 3.0 per million in the pediatric population (Fogo & Kon, 1994). The etiology of CRF and ESRF varies but may be caused by prematurity, use of nephrotoxic medications such as aminoglycosides, genetic syndromes with congenital urinary or renal obstructions, hemolytic uremic syndrome, glomerulonephritis, pyelonephritis, and other systemic infections. Some children experience CRF or ESRF as a result of immunologic dysfunction that causes actual injury to renal tissue.

Pathophysiology

The exact pathophysiology depends on the etiology of the condition that began to disrupt the kidney function. In any case, eventually the renal system is compromised, as is renal blood flow through the kidney, leading to loss of oxygen to the tissues and ultimately to destruction of portions of the nephron. The nephron is the working unit of the kidney and functions to create urine, filter substances through the kidney, and reabsorb and excrete solutes in the body. The nephron is composed of the glomerulus and the renal tubule. Nephrons once destroyed cannot be regenerated. As portions of the nephrons die, the renal function becomes less efficient. The remaining nephrons attempt to take over the complete function so they hypertrophy. The glomerular pressure increases, as does the arterial pressure in the glomerular capillaries and renal arteries. Eventually the glomeruli sclerose and die. If this cycle is not stopped and the arterial pressure lowered, ESRF results.

Clinical Manifestations

As with acute renal failure, the main clinical manifestations of CRF and ESRF include fluid and electrolyte imbalance, dehydration or edema, metabolic acidosis, and systemic hypertension. The child may also experience anemia, pallor, fatigue, anorexia, vomiting, slowed linear growth, organic failure to thrive, and renal bone disease or osteodystrophy (Watkins, 1997).

Diagnosis

The diagnosis is based on the history of either long-standing renal problems or growth problems accompanied by altered laboratory values. The child's presentation may be one of dehydration, edema, hypertension, electrolyte imbalance, altered calcium phosphorus ratios, elevated BUN and creatinine levels, low hematocrit and hemoglobin, and long bone X rays revealing osteodystrophy. Pallor, lethargy, anorexia, and vomiting may or may not be present.

Treatment

Treatment for the child with CRF and ESRF is aimed at restoring or maintaining fluid and electrolyte balance. If edema is present, then fluid restriction and sodium and potassium restriction may be necessary. Diuretics are used if edema is significant. Antihypertensive medications are given if hypertension is present. Protein intake may be restricted because of the kidney's inability to rid the body of waste products. Phosphorus is restricted in order to increase the calcium levels. If calcium levels are maintained, then there is less chance of bone disease that can result when calcium levels are low. Vitamin D supplementation may be given. The result is that vitamin D will be present to boost the calcium levels to prevent bone disease. Aluminum hydroxy gel may be given to bind with phosphorus and decrease the gastrointestinal absorption. This medication should only be used on a short-term basis as aluminum levels can become high and result in seizures. Calcium carbonate will achieve the same result and is not toxic even to infants.

Experimental therapies include erythropoietin to combat anemia and growth hormone to boost linear growth. Immunosuppressive therapy is also used especially if the child is going to require renal transplantation. While this immunosuppressive therapy is not experimental, the combination of medications (more than one immunosuppressive medication at a time) is undergoing research. For those children with

ESRF, dialysis and/or renal transplantation are the only treatment options.

Renal transplantation is usually reserved for children for whom medication and dietary management of fluid and electrolyte balance and hypertension have been unsuccessful. These children have ESRF. They may or may not have been maintained on dialysis for a long period of time prior to the transplant. Transplants can be performed on infants. The surgical team and the family make the determination of the candidate for a transplant. In some institutions an ethics committee also looks at quality of life issues to help in the decision-making process. The question they usually ask is "What will the long-term quality of life be for this child if the transplant is done?" Unfortunately there are no guarantees with this type of surgery. The usual candidates for transplants are those who can withstand a surgical intervention, are in good nutritional status, and are not severely immunocompromised (Ryckman & Pedersen-Ryckman, 1998; Tyden, Berg, Bohlin, & Sandberg, 1997).

Kidneys for transplantation are obtained either through living donors—usually close relatives—or cadavers. Tissue typing to determine a match requires meticulous tests similar to crossmatching for blood transfusions. Close relatives are most likely to be a very good tissue match, but even then there is a chance of graft (the transplanted kidney) or organ rejection. Cyclosporine, azathioprine (Imuran) and prednisone or prednisolone are used to suppress the natural immune response. Organ rejection is known as **graft versus host disease,** which occurs when the transplanted organ fights against its host, creating an exaggerated immune response to rid the body of the foreign organ. This reaction can be life-threatening. Most renal transplants are not lost by rejection but the tissue dies from vascular thrombus or clots in the renal vessels (Singh, Stablein, & Tejani, 1997).

Transplantation is just one aspect of ESRF treatment. Post-transplantation, immunosuppressive medications are required for life. Dietary restrictions may still be necessary especially regarding protein intake. Medications for hypertension and diuretics may still be needed following surgery.

REFLECTIONS FROM FAMILIES

I was so angry when I learned that my son was acutely ill. I knew that he was going to have a renal transplant and I did not know if I was up to the challenge. I resented the fact that my life was going to dramatically have to change. What impact was this going to have on my younger daughter? I have never been so frightened in my life and so angry with myself for sounding so selfish!

Critical Thinking

Cushing Syndrome Secondary to ESRF

What is the physiological process involved in the development of Cushing syndrome when steroids are administered? What other effects may this child exhibit from steroid therapy? What is the nurse's role in working with the child and family in terms of teaching about steroids?

These clients need to be followed for serum and urine chemistries, immunologic examination for signs of rejection and aggressive infections, and growth and development follow-up care. As they are on immunosuppressive medication along with steroids to decrease the chance of rejection, these children must be followed for any side effects of the steroids.

There are several concerns about the long-term effects of steroid or cyclosporine therapy. Both of these medications increase the susceptibility to infection as mentioned above. They both affect other glucocorticosteroids that in turn alter serum glucose and insulin levels. Adrenal suppression is common often resulting in glucose intolerance (Haffner, Blum, Heinrich, Mehls, & Tonshoff, 1997). Cushing syndrome or round moon face and deposition of fat around the scapular region caused by the glucocorticosteroid effects has most often been associated with long-term steroid therapy, but can also come from cyclosporine use. Other effects from steroids are seen in bone mineralization and strength, which are concerns for a growing, active child. The effects on growth hormone of the renal disease itself are made worse by some of the therapies. All these questions need further research to either substantiate or refute these clinical observations. Use of growth hormone is just becoming popular to stimulate continued growth, but again the long-term effects are in need of research (Watkins, 1997).

Nursing Management

This section will be divided into two sections. The first will be the management of the child and family with CRF or ESRF. The second part will be the management of the child and family undergoing a renal transplant. The goals of the nursing care are to restore and maintain fluid and electrolyte balance; restore and maintain nutrition and growth; and decrease the anxiety of the child and family. Most of the nursing management is the same as with acute renal failure. Other points of nursing management are discussed below.

Nurses should administer medications (diuretics, steroids, or immunosuppressive agents) as ordered, and assess for signs of infection: elevated temperature, changing

Nursing Alert:

Recognizing Need for Dialysis

The signs or indicators for dialysis are BUN >120 mg/dl, increasing metabolic acidosis, hyperkalemia, fluid overload with pulmonary edema and/or congestive heart failure, and severe systemic hypertension.

CBC with differential, cough, sore throat, or other systemic complaints. The child should be protected from visitors or personnel who may have infections. Antibiotics are administered as ordered. Nurses should always consider if these medications are cleared through the kidney, and if so, then peak and trough levels must be monitored as some medications are nephrotoxic.

If anemia is severe, blood transfusions with packed red blood cells may be administered, but this presents the danger of fluid overload. Newer therapies include the use of erythropoietin to boost the reticulocyte development. This therapy is used in the predialysis phase and is associated with delaying renal function deterioration. Erythropoietin boosts the hemoglobin by about 3 g/dl when a maintenance dose of between 70 and 300 U/kg per week is given (Krmar, Gretz, Klare, Wyhl, & Scharer, 1997). Many practitioners consider this treatment to be experimental and the long-term effectiveness has not been widely studied. This child may also need dialysis and should be assessed for signs indicating the need for this form of treatment.

The assessment and care remains the same as that described for the child and family with CRF and ESRF. These children are at risk for the development of vesicourethral reflux in the graft, which may lead to pyelonephritis (Neuhaus, et al., 1997). Signs of a kidney infection such as fever, flank pain, burning on urination, cloudy or blood-tinged urine, and sometimes abdominal cramping, must be monitored, and the caregivers must be taught these signs as well.

Reflective Thinking

How Would You Feel If Your Child Had a Renal Transplant?

As nurses we must try to imagine what it is like for caregivers to face seeing their child first have a life-threatening disease such as chronic renal failure, then to have to choose a treatment that may or may not be effective. They also know that this treatment will have risks and change their child's life as well as their own forever. These are very emotional-laden decisions and require a lot of empathy and support from health care professionals. Explore your feelings. What would you consider in making your decision?

Family Teaching

Because either CRF or ESRF is a chronic, life-long problem, the family will have many learning needs, especially related to the need for meticulous follow-up care. They need to understand the etiology of the problem and the course of treatment. They will need to be taught about dietary restrictions, use and side effects of medications, signs of further deterioration of the renal function, and possibly how to perform dialysis in their homes. The side effects from steroids and immunosuppressive therapies include a depressed immune system so the child is more vulnerable to infection, growth retardation, and bone demineralization. There is a greater risk for fractures. Some children will feel hyperactive with high doses of steroids. If they take the steroids for a long time, they may develop a moon face, fat deposits along the shoulders, and generally gain weight. If the child is on diuretics, the individual may lose potassium and feel weak or faint or experience heart palpitations. Caregivers need to know that these side effects are possible but do not always occur.

They may benefit from financial counseling as these are costly problems and are not always covered by health insurance policies or managed care contracts. They need to understand the impact that a chronic illness has on themselves and their child. They should be encouraged to take advantage of psychological counseling or participate in a support group. For the family whose child has undergone a transplant additional teaching is needed. The family must be taught signs of rejection and a kidney infection. They must also understand the need for lifelong follow-up care and medications given on the established schedule. It will be necessary to arrange for home care and nursing follow-up in the home. Quality of life issues need to be addressed. The child and family can be reassured that current research indicates that childhood transplant recipients can achieve a good

Nursing Alert:

Signs of Renal Transplant Rejection

Acute rejection usually occurs within the first 6 months after transplantation.

Signs of rejection are:

Fever, graft pain, decreased urine output, weight gain, and hypertension.

Laboratory signs of rejection are:

Increasing BUN and creatinine

Research Highlight

Immunizations in Children with Renal Disease

Study Purpose

The purpose of this study was to determine the current immunization recommendations of practicing pediatric nephrologists.

Methods

A questionnaire was sent to the members of the North American Pediatric Renal Transplant Cooperative Society.

Findings

With a 62% response rate, the results suggested that, although consensus for approaching immunization guidelines does exist, recommendations do vary from center to center. The majority of the respondents recommended standard vaccines (DTP, oral poliovirus–OPV, hepatitis B–Hep B, and Haemophilus influenzae B–Hib) for their renal insufficiency and dialysis patients. Although standard killed vaccines (DTP, Hep B, Hib) are not infectious, they are recommended less frequently for transplanted patients (86%) than their renal insufficiency (98%) and dialysis (near 100%) patients. Also, OPV and measles/mumps/rubella (MMR), which are live viral vaccines, are rarely recommended post-transplant. Almost 90% of the centers recommend the use of influenza vaccine, while only 60% of the centers recommend pneumococcal vaccine for children with renal disease. Over 70% of the centers recommend the newly licensed varicella vaccine for patients on dialysis and those with renal insufficiency.

Implications

This information is extremely important for the nurse working with pediatric patients. Although this information is very useful in providing education to the family of a child with renal insufficiency, there are several research issues that need to be examined further. The nursing research areas to consider are:

1. What are the educational needs of children diagnosed with renal insufficiency and their families?
2. What preventive health measures are important for these children?
3. How do the health beliefs of the parents affect the care provided to a child with renal disease?
4. What are the implications associated with immunization risk for children with renal disease over time?
5. Is there a model of care that is predictive of quality health outcomes for children with renal disease and their families?

Citation

Furth, S. L., Neu, A. M., Sullivan, E. K., Gensler, G., Tejani, A., & Fivush, B. A. (1997). Immunization practices in children with renal disease: A report of the North American Pediatric Renal Transplant Cooperative Study. *Pediatric Nephrology, 11*(4), 443–446.

quality of life in their adult years (Krmar, Eymann, Ramirez, & Ferraris, 1997). Families also need to know that generally the immunizations should be given and that there is no adverse affect on the kidney (Enke, Bokenkamp, Offner, Bartmann, & Brodehl, 1997). The rationale is that while these children may be immunosuppressed, their immune system still can respond to the vaccines in the immunizations. It is better to have the children challenged by a laboratory, controlled dose of the "disease" than to actually acquire the childhood disease itself.

BLADDER EXSTROPHY-EPISPADIAS COMPLEX

Bladder exstrophy-epispadias complex is a rare serious congenital anomaly affecting the urologic and musculoskeletal systems. In early fetal life the abdominal wall and underlying structures fail to fuse producing an exposed bladder and urethra, pubic bone separation, and associated genital and anal abnormalities. This complex occurs in males more frequently than in females. Epispadias is considered a mild form of bladder exstrophy, and in more severe cases the two coexist (McAninch, 1995). In males, epispadias is characterized by the urethral opening on the dorsal side of the penis in contrast to hypospadias where it is on the ventral surface (Figure 22-11). Females with epispadias present with separation of the labia and a **bifid** (split into two parts) clitoris. If the internal bladder sphincter is affected, total incontinence results. In exstrophy the lower urinary tract is exposed, and the everted bladder appears bright red through the abdominal opening. There is also a widening of the symphysis pubis.

Musculoskeletal anomalies seen in these children include an outward rotation of the hips and widening of the pelvis. Male infants have a short penis with dorsal chordee, or upward curvature, and a ventral prepuce. Females present with a bifid clitoris and nonfused labia. At birth the bladder mucosa is thin, reddened, and susceptible to injury. Various techniques are utilized to protect the mucosa and preserve hydration.

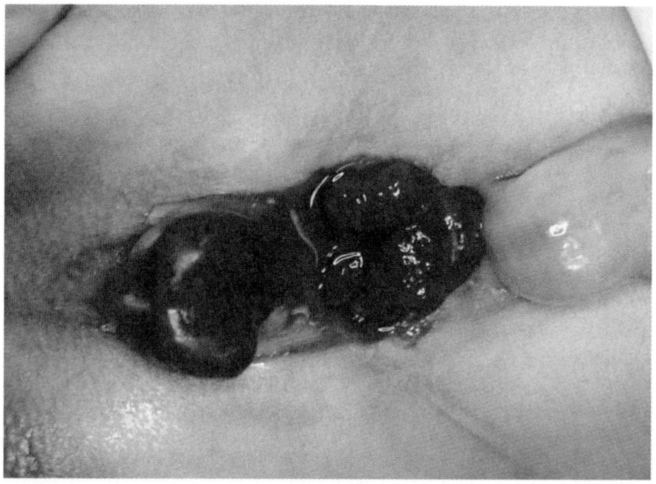

Figure 22-11 Bladder Exstrophy with Epispadias. Photo courtesy of Casimir Firlit, MD, PhD, William E. Kaplan, MD, Max Maizels, MD, and Jeffrey Palmer, MD, Children's Urology Ltd.

Surgical management of bladder exstrophy is usually performed within the first 48 hours of life but may be deferred secondarily to the infant's stability or until further testing is performed. Goals of management include preservation of the primary bladder and abdominal wall and provision of an adequate pelvic structure to support the bladder. Other goals include the achievement of a functional bladder and cosmetic reconstruction (Bowers, Hannigan, & Kushner, 1995). Initially, the bladder, abdominal wall, and symphysis are closed surgically.

Long-term care focuses on continence issues and social adjustment. In its severest forms continence may only be achieved through augmentation of the bladder to increase its storage capacity and in some cases a urinary diversion procedure. Issues of sexuality need to be addressed as the child approaches adolescence, including information regarding reproduction. Research indicates that most clients with exstrophy do not develop long-standing maladjustment and have a high level of sexual functioning (Bowers, Hannigan, & Kushner, 1995). Management of exstrophy is one of the most complex of all urologic disorders.

In the Real World

As a student nurse, I found caring for a 2-year-old child with hemolytic uremic syndrome to be quite scary. I knew that the child might not recover or at the very least have some lifelong problems. The family was devastated as they were on a family vacation and had eaten at fast-food restaurants, where the child more than likely had contracted E. coli. *While empathetic with the family and their situation, all I could think about was my own 2-year-old. I talked with a colleague about my mixed feelings about getting too close to this family. She suggested that rather than being scared of my feelings to let them help me work with the family as I would hope a nurse would if it were my child. This perspective gave me renewed strength so that instead of feeling anxious and guilty I could use this positive "energy" to be more empathetic with the family.*

Key Concepts

- The genitourinary system of the infant and child is immature compared to an adult's; therefore, medications and therapies must be considered in terms of renal maturation.
- Embryologically, the genital and urinary systems are interrelated; hence, any insult during fetal development can have devastating consequences for the child and family.

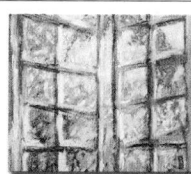

- Common manifestations of genitourinary alterations in children include vague symptoms such as abdominal pain, nausea, vomiting, and diarrhea.
- Nursing assessment of the child with genitourinary alterations includes a history about diet and feeding/eating pattern, elimination pattern (stool and urine), growth pattern, gastrointestinal symptoms, and a physical examination.
- Untreated UTIs can lead to progressive infections with kidney involvement, subsequent renal scarring, and decreased kidney function.
- Enuresis is the involuntary voiding of urine in children over the age of 5 years without a structural defect. Incontinence is wetting that results from a structural defect or abnormality.
- Vesicoureteral reflux is the backflow of urine from the bladder into the upper urinary tract. Clinically these children may be diagnosed only after a full radiographic workup after UTI.
- Hypospadias is a congenital malformation and displacement of the urethra to the underside or ventral surface of the penis, requiring surgical repair.
- Cryptorchidism is synonymous with undescended testes. It may be unilateral or bilateral and is often treated before the age of 2 in an attempt to preserve spermatogenesis. Children with UDT must be followed through puberty and into adulthood secondary to issues regarding fertility and increased tumor potential.
- Hernias present as a bulge or a swelling in the scrotum or groin and may fluctuate with increased intra-abdominal pressure such as crying.
- Acute glomerulonephritis is an inflammation of glomeruli within the kidney caused by a viral or bacterial agent.
- Nephrotic syndrome manifests as massive proteinuria and hypoalbuminemia that leads to edema and hyperlipidemia.
- Hemolytic uremic syndrome though rarely seen in children has been found to be secondary to *E. coli* infection.
- The three types of acute renal failure are prerenal, intrarenal, and postrenal.
- Chronic renal failure is a progressive disease that can lead to end-stage renal failure.
- Nursing management of children undergoing urologic procedures generally involve extensive family education and anticipatory guidance preoperatively along with postoperative issues of accurate fluid management, care of various drainage tubes, and meticulous wound care and assessment.
- Teaching for the child and family undergoing dialysis must include dietary needs, infection control, and performing the dialysis. The nurse must also emphasize the signs and symptoms of worsening renal failure and the need for close follow-up.
- Nursing management for the child with a renal transplant is directed toward teaching the family about dietary needs, infection control, and signs and symptoms of rejection.

Review Questions

1. Identify the signs and symptoms of urinary tract infections including the standard clarification between cystitis or bladder infection and pyelonephritis.
2. Describe the necessary urologic workup for a child post-first-documented UTI and the rationale for this further testing.
3. Describe the differences between the terms enuresis and incontinence. What questions should be asked when obtaining a history for a child with wetting problems?
4. Describe the conservative medical management for a child with vesicoureteral reflux.
5. Describe the clinical manifestations of hypospadias in the newborn period and nursing interventions that should be instituted.
6. Develop a teaching plan regarding the importance of long-term follow-up for a boy with UDT.
7. Develop a teaching plan for caregivers regarding signs and symptoms of increasing problems and risk of incarceration in a child with hernias and/or hydrocele.
8. Describe the pathophysiology of hemolytic uremic syndrome.
9. What should the nurse advise caregivers about fluid restrictions and dietary restrictions for the child with acute or chronic renal failure?
10. List the clinical indicators for dialysis.

References

American Academy of Pediatrics Committee on Quality Improvement and Subcommittee on Urinary Tract Infection. (1999). Practice parameter: The diagnosis, treatment, and evaluation of the initial urinary tract infection in febrile infants and young children. *Pediatrics, 103*(4), 843–852.

Belman, A. B. (1995). A perspective on vesicoureteral reflux. *Urologic Clinics of North America: Common Problems in Pediatric Urology, 22*(1), 139–159.

Bergstein, J. (1996). Nephrology. In R. Behrman, R. Kliegman, & A. Arvin (Eds.), *Nelson textbook of pediatrics* (15th ed., pp. 1480–1506). Philadelphia: W. B. Saunders.

Bowers, V., Hannigan, K. F., & Kushner, K. L. (1995). Bladder exstrophy and epispadias. In K. A. Karlowicz (Ed.), *Urologic nursing: Principles and practice* (pp. 565–592). Philadelphia: W. B. Saunders.

Constantinescu, A., Shah, H., Foote, E., & Weiss, L. (2000). Predicting first-year relapses in children with nephrotic syndrome. *Pediatrics, 105*(3), 492–495.

Craig, J., Irwig, L., Knight, J., & Roy, L. (2000). Does treatment of vesicoureteric reflux in childhood prevent end-stage renal disease attributable to reflux nephropathy? *Pediatrics, 105*(6), 1236–1241.

Enke, B. U., Bokenkamp, A., Offner, G., Bartmann, P., & Brodehl, J. (1997). Response to diphtheria and tetanus booster vaccination in pediatric renal transplant recipients. *Transplantation 1997, 64*(2), 237–241.

Fogo, A., & Kon, V. (1994). Pathophysiology of progressive renal disease. In M. A. Holliday, T. Barratt, & E. Avner (Eds.), *Pediatric nephrology* (pp. 1228–1240). Baltimore: Williams & Wilkins.

Furth, S. L., Neu, A. M., Sullivan, E. K., Gensler, G., Tejani, A., & Fivush, B. A. (1997). Immunization practices in children with renal disease: A report of the North American Pediatric Renal Transplant Cooperative Study. *Pediatric Nephrology, 11*(4), 443–446.

Gonzalez, R. (1996). Urologic disorders in infants and children. In R. Behrman, R. Kliegman, & A. Arvin (Eds.), *Nelson textbook of pediatrics* (15th ed., pp. 1548–1549). Philadelphia: W. B. Saunders.

Haffner, D., Blum, W. F., Heinrich, U., Mehls, O., & Tonshoff, B. (1997). Impaired postprandial regulation of insulin-like growth factor binding protein-1 in children with chronic renal failure. *Journal of Clinical Endocrinology & Metabolism, 82*(9), 2832–2835.

Hogg, R., Portman, R., Milliner, D., Lemley, K., Eddy, A., & Ingelfinger, J. (2000). Evaluation and management of proteinuria and nephrotic syndrome in children: Recommendations from a pediatric nephrology panel established at the National Kidney Foundation Conference on Proteinuria, Albuminaria, Risk, Assessment, Detection, and Elimination (PARADE). *Pediatrics, 105*(6), 1242–1249.

Johnson, C. (1999). New advances in childhood urinary tract infections. *Pediatrics in Review, 20*(10), 335–342.

Kaefer, M., Curran, M., Treves, S., Bauer, S., Hendren, W., Peters, C., Atala, A., Diamond, D., & Retik, A. (2000). Sibling vesicouretereal reflux in multiple gestation births. *Pediatrics, 105*(4), 800–804.

Karlowicz, K. (1995). Pediatric voiding disorders. In K. Karlowicz (Ed.), *Urologic nursing: Principles and practice* (pp. 599–604). Philadelphia: W. B. Saunders.

Kelleher, R. (1997). Daytime and nighttime wetting in children: A review of management. *Journal of the Society of Pediatric Nurses, 2*(2), 73–82.

Kenner, C. (1998). Assessment and management of genitourinary dysfunction. In C. Kenner, J. W. Lott, & A. A. Flandermeyer (Eds.), *Comprehensive neonatal nursing care: A physiologic perspective.* (2nd ed.). Philadelphia: W. B. Saunders.

Kohli, H. S., Barkataky, A., Kumar, R. S., Sud, K., Jha, V., Gupta, K. L., & Sakhuja, V. (1997). Peritoneal dialysis for acute renal failure in infants: A comparison of three types of peritoneal access. *Renal Failure, 19*(1), 165–170.

Krmar, R. T., Eymann, A., Ramirez, J. A., & Ferraris, J. R. (1997). Quality of life after kidney transplantation in children. *Transplantation, 64*(3), 540–541.

Krmar, R. T., Gretz, N., Klare, B., Wuhl, E., & Scharer, K. (1997). Renal function in predialysis children with chronic renal failure treated with erythropoietin. *Pediatric Nephrology, 11*(1), 69–73.

MacPhee, M. (1995). The family systems approach and pediatric nursing care. *Pediatric Nursing, 21*(5), 417–423.

Madder, S. M., & Milberger P. M. (1996). Renal critical care problems. In M. A. Q. Curley, J. B. Smith, & P. A. Maloney-Harmon (Eds.), *Critical care nursing of infants and children.* (pp. 695–723). Philadelphia: W. B. Saunders.

Maizels, M., Rosenbaum, D., & Keating, B. (1999). *Getting to dry: How to help your child overcome bedwetting* (pp. 32, 180–181, 200–201, 208–210). Boston: Harvard Common Press.

McAninch, J. W. (1995). Disorders of the penis and male urethra. In E. A. Tanagho & J. W. McAninch (Eds.), *Smith's general urology* (14th ed., pp. 658–669). Norwalk, CT: Appleton & Lange.

Mosier, W. A. (1998). Update on childhood enuresis. *The Clinical Advisor, 1*(4), 34.

Neuhaus, T. J., Schwobel, M., Schlumpf, R., Offner, G., Leumann, E., & Willi, U. (1997). Pyelonephritis and vesicourethral reflux after renal transplantation in young children. *Journal of Urology, 157*(4), 1400–1403.

Neumann, M. A., & Urizar, R. E. (1994). Hemolytic uremic syndrome: Current pathophysiology and management. *American Nephrology Nurses Association Journal, 21*(2), 137–143.

Paulozzi, L., Erickson, J., & Jackson, R. (1997). Hypospadias trends in two US surveillance systems. *Pediatrics, 100*(5), 831–834.

Reynolds, E., & Hoberman, A. (1995). Diagnosis and management of pyelonephritis in infants. *Maternal Child Nursing, 20,* 78–84.

Riley, K. (1997). Evaluation and management of primary nocturnal enuresis. *Journal of the American Academy of Nurse Practitioners, 9*(1), 33–39.

Rozanski, T. A., & Bloom, D. A. (1995). Common problems in pediatric urology: The undescended testis, theory and management. *Urologic Clinics of North America, 22* (1), 107–117.

Rushton, H. G. (1995). Voiding and functional voiding disorders. *Urologic Clinics of North America, 22*(1), 75–91.

Rushton, H. G. (1997). Urinary tract infection in children: Epidemiology, evaluation, and management. *Pediatric Clinics of North America, 44,* 1133–1169.

Ryckman, F. C., & Pedersen-Ryckman, S. (1998). Hepatic and renal transplantation in infants and children. In C. Kenner, J. W. Lott, & A. A. Flandermeyer (Eds.), *Comprehensive neonatal nursing care: A physiologic perspective.* (2nd. ed., pp. 838–849). Philadelphia: W. B. Saunders.

Shaw, K., Gorelick, M., McGowan, K., Yakscoe, N., & Schwartz, J. (1998). Prevalence of urinary tract infection in febrile young children in the emergency department. *Pediatrics, 102*(2), e16.

Simckes, A., & Spitzer, A. (1995). Poststreptococcal glomerulonephritis. *Pediatrics in Review, 16*(7), 278–279.

Singh, A., Stablein, D., & Tejani, A. (1997). Risk factors for vascular thrombosis in pediatric renal transplantation: A special report of the North American Pediatric Renal Transplant Cooperative Study. *Transplantation, 63*(9), 1263–1267.

Skoog, S. J., & Conlin M. J. (1995). Common problems in pediatric urology: Pediatric hernias and hydroceles, the urologist's perspective. *Urologic Clinics of North America, 22*(1), 119–129.

Stewart, C. L., & Barnett, R. (1997). Acute renal failure in infants, children and adults. *Critical Care Clinics, 13*(3), 575–590.

Stock, J., Scherz, H., & Kaplan, G. (1995). Distal hypospadias. *Urologic Clinics of North America, 22*(1), 205–219.

Sugar, E. C., Firlit, C. F., & Reisman, M. (1993). Pediatric hypospadias surgery. *Pediatric Nursing, 19*(6), 585–588.

Sugar, E., & Hoyler-Grant, C. (1995). Disorders of the external genitalia in children. In K. A. Karlowicz (Ed.), *Urologic nursing: Principles and practice* (pp. 498–525). Philadelphia: W. B. Saunders.

Tanagho, E. A. (1995). Neuropathic bladder disorders. In E. A. Tanagho & J. W. McAninch (Eds.), *Smith's General Urology* (pp. 17–30). Norwalk, CT: Appleton & Lange.

Tyden, G., Berg, U., Bohlin, A. B., & Sandberg, J. (1997). Renal transplantation in children less than two years old. *Transplantation, 63*(4), 554–558.

Watkins, S. L. (1997). Growth failure in the pediatric ESRD patient. *Peritoneal Dialysis International, 17 Suppl, 3,* S12–S14.

Zaontz, M., & Packer, M. (1997). Abnormalities of the external genitalia. *Pediatric Clinics of North America, 44,* 1267–1297.

Suggested Readings

Fangmann, J., Oldhafer, K., Offner, G., Neipp, M., & Pichlmayr, R. (1997). Factors contributing to successful renal transplantation in children less than 5 years of age: Experience of the last two decades. *Transplantation Proceedings, 29*(1–2), 255–256.

Hoberman, A., Wald, E., Hickey, R., Baskin, M., Charron, M., Majd, M., Kearney, D., Reynolds, E., Ruley, J., & Janosky, J. (1999). Oral versus initial intravenous therapy for urinary tract infections in young febrile children. *Pediatrics, 104*(1), 79–86.

Holm, A., Vicente, A., Soberanes, A., Lagunas, J., Espinosa, A., Diliz, H., Caleron, M., Zarate, A., & Madrazo, M. (1997). Immunosuppression (Neoral v. Sandimmune) in pediatric kidney transplantation. *Transplantation Proceedings, 29*(1–2), 300–302.

Hoyler-Grant, C. (1995). Health assessment of the pediatric urology patient. In K. Karlowicz (Ed.), *Urologic nursing: Principles and practice* (pp. 439–463). Philadelphia: W. B. Saunders.

Longstaffe, S., Moffatt, M., & Whalen, J. (2000). Behavioral and self-concept changes after six months of enuresis treatment: a randomized, controlled trial. *Pediatrics, 105*(4), S935–940.

Ribby, K. J. (1997). Organization and development of a pediatric end stage renal disease teaching protocol for peritoneal dialysis. *Pediatric Nursing, 23*(4), 393–399.

Shaw, K., McGowan, K., Gorelick, M., & Schwartz, J. (1998). Screening for urinary tract infection in infants in the emergency department: which test is best? *Pediatrics, 101*(6), e1.

Spital, A. (1997). Should children ever donate kidneys? Views of U.S. transplant centers. *Transplantation, 64*(2), 232–236.

Resources

Organizations and Websites

American Association of Kidney Patients
100 S. Ashely Dr., Ste. 280
Tampa, FL 33602
(800) 749-2257
www.aakp.org

American Kidney Fund
6110 Executive Blvd., Ste. 1010
Rockville, MD 20852
(800) 638-8299
www.akfinc.org

American Nephrology Nurses Association
East Holly Ave., Box 56
Pitman, NJ 08071-0056
(856) 256-2320
(888) 600-ANNA (2662)
www.annanurse.org

General renal information:
www.medweb.emory.edu/MedWeb/

The National Association for Continence
P. O. Box 8310
Spartanburg, SC 29305
(800) 252-3337 (1-800-BLADDER)
www.nafc.org

National Institute of Diabetes & Digestive & Kidney Diseases
National Institutes of Health
31 Center Drive
MSC 2560
Bethesda, MD 20892
www.niddk.nih.gov

National Kidney Foundation
30 E. 33rd Street, Ste. 1102
New York, NY 10016
(800) 622-9010
www.kidney.org

National Kidney Foundation Enuresis Hotline
(800) 622-9010

Pediatric renal information:
www.mc.vanderbilt.edu/peds/pidl/nephro

United Network for Organ Sharing
1100 Boulders Pkwy., Ste. 500
P. O. Box 13770
Richmond, VA 23225
(804) 330-8500
(800) 894-6361
www.unos.org

CHAPTER 23

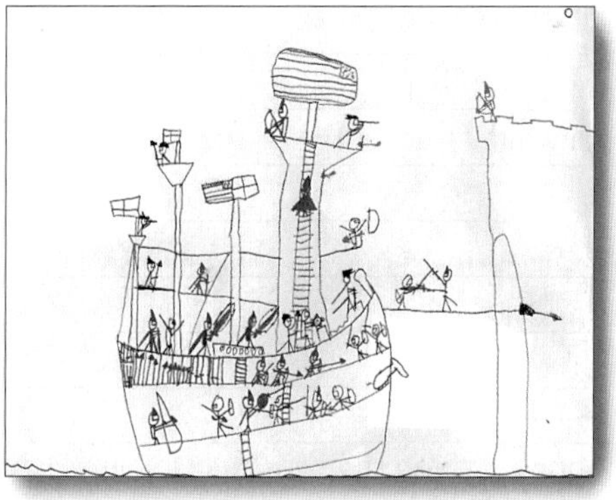

GASTROINTESTINAL ALTERATIONS

Nicki Potts, PhD, RN

The "horrible threes"! I thought my wife and I were prepared for this stage of our son trying to exert his independence. He is almost four years old and we thought he would be toilet trained by now. He does very well with urinating but he just will not "poop" in the toilet. He holds in the stool until he is in incredible pain. When he finally does go it is accompanied by pain as he strains to push the stool out. What we did not realize is that his holding in has led to the compounded problem of constipation.

COMPETENCIES

Upon completion of this chapter, the reader will be able to:

- *Describe the anatomy and physiology of the gastrointestinal (GI) system of the infant and child and how it differs from the adult GI system.*
- *Describe the etiology, pathophysiology, clinical manifestations, diagnosis, and treatment of common GI alterations.*
- *Explain how the pathophysiology is associated with the clinical manifestations of common GI alterations.*
- *Discuss nursing management and interventions appropriate for children requiring abdominal surgery for specific disorders.*
- *Identify the educational needs for families and describe appropriate content to be taught by the nurse.*

Alterations of the gastrointestinal system can involve the esophagus, stomach, small and large intestine or the accessory organs, the liver, gallbladder, and pancreas. The primary function of the system is ingestion, digestion, absorption of nutrients essential for normal growth and maintenance of fluid and electrolyte balance, and elimination of waste products. These functions are vital for normal growth and development of infants and children. Gastrointestinal complaints are common in this age group. Alterations of function can be expressions of congenital anatomic abnormalities or alterations acquired after birth from disease or infection. The severity of gastrointestinal problems ranges from minor illnesses causing inconvenience to severe, life-threatening disorders such as intestinal obstruction.

This chapter presents a discussion of the anatomy and physiology of the GI system and how it compares to the adult system and the most common GI alterations and disorders. These include upper and lower gastrointestinal alterations, alterations in motility, inflammatory disorders, malabsorption disorders, poisoning and hepatic disorders.

ANATOMY AND PHYSIOLOGY

In comparison with adults, the newborn has a very ineffective gastrointestinal system because of its immaturity at birth. Sucking and swallowing are automatic reflexes initially, gradually coming under voluntary control as the nerves and muscles develop by 6 weeks of age. The newborn's stomach capacity is only 10 to 20 ml, but expands rapidly to 200 ml by one month of age and reaches adult capacity of 2000–3000 ml by late adolescence. **Peristalsis,** the coordinated, rhythmic, serial contraction of the smooth muscle of the GI tract, is greater in the infant than in the older child. The emptying time of the stomach increases from 2 to 3 hours in the newborn to 3 to 6 hours by one to two months of age. These factors, the small stomach capacity, increased peristalsis, and increased stomach emptying rate, result in the need for small, frequent feedings. The infant's metabolic rate is faster than an adult's, thus requiring approximately 100 calories per kilogram of body weight compared with 30 to 40 for an adult. Regurgitation is common in the infant because the lower esophageal sphincter tone is decreased or relaxed.

The length of the small intestine is proportionately greater in an infant than an adult: six times the body length in infancy as opposed to four times the height of the adult. However, the infant's intestine is supplied with an adult's proportion of functional secretory glands per unit of area; therefore, an infant secretes proportionately more fluids and electrolytes into the intestine than does an adult. Similarly, the infant's small intestine has a larger surface for absorption relative to body size than does an adult's. Therefore, if diarrhea develops, more electrolytes will be lost from the intestinal secretions. In contrast, the large intestine of the infant is proportionately shorter than an adult's, resulting in less epithelial lining available for absorption of water from the feces. These two characteristics, more secretions and less absorption, are responsible for the soft, frequent stools of infants. Liver functions are also immature at birth; therefore, toxic substances are inefficiently detoxified and medications are inefficiently processed. Hence, the therapeutic dosage of drugs must be adjusted during the first few months of life to prevent them from reaching toxic levels. The processes of gluconeogenesis, deamination, plasma protein and ketone formation, and vitamin storage are immature during the infant's first year.

The infant is deficient in several digestive enzymes that are usually not sufficient until 4–6 months of age. The pancreatic enzyme *amylase,* responsible for the initial digestion of carbohydrates, is insufficient resulting in an intolerance of starches. If cereals are given before 4–6 months, the infant may develop gas and diarrhea. The enzyme *lactase* breaks down or hydrolyzes lactose, the primary source of carbohydrates in infant formula and breast milk. Lactase levels are low in the preterm infant, increase in infancy, and decline after early childhood. This initial decreased level results in incomplete absorption of lactose, which can cause gas, abdominal distention, and diarrhea. Digestion and absorption of fats is impaired because of low levels of the enzyme *lipase.* Fat in breast milk is absorbed more readily than in formula because human milk contains lipase. Protein digestion and absorption are fairly efficient in the newborn and infant. The infant intestine is more permeable to proteins than the older child or adult, thus allowing passage into the bloodstream of cow's milk protein and other potential allergens. Therefore, infants ingesting formula instead of breast milk are more susceptible to food protein allergens. Breastfed infants receive protective immunoglobulin proteins from human milk whereas formula-fed infants do not. Figure 23-1 illustrates the gastrointestinal tract of the child.

UPPER GASTROINTESTINAL ALTERATIONS

Upper gastrointestinal alterations commonly found in children include hypertrophic pyloric stenosis, cleft lip and cleft palate, and esophageal atresia and tracheoesophageal fistula.

Hypertrophic Pyloric Stenosis

Hypertropic pyloric stenosis (HPS) is the most common intra-abdominal condition requiring surgery during the neonatal period. Figure 23-2A illustrates a normal pyloric opening; Figure 23-2B shows pyloric stenosis.

Incidence and Etiology

HPS affects 1 to 3 per 1,000 live births and four to five times as many males as females. Caucasian males, especially first born, are the group most commonly affected. It is more common among Caucasians of Northern European ancestry, less common among African-Americans, and rare in Asians. The exact cause is not known; however, several theories have been proposed to explain the etiology. Environmental

REFLECTIONS FROM FAMILIES

My son, Robert, is three weeks old and had been healthy since he was born. I am breastfeeding him, and he feeds vigorously and has gained weight. All that changed two days ago when he began vomiting after every feeding. The vomiting has become more forceful, and it looks like curdled milk. He always seems hungry and eagerly sucks when I feed him. He feeds for about five minutes before he starts vomiting. He cried almost all night, and his diaper was dry this morning. I'm so upset and worried that something is seriously wrong with him. I feel so guilty because I can't console him for long. I can't even satisfy his hunger. What have I done to cause him to be so sick?

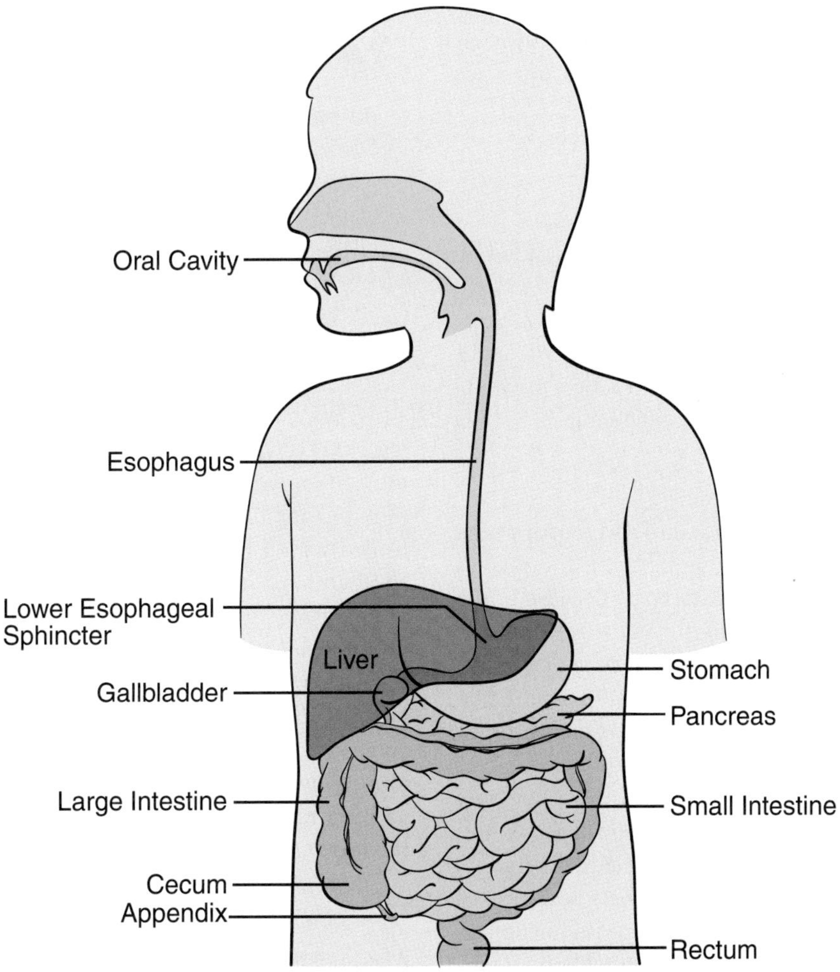

Figure 23-1 Gastrointestinal Tract of a Child

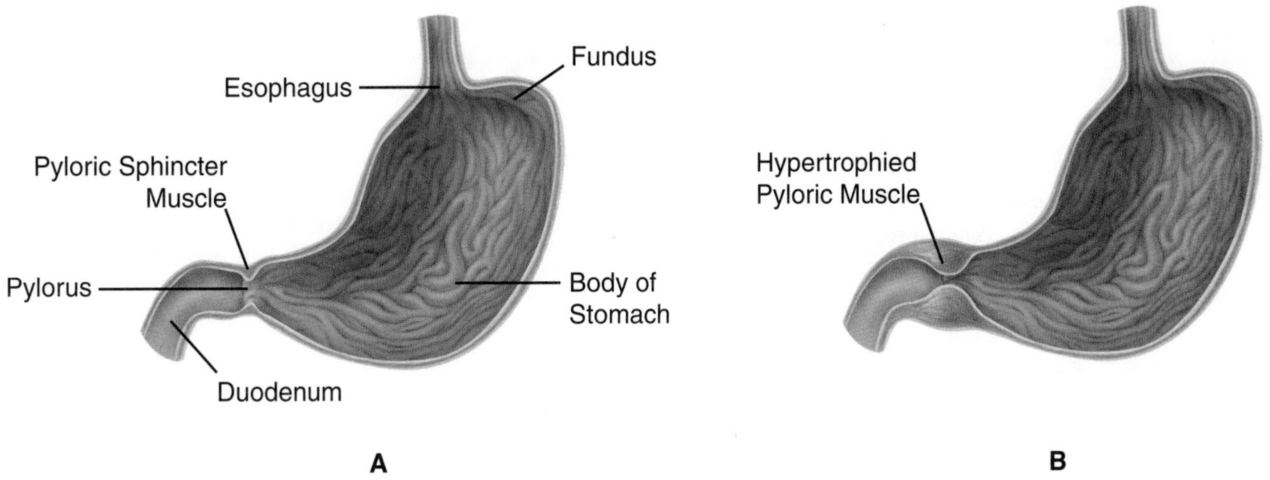

Figure 23-2 (A) Normal Pyloric Opening; (B) Pyloric Stenosis

factors, allergies, pylorospasm, and muscle enzymes are just a few of the unproven etiologies. Genetic predisposition seems to increase the risk of HPS (Cook, Lopez, & Manfredi, 1996).

Pathophysiology

The pylorus is the opening through which food passes from the stomach to the intestines. This opening is surrounded by a muscular ring, the pyloric sphincter. In HPS the pyloric sphincter hypertrophies and increases to four times its normal width, resulting in a narrowed opening and gastric outlet obstruction (Cook, et al., 1996). This obstruction prevents gastric contents from emptying into the duodenum.

Clinical Manifestations

Symptoms usually develop during the third and fourth weeks of life. Nonbilious vomiting beginning between the second and fourth week of life is the initial symptom. Because of the progressive nature of the obstruction, the vomiting increases in frequency and eventually becomes projectile with vomitus being propelled up to several feet. The emesis is not bile stained because the obstruction occurs above the outlet of the bile duct. The infant is hungry in spite of the vomiting and will usually feed again. Because food does not pass through the pylorus, bowel movements are small. As vomiting continues, there is loss of fluid, leading to dehydration, and hydrogen and chloride ions are lost, leading to hypochloremic metabolic alkalosis. Serum potassium levels are usually maintained, but there may be a total body potassium deficit. The infant has poor weight gain or experiences weight loss and becomes increasingly irritable and lethargic as dehydration and electrolyte imbalances worsen.

Diagnosis

Diagnosis may be made on history and physical identification of the hypertrophic pylorus, which can usually be palpated as an olive-shaped mass in the epigastrum, above and to the right of the umbilicus. If the olive-shaped mass is felt, the diagnosis is confirmed. However, in many cases the enlarged muscle cannot be felt and prompt diagnostic imaging is required for further evaluation. The diagnosis may be confirmed with a barium upper gastrointestinal (UGI) series or an abdominal ultrasound. The UGI, if positive, will reveal a delay in gastric emptying and a narrow, elongated pyloric channel, referred to as a "railroad track" sign (two narrow channels) or a "string sign" (one narrow channel). Ultrasonography is becoming the diagnostic method of choice because it is highly accurate (direct visualization of the muscle hypertrophy and the pyloric channel) and lacks the ionizing radiation inherent in a radiologic procedure such as the upper gastrointestinal contrast series (Deluca, 1993).

Nursing Alert:

Warning Signs of Hypertrophic Pyloric Stenosis

To prevent the infant from losing excessive fluid, nutrients, and calories, watch for early signs of HPS, which include:

1. The infant is hungry and wants to be fed again, in spite of feeding and vomiting.
2. The infant does not act or look sick.
3. The vomiting becomes more and more forceful, sometimes ejected several feet. This is the clue that it is structural in nature and not from other causes such as an infection.

Nursing Tip:

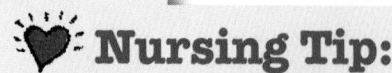

Palpating the olive-shaped mass

Successful palpation of the olive-shaped mass requires a relaxed abdominal musculature and an empty stomach. The abdominal muscles will relax by holding the infant, offering a bottle of warm sugar water, and elevating the baby's feet or flexing the knees and hips.

Treatment

A surgical procedure called a **pyloromyotomy** is the treatment of choice in which the circular muscle fibers are released opening the passage from the stomach into the duodenum. Preoperatively, a nasogastric (NG) tube may be inserted, and the stomach emptied. Fluid, acid-base, and electrolyte losses must be corrected for 24 to 48 hours before surgery. Intravenous fluids and electrolytes are administered until the infant is rehydrated and the serum bicarbonate concentrations are less than 30 mEq/dl, indicating that the alkalosis has been corrected.

Postoperatively, the NG tube should be removed, unless there is a reason to keep it in place, such as injury to or perforation of the duodenum. The blood glucose, electrolytes, and complete blood count (CBC) should be monitored. Intravenous glucose should be continued until the infant is able to feed normally. Gastric motility is delayed for up to 24 hours following anesthesia. Therefore, feeding should begin slowly and advance cautiously. The surgical treatment for HPS has a high success rate and is considered curative.

Nursing Management

Assessment

In the nursing history the relationship of feeding to vomiting is determined, and the frequency, color, and amount of emesis is documented. Strict intake and output records are essential to assess the status of the infant's hydration. Signs of dehydration are noted such as inelastic skin turgor, crying without tears, dry mucous membranes, a depressed anterior fontanel, urine output <1 cc/kg/hr, increased pulse, decreased blood pressure, and weight loss. The infant is observed for evidence of pain or discomfort, which does not occur except that of chronic hunger.

Nursing Diagnoses

Nursing diagnoses for the infant with HPS include:

1. Deficient fluid volume related to the effects of frequent vomiting.
2. Imbalanced nutrition: Less than body requirements related to vomiting and gradual reintroduction of feedings.
3. Pain related to surgical trauma.
4. Risk for infection related to surgical incision.
5. Deficient knowledge (caregivers) related to care of infant after discharge.

Outcome Identification

1. The infant will demonstrate improved fluid and electrolyte balance.
2. The infant will tolerate feedings and will demonstrate adequate nutrition by maintaining or regaining preadmission weight.
3. The infant will experience minimal postoperative pain.
4. The infant's surgical incision will remain free of infection as evidenced by decreased swelling without redness or purulent discharge.
5. Caregivers will verbalize an understanding of incision care, feeding techniques, and signs and symptoms of complications (recurrent vomiting, wound infection, failure to gain weight).

Planning/Implementation

Preoperative nursing care focuses on rehydration and correction of the electrolyte imbalance. Daily weights obtained at the same time of day using the same scale are the best indicator of extracellular deficient fluid volume. Because vomiting will continue until surgical correction, the infant is given nothing by mouth; thus, maintaining a patent intravenous infusion is essential. Monitoring the infusion, intake and output, and urine specific gravity are important nursing activities in fluid replacement. Family members need to be reminded to save diapers for weighing to measure urine output. If NG suction is used to decompress the stomach preoperatively, the nurse's responsibility is to maintain its patency and record the amount, color, and type of drainage. Laboratory data are assessed for electrolyte abnormalities. The nurse continually assesses the infant's hydration status.

Postoperative care includes maintaining fluid and electrolyte balance by (1) monitoring intravenous infusion until oral fluids are tolerated; (2) monitoring infant's response to feedings by mouth; and (3) assessing for signs of dehydration. Appropriate analgesics are given for pain. The incision site is monitored for signs of infection, such as redness, inflammation, purulent drainage, or temperature of 101°F or higher. Most surgeons remove the NG tube immediately after surgery and begin feeding within 4 to 6 hours if bowel sounds are normal. Initial feedings consist of small amounts of an electrolyte solution such as Pedialyte, and the volume is gradually increased. If greater volumes are tolerated without vomiting, formula or breast milk is offered. Most infants experience some vomiting in the first 24 to 36 hours after surgery; therefore, intravenous fluids are administered until full feedings are tolerated.

Evaluation

Evaluation of nursing care is based on how effectively the identified outcomes were met. When feedings are resumed, the infant should be able to tolerate feedings without vomiting, and weight should be gained to the pre-illness amount. The surgical incision should heal without signs of infection. The caregivers need to be able to demonstrate correct care of the incision, state plans for feeding and caring for the infant at home, and verbalize the signs and symptoms of complications and when to contact their health care provider.

Family Teaching

Caregivers often feel ineffective because their baby has been hungry and, yet, they have not been able to satisfy this hunger. They may believe they have done something wrong. Nurses can support them by explaining that they are not at fault and the condition is caused by a structural defect. They need to be encouraged to be involved in caring for the baby before and after surgery. Prior to surgery the infant is irritable, hungry, and cries often. Caregivers can be involved by holding, rocking, and cuddling their baby. A pacifier may satisfy the infant's sucking needs.

Nurses should instruct caregivers about the care of the incision (if any is required) and signs of infection. The infant's response to feedings should be observed. Vomiting may still be present; however, if it persists beyond 48 hours, the health care provider should be notified.

Cleft Lip (CL) and Cleft Palate (CP)

A cleft is a fissure or elongated opening. A cleft of the lip, palate, or both is one of the most common congenital anomalies of newborns. Most afflicted will have both cleft lip and palate; some have only a cleft of the lip and others only of the palate. Any type of cleft interferes with the development

Reflective Thinking

The Importance of Facial Attractiveness

The face is often viewed as a "reflection of the self." The birth of an infant with a cleft lip and palate brings to the forefront just how much facial attractiveness is valued. Not only must caregivers deal with questions, stares, and comments from others, but eventually they must answer the child's questions, "What happened to my face? Why don't I look like everyone else?" How would you respond if it was your child? What types of emotions would you feel?

of the normal anatomic structures of the lips, nose, muscles, and palate. The degree to which these structures are incomplete or malformed depends on the type, placement, and severity of the cleft(s).

Incidence and Etiology

The incidence of cleft lip and/or palate (CL/CP) is 1.5 in 1,000 births (Czeizel, Timar, & Sarkozi, 1999). The incidence is highest in Asians, followed by Caucasians, and is lowest in African-Americans. Clefts of the lip with or without cleft palate are more common in males, while clefts of the palate alone are more common in females.

Possible etiologies include genetic and environmental factors. If there is a family history of a cleft, the risk of other children also having a cleft is higher. Environmental factors have also been identified as a possible etiology of CL/CP including parental age, maternal intake of excessive alcohol, maternal drug exposure to phenytoin (Dilantin) or diazepam (Valium), and dietary factors such as folic acid and vitamin deficiencies.

Pathophysiology

The hard palate is the bony front part of the roof of the mouth. The soft palate lies behind the hard palate and is composed of muscle and fibrous tissue. The flap of mucosa that hangs down from the soft palate is the uvula. Cleft lip is caused by a failure of the nasal and maxillary processes to fuse between the 5th and 8th week of gestation. The lip and palate develop independently; therefore, it is possible to have either a cleft of the lip or the palate separately or together. Cleft palate is caused by the failure of the palatine plates to fuse between the 7th and 12th weeks of gestation.

Clinical Manifestations

Cleft lip can occur as either unilateral (only on one side) or bilateral (both sides) and can vary from a slight notch in the red portion of the lip to a complete separation extending into the nostril. Cleft palate can occur in the hard or bony palate and/or in the soft palate, with or without a cleft lip being present (Figures 23-3A and 23-3B).

Diagnosis

Cleft lip, and in most cases, cleft palate are obvious at birth. Even a small cleft of the palate can be detected by visual inspection and palpation. When cleft palate is not diagnosed at birth, formula coming from the nose may be the first sign. Both of these defects can be diagnosed in utero by ultrasound, and if present, the family will be referred to a multidisciplinary team at a cleft palate, craniofacial, or orofacial center.

Treatment

The treatment for a child with a cleft lip and palate is complex and involves many specialists, including a plastic surgeon, neurosurgeon, orthodontist, otolaryngologist, pediatrician, nurse, speech pathologist, and audiologist. Reconstruction begins in infancy and can continue through adulthood. Wide variations exist in the timing and technique for surgical repair. Closure of the lip is usually performed when the infant is approximately 3 months of age or 12 pounds. The goal of surgery is to close the cleft so scarring

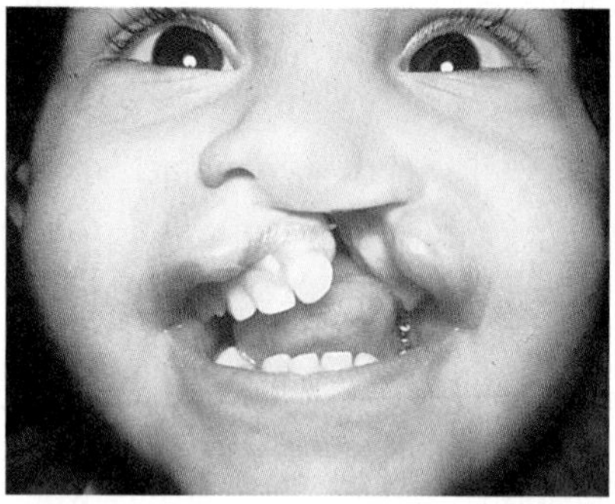

A

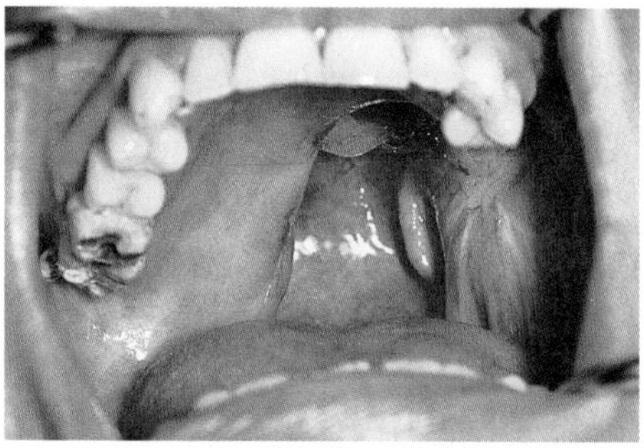

B

Figure 23-3 (A) Cleft Lip. Courtesy of Dr. Joseph Konzelman, School of Dentistry, Medical College of Georgia. (B) Cleft Palate. Courtesy of Dr. Joseph Konzelman, School of Dentistry, Medical College of Georgia.

will be minimal, and the face will have an increased chance to develop normally. Clefts of the hard and/or soft palate are surgically closed at approximately one year of age to assist feeding and to promote speech and language development. Additionally, good nutritional status and general health are essential factors influencing timing for surgery. Long-term consequences of cleft lip and palate may include speech difficulties, malocclusion problems (abnormal tooth eruption pattern), and hearing problems from recurrent otitis media caused by abnormalities of the eustachian tube.

Nursing Management

Assessment

A cleft of the lip and usually the palate are observable at birth. During the newborn assessment the nurse examines the palate by visualization and palpation with a gloved finger. A description of the location and extent of the defects is documented. The neonate's ability to suck, swallow, and feed are also noted. Nurses must also assess the caregiver's reactions as the birth of a baby with a cleft may be devastating.

Nursing Diagnoses

Nursing diagnoses for the infant with cleft lip and/or palate include:

Preoperative:

1. Imbalanced nutrition: Less than body requirements related to feeding difficulties.
2. Altered parenting related to interruption in the bonding process.

Postoperative:

3. Risk of injury and infection to the surgical site related to surgical procedure.
4. Pain related to surgical correction of clefts.
5. Deficient knowledge related to the condition, treatment, and long-term care.

Outcome Identification

1. Infant will consume adequate nutrients.
2. Caregivers will demonstrate feeding techniques that provide adequate nutrients.
3. Caregivers will begin to adjust and bond to their infant.
4. Infant will maintain optimum comfort.
5. Infant's incision will heal without disruption or infection.
6. Caregivers will verbalize understanding of treatment plan, feeding and restraint techniques, surgical site care, and need for possible later surgeries and speech therapy.

Planning/Implementation

Preoperatively, nursing care focuses on providing support for the caregivers, preventing aspiration and infection, and ensuring adequate nutrition. The birth of a child is usually a time of joy and celebration; however, the birth of a child with craniofacial anomaly has potentially devastating effects on a family. The initial reactions are shock, grief, feelings of isolation, feelings of failure or inadequacy. Shock is usually followed by anger, guilt, frustration, and depression. Caregivers may become preoccupied with the baby's appearance and experience negative feelings toward the infant, which may disrupt or delay attachment. Nurses working with these families must realize that these are normal reactions and that they can aid in the bonding process by demonstrating acceptance of the baby and by encouraging the caregivers to hold and touch their infant. Fears may be allayed by seeing before and after photographs of successful surgical repairs. Providing an opportunity to talk with other families who have a child with a cleft is also important. Agencies such as the Cleft Palate Foundation provide information and support for children and their families (see Resources).

Once the initial shock has been dealt with, the caregivers usually have many questions pertaining to the child's condition. The four most frequently asked are:

1. Why did this happen?
2. Is this hereditary?
3. What can be done? Can anything be done right away?
4. What about our baby's future? Will my child be normal?

Feeding problems, such as poor or inadequate suction, prolonged feeding time, frequent nasal regurgitation, and inadequate weight gain, can be a frustrating and exhausting experience for many caregivers. Early teaching by nurses about the anatomy and functioning of the palate and successful feeding techniques can decrease caregiver anxiety. When an infant sucks, the soft palate rises up closing off the nasopharynx from the oropharynx, thereby creating negative pressure. This mechanical vacuum draws liquid into the

> **Nursing Tip:**
>
> **Caring for families whose child has a cleft lip/palate**
>
> Help caregivers to understand this condition by explaining that:
>
> 1. Clefting occurs by the 35th day after conception, which is often before a woman knows she is pregnant.
> 2. The mother needs reassurance that she did nothing wrong during the pregnancy.
> 3. Many caregivers feel guilty about having a child with this disorder. Counsel caregivers appropriately.
> 4. Nothing is missing from their child's face. The pieces just need to be put together.

Nursing Tip:

Breast feeding an infant with a cleft lip/palate
The infant usually feeds best when the breast is full; therefore, teach the mother to place a warm washcloth on the breast to encourage the milk let-down prior to having the infant latch on.

mouth and delivers it to the back of the throat where it is swallowed.

Breastfeeding an infant with a CL/CP is one option for the mother. The infant with only a CL will probably have no more difficulty than other babies in achieving effective breastfeeding. The breast itself tends to fill the opening in the lip because it has the capacity to mold to the shape of the oral cavity. It may be possible to breastfeed an infant with both CL and CP; however, if this method is unsuccessful, a breast pump may be used to express the milk and bottle feeding with special nipples should be used.

If the method chosen is bottle feeding, it is important for caregivers to initially try a regular nipple and bottle as some infants with small clefts may feed satisfactorily without special adaptations. One method using readily available standard nipples and bottles that is inexpensive and convenient is the ***E***nlarge, ***S***timulate, ***S***wallow, and ***R***est (ESSR) method. Enlarging the nipple hole by making a cross cut allows the infant to receive formula in the back of the throat for swallowing, thus bypassing the sucking problem. The next step, stimulate, refers to stimulating the sucking reflex by rubbing the nipple on the lower lip. The nipple is inserted into the mouth, and then the bottle is inverted. The infant swallows the fluid normally. The last step is a rest.

Reflective Thinking

Caring for Children with Facial Disfigurement

To increase self-awareness about children with facial disfigurements, ask yourself:

1. How do I feel about caring for children with facial abnormalities?
2. Is my care affected by the child's appearance?
3. Do I unconsciously consider the disfigured child as less desirable?
4. Do I spend less time interacting with this child?
5. How can I ensure that children who have this anomaly receive the same quality health care as those who do not have this anomaly?

Shortly before infants choke or gag, their facial expression will signal a need for a short break to finish swallowing formula already in their mouth. The signal consists of elevating eyebrows and wrinkling of the forehead. The nipple should be removed slowly and gently from the mouth. Frequent burping is needed. These steps are repeated until the infant has consumed normal amounts of formula, 3 or 4 ounces, in a normal amount of time, 15 to 30 minutes (Richard, 1991). Figure 23-4 illustrates a cross-cut nipple.

If standard nipples are ineffective for feeding, a variety of special nipples, for example, soft, "preemie," or elongated, are commercially available. If the infant is unable to ingest adequate milk using any of these types of nipples, an asepto syringe with a rubber tip may be effective.

The major emphasis after surgery for cleft lip repair is the protection of the operative area. A small metal strip called a Logan bow or a butterfly adhesive may be placed over the upper lip and taped to the infant's cheeks to prevent tension on the suture line (Figure 23-5). The infant should be placed only on the back or side and arm or elbow restraints applied to prevent touching or pulling the site. These restraints should be removed periodically to exercise the arms (Figure 23-6). Adequate pain medication needs to be administered to minimize crying and stress on the suture line.

Evaluation

Evaluation is based on how effectively the outcomes of nursing management are met. The infant consumes adequate nutrients and gains weight along a normal growth curve. Caregivers demonstrate increased feelings of confidence with feeding techniques and routine. Caregivers begin to

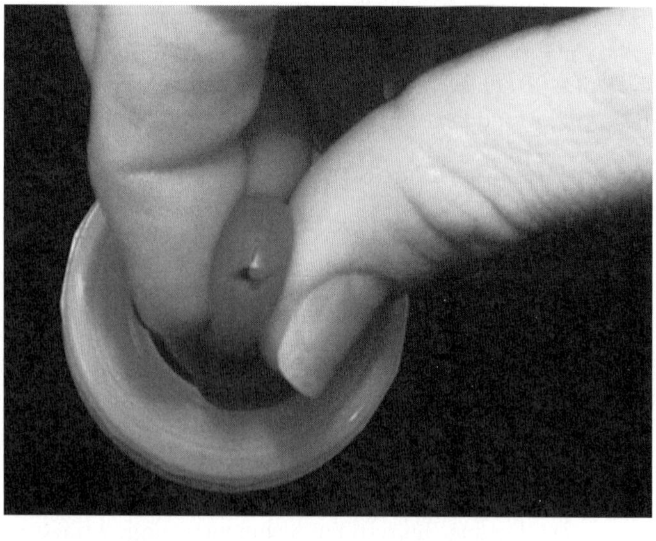

Figure 23-4 Cross-cut in Nipple. When the nipple is squeezed, the hole can be seen to have been enlarged slightly. From Golding-Kushner, K. J. (2001). *Therapy techniques for cleft palate, speech, & related disorders.* San Diego, CA: Singular Thomson Learning.

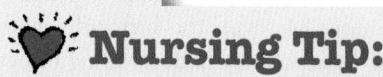

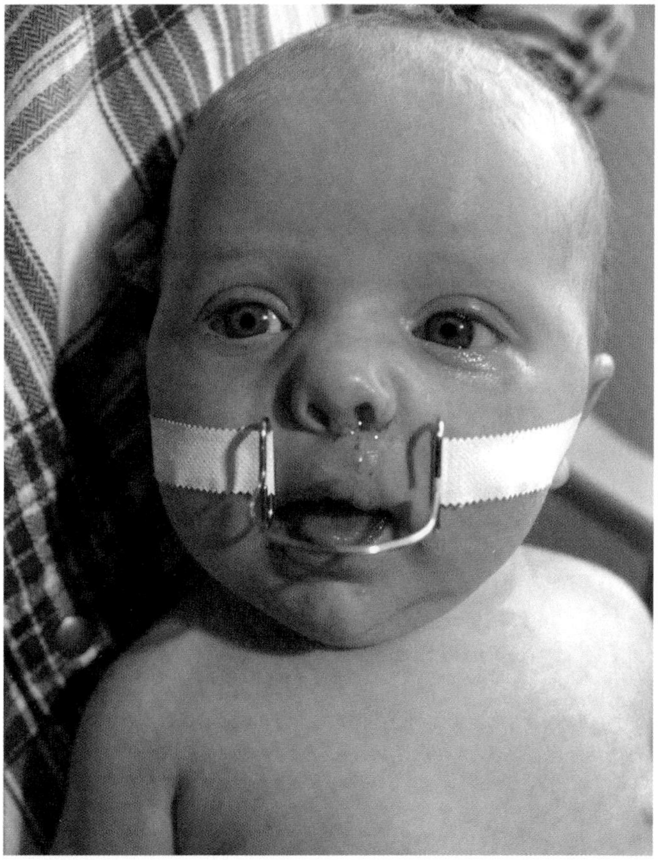

Figure 23-5 Infant with Logan Bow to Protect Suture Line After Repair of Unilateral Cleft Lip

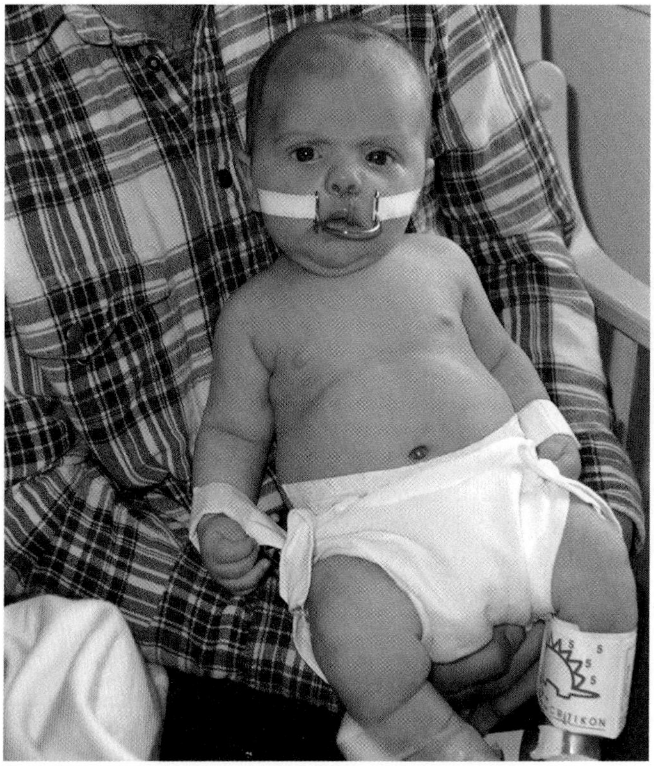

Figure 23-6 Infant with Arm Restraints to Prevent Injuring Operative Site

bond with their infant by stroking, touching, and nurturing appropriately. The infant appears content while resting and displays behaviors consistent with comfort. Caregivers verbalize understanding of CL/CP pathology, treatment plan, home care, and long-term care.

Family Teaching

Family teaching includes information about feeding techniques and care of the operative site. Nurses should instruct caregivers to clean the suture line after feeding and as necessary with cotton tipped applicators dipped in diluted hydrogen peroxide. Small amounts of water should be offered after feedings to rinse away any milk residue that could lead to bacterial growth. The elbow restraints should be removed one at a time several times each day for about 10 minutes. If the infant had a cleft lip repair, a side or back lying only position should be used. Nurses should discuss the possibility of additional surgeries on the lip, nose, and palate as the child grows and matures.

Esophageal Atresia and Tracheoesophageal Fistula

Esophageal atresia (EA) and tracheoesophageal fistula (TEF) are congenital defects of the esophagus. They can each occur as a single entity, but usually occur together. EA is characterized by incomplete formation of the esophagus so it terminates before reaching the stomach. It is usually associated with a fistula between the trachea and the esophagus (TEF). Many anatomic variations of EA with or without TEF have been described and are illustrated in Figure 23-7. The five types are (1) esophageal atresia with distal tracheoesophageal fistula (upper segment of the esophagus ends in a blind pouch; lower segment is connected to the trachea by a fistula) (87%); (2) isolated or pure esophageal atresia (blind pouch of upper and lower segments of the esophagus without a connection to the trachea) (8%); (3) tracheo-esophageal fistula without esophageal atresia (intact esophagus with fistula between the esophagus and trachea; "H-type") (4%); (4) esophageal atresia with proximal tracheoesophageal fistula (blind pouch at each end of the esophagus with a fistula from the trachea to upper segment of the esophagus) (<1%); (5) esophageal atresia with proximal and distal tracheoesophageal fistula (both upper and

Nursing Alert:

Avoiding Hard Objects in the Oral Cavity

Hard objects such as thermometers, tongue depressors, straws, and forks should not be allowed in the child's mouth until healing has adequately progressed after repair of a cleft palate.

Research Highlight

Short Stature in Children with Orofacial Clefts (Cleft Lip/Cleft Palate)

Study Purpose

To assess stature in children with orofacial clefting to determine whether this population is at risk for short stature. In subjects with growth failure (less than the 5th percentile in height), the purpose was to assess hypothalamic-pituitary function and ascertain whether growth failure or hypothalamic dysfunction was related to age, sex, or type of cleft.

Methods

Forty children, ranging in age from 3 to 12 years, with orofacial clefts were measured. Those who demonstrated growth failure were to have further evaluation to determine if hypothalamic-pituitary dysfunction was the cause of the short stature. Data were also collected on age, sex, and type of cleft.

Findings

The group of children with orofacial clefting contained significantly more individuals than expected whose heights were less than the 10th percentile for age and sex. Five children in this study were less than the 5th percentile for height. The parents of four of the five children with growth failure refused further evaluation. The one child who was evaluated had normal hypothalamic-pituitary function. Growth failure was not related to age or type of cleft; however, it was related to sex. More girls exhibited growth failure than boys.

Implications

The high rate of growth failure in this population emphasizes the need for nurses caring for these children to incorporate measurement of growth into their assessment. If growth failure is demonstrated, these children should be referred for evaluation of the etiology of their short stature. Additionally, all health care providers should monitor growth as a component of a child's assessment, regardless of the health care setting. Short stature should not be ignored or minimized in populations of children having other significant health care problems.

Citation

Lipman, T., Rezvani, I., Mitra, A., & Mastropieri, C. (1997). Assessment of stature in children with orofacial clefting. *Journal of Maternal Child Nursing, 24*(5), 252–256.

lower segments of esophagus connect to the trachea) (<1%) (Herbst, 1996).

Incidence and Etiology

Esophageal atresia with TEF occurs in 0.2 in 1,000 births, with an equal incidence in the sexes (Clark, 1999). The birth weight of infants with this anomaly is significantly lower than average. Esophageal atresia has been associated with prematurity. Associated congenital anomalies occur in approximately one-half of these infants. The presence and severity of these anomalies are thought to be the most important factor influencing mortality. Cardiac anomalies, such as ventricular septal defect, patent ductus arteriosus, and tetralogy of Fallot are encountered in approximately 30% of all cases. Refer to Chapter 25 for a discussion of these anomalies. Gastrointestinal anomalies including imperforate anus and malrotation may occur in 25% of these infants. Musculoskeletal defects are also common and include vertebral malformations. The acronym VACTERL has been used to describe the condition of multiple anomalies in infants with tracheoesophageal defects:

V—**V**ertebral defect

A—**A**norectal malformation

C—**C**ardiac defects

T—**T**racheoesophageal fistula

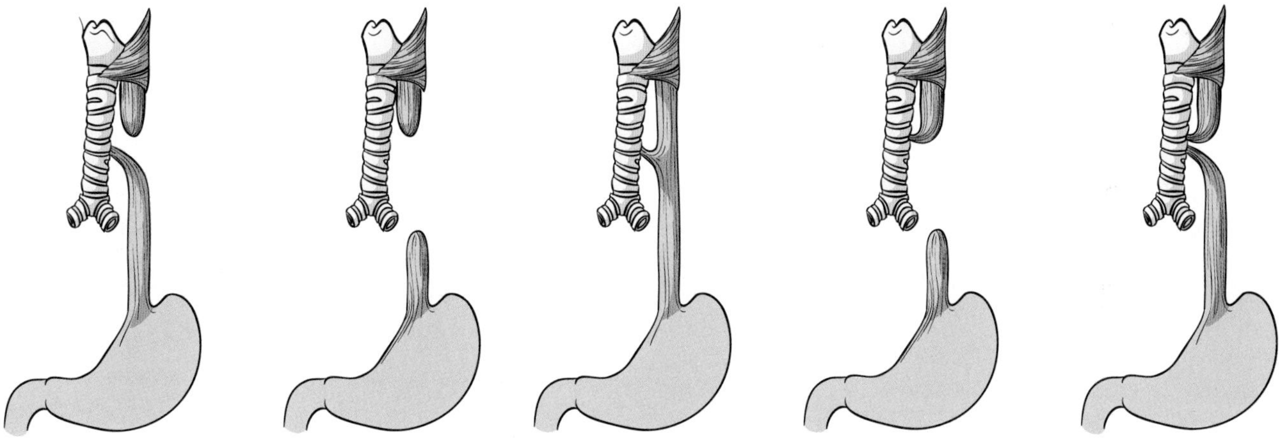

Figure 23-7 Types of Esophageal Atresia and Tracheoesophageal Fistula. (A) Esophageal atresia with distal tracheoesophageal fistula; (B) isolated or pure esophageal atresia; (C) tracheoesophageal fistula without esophageal atresia; (D) esophageal atresia with proximal tracheoesophageal fistula; and (E) esophageal atresia with proximal and distal tracheoesophageal fistula.

E—**E**sophageal atresia
R—**R**enal anomalies
L—**L**imb defects (Clark, 1999)

Pathophysiology

The esophagus and trachea derive from the common primitive foregut (embryonic digestive tube from which the pharynx, esophagus, stomach, and duodenum form) during the fourth and fifth weeks of embryonic development. This foregut lengthens and separates the esophagus from the trachea during the sixth to eighth week. EA and TEF are caused by defective separation. EA as an isolated anomaly occurs rarely. The atresia is attributable to failure of the recanalization of the esophagus.

Clinical Manifestations

Typically, the neonate with EA/TEF presents with copious, fine, frothy bubbles of mucus in the mouth and sometimes the nose. These secretions may clear with aggressive suctioning but eventually return. The infant may have rattling respirations and episodes of coughing, choking, and cyanosis. These episodes may be exaggerated during feeding. If a fistula between the esophagus and the trachea is present, abdominal distention develops as air builds up in the stomach.

Diagnosis

A history of maternal **polyhydramnios,** an excessive amount of amniotic fluid, should suggest the possibility of a high gastrointestinal obstruction, which prevents the fetus from swallowing and absorbing the fluid. The inability to identify the fetal stomach bubble on a prenatal sonogram in a mother with polyhydramnios makes the diagnosis of EA more likely. If it is suspected, after birth a radiopaque nasogastric or feeding tube should be passed through the nose to the stomach. In infants with atresia, the tube typically stops at 10–12 cm. The normal distance is 17 cm (Clark, 1999). The type of esophageal abnormality is further determined by radiographic studies. When present, curling of the tube in the upper esophageal segment is shown on radiography. If TEF is present, air will be seen in the stomach because of the connection between the esophagus and trachea. The absence of air in the stomach indicates EA without TEF.

Treatment

Before the performance of the first successful repair in 1939, this condition was fatal. However, over the past 50 years, refinements in neonatal surgical technique, preoperative support, anesthesia, and neonatal intensive care have improved the outcome (Clark, 1999). Treatment is aimed at preventing aspiration pneumonia until surgical repair of the defect is completed. Healthy infants without pulmonary complications or other major anomalies usually can undergo surgery in the first few days of life. The type of surgical correction depends on the esophageal abnormality. A one-stage repair to connect both ends of the esophagus and close the fistula is preferred in all infants with TEF.

Occasionally, the infant's condition (preterm, low birth weight, pneumonia, other major anomalies) requires that surgery be performed in stages. The first is closing of the fistula and inserting a gastrostomy tube for feeding. The second stage involves **anastomosis** (surgical connection of two tubular structures) of the two ends of the esophagus. Eight to ten days after this procedure, oral feedings are begun and usually tolerated.

Nursing Management

The goals preoperatively are prevention of aspiration of secretions from the upper esophageal pouch and prevention of regurgitation of stomach contents through the fistula into the trachea. Nursing care initially includes maintaining hydration status by allowing nothing by mouth and administering intravenous fluids. The infant is positioned with the head elevated to decrease pressure against the thoracic cavity and minimize reflux of gastric secretions into the trachea and bronchi. The patency of intermittent or continuous suction of the esophageal segment, if ordered before surgery, is essential.

In the postoperative period the nurse's goals are to maintain a patent airway and prevent trauma to the anastomosis. Suctioning must be performed gently to avoid trauma to the tissues to maintain the airway. The nurse observes the infant for early signs of airway obstruction, such as an anxious expression on the infant's face, tachypnea (increase in respiratory rate), and the presence of abnormal breath sounds. In the immediate postoperative period the gastrostomy tube is elevated to allow gastric secretions to flow into the small intestine and air to escape. A pacifier is offered to meet the infant's sucking needs and to prepare for oral feeding. The infant remains fluid restricted (NPO) until bowel sounds return and there is no danger of disturbing the surgical site. Nutrients are obtained through intravenous fluids. When the infant is begun on gastrostomy feedings, glucose water is given, and if tolerated, followed by formula or breast milk

Family Teaching

Infants who have the single-stage repair need to be observed for signs of esophageal stricture. The nurse explains and provides a written list of these and instructs the caregivers to contact their health care provider if any occur. Signs include dysphagia, inability or difficulty swallowing, increased drooling, and frequent coughing and choking that appear to be related to swallowing. The family of infants who require multiple stage surgery need to learn how to perform the necessary procedures for gastrostomy feeding and care and oral feeding.

LOWER GASTROINTESTINAL ALTERATIONS

Lower gastrointestinal alterations in infants and children include obstructive disorders in which nutrients and secretions are unable to pass through the GI tract, and elimination disorders. The alterations that will be presented include intussusception, Hirschsprung's disease, and anorectal malformations.

Intussusception

Intussusception is a common pediatric condition that occurs when one segment of the bowel telescopes into the lumen of an adjacent segment of intestine.

Incidence and Etiology

Intussusception is the most frequent cause of intestinal obstruction in infants and young children. The incidence is 1–4 in 1,000 live births with the peak in the third to ninth month of life and occurring two times more frequently in boys compared with girls (Birkhahn, Fiorini, & Gaeta, 1999). In most cases the cause cannot be identified. In a minority of cases, a specific lesion, such as a polyp or foreign body, or a viral infection can be identified as a possible trigger. Figure 23-8 illustrates intussusception.

Pathophysiology

As one segment of the bowel telescopes or invaginates into another, the walls of the bowel press against each other and compromise the blood and lymph flow. The involved intestine becomes inflamed and edematous and bleeding occurs resulting in blood and mucus in the stool. Eventually, complete bowel obstruction develops producing abdominal distention and vomiting. If untreated, it may progress to necrosis and perforation.

Clinical Manifestations

Four signs and symptoms are classically described in the infant with intussusception: colic, intermittent abdominal pain, vomiting, and currant jelly-like stools. However, these are present in fewer than one-half of infants with the disease

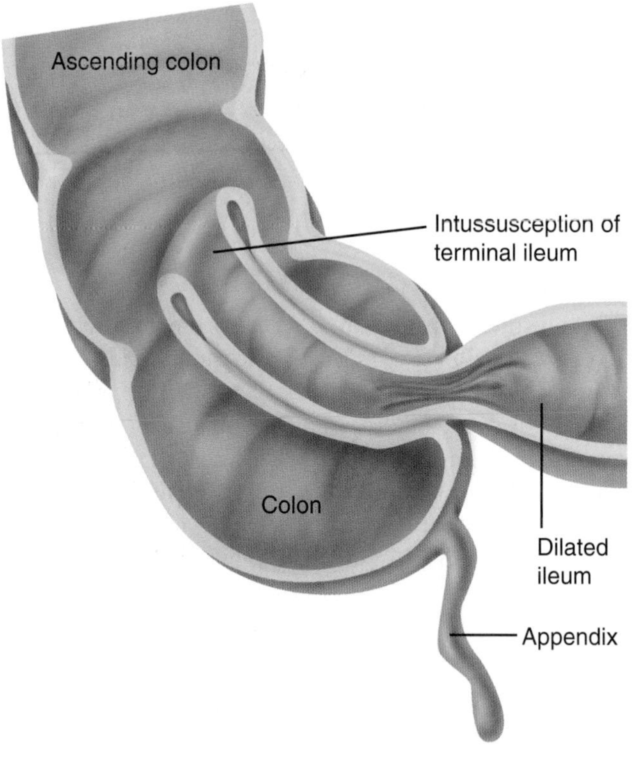

Figure 23-8 Intussusception of Terminal Ileum into the Ascending Colon

(Kuppermann, O'Dea, Pinckney, & Hoecker, 2000). Characteristically, a previously healthy, thriving infant has a sudden onset of severe and intermittent abdominal pain. Non-bilious vomiting is the predominate sign in neonates and is usually seen early in the illness. In the later phase the vomitus becomes bile stained. Blood and mucus appear in the stool, resulting in the red, currant jelly-like appearance. The abdomen is tender, and a sausage shaped mass may be felt in the right upper quadrant. As the intussusception progresses, the infant becomes listless and lethargic. Eventually a shock-like state may develop with a weak and thready pulse, shallow respirations, and a marked elevation of body temperature.

Diagnosis

An X ray of the abdomen is non-specific in the diagnosis; however, it will reveal intraperitoneal air if present, which indicates bowel perforation. The definitive test for diagnosing intussusception has been the barium or air contrast enema. Contrast enema is a safe procedure with minimal risk of bowel perforation. Nonetheless, it is invasive and presents the potential risk of radiation exposure. In addition, this test may be unnecessary if a less invasive technique can be used to accurately rule out intussusception. In recent years, abdominal ultrasound has been found to be a reliable and noninvasive screening tool for this disease (Harrington, et al., 1998).

Treatment

The treatment of choice for intussusception is non-surgical hydrostatic reduction using barium, a water-soluble contrast agent, or air enema. The water-soluble contrast and air **insufflation** (blowing air into a cavity) are believed to be safer than barium, with less risk of bowel perforation. Successful reduction rates have been reported as high as 90% for air and 65–85% for barium or the water-soluble contrast agent (Birkhahn, et al., 1999). If there is evidence of intestinal perforation, peritonitis, or shock or if hydrostatic reduction is unsuccessful, prompt surgical intervention is indicated to manually reduce the intussuscepted bowel.

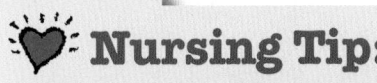

> **Nursing Tip:**
>
> **Helping families visualize intussusception**
> Comparing the anatomy of intussusception to a folding telescope may help caregivers and families understand the diagnosis. A rubber glove with one finger inverted into the glove can be used as a visual aid. To demonstrate the principle of reduction by hydrostatic pressure, fill the glove with water until the inverted finger resumes its normal position.

Nursing Management

Because the onset of this disorder is so abrupt, most caregivers need much reassurance regarding the effectiveness of treatment and excellent prognosis. Preparation for hydrostatic reduction involves placing the infant on NPO status, inserting a nasogastric tube that is connected to low suction, and administering intravenous fluids. The nurse monitors the infant's vital signs for changes that might indicate perforation, peritonitis, or shock, assesses for worsening abdominal pain, and examines and records all stools. The passage of normal stool may indicate spontaneous resolution of the obstruction. For a few hours after reduction, the child should remain in the hospital and be observed for the passage of stool and barium or water-soluble contrast, as indicated, and for the recurrence of the intussusception. Recurrence develops in about 10% of children following hydrostatic reduction. If hydrostatic reduction is unsuccessful, surgical treatment is indicated. For the child undergoing surgery, postoperative care is similar to that described in the nursing care plan for a child having an appendectomy.

Family Teaching

When the child is discharged, the nurse should instruct the caregivers to observe for signs of intestinal obstruction and recurrence. These include increasing abdominal pain, abdominal distention, blood in the stools, bile stained vomiting, and decreased or absent stools, all of which should be reported to their health care provider.

Hirschsprung's Disease

Hirschsprung's disease (HD), also called congenital aganglionic megacolon, is a motility disorder of the bowel caused by the absence of parasympathetic ganglion cells in the large intestine. This absence prevents peristalsis and causes feces to accumulate proximal to the defect, leading to bowel obstruction. It is the most common cause of distal bowel obstruction in the newborn; however, it may not be diagnosed until infancy or childhood.

Incidence and Etiology

The incidence is 0.2 in 1,000 live births, with males affected three to four times more often than females; the racial distribution is equal. HD is not a hereditary condition, but an inherited predisposition is relatively strong. A family history can be obtained in about 7% of cases, and the incidence in siblings is about 3.5% (Rudolph & Benaroch, 1995). Other associated congenital anomalies include imperforate anus, urinary tract abnormalities, cardiac defects, seizure disorders, and Down syndrome (Quinn & Shannon, 1996).

Pathophysiology

The disease is caused by an absence of parasympathetic ganglion cells in the colon. The aganglionic segment is most frequently located in the rectosigmoid area. Defecation is controlled by the parasympathetic nervous system (the ganglion cells), to which the lower colon, the internal and external anal sphincters, and the anus respond in a coordinated manner. The affected bowel (absence of ganglion cells) is unable to transmit coordinated peristaltic waves and to pass fecal contents along its length, resulting in an accumulation of fecal material and distention proximal to the defect. The normal portion of the bowel becomes hypertrophied and dilated, hence, the name megacolon (Allen, 1995). Figure 23-9 illustrates the bowel in HD.

Clinical Manifestations

In the newborn the primary manifestations are failure to pass **meconium** (the first feces of the newborn) within 24 to 48 hours after birth, abdominal distention, bile stained vomitus, refusal to feed, and intestinal obstruction. In older infants and children, the initial symptom is chronic constipation. Abdominal distention, episodes of explosive passage of stools, inadequate weight gain, ribbon-like or pellet shaped, foul-smelling stools, vomiting, and an easily palpable fecal mass are also present.

The most ominous presentation is **enterocolitis,** inflammation of the small intestine and colon. An otherwise well infant who has a history of constipation has an abrupt onset of foul-smelling diarrhea, abdominal distention, and fever. The illness may progress rapidly, with perforation of the bowel and sepsis, and may occur before, during, or after surgery. Enterocolitis and sepsis remain the major causes of death in HD, occurring in about 30% of cases (Rudolph & Benaroch, 1995).

Diagnosis

Hirschsprung's disease is diagnosed in 15% of infants within the first month of life, in 60% by the third month, and in 80% by 1 year of age (Rudolph & Benaroch, 1995). It can present with symptoms varying from complete intestinal obstruction with enterocolitis to simple constipation. In the neonate who does not pass meconium and has abdominal distention the diagnosis of HD is suspected. In older infants and children a history of chronic constipation should raise the question of HD. A rectal examination reveals the absence of stool in the rectum, and the internal anal sphincter is tight. A barium enema documents a transition zone between the narrowed aganglionic segment of the colon and the dilated, hypertrophied section. This sign may be absent in the first few weeks of life because it takes some time for normal ganglionic bowel to dilate with stool; therefore, the barium enema may not be diagnostic in newborns. For a definitive diagnosis, a rectal biopsy is required. The absence of ganglionic cells in the tissue confirms the diagnosis.

Treatment

The surgical treatment is usually performed as a two-stage procedure. In the first stage a temporary colostomy is created in the normal bowel. The purpose of the colostomy is to provide a means for the infant to defecate, to allow the bowel to rest and the infant to gain weight (Figure 23-10).

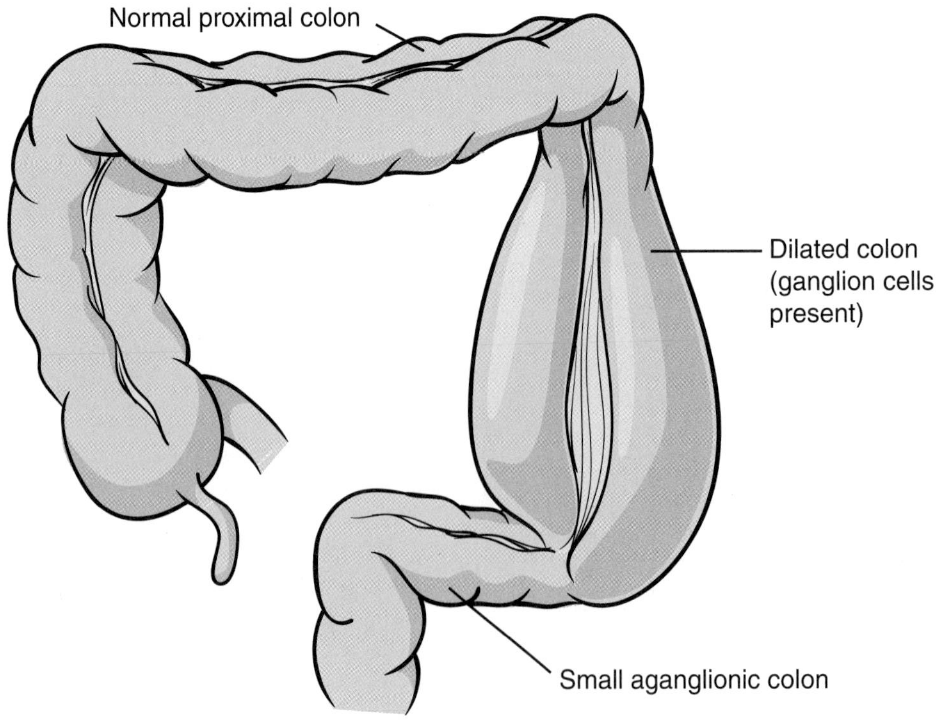

Figure 23-9 Hirschsprung's Disease with Dilation of the Colon Proximal to the Aganglionic Section

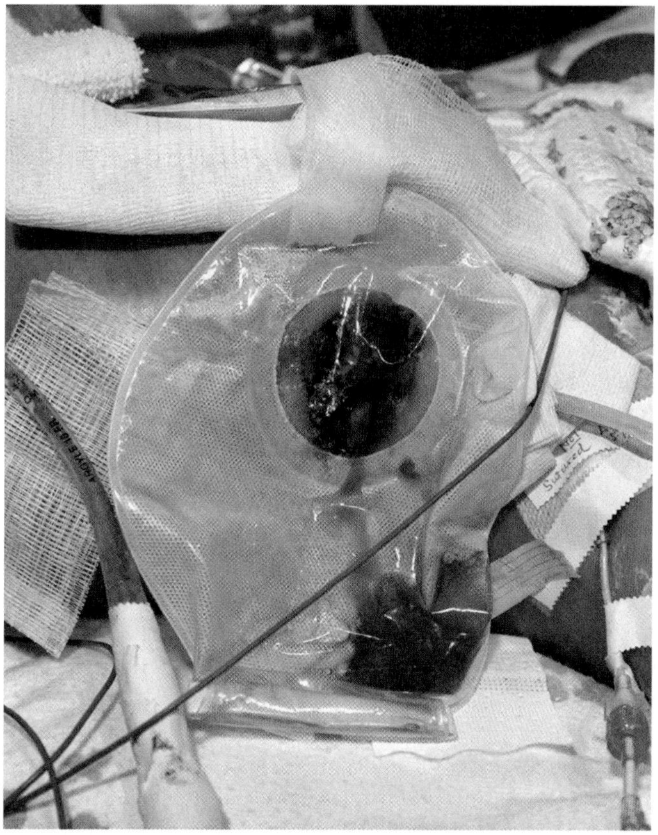

Figure 23-10 Child with Colostomy After the First Stage of Surgical Repair of Hirschsprung's Disease

The second stage involves a pull-through procedure in which the affected, aganglionic segment is resected or removed and normal bowel is anastomosed to the rectum. The temporary colostomy is also closed at this time. This definitive surgical repair is performed when the infant is between 6 and 15 months of age or weighs between 18 and 20 pounds (George, Hammes, & Schwartz, 1995).

In recent years, the treatment has been changing from a two-stage surgical repair to a one-stage pull-through without a temporary colostomy with excellent results. The timing of the definitive procedure also has been changing from approximately 12 months to early neonatal surgery. Benefits of the one-stage correction include avoidance of multiple operations, reduction in the number of hospital admissions and the cost of treatment, elimination of the problems in colostomy care, and completion of treatment at an earlier age (Ramesh, Ramanujam, Yik, & Goh, 1999).

Another advancement in the treatment is a procedure called the laparoscopic-assisted pull-through. The laparoscope allows surgeons to enter the child's body through the anus and pull the affected segment of bowel through the opening, thereby eliminating major abdominal surgery. Because the laparoscope only requires a few small incisions, the length of hospital stay is decreased, the scar is minimal, and complications are fewer (Ramesh, et al., 1999).

Nursing Management

Preoperative assessment of the infant's fluid and electrolyte status is essential because preparation for surgery involves extensive bowel cleansing with repeated saline enemas. The infant is NPO, and an NG tube is inserted. Intravenous fluids and electrolytes are administered to prevent dehydration and correct electrolyte deficiencies if they occur. Oral administration of antibiotics may be ordered in conjunction with antibiotic enemas to reduce intestinal flora.

Postoperative nursing care includes routine post-abdominal surgery interventions, such as maintaining patency of the NG tube, monitoring for abdominal distention, and assessing for return of bowel sounds. The nurse measures and records the amount of colostomy and NG drainage. An enterostomal therapist (ET) fits the ostomy with an appropriate appliance and begins education with the family about colostomy care.

Family Teaching

The nurse explains to the caregivers about the need for the surgery and the temporary colostomy and how to care for it. Instructions include skin care, appliance application, and information about community resources for obtaining supplies. Referral to an ET is important for assistance if problems occur with the appliance or stoma. The nurse teaches the family signs and symptoms of complications such as enterocolitis and leaks or strictures at the site of the anastomosis. Signs of leaks are abdominal distention and irritability, and signs of strictures are constipation, vomiting or diarrhea. These indications of complications should be reported to their health care provider. Families will usually require encouragement, understanding, and support, especially with the idea of the colostomy. They should be informed that with proper management their child can return to a normal lifestyle in a short time.

Anorectal Malformations

Anorectal malformations are defined as an arrest of rectal descent resulting in absence of an anal opening and occur during the 4th–16th week of gestation. Examples of these malformations include anorectal agenisis (imperforate anus), rectal atresia, and anal agenesis.

Incidence and Etiology

Anorectal malformations occur in 0.2 in 1,000 live births and are more common in males. The etiology is unknown; however, these defects are associated with several other congenital anomalies of the urinary tract, esophagus, and intestines.

Pathophysiology

The origin of the anus and rectum is an embryonic structure called the cloaca, which is the precursor of the anorectal and genitourinary structures. Both the rectum and the urinary structures become completely separated by the 7th week of gestation. Any abnormality in the development of these systems results in anorectal and genitourinary malformations. Depending on the week of gestation when the embryonic development is disrupted and on the level to which the rectal pouch has descended, the anomaly will be either low or high. Low malformations occur between the 10th and 12th week; high ones occur during the 4th week. In low anomalies the rectal pouch has descended below the rectal sphincter muscle complex. For rectal continence to occur the rectum must descend to this point. In high defects the rectum terminates above the sphincter muscle complex, making continence more difficult to establish (Quinn & Shannon, 1996).

Clinical Manifestations

Anorectal malformations are usually obvious at birth. Low defects vary from a normal appearing anus, to a thin translucent anal membrane, to a deep anal dimple. The anal dimple will demonstrate strong muscular contractions when pricked with a pin. High defects present as a flat perineum, absence of an anal dimple, and no muscular contraction to a pin prick. If meconium is noted in the urine, a fistula is present between the bowel and the urinary tract.

Diagnosis

Diagnosis is made by physical exam of the anal features and by radiologic imaging of the abdomen. The level of the defect and presence and location of any fistulas are determined by these tests. During the abdominal X rays the neonate is held in an inverted position for a few minutes to allow air to fill the blind colonic pouch and permit identification of the level of the defect. The presence of gas in the bladder or urethra during imaging indicates a fistula between these structures and the bowel.

Treatment

Treatment depends on the extent of the malformation. Anal stenosis is managed with repeated manual dilatation of the anus. All other defects require surgery. Low defects are corrected by creating an anal opening, followed by anal dilation to prevent stenosis. High malformations are treated with a two-stage repair, the first involving creation of a temporary colostomy. The second stage includes closure of the colostomy and a pull-through procedure in which the blind pouch of the rectum is anastomosed to the anus (Quinn & Shannon, 1996).

Nursing Management

During the newborn examination, the nurse assesses the patency of the anus by inserting a rectal thermometer. The defect is obvious when there is an absence of a normal anal opening. Nursing observations that should be documented and reported include failure of the neonate to pass meconium within the first 24 hours of life, inability to insert a rectal thermometer, and the presence of an anal dimple. Nursing care depends on the type of lesion corrected. For low defects with the anoplasty, the main focus is on preventing infection of the perineal and anal wounds. Because of the location of the surgical incisions, they are at high risk for infection from urine and stool; therefore, meticulous skin care is essential. For high lesions, postoperative care initially includes colostomy care, perineal wound care, IV fluid management, and NG tube maintenance. Oral feedings are begun when stooling has started through the stoma. Oral feedings following the pull-through are begun when peristalsis resumes, stooling occurs through the anus, and initial healing has taken place.

Family Teaching

Caregivers are instructed in colostomy care, perineal wound care, and anal dilations as appropriate. Prevention of constipation is stressed in family education. Adequate fluid, dietary fiber, and stool softeners or bulk agents help the child to achieve normal bowel activity. It is important to advise caregivers that toilet training may be delayed and children may have difficulty with this developmental task. Their patience and understanding of their child is essential. Encouraging the family and child during this stressful time is a key nursing intervention.

ALTERATIONS IN MOTILITY

Disorders discussed in this section include gastroesophageal reflux and constipation.

Gastroesophageal Reflux

Gastroesophageal reflux (GER) is the most common esophageal disorder of infants and the most frequently referred condition to a pediatric gastroenterologist (Orenstein, Izadnia, & Khan, 1999). GER is defined as the return of gastric contents into the lower esophagus through the lower esophageal sphincter (LES). The LES is a distinct area formed by the union of the muscle fibers from the esophagus and stomach (Figure 23-11).

Physiological GER is a common occurrence in many healthy infants. Improvement is usually seen between 6 and 12 months of age as the infant matures. The esophagus elongates and the LES moves down below the diaphragm decreasing the chance of reflux. Pathologic GER is reflux that manifests as respiratory disorders, esophagitis or its complication (strictures), and malnutrition.

Incidence and Etiology

GER is known to occur in 5 in 1,000 live births. Boys are affected 3 times more frequently than girls. GER is more

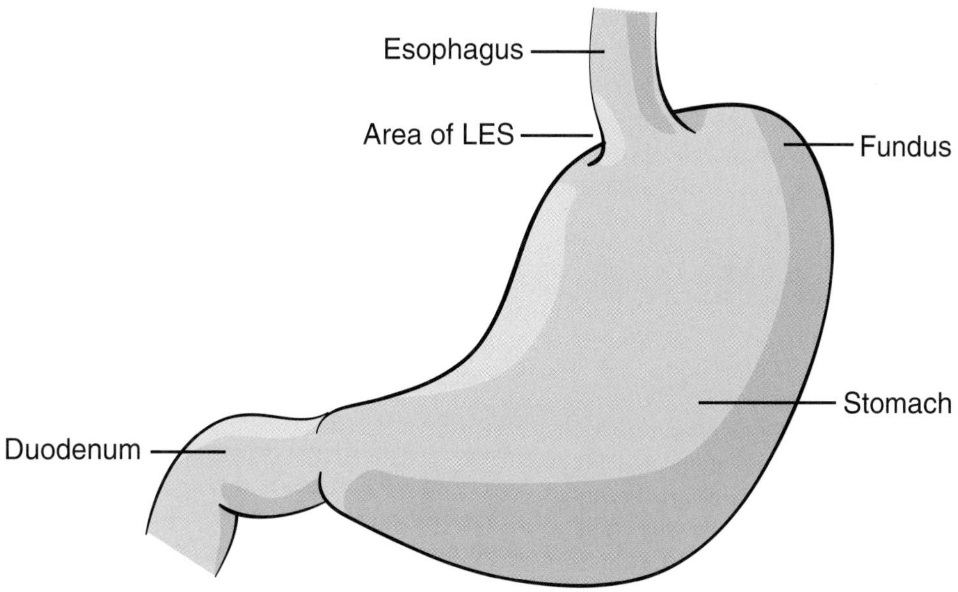

Figure 23-11 Stomach contents are refluxed into the esophagus through the lower esophageal sphincter (LES) in GER.

common in premature infants and those with neurologic impairment. The exact cause is unknown although it is thought to result from the delayed maturation of the lower esophageal neuromuscular function or impaired local hormonal control mechanisms.

Pathophysiology

The LES acts as a physiological barrier to reflux of stomach contents into the esophagus. It is innervated by the vagal nerves, so a defect in this nerve transmission may result in inappropriate relaxation of the LES. This allows the reflux of gastric contents into the esophagus. Delayed gastric emptying also occurs in infants caused by hypomotility or retrograde peristalsis of the duodenum (Ault & Schmidt, 1998).

Clinical Manifestations

Vomiting and regurgitation are the most common symptoms. The regurgitated matter is typically non-bilious and consists of undigested formula and mucus. The infant displays excessive crying and irritability from esophagitis, which is caused by recurrent reflux of acidic gastric contents into the esophagus. Refusal to feed may develop in infants with esophagitis as they learn to associate feeding with pain. Esophagitis can cause bleeding in the gastrointestinal tract, which produces anemia and is seen as blood in the stools. Insufficient caloric intake resulting from caregivers' hesitancy to feed infants who are repeatedly spitting up and nutrient losses in emesis contribute to malnourishment. Complications of GER include apnea, choking spells, recurrent aspiration pneumonia, and frequent respiratory infections.

Critical Thinking

What's the Difference Between Gastroesophageal Reflux and Hypertrophic Pyloric Stenosis?

Vomiting is a classic symptom of GER and HPS. Based on the clinical manifestations of each disorder, how would you distinguish between the two?

Diagnosis

The diagnosis of GER is established by taking a history, performing a physical examination, observing the infant's feeding habits, and conducting several diagnostic tests. The first goal is to rule out other possible causes for the symptoms such as gastrointestinal tract obstructions, neurologic disease, or metabolic disorders. Several diagnostic tests exist to help confirm GER. Initially an upper GI barium series is performed to eliminate anatomic abnormalities (esophageal stricture, pyloric stenosis, and intestinal malrotation) from consideration. Upper GI endoscopy allows direct visualization of the esophageal mucosa to detect inflammation and ulceration, which are indicative of esophagitis. Another test is the esophageal pH probe study. A small catheter is placed through a nostril into the distal third of the esophagus and is left in place for 18 to 24 hours. It measures the pH of the distal esophagus, indicating the number of reflux episodes and the time it takes for acid to clear from the esophagus. Although a sensitive test, the pH probe is not needed for routine diagnosis. Because of the cost and the need for hospitalization, this test is best used for infants who have complicated courses or who present diagnostic dilemmas.

Treatment

Medical management involves dietary modifications, positioning, and medications. Small, frequent feedings are recommended because of the probable relationship between gastric volume and reflux. This feeding method decreases the duration of reflux episodes. However, increased frequency causes more frequent stimulation of stomach acids. Therefore, the advantages must be weighed against the disadvantages. Many infants have benefited from this traditional approach. Another dietary adjustment that is recommended is the thickening of formula with cereal. This approach has major benefits for the regurgitating infant, particularly when there has been poor weight gain. These include increased caloric density, decreased time spent crying, and decreased episodes of emesis.

Controversy surrounds positioning therapy in the medical treatment for GER. Recommendations for positioning have changed from the upright or seated position prior to the early 1980s, to the 30 degrees prone or head elevated prone in the middle 1980s, to the flat prone in the early 1990s (Orenstein, 1990). One aspect of the controversy involves positioning to prevent sudden infant death syndrome (SIDS). The American Academy of Pediatrics (1996) recommends that infants be placed in the supine (on their back) position for sleep. Most of the SIDS deaths in the prone position are attributable to suffocation because of puffy bedding materials, such as comforters. If these materials are eliminated from the infant's bed, the superiority of the prone position for GER is clear and has been recommended by the American Academy of Pediatrics (Orenstein, et al., 1999). Currently either the flat prone or head elevated prone position is suggested for infants with GER.

Medications may also be used to treat GER. Antacids act to buffer existing gastric acids that may irritate the esophageal mucosa. Adverse effects of antacids include diarrhea (with magnesium based products, Mylanta) and constipation (with aluminum based products, Amphogel). Prokinetic drugs are often used before acid suppression therapy in infants who have no evidence of esophagitis. Prokinetic agents increase gastric motility and LES pressure, and enhance gastric emptying. Cisapride (Propulsid) has become the first choice prokinetic for infants because of its minimal side effects such as transient diarrhea and increased psychomotor activity. Metoclopramide (Reglan), also a prokinetic, has the same action as cisapride; however, its adverse side effects are common and include restlessness, insomnia, and extrapyramidal movements. Acid suppression medications are added if esophagitis is suspected or demonstrated. This action is achieved with histamine-2 receptor antagonists such as cimetidine (Tagamet) or ranitidine (Zantac). There are few adverse effects with these medications, primarily diarrhea or constipation, headache, and rash. Some infants likely to require the more complete acid suppression achievable with proton-pump inhibitors are those with chronic respiratory disease (cystic fibrosis, steroid-dependent asthma), or neurologic disabilities (cerebral palsy). Omeprazole (Prilosec) has minimal side effects that are similar to those of H-2 receptor antagonists.

The role of surgical treatment has decreased as pharmacotherapy has improved. Repeated episodes of pneumonia, failure to gain weight, recurrent esophagitis with stricture, severe apnea, and failure to respond to 4 to 6 weeks of medical management are indications for surgery. The Nissen fundoplication in which the fundus of the stomach is wrapped around the lower part of the esophagus is the procedure of choice. A temporary gastrostomy tube may be inserted to allow for venting of the stomach and initial feedings. The success rate with surgery is high, but recurrences are common. Less invasive fundoplication performed laparoscopically is available in a limited number of hospitals.

Nursing Management

Assessment

An in-depth assessment of the infant's feeding pattern should include the amount, type, and frequency of feedings, and the timing of emesis afterwards. The nurse inquires about the positioning of the infant during feeding and the frequency of burping. It is important to obtain height, weight, and head circumference measurements and to plot them on a growth chart to assess current and potential growth problems. Infants with GER are at high risk for aspiration; therefore, assessment of a baseline respiratory status is imperative, such as lung sounds, respiratory rate, and effort.

Nursing Diagnoses

1. Risk for aspiration related to vomiting and reflux of gastric contents into the esophagus
2. Imbalanced nutrition: Less than body requirements related to reduced nutrient intake and vomiting
3. Deficient knowledge related to infant's condition and care including feeding, positioning, and home management

Outcome Identification

1. Infant maintains normal respiratory status (respiratory rate appropriate for age, oxygen saturation within normal limits, clear, bilateral breath sounds).
2. Infant will maintain normal growth pattern and will ingest adequate number of calories.

3. Caregivers will verbalize and/or demonstrate understanding of GER, feeding and positioning of infant, and home care.

Planning/Implementation

Nursing management focuses on caregiver education including dietary modifications, positioning, medication administration, and developmental needs of the infant, and on peri-operative care if surgery is performed. Dietary modifications include small, frequent feedings, thickened feedings, and avoidance of foods that irritate the GI tract. Small, frequent feedings can cause additional stress on caregivers; therefore, they need to know that higher volume and less frequent feedings can be tolerated as the infant grows. The infant should be burped frequently during feeding. Thickening of formula with rice cereal increases consistency and retention, and supplies needed calories for the infant who vomits frequently. If the health care provider has recommended the head elevated prone position after feedings and during sleep, maintaining this can be challenging for caregivers. This position can be achieved by using a wedge, sling, harness, and towel rolls, some of which are commercially available.

Nursing interventions related to the treatment of GER with pharmacotherapy include caregiver education about dosages, proper administration and scheduling, and potential side effects. Verbal information should be augmented by written material to assure proper understanding. The nurse can support the caregivers by encouraging them to identify and verbalize their fears and concerns. They often feel guilt and inadequacy because of the frequent vomiting of feedings and weight loss of the infant. They may feel overwhelmed with doubt and anxiety about their ability to adequately care for the child. Nurses can be instrumental in forming a network of caregivers of children with GER to provide support, share experiences, and foster confidence.

Evaluation

The effectiveness of the nursing interventions is evaluated by the infant experiencing no respiratory difficulty or aspiration. A decrease in the frequency of vomiting and improvement in growth and development are also evaluated. Most important is the caregivers' comfort with the diagnosis, treatment plan, and their confidence in being able to care for the infant at home.

Nursing Alert:

Infant Seats for Positioning

Infants with GER should not be placed in an infant seat as a mode of treatment. The reduced truncal tone in infants raises their intra-abdominal pressure and actually promotes reflux.

Family Teaching

Family teaching includes an explanation of the physiology of GER so caregivers understand their feeding technique is not the cause of the frequent vomiting. In order to accommodate the thickened feedings, the nurse should demonstrate how to enlarge the hole in the nipple. Caregivers need information about spicy and acidic foods and beverages to avoid feeding their infant because they increase secretion of gastric acid. These include citrus fruits and fruit drinks and tomato products such as tomato juice. Esophageal irritants such as chocolate and caffeine (tea, coffee, and colas) for older infants and children should also be avoided. Because of the infant's limited mobility, adequate stimulation becomes essential. Bright and colorful objects, wrist rattles, mobiles, and mirrors are all appropriate. Touching and stroking the infant provide tactile stimulation. Family teaching should also include an explanation about avoiding vigorous playing with their infant after feeding to prevent reflux.

Constipation

Constipation is the difficult passage of stool or infrequent passage of hard stool, associated with straining, abdominal pain, or withholding behaviors. Children vary widely in the frequency with which they have a bowel movement; therefore, frequency alone is not a good diagnostic criterion.

Incidence and Etiology

Constipation is common in children, accounting for 3% of office visits to pediatricians and 25% of pediatric gastroenterologist's visits (Van der Plas, et al., 1996). It is more common in males during early childhood; however, during adolescence it is seen more frequently in females. The cause of constipation can be organic or non-organic, also called functional. Organic causes include:

1. Dietary (e.g., low fiber, inadequate fluid intake, excessive dairy intake)
2. Structural disorders of the gastrointestinal tract (e.g., Hirschsprung's disease, intestinal strictures)
3. Metabolic and endocrine disorders (e.g., hypothyroidism, diabetes mellitus, lead poisoning)
4. Neurogenic diseases (e.g., cerebral palsy, myelo meningocele)
5. Medications (e.g., opiates, antidepressants, anticholinergics, antacids)

For the majority of children, non-organic or functional problems are the cause.

Constipation during infancy is rare and usually caused by excessive milk intake or the transition from formula to cow's milk. In toddlers, constipation is often caused by toilet training practices. Forced training may cause the child to withhold stool. Bowel and feeding issues are common manifestations of intense autonomy struggles with toddlers.

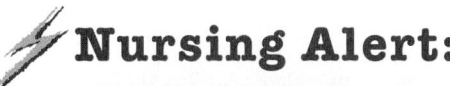

Additionally, a previously painful bowel movement because of a hard stool or anal fissures can result in fear of having a bowel movement. Magical thinking is a characteristic of toddlers' cognitive development, which can result in their fear of the toilet and cause difficulty in having a bowel movement. For example, a two-year-old boy who had developed a fear of having a bowel movement, admitted he was worried that his "poo would drown." Another child wanted to know "do poos have brains?" Fear of the toilet may be initiated by television. Commercials for toilet cleaners, for example, contain images of "germs and monsters" climbing out of the toilet. This can seem very real in a young child's imagination.

The older toddler, preschooler, and school-aged child may develop problems when starting nursery school, kindergarten, or 1st grade. Bathrooms in these settings may lack privacy and tend not to have soft toilet paper. As a result, the urge to defecate is suppressed during school hours. Continual suppression of defecation can lead to constipation.

Pathophysiology

Normal defecation occurs when stool moves into the rectum, causing rectal distention and relaxation of the internal anal sphincter. The conscious awareness of rectal distention results in contraction of the voluntary muscles of the external anal sphincter. Voluntary relaxation of the external sphincter and increased intra-abdominal pressure result in defecation. Constipation tends to be self-perpetuating. As stool is retained, the simultaneous process of stretching the rectal wall and decreasing sensory feedback leads to less frequent bowel movements, which result in further stool retention and larger stools. As water is reabsorbed, the stool becomes harder, and bowel movements may become painful. As this cycle progresses, the external and internal sphincters become compromised. Sensitivity to rectal distention and control of rectal evacuation diminish, and the child soon loses the urge to have a bowel movement.

Clinical Manifestations

The child who is constipated will have hard, small stools that may be passed at regular intervals or large masses of stool at intervals of days to weeks. Soiling of underwear in a child who is toilet trained is possible. Abdominal pain and/or distention develop as more stool accumulates in the bowel. The child may become irritable and experience a loss of appetite. Often a palpable fecal mass is felt on physical exam.

Diagnosis

Diagnosis is based on the history and physical exam. When attempting to determine the cause, it is important to rule out any organic causes. A thorough dietary history is obtained. A description of stool pattern, such as frequency, consistency, and size of stools, and toilet training history is elicited. Certain medications can cause constipation; therefore, it is important to determine if the child is taking any of these. An abdominal X ray shows a colon enlarged with stool and gas.

Treatment

Constipation is treated with a combination of therapies, which include cleansing the bowel, establishing a regular pattern of defecation, and modifying the diet. Cleaning the bowel of hardened or impacted stool is accomplished with enemas, oral medications, and suppositories. There are many types of oral medications that can be used. The choice depends on the child's ability to take the medication, the ease of giving it, and how well it works. Occasionally, if feces are impacted, they may need to be removed manually.

Modification of the diet includes increasing the intake of fiber and fluids. Establishing a regular pattern for defecation is largely a matter of caregiver education about normal defecation and bowel training techniques.

Nursing Management and Family Teaching

Nursing intervention focuses on education. Caregivers need instruction in the appropriate way to administer an enema (See the *Pediatric Nursing* Skills CD-ROM). Dietary modifications include increasing dietary fiber and fluids. The nurse should teach caregivers about high fiber foods and diet planning. High fiber foods include: whole grain breads and cereals, bran, high fiber snack bars, raw vegetables, fruits, especially raisins, prunes, cherries, and apricots, beans, popcorn, nuts, and seeds.

Establishing a regular pattern of defecation is accomplished by requiring the child to sit on the toilet after a meal for a reasonable amount of time, 5–10 minutes. Positive reinforcement with star charts or small prizes can be used to reward success and adherence with the toileting schedule and taking of medications.

INFLAMMATORY DISORDERS

Disorders caused by chronic inflammation of the GI tract can occur at any age, newborns through adolescents. Some of these disorders are short term and readily resolved like appendicitis; others are chronic and affect growth and development. Appendicitis, inflammatory bowel disease (ulcerative colitis and Crohn's disease), peptic ulcers, and necrotizing enterocolitis will be discussed in this section.

Appendicitis

Appendicitis, the inflammation of the vermiform appendix or the small sac at the end of the cecum, is the most common condition requiring abdominal surgery in children. Although appendicitis was first described over 100 years ago, the vagueness of its signs and symptoms in children poses a continuing challenge for health care providers to arrive at a timely and accurate diagnosis. Failure to diagnose appendicitis is the most frequent subject of malpractice suits and the fifth most expensive source of claims for emergency department physicians (Pisarra, 1999).

Incidence and Etiology

Appendicitis is the most common condition requiring abdominal surgery in childhood, occurring at a rate of 4 per 1,000 children younger than 14 years of age. It is more common in summer, has a higher incidence in males than females, Caucasians than non-Caucasians. Although the exact cause is poorly understood, the appendix becomes inflamed usually because of obstruction between the appendix and cecum or a systemic or enteric infection. Appendicitis is rare in third-world countries where diets are high in fiber; however, no causal relationship has been established between dietary fiber and the prevention of appendicitis (Higgenbotham & Gottlieb, 1998).

Pathophysiology

The appendix is vermiform (wormlike) in shape, with a diameter similar to a lead pencil. It rises from the wall of the cecum portion of the large intestine, below the ileocecal valve. However, its location can vary among individuals. As food passes through the cecum, the appendix also fills and empties. In 70% of cases, the lumen between the appendix and the cecum becomes obstructed with agents such as a **fecalith,** fecal matter that becomes petrified and stone-like, calculi, tumors, parasites, and foreign bodies. In the remaining 30% with no evidence of obstruction, the inflammation may be caused by a bacteria, virus, trauma, or postoperative fecal stasis (Pisarra, 1999).

Eye On:

Empacho

Empacho is a Spanish word that means indigestion, stomach pains, and abdominal cramps. Some Hispanics believe these symptoms are caused by a ball of undigested food clinging to some part of the gastrointestinal tract and are due to being forced to eat against one's will or lying about the amount of food eaten. Treatment is to massage and gently pinch the spine. This therapy can be problematic if the cause of symptoms is something serious such as appendicitis.

Nursing Tip:

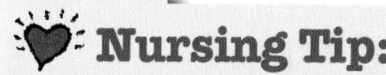

Assessing for appendicitis

When appendicitis is suspected, ask the child if she/he is hungry. If the answer is yes, chances of the child having appendicitis are slim. In most cases, the child who has this disorder does not feel like eating since symptoms began.

Clinical Manifestations

Abdominal pain is the first symptom in typical cases of appendicitis. Initially, the pain may be vague and poorly localized to the periumbilical area; gradually migrating to the right lower quadrant (RLQ). Anorexia and nausea with or without vomiting may also be present, but occur after the initial symptom of pain. The most reliable information gained from the history is the sequence of symptoms. Pain nearly always precedes anorexia, nausea, or vomiting. Nausea and vomiting that precedes abdominal pain often indicates gastroenteritis. Additional clinical manifestations that may be present are constipation or diarrhea. The child's temperature is usually normal or slightly elevated. A temperature of 101°F or higher suggests the presence of peritonitis.

Diagnosis

Appendicitis remains a diagnosis made largely on the basis of the history and physical examination. Diagnosis is challenging in children because the clinical manifestations can present atypically. Children who are misdiagnosed have an increased incidence of perforation, abscess, wound infection, and even mortality. Abdominal tenderness on palpation is a common, important, and reliable symptom. Tenseness of the muscles (muscle rigidity) over the tender area may be felt. Rigidity over the entire abdomen, accompanied by tense positioning and **guarding** (involuntary contraction of abdominal muscles caused by fear of impending pain), indicates a perforated appendix with peritonitis. **Rebound tenderness** describes a sensation of severe pain that occurs after deep pressure is applied and released and is indicative of peritonitis. However, many practitioners consider the elicitation of rebound tenderness to be a crude and unnecessarily painful technique. The resultant severe pain may adversely affect the element of trust with the child. Palpation with a stethoscope is a preferred method for children in order to identify areas of tenderness.

Laboratory findings do not establish the diagnosis, but there is often a moderate elevation of the white blood cell (WBC) count, seldom higher than 15,000 to 20,000/mm^3, with a "shift to the left" (an increased number of immature WBCs). However, some children with appendicitis have a

Nursing Tip:

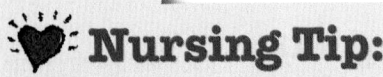

Assessment of peritoneal irritation

One way to check for peritoneal irritation in a toddler or preschooler is to have the child jump up and down with you. If the child does so several times without bending over in pain, you can confidently rule out peritoneal irritation.

Nursing Tip:

Palpating the abdomen for pain

Children frequently tense their abdominal muscles when they are being examined. Warm your hands and stethoscope before touching their abdomens. Maintain eye contact with them while palpating their abdomens, and they will watch your face rather than your hands and relax. This technique provides more reliable information about the presence of pain.

normal white blood cell count. Abdominal X rays may reveal a fecalith or some other cause of obstruction, although this rarely confirms the diagnosis. Other causes of acute abdominal pain must be ruled out, including severe constipation, urinary tract infection, acute gastroenteritis, pelvic inflammatory disease, and discomfort associated with ovulation. Abdominal ultrasound has been employed in an attempt to increase accuracy of appendicitis diagnoses. However, it may be more appropriate in verifying other causes of abdominal pain than in diagnosing appendicitis (Pisarra, 1999).

Delay in diagnosing appendicitis in children is a factor contributing to perforation rates of 30% to 60%. Young children have a thinner appendiceal wall, so progress from inflammation to perforation is more rapid than in adults. Children also have a poorly developed omentum, so local perforation is not usually confineable, and peritonitis develops. The close proximity of abdominal and pelvic organs further favors the spread of peritonitis to other structures. The inflammatory process associated with perforation may lead to intestinal obstruction or paralytic ileus. The signs and symptoms of peritonitis can be remembered by using the mnemonic *PERITONITIS* (Box 23-1).

Treatment

Once the diagnosis of appendicitis has been made, surgery is required as soon as possible. In an uncomplicated appendectomy, an incision approximately 2–3 inches is made in the right lower quadrant. If perforation is suspected, has

BOX 23-1 A mnemonic for peritonitis

P Pain: front, back, sides, shoulders
E Electrolytes fall, shock ensues
R Rigidity or rebound of abdominal wall
I Immobility
T Tenderness
O Obstruction
N Nausea and vomiting
I Increasing pulse, decreasing blood pressure
T Temperature falls, then rises
I Increasing girth of abdomen
S Silent abdomen (no bowel sounds) (Shipman, 1984)

Nursing Alert:

Treatments to Avoid in Suspected Appendicitis

Caregivers should be told to avoid giving their child laxatives or enemas and applying heat to the abdomen if appendicitis is suspected. These measures may stimulate bowel motility and increase the danger of perforation. Additionally, pain medication should be avoided because it can mask the signs of intraperitoneal inflammation.

Kids Want To Know

What will the scar look like after my appendectomy?

Maria, a 14-year-old girl, has been diagnosed with appendicitis and is scheduled for an appendectomy tomorrow. She asks her nurse "What will the scar look like? How big will it be? Will I still be able to wear my bikini swimming suit?" Because Maria's appendix has not perforated prior to surgery, the nurse can explain that the surgical incision will be small, about one-inch long, and to the right and slightly below the level of the umbilicus. She will be in the hospital for approximately three days if no complications occur and should be able to wear her bikini. She can further explain that if her appendix had ruptured and peritonitis had developed before surgery, the abdominal incision would be larger, and a drain would be placed in the abscess site. The incision may be closed only through the fascia with the skin left open and the wound packed to decrease the potential for infection or problems with healing.

occurred, or the appendix is in an atypical position, the incision is larger. An uncomplicated appendectomy may also be performed via laparoscopy. Preoperatively, the child is managed with an NPO status, intravenous fluids to replenish fluid volume and to correct electrolyte or acid-base imbalances, and pain medication. Postoperatively in an uncomplicated appendectomy, the child will receive antibiotics for 24 hours, remain NPO until intestinal peristalsis returns, and is discharged in 2–3 days. If perforation occurred, drains may protrude from the incision site or the incision may remain open and allowed to heal by secondary intention to prevent infection. Figure 23-12 illustrates an incision healing by secondary intention after an appendectomy for a perforated appendix. Additional treatment includes IV antibiotics for 7–10 days, NPO status, NG tube suction, IV fluids, and pain medication. The child remains NPO until bowel function returns and is discharged when wound drainage is minimal and oral intake satisfactory. If a laparoscopic procedure was

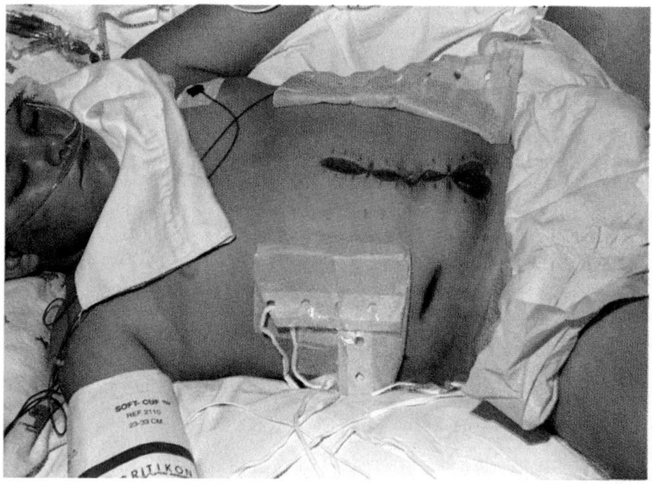

Figure 23-12 Incision Healing by Secondary Intention After Appendectomy of a Ruptured Appendix

Case Study/Care Plan

A Child with Appendicitis

Andrew is a 12-year-old boy who is being seen in the emergency department with a complaint of abdominal pain, vomiting, fever, and anorexia. Four days ago he awoke complaining of a dull stomach ache and not feeling well. He went to school but returned by noon and went back to bed. By early evening the pain was sharp and he could indicate the umbilical area as hurting. He refused to eat all day but did drink water and juices. The next morning he vomited yellow emesis, and the pain was periodically severe. His temperature was 100.5°F, and he vomited several more times that day. In the middle of the night he awoke with pain so severe he was crying and would not stand up straight. He was diagnosed with acute appendicitis and admitted to the hospital for surgery.

Nursing Care Plan

Assessment Because prompt and accurate diagnosis of appendicitis is important, nurses need to assess any child presenting with abdominal pain for the early signs and symptoms. Nurses in a variety of settings, such as emergency departments, school and school-based clinics, and ambulatory care clinics, are in an ideal position to recognize these early indicators of appendicitis. The nursing assessment should include detailed information about the child's pain (onset, location, intensity), changes in behavior (refusing to attend school or play outside, loss of appetite), and vomiting. If the symptoms of appendicitis are present, the child should be referred for further evaluation.

Nursing Diagnosis #1

Acute pain related to inflamed appendix and postoperative surgical incision (refer to Chapter 18)

Expected Outcomes

1. Andrew states and/or exhibits reduced pain

Interventions/*Rationales*

1. Use a pain assessment scale appropriate for child's developmental level to determine severity of pain. *The pain scale provides objective data and the child's input.*

continues

continued

2. Assess behavioral cues (crying, movement, facial grimace) that indicate discomfort or pain. *Behavior of child provides clues to pain experience.*

3. Use non-pharmacologic approaches such as distraction with toys and games or relaxing music. *Concentration on something other than pain directs the discomfort from conscious thought.*

4. Administer pain medication by continuous infusion or every 3–4 hours around the clock as prescribed. *Pain breakthrough occurs even during sleep; pain is continuous for 1–2 days postop.*

5. Assist child to assume position of comfort. *Fowler's position with knees flexed avoids strain on the abdomen.*

Evaluation

Andrew will experience no pain or reduced pain as evidenced by relaxed body posture and facial expression; heart and respiratory rate and blood pressure within appropriate range for age; naps and sleeps appropriately for age undisturbed by pain; and ambulation without undue resistance.

Nursing Diagnosis #2

Risk for deficient fluid volume related to inadequate intake and losses secondary to vomiting, diarrhea, and NPO status

Expected Outcomes

1. Andrew will regain adequate hydration status.

Interventions/*Rationales*

1. Administer IV fluids as prescribed. *Inadequate oral intake, vomiting, and diarrhea deplete total body water.*

2. Replace NG output with additional IV fluids as prescribed. *NG suction removes gastric contents that contain water, hydrochloric acid, and potassium.*

3. Maintain accurate intake and output; estimate wound drainage and include as output. *Provides an ongoing assessment of hydration status.*

Evaluation

Andrew has adequate fluid volume as evidenced by appropriate intake of IV and oral fluids and urine output (minimum of 1 to 2 ml/kg/hr); moist mucous membranes, elastic skin turgor, and normal vital signs for age.

Nursing Diagnosis #3

Risk for infection related to possible or actual rupture of appendix and surgical incision

Expected Outcomes

1. Andrew will be free of infection.

Interventions/*Rationales*

1. Preoperative

   a. Assess child for clinical and laboratory manifestations of appendicitis. *Successful treatment is dependent on timely diagnosis of the disorder.*

   b. Assess for and immediately report symptoms of peritonitis (initial relief of pain at time of perforation followed by increased intensity, abdominal distention, guarding, decreased or absent bowel sounds, elevated temperature, and shock-like symptoms). *Perforation occurs in a high percentage of children with acute appendicitis, which greatly increases the risk of serious complications.*

continues

continued

2. Postoperative
   a. Monitor incision for signs of infection. *Postoperative infection may increase length and cost of hospitalization and prolong child's recovery time.*
   b. Maintain intact abdominal dressing, change and/or reinforce per hospital routine. *To prevent infection.*
   c. Monitor temperature every 4 hours and prn; watch WBC count for leukocytosis. *Temperatures that exceed 101°F and elevated WBC suggest the presence of infection.*

Evaluation

The surgical incision is free from edema, excessive redness, warmth, or purulent drainage. The incision has minimal clear to serosanguineous drainage. Andrew is afebrile with WBC within normal limits. Andrew's heart rate is within an acceptable range for age.

performed, the child may remain in the hospital overnight or be discharged on the day of surgery.

Inflammatory Bowel Disease

Inflammatory bowel disease (IBD) refers to a group of chronic disorders that cause inflammation or ulceration in the small and large intestine and include ulcerative colitis (UC) and Crohn's disease (CD). Ulcerative colitis involves inflammation of the mucosa and submucosa of the colon and rectum, while CD is an inflammation that may involve the entire gastrointestinal tract and all layers of the bowel wall (transmural) (Orloski, 1998).

Incidence and Etiology

Once considered rare in children and adolescents, IBD is now being recognized with increasing frequency in this age group. In fact, 20% of all individuals with UC and 25–30% of those with CD present before age 20. Peak onset is in late adolescence. With increasing recognition of IBD, it has become one of the most significant chronic diseases affecting children and adolescents (Baldassano & Piccoli, 1999).

The incidence of IBD is similar in males and females, is higher among the Caucasian population of developed Western countries, and lower among African-Americans and Asians. The incidence of UC is 0.05 per 1,000; the incidence of CD is 0.04 per 1,000. The etiology of IBD is unclear; however, infectious agents, autoimmune, genetic, and environmental factors have been implicated. Current thinking suggests that a triggering factor, possibly a virus or an atypical bacterium, interacts with the body's immune system to induce an inflammatory reaction in the intestinal wall. About 15% to 20% of individuals with IBD have a close relative with one of these diseases, suggesting a genetic factor (Baldassano & Piccoli, 1999).

Pathophysiology

The bowel responds to an environmental trigger that the immune system identifies as dangerous and causes an injury resulting in vasoconstriction. This is followed by localized release of cellular mediators, including histamine, which produce a marked vasodilation. Capillaries become distended with blood and begin to contract, causing ruptures in the walls. The swollen engorged bowel is fragile and is, therefore, inclined to ulcerate, causing a break in the mucosal barrier. Digestive enzymes and intestinal bacteria act on this exposed tissue, causing further irritation, inflammation, ulceration, and bleeding. Ulcers can become fissures as they penetrate more deeply into the intestinal wall. Fistulas can occur into the bladder and /or vagina (more common in CD). Inflammatory exudate consisting of plasma proteins draws more fluid into the bowel resulting in diarrhea that may be bloody. Healing lesions result in scar tissue formation and subsequent scarring of bowel may lead to strictures and bowel obstruction.

Clinical Manifestations

The most common symptoms of UC are rectal bleeding, diarrhea, and abdominal pain. Multiple patterns of presentation occur in children and adolescents. Mild disease is seen in 50–60% of cases. The onset of diarrhea is insidious, and there are no extra-intestinal or systemic signs of fever, weight loss, or hypoalbuminemia. Thirty percent present with moderate disease characterized by bloody diarrhea, abdominal cramping and tenderness, and the urgency to defecate. These individuals have associated systemic signs such as anorexia, weight loss, low-grade fever, and mild anemia. Severe cases occur in 10% of clients. Clinical manifestations in these cases are more than six bloody stools per day, abdominal tenderness, fever, anemia, leukocytosis, and hypoalbuminemia. Occasionally, children with UC may have predominately extra-intestinal manifestations such as growth failure, arthritis, and skin lesions (Baldassano & Piccoli, 1999).

In contrast to UC, CD may occur in any segment of the gastrointestinal tract. The clinical manifestations are determined primarily by the location and extent of disease involvement. The majority of children (50–70%) have disease involving the terminal ileum. In these children symptoms of malabsorption predominate including diarrhea, abdominal pain, anorexia, weight loss, and growth failure. CD that occurs in the colon may be indistinguishable from UC, with symptoms of bloody diarrhea, crampy abdominal pain, and urgency to defecate. Perianal involvement includes painful defecation, bright red rectal bleeding, skin tags, hemorrhoids, fistulas, and abscesses.

Growth failure occurs more frequently in children with CD than with UC. Children with either disorder tend to reduce dietary intake below that recommended for age to diminish symptoms induced by eating, which results in growth failure, characterized by an abnormally slow growth velocity. A major consequence of prolonged reduction in growth velocity is permanent short stature, frequently seen in adults who had CD during childhood. Additionally, delayed sexual development is frequently seen. More importantly, growth failure and delayed puberty are often debilitating symptoms for adolescents, potentially affecting their self-esteem, social interactions, and school performance (Ruemmele, Roy, Levy, & Seidman, 2000). Systemic or extra-intestinal symptoms are more common in children with CD than UC. Some of these symptoms tend to be more severe in children than in adults. For example, children have higher fevers, more joint pain, nausea, and in general feel sicker than do adults with CD. See Table 23-1 for a comparison of UC and CD.

Diagnosis

Presenting symptoms and clinical course of UC and CD are similar enough that they often elude a differential diagnosis sometimes for years. Diagnosis is based on history and physical exam and endoscopic or radiologic examination of the colon to evaluate the character and location of lesions. Endoscopy includes either a sigmoidoscopy or a colonoscopy and biopsies of the mucosa are obtained and examined. Radiologic studies include a barium enema and an upper gastrointestinal contrast examination. Laboratory studies may indicate anemia, hypoproteinemia, fluid and electrolyte imbalances, and an elevated sedimentation rate.

Treatment

Treatment for inflammatory bowel disease involves pharmacologic, nutritional, and surgical approaches. The goals include controlling the disease, inducing remission and preventing relapses, providing adequate nutrition for growth and development, and assisting the child to function as normally as possible (e.g., school attendance, participation in sports). Pharmacotherapy is aimed at either decreasing inflammation or directly suppressing the immune system. Categories of medications include corticosteroids, aminosalicylates, antibiotics, and immunosuppressants. Corticosteroids are used during acute episodes for treating moderate to severe IBD. The aminosalicylate azulfidine (sulfasalazine) acts directly on the bowel mucosa to reduce inflammation. Metronidazole (Flagyl), an anti-infective, has been helpful in the treatment of perianal complications in CD. Immunosupressive medications such as cyclosporine have been useful in children with corticosteroid-resistant CD.

The goal of nutritional support is to replace lost nutrients and to provide adequate caloric intake for growth and normal metabolic functions. While no special diet has been

TABLE 23-1 Comparison of Ulcerative Colitis and Crohn's Disease

	Ulcerative Colitis	Crohn's Disease
Pathology		
Area of involvement	Colon and rectum	May affect entire GI tract from mouth to anus
Bowel wall involvement	Superficial (mucosa and submucosa)	All layers of bowel wall (transmural)
Distribution of lesions	Symmetric, continuous	Asymmetric, segmented (disease-free skip areas)
Clinical Manifestations		
Alteration in bowel pattern	Severe diarrhea	Mild to moderate diarrhea
Abdominal pain	Mild, lower abdominal	Common, severe
Rectal bleeding	Common	Uncommon
Weight loss	Mild to moderate	Common, severe
Growth retardation	Mild	Often severe
Perianal disease	Rare	Common
Fistulas	Rare	Common

proven effective for treating IBD, some individuals find their symptoms are aggravated by milk, highly seasoned foods, and fiber. The lactose in milk and milk products is usually poorly tolerated when IBD is active, resulting in bloating, pain, and increased diarrhea. This is a problem because dairy products constitute the largest source of calories in the diets of most children. Lactase hydrolyzed milk such as Lact-Aid can be helpful in providing extra calories for lactose intolerant children. High calorie liquid nutritional supplements such as Ensure may be recommended for children with growth failure. Vitamins and minerals are often deficient and replacements are necessary. Since fats are digested and assimilated in the small intestine, children with CD have a deficiency of the fat-soluble vitamins, A, D, E, and K. Elemental formulas, which are almost completely absorbed in the small intestine and leave little residue, have been useful in inducing remission and improving nutritional status. These formulas can be given either by mouth or nasogastric tube feeding at night. Total parenteral nutrition (TPN) in children with severe CD can help to reverse growth failure. Most individuals with IBD find that a low-fiber, low-residue diet is therapeutic.

Another approach to treatment is surgery. When children experience severe complications of UC, surgery may be indicated. Severe complications are bowel perforation, hemorrhage, and conventional treatment failure. Surgical removal of the entire colon and rectum (proctocolectomy) provides a permanent cure. A permanent ileostomy is created at the same time. Indications for surgery in cases of CD are disease that is unresponsive to medical treatment, bowel strictures, obstruction, or perforation, and intractable bleeding or diarrhea. The diseased segment of the intestine is removed or resected, and the two ends of healthy intestine are reattached or anastomosed. CD is not cured with surgery because the lesions tend to recur in other parts of the bowel.

Nursing Management

The focus of nursing care includes medication and nutritional management, emotional support, and community referrals. An area for potential strife between the child and caregivers is the medication regimen. When IBD is in remission, the child may see no reason for taking medications. The concept that the disease is still present although no symptoms are evident is often difficult for children to understand. The nurse should emphasize continuation of medications despite remission of symptoms. The nurse can provide information about medications used to treat IBD and their side effects, emphasizing that they be continued despite remissions of symptoms. The side effects of corticosteroids include increased appetite and weight gain, increased susceptibility to infections, increased risk for osteoporosis and aseptic necrosis of the hip, acne, rounding of the face, and personality changes. Side effects of the sulfasalazine (Azulfidine) include gastric upset, nausea, vomiting, allergic reactions, **crystalluria** (crystals in the urine), and bone marrow suppression. The total dose of the medication should be given in evenly spaced doses and after meals to minimize gastrointestinal upset. The child should be encouraged to drink a full glass of water with each dose to prevent crystalluria.

> **Nursing Alert:**
>
> **Side Effects of Sulfasalazine**
>
> *Warn the child and family that the child's urine or skin may be yellow-orange in color. Instruct caregivers to notify their health care provider if skin rash, fever, sore throat, mouth sores, bruising, bleeding, fatigue, or joint pain occur. These are signs and symptoms of blood dyscrasias resulting from bone marrow suppression, a serious side effect of sulfasalazine.*

Providing emotional support is an important nursing intervention in IBD. In addition to the expected effects of chronic illness, depression, anxiety, and low self-esteem appear to be more common in children and adolescents with IBD (Mascarenhas & Altschuler, 1997). Early detection of psychological problems is invaluable because appropriate referral and psychological therapy can help prevent further psychopathology. Often both the child and the family require counseling. Support groups are also useful in helping the child and caregivers deal with the diagnosis and disease. The nurse should assess the impact of the disease as reflected by impaired social activities and school absences. School activities (e.g., gym and bathroom privileges) may need to be modified.

Peptic Ulcers

Peptic ulcers occur when there is erosion of the mucosal wall of the gastrointestinal tract. They develop most often in the stomach and duodenum. They are classified as primary or secondary, gastric or duodenal. Primary ulcers occur in the absence of another underlying disease and often in individuals with a family history of the disorder. Secondary or stress ulcers are associated with severe physiological stress of an underlying systemic disease or injury such as shock, sepsis, burns, or surgery. Certain drugs also contribute to secondary ulcers. Gastric ulcers are usually located at the junction of the fundus and the pylorus on the lesser curvature of the stomach. Duodenal ulcers occur in the pylorus or duodenum. Figure 23-13 illustrates the most common sites for peptic ulcers.

Incidence and Etiology

The true incidence of peptic ulcers in children is unknown; however, with the advent of endoscopy, more cases have been detected and diagnosed. Primary ulcers are most common in

Family Teaching

Inflammatory Bowel Disease

HOME:

- Teach the child and family about medication regimen, side effects of drugs, and the need to continue drug therapy despite remission of symptoms.
- Instruct the child and family about the dietary plan. A low-fiber, low-residue diet generally provides some relief of symptoms such as diarrhea and abdominal pain.
- Teach caregivers methods to increase oral caloric intake such as (1) eating 3 meals plus 3 "mini-meals" each day; (2) including a source of protein at each meal; (3) ingesting milk products as tolerated (yogurt with live cultures and aged, hardened cheeses are tolerated by many children with lactose intolerance); (4) using extra fats as tolerated, such as butter, margarine, vegetable oil, mayonnaise, cream, and cream cheese; and (5) limiting low-calorie foods and beverages.

SCHOOL:

- Instruct the family that the child can be as active as she or he feels like being.
- Encourage caregivers to try giving the child the responsibility of determining whether she/he is able to go to school during flare-ups.
- Encourage the child to find practical ways of dealing with the illness in school, such as locating the nearest bathrooms, carrying extra underclothes, and visiting the school nurse as needed.
- Assess for school avoidance because of embarrassment of diarrhea. If the child is not active in school, some element of the program should be adjusted.
- Allow the child to make the decision whether to tell friends and teachers about the illness. If there are frequent hospitalizations or frequent absences from school, teachers and school administrators should be told about the illness.
- Have caregivers contact the school district to arrange for tutoring if extended absences from school become necessary.

COMMUNITY:

- Refer the family to the Pediatric Crohn's and Colitis Association and the Crohn's and Colitis Foundation of America (see Resources). Both organizations provide information and support that families may find helpful.
- Refer caregivers to social services, the visiting nurse association, and home health care agencies.

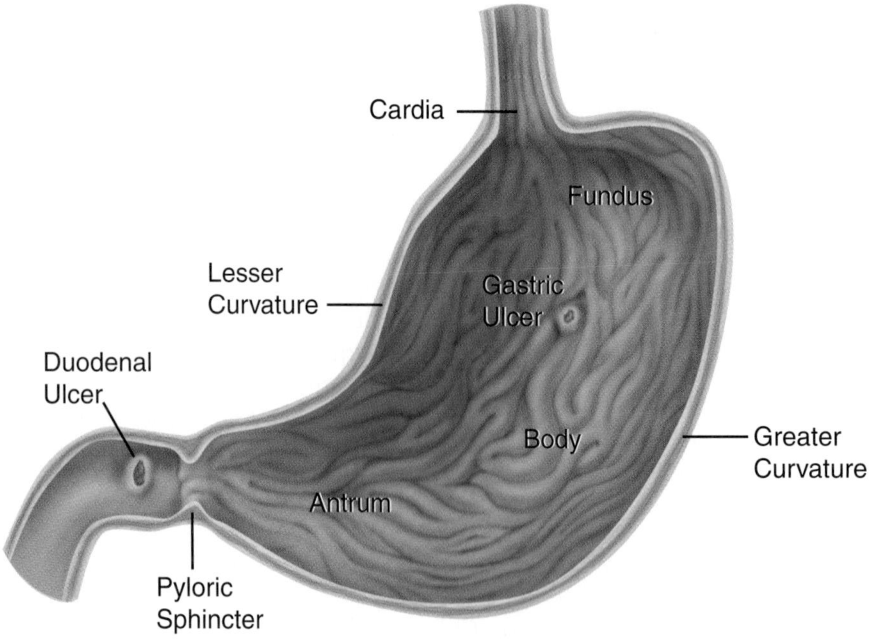

Figure 23-13 Most Common Sites for Peptic Ulcers

older children and adolescents. Up to the age of 6, most ulcers are secondary (Sondheimer & Silverman, 1995). Gastric ulcers are uncommon in children, whereas duodenal ulcers are seen most frequently. Males are affected with peptic ulcers more than females.

The exact etiology is unknown; however, several factors have been implicated. There is a close association between the bacilli *Helicobacter pylori* (*H. pylori*) and duodenal ulcers. This organism is transmitted by the fecal-oral route and is more common in lower socioeconomic areas and in developing countries (Heslin, 1997). Certain drugs contribute to peptic ulcers, for example, nonsteroidal anti-inflammatory agents such as aspirin and ibuprofen (Advil), corticosteroids, tobacco, and alcohol. For many years, diet and psychological factors were suggested as important etiologic factors; however, there is no conclusive evidence that they cause peptic ulcers.

Pathophysiology

The parietal cells of the stomach secrete hydrochloric acid (HCl) in the digestive process; other cells secrete pepsinogen. Pepsinogen converts to pepsin when activated by HCl, which adds to the acidity of the stomach. Gastric epithelial cells secrete a mucus-bicarbonate barrier to provide protection from the acid and pepsin. Ulcers occur when a substance stimulates excessive HCl production, damages the mucus barrier, or decreases mucus production.

Clinical Manifestations

The signs and symptoms of peptic ulcers in children vary depending on their age. The clinical manifestations according to age are illustrated in Table 23-2.

TABLE 23-2 Clinical Manifestations of Peptic Ulcers According to Age

Age	Clinical Manifestations
0–3 years	Primary ulcers: anorexia, vomiting, melena, hematemesis, crying after meals Secondary ulcers: hemorrhage and perforation
3–6 years	Primary ulcers: vomiting related to eating, periumbilical or generalized pain Secondary ulcers: melena, hematemesis, perforation
6–18 years	Melena, hematemesis, occult bleeding, anemia

Diagnosis

An upper GI barium series is often the initial test for a child suspected of having peptic ulcers. With this exam the ulcer crater is detected; however, the practitioner is not able to biopsy the mucosa to determine if *H. pylori* is present. A more definitive test is an endoscopy of the upper GI tract. The ulcer crater can be directly visualized, and a biopsy can be obtained to detect the organism. A blood test is also available that detects *H. pylori* antibodies. A stool exam for occult blood may be performed to diagnose GI bleeding.

Treatment

The goals of treatment are to relieve pain, hasten healing, and prevent complications. Medications are the primary method for managing ulcers. The rationale for medication therapy involves different mechanisms:

- Neutralization or buffering of gastric acid (antacids)
- Reduction of gastric acid secretions (histamine receptor antagonists)
- Suppression and blockage of gastric acid secretions (proton pump inhibitors)
- Protection of the mucus barrier (mucosal barrier fortifiers) by decreasing the activity of pepsin and HCl
- Treatment of *Helicobacter* infections (antibiotics and bismuth preparations)

Antacids decrease discomfort and pain but do not affect healing of the ulcer or prevent recurrence. A common antacid dosage schedule is 1 to 3 hours after each meal and at bedtime. The most common histamine (H) receptor antagonists for peptic ulcers are ranitidine (Zantac), cimetidine (Tagamet), and famotidine (Pepcid), all of which have few side effects, primarily diarrhea or constipation, headache, and rash. In some cases, proton pump inhibitors, which effectively suppress or block all gastric acid secretions are used in children. Omeprazole (Prilosec), the most commonly prescribed proton pump inhibitor, has minimal side effects that are similar to H-receptor antagonists. Mucosal barrier fortifiers such as sucralfate (Carafate) coat the stomach, adhere to the ulcer surface, and reinforce the mucosal protective coat of the stomach to prevent further digestive action of HCl and pepsin. It is administered on an empty stomach 1 hour before or 2 hours after meals and at bedtime, and constipation is the more common side effect. Cure of peptic ulcers associated with *H. pylori* requires eradication of the organism. The optimal therapeutic regimen is still undetermined; yet, in children, the antibiotics metronidazole (Flagyl) and ampicillin in combination with bismuth salicylate (Pepto-Bismol) is most often prescribed. Diet therapy is not indicated in the treatment of ulcers because restriction of diet does not promote or accelerate healing. Surgery is rarely needed in children but is indicated if perforation, hemorrhage, or gastric outlet obstruction occurs.

Nursing Management and Family Teaching

Because peptic ulcers are usually managed at home by caregivers, a major nursing intervention is caregiver education. Adherence with the medication regimen is important in healing the ulcer and preventing recurrences; therefore, the child and caregivers need to understand the rationale for each drug, the administration schedule, and side effects. The nurse explains that a special diet is not necessary, but the child should avoid substances that increase acid secretion such as caffeine-containing beverages (coffee, tea, cola). Any food or beverage that causes discomfort or pain needs to be avoided. Older children and adolescents need information about how alcohol and cigarette smoking cause gastric irritation and contribute to ulcer formation. It is important that caregivers know the signs and symptoms of ulcer complications, which must be reported to their health care provider immediately. **Melena** (black or tarry stool indicating presence of blood) or **hematemesis** (vomiting of blood) indicate hemorrhage; severe abdominal pain and a rigid abdomen may signal perforation.

The nurse can be instrumental in preventing secondary or stress ulcers that are due to physiological stress or certain medications by identifying infants and children who may be at risk for developing these ulcers. For critically ill individuals, maintaining gastric pH above 3.5 will help prevent ulcer formation. Thus, gastric pH values should be checked frequently and treated if too low. Additionally, histamine-2 blockers may be given as prophylaxis therapy in those identified at high risk for stress ulcers.

Necrotizing Enterocolitis

Necrotizing enterocolitis (NEC), a life-threatening condition of preterm neonates, is characterized by necrosis of the mucosa of the small and large intestine, most frequently the distal ileum and proximal colon. It is the most common surgical emergency in this age group. The necrosis may be very superficial and only detectable microscopically, or it may be through the bowel wall. Mild disease may be completely reversible, but neonates with extensive involvement may not survive.

Incidence and Etiology

NEC commonly occurs in preterm, low birthweight neonates and is rarely seen in term infants. It equally affects all races and both sexes. The incidence has been rising in recent years because of the improved survival of this high-risk group. The exact etiology of NEC is unclear; however, several factors are associated with its development. These risk factors include intestinal ischemia, bacterial colonization of the bowel, and the presence of hypertonic solutions in the intestinal lumen, usually formula (Kamitsuka, Horton, & Williams, 2000). Perinatal asphyxia, respiratory distress syndrome, exchange transfusions, and umbilical artery catheters may all contribute to ischemia of the bowel. Controversy exists about various aspects of feeding practices as a possible etiologic factor. These include feeding neonates within the first 48 hours after birth, the use of formula rather than breast milk, and enteral feedings of hypertonic solutions, for example, formula (Kamitsuka, et al.., 2000).

Pathophysiology

NEC appears to occur in preterm neonates whose bowel has experienced an injury, resulting in vascular compromise. This leads to decreased blood flow to the bowel and ischemia of the intestinal mucosa. The disruption of the intestinal mucosal barrier introduces significant vulnerability to infection. Then normal intestinal bacteria **hydrolyze** (to cause a substance to break down into its component parts by adding water) formula in the intestine, forming gas or air in the bowel wall called **pneumatosis intestinalis.** The bowel becomes edematous and distended. Progressive infiltration of the bowel wall with bacteria leads to more extensive tissue inflammation, destruction, and necrosis. Sepsis and perforation of the bowel may occur.

Clinical Manifestations

The classic clinical presentation of the neonate with NEC includes the symptom group of abdominal tenderness, distention, and erythema of abdominal wall, bloody stools, decreased bowel sounds, increased **gastric residuals** (feeding retained in stomach following tube feeding), and bilious vomiting after feeding. Manifestations of clinical deterioration include apnea and bradycardia, lethargy, temperature instability, decreased urine output, further abdominal distention, and evidence of shock (cool, mottled skin, pallor, decreased intensity of peripheral pulses). Hypotension is a late sign of deterioration. Acidosis, sepsis, and death may occur if NEC is not treated.

Diagnosis

Diagnosis is based on clinical findings and abdominal X rays. Radiographic findings associated with NEC are dilated bowel loops and pneumatosis intestinalis. **Pneumoperitoneum,** free air in the peritoneal cavity, or air in the portal circulation indicate severe disease and perforation of the bowel.

Treatment

If NEC is diagnosed in its early stages and treatment is initiated promptly to prevent perforation, the infant may improve without surgical intervention. Initial treatment includes:

- Cessation of oral feedings
- Continuous gastric drainage and decompression via an NG tube

- Maintenance of oxygenation; ventilation if necessary
- Administration of IV fluid therapy for parenteral nutrition and broad spectrum antibiotics, and to restore acid-base and electrolyte balance

Frequent monitoring of laboratory data is essential in order to detect deterioration in the infant's condition. Commonly ordered tests include blood gases, white blood cell count, hematocrit, platelet count, electrolytes, and abdominal X rays.

Despite appropriate medical treatment, surgical intervention becomes necessary in 40% to 50% of cases (Maalouf, et al., 2000). Surgery is required if the infant demonstrates evidence of perforation, localized peritonitis, persistent metabolic acidosis, or clinical deterioration unresponsive to vigorous medical management (see Box 23-2).

Resection of the necrotic bowel is necessary, and in cases of extensive removal, intestinal diversion is performed by creating a temporary ileostomy, jejunostomy, or colostomy. Postoperative complications include intestinal obstruction secondary to stricture of the ischemic portions of the bowel and short bowel syndrome characterized by malabsorption, malnutrition, and growth failure.

Nursing Management

The nurse has a major responsibility to be aware of and continually assess for early warning signs of NEC.

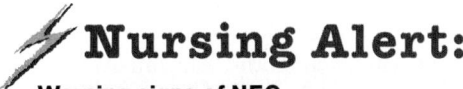

Nursing Alert:

Warning signs of NEC

- Abdominal distention
- Residual gastric contents
- Feeding intolerance
- Decreased bowel sounds
- Bloody stools

BOX 23-2 Indications for surgical intervention of necrotizing enterocolitis

1. Free intraperitoneal air (pneumoperitoneum)
2. Persistent and visible bowel loops
3. Radiographic evidence of peritonitis
   a. Increased free peritoneal fluid
   b. Increased bowel wall edema
4. Clinical deterioration despite medical treatment
   a. Irreversible metabolic acidosis
   b. Shock
   c. Respiratory failure

Frequent measurement of abdominal girth is performed to assess for distention. Prior to feedings gastric residual contents are measured to determine if the volume is increasing, which indicates malabsorption. The presence of bowel sounds is also noted to evaluate for decreased intestinal activity, and all stools are tested for blood. When NEC is diagnosed, nursing interventions include accurate intake and output measurements, frequent assessment of vital signs, maintenance of IV therapy, and ongoing assessment for changes in the infant's condition. Vital signs are monitored for changes that may reveal impending sepsis or shock from perforation and peritonitis. When oral feedings are restarted, the nurse must observe the infant's response and tolerance because NEC can recur.

MALABSORPTION ALTERATIONS

Malabsorption occurs when there is a disruption in the digestive process causing insufficient assimilation of nutrients. Common causes of problems in absorption in infants and children that will be discussed are celiac disease and lactose intolerance.

Celiac Disease

Celiac disease, also known as gluten-sensitive enteropathy, is a disorder caused by permanent intolerance to gluten, the protein component of wheat, barley, rye, and oats. It is second only to cystic fibrosis as the most common cause of malabsorption in children.

Incidence and Etiology

Celiac disease is a genetic disorder that occurs in all races but is more common in Caucasians. The incidence varies in different regions and is more common in Europe than the United States. In the U.S. it is 0.1 in 1,000 live births, and the disease coincides with the introduction of foods containing gluten (Ulsben, 1996).

Pathophysiology

The exact mechanism by which gluten damages the mucosa of the small intestine is unclear. One theory postulates that gluten toxicity results in an alteration in immunologic response. Gluten consists of two protein components, glutenin and gliadin. The harmful protein appears to be gliadin. Gliadin plays the role of antigen and causes an immune response that results in inflammation of and damage to the finger-like projections called villi in the small intestine. The villi flatten out and atrophy, leading to a decrease in the absorptive surface area. Initially, fat absorption is impaired, followed by protein, carbohydrates, and fat-soluble vitamins (A, D, E, K).

Clinical Manifestations

Early clinical manifestations of celiac disease are subtle and include anorexia, irritability, listlessness, and weight loss. As the disease progresses, abdominal distention and chronic diarrhea appear with large amounts of unabsorbed fats being excreted in the stools (**steatorrhea**). The stools are bulky, putty colored, foul-smelling, greasy, and often float because of the high fat content. Signs of progression include a protuberant abdomen, loss of subcutaneous fat, and muscle wasting secondary to hypoproteinemia. The child may appear pale because of anemia, and bruising may develop secondary to inadequate vitamin K absorption. Late signs include severe growth retardation, osteoporosis, and in the adolescent, delayed menses or puberty.

Diagnosis

The definitive diagnostic test is a small bowel biopsy, which will reveal atrophy of the villi and deep crypts on the intestinal mucosa. These characteristic lesions return to normal after dietary restriction of gluten, which help confirm the diagnosis. Serologic tests to detect antigliadin and antiendomysial antibodies are commonly ordered. Laboratory tests may be used to evaluate malabsorption and nutritional deficiencies (Stark, 1999).

Treatment

Medical management consists of a lifelong adherence to a gluten-free diet. Education about the diet is the main goal of treatment and involves the health care provider, nurse, dietician, caregivers, other family members, and the child. All wheat, barley, rye, and oats are eliminated and substituted with rice, corn, and millet. Specific nutritional supplements may be used to correct deficiency states. The most common are supplements of iron, folate, calcium, and fat-soluble vitamins. The intolerance to gluten is permanent, and lack of adherence to a gluten-free diet can cause exacerbation of symptoms.

Nursing Management and Family Teaching

The long-term goal of nursing care is to provide dietary education and supervision. The nurse explains to the caregivers the disease process, the signs and symptoms, and the rationale behind the gluten-free diet. A dietician should be involved in diet planning and nutrition education, and serves as a resource for gluten-free foods and recipes. Families are taught to read labels of all commercially prepared foods for the presence of gluten or gluten-containing additives such as hydrolyzed vegetable protein.

Children and their families often react to the necessity of a gluten-free diet with grief and may have a hard time accepting that something so fundamental to their diet could be injuring the child. Caregivers should be forewarned that many adolescents specifically have a difficult time accepting the dietary restrictions and may experiment with foods containing gluten. They may be motivated to adhere to the restrictions by the expectation of dramatic improvements in gastrointestinal symptoms such as bloating, abdominal pain, and diarrhea, and in their general well-being (Murray, 1999). Referrals to community resources for dietary and peer support organizations are important (see Resources).

Lactose Intolerance

Lactose intolerance is the inability to digest lactose, a sugar (disaccharide) present in human and cow's milk, standard infant formulas, and dairy products such as cheese and ice cream. Lactose is also added to many prepared foods, including bread and other baked goods, breakfast cereals, and mixes for cakes, cookies, pancakes, and biscuits. This disorder results from a deficiency or absence of lactase, an enzyme in the small intestine required for the digestion and absorption of lactose. Lactose intolerance can be congenital or acquired. In the congenital type, which is extremely rare, the newborn is born with a complete absence of lactase. Acquired lactose intolerance involves the gradual loss of lactase, is more common, and appears from early childhood to late adolescence.

Incidence and Etiology

The incidence appears to vary widely among different ethnic and racial groups. Low lactose levels are least common among northern and western Europeans and highest among populations from the Far East. In the United States the incidence is lowest in Caucasians and highest in Vietnamese-Americans, Native Americans, and African-Americans. Lactose intolerance is most often secondary to other disorders. Diarrheal disease, particularly when caused by rotovirus, other infections of the small intestine, and acquired immune deficiency syndrome (AIDS) may decrease the activity of lactase. Another cause may be mucosal damage to the small bowel induced by dietary components such as gluten sensitivity (celiac disease), and sensitivity to soy protein and cow's milk (Castiglia, 1994).

Pathophysiology

The absence or deficiency of lactase results in the inability of the small intestine to digest lactose. Subsequently, the undigested lactose moves into the colon where GI bacteria break down the lactose and release hydrogen, methane, and carbon dioxide. This process causes excessive gas production and abdominal bloating and pain. The undigested lactose also causes an increased number of solutes in the colon, resulting in an increase in the osmotic pressure. Therefore, water is drawn into the colon causing watery diarrhea.

Clinical Manifestations

Symptoms occur in response to ingestion of lactose and include explosive, watery diarrhea, abdominal distention, abdominal pain, and excessive flatus. Symptoms develop rapidly after the child ingests milk or foods containing lactose. Some children are able to tolerate small amounts of lactose without symptoms; yet, when larger amounts are consumed, severe symptoms occur.

Diagnosis

Diagnosis is usually made using a hydrogen-breath test that measures the amount of hydrogen left after fermentation of undigested and unabsorbed carbohydrates such as lactose.

Treatment and Nursing Management

Treatment consists of reducing or eliminating lactose from the child's diet. In most cases, total elimination is unnecessary. For infants, switching to a soy based formula (Isomil, Nutramigen, Prosobee) is effective. For older infants and children, when fluids or foods containing lactose are consumed, a commercial lactose preparation (Lact-Aid, Dairy-Ease) can be ingested or sprinkled on the items to improve tolerance. Additionally, milk products that have been commercially pretreated with microbial derived lactase are available (McBean & Miller, 1998).

POISONING

A poison is any substance that harms the body and interferes with the body's normal functioning. A poisoning can occur through ingestion, inhalation, skin exposure, eye contact, or any other mode that causes adverse effects. Ingestion accounts for the majority of poisonings.

Incidence and Etiology (Pathophysiology)

In 1998 approximately 1.1 million cases of ingestion of a toxic substance by children less than six years of age were reported to poison control centers (Shannon, 2000). Since many children with toxic ingestions are managed without contact with poison control centers or emergency facilities, the total number of cases is much larger than the numbers reported by these centers. Poisoning is the leading cause of injury and the fourth leading cause of death in toddlers and preschoolers. In infants their tendency to explore objects with their mouth puts them at high risk for accidental ingestion of toxic substances. In toddlers and preschoolers, poisoning is more often a result of curiosity. Older children may experiment with drugs and household products to produce hallucinogenic effects (Dunn & Burns, 2000). Because ingestions in children under the age of six are most commonly accidental, they rarely ingest enough poison to cause death. In contrast, adolescents are less frequently exposed to poisons but their exposure is more commonly intentional and results in more fatalities than in younger children. The incidence of childhood poisoning has decreased significantly in the past 50 years because of federal regulation of products and product safety, child-resistant containers, and safe storage of toxic substances in the home and elsewhere (Shannon, 2000).

Although the majority of poisonings occur in the home, incidents may occur anywhere medications and toxic substances are stored. Substances commonly ingested by children less than six years of age are listed in Table 23-3. Adolescents tend to ingest psychopharmacologic drugs such as tranquilizers, sedatives, and antidepressants.

Clinical Manifestations

Clinical manifestations are dependent on the specific poison ingested. Table 23-4 lists the signs and symptoms associated with toxins that are frequently ingested and/or that cause significant mortality.

Diagnosis

Identification of the type and amount of the exposure is important. Physical findings, a detailed history, and examination of

TABLE 23-3 Agents Most Commonly Ingested by Children Less Than Six Years of Age

Type	Examples
Cosmetics and personal care products	• Perfume • Cologne • Aftershave lotion
Cleaning products	• "Household" bleach • Pine oil disinfectants
Plants	• Azalea • Buttercup • English ivy • Holly • Mistletoe • Philodendron
Foreign bodies/toys/miscellaneous	• Thermometers • Bubble-blowing liquid
Hydrocarbons	• Gasoline • Kerosene • Lighter fluid • Turpentine • Paint thinner

Source: Adapted from Litovitz, T., Smilkstein, M., & Felbert, L. (1997). 1996 annual report of the American Association of Poison Control Centers toxic exposure surveillance system. American Journal of Emergency Medicine, 15(5), 447–500.

TABLE 23-4 Clinical Manifestations of Commonly Ingested Poisonous Substances

Substance	Clinical Manifestations
Acetaminophen (Tylenol)	Nausea, vomiting, malaise, right upper quadrant abdominal pain, jaundice, confusion, somnolence; coma may develop later
Salicylates	Nausea, vomiting, hyperpnea, tinnitus, fever, disorientation, lethargy, coma, seizures, diaphoresis, abdominal pain
Cyclic antidepressants	CNS excitability, confusion, blurred vision, dry mouth, fever, mydriasis, seizures, coma, arrhythmias, hypotension, tachycardia, respiratory depression; physical condition can rapidly change
Benzodiazepines	Drowsiness, lethargy, dysarthria, ataxia, hypotension, hypothermia, coma, respiratory depression with severe overdoses
Cocaine	Anxiety, euphoria, nausea, headache, chest pain, fever, hypertension, tachypnea, tachycardia, vomiting, agitation, mydriasis, diaphoresis, twitching, confusion, hallucinations, abdominal cramps, seizures, hypotension, dysrhythmias, cardiopulmonary arrest
Narcotics	Drowsiness, nausea, vomiting, miosis, respiratory depression, cyanosis, coma, seizures, bradypnea, noncardiac pulmonary edema
Hydrocarbons	Coughing, gagging, and choking; altered level of consciousness; tachypnea, grunting, retractions, and cyanosis because of pulmonary aspiration; nausea, vomiting
Corrosives (toilet drain and oven cleaners; mildew remover; ammonia)	Severe chemical burns and burning in mouth, throat, and stomach; edema of lips, pharynx, and tongue; violent vomiting; difficulty swallowing; white, swollen mucous membranes

the medication containers may suggest the type of toxin. In the history the following information should be obtained: who—the child's age and weight; what—the name and dosage of the medication or substance ingested; when—the time of ingestion; how—the route of poisoning (ingested, inhaled, absorbed, or injected); and why—whether intentional or unintentional. Information about signs and symptoms that have appeared since the poisoning, emergency care given, and whether vomiting was induced or occurred spontaneously should be determined. A detailed past medical history should also be obtained including previous poisonings, medical conditions, and medications currently taken that might affect the child or adolescent's response to and metabolism or elimination of the toxic substance. Analysis of specimens such as emesis can be helpful in determining the type of poison. Laboratory evaluation may be performed when the poison is unknown, if the poison has the potential to produce moderate to severe toxicity, and if the ingestion was intentional (Larsen & Cummings, 1998).

Treatment

Treatment approaches vary with the type of poison, amount of exposure, time elapsed since exposure, and susceptibility of the child. Stabilization of the child is the first priority in managing toxic ingestions and should address the ABCs (airway, breathing, circulation). Vital body functions must be maintained regardless of the poison. Oxygen may be administered. Maintenance of respiratory function may require endotracheal intubation and/or mechanical ventilation.

Following stabilization of the individual, attention is directed toward gastric **decontamination** (decreasing absorption of the ingested poison from the GI tract). This includes use of emesis (syrup of ipecac), gastric lavage, an absorbent agent (activated charcoal), or a cathartic agent. Gastric emptying with an emetic or lavage should not be used routinely in all oral poisonings because it is ineffective when used at a late stage, may delay more effective interventions, and may cause complications such as aspiration (Herrington & Clifton, 1995). Yet, it is beneficial when used early in the treatment of potentially severe poisonings and is most effective when used within one hour of the ingestion (Larsen & Cummings, 1998). The stomach may be emptied by inducing emesis with syrup of ipecac or gastric lavage.

Syrup of Ipecac

Syrup of ipecac may be used to induce vomiting; however, the absorption of the poison is only reduced by about 30 percent when it is administered within one hour of ingestion

Nursing Alert:

Contraindications to Use of Syrup of Ipecac

Ipecac should not be given to children less than six months of age; individuals who are already vomiting, with altered level of consciousness (LOC) or impaired gag reflexes, and who have ingested seizure-inducing medications or depressants. It should also be avoided following ingestion of acids, alkalis, most hydrocarbons, or sharp objects.

(Shannon, 2000). Vomiting will usually occur within 20 minutes and may last for several hours. Any emesis should be inspected for pill fragments and/or saved for analysis. The child should be closely observed and positioned on the left side to prevent aspiration.

Gastric Lavage

In most situations, gastric lavage is preferable to administration of ipecac, particularly in emergency departments where prolonged ipecac-induced vomiting may delay more effective interventions. Lavage is used for gastric emptying in the first 1 to 2 hours after the ingestion. It is indicated when the substance ingested is highly toxic (large ingestions or substances associated with high morbidity and/or mortality); when the toxin is not well absorbed by activated charcoal (i.e., lithium, iron, lead, methanol); or in children with the potential for a jeopardized airway (e.g., altered alertness) (Phillips, Gomez, & Brent, 1993). Contraindications to gastric lavage include ingestion of corrosives and ingestions by children with depressed gag reflexes who are not intubated. Complications of lavage are aspiration and perforation of the esophagus or bronchus. The procedure involves insertion of a nasal or orogastric tube and administration of small amounts of normal saline through the tube until the fluid returned is clear.

Activated Charcoal

Activated charcoal is effective for most oral poisonings when given alone or following the use of ipecac or gastric lavage. The use of activated charcoal decreases the amount of the toxic agent available for absorption by the gastric mucosa by up to 75 percent. It can be given when the ingestion has occurred up to two hours prior to treatment. The main concern with activated charcoal is vomiting, which occurs in approximately 15% of children and increases the risk of aspiration and pneumothorax (Shannon, 2000).

Cathartic Agents

Administration of cathartic agents increases GI motility and hastens the expulsion of the toxin. Magnesium citrate and sorbitol are the two most commonly used agents.

Antidotes

Antidotes are available for several of the common and dangerous poisons. They are typically given once the child has been stabilized, usually within a few hours of the ingestion. Examples of antidotes for some common toxins include (1) N-Acetylcysteine (Mucomyst) for acetaminophen, (2) bicarbonate for tricyclic antidepressants, (3) deferoxamine (Desferal) for iron, (4) EDTA for lead, (5) ethanol for methanol and ethylene glycol, (6) flumazenil (Romazicon) for benzodiazepines, and (7) naloxone (Narcan) for narcotics such as opiates.

Nursing Management

The solution to the problem of childhood poisonings is prevention. The nurse can discuss various preventive measures. To facilitate protection of the child, the environment should be modified during infancy before she or he crawls. The nurse should teach caregivers to call the poison control center before instituting treatment if their child has been exposed to a toxic substance. Box 23-3 lists poison prevention guidelines to teach caregivers.

LEAD POISONING

Even though there has been a decline in the average blood lead level (BLL) among the population, children continue to be exposed to lead, and it is still a major environmental health problem that could harm their health and impair their ability to learn (CDC, 2000). Based on data from Phase II of the 1991–1994 National Health and Nutrition Survey

BOX 23-3 Poison prevention guidelines

- Store potentially toxic substances such as household cleaning products, medications, and vitamins out of reach of children.
- Return toxic substances immediately after use to safe storage.
- Store products in their original containers. Never put potentially harmful products in food or beverage containers.
- Refer to medications by their proper names. Avoid calling them candy.
- Buy products with child-proof caps.
- Avoid having poisonous plants in the home.
- Have syrup of ipecac available. Administer it only after consulting with a health care practitioner or a poison control center.
- Keep the telephone number of the poison control center beside each phone.

(NHANES) III, the CDC estimated that 890,000 (4.4%) children between 1 and 5 years of age had elevated BLLs, above 10µg/dl (CDC, 1997). The BLL rate was 5.9% among children aged 1–2 years and 3.5% among children 3–5 years. Children between 1 and 5 were more likely to have elevated BLLs if they were of non-Hispanic, African-American heritage, were poor, or lived in older housing. 21.9% of non-Hispanic African-American children and 13% of Mexican-American children living in housing built before 1946 had higher BLLs than non-Hispanic Caucasian children (5.6%) living in similar housing (CDC, 2000).

Due to these figures, in 1997 the CDC changed its national blood lead screening recommendations to an approach that was state-based (CDC, 2000). *Screening Young Children for Lead Poisoning: Guidance for State and Local Public Health Officials,* (1997), suggested state health departments assess risk factors and local data on BLLs. The CDC also recommended screening children receiving Medicaid for lead unless "reliable, representative blood lead data that demonstrate the absence of lead exposure among this population" exists. Specifically, the recommendations to health care providers were to screen BLLs of all children between 1 and 2 years of age enrolled in Medicaid, refer children identified as having elevated BLLs to environmental and public health services, and provide medical management that is appropriate if the blood levels were elevated (CDC, 2000).

HEPATIC ALTERATIONS

The liver performs a wide variety of vital functions; therefore, hepatic alterations can result in life-threatening severe illness. Viral hepatitis, the most common of these disorders, will be discussed.

Hepatitis

Hepatitis is an acute or chronic inflammation of the liver caused by several viral or bacterial infections, fungal or parasitic infections, or chemical and drug toxicity. Five distinct viruses have been identified as causing hepatitis: hepatitis A virus, hepatitis B virus, hepatitis C virus, hepatitis D virus, and hepatitis E virus. In this section hepatitis A, B, and C will be discussed. Hepatitis D and E are very uncommon in children.

Hepatitis A causes only acute hepatitis, whereas hepatitis B and C cause chronic infections. Hepatitis viruses are classified as enteral or parenteral, in reference to their mode of transmission. The enteral form, hepatitis A, is transmitted by the fecal-oral route. Parenteral forms, hepatitis B and C, are transmitted via venous blood transfer or through intimate sexual contact. Currently vaccines are available to prevent hepatitis A and B.

Incidence and Etiology

Hepatitis A

Hepatitis A (HAV) is responsible for most cases of hepatitis in children and occurs most frequently in children 5 to 14 years of age. It is caused by oral ingestion of the hepatitis A virus, which is found in the stool of infected individuals. Because the virus is transmitted via the oral-fecal route, it is easily spread in areas where there are poor sanitary conditions or where good personal hygiene is not observed. Employees and children in daycare settings are at high risk for developing the disease. The risk of spread and an outbreak in this setting is related to the number of infants and children in diapers (American Academy of Pediatrics, 1997). The source of infection is either contact with an infected person or direct contact with infected fecal material that has entered food or water supplies. Outbreaks have been related to sewage-contaminated water, infected food handlers (who do not wash their hands after defecting), and shellfish caught in waters contaminated by sewage. In children, HAV is characterized by either a mild course similar to that of influenza or is asymptomatic.

Hepatitis B

Hepatitis B (HBV), previously called serum hepatitis, is spread parenterally via direct contact with infected blood or body fluids. It can be an acute and/or chronic infection and is potentially lethal. Most cases of HBV in children are acquired perinatally from an infected mother during preg-

Nursing Alert:

Risk Factors for Hepatitis A

- *Overcrowded living conditions*
- *Poor personal hygiene (poor handwashing especially after defecation)*
- *Poor sanitation (sewage disposal)*
- *Food and water contamination*
- *Ingestion of shellfish caught in contaminated water*

Nursing Alert:

Risk Factors for Hepatitis B

- *Perinatal transmission to infant from HBV infected mother*
- *IV drug use with shared needles*
- *Receipt of multiple transfusions of blood or blood products (hemophiliacs, oncology and hemodialysis clients)*
- *Heterosexual activity or sexual activity with homosexual males*

nancy and/or delivery. The disease can also be acquired from contaminated needles, especially affecting IV drug users, through sexual activity, and from blood transfusions. The clinical course of hepatitis B may be varied. It may have an insidious onset with mild or no symptoms, which is common in children, or it may result in serious complications such as fulminant or chronic hepatitis.

Hepatitis C

Hepatitis C (HCV) in children has been observed most frequently after transfusion with blood and blood products; therefore, the incidence is highest in hemophiliacs. Similar to HBV, HCV can be transmitted perinatally. The average rate of HCV infection among infants born to HCV positive mothers is 5–6%. Because HCV can be transmitted through blood transfusions or perinatally, the American Academy of Pediatrics recommends screening for the following groups: (1) infants born to HCV infected mothers; (2) drug users (injecting); (3) recipients of 1 or more units of blood or blood products prior to 1990; (4) individuals receiving hemodialysis; and (5) individuals receiving clotting factor concentrates before 1987 when effective inactivation procedures were introduced. HCV can also be transmitted sexually; however, it does not appear to be acquired as easily by sexual contact as does HBV. In sexually promiscuous individuals, the risk of infection is related to the number of sexual partners (Rajan-Mohandas, 1999).

Pathophysiology

After exposure to the hepatitis virus, the liver becomes inflamed, causing damage to the cells. As the liver becomes edematous, bile channels from the liver into the intestine become obstructed, causing biliary stasis and further destruction of cells. In most cases the disease is self-limiting and liver cells regenerate completely within 2–3 months. However, hepatitis B and C may be associated with continued degeneration of liver cells and chronic hepatitis. Chronic hepatitis is characterized by progressive liver failure, cirrhosis, and/or liver cancer. Fulminant hepatitis, a rare but often fatal complication of HBV and HCV, can also occur. It results from failure of the liver cells to regenerate, causing massive hepatic necrosis. Death can occur within 1–2 weeks.

Clinical Manifestations

The manifestations of viral hepatitis are similar. Generally, children have mild, nonspecific symptoms without jaundice or are asymptomatic. Initially, the child experiences nausea and vomiting, anorexia, slight fever, fatigue, headache, and abdominal pain in the epigastrium or upper right quadrant. These flu-like symptoms last approximately 1 week and may be so mild that they go unnoticed in infants and young children. Following this period, jaundice may develop, beginning with darkening of the urine and gray-colored stools, followed by yellowing of the skin and sclera. However, many children with acute hepatitis never develop jaundice. The liver usually is enlarged and tender to palpation. Children with HBV and HCV may also present with dermatologic symptoms such as rashes and pruritus or severe itching. Refer to Table 23-5 for a comparison of hepatitis A, B, and C.

Diagnosis

Diagnosis of hepatitis is based on history, specifically exposure to the hepatitis virus, physical examination, serologic testing for markers of hepatitis A, B, and C, and liver function tests. Diagnosis is confirmed by the presence of antigens or antibodies formed in response to specific hepatitis viruses. In hepatitis, liver enzymes are elevated, specifically ALT, AST, and serum total bilirubin, indicating liver damage.

Treatment

There is no specific treatment for hepatitis, which is generally supportive. The management for children is based on measures to rest the liver, promote cellular regeneration, and prevent complications. Rest is an essential focus of treatment to reduce the liver's metabolic demands and increase its blood supply. Treatment is aimed at maintaining comfort and providing adequate nutrition.

Once the diagnosis of hepatitis is made, attention should be directed to prevention. Vaccines have been developed to prevent HAV and HBV. Children who have been exposed to a person with HAV should receive standard immune globulin (IG) within 2 weeks of exposure. Immune globulin when given in this time period is 80–90% effective in preventing the disease. Hepatitis A vaccine is approved for children at risk aged 2 through 18 years of age. The vaccine is routinely recommended for children living in communities with high HAV rates or periodic outbreaks of infection (AAP, 1997).

Hepatitis B vaccine is recommended for all newborns as part of the routine childhood immunization schedule. All children who have not received the vaccine previously should be immunized by or before 11 to 12 years of age. Additionally, administration of hepatitis B immune globulin (HBIG) is recommended for individuals exposed to HBV. If given within 2 weeks of exposure, HBIG is effective in preventing the infection (AAP, 1997).

Nursing Management and Family Teaching

Nursing care is directed toward supportive care and education of the family about prevention measures. Most children with mild or uncomplicated hepatitis are cared for at home. Because fatigue and listlessness can last for weeks, children usually limit their own activity during the early stages of the disease. Anorexia is common; therefore, small, frequent

TABLE 23-5 Comparison of Hepatitis A, B, and C

Type	Incubation Period	Mode of Transmission	Prevention	Possible Complications
A	15–30 days	Fecal-oral through contaminated food or water Poor hygiene	Immunization Education on proper food handling	
B	45–180 days	Perinatally Unsafe sex Poor hygiene Blood transfusions Body secretions Contaminated needles	Immunization Education to prevent exposures to blood and body fluids Needle exchange program Identification of carriers	Potential chronicity Cirrhosis Liver cancer
C	2 weeks–6 months	Blood transfusions IV drug use	Education to prevent exposure to blood and body fluids Needle exchange program Identification of carriers	Potential chronicity Cirrhosis Liver cancer

Source: Hitchcock, J., Schubert, P., & Thomas, S. (Eds.). (1999). Community health nursing: Caring in action. *Albany, NY: Delmar.*

meals and snacks are tolerated well. The nurse should instruct caregivers to contact their health care provider prior to administering over-the-counter medications since normal doses of many drugs may be toxic. A primary focus of education is prevention of the spread of the infection as delineated in Box 23-4. Additionally, the nurse should educate the family about the method of transmission of hepatitis and about the availability of immunoprophylaxis after exposure and of vaccines for HAV and HBV.

BOX 23-4 Prevention of viral hepatitis

- Wash hands carefully after changing diapers, using the toilet, and before food preparation and eating.
- Wash linen or clothing contaminated with stool or blood separately in hot water.
- Dispose of diapers, tampons, and sanitary napkins in plastic bags.
- Wear gloves to clean up a child's emesis, blood, or loose stool.
- Clean contaminated household surfaces with a solution of bleach and water (1/4 cup bleach to 1 gallon water).
- Avoid sharing personal items that can get contaminated with infected blood such as razors, pierced earrings, toothbrushes.

ADDITIONAL GASTROINTESTINAL DISORDERS

The following disorders are rare in children; therefore, they are discussed briefly.

Abdominal Wall Defects: Gastroschisis and Omphalocele

Gastroschisis and omphalocele are congenital malformations in which a defect in the abdominal wall allows portions of the abdominal contents to herniate outside the abdominal cavity. Their incidence is 0.1 to 0.3 in 1,000 live births (Howell, 1998). In gastroschisis the defect in the abdominal wall permits extrusion of the abdominal contents, primarily the small and large intestines, without involving the umbilical cord. The defect is usually to the right of the umbilicus, and there is no protective sac covering the intestines. The etiology is unclear, although one theory explains gastroschisis as resulting from an incomplete lateral infolding of the embryonic disc, which allows herniation of the bowel.

An omphalocele is centrally located, includes the umbilical cord, and the abdominal viscera and are covered by a protective sac. Omphalocele results from failure of the intestines to re-enter the abdominal cavity at approximately the 7th week of gestation. The size of the defect is variable, ranging from one cm in diameter to a large mass containing all the abdominal contents.

Clinical Manifestations

In gastroschisis the bowel eviscerates into the amniotic cavity, and exposure to the amniotic fluid results in thickened, beefy-red, edematous intestines. The bowel is normal in appearance in the neonate with omphalocele; however, the abdominal cavity is small and underdeveloped.

Treatment

Goals of initial management of the newborn with either of these disorders are to prevent hypothermia, maintain a sterile environment, and maintain tissue perfusion. Two accepted surgical techniques for these defects are a primary and a staged repair. Primary repair is the procedure of choice if the exposed abdominal contents will fit into the abdominal cavity. If not, a staged repair is performed. A synthetic material is used to create a sac to cover the abdominal contents. The bowel is then gradually returned to the abdomen over 7–10 days. The abdominal wall is closed in the second surgery.

Biliary Atresia

Biliary atresia is characterized by congenital absence or obstruction of bile ducts outside the liver (extrahepatic), thus preventing flow of bile from the liver to the intestines. There is no known cure for the disease. Females appear to be slightly more at risk for developing the disease than males. It is the single most frequent indication for liver transplantation in children. The cause is unknown; however, one theory postulates that a viral or other injury affected the developing bile duct system in utero or immediately after birth (Yoon, Breseet, Olney, James, & Khoury, 1997).

Clinical Manifestations

The newborn with biliary atresia is asymptomatic at birth; however, between 2 weeks and 2 months of age, jaundice appears. The infant's urine is tea colored because of the excretion of bilirubin and bile salts. Stools are light in color because of the absence of bile pigments. Hepatomegaly may be present from the pathologic processes occurring, such as fibrosis of the liver. Failure to thrive and malnutrition eventually develop.

Treatment

Treatment involves surgery to correct the obstruction and allow for drainage of bile from the liver directly into the intestines. Hepatic portoenterostomy, such as the Kasai procedure, may be performed, thereby attempting to slow the pathologic processes that occur in the biliary duct. This surgery is not a cure, and not all surgeries are successful in delaying biliary duct injury. Complications of liver disease continue to develop and eventually result in end stage liver disease. A liver transplant is required at this point.

Cirrhosis

Cirrhosis is a pathologic condition of the liver that occurs secondary to liver disease or inflammation. Viral hepatitis, inborn errors of metabolism (galactosemia), congenital anomalies of the bile ducts (biliary atresia), and chronic diseases such as cystic fibrosis are the main disorders that cause severe liver disease and cirrhosis in infants and children. Cirrhosis is rare in the pediatric population. Fibrotic scar tissue develops in the liver as a result of chronic inflammation or disease, and the organ assumes an irregular, nodular appearance.

Clinical Manifestations

Clinical manifestations vary depending on the cause of cirrhosis. When the etiology is viral hepatitis, inborn errors of metabolism, or chronic disease, initially the child demonstrates vague symptoms of GI dysfunction, including lethargy, anorexia, and nausea. Steatorrhea is frequently present caused by disordered fat metabolism. In cases caused by biliary anomalies, ascites (accumulation of fluid in the peritoneal cavity) and portal hypertension develop. The most important sign of portal hypertension is splenomegaly, which produces anemia, leukopenia, thrombocytopenia, and often esophageal varices. The child may demonstrate easy bruising or epistaxis (nose bleeds), or GI hemorrhage. Jaundice and dark urine, and pruritis are other symptoms that occur with biliary malformations.

Treatment

Medical management focuses on preventing and treating the complications of cirrhosis. Nutritional treatment of malabsorption problems consists of a low-fat, low-protein diet and supplemental vitamins, especially fat-soluble ones. Ascites is treated with fluid restriction, decrease in sodium content of food, and diuretics. Hepatic encephalopathy is treated with reduction of protein intake and administration of lactulose (to control increased ammonia levels) and an antibiotic such as neomycin. Bleeding complications may necessitate administration of blood and blood products. Definitive treatment for cirrhosis and end stage liver disease is a liver transplant.

Umbilical Hernia

An umbilical hernia results from incomplete closure of the umbilical ring, which allows the intestines to protrude through the defect, especially during crying or straining. It is most common in African-American low birth weight females.

Clinical Manifestations

The size of the defect varies from less than 1 cm in diameter to as much as 5 cm; however, large ones are rare. It appears as a soft swelling covered by skin.

Treatment

The use of binders, tape, or other materials to flatten the protrusion do not aid in closing the defect. Most umbilical hernias disappear spontaneously by 3 to 4 years of age. If the hernia persists beyond this age; if it becomes strangulated; or if it grows larger, it is surgically corrected.

Congenital Diaphragmatic Hernia

Congenital diaphragmatic hernia (CDH) involves herniation of the abdominal contents through a defect in the diaphragm into the chest cavity and usually develops on the left side. All degrees of protrusion of the abdominal viscera through the diaphragmatic opening into the thoracic cavity may occur. The extent of herniation determines the severity and timing of the symptoms. The incidence is 0.2 in 1,000 live births (Hartman, 1996). Separation of the developing thoracic and abdominal cavities is accomplished during the 8th week of gestation by closure of the pleuroperitoneal (opening between the chest and abdomen) canal. CDH occurs when this canal fails to close.

Clinical Manifestations

Newborns will have severe respiratory distress, cyanosis, tachypnea, and retractions at birth because the lung on the side of the defect is usually **hypoplastic** or underdeveloped. Breath sounds are decreased or absent on the affected side, and the chest is barrel-shaped. Heart sounds are shifted to the right. Bowel sounds may be heard over the chest. The abdomen is scaphoid.

Treatment

Mortality rate is high (40% to 60%) despite advances in current treatment modalities (Hartman, 1996). Some fetuses are diagnosed prenatally by ultrasound in which case surgical repair is performed in utero. If not diagnosed and repaired at this time, the newborn is stabilized before surgery. Ventilatory support is required to manage respiratory compromise. Metabolic acidosis is corrected with the administration of bicarbonate. If stabilization is not possible, extracorporeal membrane oxygenation is required in most cases. The surgery involves repositioning the abdominal contents into the abdomen and closing the defect.

Malrotation and Volvus

Malrotation is the incomplete normal rotation of the midgut during fetal development as it returns from the umbilical pouch to the abdominal cavity. During early gestation the midgut grows extensively and protrudes into the umbilical cord pouch until it lies completely outside the abdominal cavity. Eventually this cavity enlarges and the midgut returns to the intra-abdominal position. Malrotation occurs when the bowel fails to rotate normally as it returns to the abdominal cavity. Volvus, a complication of malrotation, occurs when the incompletely rotated bowel twists on itself, leading to arterial obstruction, ischemia, and necrosis.

Clinical Manifestations

Most infants with this anomaly experience symptoms of bowel obstruction, abdominal distention, and bilious vomiting in the first year of life. Diarrhea may be an early symptom in infants under the age of six months. If volvus occurs, bloody stools may be followed by perforation and peritonitis. Older children may have intermittent abdominal cramping, pain, vomiting, and diarrhea or constipation.

Treatment

Treatment for malrotation is surgical. The intestine is rotated and placed into the abdominal cavity with the cecum in the left lower quadrant. If volvus and bowel necrosis are present, the affected area is removed.

Meckel's Diverticulum

Meckel's diverticulum, the most common congenital malformation of the GI tract, is a blind sac or pouch protruding from the wall of the ileum. It results when a duct connecting the embryonic yolk sac to the primitive gut fails to atrophy. It occurs in 2–3% of the population and is usually asymptomatic (Sondheimer & Silverman, 1995).

Clinical Manifestations

Most symptomatic cases appear within the first 2 years of life. Painless rectal bleeding is the most common clinical manifestation. Bleeding occurs because the tip of the pouch of the ileum contains ectopic gastric mucosa rather than ileal mucosa. The gastric mucosa secretes acid and pepsin, causing irritation, ulceration, and eventually lower GI bleeding. Rectal bleeding is massive and dark or bright red in color.

Treatment

Treatment is surgical removal of the diverticulum or pouch to prevent hypovolemic shock from hemorrhage. In most cases, intestinal resection is not required, and the child recovers rapidly.

Short Bowel Syndrome

Short bowel syndrome (SBS) is a disorder characterized by inadequate surface area of the small intestine and usually occurs after surgical resection of the intestine in cases of necrotizing enterocolitis, volvus, or Crohn's disease. The small intestine may be congenitally short in conditions such as gastroschisis, omphalocele, and intestinal atresia. SBS may not be a permanent disorder because the intestine can grow and adapt. This process of adaptation is gradual, requiring months to years.

Clinical Manifestations

The most common clinical manifestations are malabsorption, malnutrition, and diarrhea. Carbohydrate malabsorption and steatorrhea also occur. Fluid and electrolyte losses may lead to dehydration, hyponatremia, hypokalemia, and acidosis. Vitamins and minerals are lost and deficiencies occur. Skin irritation and breakdown on the buttocks and perineum are caused by the frequent loose, watery stools. Bacterial overgrowth in the remaining small intestine is common and occurs when the ileocecal valve is absent or when there is impaired motility in the bowel and stasis. This overgrowth leads to increased diarrhea and intestinal gas.

Treatment

Medical management focuses on maintaining optimum nutrition and preventing complications. Nutritional therapy initially includes total parenteral nutrition (TPN) via a central line and enteral feedings via an NG or gastrostomy tube. The main purpose of enteral nutrition is to stimulate the adaptive growth of the small intestine. Oral feedings are given when tolerated so the infant can learn to suck and swallow. Additionally, to maintain an interest in oral feeding and to stimulate sucking a pacifier may be used. When enteral and oral feedings are increased, TPN is gradually decreased proportionately. Several complications may occur as a result of long-term use of TPN, including central catheter infection, occlusion, and thrombosis; liver disease; and **cholestasis** (interruption in the flow of bile). Therefore, when TPN is initiated and regularly used throughout therapy, certain laboratory values are obtained. These include liver and renal function tests, liver enzymes, calcium, magnesium, and phosphorus.

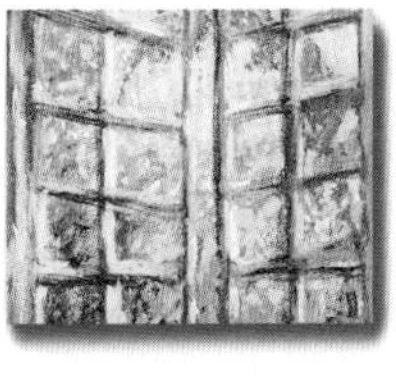

In the Real World

I was totally unprepared for what I saw when I cared for my first infant with a bilateral cleft lip and palate. I was a new graduate working on a pediatric unit and had studied this defect in school. I had even seen pictures of it in my textbook. But what I saw horrified me. My client, a 2-month-old girl, had a gaping hole in the middle of her face. All I could feel was pity for this tiny baby. She would be stared at when her parents took her out in public. I then thought of them and how disappointed they must be because their daughter was imperfect. All parents hope for and expect a perfect baby. Neither of them was in the room when I entered, and I was glad I did not have to see them right then. I soon came to my senses and remembered I was a "real" nurse now and had to care for this infant. So I began my nursing assessment and was gradually able to look at her face without dreading it. Eventually I noticed her other features, like lots of beautiful black curly hair and sky blue eyes.

Key Concepts

- The gastrointestinal system of the infant and child is immature compared to an adult; therefore, feeding must be in smaller amounts, more frequent, and consist of a greater number of calories per kilogram of weight.
- Pyloric stenosis is characterized by projectile vomiting without loss of appetite, poor weight gain, dehydration, and a palpable olive-shaped mass in the epigastrium.
- Clefts of the lip and palate are some of the most common congenital anomalies. Initial reactions of caregivers to an infant with this defect include shock, grief, feelings of failure, inadequacy, and isolation.
- Nursing management for the infant with a cleft palate or lip focuses on adapting feeding methods, providing preoperative and postoperative care, educating caregivers, and providing emotional support.
- The typical presentation of an infant with esophageal atresia includes copious, fine, frothy bubbles of mucus in the mouth and sometimes the nose.
- Intussusception is one of the most common causes of intestinal obstruction in infancy and presents with severe abdominal pain, vomiting, and blood and mucus in stools.
- Hirschsprung's disease, the most common cause of distal bowel obstruction in the newborn, is treated with surgical removal of the aganglionic portion of the bowel.
- Anorectal malformations are usually noted at birth, and after surgical repair, these infants may have difficulty with toilet training.
- Nursing care for gastroesophageal reflux is directed toward teaching caregivers methods to prevent or reduce reflux by feeding and positioning.
- For the child with chronic constipation nursing management is directed toward cleansing the bowel, diet therapy, and establishing a regular elimination pattern.
- Signs and symptoms of appendicitis include abdominal pain that begins in the periumbilical area and migrates

to the right lower quadrant, low-grade fever, nausea, and sometimes vomiting.

- Prompt and accurate diagnosis of appendicitis is essential to prevent perforation and peritonitis, which are common in children.
- Inflammatory bowel disease includes ulcerative colitis and Crohn's disease and is characterized by persistent diarrhea, abdominal pain, and growth failure. Treatment focuses on reducing the symptoms with medications, nutritional therapy, and often surgery.
- Nursing management for a child with a peptic ulcer includes teaching caregivers about medication therapy and dietary modifications.
- The nurse has a significant role in early detection of NEC, assessing for signs of complications, and providing emotional support for the family.
- For the child with celiac disease, nursing management focuses on education about the gluten-free diet and referral to community resources for emotional and dietary support.
- For a child with lactose intolerance, treatment and nursing management focuses on educating the child and caregivers about dietary needs.
- Nursing management for the child with hepatitis is directed toward teaching about dietary needs, infection control, and signs and symptoms of severely impaired liver function.

Review Questions

1. Differentiate between hypertrophic pyloric stenosis and gastroesophageal reflux.
2. Outline a teaching plan for caregivers related to feeding an infant born with bilateral CL/CP.
3. List the clinical manifestations of an infant with esophageal atresia and tracheoesophageal fistula.
4. Discuss the non-surgical treatment for intussusception.
5. Explain the pathophysiology of Hirschsprung's disease.
6. Describe the nurse's role in detecting an anorectal malformation in a newborn infant.
7. Explain the American Academy of Pediatrics recommended position for the infant with gastroesophageal reflux.
8. Discuss why appendicitis in children frequently progresses to perforation.
9. List the clinical manifestations of appendicitis.
10. Compare ulcerative colitis and Crohn's disease in the following areas: a) pathologic changes in intestine and (b) clinical manifestations.
11. Outline a plan for teaching the child with celiac disease and the child's family.
12. Identify strategies to enhance compliance with dietary restrictions for the child with celiac disease.
13. Compare the methods of transmission and clinical manifestations of hepatitis A, B, and C.

References

Allen, K. (1995). Differential diagnosis: A case study. *Neonatal Network, 14*(4), 41–45.

American Academy of Pediatrics, Task Force on Infant Positioning. (1996). Positioning and sudden infant death syndrome (SIDS): Update. *Pediatrics, 98*(6), 1218–1220.

American Academy of Pediatrics. (1997). In Peter, G. (Ed.), *Red Book: Report of the Committee on Infectious Diseases* (24th ed.). Elk Grove Village, IL: American Academy of Pediatrics.

Ault, D., & Schmidt, D. (1998). Diagnosis and management of gastrointestinal reflux in infants and children. *The Nurse Practitioner, 23*(6), 78–100.

Baldassano, R., & Piccoli, D. (1999). Inflammatory bowel disease in pediatric and adolescent patients. *Gastroenterology Clinics of North America, 28*(2), 445–458.

Birkhahn, R., Fiorini, M., & Gaeta, T. (1999). Painless intussusception and altered mental status. *American Journal of Emergency Medicine, 17*(4), 345–347.

Castiglia, P. (1994). Lactose intolerance. *Journal of Pediatric Health Care, 8*(1), 36–38.

Centers for Disease Control. (1997). Update: blood lead levels—United States, 1991–1994. *MMWR, 46*(7), 141–146.

Centers for Disease Control. (2000). Recommendations for blood lead screening of young children enrolled in Medicaid: Targeting a group at high risk. *MMWR, 49*, RR-14.

Clark, D. (1999). Esophageal atresia and tracheoesophageal fistula. *American Family Physician, 59*(4), 910–916.

Cook, M., Lopez, J., & Manfredi, O. (1996). Contemporary imaging and management of infantile pyloric stenosis. *Applied Radiology, 25*(3), 24–29.

Czeizel, A., Timar, L., & Sarkozi, A. (1999). Dose-dependent effects of folic acid on the prevention of orofacial clefts. *Pediatrics, 104*(6), e66.

Deluca, S. (1993). Hypertrophic pyloric stenosis. *American Family Physician, 47*(8), 1771–1773.

Dunn, A., & Burns, C. (2000). Environmental health issues. In C. Burns, M Brady, A. Dunn, & N. Starr (Eds.), *Pediatric primary care: A handbook for nurse practitioners* (2nd ed., pp. 1283–1309). Philadelphia: W. B. Saunders.

George, C., Hammes, M., & Schwarz, D. (1995). Laparoscopic Swenson pull-through procedure for congenital megacolon. *AORN (Association of Operating Room Nurses) Journal, 62*(5), 727–736.

Hartman, G. (1996). Diaphragmatic hernia. In R. Behrman, R. Kliegman, & A. Arvin (Eds.), *Nelson textbook of pediatrics* (15th ed., pp. 1161–1163). Philadelphia: W. B. Saunders.

Harrington, L., Connolly, B., Hu, X., Wesson, D., Babyn, P., & Schub, S. (1998). Ultrasonographic and clinical predictors of intussusception. *The Journal of Pediatrics, 132*(5), 836–839.

Herbst, J. (1996). Atresia and tracheoesophageal fistula. In R. Behrman, R. Kliegman, & A. Arvin (Eds.), *Nelson textbook of pediatrics* (15th ed., pp. 1052–1053). Philadelphia: W. B. Saunders.

Herrington, M., & Clifton, G. (1995). Toxicology and management of acute drug ingestions in adults. *Pharmacotherapy, 15,* 182–200.

Heslin, J. (1997). Peptic ulcer disease. *Nursing 97,* 34–39.

Higginbotham, P., & Gottlieb, A. (1998). Improving care with a pediatric appendicitis pathway. *Nursing Care Management, 3*(1), 26–35.

Howell, K. (1998). Understanding gastroschisis: An abdominal wall defect. *Neonatal Network, 17*(8), 17–25.

Kamitsuka, M., Horton, M., & Williams, M. (2000). The incidence of necrotizing enterocolitis after introducing standardized feeding schedules for infants between 1250 and 2500 grams and less than 35 weeks of gestation. *Pediatrics, 105*(2), 379–384.

Kuppermann, N., O'Dea, T., Pinckney, L., & Hoecker, C. (2000). Predictors of intussusception in young children. *Archives of Pediatric and Adolescent Medicine, 154,* 250–255.

Larsen, L., & Cummings, D. (1998). Oral poisonings: Guidelines for initial evaluation and treatment. *American Family Physician, 57*(1), 85–92.

Lipman, T., Rezvani, I., Mitra, A., & Mastropieri, C. (1997). Assessment of stature in children with orofacial clefting. *Journal of Maternal and Child Nursing, 24*(5), 252–256.

Litovitz, T., Smilkstein, M., & Felbert, L. (1997). 1996 Annual report of the American Association of Poison Control Centers toxic exposure surveillance system. *American Journal of Emergency Medicine, 15*(15), 447–500.

McBean, L., & Miller, G. (1998). Allaying fears and fallacies about lactose intolerance. *Journal of the American Dietetic Association, 98*(6), 671–676.

Maalouf, E., Fagbemi, A., Duggan, P., Jayanthi, S., Counsell, S., Lewis, H., Fletcher, A., Lakhoo, K., & Edwards, D. (2000). Magnetic resonance imaging of intestinal necrosis in preterm infants. *Pediatrics, 105*(3), 510–514.

Mascarenhas, M., & Altschuler, S. (1997). Treatment of inflammatory bowel disease. *Pediatrics in Review, 18*(3), 95–98.

Murray, J. (1999). The widening spectrum of celiac disease. *American Journal of Clinical Nutrition, 69,* 354–365.

Orenstein, S. (1990). Prone positioning in infant gastroesophageal reflux: Is elevation of the head worth the trouble? *Journal of Pediatrics, 117*(2), 184–187.

Orenstein, S., Izadnia, F., & Khan, S. (1999). Gastroesophageal reflux disease in children. *Gastroenterology Clinics of North America, 28*(4), 947–969.

Orloski, L. (1998). Pediatric ulcerative colitis: A review of the disease and current therapy. *Pediatric Nursing, 24*(2), 165–167.

Phillips, S., Gomez, H., & Brent, J. (1993). Pediatric gastrointestinal decontamination in acute toxin ingestion. *Clinical Pharmacology, 33,* 497–507.

Pisarra, V. (1999). Recognizing the various presentations of appendicitis. *The Nurse Practitioner, 24*(8), 42–53.

Quinn, D., & Shannon, L. (1996). Congenital anomalies of the gastrointestinal tract—Part III: The colon and rectum. *Neonatal Network, 15*(2), 63–67.

Rajan-Mohandas, N. (1999). In brief: Hepatitis C. *Pediatrics in Review, 20*(9), 323.

Ramesh, J., Ramanujam, T., Yik, Y., & Goh, D. (1999). Management of Hirschsprung's disease with reference to one-stage pull-through without colostomy. *Journal of Pediatric Surgery, 34*(11), 1691–1694.

Richard, M.E. (1991). Feeding the newborn with cleft lip and /or palate: The enlargement, stimulate, swallow, rest (essr) method. *Journal of Pediatric Nursing, 6*(5), 317–321.

Rudolph, C., & Benaroch, L. (1995). Hirschsprung's disease. *Pediatrics in Review, 16*(1), 5–10.

Ruemmele, F., Roy, C., Levy, E., & Seidman, E. (2000). Nutrition as primary therapy in pediatric Crohn's disease: Fact or fantasy? *The Journal of Pediatrics, 136*(3), 285–291.

Shannon, M. (2000). Ingestion of toxic substances by children. *New England Journal of Medicine, 342,* 186–191.

Shipman, J. (1984). *Mnemonics and tactics in surgery and medicine.* Chicago, IL: Mosby.

Sondheimer, J., & Silverman, A. (1995). Gastrointestinal tract. In W. Hay, J. Groothuis, A. Hayward, & M. Levin (Eds.), *Current pediatric diagnosis and treatment* (12th ed., pp. 608–642). Norwalk, CT: Appleton & Lange.

Stark, S. (1999). Living with celiac disease. *American Journal of Nursing, 99*(3), 24B, 24D.

Ulsben, M. (1996). Malabsorptive disorders. In R. Behrman, R. Kliegman, & A. Arvin (Eds.), *Nelson textbook of pediatrics* (15th ed., pp. 1095–1096). Philadelphia: W. B. Saunders.

Van der Plas, R., Benninga, M., Bueller, H., Bossuyt, P., Akkermans, L., Redekop, W., & Taminiau, J. (1996). Biofeedback training in treatment of childhood constipation: A randomized controlled study. *The Lancet, 348,* 776–780.

Yoon, P., Breseet, J., Olney, R., James, L., & Khoury, M. (1997). Epidemiology of biliary atresia: A population-based study. *Pediatrics, 99*(3), 376–382.

Suggested Readings

Aach, R.D., Yomtovian, R., & Hack, M. (2000). Neonatal and pediatric posttransfusion hepatitis C: A look back and a look forward. *Pediatrics, 105*(4), 836–842.

Belkengren, R., & Sapala, A. (1998). Pediatric management problems. *Pediatric Nursing, 24*(6), 590–591.

Berube, M. (1997). Ask the expert: Gastroesophageal reflux. *Journal of the Society of Pediatric Nurses, 2*(1), 43–46.

Castiglia, P. T. (1996). Hepatitis in children. *Journal of Pediatric Health Care, 10,* 286–288.

D'Epiro, N. W. (1998). Hepatitis C: Containing an invisible epidemic. *Patient Care Nurse Practitioner, 1*(8), 18–27.

Griffin, G., Roberts, S., & Graham, G. (1999). How to resolve stool retention in a child. *Postgraduate Medicine, 105*(1), 159–173.

Hillemeier, A. (1996). Gastroesophageal reflux: Diagnostic and therapeutic approaches. *Pediatric Clinics of North America, 43*(1), 197–209.

Honein, M., Paulozzi, L., Himelright, I., Lee, B., Cragan, J., Patterson, L., Correa, A., Hall, S., & Erickson, J. (1999). Infantile hypertrophic stenosis after pertussis prophylaxis with erythromycin: A case review and cohort study. *Lancet, 354,* 2101–2105.

Jack, D. B. (1997). Diagnosis of appendicitis: Getting it right every time. *Lancet, 349*(9058), 1076.

Kirschner, B. S. (1996). Ulcerative colitis in children. *Pediatric Clinics of North America, 43*(1), 235–254.

Miller, D. (1998). Appendicitis: Unmasking the great masquerader. *Patient Care Nurse Practitioner, 2*(5), 11–15.

Richter, J. (1996). Typical and atypical presentations of gastroesophageal disease: The role of esophageal testing in diagnosis and management. *Gastroenterology Clinics of North America, 25*(1), 75–102.

Shararara, A., Hunt, C., & Hamilton, J. (1996). Hepatitis C. *Annals of Internal Medicine, 125*(8), 658–668.

Wyszinski, D., Duffy, D., & Beatty, T. (1997). Maternal cigarette smoking and oral clefts: A metaanalysis. *Cleft Palate-Craniofacial Journal, 34*(3), 206–210.

Resources

Organizations and Websites

American Liver Foundation
1425 Pompton Ave.
Cedar Grove, NJ 07009
(800) 465-4837
www.liverfoundation.org

American Pseudo-Obstruction and Hirschsprung's Disease Society
158 Pleasant Street North
Andover, MA 01845-2797
(800) 394-APHS
aphs@mail.tiac.net

Celiac Disease Foundation
13251 Ventura Blvd., Suite 1
Studio City, CA 91604-1838
(818) 000-2054
www.celiac.org

Celiac Sprue Association/USA, Inc.
P.O. Box 31700
Omaha, NE 68131-0700
(402) 558-0600
www.csaceliacs.org

The Cleft Palate Foundation
104 South Estes Drive, Suite 204
Chapel Hill, NC 27514
(800) 24-CLEFT
www.cleftline.org

Crohn's and Colitis Foundation of America, Inc.
386 Park Ave. South, 17th floor
New York, NY 10016-8804
(212) 685-3440
(800) 932-2423
www.ccfa.org

Pediatric Crohn's and Colitis Association
P.O. Box 188
Newton, MA 02168
(617) 244-6678

Wound, Ostomy and Continence Nurses Society
1550 South Coast Highway, Suite 201
Laguna Beach, CA 92651
(800) 224-WOCN (800-224-9626)
Fax (949) 376-3456

UNIT V

Alterations in Oxygen Transport

CHAPTER 24

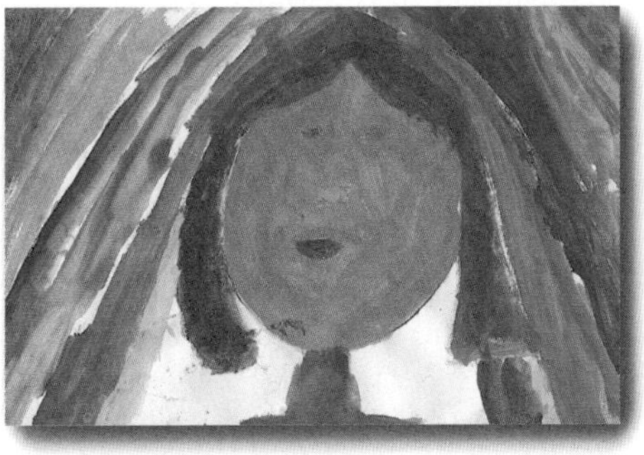

RESPIRATORY ALTERATIONS

Susan G. Fister, PhD, RN

John and I were ecstatic when we brought Joseph home from the hospital. We had recently completed adoption classes through a local agency when we were told that we were chosen as his adoptive parents. Those first weeks as new parents were near-perfect. However, when Joseph was a month old he developed an upper respiratory infection. Within a week of his initial symptoms, Joseph started breathing fast, was restless, and had little interest in eating. We took him to his pediatrician who said Joseph needed to be hospitalized. Her examination revealed wheezing, a high-pitched musical sound produced by air flow through a narrowed airway, retractions, and tachypnea. She suspected Joseph had a respiratory illness called bronchiolitis.

Joseph's chest X ray revealed bronchiolitis with pneumonia. He was started on intravenous fluids and was placed under a 50% oxygen hood. He was placed on oxygen saturation and cardiac monitoring. He was also started on bronchodilators, steroids, and antibiotics. Over the next 24 hours Joseph's condition became worse. His heart rate was 190–220, his respiratory rate was 80–100, and his oxygen saturation was 84–90. We were very scared. He was so tiny, so vulnerable. We had waited so long for him to be part of our family, and now we were afraid he was going to die.

Joseph's pediatrician suspected his infection was caused by respiratory syncytial virus (RSV). A test of his nasal secretions confirmed the doctor's suspicions. The doctor started him on Ribavirin, which is an aerosol antiviral medication used to treat RSV bronchiolitis in infants and children who are at risk for developing respiratory failure. A day or so after the medication was started, Joseph's condition improved. Within the week he was back to his cute, happy self. We were so thankful to his doctor and the nurses that took such good care of him, and us, through the ordeal.

COMPETENCIES

Upon completion of this chapter, the reader will be able to:

- *Explain differences in the anatomy, physiology, and functioning of the respiratory system of children and adults.*
- *Discuss measures to prevent respiratory alterations in children.*
- *Describe the pathophysiology, clinical manifestations, treatment, and nursing management of common acute respiratory alterations: nasopharyngitis, pharyngitis, tonsillitis, otitis media, croup, bronchiolitis, and pneumonia.*
- *Describe the pathophysiology, clinical manifestations, treatment, and nursing management of common chronic respiratory alterations: allergic rhinitis and asthma.*
- *Discuss the pathophysiology, clinical manifestations, treatment, and nursing management of less common respiratory alterations: cystic fibrosis, bronchopulmonary dysplasia, tuberculosis, and sinusitis.*
- *Discuss the manifestations and treatments of additional, rarely occurring respiratory alterations: foreign body aspiration, smoke inhalation injury, adult/acute respiratory distress syndrome, and apnea.*

The primary function of the respiratory system is to facilitate gas exchange in the body. Several elements are necessary for this gas exchange to occur. Neurochemical controls, for example, regulate the rate, depth, and rhythm of breathing. These controls signal the respiratory muscles to contract and expand the thoracic cavity. This expansion creates negative pressure in the airways, which causes air to flow into the lungs. As the respiratory muscles relax, the chest falls, and air flows from the lungs. Oxygen is taken into the lungs during inhalation and carbon dioxide waste is removed from the body during exhalation. Another critical component of this gas exchange process is a patent airway. Other essential elements include sufficient alveolar-capillary diffusion, circulation, and gas transport (Weinberger, 1998).

A respiratory system dysfunction is a frequent health concern for individuals across the life span. Infants and young children are particularly vulnerable to respiratory related diseases because of specific age-related physical differences. The purpose of this chapter is to describe these physical differences, examine varying respiratory alterations that occur in infants and children, and explore the role of the nurse in optimizing the health of the pediatric population.

ANATOMY AND PHYSIOLOGY

Several developmental variations increase the pediatric population's risks for acquiring a respiratory system dysfunction. Small airways, fewer alveoli, and increased chest compliance are leading factors that predispose them to respiratory alterations. Figure 24-1 illustrates the pediatric respiratory tract.

The size of an infant's trachea and lower airway are approximately one-third to one-half that of an adult's airway (Lewis, 1999; O'Brodovich & Haddad, 1998). Even small reductions in the lumen of an infant or young child's airway can significantly increase airway resistance and the work of breathing. Figure 24-2 provides a comparison of infant and adult airways that have become inflamed and edematous. The effect is similar when secretions collect in the airways. The negative impact of this structural difference decreases after five years of age as the lumen of the airway begin to increase in size (Lewis, 1999).

The infant and young child's nose, nasopharynx, and pharynx are also smaller and more vulnerable to obstruction. Further, infants are typically nose breathers. This causes them to have difficulty breathing when their nasal passages become blocked by the edema and mucus associated with upper respiratory infections. An infant has a more limited alveolar surface for gas exchange, in relation to height and weight, than at any other stage in life. Infants have about 20 million alveoli. By 3–8 years of age, children's lungs contain more than 300 million alveoli, the same number as in adult lungs (Lewis, 1999; O'Brodovich & Haddad, 1998).

At birth the chest wall is soft and pliable and the infant's respiratory muscles are underdeveloped. These factors lead to poor expansion of the chest and decreased lung volumes at the end of exhalation (Lockridge, 1999). These structural variations contribute to the respiratory distress infants experience when they have a respiratory alteration. When infants in distress attempt to increase lung volumes, their pliable chest wall moves inward instead of expanding. **Retractions** (inward movement of the soft tissues of the chest wall during

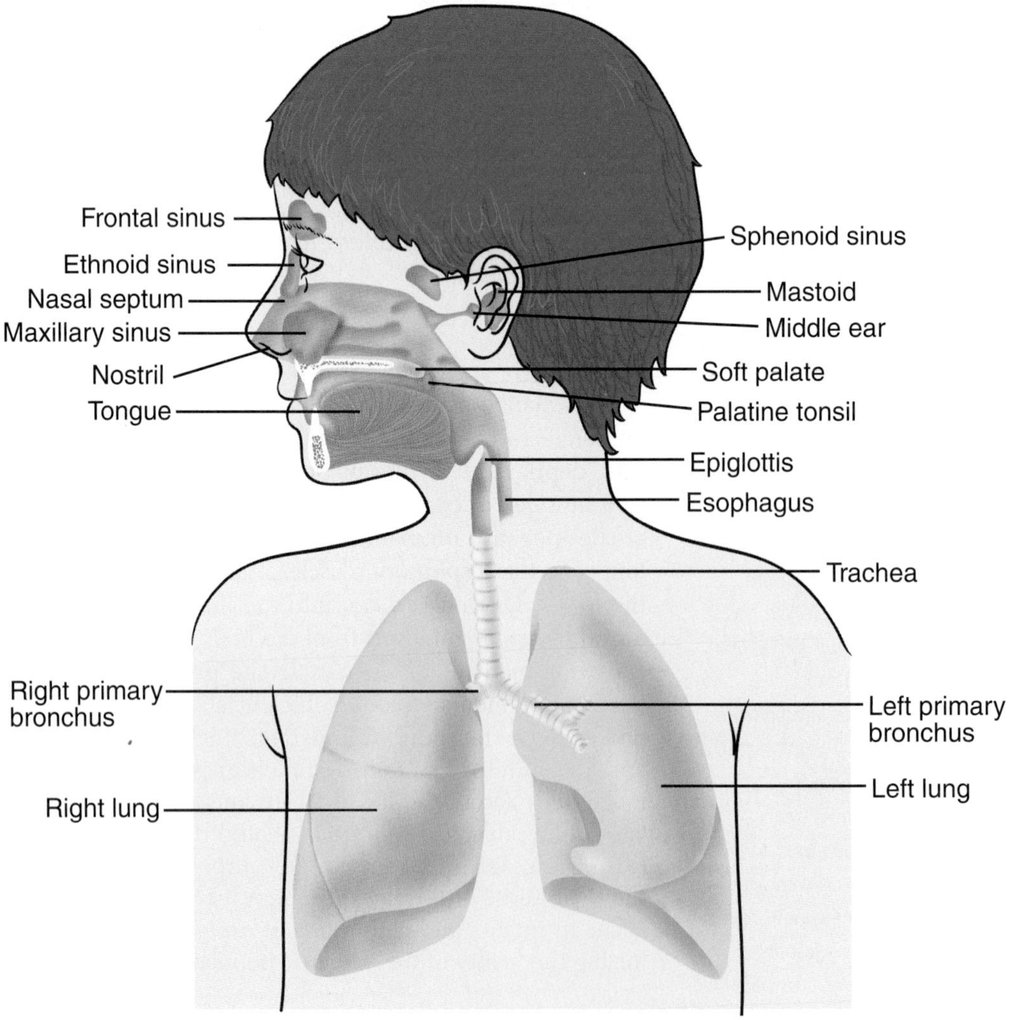

Figure 24-1 Pediatric Respiratory Tract

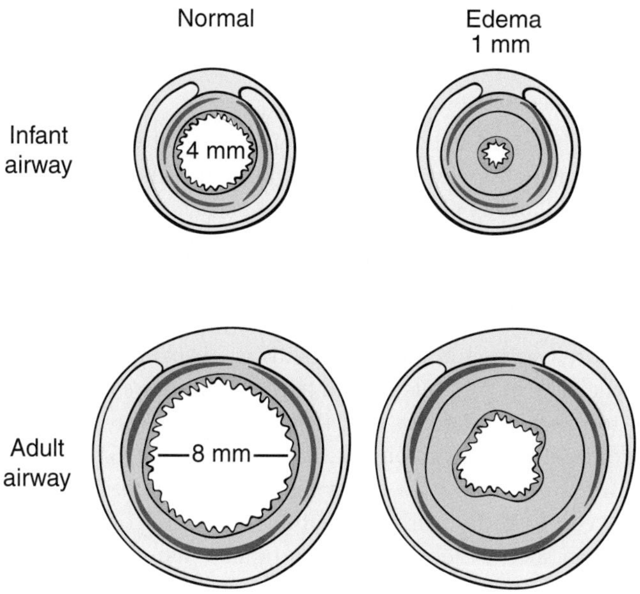

Figure 24-2 Comparison of Edema in Pediatric and Adult Airways

inspiration) occur as the soft tissue surrounding the ribs and sternum are drawn inward during inhalation. They are associated with increased respiratory effort. These movements cause a reduction, rather than an increase, in lung volumes (Lewis, 1999). The result is a decrease in ventilation of an already compromised infant.

Other developmental factors exist that may increase the pediatric population's risk for acquiring a respiratory alteration. Infants and young children have immature immune systems that make them more susceptible to a microorganism invasion. They also tend to be around other infants and children with respiratory infections. Further, hand-to-mouth activity characteristic of infants and young children may increase this population's opportunity for acquiring a respiratory system infection or injury.

Surfactant production begins around 24 weeks of gestation. By the end of gestation the surfactant production equals that of an adult. Preterm infants lack sufficient surfactant for effective lung functioning. Without adequate surfactant these infants are at high risk for developing respiratory distress syndrome and bronchopulmonary dysplasia. Treatment with exogenous surfactant therapy at birth effectively decreases the incidence of these respiratory alterations (Lockridge, 1999).

Metabolic demands, and thus oxygen consumption, are greater in infants and young children than in adults. Children's oxygen consumption is estimated to be 200% higher than adults. Additionally, infants and children have limited oxygen stores. For this reason, they tend to get hypoxic quickly and develop respiratory distress when their oxygen demand exceeds the supply (Lewis, 1999).

Nursing Alert:

Signs of Impending Respiratory Failure

Restlessness, altered sensorium, ***tachypnea*** *(rapid respirations), tachycardia, diaphoresis, and use of* ***accessory muscles*** *(neck, back, and abdomen) are signs of impending respiratory failure.*

COMMON ACUTE RESPIRATORY ALTERATIONS

Pediatric respiratory alterations can be categorized as acute or chronic conditions. Common acute alterations include nasopharyngitis, pharyngitis, tonsillitis, otitis media, croup, bronchiolitis, and pneumonia. Common chronic alterations include allergic rhimitis and asthma and will be discussed in the next section.

Nasopharyngitis

Nasopharyngitis is a frequently occurring pediatric respiratory alteration. Generally caused by an infectious agent, this respiratory condition accounts for up to 80% of missed school days (Phipps, 1995).

Incidence and Etiology

Nasopharyngitis, one of the most frequently encountered complaints in ambulatory pediatric care, is almost always caused by an infectious agent. Viruses are the etiologic agents 90% of the time (Berman, 1997). Viral nasopharyngitis, a term analogous to the common cold, is most commonly caused by a rhinovirus (Murray, Rosenthal, Kobayashi, & Pfaller, 1998). Other agents responsible for viral nasopharyngitis are respiratory syncytial virus, adenoviruses, influenza viruses, coxsackieviruses, and parainfluenza viruses. Nasopharyngitis can also be caused by bacterial agents. Streptoccocal infections are the major cause of bacterial nasopharyngitis in children (Berman, 1997; Murray, et al., 1998).

Pathophysiology

The nasopharynx is positioned behind the nasal cavities and is bordered by the soft palate and the skull (Fink, 1999). Nasopharyngitis is an inflammation of the involved tissue. The inflammatory process is associated with tissue swelling and the formation of **exudate** (fluid, cells, or other substances released from the body). Nasal congestions caused by edema and secretions impede airflow through the nasal passages.

Clinical Manifestations

Manifestations of viral nasopharyngitis include nasal stuffiness, rhinitis, sneezing, nasal discharge, coughing, sore throat, fever, irritability, and malaise. Infants may be poor

Nursing Alert:

Use of Decongestants for Nasopharyngitis

Decongestants shrink nasal passages by vasoconstricting vascular beds of nasal mucosa. The vasoconstriction effects of decongestants occur throughout the body and should, therefore, be used with caution in children with diabetes (Karch, 2000).

feeders. Children may have poor appetites. Either can have vomiting and diarrhea.

Diagnosis

Diagnosis of nasopharyngitis is based on client history and physical exam. The presence of associated manifestations leads to the diagnosis. Affected individuals generally are afebrile and have a normal WBC count.

Treatment

There is no specific treatment for viral nasopharyngitis. Management is supportive. Non-aspirin analgesics and antipyretics may be given to reduce fever and relieve discomfort. Saline nasal drops may be instilled every three to four hours, particularly before feeding infants, to relieve nasal congestion. Decongestant nose drops and cough suppressants may also be used in older infants and children. Older children may find relief by gargling with a saline solution. Antihistamines tend to dry mucous membranes so are not used in the management of nasopharyngitis (Karch, 2000). Antibiotics are not effective in the treatment of viruses and are not indicated in the treatment of viral nasopharyngitis.

Nursing Management

Assessment

The nursing assessment for a child with nasopharyngitis includes collecting information about the degree and duration of the child's signs and symptoms. Specifically, the nurse needs to know how well the individual has been drinking and eating and if the child has had a fever or cough. It is also important to note the amount and color of any nasal secretions and degree of discomfort the child has had. The physical examination includes assessing the character of nasal discharge, hydration status, and presence of any respiratory distress.

Nursing Diagnosis

1. Ineffective airway clearance related to inflammation of the nasopharynx.
2. Deficient fluid volume related to poor fluid intake caused by discomfort associated with nasal congestion, mouth breathing, and sore throat.
3. Pain related to inflammatory process.

Outcome Identification

1. The child will have a patent airway and be free from signs of respiratory distress.
2. The child will consume fluids adequate to maintain balance as evidenced by moist mucous membranes and urine output of at least 1 ml/kg/hr.
3. The child will achieve an acceptable level of comfort.

Planning/Implementation

Children with viral nasopharyngitis are usually managed at home. The nurse's role related to these children's health care is to provide education and support to their caregivers. In addition to the treatments outlined above, they may want to position the child with his or her head elevated. This position can ease the work of breathing. A bulb syringe can be used to suction secretions from infants' nares. Caregivers also need to ensure that their child consumes adequate fluids. Offering favorite beverages at regular intervals is a helpful strategy to ensure that hydration is not overlooked. Feeding young infants is particularly challenging because nasal congestion forces mouth breathing, which impedes the coordination of breathing, sucking, and swallowing. A calm approach and frequent rest periods during feedings are methods to maximize affected infants' fluid and nutrition intake.

Preventing the spread of nasopharyngitis is also an important health intervention. Facial tissues should be used when the child sneezes or when wiping away nasal secretions. Soiled tissues need to be discarded promptly to minimize the spread of the organisms to others in the home. Soiled handkerchiefs, if used, need to be contained until they can be washed. Regular handwashing following sneezing or nose blowing also deters the spread of the infection.

Evaluation

Children with nasopharyngitis are typically managed in the home. Caregivers must have the requisite knowledge to care for the ill child in order for identified outcomes to be met. Whether a child has a patent airway, adequate fluid intake, and acceptable level of comfort depends largely on the effectiveness of the family education the nurse provides.

Nursing Alert:

Early Manifestations of Respiratory Complications

Caregivers should notify their child's health care practitioner if any of these signs or symptoms are present: use of accessory muscles, dysphagia, listlessness, persistent cough, earache, headache, or fever over 101.5°F. These signs and symptoms could be early manifestations of respiratory complications.

Family Teaching

As discussed, caregivers are the primary care providers for children with nasopharyngitis. Providing comfort measures, ensuring adequate hydration, alerting the health care provider of complications, and preventing the spread of infection are the focus for family teaching.

Tonsillitis and Pharyngitis

Tonsillitis and pharyngitis are common co-morbidities of childhood and are generally attributed to a viral infection. Bacterial infections, on the other hand, can lead to serious health problems if left untreated.

Incidence and Etiology

Bacteria, primarily group A beta-hemolytic streptococci (GABHS), cause up to 20% of acute pharyngitis and tonsillitis and can lead to significant health problems (Berman, 1997; Phipps, 1995). Untreated streptococcal tonsillitis and pharyngitis infections may lead to health problems such as scarlet fever, otitis media, and **suppurative** (pus forming) infections of surrounding tissues. More serious complications of untreated streptococcal infections include acute glomerulonephritis, meningitis, and rheumatic fever (Berman, 1997; Murray, et al., 1998).

Pathophysiology

Tonsils are lymphoid tissue located in the oropharynx that serve to protect the body from invading organisms. Figure 24-3 illustrates the location of tonsils in the pharyngeal cavity. Tonsillitis refers to an inflammation, and frequently an infection, of the palatine tonsils. Adenoiditis refers to inflammation or infection of the pharyngeal tonsils, or adenoids. Children are prone to tonsillitis because they have a large amount of lymphoid tissue in the pharyngeal cavity, tend to have frequent upper respiratory tract infections, and are around other children who may be infected.

Clinical Manifestations

Manifestations of tonsillitis and pharyngitis include sore throat, difficulty swallowing, and fever. Nasal congestion that accompanies upper airway infections leads to mouth breathing and causes drying of the mucous membranes. This dryness further aggravates the pain associated with the tonsillitis and pharyngitis. Children with GABHS pharyngitis and tonsillitis may also experience a headache, abdominal pain, nausea, vomiting, and diarrhea (Murray, et al., 1998). Inflamed tonsils and oropharynx, generally with exudate, will be evident with inspection. Cervical adenopathy is also present.

Diagnosis

The diagnosis of tonsillitis and pharyngitis is based primarily on the child's symptoms and visual inspection of the throat. Throat cultures and rapid strep screening are used to determine etiologic agents.

Treatment

If a virus is the suspected cause of infection, the child is managed with supportive care. Warm saline gargles may be used to soothe the inflamed mucous membranes. Non-aspirin

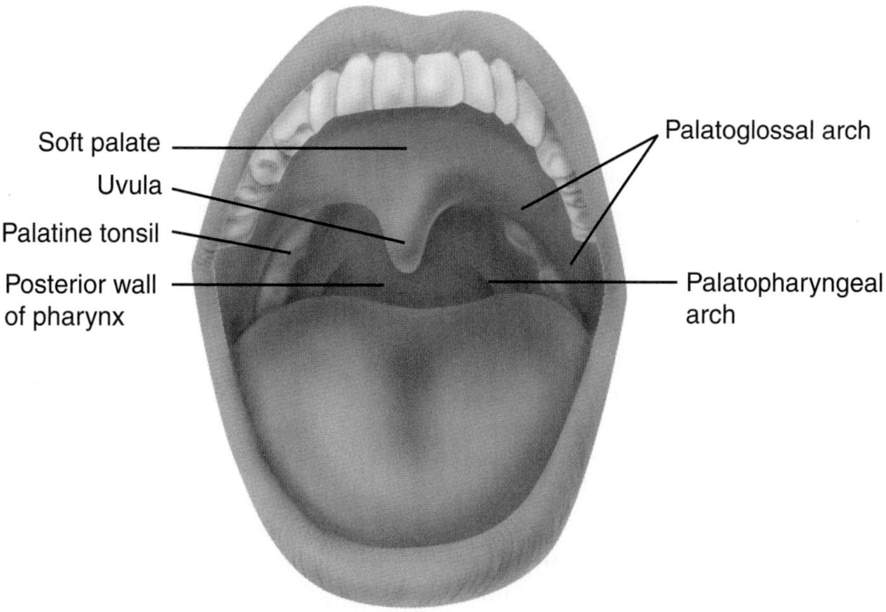

Figure 24-3 Tonsils are lymphoid tissue located in the pharyngeal cavity.

analgesics and antipyretics may be used to reduce pain and fever. If a bacterial source is identified as the etiologic agent, the child needs to be treated with an antibiotic such as penicillin or cefuroxime (Holm, 2000). A tonsillectomy, with or without an adenoidectomy, may be indicated for recurrent streptococcal tonsillitis or when hypertrophied tonsils interfere with eating or breathing. Tonsillectomies are performed on children over three years of age since excessive blood loss is more apt to occur in younger children. Also, there is a potential for the tonsils to grow back or other lymphoid tissue to hypertrophy when the surgery is performed on the very young. The surgical removal of the adenoids, or adenoidectomy, is indicated when a child's enlarged adenoids block air flow through nasal passages.

Nursing Management

Assessment

The nursing assessment for a child with tonsillitis and pharyngitis includes gathering information about the course of the child's illness and completing a physical exam. Clinical findings consistent with tonsillitis and pharyngitis include sore throat, difficulty swallowing, and fever. If the child also experiences headache and abdominal pain, GABHS is suspected, and a rapid strep screening test needs to be conducted. Children requiring a tonsillectomy need baseline assessments prior to surgery. Postsurgical assessments include monitoring for bleeding and infection and assessing the child's pain level.

Nursing Diagnosis

1. Risk for deficient fluid volume related to decreased intake because of throat pain when swallowing.
2. Pain related to surgical excision of tonsils.
3. Risk for injury: bleeding related to surgical incision.

Outcome Identification

1. The child will have moist mucous membranes and elastic skin turgor.
2. The child will achieve an acceptable level of comfort and swallow without difficulty.
3. The child will be free from bleeding.

Planning/Implementation

The nursing management for children with tonsillitis and pharyngitis is similar to the care for nasopharyngitis. If an antibiotic is prescribed, the nurse needs to remind caregivers that the antibiotic course should be completed as prescribed even if the child begins to feel better. The care for a child with a tonsillectomy is more specific.

As with other operative procedures, a complete history, physical, and baseline assessments should be obtained before a tonsillectomy and/or adenoidectomy is performed. Preoperative laboratory tests need to include clotting and bleeding times as the operative site is considerably vascular and prone to postoperative bleeding. Preoperative care also includes client and family education.

The nursing care following a tonsillectomy is centered around supportive care and ensuring client safety. Postoperatively, the child is positioned on the abdomen or side to facilitate drainage of secretions. Suctioning, if required, is done gently to avoid injury to the oropharynx. Once fully awakened, the child may sit up if so desired. The nurse reminds the child not to cough often or blow the nose, as this can disrupt an operative clot and cause bleeding. Secretions and emesis are examined for any sign of fresh bleeding. The family should be taught the difference between fresh and old blood. Old blood, dark-brown in color, is commonly in the mouth, nose, and emesis. Bright red, or fresh blood, dictates an investigation. Although postoperative hemorrhage is uncommon, the health care provider is contacted if this is suspected.

Initially, cool noncarbonated, non-acidic liquids are encouraged. The liquids are soothing and help maintain hydration. Red and brown liquids are avoided as they interfere with assessment of bleeding. A soft diet is indicated until the throat has healed. Healing of the operative site takes approximately three weeks (Phipps, 1995). Cool humidification assists in moistening mucous membranes, which become dried during mouth breathing. Opioids are typically given in the early postoperative period in order to relieve the initial moderate to severe pain generally associated with the surgery. This intensity of pain generally decreases between 4 and 7 days (Warnock & Lander, 1998). Acetaminophen is usually sufficient once the pain has diminished to a mild level.

Health care providers need to remember that children who are under-medicated are less likely to want to drink and eat. An ice collar may provide some pain relief. When fully alert, the child can be offered crushed ice or sips of water. Citrus juices are avoided since they cause discomfort to the operative site.

Evaluation

The achievement of outcomes is dependent on the appropriate care by nurses and caregivers. Moist mucous membranes and elastic skin turgor indicate the child is adequately hydrated. Pain control is achieved when the level of comfort

Nursing Alert:

Postoperative Bleeding

Frequent swallowing is the earliest manifestation of bleeding, as the child swallows more often because of trickling blood. The health care provider should be called immediately if bleeding is suspected.

is such that swallowing occurs without difficulty and the child indicates that the level of comfort is acceptable. No postoperative bleeding is a critical outcome for these children because of the risk for hemorrhage following tonsillectomies. Evaluation of this outcome is made based on visual inspection of the operative site and the absence of frequent swallowing.

Family Teaching

Family teaching includes promoting adequate fluids and rest for the ill child, administering analgesics for discomfort and antipyretics for fever, and seeking medical attention if manifestations persist or signs of a bacterial infection are present. Preoperative education includes information related to the surgery and postoperative care. Discharge instructions include teaching the caregivers about the need for providing their child with appropriate fluids and diet, pain management, activity limitations, and potential complications of the postoperative period. A membrane that forms over the operative site during the first few hours after surgery begins to pull apart around 4–10 days. During this time the surgical site may hemorrhage. Caregivers and children need to aware of this critical period and be ready to seek medical treatment as indicated (Phipps, 1995).

Otitis Media

Otitis media (OM) is an inflammation of the middle ear. The inflammation can be acute or chronic, infectious or noninfectious, and can occur with or without an **effusion** (accumulation of fluid such as in the middle ear or pleural cavity). Bilateral involvement occurs in 50% of diagnosed cases of OM (Faden, Duffy, & Boeve, 1998). There are several types of OM: acute otitis media, otitis media with effusion, and chronic otitis media. Acute otitis media (AOM) is an infectious process caused by pathogen invasion through the eustachian tube and into the middle ear with a sudden onset and short duration. Otitis media with effusion (OME) is an inflammation of the middle ear with fluid (effusion) behind the tympanic membrane and without signs of infection. While an AOM is generally associated with ear pain, OME can be found on examination of an asymptomatic child. Chronic OM is an inflammation of the middle ear that persists beyond 3 months and may or may not have effusion.

Incidence and Etiology

OM is one of the more common diseases of childhood. For example, more than 24 million cases are reported in this country annually (Faden, et al., 1998). It is estimated that otitis media accounts for 20–40% of the pediatric office visits for children under the age of five years. The peak incidence occurs in children ages 6–18 months with most having had at least one episode of OM during their first year of life (Faden, et al.; Huether, 2000a).

AOM is an infectious process generally caused by *Streptococcus pneumoniae*, *Haemophilus influenzae*, and *Moraxella catarrhalis* (Deeks, et al., 1999; Faden, et al., 1998; Heuther, 2000a; Murray, et al., 1998). Additional etiologic agents are viruses and other bacteria. AOM is diagnosed primarily in the winter months when influenza and respiratory syncytial viral infections are prevalent. As many as 93% of children with AOM have signs and symptoms of an upper respiratory infection. OME peaks during the spring and fall when allergy symptoms, parainfluenza, and rhinovirus respiratory infections are prevalent (Faden, et al., 1998). Predisposing factors, other than upper respiratory infections, include allergic rhinitis, sinusitis, cleft palate, and immune deficiency (Huether, 2000a). Associated factors include passive smoking and poor feeding techniques (Faden, et al., 1998). Immunizations and breastfeedings have been identified as preventive measures.

Pathophysiology

Children under the age of three years are especially vulnerable to OM since they have eustachian tubes that are wider, shorter, and straighter than those of older children and adults. Their eustachian tubes are also positioned horizontally. These anatomic differences are significant because they allow microorganisms and nasopharyngeal secretions easy access into the middle ear. This invasion creates the right environment for inflammation with or without infection. The inflammatory process leads to an accumulation of exudate in the middle ear. This stagnant fluid impedes the middle ear's ability to transmit sound and creates an environment conducive to pathogen colonization. The fluid can also readily block the connection between the middle ear and the pharynx, interrupting the eustachian tube's pressure equalizing function. Enlarged lymphoid tissue can further obstruct the flow of drainage from the middle ear. As the volume of fluid in the middle ear increases, the pressure in the middle ear increases. If unrelieved, this process can lead to a rupture of the tympanic membrane (Berman, 1997).

Clinical Manifestations

A primary characteristic of AOM is pain. Verbal children can readily express their pain through oral communication. Nonverbal and preverbal children may express pain by tugging or pulling at their ears. Fever, irritability, diarrhea, and vomiting are other common manifestations of AOM (Berman, 1997; Murray & Zentner, 2000; Schuring, 1995). As discussed, manifestations of an upper respiratory infection may also be present. If the OM creates a conductive hearing impairment the children may become inattentive to voices and other noises.

Diagnosis

Normally, the tympanic membrane (TM) is pearly gray with clearly visible bony landmarks and light reflex. Figure 24-4

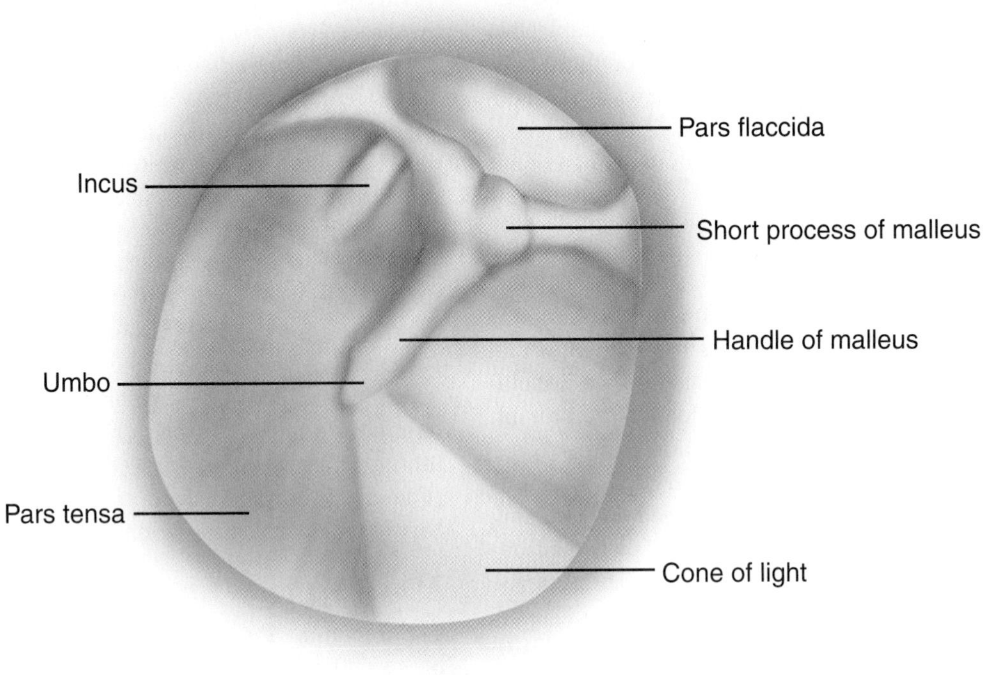

Figure 24-4 Middle Ear Landmarks

demonstrates the middle ear landmarks. An otoscopic examination of a child with an AOM reveals a red and bulging TM. The short process and handle of the malleus are prominent and the light reflex is dull or absent. Purulent or serous fluid is visible behind the TM. Figure 24-5 shows a comparison of a normal tympanic membrane and AOM. Pneumatic otoscopic assessment of TM mobility reveals diminished movement with AOM and diminished or absent movement with chronic OM. A diagnosis of OM is made based on these abnormal otoscopic examination findings (Bates, 1995; Murray & Zentner, 2000). In addition, culture with sensitivity testing is conducted if drainage in the external canal is present. The results of this testing help determine appropriate antibiotic therapy.

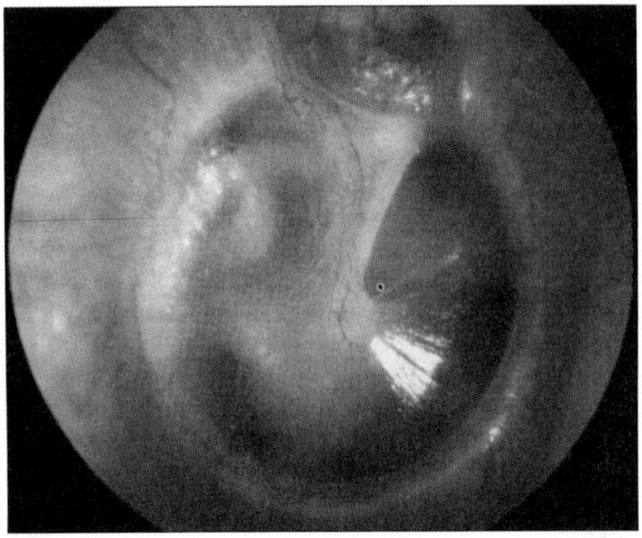

A.

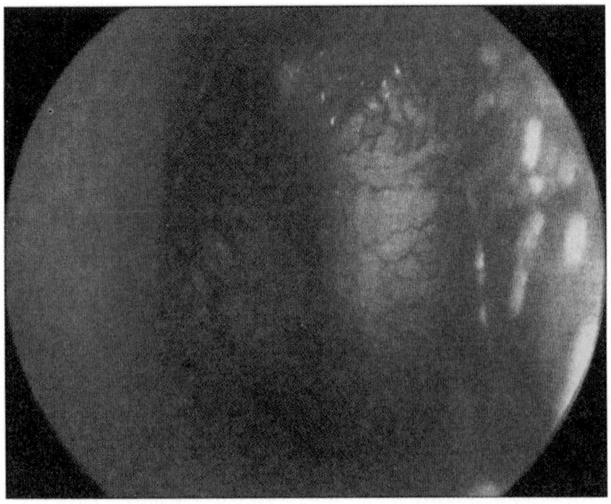

B.

Figure 24-5 Comparison of (A) Normal Tympanic Membrane and (B) Acute Otitis Media

Treatment

Amoxicillin (Amoxil), cefaclor (Ceclor), and co-trimoxazole (Bactrim) are common antibiotics used to treat AOM. Sometimes antibiotics, such as sulfonamides with penicillin or erythomycin, are prescribed in combination (Karch, 2000). Newer antibiotics such as cefixime (Suprax), cefprozil (Cefzil), and loracarbef (Lorabid) are effective in treating the primary causes of AOM (Karch, 2000). Additionally, these antibiotics are given every 12 hours instead of every 6–8 hours. This dosing is associated with increased compliance. Unfortunately, these medications are more expensive than traditional ones. Antibiotics are generally prescribed for 5–10 days. For children who have problems with GI absorption of oral antibiotics or who, for varying reasons, have poor compliance, a single intramuscular injection of ciftriaxone (Rocephin) has been shown to be effective in treating AOM (Berman, 1997).

When treated with antibiotics, an AOM begins to resolve in 2–3 days. Within a week the purulent fluid in the middle ear changes to serous fluid. At this point the OM is considered an OME. Effusions may take weeks to months to resolve. Antibiotics are not indicated during this resolution stage (Faden, et al., 1998).

The primary complication of OM is conductive hearing loss and related speech problems. Less common complications include abscess formation in the tissues adjacent to the middle ear, meningitis, and septicemia. Follow-up visits for children treated with AOM are scheduled 2–4 weeks post-treatment to evaluate the effectiveness of the antibiotic treatment and to determine if further treatment or testing is necessary. Follow-up visits should be earlier if complications arise.

A diagnosis of recurrent otitis media is made if a child has three or more episodes of AOM within a 6-month period. Prophylactic antibiotics, early management of respiratory infections, and/or influenza and pneumoccocal immunizations are treatment options shown to decrease the incidence of OM in children with recurrent infections (Berman, 1997). Chronic OME treatment involves ongoing assessment and antibiotics with or without steroid treatment. **Tympanostomy** (surgical incision in the tympanic membrane for draining fluid) tubes are indicated if an episode of OME lasts for longer than 3–4 months and is associated with a hearing loss of at least 20 decibels (Berman, 1997). Tympanostomy tubes allow for fluid drainage and middle ear ventilation, with resultant resolution of the effusion. The primary reason for treating children with chronic OME is to minimize the risks for hearing loss and related speech delays. Children with severe recurrent or chronic OM should be referred to an otolaryngologist and followed by an audiologist for hearing evaluation.

Tympanostomy, or pressure equalizing (PE), tubes create an opening between the external canal and middle ear. Care should be taken to minimize the amount of water that enters the ear as long as the tubes are in place. Ear plugs are recommended when children with PE tubes swim or bathe.

Nursing Management

Assessment

The nursing assessment of OM includes collecting information about the child's signs and symptoms. The nurse needs to know if the child has ear pain, fever, or other manifestations suggestive of an OM. An otoscopic examination provides the definitive assessment data that leads to the diagnosis of OM.

Diagnosis

The nursing diagnoses for a child with OM include:

1. Pain related to middle ear inflammation and pressure on the eardrum.
2. Infection related to presence of infective organisms (AOM).
3. Potential for delayed growth and development related to hearing impairment.
4. Potential for deficient fluid volume related to decreased fluid intake and fever.

Outcome Identification

1. The child will be free from pain.
2. The child will be afebrile.
3. The child will maintain hearing function.
4. The child will have moist mucous membranes and elastic turgor.

Planning/Implementation

Occasionally, children with chronic OM require hospitalization; however, the majority of those with OM are managed at home. The focus of nursing care for a child with OM is on family education. The ultimate goal of the education is for the child to meet identified outcomes. Alleviating the pain associated with OM is a primary concern for caregivers. Acetaminophen or ibuprofen are commonly used medications that reduce children's pain. Elevating the head and positioning children on the unaffected side may also help minimize pain. Individuals in pain from an OM are frequently uninterested in eating or drinking. Implementing pain relief measures promotes adequate hydration, as well as comfort. Offering children their favorite clear liquids at regular intervals also encourages them to consume adequate fluids.

The importance of administering antibiotics as prescribed is a critical factor in the management of AOM. This includes completing the full course of antibiotics even if the OM symptoms resolve. The child's health care provider needs to be contacted if the OM symptoms have not lessened within the first 24–48 hours after initiation of an antibiotic, or if manifestations of complications exist. Antipyretics may be used to reduce the child's fever. Antihistamines and decongestants are not indicated as they are ineffective in treating OM (Berman, 1997). Children with chronic or recurring OM need to be observed for signs of impaired hearing. Hearing testing is performed if a deficit is suspected. These children also need regular follow-up visits in order to evaluate the resolution of their OM.

Family Teaching

An assessment of caregivers' understanding about the prevention and management of OM is a fundamental component of family education. They need to recognize the benefits of controlling factors that increase their child's risk for developing an OM. For example, children exposed to second-hand smoke are at an increased risk for developing OM. Tobacco smoke irritates the eustachian tube. This irritation can cause an inflammatory process and resultant OM. Feeding practices also influence a child's risk for developing an OM. Horizontal positioning during bottle feedings allows formula to trickle into the eustachian tube, which can act as an irritant or block the tube. Either effect can lead to OM. Breastfeeding is beneficial because it provides infants with immune factors and facilitates a more upright position during feedings.

Croup

Croup is a common viral syndrome manifested by a croupy or "barking" cough, inspiratory **stridor** (a high-pitched sound produced by an obstruction of the trachea or larynx that can be heard during inspiration and/or expiration), and some degree of respiratory distress. The syndrome is an infection of the larynx, trachea, and large bronchi. The inflammatory process associated with the infection leads to airway obstruction. The primary types of croup are laryngotracheobronchitis (LTB) and spasmodic laryngitis (spasmodic croup).

Incidence and Etiology

Croup is the most common acute upper airway obstruction and is seen predominately in children between 6 months and 3 years of age (Orlicek, 1998; Wilkins & Dexter, 1998). The primary etiologic agents are parainfluenza and influenza viruses, respiratory syncytial virus, and adenovirus (Kaditis & Wald, 1998; Murray, et al., 1998; Orlicek, 1998; Wilkins & Dexter, 1998). Croup is diagnosed primarily in the winter months. Before systemic steroids became standard treatment in at least moderate to severe disease, an estimated 20–25% of children with LTB required hospitalization (Kaditis & Wald, 1998). Now most children with croup are managed in the home.

Pathophysiology

The inflammatory process in the airway creates swelling of the mucosa, secretions, and muscle spasms. Varying degrees of airway obstruction occur because of the combined factors associated with the inflammatory process and the narrow lumen of the child's airway. Additionally, the glottis has a tendency to collapse during inspiration in response to edema and muscle spasms. This further obstructs the airway. The obstruction creates turbulence during inspiration causing the characteristic inspiratory stridor associated with croup (Huether, 2000a). Other signs of respiratory distress occur as the child works to inhale sufficient oxygen.

> **Nursing Alert:**
>
> **Acute Epiglottitis is a Life-threatening Bacterial Infection**
>
> *Acute epiglottitis, sometimes classified as a croup syndrome, is a life-threatening bacterial infection that can lead to complete airway obstruction. Classic manifestations include respiratory distress, fever, sore throat, dysphagia, drooling (from edema/pain), agitation, and lethargy. The hallmark of epiglottitis is known as the tripod position. The child prefers to sit upright and lean forward, supported by the arms. The chin is thrust out and the mouth is open to attain the best airway possible. Affected children generally have no spontaneous cough. Examination of the throat by depressing the tongue is contraindicated because it has the rare possibility of causing complete airway obstruction. Children with epiglottitis are managed with antibiotics, fluids, and supportive care. Necessary equipment should be on hand in the event that a child's condition progresses to the point of requiring an emergency tracheotomy.*

Clinical Manifestations

Manifestations of LTB include a hoarse or "barking" cough, nasal drainage, sore throat, and low-grade fever. Tachycardia and tachypnea also accompany croup and point to the severity of the child's illness (Wilkins & Dexter, 1998). Manifestations of central nervous system depression may be present in children who have become **hypoxic** (decreased oxygen to body tissue) from respiratory failure (Kaditis & Wald, 1998). Inspiratory stridor is a classic feature associated with croup. Depending on the severity of the airway obstruction, stridor may be audible with inspiration and expiration without the aid of a stethoscope (Wilkins & Dexter, 1998). Retractions of the soft tissues of the neck, intercostal muscles, and sternum also may be present. **Wheezing** (a high-pitched musical sound produced by air flow through a narrowed airway) is audible in children with lower airway obstruction. While children with croup are generally not seriously ill, the increased work of breathing may cause their energy stores to become depleted and their respiratory muscles to become fatigued. Endotracheal intubation and artificial ventilation are indicated in the rare instance that ventilation becomes insufficient to sustain life.

Diagnosis

The diagnosis of croup is based on the child's history and physical examination findings. Results from the child's chest film and WBC with differential count are also used in the diagnosis of this alteration.

Treatment

The treatment of croup includes nebulized racemic epinephrine, systemic or nebulized corticosteriods, fluids, rest, and comforting measures. The **nebulizer** works by producing spray or mist with the forcing of air through a liquid. Epinephrine is a short-acting bronchodilator. It also decreases congestion in the airway, thus reducing tissue edema (Spratto & Woods, 2001). Nebulized epinephrine is used for children with hypoxia who have some degree of respiratory distress. Corticosteroids, which may be systemic or nebulized, are indicated for mild to severe croup (Kaditis & Wald, 1998). The anti-inflammatory action of these medications reduces airway edema. Nebulized corticosteriods are noted to be as effective as those given systemically and have fewer side effects (Kaditis & Wald, 1998). Fluids serve to keep airway secretions moist, and facilitate their removal from the airway. Rest reduces metabolic demands and comforting minimizes anxiety; these effects lower the demands on the respiratory system.

The benefits of cool mist therapy, a traditional treatment for croup, is debated. Many health care professionals believe that cool mist therapy moistens secretions, facilitates expectoration, and has vasoconstriction benefits (Kaditis & Wald, 1998). However, these benefits have not been substantiated through research. Additionally, children in mist tents become wet, cold, and uncomfortable. They are separated from their caregivers, which may serve to increase their anxiety and their respiratory distress. Mist reservoirs can also serve as a medium for bacterial growth. Further, humidified air increases airway resistance and results in increased work of breathing (Orlicek, 1998).

Case Study/Care Plan

A Child with Laryngotracheobronchitis (LTB)

Avery is a 10-month-old admitted to the pediatric hospital for LTB. His caregivers report that he has had a runny nose, cough, and mild fever for about two days. He also has been fussy, not interested in eating or drinking, and has not slept well for two days. They became increasingly concerned about their son because he seemed to be having difficulty breathing. Physical assessment findings reveal inspiratory stridor, **nasal flaring** (the widening of nostrils during inspiration; indicates air hunger), use of accessory muscles, muscles used to increase ventilation in individuals with labored breathing, including those in the neck, back, and abdomen, mild wheezing, and a hoarse, croupy cough. His heart rate was 164, his respiratory rate was 46, and his temperature was 100.4°F. Avery is pale, irritable, and somewhat lethargic. He has upper airway congestion and large amounts of cloudy nasal secretions.

Nursing Care Plan

Assessment Close observation and ongoing respiratory assessment for Avery are critical because he may develop respiratory insufficiency. This complication may occur if he becomes fatigued from the work of breathing or develops a superimposed bacterial infection that is left untreated (Wilkins & Dexter, 1998). Necessary assessment includes monitoring vital signs, respiratory effort, lung sounds, use of accessory muscles, and skin perfusion. Skin moisture is assessed because diaphoresis is associated with increased respiratory effort. Assessment also involves assessing Avery's oxygenation via pulse oximetry. Irritability and lethargy may suggest central nervous system depression and hypoxia. Gathering information from caregivers related to Avery's current illness and prior illnesses is important. This information provides health care providers with data that influences decisions about treatment.

Nursing Diagnosis #1

Ineffective airway clearance related to inflammatory response causing obstruction of airway from secretions, edema, and muscle spasms.

continues

continued

Expected Outcomes

1. Avery will have a respiratory rate less then 32 and be free from use of accessory muscles.
2. Avery will be free from respiratory stridor and have clear and symmetric lung sounds.

Interventions/*Rationales*

1. Assess respiratory status and vital signs (respiratory and heart rates) frequently or continuously for signs and symptoms of increased respiratory distress (extreme restlessness, cyanosis, nasal flaring, increasing tachypnea and tachycardia, diminishing breath sounds, increased stridor, retractions). *Signs and symptoms of increased respiratory distress indicate increasing airway obstruction.*
2. Administer oxygen and humidity as ordered. *Oxygen may be ordered to relieve hypoxia. Humidity helps to liquefy secretions.*
3. Administer nebulized epinephrine as ordered. *Epinephrine relieves airway obstruction by causing vasoconstriction of the airway.*
4. Administer systemic or nebulized corticosteroids as ordered. *Corticosteroids serve to decrease airway obstruction by reducing the edema of the respiratory mucosa.*
5. Have emergency equipment closely available. *If intubation is required, delay may be life-threatening.*
6. Assist child to maintain upright position with head of bed elevated. *Upright position facilitates diaphragmatic movement and air intake.*
7. Provide calm, supportive environment. Encourage caregiver participation in care. *Supportive care by familiar caregivers, in a calm atmosphere, decreases anxiety and reduces demands on the respiratory system.*

Evaluation

The goal of the nursing plan is for Avery to have adequate airway clearance. As his respiratory distress resolves, he moves closer toward meeting the identified outcomes. Clear lung sounds, resolution of the inspiratory stridor, a normal respiratory rate, and the absence of retractions are indications that the airway obstruction is resolving and the client's outcomes are met.

Nursing Diagnosis #2

Deficient fluid volume related to poor fluid intake caused by sore throat and increased fluid loss from increased work of breathing.

Expected Outcomes

Avery will maintain fluid balance, will drink adequate fluids for age and weight, and will have urine output of at least 1–2 ml/kg/hr.

Interventions/*Rationales*

1. Assess hydration status at least every 8 hours. The assessment includes measuring intake and output, assessing mucous membranes and skin turgor, and weighing daily on same scale at same time of day. *Assessment data provides information necessary for guiding and evaluating the plan of care.*
2. Administer and monitor IV fluids as ordered. *IV fluids may be ordered to prevent dehydration and to decrease the physical effort associated with oral fluids during the acute phase of croup. Oral fluids are contraindicated in children with severe respiratory distress because of risk of aspiration.*
3. Encourage oral fluids as long as respiratory rate is less than 60/minute. *Sore throat pain reduces child's interest in drinking. Increased respiratory effort and fever increase fluid demands. Fluids decrease edema and viscosity of secretions. Aspiration risks are increased when respiratory rate exceeds 60/minute.*

continues

continued

Evaluation

Avery will demonstrate adequate hydration. He will have sufficient urine output, his skin will have elastic turgor, and his mucous membranes will be moist. The nurse needs to revise the plan of care if the outcomes identified for Avery are not met.

Nursing Diagnosis #3

Fear/anxiety related to dyspnea, hospitalization, and lack of knowledge concerning child's condition.

Expected Outcomes

1. Caregivers will be less anxious as evidenced by verbalizing an understanding of Avery's condition and ability to remain with child and provide comfort.
2. Avery will be less fearful and anxious as evidenced by having restful sleep periods, crying less, and cooperating with nursing interventions as appropriate for age.

Interventions/*Rationales*

1. Explain to caregivers (and child if age-appropriate) about child's condition, and all procedures, treatments, and equipment. *Anxiety related to lack of knowledge can be lessened if explanations are provided beforehand and throughout the child's hospitalization.*
2. Encourage caregiver's participation in child's care. Provide them with breaks as needed. Assure them that child will be observed closely in their absence. *Participation and presence of caregivers promotes comfort and rest. Emotional support for caregivers helps them cope with the crisis of hospitalization.*
3. Encourage family to personalize child's room and to provide familiar objects for child such as toys, stuffed animals, blankets. *Familiar surroundings and objects provide a sense of security and help relieve some of the anxiety associated with the new and strange environment.*

Evaluation

Avery will exhibit no signs of respiratory distress. He will cry less, engage in age-appropriate play, and will have adequate sleep and rest. Caregivers will be able to explain appropriate treatment of croup. They will participate in Avery's care and will comfort him.

Nursing Tip:

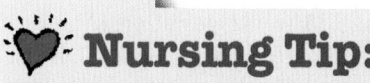

Helping the child to drink the needed amount of fluid

For many children, the amount of fluid necessary to loosen secretions seem overwhelming. The nurse can assist the child to reach the desired goal by offering a medicine cup full of liquid and then charting the data on a tracking board in her or his room. The intervention can be introduced as a game with the child ever trying to exceed the previous record. Stickers or other "prizes" may be awarded as records are broken.

Bronchiolitis

Bronchiolitis is an acute, typically viral, infection of the bronchioles. Occurring most often in young children, the infection causes inflammation in the bronchioles. Wheezing is a classic manifestation of bronchiolitis and is caused by airway obstruction from edema and secretions.

Incidence and Etiology

Approximately 95% of children have had bronchiolitis by the time they are 3 years old (Kercsmar, 1998; Sciacqua, 1998). Seasonal outbreaks are common in the winter and early spring when causative agents are most prevalent (Dolan, 2000; Kercsmar, 1998; Sciacqua, 1998). RSV is the cause of most cases of bronchiolitis (Murray, et al., 1998). Other causative agents include adenovirus, parainfluenza, and influenza (Kercsmar, 1998; Sciarqua, 1998).

Pathophysiology

The inflammation created by the infectious process leads to airway edema and the accumulation of mucous and cellular debris (Wohl, 1998). These effects result in a narrowing or occlusion of the bronchioles. The occlusion causes air trapping, which leads to hyperinflation of some alveoli and **atelectasis** (collapse of lung tissue) in others (Murray, et al., 1998; Wohl, 1998). The overall effect is hypoventilation of the affected child.

Clinical Manifestations

Initially, children with bronchiolitis exhibit symptoms of an upper respiratory illness (URI) such as rhinorrhea, sneezing, decreased appetite, a low-grade fever, and coughing. After several days the symptoms worsen. Characteristic wheezing and tachypnea become apparent (Wohl, 1998). Other manifestations include poor feeding, nasal flaring, retractions, **crackles** (an adventitious lung sound caused when air passes over airway secretions or collapsed airways are suddenly opened), prolonged expiratory phase, and intermittent cyanosis. Complications include apnea, atelectasis, secondary bacterial infection, and respiratory failure (Sciacqua, 1998). Uncomplicated bronchiolitis usually resolves in 7–10 days (Kerscmar, 1998).

Diagnosis

The physical examination and medical history are the main diagnostic tools for bronchiolitis. The white blood cell count is typically normal. Chest films show air trapping, **infiltrates** (exudate, blood, or other substances that pass into lung tissues), and atelectasis (Kercsmar, 1998; Kirchner & Abman, 1997; Wohl, 1998). Nasopharygeal secretions may be obtained for culture or antigen assay to determine the etiologic agent (Wohl, 1998).

Reflective Thinking

Parenting an Infant with an Upper Respiratory Infection

Upper airway viral infections are common in pediatric clients. These infections are of particular concern when they occur in infants. Imagine being the caregiver of a one-month-old with nasopharyngitis. What concerns would you have? What questions would you have? Would you feel different if this was your first child, if you were a teen-age parent, if you were a single parent? What information do you think you would need or want? What if your infant had croup? What if your infant had bronchiolitis? Would your concerns be different?

Treatment

The treatment of bronchiolitis is dependent upon the severity of the symptoms. Approximately 95% of children with bronchiolitis are managed in the home (Kerscmar, 1998; Kirchner & Abman, 1997). Home management includes promoting rest, ensuring adequate fluid intake, and managing the child's fever. Children who demonstrate signs of respiratory distress or who become dehydrated require hospitalization. Treatment instituted in the hospital setting generally includes bronchodilators, steroids, humidified oxygen, and intravenous fluids. Mechanical ventilation is indicated for children in respiratory failure. Antibiotics are used when a secondary bacterial pneumonia is present.

Ribavirin (Virazole), the only specific therapy for RSV bronchiolitis, is an aerosol antiviral medication reserved for severely ill infants and children with conditions such as bronchopulmonary dysplasia, cystic fibrosis, congenital heart defects, prematurity, and immunodeficiency who are at high risk for developing respiratory failure from the infection (Dolan, 2000; Sciacqua, 1998; Spratto & Woods, 2001). The drug is restricted to this population for several reasons. It may be hazardous to those who come in contact with it (Sciacqua, 1998). The particles of the medication may precipitate on contact lenses, damaging them and causing conjunctivitis. Additionally, ribavarin is expensive and has proven to be teratogenic in animals. Although there have been no documented adverse effects on the human fetus, it is recommended that pregnant health care providers not care for children on ribavarin therapy.

Two drugs are currently available for prevention of RSV: RSV immune globulin intravenous (RSV-IGIV or RespiGam) and palivizumab (Synagis). RespiGam is used for prevention of severe RSV in infants and children younger than 24 months with bronchopulmonary dysplasia or a history of premature birth, <35 weeks gestation (American Academy of Pediatrics Committee on Infectious Diseases and Committee on Fetus and Newborn, 1998). It is given monthly in an IV infusion over 3–4 hours, and recipients must delay getting measles-containing (measles-mumps-rubella) and varicella vaccines. Synagis, a monoclonal antibody to treat RSV, is indicated for children at high risk for developing complications with RSV bronchiolitis. It is administered monthly as an IM injection and does not interfere with measles-containing vaccines. The first dose of both medications is given prior to initiation of the RSV season with following doses administered monthly throughout the season (Spratto & Woods, 2001).

Nursing Management

Assessment

Ongoing and thorough respiratory system assessment, including oxygen saturation monitoring, is critical for children with bronchiolitis. Vigilant observation for these children allows for early recognition and treatment of increasing respiratory distress. Early intervention is important in minimizing the child's risk for developing respiratory failure.

Nursing Diagnosis

1. Ineffective airway clearance related to air trapping and increased mucous production.
2. Deficient fluid volume related to poor fluid intake and fever.
3. Deficient knowledge, caregivers, related to unfamiliarity with disease and its management.

Outcome Identification

1. The child will have clear lung sounds.
2. The child will have moist mucous membranes and a urine output of at least 1 ml/kg/hr.
3. The caregivers will verbalize an understanding of the disease and its management.

Planning/Implementation

Nursing care of the child managed in the home is focused on family teaching. In the acute care setting nursing care is focused on promoting adequate ventilation and fluid balance. Effective airway clearance is facilitated through nasopharyngeal suctioning with either a suction catheter or bulb syringe. Supplemental oxygen is administered through a nasal cannula. An oxygen hood may be used for young infants. Other strategies that foster adequate ventilation include raising the head of the bed, consolidating care, and encouraging caregiver involvement in the child's care. Raising the head of the bed allows for improved chest expansion, consolidating care provides the child with periods of rest, and caregiver presence reduces stress and the child's the work of breathing.

Intravenous fluids are administered until the child can drink an adequate amount of oral fluids. Antipyretics may be ordered to reduce fever. Nursing management also involves ensuring that ordered nebulized pulmonary medications and chest physiotherapy have been implemented. Another most important aspect of care of children with RSV bronchiolitis is consistent handwashing; the most effective means of preventing the spread in health care facilities.

Evaluation

The evaluation of the outcomes is a critical step in determining if the plan of care was effective in meeting the child and family's needs. Clear lung sounds is a primary criteria for evaluating the resolution of ineffective airway clearance. Moist mucous membranes and adequate urine output are measures of adequate fluid intake. Children in respiratory distress and those with fever are at risk for becoming fluid depleted. Finally, caregiver understanding of bronchiolitis and its management is a necessary step in their ability to provide appropriate care for their ill child.

Family Teaching

The nurse needs to provide information necessary for caregivers to understand their child's disease and the treatment plan. Specific information is dependent on the severity of the symptoms and whether the child is managed at home or in the hospital. Caregivers of children cared for at home are taught to alert the health care provider if signs of respiratory distress occur or if the child becomes dehydrated. Beyond being necessary for normal body functioning, fluids help liquify thick airway secretions. Caregivers also need to know how to use a bulb syringe.

Pneumonia

Pneumonia is an acute inflammation of the pulmonary **parenchyma** (the functional tissue of an organ as distinguished from supporting or connective tissue) associated with alveolar consolidation. Pneumonia can appear as a primary disease or a complication of another dysfunction.

Incidence and Etiology

Pneumonia is seen frequently in childhood, occurring most often in infancy and early childhood. Viruses, such as cytomegalovirus, RSV, influenza, and adenovirus, are the primary causative agents except in neonatal cases of pneumonia, which are most often bacterial (Correa & Starke, 1998; Glezen, 1998; Kercsmar, 1998). Bacterial pneumonia occurs infrequently in older infants and children and is generally preceded by a viral upper respiratory illness. Other etiologic agents are rare in children.

Pathophysiology

Defense mechanisms including the cough reflex, mucociliary action, phagocytosis by alveolar macrophages, the inflammatory response, and the immune response protect individuals from inhaled pathogens (Brashers, 2000). Pathogens that manage to invade a susceptible individual release toxins and stimulate secondary and tertiary defense mechanisms. The toxins and by-products of the body's defenses damage pulmonary mucous membranes and cause the accumulation of debris and exudate in the airways. These effects lead to **ventilation/perfusion ratio** (the ratio of alveolar ventilation to capillary perfusion) abnormalities. Pneumonia is frequently classified as lobar, interstitial, or bronchial (Brashers, 2000).

Lobar pneumonia involves a major portion of one or more lobes of a lung. Interstitial pneumonia includes the alveolar walls and peribronchial and interlobular tissues. Bronchial pneumonia is more diffuse and involves the bronchi and lung fields.

Clinical Manifestations

Common manifestations of pneumonia include cough, malaise, pleuritic pain, fever, and anorexia. Other signs and symptoms may include headache, tachypnea, wheezing, and gastrointestinal complaints (Brashers, 2000; Correa & Starke, 1998; Kercsmar, 1998). Affected children also frequently have manifestations associated with an upper respiratory infection.

Diagnosis

The diagnosis of pneumonia is based on physical findings and sputum culture. The WBC count in viral pneumonia is generally normal, whereas in bacterial pneumonia it may be elevated with an increased number of neutrophils (Correa & Starke, 1998). Chest radiographs show the extent and location of involvement and give clues to the etiology of the pneumonia (Brashers, 2000; Glezen, 1998; Kercsmar, 1998).

Treatment

The treatment of pneumonia depends on the etiologic agent. The management for viral pneumonia is supportive. In addition, children with bacterial pneumonia are treated with antibiotics. Most children with pneumonia are managed in the home. The aim of treatment is to maximize ventilation and prevent dehydration. Children needing to be hospitalized also require oxygen therapy and chest physiotherapy. Intravenous fluids may be necessary to maintain hydration. Antipyretics may be administered to control fever.

Nursing Management

Assessment

As with other respiratory alterations, a thorough respiratory assessment is a critical step in the nursing process. This includes monitoring for manifestations of pneumonia and signs that suggest increasing respiratory distress. Assessing for fever, pain, and hydration are also important when caring for children with pneumonia.

Diagnosis

1. Impaired gas exchange related to ventilation/perfusion abnormalities caused by pulmonary infection.
2. Ineffective airway clearance related to edema and exudate.
3. Ineffective breathing pattern related to an inflammatory infection of the lower airway.

Outcome Identification

1. The client will have pink mucous membranes and a normal respiratory rate.
2. The client will have clear lung sounds and be free from signs of dyspnea.
3. The client will demonstrate and maintain an improved breathing pattern as evident by decrease in or absence of tachypnea, retractions, cough, wheezing, grunting, and nasal flaring.

Planning/Implementation

The nursing care for children with pneumonia depends on the severity of the symptoms and the etiologic agent. Supportive care is indicated if a child has viral pneumonia. If the pneumonia is caused by a bacterial agent, antibiotics are administered as prescribed. Nursing care also includes interventions such as administering intravenous therapy and encouraging fluids to help restore and maintain hydration. Children who are able to tolerate oral fluids are offered those they like at regular intervals. Adequate fluids help liquefy and facilitate the removal of secretions from the airway. Chest physiotherapy is another intervention that may be indicated.

Pain assessment is an important nursing intervention, particularly for the child with pneumonia, because pleuritic pain is increased with coughing or deep breathing. In an attempt to minimize pain, children with pneumonia may take shallow breaths and resist coughing. For these children, pain medications not only promote comfort, they also may facilitate deep breathing.

Evaluation

As the pneumonia improves, the child's respiratory assessment findings will become normal. Although X rays may not be normal for several weeks, manifestations associated with the infection will resolve much sooner.

Family Teaching

Because most children with pneumonia are managed at home, the nurse must provide adequate instructions and teaching regarding the child's care. Caregivers are instructed to offer small amounts of liquids frequently to help promote hydration. They can also ensure that the child's position is changed at least every two hours to promote pulmonary drainage. Should the child require percussion and postural drainage, they need to be taught the technique and provide a return demonstration to the nurse. If the child requires inhaled medications, information related to the use of equipment must also be included as part of the family teaching. If the child has bacterial pneumonia, the nurse needs to instruct the caregivers about the child's antibiotic and its administration. Additionally, they

Eye On:

Herbal Remedies

Individuals in various cultures believe that diseases or conditions result from a cold/hot or wet/dry imbalance in the fluids of the body. They believe that the remedy for disease lies in restoring balance. Pneumonia, for example, is considered a "cold" disease that should be managed with "hot" treatments. Other respiratory illnesses also fall into this "cold" category. Herbal remedies may be used to achieve balance in the body. These remedies are used in different forms such as a poultice or tea. Some examples of herbs used to treat respiratory illnesses are:

Garlic–treats coughs and serves as an antibiotic (eaten raw).

Eucalyptus–clears stuffy nasal and sinus congestion; used for asthma, bronchitis, and tuberculosis (boil in water and breathe in steam).

Mullein–soothes and relaxes the airway and relieves cough; used for asthma, tuberculosis, and as a cough suppressant (mixed with water and taken orally).

Health care professionals need to incorporate questions about the use of herbal remedies in their history taking. This is important because some of these remedies are not considered safe and others may have adverse interactions with prescribed medications.

are reminded that the child's energy level will be reduced until completely recovered.

COMMON CHRONIC RESPIRATORY ALTERATIONS

Some respiratory alterations are chronic, requiring the nurse to give acute care to the child while in the hospital and coordinate long-term care with caregivers and other health professionals. These respiratory alterations are important from an epidemiologic standpoint because of the staggering numbers of children and families affected by the disorders and the exorbitant costs associated with treatment. The most common chronic alterations are allergic rhinitis and asthma.

Allergic Rhinitis

Allergic rhinitis, also known as hay fever, predisposes children to otitis media, sinusitis, and asthma (Opperwall, 2000; Pearlman, 1997; Umetsu, 1998). Left untreated, chronic allergic rhinitis can lead to chronic nasal inflammation, obstruction, and postnasal drainage (Opperwall, 2000). Seasonal allergic rhinitis is generally related to outdoor allergens such as tree, grass, and weed pollens. Perennial allergic rhinitis is most often related to sensitivity to indoor allergens such as dust mites and mold. Children may have sensitivity to both outdoor and indoor offenders.

Incidence and Etiology

Allergic rhinitis affects 5–10% of children (Umetsu, 1998). It is the sixth most common chronic illness in children (Opperwall, 2000). It is significant in terms of morbidity because of its association with other health problems. For example, approximately 40% of individuals with allergic rhinitis also have asthma (Opperwall, 2000). Asthma is associated with school absenteeism, activity intolerance, and life-threatening exacerbations. Chronic otitis media, another health alteration linked with allergic rhinitis, may cause hearing and speech delays.

Pathophysiology

Allergic rhinitis is caused by a type I allergic response to indoor and outdoor allergens. Pollens, dust mites, pet dander, and mold spores are examples of causative agents (Umetsu, 1998). Allergen exposure stimulates the release of IgE. The IgE binds to mast cells, which then become receptors for allergen antigens, a process that leads to mast cell degranulation. During this process varying mast cell products are released (Rote, Huether, & McCance, 2000). A primary mediator released is histamine. Histamine has varying effects, including increasing vascular permeability, which causes edema, increasing mucous production, and narrowing of the airway (Fink, 1999; Rote, et al., 2000). Ongoing or repeated exposure of sensitized membranes to allergens may lead to chronic nasal congestion.

Clinical Manifestations

Manifestations of allergic rhinitis include chronic sneezing, nasal congestion, serous to mucoid rhinorrhea, mouth breathing, and itching of the eyes, nose, and ears (Opperwall, 2000; Pearlman, 1997; Umetsu, 1998). An allergic salute is common in children with allergic rhinitis as they scratch their noses with the palms of their hands. This allergic salute may lead to a transverse line across the child's nose (Pearlman, 1997; Umetsu, 1998). The child's sclera may be injected and the lower lids may be darkened from venous stasis (Opperwall, 2000; Umetsu, 1998).

Diagnosis

The diagnosis of allergic rhinitis is based on the history and physical examination. The presence of associated manifestations and enlarged, purplish, and pale turbinates are findings that lead to a diagnosis (Pearlman, 1997; Umetsu, 1998).

Nursing Alert:

Safety with Allergy Testing and Immunotherapy

Skin testing and ***immunotherapy*** *(the use of synthetic or natural elements to stimulate or suppress the body's immune response) may cause severe and life-threatening reactions. For this reason, testing and injections are only administered in facilities equipped to manage allergic and anaphylactic responses. Additionally, the child should remain in the facility for at least twenty minutes following injections. Children considered at high risk for developing an untoward reaction should be observed for as long as two hours. Symptoms may be mild (local pruritus) to severe (flushing and shortness of breath). Life-threatening reactions include airway obstruction, chest pain, hypotension, cardiac arrythmias, loss of consciousness, and death.*

The child may also have an otitis media and wheezing or crackles. Elevated serum IgE and eosinophil levels indicate the presence of allergic disorder (Umetsu, 1998). Skin tests may be conducted to identify specific allergens to which the child is sensitive. Children undergoing skin testing need to avoid antihistamines for several days to weeks before the testing is conducted (Opperwall, 2000).

Treatment

Management of allergic rhinitis includes environmental control and avoidance of allergens. Reducing dust mites in the home, controlling mold counts through use of a dehumidifier, using air conditioners, and keeping windows closed during peak pollen seasons are examples of ways to minimize allergen exposure (Umetsu, 1998). Antihistamines, with or without decongestants, and nasal cromolyn sodium are the primary pharmacologic agents used to manage allergic rhinitis (Pearlman, 1997). Cromolyn sodium acts locally to inhibit the degranulation of mast cells, thereby inhibiting the inflammatory response (Spratto & Woods, 2001). Topical steroids and immunotherapy are indicated when other interventions have failed (Pearlman, 1997).

Immunotherapy is used as a last resort for young children because of the emotional trauma associated with the injections. Local analgesics may be used to minimize the discomfort associated with injections and may, therefore, lower the child's anxiety related to the therapy. Immunotherapy involves serial injections of extracts from the allergens to which the child is sensitive. The amount of extract gradually increases, as tolerated, with each injection. The process may involve giving the child 1–2 injections per week for several months to a year or two. Once the maximum dose is reached the child receives maintenance injections once every few weeks. Immunotherapy is most effective in children with seasonal allergies.

Nursing Management

Assessment

Children with allergic rhinitis have frequent runny noses, sniffles, and sneezing. Their nasal drainage is generally clear and thin. Additionally, nasal congestion may force children to be mouth breathers. Beyond assessing for the manifestations associated with this alteration, the nurse needs to also assess the child's family history. There is a familial predisposition to developing certain allergies. Additionally, the child's environment also needs to be assessed for environmental allergens such as pets, wood-burning stoves, house plants, and cigarette smoking. Because allergic rhinitis is associated with other health problems such as otitis media, upper respiratory infections, sinusitis, and asthma, the nurse should also assess the child for manifestations of these alterations.

Diagnosis

1. Impaired oral mucous membranes related to mouth breathing.
2. Deficient knowledge, caregiver, related to child with environmental allergies.

Outcome Identification

1. The child's lips and oral mucous membranes will be moist and intact.
2. The child's caregivers will verbalize a commitment to reduce possible allergens in the environment.

Planning/Implementation

Children with allergic rhinitis are managed in the home. Caregivers are taught ways to reduce the allergens in the home and to minimize the child's exposure to seasonal allergens. Box 24-1 lists strategies for reducing allergen exposure indoors and outdoors.

The family is also taught that adequate oral fluids help liquefy secretions that accumulate in the nasopharynx in children with allergic rhinitis and help to maintain fluids lost through mouth breathing. Lip balm is recommended to keep the child's lips from becoming chapped and dried.

Nurses may also be involved in skin testing and administering immunotherapy. Those involved in these interventions must be meticulous with regards to safety during testing and injection therapy and be prepared to initiate emergency treatments as indicated. Nurses may also be involved in screening children for health problems associated with chronic allergic rhinitis. Hearing, speech, and developmental screening may be conducted to assess for complications of this chronic alteration.

Evaluation

The nurse evaluates whether the child's mucous membranes are moist and intact and if the caregivers commit to reducing

BOX 24-1 Reducing allergen exposure in the home and outdoors

In the bedroom:

- Encase mattress, box springs, and pillows in vinyl covering or other similar barrier
- Tape over zippers of barriers of bedding covers
- Launder curtains, blankets, mattress pads, and comforters every two weeks
- Launder bed linens and favorite stuffed animals weekly
- Maintain laundry water at 130°F
- Avoid nonessential fabric items and those made with feathers
- Wash down the bedroom and closet every couple of months

Pets and pests:

- Keep animals outside the home
- Clean the home thoroughly if animals have lived indoors
- Keep the indoor pet in uncarpeted areas that are easily cleaned
- Premedicate the child before visiting a home with an animal
- Eradicate cockroach populations in the home
- Clean the home thoroughly if cockroaches have been present

Throughout the house:

- Clean moldy surfaces with 1:10 solution of bleach and water
- Use a dehumidifier to reduce mold growth in damp houses; keep humidity <45%
- If humidifier is used, change water regularly and clean with bleach solution
- Avoid house plants
- Damp mop and damp dust at least once per week
- Vacuum carpets and upholstery at least once per week
- Dry clean drapes and carpets
- Remove carpeting and replace if possible with wood or vinyl
- Replace furnace filters or use an electrostatic filter
- Filter furnace vents
- Close windows and use air conditioners when outdoor air quality is poor
- Keep home a smoke-free environment (tobacco or wood)
- Avoid use of strong odors or sprays

Outdoors:

- Keep child from compost or leaf piles, woods, and other high mold areas
- Keep child indoors when air quality is poor and when mold/pollen counts are high
- Keep child from wood smoke, animals, and agriculture chemicals
- Avoid exercise in cold, dry air

allergens in the child's environment. If these outcomes are not met, the nurse revises the plan of care as indicated. The ultimate goal is for the child to become asymptomatic. This should be achieved if the allergens are controlled.

Family Teaching

Allergic rhinitis is a chronic alteration that requires ongoing attention on the part of the child's caregivers. Environmental reduction of allergens is a critical factor in minimizing the affected child's symptoms. Families need teaching to identify possible sources for their child's allergies. Should the health care provider recommend skin testing and/or immunotherapy, they need information related to these interventions and their potential risks. The family also needs to understand that immunotherapy works best if the injection schedule is maintained. Missed injections require that the series of injections be restarted or that the next injection contain a reduced amount of allergens. The overall result is that the treatment period is lengthened.

Asthma

Asthma is a common respiratory illness characterized by chronic inflammation, bronchoconstriction, and bronchial hyperresponsiveness (Opperwall, 2000; Umetsu, 1998; Velsor-Friedrich & Srof, 2000). The primary manifestations of the disease, wheezing, coughing, and dyspnea, are caused by airways obstruction from edema, mucous, and bronchoconstriction. Once thought to be reversible, it is now believed that asthma causes airways to become damaged over time as a result of chronic inflammation (Owen, 1999).

Incidence and Etiology

Asthma is the most common pediatric chronic illness. The costs associated with the disease are approximately $3 billion annually. Asthma affects approximately 5 million children and is the leading cause of pediatric admissions to the emergency room and hospital (Brashers, 1998; Umetsu, 1998; Velsor-Friedrich & Srof, 2000). As many as 17% of the children in some urban areas of the country have asthma (Fink & Fahey, 1999). Asthma is also the leading cause of missed school days. Approximately 10 million absences from school are attributed to asthma each year (Velsor-Friedrich & Srof, 2000).

The incidence of asthma, and mortality rates associated with the disease, are rising. Between 1980 and 1995 the number of children diagnosed with asthma increased 75–160%. Each year approximately 5,000 children die as a result of the disease (Sydnor-Greenberg & Dokken, 2000). Inner-city African-American and Hispanic youth have the highest morbidity and mortality rates associated with the disease (Huether, 2000b). The death rate of African-American children with asthma, for example, is approximately three times that of Caucasian children (Yoos & McMullen, 1999).

Pathophysiology

The inflammatory response associated with asthma is triggered by agents such as antigens (e.g., dust mites, roaches), irritants (e.g., pollution, tobacco smoke, cold air), infection, medications (e.g., aspirin, nonsteroidal anti-inflammatory drugs), gastroesophageal reflux, foods and food preservatives, physical and emotional stress, and exercise (Opperwall, 2000; Umetsu, 1998). These triggers stimulate a cascade of events that affect the entire respiratory tract. Allergens stimulate an increase in circulating IgE, mast cells, and macrophages. These products cause the release of other substances such as histamine, basophils, eosinophils, neutrophils, platelets, T lymphocytes, and prostaglandins. The result of this inflammatory cascade is bronchoconstriction, mucosal edema, and an increased mucous production (Huether, 2000b; Opperwall, 2000; Owen, 1999). Figure 24-6 illustrates the effects of this alteration on the airway. These effects cause airway obstruction and air trapping, which lead to ventilation/perfusion alterations, an increased work of breathing, hypercapnia, and hypoxemia. If left untreated, respiratory failure and death can result.

Clinical Manifestations

The classic manifestations of asthma are expiratory wheezing, chronic cough, and **dyspnea** (shortness of breath or difficulty in breathing) (Huether, 2000b; Opperwall, 2000). Other signs and symptoms include recurrent chest tightness, greater than 20% variation in morning and evening peak flow volumes, tachypnea, chest pain, irritability, restlessness, use of accessory muscles, nasal flaring, and **orthopnea** (an increase in difficulty breathing when lying flat) (Opperwall, 2000). Older children may sit upright with shoulders in a hunched-over position with their arms braced (Figure 24-7). Children in severe distress also will experience diaphoresis, cyanosis, and pallor. Growth and development retardation may occur in children with severe, persistent asthma (Huether, 2000b).

Diagnosis

The diagnosis of asthma is made based on the client history, physical assessment findings, and pulmonary function studies. Peak expiratory flow rates (PEFR) are also particularly helpful in determining the extent of a child's asthma (Umetsu, 1998). The PEFR is the fastest speed at which air is forced from the lungs during expiration. It is measured with a peak flow meter in liters per minute. The PEFR is lowered during acute episodes because of impaired expiration and air trapping that occurs as a result of airway obstruction. Chest films may be used to rule out other diseases.

Treatment

Avoidance of triggers, regular peak flow monitoring, medications including inhalation therapies, family education, ongo-

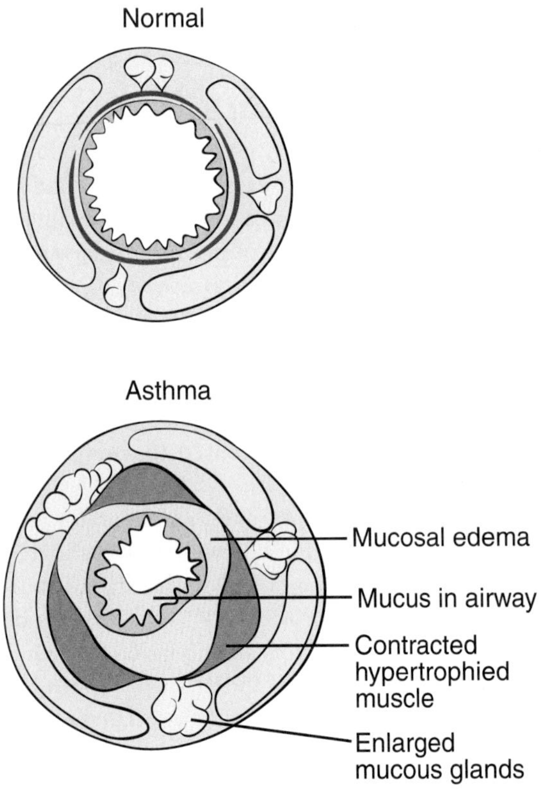

Figure 24-6 Pathophysiology of Asthma

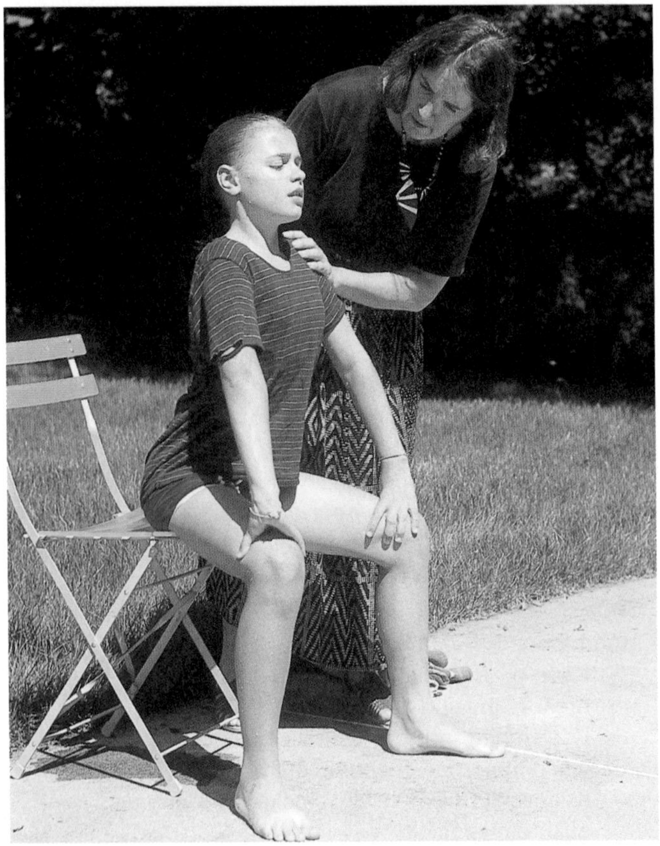

Figure 24-7 This position in an older child is a classic sign of an asthma episode.

ing follow-up, and rapid access to medical care are the chief components of successful asthma management (Capen & Sherman, 1998; Opperwall, 2000; Velsor-Friedrich & Srof, 2000). Avoidance of triggers is the primary means for preventing the symptoms of asthma. Box 24-1 (found within allergic rhinitis discussion) provides a listing of steps that can be taken to lower allergen exposure. Other preventative actions include warm-ups before exercising, short-term beta-2 agonist 15–30 minutes before exercising, and avoiding outdoor exercising when the air is cold and dry. Children with asthma need to have a good night's sleep and adequate nutrition. It is also important for them to avoid being around others with infections, particularly respiratory infections. Yoga and relaxation exercises are also beneficial in reducing asthma symptoms.

Regular monitoring of PEFR provides a guide to how well the asthma is controlled. Lowered flow rates alert the child and family that the asthma symptoms are worsening. As the Research Highlight indicates, affected children and

Nursing Alert:

Treatment of an Asthma Episode

The emergency treatment of an asthma episode includes inhaled short-acting beta-2 agonists, subcutaneous beta-2 agonists, and systemic corticosteroids. Inhaled ipratropium bromide (Atrovent) and supplemental oxygen therapy may also be administered.

Research Highlight

Symptom Perception and Evaluation in Childhood Asthma

Study Purpose

The purpose of this study was to examine the accuracy of child and parent perceptions of asthma symptoms and evaluate the participants' decision making based on their understanding of the symptoms.

Methods

A convenience sample of 28 patient/parent pairs were enrolled in the study. The sample included racially and economically diverse children from urban and suburban communities. The children ranged in age from 6–18 years. Subjective and objective assessments of asthma severity were completed. A visual analog scale was used to ascertain perceptions about the best and worst breathing. Objective assessments of the child's pulmonary function included peak expiratory flow rate measurements, office spirometry findings, and a functional assessment scale used to evaluate overall severity of the child's disease. Demographic data, the child/parent pair understanding of the child's specific symptoms and exacerbation triggers, and styles related to illness management were also examined.

Findings

Children and parents missed early symptoms of asthma and waited too long before intervening during an exacerbation. Adolescents were more accurate than school-aged children, and African-American parents were more accurate than Caucasian parents, in their perceptions of asthma symptoms. Socioeconomic levels did not affect perceptions of symptoms.

Implications

Inaccuracies on the part of children and their parents to recognize early symptoms of an asthma attack can increase the morbidity and mortality related to the disease. This study has direct implications for family education. Children with asthma and their families need to be taught to recognize the early symptoms associated with asthma (wheezing, coughing, and shortness of breath) and to intervene as appropriate when these symptoms are present.

Citation

Yoos, H. L., & McMullen, A. (1999). Symptom perception and evaluation in childhood asthma. *Nursing Research, 48*(1), 2–8.

their families may not recognize early symptoms of asthma exacerbation. Peak expiratory flow rate monitoring provides important data that can be used to guide decision making.

The pharmacologic management of asthma depends on the severity and the frequency of the child's symptoms. Table 24-1 provides a listing of the pharmacologic management for different categories of asthma. Short-acting bronchodilators such as inhaled beta-2 agonists are typically the only treatment indicated for children with mild intermittent asthma. Inhaled corticosteroids, inhaled anti-asthmatics (e.g., cromolyn, nedocromil), and/or oral anti-asthmatics (e.g., leukotriene modifiers) are the drugs of choice for long-term management of mild persistent asthma (Karch, 2000; Spratto & Woods, 2001; Velsor-Friedrich & Srof, 2000; Wever-Hess, Kouwenber, Duverman, Hermans, & Wever, 2000). Short-acting inhaled beta-2 agonists are used as needed to manage acute symptoms in children with mild persistent asthma. For children with moderate and severe persistent asthma, a long-acting bronchodilator is also used. Box 24-2 summarizes common medications used to treat asthma in children.

Inhaled medications are administered via a metered-dose inhaler (MDI). For instructions on using a MDI, read Nursing Tip: Proper MDI technique with spacer. Children are taught to use a spacer with their MDIs. Spacers make the administration of the inhaled medication easier and facilitate better distribution and inhalation of the medication. Spacers

BOX 24-2 Common medications used to treat asthma in children

Short-acting beta-2 agonists: albuterol (Proventil, Ventolin), pirbuterol (Maxair)

Inhaled corticosteroids: beclomethasone (Beclovent, Vanceril), budesonide (Rhinocort), flunisolide (AeroBid, Nasalide), and fluticasone (Flonase)

Systemic corticosteroids: methylprednisolone, prednisolone, prednisone

Inhaled non-steroidal anti-inflammatory (inhaled anti-asthmatic agents): cromolyn sodium (Intal), nedocromil sodium (Tilade)

Antileukotrienes (oral anti-asthmatic agents): zafirlukast (Accolate), montelukast (Singulair), zileuton (Zyflo)

Long-acting bronchodilators: salmeterol (Serevent), sustained-release albuterol theophylline (Theo-dur, Slo-bid)

Anticholinergics (increase effectiveness of beta-2 agonists): ipratropium bromide (Atrovent); and in combination with albuterol (Combivent)

Systemic beta-2 agonists: epinephrine, terbutaline (Brethine)

TABLE 24-1 Asthma Severity Categories and Treatment in Children 5 Years of Age and Older

Asthma Category	Pharmacologic Management
Mild Intermittent Symptoms no more than twice per week; night-time symptoms less than once per month. Episodes brief with varying intensity; PEFR ≥ 80%.	Short-acting bronchodilator: inhaled beta-2 agonist; no long-term treatment indicated.
Mild Persistent Symptoms more than twice per week, but less than once per day. Night-time symptoms more than twice per month. Asthma may affect activity level; PEFR ≥ 80%.	Short-acting bronchodilator: inhaled beta-2 agonist. Long-term control with low dose inhaled corticosteroid, inhaled anti-asthmatic, or oral anti-asthmatic.
Moderate Persistent Daily symptoms with night-time symptoms more than twice a month. Attacks may last days, activity levels are affected; PEFR 60–80%.	Daily use of inhaled short-acting beta-2 agonist. Long-term control with medium dose inhaled corticosteriod with or without a long-acting bronchodilator. A leukotriene modifier may also be part of treatment.
Severe Persistent Continuous daytime symptoms with frequent night-time symptoms. Frequent attacks, limited physical activity, and PEFR < 60%.	Inhaled short-acting beta-2 agonist 3–4 times/day. Long-term control with high dose inhaled corticosteroid, a long-acting bronchodilator, and an oral corticosteroid.

Adapted from: National Asthma Education and Prevention Program. (1997). Expert panel report II: Guidelines for the diagnosis and management of asthma *(NIH Publication No. 974051). Bethesda, MD: National Heart, Lung, and Blood Institute, National Institutes of Health.*

Nursing Tip:

Proper MDI technique with spacer

1. Attach MDI canister to mouthpiece.
2. Shake to increase pressure in canister.
3. Expire to functional residual capacity (if coughing occurs, exhale less vigorously).
4. Place mouthpiece in mouth and make a seal with lips.
5. Activate the canister.
6. Inspire slowly to total lung capacity.
7. Hold breath for 5–10 seconds, then breathe normally. For infants, and children unable to hold their breath, a mask should be used and remain in place until they have taken 5–6 breaths.
8. Wait 60 seconds.
9. Repeat steps 2–7.

minimize large droplets from being deposited in the mouth which, in the case of corticosteroid MDIs, can cause candidal mouth infections (Hunter, 2000). Figure 24-8 shows a child using a spacer with a mouth piece. Mouth pieces require the child to be able to hold his or her breath for 5–10 seconds once the medication is released from the MDI canister. Figure 24-9 presents a child using a mask with her spacer.

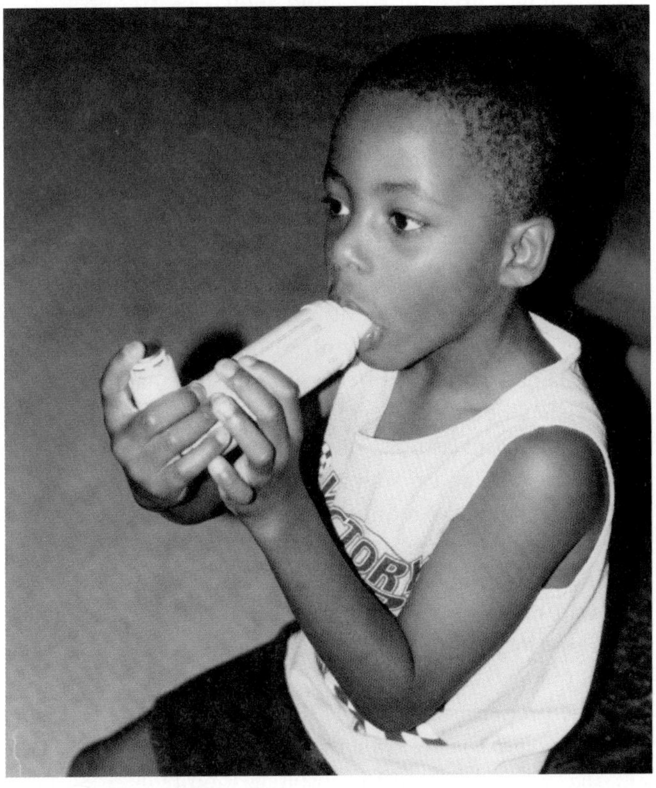

Figure 24-8 Child Using an MDI with a Spacer and Mouthpiece

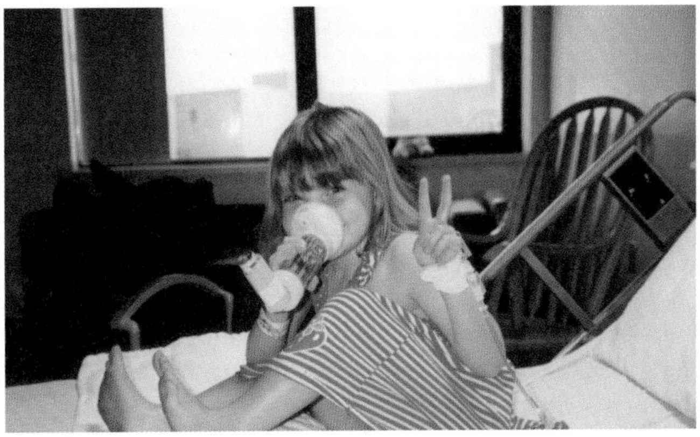

Figure 24-9 Child Using an MDI with a Spacer and Mask

When a mask is used, the canister is activated, and the mask is left in placed until the child has taken 5–6 breaths. Oral or intravenous corticosteroids and one or more hours of continuous short-acting beta-2 agonist nebulizer treatments may be used for children in severe distress. Inhaled ipratropium bromide, an anticholinergic drug that potentiates the action of beta-2 agonists, may also be used for the emergency management of symptoms. Children receiving continuous nebulizer treatments need close observation not only because of the degree of their respiratory distress, but also because of increased risks for side effects association with the medications. Figure 24-10 illustrates a child at home receiving short-acting beta-2 agonist via a nebulizer.

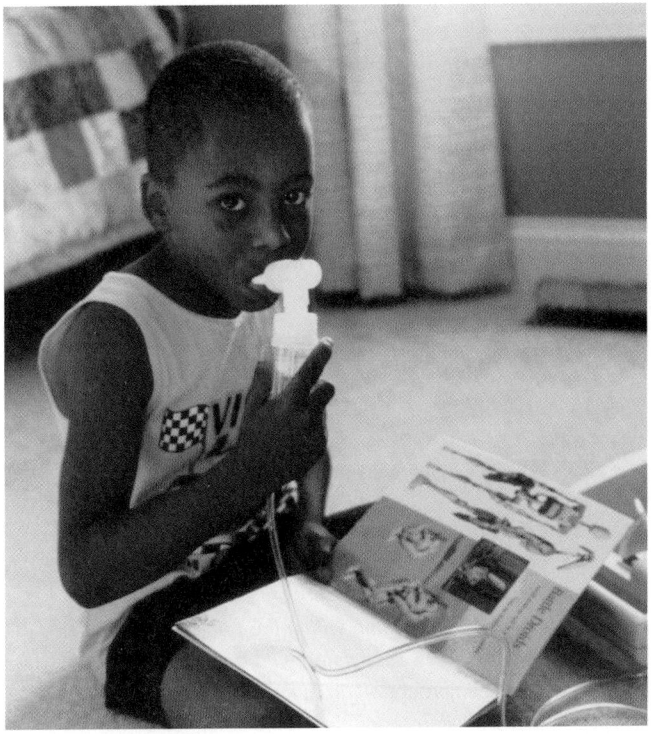

Figure 24-10 Administration of a Short-Acting Beta-2 Agonist Via Nebulizer

Nursing Management

Assessment

A critical component of the nursing management of asthma is the recognition of common early symptoms associated with an exacerbation. Of particular importance is the identification of children at risk for life-threatening attacks. Characteristics associated with an increased risk for a fatal asthma attack are repeated emergency room or hospital admissions, marked morning and evening fluctuations in lung functioning, and a prior life-threatening asthma attack (Capen & Sherman, 1998).

A thorough respiratory assessment is clearly indicated for children with asthma symptoms. Assessment of activity tolerance, cardiovascular functioning, and fluid balance are also important. Additionally, the nurse needs to assess the child and family's understanding related to asthma and its treatment. Ongoing management, early recognition of symptoms, and the initiation of emergency intervention for acute attacks are skills the child and family need in order to successfully manage the disease. Clarification of information and teaching directed to resolving deficient knowledge are critical for the safety of the child.

Diagnosis

1. Risk for suffocation related to airway obstruction.
2. Ineffective airway clearance related to allergic and inflammatory processes.
3. Interrupted family processes related to child with chronic illness.

Outcome Identification

1. The child will be free from life-threatening asthma exacerbations.
2. The child will have clear lung sounds, normal respiratory effort, and be free from cough.
3. The family will demonstrate positive adaptation in meeting the child's needs.

Nursing Alert:

Fatal Asthma Attacks

The most predictive characteristics associated with fatal asthma are prior occurrence of a life-threatening attack and a hospital admission within the prior 2 years. Fatal asthma attacks are associated with delayed onset of treatment. Early recognition of symptoms and interventions are crucial in reducing a child's risk for a fatal attack.

Planning/Implementation

While nurses are in a position to provide acute and emergency asthma-related care, most children with asthma are managed at home. Family education related to self-management of asthma is a primary focus of nursing care. The family may need help in identifying possible triggers and exploring feasible ways of limiting the affected child's exposure to these. They also need to ensure the child has appropriate follow-up care and that they have quick access into the health care system in case the child has an asthma attack. The nurse should collaborate with social services and other agencies when families need help with resources to meet their child's health needs.

Language or cultural barriers that prohibit the child from getting appropriate and timely health care need to be addressed. Different cultural practices that do not create potential health problems should be supported and integrated with necessary conventional treatments. Interpreters need to be utilized to ensure the family has the information they need to meet the child's health needs. If possible, reading materials in the family's native language should be made available to literate families. Additionally, it is important that the family acquire the language needed to access emergency care in the event of an attack.

Evaluation

The effectiveness of the nursing care plan is based on the client's achievement of outcomes. If the education the family receives is effective, the child's asthma should be managed successfully. Certainly, the child should be free from life-threatening attacks. Effective management also means the child will be free from the classic manifestations of wheezing, shortness of breath, and cough. Support, education, and referrals for needed services are ways the nurse can help the family make the adaptations necessary to meet the child's needs.

Family Teaching

Family education is focused on prevention of attacks, early recognition of attacks, treatments, and the use of PEFR monitoring devices and metered-dose inhalers (Umetsu, 1998). The importance of education in the management of asthma has been discussed. Caregivers need a thorough understanding of asthma, including learning to identify the child's triggers, and maintenance of optimal health to prevent asthma attacks requiring hospitalization. Peak expiratory flow rates can be monitored at home and school. The PEFR data provide a means of evaluating the child's condition and response to therapy and detecting asymptomatic deterioration of lung function. Figure 24-11 illustrates a PEFR meter.

The proper use of the PEFR meter allows the child and family greater control over the management of the disease and decreases the need for hospitalization by alerting them when adjustments to therapy are needed. The child identifies his or her personal best value, based upon a daily mea-

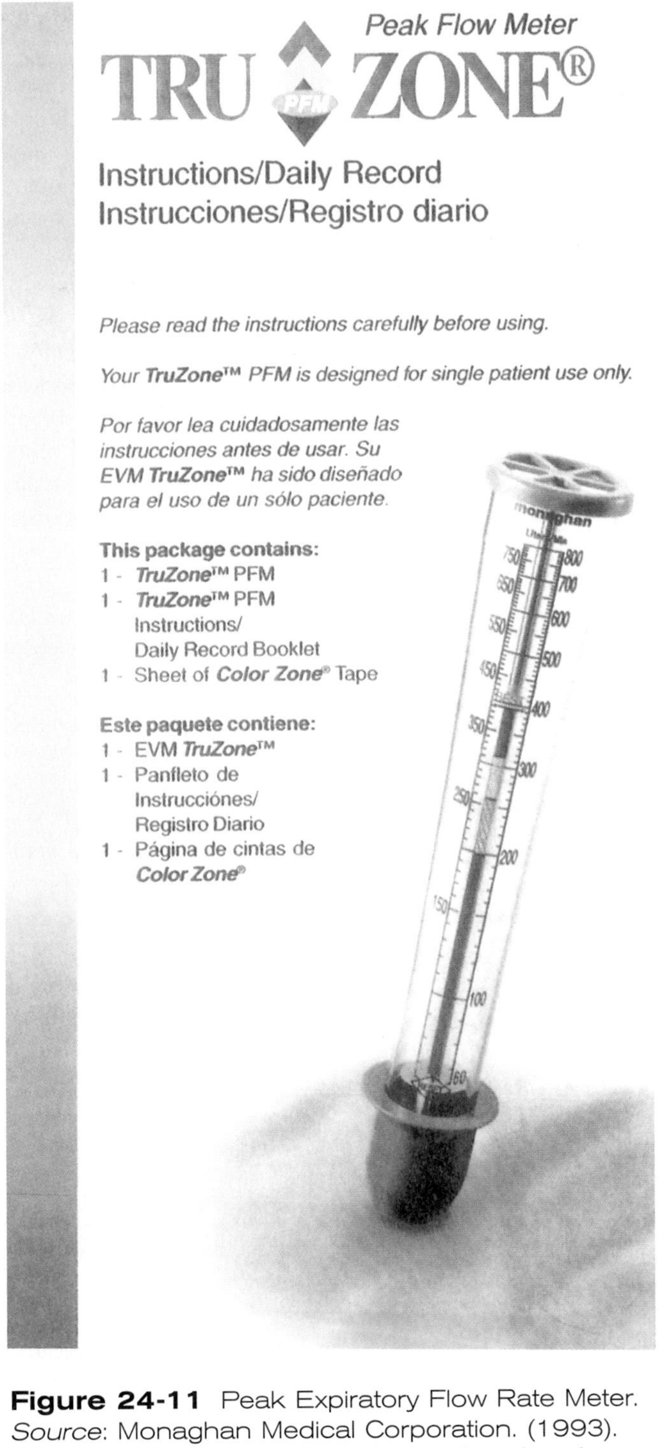
Peak Flow Meter
TRU ZONE®
PFM
Instructions/Daily Record
Instrucciones/Registro diario
Please read the instructions carefully before using.
Your TruZone™ PFM is designed for single patient use only.
Por favor lea cuidadosamente las instrucciones antes de usar. Su EVM TruZone™ ha sido diseñado para el uso de un sólo paciente.
This package contains:
1 - TruZone™ PFM
1 - TruZone™ PFM Instructions/ Daily Record Booklet
1 - Sheet of Color Zone® Tape
Este paquete contiene:
1 - EVM TruZone™
1 - Panfleto de Instrucciónes/ Registro Diario
1 - Página de cintas de Color Zone®
monaghan

Figure 24-11 Peak Expiratory Flow Rate Meter. *Source*: Monaghan Medical Corporation. (1993). *Truzone Instructions/Daily Record.* Plattsburgh, NY: Author. Used with permission.

suring and recording of the PEFR. The meter has three zones of measurement, green, yellow, and red, which are correlated to the child's personal best PEFR. When subsequent PEFR readings fall within the green zone, the child's asthma is effectively controlled. Readings falling in the yellow zone alert the family that the child may be in the early stages of an attack. Readings falling in the red zone signal a medical emergency.

Nursing Tip:

Directions for use of PEFR meters

- Make sure the sliding marker on the monitoring device is at the bottom of the scale.
- Sit up straight or stand.
- Take a deep breath and seal lips around mouthpiece.
- Blow out as hard and fast as possible into the device.
- Repeat these steps 2 more times. Record the highest of the three readings.
- Readings should be taken in the morning, evening, and other times as directed.

The child and family also need to be competent using MDIs. As previously discussed, MDIs allow for bronchodilators and steroids to be administered via inhalation. This route produces a more rapid onset than oral administration and has fewer associated side effects. Sometimes children with asthma are discharged home with nebulizer treatments, another form of aerosolized medication administration. When this happens, education about the nebulizer needs to be included in the family education.

Exercise is another focus of family education. Most children with asthma can participate in physical exercise and athletic activities as long as their asthma is under control. The ability to participate in specific sport activities is based on individual responses to the activity. Premedication with a

REFLECTIONS FROM FAMILIES

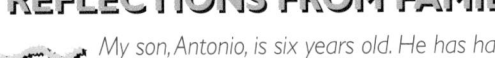

My son, Antonio, is six years old. He has had asthma since he was a baby. When he was six months old, he had to be hospitalized because he had such a hard time breathing. He was very sick for several days. I was so worried, so scared that he would die. Since then, whenever he gets a cold, I wonder if he has just a cold or the beginnings of a full-blown attack. When you have a child with asthma, you worry a lot. You also miss a lot of sleep. Antonio has problems breathing at night sometimes. I am also afraid to travel with him. Even though we take all his medicines and equipment with us on trips, we are still away from his doctor and from the hospital. And he always seems to get sick when we travel. Will the worrying ever end?

short-term beta-2 agonist may be used prophylactically before physical exercise to minimize exacerbation of symptoms. Asthma triggers are child specific. Recognizing these specific triggers is an important step in minimizing exposure. The child should avoid his or her triggers as much as possible. The nurse is positioned to help the child and family adjust to necessary environmental and lifestyle changes dictated by the child's health needs. The reinforcement of asthma education should be ongoing. Warning signs should be reviewed regularly. The family is counseled to notify the child's health care provider if symptoms such as wheezing, frequent coughing, shortness of breath, tightness in the chest, and drop in peak expiratory flow rates are present.

LESS COMMON RESPIRATORY ALTERATIONS

Less common pediatric respiratory alterations include cystic fibrosis, bronchopulmonary dysplasia, tuberculosis, and sinusitis. Nurses must have a thorough understanding of these alterations in order to effectively care for affected children and their families.

Cystic Fibrosis

Cystic fibrosis (CF) is an inherited disorder that affects the exocrine glands of the body. Alterations in sweat electrolytes and mucous production in the body lead to multiple system damage. While advances in medical and genetic research have prompted the development of new treatments for CF, a cure for the disease remains ellusive. With aggressive therapy, however, most children with CF live until they are 30 or older (Kirchner & Abman, 1997; Specht, 1998).

Incidence and Etiology

Cystic fibrosis is an autosomal recessive disease that affects 0.4 in 1,000 Caucasian children (Huether, 2000b; Kercsmar, 1998; MacLusky & Levison, 1998). Approximately 5% of the white population are carriers for the disease. The disease is uncommon in non-Caucasian children. The gene responsible for CF is on chromosome 7. The gene may be mutated in hundreds of ways. Several of these mutations cause CF (Specht, 1998). The most common mutation, the loss of an amino acid from the protein encoded by the gene, accounts for 70–75% of CF cases (Kirchner & Abman, 1997; Specht, 1998). The severity of a child's disease is related to the specific genetic form he or she inherits (Specht, 1998).

Pathophysiology

Cystic fibrosis is an exocrine gland dysfunction that leads to abnormal levels of sodium and chloride, an increase viscosity of mucous secretions, and increased susceptibility to pulmonary colonization of bacteria (MacLusky & Levison, 1998).

The epithelium of body tissues exhibits marked impermeability to chloride and an excessive reabsorption of sodium (Kercsmar, 1998). These ion alterations lead to dehydration of airway secretions, causing impaired expectoration and airway obstruction. In addition to causing airway obstruction, the stasis of thick, sticky pulmonary secretions increases the risk for pathogen invasion. Most children with CF become colonized with multiple organisms such as *H. influenzae, Staphylococcus aureus, Pseudomonas aeruginosa, Pseudomonas cepacia, Serratia, Actinobacilli,* and *Klebsiella* (Kercsmar, 1998; MacLusky & Levison, 1998; Specht, 1998). Bacterial infections cause the release of toxins and other products that generate an inflammatory response in the airway (MacLusky & Levison, 1998). Chronic infection and airway obstruction lead to bronchial epithelium destruction and **bronchiectasis** (a lung condition characterized by irreversible dilation and destruction of the bronchial walls). Atelectasis and **pneumothorax** (a collection of air or gas in the pleural cavity) are complications of this process. The chronic hypoxia associated with the disease also triggers pulmonary vasculature changes that result in pulmonary hypertension and **cor pulmonale** (right-sided heart failure).

Thick mucous leads to obstructions in other body system structures as well. The gastrointestinal tract and genitourinary tract are additional primary systems affected by the disease. The obstruction of pancreatic ducts blocks enzyme release into the gastrointestinal tract. The lack of pancreatic enzymes to aid digestion leads to malabsorption of nutrients and impaired growth (MacLusky & Levison, 1998). Pancreatitis and diabetes mellitus are complications associated with pancreatic involvement in children with CF (MacLusky & Levison, 1998). Other examples of gastrointestional complications that children with CF may experience include meconium ileus, rectal prolapse, gastroesophageal reflux, and hepatic disease (MacLusky & Levison, 1998). The thickened mucous in the reproductive tract leads to fertility problems. Female fertility is low, and males are almost always azoospermic (Kercmar, 1998; MacLusky & Levison, 1998). Puberty is delayed for most children with CF because of chronic ventilation and nutritional alterations.

Clinical Manifestations

Chronic respiratory infections are a hallmark of CF. Manifestations associated with these infections are cough, sputum production, hyperinflation of the alveoli, bronchiectasis, and eventually, pulmonary insufficiency and death (Kercsmar, 1998). Pneumothorax, **hemoptysis** (coughing up blood from the respiratory tract), and atelectasis are complications that occur as a result of airway obstruction and tissue damage. Digital clubbing occurs as a result of chronic hypoxia. Blood streaked secretions typically indicate the presence of infection.

Nursing Alert:

Signs of a Pneumothorax

A pneumothorax is suspected if a child with CF experiences acute signs of respiratory distress such as tachypnea, tachycardia, dyspnea, and pallor or cyanosis.

The majority of children with CF have some exocrine pancreatic insufficiency as a result of obstruction of the pancreatic ducts and consequent autoingestion of the pancreas (Kercsmar, 1998). Insulin deficiency may develop in adolescents with CF. Malabsorption of nutrients caused by the lack of pancreatic enzymes leads to steatorrhea and deficiency states, particularly vitamins A, D, E, and K deficiencies, in untreated children. Failure to thrive is evident even in children who have a good appetite. Approximately 10% of children with CF had a meconium ileus at birth (Kercsmar, 1998). Other effects of CF include heat exhaustion or hypochloremic alkalosis from salt wasting (Kercsmar, 1998).

Diagnosis

Diagnosis is based on history, physical examination, laboratory findings, chest films, sweat tests, and DNA analysis (Kercsmar, 1998). Genetic testing may be used to screen newborns for the disease or identify carriers (Baroni, Anderson, & Mischler, 1997). Testing of potential carriers is generally restricted to individuals who have family members with known CF. Genetic testing can also be used to determine the genetic form of a child's CF (Specht, 1998).

Treatment

The treatment of CF is aimed at maximizing lung functioning and nutritional intake. Aggressive management of the lung disease includes promoting the removal of secretions from lungs, preventing and treating infections, and managing related pulmonary complications. Specific therapies to promote the expectoration of secretions include recombinant human deoxyribonuclease (DNase) and chest physiotherapy (Kercsmar, 1998). Inhaled DNase causes the breakdown of mucous in the airway by interrupting its DNA structure (Karch, 2000). Chest physiotherapy is frequently accomplished through the use of a ThAIRapy vest (Figure 24-12). This vest provides high-frequency oscillation, which loosens airway secretions and facilitates their removal. Manual percussion using a cupped hand and postural drainage are other means for removing pulmonary secretions. Many children with CF also have manifestations of asthma. For these children, medications used to treat asthma are added to their therapy (see Box 24–2).

Antibiotics are used to manage infections. As a result of frequent respiratory infections requiring repeated antibiotic therapy, children with CF tend to develop multiple antibiotic-resistant organisms. Sputum cultures and sensitivity testing are conducted to help ensure that appropriate antibiotics are used. Antibiotics are generally administered intravenously, although some inhaled antibiotics are used (Specht, 1998).

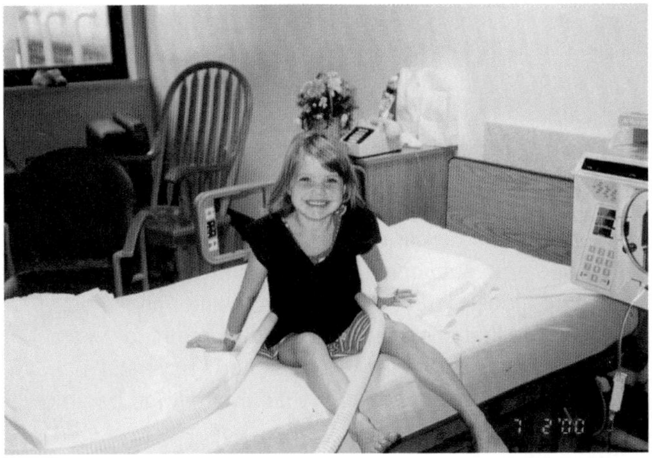

Figure 24-12 Child Demonstrating Use of a ThAIRapy Vest

Exacerbations of CF symptoms are generally the result of a pulmonary infection. Treatment during an exacerbation may include supplemental oxygen therapy, cardiopulmonary and oxygen saturation monitoring, bronchial washings, and mechanical ventilation. Chest tubes are indicated if the child has a pneumothorax. Surgical interventions may be necessary to repair eroded blood vessels or remove severely diseased or necrotic lung tissue (MacLusky & Levison, 1998).

Pancreatic enzymes are given, along with vitamins A, D, E, and K, to manage the pancreatic insufficiency associated with CF. The management of associated malabsorption includes a diet high in protein and carbohydrates. The addition of liquid nutritional supplements three or four times per day is also generally indicated. Infants, particularly during warm weather, may need a salt supplement added to their diet (Kercsmar, 1998; MacLusky & Levison, 1998).

Infants with a meconium ileus may be treated by digital removal of stool and enemas, but generally surgical intervention is required. Laxatives are typically used to manage intestinal obstructions in older infants and children (Kercsmar, 1998). Lung transplantation is an end-stage treatment that offers promise to children and young adults facing death because of respiratory insufficiency (Specht, 1998). Gene therapy research offers hope that a cure may soon become available.

Nursing Management

Cystic fibrosis, like other chronic illnesses, has enormous physical, financial, social, and emotional consequences for the child and family. Ongoing extensive treatment regimens,

Kids Want To Know

Does CF affect my ability to have a family?

Michelle is a 15-year-old with CF. She is being seen in the pediatric pulmonary clinic for a routine check-up. She confides to Lori, the pediatric pulmonary nurse specialist, that she's worried about something. "My friends have started their periods and I haven't. I'm feeling left out and wondering if I am going to be able to have children when I get older." Lori tells Michelle that while puberty is frequently delayed in children with CF, she sees signs that Michelle's sexual development is on target. Lori explains that the development of breast tissue and pubic hair are mid-puberty indicators. Since Michelle has developed these signs, Lori believes she will begin her menstrual periods soon. Lori further explains to Michelle that almost all boys, and some girls, with CF are infertile. Michelle can be tested later if fertility problems are suspected. Until then, Michelle needs to recognize that if she engages in unprotected intercourse she runs the risk of acquiring a sexually transmitted disease or having an unwanted pregnancy. Additionally, before Michelle and a future partner plan a pregnancy, they need to understand the increased cardiopulmonary demands pregnancy has on the mother. For this reason, they should explore associated health risks and family planning options with Michelle's health care provider. Having addressed Michelle's immediate concerns, the two turned to a discussion surrounding dating, relationships, and intimacy.

aggressive therapies required during exacerbations, interruptions in life routines, and an ever present awareness of the serious and fatal nature of the disease are sources of stress on the family. Assisting the family to develop strategies for successful adaptation to the demands of the disease is an integral component of the nursing management for CF. Nursing management also includes making social and community service referrals, providing direct care, and conducting ongoing family education.

Home health referrals are indicated to help facilitate transitions between inpatient and home care. This is particularly important, for example, when IV antibiotics need to be continued at home or when a new venous access device has been placed. Collaboration with social services is needed when families are unable to manage the costs associated with a child's medical care. Nurses can link families with additional sources of support through referrals to support groups and other community resources.

For the most part, children with CF are managed at home. Inpatient care, however, is commonly required during periods of exacerbation or when a "tune-up" is indicated. "Tune-ups," which involve aggressive chest physiotherapy (CPT), IV antibiotic therapy, and nutritional support, promote optimal lung functioning and decrease the potential for an exacerbation. Inpatient treatment of exacerbations also includes aggressive chest physiotherapy and the administration of IV antibiotics. Depending on the needs of the child, additional interventions, such as supplemental oxygen, are implemented.

Typically, the child's CPT is performed in the morning and in the evening. During "tune-ups" and exacerbations, CPT is performed before meals and at bedtime. Inhaled medications are administered before beginning the treatment. One of the roles of the nurse is to ensure that the child's CPT is completed as prescribed. Nursing management also involves conducting respiratory, cardiovascular, nutritional, and developmental assessments. Other nursing interventions include managing the child's IV or long-term venous access device, administering IV antibiotics and other medications, providing nutritional support, and reinforcing teaching about the child's disease and medical regimen.

Pancreatic enzymes are taken before meals and snacks or sprinkled on the first few bites of food. Favorite foods are incorporated into the child's diet and nutritional shakes between meals are encouraged. Collaboration with a nutritionist is recommended if the child's growth is impaired. Nursing management may also include administering tube feedings to children who are significantly malnourished.

Facilitating family development of coping strategies to address anxiety and stress related to the CF diagnosis and its management is another important nursing intervention. Families also need to understand the child's treatment plan and be competent with related care. Anticipatory guidance should include information related to general parenting and child developmental needs and address issues related to chronic illness, feelings of guilt, sibling reactions, and anticipatory grieving.

Family Teaching

The educational needs of families who have children with CF evolve as the children grow and develop and health states change. Teaching is based on these needs. Clearly, families need to understand the disease, its management, and measures to prevent exacerbations. Minimizing exacerbations primarily depends on reducing infection risks and aggressively treating respiratory infections that develop. Good handwashing is one of the most important ways to decrease the incidence of infections. Children with CF also need to avoid being around others with infections. This may include other children with CF. Peers with CF may be excellent sources of support, however, they may also be infected with antibiotic resistant organisms. Other ways of reducing infection risks include adhering to the prescribed medical regimen and getting adequate nutrition and rest. Families need to appreciate the need for ongoing follow-up care. They also need to be able to recognize complications and determine when medical intervention is required. Follow-up visits not only serve to address the medical needs of the child, they also provide an excellent opportunity for reviewing previously taught information, clarifying family understanding, and presenting new information (Figure 24-13).

Bronchopulmonary Dysplasia

Bronchopulmonary dysplasia (BPD) is a chronic lung disease that primarily affects premature infants with respiratory distress syndrome (RDS). Respiratory distress syndrome occurs as a result of premature infants' pulmonary system immaturity and surfactant insufficiency. Without medical intervention, premature infants require treatments to ensure adequate ventilation. Mechanical ventilation, the primary treatment modality, causes trauma to the infant's lungs. The combined effects of mechanical ventilation and a fragile pulmonary system predispose premature infants to BPD.

Incidence and Etiology

The incidence of BPD is inversely proportional to gestation age and birth weight. Infants with a birth weight of 500–700 grams have an 85% risk of developing BPD. The risks are significantly lower, about 5%, in infants whose birth weight is at least 1,500 grams (Malinowski, 1998). As a rule, infants who develop BPD have been artificially ventilated for at least three days within their first two weeks of life (Miller, Rice, DeVoe, & Fos, 1998). The rate and severity of the disease are directly related to the levels of the peak inspiratory pressures (PIPs) required to adequately ventilate an infant. The mortality associated with BPD can be as high as 40% (Malinowski, 1998). The incidence of BPD has decreased with advances in medical care for premature infants. Specifically, the use of prenatal steroids, surfactant replacement and, when needed, gentle mechanical ventilation are the primary changes that have led to improved respiratory outcomes for premature infants (Lockridge, 1999; Malinowski, 1998).

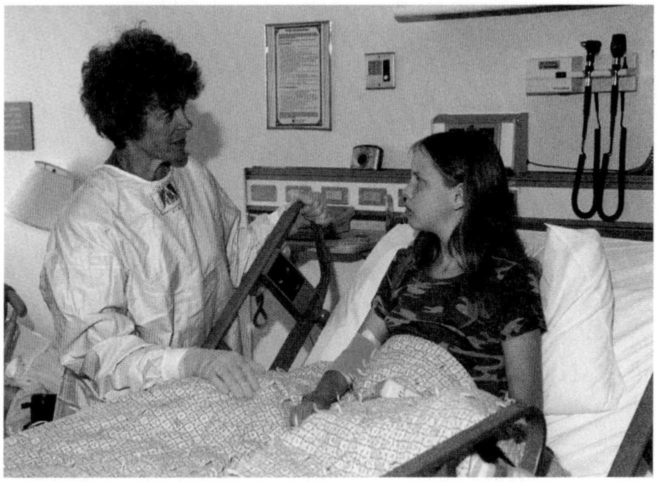

Figure 24-13 Client education for CF should include the need for adequate nutrition, rest, and ongoing follow-up care.

Pathophysiology

Infants with RDS have poor lung compliance. As a result, they generally require mechanical ventilation and supplemental oxygen (Malinowski, 1998). The result is trauma to pulmonary structures, which leads to interstitial edema and epithelial destruction (Kleigman, 1998; Malinowski, 1998). The inflammatory response and accumulation of cellular debris from tissue necrosis causes airway obstruction. Hyperinflation, atelectasis, and tissue fibrosis result. The process may also damage pulmonary vasculature (Malinowski, 1998). The overall effect of the disease process is a ventilation/perfusion ratio imbalance that leads to **hypercapnia** (an excess of carbon dioxide in the blood) and hypoxemia.

Clinical Manifestations

Infants with BPD have varying degrees of respiratory distress depending on the severity of their illness. Characteristic manifestations include dependency on supplemental oxygen for more than 28 days and compensated respiratory acidosis (Kleigman, 1998; Lewis, 1999; Miller, et al., 1998). Affected infants also have symptoms associated with pulmonary edema and cor pulmonale. Crackles and wheezing are commonly audible with auscultation. Fluid retention occurs as a result of the infant's heart failure.

Diagnosis

The diagnosis of BPD is based on the infant's history, physical examination, laboratory results, and chest X rays (Malinowksi, 1998). The diagnosis is suspected when the RDS has not improved within two weeks, oxygen therapy is required beyond 28 days, or prolonged mechanical ventilation is necessary. The diagnosis is made only after other illnesses, such as pneumonia and patent ductus arteriosus, have been ruled out. Chest radiography reveals alveolar hyperinflation, atelectasis, and **fibrosis** (the repair and replacement of injured or infected tissue with scar tissue) (Kliegman, 1998; Lewis, 1999; Malinowski, 1998; Miller, et al., 1998).

Treatment

Prevention is the primary focus of medical management of BPD. Prenatal steroids promote the maturation of fetal lungs. The administration of exogenous surfactant lowers alveolar surface tension, allowing the alveoli to open more easily with inspiration and preventing collapse on expiration (Hazinski, 1998; Lockridge, 1999). The result is more effective ventilation. Pharmacologic agents used to treat BPD include diuretics, steroids, and bronchodilators (Kliegman, 1998; Malinowski, 1998). Diuretics are used to help manage the infant's pulmonary and systemic edema. Steroids are used to reduce the inflammatory response associated with the disease and its treatment. Mechanical ventilation may be necessary for weeks to months. Preferred methods of ventilation include high-frequency ventilation and client triggered ventilation (Lockridge, 1999). A tracheostomy is indicated for infants requiring long-term ventilation. Many infants with BPD are discharged to home still requiring oxygen therapy.

Nursing Management and Family Teaching

Nursing management for infants with BPD includes addressing physical needs and providing family support and education. Family centered, developmentally supportive care is also an important aspect of nursing management of this respiratory alteration. Physical care includes conducting ongoing physical assessment and providing respiratory, nutritional, and developmental support. Respiratory support generally includes managing the infant's artificial airway, ensuring appropriate settings and functioning of the ventilator, monitoring the child's oxygenation and laboratory data, and performing endotracheal suctioning on an as-needed basis. Premature infants, particularly those in respiratory distress, tend to become further compromised with frequent handling. Noninvasive monitoring and coordination of care are measures that help promote the infant's rest, conserve energy, and ease the work of breathing.

A significant challenge for nursing is ensuring that infants with BPD have sufficient nutritional intake. These infants tire easily and their increased work of breathing impairs the coordination of sucking, swallowing, and breathing during feedings. Further, infants with BPD have increased nutritional requirements because of the elevated metabolic rate associated with their illness. They also tend to have gastroesophageal reflux, which further interferes with their nutritional intake. Nasogastric feedings are indicated until infants with BPD are stable and can tolerate breastfeeding or bottle feeding. Breast milk is preferred over formula because it is more easily digested and has immunologic benefits. Additionally, small, more frequent feedings are generally better tolerated than large volume feedings.

Infants with BPD have an increased risk for developing respiratory infections and usually continue to have chronic respiratory problems into childhood. Families are taught to recognize early signs of respiratory infection or compromise and to seek medical care for their infant should these signs develop. They are also taught the importance of immunizations as a primary prevention measure. In addition to routine immunizations, infants with BPD frequently receive respiratory syncytial virus immune globulin to lower their risk for developing an RSV infection. Infants with BPD are commonly hospitalized for an extended period of time. The combined effects of this hospitalization, inappropriate environmental stimulation, inadequate nutrition, and respiratory insufficiency place these infants at risk for developmental delays. Developmental considerations must be incorporated into the infants' care in order to maximize their long-term outcomes. This includes minimizing noxious stimuli associated with neonatal nurseries and providing stimuli appropriate for their developmental needs. Caregivers are encouraged to communicate and have physical contact with their infants. They are also encouraged to participate in their infants' care.

Infants with BPD are discharged to their families as soon as they are stable, meet weight requirements, and the family demonstrates its ability to care for the infant. Home care is clearly preferred for infants because of caregiver–infant attachment, developmental, health, and cost containment benefits. In addition to general anticipatory guidance, family education for infants with BPD includes teaching related to medications, oxygen therapy, cardiopulmonary monitoring and resuscitation, and follow-up care. Families are reminded that their infants should not be exposed to air pollutants such as smoke or be around individuals with respiratory infections.

Tuberculosis

Tuberculosis (TB) is a bacterial infection associated with significant global morbidity and mortality. If untreated the disease can lead to organ damage and central nervous system (CNS) complications. The most dreaded complication of TB is tuberculosis meningitis, which can cause CNS damage, coma, and death (Berman, 1997; Leung & Tregoning, 2000; Lopez & Marshak, 1998).

Incidence and Etiology

While the incidence of TB is low in the United States, it is the leading cause of infection related death in the world (Lopez & Marshak, 1998). The highest incidence of TB is in developing countries (Berman, 1997). In the United States, minorities and immigrants have the highest rates (Berman, 1997; Lopez & Marshak, 1998). It is estimated that over 50% of cases of TB in the United States are attributed to foreign-born residents. Individuals who are immunocompromised or have HIV infection are also at high risk for developing TB (Berman, 1997). When a child becomes infected with the pathogen, it is usually because he or she has been in close contact with an adult who has active TB. Tuberculosis is caused by the acid-fast bacillus *Mycobacterium tuberculosis* (Berman, 1997; Lopez & Marshak, 1998; Stanhope & Knollmueller, 1997).

Pathophysiology

The transmission of TB occurs through droplets from the respiratory tract of individuals with active pulmonary infections (Berman, 1997). The bacilli enter the respiratory tract on droplets of air. Once in the lung, the pathogen reproduces and spreads through the body via the lymph and circulatory systems. Granulomas are formed in the lungs as an inflammatory response to the initial pathogen invasion. These granulomas serve to contain and consume areas of infection. They are eventually replaced by scar tissue as the body heals itself (Lopez & Marshak, 1998). Pockets of infection in the primary or metastatic sites, however, may survive the immune response and lie dormant until something precipitates its reactivation. The disease causes destruction of the lung parenchyma and pulmonary vasculature, which impairs ventilation and pulmonary blood flow (Lopez & Marshak, 1998).

Clinical Manifestations

During the initial period of infection individuals are asymptomatic and cannot pass the organism to others. The TB infection will progress to TB disease if the body's defenses are unable to fight the disease. Individuals who do not receive preventive pharmacologic therapy are at risk of developing the disease later in life.

As the TB infection progresses to TB disease, pulmonary symptoms such as chronic coughing, sputum production, hemoptysis, pleuritic pain, and abnormal and adventitious lung sounds occur. Fatigue, low-grade fevers, chills, night sweats, and weight loss are general symptoms associated with TB (Lopez & Marshak, 1998). Symptoms associated with a metastatic infections are specific to the area of involvement. Complications of the disease include TB meningitis, pericarditis, ocular TB, and GI infections (Berman, 1997).

Diagnosis

The diagnosis of TB is based on the combined findings from physical examinations, X rays, and positive PPD skin tests or the isolation of the *Mycobacterium tuberculosis* organism in body fluids such as sputum (Berman, 1997). Bronchial lung sounds and course crackles are associated with active pulmonary TB. Pain may present with metastatic infections in the body. Atelectasis, pleural effusion, **empyema** (accumulation of infected fluid in a body cavity), scarring, and calcification are possible X-ray findings (Lopez & Marshak, 1998). The definition of a positive PPD depends on the child's risk factors (Stanhope & Knollmueller, 1997). Box 24-3 describes the significance of PPD readings. A false negative reaction to the skin testing can occur in immunocompromised individuals, in clients with early infections, and in infants younger than 6 months of age (Berman, 1997). Early morning sputum samples provide the best sample for stain and culture (Lopez & Marshak, 1998).

BOX 24-3 Positive TB skin test results

Tuberculin reactions are considered positive in the following cases:

A reaction of 5 mm:

- children with recent close contact with an adult with TB disease
- children with chest films suspicious for TB
- children with known or suspected HIV infection

A reaction of 10 mm:

- children born in or living in high-prevalence areas
- children using intravenous drugs
- children in long-term care facilities or prisons
- children identified as at risk: medically underserved, minority/immigrant, low-income, malnourished, immunocompromised, and those with specific diseases such as diabetes mellitus, Hodgkin's, and end-stage renal disease.

A reaction of 15 mm:

- any child not described above

Adapted from Maguire, M. (1997). Tuberculosis skin testing at the end of a century. *Pediatric Nursing, 23*(2), 209–211; Lopez, D. and Marshak, A. (1998). Tuberculosis. In R. Wilkins & J. Dexter (Eds.) *Respiratory disease: A case study approach to patient care* (2nd ed.). Philadelphia: F. A. Davis Company.

Treatment

The treatment for TB depends on the severity of the disease. For example, uncomplicated TB disease may be treated for 2 months of isoniazid, rifampin, and pyrazinamide followed by 6 months of isoniazid and rifampin. Severe TB with metastatic involvement may be treated with 4 months of isoniazid, rifampin, pyrazinamide, and streptomycin, followed by 12 months of isoniazid and rifampin. Drug-resistant organisms are treated with a combination of varying drugs for a period of 12–18 months (Berman, 1997).

Nursing Management and Family Teaching

The nursing management for TB is centered around family and community education. This education should include information related to the prevention and treatment of the disease. Prevention measures include teaching the public about infection control measures and promoting routine PPD skin testing. Health teaching also needs to include information about drug therapy used for prophylaxis or treatment regimens. Children generally become infected through contact with adults with active pulmonary disease. Therefore, the most effective way to minimize children's risk for becoming infected is to identify and treat adult contacts.

Annual TB testing is recommended for high-risk groups, including minorities, families with immigrants from developing countries, individuals who have close contact with high-risk populations, and those known to have had contact with an infected individual (Berman, 1997). Testing every six months is also recommended for health providers working with infected individuals. Positive PPD results should be reported to the health department (Stanhope & Knollmueller, 1997).

Children with positive skin testing, who have no evidence of TB disease, are treated with prophylactic isoniazid for 9 months (Berman, 1997; Lopez & Marshak, 1998). This prophylaxis is also used for children who have had close contact with an individual with active pulmonary disease. If the child's PPD testing is negative after two months, the treatment is discontinued (Berman, 1997). A vaccine, the Bacillus Clamette-Guerin or BCG vaccine, is used for individuals with repeated exposure to TB. This vaccine is contraindicated in immunocompromised children (Berman, 1997; Stanhope & Knollmueller, 1997).

Migrant and minority families may benefit from additional education and support regarding TB prevention and treatment. Their care needs to be culturally appropriate. Nursing care also should address environmental, structural, and language barriers that may exist. These barriers are thought to play a primary role in disproportionate rates of TB in these populations (Poss, 2000).

Sinusitis

Acute sinusitis results when mucociliary function is impaired by the accumulation of thick mucous in the nasal passages. If left untreated, sinusitis can lead to serious and life-threatening conditions such as periorbital cellulitis, osteomyelitis, meningitis, brain abscess, and **cavernous sinus thrombosis** (a syndrome caused by an infection of the eye resulting in venous congestion of the eye and paralysis of the extraocular muscles) (Berman, 1997; Klein, 2001).

Incidence and Etiology

Sinusitis in children is usually triggered by an upper respiratory infection or allergic rhinitis (Berman, 1997; Klein, 2001). The most common bacterial agents associated with sinusitis are *Streptococcus pneumoniae*, *H. influenzae*, and *Morazella catarrhalis* (Belkengren & Sapala, 1999; Klein, 2001). Other possible causes include facial trauma, swimming, nasal septum deviation, foreign bodies, and tumors. Otitis media is a co-morbidity in 50% of sinusitis cases. Asthma also has a strong association with sinusitis (Belkengren & Sapala, 1999).

Pathophysiology

Sinusitis occurs when thick mucous impairs the ciliary action in the nasal passages. The cilia are unable to effectively clear the sinuses, and the passages become obstructed. An accumulation of mucous and foreign particulate in these passages promotes pathogen growth leading to infection. Acute bacterial sinusitis generally involves the maxillary or ethmoidal sinuses (Berman, 1997; Klein, 2001). Figure 24-14 demonstrates the location of the sinuses.

Clinical Manifestations

The classic manifestations of sinusitis, headache, facial pain, and tenderness, may be present in older children. Younger children more often have postnasal drip, malodorous breath, and periorbital swelling (Belkengren & Sapala, 1999; Berman, 1997). Rhinorrhea, which may range from clear to purulent, cough, low-grade fever, headache, and a mild sore throat are other common manifestations (Prince, 1998).

Diagnosis

The diagnosis of sinusitis is generally based on the child's medical history and physical examination. The most important finding in the clinical diagnosis of sinusitis is cold symptoms that last longer than ten days. Transillumination of the sinuses reveals clouding and an air-fluid level when sinusitis is present (Prince, 1998). Cultures are invasive and X rays are inconclusive (Belkengren & Sapala, 1999; Klein, 2001). For these reasons, they are rarely used to diagnose sinusitis.

Treatment

Antibiotics are prescribed for 10–14 days if bacterial sinusitis is suspected (Klein, 2001). Amoxicillin and trimethoprim sulfamethoxazole (Bactrim) are the first line antibiotics used (Belkengren & Sapala,1999; Klein, 2001; Prince, 1998). Cephalosporins may also be prescribed. Intranasal cromolyn or corticosteriod nasal sprays may be used to manage the child's sinusitis if allergic rhinitis is thought to be the underlying cause. Antihistamines may also be beneficial. The usefulness of decongestants is debated because their effectiveness has been challenged and they may impair circulation and antibiotic distribution to the nasal passages (Belkengren & Sapala, 1999; Berman, 1997; Klein, 2001). Saline drops and sprays are also useful in treating sinusitis. They help liquefy nasal secretions, which facilitates their movement and clearance out of the sinuses (Klein, 2001).

Nursing Management and Family Teaching

The nursing management of sinusitis is focused on family education. This teaching includes informing the family about sinusitis and their child's treatment regimen. This includes instructing them on the proper administration of any medications prescribed for the child. Families may need to be reminded that antibiotics are useful only for bacterial infections. Children also should be taught not to block one nostril when blowing their nose. This practice forces mucous into the sinus cavities and furthers the spread of infection.

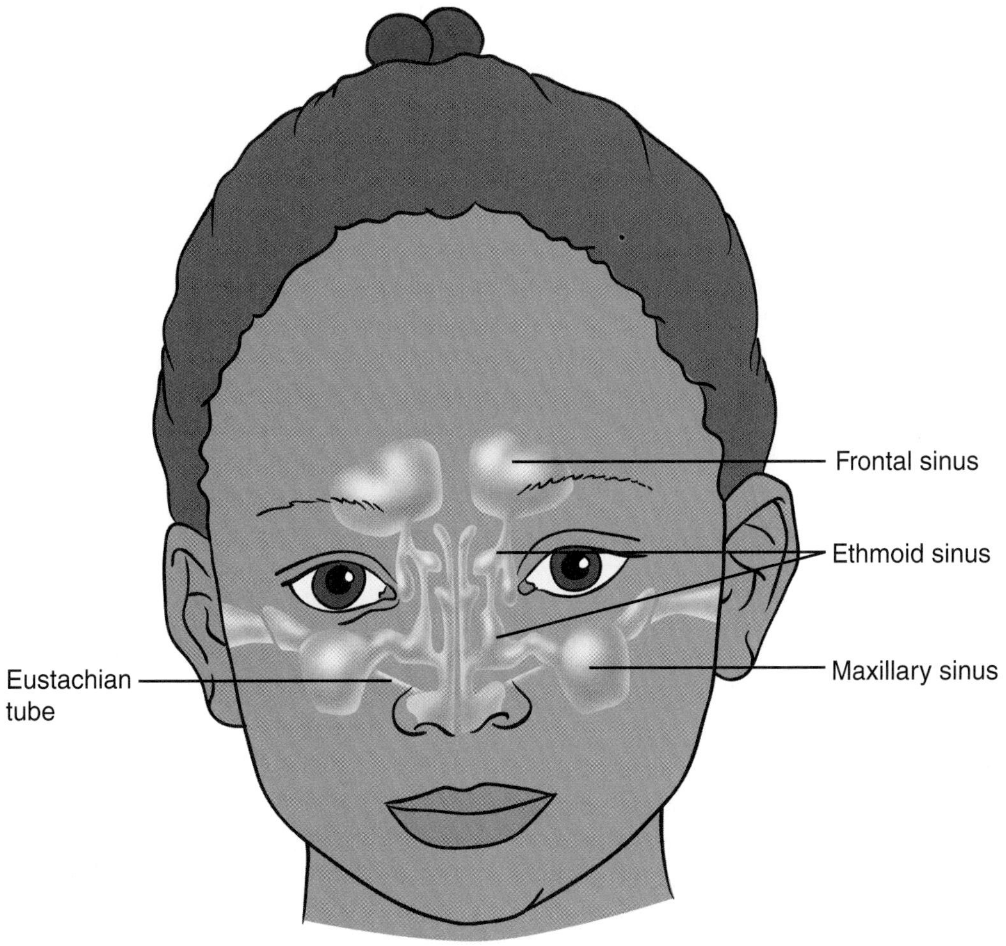

Figure 24-14 Diagram of Sinuses

ADDITIONAL RESPIRATORY ALTERATIONS

Additional respiratory alterations include foreign body aspiration, smoke inhalation injury, adult/acute respiratory distress syndrome, and apnea. Although their epidemiologic impact is limited, a discussion of these conditions is warranted because of their serious, life-threatening potential.

Foreign Body Aspiration

Foreign body aspiration is most common in children 6 months and 4 years (Huether, 2000b; Kirchner & Abman, 1997). The cough reflex generally protects the airway from foreign body obstruction. When objects do become lodged in the airway, they cause partial or complete airway obstruction. Partial airway obstruction can cause atelectasis and hyperexpansion of the alveoli and resultant respiratory distress (Huether, 2000b). Complete airway obstruction leads to hypoxia and death. Over 3,000 deaths per year are attributed to foreign body aspiration (Kirchner & Abman, 1997).

Clinical Manifestations

Acute manifestations of foreign body aspiration include coughing or gagging spells, cyanosis, and restlessness or panic (Cotton, 1998; Huether, 2000b). Other signs related to incomplete obstruction include hoarseness, dyspnea, wheezing, and stridor. Children may experience fever if they develop pneumonia as a result of the foreign body in their airway (Cotton, 1998). Children with complete obstructions are unable to cough, speak, or make vocalization. Cyanosis, loss of consciousness, and death will result if the obstruction is not relieved.

Nursing Alert:

Common Causes of Choking in Infants and Young Children

Common items that cause choking in infants and young children are nuts, hot dogs, latex or rubber balloons, peanut butter, pieces of raw vegetables or fruit, chips, and small toys.

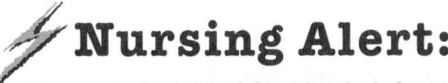

Critical Thinking

Oxygen Journey

Imagine yourself as an oxygen molecule. You and your oxygen buddies are going on a trip to a dark and unfamiliar territory. Your point of destination is the bloodstream. Before you begin, you must plan your trip and anticipate "traffic problems" encountered on the journey.

1. "Map" your path and describe some of the major landmarks you'll see on your trip.
2. Describe some "traffic problems" you may encounter and what might cause the problems.

Treatment

Prevention is the key focus in the treatment of foreign body obstruction. Infants and young children learn about their environment through oral exploration (Cotton, 1998). They also have fewer teeth, which affects their ability to safely manage foods such as raw fruits and vegetables. Their limited motor and cognitive skills also play a role in their increased risk for foreign body aspiration. Caregivers need to understand these developmental factors and make necessary adjustments in their environments to protect children from harm.

Recognizing signs of foreign body aspiration is a critical first step in relieving the problem. If the child is conscious, pink, and able to cough, observation is indicated. If the child is not able to cough or make vocalizations, loses consciousness, and/or turns cyanotic, the Heimlich maneuver should be implemented. Caregivers need to know this basic first-aid intervention. Objects that are lodged in the airway may be removed through endoscopy or surgery (Cotton, 1998).

Smoke Inhalation Injury

Smoke inhalation injury causes lung damage because of thermal and chemical factors (Bye & Mellins, 1998). These factors result in tissue destruction and inflammation. Edema, excessive mucous production, and cellular debris lead to airway obstruction, pneumonia, and impaired surfactant production (Tortorolo, Chiaretti, Piastra, Viola, & Polidori, 1999). The effects of smoke inhalation injury lead to severe acute respiratory distress syndrome (ARDS). The mortality rate in children with ARDS associated with smoke inhalation is 50–80% (Tortorolo, et al., 1999).

Clinical Manifestations

Immediate manifestations of smoke inhalation are related to inflammatory response from the thermal and chemical injury. Varying degrees of respiratory distress are related to the degree of injury. Severe injury can cause airway obstruction, hypoxia, organ damage, altered central nervous system functioning, and death (Bye & Mellins, 1998; Hicks, 1998).

Treatment

The treatment for smoke inhalation depends on the degree of injury. Ongoing assessment and monitoring, oxygen therapy, and supportive care are commonly indicated. Artificial airways and positive pressure ventilation are used to treat significant injuries (Bye & Mellins, 1998). Permissive hypercapnia is accepted as a way to lower ventilator pressures (Hicks, 1998). Exogenous surfactant is also effective in improving lung compliance and allowing for more gentle ventilation (Tortorolo, et al., 1999). Gentle ventilation minimizes **barotrauma** (physical injury sustained as a result of exposure to increased environmental air pressure) and improves outcomes.

Adult/Acute Respiratory Distress Syndrome

Acute (or adult) respiratory distress syndrome occurs as the result of direct and indirect injury to the lung. Examples of etiologic factors include sepsis, trauma, smoke inhalation injury, and pneumonia. The syndrome is characterized by increased alveolar-capillary permeability that leads to pulmonary edema. The mortality rate associated with ARDS ranges from 40–60% (Brashers, 2000; Kirchner & Abman, 1997).

Clinical Manifestations

Initial manifestations associated with ARDS are hyperventilation, retractions, and cyanosis. The affected child's hypoxemia is unresponsive to oxygen therapy, and within 6–48 hours affected children are in respiratory failure (Brashers, 2000; Kirchner & Abman, 1998). Other associated manifestations include respiratory and metabolic acidosis, hypotension, decreased cardiac output, and death (Brashers, 2000). Diminished lung sounds and crackles are noted on auscultation (Kirchner & Abman, 1998).

Treatment

The overall goal of the management of ARDS is to maximize the affected child's ventilation (Kirchner & Abman, 1998). Surfactant therapy is used to increase lung compliance and low ventilator pressures (Tortorolo, et al., 1999). Other therapies include nitric oxide, liquid ventilation, **extracorporeal membrane oxygenator (ECMO)** (a device that oxygenates the blood outside the body), and immunotherapy (Redding, 1998).

Apnea

Apnea is defined as a respiratory pause of at least 20 seconds. A shorter pause may also be defined as apnea if it is accompanied by cyanosis and bradycardia. Apnea occurs primarily in premature infants. This population is vulnerable to periods of apnea because their central respiratory centers are immature. Premature infants with apneic episodes may be responsive to cutaneous stimulation. Frequent or severe apnea may require endotracheal intubation and mechanical ventilation. Common pharmacologic agents used to manage apnea are theophylline and caffeine (Aldoretta & Spedale, 1997).

PREVENTION OF RESPIRATORY ALTERATIONS

Various health promotion strategies can be implemented to reduce the pediatric population's risk for developing respiratory alterations. These strategies include controlling environmental hazards such as second-hand smoke, air pollution, and allergens; minimizing the risk of infection through immunizations and infection control practices; genetic counseling; prenatal care; and anticipatory guidance. Nurses, as child and family advocates, need to educate families about these health promotion strategies. Caregivers are better equipped to create healthy environments for their children when they have the requisite knowledge to create such an environment.

Maternal smoking during pregnancy has been associated with increased childhood mortality and morbidity. Increased rates of spontaneous abortion, prematurity, SIDS, learning disabilities, and behavioral problems during childhood are reported effects of maternal smoking (Group Health Cooperative, 1999; Murray & Zentner, 2000). Second-hand smoke, or passive smoking, has been demonstrated to increase the numbers of respiratory infections in infants and children. Specifically, an increased incidence of pneumonia, otitis media, bronchitis, asthma, allergies, pharyngitis, and colds are connected with passive smoking (Group Health Cooperative, 1999). Children with asthma who live in homes where there are smokers are twice as likely to be admitted to an emergency room with a respiratory emergency than those living in homes without smokers (Lewis, 1999). These children also have a slower recovery from their illness.

Pollution in the air resulting from automotive and industrial air emissions can cause or exacerbate certain respiratory conditions (Loughlin, 1998; Murray & Zentner, 2000). Allergens in the air, such as pollen and mold, can also trigger alterations. At-risk children, such as those with chronic lung disorders, should avoid being outdoors when pollution and allergen indexes are high (Murray & Zentner, 2000).

Ensuring that children are properly immunized will help decrease their risk for developing a respiratory alteration. Several pediatric respiratory conditions, such as otitis media, pneumonia, pertussis, and diphtheria, can be either prevented or minimized with the appropriate immunizations (Collett, Pappas, Evans, & Hayden, 1999; Correa & Starke, 1998; Embree & Chernick, 1998; Kaditis & Wald, 1998; Law, 1998). Additional immunizations may be used to prevent respiratory alterations in high-risk children such as those with immune, cardiac, or lung disorders. Regular handwashing is a primary strategy for minimizing the spread of pathogens. Limiting the transmission of pathogens decreases a child's risk for developing a respiratory infection (Harkreader, 2000). Other common infection control methods include teaching children to cover their mouth and nose when sneezing and to avoid sharing eating utensils, drinks, and towels.

Genetic counseling is indicated when a child is born with an inherited respiratory disorder or when parents are known carriers. For example, a couple who has a child with cystic fibrosis needs to understand that there is a 25% probability that each additional child they have will have the disorder. This information is critical for parents as they make

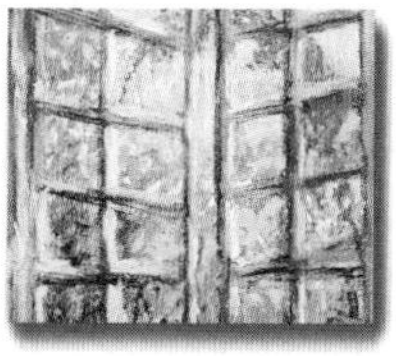

In the Real World

I was assigned to care for Khalil, age 3, the day after his tonsillectomy. He had been admitted to the hospital because he was refusing oral fluids. When I performed my initial assessment I noted that he was congested, mouth breathing, and crying. His father stated he could not get his son to eat or drink. He was also quite concerned because he was not able to calm his son. I noted that Khalil had received no pain medication since surgery. His father, who was an ear, nose, and throat (ENT) physician, indicated that his son had been refusing his pain medication because it burned his throat. Clearly, Khalil needed to get his pain under control. I collaborated with Khalil's father and physicians to get an order for IV morphine. Once Khalil's pain was controlled he stopped crying, started drinking, and was able to take his oral pain medication. Within four hours he was discharged from the hospital. I was surprised that Khalil's dad had not solved the problem situation beforehand. I was even more surprised that the nursing staff had not gotten the child's pain under control.

This experience, and later personal experiences, taught me that we, as health care providers, sometimes make assumptions about the understanding and coping of health professionals that are on the receiving end of health care. Khalil's father was not his son's health care provider. He was a father. And like other fathers, his focus was on meeting the needs of his son, juggling family and job responsibilities, and dealing with the overwhelming fatigue of being up all night and worrying about his child. The nursing staff and the father's ENT colleagues, yielding to the father's expertise, had stepped away from the situation and were unaware of the need for an intervention. Instead, what we needed to remember was that Khalil's father was not an expert in providing postoperative care to his son. This was a new experience. As health care providers, it is our responsibility to collaborate with families to ensure that interventions are employed that optimize the health outcomes for children. In addition to planning and providing care for children, we also have a responsibility to support and educate the families.

decisions about future children. Prenatal care is a critical health promotion strategy that optimizes health outcomes for children. Comprehensive prenatal care is associated with a decreased incidence of prematurity. Reducing prematurity is important because it is linked to several health alterations including respiratory distress syndrome, bronchopulmonary dysplasia, apnea, and respiratory infections (Johnson & Malinowski, 1998; Malinowski, 1998).

Anticipatory guidance about the care and safety of infants and children in the home is another important strategy for preventing respiratory alterations. Positioning infants on their backs to sleep reduces their risk for sudden infant death syndrome. The incidence of otitis media can be diminished through immunizations, breastfeeding, not propping bottles, and keeping the infant away from those who smoke. Breastfeeding provides immune complexes that can protect infants from respiratory infections. Further, caregivers can help protect their children from asthma exacerbations and allergic rhinitis by controlling the amount of allergens in the home. Establishing a fire evacuation plan in the home, and ensuring that children understand the plan, can lower a child's risk for burns and smoke inhalation injuries. Water safety education can help prevent drowning or near-drowning incidents. Finally, keeping small toys and other items away from infants and young children minimizes choking and the risk of foreign body aspirations.

Key Concepts

- The primary function of the respiratory tract is to facilitate gas exchange.
- Several anatomic and physiological variations increase infants' and young children's risk for developing a respiratory system dysfunction. These variations include smaller airways, fewer alveoli, increased chest compliance, immature immune systems, and increased oxygen demands.
- Viral respiratory infections are treated with supportive care. Antibiotics are not indicated for these infections unless a secondary bacterial infection has developed.
- A serious complication following a tonsillectomy is hemorrhage. Frequent swallowing is the earliest manifestation of bleeding during the postoperative period.
- Otitis media is a common complication of an upper respiratory tract infection and one of the most common infectious diseases of childhood.
- Croup is characterized by hoarseness, a "barky" or croupy cough, inspiratory stridor, and varying degrees of respiratory distress.
- Acute epiglottitis is a life-threatening bacterial infection that can lead to complete airway obstruction. Respiratory distress, dysphagia, drooling, fever, agitation, and lethargy are classic manifestations of this condition.
- Bronchiolitis is an acute infection of the bronchioles. The respiratory syncytial virus is the most common etiologic agent. Symptoms include labored respirations, wheezing, prolonged expiratory phase, and intermittent cyanosis.
- The accumulation of secretions, cellular debris, and other exudate resulting from airway infection and inflammation leads to ventilation/perfusion ratio disturbances, which is seen in pneumonia.
- Allergy skin testing and immunotherapy are utilized with allergic rhinitis and can cause life-threatening immune responses. For this reason, testing and allergy injections should be managed in a facility with resuscitation equipment.
- Asthma is the leading cause of chronic illness in children. Nursing management is focused on identifying and avoiding triggers and educating the family and child regarding medications, the use of PEFR meters, and the importance of follow-up care.
- Cystic fibrosis is an autosomal recessive disorder that primarily affects the lungs and digestive tracts. The disorder is managed with aggressive pulmonary treatment and digestive enzymes and supplements. The life expectancy of children with CF is 30 years.
- Bronchopulmonary dysplasia is a chronic lung alteration associated with prematurity and the treatment of respiratory distress syndrome. Treatment of BPD includes gentle ventilation, bronchodilators and diuretics, and nutritional and developmental support.
- Tuberculosis is significant in terms of global morbidity and mortality. Prevention is a prime focus of care.
- Health promotion strategies that can reduce the pediatric population's risk for developing respiratory alterations involve controlling environmental pollutants, routine immunizations, prenatal care, genetic counseling, infection control practices, and anticipatory guidance related to care and safety in the home.

Review Questions

1. Describe the anatomic differences in a child's respiratory tract from those in the adult's tract that make the child more susceptible to respiratory tract infections.
2. Develop a family teaching plan for care of a child during the pre- and post-tonsillectomy periods.
3. Compare the various croup syndromes in relation to symptoms, treatment, and nursing management.
4. Describe the clinical manifestations of nasopharyngitis.
5. Differentiate between OME and AOM.
6. Develop a family teaching plan for the care of a child with OME.
7. Discuss the clinical manifestations of pneumonia in a child.
8. Explain the treatment approaches for the different categories of asthma.
9. Describe some of the latest advances in therapy for children with cystic fibrosis.
10. Identify 5 ways to minimize a child's risk for developing a respiratory alteration.

References

American Academy of Pediatrics Committee on Infectious Diseases and Committee on Fetus and Newborn. (1998). Prevention of respiratory syncytial virus infections: Indications for the use of palivizumab and update on the use of RSV-IGIV. *Pediatrics, 102*(5), 1211–1216.

Aldoretta, P., & Spedale, S. (1997). Care of the newborn. In G. Merenstein, D. Kaplan, & A. Rosenberg (Eds.), *Handbook of pediatrics* (18th ed.). Stamford, CT: Appleton & Lange.

Baroni, M., Anderson, Y., & Mischler, E. (1997). Cystic fibrosis newborn screening: Impact of early screening results on parenting stress. *Pediatric Nursing, 23*(2), 143–151.

Bates, B. (1995). *A guide to physical examination and history taking* (6th ed.). Philadelphia: Lippincott.

Belkengren, R., & Sapala, S. (1999). Pediatric management problems. *Pediatric Nursing, 25*(1), 104–105.

Berman, S. (1997). Ear, nose & throat. In G. Merenstein, D. Kaplan, & A. Rosenberg (Eds.), *Handbook of pediatrics* (18th ed.). Stamford, CT: Appleton & Lange.

Brashers, V. (2000). Alterations of pulmonary function. In S. Huether & K. McCance (Eds.), *Understanding pathophysiology* (2nd ed.). St. Louis: Mosby.

Bye, M., & Mellins, R. (1998). Lung injury from hydrocarbon aspiration and smoke inhalation. In V. Chernick & T. Boat (Eds.), *Kendig's Disorders of the respiratory tract in children* (6th ed.). Philadelphia: W. B. Saunders.

Capen, C., & Sherman, J. (1998). Fatal asthma in children: A nurse managed model for prevention. *Journal of Pediatric Nursing, 13*(6), 367–375.

Collett, C., Pappas, D., Evans, B., & Hayden, G. (1999). Parental knowledge about common respiratory infections and antibiotic therapy in children. *Southern Medical Journal, 92* (10), 971–976.

Correa, A., & Starke, J. (1998). Bacterial pneumonias. In V. Chernick & T. Boat (Eds.), *Kendig's disorders of the respiratory tract in children* (6th ed.). Philadelphia: W. B. Saunders.

Cotton, R. (1998). Foreign body aspiration. In V. Chernick and T. Boat (Eds.), *Kendig's disorders of the respiratory tract in children* (6th ed.). Philadelphia: W. B. Saunders.

Deeks, S., Palacio, R., Ruvinshy, R., Kertesz, D., Hortal, M., Rossi, A., Spika, J., Di Fabio, J., & The *Streptococcus pneumoniae* Working Group. (1999). Risk factors and course of illness among children with invasive penicillin-resistant Streptococcus pneumoniae. *Pediatrics, 103*(2), 409–413.

Dolan, S. (2000). Tis the season. *Journal of the Society of Pediatric Nurses, 5*(1), 41–45.

Embree, J., & Chernick, V. (1998). Measles and giant cell pneumonia. In V. Chernick & T. Boat (Eds.), *Kendig's disorders of the respiratory tract in children* (6th ed.). Philadelphia: W. B. Saunders.

Faden, H., Duffy, L, Boeve, M. (1998). Otitis media: Back to basics. *Pediatric Infectious Disease Journal, 17*(12), 1105–1113.

Fink, J. (1999). Respiratory anatomy and physiology. In J. Fink & G. Hunt (Eds.), *Clinical practice in respiratory care*. Philadelphia: Lippincott, Williams & Wilkins.

Fink, J., & Fahey, P. (1999). Respiratory pathophysiology. In J. Fink & G. Hunt (Eds.), *Clinical practice in respiratory care*. Philadephia: Lippincott, Williams & Wilkins.

Glezen, W. P. (1998). Viral pneumonia. In V. Chernick & T. Boat (Eds.) *Kendig's disorders of the respiratory tract in children* (6th ed.). Philadelphia: W. B. Saunders.

Group Health Cooperative. (1999). *Secondhand smoke: Effects on adults and children*. [On-line]. Available: www.ghc.org.

Harkreader, H., (Ed.). (2000). *Fundamentals of nursing: Caring and clinical judgement*. Philadelphia: W. B. Saunders.

Hazinski, T. (1998). Bronchopulmonary dysplasia. In V. Chernick & T. Boat (Eds.), *Kendig's disorders of the respiratory tract in children* (6th ed.). Philadelphia: W. B. Saunders.

Hicks, G. (1998). Smoke inhalation and burns. In R. Wilkins & J. Dexter (Eds.), *Respiratory disease: A case study approach to patient care* (2nd ed.). Philadelphia: F. A. Davis Company.

Holm, S. (2000). Treatment of recurrent tonsillopharyngitis. *Journal of Antimicrobial Chemotherapy, 45*, 31–35.

Huether, S. (2000a). Pain, temperature, sleep, and sensory function. In S. Huether & K. McCance (Eds.), *Understanding pathophysiology* (2nd ed.). St. Louis: Mosby.

Huether, S. (2000b). Alterations of pulmonary function in children. In S. Huether & K. McCance (Eds.), *Understanding pathophysiology* (2nd ed.). St. Louis: Mosby.

Hunter, J. (2000). Nurse practitioner intervention to improve the use of metered-dose inhalers by children with asthma. *Nurse Practitioner Forum, 11*(1), 32–37.

Johnson, P., & Malinowski, C. (1998). Respiratory distress syndrome in the newborn. In R. Wilkins & J. Dexter (Eds.), *Respiratory disease: A case study aprroach to patient care* (2nd ed.). Philadelphia: F. A. Davis Company.

Kaditis, A., & Wald, E. (1998). Viral croup: Current diagnosis and treatment. *Pediatric Infectious Disease Journal, 17*(9), 827-834.

Karch, A. (2000). *Lippincott's nursing drug guide*. Philadelphia: Lippincott.

Kercsmar, C. (1998). Asthma. In V. Chernick & T. Boat (Eds.), *Kendig's disorders of the respiratory tract in children* (6th ed.). Philadelphia: W. B. Saunders.

Kirchner, K., & Abman, S. (1997). Respiratory tract. In G. Merenstein, D. Kaplan, & A. Rosenberg (Eds.), *Handbook of pediatrics* (18th ed.). Stamford: Appleton & Lange.

Kleigman, R. (1998). Fetal and neonatal medicine. In R. Behrman & R. Kliegman (Eds.), *Nelson essentials of pediatrics* (3rd ed.). Philadelphia: W. B. Saunders.

Klein, L. (2001). Sinusitis: When to treat and how. *RN, 64*(1), 42–48.

Law, B. (1998). Pertusis. In V. Chernick and T. Boat (Eds.), *Kendig's disorders of the respiratory tract in children* (6th ed.). Philadelphia: W. B. Saunders.

Leung, W-C., & Tregoning, D. (2000). Issues arising from two related cases of childhood tuberculosis meningitis. *Public Health, 114*, 57–59.

Lewis, R. (1999). Pediatric considerations. In J. Fink & G. Hunt (Eds.), *Clinical practice in respiratory care*. Philadelphia: Lippincott, Williams & Wilkins

Lockridge, T. (1999). Following the learning curve: The evolution of kinder, gentler neonatal respiratory technology. *Journal of Obstetric, Gynecologic, & Neonatal Nursing, 28*(4), 443–453.

Lopez, D., & Marshak, A. (1998). Tuberculosis. In R. Wilkins & J. Dexter (Eds.), *Respiratory disease: A case study approach to patient care* (2nd ed.). Philadelphia: F. A. Davis Company.

Loughlin, G. (1998). Bronchitis. In V. Chernick & T. Boat (Eds.), *Kendig's disorders of the respiratory tract in children* (6th ed.). Philadelphia: W. B. Saunders.

MacLusky, I., & Levison, H. (1998). Cystic Fibrosis. In V. Chernick & T. Boat (Eds.), *Kendig's disorders of the respiratory tract in children* (6th ed.). Philadelphia: W. B. Saunders.

Maguire, M. (1997). Tuberculosis skin testing at the end of a century. *Pediatric Nursing, 23*(2). 209–211.

Malinowski, C. (1998). Bronchopulmonary dysplasia. In R. Wilkins & J. Dexter (Eds.), *Respiratory disease: A case study aprroach to patient care* (2nd ed.). Philadelphia: F. A. Davis Company.

Miller, V., Rice, J., DeVoe., M., & Fos, P. (1998). An analysis of program and family costs of case managed care for technology-dependent infants with bronchopulmonary dysplasia. *Journal of Pediatric Nursing, 13*(4), 244–251.

Murray, P., Rosenthal, K., Kobayashi, G., & Pfaller, M. (1998). *Medical Microbiology* (3rd ed.). St. Louis: Mosby.

Murray, R., & Zentner, J. (2000). *Health assessment promotion strategies through the life span* (7th ed.). Stamford, CT: Appleton & Lange.

National Asthma Education and Prevention Program. (1997). *Expert panel report II: Guidelines for the diagnosis and management of asthma* (NIH Publication No. 974051). Bethesda, MD: National Heart, Lung, and Blood Institute, National Institutes of Health.

O'Brodovich, H., & Haddad, G. (1998) The functional basis of respiratory pathology and disease. In V. Chernick & T. Boat (Eds.), *Kendig's disorders of the respiratory tract in children* (6th ed.). Philadelphia: W. B. Saunders.

Opperwall, B. (2000/September). Allergies and asthma. Don't overlook the missing link. *Advance For Nurse Practitioners*, 35–38.

Orlicek, S. (1998/December). Management of acute laryngotracheobronchitis. *Concise Reviews of Pediatric Infectious Diseases*, 1164–1165.

Owen, C. (1999). New directions in asthma management. *American Journal of Nursing, 99*(3), 26–34.

Pearlman, D. (1997). Allergic disorders. In G. Merenstein, D. Kaplan, & A. Rosenberg (Eds.), *Handbook of pediatrics* (18th ed.). Stamford: Appleton & Lange.

Phipps, W. (1995). Management of persons with problems of the upper airway. In W. Phipps, V. Cassmeyer, J. Sands, & M. Lehman (Eds.), *Medical-surgical nursing: concepts and clinical practice* (5th ed.). St. Louis: Mosby.

Poss, J. (2000). Factors associated with participation by Mexican migrant farmworkers in a tuberculosis screening program. *Nursing Research, 49*(1), 20–28.

Prince, A. (1998). Infectious Diseases. In R. Behrman & R. Kliegman (Eds.), *Nelson essentials of pediatrics* (3rd ed.). Philadelphia: W.B. Saunders.

Redding, G. (1998). ARDS in the pediatric patient. In V. Chernick & T. Boat (Eds.), *Kendig's disorders of the respiratory tract in children* (6th ed.). Philadelphia: W. B. Saunders.

Rote, N., Huether, S., & McCance, K. (2000). Hypersensitivities, infection, and immunodeficiencies. In S. Huether & K. McCance (Eds.), *Understanding pathophysiology* (2nd ed.). St. Louis: Mosby.

Schuring, L. (1995). Management of persons with problems of the ear. In W. Phipps, V. Cassmeyer, J. Sands, & M. Lehman (Eds.), *Medical-surgical nursing: concepts and clinical practice* (5th ed.). St. Louis: Mosby.

Sciacqua, V. (1998). Respiratory syncytial virus. In R. Wilkins & J. Dexter (Eds.), *Respiratory disease: A case study approach to patient care* (2nd ed.). Philadelphia: F. A. Davis Company.

Specht, N. L. (1998). Cystic fibrosis. In R. Wilkins & J. Dexter (Eds.), *Respiratory disease: A case study approach to patient care* (2nd ed.). Philadelphia: F. A. Davis Company.

Spratto, G., & Woods, A. (2001). *PDR Nurse's drug handbook*. Montvale, NJ: Medical Economics Co.

Stanhope, M., & Knollmueller, R. (1997). *Public and community health nurse's consultant*. St. Louis: Mosby.

Sydnor-Greenberg, N., & Dokken, D. (2000). Communicating information at diagnosis: Helping families and children manage asthma. *Journal of Child and Family Nursing, 3*(4), 290–295.

Tortorolo, L, Chiaretti, A., Piastra, M., Viola, L., & Polidori, B. (1999). Surfactant treatment in a pediatric burn patient with respiratory failure. *Pediatric Emergency Care, 15*(6), 410–411.

Umetsu, D. (1998). Immunology and allergy. In R. Behrman & R. Kliegman (Eds.), *Nelson essentials of pediatrics* (3rd ed.). Philadelphia: W.B. Saunders.

Velsor-Friedrich, B., & Srof, B. (2000). Asthma self-management programs for children, Part I: Description of the programs. *Journal of Child and Family Nursing, 3*(2), 85–97.

Warnock, F., & Lander, J. (1998). Pain progression, intensity, and outcomes following tonsillectomy. *Pain, 75*, 37–35.

Weinberger, S. (1998). *Principles of pulmonary medicine*. Philadelphia: W. B. Saunders.

Wever-Hess, J., Kouwenber, J. M., Duverman, E. J., Hermans, J., & Wever, A. (2000). Risk factors for exacerbations and hospital admissions in asthma of early childhood. *Pediatric Pulmonology, 29,* 250–256.

Wilkins, R., & Dexter, J. (1998). *Respiratory disease: A case study approach to patient care* (2nd ed.). Philadelphia: F. A. Davis Co.

Wohl, M. (1998). Bronchiolitis. In V. Chernick & T. Boat (Eds.), *Kendig's disorders of the respiratory tract in children* (6th ed.). Philadelphia: W. B. Saunders.

Yoos, H. L., & McMullen, A. (1999). Symptom perception and evaluation in childhood asthma. *Nursing Research, 48*(1), 2–8.

Suggested Readings

Block, M. A. (1998). *No more amoxicillin: Preventing and treating children's ear and respiratory infections without antibiotics.* New York: Kensington Publishing.

Bluebond-Langner, M. (1996). *Parents and siblings of the chronically ill child.* Princeton: Princeton University Press.

Chumbley, J. (1999). *Cystic fibrosis: A family affair.* London, UK: SPCK.

Gosselin, K., & Michell, B. (Eds.). (1998). *An asthma alphabet book for kids of all ages.* Valley Park, MO: JayJo Books.

Grad, R. (1998). Acute infections producing upper airway obstruction. In V. Chernick & T. Boat (Eds.), *Kendig's disorders of the respiratory tract in children* (6th ed.). Philadelphia: W. B. Saunders.

Harrington, G. (1999). *The asthma self-care book: How to take care of your asthma.* Santa Clara, CA: Harper Collins.

Harrison, C. (2001). *Diagnosis and management of acute otitis media.* Pittsburgh: Professional Communications.

Henry, C., & Gosselin, K. (Eds.). (2000). *Taking cystic fibrosis to school.* Valley Park, MO: JayJo Books.

Schmidt, M. (1996). *Healing childhood ear infections: Prevention, home care, and alternative treatment.* Berkeley: North Atlantic Books.

Weller, T. (1999). Inhaler devices for use in asthma care. *Professional Nurse, 15*(3), 187–192.

Zevy, A. (1999). *Once upon a breath: A story of a wolf, 3 pigs, and asthma.* Toronto, Ontario: Tumbleweed Press.

Resources

Organizations and Websites

Allergy and Asthma Network (Mothers of Asthmatics, Inc.)
2751 Prosperity Avenue, Suite 150
Fairfax, VA 22031
(703) 641-9595
(800) 878-4403

American Academy of Allergy, Asthma & Immunology
611 East Wells Street
Milwaukee, WI 53202
(414) 272-6071
(800) 822-2762
www.aaaai.org

American Lung Association
1740 Broadway
New York, NY 10019
(212) 315-8700
(800) Lung-USA (800-586-4872)
www.lungusa.org

Asthma & Allergy Foundation of America (AAFA)
1233 20th St., NW, Suite 402
Washington, DC 20036
(202) 466-7643
(800) 7-Asthma (800-727-8462)
www.aafa.org

Cystic Fibrosis Foundation
6931 Arlington Rd.
Bethesda, MD 20814-3205
(301) 951-4422
(800) FIGHT-CF (800-344-4823)
www.cff.org

Johns Hopkins University Asthma Home Study
www.jhsph.edu/homestudy/home.html

Mayo Clinic Web Site
www.mayohealth.org

National Heart, Lung and Blood Institute (NHLBI)
NHLBI Information Center
National Asthma Education & Prevention Program
P.O. Box 30105
Bethesda, MD 20824-0105
(301) 496-4236
www.nhlbi.nih.gov

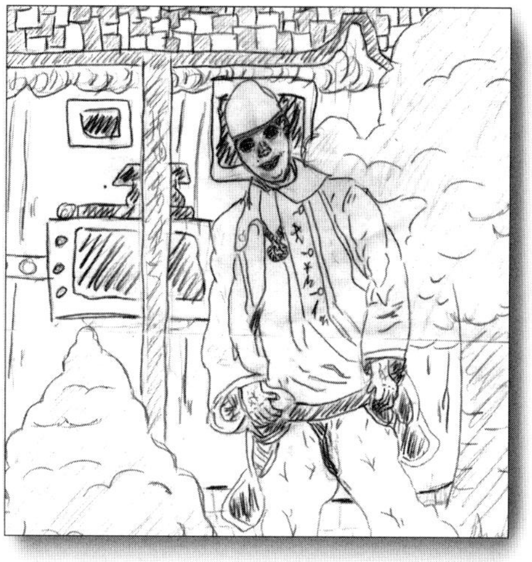

My whole life I have been different from all the other kids. I have had three heart operations. I only remember one—it was the worst thing in the world. I remember waking up from the operation, I didn't know where I was. . . I tried to talk but I couldn't. There was a tube in my throat that made me cough and gag. Finally they took it out, but I still had to stay in the PICU for a long time. It was really noisy and I couldn't get any sleep. I got to go home three days before Christmas. That was five years ago. Now I am eight. Last summer I got to play soccer for the first time. It was really fun even if I could only play a little.

A child is a precious gift that should not be taken for granted. When that precious gift is diagnosed with a heart problem it becomes a parent's nightmare. They become numb to reality, living in a world of disbelief, and sleep deprival, a form of denial. The denial heightens to a state of anxiety, consisting of a million questions, the most important one "why?" Parents don't want statistics and evasive answers. They want empathy and education. They need to understand the quality of life their child will have based on the decisions they make. Parents stop and ask how and why this happened to a family that leads a decent lifestyle. No matter what is decided the stress causes instability in the family structure, and tears at everyone's heart strings. Leaving them still looking for someone to answer "why?" and someone to make it all right again.

CARDIOVASCULAR ALTERATIONS

Janet Craig, RN, MS, CCRN, PNP
Bonnie Clay, RN, MS, CCRN, PNP

COMPETENCIES

Upon completion of this chapter the reader will be able to:

- *Explain differences in anatomy and physiology of child's cardiovascular system as compared to adults.*
- *Perform an assessment of the child with heart disease.*
- *Describe the clinical symptoms of congestive heart failure and identify appropriate interventions.*
- *Identify two congenital heart lesions that increase pulmonary blood flow.*
- *Identify two congenital heart lesions that decrease pulmonary blood flow resulting in cyanosis.*
- *Develop a plan of care for the child who has undergone open heart surgery.*
- *Describe the disorder and treatment for acute rheumatic fever, Kawasaki disease, and infectious endocarditis.*
- *Identify the three forms of shock.*
- *Identify interventions to support the psychosocial well-being of the child with heart disease and caregivers.*

The heart is the symbol for love, emotion, and mortality. In other words, it is the essence of well-being. Therefore the diagnosis of possible or real heart disease in a child is particularly trying for the family. There are a number of misperceptions about the significance of murmurs, cyanosis, and activity level. Indeed the presence of an asymptomatic simple cardiac diagnosis can evoke fears and concerns that are unfounded, although very real to the family. Many times family concerns over a simple cardiac condition exceed those raised by a more life-threatening condition in another body part.

Some 35,000 children are born per year in the United States with congenital heart disease. This number does not include those children who develop acquired heart disease. Over the last fifty years significant advances have been made in the diagnosis, treatment, and evaluation of the child with heart disease. As a result of these advances 85% will survive into adulthood (Moodie, 1994). Nevertheless, concerns about treatment plans, possibility of death, lifestyle changes, and finances remain for the child and family.

Pathophysiology in pediatric heart disease is widely variable and challenging to even the most experienced clinician. Care of the child with heart disease requires a multidisciplinary approach. A sound knowledge of normal and abnormal physiology is critically important to the understanding of pathology, therapeutic intervention, and evaluation.

Caring for children with heart disease can be challenging and rewarding. Innovations and technological advances continue to improve outcomes. However, a number of life issues remain for the family and child. The nurse is in a pivotal position to support innovative technologies, assess response to intervention, provide education, and facilitate growth and development. Often the nurse serves as the liaison between the family and health care team. A sound understanding of anatomy, physiology, and pathophysiology provides the basis for nursing intervention. Exciting opportunities await those who are interested in participating in this specialty. Opportunities are available for nursing research in a number of areas, including physiological responses, psychosocial effects, and development of children with heart disease.

As more of these children survive into adulthood a whole new subspecialty has emerged—the adult with congenital heart disease. These clients require knowledgeable, skillful nurses who understand congenital heart disease as well as the normal life issues that young adults face. Concerns regarding pregnancy, work, insurance, parenting, and healthy lifestyles become paramount. Life is a continuum; therefore, we can no longer afford to segregate pediatric cardiac issues from adult health issues. Nurses are the key to improved outcomes in *all* clients with congenital and acquired heart disease.

This chapter will review normal cardiovascular anatomy and physiology, congestive heart failure, congenital and acquired heart disease, and shock. Nursing concerns specific to this population will be addressed providing a sound basis for future practice and stimulating further investigation into the nursing care of the child with heart disease. Box 25-1 provides a list of common terms and abbreviations used in the discussion of cardiovascular alterations.

BOX 25-1 Common abbreviations in cardiovascular alterations

AS = aortic stenosis
ASD = atrial septal defect
AV = atrioventricular
CHD = congenital heart defect
CHF = congestive heart failure
CO = cardiac output
CPB = cardiopulmonary bypass
EKG = electrocardiogram
HLHS = hypoplastic left heart syndrome
HR = heart rate
LA = left atrium
LV = left ventricle
PA = pulmonary artery
PDA = patent ductus arteriosus
PFO = patent foramen ovale
PS = pulmonary stenosis
PVR = pulmonary vascular resistance
RA = right atrium
RV = right ventricle
SA = sinoatrial
SVR = systemic vascular resistance
TA = truncus arteriosus
TGA = transposition of the great arteries
TOF = tetralogy of Fallot
VSD = ventricular septal defect

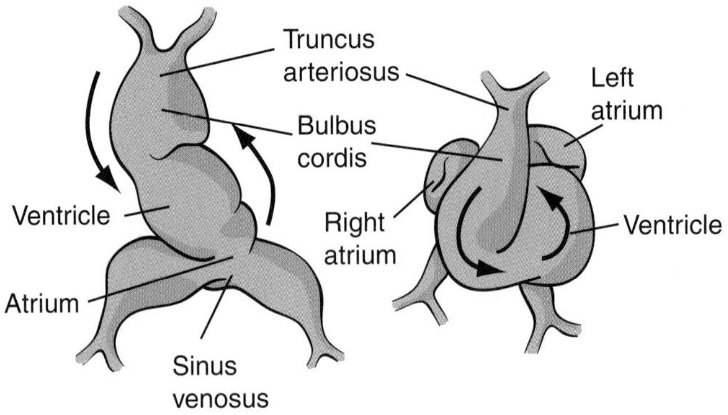

Figure 25-1 Normal Folding of the Heart Tube That Occurs Between 23 and 28 Days of Gestation

ANATOMY AND PHYSIOLOGY

Normal Cardiac Anatomy

The cardiovascular system is the first system to function in the developing fetus. The heart begins as a tube by the third week of gestation. This tube loops to the right and begins to fold into itself (Figure 25-1). Incomplete partitioning of the atria leaves a small opening called the **foramen ovale** (normal in utero connection in the atrial septum), which normally closes after birth. In addition the **ductus arteriosus** (a blood vessel connecting the aorta with the pulmonary artery) serves to divert blood from the fetal lungs to the fetal aorta as the lungs do not participate in gas exchange in utero. This structure usually closes after birth. Final formation of the ventricular septum occurs by the seventh week of gestation (Figure 25-2) (Clark, 1995). Cardiac development is fairly complete by eight weeks of gestation. Cardiac abnormalities account for about 25% of all congenital malformations. Most malformations are multifactorial secondary to genetic defects, abnormal fetal hemodynamics, and environ-

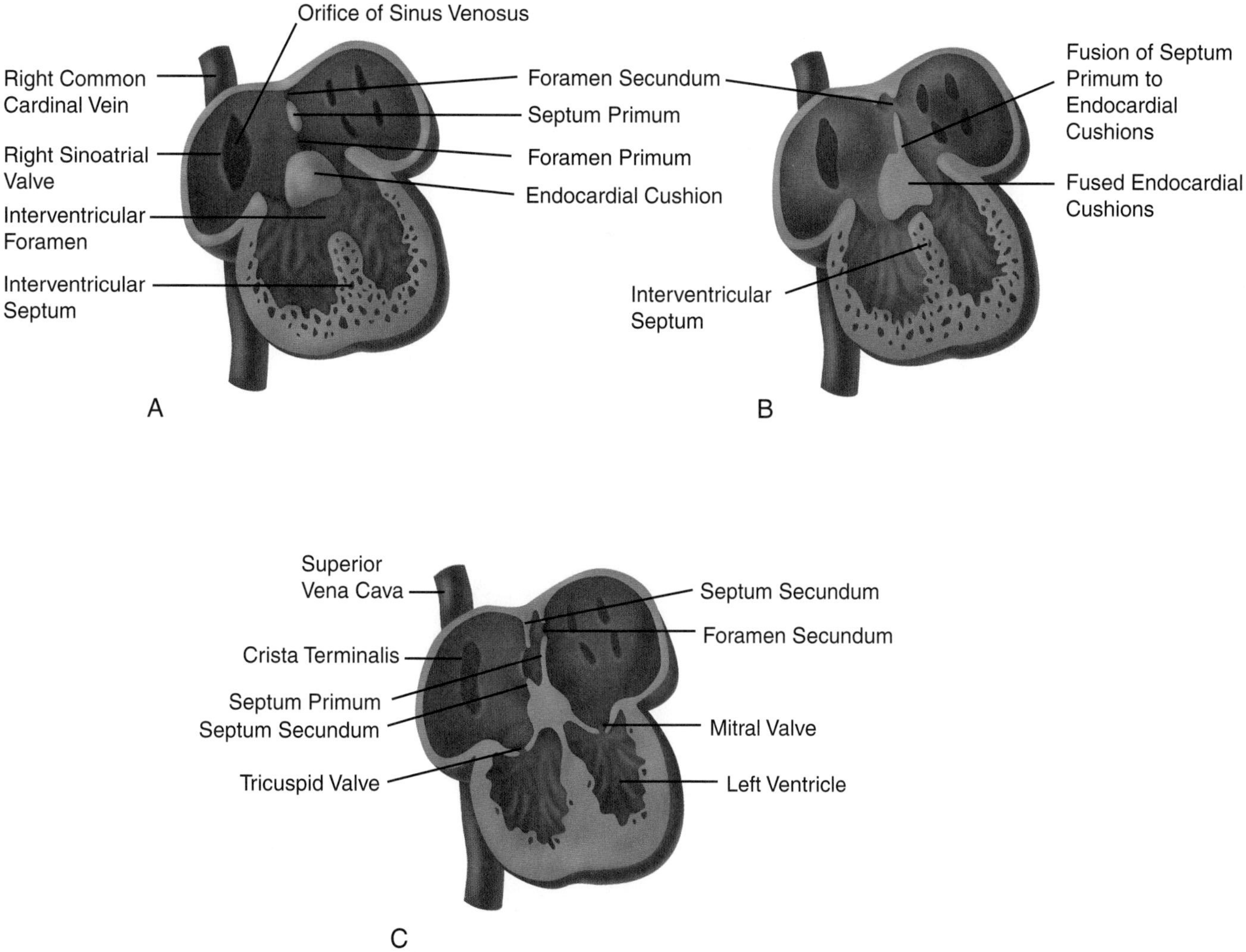

Figure 25-2 Sequential development of the heart tube (A, B, C). Final development occurs by 7 weeks gestation.

mental factors. Many defects occur before the pregnant woman knows she has conceived.

The fully developed heart is a four chambered structure that lies between the lungs in the mediastinum. Heart size corresponds with the size of the child's fist; this correlation continues into adulthood. Normal position is distinguished by the ventricular apex, which is directed downward and toward the left (Figure 25-3). The atria are thin walled low pressure chambers that serve as reservoirs for the ventricles. The ventricles are the cardiac pumps. The right ventricle is a low pressure chamber that drives blood to the low resistance pulmonary circulation (lungs) via the pulmonary artery. The left ventricle is a high pressure chamber that drives blood to the high resistance systemic circulation (body) via the aorta (Edwards, 1995; Callow, Suddaby, & Slota, 1998). There are four cardiac valves: the tricuspid, mitral, pulmonary, and aortic, which allow for unidirectional blood flow during contraction and relaxation (Callow, et al., 1998). The great vessels of the heart are the pulmonary artery and aorta. After birth the pulmonary artery is the only artery in the body that carries deoxygenated blood; all other arterial beds including the aorta carry oxygenated blood. Under normal conditions in children (outside of the newborn) the pulmonary vascular bed is a low pressure, low resistance circuit. Refer to Figure 25-4 to review normal anatomy and hemodynamics.

The conduction system is responsible for the electrical activity that initiates mechanical activity of the heart. It consists of the sinoatrial (SA) node, internodal pathways, atrioventricular (AV) node, bundle of His, bundle branch system, and Purkinje fibers (Figure 25-5). The normal cardiac electrical impulse originates in the SA node. The impulse is then sent through the atrium to the AV node. Under normal circumstances the AV node is the only area in the heart that allows transmission of an impulse from the atria to the ventricle. It controls the speed of conduction and number of impulses allowed to enter the ventricle. The Purkinje fibers

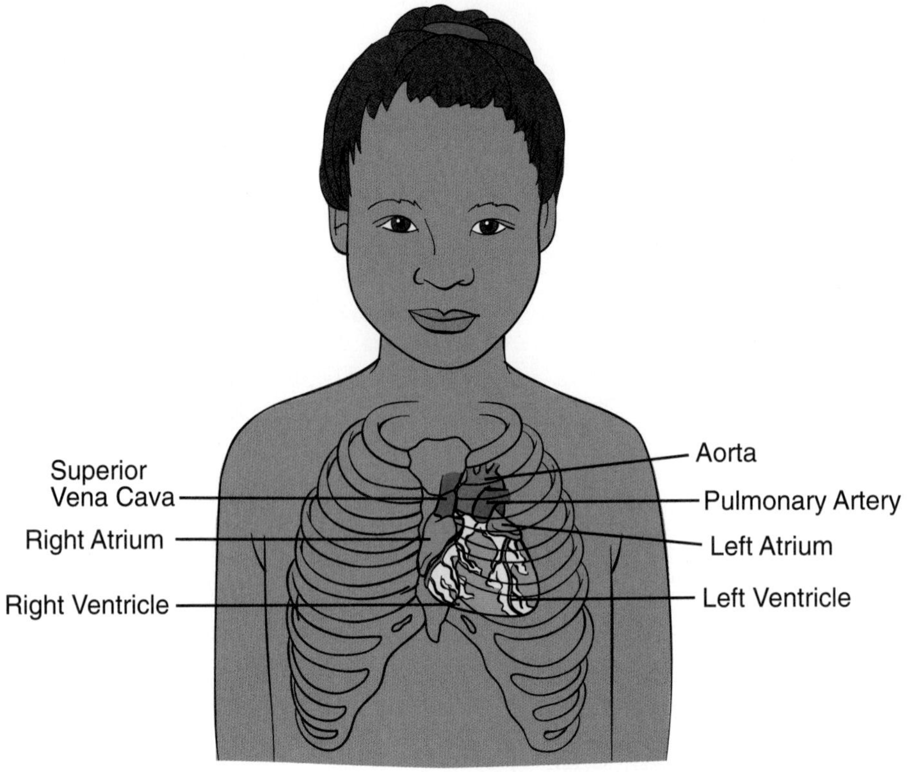

Figure 25-3 Normal Placement of the Heart in the Chest

infiltrate and transmit the electrical impulses into the ventricle. This well orchestrated process results in a uniform cardiac contraction.

Normal Hemodynamics

An understanding of transitional and normal hemodynamics is critical for the nurse caring for the child in shock or with heart disease. Abnormal hemodynamics are usually the basis for clinical pathology. A couple of key caveats to remember will help the nurse to interpret and understand diagnostic tests and therapeutic interventions. First and foremost blood flows from a higher pressure to a lower pressure, some refer to this as flowing "down hill." Second, blood flow will take the path of least resistance. For example, if a defect is present that allows blood to flow either to the pulmonary bed or systemic bed, it will preferentially flow through the low resistance pulmonary bed. With increasing expertise the nurse will be able to apply these simple concepts to more complex defects in clinical practice.

Fetal and Postnatal Circulation

Fetal circulation is distinctly different from postnatal circulation. In some cases persistence of fetal circulation can occur after birth. Refer to Chapter 7 for a discussion of fetal and postnatal circulation.

Cardiac Output

Cardiac output (CO) is the volume of blood ejected by the heart in one minute. It is calculated by multiplying the heart rate (HR) by the stroke volume (SV). Stroke volume is the amount of blood ejected by the ventricles per contraction in milliliters (ml).

$$CO = HR \times SV$$

This is one measurement of blood flow. Normal CO in an infant is 200 ml/kg/min; in adolescents it is 100 ml/kg/min.

The determinants of stroke volume are preload, afterload, and contractility. Preload is the amount of blood in the ventricle at the end of diastole and just prior to systole. It is the volume of blood returning to the heart. Preload is responsible for the stretching of the cardiac muscle and is primarily influenced by intravascular volume and the compliance of the ventricle.

Afterload is the resistance that the ventricle must overcome when ejecting blood. Clinically this value is used during cardiac catheterization to measure the degree of ventricular work. Afterload is influenced by the size of the

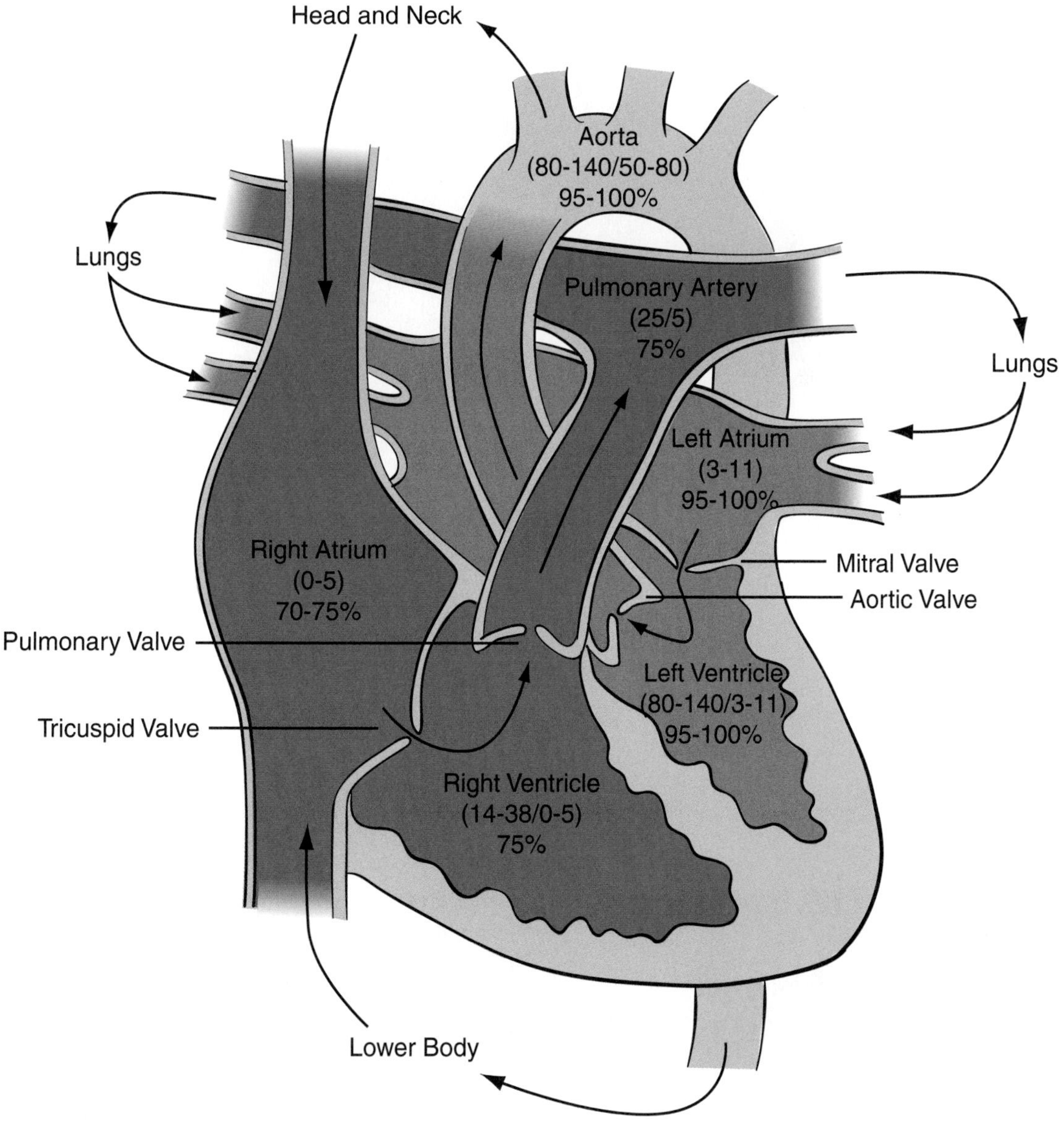

Figure 25-4 Normal Anatomy of the Heart and Blood Flow. Percentages are intracardiac oxygen saturations. Normal pressures are in parentheses.

ventricular outflow tract and accompanying semilunar valve, resistance of the associated vascular bed, and blood viscosity (hematocrit). Right ventricular afterload is subject to pulmonary vascular resistance, which is normally low after about eight weeks of life. In utero the pulmonary vascular resistance is very high to divert blood away from the fetal lung. In general it takes up to eight weeks after birth for this resistance to fall to normal levels that are maintained into adulthood. Left ventricular afterload is subject to systemic vascular resistance, which is high relative to the pulmonary bed.

Contractility is the intrinsic ability of the myocardial fiber to shorten and produce a forceful contraction. It is influenced by preload, oxygen supply, circulating catecholamines (epinephrine and norepinephrine), maturity of the **myocardium** (the cardiac muscle; middle layer of the heart,) and serum calcium. It should be noted that the newborn and infant myocardium is immature with fewer contractile fibers and limited intracellular calcium stores (Furdon, 1997).

Heart rate is also important in determining cardiac output. Rates that are too fast result in decreased diastolic filling because the resting phase of the heart is shortened. Rates that are too slow will result in low cardiac output because there are fewer beats per minute in which to eject blood. Abnormal rhythms can also interfere with cardiac output. The newborn is more sensitive to changes in heart rate than the older child (Kohr & O'Brien, 1995).

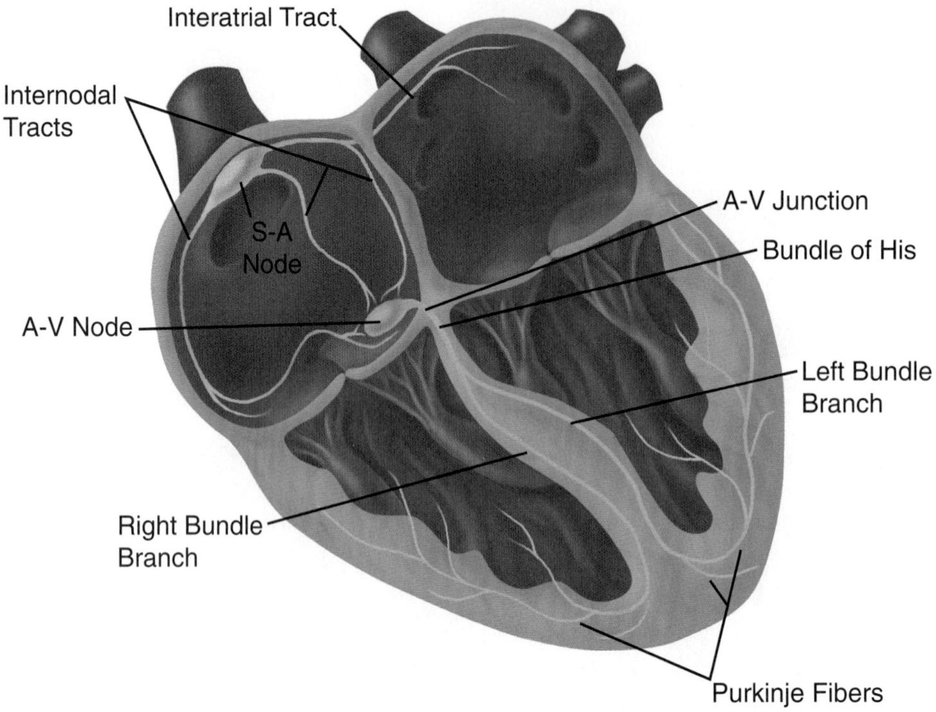

Figure 25-5 Normal Conduction System

ASSESSMENT OF THE CHILD WITH A CARDIOVASCULAR ALTERATION

History

A concise thorough history is crucial to the assessment, diagnosis and evaluation of the response to therapeutic intervention. Many caregivers have obvious concerns about the implications of cardiac symptomatology. An important outcome of history taking is the opportunity to assess caregiver/child interaction and coping skills. The chief complaint should be elicited, particularly in children who are being evaluated for the first time. Presenting symptoms such as when a murmur was first heard can help with the establishment of a possible diagnosis.

When evaluating an infant a prenatal and postnatal history must be obtained. Pertinent data include maternal infections (rubella, HIV), lifestyle, prenatal drug and alcohol exposure, complications of pregnancy, gestational age at birth, and birth complications. Eating is the exercise of the neonate, therefore feeding behaviors should be evaluated. Does the infant exhibit excessive diaphoresis, shortness of breath, fatigue, or cyanosis (a bluish tinge to the skin and mucous membranes) with feeding? The nurse should specifically determine where cyanosis is observed. Peripheral cyanosis of the extremities is usually caused by vasomotor instability typically seen in the young infant. Cyanosis of the lips (not perioral, which is the skin around the lips) and tongue is worrisome, and the presence of **hypercyanotic** (extreme cyanosis that results in a deep blue or purple color of the entire body) spells requires further investigation. Often infants with heart disease will be irritable, inconsolable, have poor weight gain, excessive diaphoresis, and poor feeding (Veasey, 1995a).

When evaluating the older child, height and weight should be documented and compared with previous trends to evaluate for growth retardation. Exercise tolerance relative to developmental norms and their peers is evaluated. Care must be taken to obtain the caregiver's as well as the child's perceptions on exercise tolerance, as these can be quite divergent. Unnecessary restrictions may have been placed on the child by the caregiver caused by anxiety about real or presumed heart disease. The presence of color changes, shortness of breath, dizziness, **syncope** (fainting), frequent respiratory infections, or **palpitations** (sensation of abnormal heart beats) should be investigated and documented (Veasey, 1995a).

When interviewing an adolescent, the primary historian should be the child, using the caregivers to corroborate information. Ability to keep up with peers while undertaking normal activities (climbing the stairs, physical education, dancing, walking in the mall) is assessed. Various limitations include shortness of breath, dizziness, fatigue, syncope, or chest pain. In addition the nurse should query the family about any genetic syndrome the child may have. It is often helpful to know if the child has been formally evaluated by a geneticist, since a number of syndromes are associated with congenital heart disease.

Obtaining a family history is very important as a number of cardiac conditions are familial. Congenital heart disease occurs in approximately 8 in 1,000 live births, and this incidence is increased when a parent or sibling has the disease (Strauss & Johnson, 1996). A number of cardiac defects are associated with various conditions and syndromes. For a list of these see Table 25-1.

Physical Examination

The following section outlines specific features that are salient to the cardiac examination. For a more detailed review of assessment of the heart and peripheral vasculature refer to Chapter 14.

Inspection

Physical abnormalities such as **dysmorphic** (abnormal or unusual) facial features, edema, chest wall deformities, and skin color (pallor, cyanosis, and/or jaundice) should be assessed. Cyanosis is best evaluated under bright natural light. Changes in skin color may be difficult to discern in children with deeply pigmented skin, so particular attention should be paid to the color of the lips, tongue, and nail beds.

The fingers should be evaluated for the presence of clubbing. This is a soft tissue deformity that is the result of chronic cyanosis with the subsequent development of the loss of the normal angle between the nail and the nail bed. The finger tips eventually become wider and rounder (Figure 25-6) (Veasey, 1995a; Callow, et al., 1998).

Auscultation for Murmurs

Refer to Chapter 14 for an in-depth review of cardiac auscultation. Murmurs are noises that occur from turbulent blood flow and they can be abnormal or "innocent." Murmurs are described by their location, timing, frequency, and intensity. When auscultating the chest four traditional areas are utilized (Figure 25-7). Location is denoted by landmarks on the chest such as left lower sternal border, left axilla, right upper sternal border, and so forth. Systolic murmurs are heard between the first and second heart sounds. Holosystolic murmurs are heard throughout systole, incorporating the second heart sound into the murmur. Diastolic murmurs are heard after S_2 but before S_1. Continuous murmurs are heard throughout the entire cardiac cycle. There is a standardized way to grade murmurs that is universally accepted (Box 25-2). Systolic murmurs that are loud (grade III or greater) are generally considered abnormal and require further evaluation by a cardiologist. Holosystolic, diastolic, and most continuous murmurs are abnormal. Pathologic murmurs associated with congenital defects are discussed with each specific defect in the congenital heart disease section.

TABLE 25-1 Conditions Associated with Congenital Heart Disease

Syndrome	Anomaly
DiGeorge syndrome	Interrupted aortic arch, tetralogy of Fallot (TOF), truncus arteriosus
Williams syndrome	Pulmonary stenosis, aortic stenosis
Trisomy 21 (Down)	Primum ASD, VSD, AV canal
Turner's syndrome	Pulmonary stenosis, coarctation of aorta
Trisomy 18	VSD, PDA
Apert syndrome	VSD
Glycogen storage disease	Cardiomyopathy
Duchenne's and Becker's muscular dystrophy	Cardiomyopathy
Noonan's syndrome	Pulmonary stenosis
Long QT	Arrhythmias
Marfan syndrome	Aortic valve regurgitation, aortic aneurysms, mitral valve prolapse
Fetal alcohol syndrome	VSD, ASD, TOF
Lithium ingestion (maternal)	Ebstein's anomaly, ASD
Amphetamines	VSD, PDA, ASD, TGA
Maternal lupus	Congenital heart block
Maternal diabetes	Cardiomyopathy, VSD, TGA
Thyroid dysfunction	Supraventricular tachycardia, cardiomyopathy

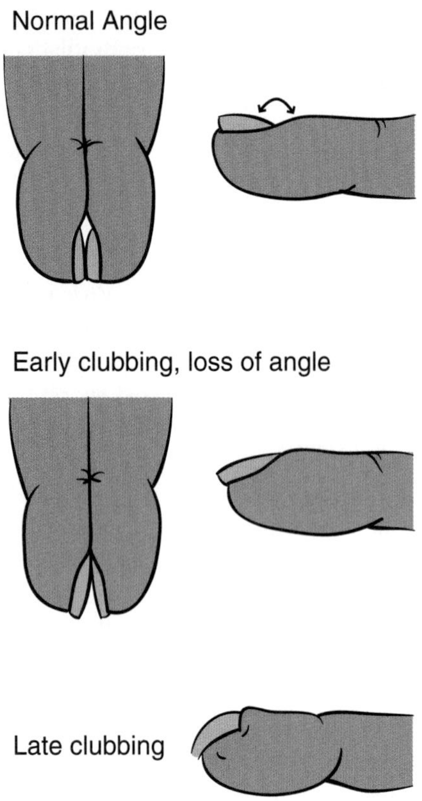

Figure 25-6 Changes in the Nailbed That Result in Clubbing

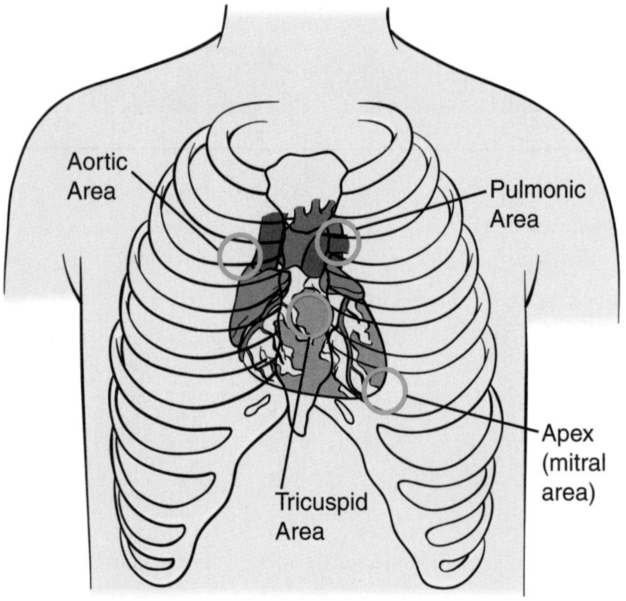

Figure 25-7 Normal Areas of Cardiac Auscultation

BOX 25-2 Classifying murmurs by grade

Grade 1–Barely audible, may require listening to several cardiac cycles to appreciate
Grade 2–Soft murmur that is readily heard
Grade 3–Moderately loud murmur without a thrill
Grade 4–Moderately loud murmur with a thrill
Grade 5–Loud murmur heard with the edge of the stethoscope touching the chest
Grade 6–Loud murmur that can be heard without the stethoscope touching the chest

It must be clarified that not all murmurs are pathologic. Many murmurs are denoted as innocent, indicating there is no structural or functional heart disease (Danford, Nasir, & Gumbiner, 1993; Du, Roguin, & Barak, 1997). Nonetheless the presence of a murmur often invokes caregivers' fears regarding their child's health and well-being. The quality of an innocent murmur is quite characteristic (soft, short, systolic, and vibratory in quality). Therefore experienced clinicians are able to determine if a murmur is innocent without obtaining special tests (Driscoll, et al., 1994; Danford, et al., 1993; Swenson, et al., 1997). Children who are found to have innocent murmurs require no intervention or specific follow-up since these murmurs often disappear with age. Activity restrictions are not necessary, and the child should be treated normally. It should be noted that the intensity of an innocent murmur will increase with fever, illness, or stress. This should be explained to the family as normal and does not indicate the sudden occurrence of heart disease. Careful education is critically important as there is evidence that some families will continue to presume their child has heart disease even though it has been determined that the murmur is innocent.

Palpation for Hepatomegaly

Refer to Chapter 14 for more in-depth review regarding palpation of the chest and extremities. The abdomen is palpated for **hepatomegaly** (liver enlargement). In normal infants the liver edge may be as far as 1–2 centimeters below the right costal margin. In older children and adolescents the liver edge may be at the right costal margin or non-palpable. Hepatomegaly is associated with congestive heart failure.

Blood Pressure Measurement

Blood pressure (BP) measurement is a common maneuver for all nurses to perform. However, in children this can be fraught with error if not executed correctly. Most important is selecting the appropriately sized cuff in order to obtain a correct measurement. Refer to Chapter 14 for information about BP cuff size and normal values for BP according to age, sex, and height. There are a number of different cuff sizes available. Arm and leg blood pressures are obtained to rule out coarctation of the aorta (the right arm and either leg are used). Normally lower extremity BP is equal to or greater than the arm BP. A right arm BP greater than a leg BP can indicate coarctation of the aorta.

Serial BP measurements must be taken on repeat visits before a child is determined to be hypertensive. Anxiety around a clinic visit, particularly with a new health care provider can elevate BP. Repeat visits will help with accommodation of the child to the environment, allowing the accurate reflection of the true BP. Body size, age, and sex are the most important determinants of BP in children (National High Blood Pressure Education Program Working Group, 1996).

Pulsus paradoxus is an excessive variation in systolic pressure with respiration. Normally the systolic BP drops no more than 10 mm Hg with inspiration (in the spontaneously breathing child). A drop of more than 10 mm Hg is pathologic and is characteristic of those conditions that interfere with cardiac filling, that is, cardiac **tamponade** (accumulation of fluid around heart that restricts filling of heart), **pericardial effusion** (collection of fluid in pericardial sac that can lead to tamponade), and **pericarditis** (inflammation of the pericardium).

Diagnostic Tests

A number of diagnostic studies can be utilized in the diagnosis and evaluation of the child with heart disease. These include laboratory tests, pulse oximetry, electrocardiogram (EKG), holter monitor, event monitoring, chest radiograph (CXR), echocardiogram (ECHO), magnetic resonance imaging (MRI), and cardiac catheterization. Not all tests are used for every child. The selection of appropriate tests is based on diagnosis and symptoms. Table 25-2 offers a listing of the most common diagnostic tests used in diagnosing cardiovascular alterations in infants and children. Figure 25-8 shows a child getting an EKG.

TABLE 25-2 Diagnostic Tests for Cardiac Alterations

Name of Test	Purpose and Description	Normal Findings	Nursing Considerations
Pulse oximetry (SpO_2)	Evaluates degree of oxygen saturation in the blood using a small infrared light probe that is placed on a finger/toe/earlobe or bridge of the nose	95–100% Clinical cyanosis is not visible until saturation is less than 85%.	• Rotate pulse oximeter probe site every 4–6 hours to prevent pressure sores. • Works best when area where probe is placed is well perfused; may have difficulty in reading oxygen saturation if area is cool or poorly perfused.
Electrocardiogram (EKG)	Detects electrical events, normal and abnormal cardiac rhythms in the heart. Waveforms are produced via the use of 12 electrodes that are placed on the chest and extremities. These waveforms can be used to assess cardiac rhythm.	P wave correlates with atrial depolarization, QRS with ventricular depolarization. There should be a P wave before every QRS, the rhythm should be regular and rate normal for child's age.	• For the best quality tracing, the child should hold still; to facilitate this the caregivers may hold the child, or distractions (toys, bubbles) can be employed. • If lotion or powder is on the skin, it should be cleansed gently with alcohol prior to placement of the electrodes. Otherwise, vigorous cleansing or shaving is not indicated in children.
Holter monitor	Continuous 24-hour EKG recorder that utilizes 5 chest leads and a tape cassette to produce a two-channel recording. This is used if symptoms or arrhythmia occur daily. A diary is kept by the caregiver or child while the holter is worn.	Normals should be similar to EKG.	• As the monitor should stay on for 24 hours the skin must be prepped with alcohol or other solvent to remove oils. The electrode adhesive is strong so adhesive remover is recommended for removal. If the skin is inflammed following removal a 1% steriod cream may be applied. • The caregiver/child should be instructed to write in the diary symptoms, activities, and sleep times so that appropriate correlation of rhythm can be made with diary entries.

continues

TABLE 25-2 *Continued*

Name of Test	Purpose and Description	Normal Findings	Nursing Considerations
Event recorder	Small pager-sized recorder that is client activated to record heart rhythm during symptoms. This is used when symptoms do not occur daily. It is generally worn for a month. Once the recorder is activated it stores the EKG; this can be transmitted via telephone at a later time.	Normal would be the same as EKG.	• Event recorder does not need to be worn during sleep (unless the symptoms occur during sleep and awaken the child). It should not be worn while bathing or swimming. • If inflammation occurs from the electrodes then the placement may be rotated slightly and 1% steriod cream applied.
Chest radiograph (CXR)	Chest X ray that is used to determine cardiac size, contour, and alterations in pulmonary vascularity.	Heart size should be no greater than 50% of widest intercostal diameter of chest. Pulmonary arteries should not appear large, lung fields should be clear.	• Best quality CXR is insured if child is still and X ray is obtained during inspiration. (The heart size is falsely increased during expiration.) Diversional activities, or caregiver assistance may be required. • Lead shields are placed over the child's gonads and are worn by any assistive personnel or family member.
Echocardiogram (ECHO)	Two-dimensional and Doppler evaluation of cardiac anatomy, size, and function. Utilizes sound waves (ultrasound) emitted by a transducer that is placed on the chest in different positions. Transesophageal echo uses a transducer that is placed in the esophagus to visualize posterior cardiac structures or to evaluate for intracardiac thrombi.	Cardiac structures should be normal without evidence of valve leakage or septal defects. Heart thickness is normal for body surface area. Function is evaluated by determining shortening fraction (normal 28–44%) and ejection fraction (normal >55%).	• Client cooperation is imperative. Children less than two years generally require sedation to hold still. Pulse oximetry and heart rate should be monitored during sedation. For patient comfort the ultrasound gel should be warmed. See Figure 25-9.
Cardiac catheterization (card cath)	An invasive procedure performed under fluroscopy that allows determination of cardiac anatomy, function, cardiac pressures, and oxygen saturations. Catheters are inserted into the heart via a large vein and/or artery. A contrast agent (dye) is sometimes injected to aid in the recording of blood flow and help evaluate the coronary arteries.	For normal intracardiac oxygen saturations and pressures, see Figure 25-4.	• Sedation or anesthesia is necessary to prevent patient movement. For pre- and post-catheterization nursing care see section under cardiac catheterization. See Figure 25-10.

continues

TABLE 25-2 *Continued*

Name of Test	Purpose and Description	Normal Findings	Nursing Considerations
Magnetic resonance imaging (MRI)	Uses large magnet that stimulates atomic nuclei in body to emit energy in form of radio waves that is then transformed into a picture of the structure(s) being evaluated. Assists in defining cardiac anatomy that cannot be well evaluated by ECHO.	Anatomic structures should be normal.	• Patient cooperation is imperative; sedation is employed with young children, toddlers, and infants. • MRI is avoided if permanent pacemaker is in place.

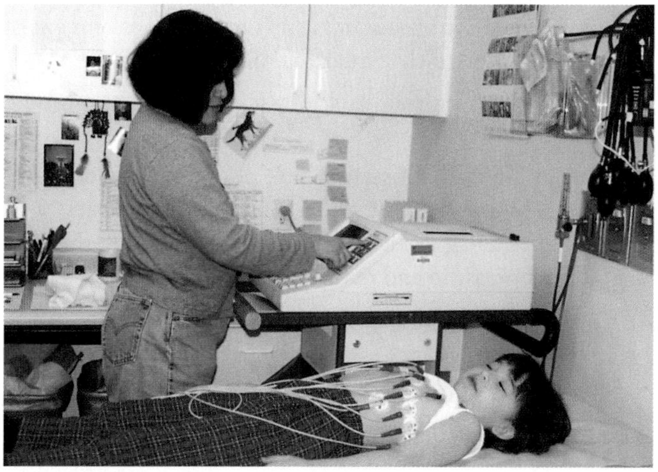

Figure 25-8 A Child with Heart Disease Getting a 12-lead EKG

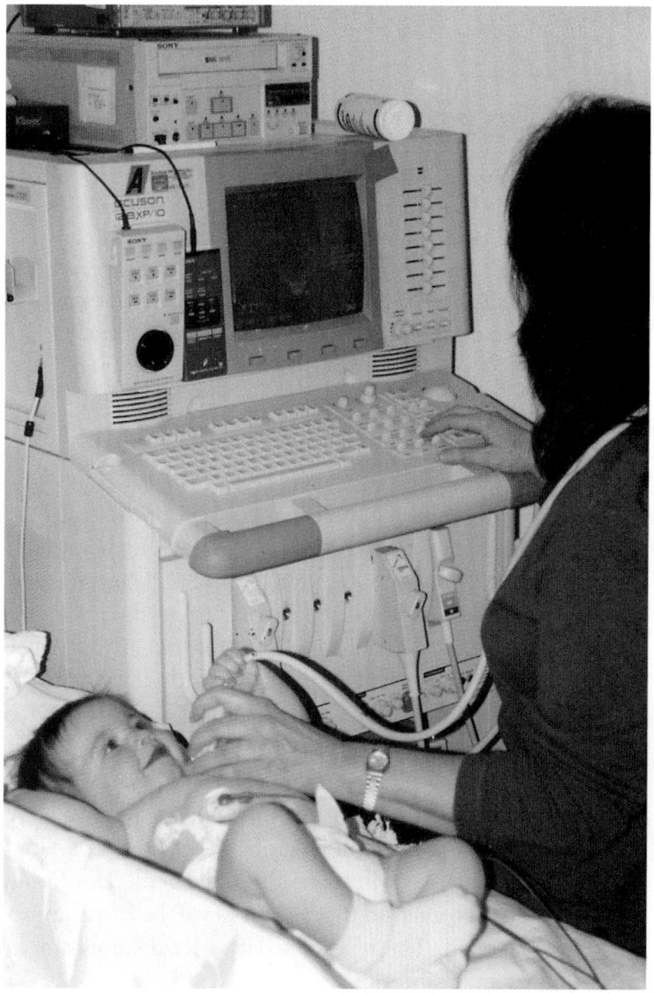

Figure 25-9 A Baby Getting an Echocardiogram

Nursing Considerations for the Child Undergoing Cardiac Catheterization

This is a routine procedure that is generally performed on an outpatient basis. Children who have undergone therapeutic cardiac cath, or small infants, may require overnight hospitalization. Even though routine this procedure can be very stressful for the child and family and is not completely risk free.

Prior to the procedure a complete nursing history must be obtained. Pretesting includes an EKG, ECHO, CBC, and platelet count. The child should be NPO for four to six hours prior to the procedure, depending on hospital policy. Assessment includes accurate height and weight as these measurements are used to determine catheter size and calculate body surface area. Obtaining a history of allergies is critically important. Many contrast materials contain iodine; therefore, allergies to iodine, contrast dyes, or shellfish must be brought to the attention of the cardiologist. Any history of fever or previous illness, as well as signs and symptoms of infection must be assessed. The presence of illness or infection may require postponement of the procedure. Baseline assessment of pedal pulses and pulse oximetry are documented so that postprocedural findings can be compared to baseline.

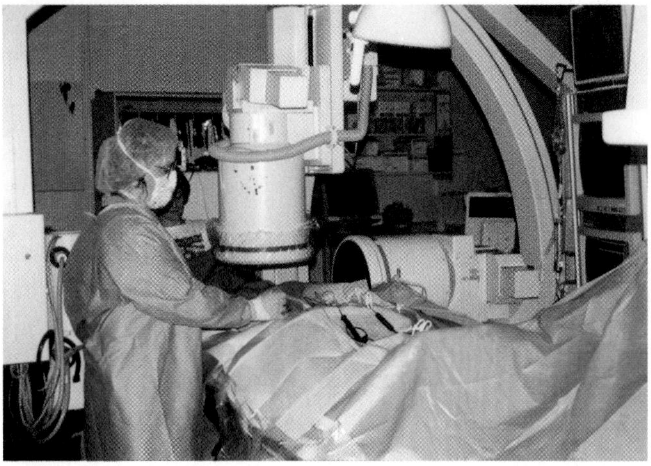

Figure 25-10 A Child Undergoing Cardiac Catheterization

Nursing Alert:

Children with Latex Allergies

The balloon used during interventional cath for balloon dilation of narrow valves or coarctation of the aorta contains latex. It is very important that the nurse determine if the child has a latex allergy prior to the cath as use of the balloon can precipitate a life-threatening reaction. If the child has a latex allergy, this intervention should be avoided and the child referred for surgical repair.

Preprocedural preparation is important for the child and family. Child life specialists, puppet therapy, or therapeutic play can all facilitate the alleviation of anxiety. The sights and sounds of the cath lab should be explained to the child, utilizing age-appropriate language. Often a tour of the lab is helpful. Specific aspects of the procedure should be explained such as the placement of the IV and the EKG electrodes, washing of the groin with betadine (brown soap), use of the numbing medicine (lidocaine) to put the skin to sleep, humming of the fluoroscopy when turned on, how injection of the contrast will create a warm flushed feeling, and how the sedative will make the child feel. The family and child must be assured that sedatives will be given appropriately as needed. The type of sedative used varies among practitioners and institutions.

Following the procedure the child is monitored for a number of hours prior to discharge, often with a cardiac monitor and pulse oximeter. It is critically important that the nurse monitor the following:

1. Temperature and color of the extremity distal to the catheter insertion.
2. Pulse of the extremity distal to the catheter insertion site.

Nursing Tip:

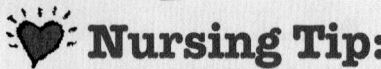

Avoid sandbags to prevent bleeding after cardiac catheterization

Sandbags should never be used to prevent or treat bleeding from the catheter site. Use of a sandbag can severely compromise distal circulation or only increase the child's agitation.

3. Vital signs frequently, for example, every 15 minutes for the first hour and hourly thereafter. Particular attention should be paid to HR and BP. The nurse must monitor trends and assess for the development of hypotension, tachycardia, and bradycardia.
4. Intake and output, as contrast material can promote brisk diuresis.
5. Bleeding at the insertion site; observe for evidence of hematoma. The nurse must inspect the dressing with each vital sign check, and if bleeding is noted, apply direct pressure and notify practitioner.
6. Oxygen desaturation. This must be compared to the child's baseline.

The child should be kept in bed with the affected extremity straight for 4 to 8 hours, depending on hospital policy. Younger children can be held by their caregiver to ensure better compliance. Diet is advanced as tolerated. The pressure dressing can be removed in 24 hours. An effort should be made to keep the dressing dry in infants and toddlers who still wear diapers. Discharge teaching includes family education on site care, observing the site for signs of inflammation and infection, monitoring for fever, restriction from strenuous activities for a few days, avoiding tub baths for 48–72 hours (showers are fine), and the use of acetaminophen or ibuprofen for pain.

CONGESTIVE HEART FAILURE

Congestive heart failure (CHF) is the inability of the cardiovascular system to provide adequate cardiac output to meet the metabolic demands of the body. To understand the pathophysiological and clinical manifestations of CHF the nurse must have a working knowledge of normal determinants of cardiac output, as well as an understanding of the normal compensatory mechanisms. Refer to the previous section on cardiac output for review of the normal determinants. A discussion of the compensatory mechanisms is located in the pathophysiology segment in this section.

Incidence and Etiology

The absolute incidence of CHF in infants and children is unknown because of the wide range of causes. Congenital heart defects are the most common causes of CHF in infants. Structural defects can impose either a volume load or pressure load on the heart. Defects with left to right shunts (ventricular septal defect) impose a volume load. Left sided obstructive defects (hypoplastic left heart syndrome, aortic stenosis, coarctation of the aorta) impose a pressure load as there is obstruction to forward flow of blood. Excessive volume and/or pressure can contribute to pulmonary edema. Most infants with significant defects will develop symptoms within weeks to months following birth (Kohr & O'Brien, 1995; Committee on Evaluation and Management of Heart Failure, 1995; Ueda, Fukushige, & Ueda, 1996).

The most common cause of CHF in infants is congenital heart disease. Acquired heart disease is the most common cause in older children or adolescents. These include **cardiomyopathy** (disease of the heart muscle resulting in poor pump function), **endocarditis** (infection of the inner lining of the heart), rheumatic fever (refer to section on rheumatic fever) and **myocarditis** (inflammation of the heart muscle). These diseases result in impaired myocardial contractility with a subsequent fall in cardiac output. This phenomenon causes volume overload and resultant pulmonary and systemic venous congestion (Kohr & O'Brien, 1995; Committee on Evaluation and Management of Heart Failure, 1995).

Tachyarrhythmias (abnormally fast heart rates) or **bradyarrhythmias** (abnormally slow heart rates) can also be responsible for CHF. Acute onset, very fast heart rates that are abnormal (supraventricular tachycardia, junctional ectopic tachycardia) will produce heart failure if not identified in a timely manner. Chronic incessant tachyarrhythmias (atrial flutter, atrial ectopic tachycardia) can produce CHF if the arrhythmia is present for greater than 10% of the day. Very slow heart rates (complete heart block) can also be an etiology for heart failure. CHF secondary to arrhythmias will resolve once the rhythm returns to normal.

Pathophysiology

The previously discussed etiologies are responsible for the hemodynamic changes and symptoms of CHF (Stewart, et al., 1995; Ueda, et al., 1996). Figure 25-11 illustrates the physiological mechanisms of CHF. Inadequate emptying of the heart caused by volume overload or poor contractility results in cardiac failure. This will generate an increase in venous volume with a subsequent increase in venous congestion. Systemic venous congestion results in liver engorgement and hepatomegaly. Pulmonary venous congestion results in pulmonary edema. Large left to right shunts result

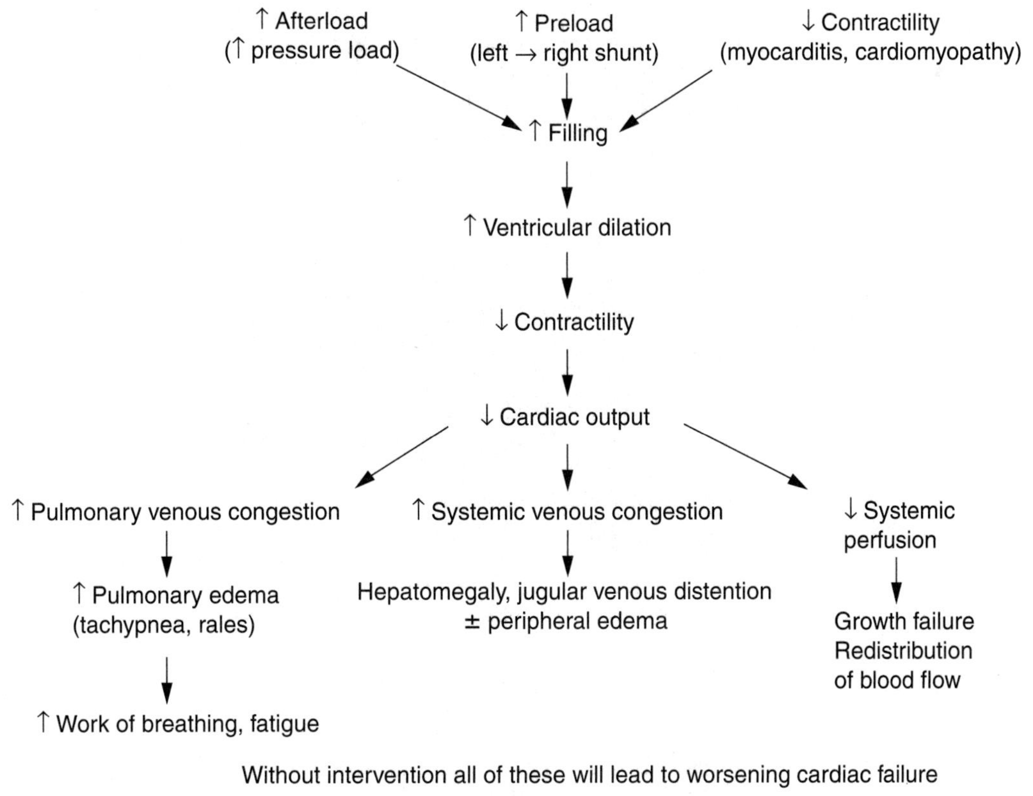

Figure 25-11 Physiological Mechanisms of Congestive Heart Failure

in an increased amount of blood circulating through the lungs, also contributing to pulmonary congestion.

Reduced ejection of the blood from obstruction or diminished contractility results in a pressure load. As the pressure in the heart increases from inadequate emptying of the heart, pulmonary and venous congestion results. The normal physiological responses to low cardiac output are increased: sympathetic activity and activation of the renin-angiotensin-aldosterone system. These compensatory responses can provide cardiovascular support for a limited period of time, but can be detrimental to the failing heart.

Epinephrine increases heart rate and cardiac output. Norepinephrine release results in vasoconstriction and elevation of BP. Both of these processes result in increased cardiac work. This is initially helpful; however, the increase in heart rate and cardiac work will eventually contribute to worsening failure.

Activation of the renin-angiotensin-aldosterone system is in response to low renal perfusion. This mechanism produces an increase in aldosterone and angiotension release. Aldosterone is responsible for reabsorption of sodium and water, which causes an increase in blood volume. Initially, this is successful in improving cardiac output, but over time it contributes to volume overload. As end diastolic volume increases so does myocardial stretch. Initially this increase in stretch improves contraction; however, as stretch progresses cardiac dilation occurs. Over time an abnormal pressure load causes the heart muscle to **hypertrophy** (become abnormally thick). A dilated or hypertrophied ventricle is a poor pump as these mechanisms interfere with normal myocardial fiber shortening.

Other mechanisms to maintain cardiovascular function include tachycardia and redistribution of blood flow. Since cardiac output is a function of heart rate times stroke volume, the body will normally increase heart rate to support cardiac output. Perfusion to major organs (heart and brain) is initially preserved. Vasoconstriction of the vessels in the skin and gut will redirect blood flow to other areas of the body. If perfusion is significantly compromised, metabolic acidosis will result from inadequate delivery of oxygen to the cells.

Critical Thinking

Relationship of Metabolic Acidosis to Pathophysiology in CHF

What is metabolic acidosis and why does it occur?
Why does metabolic acidosis occur with CHF?
What laboratory blood test is used to evaluate acid/base balance?

Clinical Manifestations

Clinical manifestations occur when mechanisms of compensatory response are exceeded and cardiac output begins to fall and can vary depending on the underlying etiology and age of the child. Box 25-3 lists clinical manifestations of CHF according to age.

Tachypnea is commonly seen in children with CHF. The respiratory rate can be ≥60 in infants and toddlers, and ≥40 in children over two years. There may be retractions, nasal flaring or rapid shallow respirations and restlessness in neonates and infants. Older children may demonstrate dyspnea with exertion and/or orthopnea. Rales and rhonchi can also be present. These symptoms commonly indicate that there is pulmonary congestion. As pulmonary congestion progresses there is a subsequent leaking of fluid into the alveoli and interstitium of the lung leading to pulmonary edema. Oxygen saturation may fall if the increase in lung fluid interferes with the diffusion of oxygen into the blood (Kohr & O'Brien, 1995; Talner, 1995).

Systemic venous congestion indicates right ventricular failure. Signs of this include hepatomegaly, jugular venous distention, and peripheral edema. Hepatomegaly is observed in children more frequently than jugular venous distention. Liver congestion reflects an increase in central venous pressure and blood volume. Jugular venous distention cannot be observed in infants because of their short necks. In the older child distention of the neck veins is evaluated when the child is sitting. Peripheral edema is a rare finding in infants, but when present, it is usually localized to the periorbital area. Rarely the older child will exhibit

BOX 25-3 Clinical manifestations of CHF

Newborns/Infants

tachycardia	tachypnea
gallop rhythm	retractions
diminished pulses	wheezing
diaphoresis	rales/rhonchi
cool, mottled extremities	hepatomegaly
pallor	low urine output
edema	
failure to thrive/poor weight gain	
restlessness	

Children/Adolescents

jugular venous distention	tachycardia
wheezing	gallop rhythm
rales/rhonchi	diminished pulses
dyspnea	pallor
orthopnea	edema
hepatomegaly	low urine output
ascites	exercise intolerance
poor weight gain	

edema of the hands and feet. Ascites indicates severely compromised cardiac function.

The cardiac symptoms of CHF include tachycardia, gallop rhythms, diaphoresis, and decreased peripheral pulses. A gallop rhythm (S_3) or extra heart beat is often heard in severe CHF. Excessive diaphoresis is caused by sympathetic stimulation. Diaphoresis is frequently noted during feeding in infants with heart failure. Cool, mottled extremities and weak, thready pulses indicate poor perfusion. The blood pressure is usually maintained; therefore, hypotension is a late and ominous sign.

Growth failure and poor weight gain is very common in infants and children with CHF. Respiratory difficulties make nursing or nippling exhausting for infants. They will demonstrate dyspnea and fatigue with feedings. Older children have exercise intolerance and excessive fatigue.

Diagnosis

A number of noninvasive tests provide supportive data for the diagnosis of CHF. Chest X ray can demonstrate cardiac enlargement, although in some instances heart size can be normal. CXR can also be used to determine if there is pulmonary overcirculation or edema. The best diagnostic tool is echocardiography, which can be used to determine if congenital defects or cardiomyopathy are present. It can also assess for heart size, hypertrophy, and dilation.

Treatment

Therapies are directed at reducing volume overload, improving contractility, reducing afterload, and decreasing cardiac work. In infants who have heart failure secondary to congenital defects, surgical correction is the primary treatment (Committee on Evaluation and Management of Heart Failure, 1995).

Diuretic therapy is the primary intervention used for volume overload. Furosemide (Lasix) is the primary diuretic used in children. These agents can decrease pulmonary and venous congestion, improving symptoms. Fluid restriction should be avoided in the infant as their primary source of calories is in formula or breast milk. Medications directed at improving contractility are referred to as positive **inotropes.** There are three classes of agents primarily used: cardiac glycosides, sympathomimetics, and phosphodiesterase inhibitors. These agents work through a number of different mechanisms of action (Table 25-3).

Digoxin is a cardiac glycoside and is currently the first line inotrope used in the infant or child. Benefits of digoxin are improved ventricular contraction, a reduction in heart rate, and a reduction of cardiac work. Dosing depends on body size and age of the child (Table 25-4). Children receiving digoxin should have their heart rate and rhythm monitored with periodic EKGs because it can cause heart block and bradycardia. Other side effects include nausea and vomiting. If any of these are noted a digoxin level should be obtained 8–12 hours after the last dose. Therapeutic levels are 0.8–2 ng/ml. It should be noted that serum digoxin levels in infants do not correlate well with clinical effect, but they are still helpful in assessing for toxicity. Digoxin should be withheld if levels are elevated above the therapeutic range or if the heart rate is lower than normal for age. Digoxin is frequently used in combination with diuretics. Because of the development of hypokalemia that is associated with diuretics, periodic serum potassium levels should be evaluated.

Nursing Alert:

Serum Potassium Levels and Digoxin Administration

Prior to the initiation of digoxin, serum potassium must be checked and levels should be normal. Hypokalemia in combination with digoxin can result in ventricular arrhythmias and can enhance digoxin toxicity. Signs and symptoms of toxicity include nausea, vomiting, bradycardia, heart block, and premature ventricular contractions. Use with caution in renal failure.

Sympathomimetics and phosphodiesterase inhibitors are generally used for acute heart failure in those children who do not respond to other medications. These agents are given intravenously by continuous infusion. Dopamine, dobutamine, and epinephrine are sympathomimetics that work via their stimulation of the sympathetic nervous system. They increase blood pressure, heart rate, and cardiac output. Amrinone (Inocor) and milrinone (Primacor) are phosphodiesterase inhibitors that improve cardiac contraction and promotion of vascular dilation. These drugs increase cardiac output without an increase in heart rate. They can also decrease cardiac work through afterload reduction.

Vasodilators augment cardiac output through a reduction in vascular resistance. If resistance is decreased then cardiac output can increase. There are a number of oral and intravenous agents. Oral agents are used in those children with mild to moderate heart failure. Intravenous agents are used in the acutely ill child in severe failure.

Angiotensin-converting enzyme (ACE) inhibitors are the primary medications used for afterload reduction. These medications inhibit the conversion of angiotensin I to angiotensin II, thus augmenting vasodilation. The end result is vasodilation with a fall in vascular resistance. The most commonly used ACE inhibitors are captopril (Capoten) and enalopril (Vasotec). Intravenous afterload reducing agents are the nitrates and phosphodiesterase inhibitors. The nitrates consist of sodium nitroprusside and nitroglycerine. These two medications produce vasodilation and a decrease in afterload.

Nutritional support is critically important in the infant or child in CHF. Because of increased work of breathing,

TABLE 25-3 Commonly Used Medications for the Treatment of CHF

Medication	Dosage	Actions	Side Effects	Nursing Considerations
INOTROPES				
Cardiac Glycosides				
Digoxin	see Table 25-4	↑ Ventricular contraction ↓ HR, ↓ cardiac work	Bradycardia, heart block Nausea, vomiting	Monitor potassium levels, should be normal before giving digoxin. Hold digoxin if PR interval greater than 0.2 on EKG or if HR is less than normal for age. Check HR prior to administration.
Sympathomimetics				
*Dopamine	1–20 μg/kg/min	↑ CO ↑ Renal blood flow ↑ BP ± ↑ HR ± ↑ SVR (high dose)	Tachycardia, arrhythmias Tissue necrosis if IV infiltrates Hypertension	Monitor HR and BP for arrhythmias or hypertension; decrease infusion for either. If infiltration occurs administer subcutaneous phenolamine.
*Dobutamine	2–20 μg/kg/min	↑ CO ↑ BP ± ↓ SVR	Arrhythmias Tachycardia	Monitor HR and BP for arrhythmias or hypertension. Decrease infusion for either. Do not mix with sodium bicarbonate.
*Epinephrine	0.05–0.3 μg/kg/min	↑ CO ↑ BP ↓ Renal blood flow ↑ SVR (high dose)	Tachycardia Hypertension ↓ Urine output Vasoconstriction	Monitor HR and BP for hypertension of arrhythmias; decrease infusion for either. Do not mix with sodium bicarbonate.
Phosphodiesterase inhibitors				
*Milrinone	50 μg/kg/load then 0.5–0.75 μg/kg/min	↑ CO ↓ Afterload ↓ Cardiac work ↓ Filling pressures	Hypotension Arrhythmias Thrombocytopenia Hepatic/GI dysfunction	If hypotension occurs administer volume, monitor for arrhythmias. Thrombocytopenia resolves when infusion is discontinued. Monitor liver function tests, discontinue infusion if values are elevated.
*Amrinone	0.75–5 mg/kg load then 5–10 μg/kg/min	Same as milrinone	Same as milrinone except greater risk of thrombocytopenia	Same as milrinone
DIURETICS				
Furosemide (Lasix)	1–2 mg/kg q 6–8 hours Oral or IV	Loop diuretic Renal loss of H_2O, sodium, and potassium	Hypovolemia Hypokalemia Hyponatremia Metabolic alkalosis	Monitor I&O and electrolytes; may require electrolyte replacement if values are low. Excessive diuresis can produce hypotension—monitor BP if urine output excessive.

continues

TABLE 25-3 *Continued*

Medication	Dosage	Actions	Side Effects	Nursing Considerations
Bumetanide (Bumex)	Oral 0.015–0.1 mg/kg/dose QD	Loop diuretic Same as furosemide	Same as furosemide	Same as furosemide
Spironolactone (Aldactone)	1–3 mg/kg/day Oral divided BID	Potassium sparing diuretic	Hypovolemia Hyperkalemia Contraindicated in renal failure	Same as furosemide; however, aldactone can cause hyperkalemia; if this occurs, discontinue.
VASODILATORS				
ACE Inhibitors				
Captopril (Capoten)	Start with 0.05–0.5 mg/kg/dose TID. Titrate up to max 6 mg/kg/day in 1–4 divided doses, oral	↓ SVR & PVR ↑ Sodium excretion	Hypotension Rash, GI upset	Monitor BP during initiation of drug—if hypotension occurs, hold next dose. Avoid concurrent administration of potassium.
Enalopril (Vasotec)	Start with 0.1 mg/kg/day BID. Titrate up to max 0.5 mg/kg/day, oral	Similar to captopril	Similar to captopril	Same as captopril
Nitrates				
*Nitroprusside (Nitropress)	0.5–10 μg/kg/min	Direct arterial and venous dilation ↓ SVR ↓ Afterload ↑ CO	Hypotension Thrombocytopenia Nitroprusside is metabolized to thiocyanate and cyanide—monitor for cyanide toxicity (i.e., metabolic acidosis) Tachypnea Tachycardia	Monitor BP continuously, stop infusion for significant hypotension (may need to administer fluids). If using high dose or long-term therapy, monitor cyanide and thiocynate levels; discontinue if elevated. Monitor serum pH; if metabolic acidosis occurs, discontinue drug.
*Nitroglycerine	0.25–3 μg/kg/min	Direct arterial dilation ↓ SVR ↓ Afterload ↑ CO	Hypotension Headache	Monitor BP continuously; decrease or discontinue for hypotension (may need to administer fluids).

** These medications are given via continuous infusion in the PICU. Dose is titrated to therapeutic effect.*

Key: CO cardiac output, SVR systemic vascular resistance, PVR pulmonary vascular resistance, GI gastrointestinal, BP blood pressure, QD daily, BID twice daily, TID three times daily, μg microgram, mg milligram, kg kilogram, min minute

Data from Taketomo, C. K., Hodding, J. H., & Kraus, D. M. (2001). Pediatric dosage handbook. *Hudson, OH: Lexi Company, Inc.*

TABLE 25-4 Digoxin Therapy in Infants and Children

Age	Digitalization Dose*	Maintenance Dose
Neonate	0.03–0.4 mg/kg IV or PO	0.01 mg/kg/day divided BID
1 mo–2 yrs	0.03–0.05 mg/kg IV or PO	0.01 mg/kg/day divided BID
2 yrs–10 yrs	0.02–0.04 mg/kg IV or PO	0.005–0.01 mg/kg/day QD or BID
>10 yrs	0.010–0.015 mg/kg IV or PO	0.005 mg/kg/day
Adolescents/Adults	0.75–1.5 mg	0.125–0.250 mg/dose QD or BID

This is total digitalization dose. Total dose is divided into three divided doses. 50% of total dose is given initially, then 8 hours later 25% of dose is given and 8 hours later final 25% of dose is given. It should be noted that not all patients are given digitalization dose, particularly when digoxin is started as an outpatient therapy.

Data from Taketomo, C. K., Hodding, J. H., & Kraus, D. M. (2001). Pediatric dosage handbook. *Hudson, OH: Lexi Company, Inc.*

tachypnea, and fatigue these fragile children may not be able to consume enough calories to meet their increased metabolic needs. Caloric density in formula can be increased by adding less water to the concentrate or powder, therefore increasing the calories per ounce. Breast milk fortifier or powdered formula can be added to expressed breast milk to increase caloric density. Increasing caloric density should be accomplished slowly over a number of days, as a sudden increase will increase the osmotic load in the gut, producing diarrhea. A maximum of 30 calories/ounce is sufficient for most infants (Norris & Hill, 1994). If the infant is a slow feeder, or is incapable of consuming an appropriate amount of formula to promote growth, then gavage feedings are implemented. A nasogastric (NG) or nasojejunal (NJ) tube can be placed to provide feedings, either bolus or continuous. It should be noted that bolus feedings should never be given in an NJ tube since the jejunum does not have the capacity to hold large volumes (as does the stomach). Continuous feedings can be given all day or only at night. Volume and calories consumed over a 24-hour period should be sufficient to promote normal growth and development (Table 25-5).

Older children are offered high calorie foods, milkshakes, or supplemental nutritional products. Fluid restriction is not necessary because of concomitant use of diuretics.

TABLE 25-5 Normal Caloric Requirements to Support Growth

Age	Calories/kg/24 hours
Neonates	100–150
1–2 years	90–100
2–6 years	80–90
7–9 years	70–80
>10 years	50–60
Adolescents/adults	50

Rarely NG or gastrostomy tube feedings are implemented in the older child. Tube feedings should be given at night to encourage normal eating habits during the day.

Many children with CHF will have low arterial oxygen saturations. The etiology for this may be congenital defects or pulmonary edema. Oxygen therapy is withheld until determination is made of the child's structural defect. Oxygen stimulates closure of the ductus arteriosus and also dilates the pulmonary vascular bed. In the presence of structural defects that depend on a patent ductus arteriosus to support life until surgical correction, oxygen therapy could be lethal. In some patients with large L→R shunts oxygen therapy can increase pulmonary blood flow, worsening congestive failure. Oxygen administration is carefully implemented only after a thorough evaluation of the patient's cardiac anatomy is completed (Committee on Evaluation and Management of Heart Failure, 1995).

Maneuvers to decrease cardiac work are used along with pharmacologic agents to help improve outcomes. Measures to limit energy expenditure are important nursing interventions. Bedrest is recommended in children in severe CHF. Client care should be clustered to allow for periods of quiet. Occasionally the extremely fussy infant or small child may benefit from small, carefully monitored doses of sedatives.

Children with severe CHF that is refractory to medical treatment and who do not have the option for surgical repair may be offered heart transplantation. In this setting heart transplantation offers the only hope of survival. Once the decision is made to transplant then a full evaluation is made by the transplant team. See the section on heart transplantation for more detail.

Nursing Management

Assessment

Negative sequela of decreased cardiac output are assessed. Physical examination includes the determination of heart rate, blood pressure, peripheral perfusion, urine output, and level of consciousness. If pharmacologic treatment has been implemented, response to therapy must be assessed. Respiratory function and oxygen saturation are evaluated and compared to the baseline assessment to monitor for trends or changes. Height, weight, and developmental milestones are determined to assess the impact CHF has had on growth and development. Nutritional assessment can be made in collaboration with a dietician.

Family supports, caregiver role, and interaction with the child are assessed. Coping skills must be determined, particularly in the family with a child who has been newly diagnosed with heart failure. Response to family teaching is evaluated to determine deficient knowledge. Reinforcement of teaching is frequently required, particularly during periods of stress.

Nursing Diagnosis

1. Decreased cardiac output related to ↓ contractility, ↑ preload, ↑ afterload as evidenced by edema, shortness of breath, ↓ urine output, hepatomegaly.
2. Excess fluid volume related to increased preload and decreased contractility secondary to CHF as evidenced by peripheral edema, hepatomegaly, and pulmonary edema.
3. Imbalanced nutrition: Less than body requirements related to poor caloric intake and increased metabolic demands as evidenced by poor weight gain, weight loss, and poor caloric intake.

Outcome Identification

- The child will have optimal cardiac output as evidenced by comfortable work of breathing, absence of edema, normal blood pressure, and normal urine output.
- The child will be alert and interactive indicating normal cerebral perfusion.
- The child will not exhibit signs/symptoms of venous congestion such as hepatomegaly or edema.
- The child will exhibit normal electrolyte levels.
- The child will ingest the appropriate number of calories for his age (see Table 25-5).
- The child will exhibit normal growth.

Planning/Implementation

Nurses should monitor vital signs, tissue perfusion, and evaluate and monitor trends and changes. Monitor heart rate and rhythm, document EKG, and treat rhythm abnormalities as indicated as many arrhythmias will adversely affect cardiac output. Administer medications as appropriate and monitor for clinical efficacy and side effects (see Table 25-3). If vasodilators are initiated or dose is adjusted, monitor blood pressure thirty minutes to one hour after dose as hypotension may occur.

Nurses should assess fluid status: mucous membranes are moist, pulses are strong, anterior fontanel is not sunken, and hepatomegaly is absent or does not worsen. Daily weight and I & O are assessed. Specific gravity is checked on urine daily. Excessive weight gain or new onset edema can mean fluid retention. Urine output is at least 1 cc/kg/hour, indicating normal renal perfusion and volume status. Diuretics are administered as ordered and electrolytes monitored if diuretic dose is increased. Potassium replacement is indicated if diuretic induced hypokalemia is present.

Nurses should document height and weight on growth chart and evaluate for changes (particularly weight loss). Weigh daily to weekly depending on acuity of child. Calorie counts help to determine if adequate calories are being consumed. Consultation with a dietician can assist in providing appropriate diet and calories. Gavage feedings are administered if necessary, and caloric density of formula is increased to maximize caloric intake if necessary.

Evaluation

Vital signs are within normal limits for age without evidence of hepatomegaly or jugular venous distention. The CXR is clear without evidence of cardiomegaly or pulmonary venous congestion. No arrhythmias are evident. Peripheral perfusion in normal; urine output is normal at 1 cc/kg/hour. The blood pressure is normal without evidence of hypotension. The medications are well tolerated without side effects. Intake and output is equal. Urine output and specific gravity are normal. Serum electrolytes are maintained within normal limits. Normal caloric intake and weight gain are supported, and feedings are tolerated without diarrhea or emesis. The family understands the rationale for dietary plan and is comfortable with NG/NJ feedings.

Family Teaching

The family is taught the signs and symptoms of worsening heart failure so that notification of the cardiologist can be made in a timely manner. They are taught how to administer all medications. The nurse must also review all medication side effects with the caregivers. Reinforcement of teaching will most likely be required, particularly upon discharge from the hospital. Questions are encouraged to clarify misconceptions.

Prior to discharge from the hospital all family members involved in the care of the child should learn CPR. Many hospitals have programs designed specifically for caregivers that are simple and straightforward. Emergency phone numbers should be provided as well. Clinic appointments are made prior to discharge from the hospital.

For many children the definitive treatment for CHF will be surgery, so outcome is somewhat less uncertain. However

CHF can also mean end stage disease and an uncertain future. Support systems must be in place in the scenario of end stage disease. If the future holds possible heart transplant, then early contact with the transplant team is critical.

Family teaching should include:

- Allow frequent short periods of time for feedings.
- Pay attention to infant cues—back arching, averting of eyes mean child wants to disengage and take a break. If disengagement cues are demonstrated allow infant to take a break.
- For tube feedings allow infant to nipple as much as possible then gavage the rest. If the infant is tube fed at night, do not awaken to try to nipple feed.
- Concentrate formula as prescribed. Teach family how to do this and have them give a return demonstration.
- If feeding the infant becomes a full-time job, get family or friends to help.
- Use home nursing to help with feeding tube placement and problem-solve tube feeding issues.
- Call health care provider if questions arise. Have family develop rapport with one health care provider who is familiar with them and their infant.

REFLECTIONS FROM FAMILIES

We waited three years to have our first baby. When she was born I thought she was the most beautiful thing I had ever seen. Then I noticed a large birth mark on her hand and thought that was no big deal and could be removed. My little girl was still perfect as far as I was concerned. Upon further examination the doctors told me she had what they called an imperforate anus and would need major surgery to correct it. I couldn't believe this was happening but I was encouraged because the doctors told me she would have a normal life after a couple of surgeries. My wife and I agreed that we could handle this. While she was being prepared for surgery they told us she had a heart murmur and needed more tests. What we heard next was very hard to handle. Our baby had two holes in the wall between the chambers of her heart and a serious narrowing of her aorta, the biggest artery in the body. She would need open heart surgery as a tiny baby and there was a chance she wouldn't live at all. Imagine how I felt being worried about her silly birthmark. I was sad, angry, worried, and hopeful that things would be okay all at the same time. As a religious man I questioned why this was happening to our precious little girl.

Our special girl has survived her open heart surgery and is doing okay. Our next step will be to have her imperforate anus surgery. My wife and I are grateful that she is doing as well as she is and have learned to love her even more and appreciate our time with her. We know the trips to the hospital are not over with but we've learned to accept life's troubles with a new attitude.

CONGENITAL HEART DEFECTS

Congenital heart defects (CHD) occur in approximately 8 in 1,000 live births (American Heart Association, 1999). There are a minimum of 35 types of recognized defects ranging from mild, easily corrected defects such as a patent ductus arteriosus to more serious and complex anomalies such as hypoplastic left heart syndrome. In the following section several of the more common congenital heart defects will be discussed.

It should be pointed out that although these defects will be presented separately, it is not uncommon for the infant to present with a combination of defects. The following section will be divided into defects that result in *increased pulmonary flow*, *decreased pulmonary blood flow*, and those with *left sided obstruction*. In the modern era the vast majority of complex defects are repaired or palliated in the first year of life (Reddy, et al., 1999; LeBlanc & Russell, 1998). Many complex defects require staged repairs, that is, more than one surgery is ultimately required for final correction. Even in this scenario completion of staged repairs occurs by age two to four. Repair of defects that impose little or no hemodynamic alteration may be deferred until age two or three. Mild isolated defects may never require surgery.

Nursing Tip:

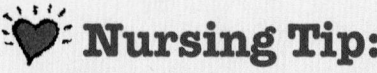

Blood flow, pressure, and resistance

Remembering that blood will always flow from an area of high pressure to an area of lower pressure and will take the path of least resistance will help the reader understand the hemodynamic effect of all congenital heart defects.

Because the heart is the size of the child's fist, intracardiac or open heart surgery can be complex. To support the child during this type of surgery, cardiopulmonary bypass (CPB) is implemented. It must be clarified that CPB is not a *treatment* but a form of life support used during open heart surgery only. Although technological advances have improved CPB, there remain a number of sequelae that have an impact on the child's condition following surgery.

CPB, which is used for the repair of many congenital defects, is a mechanical pump and artificial oxygenator that provides, for a short period, substitution for the heart and lungs. The general principles of CPB include the removal of unoxygenated blood via a venous cannula and the delivery of oxygenated blood back to the patient via an aortic cannula. The work of the heart and lungs is therefore performed by the bypass pump allowing the surgeon to work on the heart in a bloodless field.

Eye On:

Interventional Procedures for Congenital Heart Disease

A number of technological innovations are in use or evolving that will allow those with congenital heart disease to avoid surgery. Treatment options include interventional procedures performed in the cardiac catheterization laboratory. These include, but are not limited to, balloon valvuloplasty, stent placement, placement of coils, and occluding devices.

Balloon valvuloplasty can be used for balloon dilation of stenotic pulmonary, aortic, and mitral valves. A catheter with a balloon tip is passed percutaneously into the femoral artery or vein and then advanced to cross the appropriate valve. The balloon is then expanded to dilate the valve subsequently relieving the stenosis. As technology and skill improve, clinical indications are continuing to expand. Balloon dilation of recurrent coarctation of the aorta can also be used in lieu of surgical correction.

Stents can be placed in narrowed vessels such as the aorta or pulmonary arteries. Again a special catheter (with the stent loaded on the tip of the catheter) is placed percutaneously in the femoral vein or artery. Once the catheter tip is in the area of narrowing the stent is deployed, resulting in widening of the narrowed area. This procedure often obviates the need for surgery to correct either peripheral pulmonary stenosis or recurrent coarctation of the aorta.

Coils can be placed in abnormal vessels or a patent ductus arteriosus to occlude the vessel without surgery. Occluding devices are currently under investigation for non-surgical treatment of some atrial septal defects and ventricular septal defects. These occluding devices are small, round mesh containing devices that are loaded into the tip of a special catheter. Once the catheter is placed across the septal defect the device is deployed and attaches to the rim of tissue around the defect thereby effectively closing the hole. With both coil and occluding devices native tissue will eventually cover the device.

Interventional cardiac catheterization represents a rapidly growing frontier in health care. As skill and knowledge increase clinical indications will continue to expand (Mandell, 1999).

Defects with Increased Pulmonary Blood Flow

Defects that increase pulmonary blood flow are caused by a shunting of the blood from the left side of the heart to the right side through an abnormal connection (left to right shunt). The blood flows from the left to the right side because the pressures are greater on the left side of the heart. The increased amount of blood in the right side leads to increased pulmonary blood flow. Infants with these defects exhibit the clinical manifestations of CHF. Atrial septal defects, ventricular septal defects, patent ductus arteriosus, atrioventricular septal defects, and truncus arteriosus are all in this category.

Atrial Septal Defect

An atrial septal defect (ASD) is an abnormal connection between the right and left atria and is illustrated in Figure 25-12.

Incidence

ASDs account for approximately 7% of all congenital heart disease (Higgins & Reid, 1994).

Pathophysiology

Because of the normal increased pressure on the left side of the heart, blood flows from the left to the right across the ASD. This leads to increased volume on the right side of the heart, with a subsequent increase in right atrial and ventricular size, as well as an increase in pulmonary artery (PA) size.

Clinical Manifestations

The infant or child with an ASD is generally asymptomatic. There is often a soft systolic murmur and more classically a widely split S_2, unaffected by respiratory pattern.

Diagnosis

Diagnosis is often made after a murmur is detected during a routine health care examination. Chest X ray will usually demonstrate increased heart size. An echocardiogram demonstrates the location and size of the defect. Cardiac cath is not routinely indicated for diagnosis of an isolated ASD.

Treatment

Preoperative intervention is only indicated in the infant or child with a large ASD that results in CHF. Diuretics are

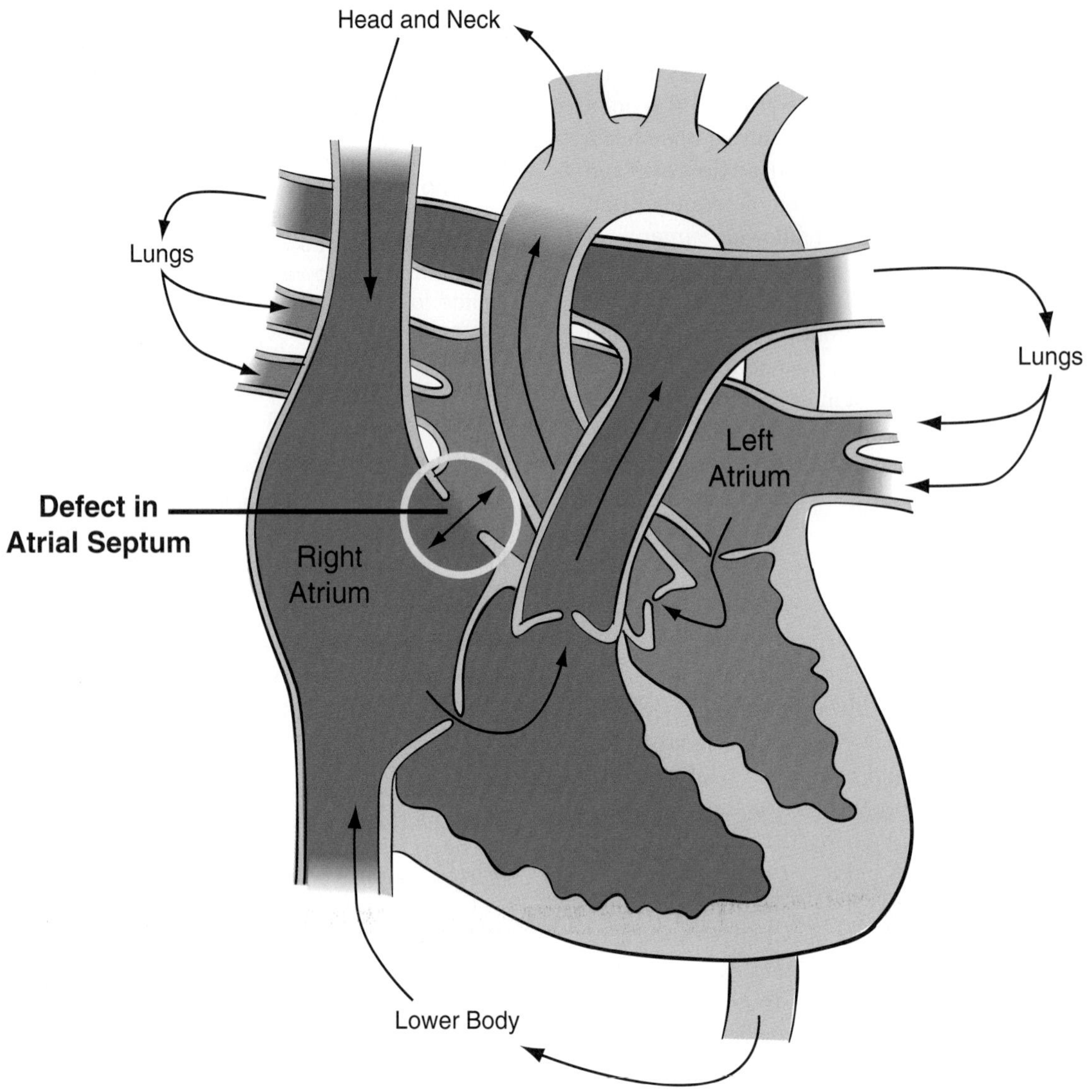

Figure 25-12 Atrial Septal Defect

given to control the symptoms of CHF until repair is performed. Surgical repair is generally performed in the preschool age period because there is a possibility of spontaneous closure in the first two years of life, and the child is usually asymptomatic. Traditionally, surgery has been performed via a median sternotomy (vertical incision along the sternum). The defect is repaired via stitch closure or patch closure through an incision made in the right atrium (Vick, 1998).

Because of what many have termed unsightly sternal incisions, several attempts have been made in recent years to close the ASD via alternative routes. A thoracotomy approach has been utilized in which the surgeon makes an incision below and to the right of the right breast (Massetti, et al., 1996) (Figure 25-13). Another surgical approach is submammary. This incision is made horizontally under the breasts and the skin is pulled upward. The sternum is then opened in

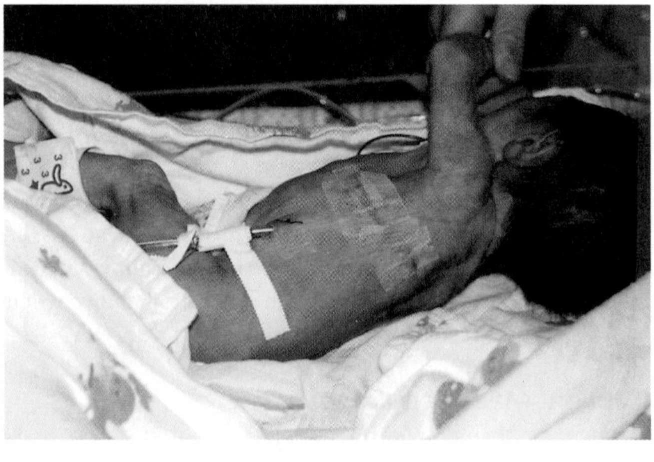

Figure 25-13 Thoracotomy Incision with a Chest Tube in an Infant After Repair of ASD

the traditional fashion and the repair is performed. The major difference is that the healing scar is below the breast line making this an attractive option for females.

Further attempts have also been made to close ASDs with an implantable umbrella via a nonsurgical approach in the cardiac catheterization laboratory. The umbrella is placed via a catheter in a large femoral vessel, threaded up into the heart and into the ASD thus occluding the opening. The major advantage of this method is simply the avoidance of open heart surgery. However, there have been some complications such as embolization (breaking off) of the device (requiring surgery to retrieve it) and residual L to R shunts (Magee & Qureshi, 1997). The future for these devices rests in their ability to effectively close the ASD with a lower complication rate than is presently seen with the surgical repair.

The main complications of an ASD repair are atrial arrhythmias or heart block secondary to edema around or surgical interruption of the conduction system. This is often temporary and normal conduction returns with time. For clients with a repaired ASD long-term survival is comparable to normal individuals when matched for age and sex. A small percentage can develop atrial arrhythmias following surgery so periodic follow-up is warranted (Vick, 1998). Natural history and resultant sequela of *unrepaired* ASD may not become apparent until the 3rd or 4th decade of life. The result of many years of increased pulmonary blood flow often leads to severe pulmonary hypertension.

Ventricular Septal Defect

A ventricular septal defect (VSD) is an abnormal connection between the right and left ventricles (Figure 25-14). The defect can be located in various positions along the septum.

Incidence

VSDs are the most common congenital heart defect accounting for approximately 20% overall (Graham & Gutgesell, 1995).

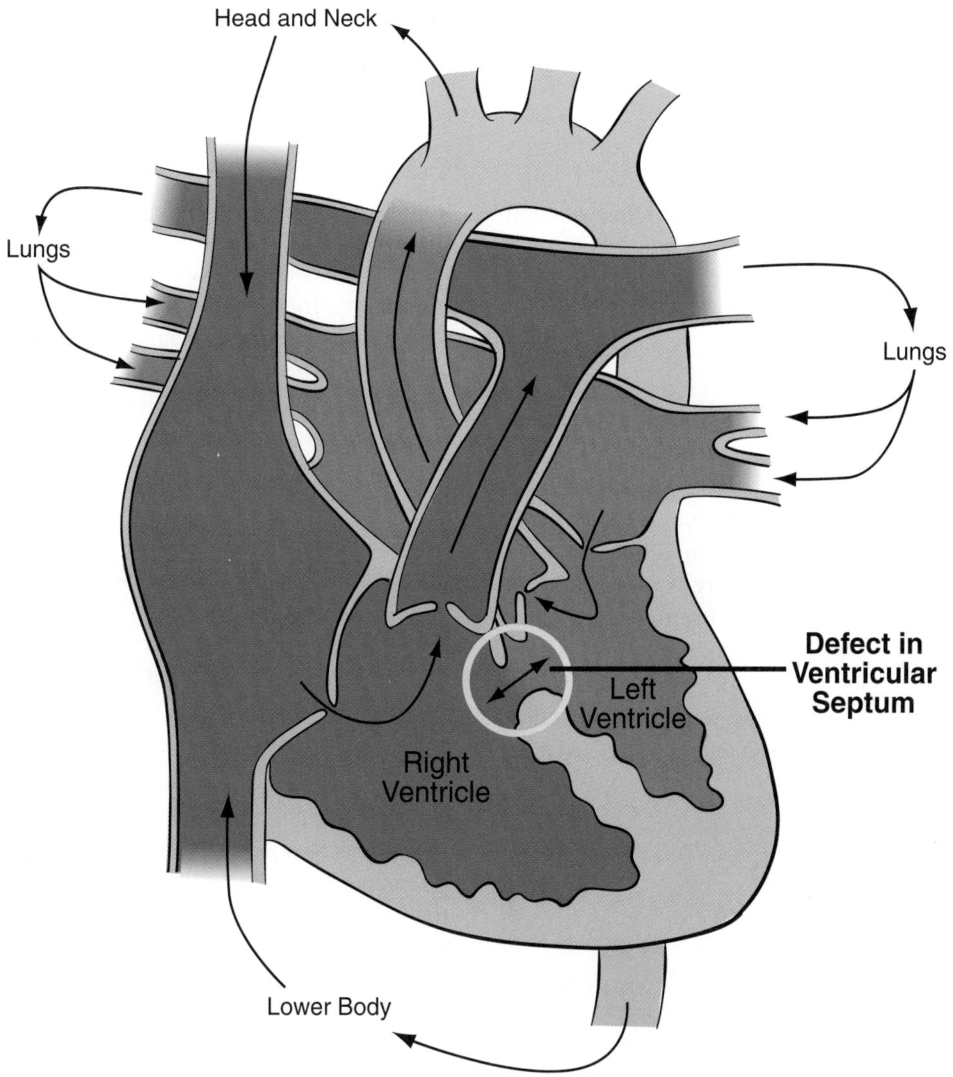

Figure 25-14 Ventricular Septal Defect

Pathophysiology

Because of normally increased pressures on the left side of the heart, blood flow through a VSD is *left to right*. The blood that flows through the VSD will recirculate through the pulmonary artery to the lungs. The increase in pulmonary blood flow leads to left heart enlargement and pulmonary venous congestion. The degree of left to right shunting depends on two major factors: *the size of the defect* and the child's *pulmonary resistance*.

Clinical Manifestations

The infant with a small VSD is likely to be asymptomatic while the infant with a moderate to large defect will demonstrate signs of CHF. The infant with a moderate to large VSD is usually tachypneic, diaphoretic, fatigues easily, and is underweight for age. Feeding history will usually reveal an infant that tires before a feeding is completed. VSDs are also seen in older children. If a VSD is detected in an older child for the first time, it is because the defect is small and the child has had no symptoms.

Diagnosis

Diagnosis of a VSD is often suspected when a loud holosystolic murmur is heard. The intensity of the murmur can reflect the size of the defect. The X ray of a child with a small VSD can be normal while the X ray of a child with a moderate to large defect will often show cardiomegaly with an increase in pulmonary blood flow. Echocardiogram is indicated to determine the size and location of the defect. Cardiac catheterization is rarely indicated.

Treatment

The infant with a small VSD usually requires no treatment because 75–80% of these defects may close in the first two years of life (Graham & Gutgesell, 1995). Many children with small hemodynamically insignificant VSDs never require surgery. These children are asymptomatic without cardiac enlargement. It is felt that the risks of surgery outweigh the benefits. Large defects are unlikely to close; therefore, the infant is treated medically for the first few months of life and watched closely for appropriate weight gain and for any signs of complicating respiratory infections (Graham & Gutgesell, 1995). Digoxin and diuretics are given to relieve symptoms of CHF. High calorie formula may be utilized to promote growth. Nasal gastric feedings are used in infants who are excessively tachypneic or who tire with feedings.

Surgical repair is indicated between 3 and 12 months of age. This is necessary to prevent the development of pulmonary vascular disease in children who have large L→R shunts (Graham & Gutgesell, 1995). Surgery is indicated earlier in the small infant who is failing to thrive. The defect is closed with a patch of the child's own pericardium or with synthetic material while on CPB. Postoperative complications include atrial arrhythmias, complete heart block, ventricular arrhythmias, and residual shunt or leaking at the sight of the VSD patch.

Children with small unrepaired VSDs exhibit life span and health similar to the unaffected population. For children with large VSDs repaired in the first two years of life, the long-term outlook for normal health is excellent. Surgical mortality is less than 5% when performed in the first year of life (LeBlanc & Russell, 1998). Those who have surgery after two years of age may have residual problems with arrhythmias and depressed myocardial function. When and if this will occur is difficult to predict.

> **Nursing Tip:**
>
> **Pulmonary vascular resistance (PVR)**
> Pulmonary vascular resistance falls in the first few weeks of life. This can dramatically change intracardiac blood flow patterns. Therefore, a newborn with a VSD may not demonstrate symptoms until after PVR falls.

Patent Ductus Arteriosus

The ductus arteriosus is a direct connection between the main pulmonary artery and the aorta (Figure 25-15). In the fetus the ductus arteriosus is necessary for survival. In the preterm infant it is a common finding simply based on developmental immaturity. In the term newborn the ductus begins to close within twelve hours and should be completely closed by 2–3 weeks. A ductus that remains open, in a full-term baby, after several weeks of life is termed a patent ductus arteriosus (PDA) (Brooke & Heymann, 1995).

Incidence

The incidence of PDA in a non-premature infant is approximately 5–10% of all CHD. The incidence in the premature infant is dramatically higher at 45% in infants who weigh less than 1,750 grams and up to 80% in infants weighing less than 1,000 grams (Brook & Heymann, 1995).

Pathophysiology

The hemodynamic effect of a PDA is similar to other defects with left to right shunts. Blood from the high pressure aorta flows directly into the low pressure pulmonary artery and pulmonary circulation. The degree of shunting depends on the size of the PDA as well as the pulmonary vascular resistance. This increase in pulmonary blood flow can contribute to CHF.

Clinical Manifestations

The degree of symptoms experienced by the infant will depend on the size of the shunt. The infant with a small

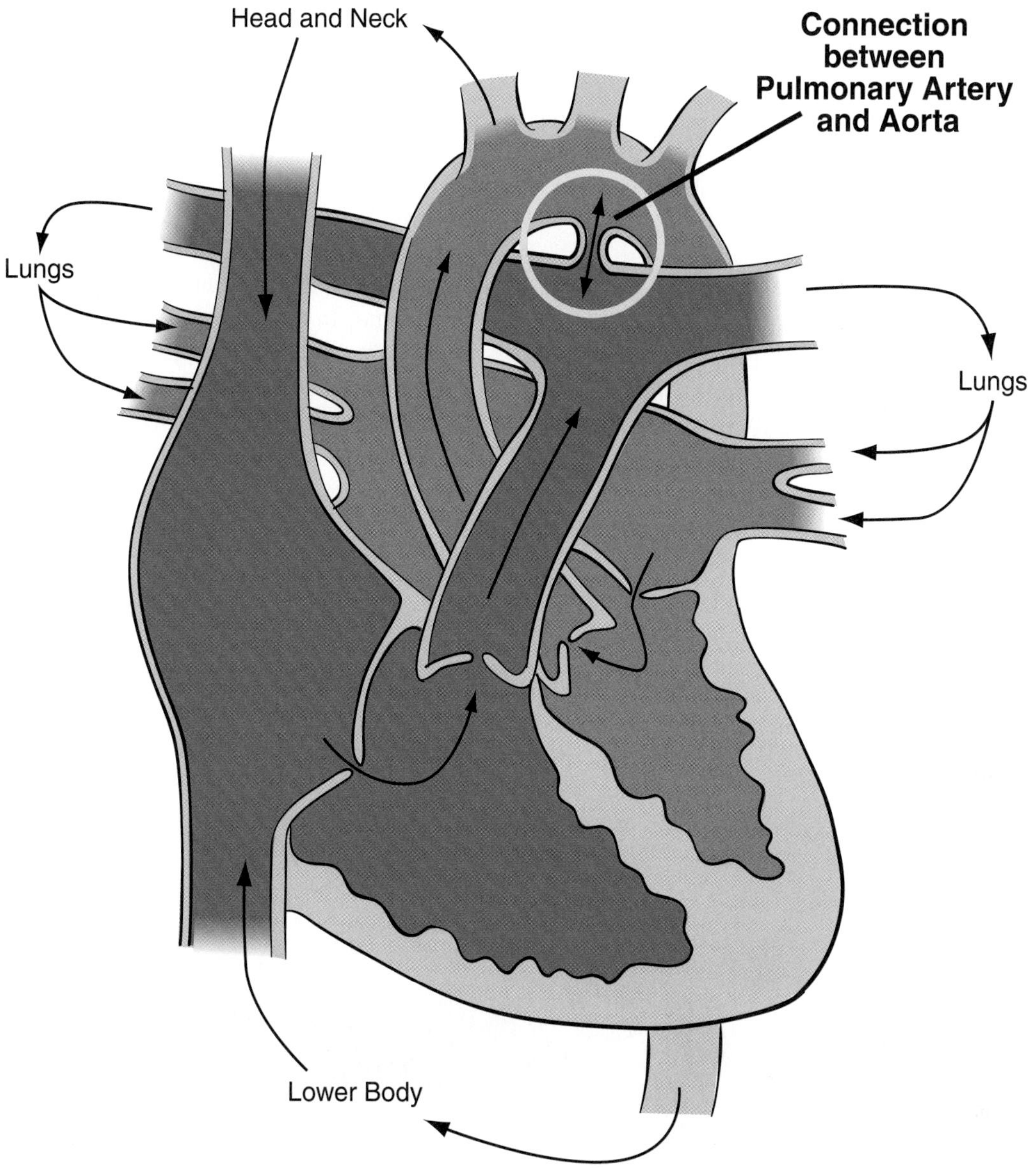

Figure 25-15 Patent Ductus Arteriosus

PDA will generally be asymptomatic. The infant with a large PDA will have signs of CHF.

Diagnosis

The murmur of a PDA is often continuous and is best heard just below the left clavicle. Chest X ray is usually normal and diagnosis is generally made with echocardiogram. Cardiac cath is not necessary for the diagnosis of a PDA.

Treatment

In the premature infant closure of the PDA is attempted by the infusion of indomethacin, which inhibits the synthesis of prostaglandin. Prostaglandins are a group of fatty acid substances present in many tissues and are responsible for a number of cellular interactions. They are responsible for maintaining patency of the ductus arteriosus. Closure is indicated in the full-term symptomatic (CHF) infant with a PDA. Indomethacin is not effective in full-term infants. Older asymptomatic children undergo elective closure before five years of age. Surgical ligation of the PDA is made via a left thoracotomy incision without the use of CPB. Technique for the nonsurgical treatment involves use of coils to occlude the PDA and is performed in the catheterization laboratory. Rare postoperative complications include injury to the recurrent laryngeal nerve causing hoarseness, or injury to the left phrenic nerve resulting in paralysis of the left hemidiaphragm.

Normal survival and quality of life are excellent for the infant and child with a repaired, isolated PDA. Because mortality approaches zero, it is therefore recommended that all PDAs without pulmonary vascular disease be closed (Chang & Wells, 1998). Individuals with large unrepaired PDAs become quite symptomatic in adulthood secondary to pulmonary complications and the development of pulmonary vascular disease (Higgins & Reid, 1994). The presence of severe pulmonary vascular disease precludes PDA closure.

Atrioventricular Septal Defect

Atrioventricular defect or atrioventricular canal (AVC) is associated with a septal defect in the atrium and ventricle, as well as involvement of the AV valves. In this defect, when the heart is developing the atrial and ventricular septums are not fully completed and never meet (Figure 25-16). This in turn causes the tricuspid and mitral valves to develop inappropriately. The severity of the defect depends on the amount of the septum that is involved as well as the degree of AV valve involvement.

Incidence

AVC accounts for about 3% of all congenital heart defects. It should also be noted that approximately 40% of children with Trisomy 21 (Down syndrome) have some form of congenital heart defect and that 40% of these are associated with some degree of AVC (Benson, Basson, & MacRae, 1996).

Pathophysiology

Because of the fact that there is free communication between all chambers of the heart, blood flow patterns are dependent on the resistance to the pulmonary and systemic circulations. In the infant whose PVR is decreasing with age, blood flow will be left to right causing increased blood flow to the lungs. Increased pulmonary blood flow will result in increased pulmonary venous return to the left side of the heart with left atrial and ventricular enlargement.

Clinical Manifestations

The infant with an AVC demonstrates signs and symptoms of CHF. The murmur can be quite variable, depending on the size of the septal defects. It is usually a long systolic or holosystolic murmur. Virtually all infants are symptomatic by their first birthday (Feldt, Porter, Edwards, Puga, & Seward, 1995).

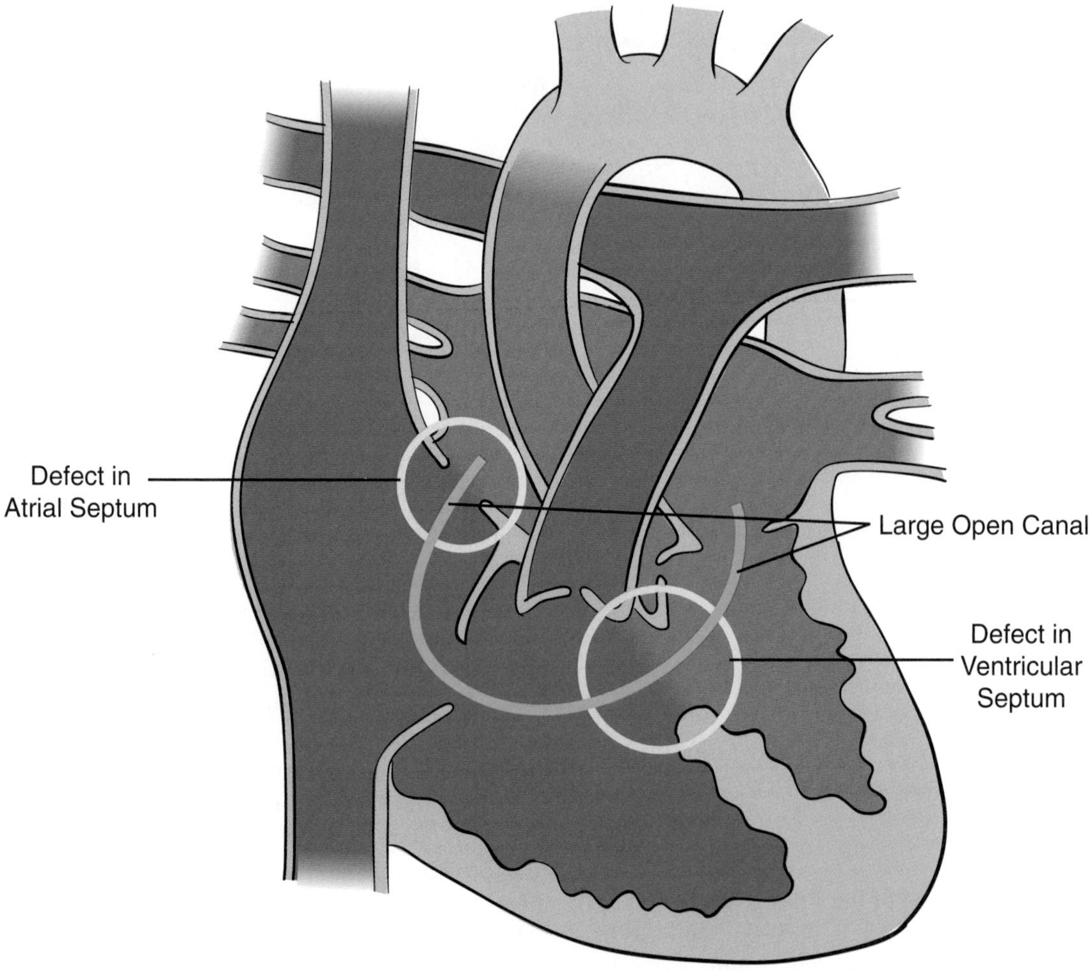

Figure 25-16 Atrioventricular Canal Defect

Diagnosis

On chest X ray the heart and main pulmonary artery are enlarged. Echocardiogram will demonstrate the degree of septal and valve involvement and is usually diagnostic. Cardiac catheterization is indicated when the diagnosis is uncertain or if hemodynamics need to be assessed (Feldt, et al., 1995).

Treatment

The infant with AVC is treated for CHF prior to surgical repair. Surgery is usually performed in the first year of life, but should always be completed by two years of age because of the potential for the development of irreversible pulmonary vascular disease. The goal of the repair is to close the atrial and septal defect and then construct new mitral and tricuspid valves from the common AV valve. This surgery is performed while the infant is on CPB. Potential postoperative complications include heart block, arrhythmias, bleeding from the multiple intracardiac suture lines, and pulmonary hypertension. Another potential postoperative problem includes poor cardiac output secondary to poorly functioning or incompetent AV valves. A postoperative echocardiogram will demonstrate the degree of incompetency of the valves and any residual ASD or VSD.

Surgical mortality rate for AVC repair is less than 10% (LeBlanc & Russell, 1998). Regurgitation through the affected AV valve (mitral or tricuspid) is not uncommon with AVC. Long-term outcomes are quite variable and are dependent upon the degree of AV valve incompetence. Natural history for the *unrepaired* AVC is quite poor with most infants dying by 15 years of age (Feldt, et al., 1995).

Truncus Arteriosus

The primary anatomical features of a truncus arteriosus result from failure of the embryologic trunk to divide into the pulmonary arteries and the aorta. Therefore, a single arterial trunk arises from the heart giving rise to the pulmonary arteries, the aorta, and the coronary arteries (Figure 25-17). There is also a single "truncal valve" in place of the aortic and pulmonary valves and a large VSD (Mair, Edwards, Julsrud, Seward, & Danielson, 1995). Following surgical repair this truncal valve serves as the aortic valve.

Incidence

The incidence of truncus arteriosus is approximately 1.4% of all CHD (Chang & Reddy, 1998). Truncus arteriosus can be associated with **DiGeorge syndrome,** which is a congenital

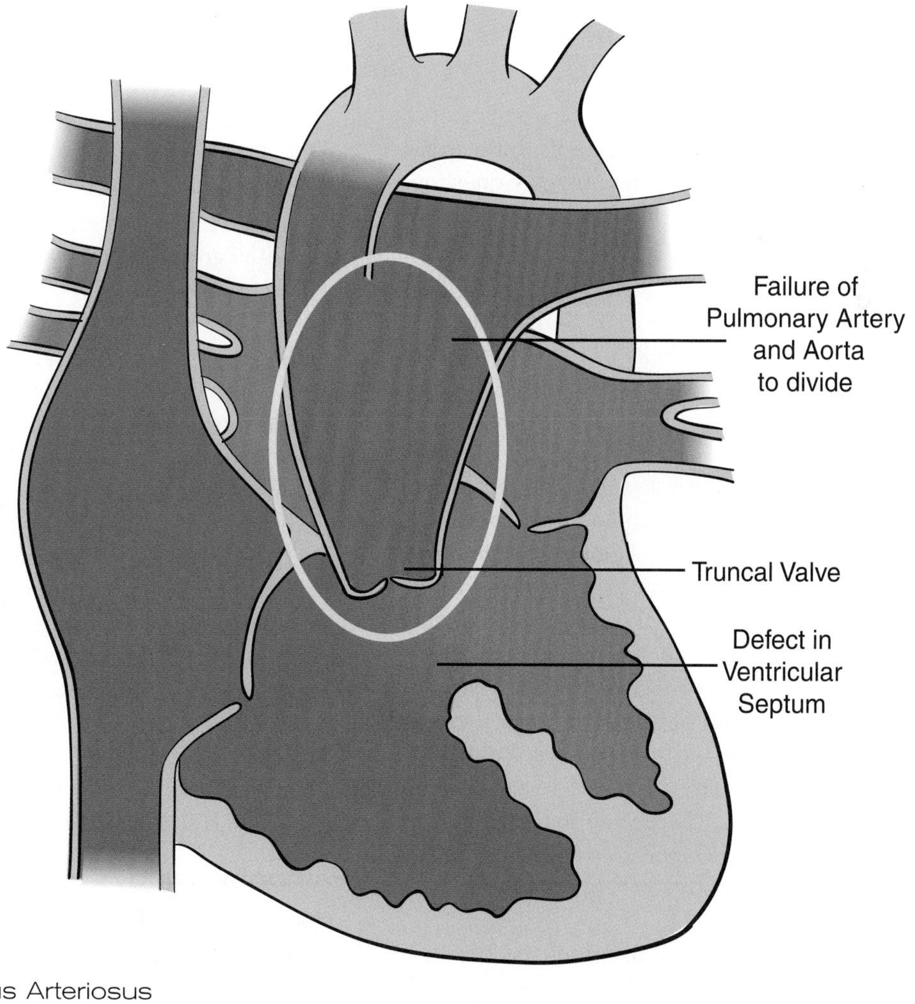

Figure 25-17 Truncus Arteriosus

syndrome associated with hypoplasia or aplasia of the thymus and parathyroid gland. Any child who is diagnosed with this lesion should have a genetic work up to evaluate for DiGeorge.

Pathophysiology

Both oxygenated and unoxygenated blood mix together and are ejected from the ventricles out the common trunk (common great vessel). Blood flow is then delivered to both the pulmonary circulation and the systemic circulation. The degree of flow to each circulation is based on vascular resistance. In the first few hours to days of life the PVR is still elevated. Thus, there will be little increase in pulmonary blood flow and unoxygenated blood is pumped through the systemic circulation making the infant mildly cyanotic. When PVR begins to fall, pulmonary flow increases making the shunt left to right. The infant will no longer be cyanotic but may develop CHF.

Clinical Manifestations

The newborn infant, as described above, may be mildly cyanotic despite supplemental oxygen. As PVR falls the newborn will develop signs and symptoms of CHF. Auscultation will reveal a loud continuous murmur along with a loud click associated with the closing of the truncal valve. Symptoms almost always develop in the first month of life.

Diagnosis

Chest X ray demonstrates moderate cardiomegaly. Echocardiogram is diagnostic for truncus arteriosus, but cardiac catheterization is still indicated to determine any questionable anatomic variations and hemodynamics.

Treatment

The infant is treated for symptoms of CHF. Surgical repair is performed within the first six weeks of life. There is an increased surgical mortality when repair is performed after six months of life (Mair, et al., 1995). The repair is performed as follows: The PAs are removed from the common trunk and the defect left in the trunk wall is sutured closed. The VSD is repaired and a valved homograft conduit is placed connecting the RV to the PAs. A **homograft conduit** is a chemically treated, human aorta or pulmonary artery, obtained from a cadaver that is placed like a tube to conduct blood from the right ventricle to the pulmonary artery. Postoperative circulation is as follows. Systemic venous return enters the RA to the RV and flows through the conduit to the pulmonary artery and to the lungs. Pulmonary venous return enters the LA to the LV and flows out through the truncal valve to the aorta. There is no longer mixing of oxygenated and unoxygenated blood so oxygen saturations should be normal. Postoperative complications include arrhythmias and low cardiac output.

Without treatment the natural history of this defect is poor. The mean age of death is 2.5 months, and 80% of children will die by their first birthday (Bengur, 1998). Those who survive infancy will often die in the first few years of life secondary to complications of pulmonary vascular disease and endocarditis (Mair, et al., 1995). In cases of surgical repair, the valved conduit will need to be replaced during the first five years of life as the child grows (Bengur, 1998).

Defects with Decreased Pulmonary Blood Flow

In these defects the amount of blood flow to the pulmonary system is decreased resulting in shunting of unoxygenated blood from the right side of the heart to the left. There is a mixing of oxygenated and unoxygenated blood in the systemic circulation. Infants with such a defect are hypoxic and cyanotic. An increase in the hematocrit (polycythemia) is frequently observed in these infants with chronic cyanosis. **Erythrocytosis** is an adaptive mechanism in which red cell production is increased in an attempt to compensate for decreased oxygen delivery, leading to an increase in hematocrit.

A hematocrit of 65–75% can lead to marked blood viscosity. Increases in viscosity will also increase afterload and ventricular work. The risk of cerebral strokes also increases if hematocrit rises above 65%. These individuals can also develop bleeding disorders caused by a decrease in circulating clotting factors and platelets. Fortunately, most children now undergo early surgical intervention, preventing or minimizing erythrocytosis. Conditions associated with erythrocytosis can still be found in adolescents and adults with residual cardiac lesions that result in long-term cyanosis (Miner & Canobbio, 1994). Defects with decreased pulmonary blood flow include pulmonary stenosis, tetralogy of Fallot, transposition of the great arteries, and tricuspid atresia.

Pulmonary Stenosis

Pulmonary stenosis (PS) refers to narrowing of the pulmonary valve and obstruction to blood flow from the right ventricle to the lungs. The obstruction can be at the valve (valvar, Figure 25-18A), just before the pulmonary valve itself (subvalvar, Figure 25-18B), above the valve (supravalvar, Figure 25-18C), or in varying places along the pulmonary artery. This discussion will focus on infants with valvar pulmonary stenosis. Valvar pulmonary stenosis results from abnormal fusion of the leaflets of the pulmonary valve. A smaller number of clients will have thickened valves known as dysplastic valves (Rocchini & Emmanouilides, 1995).

Incidence

The incidence of pulmonary stenosis is approximately 8% to 10% of all CHD (Higgins & Reid, 1994).

Pathophysiology

Secondary to the obstruction of blood flow from the RV to the PA, there is a significant increase in the right ventricular pressure. This may eventually lead to RV failure. There is

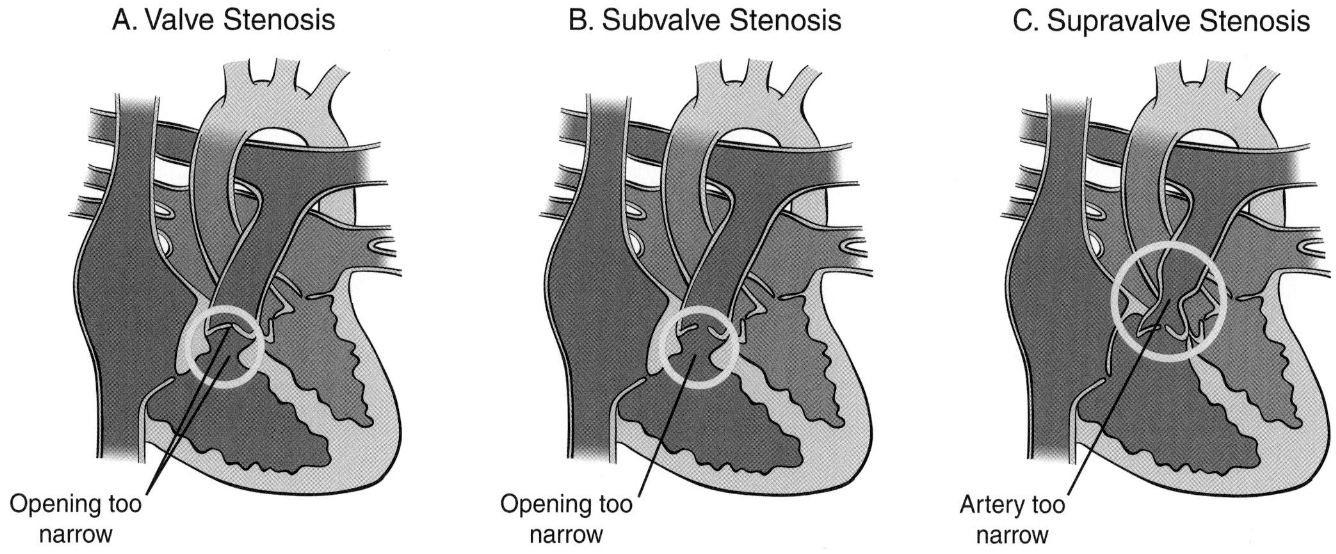

Figure 25-18 Pulmonary Stenosis: (A) valvar, (B) subvalvar, and (C) supravalvar

also a decreased amount of blood flow that is able to get to the lungs. At rest the body can compensate for this decrease in pulmonary blood flow so there are no symptoms. However, with increase in exertion, such as crying or feeding in the infant, or exercise in the child, exertion compensation is no longer effective, and the individual may develop exercise intolerance or, occasionally, cyanosis. The amount of exercise that promotes intolerance and cyanosis is dependent on the individual infant or child and could be something as simple as walking up a flight of stairs.

The degree of PS is determined by the RV systolic pressure at rest. If the pressure is low then the defect is considered mild. If the RV and LV pressures are equal, the defect is classified as moderate. The infant with an RV pressure greater than LV is considered to have severe pulmonary stenosis (Rochinni & Emmanouilides, 1995).

Clinical Manifestations

The infant with mild to moderate PS is asymptomatic, and generally a murmur is discovered on routine examination. Growth is generally normal for infants and children with PS, and symptoms are usually present only in those with severe PS. The symptoms of severe PS include dyspnea upon exertion and fatigue. Cyanosis is common with *severe* PS but is not usually seen with the milder forms.

Diagnosis

The diagnosis can often be made on clinical examination alone. Supportive diagnostic tests are usually obtained to confirm the diagnosis. The chest X ray of the client with mild to moderate PS is generally normal, while the client with severe PS may have cardiomegaly. Echocardiogram will demonstrate the size and function of the RV and the anatomy of the pulmonary valve. Cardiac cath is not necessary for diagnosis of PS.

Treatment

Treatment for PS is recommended for those with moderate to severe forms. Preoperative management with medications or exercise restriction is rarely required. The exception to this is the neonate with what is termed *critical PS*. These infants are critically ill and require the infusion of prostaglandins to maintain patency to the ductus arteriosus. This provides adequate blood flow to the lungs until surgery can be performed.

In most children with valvar PS a balloon **valvuloplasty** can be performed. This is done in the cardiac catheterization laboratory. A valvuloplasty involves using a balloon-tipped catheter to dilate a cardiac valve (the pulmonary). If a valvuloplasty cannot be performed, a surgical **valvotomy** (an incision into a cardiac valve to correct a defect) is the treatment of choice. During surgery the pulmonary valve is exposed and then surgically opened relieving the obstruction (Doty, 1997). Short-term complications of valvuloplasty include ventricular arrhythmias *during* the procedure, and long-term, the child may develop pulmonary valve insufficiency. This is often mild and requires no intervention.

Infants with mild PS are unlikely to have progression of their obstruction and are therefore not treated. However, it is recommended that they be monitored with several echocardiograms during their childhood (Driscoll, et al., 1994). Because of the safety and effectiveness of balloon valvuloplasty, this treatment is recommended for those with moderate to severe PS as the obstruction may worsen over time.

Tetralogy of Fallot

Tetralogy of Fallot (TOF) is made up of four components: (1) VSD, (2) pulmonary stenosis, (3) right ventricular hypertrophy, and (4) an overriding aorta (Figure 25-19). The degree of PS is the most important component of TOF, as its severity will determine clinical presentation, timing of surgery, and preoperative management. The right ventricle is hypertrophied because of resistance to pumping its blood through the pulmonary artery, which is stenosed or narrowed. The placement of the aorta, overriding the VSD, is of little clinical importance but is part of the anatomic features of this defect.

Incidence

TOF is the most common cyanotic heart defect accounting for approximately 10% of all CHD (Higgins & Reid, 1994).

Pathophysiology

The large VSD associated with this defect leads to equal pressures in the R and L ventricles. The amount of pulmonary blood flow and, therefore, the amount of cyanosis, will depend on the degree of pulmonary stenosis. Even with mild PS there is usually enough obstruction to pulmonary flow that these infants have some decrease in pulmonary blood flow. In some individuals there is such minimal obstruction that they are not cyanotic; thus, the term "pink tet" is often used to describe them.

Clinical Manifestations

Clinical symptoms vary greatly depending on the degree of PS. The infant or child may be profoundly cyanotic, or they may display no signs of cyanosis and be growing normally. A loud systolic murmur is usually noted at birth (Zuberbuhler, 1995). One of the most common conditions associated with TOF is hypercyanotic episodes. These episodes are also known as "tet spells" and are usually initiated by some type of activity such as crying, feeding, or defecating. There are several theories as to the cause of hypercyanotic spells but in general the following occurs. There is likely a decrease in pulmonary blood flow caused by spasm of the cardiac muscle at some point within the right ventricular outflow tract. This leads to an increase in R→L shunt, worsening cyanosis and development of **hyperpnea,** deep, rapid respirations. In the normal individual this increase in respiratory rate leads

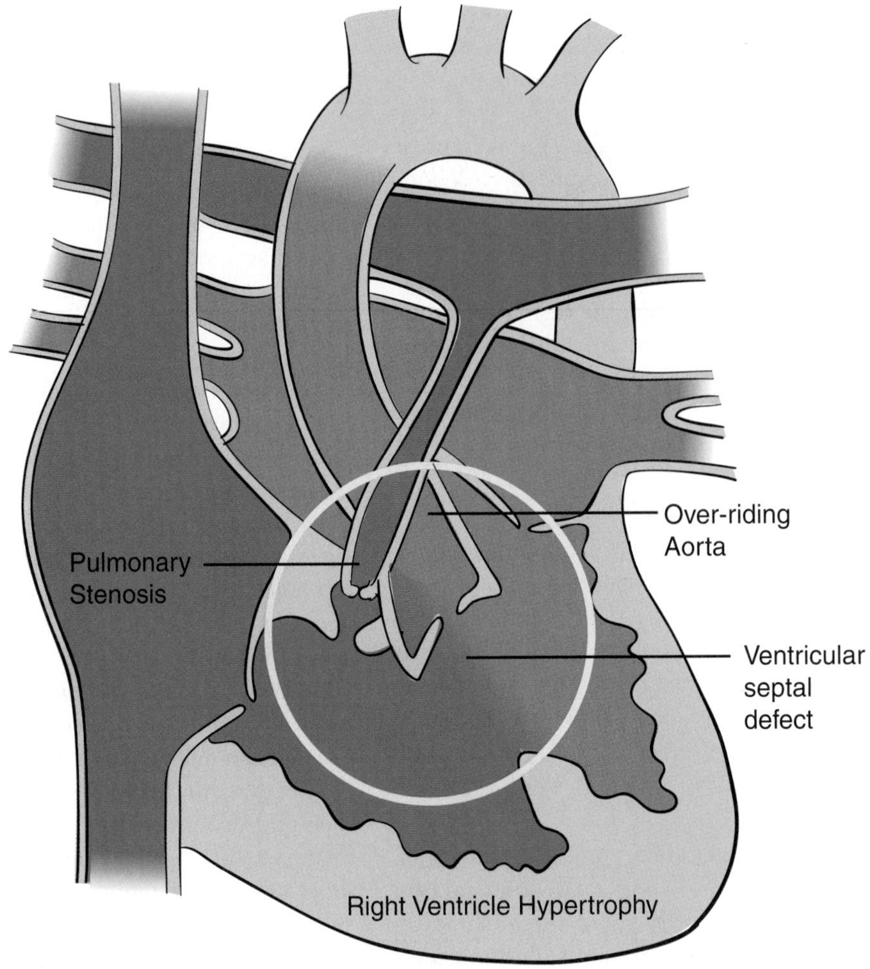

Figure 25-19 Tetralogy of Fallot

to an increase in venous return to the heart (systemic venous return). In the client with TOF increased systemic venous return of a large amount of unoxygenated blood leads to a decrease in arterial saturation (caused by R→L shunt) with continuation of profound cyanosis. If left untreated the infant or child may become unconscious or die.

Diagnosis

Chest X ray of the child with TOF is often within normal limits although sometimes the classic boot-shaped heart (caused by hypertrophy of the right ventricle) is observed. Echocardiogram will demonstrate the clinical features of TOF and is the best diagnostic tool.

Treatment

Management of the infant and child with TOF is definitive surgical correction, but preoperative medical management is important as well. A hypercyanotic spell can be frightening to watch and difficult to manage. Caregivers should be taught simple measures to alleviate these symptoms. The simplest treatment for a hypercyanotic spell is to place the infant in the knee-chest position (Figure 25-20). The older child will squat. This measure will decrease systemic venous return of unoxygenated blood as well as increase systemic vascular resistance in the hope of decreasing R→L shunt, allowing more blood flow to the lungs. In the hospital, acutely ill clients are also treated with morphine sulfate to relieve symptoms of agitation and break the cycle of hyperpnea. Other interventions include volume resuscitation to decrease blood viscosity, supplemental oxygen and, if necessary, medications such as phenylephrine (administered intravenously) to increase systemic vascular resistance. An increase in the number and severity of spells should lead to surgical palliation or complete repair.

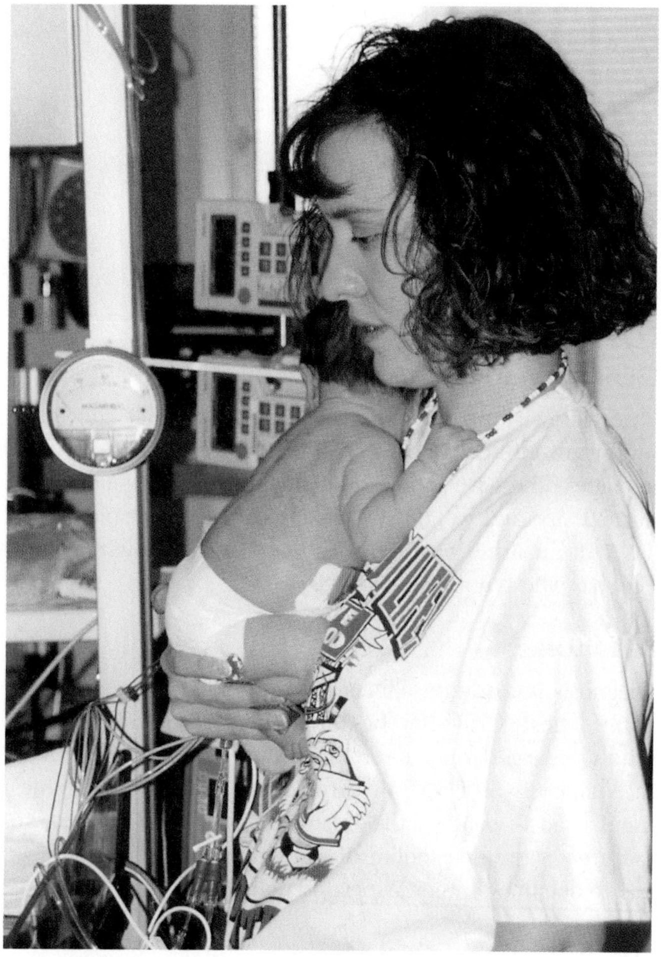

Figure 25-20 An Infant with Tetralogy of Fallot in Knee-Chest Position

For the infant with multiple hypercyanotic spells, a palliative modified Blalock-Taussing (BT) shunt is often performed to assure pulmonary blood flow until complete surgical repair is performed. A **palliative** procedure relieves or reduces the symptoms of a cardiac defect but does not correct the defect. The shunt provides a fixed amount of blood flow to the pulmonary bed and cannot grow with the child. Complete repair for the child with TOF is usually performed between 6 and 12 months of age. The goals of the repair are to widen the right ventricular outflow tract and to close the VSD. If a BT shunt is present, it is taken down or occluded at the time of the definitive repair.

Postoperative complications include low cardiac output and arrhythmias. Long-term complications include residual VSD (leaking at the patch of the VSD) and pulmonary regurgitation across the patch. TOF accounts for the largest number of adults with congenital heart disease. Approximately 11% of patients who have not had any surgical repair will live past 20 years of age, but this decreases to 3% by age 40. Death is secondary to ventricular failure. Surgical mortality for repair of TOF is approximately 2–5% during the first two years of life (Park, 1996). Long-term complications include ventricular arrhythmias, cardiac failure, and sudden death. As surgical technique evolves long-term outcomes continue to improve.

Transposition of the Great Arteries

Transposition of the great arteries (TGA) is a defect in which the great vessels (aorta and the pulmonary artery) are transposed or reversed. The aorta comes off the right ventricle and the pulmonary artery comes off the left ventricle (Figure 25-21). There is almost always a patent foramen ovale (PFO) present.

Incidence

The incidence of TGA is approximately 5–7% of all CHD, with a male predominance of 60–70% (Milton & Wernosky, 1995).

Pathophysiology

In the infant with TGA, unoxygenated blood enters the RA to RV then flows out the aorta to the body. Oxygenated

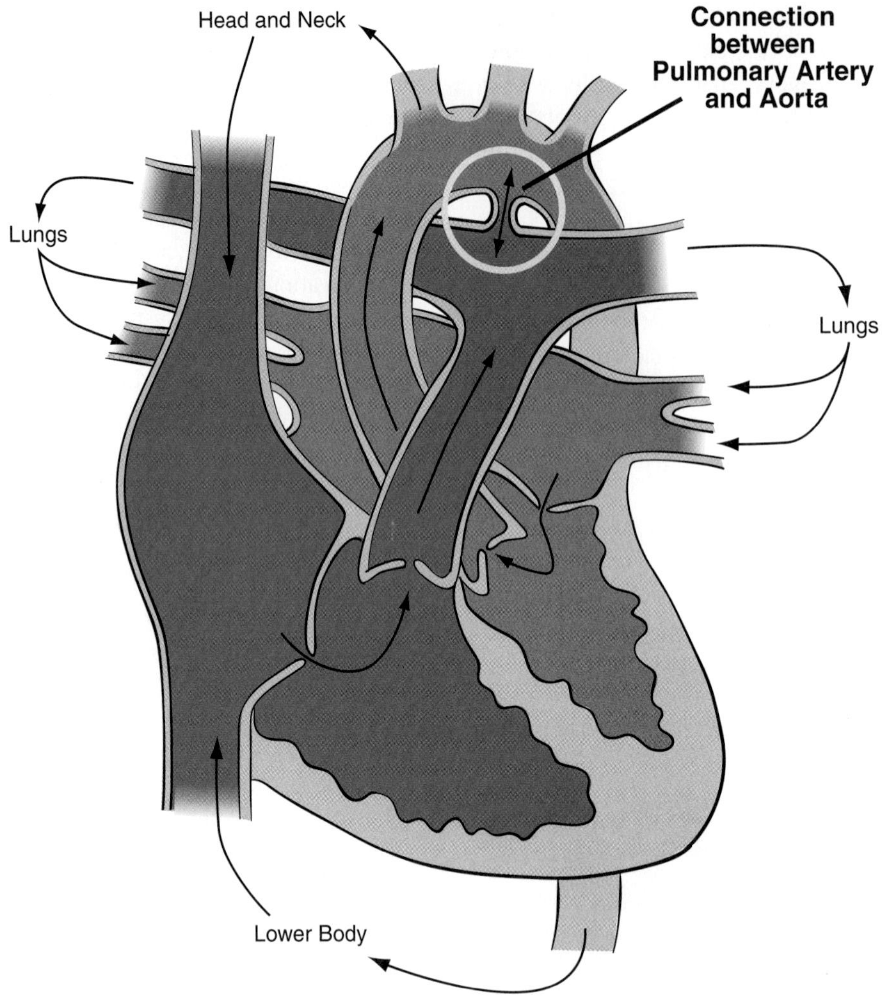

Figure 25-21 Transposition of the Great Arteries

Critical Thinking

How Does the Blood Flow in TGA?

Think about the anatomy of TGA when the PDA is still open. Draw a picture of blood flow while the PDA is open keeping in mind the role normal pulmonary and systemic vascular resistance has on hemodynamics. Then draw a picture of blood flow after the PDA closes. Would this be compatible with life? Why?

blood from the lungs enters the LA to the LV and then flows out the pulmonary artery back to the lungs. Therefore, there is a parallel circulation with no oxygenated blood getting to the systemic circulation. The infant's only chance for survival is an intra-atrial connection such as an ASD, PFO, or a PDA that will allow mixing of oxygenated and unoxygenated blood.

Clinical Manifestations

Cyanosis within the first few hours of birth is the most important clinical finding in the infant with TGA. These neonates otherwise appear quite healthy and are generally of normal size and weight. Clinicians should be suspicious of TGA in an otherwise healthy male newborn with acute cyanosis who is not responsive to oxygen.

Diagnosis

Diagnosis is made on clinical presentation and echocardiogram. Chest X ray may be within normal limits or have a mildly enlarged right heart. Echocardiogram will confirm the diagnosis of TGA but cardiac catheterization is sometimes used to confirm the relationships of the ventricles to the great vessels, to delineate the coronary artery anatomy, and to document other associated defects.

Treatment

Once diagnosis is made, stabilization of the infant is essential. Often these neonates are placed on mechanical ventilation; some will need pharmacologic support for poor cardiac output and correction of metabolic acidosis. Prostaglandin (PGE_1) is initiated to promote oxygenated blood flow from the pulmonary artery to the aorta via **retrograde** (backward) blood flow through a PDA.

In many centers a balloon **atrial septostomy** is performed. During this procedure a balloon-tipped catheter is threaded via a femoral vein into the RA. It is then passed through the PFO to the left atrium. Once in position the balloon is inflated and then rapidly pulled back across the atrial septum creating a tear in the septum creating an ASD. This will ensure enough intra-atrial mixing to provide adequate oxygenation until the child can be surgically repaired. Once adequate results are obtained from the balloon septostomy, PGE_1 can be discontinued.

The arterial switch has become the treatment of choice for the neonate with TGA. This procedure is performed via median sternotomy with the infant on CPB. The aorta is resected from the aortic trunk and similarly the pulmonary artery is resected from the pulmonary trunk. These great vessels are then switched resulting in anatomic correction. One of the more difficult tasks during this procedure is the removal and reimplantation of the coronary arteries from the old aortic trunk onto the newly created aorta (previous pulmonary trunk). Timing of this procedure is important and is normally done within the first week or two of life.

Postoperative bleeding is common after surgery. Another significant complication of the arterial switch procedure is occlusion or kinking of the coronary arteries, which will manifest as an acute decrease in cardiac output or sudden death. Long-term complications include supravalvar pulmonary stenosis that in some individuals requires re-operation. Surgical mortality for the arterial switch procedure is approximately 3–5%.

Tricuspid Atresia

Tricuspid atresia is characterized by absence of or complete closure of the tricuspid valve and therefore no connection between the RA and the RV (Figure 25-22). Other associated defects include ASD, VSD, and varying degrees of RV **hypoplasia.** Hypolpasia refers to incomplete or underdevelopment of an organ, in this case the RV.

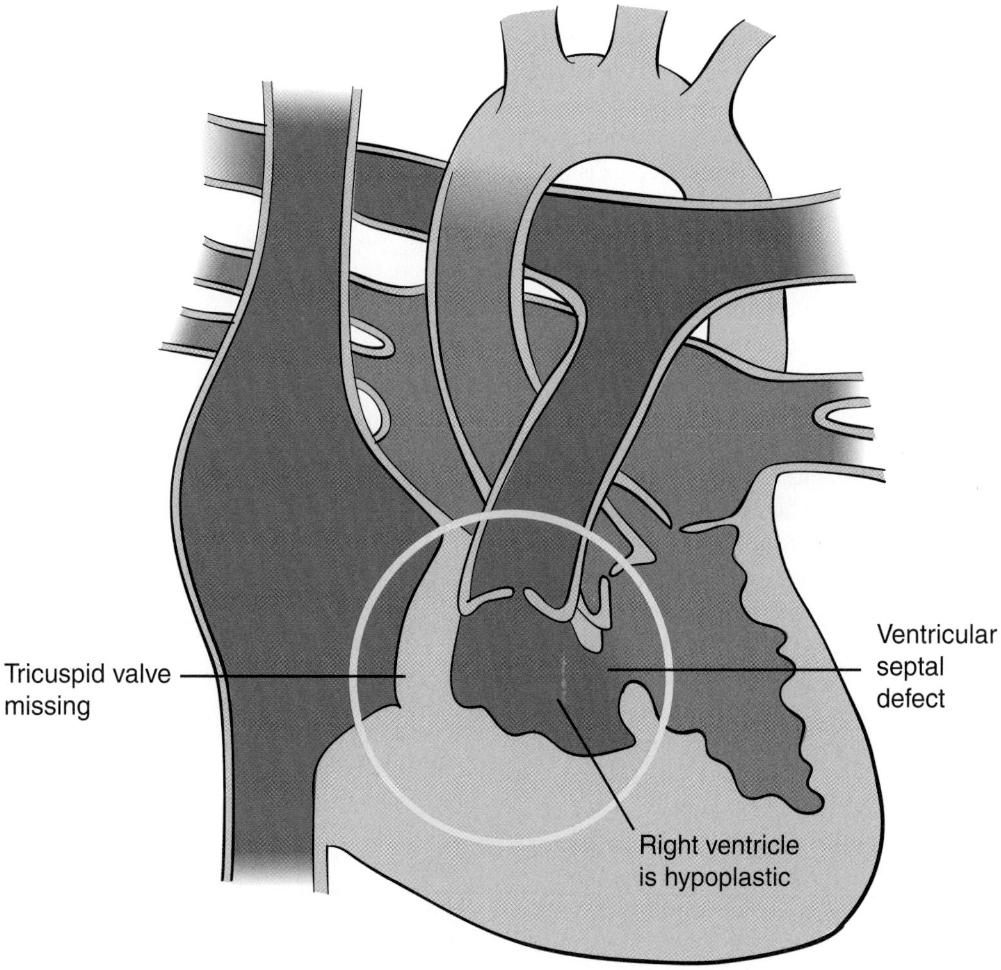

Figure 25-22 Tricuspid Atresia

Incidence

The incidence of tricuspid atresia is approximately 1–3% of all CHD (Park, 1996).

Pathophysiology

In infants with tricuspid atresia there is complete mixing of systemic and pulmonary venous return at the atrial level. Blood flow is as follows: Systemic venous return enters the RA but cannot pass to the RV through the tricuspid valve and must flow through an intra-atrial connection to the LA. Blood then flows to the LV and if there is a VSD, some blood flows through the VSD to the PA. The remainder of the blood in the left ventricle will flow out the aorta. If there is no associated VSD, then blood flow to the lungs must be through a PDA.

Clinical Manifestations

The infant with tricuspid atresia is generally cyanotic within the first day of life. Cyanosis is secondary to a R→L shunt at the atrial level. Severe hypoxic spells can occur and are related to closure of the VSD or closure of the PDA.

Diagnosis

CXR in these infants usually demonstrates enlargement of the RA, LA, and LV with decreased pulmonary markings suggestive of decreased pulmonary blood flow. Diagnosis is made with echocardiogram but cardiac cath is indicated to determine the size of the RV. Unfortunately, in many clients with tricuspid atresia the right ventricle is so small that it will never function normally, so a univentricular repair is indicated. This will be described in the following section.

Treatment

Definitive treatment for the infant with tricuspid atresia is surgical. In the preoperative period the neonate with no VSD (and therefore no pulmonary blood flow) is treated with PGE_1 to keep the ductus arteriosis open or patent until surgery can be performed. Surgical repair for the infant with a small or no VSD and a hypoplastic RV is considered palliative, as complete correction is not possible. This is true with any defect that will require the child to live his or her life with only one functioning ventricle, known as a univentricular repair.

The first stage of the repair is the placement of a BT shunt as previously described. Over the next several months as the infant begins to grow, the amount of pulmonary blood flow will decrease secondary to the fixed diameter of the BT shunt. When the infant is approximately six months old, the next palliative procedure will be performed. This is known as the **Glenn shunt.** In this procedure the superior vena cava (SVC), which normally carries unoxygenated blood back to the RA, is disconnected from the RA and sutured directly to the right pulmonary artery. This allows for all the venous return from the upper body to flow directly to both lungs, thus providing the infant with more pulmonary blood flow. At the time of this procedure the BT shunt is closed.

The final palliative procedure for children with tricuspid atresia is the **Fontan** procedure. It is performed in a variety of ways, but the general goal is to connect the inferior vena cava blood return to the pulmonary artery, thereby directing all the systemic venous return to the lungs. This will result in near normal systemic oxygen saturation. Blood flow after the Fontan is as follows. The inferior vena cava and superior vena cava bood flow directly to the pulmonary artery. Pulmonary venous return flows to the LA to the LV and out the aorta. There are in effect two separate circulations. The Fontan is generally performed when the child is greater than two years of age.

The natural history of the unrepaired infant with tricuspid atresia without a VSD is poor with few infants surviving past six months (Park, 1996). Survival and better quality of life are improving for the infant who has undergone the three palliative phases associated with this defect. Long-term complications include arrhythmias, need for pacemakers, stroke, and exercise intolerance (Driscoll, et al., 1992). Ventricular failure is not unexpected during adolescence or adulthood. Many of these individuals go on to heart transplantation.

Defects that Obstruct Left Ventricular Outflow

These defects increase afterload to the left ventricle in varying degrees. Therefore, systemic cardiac output can be limited is some individuals. Defects in this category that will be discussed are coarctation of the aorta, aortic stenosis, and hypoplastic left heart syndrome.

Coarctation of the Aorta

Coarctation of the aorta is a stenosis or narrowing located most commonly within the thoracic aorta. The area of stenosis as well as the degrees of obstruction may vary. The most common position of the coarctation is opposite the insertion of the PDA (Figure 25-23).

Incidence

The incidence of coarctation is approximately 8–10% of all CHD (Park, 1996).

Pathophysiology

Coarctation causes narrowing of the aorta and therefore increases resistance to blood flow out the left ventricle. Because all the systemic blood flow must go past the stenotic area of the aorta, an increase in left ventricular pressure and work occurs with resulting LV hypertrophy.

Clinical Manifestations

The symptomatic infant with severe coarctation is likely to present in CHF once the PDA has closed. This is secondary to the inability of the LV to eject its contents with a subsequent backup of blood from the left side of the heart to the

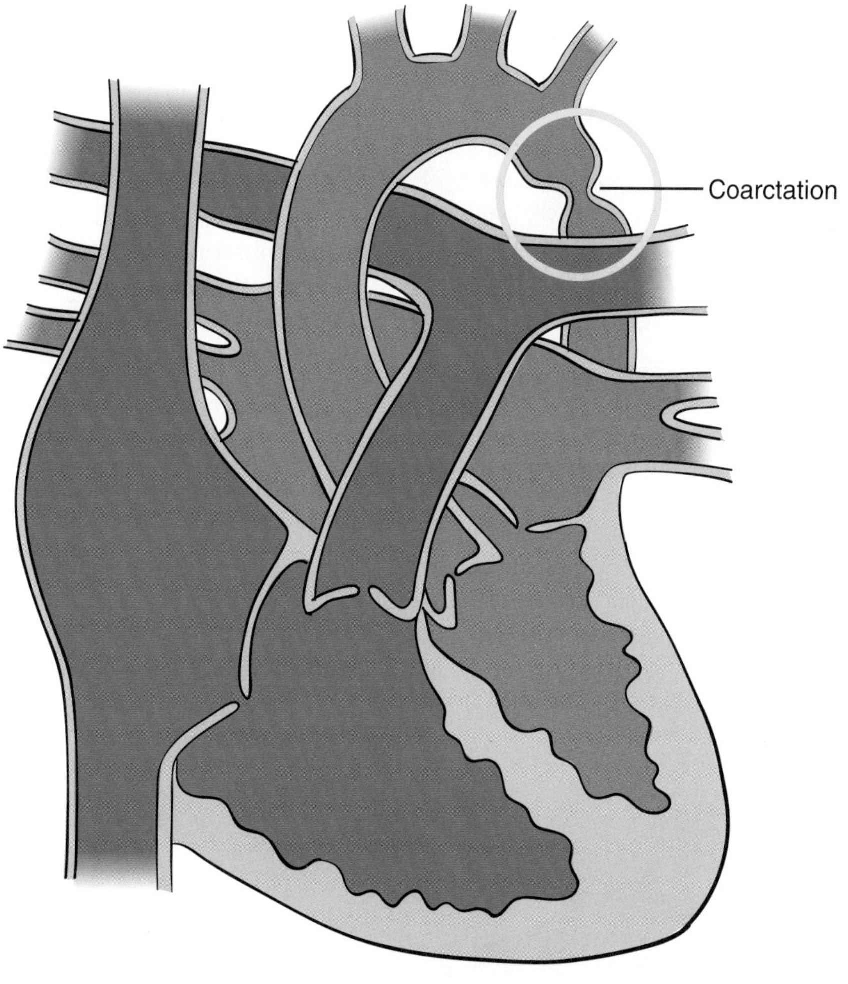

Figure 25-23 Coarctation of the Aorta

lungs. A decrease in systemic cardiac output will lead to shock, acidosis, and death unless medical intervention is initiated.

The older child with coarctation is generally asymptomatic, and the diagnosis is made when the child is sent for evaluation of a murmur or hypertension. The classic clinical finding in the child with coarctation is upper extremity hypertension and a noticeable difference in blood pressure between the arms and legs. There are also diminished pulses in the lower extremities. The simple tasks of palpating four extremity pulses and taking four extremity blood pressures should be part of all routine pediatric examinations.

Diagnosis

Diagnosis of coarctation is made on clinical examination and echocardiogram. Chest X-ray of the infant may be normal or there may be cardiomegaly. Cardiac catheterization is not indicated for diagnosis. MRI is indicated if there is need to define associated defects or **collateral** circulation. The severity of coarctation is determined by the arm/leg pressure gradient. Upper extremity blood pressure should be measured in the right arm, as this will always be the proximal pressure. A lower extremity blood pressure will always be the distal pressure. Measurements less than 20 mm Hg are associated with mild coarctation (Beekman, 1995).

Treatment

Definitive treatment for the child with coarctation is relief of the obstruction by either surgical or balloon dilation. The most common surgical repair for the infant with coarctation of the aorta is dissection of the stenotic area and end-to-end **anastomosis** (or bringing together) of the two segments of the aorta. Surgical timing for the infant with coarctation depends on his or her hemodynamic stability. The older child should have an elective repair after three to five years of age as there appears to be a decreased risk of recoarctation when the repair is performed at this age (Beekman, 1995).

Balloon angioplasty can be used to dilate the stenotic area. During this procedure a catheter with a balloon at the tip is passed via the femoral artery to the area of coarctation. The balloon is then inflated and the area of stenosis dilated

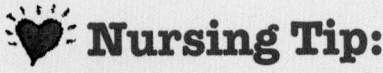

> **Nursing Tip:**
>
> **How to determine arm/leg gradients**
>
> To determine pressure gradient across a coarctation: Take right arm and leg BP; it is very important to use the appropriate size cuff. Subtract the *leg systolic* pressure from the *arm systolic* pressure; this will equal the gradient. Example: Right arm 150/70, left arm 100/68 gradient is 150–100 = 50 mm Hg.

reducing the obstruction. Angioplasty is most often used for correction of recurrent coarctation.

Medications are used in the postoperative period to control the residual hypertension that is often present in children with coarctation of the aorta. It is essential to control postoperative hypertension to prevent bleeding from the multiple sutures at the area of repair in the high pressure aorta. Long-term complications after repair include re-coarctation (particularly when the original procedure was performed during infancy) and residual hypertension. The latter complications appears to be more significant when the repair is performed in patients over six years of age (Beekman, 1995).

Aortic Stenosis

Aortic stenosis (AS) is a narrowing of the aortic valve that causes obstruction to the left ventricular outflow and decreases the amount of blood that can be ejected from the LV. Similar to pulmonary stenosis, there are three types of AS: subvalvar, valvar, or supravalvar (Figure 25-24).

Incidence

The incidence of AS is approximately 3–6% of individuals with CHD with a 4:1 ratio of males to females (Friedman, Collins, & Fenrich, 1995).

Pathophysiology

The primary hemodynamic impacts of this lesion are an increase in afterload, increased ventricular work, and left ventricular hypertrophy.

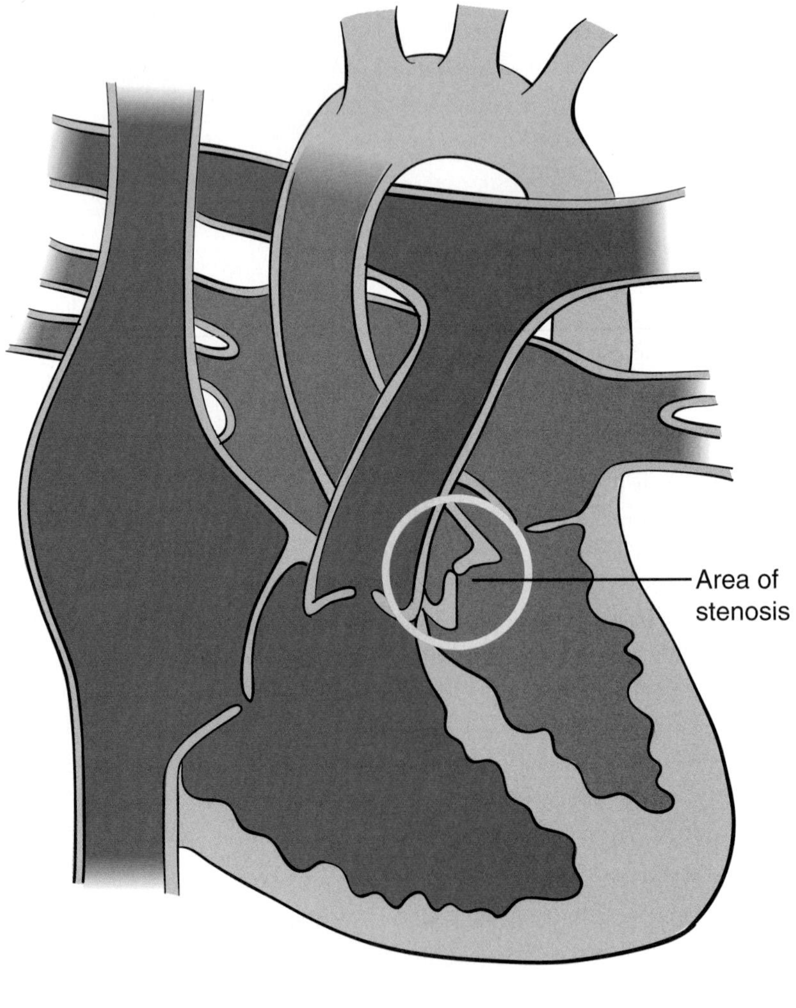

Figure 25-24 Aortic Stenosis

Clinical Manifestations

Most infants with AS grow normally, and the diagnosis is often not made until the older child is referred for evaluation of a murmur. The exception to this is the infant with *critical aortic stenosis*. Critical AS is a very serious form of AS diagnosed in the newborn. These infants present critically ill and in shock. Critical AS in an infant is a medical emergency, and death will occur without intervention.

Symptoms of AS in the older child are subtle with exertional fatigue, dyspnea, and angina. Severe AS may present with syncope. Syncope in these clients may be related to the inability of the LV to increase cardiac output during exercise and thus limiting blood flow to the brain.

Diagnosis

Diagnosis is made by clinical examination and is corroborated by diagnostic tests. Chest X-ray may be normal or demonstrate cardiomegaly. Echocardiogram is diagnostic in the patient with AS. The pressures of the LV and the aorta are measured during systole and the difference between the two is the gradient. (Example: Systolic LV pressure is 150, systolic aortic pressure is 90; gradient is 150–90 = 60 mm Hg.) Gradients less than 25 mm Hg are considered mild. Cardiac catheterization is not necessary for diagnosis but is used in treatment with balloon valvuloplasty.

Treatment

For the infant with critical AS, hemodynamic stabilization is indicated prior to correction. PGE_1 is initiated to promote retrograde blood flow from the ductus arteriosus to the distal aorta past the aortic valve. Once the infant has been stabilized, surgical correction is performed with an aortic valvotomy (Friedman, et al., 1995). In the older child the procedure of choice is balloon valvuloplasty, which is indicated when the degree of AS is severe enough to warrant correction (gradients greater than 50 mm Hg). This procedure is performed in the cardiac catheterization lab, and afterwards, the nurse monitors closely for signs of poor perfusion in the extremity where the catheterization was performed (see Nursing Care for the Child Undergoing Cardiac Cath). The main complication of valvuloplasty is aortic regurgitation. If this becomes severe, the aortic valve may need to be replaced.

Valve replacement can be performed with an artificial valve or a pulmonary autograft. Children who are recipients of artificial valves must be on anticoagulation medications such as warfarin (Coumadin) to prevent clot formation on the valve. This is a lifetime requirement. An alternative to artificial valves is to use the child's own pulmonary valve to replace the abnormal aortic valve. The main advantage of this approach is that long-term systemic anticoagulation is not required. Postoperative complications include arrhythmias, heart block, and bleeding.

Natural history of unrepaired AS varies depending on the severity of the stenosis. In general, gradients of less than 25 mm Hg are followed medically and do not require intervention. If gradients are between 25 and 50 mm Hg, the child is followed for potential progression. Unrepaired children with a gradient of greater than 50 mm Hg are at risk for **arrhythmias** (abnormal heart rhythm) and sudden death. Based on this, and with the safety of balloon valvuloplasty, those with moderate to severe AS should be corrected.

Hypoplastic Left Heart Syndrome (HLHS)

HLHS encompasses a variety of deformities characterized by lack of development of the left ventricle secondary to mitral valve atresia or aortic atresia. The left ventricle is essentially small, **hypoplastic,** and not capable of any cardiac function (Figure 25-25).

Incidence

The incidence of HLHS is approximately 1% to 2% of CHD. HLHS is the leading cause of cardiac death in the infant less than one month old (Park, 1996).

Pathophysiology

Blood flow with HLHS is as follows. Systemic venous return enters the RA and flows to the RV, out the PA to the lungs, and then returns to the LA. Secondary to atresia of the mitral valve and resulting hypoplasia of the LV, blood cannot pass into the LV and must cross the patent foramen ovale into the RA via a left to right shunt. The only way blood can enter the aorta is through retrograde flow across the PDA.

Clinical Manifestations

The infant with HLHS is generally cyanotic within hours of birth; one-third will present in cardiovascular collapse (Freedom & Benson, 1995). The infant will present with hypotension, tachycardia, cyanosis, and tachypnea.

Diagnosis

Diagnosis is made by clinical presentation and echocardiogram. Chest X ray of the infant with HLHS is generally not diagnostic but may show increased right heart size. Echocardiogram will demonstrate the structural defects and is diagnostic.

Treatment

In the recent past HLHS was an inoperable cardiac defect, and the infant was offered only comfort measures until death occurred. These infants died because the PDA closed, resulting in no systemic blood flow. Presently there are three treatment options that are presented to the family: no intervention, cardiac transplantation, or palliative surgery. These should be presented with no bias on the part of the health care provider and in no particular order of preference. The

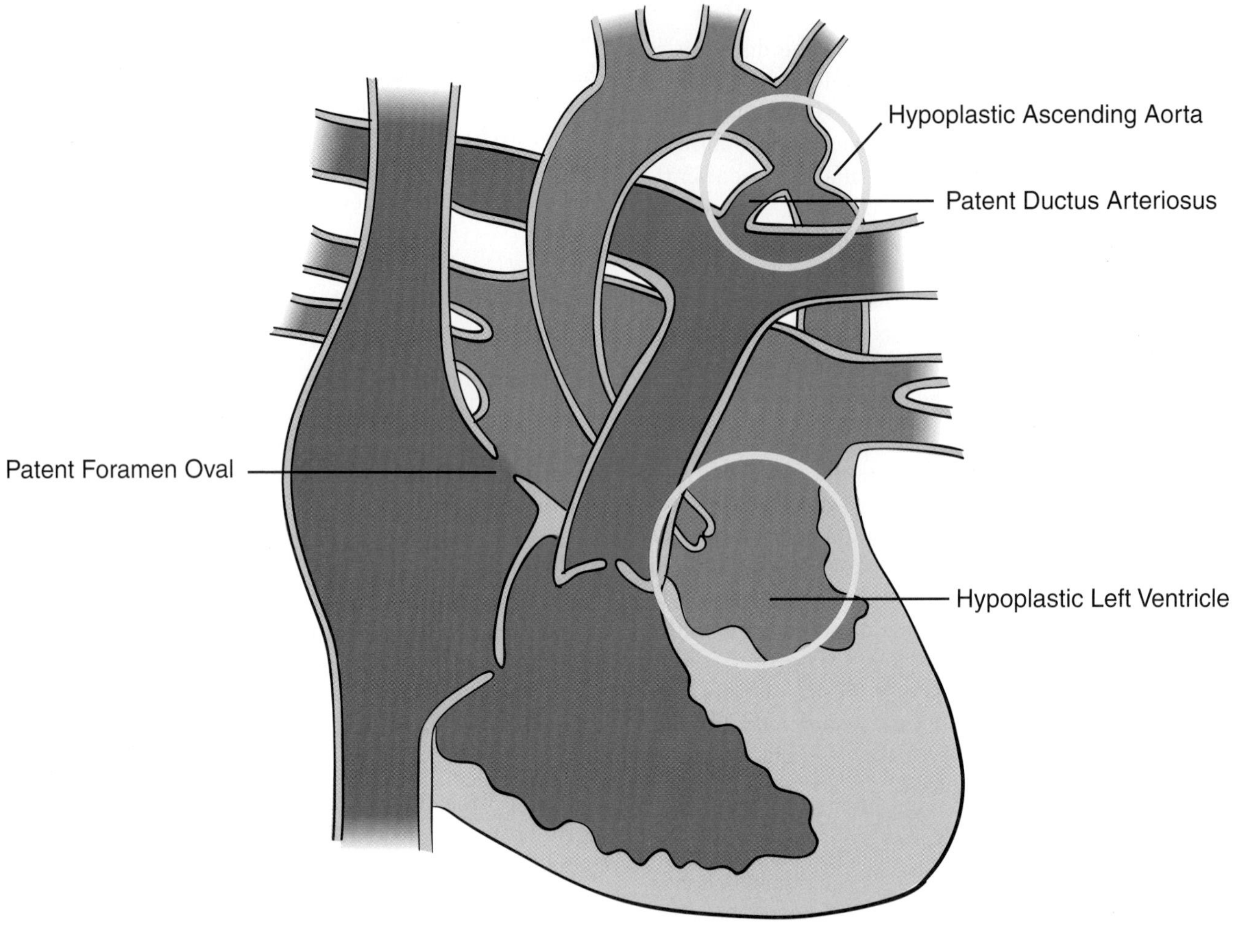

Figure 25-25 Hypoplastic Left Heart Syndrome

first is to allow the infant to die without surgical intervention, although this remains controversial. The second option is cardiac transplantation. The final choice is a three-staged palliative procedure. These procedures include the modified Norwood procedure, the Glenn shunt, and the modified Fontan. The latter two procedures were discussed in the section on tricuspid atresia and are performed in a similar fashion in infants with HLHS.

If the caregivers decide to pursue surgical transplant or palliation, medical management in the preoperative stage is extremely important in the attempt to keep the infant alive. For infants having either heart transplantation or the modified Norwood procedure, it is mandatory to maintain patency of the ductus arteriosus. Therefore, all of these infants are started on PGE_1. Preoperative support of these critically ill infants is often difficult, with little margin for error. Survival depends on the appropriate balance between systemic and pulmonary blood flow. This balance is a function of an adequately sized PDA and the pulmonary/systemic vascular resistances. These infants are sometimes maintained on 21% oxygen or inhaled carbon dioxide in an attempt to mildly vasoconstrict the pulmonary bed and prevent excessive pulmonary blood flow. The infant should have an oxygen saturation of approximately 70–75%. Alkalosis should also be avoided because this can result in too much pulmonary blood flow.

The following discussion will focus on staged repair. The initial stage of palliation is the Norwood procedure and is performed within the first week of life. The goals of this procedure are to provide systemic blood flow independent of the PDA, to provide consistent pulmonary blood flow, and to eliminate any obstruction to pulmonary venous return by eliminating the atrial septum. During the procedure the main pulmonary artery is transected and attached to the ascending aorta, creating a new aorta. A modified BT shunt is then performed to supply pulmonary blood flow, and an atrial septectomy, or complete removal of the atrial septum is performed. The other palliative procedures for HLHS are the Glenn and the modified Fontan, as previously discussed in the section on tricuspid atresia. The Glenn is generally performed at 4–6 months of age and the Fontan at approximately 2–3 years of age.

Despite astute medical and nursing care these infants or children can deteriorate rapidly with maneuvers as simple as suctioning the endotracheal tube. Sudden death is not uncommon in the immediate postoperative period and remains a potential complication when the individual has been discharged. Other complications include arrhythmias, bleeding, and poor cardiac output secondary to circulatory arrest.

Survival data for the infant who has undergone the modified Norwood procedure are evolving. Five-year survival for all three palliative procedures was 61%. Long-term survival data for the infant with HLHS who has undergone palliative repair remains to be seen. One of the most important factors that will influence long-term survival is that the right ventricle will be the systemic ventricle for life. The right ventricle is not designed to be the "high pressure" pump for a lifetime, so it may fail. These children may present for transplantation in the future.

Case Study/Care Plan

Infant with Surgical Repair of Ventricular Septal Defect

Jack is an eight-month-old infant who was noted to have a murmur at two months of age. He was not cyanotic, he fed well, and was gaining weight appropriately. Echocardiogram demonstrated a large VSD, CXR showed cardiomegaly and increased pulmonary blood flow, and ECG demonstrated ventricular hypertrophy. Over the ensuing couple of months he developed tachypnea, retractions, diaphoresis, poor feeding, and poor weight gain. His physical exam and CXR were consistent with congestive heart failure. He was placed on lasix, aldactone, and digoxin. In addition caloric density of his formula was slowly increased to 30 cal/oz. Nighttime continuous feedings were implemented so that his total caloric intake was 150 cal/kg/day. In spite of these interventions he did not gain weight, and his symptoms were only moderately controlled, so captopril was added. The decision to close his VSD was made.

He underwent patch closure of his VSD; the surgery went well without complications. He was in the PICU for three days after which he was transferred to a pediatric unit.

Nursing Care Plan

Assessment Accurate and frequent ongoing assessment of the cardiovascular system in the postoperative child is an essential part of care. Nurses should monitor for signs of decreased cardiac output such as tachycardia, poor perfusion, mottling of the skin, decreased or absent distal pulses, and poor urine output. Listen to the child's heart sounds to note changes in heart tones or murmurs. Assess the rhythm strip for arrhythmias.

Nurses should auscultate breath sounds bilaterally. Listen to the quality of the breath sounds; listen for rales, coarse rhonchi. Observe the child's color and work of breathing either spontaneously or while on mechanical ventilation. Monitor for tachypnea, retractions, and nasal flaring. Monitor oxygen saturations, keeping in mind the child's anatomy. It is essential that the nurse understand the surgical repair and the expected norm for each defect. When the child has awakened from anesthesia, the nurse assesses the neurologic function by noting equal movement of all extremities, absence of any signs of seizures, and pupillary function. Pain in the nonverbal child is expressed by an increase in heart rate and blood pressure and by grimacing and crying. Older children can convey their degree of pain by verbalization or through the use of one of the multiple pain scores and charts available to nurses. Refer to Chapter 18 for more information about pain assessment.

Many cardiac repairs involve multiple suture lines in and around a very small heart. These sutures combined with the destruction of platelets secondary to cardiopulmonary bypass can lead to excessive bleeding in the postoperative period. The child is monitored for signs of bleeding from surgical incisions and intravenous insertion sites.

Nursing Diagnosis #1

Ineffective breathing pattern related to pulmonary edema, pleural effusions, poor respiratory effort, atelectasis and/or phrenic nerve damage, as indicated by prolonged intubation, tachypnea, increased work of breathing.

continues

continued

Expected Outcomes

1. Child will have adequate respiratory function as evidenced by respiratory rate normal for age and comfortable respiratory pattern.
2. Child will have no increased work of breathing.

Interventions/*Rationales*

1. Provide analgesia and sedation. *A child who is in pain related to a sternal or thoracotomy incision is unlikely to take deep breaths.*
2. Frequently reassess breath sounds. *Unequal aeration may signal pleural effusion, pneumothorax, or damage to the phrenic nerve.*
3. Obtain chest X-ray as ordered. *To evaluate for presence of pneumothorax or pleural effusion.*
4. Administer scheduled diuretics. *To prevent interstitial fluid from accumulating in the lungs.*
5. Provide good pulmonary toilet (i.e., deep breathing, coughing, head of bed elevated, early ambulation) to prevent atelectasis. *Will assist in establishing good respiratory function.*
6. Provide supplemental oxygen as needed. *To maintain oxygen saturations in desired range.*
7. Obtain arterial blood gases as ordered. *To evaluate for CO_2 retention and hypoxia.*

Evaluation

Supplemental oxygen is weaned over the expected time period. Oxygen saturations are within normal limits for child's physiology. There is no increased work of breathing, and arterial blood gases are within normal limits.

Nursing Diagnosis #2

Decreased cardiac output related to decreased stroke volume as a result of mechanical, structural, or electrophysiological problems as demonstrated by poor perfusion, hypotenison, arrhythmias, decreased urine output, or increased chest tube output.

Expected Outcomes

1. The child will have warm, well-perfused extremities, strong peripheral pulses, and normal blood pressure.
2. The child's cardiac rhythm will be normal.
3. The child's urine output will be at least 1 cc/kg/hour.
4. Child's chest tube output will gradually decrease over 24–48 hours.

Interventions/*Rationales*

1. Administer volume resuscitation for hypovolemia. *Prevent hypotension.*
2. Monitor ongoing losses through chest tubes and dressings. *Normal chest tube output is approximately 2–3 cc/kg/hr over the first few hours and should then slowly taper off.*
3. Monitor for an abrupt cessation in chest tube output, tachycardia, narrow pulse pressure, and/or acute deterioration in cardiac output. *May indicate cardiac tamponade.*
4. Add pharmacologic support if the child shows signs of decreased cardiac output. *Maintain normal perfusion.*
5. Record rhythm strip upon arrival and anytime there is a change in rhythm. *Document any arrhythmia.*
6. Use temporary external pacemaker as needed. *Temporary external pacing will be initiated for bradycardia, complete heart block, or any abnormal rhythm that results in poor cardiac output.*

continues

continued

7. Monitor calcium, magnesium, and potassium levels and infuse ordered replacements for low levels. *Maintaining normal electrolytes will help prevent arrhythmias and support cardiac output.*

Evaluation

Extremities are warm and well-perfused. Urine output is within normal limits. Heart rate and rhythm are normal and cardiac tamponade is avoided.

Nursing Diagnosis #3

Acute pain related to operative site as evidenced by crying, verbalization of pain, tachycardia, diaphoresis, hypertension.

Expected Outcomes

1. The child's pain will be adequately controlled.

Interventions/*Rationales*

1. Perform neurologic checks upon arrival and frequently until fully awake. *Evaluate baseline and observe for trend in neurologic function.*

2. Administer ordered analgesics. *To prevent postoperative pain. Opiates can cause respiratory depression and are used with caution in the extubated child.*

3. Administer sedatives as ordered while on mechanical ventilation. *To alleviate anxiety and provide amnesia. These medications can cause respiratory depression and are generally not administered once the child is extubated.*

4. Provide non-pharmacologic pain relief measures. These can include soft music, audio tapes from home, a favorite toy or blanket, and relaxation exercises. *To augment pharmacologic intervention.*

Evaluation

The child demonstrates adequate anxiety and pain control. There are no abnormal neurologic sequelae.

Nursing Diagnosis #4

Ineffective family coping related to illness and hospitalization, as demonstrated by prolonged, disabling feelings of guilt or sadness and lack of involvement in child's care.

Expected Outcomes

1. Caregivers will have their questions answered and will be kept aware of their child's progress and complications.

2. The family will be prepared for their child's postoperative course and will be better able to handle the stress.

3. Family will be actively involved in the plan of care for their child.

Interventions/*Rationales*

1. Encourage participation in preoperative tour or teaching session. *Decrease anxiety and help answer questions and allay fears.*

2. Allow caregivers to visit as soon as possible after surgery. *Support family unit. Caregivers provide support for the child and decrease his anxiety.*

3. Explain all lines and tubes. *Educate caregivers to prevent deficient knowledge.*

4. Encourage caregivers to participate in child's care when possible. These times include diaper changes, bathing, and feeding. *Support caregiver role and family unit.*

continues

continued

5. Encourage home routines when possible. *Normalize routine for child.*
6. Involve child life team to assist with relaxation prior to painful procedures. *Provide strategies for mastery of difficult situations.*
7. Involve social workers or clergy if family continues to have problems coping with the child's illness. *Support family to help with crisis intervention.*
8. Encourage caregivers to ask questions and *listen* to their concerns. No one knows a child as well as their caregivers. *Educate caregivers and provide support.*

Evaluation

Caregiver role is maintained, and the caregiver/child interaction is normal. Stress of hospitalization will be minimized and family unit will be maintained.

Family Teaching for Postoperative Congenital Heart Surgery

Preparing caregivers for their child's discharge should begin in the early postoperative period. The usual progression toward discharge includes a transfer from the ICU to the general pediatric ward before going home. While on the ward caregivers should resume care of their child. Prior to discharge the following should be taught and clearly understood by the caregivers and (when appropriate) the child.

Activities

Infants and children will generally limit their own activity if it is uncomfortable for them. Caregivers are taught to monitor for tiring and fatigue in their child. Caregivers should encourage a return to normal feeding and sleeping schedules. Rough play and strenuous activities are avoided until six weeks following discharge. Children may return to school within approximately two weeks, but home tutoring is encouraged prior to this time. The child should be excused from physical education classes during the six weeks following surgery. Nurses should encourage involvement in nonstrenuous community activities such as scouting, church, and after-school programs.

Diet

Infants should return to breastfeeding or formula. To assess whether the infant is taking in adequate fluids, she/he should have at least 5 wet diapers/day. Since formula contains more calories than cereal or baby food, families are encouraged to limit these foods and give additional formula/breast milk. Older children are encouraged to eat a regular diet.

Wound Care

Generally the sutures used to close either the sternal incision or the thoracotomy incision are absorbable and do not need to be removed. Children may sit in a shallow tub. Caregivers should cleanse around the wound and pat the area dry. The wound should not be soaked for the first week. Showers and normal baths can resume in approximately two weeks. Caregivers are instructed to inspect the wound looking for signs of redness, swelling, drainage, or tenderness.

General Considerations

Caregivers, teachers, and other family members should be instructed to watch for signs of heart failure. Puffiness of the eyes, swelling of the feet, shortness of breath, poor feeding, and excessive irritability all warrant further investigation by the medical team.

Medications

Many children are discharged on medication to promote cardiac function. Frequently these medications are similar to those the child was taking before surgery. Refer to Table 25-3 for a listing of cardiac medications and their side effects. Schools should be notified of any medications (and possible side effects) the child is on.

Finally, before discharge the family must demonstrate an understanding of these instructions and know how to reach the health care provider's office if needed. A follow-up appointment should be in place before the family leaves the hospital. If the child develops syncope, poor perfusion, increased work of breathing, or high fever, caregivers should be instructed to go to the emergency room.

ACQUIRED HEART DISEASE

Acquired heart disease refers to disease processes or disorders that develop after birth and affect the functioning of the heart and cardiovascular system. Acute rheumatic fever,

Kawasaki disease, and infective endocarditis are the acquired heart diseases discussed in this section.

Acute Rheumatic Fever

Acute rheumatic fever (ARF) is the leading cause of acquired heart disease in developing countries. With the advent of penicillin, the incidence of ARF has decreased substantially in the United States; however, a frightening resurgence has been noted in the Rocky Mountain states.

Incidence and Etiology

An estimated 10–20 million new cases of rheumatic fever occur yearly in developing countries (Veasey & Hill, 1997). In the United States, rheumatic fever is most frequently observed in the age group most susceptible to group A streptococcal infections, children aged 5–15 years. It is estimated that 1.8 million Americans are afflicted with rheumatic fever, killing over 5,000 people in 1995. ARF follows an untreated or partially treated group A streptococcal **pharyngitis** (sore throat) (AAP, 2000). Although group A streptococci can produce infection in any number of bodily tissues, rheumatic fever will only follow a throat infection. It has never been identified subsequent to a group A streptococci skin infection (impetigo) (Veasey & Hill, 1997). With the advent of antibiotic therapy the mortality has been reduced substantially.

Pathophysiology

The exact pathogenesis of ARF is unknown. It is generally felt to be an autoimmune response to untreated group A streptococcal pharyngitis in genetically predisposed individuals (Veasey & Hill, 1997). The three organ systems primarily affected by this autoimmune response are the heart, central nervous system, and the joints.

The entire heart can be affected during the acute inflammatory phase of illness. Pericarditis, myocarditis, and **valvulitis** (inflammation of the heart valves) can occur. The most significant cardiac pathophysiological phenomena is valvulitis. The most frequently affected valve is the mitral valve. Valvulitis is responsible for mitral valve deformity that results in mitral regurgitation. The aortic valve can also be affected and develop insufficiency; however, isolated aortic insufficiency without mitral regurgitation is uncommon in ARF (Committee on Rheumatic Fever, 1992). Myocarditis and pericarditis are never encountered in rheumatic fever without valvar involvement. Therefore myocarditis or pericarditis in isolation should not be considered rheumatic in origin. (Veasey, 1995b; Committee on Rheumatic Fever, 1992)

Joint involvement consists of **polyarthritis.** Unfortunately, polyarthritis can also mimic many childhood illnesses such as juvenile rheumatoid arthritis. The involved joints are usually the larger ones, such as the knees, ankles, hips, and shoulders. Presentation of arthritis is quite variable. The pain can be mild or so severe the child is unable to bear weight. The arthritis of ARF does not result in permanent disability.

Central nervous systems manifestations often present late, sometimes years after the initial illness. Inflammatory changes in the neurons result in **chorea** (classically known as Sydenham's chorea). Chorea is characterized by involuntary, purposeless movements of the extremities and the trunk. Because this is a late manifestation of rheumatic fever there may be no antecedent evidence of recent group A streptococcal pharyngitis.

Chronic changes in the heart are responsible for the long-term sequela of ARF. Valvar regurgitation can progress to stenosis. In many situations evidence of a previous episode of rheumatic fever is not uncovered until an adult develops valvar stenosis, requiring replacement with an artificial valve.

Clinical Manifestations

The clinical presentation of rheumatic fever can be quite varied. The American Heart Association (AHA, 1998) has established clinical criteria for ARF and has categorized these into major and minor manifestations. These criteria are the Jones Criteria, in honor of T. Duchett Jones who first set forth diagnostic standards for rheumatic fever in 1944 (Veasey, 1995b). *These criteria are currently being revised and are not yet available for inclusion in this chapter. Refer to the American Heart Association website (www.americanheart.org) for current updates of the Jones Criteria for ARF.* Generally the child presents with a nondescript febrile illness and antecedent group A streptococcal throat infection. Unfortunately, some children have no history of febrile illness or pharyngitis.

The manifestations of valvulitis are the most significant clinical features. In the presence of mitral regurgitation a new systolic murmur is appreciated. If aortic insufficiency is present there will be a diastolic murmur. Sometimes the murmur is soft. Occasionally there can be "silent" mitral regurgitation with no appreciable murmur, although it will be identified on echocardiogram.

Polyarthritis is the most frequent benign major manifestation. The arthritis is migratory, meaning the joint pain moves from one joint to another. There is tenderness, pain, swelling, heat, and limitation of movement in the affected joints. An isolated severely swollen red joint that is not migratory in nature must be considered septic until proven otherwise, as this is not characteristic of ARF.

Erythema marginatum is a distinctive, fine, pink rash noted on the trunk and extremities, never on the face. It becomes more pronounced with heat, such as when the child first comes out of a hot bath. This is always seen with **carditis** (inflammation of the heart) or polyarthritis. Subcutaneous nodules are firm painless nodules over the extensor surfaces of the elbows, knees, and wrists. The skin over the nodules is not inflamed. These are rare and are never seen in isolation; they always accompany carditis. Arthralgia and fever are frequently present but are nonspecific for rheumatic fever.

Diagnosis

Those who have had a previous episode of ARF are at higher risk for a recurrent episode. The diagnosis is made on the presence of the clinical manifestations, supported by laboratory data. There is a high probability of rheumatic fever if there are evidence of antecedent group A streptococcal throat infection, and either two major manifestations of ARF or one major and two minor manifestation (Committee on Rheumatic Fever, 1992).

Laboratory findings support the presence of an inflammatory process and document an antecedent group A streptococcal infection. Elevation of sedimentation rate and C-reactive protein are nonspecific blood tests used to document an inflammatory process. A throat culture can document the organism responsible for pharyngitis; unfortunately, many children will have recovered by the time rheumatic fever is suspected, therefore a throat culture may be negative. In addition a number of asymptomatic children can be carriers of group A streptococci, hence a positive culture would result.

Fortunately there are blood tests that are sensitive and reliable in establishing a previous streptococcal infection. These are antibody determinations that can be elevated for weeks following the initial infection. Antistreptolysin O-titer (ASO) and anti-DNAse B are obtained together. In combination these two tests will increase the confirmation of rheumatic fever to 92% (Veasey, 1995b).

EKG can demonstrate PR interval prolongation with first degree heart block, although this is nonspecific and not always observed. Echocardiogram is the most sensitive tool for the diagnosis of valvar disease. The echocardiographic findings of mitral regurgitation in rheumatic fever are quite characteristic, so a firm diagnosis can be made. An ECHO should be obtained in any child suspected of having rheumatic fever because mitral regurgitation and aortic insufficiency may be "silent."

Treatment

The treatment of ARF during the acute phase is directed at eradicating the organism and implementing anti-inflammatory agents. Oral penicillin is used for the initial treatment. Aspirin is implemented as an anti-inflammatory agent because the polyarthritis of ARF does not respond to acetamenophen or ibuprofen. Aspirin in high doses is begun at 100 mg/kg/day for two days, then decreased to 70 mg/kg/day until the sedimentation rate returns to normal. Polyarthritis responds very quickly to high dose aspirin. Once acute phase reactants (sedimentation rate) are normal then aspirin can be discontinued. If aspirin side effects are noted, then the dose can be decreased slightly. Concurrent administration of antacids helps with the stomach pain associated with high dose aspirin.

Initially the child should be placed on bedrest until inflammation has resolved; this can be done as an outpatient. In the presence of new mitral/aortic regurgitation, activities should be restricted for a number of weeks to months. Compliance in this area can be quite difficult, particularly when the child begins to feel better. Frequent follow-up with a pediatric cardiologist is essential. Repeat ECHOs are obtained to evaluate for resolution of valvar involvement. Unfortunately, in many cases the valves do not completely return to normal.

Secondary prophylaxis is essential in all cases of rheumatic carditis. This consists of oral penicillin 250 mg BID, or monthly intramuscular injections of penicillin. Secondary prophylaxis is carried out for at least ten years or well past young adulthood. This is critically important as a recurrence of rheumatic fever can induce severe cardiac damage. Those children with residual valvar disease must also follow endocarditis prophylaxis (see section on endocarditis). However, because these children are on chronic penicillin therapy a different antibiotic agent must be used. Compliance with secondary prophylaxis is very difficult. Many clients either forget to take their medication or feel it is unnecessary since they are not "sick." Although traumatic for young children, intramuscular injections allow for more individual freedom resulting in better compliance.

Over the last decade death rates from rheumatic fever in the United States have dropped significantly. This is because of timely identification and antibiotic therapy. However, because the incidence has been declining some children are missed because of lack of experience on the part of the health care provider. Although mortality has dropped, morbidity remains a risk for many. This is in the form of chronic valvar disease and progressive mitral stenosis. Many individuals will require either aortic valve or mitral valve replacement for treatment of rheumatic heart disease in adulthood.

Nursing Management

Unless the child is in severe heart failure the management of acute rheumatic fever is handled as an outpatient. The treatment of congestive heart failure has been discussed previously. Timely identification and diagnosis of rheumatic fever is essential to the prevention of adverse sequelae. Community and family education is critical to the prevention and recurrence of ARF. The community must be made aware that strep throat infections must be treated in a timely manner, and the full course of antibiotics completed (to prevent undertreatment).

Family Teaching

Education is the most important nursing intervention with this disease. The family is educated on the importance of antibiotic therapy, both in the acute phase and for secondary prophylaxis. If the child is on aspirin, the family must be made aware of the side effects. Compliance with activity restrictions is important; the nurse can offer suggestions for diversional activities or home schooling can be instituted. The length and type of restriction varies between clients and is determined by clinical condition. For any child who has had an episode of ARF, the family must be vigilant in looking for the signs and symptoms of group A streptococcal throat infection in order to facilitate timely treatment. Even those children on chronic penicillin therapy can have a recurrent streptococcal infection. Adolescents must be made accountable for their own treatment. This is a high risk group for non-compliance with secondary prophylaxis. Ongoing education with frequent reinforcement is of prime importance. The importance of follow-up must also be stressed.

Kawasaki Disease

Kawasaki disease (KD) was first described by Tomisaku Kawasaki in 1967 in Japan. Since that time KD has been widely recognized through out the world, and is currently the leading cause of acquired heart disease in the United States (Barron, 1998; Takahashi, 1997).

Incidence and Etiology

Peak incidence occurs in children two years of age and younger; 80% of cases occur in children less than five years old (Barron, 1998; Shulman, De Inocencio, & Hirsch, 1995). Boys are affected more commonly than girls, and prevalence is increased in those children of Asian descent. Incidence rates in Japan approximate 100 cases/100,000 children, in the United States incidence approximates 10 cases/100,000 children (0.1 per 1,000) (Melish, 1996).

To date, a specific etiology is unknown. A number of researchers have advanced various hypotheses on the etiology of KD. These hypotheses include, but are not limited to, a superantigenic exotoxin produced by *Staphylococcus aureus* similar to the exotoxin found in toxic shock syndrome, dust mites, exposure to rug shampooing, and rickettsiae. However, none of these hypotheses has been corroborated by subsequent investigators (Todome, et al., 1995; Kawasaki, 1995; Melish, 1996). Most clinicians believe that the etiology is microbial because of the clinical presentation, response to treatment, and epidemiology. Nonetheless, viral and bacterial cultures do not reveal consistent findings.

Epidemiologic evidence suggesting an infectious etiology is as follows. It is uncommon for KD to manifest in infants less than three months of age, inferring protection from acquired immunity from the mother (Takahashi, 1997). KD in children over twelve years of age is almost unheard of, suggesting the possibility of natural immunity through subclinical infection. Epidemics occur in the winter and spring (Melish, 1996; Shulman, et al., 1995; Bradley & Glode, 1998). Past epidemiologic studies have identified community-wide outbreaks of KD at regular 3–5 year intervals, although this trend may be subsiding. To date, the most attractive hypothesis for the etiology of KD is one of a widespread infectious agent that is responsible for disease in susceptible (possibly genetically predisposed) individuals.

Pathophysiology

KD is a multisystem **vasculitis** (inflammation of the blood vessels) with a proclivity to affect the coronary arteries. The pathogenesis is felt to be an antibody-mediated vascular injury, in which the vascular endothelium plays a major role (Athreya, 1995). Infiltration of the vessel wall with inflammatory cells is responsible for the early manifestations and symptoms found in KD.

During the first ten days of illness there is infiltration and hypertrophy of the vascular vessel. At this stage aneurysms do not form, although **ectasia** (larger than normal for age) of the coronary arteries can be seen on ECHO. The vascular changes that occur lay the groundwork for possible aneurysm formation in the future. During this stage of illness there is **pancarditis** (inflammation of entire heart) and pericardial inflammation often with effusion. Some clients can develop congestive heart failure (Melish, 1996; Shulman, et al., 1995).

From day ten to day forty of the illness there is a decrease in the inflammatory process. Because of earlier pathophysiological processes, vessels have undergone destructive changes. It is during this period that coronary artery aneurysm can develop. Coronary artery abnormalities and aneurysms are more pronounced at the origins of the coronaries, proximal segments, and distal branching segments. Other arteries such as the iliac, femoral, axillary, and renal arteries can be involved, although this is rare (Takahashi, 1995).

After forty days there is progressive fibrosis and healing of coronary artery abnormalities. Aneurysms and dilation usually regress in one to two years. Individuals with aneurysms can develop progressive stenosis and calcification of the affected coronary arteries. Death can occur caused by myocardial ischemia (Fukushige, et al., 1996; Ogawa, et al., 1997).

Clinical Manifestations

The onset of illness is abrupt and begins with the first day of fever. There is no prodrome and the majority of children are healthy prior to illness. The first symptom is a high (38°–41°C; 100.4°–105.8°F) remittent fever lasting more than five days. Within two to five days other signs of KD manifest. These include **conjunctival infection** (redness of conjunctiva), **erythematous** (diffuse redness) rash, oral changes, unilateral cervical swollen lymph nodes (**lymphadenopathy**), and changes in the feet and hands.

Eye involvement consists of nonexudative conjunctival injection with photophobia, which occurs within the first five days of illness. The rash is **polymorphous** erythematous without vesicles, and appears within five days of fever. There is extensive involvement of the trunk and limbs and perineal **desquamation** (peeling of skin) may occur in 10% of individuals. Changes in the oral mucosa consist of erythema and cracking of the lips, strawberry tongue, and diffuse erythema of oropharyngeal mucosa.

The most characteristic findings of this disease are changes of the hands and feet. The hands and feet become tensely edematous and very erythematous. By the tenth day of illness desquamation begins. This starts just under the finger and toenails and progresses to involve the palms and soles, with skin peeling in sheets (Melish, 1996; Takahashi, 1995).

Cervical lymphadenopathy, although a widely recognized clinical finding, remains the least consistent manifestation, occurring in only 50% of clients. (Previously described symptoms occur in 90% of clients.) When present the enlarged lymph node is nontender and nonfluctuant. It can occur on the first day of fever.

Associated findings of KD include marked irritability, arthralgia, arthritis, aseptic meningitis, sterile **pyuria** (white cells in the urine), and diarrhea. Hepatic dysfunction with elevated liver function tests is observed in up to 40% of clients, although it is transitory and requires no intervention. White cell count and sedimentation rate are elevated secondary to the overwhelming inflammatory response. Platelet counts are significantly elevated: 450,000/mm^3 by day ten of illness to 650,000–2,000,000/mm^3 by day twenty of illness (Melish, 1996).

Cardiac manifestations are the most serious, contributing to morbidity and mortality. Sixty percent of clients will develop tachycardia and gallop rhythm. Up to 20% can develop congestive heart failure. Coronary artery lesions are seen in 25% of those *not treated* with intravenous gamma globulin (IVIG). This has dropped to 5% with the advent of gamma globulin therapy (Dajani, et al., 1994). Coronary artery ectasia is transient and usually disappears during the acute phase of illness. Coronary artery aneurysms generally develop after day ten of illness; prognosis differs according to size. Small aneurysms are less than 4 mm, medium 4–8 mm, and giant >8 mm. Small and medium aneurysms regress by one year, albeit medium aneurysms may develop local stenosis in the future. Giant aneurysms have a tendency to develop stenosis and calcification, even though regression occurs within 1 to 2 years (Kawasaki, 1995). Those children at the highest risk for the development of giant aneurysms include males, infants less than one year, and those not treated before the tenth day of illness or are refractory to treatment (Rosenfeld, Corydon, & Shulman, 1995; Melish, 1996).

Diagnosis

Kawasaki disease is a clinical diagnosis augmented by laboratory findings. Other entities that may have a similar presentation must be excluded. The diagnosis is made in children with a high fever who meet four or five of the clinical diagnostic criteria (see Box 25-4). Infants may not meet diagnostic criteria and manifestations may be subtle. "Atypical" KD may be diagnosed if coronary artery aneurysms are noted on ECHO in the absence of criteria (Barron, 1998). ECHO is the primary tool for the initial evaluation and follow-up of children with coronary artery lesions. Unfortunately, it cannot evaluate for the presence of stenosis in aneurysms that have regressed.

Differential diagnoses include bacterial infection, measles, toxic shock syndrome, and scarlet fever. Laboratory data and cultures are helpful in supporting the diagnosis. Unfortunately, there is no specific laboratory test to diagnose KD.

Treatment

Intravenous immune globulin (IVIG) and aspirin therapy provide the mainstay in the therapeutic intervention for KD. These interventions are the most beneficial if administered during the first ten days of illness, as they have demonstrated significant improvement in outcome (Yanagawa, Nakamura, Sakata, & Yashiro, 1997; Durongpisitkul, Guraraj, Park, & Martin, 1995). The child who has been ill for longer than ten days, or has become afebrile, may not benefit from IVIG.

IVIG should be administered 2 gm/kg over 10–12 hours intravenously. IVIG usually results in rapid resolution of CHF, defervescence of fever, and normalization of sedimentation rate. IVIG markedly reduces the incidence of coronary artery aneurysms (Barron, 1998). Some children will not initially respond to IVIG, so a repeat dose of 1 gm/kg may be administered. Methylprednisolone has been used in select clients who were refractory to multiple doses of IVIG in combination with aspirin (Wright, Newburger, Barker, & Sandel, 1996).

Initial aspirin therapy consists of 100 mg/kg/day in four divided doses until fever subsides; the dosage is then changed to 3–5 mg/kg/day as one dose for 6–8 weeks. If small or medium coronary artery aneurysms are present aspirin is continued until they resolve; long-term therapy is indicated in those with giant aneurysms. If the child is exposed to varicella or influenza, the aspirin should be tem-

BOX 25-4 Principal diagnostic clinical criteria for Kawasaki disease

Remittent fever of 38° to 41°C (101° to 104°F), lasting longer than five days
Conjunctival infection
Oral changes: strawberry tongue, erythema of lips & oropharynx, cracked lips
Polymorphous erythematous rash
Changes in hands and feet: tense edema, diffuse erythema, desquamation
Unilateral cervical lymphadenopathy

Nursing Tip:

Administration of aspirin

Give aspirin with meals or an antacid to prevent GI upset. If flu or chickenpox is suspected in the child on aspirin it should be discontinued or changed to dipyridamole (Persantine).

porarily discontinued, and dipyridamole substituted, to minimize the risk of Reye's syndrome.

Anticoagulation with warfarin is recommended in children with giant aneurysms to prevent coronary artery thrombosis and occlusion. Those with acute coronary artery occlusion may be treated with thrombolytics such as tissue plasminogen activator or streptokinase (Tsubata, et al., 1995; Melish, 1996). Novel interventions such as percutaneous transluminal coronary angioplasty, coronary artery bypass and graft, and heart transplant have been used on select patients with severe ischemic coronary artery disease (Sugimura, et al., 1997; Checchia, Pahl, Shaddy, & Shulman, 1997; Mavroudis, et al., 1996).

Most patients do quite well if diagnosed and treated in a timely manner. The occurrence of aneurysms, most notably giant aneurysms, has decreased markedly with the use of IVIG. Currently the mortality rate is less than 1%. Long-term issues remain unsolved. The coronary arteries in patients with a history of aneurysms demonstrate abnormalities in dilation and flow (Dhillon, et al., 1996; Hamaoka & Onouchi, 1996). Giant aneurysms can become stenotic and calcified, contributing to ischemic heart disease years after the initial illness (Kato, et al., 1996). Children who have suffered from KD may be at high risk for the development of coronary artery disease as adults (Burns, et al., 1996). Longitudinal studies are ongoing to evaluate long-term sequelae in Kawasaki disease.

Nursing Management

It is recommended that children with KD be admitted to the hospital during the acute phase (days 1–10) of illness.

Nursing Alert:

Administration of Warfarin (Coumadin)

Warfarin has a multitude of drug and food interactions. Antibiotics, vitamin K, birth control pills, and soy-based formulas can all affect International Normalization Ration (INR). INR is the blood test used to determine the degree of anticoagulation present. Family education is imperative; monitoring of INR should be adjusted accordingly.

Nursing Alert:

Administration of Intravenous Immune Globulin (IVIG)

IVIG is a blood product. The nurse should be familiar with hospital guidelines prior to administration. Frequent monitoring of vital signs should occur during the first hour or two of administration. If an adverse reaction is noted (rash, fever, shaking, chills) discontinue infusion immediately and notify practitioner.

During this period close observation and assessment of cardiac status are important. Vital signs, intake and output, and daily weights are recorded. The child should be frequently assessed for signs and symptoms of CHF (see section on CHF) such as tachycardia, gallop rhythm, poor perfusion, and decreased urine output.

Guidelines for the administration of IVIG should be the same as blood product administration. Vital signs and perfusion are assessed and documented frequently according to hospital policy. Adverse reactions include hypotension, tachycardia, chills, nausea, and hypersensitivity reaction (rare). Most side effects can be minimized by slowing the rate of infusion, or with the concurrent administration of benadryl. The infusion should be discontinued and the physician notified immediately in the case of hypersensitivity.

Most nursing care is supportive, focusing on symptomatic relief. These young children are usually miserable and very irritable. The child should be cared for in a quiet, soothing environment to minimize the extreme discomfort of fever, edema, and joint pain. Timely administration of aspirin and analgesics is critically important. Lip balm, skin lotions, cool cloths, and tepid baths may provide temporary alleviation of symptoms. The parent or primary caregiver should be allowed to stay throughout the hospitalization, and the family should be included into the plan of care. Because of oral lesions soft foods and fluids should be offered frequently. Adequate fluid intake, intake and output, and calorie counts should be monitored closely. As the child improves child life therapists, occupational therapists, and physical therapists can be utilized as appropriate.

Family Teaching

Discharge planning includes family education for aspirin administration, warfarin administration if warranted, and follow-up with pediatric cardiology. Clinic appointments are best made prior to discharge from the hospital. In addition, families should be given a phone number for the cardiology clinic in case they have questions following discharge.

Infective Endocarditis

Infective endocarditis (IE) is an infection with subsequent inflammation of the heart valves and lining of the heart.

Although it is relatively uncommon it can be life-threatening. Considerable morbidity and mortality continue to result from this disease process, in spite of advances in diagnosis and treatment.

Incidence and Etiology

Absolute incidence of IE is difficult to determine. In pediatrics most children who develop endocarditis have underlying structural heart disease. Those at the highest risk are children with complex cyanotic heart disease, prosthetic cardiac valves, and a previous history of endocarditis. The second most common group of clients to develop endocarditis are critically ill infants and children with normal hearts who have multiple invasive lines and tubes. School-aged children and adolescents who are IV drug abusers are also at high risk for the development of IE. Although uncommon, previously healthy children with normal hearts can develop IE as well (Gewitz, 1997).

IE is caused by an initial **bacteremia** (bacteria in the blood) that can occur spontaneously, following an invasive procedure (dental work, GI/GU surgery, instrumentation) or be secondary to a focal infection (abscess or urinary tract infection) (Dajani, et al., 1997). The most common organisms are group A streptococci, *Staphylococcus aureus*, enterococci, and *Candida*. However, any number of infectious agents have been reported to cause endocarditis (Sandre & Shafran, 1996; AAP, 2000).

Pathophysiology

Infectious organisms enter the blood and can lodge on areas of the heart that are irregular or where there is turbulent blood flow (abnormal valves, VSD). See Box 25-5 for procedures commonly associated with bacteremia and subsequent endocarditis.

BOX 25-5 Procedures associated with infective endocarditis

- Dental work: teeth cleaning, extractions, periodontal procedures, root canal, initial placement of orthodontic bands.
- Tonsillectomy/adenoidectomy
- Rigid bronchoscopy
- Surgical procedures involving respiratory mucosa
- Esophageal stricture dilation
- Surgery involving biliary tract or intestinal mucosa
- Genitourinary tract procedures: cystoscopy, urethral dilation

Adapted from Dajani, et al. (1997). Prevention of bacterial endocarditis. Recommendations by the American Heart Association. *Journal of the American Medical Association, 277,* 1794–1801.

The invading organism will lodge and grow on the **endocardium** (serous inner membrane of the heart) forming **vegetations,** or abnormal growths, contributing to inflammation. Fibrin deposits and platelet thrombi form on the vegetations. Vegetations can break off and embolize to other parts of the body. Adjacent tissues and valves may be invaded contributing to progressive cardiac damage.

Clinical Manifestations

Early symptoms can be quite mild; sometimes the only symptom is prolonged fever. On the other end of the spectrum the child can experience an acute onset of very high fever and exhaustion. However, most symptoms are nonspecific consisting of low-grade fever, fatigue, headache, nausea, vomiting, and cyclic afternoon chills. A new or changing murmur may be noted on auscultation, particularly in a child with known structural heart disease (Del Pont, et al., 1995). Tachycardia can be seen, and, infrequently, arrhythmias or heart failure.

There are some fairly classic skin lesions seen with IE. However, these usually appear late in the illness and are seldom seen if the child is treated in a timely manner. The lesions include Osler nodes and Janeway lesions. Osler nodes are tender pea-sized nodules on the pads of the fingers and toes. Janeway lesions are small areas of hemorrhage on the soles and palms (Callow, et al., 1998).

Diagnosis

The diagnosis of IE is based on a high index of suspicion in concert with clinical and laboratory findings. The most important diagnostic tools are blood cultures and ECHO. Blood cultures are obtained immediately prior to the administration of antibiotics. Careful antiseptic preparation of the phlebotomy site will help prevent contamination of the cultures with normal skin flora. Serial cultures may need to be obtained for definitive diagnosis (Del Pont, et al., 1995). ECHO can identify the presence, location, and size of vegetations. ECHO is also helpful is predicting whether a vegetation is at risk for embolization.

Treatment

Prevention is the best treatment of IE. The American Heart Association (AHA, 1999) has set forth guidelines for antibiotic prophylaxis of children with congenital heart disease (Dajani, et al., 1997; Gewitz, 1997). Cardiac conditions at the highest risk for IE include complex cyanotic lesions and prosthetic valves. Those at the lowest risk include isolated secundum ASD and mitral valve prolapse without regurgitation (Box 25-6). Prophylaxis is recommended prior to those procedures associated with endocarditis. Amoxicillin is the primary drug used for prophylaxis; for those children with penicillin allergies clindamycin is used. For dosage recommendations see Box 25-7.

In those individuals who have documented endocarditis, antibiotic treatment should be instituted immediately (after

BOX 25-6 Cardiac conditions associated with infective endocarditis

Prophylaxis Recommended

High risk category
- Prosthetic cardiac valves
- Previous history of infective endocarditis
- Complex cyanotic heart disease (TGA, TOF, TA, HLHS)
- Surgically constructed arterial to pulmonary shunts (BT shunt)

Moderate risk category
- Acquired rheumatic valvar disease
- Hypertrophic cardiomyopathy
- Mitral valve prolapse with regurgitation

Prophylaxis Not Recommended (Risk is no greater than general population)
- Isolated secundum ASD
- Surgical repair of ASD, PDA without residual shunt six months after surgery
- Mitral valve prolapse without regurgitation
- Innocent murmurs
- Previous history of rheumatic fever without heart involvement
- Isolated cardiac pacemakers without structural heart disease

Adapted from Dajani, et al. (1997). Prevention of bacterial endocarditis. Recommendations by the American Heart Association. *Journal of the American Medical Association, 277,* 1794–1801.

BOX 25-7 Prophylactic regimens for dental, oral, respiratory, and esophageal procedures

Amoxicillin	50 mg/kg up to the adult dose of 2 grams taken orally one hour prior to procedure.
Ampicillin	50 mg/kg up to adult dose of 2 grams IV 30 minutes prior to procedure.
Clindamycin	20 mg/kg up to adult dose of 600 mg orally one hour prior to procedure, or 20 mg/kg up to adult dose of 600 mg IV 30 minutes prior to procedure.

*A second dose six hours after the procedure is no longer required. If the preprocedure dose is missed it can be given within two hours after the procedure to infer some protection. Pediatric dose should not exceed adult dose. Cephalosporins (cephalexin, cefadroxil, cefaxolin) can be used in select patients who do not have hypersensitivy reactions to penicillin.

Adapted from Dajani, et al. (1997). Prevention of bacterial endocarditis. Recommendations by the American Heart Association. *Journal of the American Medical Association, 277,* 1794–1801.

appropriate blood cultures have been obtained). The most frequently used antibiotic is penicillin, however antibiotic therapy is determined by the causative organism and its sensitivity to antibiotic therapy. The course is 4–6 weeks of intravenous drug therapy. Amphotericin B is administered to treat fungal endocarditis.

Rarely, surgical intervention is undertaken to replace severely abnormal leaking valves. The ideal is to provide antibiotic administration for as long as possible prior to surgery. Active infection (persistent positive blood cultures) is a contraindication for surgery.

If preprocedural antibiotic prophylaxis is instituted appropriately, the incidence of endocarditis will remain low. Unfortunately, IE is difficult to treat, and mortality can be as high as 20% (Sandre & Shafran, 1996). Morbidity in the form of persistent valvar disease can be as high as 50%. Clearly the best intervention is prevention.

Nursing Management

It is imperative that the nurse caring for the child with suspected IE obtain blood cultures and institute antibiotic therapy in a timely manner. Early treatment is critically important to improving outcomes. Because of the need for long-term intravenous therapy a percutaneous peripherally inserted catheter (PICC line) should be inserted early in the hospitalization. These are small (2.0–4.0 french) silastic catheters that can be left in place long-term (weeks to months), have low risk for infection, and allow for client mobility. It is very important that antibiotic doses are *not missed*. Therefore, if intravenous access is interrupted, a new line is inserted immediately. Bedrest is implemented early in the illness. Quiet diversional activities (video games, board games, books) are offered at age-appropriate levels. If CHF is present, it is treated appropriately (see section on CHF).

Family Teaching

Family education regarding the need for endocarditis prophylaxis is done when the initial diagnosis of congenital heart disease is made. Follow-up reinforcement is mandatory. It has been demonstrated that many children and adults with congenital heart disease have inadequate knowledge of endocarditis prophylaxis (Cetta & Warnes, 1995). The AHA has developed wallet-sized cards for individual use. These should be given to every child requiring prophylaxis.

In the child who has contracted endocarditis the family and child should be educated regarding the treatment plan, including the need for prolonged hospitalization and intravenous antibiotic therapy. Reinforcement of AHA recommendations for prophylaxis should be made prior to discharge in children with congenital defects.

HYPERTENSION

Hypertension is defined as systolic and/or diastolic blood pressure equal to or greater than the 95th percentile for age, sex, and height on at least three separate occasions. High normal or borderline BP elevation is defined as systolic and/or diastolic BP between the 90th and 95th percentile for age, sex, and height. Normal BP is defined as systolic and diastolic BP below the 90th percentile for age, sex, and height (National High Blood Pressure Education Program [NHBPEP], 1996) (see Chapter 14 for tables of norms). Although clinical hypertension occurs less frequently in children than adults, evidence is accumulating that the roots of essential hypertension extend back to childhood. Children and adolescents whose BPs are in the upper percentiles are more likely to become young adults who have elevated BP, which is asociated with an increased risk of cardiovascualr disease morbidity and mortality (Daniels, 1997).

Incidence and Etiology (Pathophysiology)

The incidence (and prevalence) of hypertension in childhood is low, only about 1%. African-Americans and Asians have higher BP levels than whites (NHBPEP, 1996).

When no known underlying disease is present, hypertension is referred to as primary or essential. When the cause of the elevated BP can be explained by an associated disease, hypertension is referred to as secondary. In infants and young children below 6 years of age, secondary hypertension is more common than primary hypertension. The main causes are renal diseases, followed by cardiovascular (coarctation of the aorta), endocrine, and some neurologic disorders. After age 6 years, primary hypertension is the more common type.

Many factors play a role in the development of primary hypertension. These include heredity, obesity, stress, smoking, physical activity, and salt intake. Most children and adolescents with BP measurements exceeding the 95th percentile are overweight and have family histories of hypertension.

Clinical Manifestations

Most children and adolescents with primary hypertension are asymtomatic until the BP elevation is detected, usually during a routine examination or during physical evaluation prior to athletic participation. These individuals tend to have mild elevation in BP and are somewhat overweight. Children with secondary hypertension will usually not have symptoms unless BP has been sustained or is rising rapidly. However, with substantial elevation headache, dizziness, changes in vision, and seizures may occur. Infants and young children cannot communicate symptoms such as a headache so observation of their behavior may provide clues. However, their behavior may not be considered abnormal until complications of hypertension are present. In retrospect, many caregivers report that their child had become increasingly irritable before the hypertension was detected (Pruitt, 1996).

Diagnosis

Elevated BP must be confirmed on repeated visits before characterizing an individual as having hypertension. In general, the younger the individual, the higher the level of BP, the presence of symptoms, and the less family history of hypertension, the more likely it is that the child has secondary hypertension. The diagnostic evaluation for children whose history or physical examination suggests a specific cause of hypertenion should be guided by the suspected problem, initially focusing on the renal system (Daniels, 1997). Physical examination should determine the presence of flank masses. Screening tests should include CBC, serum electrolytes, urinalysis, blood urea nitrogen (BUN), serum creatinine, and uric acid. Renal ultrasonography may be useful to evaluate structural renal abnormalities. Diminished femoral pulses suggest the presence of coarctation of the aorta, and measurement of BP in the legs should be performed to determine if it is substantially lower than in the arms. Imaging studies such as echocardiography should be obtained on these children.

Children suspected of having primary hypertension require few diagnostic tests other than a urinalysis and blood profiles to examine serum creatinine. A lipid profile may provide useful information as many overweight children and adolescents with hypertension have elevated triglycerides and low high-density lipoprotein (HDL) cholesterol and high low-density liproprotein (LDL) cholesterol.

Treatment

Both nonpharmacologic and pharmacologic approaches to treatment are useful in managing children and adolescents with hypertension. Nonpharmacologic therapy includes weight reduction, dietary intervention, and exercise. This approach should be used not only with individuals with hypertension but also in children with high-normal BPs (90th to 95th percentile BP distribution) and those with severe hypertension to complement drug therapy. If the child is obese, efforts should be directed at reducing obesity by lowering excessive calorie intake and increasing physical exercise. Dietary intervention includes ingestion of a low-fat, high-fiber diet with an increase in fresh fruits and vegetables, and elimination of foods high in sodium and salt added to foods. Increased physical exercise, especailly aerobic exercise, and sports participation help with weight reduction and stress management.

Because of the lack of data on drug therapy outcomes in children, guidelines for treatment are conservative. Children with mild hypertension should include lifestyle changes such as weight reduction and physical activity. For those with secondary hypertension treatment should focus on the underlying cause. Drug therapy is considered for children with significant elevation of BP that has not responded to lifestyle changes. When drugs are used, the goals are to reduce BP to below the 95th percentile (NHBPEP, 1996). The oral antihypertensive drugs used most often in children include diuretics, beta blockers such as propranolol (Inderal), angiotensin-converting enzyme inhibitors such as captopril (Capoten) and enalapril (Vasotec), and calcium channel blockers such as nifedipine (Adalat).

Nursing Management and Family Teaching

The nurse focuses on teaching the child and family and supporting them in adhering to the treatment plan. Education about lifestyle habits and changes such as diet, exercise, weight control, and attitudes about smoking should include the entire family. When all members paritcipate in any of the treatment strategies, lifestyle changes tend to be more consistent and long-lasting and the child's compliance is likely to be greater. An exercise program should include physical activities the child likes. School-aged children and adolescents may prefer team sports rather than solitary activities such as running, swimming, and bicycling. Praise and encouragement for even minor changes are important for motivation to continue to follow the prescribed program. Blood pressure measurements should be performed as part of all routine physical examinations on all children older than 3 years of age. Baseline and serial measurement need to be documented in the child's record.

HEART TRANSPLANTATION

Heart transplantation is the process by which a failing heart is removed from a recipient and replaced with a functional heart from a brain dead donor. While heart transplantation offers a chance for reasonable quality of life for the recipient it must be remembered that this procedure is not a cure, but a palliation and with it come a host of potential and real complications. Heart transplantation is a lifelong commitment for the child and family.

Indications

Heart transplantation is indicated in children with heart failure who have a significant decrease in their quality of life related to their heart failure. It is also indicated in those who have failed medical management or would otherwise not survive for more than 1–2 years (Wong & Starnes, 1998). Unfortunately, not all clients are deemed physically or emotionally capable of withstanding the lifelong issues associated with transplantation.

There are two major groups in whom heart transplant is indicated. The first group are individuals with dilated cardiomyopathy, and the second group are those children with complex congenital heart disease. HLHS is the leading indication for heart transplantation in the infant population. Dilated cardiomyopathy is the most common cause in children over the age of one year (Boucek, et al., 1997). Dilated cardiomyopathy can be caused by a number of etiologies (ischemia, familial conditions, or viral infections) that result in a thin-walled poorly contractile ventricle. Contraindications to transplantation include malignancy, serious infection, or systemic disease such as diabetes. Psychosocial instability within the family may preclude heart transplantation because of inability to follow the lifelong treatment plan.

Transplant Listing

Once the extensive pretransplant work up has been completed, the child is listed with the United Network for Organ Sharing. This is a national organization that oversees transplant activity. Children are listed by their blood type and weight and are prioritized according to their severity of illness.

The waiting period can be a very stressful time for both the child and the family. Relocation may be necessary so the family will be in closer proximity to the transplant center. This can result in major disruption for the whole family. The waiting period may be quite extensive and the possibility exists that the child may die before a donor organ becomes available.

Surgical Process

When a child has been declared brain dead, he or she is considered a potential organ donor. If the donor family agrees to organ donation the local transplant organization is notified. A member of the organization will evaluate the donor to determine if he or she is suitable for organ donation. Donor organs are removed in the operating room by the procurement team. Once the donor heart has been removed the maximum time before re-implantation into the recipient should be less than 6–8 hours to prevent cardiac dysfunction. The recipient's heart is explanted and the donor heart is implanted into the recipient.

Posttransplant Issues

Postoperative complications include decreased cardiac function, rejection, and infection. Cardiac function is supported by medications to improve cardiac output (refer to Table 25-3) The new heart is perceived by the recipient's immune system as foreign, stimulating the immune system that results in rejection. Therefore, the use of anti-rejection medications is the mainstay of therapy for the heart transplant recipient.

Reflective Thinking

What Is It Like for the Nurse Caring for the Child Awaiting Heart Transplant?

Once a child has been listed for heart transplantation the family and the child begin a long process of waiting and hoping. Will a donor heart become available in time? This waiting period can similarly be very stressful and emotional for the nurse caring for the client. It is not unusual for the pediatric nursing staff to get to know the client and family quite well, especially when the child has a chronic condition.

W. H. is an 11-year-old female admitted to the PICU with heart failure. Her diagnosis includes TGA, palliated with a **Mustard procedure** (intra-atrial baffling) during infancy. She had done well until 6 months ago, at which time she became more tired and unable to keep up with her peers. Echocardiagram demonstrated a dilated RV and very poor RV function. Despite maximal medical therapy her heart failure is worsening and she has been listed for heart transplant. On the day of admission she is pale, nauseated, short of breath, and not anything like the little girl the staff was so familiar with. She is started on dobutamine in the hope of improving cardiac output. She is listed as Status I for heart transplant.

The waiting game now begins for this child, her family, and the staff. As the days go by the staff find themselves getting closer to this child. She feels better on inotropic support so is easily engaged in games and schoolwork. What could be wrong with this picture? The reality is that the girl, the family, and the staff are all waiting for another child to die so that W.H. can have her chance to live. There is even talk that it is summer time and the number of accidents increases during this time. Will this make it easier for her to get a heart?

Down at the other end of the PICU an 8-year-old boy has been admitted after being hit by a car. He has suffered a severe head injury with dismal hope for recovery. His devastated family is holding on for any hope of recovery. The nurses caring for this child are dealing with the emotions of the family and the reality that this child will not survive. Once he has been declared brain dead the parents are left to grieve, reconcile his death, and ask themselves if their son should be an organ donor.

W.H. received this little boy's heart and has done very well to this point. Nurses in these situations must be prepared to deal with a wide range of emotions themselves as well as be supportive of the families they care for. Nurses must be nonjudgmental toward families that do not believe in or support organ donation. This can be very difficult when we have so many waiting for this special gift. The nurse must be able to answer these very personal questions when faced with this situation.

1. How will confidentiality be maintained when both the donor and the recipient families are in the same unit?
2. How do you feel when caring for a child that is brain dead? Do you alter your level of care? Do you continue to talk to him/her as if he/she can hear you?
3. Do you have religious or personal beliefs for or against transplantation?
4. How do you feel about organ donation?
5. Can you respect the wishes of both families even if they are not consistent with your views?

Despite the initiation of anti-rejection medications such as cyclosporin and FK503 (Prograf) in the immediate postoperative period, rejection does occur and is the leading cause of death during the first 6–12 months posttransplant. Acute rejection is seen in the first few days while chronic rejection is seen after months and years (Wong & Starnes, 1998). Signs and symptoms of rejection are unfortunately subtle and often nonspecific. Clients can have fever, tachycardia, arrhythmias, hypotension, shortness of breath, and irritability. Because of the nonspecific nature of the signs of rejection, routine heart biopsies are scheduled to monitor for rejection.

All clients receiving immunosuppressive medications are at increased risk for infection. Strict handwashing is essential before contact with these children. Prophylactic medications are given to prevent infections from organisms such as CMV, **Pneumocystis carinii,** and **Candida** infections. Acyclovir, trimethoprim/sulfamethoxazole (Septra) and nystatin are used respectively to prevent the above infections. Fevers are treated aggressively.

Long-term complications include the development of coronary artery disease requiring re-transplantation, poor growth and development secondary to steroids, and lymphoproliferative disease (LPD). LPD is a form of cancer that can occur in any type of solid organ transplant. Mortality for heart transplantation is 15–20% in the first 30 days. Survival at one year is approximately 75–80% and at five years it is approximately 60–75% (Boucek, et al., 1997; Morrow, et al., 1997). Outcomes for those awaiting heart transplant is suboptimal. Approximately 24% of patients listed for a heart transplant will die waiting for a donor to become available (Davenport, 1995).

Heart transplantation is a viable palliation for the failing heart that may provide the recipient with years of quality life. The major roadblock to transplantation at this time is the lack of available organs to meet the needs of the listed recipients. As members of the health profession we must examine our own feelings regarding transplantation and let our families and loved ones know how we feel. Many nurses will find themselves taking care of both potential organ donors and children who need organs at some time during their careers. In dealing with families who are faced with the question of whether or not to donate their child's organs we must be nonjudgmental and supportive. Education regarding the process of transplantation for both medical and nonmedical people must continue if we are to decrease the number of individuals that will die before an organ becomes available.

Family Teaching

It cannot be emphasized enough that transplantation is a lifetime commitment. The child must remain on anti-rejection medications for his or her entire life. Lifetime follow-up is necessary to identify noncompliance and complications in a timely manner. Immunizations should be administered as scheduled, but no live viruses are to be given. Large crowds should be avoided for the first several months after transplant and children are permitted back in school approximately six months after successful transplant. Children who are still at home should always be encouraged to participate in school assignments and home education. Community resources that can be utilized include home schooling and home nursing visits to minimize exposure to infection. Many communities have heart transplant support groups that are helpful to both the child and caregivers.

Once the child returns to school, the teachers should be apprised of the treatment regimen and any precautions. The medications are taken frequently throughout the day so assistance from the school is imperative. If any child in the class comes down with varicella the family of the transplant client should be notified immediately. During periods of seasonal illness it may be beneficial for the child to be home schooled to prevent infection secondary to immunosuppression.

CARDIAC ARRHYTHMIAS

A number of children with acquired or congenital heart disease can develop cardiac arrhythmias. Many cardiac rhythm abnormalities in children are not life-threatening; however, some require close monitoring and treatment. It must be remembered that several important differences exist between children and adults, although they may have the same rhythm abnormality. Although an in-depth review of EKG interpretation is beyond the scope of this text, a brief review is warranted.

The P wave correlates with atrial depolarization and the QRS with ventricular depolarization. The PR interval is the time it takes an electrical impulse to travel from the normal pacemaker of the heart (SA node) to the AV node. The QT interval represents ventricular repolarization. Every normal beat should have a P wave before every QRS and the rhythm should be regular. Heart rates are faster in infants and children. PR interval and QRS duration are generally shorter and increase with age as the heart rate slows.

Many arrhythmias are caused by the conduction system changes that occur as a consequence of heart surgery, and may not be appreciated until adolescence. Early postoperative arrhythmias may be transient, resolving in the first few weeks after surgery. The following is a discussion of the more significant arrhythmias found in infants and children.

Supraventricular Tachycardia

Supraventricular tachycardia (SVT) is the most common arrhythmia seen in infants and children. It usually occurs in the presence of a structurally normal heart; however, it can occur in individuals with congenital heart disease. Up to 50% of children who present with this rhythm are less than four months of age (Etheridge & Judd, 1999). Half of all infants who develop this in the first few months of life will outgrow it by one year of age. The other most common period for the occurrence of SVT is during adolescence. SVT is characterized as a narrow QRS tachycardia that is abrupt in onset and termination (Figure 25-26). Heart rates in infants can be as high as 300 beats per minute, older children are >220 beats per minutes. Although this arrhythmia is not life-threatening it can cause significant symptoms (Deal, 1998).

Presentation is quite variable. Some children will have infrequent episodes that terminate spontaneously. Others

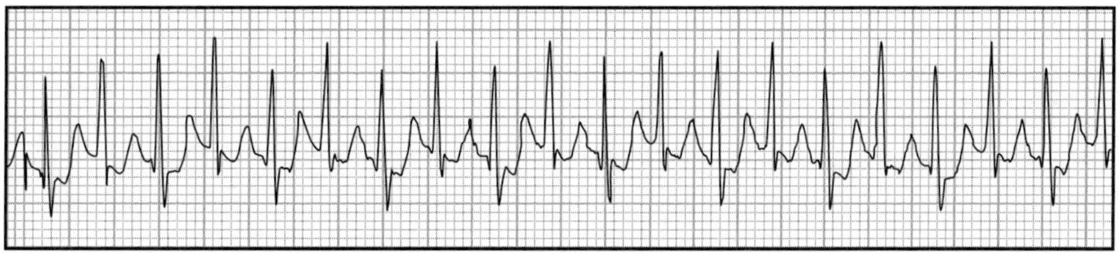

Figure 25-26 Supraventricular Tachycardia in a 12-Year-Old Boy. Heart rate is 240.

can have incessant tachycardia that is difficult to treat. Symptoms in infants are nonspecific, so frequently this diagnosis is initially missed. Symptoms include poor feeding, irritability, fussiness, and pallor. If SVT persists then cardiac failure will ensue. Once the tachycardia is terminated cardiac function returns to normal.

Older children can often identify the sudden onset of SVT. Therefore, intervention is much more timely. SVT can produce chest pain and dizziness, and syncope rarely occurs. SVT is sudden in onset and termination. It is often not associated with any specific activity, and can occur at rest or with exercise.

Diagnosis is made by EKG while the patient is in SVT. The decision to treat SVT is determined by client choice (in that SVT episodes are frequent and interfere with lifestyle), syncope associated with SVT, or presence of structural heart disease (Deal, 1998).

Initial maneuvers to treat SVT are quite simple in the stable child. Vagal maneuvers are quite successful in terminating tachycardia if implemented shortly after onset. These include valsalva maneuver (holding their breath and then bearing down), headstand for a few minutes, or placing their face in a tub of ice water for as long as tolerated. Application of an ice bag to the face of an infant is often successful in tachycardia termination. Care must be taken to avoid prolonged application of the ice bag to prevent fat necrosis from profound vasoconstriction (Craig, Schloz, Vanderhooft, & Etheridge, 1998).

If vagal maneuvers are not successful in tachycardia termination, or if the tachycardia does not terminate spontaneously, then the child should be taken to the nearest emergency room for treatment. The first line intervention for hard-to-treat SVT is intravenous adenosine. This medication blocks conduction at the AV node for 10–15 seconds, thus terminating the rhythm. Although transient, there can be a short period of asystole following administration (Figure 25-27). This can make the child lightheaded without loss of consciousness. Other side effects include a tightness in the chest and difficulty breathing. All symptoms are very transient. The child should be warned ahead of time of the effects of adenosine to prevent undue anxiety.

Infrequently a child will develop re-onset of SVT after termination with adenosine, or the child may have frequent episodes that interfere with lifestyle. In these situations, chronic therapy can be implemented. Medications used to treat SVT include beta blockers (propranolol, atenolol), procainamide, or amiodarone. All have different mechanisms of action and different side effects. The nurse should become familiar with both when administering these medications.

Acute management for unstable children who do not respond to adenosine includes overdrive pacing or **synchronized cardioversion.** For overdrive pacing esophageal pacing is utilized. A special pacing electrode is passed down the esophagus to the level of the heart. Short bursts of rapid pacing, faster than the tachycardia rate, are applied. This maneuver can break the tachycardia and is the most effective treatment in younger children.

Synchronized cardioversion uses the defibrillator to produce an electrical shock to convert the arrhythmia to sinus rhythm. Prior to cardioversion the child must be NPO for 4–6 hours and *must be well sedated,* as this is *very* painful. Following the procedure the nurse should document the subsequent rhythm with an EKG. Overall outcomes are very good with SVT. Many infants will have no recurrence of SVT after the first year of life. A number of older children learn to terminate their tachycardia without pharmacologic intervention by vagal maneuvers as previously discussed.

Complete Heart Block (CHB)

Complete heart block can be either acquired or congenital. CHB is diagnosed on EKG. There is no conduction through

Nursing Alert:

How to Safely Perform Cardioversion

The nurse must be familiar with the defibrillator prior to use. The child is placed on the defibrillator EKG; a consistent upright R wave must be present on the EKG. The "synch" button must be on, and the nurse must assess for the synch mark on the R wave. Usual output for synchronized cardioversion is $^1/_2$–1 joule/kg. Multifunction pads are recommended rather than the paddles, as these allow for pacing in cases of asystole. Prior to discharge make sure no one is touching the child or the bed, and shout "clear" prior to discharge.

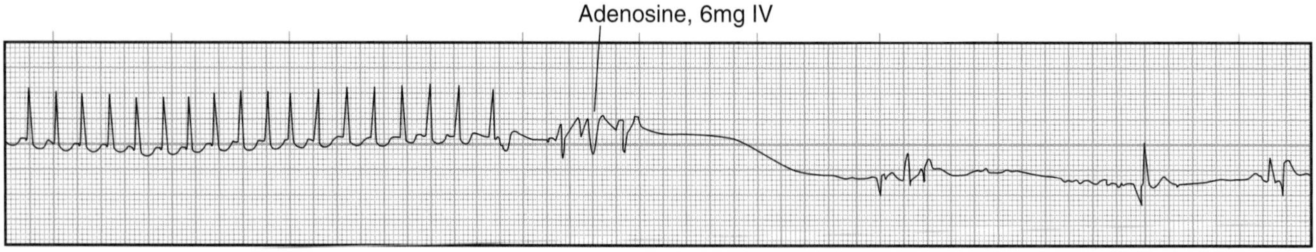

Figure 25-27 Cardioversion of SVT to Normal Sinus Rhythm with IV Adenosine; Note Long Pause of Heart Block.

the AV node so there is complete atrial and ventricular dissociation, and the atrial rate is much faster than the ventricular rate (Figure 25-28).

Acquired heart block can be secondary to myocarditis, endocarditis, or cardiac surgery. Congenital heart block is diagnosed in utero on fetal echocardiogram or in the immediate neonatal period. The most common reason for congenital heart block is maternal systemic lupus erythematosus. Other maternal connective tissue diseases can cause heart block as well.

The treatment for heart block is a permanent pacemaker. The need for a pacemaker in congenital heart block is determined by the child's resting heart rate, presence of symptoms, CHF, or ventricular arrhythmias. Heart rates lower than 55 when awake are associated with increased risk for death. Children with syncope, dizziness, PVCs, or VT also require a pacemaker (Friedman, et al., 1995). Without a permanent pacemaker the mortality rate is estimated to be 5%. Long-term sequelae include CHF and mitral regurgitation. Once a pacemaker is implanted, and sinus rhythm is restored, outcome is excellent. The pacemaker system consists of leads attached to the heart and a generator. The generator contains the battery and the microcircuitry needed to

Nursing Tip:

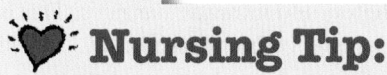

Education of the child and family with a pacemaker

The child should avoid competitive contact sports. Normal childhood play and rough-housing is unavoidable, and the child should not be restricted unnecessarily. Microwave ovens are safe. Cell phones are used on the side opposite the generator. A child with a pacemaker can *never* have an MRI scan. Some anti-theft devices interfere with pacemaker function. If the child feels abnormal heart beats or dizzy when near any of these devices, he or she should leave the area immediately. A distance of 10–15 feet away from any interfering device is sufficient.

Kids Want To Know

Life with a Pacemaker

1. What can I do after I get my pacemaker?
   - The only restrictions are no contact sports (tackle football, ice hockey, karate).
   - Other competitive and recreational sports are safe.
   - No scuba diving deeper than 100 feet.
2. What equipment is dangerous for a pacemaker?
   - Microwave ovens are safe.
   - Cell phones should be used on the side opposite where the generator has been implanted.
   - No arc welding, as this interferes with pacemaker function.
   - Some anti-theft devices and metal detectors can temporarily affect pacemaker function; avoid these if possible or pass through detectors quickly.
   - No MRI scans.
   - Avoid being around large electric generators (power plants).
3. Can the pacemaker ever be turned off by accident?
   - No. Although some of the equipment mentioned above can temporarily affect function or set the pacemaker to the default settings, it will never be turned off. If you feel like your pacemaker is not working right or your heart rate is too slow, leave the area immediately. This should rectify the problem. If you still feel bad call your health care provider immediately.
4. How long does the battery in the generator last?
   - 2–10 years, depending on how much you use the pacemaker.
5. How do you change the battery?
   - The battery is not changed like you would a flashlight; it is sealed into the generator so the whole generator must be changed when the battery gets low.
6. How can you tell when the battery is low?
   - At your clinic visits your health care provider will check the pacemaker and find out how much voltage is left.

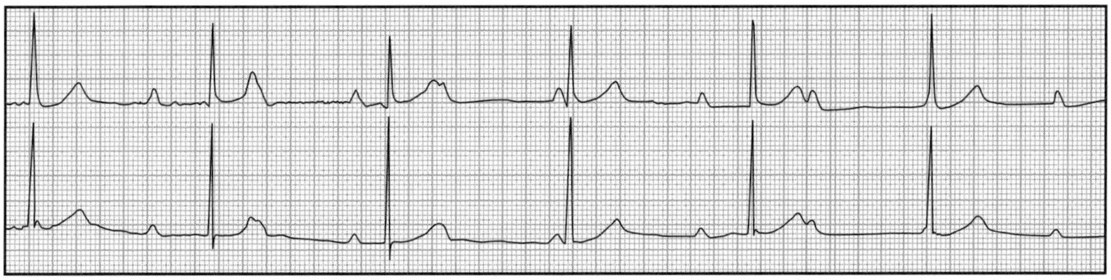

Figure 25-28 Complete Heart Block in a 14-Year-Old Girl. Atrial rate is 65. There is complete atrial and ventricular dissociation; ventricular rate is 39.

pace the heart. The generator is changed when the battery voltage is low.

Nursing Management

The care of the child with arrhythmias can be challenging for the nurse. Most rhythm abnormalities are not life-threatening. The nurse should become familiar with the identification and treatment of life-threatening arrhythmias. First and foremost hemodynamic status is assessed in any child who is experiencing an arrhythmia. Check for BP, pulses, perfusion, and level of consciousness. If the child is unstable, get help immediately and institute resuscitative measures. If the child is in cardiac arrest start CPR.

If the individual is stable obtain BP and assess perfusion. Obtain a rhythm strip or EKG of any rhythm abnormality to document in the chart. An EKG will help to finalize the diagnosis. Treatment depends on the underlying etiology and type of rhythm abnormality.

SHOCK

Shock is present when there is significant cardiovascular dysfunction leading to inadequate oxygen delivery and perfusion of vital organs. This results in anaerobic metabolism and production of lactic acid. If left untreated the final pathway will be cell destruction, multi-organ system failure, and death. Because of the morbidity and mortality of untreated or inadequately treated shock in the pediatric population it is essential that clinicians caring for these children learn to recognize the early signs and symptoms of impending shock. Early and aggressive management is likely to improve outcome and survival.

Generally shock can be divided into three major classifications: *hypovolemic*, *distributive*, and *cardiogenic*. Hypovolemic shock is secondary to intravascular volume loss. Distributive shock is a **maldistribution** of blood flow secondary to vasomotor instability or capillary leak. Cardiogenic shock is caused by cardiac pump dysfunction. When providing therapy for shock of any form all caretakers must remember to follow the principles of basic life support and the ABCs of resuscitation. These include airway, breathing, and circulation. Only then should one proceed to more specific treatment of the child in shock.

Incidence and Etiology

Hypovolemic shock is by far the most common form of shock in the pediatric population. In developing nations, hypovolemic shock continues to claim millions of lives secondary to illnesses leading to severe diarrhea. In the United States this trend has decreased in the last 30 years because of many factors; these include early recognition and aggressive fluid management in sick children. The etiology of hypovolemic shock varies. Box 25-8 lists the common causes.

In the general pediatric population, the most common cause of fluid and electrolyte loss is gastroenteritis. This is associated with vomiting, diarrhea, and inadequate oral intake with concomitant ongoing losses. Severe diarrhea leading to hypovolemic shock is a major cause of death in emerging countries (Thomas & Carcillo, 1998). Traumatic injury and hemorrhage is another cause of hypovolemic shock in children. The incidence of liver and/or spleen lacerations is significant in trauma clients. Large amounts of blood can also be lost from long bone fractures and deep lacerations (Morgan & O'Neill, 1998). Intracranial hemorrhages from subdural hematomas in the neonate and newborn, such as those associated with shaken baby syndrome, can also cause significant blood loss. Plasma losses from extensive burns can quickly lead to shock as intravascular fluid leaks into the damaged tissues. Sepsis will also lead to extensive plasma loss or "capillary leak" of fluid into the extravascular space.

The most common cause of distributive shock is sepsis, generally caused by systemic infection from a variety of bacteria, viruses, or fungi. The incidence of sepsis in the hospitalized child is much higher than the general population. These children are at increased risk from nosocomial infection from indwelling catheters and intravascular lines. This is particularly true for the immunocompromised or critically ill child. Anaphylactic shock is another form of distributive shock and is caused by the exposure of an allergic individual to a specific antigen. As this individual is exposed to an anti-

BOX 25-8 Common causes of hypovolemic shock

Fluid and electrolyte losses
- Vomiting
- Diarrhea
- Excessive use of diuretics
- Heat stroke
- Inadequate water

Hemorrhage
- Trauma
- Surgical blood loss
- Fractures

Plasma Losses
- Burns
- Sepsis
- Intestinal obstruction

Endocrine
- Diabetes mellitus
- Diabetes insipidus

gen (food, medication, insect bite) the antigen-antibody response causes massive vasomotor tone abnormalities and widespread vasodilation.

Major causes of cardiogenic shock include pre-existing congenital heart disease, cardiomyopathy, myocarditis, arrhythmias, and drug toxicity. Cardiogenic shock is seen less frequently in children than other forms of shock.

Pathophysiology

Although specific etiologies can vary, there are a number of common pathophysiological phenomena found in all children suffering from shock. A decrease in intravascular volume leads to a decrease in venous return to the heart with a subsequent fall in preload. This will lead to inadequate cardiac output. The normal compensatory mechanism is to increase heart rate. Therefore an early sign of shock is tachycardia. Anti-diuretic hormone is released by the hypothalamus to facilitate the reabsorption of free water by the kidney in a compensatory attempt to increase intravascular volume.

If infection or inflammation is present then subsequent release of toxins produces a decrease in sympathetic tone with resulting vasodilation and a decrease in systemic vascular resistance (SVR). Endothelial damage also occurs leading to the leaking of fluid from the intravascular to the interstitial space. This is known as capillary leak syndrome and can be a source of significant fluid loss internally. The initial response to vasodilation and decreased SVR is an increase in cardiac output to support blood pressure. Excessive vasodilation leads to a relative hypovolemia and hypotension.

In distributive shock the child may develop disseminated intravascular coagulopathy (DIC) secondary to the inflammatory process. DIC is an abnormal response of the clotting system leading to prolonged and inappropriate clotting. This is often seen as petechiae, small purplish hemorrhagic spots on the skin, and bleeding from IV sites and puncture wounds.

Ventricular pump dysfunction is frequently seen and is caused by a number of etiologies (structural heart disease, myocarditis, ischemia, or inflammatory mediators of septic shock). Contractility is depressed so cardiac output falls. This phenomena triggers sympathetic activation and the renin-angiotension-aldosterone system previously discussed in the section on congestive heart failure.

If cardiac output remains low, oxygen delivery to the tissues will decrease. This will result in conversion of metabolism from aerobic to anaerobic with ensuing metabolic acidosis. The lungs will attempt to compensate for metabolic acidosis by increasing the respiratory rate to exhale CO_2, so respiratory alkalosis may develop as well. If left untreated, metabolic acidosis will depress myocardial function. Therefore cardiac output decreases further, and compensatory mechanisms fail resulting in cardiovascular collapse and death.

Nursing Alert:

One of the hallmarks of septic shock *is* severe hypotension *in the face of increased cardiac output. Frequently it is the diastolic blood pressure that is most affected secondary to vasodilation. Therefore, a low diastolic pressure and wide pulse pressure is seen.*

Clinical Manifestations

Cardiovascular signs are often the most prominent. Poor perfusion will manifest as cool extremities, diminished or absent distal pulses (radial, dorsalis pedis), a capillary filling time of greater than three seconds, and mottling of the skin. Blood flow shunted away from the skin will cause extensive mottling of the extremities and eventually the trunk. However, in distributive shock skin will be warm and flushed because of intense vasodilation. Tachycardia and tachypnea are common in the child with early shock. Blood pressure should be measured. Although, because of compensatory mechanisms, blood pressure can be normal until the child deteriorates. Children can have a 30–40% reduction in intravascular volume before there is a notable decrease in BP (Chameides & Hazinski, 1997).

From a respiratory standpoint the child initially will be mildly tachypneic with a minimal need for supplemental oxygen. As acidosis worsens, work of breathing will increase. Increased work of breathing is manifested by increased respiratory rate, retractions, and nasal flaring. Neurologically, the child in early shock may be irritable and hard to console. In the face of shock, compensatory mechanisms will attempt to deliver oxygen to the brain; therefore, the development of lethargy is a ominous sign. Clients with anaphylactic shock often present with severe hypotension immediately after exposure to an antigen. Often the child will develop urticaria (hives), have swollen lips, and develop respiratory difficulties secondary to airway swelling.

Diagnosis

The diagnosis is based on clinical findings, history of preceding illness, and results of diagnostic tests. Laboratory studies

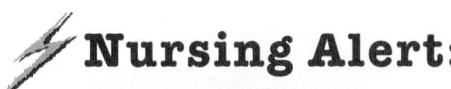

Nursing Alert:

Blood Pressure in Shock

A fall in blood pressure is a very late sign of shock. Do not be falsely reassured by a child who appears ill but has a normal BP.

Critical Thinking

The Three Types of Shock

Compare the pathophysiology and clinical manifestations of all three types of shock. Identify similarities for all three and identify appropriate interventions. Then identify specific interventions that are unique to each type of shock.

including complete blood count, electrolytes, blood gases, and blood cultures are commonly obtained. Chest X ray is obtained to evaluate heart size. In a child with hypovolemia the heart silhouette will be quite small and narrow. If the heart is larger than normal (**cardiomegaly**), the concern of cardiogenic shock must be ascertained. Echocardiogram can evaluate cardiac size and function.

Treatment

Early recognition and therapy can make the difference in the survival of the child with shock. Clients should be treated with supplemental oxygen via nasal cannula or oxygen mask. If the child's respiratory status has deteriorated to the point that he or she is unable to support him or herself, endotracheal intubation and mechanical ventilation must be initiated.

Once the airway is established, management is directed toward volume replacement, particularly in hypovolemic and septic shock. Intravenous lines are placed in any number of locations in the infant and child. For rapid fluid resuscitation a large bore, short catheter is preferable to small scalp or extremity IV. If perfusion is very poor, a femoral or subclavian line may be required as peripheral veins may be difficult to visualize and palpate in the child with shock. In the severely ill child intraosseous (IO) access may be necessary to save the child's life. In this case a special needle is placed in the anterior surface of the tibia 1–3 cm below the tibial tuberosity (Figure 25-29). Fluid and medications may be administered through an IO line. Fluid replacement begins with a minimum of 20 cc/kg of crystalloid fluid such as lactated Ringer's or normal saline (Tobias, 1996). Dextrose containing fluids are *initially avoided* as a rapid increase in the glucose level may lead to an osmotic diuresis, further complicating the hypovolemic state. If the child is a trauma victim and blood loss is documented it must be replaced. This is usually in the form of whole blood or packed red blood cells. Normal saline or lactated Ringer's is given until blood is available. Until proper typing and crossmatching can be performed O negative blood (universal donor) should be given. Therapy for the hypovolemic client continues with ongoing and frequent reassessment of initial clinical signs. Fluid boluses are repeated if perfusion does not improve. It is not unusual for the child in hypovolemic shock to require up to 100 cc/kg of fluid to improve cardiac output and perfusion. The clinician must also be vigilant in assessing any ongoing losses (i.e., bleeding, vomiting, diarrhea, chest tube drainage) that have not been controlled.

Once adequate volume resuscitation has been provided, inotropic support may be indicated for the client who continues to have decreased cardiac output. Dopamine and dobutamine are frequently used in the pediatric setting to improve cardiac output. In distributive shock epinephrine or norepinephrine is used to increase systemic vascular resistance and support blood pressure. The therapeutic approach to distributive and cardiogenic shock requires the identification and treatment of underlying etiologies. Antibiotics must be administered in a timely manner if sepsis is suspected. Specific interventions for cardiogenic shock are driven by the pathophysiology of the underlying etiology.

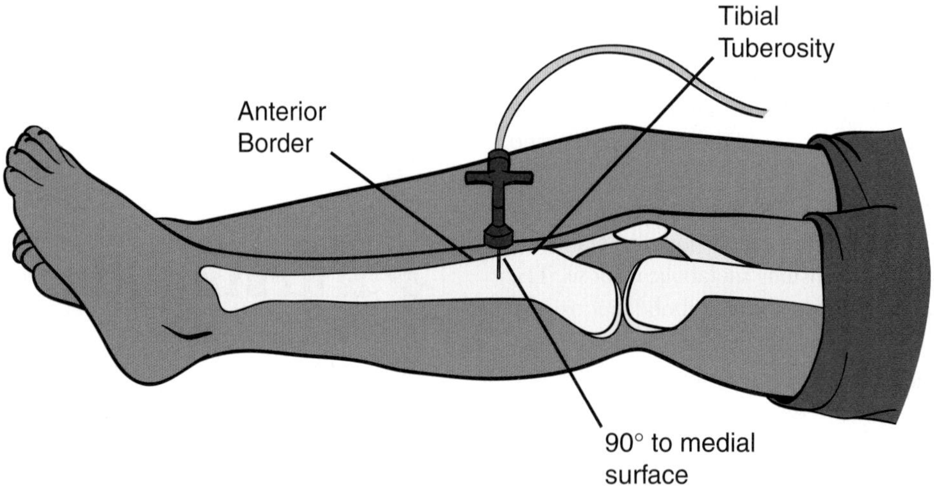

Figure 25-29 Placement of Intraosseous Needle

Nursing Alert:

Volume Replacement in Shock

A frequent error in the management of shock in pediatric clients is insufficient volume replacement.

Anaphylaxis is a true life-threatening emergency and must be recognized immediately. Once an airway is secured, or if the client is adequately breathing spontaneously, treatment is aimed at increasing blood pressure by systemic vasoconstriction. The use of epinephrine either subcutaneously or intravenously is the treatment of choice. Airway management and hemodynamic support are the mainstays of treatment until airway swelling has subsided and the cardiovascular system has returned to normal.

Children with hypovolemic shock who are appropriately resuscitated have an excellent chance to return to their previous state of health. The child in sepsis-induced distributive shock unfortunately continues to have a high rate of morbidity and mortality. Ongoing research in this area continues. Research in progress is investigating specific pathophysiological responses to sepsis to better delineate therapeutic intervention. Studies have also been done to look at specific indicators to predict survival in the pediatric population. Such parameters as heart rate, arterial blood pressure, serum lactate levels, and degree of acidosis have been studied as potential indicators (Duke, Butt, & South, 1997). Outreach education is also important to teach emergency and clinic staffs the early signs of impending shock and the deleterious effects of failing to recognize these signs with adequate treatment. Survival for the child in cardiogenic shock will depend on accuracy of diagnosis, the underlying etiology, and the ability to provide surgical and/or medical support. Refer to the sections on acquired and congenital heart disease for specific outcomes for these conditions.

Nursing Management

Assessment

Ongoing and frequent assessment of the child in shock is essential. The nurses assess pulses, perfusion, CFT, color and temperature of skin, vital signs, urine output, level of conciousness, and respiratory effort. Frequent reassessment after intervention is critical to evaluate for therapeutic response.

Nursing Diagnosis

1. Decreased cardiac output related to decreased cardiac function or inadequate intravascular volume as evidenced by hypotension, tachycardia, poor urine output, lethargy, and/or poor perfusion.
2. Ineffective peripheral tissue perfusion related to vasodilation and coagulopathy as evidenced by altered neurologic status, decreased urine output, and metabolic acidosis.

Outcome Identification

- The child will show restoration of normal volume status, heart rate, urine output, blood pressure, and level of conciousness within 24–48 hours.
- The child suffering from sepsis-induced distributive shock will exhibit restoration of normal vascular tone.
- The child's blood cultures will be negative for sepsis.
- The child's coagulation studies will be normal without evidence of bleeding disorders.

Planning/Implementation

Vital signs, perfusion, and pulses are assessed on presentation and followed for changes. These paramaters are also monitored to evaluate clinical response to therapeutic intervention. IV access is maintained for the administration of fluids and medications. Many of these children require continuous infusions of inotropes to maintain heart rate and blood pressure. The nurse should ensure accurate delivery of these medications and monitor for efficacy. The nurse should record accurate intake and output and any ongoing losses such as vomiting, diarrhea, chest tube or surgical drain output.

Nurses should monitor for any changes in respiratory status that may indicate the child is becoming fatigued. Interventions such as oxygen administration and endotracheal intubation may be necessary to support respiratory function during the acute illness.

Neurologic status should be closely monitored as changes in level of orientation may indicate poor cerebral perfusion. Any child with decreased level of conciousness requires airway protection with either an artifical airway or endotracheal intubation. Airway suction is implemented if there is a poor cough, as this will facilitate clearance of secretions.

Many of these children (particularly those suffering from septic shock) will have positive blood cultures and coagulation disorders. Blood cultures are obtained for the identification of infectious organisms and should be obtained prior to the initiation of antibiotics. As determined by blood culture and sensitivities, appropriate antibiotics will be administered as ordered. If coagulopathy is present, interventions such as fresh frozen plasma, cryoprecipitate, and vitamin K are administered as ordered. Careful inspection of the skin to monitor for worsening petechia and skin breakdown is imperative. To prevent breakdown the child should be turned every two hours, heels/elbows should be protected, and mobility encouraged as soon as tolerated. Fever should be treated with antipyretics or tepid sponge baths.

Evaluation

The child will be hemodynamically stable with good respiratory function and appropriate level of consciousness.

Ongoing losses will be accounted for and adequately replaced. Cardiac output and BP will be normal. There will be no evidence of bleeding from intravascular lines or orifices. All lab work will be normal. Fever will diminish to normal and white count will be normal.

Family Teaching

To prevent hypovolemic shock caregivers should be taught the signs of dehydration as well as potential causes. Infants are at high risk for dehydration and hypovolemic shock if diarrhea/vomiting becomes protracted. All caretakers should be taught good handwashing techniques and proper mixing of formulas. It is not uncommon for an infant to become severely dehydrated because not enough water was mixed with powdered formula. Caregivers should also be instructed on appropriate diets for clients with gastroenteritis clients (Refer to Chapter 23).

For the child with anaphylactic shock the caregivers are educated to avoid the triggering antigen. Caregivers and the child (when old enough) should be instructed in the use of an *epi–pen.* These are precalculated doses of epinephrine that the child should have with him/her at all times in the case of accidental exposure to a known allergen. They are administered subcutaneously or intramuscularly in the event of exposure. Medical alert bracelets should also be worn by all these clients.

It is every nurse's responsibility to be aware of medication and food allergies that a child may be exposed to while in the hospital setting. Nurses should always check clients' charts and ID bracelets prior to the administration of any medication. This is especially true in pediatrics where the individual is often too young to know his/her own allergies. For the child with a newly diagnosed heart disease, whether acquired or congenital, child and family education will center on the specific disease or defect. Interventions generally involve a combination of medications and nutritional support.

PSYCHOSOCIAL ISSUES FOR CHILDREN WITH HEART DISEASE

A number of issues become apparent when a child is born with, or develops, heart disease. At birth the parents must grapple with the fact that their newborn is not perfect. If the newborn is in distress it is quickly taken away from the parents in the delivery suite, interrupting the normal bonding that occurs in the immediate post partum period. If the child remains ill and on life support, the parents are not afforded the opportunity to hold or nourish their newborn. Parents frequently feel grief at their loss of an anticipated healthy infant. Inability to form an attachment to the infant and marital stress can result (Hinoki, 1998).

As the child grows, the family must deal with the dilemma of normality. After the family adjusts to the initial shock of having something wrong with their infant, they must be able to incorporate the child into the family and society. Health care providers advise parents to treat their child "normally," as if there were no existing heart disease. Unfortunately, health care providers do not always offer tools to the family on how to do this. Some families are able to look past their child's condition, while others continue to impose unnecessary restrictions. As the child grows, physical limitations become more apparent, and the child may withdraw from peer interactions. Support groups can be helpful in this situation. Many congenital heart programs have an ongoing cardiac support group facilitated by social workers who can offer therapeutic strategies. Nurses working with these children must be able to listen, and apply reflective feedback and support for both the child and family. Creative solutions for such necessary treatments as oxygen, medication administration, and exercise restrictions can be implemented in concert with school nurses or community agencies. Cyanotic children, particularly adolescents, benefit from fashion consultants who can select colors for makeup and clothing that will minimize the appearance of cyanosis.

Caregivers of newly diagnosed children, and adolescents with heart disease must decide who they disclose medical information to. How information regarding heart disease is transmitted to family and friends is an early issue for caregivers (Sparacino, et al., 1997). Extended family can pressure the family to not disclose information to the child. When the child enters school this issue re-emerges. Should the family tell teachers about the child's condition? On the surface the answer would be yes, as a logical means to keep the school informed and treat emergencies. However this frequently backfires because teachers and principals can form incorrect judgments about the child's capabilities. As teenagers are struggling to develop their own identity, peer acceptance is very important. Many teenagers prefer not to tell friends and peers of their condition. Some will avoid group activities, dances, dating, or swimming. Surgical scars and/or exercise intolerance can become a source of embarrassment.

As adolescents gain independence, they must be able to assume their own care. Many caregivers struggle with this issue, and do not allow normal self-determination to develop. Therefore, the chronically ill adolescent may never achieve true mastery of life skills. Caregivers must be encouraged to allow their teenagers to care for themselves. Teenagers should become responsible for taking their own medicines, limiting their own activities, and paying attention to their bodies' cues. The primary historian during follow-up clinic visits must be the adolescent. Teenagers must never be excused to allow private discussion with the caregivers, as this will hinder the development of a trusting relationship.

Family lifestyles and activities change. Because of the extra attention received by the child with heart disease sibling rivalry and jealousy are common. Older siblings can feel displaced and resentful. These feelings can carry on throughout childhood and adolescence. Previously enjoyed athletic activities such as hiking, skiing, or camping are no longer pursued. Divorce is a possible consequence in some families. Coping with uncertainty is difficult for caregivers and child. There is always the uncertainty of another operation, worsening symptoms, or an untimely death. Support systems must be identified. Social workers, therapists, church leaders, community services, and support groups can all be accessed to provide support. Each family must be assessed individually to make the appropriate fit. Financial stresses are almost inevitable. Early referral to financial counselors can be made on a proactive basis to prevent financial catastrophes.

Family issues are multifaceted. Some families have the personal resources to effectively deal with the stresses and uncertainties of a child with heart disease. Others can decompensate over minor issues. Every child and family is assessed individually to determine suitable intervention. A multidisciplinary team is best suited to meet the needs of these families. Health care providers, nurses, social workers, and therapists work together to develop an individualized plan of care. Community and national organizations such as the American Heart Association can be tapped to provide ancillary support.

Physical activity is necessary for psychological as well as physical well being. Today's society places much well-deserved

Research Highlight

The Dilemmas of Adolescents and Young Adults with Congenital Heart Disease

Study Purpose

Parents of children with heart disease are faced with many psychological and social dilemmas, in addition to the dilemma of their child's physical health. The purpose of this study was to provide a better understanding of parental experiences during normal maturation of their children with congenital heart disease.

Methods

Qualitative pilot study utilized a semi-structured interview of eight parents of adolescents and young adults with congenital heart disease. Parents' experiences of learning the diagnosis, concerns, perceptions of their child's relationships and activities were explored.

Findings

Seven themes were identified that were struggles for parents as their child grew into young adulthood. These themes were: dilemma of normality, dilemma of disclosure, uncertainty, illness management, social integration, impact on the family, and coping.

Implications

Parents need assistance from health care providers to help each individually determine what is "normal" and how to best monitor their child's health and safety. The authors acknowledged that further research is needed to develop specific interventions.

Citation

Sparacino, P. S., Tong, E. M., Messias, D. K., Foote, D., Chesla, C. A., & Gillis, C. (1997). The dilemmas of adolescents and young adults with congenital heart disease. *Heart & Lung, 26,* 187–195.

significance on the positive effects of regular exercise. Technological and surgical advances have improved the physical status of children with heart disease. Consequently more and more of these children will be participating in both recreational and competitive athletics. However, families and health care providers continue to place restrictions on children with heart disease, regardless of the severity of disease (Tong & Sparacino, 1994).

Exercise can be divided into two types: static (isometric) or dynamic. Static exercise generates a large intramuscular tension with little muscular movement. High static activities include weight lifting, rock climbing, and gymnastics. This form of exercise primarily increases blood pressure and afterload. Dynamic exercise is aerobic in that muscle length and movement change rhythmically. Dynamic activities include running, soccer, basketball, and swimming. This form of exercise increases oxygen consumption, heart rate, and cardiac output. It also decreases systemic vascular resistance (afterload) (Kaminer, Hixon, & Strong, 1995).

The child is evaluated on a individual basis as to which form of exercise is appropriate and safe. The potential risks as well as the benefits must be considered. Recreational activities versus competitive athletics must be evaluated separately for each patient. The nurse must remember that many forms of competitive athletics incorporate both static and dynamic levels of training (e.g., football employs weight training and running as part of training).

Most congenital defects are minor, therefore imposing no limitation on physical performance. Children with more complex defects will often limit their own level of activities, especially when they are young. However many adolescents wish to participate with peers in a variety of physical activities. Simples defects such as repaired ASD, VSD, or PDA impose little or no limitation. Children with obstructive lesions such as severe AS or coarctation of the aorta should not participate in static exercise, or those competitive sports requiring weight lifting for training. The increase in afterload imposed by this form of exercise in combination with their obstructive lesion will significantly impede cardiac output and increase ventricular work. Over the long run this will affect myocardial function.

Cyanotic children will have severe exercise limitations because of decreased cardiovascular function as well as pulmonary abnormalities. This is also true for children with single ventricle physiology following a Fontan procedure (Paridon, 1997). These children should be allowed to participate in recreational activities to the best of their abilities, but competitive athletics are discouraged. Of note, altitude is generally not well tolerated by these children so caution must be used when planning activities in the mountains.

Children with cardiac arrhythmias are evaluated with an exercise test to ensure that abnormal heart rhythms are suppressed with exercise. If rhythm abnormalities persist or worsen with exercise, then the child is restricted from vigorous competitive sports. An inability to increase heart rate (chronotropic incompetence) with exercise will also impose physical limitations. Many times these children will benefit from a permanent pacemaker (Paridon, 1997).

A small group of individuals is at high risk for sudden death with exercise so these children are restricted from physical education classes, competitive sports, and strenuous activities. These include hypertrophic cardiomyopathy, long QT syndrome, pulmonary hypertension, syncope with exercise, and exercise-induced ventricular tachycardia. Contact sports are prohibited for those on warfarin therapy and those with artificial conduits placed under the sternum. Nonstrenuous recreational activities with friends, family, community, or church groups are generally safe.

As longevity of children with heart disease improves, so must quality of life. Exercise is important to a sense of well-being. Unfortunately there are few objective data to make judgments about exercise in this population; most recommendations are based on collective experience. Nonetheless, physical activity should be encouraged to the best of the child's abilities. Emphasis should be on the enjoyable and fun aspects of regular exercise, and not on competitive rewards.

Congenital heart disease can affect normal growth and development in infants and children. The impact of early parental stress, multiple hospitalizations, cyanosis, child temperament, parent-child relationships, and health status all play a role in development. It is also well known that children with chronic illnesses are at high risk for the development of behavioral problems.

Early maternal interaction and bonding are critical to the development of the infant. This includes the mother's ability to read her infant's cues and respond appropriately. Frequently postnatal growth is compromised by cardiac disease. Social interactions around feedings can be hampered by respiratory difficulties, infant fatigue, and poor stamina. These infants are frequently irritable and difficult to console. Mothers of infants with heart disease report high levels of stress, frustration, and inadequacy. If these difficulties become prolonged, then the infant will have low levels of engagement and will demonstrate more aversion behaviors (arching the back, lack of eye contact) (Gardner, Freeman, Black, & Angelini, 1996). If the mother is sensitive to these cues, she will allow the infant time to rest and regroup cognitive processes. Unfortunately, many mothers respond to these behaviors by overstimulating their infant in an attempt to regain their attention. Unfortunately this will only serve to aggravate the infant further. Sensitive and responsive interaction must be developed. The nurse is in a crucial position to assist caregivers by giving them the tools they need to provide a solid foundation for infant attachment. Educating caregivers about common aversion behaviors is helpful. Continuous support will help strengthen maternal sensitivity to her infant's cues. This can be started early in the neonatal period with positive feedback and encouragement.

Unfortunately a number of physiological phenomena also unfavorably affect development. Poor nutritional intake and weight gain adversely affect brain growth and psychosocial development. Chronic cyanosis has been long recognized to adversely affect cognitive function and intelligence. Other neurologic complications of cyanosis include risk for stroke, cerebral abscessess, and abnormal cerebral metabolism (Walsh, Morrow, & Jonas, 1995). Chronic illness with associated hospitalizations will slow achievement of developmental milestones, or in some cases, cause regression.

Other significant factors in developmental dysfunction in this population are the intraoperative events that can cause damage to the central nervous system. Cardiopulmonary bypass is associated with microthrombi and inflammatory response that can affect the whole body, including the brain. Hypothermia is intended to decrease the metabolic rate of the body therefore protecting it from adverse sequela of ischemia. The organ most sensitive to ischemic injury is the brain. If cooling occurs too slowly, there is an associated delay in subsequent developmental achievements (Oates, Simpson, Turnbull, & Cartmill, 1995).

As the child approaches preschool and school age, behavior problems may become apparent. A sense of well-being, physical health and activity, child-parent relationships, and family environment all contribute to a child's psychosocial development. Children with congenital heart disease also have adjustment problems, possibly caused by low self-esteem. Caregiver stress can contribute to family dysfunction and inadequate coping, but is not always related to the severity of illness. Frequently less severe illness is associated with high stress. This may be caused by perceived uncertainty of medical outcome and lack of control. If caregivers make extensive accommodations for perceived illness and overestimate severity, then the risk for future behavior problems is very high (Goldberg, et al., 1997). All these issues can manifest as behavioral problems in the child or adolescent.

Developmental issues for the adolescent are compounded by peer pressures. Frequently these young people have struggled with motor and language delays, learning disabilities, insecurities, exercise intolerance, and social withdrawal. It is not uncommon for teenagers with heart disease to act out and test limits during this period. Experimentation with alcohol, drugs, and alternative lifestyles are not uncommon. Frequently peer support groups with other teens who have similar illnesses is very helpful during this time.

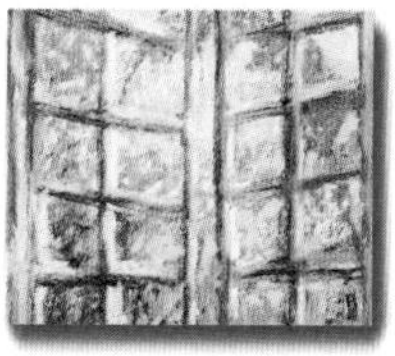

In the Real World

As a student nurse, nothing can prepare you for when you see your first patient coming back from having a cardiac procedure. My first patient scared and overwhelmed me. The infant came to the pediatric intensive care unit following an intensive cardiac procedure. The infant had four chest tubes, numerous IV pumps, and an external pacemaker. This poor infant was so sick and had so many things happening to him at once. No matter how much theory we are taught as students the complexity of these patients is terrifying. The heart is not the only organ that potentially is affected and luckily I had a great nurse mentor me on what this child was going through. She sat and explained everything to me and the more she talked the less frightened I was. From this experience I decided I really enjoyed learning about cardiac patients and I look forward to taking care of these patients.

Caregivers have more difficulty allowing their teen increasing freedom if there are concerns about chronic illness. They should be counseled to allow their teenager more autonomy and freedom, as long as health care interventions (medications) are not ignored. Teenagers should be expected to begin assuming their own health care.

Issues continue into adulthood. Professional achievement, job ability, and livelihood become significant issues for the young adult. Many adults with congenital heart disease can go on to be productive members of society. Others, because of physical limitations, may only be able to work part time or not at all. Job counseling, occupational therapy, and financial planning are beneficial and should be offered. Health insurance may be denied because of pre-existing conditions. Ongoing medical expenses can be quite high so referral must be made to social service agencies when needed. Frank and open discussions about contraception and pregnancy should first occur during adolescence. Many women with heart disease can have children without complications; unfortunately for many others pregnancy can be life-threatening. This must be discussed prior to conception so the woman is well informed about potential complications and choices.

As one can see, pediatric heart disease imposes physiological, psychological, and social concerns. Some can be quite small and insignificant, others seemingly insurmountable. As with other life problems, perceived severity of these concerns influences coping and outcomes. Nurses are in a pivotal position to assist families with all these issues. Continuity of care allows for timely problem identification and intervention.

Key Concepts

- Normally, the three fetal shunts (ductus venousus, foramen ovale, ductus arteriosus) close at birth or shortly thereafter. The cardiac output of an infant is normally 200 ml/kg/min. Cardiac output per minute decreases during childhood and by the age of 15 years, it is the same level as an adult, 100 ml/kg/min.
- Normal determinants of cardiac output are heart rate and stroke volume. The determinants of stroke volume are preload, afterload, and contractility.
- Assessment of the child with a cardiovascular alteration should include health history and a physical examination.
- The physical exam of a child with a cardiovascular alteration should include an inspection of facial features, edema, chest wall deformities, skin color, presence of finger clubbing, auscultation for murmurs, palpation for hepatomegaly, and blood pressure along with other routine exam procedures.
- Congestive heart failure can be caused by volume overload, pressure overload, or poor contractility. Many different cardiac lesions can produce CHF for one or more of these reasons.
- Clinical manifestations of CHF are numerous and can include gallop rhythm, diaphoresis, jugular venous distention, tachycardia, and poor weight gain.
- The primary treatments of CHF are diuretics, intropes, and afterload reducing agents. Infants with structural heart defects responsible for CHF should have surgical repair.
- Nutritional support and maneuvers to decrease metabolic demands of CHF clients are important nursing interventions to promote growth and development.
- Congenital defects that produce L→R shunt result in excessive pulmonary blood flow (ASD, VSD, PDA, AV canal).
- Congenital defects with R→L shunt result in decreased pulmonary blood flow and are associated with cyanosis (Tetralogy of Fallot, Tricuspid atresia).
- Acquired rheumatic fever follows an untreated or partially treated group A streptococcal pharyngitis.
- Kawasaki disease is the number one reason for acquired heart disease in pediatrics.
- Children with structural heart defects require prophylaxis against endocarditis before surgical or dental procedures.
- Heart transplantation is not a cure, it is trading one chronic disease for another.
- There are three major classifications of shock: hypovolemic, distributive, and cardiogenic.
- If an abnormal heart rhythm is noted, check the client's blood pressure and perfusion to ensure stability. Document with an EKG.
- Psychosocial issues surrounding a child with heart disease and their families include grief and loss, dilemma of normality, and marital and family stress.

Review Questions

1. What are the determinants of cardiac output? Define preload, afterload, and contractility.
2. Draw a diagram of fetal circulation and identify those structures that close after birth.
3. What diagnostic tests would be ordered in a child you suspect of having congenital heart disease?
4. What are the clinical manifestations of congestive heart failure? What are the corresponding treatments?
5. Draw the blood flow for a VSD.
6. Draw the blood flow for transposition of the great arteries.
7. Why is it necessary to keep the ductus arteriosus open in children with severely decreased pulmonary blood flow? How is it kept open?
8. Write a nursing care plan for an infant with coarctation of the aorta.
9. What are the criteria for the diagnosis of rheumatic fever?
10. Describe the treatment for Kawasaki disease; include nursing interventions.
11. What are the three types of shock? Compare physiology and treatment of the three types of shock.
12. What are some of the psychosocial concerns for the family with a child who has heart disease?

References

American Academy of Pediatrics, Committee on Infectious Diseases. (2000). *2000 Red Book: Report of the Committee on Infectious Diseases* (25th ed.). Elk Grove, IL: Author.

American Heart Association. (1998). *Rheumatic heart disease statistics*. [On-line]. Available: www.americanheart.org/Heart_and_Stroke_A_Z_Guide/rhds.html.

American Heart Association. (1999). *Congenital cardiovascular disease statistics*. [On-line]. Available: www.americanheart.org/Heart_and_ Stroke_A_Z_Guide/conghds.html.

Athreya, B. H. (1995). Vasculitis in children. *Pediatric Clinics of North America, 5*, 1239–1261.

Barron, K. S. (1998). Kawasaki disease in children. *Current Opinion in Rheumatology, 10*, 29–37.

Beekman, R. (1995). Coarctation of the aorta. In G. C. Emmanouilides, T. A. Riemenschneider, H. G. Allen, & H. P. Gutgesell (Eds.), *Moss & Adams' heart disease in infants, children and adolescents* (5th ed.). Baltimore: Williams & Wilkins.

Bengur, A. R. (1998). Truncus arteriosus. In A. Garson, J. T. Bricker, D. J. Fisher, & S. R. Neish, (Eds.), *The science and practice of pediatric cardiology*. Baltimore: Williams and Wilkins.

Benson, D. W., Basson, C. T., & MacRae, C. A. (1996). New understanding in the genetics of congenital heart disease. *Current Opinion in Pediatrics, 8*, 505–511.

Boucek, M. M., Novick, R. J., Bennett, L. E., Fiol, B., Keck, B.M., & Hosenpud, J. D. (1997). The registry of the International Society of Heart and Lung Transplantation: First official pediatric report—1997. *Journal of Heart Lung Transplant, 16*, 1189–1206.

Bradley, D. J., & Glode, M. P. (1998). Kawasaki disease: The mystery continues. *Western Journal of Medicine, 168*, 23–29.

Brook, M., & Heymann, M. (1995). Patent ductus arteriosus. In G. C. Emmanouilides, T. A. Riemenschneider, H. G. Allen, & H. P. Gutgesell (Eds.), *Moss & Adams' heart disease in infants, children and adolescents* (5th ed.). Baltimore: Williams & Wilkins.

Burns, J. C., Shike, H., Gordon, J. B., Malhotra, A., Schoenwetter, M., & Kawasaki, T. (1996). Sequelae of Kawasaki disease in adolescents and young adults. *Journal of the American College of Cardiologists, 28*, 253–257.

Callow, L., Suddaby, E. C., & Slota, M. C. (1998). Cardiovascular system. In M. C. Slota (Ed.), *Core curriculum for pediatric critical care nursing*. Philadelphia, PA: W. B. Saunders.

Cetta, F., & Warnes, C. A. (1995). Adults with congenital heart disease: Patient knowledge of endocarditis prophylaxis. *Mayo Clinic Proceedings, 70*, 50–54.

Chameides, L., & Hazinski, M. F. (Eds.). (1997). *Pediatric advanced life support*. Dallas, TX: American Heart Association.

Chang, A., & Reddy, M. (1998). Truncus arteriosus. In A. Chang, F. Hanley, G. Wernosky, & D. Wessel (Eds.), *Pediatric cardiac intensive care*. Baltimore: Williams & Wilkins.

Chang A., & Wells, W. (1998). Patent ductus arteriosus. In A. Chang, F. Hanley, G. Wernosky, & D. Wessel (Eds.), *Pediatric cardiac intensive care*. Baltimore: Williams & Wilkins.

Checchia, P. A., Pahl, E., Shaddy, R.E., & Shulman, S. T. (1997). Cardiac transplant for Kawasaki Disease. *Pediatrics, 4*, 695–699.

Clark, E. B. (1995). Morphogenesis, growth and biomechanics: Mechanisms of cardiovascular development. In G. C. Emmanouilides, T. A. Riemenschneider, H. G. Allen, & H. P. Gutgesell (Eds.), *Moss & Adams' heart disease in infants, children and adolescents* (5th ed.). Baltimore: Williams & Wilkins.

Committee on Evaluation and Management of Heart Failure. (1995). Guidelines for the evaluation and management of heart failure. Report of the American College of Cardiology/American Heart Association Task Force on Practice Guidelines. *Journal of the American College of Cardiologists, 26*, 1376–1398.

Committee on Rheumatic Fever. (1992). Guidelines for the diagnosis of rheumatic fever. *Journal of the American Medical Association, 268*, 2069–2073.

Craig, J., Scholz, T. A., Vanderhooft, S. L., & Etheridge, S. P. (1998). Fat necrosis after ice application for supraventricular tachycardia termination. *Journal of Pediatrics, 133*, 727.

Dajani, A. S., Taubert, K. A., Takahashi, M., Bierman, F. Z., Freed, M. D., Ferrieri, P., Gerber, M., Shulman, S. T., Karchmer, A. W., Wilson, W., Peter, G., Durack, D. T., & Rahimtoola, S. H. (1994). Guidelines for long term management of patients with Kawasaki Disease. *American Heart Association Medical Scientific Statement*. www.americanheart.org/Scientific/statements/1994/029402.html.

Dajani, A. S., Taubert, K. A., Wilson, W., Bolger, A. F., Bayer, A., Ferrieri, P., Gewitz, M. H., Shulman, S. T., Nouri, S., Newburger, J. W., Hutto, C., Pallasch, T. J., Gage, T. W., Levison, M. E., Peter, G., & Zuccaro, G. (1997). Prevention of bacterial endocarditis: Recommendations by the American Heart Association. *Journal of the American Medical Association, 257*, 1794–1801.

Danford, D. A., Nasir, A., & Gumbiner, C. (1993). Cost assessment of the evaluation of heart murmurs in children. *Pediatrics, 91*, 365–368.

Daniels, S. (1997). Consultation with the specialist: The diagnosis of hypertension in children: An update. *Pediatrics, 19*, 131–135.

Davenport, Y. (1995). Advanced technology within the cardiac transplant process. *Intensive Critical Care Nursing, 11*, 170–174.

Deal, B. J. (1998). Supraventricular tachycardia mechanisms and natural history. In B. J. Deal, G. S. Wolff, & H. Gelband (Eds.), *Current concepts in diagnosis and management of arrhythmias in infants and children*. Armonk, NY: Future Publishing.

Del Pont, J. M., De Cicco, L. T., Vartalitis, C., Ithurralde, M., Gallo, J. P., Vargas, F., Gianantonio, C. A., & Quiros, R. E. (1995). Infective endocarditis in children: Clinical analysis and evaluation of two diagnostic criteria. *Pediatric Infectious Disease Journal, 14*, 1079–1086.

Dhillon, R., Clarkson, P., Donald, A. E., Powe, A. J., Nash, M., Novelli, V., Dillon, M. J., & Deanfield, J. E. (1996). Endothelial dysfunction late after Kawasaki disease. *Circulation, 94*, 2103–2106.

Doty, D. (1997). Right heart valve lesions. In D. Doty (Ed.), *Cardiac surgery; Operative technique*. St. Louis: Mosby.

Driscoll, D., Allen, H. G., Atkins, D. L., Brenner, J., Dunnigan, A., Franklin, W., Gutgesell, H. P., Herndon, P., Shaddy, R. E., Taubert, K. A., Zahka, K., Garson, A., Skorton, D. J., & Danielson, G. K. (1994). Guidelines for evaluation and management of common congenital cardiac problems in infants, children, and adolescents. *Circulation, 90*, 2180–2188.

Driscoll, D., Offord, K. P., Feldt, R. H., Schaff, H. V., Puga, F. J., & Danielson, G. K. (1992). Five to fifteen year follow up after Fontan operation. *Circulation, 85*, 469–496.

Du, Z. D., Roguin, N., & Barak, M. (1997). Clinical and echocardiographic evaluation of neonates with heart murmurs. *Acta Paediatrics*, 86, 752–756.

Duke, T. D., Butt, W., & South, M. (1997). Predictors of mortality and multiple organ failure in children with sepsis. *Intensive Care Medicine, 23*, 684–692.

Durongpisitkul, K., Gururaj, V. J., Park, J. M., & Martin, C. F. (1995). The prevention of coronary artery aneurysm in Kawasaki disease: A meta-analysis on the efficacy of aspirin and immunoglobulin treatment. *Pediatrics, 96*, 1057–1061.

Edwards, W. D. (1995). Cardiac anatomy and examination of cardiac specimens. In G. C. Emmanouilides, T. A. Riemenschneider, H. G. Allen, & H. P. Gutgesell (Eds.), *Moss & Adams' heart disease in infants, children and adolescents* (5th ed.). Baltimore: Williams & Wilkins.

Etheridge, S. E., & Judd, V. E. (1999). Supraventricular tachycardia in infancy: Evaluation, management and follow up. *Archives of Pediatric Adolescent Medicine, 153*, 267–251.

Feldt, R., Porter, C., Edwards, W., Puga, F., & Seward, J., (1995). Atrioventricular septal defects. In G. C. Emmanouilides, T. A. Riemenschneider, H. G. Allen, & H. P. Gutgesell (Eds.), *Moss & Adams' heart disease in infants, children and adolescents* (5th ed.). Baltimore: Williams & Wilkins.

Freedom, R., & Benson, L. (1995). Hypoplastic left heart syndrome. In G. C. Emmanouilides, T. A. Riemenschneider, H. G. Allen, & H. P. Gutgesell (Eds.), *Moss & Adams' heart disease in infants, children and adolescents* (5th ed.). Baltimore: Williams & Wilkins.

Friedman, R., Collins, E., & Fenrich, A. (1995). Pacing in children: Indications and techniques. *Progress in Pediatric Cardiology, 4*, 21–29.

Fukushige, J., Takahashi, N., Ueda, K., Hijii, T., Igarashi, H., & Ohshima, A. (1996). Long term outcome of coronary abnormalities in patients after Kawasaki disease. *Pediatric Cardiology, 17*, 71–76.

Furdon, S. A. (1997). Recognizing congestive heart failure in the neonatal period. *Neonatal Network, 16*, 5–13.

Gardner, F. V., Freeman, N. H., Black, A. M. S., & Angelini, G. D. (1996). Disturbed mother infant interaction in association with congenital heart disease. *Heart, 76*, 56–59.

Gewitz, M. H. (1997). Prevention of bacterial endocarditis. *Current Opinion in Pediatrics, 9*, 518–522.

Goldberg, S., Janus, M., Washington, J., Simmons, R. J., MacLusky, I., & Fowler, R. S. (1997). Prediction of preschool behavioral problems in health and pediatric samples. *Developmental and Behavioral Pediatrics, 18*, 304–313.

Graham, T., & Gutgesell, H. (1995). Ventricular septal defect. In G. C. Emmanouilides, T. A. Riemenschneider, H. G. Allen, & H. P. Gutgesell (Eds.), *Moss & Adams' heart disease in infants, children and adolescents* (5th ed.). Baltimore: Williams & Wilkins.

Hamaoka, K., & Onouchi, Z. (1996). Effects of coronary artery aneurysms on intracoronary flow velocity dynamics in Kawasaki Disease. *American Journal of Cardiology*, 77, 873–875.

Higgins, S., & Reid, A., (1994). Common congenital heart defects: Long term follow-up. *Nursing Clinics of North America, 29*(2), 233–248.

Hinoki, K. W. (1998). Congenital heart disease: Effects on the family. *Neonatal Network, 17*, 7–10.

Kaminer, S. J., Hixon. R. L., & Strong, W. B. (1995). Evaluation and recommendations for participation in athletics for children with heart disease. *Current Opinion in Pediatrics, 7*, 595–600.

Kato, J., Sugimura, T., Akagi, T., Sato, N., Hashino, K., Maeno, Y., Kazue, T., Eto, G., & Yamakawa, R. (1996). Long term consequences of Kawasaki disease. *Circulation, 94*, 1379–1385.

Kawasaki T. (1995). Kawasaki disease. *Acta Paediatrics, 84*, 713–715.

Kohr, L. M., & O'Brien, P. (1995). Current management of congestive heart failure in infants and children. *Nursing Clinics of North America, 30*, 261–290.

LeBlanc, J. G., & Russell, J. L. (1998). Pediatric surgery in the 1990's. *Surgical Clinics of North America, 78*(5), 729–747.

Magee, A. G., & Qureshi, S. A. (1997). Closure of atrial septal defects by transcatheter devices. *Pediatric Cardiology*, 18, 326–325.

Mair, D., Edwards, W., Julsrud, P., Seward, J. & Danielson, G. (1995). Truncus arteriosus. In G. C. Emmanouilides, T. A. Riemenschneider, H. G. Allen, & H. P. Gutgesell (Eds.), *Moss & Adams heart disease in infants, children and adolescents* (5th ed.). Baltimore: Williams & Wilkins.

Mandell, V. S. (1999). Interventional procedures for congenital heart disease. *Radiologic Clinics of North America, 37*(2), 439–461.

Massetti, M., Babatasi, G., Rossi, A., Neri, E., Bhoyroo, S., Zitouni, S., Maragnes, P., & Khayat, A. (1996). Operation for atrial septal defect through a right anterolateral thoracotomy: Current outcome. *Annals of Thoracic Surgery, 62*, 1100–1103.

Mavroudis, C., Backer, C. L., Muster, A. J., Pahl, E., Sanders, J. H., Zales, V. R., & Gevitz, M. (1996). Expanding indications for pediatric coronary artery bypass. *Journal of Thoracic Cardiovascular Surgery, 111*, 181–189.

Melish, M. (1996). Kawasaki disease. *Pediatrics in Review, 17*, 153–162.

Milton, P., & Wernosky, G. (1995). Transposition of the great arteries. In G. C. Emmanouilides, T. A. Riemenschneider, H. G. Allen, & H. P. Gutgesell (Eds.), *Moss & Adams' heart disease in infants, children and adolescents* (5th ed.). Baltimore: Williams & Wilkins.

Miner, P. D., & Canobbio, M. M. (1994). Care of the adult with cyanotic congenital heart disease. *Nursing Clinics of North America, 29*, 249–267.

Moodie, D. S. (1994). Adult congenital heart disease. *Current Opinion in Cardiology, 9*, 137–142.

Morgan, W., & O'Neill, J. (1998). Hemorrhagic and obstructive shock in pediatric patients. *New Horizons, 6*(4), 150–154.

Morrow, R., Naftel, D., Chinnock, R., Canter, C., Boucek, M., Zales, V., McGriffin, D., Kirklin, J., & the Pediatric Heart Transplant Study Group. (1997). Outcome of listing for heart transplantation in infants younger than six months: Predictors of death and interval to transplantation. *Journal of Heart and Lung Transplantation, 16*, 1255–1265.

National High Blood Pressure Education Program Working Group. (1996). Update on the 1987 Task Force on High Blood Pressure in Children and Adolescents. A Working Group Report from the National High Blood Pressure Education Program. *Pediatrics, 98*, 649–657.

Norris, M. K. G., Hill, C. S. (1994). Nutritional issues in infants and children with congenital heart disease. *Critical Care Nursing Clinics of North America, 6*, 153–163.

Oates, R. K., Simpson, J. M., Turnbull, J. A. B., & Cartmill, T. B. (1995). The relationship between intelligence and duration of circulatory arrest with deep hypothermia. *Journal of Thoracic and Cardiovascular Surgery, 110*, 786–792.

Ogawa, S., Fukazawa, R., Ohkubo, T., Zhang, J., Takechi, N., Kuramochi, Y., Hino, Y., Jimbo, O., Katsube, Y., Kamisago, M., Genma, Y., & Yamamoto, M. (1997). Silent myocardial ischemia in Kawasaki Disease. *Circulation, 96*, 3384–3389.

Paridon, S. M. (1997). Congenital heart disease: Cardiac performance and adaptations to exercise. *Pediatric Exercise Science, 9*, 308–323.

Park, M. K. (1996). *Pediatric cardiology for practitioners*. St. Louis, MO: Mosby Year Book.

Pruitt, A. (1996). Systemic hypertension. In R. Behrman, R. Kliegman, & A. Arvin (Eds.), *Nelson textbook of pediatrics* (15th ed., pp. 1368–1374). Philadelphia: W. B. Saunders

Reddy, V. M., McElhinney, D. B., Sagrado, T., Parry, A. J., Teitel, D. F., & Hanley, F. L. (1999). Results of 102 cases of complete repair of congenital heart defects in patients weighing 700 to 2500 grams. *Journal of Thoracic Cardiovascular Surgery, 117*, 324–331.

Rocchini, A., & Emmanouilides, G. (1995). Pulmonary stenosis. In G. C. Emmanouilides, T. A. Riemenschneider, H. G. Allen, & H. P. Gutgesell (Eds.), *Moss & Adams heart disease in infants, children and adolescents* (5th ed.). Baltimore: Williams & Wilkins.

Rosenfeld, E. A., Corydon, K. E., & Shulman, S. T. (1995). Kawasaki disease in infants less than one year of age. *Journal of Pediatrics, 126*, 524–529.

Sandre, R. M., & Shafran, S. D. (1996). Infective endocarditis: Review of 135 cases over 9 years. *Clinical Infectious Diseases, 22*, 256–286.

Shulman, S. T., DeInocencio, J., & Hirsch, R. (1995). Kawasaki Disease. *Pediatric Rheumatology, 42*, 1205–1222.

Sparacino, P. S. A., Tong, E. M., Messias, D. K. H., Foote, D., Chesla, C. A., & Gillis, C. L. (1997). The dilemmas of parents of adolescents and young adults with congenital heart disease. *Heart & Lung, 26*, 187–195.

Stewart, J. M., Hintze, T. H., Woolf, P. K., Snyder, M. S., Seligman, K. P., Gewitz, M. H. (1995). Nature of heart failure in patients with ventricular septal defect. *American Journal of Physiology, 269*, H1473–1480.

Strauss, A. W., & Johnson, M. C. (1996). The genetic basis of pediatric cardiovascular disease. *Seminars in Perinatology, 20*, 564–576.

Sugimura, T., Yokoi, H., Sato, N., Akagi, T., Kimura, T., Iemura, M., Nobuyoshi, M., & Kato, H. (1997). Interventional treatment for children with severe coronary artery stenosis with calcification after long term Kawasaki Disease. *Circulation, 96*, 3928–3933.

Swenson, J. M., Fischer, D. R., Miller, S. A., Boyle, G. J., Ettedgui, J. A., & Beerman, L. B. (1997). Are chest radiographs and electrocardiograms still valuable in evaluating new pediatric patients with heart murmurs or chest pain? *Pediatrics, 99*, 1–3.

Takahashi, M. (1995). Kawasaki disease. In G. C. Emmanouilides, T. A. Riemenschneider, H. G. Allen, & H. P. Gutgesell (Eds.), *Moss & Adams' heart disease in infants, children and adolescents* (5th ed.). Baltimore: Williams & Wilkins.

Takahashi, M. (1997) Kawasaki Disease. *Current Opinion in Pediatrics, 9*, 523–529.

Taketomo, C., Hodding, J., & Krause, D. (2001). *Pediatric dosage handbook*, Hudson, OH: Lexi Company Inc.

Talner, N. S. (1995). Heart failure. In G. C. Emmanouilides, T. A. Riemenschneider, H. G. Allen, & H. P. Gutgesell (Eds.), *Moss & Adams heart disease in infants, children and adolescents* (5th ed.). Baltimore: Williams & Wilkins.

Thomas, N., & Carcillo, J. A. (1998). Hypovolemic shock in pediatric patients. *New Horizons, 6*(4), 120–129.

Tobias, J. D., (1996). Shock in children: The first 60 minutes. *Pediatric Annals, 25*, 330–338.

Todome, Y., Ohkuni, H., Mizuse, M., Okibayashi, M. F., Ohtani, N., Suzuki, H., Song, C., Igarashi, H., Harada, K., Sakurai, S., & Kotani, S. (1995). Superantigenic exotoxin production by isolates of *Staphylococcus aureus* from Kawasaki syndrome patients and age matched control children. *Journal of Medical Microbiology, 42*, 91–95.

Tong, E., & Sparacino, P. S. A. (1994). Special management issues for adolescents and young adults with congenital heart disease. *Critical Care Nursing Clinics of North America, 6*, 199–214.

Tsubata, S., Ichida, F., Hamamichi, Y., Miyazaki, A., Hashimoto, I., & Okada, T. (1995). Successful thrombolytic therapy using tissue type plasminogen activator in Kawasaki disease. *Pediatric Cardiology, 16*, 186–189.

Ueda, Y., Fukushige, J., & Ueda, K. (1996). Congestive heart failure during early infancy in patients with ventricular septal defect relative to early closure. *Pediatric Cardiology, 17*, 382–386.

Veasey, L. G. (1995a). History and physical examination. In G. C. Emmanouilides, T. A. Riemenschneider, H. G. Allen, & H. P. Gutgesell (Eds.), *Moss & Adams heart disease in infants, children and adolescents* (5th ed.). Baltimore: Williams & Wilkins.

Veasey, L. G. (1995b). Rheumatic fever—T. Duckett Jones and the rest of the story. *Cardiology in the Young, 5*, 293–301.

Veasey, L. G. & Hill, H. R. (1997). Immunologic and clinical correlations in rheumatic fever and rheumatic heart disease. *Pediatric Infectious Diseases Journal, 16*, 400–407.

Vick, G. W. (1998). Defects of the atrial septum including atrioventricular septal defects. In A. Garson, J. T. Bricker, D. J. Fisher, & S. R. Neish (Eds.), *The science and practice of pediatric cardiology*. Baltimore: Williams & Wilkins.

Walsh, A. Z., Morrow, D. F., & Jonas, R. A. (1995). Neurologic and developmental outcomes following pediatric cardiac surgery. *Nursing Clinics of North America, 30*, 347–364.

Wong, P., & Starnes, V. (1998). Heart transplantation. In A. Chang, F. Hanley, G. Wernosky, & D. Wessel (Eds.), *Pediatric cardiac intensive care*. Baltimore: Williams & Wilkins.

Wright, D. A., Newburger, J. W., Baker, A., & Sundel, R. P. (1996). Treatment of immune globulin resistant Kawasaki disease with pulsed doses of corticosteroids. *Journal of Pediatrics, 128*, 146–149.

Yanagawa, H., Nakamura, Y., Sakata, K., & Yashiro, M. (1997). Use of intravenous γ-globulin for Kawasaki disease: Effects on cardiac sequelae. *Pediatric Cardiology, 18*, 19–23.

Zuberbuhler, J. (1995). Tetralogy of Fallot. In G. C. Emmanouilides, T. A. Riemenschneider, H. G. Allen, & H. P. Gutgesell (Eds.), *Moss & Adams heart disease in infants, children and adolescents* (5th ed.). Baltimore: Williams & Wilkins.

Suggested Readings

Devine, S., Anisman, P., & Robinson, B. (1998). A basic guide to cyanotic congenital heart disease. *Contemporary Pediatrics, 15*(10), 133–139.

Feit, L. (1997). The heart of the matter: Evaluating murmurs in children. *Contemporary Pediatrics, 14*, 97–122.

Higgins, S., & Kayser-Jones, J. (1996). Factors influencing parent decision making about pediatric cardiac transplantation. *Journal of Pediatric Nursing, 11*(3), 152–160.

Hohn, A. (1997). Diagnosis and management of hypertension in childhood. *Pediatric Annals, 26*, 105 –110.

Hussein, T. (1998). Patients waiting for heart transplant: An analysis of vulnerability. *Critical Care Nurse, 18*, 40–48.

Kuel, K., Loffredo, C., & Ferencz, C. (1999). Failure to diagnose congenital heart disease in infancy. *Pediatrics, 103*(4), 743–747.

Kugler, J. (1998) Benign arrhythmias: Neonate throughout childhood. In B. Deal, G. Wolff, & H. Gelband (Eds.), *Current concepts in diagnosis and management of arrhythmias in infants and children*. Armonk, NY: Future Publishing.

Lehrer, S. (1992). *Understanding pediatric heart sounds*. Philadelphia: W. B. Saunders.

Mahle, W., Clancy, R., McGaurn, S., Goin, J., & Clark, B. (2001). Impact of prenatal diagnosis on survival and early neurologic morbidity in neonates with the hypoplastic left heart syndrome. *Pediatrics, 107*(6), 1277–1282.

North American Nursing Diagnosis Association (1996). *NANDA nursing diagnoses: Definitions and classification 2001–2002*. Philadelphia, PA: NANDA.

Steinberger, J., Moller, J., Berry, J., & Sinaiko, A. (2000). Echocardiographic diagnosis of heart disease in apparently healthy adolescents. *Pediatrics, 105*(4), 815–818.

Tuite, P. (1997). Recognition and management of shock in the pediatric patient. *Critical Care Nurse, 20*(1), 52–61.

Wood, M. (1997). Acyanotic lesions with increased pulmonary blood flow. *Neonatal Network, 16*(3), 17–28.

Resources

Organizations and Websites

American Association of Critical Care Nurses
101 Columbia
Aliso Viejo, CA 92656
(800) 899-2226
www.aacn.org

American Heart Association
National Center
7272 Greenville Ave.
Dallas, TX 75231-4596
(800) 242-8721
www.americanheart.org

American Society of Hypertension
515 Madison Ave., Suite 1212
New York, NY 10022
(212) 644-0650
www.ash-us.org

International Long QT Syndrome Registry
University of Rochester Medical Center
P.O. Box 653
Rochester, NY 14642-8653
(716) 275-5391

National Down Syndrome Congress
7000 Peachtree-Dunwoody Rd., N.E.
Lake Ridge 400 Office Park
Bldg. 5, Suite 100
Atlanta, GA 30328
(800) 232-NDSC
www.ndsccenter.org

National Heart, Lung and Blood Institute
P.O. Box 30105
Bethesda, MD 20824-0105
(800) 757-9355
www.nhlbi.nih.gov

Sudden Arrhythmia Death Syndromes Foundation
508 E. South Temple, Suite 20
Salt Lake City, UT 84102
(800) 786-7723
www.sads.org

United Network of Organ Sharing
1100 Boulders Parkway, Suite 500
P.O. Box 13770
Richmond, VA 23225-8770
(804) 330-8500
www.unos.org

Patient Education Materials

American Heart Association
National Center
7272 Greenville Ave.
Dallas, TX 75231-4596

Abnormal heart rhythms, what parents should know.
If your child has a congenital heart defect.
Innocent heart murmurs.
You, your child and rheumatic fever.
Mitral valve prolapse.
Living with your pacemaker.
Kawasaki disease.
Your heart and anticoagulants.

Heartwise Patient Education Series
Health Trend Publishing
P.O. Box 7390
Menlo Park, CA 94026
(800) 747-1606

Arrhythmias.
Catheter Ablation.
Holter monitoring.
Electrophysiology study.
Tilt table testing.
Cardiac catheterization.

CHAPTER 26

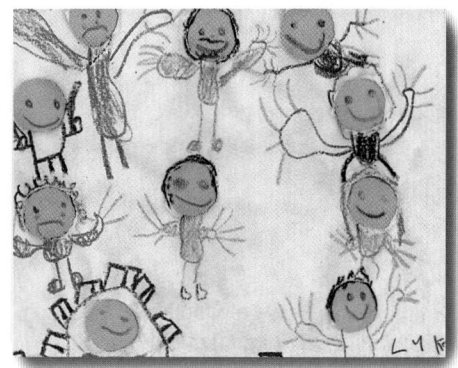

HEMATOLOGICAL ALTERATIONS

Christina P. Linton, RN, MSNc
Lisa Nicole Sessoms Kaplan, RN, MSN

At first we ignored the bruises on Denise's arms and legs, thinking that she was just an active 3-year-old girl. When we mentioned them to her doctor he ran some blood tests and found Denise has aplastic anemia—a fatal disease. Our lives changed completely that day. The doctors have placed her on medications that make it very hard for her to fight infections, and we have to be very careful so she does not get sick. We are actively looking for a bone marrow donor, because the doctors told us that that would give Denise the best chance for survival, but we have not found anyone yet. So, we just wait, watching our sweet little angel become weak and vulnerable. We long for her to have a long and happy life, but do not know what the future holds.

COMPETENCIES

Upon completion of this chapter, the reader will be able to:

- *Discuss the anatomy and physiology of the hematological system.*
- *Identify differences between child and adult hematological systems.*
- *Explain and identify different types of anemia and discuss the etiology, treatment, and nursing care of those types.*
- *Identify several types of coagulation disorders and discuss the etiology, treatment, and nursing care of those disorders.*

In a healthy child, the hematological system enables the body to transport oxygen, fight infection, and minimize hemorrhage. These functions, which are essential for survival, are a direct result of the functions of the cellular components of the blood. Alterations involving these cellular components can cause illnesses such as iron deficiency anemia, sickle cell anemia, beta-thalassemia major, hemophilia, von Willebrand's disease, immune thrombocytopenic purpura, and disseminated intravascular coagulation. The etiology of each alteration is discussed in this chapter, along with the treatment and nursing care for children with these disorders.

ANATOMY AND PHYSIOLOGY

Human blood has two major components: the plasma, which consists primarily of water with a small percentage of solutes, and the formed elements, which consist of cells and proteins. The **cellular elements** of the blood are the erythrocytes or red blood cells, the leukocytes or white blood cells, and the thrombocytes or platelets. During fetal development blood cells are produced in the liver and the spleen. After birth, new blood cells are synthesized from stem cells in the bone marrow through the processes of hematopoiesis. RBC volume varies with age. A unique circumstance exists in newborns immediately following birth. At this time there is a period of inactive erythropoiesis during which the iron obtained from catabolized RBCs is stored as hemosiderin in the bone marrow and the liver tissue. These stores are greatest at 4 to 8 weeks of age and function to protect the infant from anemia because the stores can be used in lieu of dietary iron intake. Premature infants use up these stores within 6 to 12 weeks, whereas the iron stores of full-term infants last up to 20 weeks. Each component of the blood has a specific purpose and together enables the blood to carry out the following functions: (1) transporting substances needed for cellular metabolism in the tissues; (2) regulating acid-base balance; and (3) protecting against infection and injury (McCance, 1998b).

Red Blood Cells

The **red blood cells'** (RBCs) primary function is to supply the tissues of the body with oxygen, made possible by the shape, size, and structure of these cells. They are the most abundant cells in the blood, although the number of RBCs varies with age (see Appendix H for normal RBC values in children). The RBCs remain in circulation for approximately 120 days and are removed from circulation, mainly by the spleen. Because RBCs are not capable of replication, the bone marrow releases new, immature erythrocytes called reticulocytes to replace the RBCs removed from circulation. The characteristic biconcave shape of RBCs allows for a maximal amount of surface area while maintaining a small volume. This feature, in addition to their small size and ability to squeeze through small spaces, allows them to reach all the tissue sites in the body (McCance, 1998b).

The ability of the RBCs to supply oxygen to the tissues is further facilitated by the oxygen-carrying protein **hemoglobin** (Hb), the most abundant protein within a RBC numbering nearly 300 molecules per cell. There are several types of Hb, the two most common being adult hemoglobin (Hb A) and fetal hemoglobin (Hb F). Hb F is the primary Hb found in newborns. This form of Hb is gradually replaced with Hb A as the child ages. Normal Hb molecules are made up of four globin components, composed of polypeptide chains, and four heme sections, composed of iron and a substance called protoporphyrin (Figure 26-1). With its unique structure, hemoglobin enables RBCs to transport 100 times more oxygen than could be transported dissolved in plasma alone (McCance, 1998b).

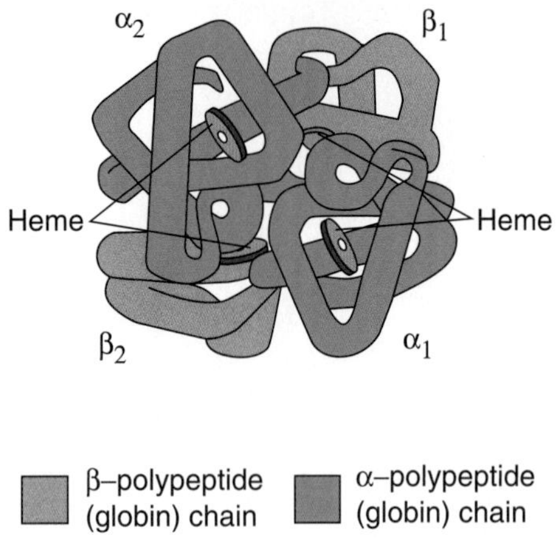

Figure 26-1 The Structure of Normal Hemoglobin

White Blood Cells

The primary function of **white blood cells** (WBCs) is to defend against invading microorganisms and remove debris. These functions are carried out primarily in the injured tissues themselves, but the circulatory system provides a method of transportation that delivers the WBCs to the site of the injury. When invasion by a foreign organism or substance occurs, the body first responds with the inflammatory response, followed by the immune response. The inflammatory response is rapid and nonspecific, whereas the immune response is slower and requires previous sensitization to the foreign organism or substance. This prior sensitization allows the body to recognize and remember the foreign organism, resulting in a more specific response. Members of a subcategory of WBCs called the lymphocytes are responsible for the immune response, whereas the inflammatory response involves other WBCs, namely, the monocytes, macrophages, neutrophils,

Kids Want To Know

What are blood cells?

Many children are curious about their bodies, especially if there is something that is different about them. When caring for a child with a hematological disorder, questions about blood cells can be answered in the following manner:

- Cells are very small parts of our bodies, so small that we cannot see them one at a time. We can only see them when they are all piled together. They are in every part of our bodies, even the blood.
- The cells in our blood are either red or white or a special kind of cell called a platelet.
- Just like us, cells need air in order to live. This is why we need red blood cells. They pick up the air from the lungs and take it to the other cells in the body. If these cells are not working right, we might get tired or dizzy.
- The white blood cells are like watchdogs. They look for anything they have not seen before and if they find something, they fight it so it cannot hurt the body. If we do not have enough cells, they may not be able to fight hard enough to stop something that could make us sick.
- The platelets are special cells that help stop bleeding. When we get hurt and start to bleed, these cells become sticky and form a big clump that blocks the hole where the blood is getting out. This is why we get a scab. If we do not have enough of these cells, it is hard for our bodies to stop the bleeding.

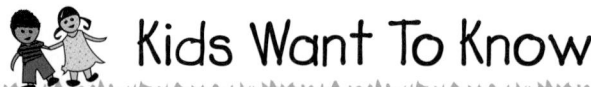

eosinophils, and basophils. Table 26-1 outlines the functions of the these cells in more detail (McCance, 1998b). The proportions of each WBC type within the blood varies with age, as does the total number of WBCs (see Appendix H for normal WBC values in children). The CBC with differential is the primary method of assessing WBC prevalence and function, and therefore is helpful in determining the presence of infection.

Platelets

The **platelets** are disk-shaped cytoplasmic fragments and are not considered cells. As such, they do not have a nucleus or DNA strands and cannot reproduce. Instead, they live for approximately 10 days and are then removed from circulation, primarily by the spleen. Their primary function is to facilitate blood coagulation in order to control bleeding. This is accomplished when platelets adhere to the injured vessel wall, release biochemical mediators, and form platelet plugs, which soon turn into clots (McCance, 1998b).

ANEMIA

Anemia is not a disease, but rather a term used to describe a decrease in the oxygen-carrying capacity of the blood caused by underlying disease or injury. Anemia is the most common blood disorder in children (Kline & Mooney, 1998). In a study of American children conducted by the CDC, approximately 18% of children under 2 years of age and nearly 17% of children age 2 to 5 years had anemia (Centers for Disease Control and Prevention, 1998). Anemia is also common in American adolescents, with a prevalence rate of 10%. (Hord, 1999). This alteration is manifested by a decrease in the hemoglobin concentration of the blood to less than 11.0 g/dl or a hematocrit (HCT) less than 33%. Anemias can be classified either by morphology or etiology. The morphology system uses the terms microcytic, normocytic, and macrocytic to describe the size of RBCs and the terms hypochromic, normocromic, and hyperchromic to describe the color and Hb content of the cells. Within this classification system, abnormally sized RBCs indicate alterations in RBC formation and abnormally colored RBCs indicate alterations in the hemoglobin content of the cells. The etiology system of classification is based on the idea that anemia develops because either production of RBCs (**erythropoiesis**) is decreased, destruction of RBCs (**hemolysis**) is increased, or blood is lost (Cohen & Close, 2000a). This system of classification according to etiology lends itself better to a discussion of the causes of anemia, and is the system used in this chapter. The types of anemia discussed in this chapter are listed according to this classification system in Box 26-1. Information regarding the morphology of specific anemias is presented in the laboratory findings section for each type of anemia.

TABLE 26-1 Functions of the White Blood Cells

Leukocyte	Function	Other important characteristics
Lymphocytes	Immune response	• Majority are located in lymphoid tissue • B cells are responsible for humoral immunity • T cells are responsible for cell-mediated immunity
Monocytes and macrophages	Phagocytosis	• Monocytes are immature macrophages in the blood stream • Macrophages reside in lymphoid tissue • Both make up the mononuclear phagocyte system (along with cells in the marrow), which destroys unwanted materials in the blood and organs
Eosinophils	Phagocytosis	• Prevalent in parasitic infections and allergic reactions • Associated with Hodgkin's disease • Involved in the recovery phase of infection
Neutrophils	Phagocytosis	• Prevalent in early phases of inflammation • Also called polymorphonuclear neutrophils (PMNs) • Immature cells are called bands or stabs • Mature cells are called segmented neutrophils
Basophils	Unknown	• Associated with allergic reactions and mechanical irritation

Adapted from McCance, K. L. (1998b). Structure and function of the hematologic system. In K. L. McCance & S. E. Huether (Eds.), Pathophysiology: The biologic basis for disease in adults and children *(3rd ed., pp. 845–877). St Louis, MO: Mosby.*

BOX 26-1 Anemias classified according to etiology

Decreased Production of RBCs
- Iron Deficiency Anemia
- Aplastic Anemia

Increased Destruction of RBCs
- Sickle Cell Anemia
- Thalassemia

Blood loss
- Iron Deficiency Anemia

Adapted from Cohen, P. S. & Close, P. (2000a). Anemia. In C. D. Berkowitz (Ed.), *Pediatrics: A primary care approach* (2nd ed., pp. 275–279). New York: W. B. Saunders.

Iron Deficiency Anemia

Iron deficiency anemia is the most common hematologic disorder of infancy and childhood.

Incidence and Etiology

The incidence of iron deficiency anemia is not innately related to race, but children with low socioeconomic status and those who are between the ages of 6 months and 2 years are particularly at risk (Kline & Mooney, 1998). Specifically, iron deficiency anemia affects 9% of toddlers 1 to 2 years of age and 4% of children 3 to 4 years of age. For these same age groups in low income families, the incidence rates are 12% and 5%, respectively (U. S. Department of Health and Human Services, 2000). After these critical years, incidence drops to 1% or less, but increases again in adolescence, particularly in adolescent girls, of whom 2% have iron deficiency anemia (Looker, Dallman, Carroll, Gunter, & Johnson, 1997). This increased incidence is predominantly because adolescence is a period of rapid growth and is often associated with poor food choices. Pregnant adolescents are particularly at risk for iron deficiency anemia because of the increased demand for iron imposed by the developing fetus (Kline & Mooney, 1998; Mansen & McCance, 1998).

Inadequate intake of dietary iron is the most common cause of iron deficiency anemia in the first few years of life and during adolescence in the United States. In school-aged children, however, the most common cause is blood loss. In developing third-world countries, the most common cause of iron deficiency anemia is hookworms. Less common causes include inadequate iron stores at birth, impaired iron absorption, and excessive demands for growth (Kline & Mooney, 1998; Mansen & McCance, 1998). No matter the cause of the iron deficiency, the result is the same. The body eventually does not have enough iron to synthesize the hemoglobin necessary to carry oxygen to the tissues and as a result, anemia develops.

Pathophysiology

In children of all ages, dietary iron is absorbed in the small intestine and either passed into the bloodstream or stored in the intestinal epithelial cells as **ferritin.** The iron in the intestinal cells is often lost when the epithelial cells slough off into the intestinal lumen, but can be used for hemoglobin synthesis if necessary. The iron in the blood stream binds to the iron-transport molecule **transferrin** and is then delivered to the RBCs in the bone marrow where it combines with the other components of hemoglobin. If the iron is not used for hemoglobin formation, it is stored as ferritin or **hemosiderin** and later excreted if it remains unused. Normally approximately 67% of the body's iron is bound to heme and 30% of the iron is stored as ferritin or hemosiderin. Iron for hemoglobin formation can also be obtained from RBCs that have been removed from the bloodstream and catabolized. Like dietary iron, this iron is either stored as ferritin or hemosiderin or released into the bloodstream where it can bind to transferrin and travel to the bone marrow to participate in hemoglobin formation (Kline & Mooney, 1998; McCance, 1998b).

When a child or adolescent does not ingest enough dietary iron, the normal process of obtaining iron for hemoglobin synthesis is impaired because there is not enough iron absorbed by the small intestine. When blood loss occurs there are fewer RBCs to be catabolized by the body and consequently, the iron contained in these cells cannot be recycled by the body for future use. One of the most common forms of blood loss in children with iron deficiency anemia is chronic intestinal blood loss caused by a heat-labile protein in cow's milk. This protein causes an inflammatory reaction in the gastrointestinal system, which damages the mucosa and results in diffuse hemorrhage (Kline & Mooney, 1998).

As mentioned earlier, because premature infants use up their iron stores within 6–12 weeks from birth, they are at greater risk for iron deficiency anemia (Kline & Mooney, 1998).

Clinical Manifestations

The signs and symptoms of iron deficiency anemia are directly related to the severity of the tissue hypoxia and the effectiveness of the compensatory mechanisms employed by the body. Iron deficiency anemia, like other types of anemia, can be classified as mild (Hb of 11 g/dl), moderate (Hb of 3–7 g/dl) or severe (Hb <3 g/dl) (Cohen & Close, 2000a). With mild anemia, caregivers commonly do not notice the gradual increase in lethargy and lassitude in their young child or adolescent. Once the child becomes moderately anemic, he/she presents with general irritability, weakness, and lack of interest in play. At this point, the compensatory mechanisms of the body (Box 26-2) are still able to make up for much of

BOX 26-2 Compensatory mechanisms for anemia

- Interstitial fluids enter bloodstream (if the anemia is caused by blood loss)
- Vasodilation occurs
- Heart rate increases
- Rate and depth of respiration increase
- Hemoglobin releases oxygen to tissues more readily
- Erythropoiesis increases
- Peripheral vasoconstriction occurs (with severe anemia)
- Renin-angiotensin system retains salt and water

Adapted from McCance, K. L. (1998b). Structure and function of the hematologic system. In K. L. McCance & S. E. Huether (Eds.), *Pathophysiology: The biologic basis for disease in adults and children* (3rd ed., pp. 845–877). St Louis, MO: Mosby; Mansen, T. J., & McCance, K. L. (1998). Alterations of erythrocyte function. In K. L. McCance & S. E. Huether (Eds.), *Pathophysiology: The biologic basis for disease in adults and children* (3rd ed., pp. 878–898). St Louis, MO: Mosby.

BOX 26-3 Signs and symptoms of anemia according to severity

Mild Anemia
- Generally asymptomatic
- May experience symptoms of moderate anemia during exertion.

Moderate Anemia
Effects of compensatory mechanisms:
- Shortness of breath
- Rapid, pounding heart beat
- Dizziness, fainting, lethargy, irritability

Severe Anemia
Effects of compensatory mechanisms:
- Cardiac murmurs
- Congestive heart failure

Effects of tissue hypoxia:
- Pale skin, mucous membranes, lips, nail beds, and conjunctiva
- Impaired healing and loss of skin elasticity
- Thinning and early greying of the hair
- Abdominal pain, nausea, vomiting, anorexia
- Low-grade fever

Other:
- Yellowish skin color (if the anemia is from increased RBC destruction)

Mansen, T. J., & McCance, K. L. (1998). Alterations of erythrocyte function. In K. L. McCance & S. E. Huether (Eds.), *Pathophysiology: The biologic basis for disease in adults and children* (3rd ed., pp. 878–898). St Louis, MO: Mosby.

the decreased oxygen-carrying capacity of the blood. Eventually the compensatory mechanisms cannot keep up with the anemia and manifestations such as pallor, anorexia, and systolic murmurs begin to appear (Kline & Mooney, 1998). Additional signs and symptoms common to all types of anemia, according to severity, are listed in Box 26-3. The distinction between these categories is not rigid and there may be an overlap of symptoms between categories.

In addition to the common manifestations of anemia, there are several specific signs and symptoms for iron deficiency anemia. These include hair that falls out, nails that are brittle and spoon shaped, and spleen enlargement. Long-standing iron deficiency anemia can also cause decreased physical growth, developmental delays, and widening of cranial sutures. Children with iron deficiency anemia can be underweight, normal weight, or overweight (Cohen & Close, 2000a; Kline & Mooney, 1998). The signs and symptoms of iron deficiency anemia generally resolve with adequate treatment, although some studies suggest that developmental delays may persist (see Research Highlight).

Diagnosis

For all ages, a diagnosis of iron deficiency anemia is made on the basis of history, clinical presentation, and laboratory data. The assessment should include questions about family history, recent blood loss, and dietary history. The child's clinical presentation should be evaluated according to the signs and symptoms listed in Box 26-3. Initial laboratory tests for a child suspected of having iron deficiency anemia are listed in Table 26-2.

Treatment

Treatment of iron deficiency anemia is twofold: correction of the underlying problem responsible for the iron deficiency and replacement of depleted iron stores. If the cause of the iron deficiency is blood loss, the bleeding must be stopped before treatment will be effective. Once the bleeding has stopped, or if the cause is purely nutritional, an adequate teaching plan for the caregiver and child needs to be implemented. For infants, breast milk should be encouraged as the exclusive source of nutrition because the bioavailability of iron in human milk is greater than the iron found in iron-fortified formulas. Once a child is started on solid foods at 4–6 months of life, he or she should be given iron-fortified cereal (Grover, 2000). For a school-aged child with iron deficiency anemia, cow's milk restriction may be implemented to increase the child's hunger for other iron-rich foods and also

TABLE 26-2 Common Laboratory Tests and Findings for Anemia

Laboratory Test	No Anemia Present	Iron Deficiency Anemia	Sickle Cell Anemia	Cooley's Anemia	Aplastic Anemia
Hemoglobin—measures the total amount of Hb in the peripheral blood	9–16 g/dl (see Appendix H)	Decreased	Decreased	Decreased	Decreased
Hematocrit—measures the percentage of RBCs in the total blood volume	28–49% (see Appendix H)	Decreased	Decreased	Decreased	Decreased
Reticulocyte count—measures immature RBCs in order to measure RBC production	Infant: 0.5–3.1% Child & Adolescent: 0.5–2%	Normal	Increased	Normal	Decreased
Mean corpuscular volume (MCV)—measures average RBC volume/size	80–95 μ^3	Decreased	Normal	Decreased	Normal
Mean corpuscular hemoglobin (MCH)—measures the average weight of Hb within a RBC	27–31 pg	Decreased	Normal	Decreased	Normal
Mean corpuscular hemoglobin concentration (MCHC)—measures the average concentration of Hb in one RBC	32–36 g/dl	Decreased	Normal	Decreased	Normal
Hemoglobin electrophoresis—enables detection of abnormal forms of Hb	Predominantly Hb A with decreasing amounts of Hb F as the child ages	Normal	Predominantly Hb S	Abnormally high Hb F	Normal
Peripheral smear—reveals variations in RBC size, color, and shape	Normocytic, normochromic	Microcytic Hypochromic	Normocytic Normochromic Sickle shaped cells	Microcytic Hypochromic	Normocytic Normochromic
Serum iron—measures the iron bound to transferrin in the blood	60–190 µg/dl	Decreased	Normal	Normal	Normal
Serum ferritin—measures available iron stores	6 mo–15 yrs: 7–142 ng/ml Male adolescents: 12–300 ng/ml Female adolescents: 10–150 ng/ml	Decreased	Normal	Normal	Normal
Total iron binding capacity (TIBC)—measures transferrin	25–420 µg/dl	Increased	Decreased	Normal	Normal

Adapted from Pagana, K. D., & Pagana, T. J. (2001). Mosby's diagnostic and laboratory test reference *(4th ed.). St Louis: MO: Mosby; Linker, C. A. (2001). Blood. In L. M. Tierney, S. J. McPhee, & M. A. Papadakis (Eds.),* Current medical diagnosis & treatment 2001 *(40th ed., pp. 505–558). New York: McGraw-Hill.*

Research Highlight

Lower Developmental Test Scores in Infants with Iron-Deficiency Anemia

Study Purpose

To determine if the lower developmental test scores typically found in infants with iron deficiency anemia would improve with the administration of extended oral iron therapy.

Methods

This was a double-blind, controlled trial in Costa Rica involving thirty-two 12- to 23-month-old infants with iron deficiency anemia and a non-anemic control group of fifty-four subjects. The anemic infants were treated with orally administered iron for 6 months. Half of the non-anemic children were treated with iron and half with a placebo. Developmental test scores and hematologic status were evaluated before treatment, after 3 months of treatment, and after 6 months of treatment.

Findings

The anemic infants demonstrated an excellent hematologic response to the oral iron therapy, but still received lower developmental test scores than non-anemic infants at all three points of assessment. There were no significant differences in motor test scores. More of the anemic infants were rated as unusually tearful and unhappy than were the non-anemic children.

Implications

When interpreting the findings of this study, it is important to note that the anemic infants came from families with lower maternal education and less support for child development. They were less likely to be breastfed, were weaned earlier, and consumed more cow's milk. All of these factors could have influenced the results; however, the suggestion that developmental delays could persist even with long-term oral iron supplementation warrants consideration and further research. This study also suggests that iron deficiency anemia may serve as a marker for a variety of nutritional and socioeconomic disadvantages adversely affecting infant development.

Citation

Lozoff B., Wolf A. W., & Jimenez, E. (1996). Iron-deficiency anemia and infant development: Effects of extended oral iron therapy. *Journal of Pediatrics 129*(3), 382–9.

to prevent blood loss in those children who have an inflammatory reaction to cow's milk proteins (Kline & Mooney, 1998). Both school-aged children and adolescents should be encouraged to increase their intake of foods high in iron (Box 26-4) and vitamin C, which increase the body's absorption of iron. Pregnant adolescents need to be especially aware of their iron intake. Iron supplementation is recommended both to prevent and treat iron deficiency anemia in this population (Wardlaw, 1999).

In addition to dietary supplementation, iron supplementation is given either orally or parenterally. However, parenteral iron is reserved for use in clients with iron malabsorption, chronic blood loss, or inability to tolerate oral iron. This is because oral iron corrects iron deficiency just as rapidly and completely as parenteral iron, with potentially less severe side effects. The recommended form of oral iron supplementation is ferrous iron because it is the most efficiently absorbed. The common side effects of oral iron supplementation are listed in Table 26-3. If a child cannot tolerate these side effects, they can often be overcome by either switching to a different type of oral iron, lowering the daily dose of iron, or by taking the tablets immediately after or with meals (Santi & Masters, 2001). The recommended dosage for oral iron supplementation is dependent

BOX 26-4 Good dietary sources of iron

High Iron Density
- Organ meat
- Spinach
- Oysters
- Peas
- Legumes
- Beef

Medium Iron Density
- Tofu
- Seafood
- Whole grains
- Enriched grains
- Wheat germ
- Oatmeal

Low Iron Density
- Peaches
- Prune juice
- Dried apricots
- Potatoes
- Green beans
- Broccoli

Adapted from Wardlaw, G. M. (1999). *Perspectives in nutrition* (4th ed.). Boston: WCB/McGraw-Hill.

on age and gender. For infants and preschool children, the dosage is 3 mg/kg/day. One 60 mg tablet daily is recommended for school-aged children and two 60 mg tablets are recommended daily for adolescent boys. For adolescent girls, the desired dosage is 60 to 120 mg per day (Morey, 1998). In order to ensure iron stores are replenished, treatment is continued for at least 2 months after RBC indexes have returned to normal. If hemoglobin levels do not increase after 1 month of oral therapy, the oral supplementation should be stopped and the child evaluated for other causes of anemia (Cohen & Close, 2000a).

Nursing Management

Assessment

The assessment of a child with iron deficiency anemia consists mainly of observing for the signs and symptoms listed in Box 26-3. A good client history will also provide valuable information, and should include a detailed dietary history along with a history of bowel movements.

Nursing Diagnosis

Appropriate nursing diagnoses for a child with iron deficiency anemia include:

- Ineffective tissue perfusion related to anemia
- Imbalanced nutrition: less than body requirements related to inadequate iron intake
- Deficient caregiver knowledge related to age-appropriate iron intake
- Activity intolerance related to decreased oxygen delivery to the tissues

Outcome Identification

The desired outcomes for these nursing diagnoses include the following: (a) the child will take daily iron supplements to increase his/her Hb and HCT; (b) the child will consume at least the minimum recommended daily allowance (RDA) of iron each day; (c) the caregiver will be able to describe the appropriate feeding guidelines for the child's age; and (d) the child will be able to engage in age-appropriate play without signs or symptoms of excessive exertion.

Planning/Implementation

In order to achieve these outcomes, the primary focus of nursing intervention is caregiver education. This education

TABLE 26-3 Common Side Effects of Iron Supplementation

Oral Iron	Parenteral Iron	
Nausea	Local pain	Back pain
Epigastric discomfort	Tissue staining	Flushing
Abdominal cramps	Headache	Urticaria
Constipation	Light-headedness	Bronchospasm
Diarrhea	Fever	Anaphylaxis (rare)
Black stools	Arthralgias	Death (rare)
	Nausea and vomiting	

Adapted from Santi, D. V., & Masters, S. B. (2001). Drugs used in anemias: Hematopoietic Growth Factors. In B. G. Katzung (Ed.), Basic and clinical pharmacology *(8th ed., pp. 549–563). New York: McGraw-Hill.*

Nursing Alert:

Iron Supplements

Although oral iron supplementation is generally perceived as a safe treatment alternative, an overdose can be lethal for children. Initial signs and symptoms of overdose include vomiting, abdominal pain, and bloody diarrhea. These manifestations are typically followed by shock, lethargy, and dyspnea. Often the child will appear to improve before the onset of severe metabolic acidosis, coma, and death. Urgent treatment is essential and includes flushing out unabsorbed pills, administration of Desferal (see beta-thalassemia section), and supportive therapy (Santi & Masters, 2001).

Eye On:

Alternative Approaches to Iron Supplementation

In at risk populations, routine iron supplementation is a method of preventing iron deficiency anemia. In addition to the iron-fortified foods and oral iron supplements used in the United States, alternative methods of iron supplementation are surfacing in other countries, with promising results.

Researchers in a Brazilian study provided 21 families of low socioeconomic status with an iron/ascorbic acid solution to be added to their domestic drinking water. Over the course of the four-month study, researchers found the iron-fortified drinking water was well received by the families and was effective in raising the hemoglobin and serum ferritin levels of the children in these families (de Oliveira, Scheid, Desai, & Marchini, 1996).

In Indonesia, researchers investigated the use of inexpensive iron-fortified candies to improve the iron status of over 100 kindergarten children. The children ate ten iron-fortified candies a week and after 12 weeks both anemia and iron deficiency had decreased. The researchers also reported most children liked the candies and caregivers expressed willingness to continue using them (Sari, Bloem, dePee, Schultink, & Sastroamidjojo, 2001).

should include a discussion of iron deficiency anemia, age-appropriate dietary guidelines, and information regarding the administration of oral iron supplements. This education, which is included in the family teaching section, will help caregivers overcome their lack of knowledge in relation to iron intake, and increase their child's iron intake, tissue perfusion, and activity tolerance.

Evaluation

Follow-up with the family should focus on evaluating the desired outcomes and reviewing education concepts as needed. The caregiver and child should be asked about how and when the child has been taking iron supplements. Laboratory work will also be helpful in determining the success of the interventions. A dietary history should be obtained to determine if the child has consumed at least the minimum RDA of iron each day. The nurse should ask the caregiver to explain the appropriate feeding guidelines for his/her child's age and observe the child's actions for any signs or symptoms of excessive exertion.

Family Teaching

The nurse should explain that adequate iron is necessary for the blood to be able to transport oxygen to the tissues. If a child does not eat enough iron, the body will use up all the extra iron it has stored. Once the stores of iron have been used, the child will have symptoms, such as weakness, irritability, pale skin, decreased appetite, and a fast heart beat. Eating more iron and taking iron supplements will help replenish the body's stores of iron and allow adequate oxygen to be transported to the tissues.

The nurse should also reinforce age-appropriate dietary guidelines. These include:

Under 12 months of age:

- Encourage exclusive breastfeeding of infants for 4–6 months after birth.
- When exclusive breastfeeding is stopped, encourage intake of approximately 1 mg/kg per day of iron, preferably from supplementary foods (see Box 26-4).
- For infants who are not breastfed or who are partially breastfed, recommend only iron-fortified infant formula as a substitute for breast milk.
- For breastfed infants who receive less than 1 mg/kg per day of iron from supplementary foods by age 6 months, suggest 1 mg/kg per day of iron drops.
- For breastfed infants who were preterm or had a low birth weight, recommend 2–4 mg/kg per day of iron drops (to a maximum of 15 mg/day) starting at 1 month after birth and continuing until 12 months after birth.
- Encourage the use of only breast milk or iron-fortified infant formula for any milk-based part of the diet (e.g., in infant cereal).
- Discourage the use of low-iron milks (e.g., cow's milk, goat's milk, and soy milk).
- At age 4–6 months two or more servings per day of iron-fortified infant cereal can meet an infant's requirement for iron.
- By approximately age 6 months, encourage one feeding per day of foods rich in vitamin C (e.g., fruits,

vegetables, or juice) to improve iron absorption, preferably with meals.

- Suggest introducing plain, pureed meats after age 6 months or when the infant is developmentally ready to consume such food.

School-aged children and adolescents:

- Suggest children aged 1–5 years consume no more than 24 oz of cow's milk, goat's milk, or soy milk each day.
- Encourage consumption of iron-rich foods (see Box 26-4).
- Recommend cooking acidic foods in iron cookware.
- Increase dietary intake of foods rich in vitamin C (e.g., fruits, vegetables, or juice) to improve iron absorption, preferably with meals.

The nurse should provide the following information about oral iron supplements:

- Give exactly the prescribed amount. More is not better and can actually harm the child.
- Keep the iron locked in a safe place to prevent accidental overdoses.
- The side effects listed in Table 26-3 are common and can be avoided by taking the tablets immediately after or with meals.
- If the child is getting enough iron, stools should be a tarry green color.
- Constipation will often persist and may require the use of stool softeners or laxatives.
- Liquid iron supplements may stain teeth. If the child is old enough, give the iron solution with a straw. Otherwise, give with a dropper or syringe in the back part of the mouth.
- Avoid giving the child flouride, antacids, tetracycline, coffee, tea, dairy products, eggs, or whole-grain breads within 1 hour before or 2 hours after the oral iron supplement because these substances interfere with iron absorption.

Much of the teaching provided to caregivers for home management of iron deficiency anemia applies in the school setting as well. If the child eats foods prepared by the school, these foods should provide adequate iron intake and include vitamin C if possible. If the iron supplements need to be given at school, instructions should also be provided concerning their proper administration and storage.

Refer the family to the Iron Disorders Institute; the National Heart, Lung and Blood Institute Information Center; or the Children's Blood Foundation (see the Resources section at the end of this chapter).

Critical Thinking

What Is the Diagnosis?

While working in the community you encounter 10-month-old Wendy, who is irritable and appears weak for her age. Her mother states she seems more tired than usual and does not play as much as she used to. She has tried giving Wendy a bottle of milk like she usually does when she appears unhappy, but that does not seem to pacify her. You ask more about dietary habits and find that when Wendy's mother stopped breastfeeding, she started her on a cow's-milk bottle. She usually uses this bottle to calm her and when it is time for meals, Wendy typically does not eat very much. What do you think Wendy's diagnosis is and what nursing interventions would be appropriate?

Sickle Cell Anemia

Sickle cell anemia (SCA) is one of three disorders that fall under the classification of sickle cell disease. Each disorder in this class is characterized by the presence of **hemoglobin S** (Hb S), also known as sickle hemoglobin. The other types of Hb inherited from the parents of a child with sickle cell disease determine which sickle cell disorder the child will manifest. In addition to SCA, the other two types of sickle cell disease are sickle cell-hemoglobin C disease and sickle cell-thalassemia disease. Of these disorders, SCA is the most severe, although every type of sickle cell disease is a lifelong disorder with no known cure (Kline & Mooney, 1998).

Incidence and Etiology

Like the other sickle cell disorders, SCA is an autosomal recessive disorder that can be transmitted to the offspring of those with the disease, as well as to the offspring of carriers. In order for either of these possibilities to occur, both parents must carry at least one of the recessive genes (Figure 26-2). If both parents do not have the gene, the child will either be a carrier for sickle cell disease or will not have the sickle cell gene. Carriers of sickle cell disease are said to have the sickle cell trait (SCT), although they generally have no symptoms (U. S. Department of Health and Human Services [DHHS], 1996).

Sickle cell disease has been traced back thousands of years to the inhabitants of Africa, the Mediterranean basin, the Middle East, and India. During this time, a deadly form of malaria was very common in these areas. However, researchers have found that children in these areas who had the sickle cell trait were able to survive the malaria epidemics more often than those who did not. Thus, the gene for sickle cell disease was passed on to the children of these survivors. At present, however, possessing the sickle cell gene may be a serious threat to those not likely to be exposed to malaria (DHHS, 1996).

(A) When both parents carry the disease gene, there is a 25% chance that each child conceived will not have the disease or carry the disease. There is a 50% chance that each child conceived will carry the gene, and a 25% chance that each child conceived will have the disease.

	B	b
B	BB 25% Normal	Bb 25% Carrier
b	Bb 25% Carrier	bb 25% Disease

(B) When one parent has the disease and the other is a carrier for the disease, there is a 50% chance that each child conceived will carry the disease and a 50% chance that each child conceived will have the disease.

	b	b
B	Bb 25% Carrier	Bb 25% Carrier
b	bb 25% Disease	bb 25% Disease

Legend
b = Recessive disease gene
B = Dominant normal gene
bb = Disease state
Bb or bB = Carrier state
BB = Normal state

Figure 26-2 Autosomal Recessive Inheritance

Sickle cell anemia affects millions of people throughout the world. However, because of the benefits of the sickle cell trait in regard to malaria exposure, SCA is particularly common among individuals whose ancestors originated in sub-Saharan Africa, South America, Cuba, Central America, Saudi Arabia, India, and Mediterranean countries. In the United States, SCA affects approximately 72,000 people and approximately 2 million Americans carry the sickle cell trait. SCA occurs in approximately 1 in every 1,000–1,400 Hispanic American births and 1 in every 500 African-American births. The sickle cell trait is even more prevalent in this group, with 1 in 12 African-Americans possessing this genotype (DHHS, 1996).

Pathophysiology

In children who have the recessive sickle cell gene one amino acid replaces another, resulting in the production of sickle hemoglobin (Hb S). This abnormal form of hemoglobin contains a semisolid gel that aggregates within the RBC, causing it to stretch into an elongated crescent or sickle shape (Figure 26-3). When compared to normal RBCs, sickled cells are more stiff and less able to change shape. As a result, they are often unable to pass through the microcirculation, causing vaso-occlusion, pain, and organ infarction. They can also cause infarction of the splenic vessels and blood pooling in the spleen because the cells are destroyed or sequestered there. This phenomenon results in an anemia of increased RBC destruction. The body tries to compensate by increasing RBC production. This anemic condition is worsened by the fact that sickled RBCs die after only about 10 to 20 days, resulting in an abnormally low number of RBCs in circulation (Kline & Mooney, 1998; DHHS, 1996).

The sickling of RBCs is occasional and intermittent, resulting from or sustained by decreased oxygen tension of the blood (i.e., hypoxemia), increased hydrogen ion concentration

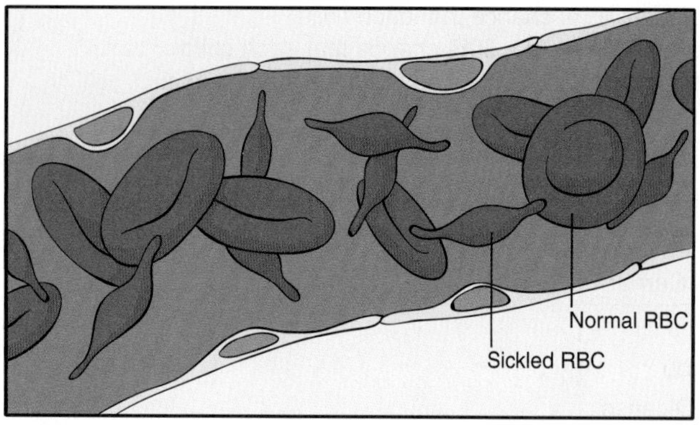

Figure 26-3 Regular and Sickled RBCs

Nursing Alert:

Children with SCA and SCT

Children with sickle cell anemia, and on rare occasions children who have the sickle cell trait, can experience vaso-occlusive episodes and severe hypoxia caused by shock, vigorous exercising at high altitudes, flying at high altitudes in unpressurized aircraft, or undergoing anesthesia (Kline & Mooney, 1998).

in the blood (decreased pH), increased plasma osmolality (increased concentration of solutes in blood), decreased plasma volume (increased viscosity), and low temperature (associated with vasoconstriction). These factors can create a self-perpetuating cycle because as sickled cells clog the vessels, hypoxemia develops and perpetuates the sickling. Both the intensity and duration of the stimulus affect the amount of sickling and when rehydrated or reoxygenated, most sickled cells regain a normal shape. However, irreversible sickling can occasionally occur because of plasma membrane damage (Kline & Mooney, 1998).

Sickle cell anemia has the highest prevalence of Hb S, with approximately 75–95% of the Hb within a RBC being Hb S. The severity of sickling is directly correlated with the percentage of Hb S, thus making SCA the most severe type of sickle cell disease. On the other end of the spectrum, children who have the sickle cell trait rarely experience RBC sickling because Hb F (fetal hemoglobin) and Hb A (adult hemoglobin) do not participate in sickling. These children may experience anemia, however, because of the prevalence of Hb F. Hb F does not live as long as Hb A and therefore causes these children to have lower Hb concentrations (Kline & Mooney, 1998). Figure 26-4 illustrates the effect on the body.

Clinical Manifestations

The clinical manifestations of SCA can vary widely in severity and frequency. During the first six months of life most newborns are asymptomatic because Hb F does not sickle. As Hb S replaces Hb F, however, sickling increases and symptoms begin to develop. The anemia of SCA is manifested by the same signs and symptoms of other anemias, including pallor, fatigue, shortness of breath, irritability, and jaundice (see Box 26-3 for additional signs and symptoms). Children with SCA also experience delayed growth and delayed onset of puberty. However, the principal symptom experienced by children with this disorder is pain. This pain can occur unpredictably in any body organ or joint and is typically associated with the occurrence of vaso-occlusive crises. These crises are the most common type of sickle cell crisis, although sequestration crisis and aplastic crisis can also occur (Dover & Platt, 1997; Kline & Mooney, 1998; DHHS, 1996).

The term **vaso-occlusive crisis** refers to the aggregation of sickled cells within a vessel, causing obstruction. If the process is not reversed, infarction of the distal tissues will ensue. This type of crisis causes extreme pain and can occur less than once a year or as often as 15 or more times a year. The duration of the pain varies from a few hours to several weeks, with an average duration of 4 to 6 days (Kline & Mooney, 1998; DHHS, 1996). The most common sites of vaso-occlusive crises are listed in Table 26-4 along with the common manifestations associated with each type of obstruction. Of particular importance in the pediatric population is the vaso-occlusive manifestation of **hand-foot syndrome** (tender, warm, and swollen hands, feet, or both) because it is typically the first manifestation of SCA in infants. The pain associated with this syndrome is severe, causing children to cry and refuse to bear weight (Dover & Platt, 1997). Another commonly occurring manifestation in children is a cerebral vascular accident (CVA). Approximately 10% of children with sickle cell disease experience CVAs, with a peak incidence between the ages of four and six years. These CVAs typically occur without warning, but may be preceded by severe headaches or a deterioration in school performance (Wethers, 2000).

The term **sequestration crisis** refers to the excessive pooling of blood in the liver and spleen. As more and more of the child's blood leaves circulation, the decreased blood volume results in shock (see Box 26-5 for the signs and symptoms of shock). This type of crisis can cause fatal cardiovascular collapse, because the spleen is capable of holding as much as one-fifth of the body's blood volume. This type of crisis is most commonly seen in children under three years of age. By four years of age most children with SCA have experienced splenic infarction. Sequestration crisis is associated with a mortality rate of up to 50% (Kline & Mooney, 1998; Wethers, 2000).

Aplastic crisis occurs when there is a decrease in erythropoiesis, despite the shortened life span of sickled RBCs and the body's need for increased RBC production. In 80%

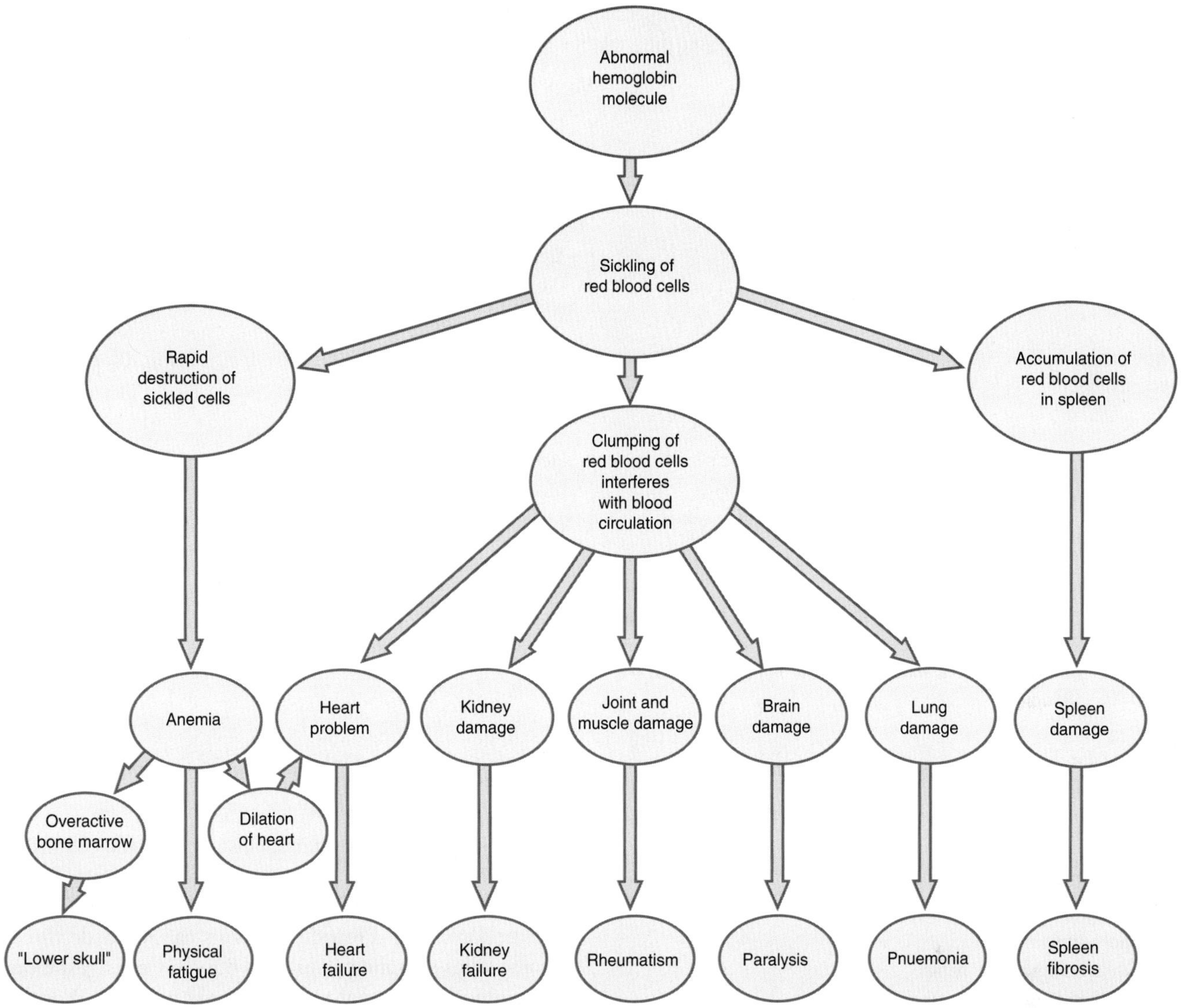

Figure 26-4 Sickle Cell Anemia: The clumping of red blood cells, rapid destruction of red blood cells, and accumulation in the spleen with their resulting effects on the body are shown.

of cases, this type of crisis is precipitated by an infection with human parovirus B19. The infection is self-limited, but highly contagious and warrants isolation from persons vulnerable to infection. Aplastic crisis results in severe anemia, manifested by the signs and symptoms listed in Box 26-3 (Kline & Mooney, 1998; Wethers, 2000).

Many children with SCA will eventually experience organ damage as a direct result of sickled RBCs reducing blood flow to the organ. Nearly every organ system of the body is affected. In addition to the common sites of vaso-occlusive crisis, sickle cells can reduce blood flow to the eyes, gastrointestinal tract, and the kidneys, and result in blindness, abdominal pain, and **enuresis** (urinary incontinence). Sickled cells can also cause damage to the spleen and reduce its ability to destroy bacteria in the blood, leaving the child immunocompromised and susceptible to serious infections, usually caused by common pathogens. For instance, the risk of pneumococcal infection in young children with SCA appears to be 400 times that of normal children. The severity of these bacterial infections can kill a child with SCA in as little as nine hours from the onset of fever (Linker, 2001; DHHS, 1996; Wethers, 2000).

Diagnosis

Although family history and clinical manifestations may raise suspicion about sickle cell disease, a definitive diagnosis can only be made through evaluating laboratory findings. If the child presents with an anemia of unknown cause, the tests listed in Table 26-2 can be helpful in determining if further testing for SCA is warranted. Further testing would begin with a sickle solubility test in order to confirm the presence

TABLE 26-4 Common Manifestations of Vaso-occlusive Crises

	Underlying Cause	Manifestations
Painful crisis	Bone marrow ischemia	• Deep, gnawing, throbbing pain of rapid onset • Normal physical and laboratory findings • Usually located in the lumbosacral spine, knee, shoulder, elbow, or femur regions.
Hand-foot syndrome	Bone marrow ischemia in the hands and feet.	• Tender, warm, and swollen hands, feet, or both. • Usually acutely ill with fever and increase numbers of WBCs
Acute chest syndrome	Infection, pulmonary infarction by sickled cells or fat emboli, or a combination of the two.	• Pain in the chest or extremities, fever, respiratory distress, and/or hypoxemia • Life-threatening
Stroke	Infarction of the carotid or cerebral arteries	• Hemiparesis, speech defects, focal seizures, and gait dysfunction.
Priapism	Obstruction of the penile veins	• Persistent penile erection • Possible urinary retention

Adapted from: Dover, G. J., & Platt, O. S. (1997). Sickle cell disease. In D. G. Nathan & S. H. Orkin (Eds.), Nathan and Oski's hematology of infancy and childhood *(5th ed., Vol. 2, 762–809). Philadelphia: W. B. Saunders; Wethers, D. L. (2000). Sickle cell disease in childhood: Part II. Diagnosis and treatment of major complications and recent advances in treatment.* American Family Physician, *62(6), 1309–1314.*

BOX 26-5 Signs and symptoms of shock

Early signs
- Tachycardia
- Delayed capillary refill
- Cool, clammy, pale, or mottled skin
- Decreased urine output

Late signs
- Altered mental status
- Weak, thready, or absent pulses
- Hypotension
- Tachycardia or bradycardia
- Delayed capillary refill
- Severely mottled or cyanotic skin
- Decreased or absent urine output

Adapted from Young, K. D. (2000). Shock. In C. D. Berkowitz (Ed.), *Pediatrics: A primary care approach* (2nd ed., pp. 163–167). New York: W. B. Saunders.

of Hb S in the blood. If this test is positive, hemoglobin electrophoresis would then be conducted to determine the amount of Hb S in the blood. The results of this test can then be used to differentiate SCA from other types of sickle cell disease. These two tests would also be appropriate in evaluating children who present with the clinical manifestations of SCA. If there is a family history of sickle cell disease, concerned parents can choose to have these tests done on their children, or can have prenatal testing conducted on their unborn fetus. Prenatal diagnosis can be made through chronic villus sampling as early as 8 to 10 weeks gestation or with amniotic fluid analysis at 15 weeks gestation. For those families without a known family history of sickle cell disease, the routine testing of newborns conducted in over 40 states is able to detect both sickle cell disease and sickle cell trait (Kline & Mooney, 1998; DHHS, 1996).

Treatment

The primary treatment for children with sickle cell disease is prevention of RBC sickling in order to prevent anemia and sickle cell crises. This entails avoiding stimuli such as fever, infection, acidosis, dehydration, constricting clothing, and exposure to cold. Adherence to the recommended childhood immunization schedule, including the hepatitis B and pneumococcal vaccines, is essential for children with this disease because of their increased risk for infection. For this reason, children with SCA are also maintained on prophylactic oral penicillin until age 5 (Dover & Platt, 1997). For children who are at high risk for CVAs, the use of routine blood transfusions every three to four weeks has been found to decrease the incidence of stroke by 90%. If this treatment is used, chelation therapy will also be necessary (see beta-thalassemia major section) (National Institutes of Health, 1997).

If a vaso-occlusive crisis does occur, pain can usually be managed with acetaminophen or ibuprofen if mild or if the child is under six years of age. For more severe pain, the use of narcotics such as morphine is appropriate. IV fluids may be necessary to achieve optimal hydration and reverse RBC sickling. A sequestration crisis requires the transfusion of red blood cells to treat the rapid decrease in circulating blood volume. If sequestration crises occur frequently, a splenectomy may be performed to alleviate the danger of cardiovascular collapse. Most aplastic crises are short, mild, and do not require therapy (Dover & Platt, 1997; Wethers, 2000).

Fortunately, the sickle cell trait is not associated with decreased life expectancy. However, sepsis and meningitis develop in as many as 10% of SCA children under the age of 5, with a mortality rate of 25%. Many children who survive past age 5 only live into their twenties, but survival is unpredictable (Kline & Mooney, 1998).

Nursing Management

Assessment

In addition to observing for the signs and symptoms of anemia listed in Box 26-3, nurses should also assess for pain related to vaso-occlusive crises or shock related to sequestration crisis.

Nursing Diagnosis

Potential nursing diagnoses for the child with sickle cell anemia include:

- Pain related to vaso-occlusive crisis
- Ineffective tissue perfusion related to impaired arterial blood flow
- High risk for infection related to splenic malfunction and chronic immunocompromised state
- Ineffective coping of child and family related to chronic and potentially life-threatening disease

Outcome Identification

The desired outcomes for these diagnoses include:

- The child will report pain relief is adequate.
- The child will not demonstrate the manifestations of anemia.
- The child will be afebrile.
- Caregivers will be aware of resources available to help them cope with difficulties inherent in having a child with SCA.

Planning/Implementation

Pain management is most commonly needed when a child experiences a vaso-occlusive crisis. In this instance, analgesics should be given around the clock, rather than on an as-needed basis. Children experiencing sickle cell crisis are often under-medicated resulting in "clock watching" and requests for additional doses occurring sooner than prescribed. Many misinformed health care professionals interpret this behavior as a sign of drug addiction, whereas the actual problem is inadequate pain control. Other nursing interventions include (a) applying heat to the painful area (cold is contraindicated because it promotes sickling), (b) allowing the child to determine the amount of activity he/she can tolerate, (c) providing passive range of motion exercises to prevent venous stasis, (d) administering intravenous fluids to maintain hydration status, (e) frequent handwashing, and (f) proper aseptic techniques. If blood transfusions are administered, hospital protocol should be followed (see beta-thalassemia section). As the nurse interacts with the child and caregivers, he/she should take the time to talk with them about their emotions related to their child's situation. The nurse should also refer the caregivers to social workers and/or community resources for the clients and their families.

Evaluation

Once nursing interventions have been implemented, the desired outcomes can be evaluated by assessing the child for pain, anemia, and fever. Assessment should also include thorough observation and discussion to determine if the

Reflective Thinking

Family Planning for a Person with Sickle Cell Disease

1. If you and your partner were carriers of the sickle cell gene, would you make a decision to attempt a pregnancy and hope for a child born without the disease?
2. If you decided to conceive, would you use prenatal testing to determine if the child you were carrying was positive for the disease or the trait? Why or why not?
3. If the fetus was positive for the disease, what would you do? Would you terminate the pregnancy? Would you carry to term? Would it make a difference if the fetus had the trait rather than having the disease? Why or why not?
4. What if you and your partner decided not to conceive but accidentally became pregnant? Would you go through prenatal testing, carry the fetus to term and hope for a healthy outcome, or abort the pregnancy without determining the sickle cell status of the fetus? Why or why not?
5. What are options two people who are both carriers for the disease might have in terms of having children?

child and caregiver are aware of the resources available to help them.

Family Teaching

Caring for a child with sickle cell anemia at home requires a clear understanding of the situations that precipitate sickling, including dehydration, infection, and exposure to cold. The child and caregivers should be taught to avoid any known sources of infection and maintain adequate nutrition and handwashing. They should also be taught to seek medical help if they notice fever, pallor, pain, or enlargement in the area of the spleen.

The child's teachers should be made aware of the child's condition, the situations that the child needs to avoid, and indications of a need for medical help. If the child participates in any school sports it is essential to maintain adequate hydration.

There are numerous agencies that provide information and support for both caregivers and children with SCA, including the Sickle Cell Disease Association of America; the Center for Sickle Cell Disease; the National Sickle Cell Disease Program; the Sickle Cell Association of Ontario; and the Joint Center for Sickle Cell and Thalassemic Disorders (see the Resources section at the end of this chapter).

Beta-thalassemia Major

The **thalassemias** are a group of inherited autosomal recessive disorders, characterized by an impaired rate of hemoglobin chain synthesis (see Figure 26-2). These lifelong disorders are classified as alpha- or beta-, according to which globin chain of hemoglobin synthesis is impaired; and as major or minor, depending on how many genes are defective. That is, thalassemia major refers to the inheritance of recessive genes from both parents and thalassemia minor refers to the inheritance of recessive genes from only one parent. Of all thalassemias, the beta-thalassemias are more common and present the most significant health concerns for children (Kline & Mooney, 1998).

Incidence and Etiology

The beta-thalassemias are common among children of Mediterranean descent, such as Italians and Greeks, and are also found in the inhabitants of the Arabic peninsula, Iran, Africa, Southeast Asia, and southern China. Children with thalassemia minor, also referred to as having the thalassemia trait, carry the gene for thalassemia without manifesting significant health problems. In these children, the lack of alpha- or beta-globin is generally not great enough to cause altered hemoglobin function, other than causing mild anemia. It is estimated that over 2 million people in the Unites States carry the genetic trait for thalassemia. In contrast, **beta-thalassemia major** (also called Cooley's anemia) is associated with a life-threatening form of anemia that requires regular blood transfusions and ongoing medical care. Death from cardiac failure usually occurs between ages 20 and 30 (Cooley's Anemia Foundation [CAF], 2001b, 2001c; Linker, 2001).

Pathophysiology

Each normal Hb A contains four globin components, or polypeptide chains. Two of these globins are alpha polypeptide chains and two are beta polypeptide chains. These four chains combine with four heme complexes, the oxygen carrying component, to form one Hb molecule (see Figure 26-1). In beta-thalassemia the synthesis of beta-globin chains is impaired, resulting in RBCs that contain less hemoglobin. In addition, these RBCs contain free alpha chains that are unstable and precipitate, causing many of the RBCs in the marrow to be destroyed. Thus, an anemia of decreased RBC production results. The RBCs that do mature and enter the bloodstream are destroyed prematurely in the spleen, resulting in a concomitant anemia of increased RBC destruction (Kline & Mooney, 1998; McCance, 1998b).

The severe anemia associated with beta-thalassemia major causes the kidneys to release **erythropoietin**, a hormone that stimulates the bone marrow to produce more RBCs. The resulting increase in hematopoiesis is ineffective, however, because of the increased rate of RBC destruction that is characteristic of the disorder. As a result of this process, the bone marrow eventually becomes hyperplastic. This **hyperplasia** (abnormal proliferation) of the bone marrow cells causes the bones themselves to enlarge in order to accommodate the increased bone marrow volume (Linker, 2001; McCance, 1998b).

Clinical Manifestations

Beta-thalassemia major typically manifests itself during the second six months of life when Hb F is replaced by Hb A. As they grow older, children with this disorder not only develop the signs and symptoms of severe anemia (see Box 26-3), but also exhibit numerous other manifestations associated with beta-thalassemia major (Table 26-5 and Figure 26-5). All these factors contribute to the impaired growth and development manifested by these children. If children with this disorder are not treated, they will die by the age of 5 to 6 years. This clinical course can be modified with transfusion therapy, which can increase life span by 1 to 2 decades. However, as will be discussed in the treatment section, severe symptoms of iron overload can develop (Kline & Mooney, 1998; Linker, 2001).

Diagnosis

The diagnosis of thalassemia is based on family disease history, clinical presentation, and laboratory findings. Thalassemia can be detected through specific newborn screening tests, which are collected according to state law. Prenatal diagnosis is also possible. The laboratory tests for

TABLE 26-5 Clinical Manifestations of Beta-thalassemia Major

Manifestations	**Underlying Cause**
Facies of beta-thalassemia major: Prominent and protruding forehead Maxillary prominence Wide-set eyes Flattened nose	Expansion of bones to accommodate hyperplastic marrow
Pathologic fractures	Expansion of bones to accommodate hyperplastic marrow
Decreased bone mineralization	Expansion of bones to accommodate hyperplastic marrow
Malocclusion	Maxillary overgrowth
Splenic enlargement	Extramedullary hematopoiesis and increased hemolysis
Jaundice	Increased RBC hemolysis
Bronze coloring of the skin	Iron accumulation in the skin

Adapted from: Kline, N. E. & Mooney, K. H. (1998). Alterations of hematologic function in children. In K. L. McCance & S. E. Huether (Eds.), Pathophysiology: The biologic basis for disease in adults and children *(3rd ed., pp. 935–967). St Louis, MO: Mosby; Linker, C. A. (2001). Blood. In L. M. Tierney, S. J. McPhee, & M. A. Papadakis (Eds.),* Current medical diagnosis & treatment 2001 *(40th ed., pp. 505–558). New York: McGraw-Hill.*

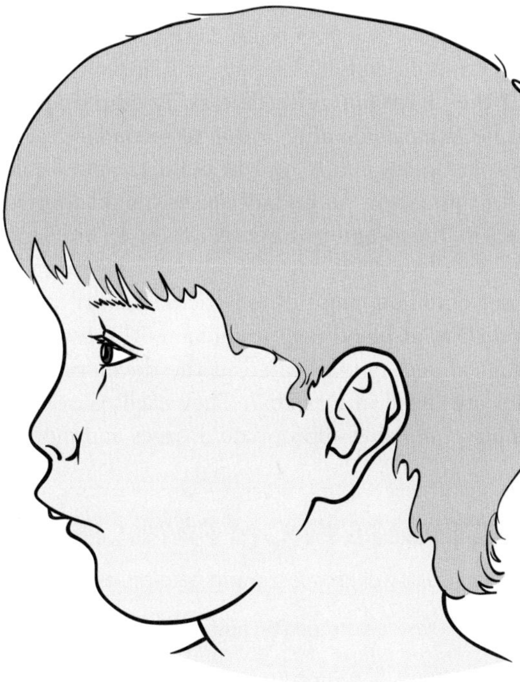

Figure 26-5 Facies of a Child with Beta-Thalassemia

children or adolescents suspected of having thalassemia are listed in Table 26-2, along with the findings typically associated with beta-thalassemia major. One of the most striking laboratory findings is the extremely low hematocrit, which can fall to less than 10% of normal if not treated with transfusions. Thalassemia minor, however, often presents with an anemia so mild that it is mistaken for iron deficiency anemia (Kline & Mooney, 1998; Linker, 2001).

Treatment

Unlike thalassemia minor, which does not require any specific treatment, beta-thalassemia major requires medical intervention to support and prolong life. There is no cure for thalassemia, so the goal of treatment is to normalize the Hb and HCT of the child, thus alleviating the symptoms of severe anemia. This is accomplished via a regular schedule of transfusions, with many children requiring transfusions every two to three weeks. Along with these transfusions, a splenectomy is often performed because eliminating the site of hemolysis can decrease the child's need for frequent transfusions (CAF, 2001b; Kline & Mooney, 1998).

Repeated transfusions eventually result in a buildup of excess iron in the body, causing iron overload or **hemosiderosis.** In hemosiderosis, the excess iron is stored as hemosiderin in the cells of many organs and tissues, particularly in the liver and heart. Iron is toxic to the tissues and organs and eventually causes organ failure and death. This condition is exacerbated by the increased rate of hemolysis that is present if the spleen has not been removed (CAF, 2001b; Linker, 2001; McCance, 1998a).

In order to reduce hemosiderosis, Desferal (Deferoxamine) is given as a chelating agent to reduce the amount of stored iron. A **chelating agent** is a drug that is used to either prevent or reverse the toxic effects of a heavy metal or to accelerate the elimination of the metal from the body. In this instance, Desferal binds to the iron and aids in removing it from the tissues. The recommended route of administration is intravenously (IV), although intramuscularly (IM) is also acceptable. Oral administration may increase iron absorption and should never be used in a child receiving repeated blood transfusions. Desferal is administered 5 to 7 times a week for up to twelve hours and may be associated with the side effects listed in Box 26-6 (CAF, 2001b; Kosnett, 2001).

In an attempt to eliminate the need for lifelong blood transfusions, both bone marrow transplants and cord blood transplants have been used in children with beta-thalassemia major. The goal of both interventions is to introduce healthy stem cells into the marrow so normal red blood cells and hemoglobin production will occur. Bone marrow transplantation is a difficult option because the bone marrow donor must be a genetic match, usually a family member (refer to Chapter 29). However, those children who find a suitable donor and who have not yet experienced iron overload or chronic organ toxicity experience long-term survival in more than 80% of cases. Cord blood transplants are similar to bone marrow transplants, except the stem cells are taken from the placenta or umbilical cord of a suitable donor. These donors do not have to be as close genetically; there appears to be a lower probability of rejection in this type of treatment (CAF, 2001a; Linker, 2001).

Nursing Management

Nursing management for the child with beta-thalassemia major is centered around family teaching and family support, as well as actual treatment of the anemia. The nurse is responsible for administering the blood transfusions and observing for transfusion reactions. Hospital protocols should always be observed when performing blood transfusions. As is the case with any chronic disease or life-threatening disorder, both the child and caregivers need special attention. Because beta-thalassemia major eventually results in death, the child and caregivers may need assistance in coping with the disease, its treatment, and its eventual outcome. Caregivers and their children should be referred to hospital social workers and/or the following agencies for further emotional support: the Cooley's Anemia Foundation; the Sibling Donor Cord Blood Program; the Northern California Comprehensive Thalassemia Center; or the Joint Center for Sickle Cell and Thalassemic Disorders (see the Resources section at the end of this chapter).

Aplastic Anemia

Aplastic anemia is a condition wherein injury to or abnormal expression of the stem cells in the bone marrow results in the production of inadequate numbers of erythrocytes, leukocytes, and platelets.

Incidence and Etiology

Aplastic anemia can be categorized as either hereditary or acquired. The hereditary form of aplastic anemia, **Fanconi's anemia** (FA), is a rare autosomal recessive disorder that develops early in life and is accompanied by multiple congenital abnormalities (see Figure 26-2). FA should be suspected in all children and adolescents with aplastic anemia, especially if they have any birth defects. Acquired aplastic anemia can be either idiopathic or due to secondary causes. Idiopathic aplastic anemia is rare in children and adolescents, and for this reason, secondary causes should always be investigated in these age groups (Mansen & McCance, 1998).

The most common cause of aplastic anemia is autoimmune suppression of blood cell production. The toxins and pharmacological agents implicated in the development of this disorder are listed in Box 26-7. They each cause direct stem cell injury, but using appropriate dosages and monitor-

BOX 26-6 Potential side effects of Desferal

Side Effects
- Hypotension with rapid IV infusion
- Orange-red colored urine
- Flushing
- Blotchy erythema
- Intestinal irritation
- Urticaria
- Pulmonary complications with infusion > 24 hrs
- Neurotoxicity after long-term therapy

Adapted from Kosnett, J. J. (2001). Heavy metal intoxication & chelators. In B. G. Katzung (Ed.), *Basic and clinical pharmacology* (8th ed., pp. 999–1010). New York: McGraw-Hill.

REFLECTIONS FROM FAMILIES

When Taylor was diagnosed with beta-thalassemia major, I was devastated. My husband and I had no idea that we carried the gene for this disease, but that is the only way she could have gotten it. I hate to think it is my fault that Taylor is so sick, but it is. She needs blood transfusions every three weeks now, but even those harm her body. I do not know how much longer she will live, but I am trying to cherish every moment that I have with her.

BOX 26-7 Common toxic and pharmacologic causes of aplastic anemia

Toxic Agents
Benzene
Toluene
Insecticides
Arsenic

Pharmacologic Agents
Antibiotics
- Chloramphenicol
- Sulfonamides

Anti-inflammatory agents
- Gold salts
- Phenylbutazone

Anticonvulsants
- Phenytoin (Dilantin)
- Mephenytoin (Mesantoin)
- Trimethadione (Tridione)
- Carbamazepine (Tegretol)

Antimalarials
- Quinacrine

Analgesics
- Pryidium

Oral hypoglycemics
- Tolbutamide (Orinase)

Adapted from Linker, C. A. (2001). Blood. In L. M. Tierney, S. J. McPhee, & M. A. Papadakis (Eds.), *Current medical diagnosis & treatment 2001* (40th ed., pp. 505–558). New York: McGraw-Hill; Mansen, T. J., & McCance, K. L. (1998). Alterations of erythrocyte function. In K. L. McCance & S. E. Huether (Eds.), *Pathophysiology: The biologic basis for disease in adults and children* (3rd ed., pp. 878–898). St Louis, MO: Mosby.

ing blood levels when using these agents are generally effective in preventing aplastic anemia. In rare instances, aplastic anemia has resulted from abnormal responses to appropriate doses of these substances. In addition to toxins and pharmacological agents, factors such as radiation, chemotherapy, and infections are also known to play a role in the development of this condition. Of the implicated infections, viral infections are the most common. The severity of the infection has not been shown to predict the severity of the resulting anemia (Linker, 2001; Mansen & McCance, 1998).

The incidence of aplastic anemia is 2 to 6 cases/million (Nathan & Orkin, 1997). The onset of acquired aplastic anemia is dependent on exposure to the causal factor. The onset of FA is quite variable although 73% of children with FA have evidence of bone marrow failure by 10 years of age, with a median age of onset of seven years. The median age of survival is 19 years, and only one-fourth of clients live beyond age 29 (Camitta, 1998; Alter & Young, 1997). Following onset, the progression of aplastic anemia may be gradual or rapid, with the severity defined by laboratory values (Box 26-8). Without treatment, children with at least three of the four criteria for severe aplastic anemia have a median survival rate of 3 months. Only 20% of children with this disorder will survive for 1 year (Linker, 2001).

Pathophysiology

In the fetus, hematopoiesis occurs in the liver and the spleen. After birth, however, hematopoiesis normally occurs only in the bone marrow. Within the marrow, the stem cells, from which all blood cells originate, proliferate and differentiate into the cellular components of the blood. If these stem cells are abnormal, as is the case with aplastic anemia, the body experiences **pancytopenia,** a condition in which all three types of blood cells are either decreased or absent. The life span of each type of blood cell affects the rate of reduction experienced by that cellular line. Thus, RBCs are the last to demonstrate a reduction in number because of their relatively long life span (Mansen & McCance, 1998).

Clinical Manifestations

Although the age of onset of varies, the clinical manifestations of both FA and acquired aplastic anemia are similar in all age groups and directly related to the decrease in each of the three cell types. Typically, the first sign noted is increased bruising caused by the decreased number of platelets. After this, the child becomes more vulnerable to infection because of the decreased number of WBCs. Once the RBCs have decreased in number, the signs and symptoms of anemia begin to manifest themselves. These typically begin with pallor, weakness, and difficulty breathing and proceed as shown in Box 26-3. Children with aplastic anemia will also experience impaired growth and development and 5–10% will develop acute myelogenous leukemia (Camitta, 1998; Linker, 2001; Mansen & McCance, 1998).

BOX 26-8 Criteria for severe aplastic anemia

Severe Aplastic Anemia
- Neutrophils <500 μl
- Platelets <20,000 μl
- Reticulocytes <1%
- Bone Marrow Cellularity <20%

Adapted from Linker, C. A. (2001). Blood. In L. M. Tierney, S. J. McPhee, & M. A. Papadakis (Eds.), *Current medical diagnosis & treatment 2001* (40th ed., pp. 505–558). New York: McGraw-Hill.

Diagnosis

History and clinical manifestations are helpful in the diagnosis of aplastic amenia, but laboratory tests are essential. A CBC with differential will show pancytopenia, although not all cell lines will be reduced early in the development of the disorder. Other initial laboratory tests and their results are listed in Table 26-2. The definitive diagnosis must be based on a bone marrow biopsy, which will typically show hypocellular marrow, although all of the cells that are seen will appear normal. To differentiate FA from acquired aplastic anemia, bone marrow chromosome studies must be done (Linker, 2001).

Treatment

If the aplastic anemia is acquired, the first line of treatment is to alleviate the underlying disorder or prevent further exposure to the causal agent. Once this has been accomplished, or if FA is present, the effects of pancytopenia may need to be treated. If any symptoms of bleeding are present or the platelet count is less than 10,000 cells/µl, platelet transfusions are used to increase the number of platelets in circulation. If the symptoms of anemia interfere with normal functioning, packed RBCs should be administered to increase the Hb level. If a fever develops in a child with decreased numbers of WBCs, an intensive work-up should be initiated in conjunction with administering broad-spectrum antibiotics (Alter & Young, 1997).

For children with acquired aplastic anemia, remission can generally be achieved with either a bone marrow transplant or immunosuppressive therapy. If a suitable donor can be found, bone marrow transplantation is a very effective treatment for aplastic amenia. In previously untransfused children and young adults with an HLA-matched sibling, the durable complete response rate exceeds 80% (Linker, 2001). Slightly less effective is the use of antithymocyte globulin (ATG) to suppress the immune system. ATG selectively attacks the immune response and can alter the course of aplastic anemia if the aplastic anemia was caused by an autoimmune process (Lake, Akporiaye, & Hersh, 2001). The recommended dose is 40 mg/kg each day for 4 days. Longer periods of treatment are associated with decreased effectiveness and serum sickness. If effective, this treatment increases blood counts within 3 months. Cyclosporine may also be used for immunosuppression, although it has potentially more severe side effects (Box 26-9). The recommended dosage for children is 15 mg/kg each day. Cyclosporine has been shown to promote remission in clients who did not respond to ATG therapy, and when used in conjunction with ATG, remission has occurred in clients who did not respond to either medication alone (Alter & Young, 1997).

The only potential cure for FA is a bone marrow transplant. Unfortunately, the chemotherapy and/or irradiation associated with the procedure may accelerate the development of cancer. For this reason, this method of treatment must be considered with caution. The other common treatment option for children with FA is androgen therapy. The most commonly given androgen is oxymetholone. The recommended dosage is 2 to 5 mg/kg each day and may cause obstructive liver disease, hepatitis, or liver tumors. Most clients respond to the treatment and relapse if the treatment is discontinued. Often the child develops resistance to the androgen being administered and must change to another androgen. On average, this treatment approach can prolong the life of a child with FA for a few years. Corticosteroids are often given in conjunction with the androgens in order to decrease bleeding and counteract the accelerated growth stimulation of the androgens. Typically, this is done with prednisone in a dosage of 5 to 10 mg every other day (Alter & Young, 1997).

BOX 26-9 Common side effects of cyclosporine

Side effects
- Hypertension
- Excessive body hair
- Urea remains in the blood
- Gingival hypertrophy
- Immunodeficiency
- Increased serum creatinine levels
- Irreversible nephrotoxicity
- *P. carinii* pneumonia

Alter, B. P., & Young, N. S. (1997). *The bone marrow failure syndromes.* In D. G. Nathan & S. H. Orkin (Eds.), *Nathan and Oski's hematology of infancy and childhood* (5th ed., Vol. 2, 237–335). Philadelphia: W. B. Saunders.

Nursing Management

The nursing management for a child with aplastic anemia begins with assessment of the child for potential health care needs. This assessment should include observation for any of the signs and symptoms of anemia listed in Box 26-3 in addition to observation for excessive bruising. A baseline temperature should be recorded and the child monitored for any fever or signs and symptoms of infection. The nurse is also responsible for implementing and teaching precautions for preventing infection including proper handwashing, aseptic technique, and adequate fluid intake. Hospital care of a child with aplastic anemia may include the administration of platelets or other blood products (see beta-thalassemia section), or bone marrow transplantation (see Chapter 29). Because this is a life-threatening illness, the emotional needs of both the child and the family should also be assessed. The child or other family members may need education about aplastic anemia, reassurance, or just a listening ear. Some of these needs can also be met by community agencies such as the Fanconi Anemia Research Fund, or the Aplastic Anemia

Reflective Thinking

Conception of a Child in Order to Benefit a Living Sibling

If you had a child with aplastic anemia or some other disorder that required a bone marrow transplant for survival, would you attempt to conceive a child who might serve as a donor? Occasionally in the news we read about a family with a living child who needs a bone marrow transplant or another type of transplant. If a suitable donor cannot be found for the child, the family may chose to conceive another child in hopes of supplying the living child with a suitable donor for the transplant. What are your feelings about this?

& MDS International Foundation (see the Resources section at the end of this chapter).

Family Teaching

If bone marrow transplantation occurs, caregivers can be a tremendous resource and support to their child if they understand each preprocedure treatment and its rationale. The child will need to be hospitalized for approximately one month prior to the actual transplant to provide adequate time to pharmacologically suppress the child's immune system. The rationale is to ensure all diseased cells are destroyed, and any immunity that could adversely affect the donor marrow is also eliminated. To achieve immune depletion, the child will receive very large doses of cyclophosphamide. If the child has already received a number of blood transfusions, total body irradiation will be performed. This severe immunosuppression carries with it a number of risks including infection, stomatitis, diarrhea, and skin breakdown. However, a successful transplant will result in the child's own bone marrow beginning to produce normal cells.

Because the most common type of transplant is allogenic, with a relative serving as the donor, caregivers also need to be educated about the procedures involved in being a donor. The donor, often a sibling, is placed under general anesthesia, and several bone marrow aspirates are taken, usually from the hip area. The donor is then recovered as a typical postoperative client. The bone marrow aspirates are washed and irradiated, then transfused to the recipient in a manner similar to a blood transfusion.

DISORDERS OF COAGULATION

Coagulation is the main mechanism of **hemostasis** (control of bleeding) and is vital in maintaining blood volume, pressure, and flow through injured vessels. The three integral components in this effort are the platelets, the clotting factors, and the vasculature. When a blood vessel is injured, it undergoes endothelial sloughing in order to expose the subendothelial tissue. The platelets are then attracted to this tissue and adhere to the vessel wall. Following adhesion, platelets release biochemical mediators such as serotonin and histamine to direct platelet activity and promote temporary vasoconstriction. The vasoconstriction minimizes blood loss and is followed by vasodilation so that WBCs can be transported to the site of injury. The platelets then aggregate into plugs, which are stabilized by blood clot formation. Blood clots are made up of fibrin strands that form around the plug and trap other blood cells. **Fibrin** is a protein that is formed through a series of reactions called the coagulation cascade. The coagulation cascade involves numerous blood clotting factors and can be initiated by either damage to body tissues or vessel walls (Figure 26-6). Although fibrin is only created when an injury occurs, all clotting factors, in addition to prothrombin and fibrinogen, circulate continually in the blood of healthy individuals (McCance, 1998b).

Conditions that alter the delicate balance of platelets, clotting factors, and vasculature can have effects ranging from bruising to life-threatening illness. Within this portion of the chapter the etiology and treatment of the following coagulation disorders are discussed: hemophilia, von Willebrand's disease, immune thrombocytopenic purpura, and disseminated intravascular coagulation. Both hemophilia and von Willebrand's disease involve a decrease in specific factors necessary for coagulation. Immune thrombocytopenic purpura is characterized by a decreased number of platelets. In disseminated intravascular coagulation, the normal mechanisms that regulate coagulation are ineffective.

Hemophilia

The **hemophilias** are a group of bleeding disorders in which one factor in the first phase of coagulation is deficient.

Incidence and Etiology

The most common type of hemophilia, **hemophilia A,** occurs in approximately 1 in 5,000 males and accounts for approximately 80–85% of hemophilia cases. Hemophilia A, also referred to as classic hemophilia, is caused by a deficiency of factor VIII. The second most common type of hemophilia is **hemophilia B,** or Christmas disease. This type of hemophilia is caused by a deficiency in factor IX (Christmas factor) and affects 10–15% of clients with hemophilia. The least common type of hemophilia is **hemophilia C,** a factor XI deficiency (Kline & Mooney, 1998; Montgomery, Gill, & Scott, 1998). Each type of hemophilia impairs the body's ability to control bleeding and can result in fatal hemorrhage. With proper monitoring and the use of prophylactic treatment, however, children with hemophilia can lead relatively normal lives.

	Intrinsic Pathway Activated by damage to blood vessels	**Extrinsic pathway** Activated by damage to body tissues
Phase 1:	Sequence of enzymatic reactions involve factors listed below in the order listed: 1) Factor XII 2) Factor XI 3) Factor IX 4) Factor VIII 5) Factor X	Sequence of enzymatic reactions involve factors listed below in the order listed: 1) Factor VII 2) Factor X

The last step of phase 1 for each pathway leads to phase 2 and the Common Pathway

	Common Pathway
Phase 2:	Prothrombin activator complex facilitates Prothrombin → Thrombin
Phase 3:	Thrombin facilitates Fibrinogen → Fibrin

Figure 26-6 Coagulation Cascade and Common Disorders of Coagulation. Adapted from Kline, N. E. & Mooney, K. H. (1998). Alterations of hematologic function in children. In K. L. McCance & S. E. Huether (Eds.), *Pathophysiology: The biologic basis for disease in adults and children* (3rd ed., pp. 935–967). St Louis, MO: Mosby.; McCance, K. L. (1998b). Structure and function of the hematologic system. In K. L. McCance & S. E. Huether (Eds.), *Pathophysiology: The biologic basis for disease in adults and children* (3rd ed., pp. 845–877). St Louis, MO: Mosby.

Both hemophilia A and hemophilia B are X-linked recessive disorders (Figure 26-7). Because the female genotype consists of two X chromosomes, a female would need two recessive genes for disease expression to occur. Males, however, only have one X chromosome and, therefore, the possession of just one recessive hemophilia gene results in disease expression. Hence, a female can only have the disorder when both the mother and the father have the recessive gene. A male, on the other hand, only needs to have a mother who carries the gene in order for the disease to be expressed in his phenotype. For this reason, hemophilia is much more commonly expressed in males. One exception is hemophilia C, an autosomal recessive disorder that occurs equally in males and females (Kline & Mooney, 1998).

Pathophysiology

Although there are several different types of gene deletions and mutations that can cause hemophilia, the genetic alteration appears to be the same among members of a given family and, therefore, the severity of symptoms among family members is typically very similar. In each child with hemophilia, regardless of the cause, there is either a missing or a deficient clotting factor. This factor, whether it is VIII, IX, or XI, is an integral part of the coagulation cascade and, as such, enables the body to create adequate fibrin for clot formation to repair damaged blood vessels (see Figure 26-6). Hence, a decreased amount, or the complete absence of any factor impairs or completely prevents the body from forming clots (Kline & Mooney, 1998).

Clinical Manifestations

The clinical manifestations of hemophilia A and hemophilia B vary, depending on the concentration of clotting factor VIII or IX in the blood. The three levels of severity, along with their associated frequency of bleeding episodes, are listed in Table 26-6. Generally, hemophilia C is less severe than either hemophilia A or hemophilia B, and presents with only mild bleeding (Kline & Mooney, 1998).

During the first year of life spontaneous bleeding in hemophiliacs is rare, although injections or firm holding of the infant can result in **hematomas,** pockets of blood under the skin caused by excessive bleeding following trauma. As the child learns to walk he may bruise easily and bleed into his joints, a condition called **hemarthrosis.** By 3 to 4 years of age, episodes of persistent bleeding from minor lacerations occur in 90% of children with this disorder. Hemarthrosis continues to be a problem, causing pain and limited movement in the elbows, knees, and ankles. Hemarthrosis also predisposes the child to degenerative

(A) When the mother is a carrier for the disease, there is a 50% chance that each child conceived will not have nor carry the disease. There is a 25% chance that each child conceived will carry the disease and a 25% chance that each child conceived will have the disease.

	Y	X
X	XY 25% Normal (Male)	XX 25% Normal (Female)
x	xY 25% Disease (Male)	Xx 25% Carrier (Female)

(B) When the father has the disease, there is a 50% chance that each child conceived will not have the disease or carry the disease and a 50% chance that each child conceived will carry the disease.

	Y	x
X	XY 25% Normal (Male)	Xx 25% Carrier (Female)
X	XY 25% Normal (Male)	Xx 25% Carrier (Female)

Legend
x = Recessive disease gene
X or Y = Dominant normal gene
xx or xY = Disease state
Xx = Carrier state
YX or XX = Normal state

Figure 26-7 X-Linked Recessive Inheritance

TABLE 26-6 Classifying the Severity of Hemophilia A and Hemophilia B

	Concentration of Clotting Factor VIII or IX in the Blood	Occurrence of Excessive Bleeding
Mild	5–35% of normal	Only after severe trauma or surgery
Moderate	1–5% of normal	Only after trauma
Severe	Less than 1% of normal	Spontaneously

Adapted from Kline, N. E. & Mooney, K. H. (1998). Alterations of hematologic function in children. In K. L. McCance & S. E. Huether (Eds.), Pathophysiology: The biologic basis for disease in adults and children *(3rd ed., pp. 935–967). St Louis, MO: Mosby.*

joint changes later in life. Other complications of hemophilia include minor occurrences of **hematuria** (blood in the urine) and **epistaxis** (nose bleed), as well as major events such as intracranial hemorrhage and bleeding into the neck or abdomen (Kline & Mooney, 1998).

Diagnosis

After a client history and/or physical examination reveals evidence of excessive bleeding, several laboratory tests can be used to determine the presence of hemophilia. These diagnostic tests and the results typically associated with hemophilia are listed in Table 26-7. Often the type of hemophilia present is determined by using the thromboplastin generation test, which can precisely identify deficiencies of factors VIII and IX. A positive family history of hemophilia can also lead to testing asymptomatic children in order to determine carrier status (Kline & Mooney, 1998).

Treatment

The treatment of hemophilia A consists mainly of replacing the missing coagulation factor through infusion of recombinant factor VII concentrates. The advent of recombinant factor concentrates replaced the previously used plasma-derived products in 1989. The new recombinant factor concentrates are similar in their treatment effect without the danger of transmitting diseases such as HIV or hepatitis to the recipient. The amount of recombinant factor concentrate given varies with the severity of the hemophilia, must be calculated for each child's situation, and is routinely given when excessive bleeding and/or hemarthrosis occurs. For many children, prophylactic treatment is administered three or four times a week. This preventive approach, which is started after the child manifests hemarthrosis, is generally effective in preventing spontaneous bleeding. As the child ages, caregivers can be taught to administer the factor concentrates at home. This is more convenient for the child and caregiver and allows for immediate administration following an injury (Montgomery, Gill, & Scott, 1998).

For many pediatric clients with mild hemophilia A, desmopressin (DDAVP) has proven to be an effective treatment for spontaneous bleeding and is also effective in preventing excessive bleeding when administered prior to dental or surgical procedures. Responses to DDAVP vary considerably and a therapeutic trial is necessary to determine the adequacy of the treatment for a specific child. The recommended dosage for bleeding disorders is one intranasal spray (1.5 mg) for young children and increases to one spray in each nostril for adolescents over 50 kg. IV doses of 0.3 mcg/kg can also be given. Potential side effects are mild and include headache, flushing, low sodium levels, and slight alterations in heart rate or blood pressure. Low sodium levels are a rare complication, but can cause seizures. Consequently, fluid intake should be monitored (Montgomery, Gill, & Scott, 1998).

Because of the propensity of children with hemophilia to experience mucosal bleeding, antifibrinolytic agents such as aminocaproic acid (Amicar) or tranexamic acid (Cyklokapron) may be used following dental extractions. These medications inhibit the breakdown of fibrin and

TABLE 26-7 Common Laboratory Tests and Findings for Coagulation Disorders

Laboratory Test	No Disorder Present	Hemophilia	Von Willebrand's Disease	ITP	DIC
Platelet count—measures the number of platelets in the blood	See Appendix H	Normal	Normal	Decreased	Decreased
Standard bleeding time (Ivy Method)—evaluates the vascular and platelet factors	1–9 minutes	Normal	Prolonged	Prolonged	Prolonged
Prothrombin time (PT or INR)—evaluates the extrinsic system and common pathway of coagulation	11.0–12.5 sec	Normal	Normal	Normal	Prolonged
Partial thromboplastin time (PTT)—evaluates the intrinsic system and common pathway of coagulation	60–70 sec	Prolonged	Prolonged	Normal	Prolonged

Adapted from Cohen, P. S. & Close, P. (2000b). Bleeding disorders. In C. D. Berkowitz (Ed.), Pediatrics: A primary care approach *(2nd ed., pp. 280–285). New York: W. B. Saunders; Pagana, K. D., & Pagana, T. J. (2001).* Mosby's diagnostic and laboratory test reference *(3rd ed.). St Louis: MO: Mosby.*

thereby delay the degradation of blood clots. The agents are administered for 7–10 days following the procedure and are generally effective in preventing recurrent bleeding from the site. Potential side effects include thrombosis, hypotension, muscle wasting, abdominal discomfort, diarrhea, and nasal stuffiness (Hambleton & O'Reilly, 2001; Montgomery, Gill, & Scott, 1998).

The treatment of hemophilia B is similar to that of hemophilia A, except factor IX concentrates are given instead of factor VIII concentrates. The factor concentrates currently in use for hemophilia B are plasma-derived, but treated to reduce the likelihood of disease transmission. DDAVP is not an effective treatment for patients with hemophilia B and subsequently should not be used (Montgomery, Gill, & Scott, 1998). Aggressive treatment of hemophilia C is rarely necessary because of the mild nature of the disease. Instead, these clients should be given supportive therapy and education about how to control minor bleeding episodes.

Nursing Alert:

Child with Hemophilia

If a child with hemophilia is showing signs and symptoms of neurological impairment such as irritability, altered level of consciousness, or vomiting, the child may have an intracranial bleed and should be taken to the hospital immediately. If head trauma occurs, a child with hemophilia should be treated as if he/she were experiencing an intracranial bleed, even if the child does not manifest these signs or symptoms.

Reflective Thinking

Adolescent Hemophiliacs with HIV: What Should Be the Focus of Sex Education?

Many of today's adolescent hemophiliacs received plasma-derived factor concentrates prior to 1989 and are infected with HIV. Education should focus on ways to prevent transmission to others. For some nurses, this may be easier said than done. Consider 16-year-old Mackensie, who contracted HIV from factor administration. What advice would you give him when he tells you he wants to become sexually active with his girlfriend, Christine? Do you think Christine would be more or less likely to have sexual intercourse with him because Mackensie contracted HIV in an "acceptable" manner? If you had the chance, what advice would you give Christine?

Case Study/Care Plan

Hemophilia Type A

Tommy is an 18-month-old diagnosed with hemophilia type A during the neonatal period. He was circumcised at two days of age in the hospital and continued to bleed from the circumcision site. He has moderate hemophilia, and has received frequent factor infusions because of falls and subsequent hemarthrosis. His caregivers now want to learn how to better manage and cope with his illness.

Nursing Care Plan

Assessment The main focus of nursing assessment in this instance is to determine the history of the child's illness and the current knowledge level of his caregivers. The history should focus on (a) any factors that precipitated the child's bleeding episodes; (b) the frequency of the bleeding episodes; and (c) how bleeding episodes have been managed in the past. Finally, the child and caregiver need to be given the opportunity to express any emotional concerns that they may have in relation to the child's illness. While having this discussion, the nurse should observe for any behaviors that indicate the child and caregiver's level of coping.

Nursing Diagnosis #1

Ineffective tissue perfusion related to bleeding episodes.

continues

continued

Expected Outcomes

1. Caregivers will be able to prevent bleeding episodes.
2. Caregivers will be able to manage mild bleeding episodes.
3. Caregivers will be able to manage an episode of hemarthrosis.

Interventions/*Rationales*

1. Educate caregivers about the following strategies to prevent bleeding episodes:
   - Make the home and play environment as safe and clutter free as possible. *Minimizes accidental injuries and falls during time when the child is learning to ambulate.*
   - Provide close supervision during the toddler years. *Prevents the child from engaging in dangerous activities.*
   - Pad the crib and playpen. *Allows for safer play and prevention of injury from accidental falls.*
   - Use protective equipment while the child learns to walk and when playing. *Prevents injuries to the joints and the head.*
   - As the child gets older, encourage participation in low contact sports such as swimming or tennis. *Prevents injuries to the joints and the head.*
   - Use soft-bristled tooth brushes, water pics, and so forth. *Prevents oral mucosal bleeding.*
   - Help the child maintain a healthy weight. *Prevents undue stress and strain on joints.*
2. Educate caregivers about the following interventions for a mild bleeding episode:
   - In preparation for bleeding episodes, contact the Medic Alert Foundation (see Resources section at the end of this chapter) and obtain a medic alert bracelet. *Ensures proper care and treatment of child in the event of a bleeding episode.*
   - Apply pressure to any bleed for ten to fifteen minutes. *Promotes clot formation.*
   - Immobilize and elevate the extremity where the bleed is occurring. *Decreases blood flow to the area of bleeding.*
   - Apply ice or cold to bleeding area. *Promotes vasoconstriction.*
3. Educate caregivers about interventions for an episode of hemarthrosis:
   - Elevate and immobilize the affected extremity. *Decreases the amount of bleeding into the joint space.*
   - Provide pain relief for joint pain. *Allows for more feasible range of motion exercises without pain.*
   - Avoid taking aspirin. *Prevents the blood-thinning effects of aspirin from exacerbating the bleeding.*
   - Institute active range of motion exercises after forty-eight hours. *Prevents joint contractures.*

Evaluation

After the nursing interventions have been completed, a follow-up visit with the family is necessary to assess the success of the interventions and the need for additional education. During this follow-up visit, the nurse should again elicit a history from the family and compare it to the baseline information collected before the interventions were started. If the desired outcomes have been met, this history will demonstrate that the number of bleeding episodes have decreased and that the family was able to manage any mild bleeding episodes or hemarthrosis that had occurred.

Nursing Diagnosis #2

Interrupted family processes related to having a child with an inherited, potentially fatal disease.

continues

continued

Expected Outcomes

1. The family members will be able to express an understanding of the disease process.
2. The family members will be able to cope effectively with the child's illness.

Interventions/*Rationales*

1. Assess caregivers' knowledge of the disease process. *Aids in delivering appropriate teaching content.*
2. Teach family members appropriate content related to the disease process. *Facilitates understanding and acceptance of the diagnosis of hemophilia.*
3. Listen to and be aware of caregivers' feelings related to the disease, remembering that if they are Tommy's biological parents they may have feelings of guilt related to the transmission of the disease to him. *Provides the caregivers with an opportunity to express and work through their emotions.*
4. Refer caregivers to social workers or community agencies that can provide additional education and emotional support (see the Resources section at the end of this chapter). *Ensures that proper support and resources are known to the family.*

Evaluation

During the follow-up visit with the family, the nurse can determine if the desired outcomes have been reached by asking caregivers to explain the disease process. The nurse should also observe the caregivers for effective coping skills and the presence of guilt. A discussion of the caregivers' emotions regarding the child's illness may also be appropriate in order to assess their current level of coping and the need for further interventions.

Von Willebrand's Disease

Von Willebrand's disease is the most common congenital disorder of homeostasis. It is a genetic disorder in which **von Willebrand's factor** (vWF), a protein that facilitates adhesion between platelets and injured vessels, is either deficient or defective.

Incidence and Etiology

This deficiency of normal vWF results in a mild bleeding disorder that is rarely as severe as hemophilia. It is estimated that 1% of the population may have this disorder, but many are undiagnosed because of the mildness of their symptoms. Therefore, the prognosis for von Willebrand's disease is excellent (Linker, 2001; Montgomery, Gill, & Scott, 1998).

As shown in Box 26-10 there are three major variants, with type I accounting for approximately 80% of cases. Both type I and type II are transmitted via autosomal dominant inheritance and affect males and females equally. With this method of genetic inheritance there can be no carriers (Figure 26-8). Type III von Willebrand's disease is a rare autosomal recessive disorder.

BOX 26-10 Types of von Willebrand's Disease

	Characteristics of vWF
Type I	Decreased amount of normal vWF
Type II	Presence of abnormal vWF
Type III	Near absence of vWF

Linker, C. A. (2001). Blood. In L. M. Tierney, S. J. McPhee, & M. A. Papadakis (Eds.), *Current medical diagnosis & treatment 2001* (40th ed., pp. 505–558). New York: McGraw-Hill.

Pathophysiology

When a person without von Willebrand's disease sustains injury to the wall of a blood vessel, the concentration of vWF in the area of the injury increases. This is important because vWF binds to the platelets and is essential in adhering them to the damaged vessel wall, one of the first steps of clot formation. Hence, when vWF is not present in sufficient quantities or is dysfunctional, as in von Willebrand's disease, the body is unable to adequately form clots and control bleeding.

(A) When both parents are heterozygous for the disease, there is a 25% chance that each child conceived will not have the disease and a 75% chance that each child conceived will have the disease.

	B	b
B	BB 25% Disease	Bb 25% Disease
b	Bb 25% Disease	bb 25% Normal

(B) When one parent is heterozygous for the disease, there is a 50% chance that each child conceived will not have the disease, and a 50% chance that each child conceived will have the disease.

	b	b
B	Bb 25% Disease	Bb 25% Disease
b	bb 25% Normal	bb 25% Normal

Legend
b = Recessive normal gene
B = Dominant disease gene
bb = Normal state
Bb or bB = Heterozygous disease state
BB = Homozygous disease state

Figure 26-8 Autosomal Dominant Inheritance

In addition to its role in facilitating platelet adhesion, vWF also carries and protects factor VIII. For this reason, children with von Willebrand's disease may also experience secondary factor VIII deficiencies (Montgomery, Gill, & Scott, 1998).

Clinical Manifestations

Children with von Willebrand's disease, unlike those with hemophilia, usually do not experience spontaneous hemarthrosis. Rather, the most common types of bleeding are mucosal such as epistaxis, **ecchymoses** (bruises), and gingival bleeding. In females abnormally long and heavy menstrual periods, referred to as **menorrhagia,** can also occur. Other possible bleeding manifestations include gastrointestinal bleeding and excessive bleeding following surgery or dental extractions. These manifestations commonly vary in severity over time, and are generally aggravated by the intake of aspirin and lessened by pregnancy or estrogen administration (Linker, 2001).

Diagnosis

Because the manifestations of von Willebrand's disease are typically mild in nature, many families dismiss their increased incidence of epistaxis or ecchymoses as normal and do not seek medical attention. For this reason, many children with von Willebrand's disease remain undiagnosed until they bleed excessively following a surgical or dental procedure. In addition to the clinical manifestation characteristic of the disease, a family history is helpful in making the diagnosis. Because most cases of von Willebrand's disease are transmitted via autosomal dominant inheritance, there will almost always be a family history of excessive bleeding. Once a suspicion of von Willebrand's disease has been raised, laboratory tests can then be conducted to make a definitive diagnosis. The laboratory tests commonly used to assess bleeding disorders, along with the results typical for von Willebrand's disease, are listed in Table 26-7. In addition to these tests, immunoassays for vWF can further differentiate von Willebrand's disease from other bleeding disorders and determine which type of the disease is present (Linker, 2001; Montgomery, Gill, & Scott, 1998).

Treatment

The first line of treatment for type I, or mild type II, von Willebrand's disease is desmopressin (DDAVP). DDAVP is believed to promote the release of stored vWF and should be given in the same dosages as for hemophilia A (refer to the Hemophilia section for dosages and side effects). In order to prevent depletion of the vWF stores, DDAVP doses should not be given more often than 24 hours apart. DDAVP should be avoided in type III von Willebrand's because of potentially adverse effects. As with hemophilia, antifibrinolytic agents such as Amicar or Cyklokapron may be used to control the bleeding associated with dental extractions (refer to the Hemophilia section) (Linker, 2001; Montgomery, Gill, & Scott, 1998).

For clients who do not respond to DDAVP or who experience adverse reactions, plasma-derived factor VIII concentrates are used. This is because the newer, disease-free recombinant concentrates do not have sufficient levels of normal vWF to be therapeutic. Cryoprecipitate is the plasma-derived factor VIII concentrate that is thought to contain the most normal vWF protein molecules, but presents the recipient with the risk of blood-borne disease transmission. Another alternative, Humate-P, does not contain as many normal vWF molecules, but it can be treated to attenuate any viruses contained in the factor concentrate. For this reason, it is often the preferred method of treatment. If either of these factor concentrates are necessary, they are given in dosages similar to those used for hemophilia (Montgomery, Gill, & Scott, 1998).

Nursing Management

The nursing management for a child with von Willebrand's is the same as a child with hemophilia.

Immune Thrombocytopenic Purpura (ITP)

As the name suggests, the thrombocytopenic purpuras are a group of acquired diseases characterized by thrombocytopenia and purpura. **Thrombocytopenia** is a decrease in the platelet count below 150,000 mm^3 (see Appendix H for normal values in children) and **purpuras** are areas of blood underneath the skin or mucous membranes.

Incidence and Etiology

The thrombocytopenic purpuras are classified as either intrinsic or immune, depending on the cause of the symptoms. In children the most common form is **immune thrombocytopenic purpura** (ITP). This disease was formerly called idiopathic thrombocytopenic purpura, but has since been found to be an autoimmune disorder. Consequently, the name was recently changed to reflect this discovery. ITP can occur at any age, but the peak incidence in children is between 2 and 4 years of age. The ITP of children differs from the ITP of adults in several ways (Table 26-8). Because of these differences, the prognosis for children is excellent, even without therapy. Approximately 75% of children recover completely in 3 months. Within 6 months of onset, 80–90% of affected children have regained normal platelet counts (Cohen & Close, 2000b; Linker, 2001; Kline & Mooney, 1998; Mansen, McCance, & Field, 1998).

Nursing Tip:

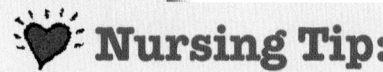

Care of a child experiencing a nosebleed
Blood coming from a child's nose can be a frightening experience for a caregiver and for the child. The most important thing to remember is to remain calm. Have the child sit up and lean forward. The child should not lean his/her head back because he/she could aspirate blood if the bleeding is profuse. The child should pinch his/her nose between two fingers and hold it with pressure for 10 minutes. This should stop the bleeding, but if it does not, the caregiver can apply ice to the bridge of the nose.

Pathophysiology

One of the essential components of maintaining hemostasis is the process whereby the platelets adhere to injured vessel walls, release biochemical mediators, and form plugs. Through these actions, platelets block the many minute ruptures occurring daily in the microcirculation. When there are inadequate numbers of platelets, these ruptures are not repaired, resulting in purpura under the skin and throughout the tissues. In ITP the inadequate supply of platelets results from an autoimmune process, which in approximately 70% of ITP cases, is triggered by a viral infection (Box 26-11). Once the autoimmune process has been triggered, antiplatelet antibodies bind to the platelets, causing them to become sequestered and destroyed prematurely in the spleen. This increased rate of platelet destruction exceeds the bone marrow's ability to create new platelets, resulting in a decreased platelet count. No other blood cell types are affected by this process (Kline & Mooney, 1998; Mansen, McCance, & Field, 1998; NIH, 1998).

Clinical Manifestations

The most common presentation of ITP is one of acute onset. With this presentation, ecchymoses and a general petechial rash (small purpuras) will often occur 1 to 4 weeks following

TABLE 26-8 Different Presentations of ITP in Children and Adults

Children	Adults
Generally preceeded by viral infection	Rarely preceeded by a viral infection
Usually self-limiting	Usually chronic (>6 months)
Affects males and females equally	Females affected 2–3 times more often than males

Adapted from: National Institutes of Health. (1998). Immune thrombocytopenic purpura (ITP). *[On-line]. Available: www.niddk.nih.gov/health/hematol/pubs/itp/itp.htm; Linker, C. A. (2001). Blood. In L. M. Tierney, S. J. McPhee, & M. A. Papadakis (Eds.),* Current medical diagnosis & treatment 2001 *(40th ed., pp. 505–558). New York: McGraw-Hill.*

BOX 26-11 Viruses associated with ITP

Cytomegalovirus (CMV)
Epstein-Barr virus (EBV)
Human immunodeficiency virus (HIV)
Parovirus
Viral respiratory infection

Adapted from Kline, N. E. & Mooney, K. H. (1998). Alterations of hematologic function in children. In K. L. McCance & S. E. Huether (Eds.), *Pathophysiology: The biologic basis for disease in adults and children* (3rd ed., pp. 935–967). St Louis, MO: Mosby.

the viral infection. The child's presenting complaint is often spontaneous bleeding of the skin or hemorrhagic blisters of the mucous membranes. Asymmetrical bleeding is typical, especially on the legs and trunk. Bleeding in gastrointestinal or urinary tracts may occur. Nose bleeding may also be present and difficult to control. These are the only manifestations of ITP, and the child otherwise appears healthy. The spontaneous hemorrhage of the acute stage lasts for 1 to 2 weeks and is associated with a platelet count below 20,000 mm^3. In some children the onset is more gradual with clinical manifestations of moderate bleeding and a few **petechiae** (small purpuras). The most severe complication is intracranial hemorrhage, which occurs in only 1% of patients (Cohen & Close, 2000b; Kline & Mooney, 1998; NIH, 1998).

Diagnosis

The diagnosis is based on history, clinical presentation and laboratory tests. The child's history should be examined for other causes of thrombocytopenia such as aspirin or heparin use. The child's clinical presentation will also demonstrate the signs and symptoms discussed previously. Enlargement of the liver, spleen, or lymph nodes suggests other causes of thrombocytopenia such as leukemia or HIV infection. The common laboratory tests and findings for a child with ITP are listed in Table 26-7. Other than the platelet count, all CBC values should be normal. A peripheral blood smear will reveal very few platelets, with normal amounts of all other cell types. The platelets seen on the smear will be large and more immature. A bone marrow aspiration will appear normal, although there may be increased numbers of megakaryocytes, the precursor cells of platelets (Cohen & Close, 2000b; Linker, 2001).

Treatment

Because ITP in children is generally a self-limiting condition with excellent prognosis, treatment is largely supportive. Children and their caregivers should receive information on how to prevent injury or trauma and control bleeding episodes (see Nursing Management section). If severe symptoms are present, the severity and duration of the initial acute phase may be lessened by administering medications that suppress the immune system. These medications, listed in Box 26-12, decrease the autoimmune process and thereby decrease the destruction of platelets. Of these medications, prednisone is the drug of choice, followed by intravenous immunoglobulin. The other medications are used only when these two safer alternatives are ineffective. Splenectomy is reserved for children with chronic ITP who do not respond to less invasive interventions. Because of the short life span of platelets, transfusion of fresh blood or platelets is ineffective unless life-threatening hemorrhage is present (Kline & Mooney, 1998; Lake, Akporiaye, & Hersh, 2001; Mansen, McCance, & Field, 1998).

Nursing Management

Nursing management for the child with ITP centers mainly around educating the child and caregivers about preventing injury and managing bleeding episodes. The amount of activity restriction placed on the child depends on illness severity, but the child should be given the opportunity to help decide what the restrictions will be. This will help the child under-

BOX 26-12 Immunosuppressive medications used in ITP

Prednisone
Vincristine (Oncovin)
Cyclophosphamide (Cytoxan)
Mercaptopurine (Purinethol)
Azathioprine (Imuran)
Gamma globulin
Danazol (Danocrine)
Cyclosporine (Sandimmune)

Adapted from Lake, D. F., Akporiaye, E. T., & Hersh, E. M. (2001). Immunopharmacology. In B. G. Katzung (Ed.), *Basic and clinical pharmacology* (pp. 959–986). New York: McGraw-Hill; Linker, C. A. (2001). Blood. In L. M. Tierney, S. J. McPhee, & M. A. Papadakis (Eds.), *Current medical diagnosis & treatment 2001* (40th ed., pp. 505–558). New York: McGraw-Hill.

stand and comply. The use of safety equipment should be emphasized to prevent trauma and bleeding. Aspirin should not be taken since it may aggravate the bleeding. If an external bleeding episode occurs, the area should be elevated while pressure is applied for at least ten minutes. Application of ice to the area will further reduce the amount of bleeding. The child and caregivers should also be taught to recognize the signs and symptoms of internal bleeding: pallor, altered level of consciousness, and increased pulse. If any manifestations occur, the child should be seen by a physician. Children with ITP and their families can also be referred to the National Organization for Rare Disorders; the NIH/National Heart, Lung and Blood Institute Information Center; and the Genetic Alliance for additional information and support (see Resources section at the end of this chapter).

REFLECTIONS FROM FAMILIES

Last winter it seemed like my daughter Jennifer was always getting sick. Every few weeks she had something new and I was starting to get used to it. About two weeks after one of her illnesses, I noticed she had several blood blisters. I was immediately worried and thought Jennifer might have something very serious—like cancer. I took her to the doctor and was relieved to find out she had a disease called ITP. It was difficult to see her suffer until the disease resolved on its own two and a half months later, but it was much better than a diagnosis of something potentially terminal.

Disseminated Intravascular Coagulation (DIC)

Disseminated intravascular coagulation (DIC) is a coagulation disorder in which the stimulus for coagulation overwhelms the control mechanisms that normally confine coagulation to the area of bleeding. This sequence of events can lead to either an acute and potentially life-threatening process of ischemia and hemorrhage, or a chronic and low-grade condition of mild hemorrhage and microcirculatory thrombosis.

Incidence and Etiology

A variety of precipitating factors can overstimulate the coagulation mechanism and cause DIC. Of these factors, which are listed in Box 26-13, infection and sepsis are the most common. Any time a child or adolescent is very ill with one of these conditions, he or she is at risk for DIC (Linker, 2001; Mansen, McCance, & Field, 1998).

Pathophysiology

When one of the precipitating factors listed in Box 26-13 abnormally stimulates the first stage of the coagulation process, thrombin is generated in greater amounts than can be neutralized by the body. This excess thrombin leads to excessive conversion of fibrinogen to fibrin, leading to excessive clot formation (see Figure 26-6). As this process continues, blood clots can eventually obstruct the blood vessels, causing ischemia, infarction, and necrosis. This necrotic tissue damage then activates the coagulation cascade and stimulates the formation of more clots. As more and more clots are formed, the components of the clotting process are consumed at an accelerated pace. The depletion of platelets and coagulation factors leads to thrombocytopenia and hemorrhage. The presence of numerous clots also triggers the release of factors to dissolve the clots. The by-products of this process are potent anticoagulants that exacerbate the hemorrhage. This process continues until the initial precipitating factor is removed or the child is treated with the appropriate therapeutic interventions (Linker, 2001; Mansen, McCance, & Field, 1998).

Clinical Manifestations

Depending on the intensity of the precipitating stimulus and the intensity of the damage incurred by the endothelium and tissues, the clinical presentation of DIC can be either acute or chronic. The acute form is associated with massive

BOX 26-13 Causes of disseminated intravascular coagulation

Sepsis
- Especially gram-negative bacteria

Any widespread infection
- Bacterial
- Fungal
- Protozoal
- Viral

Severe tissue injury
- Especially burns and head injury

Obstetric complications
- Amniotic fluid embolus
- Septic abortion
- Retained fetus

Cancer
- Acute promyelocytic leukemia
- Mucinous adenocarcinomas

Major hemolytic transfusion reactions
- Anaphylaxis

Hypotension/Hypoxia
- Shock
- Cardiopulmonary arrest

Snake bites
- Snake venom

Organ injury
- Pancreatitis
- Liver Disease

Adapted by Linker, C. A. (2001). Blood. In L. M. Tierney, S. J. McPhee, & M. A. Papadakis (Eds.), *Current medical diagnosis & treatment 2001* (40th ed., pp. 505–558). New York: McGraw-Hill; Mansen, T. J., McCance, K. L., & Field, R. B. (1998). Alterations of leukocyte, lymphoid, and hemostatic function. In K. L. McCance & S. E. Huether (Eds.), *Pathophysiology: The biologic basis for disease in adults and children* (3rd ed., pp. 899–934). St. Louis, MO: Mosby.

hemorrhage and thrombosis. This is manifested by oozing from venipuncture sites, arterial lines, or surgical sites. Bleeding may also occur in the nose, gums, and sclera or conjunctiva of the eyes. Typically the bleeding will be apparent in at least three unrelated sites and will be accompanied by purpura, petechiae, and hematomas. Bleeding can also occur in closed compartments of the body, but will often be less obvious. The damage resulting from thrombosis may be localized to one organ, or generalized to many organs. The organ systems most commonly damaged are the cardiovascular, pulmonary, central nervous, renal, and hepatic systems. The resulting alterations in organ function result in a variety of clinical manifestations (Box 26-14). If not treated, children with acute DIC can also develop end organ failure. Children with chronic DIC do not present with these overt manifestations of hemorrhage and thrombosis because the pathological mechanisms are partially compensated for by the body. Instead these children experience mild hemorrhage and thrombosis that is confined to the microcirculation. As a result, these children may present with confusion, jaundice, hypoxia, and **oliguria** (a decreased ability to form and excrete urine) (Linker, 2001; Mansen, McCance, & Field, 1998).

Diagnosis

A diagnosis of DIC is based on the clinical manifestations already discussed, in addition to several laboratory findings. The preliminary tests used to distinguish between various bleeding disorders are listed in Table 26-7, along with the findings typically associated with DIC. Because no one test exists to definitively diagnose DIC, a combination of several laboratory findings needs to be used. Additional tests may include serum fibrinogen levels, which will be decreased, and measures of fibrin degradation products, which will be increased (Linker, 2001; Mansen, McCance, & Field, 1998).

Treatment

The first step in treating acute DIC is identification and correction of the underlying cause. The next step, replacement

BOX 26-14 The clinical manifestations of organ damage in DIC

- Altered level of consciousness
- Behavioral changes
- Mental activity changes
- Confusion
- Seizure activity
- Oliguria
- Hematuria
- Hypoxia
- Hypotension
- Coughing up blood
- Chest pain
- Tachycardia

Adapted from Mansen, T. J., McCance, K. L., & Field, R. B. (1998). Alterations of leukocyte, lymphoid, and hemostatic function. In K. L. McCance & S. E. Huether (Eds.), *Pathophysiology: The biologic basis for disease in adults and children* (3rd ed., pp. 899–934). St. Louis, MO: Mosby.

therapy, provides the client with adequate amounts of platelets, fibrinogen, and possibly coagulation factors. The platelets are replaced via platelet transfusion. Cryoprecipitate administration is effective in increasing fibrinogen levels (see von Willebrand's disease for a discussion of cryoprecipitate). The liver generally is able to restore coagulation factors, but fresh-frozen plasma can be used for replacement if necessary. The use of heparin in the treatment of DIC is controversial, but if given it should be administered in conjunction with the replacement of these coagulation components (Linker, 2001; Mansen, McCance, & Field, 1998).

Nursing Management

The nursing management for a child with DIC takes place in an intensive care setting and involves assessment, the administration of blood products, and supportive care. Because of the potential for severe hemorrhage, the nurse must frequently assess for overt bleeding, manifestations of internal bleeding such as pallor and tachycardia, and signs and symptoms of shock (see Box 26-5). The administration of blood products should be done in accordance with hospital policy (see beta-thalassemia section). The supportive role of the nurse focuses on the anxiety and fear likely to be present in both the child and caregivers. Some nursing interventions that can help calm the child and their caregivers are to (a) explain all procedures to the family; (b) allow the child to make choices about care when possible; (c) encourage open conversation about the situation; and (d) offer to listen to and address the family's questions and concerns.

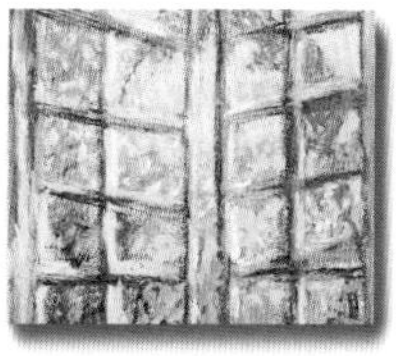

In the Real World

When I entered nursing school, I never imagined that there were so many children in the prosperous country of America whose health care needs were not being met. Before I started working with poor families in the clinics, I thought that those individuals with inadequate nutrition either chose not to or did not know any better. Now I know that even with education many families cannot provide the nutrition necessary to keep their children healthy. I have also learned a great deal about the difficulties faced by children trying to find suitable bone marrow donors. It seems amazing that with our advanced system of medical care we are unable to match potential donors and recipients more efficiently, but that is a reality that many potential recipients must face.

Key Concepts

- Human blood has two major components, plasma and formed elements.
- The formed elements of the blood include red blood cells, white blood cells, and platelets.
- During fetal development blood cells are produced in the liver and spleen. After birth new blood cells are synthesized from stem cells in the bone marrow.
- RBC, WBC, and platelet counts vary with age.
- Iron deficiency anemia, the most common pediatric hematological disorder, occurs when there is not enough iron available for adequate hemoglobin production and can usually be treated with age-appropriate dietary modification and oral iron supplementation.
- Sickle cell anemia, a genetic disorder, is characterized by red blood cells that undergo sickling and cause an anemia of increased red blood cell destruction.
- Beta-thalassemia major, a genetic disorder resulting in altered hemoglobin formation, causes a life-threatening anemia requiring regular blood transfusions to sustain life.
- Aplastic anemia can be either an inherited or an acquired disorder characterized by altered stem cells in the bone marrow. The resulting pancytopenia may need treatment with platelet transfusions, red blood cell transfusions, and/or broad spectrum antibiotics.
- Hemophilia A is an inherited coagulation disorder in which there is a deficiency of coagulation factor VIII. The episodes of excessive bleeding that result from this deficiency are treated with either recombinant factor VIII concentrates or DDAVP.
- Von Willebrand's disease is the most common pediatric coagulation disorder. This genetic disorder is characterized by a deficiency of von Willebrand's factor, which causes a mild anemia that is often undiagnosed. If necessary, DDAVP and plasma-derived factor VIII concentrates can be used for treatment.
- Immune thrombocytopenic purpura is an autoimmune disease wherein the platelets are destroyed prematurely. The associated bleeding is usually mild enough to only require supportive treatment, and spontaneous resolution generally occurs in affected children within a few months of onset.
- Disseminated intravascular coagulation occurs when a stimulus for coagulation overwhelms the control mechanisms that normally confine coagulation to the area of bleeding, resulting in a potentially life-threatening combination of hypercoagulation and hemorrhage. Treatment may include platelet transfusion, cryoprecipitate administration, and the use of fresh-frozen plasma.

Review Questions

1. Which of the anemias are inherited disorders?
2. Describe the signs and symptoms associated with mild anemia, moderate anemia, and severe anemia.
3. Discuss the most common cause of iron deficiency anemia in young children and adolescents, in school-aged children, and in children living in third-world countries.
4. What are ten points discussed when educating a child or caregiver about iron supplementation and dietary modification for iron deficiency anemia?
5. Describe the type of hemoglobin characteristic of sickle cell disease. What change does it cause in the red blood cells?
6. Describe five situations that could cause red blood cells to sickle in a child with sickle cell anemia. Which syndrome is usually the first manifestation of sickle cell disease in an infant?
7. What treatment is necessary to sustain the life of a child with beta-thalassemia disease?
8. What condition develops after repeated blood transfusions? How is it treated?
9. Which cells are affected by aplastic anemia?
10. What condition may occur in the joints of a child with hemophilia?
11. What should a child or caregiver do to stop a bleeding episode in a child with hemophilia or von Willebrand's disease?
12. Describe the most common coagulation disorder in children. How severe is this condition?
13. What cells are destroyed in immune thrombocytopenic purpura? What manifestations result?
14. How is immune thrombocytopenic purpura treated?
15. Describe the two paradoxical conditions present in disseminated intravascular coagulation.

References

Alter, B. P., & Young, N. S. (1997). The bone marrow failure syndromes. In D. G. Nathan & S. H. Orkin (Eds.), *Nathan and Oski's hematology of infancy and childhood* (5th ed., Vol. 2, pp. 237–335). Philadelphia: W. B. Saunders.

Camitta, B. M. (1998). *Aplastic anemia: Introduction for the general physician.* Annapolis, MD: Aplastic Anemia Foundation of America, Inc.

Centers for Disease Control and Prevention. (1998). *Pediatric nutrition surveillance 1997: Full report.* Atlanta: U. S. Department of Health and Human Services.

Cohen, P. S. & Close, P. (2000a). Anemia. In C. D. Berkowitz (Ed.), *Pediatrics: A primary care approach* (2nd ed., pp. 275–279). New York: W. B. Saunders.

Cohen, P. S. & Close, P. (2000b). Bleeding disorders. In C. D. Berkowitz (Ed.), *Pediatrics: A primary care approach* (2nd ed., pp. 280–285). New York: W. B. Saunders.

Cooley's Anemia Foundation. (2001a). *Focus on a cure.* [On-line]. Available: http://www.cooleysanemia.org/sections.php.

Cooley's Anemia Foundation. (2001b). *What is thalassemia?* [On-line]. Available: http://www.cooleysanemia.org/sections.php.

Cooley's Anemia Foundation. (2001c). *What is thalassemia trait?* [On-line]. Available: http://www.cooleysanemia.org/sections.php.

de Oliveira, J. E., Scheid, M. M., Desai, I. D., & Marchini, S. (1996). Iron fortification of domestic drinking water to prevent anemia among low socioeconomic families in Brazil. *International Journal of Food Sciences and Nutrition, 47*(3), 213–9.

Dover, G. J., & Platt, O. S. (1997). Sickle cell disease. In D. G. Nathan & S. H. Orkin (Eds.), *Nathan and Oski's hematology of infancy and childhood* (5th ed., Vol. 2, pp. 762–809). Philadelphia: W. B. Saunders.

Grover, G. (2000). Nutritional needs. In C. D. Berkowitz (Ed.), *Pediatrics: A primary care approach* (2nd ed., pp. 34–39). New York: W. B. Saunders.

Hambleton, J., & O'Reilly, R. A. (2001). Drugs used in disorders of coagulation. In B. G. Katzung (Ed.), *Basic and clinical pharmacology* (pp. 564–580). New York: McGraw-Hill.

Hord, J. D. (1999). Anemia and coagulation disorders in adolescents. *Adolescent Medicine, 10*(3), 359–367.

Kline, N. E., & Mooney, K. H. (1998). Alterations of hematologic function in children. In K. L. McCance & S. E. Huether (Eds.), *Pathophysiology: The biologic basis for disease in adults and children* (3rd ed., pp. 935–967). St Louis, MO: Mosby.

Kosnett, J. J. (2001). Heavy metal intoxication & chelators. In B. G. Katzung (Ed.), *Basic and clinical pharmacology* (pp. 999–1010). New York: McGraw-Hill.

Lake, D. F., Akporiaye, E. T., & Hersh, E. M. (2001). Immunopharmacology. In B. G. Katzung (Ed.), *Basic and clinical pharmacology* (pp. 959–986). New York: McGraw-Hill.

Linker, C. A. (2001). Blood. In L. M. Tierney, S. J. McPhee, & M. A. Papadakis (Eds.), *Current medical diagnosis & treatment 2001* (40th ed., pp. 505–558). New York: McGraw-Hill.

Looker, A. C., Dallman, P. R., Carroll, M. D., Gunter, E. W., & Johnson, C. L. (1997). Prevalence of iron deficiency in the United States. *Journal of the American Medical Association, 277*(12), 973–976.

Lozoff, B., Wolf, A.W., & Jiminez, E. (1996). Iron-deficiency anemia and infant development: Effects of extended oral iron therapy. *Journal of Pediatrics, 129*(3), 382–389.

Mansen, T. J., & McCance, K. L. (1998). Alterations of erythrocyte function. In K. L. McCance & S. E. Huether (Eds.), *Pathophysiology: The biologic basis for disease in adults and children* (3rd ed., pp. 878–898). St. Louis, MO: Mosby.

Mansen, T. J., McCance, K. L., & Field, R. B. (1998). Alterations of leukocyte, lymphoid, and hemostatic function. In K. L. McCance & S. E. Huether (Eds.), *Pathophysiology: The biologic basis for disease in adults and children* (3rd ed., pp. 899–934). St. Louis, MO: Mosby.

McCance, K. L. (1998a). Altered cellular and tissue biology. In K. L. McCance & S. E. Huether (Eds.), *Pathophysiology: The biologic basis for disease in adults and children* (3rd ed., pp. 44–81). St. Louis, MO: Mosby.

McCance, K. L. (1998b). Structure and function of the hematologic system. In K. L. McCance & S. E. Huether (Eds.), *Pathophysiology: The biologic basis for disease in adults and children* (3rd ed., pp. 845–877). St. Louis, MO: Mosby.

Montgomery, R. R., Gill, J. C., & Scott, J. P. (1998). Hemophilia and von Willebrand disease. In D. G. Nathan & S. H. Orkin (Eds.), *Nathan and Oski's hematology of infancy and childhood* (5th ed., Vol. 2, pp. 1631–1659). Philadelphia: W. B. Saunders.

Morey, S. S. (1998). CDC issues guidelines for prevention, detection and treatment of iron deficiency. *American Family Physician, 58*(6), 1475–1477.

Nathan, D. G., & Orkin, S. H. (Eds.). (1997). *Nathan and Oski's hematology of infancy and childhood.* (5th ed.). Philadelphia: W. B. Saunders.

National Institutes of Health. (1997). *New treatment prevents strokes in children with sickle cell anemia.* [On-line]. Available: www.nhlbi.nih.gov/new/ press/nhlbi-18.htm.

National Institutes of Health. (1998). *Immune thrombocytopenic purpura (ITP).* [On-line]. Available: www.niddk.nih.gov/health/hematol/pubs/itp/itp.htm.

Pagana, K. D., & Pagana, T. J. (2001). *Mosby's diagnostic and laboratory test reference* (4th ed.). St. Louis, MO: Mosby.

Santi, D. V., & Masters, S. B. (2001). Drugs used in anemias. Hematopoietic growth factors. In B. G. Katzung (Ed.), *Basic and clinical pharmacology* (8th ed., pp. 549–563). New York: McGraw-Hill.

Sari, M., Bloem, W., dePee, S., Schultink, W. J., & Sastroamidjojo, S. (2001). Effect of iron-fortified candies on the iron status of children aged 4–6 y in East Jakarta, Indonesia. *American Journal of Clinical Nutrition, 73*(6), 1034–1039.

U. S. Department of Health and Human Services. (1996). *Facts about sickle cell anemia* (NIH Publication No. 96-4057). Bethesda, MD: National Institutes of Health.

U. S. Department of Health and Human Services. (2000). *Healthy People 2010: Volume II* (2nd ed.). Washington, DC: U. S. Government Printing Office.

Wardlaw, G. M. (1999). *Perspectives in nutrition* (4th ed.). Boston: WCB/McGraw-Hill.

Wethers, D. L. (2000). Sickle cell disease in childhood: Part II. Diagnosis and treatment of major complications and recent advances in treatment. *American Family Physician, 62*(6), 1309–14.

Young, K. D. (2000). Shock. In C. D. Berkowitz (Ed.), *Pediatrics: A primary care approach* (2nd ed., pp. 163–167). New York: W. B. Saunders.

Suggested Readings

Adams, R. J. (2000). Lessons from the stroke prevention trial in sickle call anemia (STOP) study. *Journal of Child Neurology, 15*(5), 344–349.

Autret, E., Jonville-Bera, A.P., Galy-Eyraud, C., & Hessel, L. (1996). Thrombocytopenic purpura after isolated or combined vaccination against measles, mumps and rubella. *Therapie, 51*(6), 677–80.

Beyer, J. E., Platt, A. F., Kinney, T. R., & Treadwell, M. (1999). Practice guidelines for the assessment of children with sickle cell pain. *Journal of the Society of Pediatric Nurses, 4*(2), 61–73.

Callen, B. L. (2000). Program of care for young women with iron deficiency anemia: A pilot study. *Journal of Community Health Nursing, 14*(4), 247–62.

Chaunsumrit, A., Hotrakitya, S., Sirinavin, S., & Supapanachart, S. (1999). Disseminated intravascular coagulation findings in 100 patients. *Journal of the Medical Association of Thailand, 82* (Suppl. 1), 63–8.

Clegg, J. B., & Weatherall, D. J. (1999). Thalassemia and malaria: New insights into an old problem. *Proceedings of the Association of American Physicians, 111*(4), 278–282.

Giardini, C. (1997). Treatment of beta-thalassemia. *Current Opinions in Hematology, 4*(2), 79–87.

Gupta, S. (1999). Childhood iron deficiency anemia, maternal nutritional knowledge, and maternal feeding practices in a high-risk population. *Preventative Medicine, 29*(3), 152–6.

Hendricks-Ferguson, V. L., & Nelson, M. (1999). Update of the health care management needs of infants with sickle cell disease. *Journal of Pediatric Health Care, 13*(5), 217–222.

Incorpora, G., Di Gregorio, F., Romeo, M. A., Pavone, P., Trifiletti, R. R., & Parano, E. (1999). Focal neurological deficits in children with beta-thalassemia major. *Neuropediatrics, 30,* 45–48.

Kuhne, T, Elinder, G., Blanchette, V. S., & Garvey, B. (1998). Current management issues of childhood and adult immune thrombocytopenic purpura (ITP). *Acta Paediatrica. Suppl., 424,* 75–81.

Margolis, D. A., & Casper, J. T. (2000). Alternative-donor hematopoietic stem-cell transplantation for severe aplastic anemia. *Seminars in Hematology, 37*(1), 43–55.

Miners, A. H., Sabin, C. A., Tolley, K. H., & Lee, C. A. (1998). Assessing the effectiveness and cost-effectiveness of prophylaxis against bleeding in patients with severe haemophilia and severe von Willebrand's disease. *Journal of Internal Medicine, 244*(6), 515–522.

National Institutes of Health. (1996). *Hemophilia.* Retrieved from the World Wide Web June 28, 2001: http://www.nhlbi.nih.gov/health/public/blood/other/hemophel.htm.

Overturf, G. D. (1999). Infections and immunizations of children with sickle cell disease. *Advances in Pediatric Infectious Diseases, 14,* 191–218.

Phillips, M. D., Santhouse, A. (1998). Von Willebrand's disease: Recent advances in pathophysiology and treatment. *American Journal of the Medical Sciences, 316*(2), 77–86.

Simon, K., Lobo, M. L., & Jackson, S. (1999). Current knowledge in the management of children and adolescents with sickle cell disease: Part I, physiological issues. *Journal of Pediatric Nursing, 14*(5), 281–295.

Tarantino, M. D. (2000). Treatment options for chronic immune (idiopathic) thrombocytopenia purpura in children. *Seminars in Hematology, 37* (1 Suppl 1), 35–41.

U. S. Department of Health and Human Services. (1998). Recommendations to prevent and control iron deficiency in the United States. *Morbidity and Mortality Weekly Report, 47*(RR-3), 1–29.

Wethers, D. L. (2000). Sickle cell disease in childhood: Part I. Laboratory diagnosis, pathophysiology, and health maintenance. *American Family Physician, 62*(5), 1013–1020, 1027–1028.

Resources

Organizations and Websites

Aplastic Anemia & MDS International Foundation, Inc.
P.O. Box 613
Annapolis, MD 21404-0613
(410) 867-0242
(800) 747- 2820
Fax: (410) 867-0240
www.aplastic.org

Canadian Hemophilia Society
625 President Kennedy Ave., Suite 1210
Montreal, Quebec H3A 1K2
(514) 848-0503
(800) 668-2686
Fax: (514) 848-9661
www.hemophilia.ca

Center for Sickle Cell Disease
Howard University
2121 Georgia Ave NW
Washington, DC 20059
(202) 806-7930

Children's Blood Foundation
333 East 38th Street, Suite 830
New York, NY 10016
(212) 297-4336

Cooley's Anemia Foundation
129-09 26th Avenue—#203
Flushing, NY 11354
(718) 321-CURE (2873)
(800) 522-7222
Fax: (718) 321-3340
www.cooleysanemia.org

Fanconi Anemia Research Fund, Inc.
1801 Willamette Street, Suite 200
Eugene, OR 97401
(541) 687-4658
Fax: (541) 687-0548
www.fanconi.org

Genetic Alliance
4301 Connecticut Avenue NW, Ste. 404
Washington, DC 20008-2304
(202) 966-5557
Fax: (202) 966-8553
www.geneticalliance.org

Iron Disorders Institute, Inc.
P.O. Box 2031
Greenville, SC 29602
(888) 565-IRON (4766)
Fax: (864) 244-2104
www.irondisorders.org

Joint Center for Sickle Cell and Thalassemic Disorders
Brigham & Women's Hospital
221 Longwood Avenue
Suite 620 LMRC
Boston, MA 02115
(617) 732-8490
www.sickle.bwh.harvard.edu

March of Dimes Birth Defects Foundation
1275 Mamaroneck Avenue
White Plains, NY 10605
(888) MOD-IMES (663-4637)
www.modimes.org

Medic Alert Foundation
2323 Colorado Avenue
Turlock, CA 95380
(888) 633-4298
www.medicalert.org

National Hemophilia Foundation
116 West 32nd Street, 11th Floor
New York, NY 10001
(212) 328-3700
(800) 42-HANDI
Fax: (212) 328-3777
www.hemophilia.org

National Organization for Rare Disorders
P.O. Box 8923
New Fairfield, CT 06812-8923
(203) 746-6518
(800) 999-6673
Fax: (203) 746-6481
www.rarediseases.org

National Sickle Cell Disease Program
National Heart, Lung, and Blood Institute
National Institutes of Health
7550 Wisconsin Ave.
Bethesda, MD 20892
(301) 496-4236

NIH/National Heart, Lung and Blood Institute Information Center
P.O. Box 30105
Bethesda, MD 20824—0105
(301) 592-8573
www.nhlbi.nih.gov

Northern California Comprehensive Thalassemia Center
Children's Hospital Oakland
Department of Hematology/Oncology
747 52nd Street
Oakland, CA 94609
www.thalassemia.com

Sibling Donor Cord Blood Program
Children's Hospital Oakland
5700 Martin Luther King Jr Way
Oakland, CA 94609
(510) 450-7605
www.siblingcordblood.org

Sickle Cell Association of Ontario
3199 Bathurst St., Suite 202
Toronto, Ontario M6A 2B2
(416) 789-2855

Sickle Cell Disease Association of America
200 Corporate Pt., Suite 495
Culver City, CA 90230-8727
(310) 216-6363
(800) 421-8453
Fax: (310) 215-3722
www.sicklecelldisease.org

UNIT VI

Alterations in Protective Mechanisms

CHAPTER 27

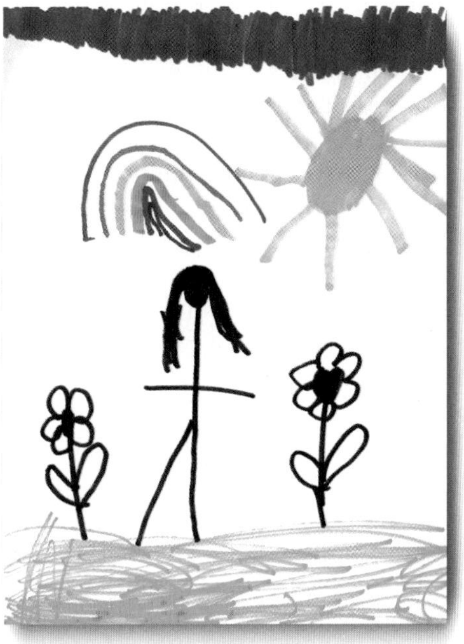

Grace is so sick. She was diagnosed with AIDS when she was nine months old and now she is two. I do not think she will see her third birthday. The family is really upset as she is such a sweet child. She was exposed to the AIDS virus during her mother's pregnancy. Lynn, her mother, was diagnosed with HIV and then AIDS right after Grace was born. As Grace's grandmother and Lynn's mother, I am overwhelmed to know that I will lose them both at a young age.

IMMUNOLOGIC ALTERATIONS

Kimberly A. Stieglitz, DNSc, RN, CS
Karen D. Peterson, MSN, RN, CPNP

COMPETENCIES

Upon completion of this chapter, the reader will be able to:

- *Describe the normal functions of the immune system.*
- *Describe the etiology, clinical manifestations, treatment, and nursing management of juvenile rheumatoid arthritis (JRA), systemic lupus erythematosus (SLE), human immunodeficiency virus (HIV), and allergic reactions to drugs.*
- *Discuss the educational needs of families with children with immune system alterations.*

The primary functions of the immune system are to prevent or ameliorate infections, recognize self from nonself, and maintain homeostasis. The immune system has two basic divisions, the innate immune system and the adaptive immune system. The **innate immune system** acts as the first line of defense against infections, and includes biochemical and physical barriers. The **adaptive immune system** produces a specific reaction to each infectious agent, remembers that agent, and can prevent a later infection by the same agent. Even though the two systems interact considerably, they are discussed separately.

The **immune system** includes the spleen, lymph nodes, and lymphoid tissue, along with cellular elements such as the white blood cells or leukocytes, phagocytes, and natural killer cells. It also includes the skin, mucus produced by the body, cilia, sebaceous gland secretions, stomach acid, normal intestinal flora, and spermine in the semen. Biochemicals such as cytokines, complement factors, and interferon also play crucial roles.

Although immune system alterations occur less commonly in children than other types of alterations, the effects are often disabling or terminal. In addition, the immune system interacts with other body systems so symptoms may not appear to be immune related but rather primarily musculoskeletal, such as in juvenile arthritis, or integumentary such as with systemic lupus erythematosus. HIV, another immune system disease, can affect all organ systems. However, much of how the immune system functions and dysfunctions is still poorly understood, so therapies described may not be clearly related to a known pathologic entity.

This chapter begins with a brief overview of the immune system to delineate a basic frame of reference for alterations. The illnesses and conditions described are examples of the most common immune system alterations, primarily immune based, but demonstrate multisystem involvement. These clinically significant immune system alterations are (1) autoimmunity, such as juvenile rheumatoid arthritis and systemic lupus erythematosus; (2) immunodeficiency, such as human immunodeficiency virus (HIV) disease; and (3) hypersensitivity reactions, such as drug sensitivities. Illnesses primarily associated with other systems, although with immune system implications (asthma, transplants), are described elsewhere (refer to Chapters 24 and 29 for more information about these topics).

ANATOMY AND PHYSIOLOGY

The immune system of neonates and young children is immature. Because of this immaturity, infants and young children are susceptible to infectious organisms that can cause illness and its associated morbidity (Behrman & Kliegman, 1998). Immunizations in early childhood can help prevent many viral and bacterial infections, thus decreasing morbidity and mortality caused by major infectious illnesses. A child's immune system matures by three to six years of age. Lymphoid tissue reaches adult size by six weeks of age, becomes larger in the prepubertal ages, and then goes back to normal by puberty. The spleen becomes full size at adulthood. The risks of being infected by invading organisms are lower when the immune system is fully functioning. However, autoimmune disorders may appear at later ages if the body incorrectly begins to recognize its own proteins as foreign.

The term **immunity** refers to all the processes used by the body to protect against foreign material from environmental sources, including microorganisms or their toxins, foods, chemicals, pollen, dander, or drugs. The processes of immunity used by the body are either innate (natural) or acquired. Although discussed separately here, it is important to remember that all facets of the immune system work together to provide the immune response; alterations in one area may stimulate changes in other areas. These changes may be beneficial, that is, compensate for a damaged function, or be harmful to a person if the response is dramatic or causes more symptoms.

Innate or **natural immunity** consists of many factors that are relatively nonspecific, but function against most threats to the body in a broad sense. These consist of physical barriers such as the skin, mucous membranes, and cough reflex; chemical barriers such as pH of the stomach, fatty acids and proteolytic enzymes of the small intestine, and fever. Innate/natural immunity also includes nonspecific immune cells such as phagocytes (macrophages, neutrophils, natural killer cells), and lymphocytes whose granules release lysing chemicals. **Inflammation** is also a nonspecific function of the innate/natural immune system, where increased vasodilation brings an increased blood supply and is responsible for chemical messengers.

Acquired immunity is specific immunity, triggered when a person has had prior contact with a foreign agent. Upon initial contact, a chain of events leads to the activation of the **humoral system,** consisting of primarily B lymphocytes, and/or the **cell mediated system** of primarily the T lymphocytes. The **B lymphocytes** are produced in the bone marrow (hence the designation of "B" lymphocytes) and differentiate into producers of one of five major classes of **immunoglobulins,** including IgG, IgM, IgA, IgE, and IgD. Each of these five classes may have the same specificity against an antigen, but have different functional properties, thereby increasing the complexity of immune response. Their essential role is to "tag" or identify an **antigen** (foreign substance capable of stimulating an immune response) or pathogen for destruction by other immune cells. Refer to Table 27–1 for specific information about the immunoglobulins.

Cell mediated immunity has an antigen-specific arm consisting of the **T lymphocytes** or cells, developed in the thymus gland (hence "T" cells), and accounting for 70–80% of all lymphocytes. There are many subclasses of T lymphocytes identified to date; each performs different functions. The four main subclass types include the **helper T-cells,** which cooperate with B lymphocytes to induce antibody production and activate cytotoxic T cells; **cytotoxic/killer T lymphocytes,** which attack infected or pathogenic cells; **suppressor cells** whose release of **cytokines** slows the immune response; and **memory cells,** distinctive for their memory and specificity in immune responses. T lymphocytes are the immune system's main defense against viruses, and direct and regulate the immunologic response by secreting lymphokines. **Lymphokines,** in turn, affect other T cells, and attract and activate mononuclear cells, particularly macrophages. Both the humoral and cell mediated systems consist of components that specifically recognize antigens, (B cells in humoral immunity and T cells in cell mediated immunity), and interact with each other and with components of the innate system to inactivate the immune challenge. Figure 27–1 illustrates acquired immunity.

The chemical mediators or messengers that communicate throughout the immune process are called cytokines or **interleukins.** These include the lymphokines, produced by lymphocytes, and the **monokines,** produced by monocytes and macrophages. **Interferons** are also important messengers, but are host specific rather than antigen specific as infected cells secrete them, inhibit replication of many viruses, and have anti-tumor effects. The final major compo-

TABLE 27-1 Immunoglobulins

Ig Type	%	Where Found	Action	When Appears
IgG	70–80	All body fluids	Longest and strongest response. Neutralizes bacterial toxins. Activates phagocytosis. Thought to influence B cell differentiation.	Crosses placenta. Disappears by 6–8 months. Reaches adult levels by 7–8 years.
IgA	10–15	Secretions of gastrointestinal, respiratory, and genitourinary tract, including breast milk	Prevents infections.	Not present at birth.
IgM	5–10	Intravascular spaces	Agglutinates antigen. Lyses cell walls. First immunoglobulin produced in response to bacterial and viral infections. Responsible for transfusion reactions in the ABO blood typing system.	Low at birth. Adult levels reached at 1 year. Produced 48–72 hours after an antigen enters the body. Presence in cord or infant blood suggests an infection in utero or during the newborn period.
IgD	0.2	Plasma	May be receptor that binds antigen to lympocyte surfaces. May influence B cell differentiation.	Not present at birth. Adult values achieved at 6–7 years.
IgE	0.004	Internal/external body fluid	Binds to mast cells on tissue surfaces. Associated with allergy and parasitic infections.	Seen in hypersensitivity reactions.

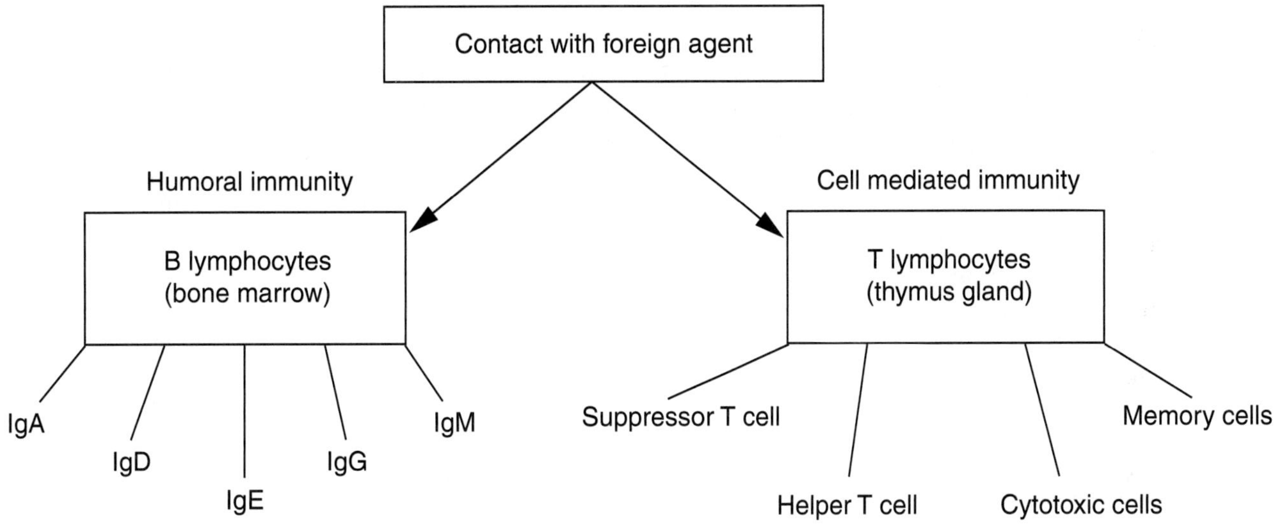

Figure 27-1 Acquired Immunity

nent of the immune response is **complement,** a group of about 25 serum proteins, activated by the onset of the immune response or chemical markers on a pathogen surface. Complement amplifies the immune response, and "complements" antibody activity by facilitating phagocytosis by macrophages or attacking the pathogen's cell membranes (Rosen, 1994; Seely, Stephens, & Tate, 2000).

Passive immunity refers to the passing or administration of preformed antibodies to someone. The transfer of maternal antibodies to an infant through breast milk is an example of passive immunization. In addition, human or animal antibodies are sometimes given to prevent or minimize the effects of an infectious disease in people with congenital or acquired B lymphocyte defects, when a person is susceptible to a disease, when there is a high risk of complications from a disease, or when there is no time for active immunization. Antibodies may also help suppress the effect of some toxins when a disease is already present (American Academy of Pediatrics, 2000).

An important factor in acquired immunity is the distinction between what is self and what is nonself. For various reasons, the identification of "self" is sometimes made as foreign and an immune response mounted. This response is called **autoimmunity,** and causes illnesses that are most difficult to treat.

Immune responses are also sometimes directed against substances that are foreign to the body, but not necessarily harmful in themselves. Examples include pollen, animal fur or dander, and food proteins. Here, the immune response is initiated just like a response to dangerous microorganisms, as these innocuous substances sensitize a person so that on re-exposure to the same substance, the person has a hypersensitive or allergic reaction that can be severely pathologic or cause death if the dose of the **allergen** (foreign antigen) is high or the antibody response is excessive.

Humoral and/or cell mediated immunity may also be involved in hypersensitivity. **Immediate hypersensitivity** results from the release of chemical mediators such as histamine and/or damage to tissue by lysosomal enzymes, and has a short duration between exposure and reaction. **Delayed hypersensitivity** is a cellular reaction involving T cells and macrophages, and has a longer duration between exposure and reaction.

RHEUMATOLOGICAL AUTOIMMUNE INFLAMMATORY DISEASES

Common rheumatological autoimmune inflammatory diseases include systemic onset juvenile arthritis, polyarticular (poly) juvenile arthritis, pauciarticular (pauci) juvenile arthritis, and systemic lupus erythematosus. Refer to Box 27–1 for a definition of autoimmunity and inflammation.

BOX 27-1 Terminology

AUTOIMMUNITY: The inability of the body to distinguish "self" from other, leads to an immune response aimed at parts of one's own body.

INFLAMMATION: Increased blood flow and permeability of blood vessels; results in increased fluid production and attraction of lymphocytes and leukocytes to the area, caused by the release of inflammatory substances called cytokines.

Juvenile Rheumatoid Arthritis

Juvenile rheumatoid arthritis (JRA), juvenile chronic arthritis (JCA), or increasingly **juvenile arthritis (JA)** are terms used for this inflammatory autoimmune disease causing many forms of arthritis in children.

Incidence and Etiology

JRA is the most common pediatric connective tissue disease with arthritis being the principal manifestation (Johnson & Oski, 1997). The incidence is 1:1,000. African-American and Asian children are less likely to suffer from JRA, with Native Americans being more frequently affected (Edgerton & DuPlessis, 2000). Even though the outcome for most children is favorable, it is almost impossible to predict an outcome for an individual child (Behrman & Kliegman, 1998).

Eighty to ninety percent of children with JRA satisfactorily recover and have no functional limitations. However, 10% of children become adults with moderate to significant functional impairment. Children at most risk for these impairments are those with polyarthritis of later age onset, prominent systemic manifestations, early symptomatic involvement of the small joints (hands, feet), or progressive hip disease (Johnson & Oski, 1997). Even though mortality is not increased, morbidity affecting functional capacity, growth, and emotional well-being may be high (Edgerton & DuPlessis, 2000). Two peak ages of onset have been identified: between 2 and 4 years of age (more commonly girls), and between 10 and 12 years of age (most often boys) (Behrman & Kliegman, 1998). Overall, girls are affected twice as often as boys. Additionally, there are variations within the subgroups. (See Table 27-2 for a comparison of JRA by onset criteria.)

The etiology is unknown, but is does involve the interactions of genetic, environmental, and immunologic factors (Edgerton & DuPlessis, 2000). The current theory is that an immunogenetic susceptibility in an individual along with an external trigger, probably viral or bacterial, are both necessary to start the inflammatory process in genetically targeted body cells. In arthritis, the lining of the joints and in the case of systemic arthritis, other organs such as the heart and skin

TABLE 27-2 Comparison of JRA by Onset Criteria

	Systemic	RF-Poly	RF+Poly	Young Pauci	Older Pauci
Incidence	**30%**	**25%**		**45%**	
Female/Male Ratio	F=M	F>M	F>M	F>M	F<M
Rheumatoid Factor	neg	pos	neg	neg	neg
Anti-nuclear Antibody	neg	neg	neg	pos	neg
Median Age of Onset	5 yr	3 yr	12 yr	2 yr	10 yr
Most Common Joints	Any	Any—usually symmetric		Knee most common	Lower extremities
Other Common Clinical Manifestation	Fever, fatigue, malaise, rash	Rheumatic. Nodules		Iritis	
Other Labs	↑ ESR* Moderate anemia ↑ WBC† ↑ Platelet	↑ ESR* Mild anemia	↑ ESR* Moderate anemia	↑ ESR*	↑ ESR* +HLA-B27‡
Course/ Prognosis	Systemic symptoms remit, progress to poly arthritis	Usually burns out	Persistent, chronic joint destruction, poor functional outcome	Bony overgrowth Good prognosis	May progress to ankylosis

** ESR – Erythrocyte Sedimentation Rate*
† WBC – White Blood Count
‡ HLA = Human Leukocyte Antigen

are affected. In susceptible individuals, the eyes can also be affected (Behrman & Kliegman, 1998; Edgerton & DuPlessis, 2000; Johnson & Oski, 1997).

Pathophysiology

Current research suggests T cell activation triggers development of antigen-antibody complexes, which cause release of inflammatory substances called cytokines in targeted organs such as joints and skin. This causes inflammation of the synovial membranes and other tissues leading to joint effusion and swelling. Chronic inflammation eventually evolves into erosion of articular cartilage and other symptoms of inflammatory diseases (Behrman & Kliegman, 1998; Johnson & Oski, 1997).

Clinical Manifestations

JRA is classified by symptoms at onset of disease: systemic, polyarticular, or pauciarticular. (See Box 27-2 and Table 27-2 for detailed information.) The classical symptom of arthritis is morning immobility and stiffness or "gelling," and joint pain (Johnson & Oski, 1997).

Diagnosis

The American College of Rheumatology has determined diagnostic criteria for JRA that include onset before 16 years of age; arthritis (objectively observed) of at least 6 weeks duration; a defined subtype (by onset characteristics); and exclusion of other conditions such as other rheumatic diseases, infectious arthritis, inflammatory bowel disease, and nonrheumatic conditions of bones and joints. Objectively observed arthritis is defined as joint swelling or effusion, *or* two of the following: warmth, pain on motion, or limited range of motion (Edgerton & DuPlessis, 2000).

The diagnosis and categorization of the disease is based on history, physical examination, the American College of Rheumatology onset criteria previously

BOX 27-2 Symptoms of JRA

Systemic Onset

- Fevers–High, quotidian/diquotidian as high as 105 degrees, returning back to baseline between spikes.
- Rash–Salmon-pink, migratory, macular/papular, most common late afternoon or early evening.
- Arthralgia/myalgia
- Arthritis (see definition under "Diagnosis" section), usually multiple joints are involved.
- Fatigue/malaise
- Lymphadanopathy–Usually cervical, epitrochlear, axillary, and/or inguinal.
- Hepatosplenomegaly
- Can also present with signs of carditis–chest pain, tachycardia.

Polyarticular Onset

- Arthritis in many joints (5 or more)–any joint can be affected, but most particularly the joints of the knees, wrists, ankles, and proximal interphalangeal joints of the fingers. Often neck and temporomandibular (TMJ) joints are affected.
- Fever–occasionally, low grade.

Pauciarticular Onset

- Arthritis in a few joints (4 or fewer)–often, though not exclusively, joints of the knees and ankles.
- Inflammation of the eyes–common in anti-nuclear antibody positive preschool girls.

described, and laboratory and radiographic testing for both inclusion and exclusion criteria. Systemic symptoms such as fevers, rash, and lymphadenopathy may complicate the diagnosis, as they can precede joint involvement by months or years and may suggest other diseases that must first be ruled out (Cassidy & Petty, 1995).

The clinical manifestations of the varied forms of juvenile arthritis are also often the presenting symptoms of many childhood diseases, both rheumatological and non-rheumatological. For instance, fever and lymphadenopathy can be symptoms of infection (Lyme disease), or certain malignancies (leukemia, lymphoma). Arthralgia and arthritis can be symptoms of many inflammatory conditions such as systemic lupus erythematosus, juvenile dermatomyositis, and inflammatory bowel disease, as well as malignancies, trauma, and infections of the bone. Other conditions that have to be ruled out are benign arthralgia of childhood (growing pains), rheumatic fever, and school phobia.

There are no specific laboratory tests for JRA. Tests reflecting inflammation are completed, but are nonspecific and can reflect other conditions causing inflammation. Nevertheless they are used to help diagnose and monitor rheumatological diseases. These tests and results include elevated erythrocyte sedimentation rate (ESR), elevated c-reactive protein (CRP), elevated white blood count, decreased hemoglobin, and increased platelet count. Antinuclear antibody (ANA) and rheumatoid factor (RF) are positive in a proportion of children with arthritis (see Table 27–2). A positive ANA is not itself diagnostic as there are positive results in about 5% of the non-arthritic population, and it is very closely associated with systemic lupus erythematosus. Positive RF is linked to adult rheumatoid arthritis and in children is associated with a poor prognosis, rheumatoid nodules, and eventual decrease in functional ability. Some feel this may be early onset of adult rheumatoid arthritis (Behrman & Kliegman, 1998; Johnson & Oski, 1997).

X rays can demonstrate characteristic changes such as soft tissue swelling and joint effusion. With continued disease activity, bony erosions and narrowing of the joint spaces are seen. Subluxations and malalignment may also be visible. Late changes include increased bone destruction and fusion. Bone scans can rule out malignancies and MRI can help evaluate both joints and soft tissues.

Treatment Approaches

Treatment is best undertaken by a multidisciplinary team, including the child and family, nurse, physician, occupational and physical therapists, and social worker. Overall goals include decreasing inflammation, maintaining joint function, and preventing psychosocial complications (Hartley & Fuller, 1997). Treatment includes medications, physical–occupational therapies, nutrition, and education.

Medications are the mainstay of treatment for arthritis in children (Edgerton & DuPlessis, 2000), and the goal is to decrease inflammation. Refer to Table 27–3 for specific information about medications prescribed. For years aspirin and prednisone were commonly used along with gold salts to slow the inflammatory process enough to relieve pain, maintain function, and promote normal growth and development. Unfortunately, there were many side effects with these medications. More recently, non-steroidal anti-inflammatory drugs (NSAIDs) have become the first line treatment. Not only do they decrease inflammation by decreasing production of the inflammatory substance prostaglandin, but they are also antipyretic, helping decrease fever. NSAIDs approved for use in children include ibuprofen, naproxen, indomethacin, tolmetin, and salicylates. NSAIDs commonly cause stomach pain and/or bleeding and medications may be needed to prevent or minimize symptoms of ulceration (Behrman & Kliegman, 1998). Aspirin has been linked to Reye's syndrome in children exposed to the flu virus and should not be administered if a child develops flu symptoms. A newer type of NSAID is the cox-2 inhibitor, which causes fewer gastrointestinal side effects.

Slow-acting anti-rheumatic drugs (SAARDs), such as sulfasalazine may also be used in combination with NSAIDs

TABLE 27-3 Common Medications Used to Control Inflammation

Medication	Action	Common Side Effects	Nursing Implication
NSAIDs	Interferes with production of prostaglandin.	Stomach upset, ulcers	Give with food or milk. Monitor for GI bleeding, blood in stool, anemia. Give GI meds as necessary.
Aspirin	Interferes with production of prostaglandins.	Stomach upset, ulcers, Reye's syndrome	Give with food D/C if develops flu symptoms.
Sulfasalazine	Antibiotic, anti-inflammatory	Allergic reaction (sulfa)	Begin slowly at low doses, gradually increase
Hydrochloroquine	Anti-malarial	Retinopathy	Eye exams q 6 months –1 yr.
Methotrexate	Folic acid antagonist	Nausea, ↑ liver enzymes	Folic acid supplement may ↓ side effects, monitor liver enzymes.
Corticosteroids	Anti-inflammatory	Round face, ↑ BP, weight gain, ↓ bone density	↓ Na, ↑ fat diet monitor bone density, encourage calcium in diet, do not abruptly D/C.
Cytotoxics	Interferes with cell production.	Hair loss, possible Fertility problems Risk of infection.	Discuss side effects before starting, protect from infection.

and other medications to control inflammation (Edgerton & DuPlessis, 2000). One of the most helpful discoveries in recent years has been the effectiveness and relative safety of methotrexate to control arthritis, first in adults and now in children (Johnson & Oski, 1997). Used in smaller doses than used for chemotherapy, this cytotoxic medication has been quite useful in controlling the white blood cell proliferation related to the inflammation associated with arthritis and other rheumatological conditions. The most common side effects are elevation of liver enzymes and nausea.

Corticosteroids such as prednisone, or increasingly intravenous "pulses" of high dose solumedrol, are often used to help control systemic onset and polyarticular disease, especially during the acute phase, to bring relief until the slower-acting medications have time to take effect. Common side effects are weight gain, round face, increased blood pressure, cataracts, decreased bone density, "buffalo hump," increased body hair, acne, and striae of skin from weight gain.

A medication that works in a completely new way is Etanercept (Enbrel), a TNF-alpha blocker (one of the inflammatory substances). Preliminary studies look promising in children, as with adults (Wargula & Lovell, 2000). This is good news for children who have not responded well to other forms of drug therapy. At issue, though, are cost and accessibility, as newer and more expensive medications are developed.

As integral members of the team, physical and occupational therapists evaluate the status of affected joints for range of motion, alignment, and strength. Approaches (heat and cold application) can then be recommended to help lessen pain. These professionals also recommend therapeutic home exercise programs for maintaining/increasing range of motion and improving strength and endurance. They can

REFLECTIONS FROM FAMILIES

Having a seven-year-old child who moves around slowly and painfully is heartbreaking. Arthritis always seemed like something you get when you are old. Emily had not been able to jump rope, play tag,, or swing on the swing set. She was sad and angry. The doctors put her on ibuprofen. I can't believe what a difference putting Emily on ibuprofen has made. Now after taking her morning dose, she is able to be much more active and can join her friends in their play. A normal childhood is what I pray for every day.

Nursing Tip:

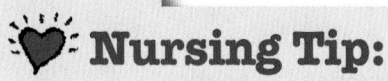

Stiffness in a child with JRA

If a child is having prolonged stiffness in the morning, recommend a warm bath or shower as warm water makes movement easier. This may require a schedule change for the family necessitating an earlier waking time.

also help if splinting is needed to protect a joint, decrease pain, or help with alignment.

Physical activity options for a child with arthritis are swimming, walking, and biking, and should continue unless a joint is acutely inflamed. High impact and contact sports should be avoided. Although activity is important, pacing and rest periods may be necessary.

It is important for children with arthritis to eat well-balanced meals and maintain a healthy body weight. Increased weight gain puts additional stress on tender joints and makes movement more difficult. Calcium intake should be 3–4 servings daily to maintain strong bones. Low fat and low sodium intake is important, especially if the child is on corticosteroids.

Family Teaching

Education for caregivers and other family members should include information about the disease and medications, diagnostic tests and their significance, physical activity, and nutrition. Because arthritis is a disease affecting the entire family, time should be spent describing the adjustment process, and addressing parental, sibling, and child issues. The nurse is an important person to coordinate and facilitate family contact with appropriate caregivers, from medical to psychosocial perspectives, and should be a leading team member.

Case Study/Care Plan

Child with JRA

Asya is a 7-year-old who was diagnosed with JRA when she was 4 years old. She currently complains of joint stiffness and swelling, and is beginning to lose mobility in the affected joints (hands, feet, knees). She "doesn't feel well" and complains of nausea.

Nursing Care Plan

Assessment Swelling, inflammation, and stiffness are noted on the joints of the fingers and knees. She limps and complains of pain when asked to walk across the examination room. Her temperature is 100°F, pulse 85, and respirations 24.

Nursing Diagnoses #1

Chronic pain and fatigue related to swollen or inflamed joints, restricted movement, physical therapy, and chronic disease state.

Expected Outcomes

Asya's pain and fatigue will be decreased and her mobility will be increased.

Intervention/*Rationales*

1. Administer medications in an accurate and timely manner. *Will minimize pain.*
2. Use heat or cold and positioning to relieve and support affected joint. *Will relieve pain.*
3. Encourage participation in activities that maximize the child's capability and allow normal involvement in family, school, and other social activities. *To facilitate growth and development and minimize fatigue.*
4. Encourage participation in occupational and physical therapy and home exercise programs. *Will prevent deformity.*
5. Maintain good body alignment. *Will prevent deformity.*

continues

continued

Nursing Diagnosis #2

Deficient knowledge related to cause, pathophysiology, and treatment of JRA.

Expected Outcomes

Asya and her family will improve their knowledge regarding JRA and the treatment prescribed.

Interventions/*Rationales*

1. Provide information to Asya and her family regarding JRA, the prescribed medications, including the time of administration, side effects, and treatment plans. *With improved knowledge they will be better able to manage JRA.*
2. Provide information to Asya and her family regarding her activity level limits and occupational and physical therapy exercises they can carry on at home. *Improves knowledge.*

Expected Outcomes

Asya's pain and fatigue will be decreased and her mobility increased. Asya and her family will learn about JRA as well as the treatment and management plan.

Systemic Lupus Erythematosus

Incidence and Etiology

Although systemic lupus erythematosus (lupus or SLE) can develop at any age, onset in childhood usually occurs after the age of 5 years or during adolescence (Johnson & Oski, 1997). Peak age of childhood onset is 11 to 15 years (White, 1994). Involving females 8 to 10 times as often as males, it also occurs more often in African-Americans than in Caucasians (Behrman & Kliegman, 1998). Average incidence rate is 5.56/100,000. This is a tripling of incidence in the last 40 years. There is also a significant increase in survival, changing lupus from a mostly fatal disease to a chronic illness, most likely because of improved treatment and earlier recognition (Uramoto, et al., 1999).

The exact etiology is unknown; however, there is general agreement that lupus is an autoimmune process requiring a genetic susceptibility and probably a viral or bacterial trigger (Behrman & Kliegman, 1998; Johnson & Oski, 1997). Because the onset of lupus often occurs during puberty, hormones are also a suspected, but not proven trigger (Rakel, 1996).

Pathophysiology

As in JA, the process is one of autoimmunity. It is thought that immune complexes recognize normal body tissues as foreign, bind complement (proteins that are a part of the body's protective immune response), and then deposit these proteins in the vascular system of targeted organs (skin, kidneys, joints, heart, lungs, bone marrow, brain) causing inflammation and damage. Because so many organs can be affected, each child's symptoms may be different (Behrman & Kliegman, 1998; Johnson & Oski, 1997).

Clinical Manifestations

Clinical manifestations depend on which organs are targeted by the immune complexes, are chronic, and characterized by remissions and exacerbations. Refer to Box 27–3 for criteria used to diagnose SLE and see Figure 27–2.

Diagnosis

Diagnosis is made by history, physical exam, and laboratory testing, and the presence of four of the eleven criteria listed in Box 27–3 (Behrman & Kliegman, 1998). If a child's ANA is negative, lupus is an unlikely diagnosis. Lab tests to monitor disease activity and side effects of medications include the CBC, UA, BUN/Creatinine, and anti-DNA antibody titer.

Nursing Tip:

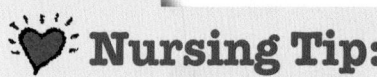

Urinalysis for SLE

It is important to note the presence of menses when obtaining urine for analysis because RBCs can be found and mistaken for renal involvement.

BOX 27-3 Diagnostic criteria for systemic lupus erythematosus

- Malar rash: Erythematous, flat or raised over the cheeks.
- Discoid rash: Erythematous raised patches with scaling.
- Photosensitivity: Skin rash from exposure to sun.
- Oral or nasal ulcers: Usually painless ulceration of the mucosa.
- Nonerosive arthritis: Two or more peripheral joints with tenderness, swelling, or effusion.
- Pleuritis or pericarditis: History of pleuritic pain or rub heard by a physician OR pericarditis documented by cardiogram OR pericardial effusion.
- Renal disorder: Persistent proteinuria OR cellular casts; can progress to hypertension, nephrotic syndrome, renal insufficiency, and end stage renal disease requiring transplantation.
- Neurologic disorder: Seizures OR psychosis without other cause.
- Hematologic disorder: Hemolytic anemia OR leukopenia OR thrombocytopenia.
- Immunologic markers: Positive antibodies to DNA, other nuclear antigens, or lupus anticoagulant.
- ANA: Positive antinuclear antibody (ANA).
- Alopecia

(Adapted from American College of Rheumatology Ad Hoc Committee of Systemic Lupus Erythematosus Guidelines. (1999). Guidelines for referral and management of systemic lupus erythematosus in adults. *Arthritis and Rheumatism, 42*(9), 1785–1796.)

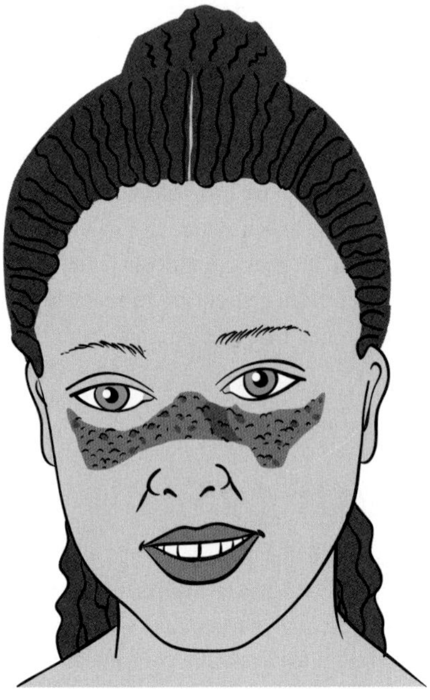

Figure 27-2 Butterfly Rash Often Seen in SLE

Treatment

Treatment is targeted at the organ(s) affected, but overall immunosuppression is usually necessary. The aim of most medications is to reduce inflammation, thus decreasing tissue damage. Corticosteroids are used in high doses during acute phases of the disease and in low, maintenance doses, when inflammation is under better control. Cytotoxic medications such as aziothiaprin (Imuran), cyclophosphamide (Cytoxan), and methotrexate can help control inflammation and are steroid-sparing, allowing use of lower steroid doses. Salicylates and non-steroidal anti-inflammatory drugs are used for arthritis, and anti-hypertensive medications are often necessary if there is kidney involvement. Seizures are controlled by anticonvulsant medications and skin rashes are helped by antimalarial drugs, such as hydrochloroquine (Behrman & Kliegman, 1998; Johnson & Oski, 1997; Rakel, 1996). Refer to Table 27–3 for medications also used in SLE.

Nursing Management

Because this is a chronic disease, nursing care needs to include support, recognition and treatment of infection, and information about the importance of adequate fluid and electrolyte balance and nutrition. Anti-inflammatory medications are the major part of the treatment plan. Therefore, it is necessary for the child and family to understand the importance of complying with timeliness, dosing, and side effects. In addition, families need to know exposure to the sun can trigger a flare up so it should be avoided (Behrman & Kliegman, 1998; Rakel, 1996).

Teenagers need to know they are more susceptible to STDs because of immunosuppressive medications; pregnancy can stress the body and increase disease activity; and cytotoxic medications increase the risk of birth defects. However, if pregnancy is planned for and closely monitored, it is more likely to be successful. As children develop into teens, they must also think of vocational issues, including interests and professions likely to include good health insurance benefits and allow for the possibility of absence in the event of serious disease flare-ups.

Reflective Thinking

SLE and Pregnancy

You are caring for 17-year-old Tena, a pregnant teen with SLE who is on corticosteroids and cyclophosphamide for disease control. Even though you have discussed the risks of pregnancy and precautions to take with her many times, she becomes pregnant. How do you feel about the situation? How will you provide support for Tena during this time? What will you recommend as she plans for the future?

It is also helpful for families to know that the course of the disease may become frustrating and discouraging at times because of its lifelong nature, remissions, exacerbations, and body image issues from medications (corticosteroids, especially). They also need to be able to identify resources to help them through the difficult times. Family members, friends, counselors and school personnel, and medical caregivers can be supportive in times of need. Participation in all normal activities for age should be encouraged.

HUMAN IMMUNODEFICIENCY VIRUS (HIV)

Incidence and Etiology

HIV, one of several retroviruses that allow viral RNA to act as a template for DNA transcription and incorporation into the host geome (Behrman & Kliegman, 1998), is the virus responsible for a range of symptoms, conditions, and **opportunistic infections** (OIs). **HIV infection** is a multisystem disease known primarily for its effects on the immune system. **HIV disease** is an illness continuum, from asymptomatic to death, with an acquired immunodeficiency syndrome (AIDS) diagnosis usually occurring in the latter part of the continuum. **AIDS** is a term used when the immune system has become compromised enough to allow one of the many diagnoses or conditions known to be associated with advanced HIV disease to occur. These diagnoses or conditions are caused by either the direct or indirect effects of the virus on the immune system, or because of HIV's affinity for other cells of the body with CD4 receptors, including the lining of the intestines causing diarrhea, or neurological cells leading to cerebral atrophy.

The diagnosis of AIDS is somewhat different for children under 13 years of age than those above or at 13 years of age. Adolescents' AIDS-defining illnesses are the same as adults. Once a person has AIDS, he or she always has AIDS, even though few symptoms and only moderately impaired laboratory values are exhibited. For children, an AIDS diagnosis often follows the progression of symptoms such as failure to thrive, an encephalopathy, or an opportunistic infection (Boland, 2000). The most common AIDS-defining condition for children is *Pneumocystis carinii* pneumonia (PCP) (33%), and accounts for 57% of AIDS-diagnoses in infants under one year (Lindgren, Steinberg, & Byers, 2000). For those acquiring HIV in adolescence, low CD4+ cell counts are the most common criteria for an AIDS diagnosis since highly active antiretroviral therapy (HAART) during pregnancy and delivery became widely available in 1996 (Luzuriaga & Sullivan, 2000).

More useful tools for monitoring and reporting HIV infection in children are the Immunologic and Clinical Categories of the revised Pediatric Classification System (CDC, 1994), which consider age as a variable, as infants' CD4+ T lymphocyte counts and percentage values are much higher than adults. Adult values are reached by the age of six (Table 27-4 and Box 27-4).

HIV is the eleventh leading cause of death among children aged 1 to 4 (Lindgren, et al., 2000). In many cities in the United States, it is the leading cause of death among 2 to 5 year olds (NIAID, 1996). For those children surviving beyond four years of age, the mean survival time is 9 to 10 years (Luzuriaga & Sullivan, 2000). Over 84% of perinatally infected children are African-American and Hispanic, demonstrating that this disease disproportionately affects children and families of color. Rates of AIDS in 1998 were 3.2/100,000 for African-American and 0.9/100,000 for Caucasian (0.2/100,000) children (Lindgren, et al., 2000).

There have been significant reductions in morbidity and mortality in recent years because of the availability of HAART, early diagnosis, and supportive treatment; some children may now live beyond adolescence (Boland, 2000; Nielsen, et al., 1997). The importance of early diagnosis and therapeutic intervention cannot be underestimated as the advances made in caring for children with HIV have been

TABLE 27-4 Revised Pediatric Classification System (AIDS): Immunologic Categories Based on Age-Specific CD4+ Lymphocyte Count and Percentage

Immune Category	Age of Child		
	<12 mo	**1–5 yr**	**6–12 yr**
1: No suppression	≥1500	≥1000	≥500
2: Moderate suppression	750–1499	500–900	200–499
3: Severe suppression	<750	<500(<15)	<200

(CDC, 1994; Working Group on ART, 1998)

BOX 27-4 Revised Pediatric Classification System (AIDS): Clinical Categories

Category N: Not Symptomatic
No signs or symptoms considered to be the result of HIV infection, or only one condition listed in category A.

Category A: Mildly Symptomatic
Two or more of the conditions listed below but none of the conditions listed in categories B and C.

- Lymphadenopathy (≥0.5 cm at more than two sites; bilateral at one site)
- Hepatomegaly
- Splenomegaly
- Dermatitis
- Parotitis
- Recurrent or persistent upper respiratory infection, sinusitis, or otitis media

Category B: Moderately Symptomatic
Symptomatic conditions other than those listed for category A or C that are attributed to HIV infection. Examples of conditions in clinical category B include but are not limited to:

- Anemia (<8 gm/dl), neutropenia (<1000/mm^3) or thrombocytopenia (<100,000 mm^3) persisting ≥30 days
- Bacterial meningitis, pneumonia, or sepsis (single episode)
- Candidiasis, oropharyngeal (thrush) persisting >2 months in children >6 months
- Cardiomyopathy
- Cytomegalovirus infection with onset <1 month age
- Diarrhea, recurrent or chronic
- Hepatitis
- HSV stomatitis, recurrent (>2 episodes within 1 yr)
- HSV bronchitis, pneumonitis, or esophagitis <1 month age
- Herpes zoster (shingles) involving at least 2 distinct episodes or >1 dermatome
- Leiomyosarcoma
- Lymphoid interstitial pneumonia (LIP) or pulmonary lymphoid hyperplasia complex
- Nephropathy
- Nocardiosis
- Persistent fever lasting >1 month
- Toxoplasmosis, onset <1 month age
- Varicella, disseminated (complicated chickenpox)

Category C: Severely Symptomatic
Any condition listed in the 1987 surveillance case definition for AIDS, with the exception of LIP, which is a category B condition.

- Serious bacterial infections, multiple or concurrent (≥2 within 2-yr period) of the following types: septicemia, pneumonia, meningitis, bone or joint infection, or abscess of an internal organ or body cavity (excluding otitis media, superficial skin or mucosal abscesses, and indwelling catheter related infections)
- Candidiasis, esophageal, or pulmonary (bronchi, trachea, or lungs)
- Coccidioidomycosis, disseminated
- Cryptococcosis, extrapulmonary
- Cryptosporidiosis or isosporiasis with diarrhea persisting >1 month
- Cytomegalovirus disease with onset of symptoms at age >1 month at site other than liver, spleen, or lymph nodes
- Encephalopathy (at least one of the following progressive findings present for at least 2 months in the absence of a concurrent illness other than HIV infection that could explain findings): 1) failure to attain or loss of developmental milestones or loss of intellectual ability, verified by standard developmental scale or neuropsychological tests; 2) impaired brain growth or acquired microcephaly demonstrated by head circumference measurements or brain atrophy demonstrated by CT or MRI (serial imaging is required for children <2 years age); 3) acquired symmetric motor deficit manifested by ≥2 of the following: paresis, pathologic reflexes, ataxia, or gait disturbance
- HSV infection causing a mucocutaneous ulcer persisting for >1 month or bronchitis, pneumonitis, or esophagitis for any duration affecting a child >1 month age
- Histoplasmosis, disseminated at a site other than or in addition to lungs or cervical or hilar lymph nodes
- Kaposi's sarcoma
- Lymphoma, primary, in brain
- Lymphoma, small, noncleaved cell (Burkitt's), or immunoblastic or large cell lymphoma of B cell or unknown immunologic origin

(CDC, 1994; Working Group on ART, 1998)

dramatic in the last decade, changing the grim statistics and offering greater quality and quantity of lives.

Children acquire HIV infection through perinatal transmission, unprotected sexual behaviors, or injection (intravenous or intramuscular) drug use. Approximately 91% of new cases and those with AIDS are acquired perinatally (Centers for Disease Control [CDC], 1999). The risk of perinatal infection may be higher if the mother acquires HIV infection during the first trimester of pregnancy, has a high viral load, or delivers a premature infant (Fowler, Simonds, & Roongpisuthipong, 2000). Contact with the mother's vaginal secretions during delivery is now thought to be the highest risk for perinatal transmission, supported in part by the reduction in transmission with elective cesarean sections (Fowler et al., 2000). The presence of maternal sexually transmitted diseases (STDs) and chorioamnionitis may increase the risk of transmission, as does the prolonged rupture of membranes prior to delivery (Bulterys & Fowler, 2000).

Postnatally, infants may become infected through breast milk (Behrman & Kliegman, 1998; Johnson & Oski, 1997). For this reason, mothers with HIV in developed countries are advised to bottle-feed formula to their infants.

It is important to note that only a very small percentage of infants born to infected mothers will be infected themselves. The incidence of perinatal HIV transmission is currently declining in the United States due to women taking combination **highly active antiretroviral therapy (HAART)** during pregnancy and delivery, and neonates receiving one or two antiretroviral drugs, such as zidovudine and epivir, for six weeks after birth (Bulterys & Fowler, 2000). The transmission rate with these regimens has decreased to less than 2% in many urban HIV care centers (Cohen, Stieglitz, & Moure, 2000), compared to a transmission rate of approximately 23% in infants whose mothers do not take antiretroviral therapy (Perinatal HIV Guidelines, 2001). Infants born to mothers with HIV are called HIV-exposed until their infection status is known.

Reflective Thinking

HIV Testing of Pregnant Women: Voluntary or Mandatory?

The United States has always placed a high value on individual rights; however, these rights are sometimes set aside for the greater good of society, such as in cases of reportable sexually transmitted diseases like syphilis. HIV continues to be an illness associated with stigma and acts of discrimination. When should the rights of a pregnant woman to choose whether or not to be tested for HIV be set aside for the potential good of her child? In what way could such a public policy be decided that would knowingly place women at risk for stigma, discrimination, and possibly acts of violence versus interventions to prevent transmission to their infants?

Eye On:

The Global Pandemic

The care of AIDS, unlike any others, changes rapidly due to the huge worldwide impact of the pandemic and the amount of research conducted internationally. HIV care in the U.S. and Europe differs dramatically from developing countries, most notably in Africa. New knowledge and therapies are rapidly integrated into care in the U.S., creating vast discrepancies in care and international debates over drug patents, drug availability, and who should receive the drugs.

Older adolescents may have acquired HIV through contaminated blood or blood products prior to 1985, when testing was first licensed for the HIV antibody in donated blood. Beginning in 1984, coagulation factors were heat treated to inactivate the virus, which also significantly decreased the number of pediatric infections (Bulterys & Fowler, 2000). Therefore, older adolescents with hemophilia, other bleeding disorders, or idiopathic thrombocytopenia may have acquired HIV during treatment for their disease.

Children and adolescents are also at risk for HIV infection through sexual contact with an infected person. Even though the number of children who acquire HIV through abuse is relatively low, it should always be considered when evaluating a child with a history of abuse. In addition, drug use among children and adolescents continues to be prevalent in some areas of the country and should be assessed as it also is a risk factor for HIV transmission because of the potential for sharing needles with an infected person, exchanging sex in return for drugs, and consensual sex with a drug-using person infected with HIV. Use of drugs, including alcohol, is known to inhibit thought, impair gross and fine motor ability, and, as a consequence, decreases the likelihood that safer sex including using condoms will be practiced.

Pathophysiology

HIV belongs to the family of lentiviruses, which are retroviruses and known to cause an illness trajectory with long periods of clinical latency and asymptomatic infection, weak humoral response, and persistent viremia (Greene, 1997). There are two known types of HIV. HIV-1, which is worldwide, and HIV-2, which exists primarily in West Africa. Both types cause primary immunodeficiency in humans. HIV-1 is highly mutant, and has a number of different subtypes based on their nucleotide sequences. Most HIV testing carried out in the United States is for HIV-1 subtypes although worldwide there are different subtypes that affect the sensitivity and specificity of antibody tests, and DNA and RNA assays, necessitating the need for using a combination of tests and the further development of broader tests (Nielsen & Bryson, 2000).

HIV is composed of inner and outer envelopes of two glycoproteins, gp120 and gp41 (gp160 together), and a viral core. The outer glycoproteins are needed to bind HIV-1 to CD4+ lymphocytes. The viral core capsule consists of the core proteins p24, p7, and p9. The viral core has two single strands of viral RNA and essential viral enzymes for replication, reverse transcriptase, RNAse, polymerase, integrase, and protease. The structure of HIV and the replication of viral components are directed by at least nine different genes with specific functions (Greene, 1997).

HIV-1 binds to a host cell with an attachment between gp120 and the host's CD4+ receptor site. The gp41 facilitates the fusion of the envelope with the CD4+ cell membrane (Barre-Sinoussi, 1996). The HIV-1 then penetrates into the host cell, uncoats its viral core, releases two single strands of viral RNA into the host cytoplasm, and makes a DNA copy from the RNA using reverse transcriptase. The other viral enzymes separate the RNA and DNA, and join two DNA strands together, which move into the host nucleus' DNA forming the HIV-1 provirus. The provirus remains quiet until CD4+ cell activation causes it to replicate (Brennan & Porche, 1997).

When activated, the CD4+ cell transcribes the proviral DNA into messenger RNA, which moves out of the nucleus facilitating the production of viral polyproteins that are precursors to the HIV envelope and core. Some polyproteins bud as immature, noninfectious HIV-1 virions, but others are changed by the enzyme protease into active glycoproteins and enzymes, which mature into infectious HIV-1 retrovirus and then bud from the CD4+ cell (Phillips, 1996).

An initial infection with HIV is marked by high levels of plasma HIV and a decrease in CD4+ lymphocytes, which fluctuate as the immune response attempts to contain the infection. These values stabilize after about six months of infection and the levels depend on a client's strength of immune response, the number of infected cells, and the virulence of the HIV strain (Staprans & Feinberg, 1997). Clients with higher plasma levels after stabilization are at higher risk of disease progression (Feinberg, 1996).

HIV infection affects the immune system directly and indirectly. Directly, the virus infects cells that possess the CD4+ marker/receptor such as the CD4+ T lymphocytes, macrophages, monocytes, follicular dendritic cells, and some bone marrow progenitor cells (Brennan & Porche, 1997). This process then results in killing the CD4+ cell, syncytia formation with cell killing, and suppression of immune cell function (Staprans & Feinberg, 1997). The CD4+ mononuclear cells (lymphocytes, macrophages, and monocytes) also travel to many tissue sites, infecting other organs, adding to its multisystem effects and variety of clinical sign and symptoms (Abuzaitoun & Hanson, 2000).

Indirect effects result from substances released as part of the immune response causing a chronic activation, which depletes the CD4+ cells, resulting in dysfunction and cellular death. The activation of B lymphocytes results in autoimmune responses to potentially any CD4+ cells, while abnormally high levels of B cell produced antibodies can also cause a variety of autoimmune disorders (Brennan & Porche, 1997). A binding of viral glycoprotein to CD4+ receptors can inactivate cells so that the immune system does not respond to infectious challenges (**anergy**). In addition, superantigens formed from an immune response can cause CD4+ cells to become more susceptible to infections by binding to them, and causing massive stimulation and destruction (Staprans & Feinberg, 1997). Hence, people with HIV have deficiencies in both cellular and humoral immunity.

Clinical Manifestations

Clinical manifestations range from being completely asymptomatic with normal CD4+ counts to having associated symptoms of the presenting OI or condition that meet the criteria for an AIDS diagnosis. The symptoms are variable depending on the mode of transmission and the age a child becomes infected. In general, the younger a child is at the time of acquisition, the more severe the symptoms, the more quickly the disease progresses, and the poorer the prognosis. However, there have been tremendous gains in understanding HIV and in developing new effective therapies that slow disease progression thus delaying the appearance of symptoms.

The severity of each clinical manifestation varies by organ system and often is the result of several factors, including viral replication in the affected tissue, an opportunistic infection of the organ, concurrent autoimmune or immunodeficiency processes in the organ, or the side effects of drug therapies for treatment of HIV or prophylaxis (Abuzaitoun & Hanson, 2000). However, the pathogenesis of many of the systemic effects of HIV is not yet clearly understood.

Infants who acquire HIV perinatally are at greatest risk of poor health outcomes and premature death. Immature immune systems and the developing organs of fetuses and infants are affected by HIV in different ways than adults. The natural history of infants shows that 15–20% are "fast progressors" because of the rapid onset of symptoms. Almost all these infants, if not treated, will have met AIDS-defining criteria by one year of age, with many dying by four years of age. Infants in this group may experience failure to thrive, developmental delays, generalized lymphadenopathy, hepatomegaly, splenomegaly, *Pneumocystis carinii* pneumonia, bacterial pneumonia, anemia, thrombocytopenia, recurrent candidiasis, nephropathy, cardiomyopathy, and cancers.

The other 80–85% of infants with perinatal transmission are termed "slow progressors." These infants demonstrate laboratory changes, such as leukopenias, and may have decreased T cell counts for their age. They may have developmental delays, but the incidence is lower. The onset of AIDS-defining OIs or conditions is delayed, often until after four years of age. It may be difficult to identify specific causes of some clinical manifestations, as symptoms may be similar to the effects of perinatal drug exposure or poor nutrition, which are often co-factors in HIV infection.

Older children may exhibit recurrent bacterial infections, generalized lymphadenopathy, hepatomegaly, splenomegaly, lymphoid interstitial pneumonitis, poor school performance, fatigue, and so forth. Laboratory data may show decreased T cells, elevated or decreased B cells, or anemia. If other organ systems are involved, lab tests pertaining to those systems may be altered. For example, in nephropathy, an elevated BUN and creatinine may be evident (Behrman & Kliegman, 1998; Berkowitz, 2000; Johnson & Oski, 1997).

Adolescents present with symptoms similar to adults, although many will be asymptomatic for many years. Many adults diagnosed with HIV are thought to have become infected during adolescence, demonstrating the initial benign course of HIV disease. Some people who become infected have an initial illness resembling the flu, who then appear to recover fully without symptoms of any illness.

Reflective Thinking

Working with Caregivers with Known HIV Infection Who Choose to Have More Children

To increase self-awareness about caregivers' choices, ask yourself:

1. How do I feel about people with HIV infection in general?
2. How do I feel about caring for a child with HIV?
3. Do I blame the caregivers for placing their child at risk for HIV? Why?
4. Do I avoid interacting with the caregivers because I do not agree with their choice? Why?
5. Do I feel uncomfortable with the caregivers because they are a different race or class, or might have done something I think is wrong in order to have acquired HIV?

Diagnosis

A careful history is important in determining whether or not testing for HIV is indicated, although testing should be offered to anyone who (a) is sexually active, (b) has drug-using sexual partners, (c) has a suspicious or documented history of sexual abuse, (d) is pregnant, (e) is an infant whose mother used drugs, (f) uses drugs, or (g) has symptoms suggestive of HIV infection.

The timing of transmission of HIV from mother to child is particularly important in the correct diagnosis of infants (Nielsen & Bryson, 2000). The standard ELISA (enzyme linked immunosorbent assay) HIV antibody test can be used for anyone older than 15–18 months of age. It cannot be used for younger infants because of the persistence of maternal antibodies (IgG) until this age, so the test would actually only be indirectly testing the mother. The antibody will be positive (i.e., antibodies are detected) from three weeks to six months after initial infection. A positive result on the ELISA is confirmed by the Western Blot test, which identifies specific proteins and glycoproteins found in antibodies specific to HIV (Table 27–5).

Infants from birth to 18 months of age should be tested by using a viral diagnostic assay, such as the HIV DNA polymerase chain reaction (PCR), plasma HIV RNA assay, or HIV whole cell viral culture. A positive test indicates probable infection, and should be confirmed on a second specimen as soon as possible. Testing for HIV by a PCR test should be done at birth or before the infant is 48 hours of age, at 14 days, at 1–2 months, and at 3–6 months of age (Working Group on ART, 1998) to determine actual infection status in an infant known to have a mother with HIV,

TABLE 27-5 Diagnosis of HIV Infection in Infants, Children, and Adolescents

Age for Test	Name of Test	Sensitivity	Comments
Birth, 1, 3–6 months	HIV DNA PCR	38% @ 48 hrs age, 93% age 14 d	Most common test
	HIV plasma RNA assay	May or may not be more sensitive	More expensive
	HIV cultures	Same as DNA PCR	More complex, expensive, results in 2 weeks
> 18 months	HIV IgG EIA "antibody test"	99%	Most commonly known test
Any	P24 antigen	Less sensitive	Very specific

and at anytime up to 18 months of age in an infant having other indications for testing. Many treatment decisions are made based on lymphocyte subsets (primarily CD4+ T lymphocytes and percentage) in conjunction with the DNA viral load level, particularly in determining when to initiate medications and when to change them.

Treatment

The management of HIV is complex, and requires a coordinated multidisciplinary team approach for the many physiological, psychosocial, and spiritual issues involved. It is a unique infectious illness because multiple family members may be infected, the course of illness is unpredictable, and the outcome is eventually death. This also means many uninfected and infected children have and will become orphans because of the deaths of their caregivers, and may be placed in foster care, or will live with extended family members. Multidisciplinary team members usually include physicians, nurses, social workers, dieticians, physical therapists, occupational therapists, pharmacists, and case managers. Care often includes mental health and chemical dependency services, which may be present at some integrated care sites. It is helpful to offer other support services, particularly in this overwhelmingly low socioeconomic group of affected clients, transportation assistance, child care, and interpreter services.

The goals of management are to slow the progression of disease and to improve the quality of life of infected persons. This is done primarily through a combination of three or four antiretroviral drugs (HAART), and the prevention and early treatment of opportunistic infections. There are fewer drugs available to young children than the older population because the medicine may not be available in liquid form, or may not be crushable. In addition, the liquid formulations often have high alcohol content, which is unpalatable to many small children (see Table 27–6 for the drugs that are used in treating AIDS).

The guidelines for initiating HAART and when to change drug regimens are updated frequently by collaborations between a number of clinicians, researchers, and health policy groups. Initial three drug regimens usually include one or two non-nucleoside reverse transcriptase inhibitors (NNRTI), possibly one nucleoside reverse transcriptase inhibitor (NRTI), and one protease inhibitor (PI). There is emerging information in the adult population regarding lipodystrophy with long-term use of protease inhibitors, so the trend by many providers is to delay their introduction by using another NNRTI or NRTI instead. The long-term effects of all antiretrovirals in children are unknown, although there seems to be no effect in children who have received antiretrovirals as prophylaxis in the newborn period. There is a great deal of research being conducted with vaccines, gene therapy, interferon, and cytokines in efforts to strengthen the immune system and eventually find a cure. New therapies have an accelerated approval process through the FDA because of the urgent need for life-saving treatments.

TABLE 27-6 Antiretroviral Agents for HIV

Nucleoside Analogs: Incorporated into Viral DNA and Block Reverse Transcriptase
Zidovudine (ZDV or AZT, Retrovir)
Stavudine (d4T, Zerit)
Zalcitabine (ddC, Hivid)
Didanosine (ddI, Videx)
Lamivudine (3TC, Epivir)
Nonnucleoside Reverse Transcriptase Inhibitors: Bind Directly to Reverse Transcriptase and Prevent Conversion of RNA to DNA
Nevirapine (Viramune)
Delavirdine mesylate (Rescriptor)
Protease Inhibitors: Prevent Assemblage and Release of HIV from Infected CD4 Cells
Saquinavir (Fortovase)
Nelfinavir mesylate (Viracept)
Ritonavir (Norvir)
Indinavir (Crixivan)

From Berkowitz, C. (2000). Pediatric HIV. In C. Berkowitz (Ed), Pediatrics: A primary care approach, *(2nd ed., p. 548). Philadelphia: Saunders.*

The prevention of opportunistic infections includes the use of sulfamethoxazole/trimethoprim as prophylaxis against *Pneumocystis carinii* pneumonia (for CD4+ cells <200), which is still the primary cause of death for both children and adults, and possibly prophylaxis for *Mycobacterium avium-intracellulare* and cytomegalovirus retinitis, which are of more concern with very low CD4+ cells (<50). These, and other OIs, are becoming less frequent with the use of HAART. Refer to Table 27–7 for medications used prophylactically to treat opportunistic infections.

Much of the remaining ongoing medical management is related to early detection of HIV clinical manifestations and opportunistic infections. Early intervention can then be initiated, often ameliorating effects of the illness through appropriate treatment and referrals (Table 27–8). It is also important to incorporate well-child care with the usual anticipatory guidance topics, which are often overlooked in many chronic illnesses. Important considerations in immunizations include following the usual schedule with the exceptions of using only the inactivated formulation for polio (IPV), receiving an annual influenza vaccine, considering varicella only for children in category N1 or A1 with a CD4% ≥25%, and excluding those with severe suppression from measles vaccine (Laufer & Scott, 2000).

TABLE 27-7 Prophylaxis for Common Opportunistic Infections in Children

Pneumocystis carinii
Trimethoprim-sulfamethoxazole
Dapsone
Pentamidine (IV or aerosolized)
Mycobacterium avium-intracellulare
Clarithromycin
Azithromycin
Rifabutin
Candida
Nystatin
Clotrimazole
Fluconazole

From Berkowitz, C. (2000). Pediatric HIV. In C. Berkowitz (Ed), Pediatrics: A primary care approach, *(2nd ed., p. 548). Philadelphia: Saunders.*

Nursing Management

Assessment

The assessment of children with HIV can be extensive, and will be revised over time. Family processes must always be considered, particularly around issues of diagnosis, disclosure, grieving, caregiver strain, involvement of extended family in care (particularly when multiple members are ill), fears, hopes or hopelessness, spiritual beliefs, support systems, loneliness or social isolation, altered parenting, and coping. The child's condition will also affect assessment and the related diagnosis, plans, and outcomes.

Nursing Diagnosis

1. Deficient knowledge related to HIV, transmission, managing acute illness, and chronic symtoms.
2. Altered nutrition related to an increased metabolic rate and a chronic disease state.
3. Increased susceptibility to infection related to inadequate immune system.
4. Altered growth and development related to effects of chronic, sometimes fatal disease.
5. Impaired care at home due to insufficient organization or planning, finances, unfamiliarity with community resources, or inadequate support systems.

Outcome Identification

1. Family will understand disease, how transmission occurs, and how to manage acute illness and chronic symptoms.
2. Child's nutritional status will be improved and kept at an optimal state.
3. Child's immunizations will be up to date; child will not develop frequent secondary/opportunistic infections.
4. Child's development will be normal and minimally affected by disease state.
5. Family care at home will be adequate and community resources and supports will be utililized.

Planning/Implementation

1. Teach family about disease, transmission, signs and symptoms of acute illness, how to manage symptoms, and when to call the doctor.
2. Teach family principles of adequate nutrition, suggest foods high in protein and calories, offer frequent small meals.
3. Teach family immunization schedule, stress importance of keeping immunizations up to date, encourage good handwashing, and avoiding contact with individuals who have a communicable disease (respiratory, etc.).
4. Teach family normal developmental milestones; encourage family to facilitate development by providing appropriate activities.
5. Listen to family verbalize concerns related to their ability to care for child; suggest community resources that may be helpful.

Evaluation

1. Family understands disease and disease transmission, and manages acute illness and chronic symptoms.
2. Child's nutritional status is improved.
3. Child's immunizations are up to date; secondary/opportunistic infections are at a minimum.
4. Child's development is normal.
5. Family provides adequate care and utilizes apropriate community resources and supports.

Nursing Alert:

Herbal and Homeopathic Therapies

HIV, like many other illnesses without a cure, often invites the use of alternative and complementary therapies in efforts to improve quality of life or even attempt to cure the disease. Some of these herbal and homeopathic therapies can interact with allopathic (traditional Western) medicines and be harmful, or cause allergic reactions. Remember to ask caregivers and clients about all therapies being utilized.

TABLE 27-8 Management of Children with HIV Infection

Evaluation	Interval
Complete history and physical examination	3 mo
Review of systems	3 mo
Immunization	See Appendix C
Developmental examination	
0–12 mo	3 mo
1–3 y	6 mo
>3 y	Annually
CT scan of the brain	Baseline and as indicated
Chest radiography	Annually
Laboratory values	
Complete blood count	3 mo
T-cell subsets	3 mo
HIV RNA PCR (quantitative)	3 mo
Liver enzymes	3 mo
Pancreatic enzymes	3 mo
Electrolytes, BUN, and creatinine	Baseline and as indicated
Quantitative immunoglobulins	6 mo
Urinalysis	Annually
Serology	
Cytomegalovirus	Baseline, annually if negative
Epstein-Barr virus	Baseline, annually if negative
Toxoplasmosis	Baseline, annually if negative
Rubella	Baseline
Varicella-zoster	Baseline
Herpes simplex	Baseline
Hepatitis B, C	Baseline
Tuberculin skin test and control	Annually*
Referrals	
Ophthalmologic examination	Annually†
Dental examination	6 mo
Cardiology (echocardiogram)	If clinically indicated
Gynecologic examination	Puberty, annually thereafter

**For control use mumps or tetanus antigen if the patient has already been immunized; otherwise use candida antigen.*
†Every 6 mo if severely immunosuppressed.
PCR = polymerase chain reaction, BUN = blood urea nitrogen.

Family Teaching

The waiting period to determine the infection status of the young infant at about four months of age is one of uncertainty, anxiety, and distress for caregivers. Encourage the family to talk to health care professionals. If diagnosis is positive, referral to support groups is warranted. The majority of children generally are healthy for a number of years. They will be closely monitored, however. Healthy infants and children will be evaluated at the usual well-child intervals, and often at three month intervals when older, instead of annual well-child visits. Children's growth and development will be closely monitored for early signs of growth failure and developmental delays. Caregivers should be encouraged to consult with their health care provider if they notice anything that doesn't seem on track. The facts about what does and does not transmit HIV should be discussed and clarified, as misconceptions continue to abound. Encourage living as normal a life as possible with the restrictions imposed by the illness processes. Family and individual development are critical, and should be supported whenever possible and in creative ways. These can be assisted through social support systems, peer networks, obtaining needed resources, ongoing formal education, and spiritual beliefs. It is important to establish strong trusting relationships with health care providers in a multidisciplinary team, as the relationships are likely to be long ones. Infants and children need to be integrated into all aspects of their respective communities and cultures to maximize their full developmental potentials.

Children with HIV or AIDS should attend school. Schools have a legal obligation to provide for a child's education, and to provide medications to the child when indicated during school hours. There is a continuing concern about transmitting HIV through biting, although there has not been a single documented case of this occurring in the United States. HIV positive children are at greater risk of contracting illnesses at school, such as varicella (chickenpox) or influenza. These common childhood illnesses can be treated or minimized, so it is important to notify the child's health provider if these exposures occur.

Stigma, discrimination, and acts of violence against people with HIV and their families, including young children, still exist today. Constant factual information must be presented by health care providers and by the popular media.

ALLERGIC REACTIONS TO DRUGS

Drug allergies are adverse reactions to drugs or their metabolites caused by immunologic responses (deShazo & Kemp, 1997). The reactions demonstrate either systemic hypersensitivity or organ-specific patterns, and usually recur on re-exposure to the same drug, but may also occur with prolonged administration.

Research Highlight

Children and Families Affected by HIV/AIDS

Study Purpose

To explore goals and the strategies families use to reach these goals when raising a child with HIV.

Methods

This ethnographic study used semi-structured and open-ended interviews. Five uninfected adult family member caregivers, nine children between 7 and 15 who were diagnosed with HIV infection, and six mothers and one father with HIV infection participated. Families were asked to talk about their family composition, symptom management, and how they disclosed information about the disease to others.

Findings

The three goals that helped families maintain stability and establish normalcy included (1) facilitating their child's participation in social and school activities, (2) staying healthy, and (3) enhancing emotional and social well-being of family members. Strategies included a balanced diet and exercise, active participation in treatment, juggling multiple responsibilities so they could care for family members, allowing and encouraging children to attend and participate in school activities, being selective about disclosing information about the infection to those outside the family group, so their children would be treated normally, having other family members help care for the child, having spiritual and religious beliefs and practices, and using supportive professionals.

Implications

Nurses should (1) be aware that families might limit information they share with others about their child's illness, (2) encourage children and families to establish goals and strategies that will help them achieve their goals, and (3) help parents raising children with HIV/AIDS realize most families impacted by chronic illness such as HIV/AIDS are able to set and meet their goals of living a "normal" life.

Citation

Rehm, R., & Franck, L. (2000). Long-term goals and normalization strategies of children and families affected by HIV/AIDS. *Advances in Nursing Science, 23*, 69–82.

Incidence and Etiology

Allergic and immunologic drug reactions account for 6–10% of adverse reactions in hospitalized patients. The risk of allergic reaction for most drugs is 1–3%. Some people may be allergic to all drugs in the same or similar class based on antigen properties. Common drug allergens are aspirin and other nonsteroidal anti-inflammatory agents, beta-lactam antibiotics, penicillamine (the most common), sulfonamides, antituberculous drugs, anticonvulsants, general anesthetics, enzymes, radiocontrast media, and antithyroid drugs (deShazo & Kemp, 1997).

Drug allergy is less common and less severe in infants, probably because of their immature immune systems. Children whose parents have antibiotic allergies may have a 15-fold increase in relative risk for allergic reactions to antibiotics (Attaway, Jasin, & Sullivan, 1991).

Pathophysiology

Drug reactions can be IgE mediated, such as in anaphylaxis, or caused by nonspecific histamine release. In the latter case, the drugs induce the release of mediators from mast cells of immediate hypersensitivity reactions, which cannot be distinguished clinically from IgE mediated responses (deShazo & Kemp, 1997).

Clinical Manifestations

Reactions can be classified into cutaneous or multiple organ system manifestations. Cutaneous reactions are the most common, while multiple organ system involvement is the more life-threatening and dramatic presentation. Cutaneous reactions include urticaria and/or **angioedema,** maculopapular exanthems, and allergic contact dermatitis. With **urticaria,** the wheal-like lesions appear after beginning the drug and resolve fairly rapidly after discontinuing the drug. Occasionally, a chronic urticaria lasting six weeks or more may persist despite drug stoppage.

Maculopapular rashes are the most common form of cutaneous reactions. They are symmetric, often confluent erythematous lesions, which typically spare the palms and soles (deShazo & Kemp, 1997), and are more common in people with concurrent viral infections. The eruptions usually appear within one week of starting the drug, may subside even with use of the drug, may not recur with repeated exposure, or may occasionally progress to an exfoliative dermatitis.

Contact dermatitis is an example of delayed-type hypersensitivity and occurs with medications applied directly to the skin. It is usually pruritic, erythematous, vesicular, or maculopapular. Contact dermatitis usually takes 5–7 days to develop, and can occur within 24 hours after re-exposure (deShazo & Kemp, 1997).

Multiple organ system manifestations include anaphylaxis, nonspecific histamine release, erythema multiforme/Stevens-Johnson syndrome, toxic epidermal necrolysis (TEN), hypersensitivity syndromes, and drug fever (deShazo & Kemp, 1997). **Anaphylaxis** is an acute, life-threatening reaction with diffuse erythema, urticaria, angioedema, pruritis, bronchospasm, laryngeal edema, hyperperistalsis, hypotension, or cardiac dysrhythmias (deShazo & Kemp, 1997). Anaphylaxis occurs rapidly, within 5 to 30 minutes after exposure. Nonspecific histamine release reactions, although having a different etiology, have the same systemic manifestations as anaphylaxis.

Erythema multiforme may be caused by drugs in 10–20% of all cases, and is an erythematous, maculopapular, vesicular, urticarial rash that may include target lesions. The most severe form is **Stevens-Johnson syndrome,** which includes mucosal and conjunctival lesions, and epidermal loss of 10% or less of the body surface area. **Toxic epidermal necrolysis** is an acute illness of fever, epidermal loss of more than 30% of the body surface area, and visceral involvement with an associated 30–40% mortality rate (deShazo & Kemp, 1997).

Hypersensitivity syndromes, such as with anticonvulsant therapy, usually occur within one to three weeks after initiating therapy, but can occur within three months or later. Manifestations include fever, erythematous papules, tender and generalized lymphadenopathy, hepatitis, nephritis, and leukocytosis. Periorbital edema, myalgias, or arthralgias may also occur. Drug fever, manifested by fever, rash, eosinophilia, leukocytosis, and elevated sedimentation rate can occur with any drug, and almost always resolves within 72 hours of discontinuing the drug.

Family Teaching

Anaphylaxis

- Know the offending drug or allergen such as latex, insect stings, drugs, or foods.
- Encourage child or caregiver to carry epi-pen.
- Remind family that prevention is critical for those susceptible to anaphylaxis.

Diagnosis

The diagnosis of allergic drug reactions is usually made by a history of drug initiation and use, onset and presentation of clinical manifestations, and improvement of symptoms after discontinuing the drug. Administering the drug again is occasionally used to confirm the diagnosis, although this can cause a serious reaction. Diagnostic skin testing is available for some drugs, which can limit the systemic symptoms.

Certain laboratory tests can be ordered, such as white cell count and sedimentation rate.

Treatment

Treatment varies based on the pathophysiology and severity of the reaction. Avoidance of contact with the offending drug is the first intervention. Anaphylaxis and histamine release reactions are an emergency, and should be treated with epinephrine, which inhibits further mediator release, reduces vascular permeability, and improves vasomotor tone (deShazo & Kemp, 1997). Oxygen should be administered if indicated, along with measurement of blood oxygen levels. An intravenous infusion of saline may be indicated for hypotension. Breathing may need to be supported through intubation or tracheostomy for laryngeal spasm or edema. Antihistamines may attenuate the reaction, although they are limited in usefulness during the acute onset of symptoms. Corticosteroids may decrease the possible late-phase reactions occasionally occurring 6 to 12 hours after the onset of anaphylaxis.

Kids Want To Know

How come I have to wear that bracelet?

Tiani, you need to wear that silver bracelet because it lets people know you are allergic to penicillin. We need to do that so you do not receive that drug.

Critical Thinking

Stevens-Johnson Syndrome

Twelve-year-old Ron was admitted to the unit with an erythematous papular rash covering his arms, legs, abdomen, the soles of his feet, and the palms of his hands. His mother Helen said that he had a sore throat, headache, fever, and "just didn't feel well" a day or two before he broke out with his rash. He also had been on penicillin for five days because of a throat infection. He was diagnosed with Stevens-Johnson syndrome. What nursing care would be appropriate?

Treatment is primarily supportive for erythema multiforme and TEN, although corticosteroids are recommended in the former to prevent visceral involvement and shorten the duration of symptoms. Corticosteroids are also indicated in hypersensitivity syndromes. Diphenhydramine relieves symptoms of most milder cutaneous reactions, and other symptoms of histamine release such as pruritis, erythema, and swelling (deShazo & Kemp, 1997).

Nursing Management

General nursing care for a child with a drug reaction involves being sure there is an effective airway if the child is having an acute reaction; providing comfort measures related to pruritis, pain, and itching; providing good oral hygiene and skin care; teaching the child and family about the treatments ordered and experienced; administering and watching for the side effects of any medications ordered; teaching the child and caregivers about drugs that should be avoided; providing opportunities for the child to rest; providing age-appropriate activities; and encouraging the child to wear a medic alert bracelet with the drug the child is allergic to listed on the back.

Family Teaching

Encourage caregivers and children to know the name of the offending drug(s) to avoid exposure or being prescribed that drug in the future. Although it cannot be known for certain the drug will cause the same reaction, it is more likely than not to cause a similar reaction.

Some drugs may be required for life-saving treatment in the future; drug sensitization may be needed, such as for penicillin, when there is a history of reactions to a particular class of drugs.

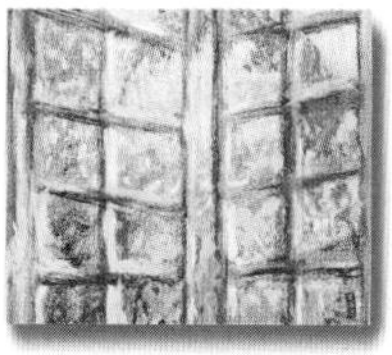

In the Real World

I was diagnosed with JRA as an early teen, around the time when I started my period. My joints really hurt and were so swollen. I was really miserable. I remember the nurses who took care of me. They were so kind and patient. I am sure I was not an easy child to care for, and at the time, thought I would never be able to lead a normal life. But, I was one of the lucky ones. I have no problems today and no residual effects from that disease. Perhaps those early experiences were why I decided to become a nurse. I hope that the children I care for feel the same way about me that I did about those nurses who cared for me so long ago.

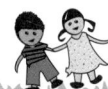

Key Concepts

- The function of the immune system is to prevent or ameliorate infections, recognize self from nonself, and maintain homeostasis.
- Immune system alterations are almost always chronic illnesses that are managed rather than cured; health care is best delivered by a multidisciplinary team.
- Immune system dysfunction demonstrates a wide variety of clinical manifestations not confined to the immune system.
- Juvenile rheumatoid arthritis, an autoimmune disorder involving joints and occasionally the eyes or heart, affects mobility and activities of daily living and has multiple psychosocial consequences.
- Systemic lupus erythematosus, a lifelong autoimmune disorder characterized by multiple system involvement, requires a delicate balance between symptoms of the disease, side effects of medication and treatment, and psychosocial aspects of both.
- HIV/AIDS is an infectious disease known for affecting primarily the immune system, but demonstrates multiple clinical manifestations directly related to its multiorgan system involvement.
- Drug reactions may vary from a mild rash to a serious systemic reaction.
- Nursing care of children with immune system alterations involves knowing about the etiology, treatment, medications, management, and educational needs of children and their families.

Review Questions

1. Describe the three subgroups of juvenile rheumatoid arthritis (JRA).
2. Discuss management goals of JRA.
3. Describe the pathophysiology of systemic lupus erythematosus (SLE).
4. Explain why pregnancy is so important to plan for in a teenage girl with SLE.
5. Discuss the two laboratory tests and the clinical criteria most often used to make treatment decisions for children with HIV.
6. Discuss the major medical management goals for children with HIV.
7. List several nursing diagnoses for the child with HIV and discuss potential nursing management issues.
8. Describe the multiple organ system patterns involved in allergic drug reactions.

References

Abuzaitoun, O.R., & Hanson, I.C. (2000). Organ-specific manifestations of HIV disease in children. *Pediatric Clinics of North America, 47*, 109–126.

American College of Rheumatology Ad Hoc Committee of Systemic Lupus Erythematosus Guidelines. (1999). Guidelines for referral and management of systemic lupus erythematosis in adults. *Arthritis and Rheumatism, 42*(9) 1785–1796.

American Academy of Pediatrics. (2000). *2000 Red book: Report of the Committee on Infectious Diseases* (25th ed.). Elk Grove Village, IL: Author.

Attaway, N. J., Jasin, H. M., & Sullivan, T. J. (1991). Familial drug allergy. *Journal of Allergy and Clinical Immunology, 87*, 227.

Barre-Sinoussi, F. (1996). HIV as the cause of AIDS. *Lancet, 348*, 31–35.

Behrman, R., & Kliegman, R. (1998). *Nelson's textbook of pediatrics* (3rd ed.). Philadelphia: Saunders.

Berkowitz, C. (2000). Pediatric HIV. In C. Berkowitz (Ed.), *Pediatrics: A primary care approach*, (2nd ed., pp. 524–529). Philadelphia: Saunders.

Boland, M.G. (2000). Caring for the child and family with HIV Disease. *Pediatric Clinics of North America, 47*, 189–202.

Brennan, C., & Porche, D. J. (1997). HIV immunopathogenesis. *Journal of the Association of Nurses in AIDS Care, 8*, 7–22.

Bulterys, M., & Fowler, M.G. (2000). Prevention of HIV infection in children. *Pediatric Clinics of North America, 47*, 241–260.

Cassidy, J., & Petty, R. (1995). *Textbook of pediatric rheumatology* (3rd ed., pp.133–198). Philadelphia: Saunders.

Centers for Disease Control and Prevention (CDC). (1994). Revised Classification system for human immunodeficiency virus infection in children less than 13 years of age. *Morbidity and Mortality Weekly Report (MMWR), 43* (RR-12), 1–10.

Centers for Disease Control and Prevention (CDC). (1999). *HIV/AIDS Surveillance Report, 11*, 22–23.

Cohen, M., Stieglitz, K., & Moure, B. (2000) [abstract ThPeB5266] Women and children with HIV program: A decade of care and change. In Program and Abstracts of XIIIth World AIDS Conference, Durban, South Africa.

deShazo, R. D., & Kemp, S. F. (1997). Allergic reactions to drugs and biologic agents. *Journal of the American Medical Association, 278*, 1895–1906.

Edgerton, E., & DuPlessis. (2000). Juvenile rheumatoid arthritis. In In C. Berkotiwz (Ed.), *Pediatrics: A primary care approach* (2nd ed. pp. 549–552). Phildelphia; Saunders.

Feinberg, M. (1996). Changing the natural history of HIV disease. *Lancet, 348*, 239–246.

Fowler, M., Simonds, R., & Roongpisuthipong, A. (2000). Update on perinatal HIV transmission. *The Pediatric Clinics of North America, 47*(1), 21–38.

Greene, W. (1997). Molecular insights into HIV-1 infection. In M. Sande & P. Volberding (Eds.), *The medical management of AIDS* (5th ed., pp. 17–28). Philadelphia: Saunders.

Hartley, B., & Fuller, C. C. (1997). Juvenile arthritis: A nursing perspective. *Journal of Pediatric Nursing, 12*, 100–109.

Johnson, K., & Oski, F. (1997). *Oski's essential pediatrics*. Philadelphia: Lippincott-Raven.

Laufer, M., & Scott, G.B. (2000). Medical management of HIV disease in children. *Pediatric Clinics of North America, 47*, 127–154.

Lindgren, M., Steinberg, S., & Byers, R.H. (2000). Epidemiology of HIV/AIDS in children. *Pediatric Clinics of North America, 47*, 1–20.

Luzuriaga, K. & Sullivan, J.L. (2000). Viral and immunopathogenesis of vertical HIV-1 infection. *Pediatric Clinics of North America, 47*, 65–78.

Nielsen, K., & Bryson, Y. (2000). Diagnosis of HIV infection in children. *Pediatric Clinics of North America, 47*, 39–64.

Nielsen, K., McSherry, G., Petru, A., Frederick, T., Wara, D., Bryson, Y., Martin, N., Hutto, C., Ammann, J., Grubman, S., Oleske, J., & Scott, G. (1997). A descriptive survey of pediatric human immunodeficiency virus-infected long-term survivors. *Pediatrics*, E4, 99.

Perinatal HIV Guidelines Working Group Members. (2001). *Public Health Service Task Force recommendations for use of antiretroviral drugs in pregnant HIV-1-infected women for maternal health and interventions to reduce perinatal HIV-1 transmission in the United States*, 1–54.

Phillips, K. (1996). Protease inhibitors: A new weapon and a new strategy against HIV. *Journal of the Association of Nurses in AIDS Care, 7*, 57–68.

Rakel, R. (1996). *Saunders' manual of medical practice*. Philadelphia: Saunders.

Rehm, R., & Franck, L. (2000). Long-term goals and normalization strategies of children and families affected by HIV/AIDS. *Advances in Nursing Science, 23*, 69–82.

Rosen, S.T. (1994). *A guide to the immune system*. Chicago: Triclinica Communications.

Seely, R. R., Stephens, T. D., & Tate, P. (2000). *Anatomy and physiology* (5th ed). pp.703–731. USA. McGraw-Hill.

Staprans, S., & Feinberg, M. (1997). Natural history and immunopathogenesis of HIV-1 disease. In M. Sande and P. Volberding (Eds.), *The medical management of AIDS* (5th ed., pp. 29-56). Philadelphia: Saunders.

Uramoto, K., Michet, C., Thumboo, J., Sunku, J., O'Fallon, W., & Gabriel, S. (1999). Trends in the incidence and mortality of systemic lupus erythematosus. *Arthritis and Rheumatism, 42*(1), 46–50.

Wargula, J., & Lovell, D. (2000). Use of etanercept in children. *Bulletin of Rheumatic Disease, 40*(12), 1–4.

White, P. H. (1994). Pediatric systemic lupus erythematosus and neonatal lupus. *Rheumatic Disease Clinics of North America, 20*, 119–127.

Working Group on Antiretroviral Therapy and Medical Management of Infants, Children and Adolescents with HIV Infection. (1998). Antiretroviral therapy and medical management of pediatric HIV infection. *Pediatrics, 102*, 1005–1062S.

Suggested Readings

Abud-Mendoza, C., Sturbaum, A. K., Vasquez-Compear, R., & Gonzalez-Amaro, R. (1993). Methotrexate therapy in childhood systemic lupus erythematosus. *The Journal of Rheumatology, 20*, 731–733.

Ackley, B. J., & Ladwig, G. B. (1997). *Nursing diagnosis handbook: A guide to planning care* (3rd ed.). St. Louis, MO: Mosby.

Barron, K. S., Silverman, E. D., Gonzales, J., & Reveille, J. D. (1993). Clinical, serologic, and immunogenetic studies in childhood-onset systemic lupus erythematosus. *Arthritis and Rheumatism, 36*, 348–354.

Beck, S.A., & Burk, A.W. (1999). Taking action against anaphylaxis. *Contemporary Pediatrics, 16*, 87–96.

Brewer, E. J., Bass, J., Baum, J., Cassidy, J., Fink, C., Jacobs, J., Hanson, V., Levinson, J., Schaller, J., & Stillman, J. S. (1977). Current proposed revision of JRA criteria. *Arthritis and Rheumatism, 20*, 195–199.

Butz, A., Joyner, M., Friedman, D. G., & Hutton, N. (1997). Primary care for children with immunodeficiency syndrome. *Journal of Pediatric Health Care, 12*, 10–19.

Cassidy, J. T. (1998). Outcomes in the therapeutic use of methotrexate in children with chronic peripheral arthritis. *Journal of Pediatrics, 133*, 179–180.

Conner, E.M. (1994). Reduction of maternal-infant transmission of human immunodeficiency virus type 1 with zidovudine treatment. *The New England Journal of Medicine, 331*, 1173–1180.

Cook, R. J., Gladman, D., Pericak, D. & Urowitz, M. (2000). Prediction of short term mortality in systemic lupus erythematosus with time dependent measures or disease activity. *Journal of Rheumatology, 27*(8), 1892–1895.

Evans, R. (1993). Epidemiology and natural history of asthma, allergic rhinitis, and atopic dermatitis. In E. Middleton, C. Reed, E. Ellis, J. Adkinson, J. Yunginger, & W. Busse (Eds), *Allergy: Principles and Practice* (4th ed., pp. 1109–1136). St. Louis, MO: Mosby.

Fox, D. A., & McCune, W. J. (1994). Immunosuppressive drug therapy of systemic lupus erythematosus. *Rheumatic Disease Clinics of North America, 20*, 265–297.

Futterman, D., Chabon, B., & Hoffman, N.D. (2000). HIV and AIDS in adolescents. *Pediatric Clinics of North America, 47*, 171–188.

Gottlieb, B. S., & Ilowite, N T. (2000). Meeting the challenge of rheumatological disease in teens. *Contemporary Pediatrics*, December, 61–93.

Hoekelman, R. A. (Ed.). (1992). *Primary pediatric care* (2nd ed., pp. 1314–1320). St Louis, MO: Mosby.

Hughes, R., & D'Ambrosia, K. (1993). Nursing management of a child with rheumatoid arthritis. *Orthopedic Nursing, 12*, 17–23.

Klippel, J. H. (1997). Primer on the rheumatic diseases (11th ed.). Atlanta, Georgia: Arthritis Foundation.

Lindsley, C. B. (1992). Lupus: A brighter outlook, a continuing challenge. *Contemporary Pediatrics, 9*, 19–44.

Lovell, D. J. (2000). Etanercept in children with polyarticular rheumatoid arthritis. *New England Journal of Medicine*, 763–769.

Lovell, D. J., Miller, M. L., & Cassidy, J. T. (2000) Treatment of rheumatic disease. In Behrman, R. (Ed.), *Nelson's textbook of pediatrics* (16th ed.). Philadelphia: Saunders.

Majchel, A., Proud, D., Kagey-Sobotka, A., Witek, T., Lichtenstein, L., & Naclerio, R. (1992). Evaluation of a bedtime dose of a combination antihistamine/analgesic/decongestant product on antigen challenge the next morning. *Laryngoscope, 102*, 330–334.

Miller, M. L., Kress, A. M., & Berry, C. A. (1999). Decreased physical function in juvenile rheumatoid arthritis. *Arthritis Care and Research, 12*(5), 309–313.

Oen, K. G., & Cheang, M. (1996). Epidemiology of chronic arthritis in childhood. *Seminars in Arthritis and Rheumatism, 26*, 575–591.

Page-Goertz, P. (1989). Even children have arthritis. *Pediatric Nursing, 15*, 11–16.

Palumbo, P.E. (2000). Antiretroviral therapy of HIV infection in children. *Pediatric Clinics of North America, 47*, 155–170.

Rosenberg, A. M. (1996). Treatment of juvenile rheumatoid arthritis: Approach to patients who fail standard therapy. *The Journal of Rheumatology, 23*, 1652–1656.

Silverman, E. (1996). What's news in the treatment of pediatric SLE. *The Journal of Rheumatology, 23*, 1657–1660.

Spencer, C. H., Fife, R. Z., & Rabinovich, C. E. (1995). The school experience of children with arthritis. *Pediatric Clinics of North America, 42*, 5.

Szer, I. S. (1986). The diagnosis and management of systemic lupus erythematosus in childhood. *Pediatric Annals, 15*, 596–604.

Tan, E.M., Cohen, A.S., Fries, J., Masi, A., McShane, D., Rothfield, N., Schaller, J., Talal, N., & Winchester, R. (1982). The 1982 revised criteria for the classification of systemic lupus erythematosus. *Arthritis and Rheumatism 25*, 1271–1277.

Theodosakis, J., & Adderly, B. (1997). *The arthritis cure*. New York: St. Martin's Press.

Resources

Organizations and Websites

Antiretroviral Pregnancy Registry
(800) 722-9292 ext. 38465

The Arthritis Foundation
1330 West Peachtree St.
Atlanta, GA 30309
(800) 283-7800
www.arthritis.org

Association of Rheumatology Health Professionals
1800 Century Place, Suite 250
Atlanta, GA 30345
(404) 633-3777

The Elizabeth Glaser Pediatric AIDS Foundation
2950 31st Street, #125
Santa Monica, CA 90405
(888) 499-HOPE
Fax: (310) 314-1469
www.pedaids.org

HIV/AIDS Treatment Information Service
P.O. Box 6303
Rockville, MD 20849-6303
(800) HIV-0440
www.hivatis.org

Information about HIV Clinical Trials for Children and Adults
ACTIS
P.O. Box 6421
Rockville, MD 20849-6421
(800) TRIALS-A
www.actis.org

Lupus Foundation of America, Inc.
1300 Piccard Drive, Suite 200
Rockville, MD 20850-4303
(800) 558-0121
www.web4.xor.com/lupus

National AIDS/HIV Hotline
TTY Service (800) 243-7889
English (800) 342-2437
Spanish (800) 344-7432
www.ashastd.org/nah

National AIDS Clearinghouse
(800) 458-5231
www.cdcnpin.org

National Association of People with AIDS
1413 K Street N.W. 7th Fl.
Washington, DC 20005
(202) 898-0414
www.napwa.org

National Pediatric & Family HIV Resource Center
University of Medicine & Dentistry of New Jersey
30 Bergen Street – ADMC #4
Newark, NJ 07103
Fax: (973) 972-0399

CHAPTER 28

ENDOCRINE ALTERATIONS

Shirley Goodman, RN, CDE

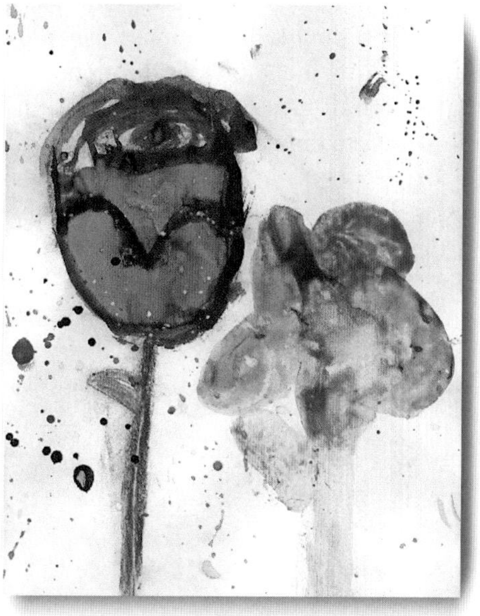

My name is Jennifer Hill and I'm 15 years old. I was diagnosed with type 1 diabetes 3 years ago. I am on the dance team in my high school, which keeps me very busy the entire school year. I have had an insulin pump for a year, and it has made it easier to manage my diabetes and keep my glucose at normal levels. I used to give myself 4 insulin injections a day. Now all I have to do is insert a new needle in my abdomen every few days. I still have to count carbohydrates in my diet and test my blood glucose several times a day, but I feel so much better when I monitor what I eat and keep my blood sugar as close to normal as possible.

COMPETENCIES

Upon completion of this chapter, the reader will be able to:

- *Describe the endocrine glands, their hormones, and functions.*
- *Explain the principle of negative feedback.*
- *Describe the etiology, clinical manifestations, treatment, and nursing management of common endocrine alterations.*
- *Discuss the management goals for the child with Type I diabetes mellitus (insulin dependent diabetes mellitus).*
- *Develop a teaching plan for a child with newly diagnosed Type I diabetes.*
- *Compare the causes, clinical manifestations, and treatment of hypoglycemia and hyperglycemia.*

The endocrine system is composed of glands that produce and secrete chemical substances called hormones, which affect multiple tissues and organs. Hormones control or regulate important body functions, such as growth, fluid and electrolyte balance, energy production, sexual maturation, reproduction, and response to stress. Endocrine disorders are related to either a deficiency (hypofunction) or an excess (hyperfunction) of a specific hormone. In children most endocrine disorders are caused by insufficient production of hormones. Additionally, disorders can be classified based on the origin of the defect that results in a malfunction. Primary disorders occur when the target gland itself is not functioning normally. Secondary disorders are ones in which the origin of the disorder is in the pituitary, resulting in inadequate stimulation of the target gland. A tertiary disorder is one in which the hypothalamus is the cause of the problem. Early identification of endocrine disorders is imperative because they can cause significant problems, some of which are life-threatening. The onset of these disorders is insidious, and most do not become clinically apparent for a long time.

This chapter will include an overview of the anatomy and physiology of the endocrine system. Common childhood endocrine disorders will be discussed including lifelong management of the diseases. Understanding the mechanisms of action of the endocrine system is essential for interpreting the various laboratory values and is helpful when providing education to a family about an endocrine abnormality.

ANATOMY AND PHYSIOLOGY

The endocrine system consists of glands that affect numerous body functions through the production of hormones. These glands include the pituitary, thyroid, parathyroids, adrenals, pancreas, ovaries, and testes (Figure 28-1). A **hormone** is a chemical substance produced by an endocrine gland, which is secreted into the bloodstream and affects other tissues or organs (target tissues or organs). Table 28-1 lists the endocrine glands and the major hormones they produce. The endocrine system is incompletely developed at birth. It is less mature than any other body system. Hormonal control of many body functions is lacking until 12 to 18 months of age.

The endocrine system has a close relationship with the nervous system, and the integration of both is necessary to maintain homeostasis. The central nervous system (CNS) receives and reacts to stimuli and transmits a message to the

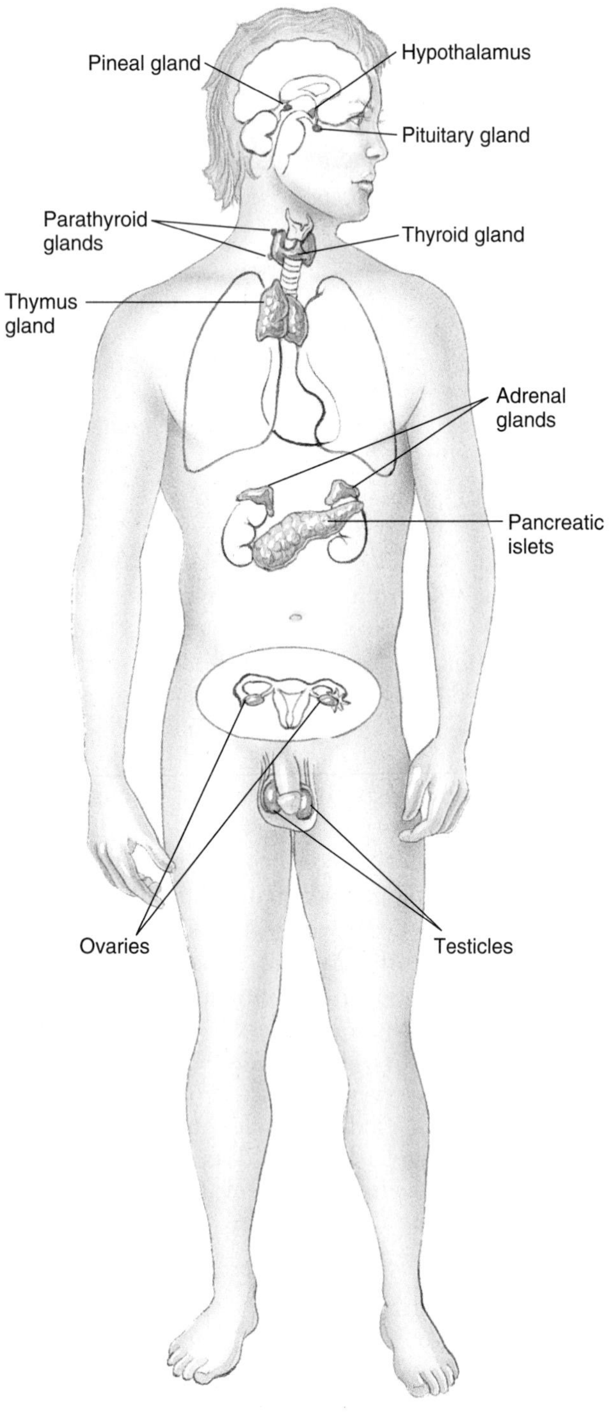

Figure 28-1 The Endocrine System

TABLE 28-1 Endocrine Glands and Hormones

Gland	Hormones
Anterior pituitary	Thyroid-stimulating hormone (TSH)
	Growth hormone (GH)
	Adrenocorticotropic hormone (ACTH)
	Luteinizing hormone (LH)
	Follicle-stimulating hormone (FSH)
	Prolactin (PL)
	Melanocyte-stimulating hormone (MSH)
Posterior pituitary	Vasopressin [antidiuretic hormone (ADH)]
	Oxytocin
Thyroid	Triiodothyronine (T_3)
	Thyroxine (T_4)
	Calcitonin
Parathyroids	Parathyroid hormone (PTH)
Adrenal cortex	Glucocorticoids (cortisol)
	Mineralocorticoids (aldosterone)
	Androgens
Adrenal medulla	Epinephrine
	Norepinephrine
Ovaries	Estrogen
	Progesterone
Testes	Testosterone
Pancreas	Insulin
	Glucagon
	Somatostatin

hypothalamus. The hypothalamus responds to the stimuli and produces either releasing or inhibiting hormones, which are transported to the pituitary gland. Box 28-1 lists the hormones produced by the hypothalamus. The anterior pituitary in response secretes **tropic hormones,** which cause the target tissue or organ to produce its hormones. An example of this process is seen in the stress response of the body. A stimulus (psychological stress) is received by the CNS, a message is conveyed to the hypothalamus, and corticotropin-releasing hormone (CRH) is produced. CRH stimulates the anterior pituitary to release adrenocorticotropic hormone (ACTH). The adrenal glands in turn secrete glucocorticoids (cortisol) and mineralocorticoids (aldosterone).

The production and secretion of hormones is controlled by a negative feedback system. The example in Figure 28-2 illustrates the hypothalamic–pituitary–thyroid gland axis. The hypothalamus secretes a hormone, thyrotropin-releasing hormone (TRH), which stimulates the anterior pituitary. The anterior pituitary then secretes thyroid-stimulating hormone (TSH), which in turns acts on the thyroid gland (target organ) to increase the production of the thyroid hormones, triiodothyronine (T_3) and thyroxine (T_4). Feedback occurs when an increased secretion of T_3 and T_4 leads directly to a decrease in the secretion of the stimulating pituitary hormone (TSH) and indirectly to a decrease in the hypothalamic production of TRH.

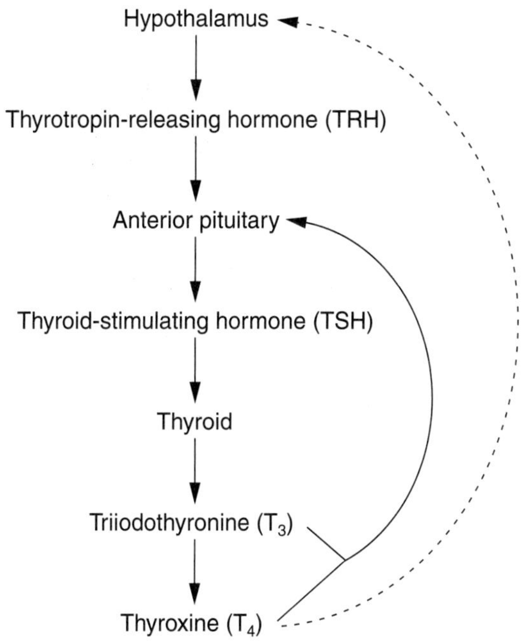

Figure 28-2 Negative Feedback System of the Hypothalmic–Pituitary–Thyroid Gland Axis. The hypothalamus secretes TRH, stimulating the anterior pituitary to release TSH. TSH stimulates the thyroid gland to release its hormones T_3 and T_4. The levels of T_3 and T_4 directly stimulate the anterior pituitary production of TSH and indirectly affect the hypothalamus production of TRH.

Pituitary Gland

Located in the sella turcica (at the base of the brain), the pituitary gland is commonly referred to as the master gland of the body. It is divided into two parts, the anterior and posterior lobes. The anterior lobe is larger, occupying 80% of the gland. It produces growth hormone (GH), lutenizing hormone (LH), follicle-stimulating hormone (FSH), ACTH, TSH, and prolactin hormone (PL). The posterior gland produces oxytocin and stores the hormone arginine vasopressin or antidiuretic hormone (ADH), which is produced in the hypothalamus. By the 4th month of gestation the pituitary gland is formed, and measurable amounts of hormones can be detected.

BOX 28-1 Hormones produced by the hypothalamus

- Corticotropin-releasing hormone (CRH)
- Gonadotropin-releasing hormone (Gn-RH)
- Growth hormone-releasing hormone (GH-RH)
- Growth hormone-inhibiting hormone (somatostatin) (GN-IH)
- Melanocyte-inhibiting hormone (MIH)
- Prolactin-inhibiting hormone (PIH)
- Thyrotropin-releasing hormone (TRH)

Thyroid Gland

The thyroid gland, composed of two lobes joined by a thin band called the isthmus, is located anteriorly in the neck, directly below the cricoid cartilage. It is regulated in feedback fashion by the pituitary gland (Figure 28-2). The thyroid gland synthesizes and secretes the hormones triiodothyronine (T_3) and thyroxine (T_4), which are essential for normal growth and development, maturation of the central nervous system, and metabolism of proteins, carbohydrates, and fat. The production of the thyroid hormones is dependent on sufficient dietary intake of protein and iodine in food and water.

Immediately after birth the newborn's TSH rises rapidly, up to 10 times higher than the levels seen in older children. Then, over the first several days of life, the TSH declines to the normal levels. The newborn's T_3 and T_4 levels will similarly rise in the first 24 hours of life in response to the stimulation by the TSH. The newborn's initial thyroid function tests cannot be interpreted using the normal standards of childhood or adults.

Parathyroid Glands

The parathyroid glands, usually four in number, are located on the posterior surface of the thyroid gland and secrete parathyroid hormone (PTH). PTH regulates calcium and phosphorus as a result of its effect on three target organs: bone, kidney, and the gastrointestinal tract. PTH secretion influences the bone mobilization of calcium, thus increasing serum calcium. In the kidneys, PTH decreases urinary excretion of calcium and increases excretion of phosphate. In the intestines, PTH causes increased absorption of calcium. Lastly, PTH influences vitamin D metabolism. PTH is secreted in response to a decrease in systemic calcium levels. Conversely, a rise in serum calcium causes decreased secretion of PTH.

Adrenal Gland

The adrenal glands are located on top of each kidney and are divided into two parts, the cortex and the medulla. Each operates independently of the other. The primary function of the cortex is to synthesize and secrete glucocorticoids, mineralocorticoids, and sex steroids. The adrenal medulla secretes catecholamines, epinephrine, and norephinephrine. Cortisol, the most potent glucocorticoid produced by the adrenal cortex, is regulated directly by the anterior pituitary hormone ACTH and indirectly by the hypothalamic corticotropin-releasing hormone. Cortisol provides feedback to the hypothalamic–pituitary–adrenal system, which regulates glucocorticoid synthesis. In a classic example of the feedback system, when serum levels of cortisol are low, the hypothalamus secretes CRH, which stimulates the anterior pituitary to secrete ACTH. ACTH then stimulates the adrenal cortex's conversion of cortisol from its substrate cholesterol. Stress and the sleep–wake cycle affect the secretion of CRH and ACTH, thereby influencing the secretion of cortisol. Aldosterone is the most important mineralocorticoid, causing sodium retention and potassium excretion. Its secretion is regulated by the renin–angiotensin system. The synthesis of the sex steroids, androgens and estrogens, produced by the adrenal cortex is mediated by events of puberty.

Pancreas

The pancreas is located behind the stomach and is both an exocrine (duct-type) and endocrine (ductless) organ. Between 4 and 8 weeks of fetal development the differentiation of cells of the exocrine and endocrine portion of the pancreas occurs. The exocrine function is to secrete enzymes that are essential for digestion. The endocrine function is the secretion of the hormones from the islets of Langerhans. The islets, clusters of endocrine cells within the pancreas, produce glucagon by its alpha cells, insulin by the beta cells, and somatostatin by the delta cells. Glucagon increases blood glucose levels by stimulating the liver to convert its stored glycogen into glucose (**glycogenolysis**). Insulin, an anabolic hormone produced by the fetus by 20 weeks gestation, promotes synthesis and storage in carbohydrate metabolism and prevents the breakdown of fat and protein. In carbohydrate metabolism, nutrients are consumed and digested. Carbohydrate is broken down into glucose through digestion and enters the peripheral system. The changes in glucose stimulate the beta cells to secrete additional insulin. Insulin promotes the transportation of glucose into muscle and fat cells. Somatostatin inhibits the release of insulin and glucagon from the islets of Langerhans.

DISORDERS OF THE ANTERIOR PITUITARY

The anterior pituitary gland regulates growth, sexual development, and metabolic activity. Common disorders of childhood that are discussed are growth hormone deficiency and precocious puberty.

Growth Hormone Deficiency

Growth hormone deficiency (GHD) is characterized primarily by poor growth and short stature caused by failure of the pituitary to produce sufficient GH. Growth hormone plays a primary role in postnatal growth. It is released in a pulsatile (pulsating) fashion throughout the day; however, most is secreted primarily after the onset of sleep.

Incidence and Etiology

Growth hormone deficiency occurs in 0.05–0.25 per 1,000 (Gotlin, Kappy, Eisenbarth, & Chase, 1995). The frequency of occurrence is equal in both sexes. Boys are evaluated for GHD more often because the social pressures placed on the short male are of greater magnitude than those placed on "petite" females. GHD may result from injury, destruction of the anterior pituitary gland by a brain tumor, infection, or irradiation, but, most commonly, no cause for the dysfunction is found (idiopathic).

Pathophysiology

The hypothalamus secretes growth hormone-releasing hormone (GRH), which stimulates the production of GH by the pituitary. GH stimulates growth and has metabolic actions. In GHD the pituitary is unable to respond and produce GH, which has an impact on growth and can result in short stature.

Clinical Manifestations

A child with GHD presents with short stature and a deteriorating (<4–5 cm/yr) or absent **rate of growth** (a calculation of the amount of growth in a defined period of time, usually a year). Children with GHD tend to have a higher weight to height ratio and a delayed **bone age,** a determination of skeletal maturation by X ray of the hand, wrist, or knee. Additional clinical manifestations include:

- Increased fat in the trunk area
- Childlike face with a large, prominent forehead
- High-pitched voice
- Hypoglycemia
- Micropenis and small testes in males
- Delayed sexual maturation
- Delayed dentition

Diagnosis

The growth concern is typically identified by the family or primary care provider in an outpatient setting. A clinician who carefully and consistently plots the growth of the child on a standardized growth chart will note the deteriorating rate of growth. The diagnostic work-up includes a review of the previous growth records, determination of growth rate, radiographic bone studies (the bone age), and baseline blood testing. Pituitary function testing is necessary to confirm the diagnosis. This testing consists of provocative tests in which a growth hormone stimulant such as glucagon, clonidine, insulin, arginine, or L-dopa is given to stimulate the pituitary to release a burst of growth hormone. Because up to 20% of non-GHD children will randomly not respond to a single provocative growth hormone test, two or more tests with peak growth hormone levels below 7–10 ng/l are used to confirm the diagnosis (American Academy of Pediatrics, Committee on Drugs and Committee on Bioethics, 1997).

Treatment

The goal of treatment is to promote normal growth rates by the administration of growth hormone. It is administered as a subcutaneous injection, typically given 6–7 days each week at a dosage of 0.15 to 0.33 mg/kg/wk divided in equal doses (MacGillivray, et al., 1998), or as an intramuscular depot injection every 2–4 weeks with a dosage of 0.75 mg/kg every 2 weeks or 1.5 mg/kg once a month. A **depot injection** is an intramuscular injection of a medication that is absorbed over an extended period of time. Response to the therapy is more pronounced in the younger child as compared to an adolescent, in the more obese child compared to the thinner individual, and in the more severely growth hormone deficient child compared to one with partial growth hormone deficiency. Growth hormone therapy is commonly discontinued the child has completed growing, that is, when the child's epiphyseal growth plates have fused.

There are potential complications to growth hormone therapy. Growth hormone is now produced through recombinant DNA technology by several different drug companies. It is essentially free from contaminants. At physiological replacement doses, side effects can include slipped femoral epiphysis, pseudotumor cerebri, edema, and sodium retention. There are also the theoretical concerns that growth hormone treatment increases the child's potential to develop cancers.

Nursing Management

Assessment

For the child on growth hormone accurate measurements are essential for evaluating the effectiveness of therapy. The child should be evaluated and measured no less than every six months. Growth charts should be maintained properly, rates of growth calculated, and drug dosage recalculated as the child gains weight to ensure that the appropriate dose of growth hormone is being prescribed.

Nursing Tip:

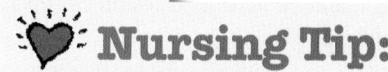

Measuring the child

- Under age 2 years and in children with motor problems who cannot stand independently, it is customary to do length measurements in the supine position, ideally using a measuring board developed for supine measurements.
- The growth charts from birth to 36 months are based on supine measurements. The 2- to 18-year-old growth charts are based on standing heights.
- A supine measurement requires 2 individuals. One person holds the child's head against the headboard of the measuring board. The child's face and pelvis are in a horizontal plane, the hips and knees are gently extended. A movable footboard is placed against the soles of the feet in a 90 degree angle.
- Standing measurements should be done on a stadiometer, a standing measuring board. The child should stand barefoot on a level surface (no inclines or carpeting). The child's back and heels are in the same vertical plane as the measuring instrument. The arms should be relaxed. The child's face should be placed with the outer canthus of the eye and the outer external auditory meatus horizontal. A gentle upward traction is exerted on the child's mastoid process.
- Height is measured to the nearest full millimeter.
- Measurement should be plotted accurately on a standardized growth chart.

From: Wales, J., Rogol, A., & Wit, J. (1996). *Pediatric endocrinology and growth*. Barcelona, Spain: Mosby-Wolfe.

Nursing Diagnosis

- Delayed growth and development related to inadequate growth hormone secretion.
- Disturbed body image related to short stature.
- Deficient knowledge (caregiver) related to treatment.

Outcome Identification

- The child will demonstrate an improvement in growth rate, yielding a minimum of 4–5 cm/yr of linear growth.
- The child will express positive feelings about his or her body image.
- Caregiver and child will demonstrate a realistic understanding of the likely response to GH replacement therapy.
- The caregiver will demonstrate correct medication preparation and injection technique.
- The caregiver will be able to identify the side effects of GH replacement therapy.

Planning/Implementation

The nurse fills the role of coordinator, teacher, and provider of support to the child and the caregivers. Nursing care initially focuses on providing the child (if appropriate) and caregivers with information about normal development, normal growth rates, bone age, and growth potential. Many caregivers and children are unaware of normal growth patterns and genetic expectations for a child's growth. The nurse should explore with the child and the caregivers their expectations of treatment, which at times are unrealistic. Counseling referrals should be considered. Many children with short stature and GHD are emotionally immature. Because these children look much younger than they are, caregivers, teachers, peers, and relatives tend to have expectations similar to those for a younger child. The nurse and other health care providers need to pay particular attention to how they talk to the child with short stature. The health care team should speak to the child in an age-appropriate manner. Discreetly provide step stools to aid the child's ability to independently get onto the exam table.

Caregivers need to be prepared for the financial implications of growth hormone therapy, which costs $25,000– 30,000 per year to treat the average 30 kg GHD child. Many third-party payers, with the appropriate documentation of the diagnosis, will cover the cost of the treatment once the child's deductible has been met. Should the third-party payer deny coverage, or in situations where the family's financial obligation for the drug exceeds their ability to pay, the numerous pharmaceutical companies that market GH have indigent drug programs that assist qualified families.

Kids Want To Know

What do growth hormone shots feel like?

An 8-year-old boy with short stature is to start daily, subcutaneous growth hormone for a new diagnosis of growth hormone deficiency. He asks "How much do the shots hurt?" "Will I have to give them to myself?" and "How soon will I be really taller?" Be honest in your reply that the injections may pinch but are given with the smallest needles into the fat areas of the body. Reassure him that when he is ready and interested, he can also learn to do the injections, but until that time, the adults in his life will be responsible for them. Reassure him that the growth hormone is expected to help him grow and he will be monitored to see how well his body responds.

Evaluation

The child shows an increase in height and acceptance of his or her body image. The child and caregivers accept the eventual height increase. Caregivers are able to correctly prepare and administer injections and know the side effects.

Family Teaching

Growth hormone is a powder that must be mixed with its packaged diluent. The nurse needs to teach caregivers how to properly dilute the medication and give the correct dose. The potential side effects of growth hormone replacement therapy need to be communicated. The caregiver should alert the health care provider of the child's complaints of headaches, rapid weight gain, or painful hip joints. Because the treatment can continue for many years, the nurse needs to prepare the child and family about this issue before therapy begins. They need guidance in setting realistic goals and expectations. For example, the child should be encouraged to choose sports activities that are not dependent on height (e.g., gymnastics, dancing, swimming, and wrestling). During adolescence, the child should dress in clothing that reflects his/her age not size. Counseling referrals for the child and family should be considered if appropriate.

Precocious Puberty

Precocious puberty is defined in Caucasian girls as breast development before the age of 7 years and before 6 years old in African-Americans. In boys less than 9 years of age, the development of secondary sex characteristics is considered precocity (Styne & Grumbach, 1998).

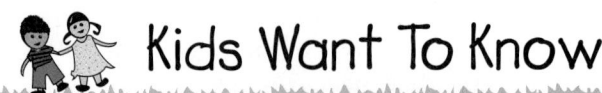

Incidence and Etiology

The incidence of precocious puberty is approximately 0.1–0.5 per 1,000 children and is five times more common in girls. The cause is most frequently idiopathic in girls. In contrast, in boys, the cause is most likely related to abnormalities in the central nervous systems such as lesions.

Pathophysiology

The normal fetus and infant's hypothalamic–pituitary–gonadal axis is activated, with the hypothalamus secreting GnRH in a pulsatile fashion. GnRH, in turn, stimulates the pituitary to produce LH and FSH, which are measurable for months after birth. By the age of four years and throughout childhood, the level of the gonadatropins is minimal. Negative feedback of sex steroids on the hypothalamus and pituitary is evident, although the exact mechanism for this inhibition of the axis is not yet understood. Puberty begins when the secretion of GnRH increases, and gonadatropins are again released.

True or central precocious puberty can be distinguished from precocious pseudopuberty. True precocious puberty results from premature activation of the hypothalamic–pituitary–gonadal axis, with GnRH, LH, FSH, and estrogen or testosterone produced (Figure 28-3). Precocious pseudopuberty occurs when there is evidence of secondary sexual characteristics (breast and/or sexual hair growth) but no activation of the axis (normal levels of GnRH, LH, and FSH).

Clinical Manifestations

The child with precocious puberty will have an accelerated growth rate, an advanced bone age, evidence of secondary sexual characteristics, acne, an adult body odor, and sometimes behavioral changes. Psychosocial development is typically age-appropriate, and not a reflection of the physical maturation. Inappropriate sexual behavior is not commonly observed in children with precocious puberty; however, emotional lability, aggressive behavior, and mood swings may occur. A child with untreated central precocious puberty is potentially fertile.

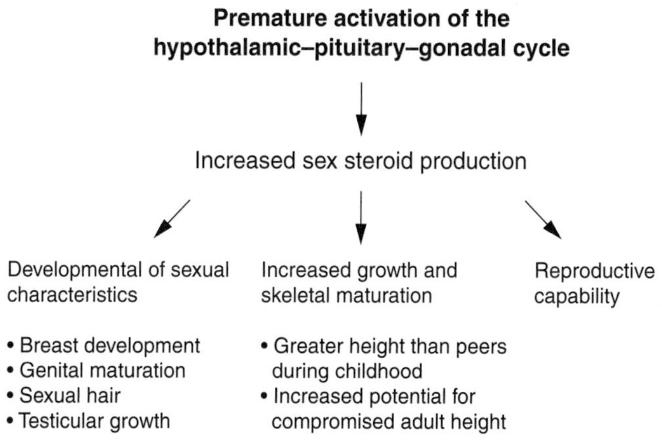

Figure 28-3 True Precocious Puberty

Nursing Tip:

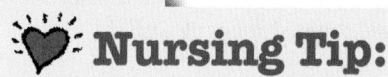

Estrogen-containing products

Many over-the-counter beauty products contain estrogen. When taking the history of a child with the complaint of precocious puberty, ask about the use of skin lotions or hair products. There are several beauty products that contain estrogen, placenta, or placental extracts in them. A child could absorb enough estrogen from one of these products to have measurable levels of estrogen and physical changes reflecting exposure to estrogen. If you are unfamiliar with a product, ask the family to bring the product with them. You may then need to contact the manufacturer to determine if there is estrogen in the product. If birth control pills are available in the house, verify that the child has not had access to them, possibly ingesting the pills to be "just like mommy." This exposure to exogenous hormones could promote the development of secondary sexual characteristics.

Diagnosis

A diagnosis of precocious puberty is based on a complete history, which includes a review of the linear growth chart to identify when growth acceleration was evident, exposure to exogenous hormones, CNS trauma or infection, and family history of pubertal development.

The physical examination should include a precise description of the child's pubertal status. Sexual maturation staging (also known as Tanner staging) of the breast, genitalia, pubic hair, and testes should be documented. Careful measurement of height, weight, **span** (a measurement from fingertip to fingertip), and **upper/lower body ratio** (a ratio calculated from a measurement from the top of the head to the top of the synthesis pubis and from the synthesis pubis to the bottom of the feet) also need to be documented. Radiological exams should be ordered and the child's bone age calculated. In girls, a pelvic ultrasound to identify size of the uterus and ovaries may be helpful. Given the high incidence of CNS lesions with boys, a CT, MRI, or skull film is usually warranted.

The child will need screening lab tests for LH, FSH, estradiol, or testosterone. Provocative testing to evaluate the child's response to GnRH stimulation will be necessary to confirm the diagnosis of central precocious puberty. This is done by administering GnRH to the child and drawing serial blood levels of LH, FSH, and estrogen or testosterone. A child whose hypothalamic–pituitary–gonadal axis has been activated will exhibit a pubertal or adult level of these hormones in response to the administration of GnRH.

Treatment

Treatment initially focuses on the underlying cause of sexual precocity. In cases of a CNS tumor, surgery, radiation, or chemotherapy is indicated. Precocious puberty itself is treated with a GnRH analog (Conn & Crowley, 1994). GnRH analog is available as a depot injection given every 3–4 weeks, subcutaneous injection given daily, or an intranasal compound given 2–3 times each day. The depot is the most common form. When the GnRH analog is initially given, it will stimulate gonadatropin release. When given on a long-term basis, it will suppress gonadatropin release.

Treatment results in a decrease in growth rate, usually to an age-appropriate level. Secondary sexual development stabilizes or regresses. In girls breasts may decrease in size, and pubic hair fails to progress. The ovaries and uterus also decrease in size. In boys there is a decrease in the size of the testes and in the frequency of erections and variable regression of pubic hair. Effectiveness of the treatment is gauged through accurate growth records and intermittent serum gonadotropin and sex steroid measurements (Styne, 1997). When therapy is discontinued, puberty resumes promptly.

The child's family will need to be prepared for the financial aspect of treatment. The GnRH analog depot cost averages $700–1,000 per injection. Third-party payers, with appropriate documentation, will frequently cover the cost of the therapy after the child's deductible has been met. In order to get fully covered by the third-party payer, some children will need to have the injectable GnRH analog administered in a health care provider's office. Others may need to obtain the drug through a specific home care company, and some children will not be eligible for coverage. In these situations, the pharmaceutical companies often have indigent drug programs to assist with the financial impact of treatment.

Case Study/Care Plan

Precocious Puberty in a Young School-aged Girl

Anna is a 6-year, 3-month-old female being seen in the ambulatory clinic setting with a complaint of breast and pubic hair. In reviewing her history, Anna had been growing at the 75th percentile on standardized growth charts until age 4 years when she experienced growth acceleration and is now above the 95th percentile. Her weight is also above the 95th percentile. Over the last 9 months, her caregivers noted breast development, with Anna frequently complaining of breast tenderness. Recently, her caregivers grew concerned when pubic hair began to develop and sought a consultation after speaking with the child's primary care provider.

On physical exam, Anna has Tanner III breasts and Tanner II pubic hair. Her bone age is read at 10 years 4 months. Screening lab tests were done, with pubertal levels of LH, FSH, and estradiol noted. Provocative testing was performed, confirming the diagnosis of central precocious puberty. Treatment options were discussed with the caregivers, who chose the depot LH-agonist.

Nursing Care Plan

Assessment The child's growth is monitored regularly after initiating treatment (every 3–4 months) and plotted accurately on a standardized growth chart. Bone age will be reevaluated periodically, assessing growth potential and success of treatment. Periodic serum hormone levels will also be necessary to evaluate the response to treatment. Additionally, the child and caregivers should be interviewed about their perception of any further changes or regression in secondary sexual characteristics. Females should be interviewed regarding their experience with any menstrual flow, including spotting. The child's and caregivers' experience with emotional or social concerns regarding early pubertal development and growth potential need to be explored.

These children may have body image concerns or impaired social relationships because of teasing from their peers and appearing different. They appear older than their chrono-

continues

continued

logical age; therefore, expectations of caregivers, teachers, coaches, etc. may be higher. These issues need to be assessed. Caregivers' feelings about their child's early sexual development and reproductive ability should be explored. The nurse should ask about episodes of moodiness and emotional lability in girls and aggressiveness in boys.

Nursing Diagnosis #1

Disturbed body image related to early development of secondary sexual characteristics.

Expected Outcomes

1. Child will exhibit normal psychosocial development.
2. Child will express concerns about body image and eventually will verbalize positive feelings about self.

Interventions/*Rationales*

1. Provide information to child and caregivers regarding the physical changes the child is experiencing. *Providing information places the precocious development in context to normal development.*

2. Approach the child in a manner appropriate to her emotional and cognitive development. *Role model for caregivers and others an appropriate developmental approach to the child based on chronological age and emotional maturity.*

3. Explore with the caregivers how they and the other significant people approach the child and what expectations they place on the child. *Expectations of caregivers and others (i.e., teachers) are often based on the physical appearance of the child. These inappropriate expectations can increase the social isolation of the child.*

4. Provide counseling referrals. *To screen for behavioral/psychological disturbances and provide interventions as appropriate.*

5. Inform caregivers that the child's dress should be appropriate for chronological age. Loose-fitting clothing will help minimize body changes. *Heterosexual sexual interest is not advanced beyond child's chronological age. Early sexual development does not indicate that the child is ready for adolescent activities.*

Evaluation

The child expresses acceptance of body changes and dresses appropriately. Caregivers and other significant individuals in the child's life have realistic expectations of her.

Nursing Diagnosis #2

Altered growth and development: advanced bone age, accelerated growth, and development of secondary sexual characteristics related to premature activation of the hypothalamic–pituitary–gonadal axis.

Expected Outcomes

1. Child will achieve appropriate physical development.
2. Child will achieve normal rate of growth for age.
3. Child's pubertal progression will be age and developmentally appropriate.

Interventions/*Rationales*

1. Obtain accurate, serial height and weight measurements, and plot on standardized growth charts. *Assessment for growth acceleration and impact of therapy on growth.*

2. Assess progression or regression of secondary sexual characteristics. *Evaluates the impact of therapy on development.*

3. Assess adherence with prescribed medication. *Evaluate medical therapy.*

continues

continued

Evaluation

During therapy the child's rate of growth decreases to an age-appropriate level. Secondary sexual development stabilizes or regresses. Caregivers correctly administer the medication and adhere to the prescribed treatment plan.

Nursing Diagnosis #3

Deficient knowledge related to diagnosis, financial impact, and home care.

Expected Outcomes

1. Caregivers and child will understand the physical and emotional changes that occur with early onset of puberty.
2. Caregivers will explain and demonstrate correct method for medication administration and list its action.
3. Caregivers will identify available resources for financial assistance if needed.

Interventions/*Rationales*

1. Provide information about normal pubertal development and child's early development. *Providing information places child's development in context.*
2. Explore with caregivers their comfort with medication administration and their options for administration. *Identify caregivers who would benefit from home health nursing care or routine appointments at physician's office for depot injections.*
3. Teach caregivers medication action, preparation, and administration techniques. *Empowers caregivers to adhere to medical plan.*
4. Explore with caregivers and third-party payers financial support for medication and follow-up needs. *Identifies potential financial limitations to recommended therapy and various options for financing care.*

Evaluation

The caregivers and child are informed about the disorder and treatment including medication regimen. Financial implications do not limit child's access to appropriate treatment.

Critical Thinking

Precocious Puberty

Draw a diagram of the activated hypothalamic–pituitary–gonadal axis, including the various hormones excreted by each endocrine gland, that would be consistent with puberty. Can this be differentiated from the axis seen in the child with precocious pseudopuberty? At what age is puberty precocious?

DISORDERS OF THE POSTERIOR PITUITARY

Disorders of the posterior pituitary are related to a deficiency or excess of vasopressin or antidiuretic hormone (ADH). Diabetes insipidus (DI) is one of these disorders.

Diabetes Insipidus

Diabetes insipidus or neurogenic DI is a disorder of water regulation. The function of ADH is to concentrate urine by stimulating reabsorption of water in the renal collecting tubules. A deficiency of ADH results in excretion of large amounts of dilute urine.

Incidence and Etiology

DI is most often seen in children as a complication following head trauma or cranial surgery to remove tumors of the hypothalamic–pituitary region. DI that develops after surgery may be transient or permanent. Other causes include vascular anomalies (cerebral aneurysms), infection (encephalitis or meningitis), and a genetic defect in the synthesis of ADH (Bayliss & Cheetham, 1998).

Pathophysiology

The posterior lobe of the pituitary gland secretes arginine vasopressin (also known as antidiuretic hormone or ADH), which is produced in the hypothalamus and stored in the pituitary gland. ADH acts at the level of the renal collecting ducts, increasing their permeability to water, in order to limit water loss. A deficiency in ADH secretion results in massive loss of water and retention of sodium in the serum.

Clinical Manifestations

In infants, failure to thrive, a history of fevers, vomiting, constipation, dehydration, and poor growth are the initial clinical manifestations. In the older child, **polyuria** (excretion of an abnormally large amount of urine) and **polydipsia** (excessive thirst) are the most common first symptoms (over 50% of children have these initial reported symptoms). Children experience nocturnal enuresis, which interrupts their sleep, and increased thirst. Urine output can range from a few liters to eighteen liters a day. Urine specific gravity is 1.005 or less, urine osmolarity is <200 mmol/l, serum sodium concentration and plasma osmolarity are elevated.

Diagnosis

An initial screen, rather than a full work-up, is valuable in a child who presents with a history that suggests DI. An outpatient screening includes obtaining a first morning urine sample for osmolarity, specific gravity, and sodium after attempting an overnight fast. Caution should be exercised in instructing the caregivers to do an overnight fast, in that the child with DI can become hypernatremic if fluids are discontinued. A child with hypernatremia is at risk for seizure. If the history of the child strongly suggests that the child has DI, an overnight fast should not be conducted. The child who does have an outpatient screening should be evaluated for hydration status, which includes a weight before the fast has been terminated. Serum osmolarity, sodium, and creatinine levels are also checked.

Further investigation is pursued should the urine be dilute (<1.005, osmolarity <200 mmol/l), especially if the serum is hypertonic and hypernatremic. A water deprivation test is commonly performed at this point. The object of the water deprivation test is to measure the vasopressin release from the pituitary in response to depriving the child of water. The test requires several hours to complete with close monitoring (I & O, weight, vital signs, hydration assessment, and urine and blood samples) most frequently by the nurse.

Treatment

As long as a child has a normal thirst drive and free access to water, treating DI is not necessary to maintain life. Treatment, however, greatly improves the quality of life because of the inconvenience of polyuria and polydipsia. The usual treatment is daily replacement of the hormone ADH (vasopressin). The drug of choice is desmopressin acetate (DDAVP), a long-acting vasopressin analog, which is given intranasally or orally. DDAVP is also available in a parenteral form. The mechanism for delivery is based on the dosage, ease of administration, and ability of the child and family to reach the treatment goals. Common goals of therapy include antidiuresis, uninterrupted sleep, and increased ability to participate in school and other programs. In order

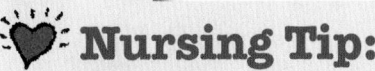

Nursing Tip:

Symptoms of DI

A common symptom of DI is the child who is much more satisfied with water in copious amounts than other liquids. The child will awaken at night to drink. Young children who have been denied fluids have been known to drink from a toilet or a puddle on the ground.

Nursing Tip:

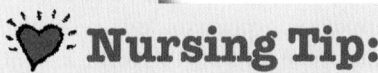

Use of rhinal tube to administer DDAVP

When using a rhinal tube to administer the DDAVP intranasally:

1. Have the child blow the nose before administering.
2. Have the child lay on a side (same side where the medication was administered) for several minutes after the medication is given.
3. Ask the child if he/she swallowed the medication, which would indicate that it "overshot" the nasal choana, and will, therefore, not be absorbed.

to avoid possible water intoxication and hyponatremia, a brief period of time each day when the DDAVP begins to wear off and unrestrained urination can occur is planned as part of the therapy (Bayliss & Cheetham, 1998).

Nursing Management

Children with a damaged thirst center provide a special challenge to both the health care providers and families. Fluid intake regimens will need to be devised, and families will need to carefully monitor the child's fluid status by measuring intake, urine output, and daily weights. A journal or log is essential for these caregivers. Infants present special treatment concerns. They excrete a more dilute urine, consume large volumes of free water, and secrete lower amounts of vasospressin than older children. Treatment typically calls for more frequent feeds or, if breastfed, supplements of water. DDAVP dosing is controversial in this age group.

A client who is NPO (i.e., pre- or postsurgery) with DI will require careful titration of the medication and fluid volumes and concentration. Frequent electrolytes, I & Os, and reassessment of the fluid management plan are necessary. Medical identification jewelry should be encouraged.

DISORDERS OF THE THYROID GLAND

The disorders of the thyroid gland are some of the most common endocrine abnormalities of childhood and include congenital hypothyroidism, acquired hypothyroidism, and hyperthyroidism.

Congenial Hypothyroidism

Congenital hypothyroidism (CH), a disorder present at birth, is a reduced rate of metabolism caused by a low concentration of circulating thyroid hormones (T_3 and T_4). The early detection and treatment of hypothyroidism can prevent **cretinism** (severe mental retardation). In North America and most of Europe and Japan, mass screening of newborns for CH is routine and identifies the majority of those affected.

Incidence and Etiology

Congenital hypothyroidism occurs in 0.25 in 1,000 live births (American Academy of Pediatrics Committee on Genetics, 1996). More female infants are affected than males. CH may develop from a variety of conditions. The majority of cases are caused by a defect in the embryonic development of the thyroid gland in which it is absent, partially present, or ectopic (in the wrong position). Other causes include an inborn error of thyroid hormone synthesis (**dyshormonogenesis**), which is inherited as an autosomal, recessive trait, and pituitary dysfunctions.

Pathophysiology

CH is caused by an absent, underdeveloped, or ectopic placement of the thyroid gland or an error of thyroid hormone synthesis. The thyroid gland is unable to produce T_3 and T_4 in response to increasingly elevated levels of TSH secreted by the pituitary gland.

Clinical Manifestations

The majority of affected infants are asymptomatic at birth. The most common neonatal clinical signs are a large posterior fontanel, an umbilical hernia, constipation, and prolonged jaundice. Other clinical manifestations may include the following:

- Pallor
- Hypothermia
- Enlarged tongue
- Hypotonia, hypoactivity
- Feeding difficulties
- Delayed mental responsiveness/dull expression
- Cool, dry, scaly skin
- Swollen eyelids (Figure 28-4)

Diagnosis

Mandatory newborn screening identifies the majority of newborns with CH and allows early treatment, thereby

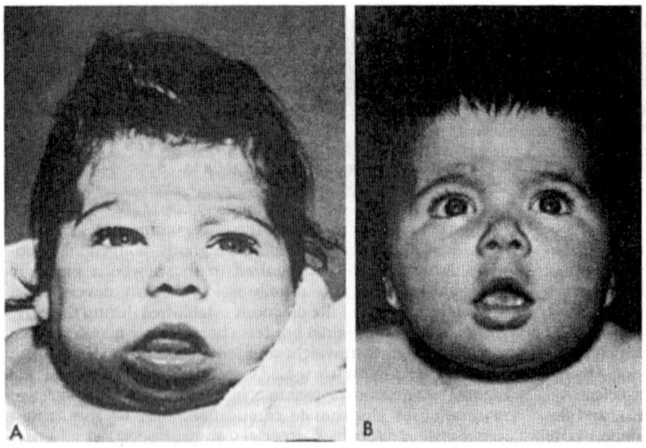

Figure 28-4 Congenital Hypothyroidism (A) Before Treatment: Note the facial puffiness, swollen eyelids, enlarged tongue, low anterior hairline, flattened nasal bridge, and dull expression, (B) Six Months After Treatment: Note the decreased facial puffiness and alert appearance. Source: Behrman, R., Kliegman, R., & Arvin, A. (Eds.). (1996). *Nelson textbook of pediatrics* (15th ed., p. 1592). Philadelphia: W. B. Saunders.

reducing the incidence of mental retardation. When the initial test is positive, the newborn should have a second confirming laboratory test performed. A T_4 level (normal=6.5 to 13 μg/dl) is determined, and if low, the TSH (normal <5 μU/ml) is measured (Vogiatzi & Kirkland, 1997). A low T_4 and a high TSH indicate CH. A thyroid scan to evaluate for absence or ectopic placement of the gland may be performed. It is the practice of some pediatric endocrinologists to have radiological films of the infant's knee to evaluate for growth retardation, a reflection of the severity of the hypothyroidism in utero.

Treatment

Thyroid hormone is vital to the growing, developing central nervous system. A delay in treatment is associated with lower mean intelligence quotients (IQ). Thyroid replacement with sodium L-thyroxine (Synthroid) is initiated as soon as possible with a recommended starting dose of 10–15 mcg/kg/day (American Academy of Pediatrics [AAP], 1993). Given in physiological doses the medication does not have side effects. There are no contraindications of or options for therapy. Thyroid function tests should be closely monitored to ensure proper dosing, initially as often as every 2 weeks. The goal of therapy is to quickly normalize thyroid function. In the newborn, the goal is to maintain the level of T_4 in the upper half of the normal range and TSH in the normal range. Lifelong thyroid replacement is necessary to maintain normal metabolism in most cases of CH.

Nursing Management

The child's growth should be accurately measured and plotted on a standardized growth chart at regular intervals, often corresponding with visits during which lab values are obtained. Lab tests are performed initially every 2–4 weeks until thyroid function is within the target range on a stabilized dose of medication. Tests will be performed every 3–4 months for the first several years of life, with the interval lengthening as the child grows older, to every 6–12 months in adolescence.

Initially, the urgency to begin treatment must be communicated to the caregivers. Most newborns with CH are asymptomatic, and the initial notification by the health care provider is unexpected. Caregivers will need reassurance that the occurrence of CH is random and not a reflection of the mother's actions during pregnancy. Developmental screening may be recommended as the child gets older.

Family Teaching

L-thyroxine is an oral medication and is available only as a pill. Caregivers will need to be instructed in the preparation and administration of the pill, which must be crushed for infants and young children. One method involves crushing the pill, placing the powder on the infant's tongue, and then feeding the infant. The crushed pill can also be mixed with a small amount of formula and placed in the nipple without a bottle attached for the infant to suck. The crushed medication should not be put in a full bottle of formula since this can lead to remnants of the drug remaining and the infant not getting the entire dose. The powder may also be mixed with a small amount of liquid and given with a dropper. Teach the caregivers about the need to continue thyroid hormone replacement for the child's life. They also need to be prepared for the importance of frequent blood tests for ongoing evaluation of thyroid function. If appropriate, nurses should help them identify a lab that is convenient for them to use for the intermittent blood draws that may be

Nursing Tip:

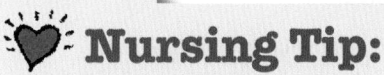

Absorption of L-thyroxine

L-thyroxine's absorption is affected by formulas that are soy based; therefore, caregivers should avoid using these. Soy formulas include Alsoy (Nestle), Gerber Soy, Isomil (Mead Johnson), Nursoy (Wyeth-Ayerst), ProSobee (Mead Johnson), and Soyalac (Loma Linda).

REFLECTIONS FROM FAMILIES

When I received a phone call from the nurse at my son's pediatrician's office a few days after he was born to tell me his newborn blood tests indicated a problem, I was shocked. He looked so healthy, right from the time he was born. His APGAR was perfect. I didn't even know that they had done blood tests before I took him home from the hospital. (I'd wished someone had told me about this while I was pregnant.) When I was told that his thyroid gland didn't seem to be working, I was sure I did something to cause it. While the nurse assured me that this was unrelated to anything I had done during pregnancy, it frightened me when she insisted that I bring him in immediately to confirm the diagnosis and start treatment. I had a million questions. Would he be slow? Would he look different? At our appointment, I was relieved that this could be managed but I worry that he will not take enough of his medicine through his bottle for it to work.

necessary. The nurse should provide information about soy-containing formulas to avoid.

Acquired Hypothyroidism

Acquired hypothyroidism, recognized after the age of 2 years, is a condition in which there are inadequate thyroid hormones.

Incidence and Etiology

Acquired hypothyroidism is categorized as primary, secondary, or tertiary. Primary is the most common form and is usually caused by autoimmune chronic lymphocytic thyroiditis, called Hashimoto's thyroiditis (Adlin, 1998). This condition occurs during childhood and adolescence and more frequently in girls. It occurs in greater frequency with other autoimmune-mediated diseases like type 1 diabetes or chromosal abnormalities such as Down syndrome. Secondary and tertiary hypothyroidism are associated with pituitary or hypothalamic dysfunction.

Pathophysiology

Acquired hypothyroidism is commonly caused by an autoimmune disorder. Antibodies are developed against the thyroid gland. The gland becomes inflamed, infiltrated by the antibodies, and is progressively destroyed. Serum T_4 levels decrease and concurrently TSH levels increase.

Clinical Manifestations

The child may present with complaints of fatigue, weakness, constipation, and dry skin. Some children will present with a **goiter,** an enlargement of the thyroid gland. The course of acquired hypothyroidism may be silent, with a subtle shift in the child's growth parameters (i.e., a decrease in the linear rate of growth, change in the linear growth percentiles evident on a standardized growth chart, and weight increase). There is often a delay in puberty and teeth eruption. Box 28-2 lists the clinical manifestations of acquired hypothyroidism.

BOX 28-2 Clinical manifestations of acquired hypothyroidism

- Decreased rate of growth
- Weight gain
- Constipation
- Dry skin
- Thinning or coarse hair
- Fatigue
- Cold intolerance
- Edema of face, eyes, and hands
- Delayed deep tendon reflexes
- Delayed puberty and tooth eruption

Diagnosis

The diagnostic evaluation for primary acquired hypothyroidism is relatively simple, requiring serum thyroid function studies (TSH, T_4, free T_4). Confirmation of autoimmune thyroiditis is made with serum thyroid antibodies.

Treatment

Treatment involves replacing thyroid hormone with L-thyroxine with the dosage based on the weight of the child and the severity of the hypothyroidism. In the newborn, the prevailing advice is a rapid restoration to a **euthyroid** (normal) state. The child or adolescent with severe or chronic hypothyroidism is more likely to experience side effects if the restoration phase is too rapid, which mimic symptoms of hyperthyroidism and can include aggressive behavior and deterioration in school performance. The initiating dose in these cases is small and titrated upwards based on symptoms and thyroid lab tests, usually every few weeks until a euthyroid state is reached.

Nursing Management and Family Teaching

Assessment

The child in the diagnostic phase is evaluated for symptoms of hypothyroidism. Nurses should interview the family and child for information regarding a change in activity tolerance and behavior. The child's growth history should be reviewed, evaluating the growth chart for information regarding when height slowed or stopped and weight increased. The caregivers' understanding of the role the thyroid plays in the body needs to be assessed.

Nursing Diagnosis

1. Delayed growth and development related to the absence or deficiency of thyroid hormone synthesis.
2. Hypothermia related to decreased basal metabolic rate.
3. Constipation related to decreased motility of the GI tract.
4. Activity intolerance related to fatigue and decreased endurance.

Outcome Identification

1. Child will return to a normal growth pattern.
2. Child will maintain normal body temperature and bowel habits.
3. Child will be able to return to previous level of function, capable of participating in activities without undue fatigue.

Planning/Implementation

Caregivers and children need to be educated about the diagnosis of primary hypothyroidism. They will need instruction on the importance of daily medication. L-thyroxine should be taken 30–60 minutes prior to a meal to optimize its absorption. Children and adolescents are usually diagnosed with hypothyroidism because of a concern about their growth or pubertal development. Many of these children will experience catch-up growth after starting therapy. The child's potential growth is related to the response to treatment and cannot be aided by specific strategies. Both caregivers and children will need support and information about the potential for catch-up growth. The child with chronic or severe hypothyroidism has an increased risk of experiencing side effects with therapy. Caregivers should be cautioned to immediately report symptoms of restlessness, inability to sleep, or irritability.

Evaluation

The child who is receiving L-thyroxine in a dose that supports normal growth and development with normal thyroid hormone levels has optimal management.

Hyperthyroidism

Hyperthyroidism or hyperfunction of the thyroid gland is characterized by excessive levels of circulating thyroid hormones.

Incidence and Etiology

Hyperthyroidism is uncommon in children and adolescents. Exact incidence rates are not available, but a peak occurs during adolescence (Dallas & Foley, 1996). The most common cause of hyperthyroidism in children is Graves' disease, which is 5 times more common in girls than in boys. There is a common genetic marker in individuals with this disease, and approximately 60% have a family history of autoimmune thyroid problems. In identical twins, the concordance rate is less than 50%, thereby suggesting that factors other than genetics play a role in the development of Graves' disease.

Pathophysiology

Graves' disease occurs when antibodies are formed against antigens in the thyroid gland, orbital tissue, and dermis. The antibodies that are directed against the thyroid gland mimic the action of TSH, thereby causing the gland to inappropriately produce thyroid hormone. A goiter is usually present in the child with Graves' disease.

Clinical Manifestations

Initially, the symptoms may be mild and easily overlooked by the child's family (Box 28-3). Growth patterns may include increased growth velocity, rapidly advancing bone age, and decreasing weight.

BOX 28-3 Clinical manifestations of hyperthyroidism

- Increased rate of growth
- Weight loss despite excellent appetite
- Warm, moist skin
- Tachycardia
- Ophthalmic changes (Box 28-4)
- Heat intolerance
- Emotional lability
- Insomnia
- Fine tremors

BOX 28-4 Ophthalmic changes with hyperthyroidism

Exophthalmos (bulging of the eyeballs) (Figure 28-5)

Proptosis (downward displacement of the eyeball) (Figure 28-5)

Lid lag

Lid retraction

Staring expression

Periorbital edema

Diplopia

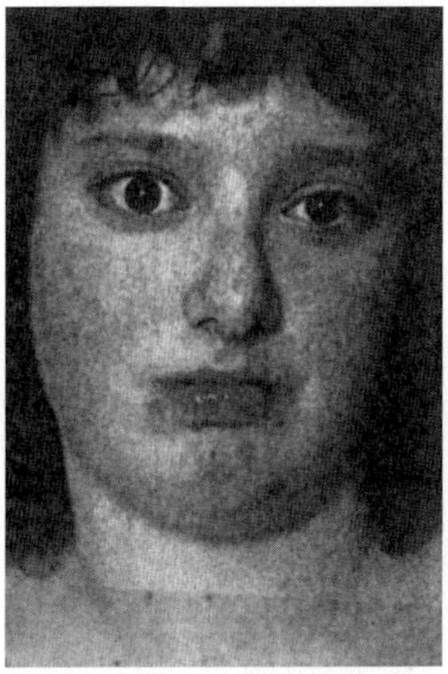

Figure 28-5 An Adolescent Girl with Hyperthyroidism. Note the exophthalmos (bulging) of the right eyeball and proptosis (downward displacement) of the left eye. *Source:* Zitelli, B., & Davis, H. (Eds.). (1997). *Atlas of pediatric physical diagnosis* (3rd ed., p. 271). St. Louis, MO: Mosby-Wolfe.

Diagnosis

The diagnosis of hyperthyroidism is confirmed with serum thyroid tests. The active circulating thyroid hormones will be markedly elevated. TSH levels will be suppressed because increased levels of T_3 and T_4 inhibit the anterior pituitary from producing TSH.

Treatment

Current treatment options include antithyroid medication, radioactive iodine therapy, and sub-total thyroidectomy. Antithyroid drug therapy has been used the longest and includes the use of propylthiouracil (PTU) or methimazole (MTZ; Tapazole), which block the synthesis of T_3 and T_4. It may be 4–8 weeks before the child becomes euthyroid on this therapy. Adjunct therapy of beta-adrenergic blockers such as propanolol (Inderal) may be considered in the individual with marked symptoms. These drugs relieve tachycardia, restlessness, and tremors. The major problems with drug therapy are the risk of toxic effects and the duration of the therapy, which may last for years. The side effects of antithyroid medication can be serious, and if suspected, therapy must be promptly discontinued (Table 28-2). Alternative drugs should be initiated when appropriate (Williams, Nayak, Becker, Reyes, & Burmeister, 1997).

The second treatment option for hyperthyroidism is radioactive iodine therapy. Used for years with adults, this therapy is becoming more acceptable for children as an alternative to long-term drug therapy. Oral radioactive iodine is administered, with tissue damage and destruction of the thyroid gland occurring in approximately 6–18 weeks. Hypothyroidism is one of the most frequent complications of this treatment, and L-thyroxine therapy is initiated if this occurs (Cheetham, Hughes, Barnes, & Wraight, 1998).

The third option, sub-total thyroidectomy, is used when adequate caregiver cooperation with drug therapy is not possible or when treatment has failed to result in permanent remission. Surgery is performed after the child has been brought to a euthyroid state, which is accomplished with antithyroid medication. Hypothyroidism frequently occurs as a complication following thyroidectomy. Hypoparathyroidism and laryngeal nerve damage are also a risk. Spontaneous remissions of Graves' disease are possible and may last for years. Others will have a disease course that is persistent.

TABLE 28-2 Side Effects of Antithyroid Medication

Mild effects	Skin rash
	Mild leukopenia
	Loss of taste
	Arthralgia
	Loss or abnormal pigmentation of hair
Severe (possibly fatal)	Agranulocytosis (manifested by sore throat, high fever)
	Lupus-like syndrome
	Hepatitis
	Hepatic failure
	Glomerulonephritis

Nursing Alert:

Academic Performance of Children with Hyperthyroidism

Children who are in school may have a change in behavior with increased difficulty staying on task, inability to sit still, and decreased academic performance. Some of these children may have been referred for evaluation of learning disabilities or attention deficit hyperactivity disorder (ADHD) (refer to Chapter 35 for information on ADHD).

Nursing Management

The majority of children with hyperthyroidism are diagnosed and treated in an ambulatory environment. A history of the child's behavior including the pattern of sleep, school performance (past and current), and distractibility need to be obtained. Nursing intervention should focus on providing information about the disorder. In the acute phase, teaching centers on providing information to the caregiver about the treatment options. If radioactive therapy or thyroidectomy is the treatment of choice, the caregivers need to be prepared with information about the procedure, goals of treatment, and complications. If surgical intervention is chosen, nurses should explore with the child and caregivers their perceptions and fears of having an incision in the neck.

Family Teaching

When working with a child with hyperthyroidism that is being treated with medication it is important to teach the family the medication regimen, the side effects of the drugs, and the need to continue with the medication despite resolution of symptoms of hyperthyroidism. The nurse must familiarize the family with the routine of blood tests and if medically appropriate, help them to identify a lab facility that is convenient for them to use for interval labs.

Nurses should teach caregivers about the symptoms of hypothyroidism and provide guidelines for contacting the health care provider (e.g., presence of symptoms of drug reaction, tachycardia, fatigue). The child with heat intolerance caused by increased basal metabolic rate may be more comfortable in light weight clothing, using fans or air conditioning if available, and taking frequent baths or showers. Until symptoms disappear with drug therapy, children need a low-stress, low-pressure environment. Emotional lability may be evidenced by sudden episodes of crying and irritability or elation. Caregivers need to be taught that these emotions are uncontrollable and can be minimized by encouraging the child to discuss these feelings.

If the child attends school, instruct the family on activity restrictions if medically appropriate. Nurses should discuss with school personnel restrictions for P.E. and when these will be reevaluated. Nurses should provide the school with information regarding the symptoms of hyperthyroidism that may have an impact on the child's ability to focus during class, and thereby affect the child's school performance. If appropriate, nurses may request that the school nurse monitor the child's pulse and blood pressure changes in response to the medication or symptoms of hyperthyroidism. Once recovery is evident, the caregivers may consider tutoring to assist the child who may have fallen behind in school work. It is important to refer caregivers to community resources, including the National Graves' Disease Foundation, the local chapters of the Pediatric Endocrine Nurse Society, or the Lawson Wilkins Pediatric Endocrine Society (an organization of pediatric endocrinologists) for any local support groups or educational opportunities.

DISORDERS OF THE ADRENAL GLAND

The adrenal glands are composed of the inner cortex and the outer medulla. The cortex produces hormones called steroids: glucocorticoids and mineralocorticoids. The main glucocorticoid, cortisol, has an effect on the metabolism of glucose, proteins, and fats, stress reactions, and inhibition of inflammation. Aldosterone is the most important mineralocorticoid. It is responsible for maintaining extracellular fluid volume and blood pressure by conservation of sodium, chloride, and water, and excretion of potassium by the kidneys. The adrenal medulla secretes the catecholamines epinephrine and norepinephrine. These hormones are produced by the sympathetic nervous system (SNS); therefore, when the adrenal supply is decreased or absent, it is not life-threatening.

Congenital Adrenal Hyperplasia

Congenital adrenal hyperplasia (CAH) is a group of inherited disorders in which a genetic defect results in the deficiency of an enzyme essential for synthesis of cortisol and, at times, aldosterone.

Incidence and Etiology

The incidence of CAH is 0.06 to 0.08 in 1,000 live births. There are several forms of CAH, the most common of which is 21-hydroxylase (21-OH) deficiency, occurring in over 90% of all cases (AAP, 2000).

Pathophysiology

In a child with CAH, cortisol synthesis is blocked by the lack of the enzyme 21-OH. This reduction of cortisol leads to increased ACTH production by the anterior pituitary. Prolonged oversecretion of ACTH causes enlargement or hyperplasia of the adrenal glands and excess production of androgens.

Clinical Manifestations

The enzyme deficiency of 21-OH exposes the fetus to excessive production of androgens. In the male fetus, this causes no physical changes; however, in the female, excessive androgens will **virilize** (to develop sexual characteristics of a male) the external genitalia, resulting in an enlarged clitoris (possibly to the extent of resembling the male phallus), fusion of the labial folds, and a rugated appearance to the labia. This is known as ambiguous genitalia or **pseudohermaphrodism.** The ovaries, fallopian tubes, and uterus are normal.

Approximately 75% of cases of 21-OH deficiency have salt wasting from a defect in ability to synthesize aldosterone. If not diagnosed at birth, the neonate with 21-OH deficiency and salt wasting will develop a life-threatening hyponatremia, hyperkalemia, and hypovolemia by day 10–14 of life. This is known as adrenal crisis.

Children with atypical 21-OH deficiency will present later (often in the toddler or preschool years) with premature **adrenarche** (pubic hair development), accelerated growth velocity, advanced bone age, acne, and **hirsutism** (excessive body hair in a masculine distribution pattern).

Diagnosis

Prenatal diagnosis and treatment of CAH is possible with the objective of preventing prenatal virilization in affected female infants and early recognition of the potential for salt wasting in newborn infants. This is performed most commonly in families with a previously affected child with CAH with a defined genetic defect (AAP, 2000). Twenty states test for 21-OH deficiency in their newborn screening programs (Pang & Shook, 1997). The major objectives of this screening are to identify infants at risk for the development of life-threatening adrenal crisis and to prevent the incorrect male sex assignment of affected female infants with ambiguous genitalia (AAP, 2000). Health care practitioners are notified of abnormal screens, similar to that for congenital hypothyroidism. Confirmation of the diagnosis through repeat blood testing, electrolytes (to screen for abnormalities associated with salt wasting), and physical examination are done immediately.

In the child who presents with clinical symptoms suggestive of CAH, hormonal testing is pursued. While the most common type of CAH is 21-OH deficiency, there are other enzyme deficiencies that cause CAH, and each type has its own unique hormonal profile. Several different adrenal steroids and their precursors should be measured to seek the most appropriate diagnosis. Bone age films should also be obtained to evaluate future growth potential and to monitor response to therapy.

Treatment

The goal of treatment is suppression of adrenal secretion of androgens and prevention of progressive virilization and includes lifelong replacement of the steroids the adrenal gland is unable to produce. The vast majority of individuals with 21-OH deficiency will take both the glucocorticoid hydrocortisone and the mineralocorticoid fludrocortisone (Florinef). At physiological replacement doses, there are no side effects related to these drugs, but at doses that are elevated, hypertension, growth impairment, and acne can occur. Regular and ongoing follow-up are essential for titrating dose of the medication and for monitoring treatment goals of normal growth and development. Medication therapy is lifelong.

The female infant with CAH is often born with ambiguous genitalia. Standard medical treatment has recommended surgical intervention for correction of external genitalia and adequate sexual functioning. A reduction of the clitoris and opening of the labial folds are done within the first several months of life, and further surgeries may be necessary during puberty.

Medical advice is currently being influenced by a growing movement in the United States, driven by individuals whose gender was previously described as ambiguous, to delay the decision of cosmetic correction of the genitalia until the child is of an age to make the decision. Surgical intervention most often results in a loss of the nerve endings in the clitoris, which has an impact on sexuality and sexual experiences later. It can also have an impact on the appearance of the genitalia. The decision to surgically intervene immediately versus delaying the decision is a complex one. The decision to raise a child with an ambiguous gender in today's society raises numerous concerns and problems. Yet, many of the individuals who have experienced surgical intervention of the genitalia are adamant that the decision is too complex to be decided solely by the caregivers and health care provider of a newborn or young child.

Reflective Thinking

The Newborn with Ambiguous Genitalia

Gender identification is most commonly based on the appearance of the external genitals. Think about one of the very first questions asked when a child is born.

"Is it a boy or a girl?" Think about the answer: "The sex of the child cannot be determined yet." When the newborn presents with ambiguous genitalia, this is the response in the delivery room. Sometimes the ambiguity of the genitalia is missed, and a sex assignment is made at birth. The caregivers announce the gender of the baby to their friends and families, yet the gender is not consistent with the child's genetic make-up or gonads.

For the child with 21-OH deficiency, gender misidentification is problematic only for the females. Most of these girls who have mildly virilized external genitalia are rapidly identified as ambiguous. However, some go home with a male sex assignment and are thought of as a male by caregivers, relatives, and friends. These children and caregivers present a special challenge.

What is your own personal view of what makes a girl a girl or a boy a boy?

Nursing Management and Family Teaching

Nursing management with the newborn in adrenal crisis is focused on interventions necessary to maintain homeostasis through administration of fluids and cortisone, and monitoring electrolytes and vital signs. Nurses need to also provide a safe environment for the caregivers to ask questions and explore their feelings. They need to address the newborn with ambiguous genitalia as "baby," not he, she, or it. The genitals should be described as sex organs, not as a penis or clitoris. Nurses should describe to the caregivers that the penis and clitoris develop from the same fetal tissue. Most infants in the United States have been assigned a sex at birth; delaying a sex assignment is stressful for the family and often the health care team. Depending on the severity of the virilization of the genitalia in the female and the sex assignment decision made by the caregivers and health care provider, corrective surgery may be immediately considered.

Nursing Tip:

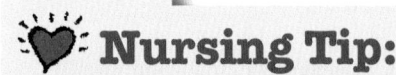

Cortisol replacement

In the event of an illness, stress, or surgery that would normally cause an increase in the production of cortisol, changes in the dose of medication will need to be made. Caregivers need to be taught when to increase the cortisol dose and by how much for common illnesses. They should be instructed that any surgical procedure will require increases in the child's medication and should be discussed with their health care provider well in advance of any planned procedure, and as soon as possible for any emergency procedure.

If the genitals remain in an ambiguous state, nurses should discuss with the caregivers how they feel about handling diaper changes in public or by other family members. If a birth certificate was issued at birth, nurses should discuss how to best change the sex identification and possibly the child's name if there is a sex reassignment. It is important to discuss with the caregivers how to best handle notifying those people whom they have already contacted about the baby and gender identification.

Medication administration and the lifelong nature of treatment need to be taught to the caregivers. Intramuscular injection technique will need to be taught. Cortisone is necessary to sustain life, and at times when the oral medication cannot be taken, intramuscular injections are given.

Nursing management for the child diagnosed later focuses on coordinating the testing for establishing the diagnosis. Most caregivers will have little understanding of adrenal function and will benefit from education. If the child who is diagnosed later has been assigned a sex that is not consistent with the child's gonads or chromosomes, the issues and focus of management will quickly include this new dilemma. The full ramifications of reassigning the sex of the child versus raising the child with the sex as assigned at birth will need to be considered.

DISORDERS OF THE PANCREAS

The most common disorder of the pancreas is diabetes mellitus, in which the islets of Langerhans fail to produce adequate insulin.

Diabetes Mellitus

Diabetes mellitus is a group of diseases in which carbohydrate and lipid metabolism is impaired. Diabetes mellitus, as a whole, is one of the leading causes of health problems and death in the United States. Type 1 diabetes (previously known as insulin dependent diabetes mellitus [IDDM], juvenile onset, or type I) is the second most common chronic disease of childhood in the United States and much of Europe. Type 2 diabetes mellitus occurs most commonly in adults over age 40 and accounts for 90% of the diagnosed cases in the United States.

Incidence and Etiology

Diabetes mellitus is an umbrella diagnosis, under which several diseases that result in an alteration in insulin mediated glucose metabolism are grouped. A differential diagnosis is established based on the pathogenesis of disease development. Type 1 is an autoimmune disease that occurs in genetically susceptible individuals. Several environmental factors, such as viruses or chemicals in the environment, have been implicated in the process of developing type 1 diabetes. In a genetically susceptible individual exposed to environmental factors, the immune system begins a T lymphocyte mediated process that damages and destroys the beta-cells of the pancreas (Figure 28-6). Islet cell antibodies (ICA), insulin autoantibodies (IAA), and other antibodies specific to the beta-cell can be measured in the serum of individuals who are in the process of developing type 1 diabetes for years before the clinical appearance. By the time symptoms are evident and diagnosis is commonly made, approximately 90% of the beta-cells have been destroyed.

Type 1 diabetes is the most common form of diabetes found in young people. The incidence is 0.14–0.17 in 1,000 Caucasians and 0.03–0.12 in African-Americans younger than 20 years of age (Tull & Roseman, 1995). There is an equal distribution between males and females. The peak age of onset is 11 years in girls and 13 in boys, coinciding with the average age of the onset of puberty. By age 20 the incidence decreases significantly.

Historically accounting for 2–3% of childhood cases of diabetes, the incidence of type 2 diabetes has been increasing in individuals under age 25 in the past 10 years, especially among children of ethnic minority populations (American Diabetes Association [ADA], 2000). It now appears to account for 16% of the childhood/adolescent diabetes diagnoses. Many of these children have a relative who has type 2 diabetes. They also tend to be overweight or obese and of African-American, Hispanic-American, Asian American, or Native American descent. They typically have low levels of physical activity. The exact mechanism and causative factors for type 2 diabetes in childhood is unknown but are under investigation (Glaser, 1997). The problem of obesity is so prevalent, that even in the type 1 diabetes population, 16% of children at diagnosis met the criteria for obesity

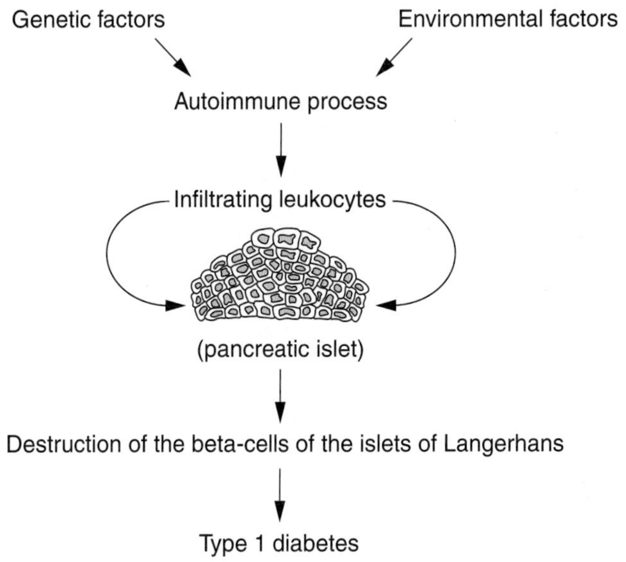

Figure 28-6 Development of Type 1 Diabetes

(Libman, Pietropaulo, Arslanian, LaPorte, & Becker, 2000). The median age for type 2 in childhood is 12–14 years. In the past, some children and adolescents with type 2 diabetes were inaccurately given the diagnosis of type 1 diabetes.

Pathophysiology

The autoimmune destruction, mediated by the T lymphocyte, of the beta-cells results in inadequate insulin secretion, and eventually insulin deficiency. When beta-cell insulin production is less than 10–20% of normal, overt clinical symptoms emerge. Insulin is unable to alter peripheral cells to aid in the transportation of glucose across the cell membranes. Hyperglycemia results from this impairment of peripheral glucose uptake. With impaired insulin production, hepatic glucose production increases, and hyperlipidemia and ketone formation occur. Counterregulatory hormones (growth hormone, cortisone, and glucagon) increase in concentration during insulin deficient states. These hormones promote insulin resistance and enhance **glyconeogenesis** (the fixation of glycogen from non-carbohydrate sources) through protein breakdown (**proteolysis**), fat breakdown (**lipolysis**), and **glycogenolysis** (the conversion of glycogen into glucose). The end result of the glyconeogenesis is more circulating glucose. The breakdown of fats increases ketone body formation, leading to ketonuria and ketonemia.

When the blood glucose exceeds 150–180 mg/dl, the renal threshold for glucose is exceeded and it is filtered out of the serum and into the urine. When glucose is excreted in the urine, an osmotic shift begins. Additional water is excreted, and polyuria, the first of the classic symptoms of diabetes, is evident. The osmotic shift and increasing fluid loss from the glucosuria stimulate the thirst center and polydipsia, the second of the classic symptoms, develops. **Polyphagia** (excessive hunger) occurs as less glucose is used for energy production and storage and the hunger center is stimulated. As the hyperglycemia becomes even more pronounced and persistent, fluid loss becomes severe, and oral consumption will not replenish the loss. Dehydration occurs, and weight loss ensues caused by fluid loss from the osmotic diuresis and inadequate storage of nutrients. Electrolyte disturbances result from the osmotic diuresis and cell death.

Ketones are acid bodies that are initially buffered by stores of bicarbonate. The kidney eventually loses its ability to buffer the ketone bodies, and bicarbonate stores are depleted, worsening the metabolic acidosis. Respiratory compensation of the metabolic acidosis begins with the clinical symptoms of increased respiratory rate, **Kussmaul respirations** (deep, slow, labored breathing), flushed cheeks, and an acetone odor to the breath, resembling nail polish remover or rotten apples.

In type 2 diabetes the pancreas usually produces enough insulin, but for unknown reasons, the body is unable to use the insulin effectively, a condition called insulin resistance. After several years, insulin production decreases. The result is the same as for type 1 diabetes: glucose accumulates in the blood and the body cannot make efficient use of its main source of fuel.

Nursing Tip:

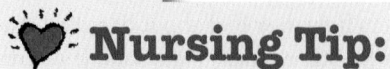

Characteristics of Kussmaul respirations

Kussmaul respirations sound like a train. They are deep and laborious. The respiratory system is attempting to eliminate excess carbon dioxide to compensate for the metabolic acidosis.

Clinical Manifestations

The individual with type 1 diabetes presents most commonly with a history of polyuria, polydipsia, polyphasia, weight loss, and dehydration. In some individuals, abdominal pain and vomiting will be present, leading to a misdiagnosis of appendicitis or gastroenteritis. In the early diagnosis of type 1 diabetes, there may a virtual lack of symptoms. Children and adolescents are sometimes diagnosed early through a routine urinalysis done in the course of a yearly physical examination by their primary care provider. The clinical manifestations of type 2 diabetes develop gradually. Children with this diabetes may also have polyuria, polydipsia, or polyphasia. Fatigue and frequent infections may be present; however, the child would not have ketosis.

Diagnosis

The individual with type 1 diabetes can present in a variety of ways, from the most critical to the most stable. In the vast majority of children, the diagnosis is immediately apparent. They present with a history of polyuria, polydipsia, and polyphagia (the classic triad of symptoms of diabetes) and a glucose in excess of 200 mg/dl. Most will also have experienced weight loss and fatigue. Some will present in diabetic ketoacidosis (DKA). Oral glucose tolerance testing (OGTT) and fasting serum glucose determination, the historical hall-

Nursing Tip:

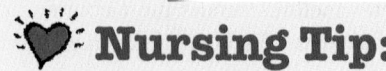

History taking in the evaluation of new onset type I diabetes

When taking a history on a child with symptoms of diabetes, explore for new onset nocturia or newly developed bed-wetting. Ask caregivers of infants and toddlers about a recent increase in frequency of diaper changes, which would indicate polyuria, a symptom of diabetes.

mark used in diagnosing type 2 diabetes, are not commonly needed in children because of their unequivocal presentation. The current diagnostic standards do not recommend the use of the OGTT for routine clinical use in the diagnosis of any type of diabetes.

Treatment

Treatment of type 1 diabetes in pediatrics ideally involves a team consisting of the child, caregivers, health care practitioner, nurse, nutritionist, and mental health professional. Each discipline brings to the management a unique and helpful perspective. The general goals for therapy include achieving normal growth and development, optimal glucose control, minimal complications, and a positive adjustment to the disease. It requires daily injections of insulin, blood glucose monitoring, following a meal plan, exercise, self-management skills, and decision making. Treatment of type 2 diabetes includes diet, exercise, home glucose monitoring, and in many cases, oral hypoglycemic medications and/or insulin. Management also includes the avoidance or minimization of complications. Table 28-3 lists the acute, intermediate, and chronic complications of diabetes.

Insulin Management

Insulin replacement is the cornerstone of management. Daily insulin is administered by subcutaneous injections or a portable insulin pump. The frequency of injection is based on the goals of management for the child. Two or three daily injections have become commonplace in the management of type 1 diabetes. The use of insulin pumps in children and teens with diabetes is rapidly growing. Types of insulin preparations are categorized by their actions as short, intermediate, or long-acting (Table 28-4). Except for Lispro

REFLECTIONS FROM FAMILIES

When my child was first diagnosed with diabetes, I was so frightened. My father had also had diabetes diagnosed when he was a young man. I can remember when I was a child that he would act so different when his blood sugar was low. (As a teenager, I found his behavior during those events so embarrassing.) When I was in my later teenage years, he started to have real problems with his vision and we learned that he might lose his eyesight. But nothing prepared me for his developing kidney failure and death when I was in my twenties. He was only 48 years old and had diabetes for twenty-five years when he died from diabetes complications.

Diabetes management is so different today than when my father was diagnosed. He never knew what his blood sugar was (he could only test his urine) and he could never adjust his insulin doses to keep himself in control. He never really knew when he was younger what kind of control he was in. When my child was diagnosed, the nurses and physicians took so much time helping me to understand that my child and I could manage the diabetes by monitoring blood sugar levels, how food affects blood sugar, and how to adapt the dose of insulin my child receives. I feel more in control, more empowered to manage the diabetes, because of the tools I have and the knowledge of the health care professionals on the diabetes team. I still worry, but my fear of the future and my child's health is not stopping me from envisioning a healthy future for my child.

Eye On:

Insulin Pumps–A Pediatric Controversy

Insulin pumps have been available for over 20 years. The current pumps are the size of a pager and contain a syringe that holds up to 30 units of insulin. The syringe is attached to tubing and a cannula. The cannula is inserted into the subcutaneous tissue, typically in the abdomen or hip. The pump is programmed to deliver small amounts of insulin constantly throughout the day and night. With each meal or snack, the wearer programs the pump to immediately deliver a dose of fast-acting insulin based on the individual's blood glucose level and amount of carbohydrate being eaten.

The controversy surrounding these pumps in pediatrics hinges on the developmental appropriateness of them in children and adolescents. Insulin pump therapy requires a motivated individual willing to test and record glucose levels, wanting to improve control, having the ability to quantify food intake, and willing to maintain medical follow-up. Abstract thinking skills are required, a competence that is usually developed in mid-adolescence. No research has been performed regarding whether pump therapy interferes with normal developmental issues of childhood and adolescence. The physical operation of the pump, learning which button to push and when, can be taught to a young child. The management objectives and problem-solving skills cannot.

TABLE 28-3 Complications of Type 1 Diabetes

Acute	Intermediate	Chronic
Ketoacidosis	Lipohypertrophy	Retinopathy
Hypoglycemia	Lipoatrophy	Nephropathy
Weight loss	Growth failure	Neuropathy
	Pubertal delay	Cardiopathy
	Menstrual disturbances	
	Impaired cognitive function	
	Hyperlipidemia	
	Emotional disturbances	
	Cataracts	

TABLE 28-4 Insulin Types and Action

Name	Type	Onset	Peak	Duration
Lispro/Humalog	Rapid-acting	5–12 min	$^1/_2$–2 hrs	3–4 hrs
Regular	Short-acting	20–30 min	2–4 hrs	6–8 hrs
NPH	Intermediate-acting	1–4 hrs	6–10 hrs	12–20 hrs
Lente	Intermediate-acting	2–4 hrs	8–12 hrs	12–20 hrs
Ultra Lente	Long-acting	3–5 hrs	10–16 hrs	18–24 hrs

insulin, all others are nonprescription. Insulin is either animal (pork) or synthetic human, produced through DNA recombinant technology. Dosage of insulin is based on the needs of the child or adolescent. Common dosage for a child more than one year post diagnosis is 0.75–1.0 u/kg/day. The insulin dose in the adolescent tends to exceed 1.0 u/kg/day, sometimes reaching 1.6–1.7 u/kg/day. Different types of insulin can be mixed together. It is common for insulin regimens to incorporate mixed insulins. Regular and Lispro insulin are stable when mixed with Lente and NPH. Lente and Ultra Lente are not stable if combined with NPH.

Blood Glucose Monitoring

Home blood glucose monitoring (HBGM) became available in the late 1970s–early 80s. Prior to its introduction daily glucose monitoring was often done through urine testing. Urine glucose monitoring did not supply quantitative data that could aid in making decisions about insulin doses or success of treatment. The introduction of HBGM facilitated the introduction of insulin regimens geared toward tighter glucose control, the use of supplemental insulin to correct or prevent hyperglycemia, and the ability of clients and care-

Nursing Tip:

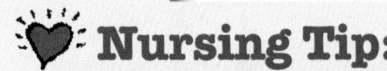

Monitoring for long-term glucose control: The hemoglobin A1c

The hemoglobin A1c (HgbA1c), or glycosolated hemoglobin, measurement reflects the average blood glucose control of the individual over the previous 8-12 weeks. It measures the amount of glucose that attaches to protein in the red blood cells. The greater the amount of glucose in the blood overall, the higher the HgbA1c will be. Acceptable control is a value of 8–8.5% in children younger than 7 years and below 8% for children over 7 and adolescents (Betschart, 2000). The national standards recommend that this be measured semiannually to quarterly for individuals with type I diabetes. It is an invaluable tool for the assessment of overall glucose control, and is an outcome measurement used to describe comparable risk for the development of the long-term (or chronic) complications.

givers to become skilled at self-management. HBGM is done by lancing the fingertip or other appropriate area (several meters today can test small samples of blood obtained from a forearm, thigh, or side of the hand) with a small lancet to obtain a blood sample. The blood sample is placed on a testing strip in a glucose meter. The glucose level is measured by the meter. Home blood glucose meters are commercially available, and are frequently covered by third-party insurers; however, the test strips can be one of the more costly items for diabetes management. Frequency of blood glucose testing is based on the goals of the individual's management.

National standards for medical monitoring are listed in Box 28-5. This monitoring reflects the ongoing needs of the individual with type 1 diabetes, and the assessment of the various body systems that are affected by the disease. The individual is monitored for immediate, intermediate, and long-term complications.

Nutrition

In 2001 new nutritional recommendations for diabetes were released by the American Diabetes Association in conjunction with the American Dietetics Association (ADA, 2001). Now known as medical nutrition management (MNT), the recommendations include evidenced-based nutritional and meal planning principles. MNT should reflect the management goals of the individual. In children, the meal plan should be updated at least annually and should reflect their growing needs. The meal plan is no longer a plan that excludes foods. The previous philosophy (pre-1994) was that foods that were simple sugars, for example candy or pie, were automatically forbidden. The new philosophy is that while some foods are better nutritional choices than others, no food is automatically excluded. The typical meal plan calls for approximately 50–60% of the calories coming from carbohydrates (grains, breads, fruit, milk, vegetables), 10–20% from protein (meat, beans, eggs, cheese, legumes), and 20–30% from fat (butter, oil, mayonnaise).

BOX 28-5 Medical monitoring recommendations for type 1 diabetes

Semiannual/quarterly exams

Height measurement (until maturity)

Weight

Blood pressure (quarterly)

Sexual maturation staging (periodically in the peripubertal client)

Foot exam with quarterly exam

Comprehensive eye exam for all clients over age 12 after 5 years of diagnosis with diabetes

Medical history: include frequency/severity of hypoglycemia HBGM results, regimen adjustments made by client, lifestyle changes, symptoms of complications, medications, psychosocial issues

Annual physical exam (any abnormality noted is reevaluated at next visit)

Laboratory evaluation: Hemoglobin A1c 2–4 times per year, annual lipid profile and urine for protein and microalbumin

Review of management plan

Eye On:

Micronutrients and Antioxidants

Many clients with diabetes are beginning to incorporate vitamins, antioxidants, and herbal supplements into their daily management. There is theoretical evidence that supplements with antioxidants may have benefits, but there is little if any confirmation of these reported benefits. Some of the reported benefits of micronutrients like chromium and magnesium are evident in deficient individuals and include a reduction of insulin resistance, a causitive factor of type 2 diabetes. Research into the benefits of antioxidants and other micronutrients continues.

Exercise

Exercise plays an important role in diabetes management as it potentiates the hypoglycemic effect of insulin. Regular activity and exercise may assist in blood glucose control. For some individuals, higher levels of activity may permit a larger meal plan or lower doses of insulin. Exercise and activity are rarely restricted, but preparation for increased activity (i.e., insulin dose changes, changes in food) may be necessary to maintain blood glucose control.

Nursing Management

Assessment

Diabetes management is fluid and should reflect the growing and changing needs of the client. The success of the management is based on achieving the established goals for the client. The nurse is vigilant for evidence of complications, problems with management, and opportunities to provide education that will expand the child and caregiver's understanding and skills for diabetes management.

Nursing Diagnosis

The following nursing diagnoses are pertinent to the child with type 1 diabetes:

1. Risk for injury related to insulin insufficiency and deficiency.
2. Risk for injury related to hypoglycemia or hyperglycemia.

3. Disturbed body image related to developing a chronic disease.
4. Deficient knowledge related to management of type 1 diabetes.
5. Interrupted family processes related to management of a chronic illness.

Outcome Identification

1. Child will have adequate insulin levels, with normalized glucose levels.
2. Child will exhibit no evidence of hypoglycemia or hyperglycemia.
3. Child will have a positive body image.
4. Child and caregiver will be capable of managing diabetes in the home environment with the support and guidance of the other team members.
5. Family members will show evidence of healthy family processes.

Planning/Implementation

Once the child is medically stable, the priority of the health care team is the education of the child and caregivers. Initial education has traditionally occurred over several inpatient hospital days, but there is a growing movement to develop ambulatory educational programs for the newly diagnosed child and family. Education does not only occur at diagnosis, but is an ongoing process. Every meeting with a family or child with diabetes is an opportunity to provide ongoing education or assessment of knowledge.

Survival Education

The initial goal is to provide survival education, which encompasses the management skills and decision-making processes necessary for the caregiver or child to be safe at home. Once basic management skills are understood and the caregiver and child are proficient, the goals of education shift. Self-management becomes the overall goal at this time, and the role of the health care team is to empower the family and child to accomplish this goal.

The following concepts and skills are considered survival level:

1. Essential nature of insulin therapy
2. Identifying prescribed insulin
3. Preparing an accurate injection
4. Giving an injection with proper technique
5. Blood glucose monitoring and documentation
6. Urine testing for ketones
7. Understanding how to obtain supplies and equipment
8. Hypoglycemia and hyperglycemia, their causes, signs and symptoms, treatments
9. Understanding whom to call and when
10. Identifying the daily routine (timing of injection, when to do blood testing, when to eat)
11. Wearing medical identification
12. Meal planning

Most families and children will want to understand the "why and how come" of type 1 diabetes. To best understand the reason for the management regimen, they will need information on the function and action of insulin, carbohydrate metabolism, and the relationship the blood glucose level has to food intake, insulin level, and exercise. Caregivers tend to have many questions. Providing answers will increase their confidence and sense of security.

Education should be given to the caregiver and also in a developmentally appropriate manner to the child. Box 28-6 identifies diabetes management skills and the common age the skill is introduced to children. The nurse and family need to clarify at the beginning of the education whom the primary caregiver will be initially. With the growing trend for short inpatient stays or ambulatory education programs, there may be insufficient time to prepare several individuals and offer them direct experience with diabetes care. Helping the primary caregiver identify who else in the family can assist with the diabetes care and incorporating that individual in the primary education sessions is an important nursing responsibility.

Insulin Preparation and Injection

Insulin preparation and injection require one-on-one time with the caregiver and child. Learning to give an injection is a task many caregivers and children approach with fear and anxiety. Both demonstration and return demonstration should be provided. Nurses should emphasize accuracy and consistency of the preparation technique. Refer to the accompanying Nursing Tip for specifics on the insulin injection.

Nurses should provide information about site selection and rotation. The sites for injections are the abdomen, arms, legs, and buttocks (Figure 28-7). The absorption of insulin is fastest in the abdomen, followed by the arms. Leg and buttock insulin injections are absorbed the slowest. Injection sites may have evidence of **lipoatrophy** (indentation or atrophy of subcutaneous fat) or **lipohypertrophy** (lumpiness or hypertrophy of subcutaneous fat). Lipoatrophy is currently

BOX 28-6 Developmental target ages for technical skill training

Urine testing—4 to 6 years
Blood testing—4 to 8 years
Insulin injections—8 to 10 years
Nutrition decision skills—10 to 14 years
Management decision skills—12 to 18 years

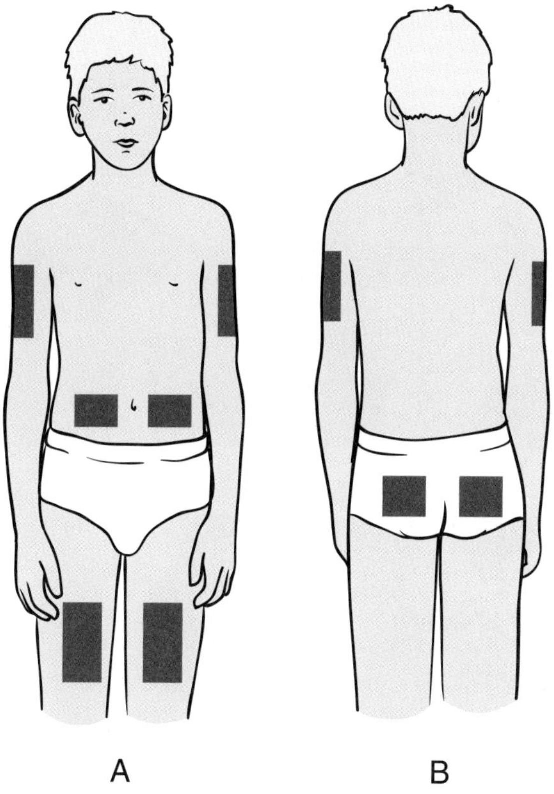

Figure 28-7 Insulin injections need to be rotated among the sites illustrated. (A) Front (B) Back.

Kids Want To Know

Do I really have to check my blood sugars so often?

The 10-year-old child you are caring for has been diagnosed with type 1 diabetes and is preparing to be discharged home. In preparing for her discharge, she asks "Do I really have to check my blood sugars so often? Can't I just test them in the morning and then test my urine the rest of the day? Every time I test, it hurts so much!"

A child of 10 has not developed an abstract cognitive thought process and may not understand the relationship between the blood glucose testing and the ongoing evaluation of the success of diabetes management. Additionally, blood glucose testing does require a small lancing of the skin, which can be uncomfortable. Review with her the techniques for doing less painful blood testing, using the sides of her upper fingers, not the tips or the pads, or using a meter that allows for less painful testing sites like the forearm. Reassure her that over the next several weeks, the discomfort will ease a bit as her fingers become slightly callused.

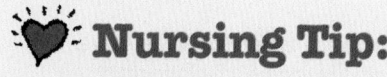

Nursing Tip:

Insulin injection

1. Encourage the caregiver and/or child (if child is doing self-injection) to receive a practice saline injection. This will help them to have knowledge about the comfort of the injection and will often allay their fear of performing the procedure. This practice session also allows caregivers an opportunity to role model for the child receiving an injection with cooperation.
2. Provide practice materials for the caregiver and child to use outside the educational sessions.
3. Initially when the caregiver is preparing the first injection, the child's anxiety may make the caregiver anxious and interfere with the ability to prepare it successfully. Should this occur, offer to have the caregiver prepare the injection in an area away from the child.
4. Insulin bottles in use can be stored at room temperature or in the refrigerator for up to 30 days or to the expiration date on the bottle, whichever comes first. Unopened bottles are stored between 50–85 degrees Fahrenheit up to the expiration date on the bottle. Insulin that is stored at temperatures that exceed 85 degrees or below 50 should be discarded. Room temperature injections are considered more comfortable.
5. Recommend and provide insulin syringes that are the smallest volume for the dose. For example, use a 30 unit (3/10 cc) insulin syringe for insulin doses that are less than 30 units. This strategy will help to ensure more accuracy with prepared doses. Syringes are also available with $^1/_2$ unit marking for clients who use $^1/_2$ unit insulin doses.
6. Insulin pens are also available. Containing small containers of insulin, these pens (the size of a magic marker) can be dialed to deliver a single dose of insulin. A needle is attached to the end of the pen, the dose dialed, needle inserted into the subcutaneous fat, and the insulin injected. Insulin pens come in Lispro, NPH, or Regular insulin, along with pre-mixed insulin (70/30 or 75/25 insulin).

uncommon with the purified insulin preparations available and is treated by injecting insulin into the edges of the area of atrophy. Lipohypertrophy occurs commonly and is caused by trauma to the injection sites from repeatedly giving injections into the same area. Lipohypertrophy results in a cosmetically unsightly area that has decreased sensation and absorption. It resolves only by avoiding the area for injections.

Blood Glucose and Urine-Ketone Monitoring

The technique of blood glucose monitoring will need to be taught to caregivers and the child (if appropriate). Specific instruction should concentrate on the technique of performing the blood-letting procedure and applying an adequate sample to the testing area of the meter to be used in the home. The instructor needs to be familiar with the glucose meter being used, aware of the volume of blood necessary for the performance of the test, how the blood sample is applied to the strip, and how the meter itself operates. Nurses should instruct and reinforce the practice of writing the results in a log, even with meters that have memories, and emphasize that the blood glucose monitoring, and its ongoing evaluation, play a major role in the success of the regimen by identifying problem areas and successful strategies for management (Figure 28-8).

Nursing Tip:

Blood glucose testing

1. The pads and tips of the finger contain many nerve endings and few capillaries. For a less painful finger puncture, use the sides of the fingertips or a meter that allows testing from a alternative site.
2. Warm the fingers by rubbing the hands together or milking the finger to aid in obtaining a blood drop. Cleaning the area with soap and warm water will help draw the blood to the surface and cleans the area at the same time. Using soap and water eliminates the need to cleanse the area with alcohol.
3. Once finger punctures are done repeatedly, small calluses form. As long as an adequate sample can be obtained from a finger puncture, using these areas with calluses is less painful and should be encouraged,
4. Finger puncture devices (lancet devices) come in many styles. Some allow the client to adjust the depth of penetration, which can be helpful for obtaining blood samples in young children.
5. Newer glucose monitors and devices are becoming available that allow for a client to lance the forearms or thighs for drops of blood to do glucose monitoring, increasing a client's options of sites for testing.

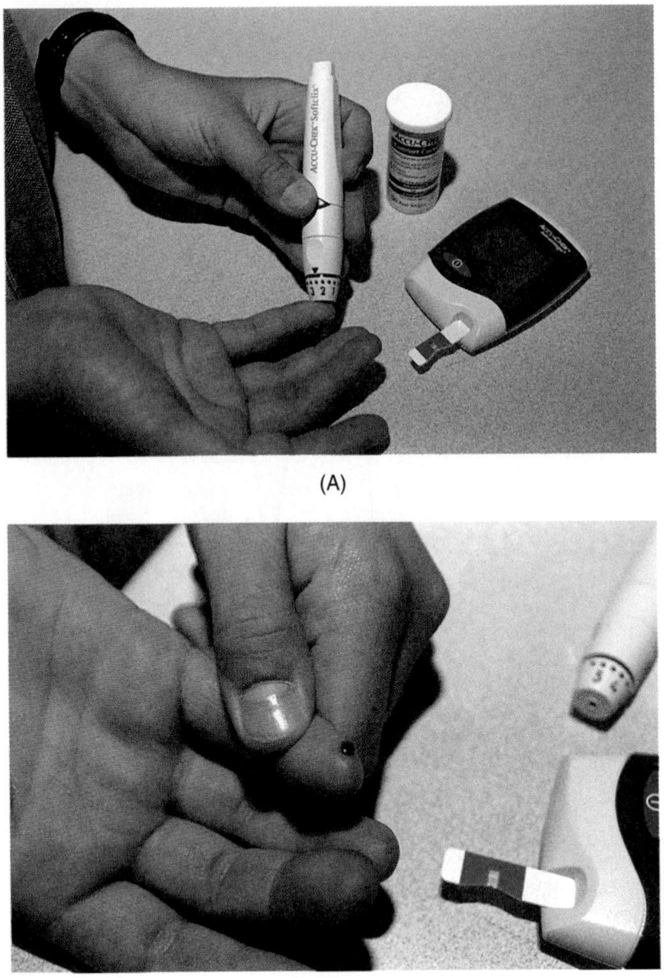

(A)

(B)

Figure 28-8 This school-aged child is able to perform his own blood glucose monitoring.

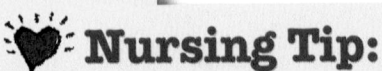

The technique and rationale for urine testing should be taught to the family. Given that most children and caregivers will be doing blood glucose testing, urine is monitored for ketones. Ketones are tested when there is a question about insulin deficiency. Common recommendations are that the urine is tested for ketones when a client is ill, has a glucose over 250 mg/dl, or is experiencing unexplained weight loss. Return demonstration should be done. Results should be documented.

Hypoglycemia

Hypoglycemia, or low blood glucose or an insulin reaction, is also a survival topic. Hypoglycemia is a short-term complication of diabetes and occurs when the blood glucose level falls below 60 mg/dl. It is caused by more insulin being available than is necessary and may result from an insulin dose that is too large, insufficient food consumed, or increased activity. The most common symptoms of mild to moderate hypoglycemia include drowsiness, lightheadedness, irritability, tremors, sweating, and confusion. Severe hypoglycemia, which is rare, may lead to unconsciousness and convulsions and, if not treated promptly, can be life-threatening. Causes, symptoms, and treatment of hypoglycemia should be taught, reviewed, and assessed for retention of knowledge. Mild episodes will typically respond to 10–15 grams of carbohydrate (e.g., 3–4 glucose tablets, 4 ounces of juice or soda, 6 ounces of milk, 6–7 lifesaver-type candies) within 10–15 minutes. Moderate episodes should also resolve with treatment of 10–15 grams of carbohydrate, but the individual will likely require assistance. Severe episodes will require IV glucose or IM glucagon. As IV glucose is an unrealistic intervention by a caregiver, glucagon preparation (which requires reconstitution) and administration will need to be taught. Caregivers should be instructed on treatment options, glucagon preparation, and injection technique. Caregivers and children should be instructed to always carry a source of oral carbohydrate for hypoglycemia.

Whom to Call and When

Caregivers will need to understand whom to call and how to reach the health care team for questions, advice, problem solving, and emergency situations. The plan of care should include guidelines for routine phone calls and for what constitutes a more urgent call. Telephone, e-mail, and fax numbers, including emergency instructions should be provided. Medical identification jewelry should be worn by the child.

Medical Nutrition Treatment: Meal Planning

Typically the instruction for meal planning is provided by a nutritionist. The extent of meal planning at diagnosis is based on the ability of the caregivers and child to understand the plan. For some families, the concept of three meals and two snacks at routine, regular times of the day is revolutionary. For other families, counting grams of carbohydrate is quickly and easily understood, and the meal plan is sophisticated. From a baseline, survival standpoint, the minimal understanding needed to be demonstrated by the caregivers are the concepts that food intake will increase blood glucose levels and that consistent times for eating are essential.

Family Teaching: Beyond the Survival Stage

As mentioned previously, the education provided to prepare a family to care for a child with type 1 diabetes at the time of diagnosis is just the beginning of the educational process. Ongoing and advanced education begin as the caregivers and child gain experience with the diabetes care. For some families, this occurs quickly, and some of these topics are addressed at the time of the initial education. Topics that are addressed after the initial diagnosis phase include:

1. Hyperglycemia, its causes, symptoms, treatment options
2. Exercise and activity
3. Sick day care
4. Community resources
5. Adjustment and adaptation process
6. Complications of diabetes
7. Hygiene
8. Meal planning
9. Areas of research
10. Anticipatory planning
11. Insulin dose adjustment and use of supplemental insulin

This level of education begins to require the skills of an individual who has experience with diabetes management, not the inpatient, unit-based nurse. The educational process is ongoing and never-ending. The goals of education are to empower the child and caregivers, and to provide them with support and knowledge to make management decisions and plans, and to evaluate their success.

Hyperglycemia

Hyperglycemia or high blood glucose occurs when the body gets too little insulin, too much food, or too little exercise. It may also be caused by stress, an illness, or surgery. The most common symptoms are thirst, polyuria, fatigue, and blurred vision. Hyperglycemia can lead to diabetic ketoacidosis if untreated over a period of several days. Table 28-5 compares hypoglycemia and hyperglycemia.

Diabetic Ketoacidosis

Diabetic ketoacidosis (DKA), a common and potentially life-threatening acute complication of type 1 diabetes, is characterized by a severe insulin deficit, hyperglycemia, acidosis,

TABLE 28-5 Symptoms of Hypoglycemia and Hyperglycemia

Hypoglycemia	Hyperglycemia
Shakiness	Polyuria
Dizziness	Polydipsia
Pallor	Flushed face
Headaches	Dry skin
Disturbed vision	Blurred vision
Hunger	Hunger
Fatigue	Weakness
Tachycardia	Weaker, slower pulse rate
Disorientation	Fruity odor to breath
Confusion	Rapid respiratory rate
Seizure	Confusion
Coma	Coma

and ketosis. While 30–40% of all newly diagnosed individuals with type 1 diabetes will present in DKA, it is also the primary reason for rehospitalization or emergency care of the previously diagnosed. DKA is also the leading cause of death in children with this type of diabetes. The basic cause of DKA is absolute or relative insulin deficiency. It may be precipitated by an illness, particularly an infection, but usually is caused by the omission of insulin (Freeland, 1998).

There usually will be a history of classic signs and symptoms of polyuria, polydipsia, and weight loss. Once the child is sufficiently acidotic and ketotic, the breath will have a fruity or acetone odor. Many will have nausea, vomiting, and abdominal pain. The individual's state of consciousness varies from alertness to coma, and the degree of compromise does not always correlate with the degree of acidosis or hyperglycemia. Kussmaul respirations and dehydration are also seen. The diagnosis of DKA, while at times readily apparent, is based on clinical presentation and laboratory data. Confirmation of the diagnosis is based on the following criteria: a blood glucose over 200 mg/dl, ketonuria or ketonemia, an arterial pH<7.30 or a serum bicarbonate <15 mEq/l.

Treatment of DKA focuses on the problems of fluid deficit, electrolyte imbalances, alteration in acid-base balance, and insulin deficiency. It is a process that does not follow a specific protocol, but requires ongoing assessment and readjustment of the plan. The ultimate goal of therapy is to restore normal hemodynamic status and acid-base balance, and to slowly reduce and stabilize the blood glucose level.

Fluids are most often the first priority. Hypovolemic shock may be imminent. Fluids should be isotonic in concentration, and the volume should be geared toward replenishing the deficit over 24–48 hours. Rehydration is a slow process, and is limited to a volume of 4 liters/m^2/day, a rate suggested as a maximum rate that will not increase the individual's risk of complications to the therapy (Plotnick, 1994).

The goal of electrolyte replacement is to correct the imbalance and is most often integrated with the fluid replacement guidelines. In DKA, potassium is depleted. The hydrogen ions circulating in acidosis will replace intracellular potassium and the serum potassium level will be falsely elevated. However, the total body potassium is depleted. Correction of potassium is initiated once there is evidence of a renal output. Other electrolytes are potentially diminished (sodium, phosphorus, magnesium, calcium), and replacement may be necessary. Correction of acid-base imbalance, by the infusion of bicarbonate, is initiated in the most severe cases of DKA, where the acid-base imbalance is not improving. Bicarbonate infusion does not cross the blood-brain barrier and can accentuate the cerebral acidosis.

Fluid, electrolyte replacement, and bicarbonate will not, in and of themselves, halt the process of DKA. Insulin is the essential intervention for the correction of DKA. Insulin is necessary to stop glucosuria and is essential to facilitate the transportation of glucose across the cell membrane to halt cellular death and loss of potassium. Acid-base imbalance will correct as insulin stabilizes counter-regulatory hormone production and halts ketosis.

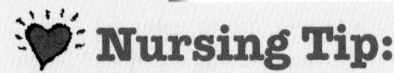

> **Nursing Tip:**
>
> **Insulin infusion**
>
> Insulin will adhere to plastic and glass tubing. When preparing an insulin infusion, some hospital pharmacies will add albumin to decrease this tendency. Flushing the tubing with the insulin infusion to saturate the binding sites is also recommended in many hospitals.

Except in mild cases of DKA, insulin is given by infusion (using Regular insulin). Insulin cannot be absorbed from subcutaneous or intramuscular injection sites in the dehydrated or acidotic individual. The rate of the infusion is titrated to achieve the established goal for the rate of glucose decline. A decrease of 100–150 mg/dl/hour is the maximum acceptable glucose drop in DKA in order to minimize the risks of therapy. When the blood glucose reaches approximately 200–300 mg/dl, stabilization of the glucose may be warranted with dextrose added to the fluid regimen.

The most serious risk associated with the treatment of DKA is cerebral edema, which occurs in less than 1% of cases but accounts for the majority of DKA-associated deaths. Cerebral edema occurs more commonly in infants and young children and in cases of new-onset type 1 diabetes. Symptoms (signs of increased intracranial pressure) include sudden complaint of a headache, confusion, difficulty in arousing the child, widening pulse pressure, tachycardia, or bradycardia. Immediate assessment and intervention are essential.

The child in DKA is often managed in the ICU. Nursing plays a vital role in the management of DKA. Time is essential, and the assessment should be done quickly. Nurses should assess: fluid status by determining recent changes in weight, skin turgor, blood pressure, and pulse rate; assess neurological function with a fundi exam and level of consciousnesss. Acidosis is assessed with complaints of back pain or abdominal pain, presence of Kussmaul respirations, flushed cheeks, and the odor of acetone on the breath of the child. Electrolytes, blood gas, serum or urine ketones, magnesium, calcium, and glucose should be drawn.

It is the nurse at the bedside who has been monitoring the child, whose concern is first heightened when the child just doesn't seem to be responding in the same way as he/she was earlier, and intervenes appropriately. This nurse needs to be skilled in assessment and understand the goals of therapy in the stabilization and treatment of DKA. Careful,

Nursing Tip:

Check for adherence to diabetes regimen

In the known client with diabetes, evaluate for adherence to the diabetes regimen. Evaluate the child's fingers for the small marks indicating blood glucose monitoring. Assess the injection sites for bruising (a benign indication of receiving injection) or hypertrophy, a lumpy appearance to the sites (indicating tissue damage caused by repeatedly giving injections to a specific area). Ask the child and/or caregivers how much insulin the child takes, how long it takes to empty a bottle of insulin, and compare the answers to determine if the child is receiving the prescribed dose of insulin.

accurate records must be maintained documenting the course of care and the child's response. These records should document the child's vital signs, fluids administered, laboratory results (electrolytes, glucose, ketones, pH), insulin infused/administered, intake and output, level of consciousness, and weight. The successful clinical course of DKA resolves in 24–48 hours, and the child is advanced to subcutaneous insulin and oral nutrition.

The ultimate, ideal goal of therapy is to develop a diabetes management plan that is user-friendly and provides the most normal glucose levels on average. Diabetes is the leading cause of blindness, kidney failure, and amputations in the U.S. Children with diabetes face these health risks as they age into adulthood. Among people with age at diagnosis <30 years, type 1 diabetes reduces life expectancy by at least 15 years (ADA, 1996). The research that has been done on the relationship between glucose control and the development of long-term complications clearly defines that near normal glucose control provides the greatest protection against the development of long-term complications (Diabetes Control and Complications Trial Research Group, 1993).

Nursing Tip:

School nursing and type I diabetes

Because type I diabetes is the second most common chronic disease of childhood, the school nurse is likely to have responsibility for a child with type I diabetes at some time. Monitoring, adherence to the meal plan, medication administration, education of school personnel, and communication with the caregivers will be part of the school nurse's plan of care. The school nurse can play a vital role in the health management of the child with type I diabetes by helping to facilitate the management regimen that may conflict with the typical school routine.

Reflective Thinking

Injections and School Policy

School policy forbids students from carrying any medication. Sally, a high school junior who has had type 1 diabetes for 6 years, has found Lispro insulin given pre-lunch is the best way to control her afternoon glucose. Her lunch period is 20 minutes in length. It takes her 4 minutes to reach the nurse's office, another 5 minutes on average to test her blood glucose and do her insulin injection, and 3 minutes to get to the cafeteria. This leaves her 8 minutes on average to consume her lunch and get on to her next class. Sally, whose nurse educator and physician have provided permission, would like to administer her insulin in the restroom outside the cafeteria. How would you, as the school nurse, approach Sally's dilemma? How would you, as her diabetes nurse educator, approach her dilemma?

ADDITIONAL ENDOCRINE DISORDERS

The following disorders are rare in children; therefore, they are discussed only briefly.

Hypoparathyroidism

Hypoparathyroidism is characterized by a deficiency in the secretion of parathyroid hormone (PTH), whose main function is maintenance of serum calcium. The impaired secretion of PTH affects calcium and phosphorus metabolism. This disorder is very rare and can be congenital or acquired. A frequent cause of congenital hypoparathyroidism is aplasia or hypoplasia of the parathyroid glands. The acquired type is primarily caused by inadvertent removal of the glands during a thyroidectomy. A deficit of PTH results in hypocalcemia and hyperphosphatemia.

Clinical Manifestations

The neonate may present with jittery movements, convulsions, apnea, lethargy, poor eating, and vomiting. Symptoms outside the neonatal period include tetany, stridor, **Chvostek's sign** (elicited by tapping the facial nerve, which produces a facial muscle spasm), **Trousseau's sign** (a carpopedal spasm that results from oxygen deficiency), complaints of tingling of the hands or around the mouth, diarrhea, seizures, papilledema, and skin and dental enamel changes. The skeleton is the storage area for calcium and phosphorus, and abnormalities of these substances will have an impact on bone formation. In the growing child, severe disease may result in permanent bone deformities and limited growth.

Treatment

Acute treatment, in cases of seizures or tetany, includes giving intravenous calcium in the form of calcium gluconate. The infusion should be given slowly except in the most dire of emergencies. Rapid infusion can lead to cardiac dysrhythmias. Calcium given IV is caustic, and extravasation will cause severe tissue burns. The nonacute treatment of transient hypocalcemia involves oral calcium gluconate. Chronic hypocalcemia is treated with an active metabolite of vitamin D, calcitriol. Calcium glucaonte orally is usually added as an adjunct to therapy, as it may help to bind phosphorus in the gut.

Addison's Disease

Addison's disease in childhood is rare. Damage or destruction of the adrenal glands caused by tuberculosis, fungal infections, autoimmune disease, and HIV result in decreased production of adrenal steroids, cortisol and aldosterone. The disease can also result from dysfunction of the hypothalamus or pituitary gland or from discontinuation of high levels of glucocorticoids for treatment of other diseases. The decrease in production of cortisol has an impact on the metabolism of glucose, fat, and protein. Aldosterone plays a primary role in sodium, potassium excretion; therefore, a deficit of this hormone has an impact on blood pressure and electrolytes.

Clinical Manifestations

The presentation of Addison's may be as an acute or chronic problem. The acute phase is life-threatening, with symptoms of severe hypotension, shock, electrolyte imbalances, dehydration, weakness, cardiovascular changes, fever, mental status changes, and hypoglycemia. An acute crisis can occur with febrile illnesses, infection, or stress.

Treatment

Treatment for Addison's involves replacing the deficient or absent hormones. In acute Addison's, IV hydrocortisone is given at regular intervals, and IV hydration is given to correct the dehydration and prevent hypovolemia. Electrolyte replacement will also be pursued in the acute phase. Chronic, nonacute treatment involves oral hydrocortisone and florinef. The dose of hydrocortisone will need to be increased with illness, stress, or surgery to meet the physiological needs of the body. If oral medication cannot be used or tolerated, intramuscular or intravenous cortisone should be used. The child and caregivers should be counseled on the essential need for lifelong treatment, with the information that untreated Addison's disease can be life-threatening. A medical identification should be worn by the individual with Addison's irrespective of age.

Cushing's Syndrome

Cushing's syndrome is a cluster of signs and symptoms caused by hypercortisolism or excessive circulating free cortisol. The most common cause of hypercortisolism in children is caused by the prolonged or excessive corticosteroid therapy. Other possible etiologies are an adrenal tumor or a pituitary tumor that produces excessive ACTH. This disorder is rare in childhood and adolescence.

Clinical Manifestations

The most obvious sign of Cushing's syndrome is rapid weight gain, particulary in the abdomen, the face (moon-shaped) and the cervical fat pad (buffalo hump). Linear growth is decreased or stops because the excessive cortisol suppresses the release of the growth hormone. The child may complain of muscle weakness and fatigue. The skin may be thin and fragile, with an increased tendency to bruise. Reddish purple striae appear in the abdomen, as might acne and increased hair growth in inappropriate locations (hirsutism). Other symptoms include poor wound healing, increased susceptibility to infections, and decreased inflammatory response.

Treatment

Treatment is based on the cause. Adrenal or pituitary tumors should be surgically removed if possible. When the cause is steroid therapy, the effects may be lessened if the medication is given early in the morning or on an alternate day schedule. Morning administration mimics the normal diurnal pattern of cortisol secretion. Alternate day administration allows the anterior pituitary to maintain a more normal hypothalmic–pituitary–adrenal control mechanism.

Syndrome of Inappropriate Antidiuretic Hormone

Syndrome of inappropriate antidiuretic hormone (SIADH) occurs when ADH (vasopressin) is secreted in the presence of low serum osmolality. Normally a decrease in serum osmolality inhibits ADH production and secretion. In children with SIADH the feedback mechanism that regulates ADH does not function properly, and ADH continues to be released. This leads to water retention, dilutional hyponatremia (decrease in serum sodium level due to dilution), and extracellular fluid volume expansion. SIADH is caused by various conditions such as CNS infection (meningitis), head trauma, brain tumors, intracranial surgery, and certain medications (analgesics, barbiturates, chemotherapy).

Clinical Manifestations

Clinical manifestations related to water retention include decreased urine output and weight gain. Gastrointestinal symptoms such as anorexia, nausea, and vomiting develop. As the sodium level continues to decrease, neurological manifestations appear, including lethargy, behavioral changes, headaches, changes in level of consciousness, seizures, and finally coma.

Treatment

Treatment consists of fluid restriction to correct the hyponatremia, raising the serum sodium level with intravenous sodium chloride, and increasing the serum osmolality. The underlying disorder is also treated.

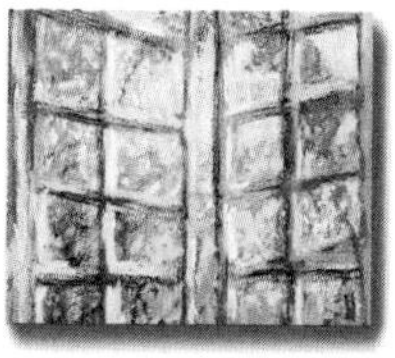

In the Real World

As a student, I became overwhelmed with the hormonal feedback loops my biology teacher diligently taught me. I remember thinking to myself, "Thank goodness I only need to learn this for the exam. I'll never need to understand this in real life." Then, I started working with children with hormonal problems. When I started to see the impact of the various hormones on the children in my practice and had to explain this to caregivers and children, I began to understand the process. Teaching them by illustrating the feedback system of the hormones produced by the various endocrine organs helped me conceptualize the information. My teaching, both of the families, children, and my colleagues became more comprehensive and accurate, helping them be fully prepared for the management of each endocrine abnormality.

Key Concepts

- The endocrine system is composed of glands that produce chemical substances called hormones in response to stimulation from the nervous system.
- Hormones have an intrinsic role in reproduction, growth and development, maintenance of the internal environment, and energy production, utilization, and storage.
- Feedback loops are characteristic of the endocrine system.
- The pituitary gland is the master gland, producing hormones that stimulate the other glands of the endocrine system.
- Growth hormone deficiency (GHD) is characterized primarily by poor growth and short stature caused by failure of the anterior pituitary to produce sufficient GH.
- Precocious puberty is a result of early or premature activation of the hypothalamic–pituitary–gonadal cycle, which causes the child to develop secondary sex characteristics.
- Diabetes insipidus is an endocrine disorder of water regulation caused by a deficiency of antidiuretic hormone. Common symptoms are polyuria, polydipsia, and dehydration.
- Thyroid dysfunction is the most common endocrine abnormality in pediatrics.
- Early diagnosis and treatment of hypothyroidism is important to prevent severe mental retardation.
- Symptoms of hyperthyroidism include nervousness, weight loss, increased growth rate, ophthalmic abnormalities, emotional lability, and heat intolerance.
- Congenital adrenal hyperplasia results from a genetic defect, which causes a breakdown in steroid synthesis and an overproduction of androgens. The goal of treatment is suppression of adrenal secretion of androgens, prevention of progressive virilization, and includes lifelong replacement of glucocorticoids and mineralocorticoids.
- Type 1 diabetes is an autoimmune form of diabetes that has its peak onset in childhood and is the second most common chronic disease of children.
- Type 1 diabetes results from damage and destruction of the beta-cells of the pancreas, resulting in insulin insufficiency and deficiency. Insulin treatment is essential to preserve the life of the affected individual.
- Diabetic ketoacidosis is a medical emergency, and in pediatric cases of diabetes, is the most common cause of death.

Review Questions

1. Describe a feedback loop system characteristic of an endocrine system.
2. Discuss the relationship between the clinical manifestations and pathophysiology of diabetes insipidus.
3. Describe the impact of neonatal screening on congenital hypothyroidism.
4. Differentiate the symptoms of hypothyroidism and hyperthyroidism.
5. List the clinical manifestations of type 1 diabetes.
6. Identify the clinical manifestations of diabetic ketoacidosis (DKA).
7. What is the most serious complication of the treatment of DKA?
8. Describe the difference in time action of Lispro, Regular, NPH, and Ultra Lente insulin.
9. Differentiate the symptoms of hypoglycemia and hyperglycemia.
10. Differentiate the diagnosis of type 1 diabetes from type 2 diabetes.

References

Adlin, V. (1998). Subclinical hypothyroidism: Deciding when to treat. *American Family Physician, 57*(4), 776–779.

American Academy of Pediatrics. (1993). Newborn screening for congenital hypothyroidism: Recommended guidelines. *Pediatrics, 91*(6), 1203–1209.

American Academy of Pediatrics Committee on Drugs and Committee on Bioethics. (1997). Considerations related to the use of recombinant human growth hormone in children. *Pediatrics, 99*(1), 122–129.

American Academy of Pediatrics Committee on Genetics. (1996). Newborn screening facts. *Pediatrics, 98*(3), 473–481.

American Academy of Pediatrics Section on Endocrinology and Committee on Genetics. (2000). Technical report: Congenital adrenal hyperplasia. *Pediatrics, 106*(6), 1511–1518.

American Diabetes Association. (1996). *Diabetes 1996 vital statistics.* Alexandria, VA: Author.

American Diabetes Association Consensus Statement. (2000). Type 2 diabetes in children and adolescents. *Diabetes Care, 22*(12), 381–398.

American Diabetes Association. (2001). Nutrition recommendations and principles for people with diabetes mellitus. *Diabetes Care, 24* (Suppl. 1), S44–S46.

Bayliss, P., & Cheetham, T. (1998). Diabetes insipidus. *Archives of Disease in Childhood, 79*, 84–89.

Betschart, J. (2000). Endocrine and metabolic diseases. In C. Burns, M. Brady, A. Dunn, & N. Starr (Eds.), *Pediatric primary care: A handbook for nurse practitioners* (2nd ed., pp. 662–688). Philadelphia: W. B. Saunders.

Cheetham, T., Hughes, I., Barnes, N., & Wraight, E. (1998). Treatment of hyperthyroidism in young people. *Archives of Disease in Childhood, 78*, 207–209.

Conn, P., & Crowley, W. (1994). Gonadotropin-releasing hormone and its analogs. *Annual Review of Medicine, 45*, 371–405.

Dallas, J., & Foley, T. (1996). Hyperthyroidism. In F. Lifshitz (Ed.), *Pediatric endocrinology* (3rd ed., pp. 401–414). New York: Marcel Dekker, Inc.

Diabetes Control and Complications Trial Research Group. (1993). The effect of intensive treatment of diabetes on the development and progression of long-term complications in insulin dependent diabetes mellitus. *The New England Journal of Medicine, 329*, 977–986.

Freeland, B. (1998). Diabetic ketoacidosis. *American Journal of Nursing, 98*(8), 52.

Glaser, N. (1997). Non insulin-dependent diabetes mellitus in childhood and adolescence. *Pediatric Clinics of North America, 44*, 307–337.

Gotlin, R., Kappy, M., Eisenbarth, G., & Chase, P. (1995). Endocrine disorders. In W. Hay, J. Groothuis, A. Hayward, & M. Levin (Eds.), *Current Pediatric Diagnosis and Treatment* (12th ed., pp. 881–925). Norwalk, CT: Appleton and Lange.

Libman, I., Pietropaulo, M., Arslanian, S., LaPorte, R., & Becker, D. H. (2000). Obese children with insulin-treated diabetes: Is it type 1 or type 2? *Diabetes Research Clinical Practice* (Suppl. 1), s9.

MacGillivray, M., Blethen, S., Buchlis, J., Clopper, R., Sandberg, D., & Conboy, T. (1998). Current dosing of growth hormone in children with growth hormone deficiency: How physiologic? *Pediatrics, 102*(2), 527–530.

Pang, S., & Shook, M. (1997). Current status of neonatal screening for congenital adrenal hyperplasia. *Current Opinions in Pediatrics, 9*, 419–423.

Plotnick, L. (1994). Insulin-dependent diabetes mellitus. *Pediatrics in Review, 15*(4), 137–148.

Styne D. (1997). New aspects in the diagnosis of pubertal disorders. *Pediatric Clinics of North America, 44*, 505–529.

Styne, D., & Grumbach, M. (1998). Puberty: Ontogeny, neuroendocrinlology, physiology, and disorder. In J. Wilson, D. Foster, H. Kroneberg, & P. Larsen (Eds.), *Williams Textbook of Endocrinology* (9th ed., pp.1509–1625). Philadelphia: W.B. Saunders.

Tull, E., & Roseman, J. (1995). Diabetes in African-Americans. In National Institute of Diabetes and Digestive and Kidney Diseases, *Diabetes in America* (2nd ed., 613–625). Bethesda, MD: National Institute of Diabetes and Digestive and Kidney Diseases.

Vogiatzi, M., & Kirkland, J. (1997). Frequency and necessity of thyroid function tests in neonates and infants with congenital hypothyroidism. *Pediatrics, 100*(3), e6.

Wales, J., Rogol, A., & Wit, J. (1996). *Pediatric endocrinology and growth.* Barcelona: Mosby-Wolfe.

Suggested Readings

American Diabetes Association. (1999). Position statement: Standards of medical care for patients with diabetes mellitus. *Diabetes Care, 22*, S32–41.

American Diabetes Association. (1999). Report of the expert committee on the diagnosis and classification of diabetes mellitus. *Diabetes Care, 22* (Suppl. 1), S5–S19.

Blethman, S. (1996). Hypopituitarism. In F. Lifshitz (Ed.), *Pediatric endocrinology* (3rd ed., pp.19–32). New York: Marcel Dekker, Inc.

Boland, E., Ahern, J., & Grey, M. (1998). A primer on the use of insulin pumps in adolescents. *The Diabetes Educator, 24,* 78–89.

Drash, A. (1996). Diabetes mellitus in the child: Classification, diagnosis, epidemiology and etiology. In F. Lifshitz (Ed.), *Pediatric endocrinology* (3rd ed., pp. 555–566). New York: Marcel Dekker, Inc.

Gumowski, J., & Loughran, M. (1996). Diseases of the adrenal glands. *Nursing Clinics of North America, 31*(4), 747–768.

Howey, D., Bowsher, R., Brunnelle, R., & Woodworth, J. (1994). [Lys(B28), Pro (B29)]-human insulin: a rapidly absorbed analog of human insulin. *Diabetes, 43,* 396–402.

Laredo, R. (2000). Carbohydrate counting: A return to basics. *Diabetes Spectrum, 13*(3) 149–151.

Lifshitz, F., & Cervantes, C. (1996). Short stature. In F. Lifshitz (Ed.), *Pediatric endocrinology* (3rd ed., pp. 1–18). New York: Marcel Dekker, Inc.

Migeon, C., & Lanes, R. (1996). Adrenal cortex: Hypo- and hyperfunction. In F. Lifshitz (Ed.), *Pediatric endocrinology* (3rd ed., pp. 321–346). New York: Marcel Dekker, Inc.

New, M., Ghizzoni, L., & Speiser, P. (1996). Update on congenital hyperplasia. In F. Lifshitz (Ed.), *Pediatric endocrinology* (3rd ed., pp. 305–320). New York: Marcel Dekker, Inc.

Perheentupa, J. (1996). Hypoparathyroidism and mineral homeostasis. In F. Lifshitz (Ed.), *Pediatric endocrinology* (3rd ed., pp. 433–472). New York: Marcel Dekker, Inc.

Rivkees, S. (1996). Hyperparathyroidism in children. In F. Lifshitz (Ed.), *Pediatric endocrinology* (3rd ed., pp. 497–506). New York: Marcel Dekker, Inc.

Romeo, J. (1996). Hyperfunction and hypofunction in the anterior pituitary. *Nursing Clinics of North America 31,* (4), 769–778.

Weissburg-Bewnchell J., & Pichert, J. (1999). Lifestyle and behavior: Counseling techniques for clinicians and educators. *Diabetes Spectrum, 12,* 103–112.

Resources

Organizations and Websites

American Association of Diabetes Educators
444 N. Michigan Avenue, Suite 1240
Chicago, IL 60611-3901
(312) 661-1700
(800) 338-DMED
www.aadenet.org

American Diabetes Association
1660 Duke Street
Alexandria, VA 22314
(703) 549-1500
(800) 806-7801
www.diabetes.org

American Dietetics Association
216 W. Jackson Blvd.
Chicago, IL 60606
(312) 899-0040
(800) 877-1600
www.eatright.org

Children with Diabetes
www.childrenwithdiabetes.com

Congenital Adrenal Hyperplasia Support Association
10 Country Highway
Wrenshall, MN 55797

Human Growth Foundation
997 Glen Cove Ave.
Glen Head, NY 11545
(800) 451-6434
www.hgfound.org

Juvenile Diabetes Foundation
432 Park Avenue South
New York, NY 10016-8013
(800) JDF-CURE
www.jdfcure.com

MAGIC (Major Aspects of Growth in Children) Foundation
1327 N. Harlem Ave.
Oak Park, IL 60302

National Diabetes Information Clearinghouse
1 Information Way
Bethesda, MD 20892
(301) 654-3327
(800) 860-8747

National Graves' Disease Foundation
320 Arlington Road
Jacksonville, FL 32211
(904) 724-0770
www.ngdf.org

Pediatric Endocrinology Nursing Society
P.O. Box 2933
Gaithersburg, MD 20886-2933

Thyroid Foundation of America
350 Ruth Sleeper Hall
40 Parkman Street
Boston, MA 02114
(617) 726-8500
(800) 832-8321
www.tsh.org

CHAPTER 29

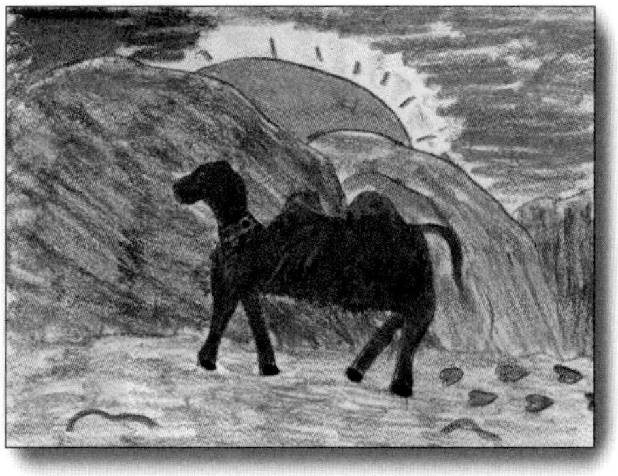

CELLULAR ALTERATIONS

Mary N. Yeaney, RN, MSN, CPNP
Ellen M. White, ARNP, MSN, OCN

After receiving the diagnosis of acute lymphocytic leukemia in our 5-year-old daughter, our first and most immediate reaction was the shock of finding our child in imminent mortal danger. When we were able to accept what we were hearing, there was a sense from the outset that, no matter what happens in the future, our life as a family will never be the same. In a few moments, with a few words, our image of ourselves as a healthy family was shattered, and our sense of stability and self-confidence as parents was destroyed.

COMPETENCIES

Upon completion of this chapter, the reader will be able to:

- *Discuss the importance of clinical trials.*
- *Identify the different treatment modalities used to treat cancer in children.*
- *Explain how the different treatment modalities affect malignant cells.*
- *Discuss the nursing management of common side effects of treatment modalities.*
- *Describe the clinical manifestations, treatment, and nursing management of common malignancies in children.*
- *Identify the emotional and educational needs of families who have children with cancer.*
- *Discuss the long-term, late effects of childhood cancer therapy.*

Cancer refers to a group of diseases in which there is out-of-control growth and spread of abnormal cells. A **tumor** is a mass that may be either benign, with slow noninvasive growth, or malignant with progressively virulent growth. Cancerous growths may be initiated at a primary localized area, as in most solid tumors, or more broadly disseminated, as in systemic cancers such as leukemia and lymphoma. Cancer, although rare in children, is the leading cause of death from disease in children, 1 to 14 years of age, in the United States. Only accidents claim more lives each year (Figure 29-1).

The most common childhood malignancy is leukemia, followed by tumors of the central nervous system, lymphoma, neuroblastoma, Wilms' tumor, bone tumors, and soft tissue sarcomas. This chapter discusses these malignancies and their treatment modalities as well as the nursing management of a child with cancer. The late effects of therapy in children who are long-term cancer survivors is also addressed.

ANATOMY AND PHYSIOLOGY

Childhood cancer differs from adult cancer in many ways. Common childhood malignancies usually arise from primitive embryonic tissue, whereas adult malignancies are of epithelial origin. In adult malignancies there is a

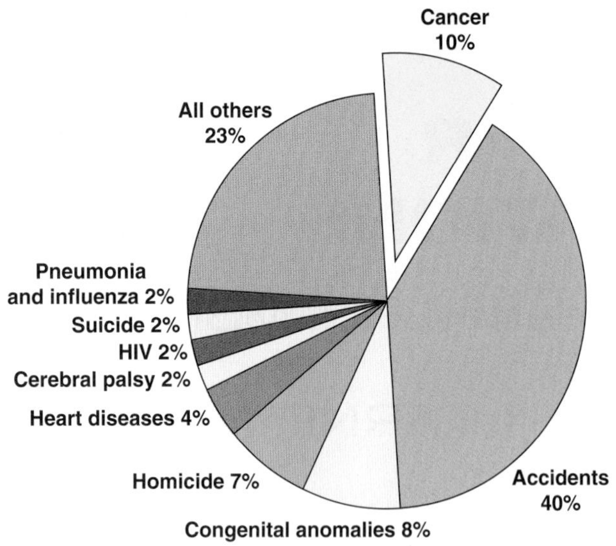

Figure 29-1 Ten Leading Causes of Death, Children Age 1–14. Adapted from Parker, S., Tong, T., Bolden, S., & Wingo, P. (1997). Cancer statistics 1997. *CA: A Cancer Journal for Clinicians, 47*(2), 68. Used with permission.

strong relationship between environmental factors and the development of cancer. Children have not lived long enough for exposure to carcinogens to cause a malignancy. Routine screening, which leads to early detection, is a key to survival in many adult cancers. The diagnosis of cancer in children is usually made when symptoms warrant a diagnostic work-up. See Table 29-1 for a summary of the differences between adult and childhood cancers.

In the 1990s more than 71% of children who were diagnosed with cancer survived their disease (Mosher & McCarthy, 1998). An organized multidisciplinary approach to providing care for these children, as well as greatly improved supportive care measures, have been essential to this success. The Children's Oncology Group (COG) and the Pediatric Oncology Group (POG) are two national collaborative study groups composed of pediatric oncology professionals. These cooperative study groups have provided an organized, coordinated approach to cancer treatment with the use of **clinical trials,** which are protocols or guidelines used to treat specific diseases. Following these guidelines and submitting treatment results to the study group provides the necessary data to improve therapy, decrease morbidity, and increase the survival of children with cancer.

Reflective Thinking

What Would It Be Like to Be Registered in a Clinical Trial?

Newly diagnosed children are eligible for front-line treatment in clinical trials where there is a comparison of the existing standard treatment to a new therapeutic approach. The decision to receive either approach is by random selection. What would it be like to be the caregiver of a child, newly diagnosed with cancer, and be asked to sign consent to participate in a clinical trial?

TREATMENT MODALITIES

The goal of cancer therapy is to rid the body of all malignant cells, thereby curing the cancer. Therapy may include

TABLE 29-1 Differences Between Adult and Childhood Cancers

Adult	Childhood
Most tumors are carcinomas of epithelial origin.	Most common tumors are lymphoma and sarcoma, which are of primitive embryonic origin.
Strong relationship to environmental factors.	Not a strong relation to environmental factors. Genetic factors may be involved.
Routine screening for certain malignancies, such as mammograms for breast cancer is recommended.	Routine screening is not recommended except in cases of known genetic abnormalities associated with a particular childhood malignancy.
Many adult cancers are preventable.	Few preventive strategies known.
Often present with localized disease.	Metastatic disease often present at diagnosis.
Less responsive to treatment.	More responsive to treatment.
Less than a 60% cure rate.	Greater than 70% cure rate.

surgery, chemotherapy, radiation therapy, bone marrow transplantation (BMT), and biological response modifiers (BRM). A combination of these modalities is frequently used (Table 29-2). The type of cancer and the extent of metastasis, known as **stage,** determine the appropriate treatment. Staging is rated from stage I (1), which is localized disease in just one area or organ, to stage IV (4), with disseminated metastatic disease.

Surgery

The goal of surgery in cancer therapy is to remove all visible and microscopic malignant cells when possible. Surgery is used to obtain a biopsy, a sample of the tumor, which is examined microscopically for diagnosis. Surgery also aids in tumor staging by noting the presence and extent of metastatic disease. Later, a "second look" surgical procedure may be performed to assess the response of therapy. Reconstructive surgery corrects defects caused by previous therapy or the tumor itself. Palliative care is given to relieve pain and improve quality of life when cancer treatment is no longer effective. It may include a surgical procedure such as the excision of an abdominal tumor that is causing severe pain and obstruction.

Chemotherapy

Chemotherapy is the most frequently used treatment modality in pediatric oncology and is unique because it is effective for systemic cancers that cannot be managed by surgery or radiation therapy. Dramatic advances in the successful use of multi-agent chemotherapy have increased the rate of survival of many children with cancer. Chemotherapy drugs are classified into six major categories according to their chemical structure. These categories are alkylating agents, antimetabolites, antitumor antibiotics, plant alkaloids, corticosteroids, and miscellaneous agents. Unfortunately, these drugs do not exclusively affect malignant cells, but also affect normal cells that reproduce rapidly such as the intestinal mucosa, blood cells, and hair follicles. Chemotherapy drugs are given in cycles to allow normal cells to recover. The child's disease and treatment regimen determine which drugs are used. The route and method of administration of a particular agent is influenced by the drug's pharmacology, side effects, classification, the child's disease, and the treatment regimen. Routes of administration include intravenous (IV), oral (PO), intramuscular (IM), subcutaneous (SC), intrathecal (IT), and intra-arterial (IA). Table 29-3 lists common chemotherapeutic agents, indications for use, route of administration, and side effects.

Side Effects of Chemotherapy

The hematopoietic, gastrointestinal, hepatic, renal, integumentary, and reproductive systems are most commonly affected by side effects of chemotherapy.

Hematopoietic Effects

The hematopoietic side effects include **myelosuppression** (transient decrease in blood cell production), anemia, thrombocytopenia, **neutropenia** (an abnormal decrease in number of neutrophils or white blood cells), and **immunosuppression** (a condition in which the patient's immune system is functioning at a lower than normal level). The lowest point in the child's blood counts or myelosuppression is called a **nadir** and occurs approximately 10 to 14 days after most chemotherapy is given. If a child becomes anemic while undergoing chemotherapy, red blood cell transfusions

TABLE 29-2 Cancer Treatment Modalities

Modality	Goal	Function
Surgery	Remove all existing cancer cells. Biopsy, excise tumor, decrease tumor burden, provide palliative procedures	Remove existing cancer, provide tissue for identification, provide comfort when cure is not possible
Chemotherapy	Kill all malignant cells and microscopic metastasis	Provide systemic treatment for cancer
Radiation therapy	Kill malignant cells and provide comfort	Eradicate all local tumor cells and provide local control of malignancy for comfort and palliation when cure is not possible
Bone marrow transplantation	Replace bone marrow that has been destroyed by disease or treatment	Provide new hematopoietic system with all its components
Biological response modifiers	Destroy cancer cells, or stimulate specific processes of hematopoiesis	Stimulate immune system to destroy cancer cells or accelerate hematopoiesis

TABLE 29-3 Chemotherapeutic Agents

Agent	Indications	Route	Side Effects
Asparaginase (L-asparaginase, Elspar) *Classification: Enzyme*	• Acute lymphocytic leukemia (ALL)	• IM	• Allergic reactions, from mild urticaria to anaphylaxis. (Have emergency medications with doses available.) • Coagulation abnormalities • Myelosuppression • Hepatotoxicity • Pancreatitis
Azacitidine (5-azacitidine, 5-Aza-C) *Classification: Antimetabolite*	• Acute myelogenous leukemia (AML)	• IV	• Myelosuppression • Nausea, vomiting, diarrhea • Mucositis, skin rash • Fever • Hepatotoxicity
Bleomycin Sulfate (Blenoxane, Bleo) *Classification: Antitumor antibiotic*	• Hodgkin's disease (HD) • Osteosarcoma	• IV • SQ • IM	• Anaphylaxis (rare) • Pulmonary toxicity • Myelosuppression • Nausea, vomiting, anorexia • Hepatotoxicity
Carboplatin (Paraplatin, CBDCA) *Classification: Heavy metal, alkylating-like agent*	• Brain tumors • Soft tissue sarcoma • Osteosarcoma • Retinoblastoma • Neuroblastoma	• IV	• Myelosuppression • Nausea, vomiting, diarrhea • Renal and liver toxicity • Ototoxicity • Alopecia • Neuropathy
Carmustine (BCNU, BiCNU) *Classification: Nitrosourea*	• Brain tumors	• IV	• Myelosuppression (delayed) • Nausea, vomiting • Pain and burning at IV site • Hepatotoxicity • Pulmonary toxicity • Alopecia
Cisplatin (Platinol, platinum, CDDP) *Classification: Heavy metal, alkylating-like agent*	• Brain tumors • Osteosarcoma • Soft tissue sarcoma • Wilms' tumor • Germ cell tumors • Neuroblastoma	• IV	• Myelosuppression • Nausea, vomiting (severe) • Nephrotoxicity with electrolyte wasting (Mg, Ca) • Ototoxicity • Peripheral neuropathies • Allergic reactions (rare)
Corticosteroids (Prednisone, dexamethasone, hydrocortisone, methylprednisolone) *Classification: Corticosteroids*	• ALL • Non-Hodgkin's lymphoma (NHL) • HD • Cerebral edema • Nausea and vomiting	• PO • IV • IT	• Immunosuppression • Weight gain • Acne, hirsutism, striae • Osteoporosis, growth delay • Cushinoid features • Hypertension • Diabetes • Pancreatitis • Mood swings

continues

TABLE 29-3 *Continued*

Agent	Indications	Route	Side Effects
Cyclophosphamide (Cytoxan, CTX, CPM) *Classification: Alkylating agent*	• NHL • HD • ALL • Neuroblastoma • Wilms' tumor • Bone and soft tissue sarcomas • Retinoblastoma	• IV • PO	• Myelosuppression • Nausea, vomiting, anorexia, and diarrhea • Hepatotoxicity • Hemorrhagic or non-hemorrhagic cystitis • Alopecia • Sterility • Syndrome of inappropriate anti-diuretic hormone (SIADH) • Cardiac toxicity (rare) • May cause second neoplasm
Cytarabine (Ara-C, Cytosine arabinoside, Cytosar-U) *Classification: Antimetabolite*	• AML • ALL • CNS leukemia	• IV • SQ • IT	• Myelosuppression • Nausea, vomiting, diarrhea • Hepatotoxicity • Fever and malaise • Alopecia, rash • Conjunctivitis • Stomatitis • Neurotoxicity
Dacarbazine (DTIC-Dome, DIC) *Classification: Alkylating agent*	• HD • Soft tissue sarcoma	• IV	• Myelosuppression • Nausea and vomiting • Venous irritant • May cause second neoplasm
Dactinomycin (Actinomycin D, Act-D, Cosmegen) *Classification: Antitumor antibiotic*	• Wilms' tumor • Soft tissue sarcoma • Ewing's sarcoma • Retinoblastoma	• IV	• Vesicant • Myelosuppression • Nausea and vomiting • Potentiation of radiation • Alopecia • Stomatitis
Daunorubicin (Daunomycin, Cerubidine) *Classification: Anthracycline antibiotic*	• ALL • AML • Osteosarcoma • Soft tissue sarcoma	• IV	• Vesicant • Myelosuppression • Cardiotoxicity, arrhythmias—acute, cardiomyopathy—delayed • Nausea, vomiting, stomatitis • Potentiation of radiation • Alopecia, rash, hyperpigmentation of nails
Doxorubicin (Adriamycin, Adria, DOX) *Classification: Anthracycline antibiotic*	• ALL • AML • Osteosarcoma • Soft tissue sarcoma • Neuroblastoma	• IV • IA	• Vesicant • Myelosuppression • Cardiotoxicity, arrhythmias—acute, cardiomyopathy—delayed • Nausea, vomiting, stomatitis • Potentiation of radiation • Alopecia, rash, hyperpigmentation of nails

continues

TABLE 29-3 *Continued*

Agent	Indications	Route	Side Effects
Etoposide (VP-16, VePesid) *Classification: Plant alkaloid*	• AML • NHL • HD • Bone and soft tissue sarcoma • ALL • Wilms' tumor • Brain tumors • Neuroblastoma • Retinoblastoma	• IV • PO	• Myelosuppression • Hypotension • Hypersensitivity reactions • Nausea, vomiting • Alopecia
Fluorouracil (5-FU, Adrucil) *Classification: Antimetabolite*	• Brain tumors • Germ cell tumors	• IV • PO	• Myelosuppression • Nausea, vomiting (mild) • Mucositis (severe) • Hyperpigmentation of nails • Dermatitis
Hydroxyurea (Hydrea, HU) *Classification: Antimetabolite*	• ALL and AML with high blast counts	• PO	• Myelosuppression • Nausea, vomiting • Stomatitis (rare)
Idarubicin (Idamycin, IDA) *Classification: Anthracycline antibiotic*	• ALL • AML	• IV	• Vesicant • See Doxorubicin
Ifosfamide (IFEX) *Classification: Alkylating agent*	• Osteosarcoma • Soft tissue sarcoma • NHL • ALL	• IV	• Mylosuppression • Nausea, vomiting, diarrhea • Neurotoxicity (encephalopathy, peripheral neuropathy) • Hepatotoxicity • Hemorrhagic cystitis • Renal tubular damage • Alopecia • Sterility potential • May cause second neoplasm
Lomustine (CCNU, CeeNU) *Classification: Alkylating agent*	• Brain tumors • HD	• PO	• Myelosuppression (severe and delayed) • Nausea, vomiting • Neurotoxicity (confusion, ataxia, and lethargy)
Mechlorethamine (nitrogen mustard, Mustargen, NH2) *Classification: Alkylating agent*	• HD	• IV	• Vesicant • Myelosuppression • Nausea, vomiting (severe) • Sterility potential • Pain and phlebitis at IV site • May cause second neoplasm

continues

TABLE 29-3 *Continued*

Agent	Indications	Route	Side Effects
Mercaptopurine (6-MP, Purinethol) *Classification: Antimetabolite*	• ALL • NHL • AML	• PO • IV	• Myelosuppression (mild) • Nausea, vomiting (mild) • Anorexia • Hepatotoxicity • Stomatitis
Methotrexate (MTX, Amethopterin) *Classification: Antimetabolite*	• ALL • Osteosarcoma • NHL	• IV • PO • IM • IT	• Myelosuppression • Nausea, vomiting, stomatitis • Alopecia • Hepatotoxicity • Neurotoxicity • Photosensitivity • Rash
Procarbazine (Matulane) *Classification: Alkylating agent*	• HD • NHL • Brain tumors	• PO	• Myelosuppression • Nausea, vomiting, stomatitis • Alopecia, pruritus, rash • CNS toxicity • Sterility potential • May cause second neoplasm
Tenoposide (VM-26) *Classification: Plant alkaloid*	• ALL • Neuroblastoma	• IV	• Myelosuppression • Hypotension • Nausea, vomiting, mucositis • Alopecia • Hypersensitivity reactions • May cause secondary leukemia
Thioguanine (6-TG, Tabloid) *Classification: Antimetabolite*	• ALL • AML	• PO	• Myelosuppression • Nausea, vomiting (mild) • Anorexia, stomatitis • Hepatotoxicity
Topotecan *Classification: Topoisomerase inhibitor*	• Soft tissue sarcoma • Osteosarcoma • Neuroblastoma	• IV	• Myelosuppression • Nausea, vomiting (mild) • Alopecia
Vinblastine (Velban, VLB) *Classification: Plant alkaloid*	• HD	• IV	• Vesicant • Peripheral neuropathy • Alopecia • Constipation • SIADH (rare)
Vincristine (Oncovin, VCR) *Classification: Plant alkaloid*	• ALL • HD • Wilms' tumor • Ewing's sarcoma • Brain tumor	• IV	• Vesicant • Peripheral neuropathy • Alopecia • Constipation • SIADH (rare) • Seizure (rare)

Nursing Alert:

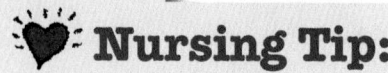

Aspirin, Aspirin-Containing Products, and NSAIDs (non-steroidal anti-inflammatory drugs)

These products are not to be given to a child receiving chemotherapy because they interfere with normal platelet function. While on chemotherapy, a child is at increased risk of developing thrombocytopenia so the function of the circulating platelets should not be further compromised.

Nursing Tip:

Neutropenic children may not show signs of infection

Children who are neutropenic will not mount an immune response to infection. They may not show signs of inflammation such as redness or the production of pus because they lack the neutrophils to do so. Some will complain of pain and swelling in the area. These symptoms are to be considered indicative of infection and should be treated promptly.

may be given. The caregivers and child should be told when to expect anemia and taught to recognize pallor, fatigue, and headache. Thrombocytopenia results in a decrease in the number of platelets, and if low, the child is at risk of bleeding. A platelet count of 50,000/mm^3 is associated with only a slight risk of bleeding, while a platelet count of less than 20,000 poses a higher risk of spontaneous bleeding. Common sites of bleeding include the skin, oral mucosa, eyes, and nose. Intracranial and visceral bleeding, although uncommon, can be life-threatening. When IM injections or venipunctures are necessary in the thrombocytopenic child, the sites require the application of direct pressure for 10 minutes to prevent bleeding. Caregivers are taught to look for signs of thrombocytopenia (easy bruising, petechiae, and purpura) and instructed when to notify the health care provider. If the platelet count is very low or if there is active bleeding, a platelet transfusion may be ordered. Children should be inspected daily for signs of bleeding. Those with low platelet counts are to be protected from trauma. Prevention measures include instructing the child and caregiver to avoid playing or engaging in any contact sports or activity that has a risk of physical injury such as roller skating or riding a bicycle. Menstruating girls who have prolonged or heavy periods may require oral contraceptives to control the vaginal bleeding.

When the neutrophil level is low the child has neutropenia and is at risk for serious life-threatening bacterial infections. To determine the severity of neutropenia a calculation is made to determine the absolute neutrophil count (ANC). The ANC is the percentage of polys and bands times the total white blood cell count (WBC) and is computed using the following formula: ANC = (% polys + % bands) × WBC. A child with an ANC of 500/mm^3 or less is at risk for serious life-threatening bacterial infections, which are usually caused by normal body flora. Infection in the neutropenic child can quickly progress to septic shock and death. Handwashing is the cornerstone of infection prevention and control (Nenstiel, White, & Aikins, 1997). When a child is neutropenic any signs of infection must be treated emergently. All children with fever and neutropenia are to have a septic work-up that includes peripheral and venous access device (VAD) blood cultures, a chest X ray, and urine and wound cultures. If the fever does not subside with IV antibiotics and if the causative organism has not been isolated, it may be necessary to start an antifungal agent. This protects the child, as fungal organisms are slow to grow in culture medium and isolate. Invasive procedures should be avoided when possible. These include rectal temperatures, and use of suppositories and urinary catheters. Infectious organisms can be introduced through the mucosal lining of these areas.

The child's immune system is suppressed (immunosuppression) and not able to respond or mount a response because of lack of lymphocytes. Management of the immunosuppressed child includes prevention and prompt treatment of infections. Also, exposure to viral diseases such as varicella (chickenpox) and measles is to be avoided if possible.

Gastrointestinal Effects

Gastrointestinal (GI) side effects are common. **Mucositis,** also called stomatitis, is an inflammation of the oral mucosa

Nursing Alert:

Varicella (Chicken pox)

Caregivers should be taught that varicella can be an overwhelming infection in the immunosuppressed child, and exposure is to be avoided, if at all possible. If the child is exposed, caregivers need to notify the health care provider and seek prompt treatment with a varicella immune globulin within 72 hours of exposure as a preventive measure. Children who present with an active case of varicella will receive antiviral therapy. It is recommended that healthy siblings of an immunosuppressed child who have not had varicella receive the vaccine (Friebert & Shurin, 1998). If the vaccinated sibling develops a rash, the individual should avoid contact with the child with cancer until the rash is no longer present. The goal is to prevent widespread dissemination of the virus to the lungs, liver, or central nervous system.

Nursing Alert:

Live Viral Vaccines

Oral poliovirus vaccine (OPV) and measles, mumps, and rubella (MMR) are live viral vaccines. Immunosuppressed children are not given these vaccines because they cannot mount an immune response to the vaccine and may be at risk of developing the actual disease. Household contacts of the child should receive inactivated poliovirus vaccine (IPV), because after OPV is given, the immunized person will shed live inactive poliovirus in their stool for a period of up to three months. If a household contact receives an OPV unknowingly, the child and caregiver must practice good handwashing after bowel movements or diaper changes. Household contacts may receive MMR either in combination or separately (U.S. Department of Health and Human Services, 1998).

that ranges from mild redness to severe painful ulceration. The entire gastrointestinal tract can be affected. Mucositis is one of the most difficult and painful side effects of cancer therapy, and usually presents several days after the administration of chemotherapy. The primary management is good oral care, which includes using a cleansing solution such as warm water or chlorhexidine to clean and rinse the oral cavity of food particles and debris several times a day, particularly after meals. Gentle cleansing with oral sponges or ultra-soft toothbrushes may be necessary to minimize pain and to prevent further trauma to the oral mucosa. Painful mouth lesions may cause a decrease in oral intake and lead to dehydration, poor nutrition, and weight loss.

Other GI side effects are nausea and vomiting, which may range from mild nausea to severe vomiting. Some children experience anticipatory vomiting, which occurs when the child associates a certain situation with chemotherapy and vomiting, such as riding to the hospital or entering the

Research Highlight

Mucositis

Study Purpose

The purpose of this research study was to compare the effectiveness of oral care done with sterile water versus chlorhexidine in preventing mucositis. There are several solutions commercially available for mouth care. Chlorhexidine is widely used but costs approximately $20.00 per pint. The cost to clients would be markedly reduced if sterile water for oral care is found to be as effective in preventing chemotherapy-induced mucositis.

Methods

Two hundred clients receiving mucositis-inducing chemotherapy were evaluated over three courses of chemotherapy. They were randomly assigned to use a mouthwash of sterile water or chlorhexidine prior to the onset of mucositis. An oral assessment guide was used to evaluate their oral cavities on a monthly basis, with each chemotherapy cycle, and when oral symptoms occurred between cycles. The assessment guide used parameters of voice, ability to swallow, lips, tongue, saliva, mucous membranes, gingiva, and teeth for clinical ratings. Data for the two solutions were compared.

Findings

There were no significant differences between the two mouthwashes.

Implications

Oral care with sterile water is cost efficient and may be as effective in preventing mucositis as chlorhexidine. Nurses should encourage use of sterile water in clients receiving chemotherapy.

Citation

Dodd, M.J., Larson, P.J., Dibble, S.L., Miaskowski, C., Greespan, D., MacPhail, L., Hauck, W.W., Paul, S.M., Ignoffo, R., & Shiba, G. (1996). Randomized clinical trial of chlorhexidine versus placebo for prevention of oral mucositis in patients receiving chemotherapy. *Oncology Nursing Forum 26*(6), 921–927.

outpatient clinic. Prolonged nausea, vomiting, and anorexia can lead to significant weight loss and weakness, which can further compromise the child's immune status. The administration of antiemetics and nonpharmacologic interventions can help to control the nausea and vomiting. Maintaining adequate hydration and monitoring fluids and electrolytes is necessary in children with severe nausea and vomiting. Nonpharmacologic interventions to reduce nausea and vomiting include relaxation, biofeedback, and distraction. Music therapy has also been shown to be effective (Potter & Schafer, 1999).

Hepatic Effects

Liver toxicity seen with different chemotherapeutic agents ranges from the elevation of hepatic enzymes to liver fibrosis caused by long-term use of these drugs. Periodic monitoring of hepatic function allows for the adjustment of liver toxic chemotherapeutic agents to prevent severe long-term liver damage. A liver function evaluation is performed routinely by examining liver transaminases and bilirubin levels prior to chemotherapy administration. The nurse, prior to administering the chemotherapy, must check the results and notify the health care provider of any abnormal findings. High transaminases and bilirubin may require a dose reduction adjustment or postponement of the chemotherapeutic agent.

Renal Effects

Various chemotherapeutic agents, especially high dose methotrexate and cisplatin, can cause significant renal toxicity. Renal toxicity will be manifest as an increase in blood urea nitrogen (BUN) and serum creatinine and decrease in urine creatinine clearance. Factors that compound renal toxicity include the use of certain antibiotics, anti-fungal agents, and radiation to the kidney area. Children receiving cytoxan and ifosfamide are at risk for **hemorrhagic cystitis** (abnormal bleeding of the bladder), which may occur during the administration of the agent or months after. To prevent stasis of the end products of these drugs, the child must be well hydrated and encouraged to void every two hours during and after the drug is given. Continued periodic urine examination for blood is recommended because it may occur months after the drug is given. Kidney function is also determined by the client's ability to handle body fluids; therefore, monitoring intake and output is essential. A discrepancy in intake and output must be reported as this may be the first indication of renal toxicity.

Integumentary Effects

Alopecia or hair loss is often the side effect most associated with cancer treatment, but not all children undergoing chemotherapy will lose their hair. When it does occur it can be devastating to the child and family. Hair loss from chemotherapy is not permanent, and re-growth often starts while the child is still receiving treatment. Children less than 5 years of age are not as concerned with hair loss as an adolescent whose body image and peer acceptance are of utmost importance. If the child requests a wig, arrangements for the purchase should be done prior to the alopecia. Many young children are bothered by wigs and prefer to use scarves and hats or to wear nothing at all. All children experiencing alopecia should protect their heads from sunburn or cold weather (Figures 29-2, 29-3, and 29-4).

Some chemotherapy drugs (daunomycin and vincristine) are **vesicants** or skin irritants and cause discomfort with the

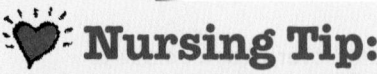

> **Nursing Tip:**
>
> **Nausea and vomiting**
>
> Giving chemotherapy at bedtime may alleviate nausea and vomiting in children. It may allow them to sleep through the emetic effects. Playing soft music, such as lullabies, or recording a caregiver singing soft songs is soothing and distracting and may alleviate symptoms of nausea and vomiting.

> **Nursing Alert:**
>
> **Nothing by Rectum**
>
> *Giving rectal medications, taking a rectal temperature, or performing a rectal examination can lead to breaks in the rectal mucosa, allowing bacteria into the bloodstream, which may lead to sepsis or a rectal abscess. Children undergoing chemotherapy have fragile intestinal mucosa and are not to receive anything per rectum.*

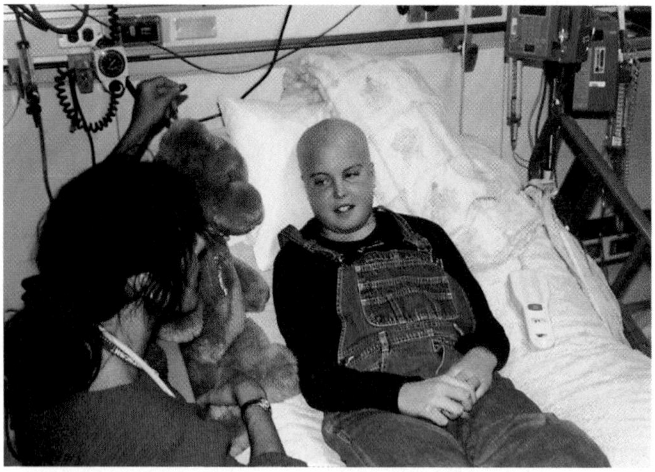

Figure 29-2 Alopecia is a common side effect of chemotherapy and a threat to body image, especially for the older child.

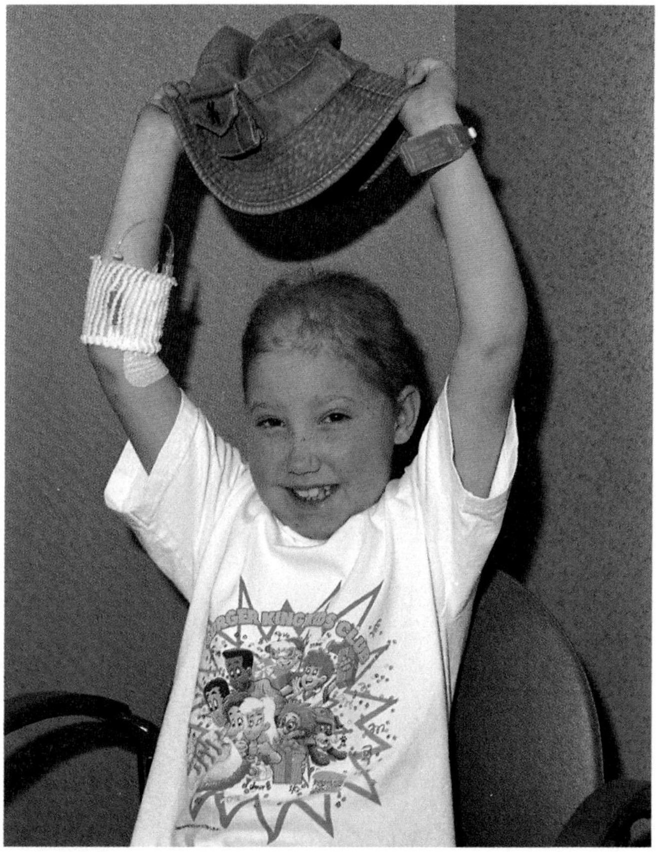

Figure 29-3 Regrowth of hair often begins when the child is still receiving chemotherapy.

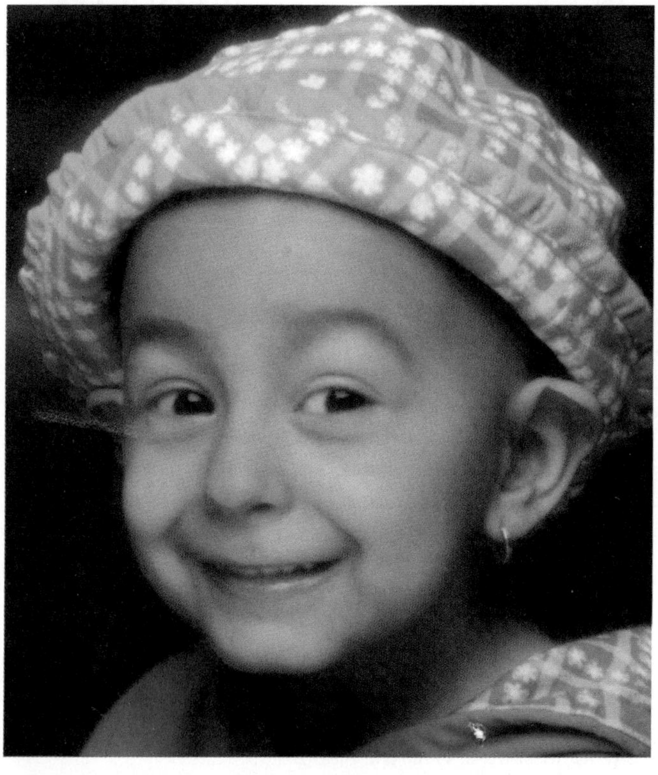

Figure 29-4 Children with alopecia must protect their heads from cold weather and sunburn.

Kids Want To Know

Will I lose my hair, and if so, when will it grow back?

A 12-year-old girl recently diagnosed with osteogenic sarcoma is admitted for her first course of chemotherapy. She says to you, "I know I need this chemotherapy to fight the tumor in my leg, but I really think it's awful that my hair is going to fall out. Will it fall out as soon as I get the chemotherapy?" This girl's worry about her appearance is a real concern. The nurse should explain that her hair will probably start to fall out in ten days to two weeks. The hair will come out over several days and it can be messy. Some clients cut the hair short to prevent this. When the chemotherapy is complete, the hair will grow back. The nurse should advise the girl of the options available (wig, hat, scarf, nothing). Emphasis should be on personal choice. Speaking with another girl of the same age who has also lost her hair may be helpful.

Nursing Tip:

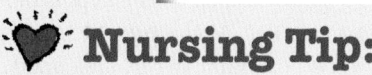

Coping with alopecia
Role-play with the child as to what to say when someone asks, "What happened to your hair?" Children returning to school have many anxieties regarding their acceptance back into their peer group because of the many changes in their appearance. This activity helps to develop coping strategies to deal with alopecia. A school visit from the oncology team nurse to speak with the child's teacher and classmates can help the transition back to school.

sensation of burning, redness, and inflammation if they **extravasate** or leak out of the vein during administration. Vesicants cause a skin reaction that may range from a slight hyperpigmentation at the area of extravasation to a severe burn leading to loss of function and mobility of the extremity where the drug was given. To prevent extravasation, the nurse should assure venous patency prior to the administration of a chemotherapeutic agent. A free-flowing intravenous access with a blood return should be present. Venous blood return is checked during the infusion, and if there is a loss of blood return, the infusion is stopped immediately, and any residual medication is aspirated to reduce the extent of extravasation. Vesicants are not to be administered over joints, bony prominences, in the anticubital fossa, or above tendons, as extravasation damage in these areas can affect limb function.

Reproductive Effects

The reproductive system is also adversely affected by chemotherapy. Most children have normal pubertal development, but fertility may still be affected. Prepubertal girls may have delayed pubertal development, and girls who have already started menstruating may develop **oligomenorrhea** (abnormally light or reduction in menstruation), amenorrhea, excessive bleeding, or menopausal symptoms. The effect of cancer treatment on male fertility is more severe than on female fertility. Sterility may result from the use of alkylating agents, which have a dramatic effect on spermatogenesis. A decrease in spermatogenesis may be reversible in months or years after completion of chemotherapy, but sterility is frequently permanent. The increased risk of infection during neutropenic episodes poses additional potential problems. Condoms should be used to reduce the risk of infection and also to prevent pregnancy. Oral contraceptive pills are sometimes ordered to control excessive menstrual bleeding. The adolescent female should be instructed to use sanitary pads instead of tampons to reduce the risk of trauma and infection. Sexually mature males can be offered the option of sperm banking if they are well enough prior to initiating chemotherapy. This is to be done as expeditiously as possible in order to not delay cancer treatment. At the present time egg banking for adolescent girls is not routinely recommended. If puberty is delayed, it may be managed with hormonal therapy in both males and females.

Venous Access Devices

The most frequent route of delivery of antineoplastic drugs is IV, which is also one of the most difficult in children. Venipuncture is painful and disturbing for children who may not have a full understanding of the importance of cancer therapy. Hundreds of venipuctures may be needed during the course of cancer treatment. For therapeutic as well as psychological reasons, most children will have a **venous access device** (VAD), which is a catheter that is usually inserted into the superior vena cava (Figure 29-5). It is utilized for chemotherapeutic drug delivery, blood sampling and blood product administration, intravenous fluids, medications, and total parenteral nutrition (TPN). The most common devices used with children are external catheters (i.e., Broviac, Hickman, Groshong), and implanted ports (i.e., Port-A-Cath, Infusaport). An external catheter requires exit site care and frequent flushing of a heparinized saline solution to maintain patency. Implanted ports are accessed with a special non-boring needle and require monthly flushing when not used more frequently. There are no restrictions on the child's activities such as swimming with ports. Complications of VADs include increased risk of infection, occlusion with fibrin sheath formation, and dislodgment.

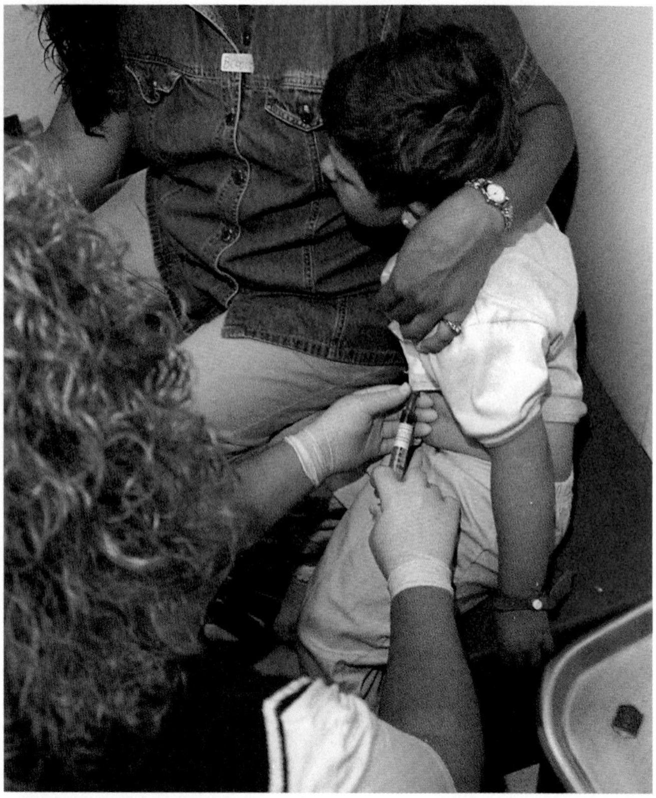

Figure 29-5 Child Receiving Chemotherapy Via VAD

Kids Want To Know

How will the other students react to my VAD?

A 17-year-old high school student is undergoing chemotherapy and has an external venous access device. While the adolescent appreciates the device and the ease it provides for blood drawing, and administration of medications and blood products, she is very concerned about returning to school with the device. "What if someone notices it? What if someone bumps into me? What if someone pulls it?" Unlike hair loss, a central venous access device is for the most part unnoticeable. It still is a constant reminder of the diagnosis, and a feature that makes the adolescent stand out as different from his or her peers. It is important to stress that a central venous device is unnoticeable when covered by clothing and would not be pulled by an unknowing person. Trauma to the device is unlikely, because of its location on the upper chest wall. Stress the importance of continuing school and maintaining friendships. Meeting another adolescent who has had a VAD will also help.

Fibrin sheath formation requires the use of a fibrinolytic agent to restore patency. A dislodged device must be surgically repaired or replaced. Figures 29-6 and 29-7 illustrate an external catheter and an implanted port, respectively.

Teaching the family to care for a VAD begins before it is surgically placed. Implanted devices require no home care once the initial incision from placement is healed. External catheters require more care. Daily assessment for signs of infection at the exit site, such as drainage, redness, or pain, is needed. To maintain patency, the catheter is flushed daily with a heparinized solution. Sterile dressing changes of the catheter site and change of catheter injection caps need to be done on a schedule. The caregiver must be instructed to

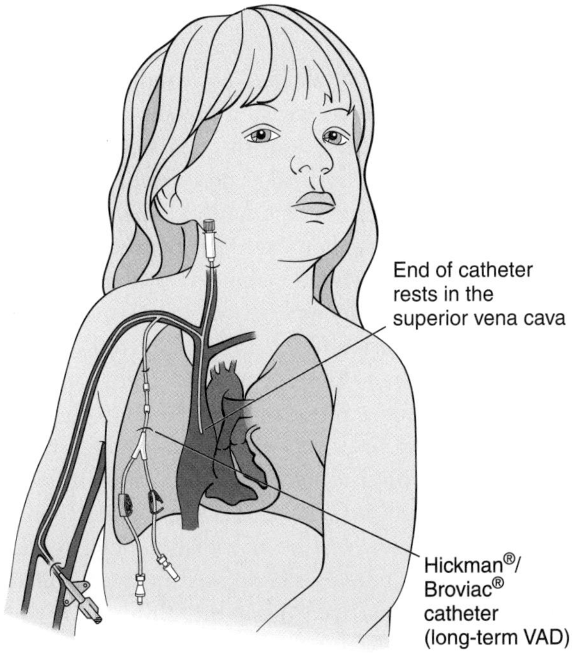

Figure 29-6a External catheters allow chemotherapy, IV medications, and TPN to be administered without piercing the child's skin with a needle.

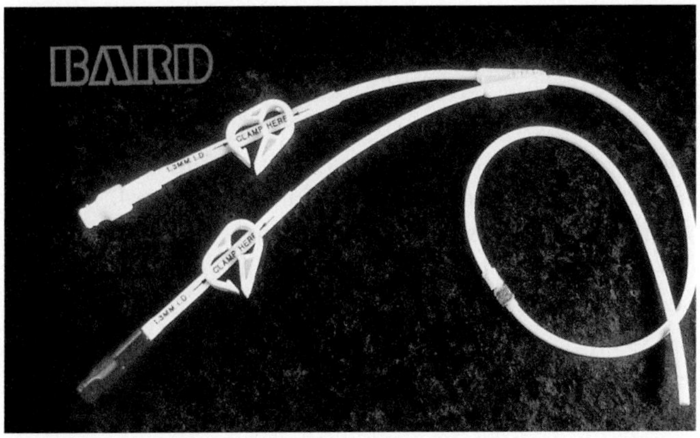

Figure 29-6b Hickman® Dual Lumen. Courtesy of Sims Deltec, Inc., St. Paul, Minnesota.

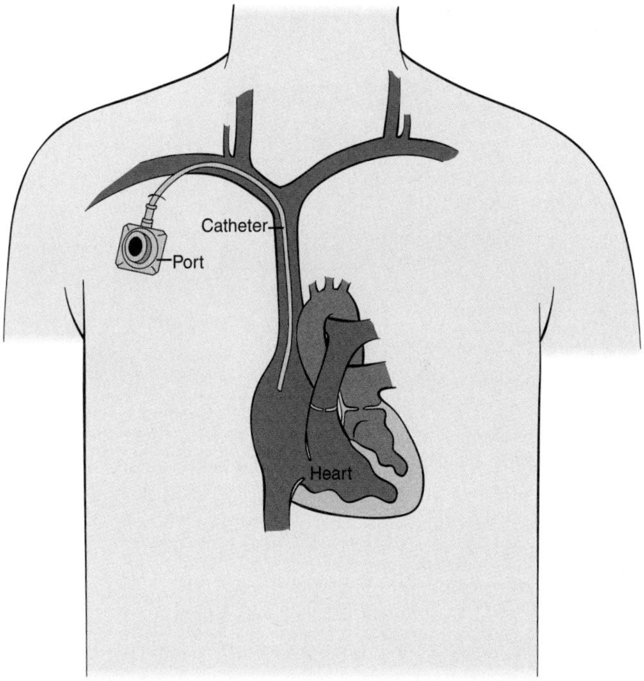

Figure 29-7 An implanted port is surgically inserted under the skin, and the catheter tip is frequently placed in superior vena cava for long-term chemotherapy administration.

Nursing Alert:

Safe Handling of Chemotherapy

Many chemotherapeutic agents have been found to be carcinogenic, mutagenic, and tetratogenic in animals, although further research is needed to determine the implications to human exposure. Nurses can be exposed to these agents through inhalation, absorption, or ingestion, while mixing, administering, or handling the body excreta of the client. Precautions must be taken for 48 hours after single-agent chemotherapy and 5 days after multi-agent chemotherapy. The Occupational Safety and Health Administration (OSHA) has developed guidelines to protect workers. Guidelines include the use of an airflow hood while mixing chemotherapy, and the use of protective gowns, gloves, masks, and eyeshields when handling the agents or excreta. All equipment and linen contaminated with chemotherapy waste must be disposed of in labeled, sealed containers (Goodman & Riley, 1997). The nurse is responsible to follow the guidelines found in the policy and procedure manual of his/her institution, and must also teach caregivers safe handling procedures (Figure 29-8).

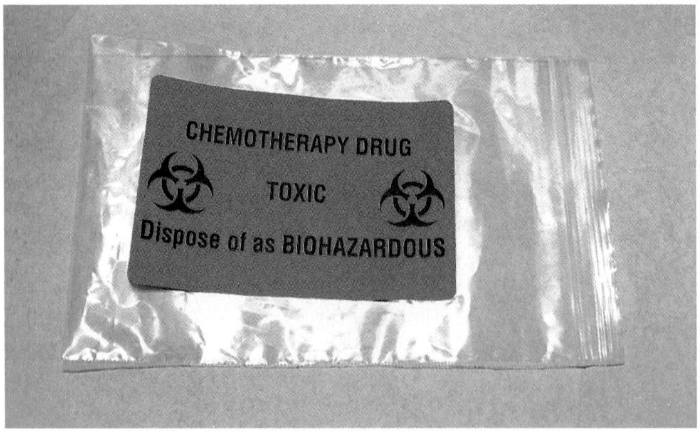

Figure 29-8 Equipment that has contained chemotherapy drugs is considered hazardous waste and should be disposed of in designated containers that are properly labeled.

Family Teaching

Chemotherapy

- Teach the child and family the chemotherapeutic regimen. Include the drug's side effects and reasons to notify the medical team, such as signs of an infection.
- Using the child's protocol roadmap as a guide, write a calendar of daily medications, clinic visits, admissions, lab tests, radiographic studies, and procedures. Update the calendar as needed.
- Familiarize the family with routine CBC results. Teach caregivers to calculate the ANC and to understand the consequences of being neutropenic.
- Teach the caregivers how to care for the child's VAD. Provide written instruction. Set up a visit from a home care nurse to reinforce home care of the VAD and reassure caregivers.
- Indicate telephone numbers to call for questions or concerns.
- Provide the school with information regarding the return to school of the child who is receiving chemotherapy. Offer a school visit to facilitate the re-entry.
- Provide instructions in writing to the school nurse and teacher regarding infection precautions, exposure to communicable diseases, and bleeding precautions.
- Give caregivers information regarding support groups such as Candlelighters.

notify the health care provider if the child has a fever or signs of infection. The inability to flush the catheter with ease may be caused by a catheter malposition, anatomical obstruction, or the formation of a fibrin sheath. The caregiver must be instructed not to force flush the catheter at any time and to call should any problems with flushing exist. Consistency of catheter care methods between the hospital and home is essential to avoid confusion and anxiety in the child and caregiver.

Radiation Therapy

Radiation therapy is used to deliver a therapeutic dose of ionizing radiation to a tumor with minimal effects to the healthy surrounding tissue. It is the primary treatment for several pediatric malignancies such as lymphomas, solid tumors, and brain tumors. Radiation therapy can also be given for pain control as a part of palliative care in terminally ill clients in which it is used to enhance the quality of remaining life.

Radiation therapy is delivered by several methods: fractionation, hyperfractionation, stereotactic, and total body irradiation. With fractionation, the conventional method, radiation is given daily in divided doses until the total prescribed dose is delivered. This method spares damage to normal tissues, allowing them to repair between doses (Lew & LaVally, 1995). Hyperfractionation is the delivery of radiation in smaller doses, divided two or three times a day, to give a higher total dose and to further reduce the effects to the surrounding tissue. Another method, stereotactic radiation therapy, is effective on small distinct tumors that are not surgically accessible or as a boost to conventional radiation therapy. In this method a single dose of radiation is delivered with pinpoint accuracy (Lew & LaVally, 1995). Total body irradiation (TBI) is external beam radiation delivered to the whole body in preparation for bone marrow transplantation.

At each radiation treatment the child must remain immobile on a hard flat surface. This may be uncomfortable for the 10–15 minutes it takes for the preparation, positioning, and delivery of the treatment. The actual treatment is quite quick. Depending upon the developmental level of the child, sedation or anesthesia may be necessary to complete the treatments. Immobilization devices such as plastic casts and molds are often necessary for children, so that accurate delivery of the treatment can be accomplished.

Nursing care of the child undergoing radiation therapy involves teaching about the process and its effects on the child. Children and caregivers need to know that radiation therapy is not painful, yet it may be frightening to the child and caregiver. Pre-radiation teaching and role-playing decrease the child's anxiety and promote more cooperation. Caregivers need to know the daily time schedule and any sedation/anesthesia protocol, if used.

Side Effects of Radiation Therapy

Children who are receiving radiation to large bones, such as the pelvis, cranium, and spine, may show signs of anemia, thrombocytopenia, and neutropenia caused by the effects of ionizing radiation on the blood producing bone marrow. Ionizing radiation suppresses the bone marrow and causes a drop in all blood cell lines. Care of the child with these hematopoietic effects is addressed in the chemotherapy section of this chapter.

Radiation therapy delivered to the head and neck area will cause an alteration of the oral mucosa. The epithelial cells of the mouth are very sensitive to ionizing radiation, leading to mucositis after the start of therapy. **Xerostomia,** or dryness of the mouth, occurs from a decreased or arrested production of salivary secretions. Pain, teeth sensitivity, and difficulty speaking may accompany this dryness. Mouth care is essential to promote comfort, prevent infection, and provide lubrication to the mucosa. Nurses should offer relief by encouraging fluids, sucking hard candy, or chewing sugarless gum to stimulate saliva production. Continued use of fluorinated water and toothpaste can help prevent caries caused from a decrease in saliva production. Esophagitis is caused by radiation to the chest and upper back area. A burning pain behind the sternum is a common complaint. Regurgitation and indigestion may accompany this side effect. Milk and milk products frequently can relieve this discomfort, but medication is sometimes necessary. Radiation to the abdomen, pelvis, or lower back may cause nausea, vomiting, and diarrhea, which may be alleviated by the use of antiemetics and antidiarrheal agents. Weight should be monitored frequently, and a loss greater than 10% is an indication for parenteral nutrition to maintain the child's nutritional needs until the effects of radiation subside.

Skin in the radiated field may exhibit changes such as dryness, erythema, or pruritus. More serious reactions with skin breakdown and desquamation may warrant a delay in treatments. Skin care is to be given daily with a mild soap with care not to wash off any skin markings made by the radiation oncologist, which identify the treatment field. Friction, tight clothing, hot water, tape, and strong soaps should be avoided because they can contribute to skin breakdown. The use of creams, lotions, or deodorants should be discussed with the radiation oncologist. All children are to avoid sun exposure in the treatment area because radiated skin may burn more easily. Moist desquamated skin requires a culture of the wound, and further skin care may be ordered by the radiologist. Good nutrition and hydration are important to maintain skin integrity, healing, and recovery.

Radiation to the scalp produces alopecia that may be permanent. The child and caregivers should be made aware of this and encouraged to obtain appropriate head coverings. A warm head covering is important during the colder months to prevent heat loss, and coverings are also necessary to prevent sunburn.

Radiation pneumonitis is an acute reaction caused by the swelling and sloughing of the endothelial cells of the small vessels of the lung, which allows fluid to accumulate in the interstitial tissues. Signs and symptoms include tachypnea, orthopnea, a dry cough, and respiratory difficulty. Radiation pneumonitis can be a serious condition that may lead to a hospital admission and at times mechanical ventilation. Caregivers need to seek medical attention if their child shows any signs of respiratory difficulty.

Whole-brain radiation can cause acute, subacute, and delayed toxicity. Acute toxicity occurs during or shortly after radiation and is caused by inflammation, edema, and increased intracranial pressure. Headache, nausea, and vomiting are common signs and symptoms of acute toxicity. Subacute toxicity is seen 5 to 7 weeks after radiation and resolves within 1 to 3 weeks. This is called **somnolence syndrome.** Children will experience drowsiness and may sleep up to 20 hours a day. Nausea and malaise frequently accompany this sleepiness, and fever, dysphasia, ataxia, and transient **papilledema,** an inflammation of the optic disk, may also occur.

Caregivers and the child may view the nausea, vomiting, and headache of acute neurological toxicity as a tumor recurrence or progression, and must be reassured that it is a side effect of the radiation treatment. Steroids may be prescribed

Family Teaching

Radiation Therapy

- Provide the caregiver with a daily schedule of appointments and sedation or anesthesia instructions. Written literature about radiation therapy is helpful and provides the caregiver the opportunity to review the details of treatment at their own pace, and to ask questions at a later time.
- Teach the child and family about acute side effects and their management.
- Provide specific instructions about the amount of fluid intake that is adequate.
- Provide instructions about when and how to contact the medical team if side effects or concerns occur.
- Plan a school visit or phone call to facilitate the child's school re-entry. A school visit will assure school staff and classmates that the child is not radioactive and no radiation precautions are necessary for children who has undergone external beam radiation therapy.
- Help to schedule the radiation treatment later in the day, so the child can continue to go to school in the morning.
- Provide written guidance for teachers and the school nurse, so they know when to contact the child's caregiver should an acute side effect occur.
- Refer the family and child to appropriate support groups such as the Childhood Brain Tumor Foundation.

to reduce the swelling and pressure on the brain and thereby alleviate the symptoms. The child and caregivers must also be prepared for somnolence syndrome because the symptoms can be very worrisome. The family often fears that there has been a recurrence. Repeated reassurance that somnolence syndrome will resolve is helpful, but occasionally imaging studies are performed to assure the child and family that there has not been a relapse.

Radiation to the bones, soft tissue, and blood vessel areas of a growing child will affect growth in the treated area. Effects of radiation include impaired growth of bone and soft tissue resulting in an asymmetry as the child grows. Children who are most susceptible are those less than 6 years of age or undergoing pubertal growth spurts. These bones are also susceptible to fractures and recurrent tumors later in life. Teaching to protect the affected bones from trauma must be repeated, even when the child's therapy has been completed.

Bone Marrow Transplantation

Bone marrow transplantation (BMT) is the replacement of hematopoietic stem cells into a person whose own bone marrow has been destroyed by disease or by the treatment of a malignant disease (Yeaney, 1995). In cancer therapy the use of bone marrow transplant has become increasingly accepted as treatment for leukemia, lymphoma, and certain solid tumors. See Table 29-4, which describes different types of bone marrow transplant.

For all types of BMT, except autologous, donor marrow must be found. A suitable donor is one whose tissue type closely matches the client's. Genetic markers on the surface of white blood cells, called human lymphocyte antigens (HLA), define a person's tissue type. These antigens are proteins that play a critical role in protecting the body against invading organisms such as bacteria, viruses, and other foreign matter. These HLA markers are inherited, so siblings are more likely to be compatible donors. If a donor must be located in the general population, the chances of finding a HLA match range from one in a thousand to one in several million, depending on the frequency of the child's tissue type in the general population (Stewart, 1995). There are several bone marrow registries in the United States with the HLA tissue types of people who are willing to donate bone marrow.

> ### Eye On:
> **Ethnic Minorities and Bone Marrow Donors**
>
> Not all clients who may benefit from a bone marrow transplant have a suitable donor. Children who are from minority racial or ethnic backgrounds have more difficulty finding suitable donors because minority groups are not well represented in the donor registries. Nursing efforts must concentrate on recruiting minority donors.

Bone marrow transplantation consists of three phases: 1) pre-transplant, 2) transplant, and 3) post-transplant. The pre-transplant phase involves thorough evaluation and testing of the child and donor to assure both are physically capable of undergoing transplant. The donor must also undergo several tests to assure that the individual is free of infectious diseases such as hepatitis or HIV.

During the transplant phase, the **cytoreduction** or conditioning regimen is initiated. Lethal doses of chemotherapy, often combined with radiation, are used to eradicate all malignant cells and to suppress the child's immune system to prevent rejection of the transplanted marrow. Cytoreduction therapy induces a profound and prolonged decrease in the production of blood cells. The toxicity associated with cytoreduction, such as immunosuppression, may appear

TABLE 29-4 Types of Bone Marrow Transplant

Type	Description
Autologous	The client receives his own marrow, which is possible if the disease afflicting the bone marrow is in remission, or if the condition does not involve the bone marrow (e.g., Hodgkin's disease lymphoma and brain tumor). The bone marrow is extracted from the client prior to transplant and may be "purged" to remove lingering malignant cells.
Allogeneic	The client receives bone marrow from a donor. The new marrow must match the genetic makeup of the client's own marrow as perfectly as possible.
Syngeneic	The donor is an identical twin, whose marrow genetically matches the client.
Umbilical cord blood	Hematopoietic stem cells collected from the placenta, after birth, are used as the source of cells for marrow regeneration. These cells must match the genetic makeup of the client as perfectly as possible.

soon after transplant and last for many months to years (Buschsel, Leum, & Randolph, 1996). After the conditioning regimen is delivered, the bone marrow infusion is given IV, similar to the transfusion of a blood product.

During the post-transplant phase, all children have a period of prolonged **pancytopenia** (a marked decrease in the number of RBCs, WBCs, and platelets) immediately after the conditioning, lasting at least 3 weeks. This period includes the greatest risk of infection, bleeding, and anemia. Clients who receive an allogeneic or cord blood BMT are also at risk for **graft versus host disease (GVHD).** This immune response is the result of disparities in the HLA match between donor and recipient. The donor white cells perceive the child's body as foreign material to be attacked and destroyed. Graft versus host disease is usually restricted to certain organs such as the skin, gastrointestinal tract, liver, and other organs. The symptoms of GVHD can be minimal to life-threatening and include skin rash beginning on the hands and feet, spreading to other parts of the body; diarrhea; jaundice; and infection. These symptoms are managed with symptomatic support and immunosuppressive drugs such as cyclosporin-A and steroids.

Nurses are responsible for the family orientation, education, and coordination of the pre-transplant evaluation. Caregivers and older children may be acutely aware that the only chance of long-term survival may rest on finding a suitable donor for transplantation. Providing emotional support to a family who is waiting for a donor before their child relapses or becomes too ill to undergo BMT is crucial. During the hospitalization for the transplant phase the nurse is responsible for monitoring the side effects of therapy, and maintaining isolation precautions to provide infection control. When the child becomes pancytopenic, he or she will be dependent upon transfusion support of both red cells and platelets. Mucositis and other side effects of the cytoreduction may make it impossible for the child to eat. Accurate monitoring of intake, output, and the child's weight are necessary. Total parenteral nutrition (TPN) is used in many cases to provide all essential nutrients by the IV route. Careful assessment for signs of infection, vigilant handwashing, and isolation technique is of the utmost importance. Family teaching about infection control should be emphasized daily. At the first sign of infection, cultures are obtained and then IV antibiotics are started. This supportive care post-transplant is a major component that affects the survival of children undergoing bone marrow transplantation (Abramovitz & Senner, 1995).

Careful nursing assessment of the child's skin, GI tract, and liver function is essential to diagnose and treat GVHD. The earliest sign of GVHD is often a skin rash, first appearing on the hands and feet. It may spread to other parts of the body and include redness and blistering. Graft versus host disease of the gastrointestinal tract presents with diarrhea stools, abdominal pain and cramping, malaise, anorexia, nausea, and vomiting. All stools are monitored for quantity, consistency, and the presence of blood and mucus. The diarrhea may be copious and the need to monitor fluids and electrolytes is essential. Jaundice may indicate that GVHD has affected the liver. The child with elevated liver transaminases and bilirubin must be evaluated for GVHD. Obtaining a biopsy of the affected tissue or organ confirms the diagnosis. Treatment is with immunosuppressive drugs such as Cyclosporin and steroids. Cyclosporin can be toxic to the kidneys, cause excessive hair growth, and in rare instances cause neurological problems. Steroid side effects include weight gain, fluid retention, elevated blood sugar, and mood swings. Clients and family members need to be reassured that these side effects are temporary and will disappear once the drugs are discontinued.

Immunosuppressive drugs increase the risk of infection. Precautions must be taken and taught to the child and family to limit the exposure to harmful bacteria, viruses, and fungi. This may include special air-filtering of the client's room,

Family Teaching

Going Home from Bone Marrow Transplant

- Obtain all medications prior to discharge. Each medication should be reviewed and a written time schedule given for the administration of each drug.
- Provide caregivers with a follow-up appointment schedule prior to discharge.
- Instruct the child and caregivers of the studies such as blood tests and bone marrow aspirates that will be needed to monitor the child's recovery status.
- Teach caregivers and the child of the signs and symptoms of GVHD, and to report these immediately to the health care provider.
- Reinforce the need to contact the health care provider immediately for fever, signs of infection, or exposure to varicella.
- Refer the child for homebound schooling if available through the local school district.
- Notify school personnel that the child may not be allowed to return for several months post-transplant. It may be facilitated by a visit from the bone marrow transplant team nurse to answer questions from the other students, school nurse, or staff.
- Refer the child and family to national BMT information and support groups, such as BMT Newsletter, BMT Family Support, or National BMT Link.
- Encourage families to ask for help from friends, church groups, and local social service agencies.

frequent handwashing, use of masks, gloves, and gowns by anyone coming in contact with the child, the elimination of fresh fruits and vegetables from the child's diet, and not permitting flowers in the room, which can harbor bacteria.

Discharge planning starts when the child's condition stabilizes. With home care nursing services now able to provide parenteral nutrition, antibiotics, and other intravenous medications, children are able to return home sooner than they used to. Hospitalizations that used to last months or years are now typically six weeks or so in duration. Understandably, given the acutely life-threatening condition from which the child is emerging, all families have concerns regarding returning home. Nursing support to prepare the family for this transition is essential.

Biologic Response Modifiers

Biologic response modifiers (BRMs), naturally occurring and synthetic agents, are a relatively new modality of cancer treatment and are used to stimulate the body's immune system to destroy cancerous cells. Examples of BRMs include colony stimulating factors (CSF), interleukins, monoclonal antibodies, interferon, and tumor necrosis factor. The use of these drugs is also referred to as immunotherapy or biotherapy.

CSF are responsible for stimulating and regulating the physiological process of hematopoiesis, which can be accelerated to accommodate the body's needs (Pitler, 1996). They are used to accelerate hematopoietic recovery after chemotherapy, which leads to the reduction of hospital admission days secondary to fever and neutropenia, and permits the use of aggressive dose intensive chemotherapy Examples of CSF are granulocyte-macrophage colony stimulating factor (GM-CSF), granulocyte-colony stimulating factor (G-CSF), and macrophage-stimulating factor (M-CSF). These factors are used to counteract the myelosuppressive effects of radiation and chemotherapy. Side effects of CSF include low-grade fever, myalgia, headache, and bone pain.

Interleukins are proteins that regulate the intensity and duration of immune responses. They do not directly kill cancer cells, but act as messengers to initiate immune defense actions that enhance the body's immune system. Clinical trials in pediatric oncology are ongoing to determine the best way these agents can aid cancer treatment in children. Side effects of interleukin therapy include fever, chills, malaise, hypotension, myalgia, and nausea and vomiting. Interleukin-11 was the first biological immune response agent to be used to treat chemotherapy-induced thrombocytopenia. This interleukin stimulates the proliferation of functioning platelets, which can decrease the child's risk of bleeding or need for platelet transfusions (Rust, Wood, & Battiato, 1999). Side effects include edema, dyspnea, tachycardia, and redness of the conjunctiva.

Monoclonal antibodies are produced in the laboratory to target cancer cells. They are used for several reasons in cancer therapy including the delivery of immunotoxins, early cancer detection, and the delivery of radioactive isotopes. The delivery of immunotoxins is achieved by attaching a toxin to the monoclonal antibody, which penetrates the malignant cell and delivers the lethal toxin. Monoclonal antibodies used to detect specific tumors can be "tagged" with radioactive isotopes. This approach can also be used for both diagnostic scans and the delivery of therapeutic radiation doses. Side effects include fever, arthralgia, pruritus, and, rarely, anaphylaxis.

Interferon is a natural human protein produced by the body in small amounts and is capable of inhibiting viral replication, modulating immune responses, and altering cellular proliferation. Research is ongoing to determine the place of the interferons in pediatric cancer treatment. Side effects of interferon therapy include fatigue, nausea and vomiting, fever, chills, and thrombocytopenia.

Tumor necrosis factor (TNF) is the product of activated macrophages and phagocytic monocytes that selectively kill cancerous cells. Exposure to TNF activates macrophages to release cytotoxic factors that mediate events leading up to the hemorrhagic necrosis of the core of the tumor (Woolery-Antill & Colter, 1993). Nurses who care for children receiving BRM must be familiar with their function and side effects. Each BRM has specific potential side effects ranging from mild fatigue to severe anaphylaxis. Caregivers must be taught about the agent and learn potential side effects. Colony stimulating factors and interferons are given subcutaneously and usually in the home; therefore, caregivers will need to learn how to administer the agent. Children who receive BRM, especially CSF, will need frequent monitoring of their CBC to make decisions regarding the discontinuation of the drug. Caregivers should be instructed to give acetaminophen prior to giving interferon to prevent the fever associated with this agent.

Family Teaching

Biological Response Modifiers

- Instruct the caregivers in subcutaneous injection technique.
- Teach the family about the medication, including the schedule, dose, and side effects. Recommend measures to alleviate symptoms of side effects such as antipyretics for fever.
- Teach family the importance of frequent monitoring of blood counts.
- Provide written information about the BRM that the child is receiving to the caregiver to share with the school.

Reflective Thinking

The Side Effects of Cancer Therapy

Caregivers of children, newly diagnosed with cancer, suddenly find themselves in a medical environment, interacting with health care providers who are asking for consent to initiate treatment on their child. By the time the diagnosis is made, many caregivers are emotionally distraught and physically exhausted. At this time of emotional stress, they are told of the potentially life-saving treatments, which have a high risk of creating new lifelong side effects. Their child may have seemed normal and healthy a short time before the diagnosis. The health care team must take the time to teach the caregivers about the disease and the proposed treatment so that a truly informed consent can be made. The treatment in some cases may seem as horrible as the cancer, but not treating will ensure the death of the child. How can you support caregivers who find themselves in this situation?

LEUKEMIA

Leukemia is a broad term describing a group of malignant diseases in which normal bone marrow elements are replaced by abnormal immature lymphocytes, known as blast cells. It is the most common childhood malignancy in those under 15 years of age. In children two forms of leukemia are generally recognized: acute lymphocytic leukemia (ALL) and acute myelogenous leukemia (AML).

Acute Lymphocytic Leukemia

Incidence and Etiology

Acute lymphocytic leukemia (ALL) accounts for 80% of all childhood leukemia and for approximately one-third of all childhood cancers (Friebert & Shurin, 1998). There are approximately 3,000 new cases each year in the United States (Robinson, 1997), and the peak incidence occurs between the ages of two and five years old (Margolin & Poplack, 1997). A variety of agents have been implicated that might increase the risk of developing leukemia, including viruses, irradiation, exposure to certain toxic chemicals or drugs such as benzene, and a genetic predisposition. The etiology of most cases of ALL is unknown.

Pathophysiology

Acute lymphocytic leukemia develops when a single lymphoid cell undergoes malignant transformation and proliferates uncontrollably. In the bone marrow of an individual with ALL the invasion of these malignant **lymphoblasts,** or immature white cells, causes a "crowding out" of normal red blood cells, platelets, and white blood cells, resulting in pancytopenia (marked reduction in the number of RBCs, WBCs, and platelets) and immunosuppression.

Clinical Manifestations

The most common presenting signs of ALL are fever, bone pain, pallor, and bruising. Most children diagnosed with ALL have been symptomatic for only one or two weeks. The clinical manifestations arise from the organs that are affected (Figure 29-9).

Diagnosis

A bone marrow aspirate (BMA) is required to make the diagnosis of ALL, and a finding of more than 25% of abnormal lymphoblasts in the bone marrow is diagnostic. Other samples of the bone marrow are sent for further testing, which can show chromosomal changes and better identify the specifics of the leukemia. The child's white blood count and age at diagnosis are the most important prognostic signs in ALL. The best prognosis is a WBC less than 5,000/mm^3 and an age of 2–9 years, and the worst prognosis an initial WBC of 50,000/mm^3 and an age younger than 2 years and older than 10 years. A lumbar puncture is done to assess for the presence of CNS disease (Figure 29-10), and a chest X ray is obtained to detect a mediastinal mass. Laboratory findings will show liver or kidney involvement.

Treatment

ALL is treated with systemic chemotherapy and includes three phases: induction, consolidation, and maintenance. The goal in the **induction phase** is to reduce the tumor burden to an undetectable level, a state known as remission. In remission there is no evidence of leukemia on physical exam, bone marrow evaluation, peripheral blood counts, in the CSF, or any other **extramedullary** (outside the bone marrow) site. Ninety-five percent of children with ALL achieve remission during induction, which usually lasts four weeks. Once remission is achieved most children will relapse within a few months if treatment is stopped, indicating the existence of undetectable blasts and the necessity of continuation of therapy. Remission induction is achieved by treating the child with the chemotherapeutic agents, vincristine (Oncovin), L-asparaginase (Elspar), and prednisone. Children, who have a poorer prognosis, will have an **anthracycline** drug (chemotherapeutic agents known to affect the heart by damaging cardiac myocytes) such as doxorubicin (Adriamycin) added to this phase. Once the child is stable, this phase of treatment is administered in the outpatient clinic. Presenting symptoms, such as anemia, infection, or bleeding are treated at the time of diagnosis. Once chemotherapy begins, the release of purines from the destroyed leukemic lymphoblasts causes an elevation of uric

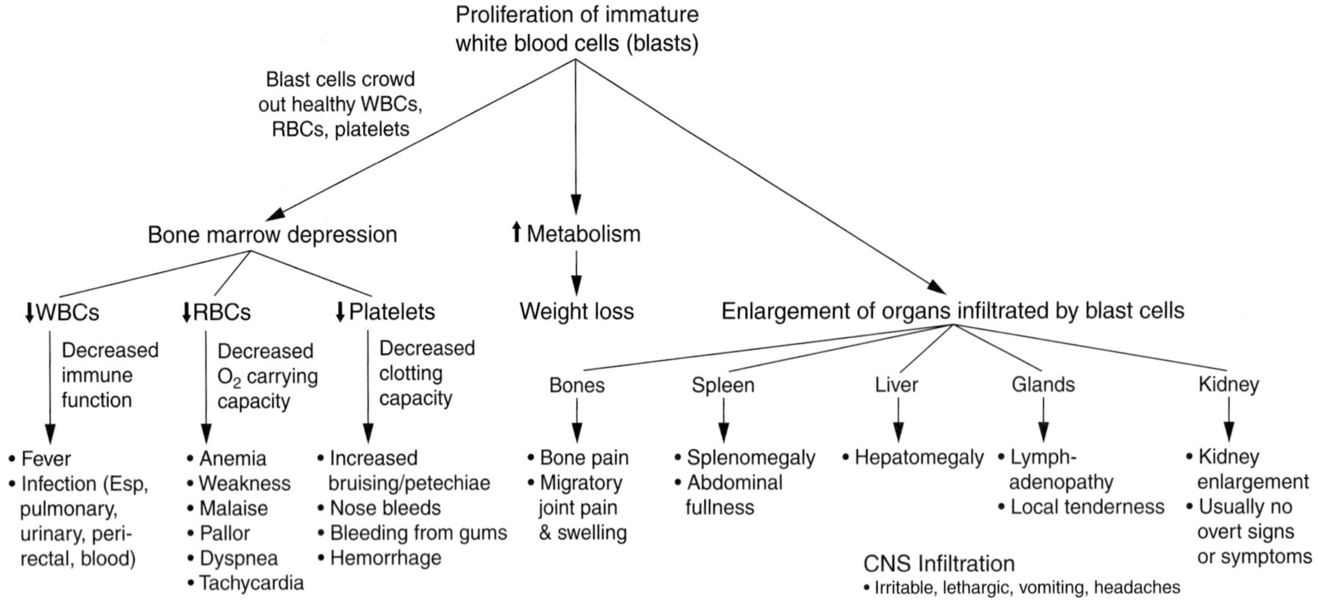

Figure 29-9 Pathophysiology Leading to Clinical Manifestations in Acute Lymphocytic Leukemia. *Source:* Adapted from Betz, C., Hunsberger, M., & Wright, S. (1994). *Family Centered Nursing Care of Children* (2nd ed., p. 1908, Fig. 42–45). Philadelphia: W. B. Saunders.

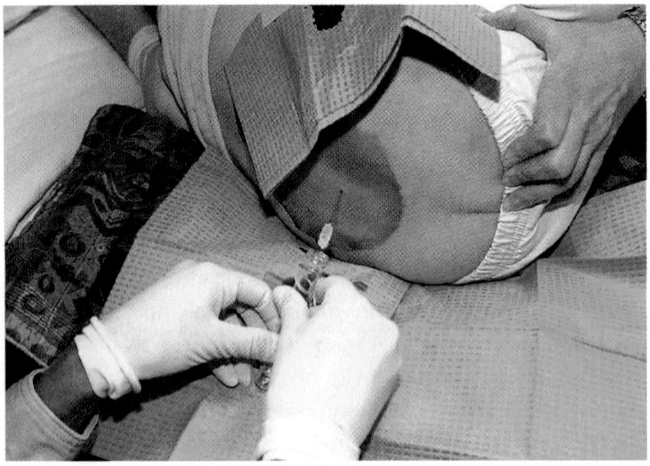

Figure 29-10 A lumbar puncture is performed to detect the presence of leukemic cells in the central nervous system of this child with acute lymphocytic leukemia.

acid, which can lead to acute renal failure. This is called **tumor lysis syndrome.** This complication is prevented with IV hydration containing sodium bicarbonate to alkalinize the urine to a pH of 7 or 8. Allopurinol (Zyloprim) is also given to aid in the excretion of uric acid through the kidneys, preventing renal obstruction and failure. Tumor lysis syndrome occurs more frequently and severely with children who have a greater tumor burden, such as those with a high WBC of 50,000 or greater, or extensive lymphadenopathy.

Leukemia cells can cross the blood-brain barrier and most drugs that are effective treatment do not. Children with ALL receive CNS prophylaxis with chemotherapy instilled **intrathecally** (IT), into the cerebral spinal fluid space during a lumbar puncture. Children who present with CNS disease at diagnosis will also receive radiation therapy to the brain and spinal cord to eradicate malignant leukemic cells. Some clinical trials treat children with radiation to the brain if they present with WBC of 50,000/mm^3 or greater, to reduce their risk of CNS disease. Radiation to the testes is reserved for males with testicular involvement of ALL.

The next phase of treatment is called **consolidation** and aims at eradicating any residual leukemic cells, and starts promptly once remission is attained. Chemotherapy is frequently given in high doses, requiring hospitalization during this phase of treatment. The administration of IT medications is frequent and radiation therapy to the brain may be given for CNS prophylaxis or treatment during this phase. Children who have extramedullary disease will receive radiation to those sites at this time. This phase of therapy is intense and lasts about six months.

The **maintenance** phase follows consolidation and maintains control of the leukemia with most chemotherapeutic agents administered by the oral, IV, or IM routes. During this phase, occasional intravenous injections of vincristine and lumbar punctures with IT chemotherapy may be given. Most centers continue therapy for two and a half to three years after diagnosis. Children who maintain a complete continuous remission during this time electively discontinue treatment. Today, remission can be induced in 95% of children, and 5-year survival rates are now nearly 80% (Smith, Ries, Gurney, & Ross, 1999).

REFLECTIONS FROM FAMILIES

My child and the entire family had been counting the admissions, spinal taps, and weeks of chemotherapy left until the treatment was complete. As the "big day" grew near, though, we were all surprised to find ourselves anxious. Although the treatment was stressful, we all felt some comfort that the chemotherapy was keeping the cancer away. What will happen when the chemotherapy isn't there?

The completion of chemotherapy is a goal that many caregivers and children look forward to with a hope to return to a "normal life" again. It is also met with high anxiety and fear that if no further therapy is given the child will promptly relapse. The family needs to be assured that there is no significant advantage to continuing therapy beyond this period. All phases of therapy depend upon guidelines set by each child's specific clinical trial.

Unfortunately, regardless of all the success in the treatment of ALL, a number of children will relapse, and those who relapse while on therapy or within six months of completing treatment have a very poor prognosis. Bone marrow transplant is a treatment option for children with ALL who attain a second remission after relapse and who have a compatible bone marrow donor.

Case Study/Care Plan

Child with Acute Lymphocytic Leukemia

Duane is a 6-year-old boy referred by his pediatrician to the Pediatric Hematology/Oncology clinic at the university medical center for severe anemia and to rule out aplastic anemia. The previous week, Duane was noted to be pale, had low-grade temperatures (<101°F), and complained of pain in his legs and over his sternum. His mother had started giving him an iron preparation. Duane had always been well and had never been hospitalized. He has no known allergies and his immunizations are up to date. He lives with his mother and father and his six siblings. He is currently in the first grade doing above average work.

A CBC done in the clinic revealed a WBC of 2.4, a hemoglobin of 2.7 g/dl, and platelet count of 17,000. The oncologist reviewed the peripheral blood smear and identified blast cells. Duane and his family were told of the probability of leukemia, and a bone marrow aspirate was performed in the clinic under local anesthesia. The bone marrow aspirate confirmed the diagnosis of acute lymphocytic leukemia. Duane was admitted, and received transfusions of packed red blood cells (PRBC) and platelets. He was started on IV hydration with sodium bicarbonate added, and Allopurinol was begun in preparation for chemotherapy to begin the next day.

Nursing Care Plan

Assessment Nursing assessment includes a physical evaluation of the child. A baseline evaluation allows the nurse to determine if improvement or deterioration of the child's physical status has occurred over the course of treatment. Physical assessments should be done at least daily in the hospital setting and at each outpatient visit. The family's cultural, spiritual, and social background must be assessed to be able to provide individualized holistic care. Emotional support is given differently to a family with strong extended member ties than to a family who is separated from this help. Families from other cultures may perceive the cause of the disease very differently than western scientific reasoning; therefore, taking time to talk with family members about the meaning of the illness is important. Many families find comfort in the support of their spiritual leaders while others would prefer the support of a team member such as the social worker. An assessment of the support systems of families should be obtained. Nursing assessment of the child's developmental level and emotional maturity will determine the appropriate approach to use during the many painful procedures involved in diagnosis and treatment. The child

continues

continued

and caregiver's ability to learn should be assessed prior to the initiation of teaching. This includes the educational and reading level of the caregiver, his/her stress level and the child's developmental level of learning. Once this assessment is made, appropriate written and verbal instructions can be given.

Nursing Diagnosis #1

Risk for infection related to neutropenia from the disease process and treatment.

Expected Outcomes

1. Duane and his caregivers will demonstrate infection prevention actions.
2. Duane will remain free of infection.

Interventions/*Rationales*

1. Use meticulous handwashing techniques at all times and teach Duane and his family about the importance of good handwashing. *The most important intervention in preventing infections is strict handwashing; educating Duane and his family allows them to observe and question all persons coming in contact with him about washing their hands.*

2. Monitor vital signs frequently for signs of infection. Report temperatures above 101°F. *Because of the risk of overwhelming infection, prompt interventions must be instituted when the child develops fever. Increased temperature, pulse, and respirations may indicate an infection.*

3. Administer antibiotics as ordered; monitor for expected and toxic effects. *Antibiotic therapy is started in the child with fever and neutropenia (ANC <500/mm^3).*

4. Assess Duane for any potential signs of infection (oral ulcerations, needle punctures, lesions/breaks in skin) and for localized sign of infection (pain, erythema, induration). *Skin is the first line of defense against infection; the child with neutropenia has no defense against infection and sepsis can develop quickly.*

5. Use aseptic technique for all invasive procedures. *To minimize exposure to infective organisms.*

Evaluation

Duane, his caregivers, and anyone entering the room will carry out measures to prevent infection. His vital signs will remain stable and within normal limits. He will be free of infection. If an infection develops, he will be promptly and effectively treated with no long-term adverse consequences.

Nursing Diagnosis #2

Risk of injury (bleeding) related to thrombocytopenia.

Expected Outcomes

1. Duane will have minimal or no bleeding episodes.
2. Duane will exhibit no signs of hemorrhage (normal BP and heart rate).

Interventions/*Rationales*

1. Monitor susceptibility to bleeding. Assess for signs of bleeding, including petechiae and bruising. Monitor urine and stool for signs of occult bleeding. Check daily platelet counts. *Decreased platelet count, bruising, petechiae, and blood in urine or stool can indicate bleeding.*

2. Take vital signs frequently. *To monitor for signs of hemorrhage (decreased BP, tachycardia, pallor, diaphoresis, restlessness).*

3. Avoid skin punctures when possible. Apply pressure if punctures necessary for 5–10 minutes. *Children with platelet counts below 20,000/mm^3 are at risk for spontaneous bleeding.*

continues

continued

4. Protect mucous membranes by using soft bristle or sponge toothbrush to avoid trauma. *Protecting membranes decreases likelihood of capillary damage and mucous membrane breakdown.*

5. Institute and teach safety precautions. *Protecting child from falls, cuts, or other trauma decreases the risk of bruising or bleeding.*

Evaluation

Duane will have no excessive bleeding or hemorrhage. Safety precautions will be followed, and he will sustain no injuries.

Nursing Diagnosis #3

Risk for injury (renal) related to tumor lysis.

Expected Outcomes

Duane will exhibit no signs of renal damage as documented by BUN, serum creatinine, and urine output remaining in the normal range.

Interventions/*Rationales*

1. Administer Allopurinol as ordered. *Allopurinol decreases the production of uric acid. During tumor lysis from chemotherapy, uric acid crystals may be deposited in the kidneys and cause obstruction leading to renal failure.*

2. Administer sodium bicarbonate as ordered to maintain alkalization of urine (pH at 7 to 8). *Uric acid is more soluble in alkaline urine.*

3. Maintain IV hydration to induce urine output of 1 cc/kg/hour or greater. *Urine output of less than 1 cc/kg/hour or urine that contains uric acid crystals can be the first sign of impending renal obstruction. Close monitoring of the child's intake and output allows the early detection of renal problems.*

4. Monitor blood urea and nitrogen (BUN), creatinine, electrolytes, and minerals (potassium, calcium, phosphorus, and uric acid). *Tumor lysis results in hyperkalemia, hypocalcemia, hyperphosphatemia, and hyperuremia, which lead to metabolic acidosis.*

Evaluation

Duane will exhibit no evidence of renal damage. He will void adequately without evidence of hyperuremia.

Nursing Diagnosis #4

Pain related to diagnosis, disease process, and treatment.

Expected Outcomes

Duane will maintain a level of comfort without significant pain.

Interventions/*Rationales*

1. Assess painful areas for location, severity, and signs of infection. *Bone pain is common in the child with leukemia who has not yet received treatment because of leukemic infiltrates in bones. Pain is also an indicator of infection, so the child must also be evaluated for infection.*

2. Provide Duane with pain medication on a preventive schedule (around the clock). *To prevent pain from recurring. Pain is easier to prevent than to treat.*

3. Reassess for relief from medication given. *To determine need for changes in drug, dosage, frequency.*

4. Implement and teach nonpharmacological pain reduction methods. *As an adjunct to analgesics.*

5. Venipunctures and procedures should be done in the treatment room and not in the child's room. *The child's room is a place for the child to feel safe from harmful events.*

continues

continued

Evaluation

Duane will report and/or exhibit no evidence of pain.

Nursing Diagnosis #5

Imbalanced nutrition: Less than body requirements related to loss of appetite, nausea, vomiting, and mucositis.

Expected Outcomes

1. Duane will ingest adequate nutrition to maintain and support normal growth.
2. Duane will maintain weight.

Interventions/*Rationales*

1. Offer small amounts of food frequently throughout the day. *Small portions are usually better tolerated.*
2. Avoid making food an issue for power/control and emphasize this to caregivers. *Child may resist eating even when he/she has an increase in appetite.*
3. Encourage high protein and high calorie foods. *To maximize nutritional quality of intake.*
4. Encourage caregivers to bring child's favorite foods from home. *To encourage eating.*
5. Make breakfast as high in caloric intake as possible. *Children often lose their appetite as the day progresses.*
6. Administer antiemetics as ordered. *To decrease nausea.*
7. Provide mouth analgesics as ordered before food and fluid intake. *Mucositis is painful and analgesics will improve comfort and increase interest in eating.*

Evaluation

Duane will experience no more than 5% weight loss and show normal growth for age.

Nursing Tip:

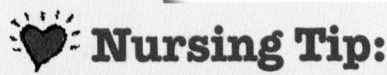

Medication swallowing

Prednisone, a frequently used medication in leukemia therapy, tastes very bitter and many children have difficulty taking it. Prednisone may be given crushed in ice cream, mixed in chocolate syrup, crushed and placed in blank capsules, mixed in applesauce, or placed in a fruit roll-up. It should be given with milk or an antacid to prevent heartburn. Enteric coated or time-released tablets and capsules should never be crushed before giving.

Acute Myelogenous Leukemia

Acute myelogenous leukemia (AML) is the second type of leukemia recognized. Children with AML have a poorer prognosis than those with ALL. Seventy to 85% of children with this type of leukemia will achieve remission, but only 30% to 40% will become long-term survivors (Smith, Ries, Gurney, & Ross, 1999).

Incidence and Etiology

AML accounts for approximately 15% to 25% of childhood leukemia (Golub, Weinstein, & Grier, 1997). The etiology is not known; however, certain predisposing factors have been associated with AML. Risk factors such as exposure to radiation and chemotherapy for the treatment of a previous cancer, exposure to benzene, and genetic predisposition in children with Down syndrome and Fanconi's anemia have been named.

Pathophysiology

As in ALL the malignant myeloid blasts crowd out the normal WBC, platelets, and red blood cells causing neutropenia and immunosuppression, thrombocytopenia, and anemia.

Clinical Manifestations

Children with AML may present with seemingly benign symptoms resembling the flu (i.e., fever, fatigue, malaise, anorexia) or may be severe and life-threatening (i.e., bleeding and severe hemorrhage). Bleeding at the time of diagnosis is usually associated with thrombocytopenia but may also be caused by disseminated intravascular coagulation (DIC). A particular subtype of AML, specifically acute promyelocytic leukemia, is associated with DIC. Children with AML may present with gingival hypertrophy caused by infiltration of the gums with malignant myeloid cells. **Chloromas** are localized collections of malignant cells. When this occurs in the skin or subcutaneous tissue, it presents as a nodular protuberance in the skin. There is a higher incidence of CNS disease at diagnosis with AML than with ALL, but the clinical manifestations are the same. In AML the CNS symptoms may also be caused by a chloroma in the brain. An epidural chloroma may manifest by difficulty walking or incontinence of urine and stool caused by spinal cord compression. Enlargement of the liver and spleen is seen at initial presentation; significant lymphadenopathy occurs less often.

Diagnosis

A bone marrow aspirate, showing >25% malignant myeloid blasts confirms the diagnosis of AML.

Treatment

Once a diagnosis is made, treatment begins promptly, attending to the presenting symptoms such as anemia, bleeding from thrombocytopenia or DIC, infection, and metabolic abnormalities such as hyperuricemia. The treatment of hyperuricemia, anemia, thrombocytopenia, and neutropenia are addressed in the ALL section of this chapter. DIC is best treated with the aggressive management of the underlying disease process. Many children will require platelet transfusions as well as the replacement of coagulation factors such as cryoprecipitate, and fresh frozen plasma to control bleeding. Red cell transfusions may be necessary to replace blood loss and maintain tissue perfusion.

Treatment of AML is with systemic chemotherapy. The phases of AML treatment are remission induction and continuation therapy. Chemotherapy drugs such as cytarabine (Ara-C) and an anthracycline agent such as daunorubicin (Daunomycin) are used in the induction phase. After remission is achieved many clinical trials call for a continuation with intense high dose chemotherapeutic agents such as cytarabine, cyclophosphamide (Cytoxin), anthracyclines, and etoposide (VePesid). Treatment of the CNS is with cytarabine and or methotrexate (MTX) given intrathecally. Radiation to the head may be part of CNS therapy and prophylaxis. Bone marrow transplantation has been used for the treatment of AML once remission is achieved and a suitable donor is available. Therapy for AML is very intense, and is usually given as an inpatient. Children who receive this intense chemotherapy often are hospitalized for lengthy periods of time because of pancytopenia and fever. Survival has improved over the last two decades from 10% to 40% in children with AML. The low relapse rate after allogeneic bone marrow transplant makes this approach to the treatment of AML attractive (Golub, et al., 1997).

Nursing Management

Nursing management is similar to that of ALL with the addition of the following interventions. Children with AML are at high risk for bleeding related to DIC. Assessment for signs of bleeding such as a change in vital signs, including a decrease in blood pressure or increase in heart rate, is important. Physical assessment of the mucous membranes and skin includes looking for petechiae or bruising. Bleeding may be seen at needle puncture sites even hours after the puncture. Trends in laboratory findings that suggest DIC include a prolongation of the prothrombin time, a decrease in platelet count, and a decrease in fibrinogen levels.

BRAIN TUMORS

Brain tumors are the most common solid tumor of childhood, and are second only to leukemia among childhood malignancies. Brain tumors are the third leading cause of death in children under 16 years, and prognosis varies depending upon the age of the child at diagnosis, pathology, and location of the tumor. Histology, or cell structure, and location determine the classification of brain tumors.

Incidence and Etiology

Approximately 2,950 children are diagnosed annually with central nervous system (CNS) tumors in the United States (American Brain Tumor Association, 1998). Brain tumors represent 16.6% of all malignancies of childhood (Gurney, Smith, & Bunin, 1999). Most brain tumors are found in children younger than 10 years of age. The cause of most pediatric brain tumors remains unknown (Shiminski-Maher & Wisoff, 1995). A strong link exists between hereditary and environmental factors and the occurrence of certain brain tumors. Certain hereditary diseases such as neurofibromatosis and tuberous sclerosis are associated with certain rare brain tumors (Heideman, Packer, Albright, Freeman, & Rorke, 1997). Environmental factors such as industrial and chemical toxins and ionizing radiation have been related to an increase in pediatric brain tumors, although epidemiologic evidence is lacking (Gurney, Smith, & Bunin, 1999). Children who received cranial irradiation for the treatment of previous malignancies have an increased risk of brain tumors.

Pathophysiology

Brain tumors are classified according to their histology and location. Sixty percent of pediatric brain tumors arise from **glial cells,** which are the supporting cell structures of the brain. These include astrocytoma, brain stem gliomas, and ependymomas. Brain tumors arising from neurons or their precursors include primitive neuroectodermal tumors (PNET) and medulloblastoma.

The location of the tumor makes a further classification and includes infratentorial, supratentorial, and midline tumors. About 50–60% of all pediatric brain tumors are **infratentorial** (in the posterior third of the brain, primarily in the cerebellum and brain stem and below the tentorium). The **tentorium** is the dura mater located between the cerebrum and cerebellum supporting the occipital lobes. These include the following types of tumors: medulloblastoma, cerebellar astrocytoma, brain stem glioma, and ependymoma. **Supratentorial** tumors occur in the anterior two-thirds of the brain above the tentorium, primarily in the cerebrum. These include cerebral astrocytomas. Other brain tumors occur in the midline (third and fourth ventricles, optic chiasm, and brain stem) and include optic nerve gliomas, craniopharyngiomas, and pineal region tumors. Astrocytomas are the most common type of CNS tumors in children (50%), followed by medulloblastomas (15–20%), brain stem gliomas (10–20%), ependymomas (7%), and others (9%) (American Brain Tumor Association, 1998). Figure 29-11 shows the location of common childhood brain tumors.

Clinical Manifestations

The initial symptoms of childhood brain tumors are often vague and mimic common childhood illnesses. They include irritability, vomiting, and anorexia. Increased intracranial pressure is frequently seen in the infratentorial tumors of the posterior fossa, caused by the tumor itself or indirectly by an obstruction of the flow of cerebrospinal fluid. Symptoms include headache and vomiting, which may be worse in the morning (Shiminski-Maher & Shields, 1995). The vomiting may temporarily relieve the headache. A child less than 3 years old may present with irritability and an increase in head circumference. Infants with increased intracranial pressure

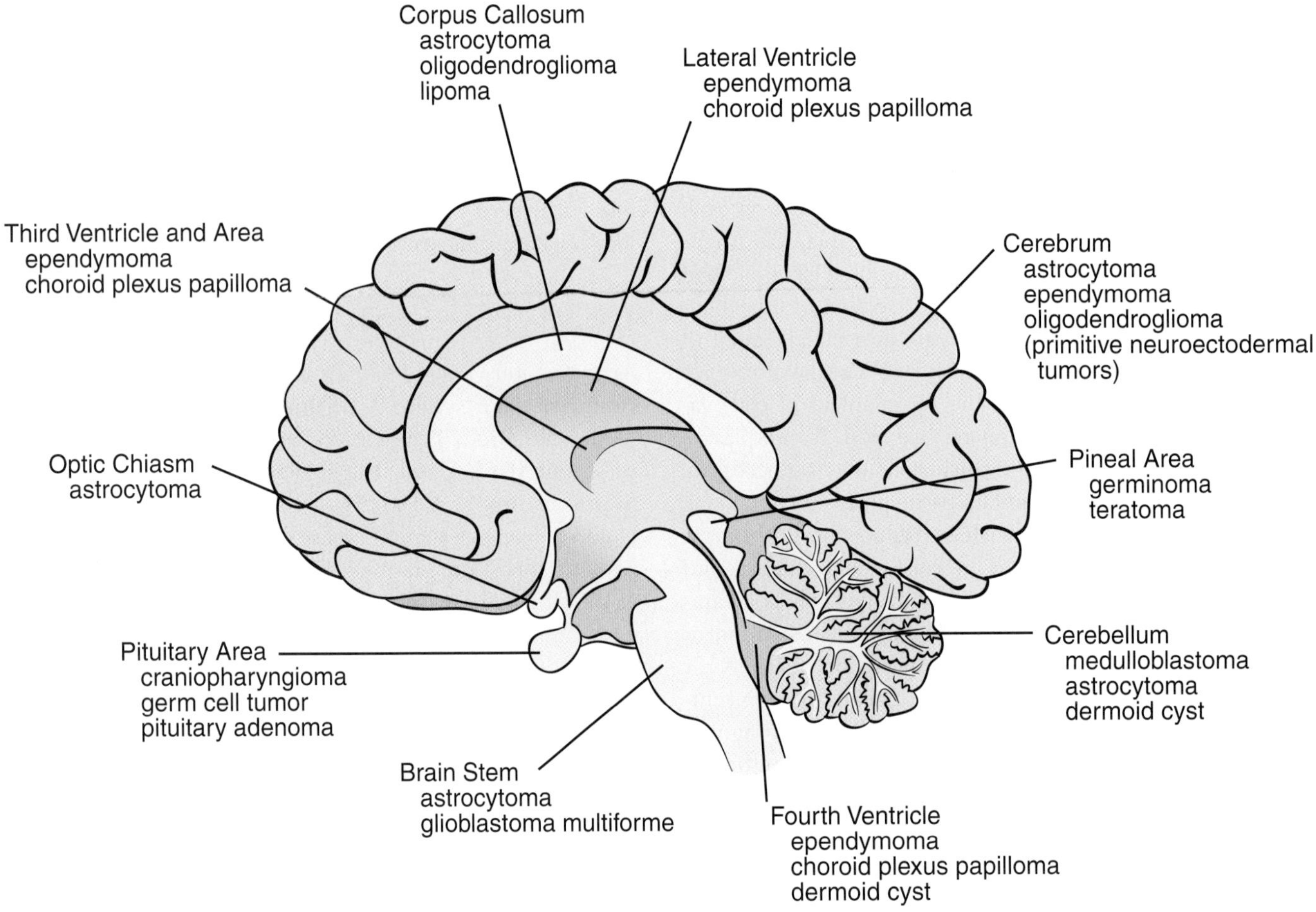

Figure 29-11 Location of Common Childhood Brain Tumors. *Source:* American Brain Tumor Association. (1998). *A primer of brain tumors.* Des Plaines, IL: Author. Used with permission.

may have a raised or tense anterior fontanel, which may not close as expected between 8 and 18 months. Infants and toddlers with brain tumors may show delay in achieving or loss of developmental milestones. A young child who no longer does an activity he or she has mastered, such as walking or sitting up, needs a careful evaluation. Diplopia or double vision may be present but is difficult to diagnose in a young child. The young child with diplopia may tilt the head or use a hand to cover one eye. Ataxia, unsteady uncoordinated movement, nystagmus, rhythmic oscillation of the eyes, and impaired upward gaze can also be signs of increased intracranial pressure (Heideman, Packer, Albright, Freeman, & Rorke, 1997).

Brain stem tumors are associated with cranial nerve abnormalities, hemiparesis, a weakness of one side of the body, and a spastic gait. A complete neurological examination will show a positive Babinski's sign. The symptoms associated with increased intracranial pressure caused by tumor growth will not appear until late in the course of the disease with brain stem tumors. Children with supratentorial tumors commonly present with a hemiparesis, **hemisensory** loss, a decrease or loss of function of a sense organ on one side of the body, seizures, visual field changes, and cognitive problems. Midline tumors are associated with visual field and acuity changes, personality changes, and endocrine system problems such as precocious puberty. The presenting symptoms of a child with a brain tumor can lead the health care providers to suspect specific locations of the tumor. See Table 29-5 for the common presenting symptoms and treatment of specific pediatric brain tumors.

Diagnosis

Any child who displays signs of increased intracranial pressure or other neurological symptoms such as ataxia, visual

TABLE 29-5 Common Pediatric Brain Tumors: Symptoms and Treatment

Tumor Type (% of incidences)	Tumor	Symptoms	Treatment
Infratentorial/ posterior fossa (50 to 60)	Medulloblastoma	Increased ICP, headache, morning vomiting, cranial nerve deficits, ataxia	Maximal surgical resection and cranial/spinal radiation* and chemotherapy
	Ependymoma	Neck pain, increased ICP, cranial nerve deficits	Maximal surgical resection and radiation* and/or chemotherapy
	Brain stem glioma	Cranial nerve deficits, increased ICP, hemiparesis, usually short history Long history, minimal symptoms, focal lesion on MRI, considered low-grade	Hyperfractionated radiation* and/or chemotherapy Low-grade tumor, surgical debulking, observation or radiation* and/or chemotherapy
Supratentorial (30 to 50)	Low-grade astrocytoma	Seizures, visual changes, endocrinopathies, incidental finding: hemiparesis	>90% surgical removal and observation <90% surgical removal, observation or radiation* or chemotherapy
	High-grade astrocytoma	Seizures, increased ICP, mental status change, hemiparesis	Maximal surgical removal and radiation and/or chemotherapy
Midline (10 to 15)	Optic-nerve chiasmal gliomas	Seizures, endocrinopathies, increased ICP, visual changes	Observation, surgical debulking, radiation* and/or chemotherapy
	Craniopharyngiomas	Seizures, visual changes, increased ICP, endocrinopathies	<95% surgical removal, observation >95% surgical removal, reoperation or radiation*
	Pineal region	Increased ICP, no upward gaze, headache	Low-grade: surgery alone; High-grade: surgery, radiation*, and chemotherapy

** Delay radiation therapy in children younger than 5 years of age.*

Source: Shiminski-Maher, T., & Shields, M. (1995). Pediatric brain tumors: Diagnosis and management. Journal of Pediatric Oncology Nursing, *12(4), 188–198.*

disturbances, or hemiparesis needs to be referred for a complete physical and neurological examination. The diagnostic work-up of a child with neurological symptoms includes magnetic resonance imaging (MRI), which has replaced computerized tomography (CT) as the most common first diagnostic test obtained (Shiminski-Maher & Wisoff, 1995). Both tests have advantages and disadvantages.

MRI creates an image of the brain in three different planes, which allows for exact localization of the tumor. MRI best defines neuroanatomy and tumor margins. This complete picture of the tumor can be helpful to the neurosurgeon in planning the surgical approach and to the oncologist in evaluating growth of the tumor over time. MRI of the spine is the diagnostic method most used to evaluate spread of the tumor to the spinal cord.

There are disadvantages of MRI, which relate to the lengthy time that the child must remain motionless inside a dark noisy tube to obtain the scan. It takes about one hour and can be frightening to a young child. Sedation or anesthesia may be needed to obtain the scan. It is difficult to safely monitor a seriously ill child during this test especially when sedation or anesthesia is required.

CT scan is still a useful diagnostic tool for the evaluation of a child with a brain tumor. It is easier and less expensive to perform than MRI. CT scan is a quick test, taking 5 to 10 minutes and is less affected by body motion than MRI. Many children can tolerate a CT without sedation. It is most useful when there is a sudden change in neurological status that needs evaluation.

Other studies are used in limited situations. Angiography contributes to preoperative evaluation of the vascularity of the tumor, which is helpful to the neurosurgeon in planning how to approach the tumor surgically. Magnetic resonance angiography (MRA) has replaced angiography in many situations because it is noninvasive and can often provide the same information. The positron-emission tomography (PET) scan and the thallium single photon emission computed tomography (SPECT) scan both provide information about residual abnormalities after treatment. They help to distinguish between recurrent tumor versus cells killed by radiation versus scar tissue. With advances in computer technology, more and more specific diagnostic tests will be made available. A biopsy is performed in all but brain stem tumors, where the risk of surgical complication is too great and the knowledge gained will add little to treatment decisions. A biopsy may be done as a separate surgical procedure or as part of the surgery to remove the tumor.

> **Nursing Tip:**
>
> **Sedation for neurodiagnostic testing**
>
> Adequate sedation is necessary in obtaining the needed neurodiagnostic information to confirm the diagnosis of a brain tumor. Sedation protocols vary from institution to institution, but sleep deprivation can enhance the effects of sedation. Advising caregivers to put the child to sleep an hour or two later the night before a procedure and then waking her or him a few hours earlier will enhance the effects of the medication. All children who are sedated must be monitored carefully with pulse oximetry and telemetry to prevent complications of oversedation.

Treatment

Pediatric brain tumors are treated on an individual basis and may include surgery, radiation therapy, or chemotherapy or a combination of all these modalities. The actual plan of treatment depends upon the location and pathology of the tumor and the age of the child. Radiation and/or chemotherapy are often major components of the plan. Surgery is used to remove as much of the tumor as possible while preserving normal brain function. Prognosis is improved when all or most of the tumor can be surgically removed. In the postoperative period intravenous steroids such as dexamethasone (Decadron) are used to prevent edema within the brain and are tapered gradually. Anticonvulsants are indicated for children with supratentorial lesions where seizures are possible.

The goal of radiation therapy is to destroy tumor cells while sparing normal brain tissue. Because of the damage that radiation causes to the developing brain, such as intellectual and growth impairment, it is avoided in children who are less than 3 years old, if possible. When radiation therapy is used to treat brain tumors, the dose is usually high, and the toxicity can be severe.

In the last decade, chemotherapy has emerged as standard care in the treatment of certain pediatric brain tumors. The drugs most commonly used in brain tumor treatment include the nitrosoureas (carmustine [BiCNU] and lomustine [CeeNU]), cisplatin, vincristine, etoposides, carboplatin, and ifosfamide. These agents are given in intense doses and are sometimes included in a regime with autologous bone marrow transplant to rescue the child from the toxic effects of the drugs. Chemotherapy is often used in children younger than 3 years of age to delay or eliminate the necessity of radiation therapy.

Nursing Management

Assessment

The focus of the physical assessment of the child with a brain tumor is dictated by the clinical manifestations. A thorough neurological assessment is performed before surgery and includes vital signs; pupil size, equality, and response to light; level of consciousness; and strength and equality of grip. Head circumference measurement and assessment of the anterior fontanel in infants is necessary to evaluate increasing intracranial pressure. Seizure precautions are instituted both preoperatively and postoperatively. The nurse assesses the child for developmental and behavioral alterations. Behavior changes, school performance, and social interactions should be ascertained.

Nursing Diagnosis

Preoperative:

1. Pain (headache) related to increased intracranial pressure.
2. Risk for injury related to altered neurological functioning.
3. Deficient knowledge regarding the diagnosis and treatment of childhood brain tumors

Postoperative:

4. Risk for infection related to the surgical procedure.
5. Risk for delayed growth and development related to the brain tumor and its treatment.

Planning/Implementation

Caregivers whose child has been diagnosed with a brain tumor as with other tumors are faced with the real concern of having their child die. They must also face the possibility that their child, who was healthy and active only a short time ago, may now have severe physical, intellectual, and growth impairments. During the pre-diagnosis period, nursing care includes providing support and coordination of the many diagnostic procedures, which can help reduce some of the stress experienced by the child and caregiver. Using role-play to teach the child about the tests can sometimes reduce the need for sedation during scans.

Once a tumor is identified, surgery is planned. Caregivers often do not have adequate time to comprehend all that is being asked of them. Being available to answer questions, providing written information, and providing emotional support are important nursing responsibilities. Preparing the child and caregivers for the postoperative stay in the intensive care unit is crucial. Postoperative care of the child who has had a craniotomy usually includes several days in an intensive care unit. Because of the surgical trauma to the brain, there is a chance of developing edema and increased intracranial pressure; therefore, frequent neurological assessment and monitoring of vital signs is essential. Careful monitoring of fluid and electrolyte balance is another important aspect of nursing care. The need to identify and prevent increased intracranial pressure is paramount. Usually the child has a MRI within a few days postoperatively to determine the extent of any residual tumor. Steroids are given intravenously at first but later changed to the oral route, and then the dosage is slowly tapered. Caregivers and the child must be made aware of the side effects of this medication, including mood swings, increased appetite, and changes in body shape and weight. Assurance that the moon face and weight gain from steroids is temporary and will disappear once the medication is withdrawn is helpful (Figure 29-12). The combination of chemotherapy and radiation can result in heightened toxicity, for example, cisplatin with radiation increases the risk of ototoxicity, resulting in severe hearing loss. After the immediate postoperative period, the child is often evaluated with audiologic, neuropsychological, and repeated scans to determine the response to therapy and side effects.

Caregivers may become overwhelmed with the physical, emotional, and financial demands that the diagnosis of a brain tumor in their child brings. Nurses can be instrumental in helping them cope by introducing them to other members of the multidisciplinary team and families who have managed a similar difficult situation. It is also important for

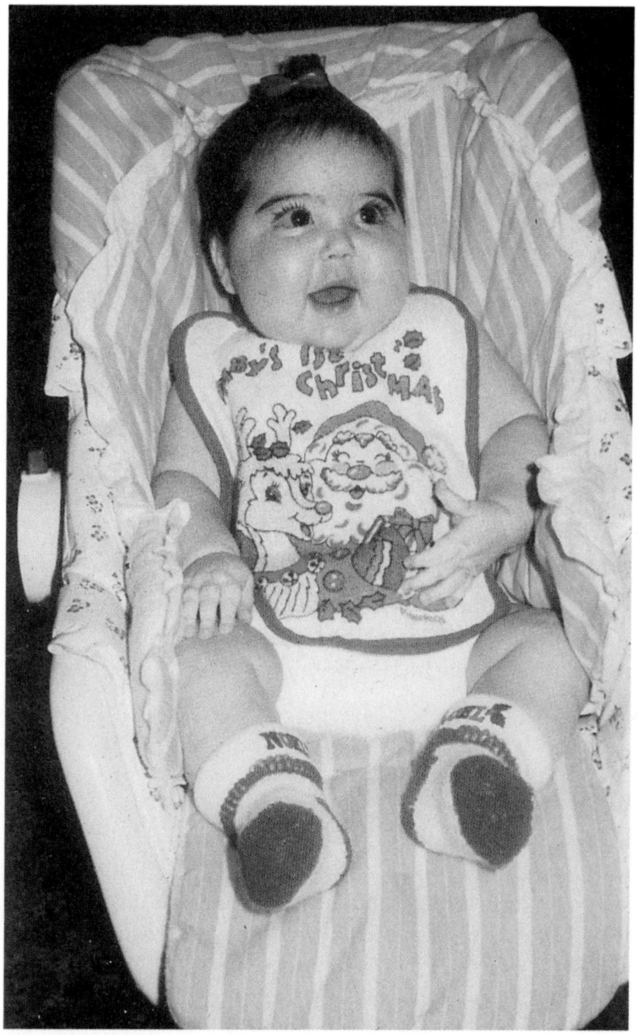

Figure 29-12 This infant is being given steroids as a chemotherapeutic agent. Notice the "moon" face and prominent cheeks, which are a side effect that will disappear when the drug is discontinued.

Nursing Alert:

Safety Precautions for children with Ataxia

Children with ataxia have difficulty walking and are at risk of falling and injury. Some children need pediatric walkers or the assistance of an adult to walk. They should be referred to physical therapy for neuromuscular retraining and muscle strengthening. Safety issues to be addressed prior to going home include gates for stairways and doors and placing pads on sharp furniture corners.

nurses to help families identify other sources of support, such as the extended family, friends, religious organizations, and childhood cancer support groups.

Outcome Identification

1. The child will experience no pain or reduction of pain.
2. The child will avoid injury from falls.
3. The family will ask questions related to diagnosis, treatment, and support needed.
4. The child will recover from surgery without infection as evident by normal body temperature and lack of erythema or discharge at the wound site.
5. The child will have minimal or no impairments in growth and development.

Evaluation

To evaluate the effectiveness of nursing interventions, the answers to the following questions should be explored. Did the child display verbal and nonverbal indications of reduction of pain? Did the child remain free of injuries such as falls from the bed or falls from ambulating? Was the family able to discuss the disease process, diagnosis, and treatment plan? Has the child remained free of infection? Did the child return to optimal functioning with minimal or no deficits?

LYMPHOMAS

Lymphoma is a malignancy that arises from the lymphoid system. Lymphatic tissue is present throughout the body and is responsible for recognizing and destroying foreign invaders. Lymphatic tissue is responsible for developing competent lymphocytes to perform this task. Lymphomas are a malignant transformation of these cells. There are two types of lymphomas seen in children, Hodgkin's disease (HD) and non-Hodgkin's lymphoma (NHL). Malignant lymphomas are the third most common type of childhood cancer.

Hodgkin's Disease

Hodgkin's disease (HD) usually originates in a cervical lymph node and spreads to other lymph node regions, and if left untreated, to the organs.

Incidence and Etiology

HD accounts for approximately 5% of childhood malignancies, with 850–900 new cases diagnosed in the United States each year (Percy, Smith, Linet, Ries, & Friedman, 1999). It is seen more frequently in boys than girls, and the incidence increases with age accounting for a greater proportion of lymphoma in older children (Shad & Magrath, 1997). HD is rare before five years of age (Hudson & Donaldson, 1997). The etiology is unknown; however, the role of an infectious agent has been implicated. Indirect associations between Epstein-Barr virus (EBV) and HD have been reported, but the DNA of EBV has not been isolated in tumor tissue.

Pathophysiology

HD originates in the lymphatic system and is differentiated from other lymphomatous diseases by its histology. The malignant cell is more differentiated than with NHL, and the pattern of infiltration is more specific. HD is classified by histology into four types: nodular sclerosing, mixed cellularity, lymphocyte predominant, and lymphocyte depleted.

Clinical Manifestations

The onset of HD is commonly not acute in nature, and the child may have had symptoms for a prolonged time prior to seeking medical attention. The disease is usually localized at the time of diagnosis. The usual presentation is painless enlarged lymph nodes. The most common sites of presentation are the cervical and supraclavicular areas. Other symptoms may include malaise, anorexia, night sweats, and fever. Most children have localized disease at the time of diagnosis, but HD can metastasize to the spleen, bone marrow, and lungs (Figure 29-13). It is necessary to obtain a staging evaluation to determine the extent of disease and to plan treatment.

Diagnosis

Diagnosis of HD is made by biopsy of an affected node and histologic classification by the pathologist. Staging of the disease helps determine the prognosis and is determined by the extent of lymph node involvement. A staging evaluation includes chest X ray and CT of the chest, abdomen, and pelvis to assess for distant lymph node involvement. Stages range from I to IV, with I having the best prognosis and IV the worst. A gallium scan may be used to assess for metastatic disease. Bone marrow aspirates and biopsies are performed to assess for marrow involvement. Laboratory tests will include a CBC and liver function tests. Abnormalities

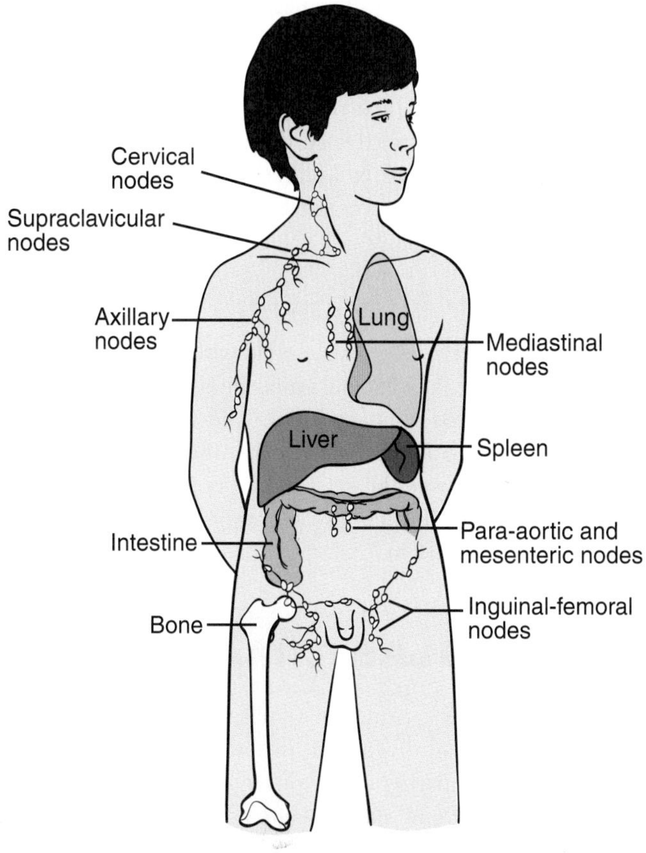

Figure 29-13 Lymph Nodes Affected by Hodgkin's Disease

noted in these tests suggest marrow or liver disease, respectively. The child's erythrocyte sedimentation rate (ESR), ferritin, and copper levels may be elevated at the time of diagnosis.

For those children who will undergo chemotherapy and/or radiation therapy, pulmonary function tests and a cardiac evaluation are needed as a baseline evaluation of these organs. Bleomycin (Bleo) and doxorubicin (adriamycin) are two commonly used drugs in HD that may affect these organs. Baseline thyroid studies are helpful, especially if the treatment plan will include radiation to the neck area.

Treatment

Depending upon the clinical stage at the time of diagnosis, HD treatment includes chemotherapy, radiation therapy, or a combination of these modalities. Traditional chemotherapeutic regimens used to treat HD include mechlorethamine (nitrogen mustard), vincristine (oncovin), prednisone, procarbazine (MOPP), adriamycin, bleomycin, and dacarbazine (ABVD). When radiation therapy is used, the lymph node areas of the neck, mediastinum, and inguinal areas are irradiated. Girls and young women often have surgery to move their ovaries out of the radiation field to help prevent sterility. When treatment is complete, the ovaries are then returned to their normal position.

Nursing Management

Nursing care of the child with HD includes the administration of chemotherapy and management of the side effects of chemotherapy and radiation. If the spleen has been removed, the child is at risk for long-term infection. The nurse observes the child for signs of infection and teaches the caregivers about the risk of serious infection after a splenectomy. Some health care providers prescribe prophylactic antibiotics. Emotional and physical support to the child and family who are experiencing cancer are always part of holistic nursing care.

Non-Hodgkin's Lymphoma

Non-Hodgkin's lymphoma (NHL) is significantly different from HD in that there is no single focal origin and, therefore, the malignant cells are rarely localized. Also, NHL has a rapid onset and presents with widespread involvement.

Incidence and Etiology

Non-Hodgkin's lymphoma is approximately one and a half times more prevalent than HD in children. Where HD is seen in older children and adolescents, NHL is seen from infancy through adolescence, with a peak between the ages of 7 and 11 years. Boys are affected more often than girls, and the incidence increases steadily throughout life (Shad & Magrath, 1997).

The cause of NHL is unknown although viral, genetic, immunologic, and environmental factors have been implicated as playing a role. Children with congenital and acquired immune deficiencies, including children post-organ transplant, have a higher risk of developing NHL. Children with AIDS often present with primary lymphoma of the CNS.

Pathophysiology

Because NHL is a malignancy of the lymph system, which is widely spread throughout the body, this disease is often generalized at diagnosis. Non-Hodgkin's lymphomas of childhood are distinct from the lymphomas of adults. Childhood NHL is extremely aggressive in its ability to proliferate and is divided into four high-grade categories: 1) Burkitt's lymphoma, 2) lymphoblastic lymphoma, 3) large B cell lymphoma, and 4) anaplastic large cell lymphoma (Percy, et al., 1999).

Clinical Manifestations

The presenting complaint of a child with NHL is usually pain or swelling with acute onset and progression (Castiglia, 1995). Children with lymphoblastic NHL commonly present with mediastinal mass, pleural effusion, and lymphadenopathy,

Nursing Alert:

Mediastinal Mass Can Cause Obstruction

A child with NHL and a large mediastinal mass may present with respiratory distress caused by compression of the trachea by the malignant lymphoma. A mediastinal mass can also cause ***superior vena cava syndrome (SVC),*** *which is obstruction of the superior vena cava resulting in edema of the face, neck, and upper trunk. Both respiratory distress and SVC syndrome are oncologic emergencies.*

and have a tendency for spread to the bone marrow and CNS. Burkitt's NHL manifests with an abdominal mass, which can mimic appendicitis, and can also spread to the CNS and bone marrow.

Because of the rapidity with which this tumor can proliferate, most children have advanced disease at diagnosis even though they may have had symptoms for only a short period of time. Most have stage III and IV disease when diagnosed. Children with advanced disease may present with CNS symptoms including headaches, nausea, and vomiting. Petechiae, bruising, bleeding, and bone pain are present if the bone marrow is involved. Those with a large mediastinal mass may present with respiratory distress.

Diagnosis

The diagnosis of NHL is made from a biopsy. The cells or tissue may be obtained from the bone marrow, pleural effusion, ascites, or an affected node or mass. The diagnostic studies and staging of NHL must be done expeditiously to avoid delay in treatment.

Staging evaluation includes a bone marrow aspirate and biopsy, and lumbar puncture to assess for marrow and CNS involvement, respectively. Radiologic studies include CT of the affected area, the chest, abdomen, and pelvis. Nuclear studies including bone and gallium scans are done to identify any other sites of disease. Laboratory evaluations include a CBC, liver and kidney function tests, electrolytes, calcium, phosphorus, magnesium, lactate dehydrogenase (LDH), uric acid, and urinalysis.

Treatment

Aggressive multi-agent chemotherapy is started as soon as possible once the diagnosis is made and the staging of the tumor is complete. Like the child with leukemia, these children are at risk for tumor lysis syndrome, and all precautions to prevent renal injury are followed. Children who have stage I and II disease receive a shorter and less aggressive course of treatment than those with stages III and IV. Intrathecal chemotherapy is given for CNS prophylaxis, and cranial radiation is used with children who have disease in their CNS. In the past, radiation therapy was commonly used in treatment, but studies have demonstrated that with intensive chemotherapy there is no benefit to adding irradiation. Children with limited disease have an excellent prognosis of 90% to 100% cure rate, and those with extensive disease with good supportive care can expect to be cured in 70–90% of cases (Shad & Magrath, 1997). Bone marrow transplant may be recommended as a treatment option for those children who relapse.

Nursing Management

The nursing management of the child with NHL is similar to the care of the child with leukemia. In NHL there is a high incidence of tumor lysis syndrome, and these children are often admitted to an intensive care unit for initiation of treatment. Because of the intense chemotherapy these children receive, side effects are common, and nursing care involves managing these.

NEUROBLASTOMA

Neuroblastoma is a tumor, originating from neural crest cells, which are embryologic precursors of the adrenal medulla and sympathetic nervous system. These cells are present in tissue found in the brain, adrenal medulla, pelvis, mediastinum, and sympathetic ganglia. A neuroblastoma tumor may occur at any of these sites.

Incidence and Etiology

Neuroblastoma is the fourth most common childhood malignancy. Because neuroblastoma is an embryonal tumor, it is usually seen in early childhood with 39% of cases diagnosed in children under 1 year of age and 79% identified in children less than 4 years of age. The true incidence of neuroblastoma is unknown because this tumor can spontaneously regress and mature. This phenomenon occurs more commonly in neonates and infants and results in cases being undetected and uncounted (Brodeur & Castleberry, 1997).

The etiology of neuroblastoma remains unknown. Studies have failed to link this tumor with sex, race, parental age and education, and complications of pregnancy, labor, or delivery. There are rare cases of neuroblastoma occurring in more than one child in a family. Children with a familial occurrence tend to be diagnosed at an early age and have multiple primary sites.

Pathophysiology

Neuroblastoma is a soft solid mass, which usually contains areas of necrosis, calcification, and hemorrhage. Within the same tumor the histology may be different with more mature cells called ganglioneuroblastoma or even benign cells called ganglioneuroma. There is a "special" group of infants less than 12 months of age who present with a localized primary tumor and dissemination limited to the liver, skin, and/or bone marrow in which the malignant neuroblastoma will spontaneously mature and disappear without treatment. These children are said to have stage 4S.

The gene that is capable of causing cells to transform to neuroblastoma has been identified. This **oncogene** is called N-*myc* and is present in the cells of human neuroblastoma. An increase in the number of copies, or amplification of N-*myc*, is related to rapid tumor progression and a poorer prognosis (Brodeur & Castleberry, 1997).

Nursing Alert:

Safety in Handling Radioactive Fluids

Because ^{131}I-MIBG contains the radioisotope, iodine^{131}, precautions by health care personnel and family members should be taken. The half-life of iodine^{131} is 8 days. Gloves should be worn when handling the child's body fluids for at least 48 hours after the injection. As always, good handwashing technique is needed. Caregivers should be instructed to not allow the child to sleep with them or siblings for at least 48 hours while the isotope is being excreted.

Clinical Manifestations

Children with neuroblastoma can present with a wide variety of initial symptoms, depending upon the location of the tumor. The most common primary site is in the abdomen with involvement of the adrenal gland or the paraspinal ganglia. Less common primary sites include the paraspinal areas in the thorax, neck, or pelvis. Metastases are found in 62% of all newly diagnosed patients and include bone marrow, bones, liver, lung, and skin (DeVitta, Hellman, & Rosenberg, 1997).

Most commonly, the tumor is detected by palpation of an abdominal mass that can be firm and irregular in shape and frequently crosses the midline. Masses of the thorax can be seen on chest X ray, and if large enough, can cause respiratory symptoms or superior vena cava syndrome. Large abdominal or pelvic tumors can cause edema to the lower extremities, caused by vascular compression. When the tumor presents in any paraspinal area, it can grow into the spinal foramen and cause spinal cord compression. When neuroblastoma presents behind the orbit, it causes ecchymosis of the eyelid and proptosis. Bone marrow involvement usually presents with pain and commonly the refusal to bear weight or limping.

Diagnosis

Although signs and symptoms, blood and urine tests, and imaging studies may indicate that a neuroblastoma is probably present, a conclusive diagnosis can be made only when neuroblastoma cells in tissue samples are seen under a microscope. Once neuroblastoma is suspected, a complete history and physical examination is done. Laboratory tests include a CBC, liver and kidney function tests, and chemistry profile. Neuroblastoma often causes an elevation in the catecholamine metabolites vanillymandelic acid (VMA) and homovanillic acid (HVA), which can be measured in the urine. With treatment leading to remission, these metabolites become undetectable in the urine and are important markers of a recurrence.

Bone marrow aspiration and biopsy from multiple sites can often confirm the diagnosis of neuroblastoma. Chest X ray may reveal thoracic or paravertebral primary tumor, and abdominal ultrasound can show the extent of any mass. In order to determine if the tumor is surgically resectable, a CT or MRI scan is done, which more accurately defines the location of the mass and identifies if other organs are being impinged upon by the tumor.

A metastatic work-up is also conducted to determine the stage of the disease. A bone scan and skeletal survey are done to determine if bony metastases are present. A nuclear medicine imaging study may also be used. The radioactive agent ^{131}I-MIBG is highly specific to neuroendocrine tissue and localizes in a variety of tumors, including neuroblastoma. After this isotope is injected, the scan can screen the body for both primary and metastatic sites.

The International Neuroblastoma Staging System (INSS) is a major system used throughout the world to standardize the definition of diagnosis, determine the extent of dissemination of the tumor, and assist in treatment (Table 29-6). The prognosis for a child with neuroblastoma is determined by four variables: the age of the individual at diagnosis, the stage of the tumor, the N-*myc* amplification, and the histology of the tumor. The most important variables are age and stage. Children with single N-*myc* amplification and stage 1 or 2 with complete tumor excision have an excellent prognosis. Children with higher N-*myc* amplification, regardless of stage, who are older than 1 year have a very poor prognosis. Infants with stage 4S only require supportive care and have a moderate risk of disease recurrence (DeVitta, Hellman, & Rosenberg, 1997). The outcome for children who present with abdominal masses is poorer than those with cervical, mediastinal, or pelvic tumors (Nemes & Donahue, 1994).

Treatment

The treatment plan is determined by the stage and prognostic markers of the disease and can include surgery, chemotherapy, radiation therapy, and possibly bone marrow transplantation. Surgery can be both diagnostic and therapeutic. The surgery can be performed before any treatment to establish a diagnosis by biopsy, stage the extent of the disease, and completely resect or partially reduce the tumor. Complete surgical resection is the only therapy needed for

TABLE 29-6 International Staging System for Neuroblastoma

Stage 1	Localized tumor confined to the area of origin; complete gross excision, with or without microscopic residual disease; identifiable ipsilateral and contralateral lymph nodes negative microscopically.
Stage 2A	Unilateral tumor with incomplete gross excision; identifiable ipsilateral and contralateral lymph nodes negative microscopically.
Stage 2B	Unilateral tumor with complete or incomplete gross excision; with positive ipsilateral regional lymph nodes; identifiable contralateral lymph nodes negative microscopically.
Stage 3	Tumor infiltrating across the midline with or without regional lymph node involvement; or, unilateral tumor with contralateral regional lymph node involvement; or, midline tumor with bilateral regional lymph node involvement.
Stage 4	Dissemination of tumor to distant lymph nodes, bone, bone marrow, liver, and/or other organs (except as defined in stage 4S).
Stage 4S	Localized primary tumor as defined for stage 1 or 2 with dissemination limited to liver, skin, and/or bone marrow.

Source: Brodeur, G., Pritchard, J., Berthold, F., Carlsen, N., Castel, V., Castleberry, R., De Bernardi, B., Evans, A., Favrot, M., & Hedborg, F. (1993). Revisions of the international criteria for neuroblastoma diagnosis, staging, and response to treatment. Journal of Clinical Oncology, 11, *1466–1477.*

the child who presents with stage 1 or 2 disease. Secondary surgery is used to evaluate the response of treatment and to excise any residual tumor. The majority of children with neuroblastoma with advanced disease at diagnosis are in a high-risk category. Multi-agent chemotherapy is the predominant modality of treatment for these children. Initial response rates are high, greater than 85%, but the disease frequently recurs. Neuroblastoma is radiosensitive, but radiation therapy is not curative when used alone. Radiation is used for tumor control in conjunction with chemotherapy and autologous or allogeneic bone marrow transplant, and is important in palliation of pain in end stage clients.

Nursing Management and Family Teaching

Nursing assessment is similar to the assessment of children with other tumors such as leukemia or lymphomas. Emphasis is on alleviating the child's discomfort associated with the presenting symptoms, and the expeditious completion of the metastatic work-up. Neuroblastoma usually causes fear and anxiety for caregivers because of the poor prognosis of advanced stage disease. The therapy is intense, and the child spends lengthy periods of time in the hospital. Radiological scans to evaluate the efficacy of treatment are frequently performed requiring the family to attend many outpatient appointments.

Nursing care focuses on supporting the child and family through the diagnostic work-up, helping with the coordination of tests and procedures, and teaching the family the importance of these to determine the extent of tumor involvement. Frequently the child and caregivers must be prepared for major surgery in a relatively short time period following the discovery of a malignant mass. Feelings of fear and uncertainty may occur in all family members, and they need support. Chemotherapy and/or radiation therapy will begin once the child is stable postoperatively. Caregivers will need to be educated about the side effects of these treatments.

Critical Thinking

Identification of Infection in the Neutropenic Child

You are caring for a 4-year-old boy who has an ANC of 300. He was admitted the previous evening with a fever of 102.3°F. He is receiving intravenous antibiotics. While you are bathing him, he complains of pain in the perianal area. You do not note any redness or inflammation in the area. You suspect the source of infection is a rectal abscess. What would you do?

WILMS' TUMOR

Wilms' tumor, also called nephroblastoma, is a tumor that arises in the kidney. It is a renal embryoma, meaning that the tumor is derived from undifferentiated primitive cells.

Incidence and Etiology

Wilms' tumor is the most common malignancy of the kidney in children and accounts for 5–6% of all childhood cancer. The tumor usually presents between 2 and 3 years of age and is seen slightly more often in females than males. There are approximately 500 new cases in the United States every year (Bernstein, Linet, Smith, & Olshan, 1999). The cause of Wilms' tumor is unknown in most cases. Rare cases are associated with certain congenital anomalies such as **aniridia** (a congenital absence of the iris), **hemihypertrophy** (a relative increase in size of one-half of the body as compared to the other), and urinary defects. Therefore, children who have these anomalies need close surveillance including frequent abdominal examination and ultrasound as part of their primary care.

Pathophysiology

Wilms' tumor grows rapidly and may be very large at the time of diagnosis. A fragile thin capsule that may be easily torn or broken usually encloses the tumor, which may be present in one or both kidneys. There are two categories to describe the histology of a Wilms' tumor, favorable and unfavorable. Favorable histology tumors are more responsive to therapy and, as the name implies, have a favorable prognosis; whereas, children having the unfavorable histology tumors have a poorer prognosis. Histology type and the stage of tumor at diagnosis determine prognosis and treatment decisions. Wilms' tumor may metastasize to the lungs, liver, brain, bones, or to the unaffected kidney.

Clinical Manifestations

An abdominal mass is the most common presentation of Wilms' tumor. A large flank mass is usually found in a healthy child by a family member. The mass presents on one side and seldom crosses the midline, as does neuroblastoma. Some children experience pain, microscopic or gross hematuria, hypertension, and general malaise.

Diagnosis

Any child with an abdominal mass needs a timely and thorough diagnostic work-up. Abdominal ultrasound is often the first test ordered and can detect a solid intrarenal mass. Rapidly growing tumors migrate toward the point of least resistance, and it is not unusual to find Wilms' tumor infiltrating the renal veins or inferior vena cava. Ultrasound will also evaluate the unaffected kidney and abdominal lymph nodes for any signs of disease. An abdominal CT scan or MRI will give a clearer preoperative view of the abdomen. Because the lungs are the most common site of distant metastatic disease, an X ray and CT scan of the chest are ordered. Laboratory studies including a CBC, urinalysis, blood chemistries, and liver function tests are performed. The diagnosis is confirmed at surgery when the mass is removed, usually with the entire kidney, and biopsied.

Nursing Alert:

Manipulation of the Abdomen in a Child with Wilms' Tumor

A precaution is to limit manipulation of the abdomen or liver in these children that might cause spread of malignant cells should the encapsulated mass rupture. A sign placed on the child's crib or bed that warns all health care providers to avoid palpation of the abdomen, and instructions to caregivers to use caution when handling and bathing their child can prevent trauma to the tumor.

Treatment

The usual treatment for Wilms' tumor is surgical resection followed by chemotherapy and, at times, radiation. The treatment used depends upon the extent of disease and histology of the mass. If surgery cannot be performed because of bilateral disease or if the mass is too large and involved to resect, then preoperative chemotherapy is given. Preoperatively, it is important to monitor the child's blood pressure. Children who have hypertension are at risk for severe life-threatening intraoperative hypotension when the renal vessels are tied off. A tumor that is completely enclosed within one kidney will be resected, and the child will receive a short course of chemotherapy. Chemotherapeutic agents used are dactinomycin (Actinomycin D) and vincristine. Children with more extensive disease will have additional chemotherapeutic agents added to their regimens and possibly radiation therapy.

Wilms' tumor is highly radiosensitive, and in the past all children received radiation. Today radiation therapy is used only in those who have metastatic disease, residual tumor after surgical resection, and recurrent tumors. When radiation is necessary, it can cause defects in the spine including a decrease in linear growth or scoliosis. Children who present with or develop bilateral kidney disease pose a special problem. Usually the most affected kidney is removed, and an excisional biopsy of the tumor in the other kidney is performed. The remaining kidney is then irradiated and followed closely for signs of recurrent disease. These children usually have "second look" surgery to determine the effectiveness of therapy.

The prognosis for children with Wilms' tumor continues to improve. The overall survival rate is 92% (Bernstein, et al., 1999). The long-term survivor must continue to have active surveillance of the remaining kidney and follow-up for late effects. Irradiation to the trunk can cause scoliosis, and pulmonary radiation can cause fibrosis of lung tissue. Survivors of Wilms' tumor are at higher risk for a second neoplasm, especially those children who received radiation.

Nursing Management

Caregivers have little time to prepare for the major surgery involved with a nephrectomy and the diagnosis of cancer.

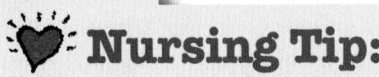

> **Nursing Tip:**
>
> **Avoid trauma to remaining kidney**
> A child who has one kidney must avoid trauma and injury to that kidney. The caregiver and the child must learn that contact sports, such as football and basketball, pose a special risk. Activities that do not have great potential for injury should be encouraged such as swimming, golf, bike riding, and hiking.

The nurse should remain available to answer questions and describe what they can expect. Chemotherapy is started soon after surgery, usually before the child is discharged postoperatively. Pain control is necessary after the nephrectomy and is given around the clock in the first 24 hours postoperatively, with a weaning of analgesia over the following few days. By discharge most children are no longer receiving pain medication. Postoperatively the nurse also needs to make certain that the child's oral fluid intake is adequate and that any nausea, vomiting, or constipation from the chemotherapy is under control before discharge. Wound care and activity restrictions should be reviewed. The surgical wound site is usually a large abdominal incision and signs of increased pain, redness, or drainage should be reported. When radiation is necessary, caregivers will be told of the potential side effects of altered growth and increased risk of second malignancies. Because these are late effects of treatment, continued education regarding the need for long-term follow-up is necessary.

BONE TUMORS

Malignant bone tumors account for approximately 5% of all childhood cancers. The two most common bone tumors are osteogenic sarcoma and Ewing's sarcoma.

Osteogenic Sarcoma

Osteogenic sarcoma, also called osteosarcoma, is a tumor of bone that usually occurs in the growth metaphysis or the end of the long bones. Trauma is frequently associated with the diagnosis of osteosarcoma. Rather than being a cause of the tumor, trauma is the event that brings the malignancy to the attention of the child, the family, and the health care team.

Incidence and Etiology

Osteogenic sarcoma is the most common bone tumor of children and adolescents and has a peak incidence in the second and third decades of life (Pearson, 1998). There are approximately 400 new cases diagnosed in the United States annually, and males are affected more often than females. The cause of most osteosarcoma tumors is unknown. Children with the hereditary form of retinoblastoma, an eye tumor, have an increased risk of developing osteogenic sarcoma (American Cancer Society, 2000).

Pathophysiology

The bones are composed of different cell types that include osteoblasts and osteoclasts. Osteosarcomas derive from primitive bone-forming cells similar to the osteoblasts that make bone matrix. These malignant cells do not function normally and have the potential to spread to other areas of the body such as the lungs and other bones. Osteogenic sarcoma occurs most frequently in the rapidly growing bones of the distal femur, proximal tibia, and proximal humerus. Children with tumors arising in sites such as the skull or vertebrae have a poorer prognosis because these bones are not surgically resectable.

Clinical Manifestations

Pain at the site of the tumor is almost always present and frequently is associated with a swelling or palpable mass. The pain increases with activity and weight bearing and may cause the child to limp. Signs and symptoms of the tumor may have a short duration but a history as long as 6 months is not unheard of. Osteosarcoma tumors that have destroyed normal bone place the child at risk for fracture. Occasionally the fractured bone is the first clinical manifestation of the tumor.

Diagnosis

A child with a suspected tumor of the bone requires a complete evaluation, including history, physical examination, and X rays of the primary site and chest. Often characteristic patterns seen on the X rays suggest the histology of the bone tumor, but a more complete evaluation and biopsy are necessary. Metastatic evaluation is necessary, as approximately 10% to 20% of children have distant lung metastasis at diagnosis (Meyers & Gorlick, 1997). The lung is the most common site of metastasis, but distant bone lesions can also be seen. Other organ involvement is rare. The presence of metastasis at diagnosis is an important prognostic indicator and helps to determine the specifics of therapy. Metastatic evaluation includes CT scan of the chest and a radionuclide bone scan to identify bone lesions. MRI of the primary lesion is performed to assess the extent of the bone and soft-tissue tumor and its relationship to blood vessels, nerves, and other bones prior to definitive surgery. Laboratory evaluation includes a CBC, blood chemistries, serum alkaline phosphatase, and lactic dehydrogenase (LDH). A biopsy is required to confirm the diagnosis of osteogenic sarcoma.

Treatment

Osteosarcoma is treated with surgical resection of the affected bone and multi-agent chemotherapy to eradicate any microscopic disease that could lead to metastasis. Many clinical trials use several courses of preoperative chemotherapy to reduce tumor size and permit a less radical surgical procedure. A complete radiographic evaluation is repeated prior to surgery.

Amputation was the surgical treatment used almost exclusively in the past, but now many children can be offered a limb-sparing procedure. Limb-sparing surgery uses a cadaver bone, grafted into place, to replace the section of bone with tumor that must be excised. Both amputation and limb-sparing surgery seek to excise the tumor completely and preserve the adjacent nerves and vessels. Limb-sparing surgery should be a consideration, over amputation, only if there is no compromise to the child's ultimate prognosis. Contraindications to limb-sparing surgery include displaced pathologic fractures at the tumor site, and skeletal immaturity, which would create problems with leg length discrepancies. The grafted bone will not grow, so a child who still has significant growth to achieve will have an unacceptable leg length discrepancy with limb-sparing surgery of the leg. The family must be educated about the advantages and disadvantages of all possible surgical procedures so they can make informed decisions. Issues of body image and the amount of function to be expected through rehabilitation must be discussed. The client, who is usually an adolescent, must be made an active participant in the discussion and decision-making process.

Research Highlight

Limb Salvage Versus Amputation for Bone Tumors in Children

Study Purpose

To assess the general satisfaction of children who underwent a surgical limb-sparing procedure or limb amputation for a pediatric bone tumor. The impact of the surgery in the areas of educational achievement and employment, functional limitations, pain, emotional distress, self-image, and social functioning and rehabilitation were also assessed.

Methods

A total of 65 clients aged 13 years or older were drawn from a cohort of children and adolescents treated at a major center caring for children with cancer. Eligibility criteria included a remission status and at least 1-year post limb-salvage procedure or amputation for a bone tumor. A 104-item questionnaire was developed for the study by a multidisciplinary group who believed to have included clinically relevant issues representing the functional outcome of bone tumor clients who underwent surgical limb-sparing procedures or amputation. Areas that were addressed included educational and employment status, functional limitations, pain intensity and interference, emotional distress, interpersonal and social functioning, self-image, and rehabilitation and general satisfaction with the surgical procedure.

Findings

Overall, the children with amputations and limb-salvage surgical procedures for bone tumors reported little or no interference or negative impact from their surgical procedure on the various functional and psychological outcomes assessed in the study.

Implications

The general satisfaction outcomes of the study indicate that the efforts of the multidisciplinary team to treat children with bone tumors accommodating for their individual needs and providing optimal treatment and rehabilitation have been relatively successful and the approach should be continued.

Citation

Hudson, M., Tyc, V., Cremer, L. K., Luo, X., Rao, B. N., Meyer, W. H., Crom, D. B., & Pratt, C. B. (1998). Patient satisfaction after limb-sparing surgery and amputation for pediatric bone tumors. *Journal of Pediatric Oncology Nursing, 15*(2), 60–69.

Aggressive chemotherapy is restarted after a few weeks of postoperative recovery. Surgery can control the local disease but 80% of clients who are treated with surgery alone develop metastasis and die within months of the surgical resection (Pearson, 1998). The combination of surgery and multi-agent chemotherapy has improved 5-year survival rates to approximately 80% (Mosher & McCarthy, 1998). Complete surgical resection of all overt metastatic disease is necessary for long-term survival. Children who develop metastatic lesions after treatment has begun have a poorer long-term prognosis. Osteosarcoma is radiation resistant and this modality is rarely used in primary treatment. Occasionally, radiation is used for pain palliation in clients who have disease that is unresponsive to chemotherapy.

Nursing Management

Adolescents and their families need ongoing explanations about the disease, treatment, equipment, and expected outcomes. Explanations before a procedure or treatment is initiated help keep the adolescent informed and take into consideration the need for autonomy. Introducing the adolescent to another adolescent who has undergone the same procedures and therapy may help alleviate some stress and provide another support system.

Pain from bone lesions of osteosarcoma in many cases requires analgesics prior to surgery. Postoperatively pain medication needs to be given around the clock the first 24 hours. Clients who undergo amputation may experience **phantom limb pain,** which is pain perceived to be coming from the amputated limb. After limb-sparing surgery the client is at risk for altered tissue perfusion and nerve damage in the affected limb. Checking nail beds for capillary refill and assessing sensation of the limb distal to the surgery site every 15–30 minutes is important to assess nerve damage. Infection risks are great in individuals who undergo extensive and lengthy orthopedic surgery such as in a limb-sparing procedure. This risk is compounded when immunosuppressive chemotherapy is instituted after surgery. Wound care must be meticulous, and signs of infection such as redness, drainage at the site, or fever should be reported.

Adolescents who have either limb-sparing surgery or amputation will have major alterations in their body image. Aside from the surgery, they will also face body changes related to chemotherapy such as alopecia. Normal activities with friends may be curtailed, and previous activities such as sports or dance may have to be given up completely. The nurse can support these adolescents by listening to their concerns, encouraging them to dress in their own clothes while in the hospital, and suggesting peer support groups.

Ewing's Sarcoma

Ewing's sarcoma is a highly malignant bone tumor with a histiologic appearance and presentation that is different from osteosarcoma. Ewing's sarcoma can present in any bone of the skeleton but is often seen in the bones of the pelvis, tibia, fibula, and femur.

Incidence and Etiology

Ewing's sarcoma represents about one-third of all childhood malignant bone tumors with approximately 200 children and adolescents diagnosed every year in the United States. Ewing's sarcoma is a disease of older children and young adults. It is rare in children less than 5 years old or in older adults. African-American children in the United States rarely develop Ewing's sarcoma, but the protective etiology has yet to be found.

Pathophysiology

Ewing's sarcoma is a highly malignant tumor that arises from primitive undifferentiated cells. These small round blue cells are also seen in tumors such as primitive neuroectodermal tumors.

Clinical Manifestations

As with osteosarcoma, pain and swelling at the site of the tumor are the usual presenting symptoms of Ewing's sarcoma. Pain may be caused by tumor under the periosteum or the tissue covering the bone, or by a fracture of the weakened bone.

Diagnosis

The diagnosis of Ewing's sarcoma is made by biopsy of the bone lesion. Ten to thirty percent of newly diagnosed clients have metastatic disease, with the lung, other bones, or the bone marrow as the most common sites. A complete staging evaluation must be done, including CT scan of the lungs, MRI of the primary site, and a radionuclide bone scan. As with other pediatric malignancies the stage of the disease at the time of diagnosis is an important prognostic factor in Ewing's sarcoma. Widespread metastatic disease to other bones and the bone marrow has a poor prognosis. Location of the primary tumor is also a significant factor with pelvic and sacral lesions having a worse prognosis because these tumors are not resectable.

Treatment

The primary lesion of Ewing's sarcoma is treated with surgical resection of the bone when possible, and radiation therapy. If the bone is expendable, such as a rib or fibula, then the entire bone is removed. Control of the primary lesion can be achieved in this fashion. Multi-agent, intense chemotherapy is used to prevent and control metastatic disease. Most current protocols use chemotherapy prior to definitive surgery and the amount of tumor decreased prior to resection is a prognostic factor, with more tumor decrease associated with a better prognosis.

When complete removal of the primary lesion cannot be achieved surgically, then radiation therapy is added to the treatment. With increases in the survival rate of Ewing's sarcoma, secondary malignancies in the radiation field have become an issue. Long-term follow-up must be stressed as an essential part of these clients' care. Since the 1990s children with Ewing's sarcoma treated with combination therapy of chemotherapy and surgery have a 5-year survival rate of 60% to 72% (Mosher & McCarthy, 1998). Nursing management is similar to the management of osteogenic sarcoma.

SOFT TISSUE SARCOMA

Soft tissue sarcomas arise primarily from the connective tissues of the body, such as fibrous, adipose, or muscle tissue. Rhabdomyosarcoma arises from tissue resembling striated muscle and contains primitive muscle cells. There are two types of rhabdomyosarcomas seen in children, embryonal, which is the most common, and alveolar. Other rhabdomyosarcoma cells are too primitive and undifferentiated to classify and are referred to as undifferentiated sarcoma. The treatment of rhabdomyosarcoma and soft tissue sarcoma is similar.

Incidence and Etiology

In the United States 850–900 children and adolescents are diagnosed with soft tissue sarcomas each year, of which approximately 350 are rhabdomyosarcomas (Gurney, Young, Roffiers, Smith, & Bunin, 1999). There is no known definitive cause of soft tissue sarcoma. Studies have suggested certain prenatal influences increase the risk of developing soft tissue sarcoma. These include parental use of marijuana and cocaine during the pregnancy and in utero exposure to diagnostic X rays. Further investigation is needed to clarify the significance of these findings (Gurney, et al., 1999).

Pathophysiology

Rhabdomyosarcoma cells resemble rhabdomyoblasts, which in the human embryo will eventually form voluntary and skeletal muscle tissue. The embryonal type of rhabdomyosarcoma usually affects infants and young children in the area of the genitourinary tract and the head and neck area. The alveolar type usually occurs in the large muscles of the trunk, arms, and legs, affecting older children and teenagers. Most often sarcomas metastasize via the blood and lymphatic systems to the lung, bone, and bone marrow.

Clinical Manifestations

As with other solid tumors, the presentation of soft tissue sarcoma depends upon the location, with the most common symptom being a hard non-tender mass. Orbital involvement may present with **ptosis,** a drooping of the eyelid, and **proptosis,** a protrusion of the eyeball. These signs may also be associated with eye movement abnormalities. Tumors in the orbit are usually detected early because of the visible physical changes. Nasopharyngeal tumors may present with nasal obstruction, chronic sinusitis, epistaxis, or pain. Tumors that arise in the paranasal sinuses or middle ear result in signs and symptoms of chronic otitis media and sinusitis. Rhabdomyosarcoma in these areas may invade through foramina and cause intracranial spread, which results in cranial nerve palsies and signs of increased intracranial pressure. Intracranial disease reduces overall survival. Tumors in the extremities are similar to traumatic hematomas, which are raised and easily palpable. The tumor is fixed to the underlying muscle and can involve the skin. When rhabdomyosarcoma arises in the retroperitoneal area, it is usually asymptomatic until the disease is widespread and the mass is very large. A tumor in this location can cause bowel and urinary obstruction. Genitourinary involvement may cause urinary obstruction, hematuria, vaginal discharge, or a mass. Pain, swelling, and limping may be seen in bone involvement. Metastatic spread of rhabdomyosarcoma is seen in about 18% of children at the time of diagnosis. Most children with bone marrow involvement have their primary tumor in an extremity or in the trunk, and usually have widespread metastatic disease to other organs.

Diagnosis

The diagnosis of rhabdomyosarcoma and soft tissue sarcoma is confirmed after tumor biopsy or resection. The diagnostic evaluation includes a history and physical examination. Radiographic studies include CT and MRI of the primary tumor site and CT scan of the lungs to assess for metastases. A radionuclide bone scan and skeletal survey look for metastatic disease of bone. Bone marrow aspirates and biopsies are usually performed at multiple sites, and lumbar puncture is performed to examine the CSF for the presence of malignant cells. Laboratory evaluation includes a CBC, urinalysis, blood chemistries, and liver function studies.

As with other malignancies, the treatment and prognosis of rhabdomyosarcoma depends upon the stage and histology of the disease. Overall, two-thirds of children diagnosed with rhabdomyosarcoma will become long-term survivors. Children with distant metastatic disease at diagnosis have a poor prognosis with only 30% surviving five years (American Cancer Society, 2000).

Treatment

The primary treatment of rhabdomyosarcoma and soft tissue sarcoma is wide surgical resection, whenever feasible. Only about one in six tumors can be completely removed because of the location or metastatic dissemination. When complete excision is done, the child will still receive adjuvant therapy to treat microscopic spread. Second-look surgery is often done to try to excise the remaining tumor completely and to evaluate the response to treatment.

Radiation therapy is used to control tumor growth byeradication of gross or microscopic disease. It usually follows surgery to treat residual disease and at times may be given preoperatively to decrease tumor size in inoperable masses or to spare radical surgical excision, as in the orbit. Radiation given to young children will cause decrease in growth in the radiated field. If the field includes a part of the face, the child may develop a noticeable asymmetry with aging.

Chemotherapy is recommended in all children with rhabdomyosarcoma and soft tissue sarcoma. The use of chemotherapy has increased the survival rate in these children whether they have metastatic disease at diagnosis or not. The regimens for advanced stage disease are severely myelosuppressive.

Nursing Management and Family Teaching

Nursing management of the child with rhabdomyosarcoma emphasizes emotional support and education of the client and family. Therapy is multimodal and intense in nature. As with other malignancies, teaching about prevention and early recognition of side effects of treatment or recurrence cannot be overemphasized. Children who receive this intense therapy are at risk for late effects.

RETINOBLASTOMA

Retinoblastoma is a rare form of cancer seen only in children. It is a tumor of the eye that develops when immature retinal cells, called retinoblasts, become malignant and grow out of control. This tumor is usually found in infants and very young children. About 40% of cases of retinoblastoma are hereditary, with 60% of this hereditary type being bilateral. The retinoblastoma cells can spread along the optic nerve to reach the brain, or through the covering layers of the globe into the eye socket. Once tissues outside the globe are affected, the cancer may then spread to lymph nodes, bones, bone marrow, or other organs. Most retinoblastoma tumors are discovered before they spread outside the globe of the eye.

Clinical Manifestations

Usually retinoblastoma is detected by the caregiver, who notices a whitish glow in the pupil (**cat's eye reflex**) instead of the red reflex typically seen in photographs. This is the most common manifestation. Other signs include strabismus and red painful eyes and blindness (late manifestations).

Treatment

Treatment of retinoblastoma depends upon whether the tumor is just in one eye or both; how good the vision is in the eyes; and whether the tumor has extended beyond the globe. Surgery, radiation therapy, laser therapy, cryotherapy (using very cold probes to freeze and kill the tumor), and chemotherapy are all used to treat this tumor. When the tumor is found in only one eye and vision has been destroyed, the usual treatment is **enucleation,** or surgical removal of the eye. If bilateral disease is present, and there is still some useful vision, then other forms of treatment are used. Chemotherapy is used when the retinoblastoma has spread beyond the eye, or when the spread within the eye is extensive, and near the optic nerve. Once retinoblastoma metastasizes, chemotherapy may control the disease, but usually is not curative. Over 90% of children with retinoblastoma survive more than five years (American Cancer Society, 2000).

LATE EFFECTS OF CANCER THERAPY

The number of childhood cancer survivors is increasing as the long-term prognosis of these children improves. Continued follow-up related to these long-term effects is necessary. Children tolerate the acute side effects of cancer therapy relatively well; however, this treatment may produce complications that are not apparent until the child grows and matures (Marina, 1997). A long-term survivor is defined as the child who has been in remission for 5 years and has been off cancer therapy for a minimum of 2 years (Hobbie, Ruccione, Moore, & Truesdell, 1993). Many survivors have complex psychosocial and physical problems that are the result of aggressive combination lifesaving therapy. These problems are to be approached by health care providers with understanding and knowledge. Childhood cancer survivors need lifelong care that monitors for the late effects of cancer treatment. Late effects of cancer therapy given during childhood have been identified in all major organs.

Children who have received radiation therapy to the brain may show growth retardation and cognitive impairments. These effects are dose and age related, with children under 5 years of age at the time of radiation being the most affected. Cognitive impairment may be manifest as a significant decrease in the child's general intelligence, or as problems with visual spatial skills, attention span, verbal fluency, and the rapidity with which information can be processed (Moore, 1995).

Musculoskeletal defects involving the bones, soft tissues, and teeth have been reported most frequently in children with solid tumors. These disabilities may include scoliosis, atrophy, avascular necrosis, and osteoporosis. These effects are usually the result of radiation therapy to the area. The higher the dose of radiation delivered to the younger child results in more pronounced late effects to the treated area (Marina, 1997).

Impaired ovarian function in women and testicular dysfunction in men are seen in clients who have received alkylating chemotherapeutic agents such as nitrogen mustard or cyclophosphamide. These findings are related to the age of the child and dose of the alkylating agents. Gonadal irradiation, including total body irradiation, affects the function of these reproductive organs. Treatment can produce sterility and decreased hormone production, leading to an absence or delay in pubertal development.

The thyroid gland is very sensitive to radiation therapy. Children who have received radiation to the head and neck area may develop primary hypothyroidism. Radiation to the head and neck may also produce abnormalities in the teeth, including incomplete calcification, tooth and root agenesis, and arrested tooth development. The most severe effects are seen in children who were radiated before six years of age. Chronic changes to the oral mucosa may be seen post-radiation, including xerostomia, loss of mucosal pliability, and chronic oral ulcers.

Radiation that includes the ear canal may lead to chronic radiation otitis. The chemotherapeutic agent, cisplatin, is known to cause hearing loss and when radiation therapy is also given the severity of the hearing loss is increased. Skin changes post-radiation may include permanent hyperpigmentation, atrophy, and hair loss, of the affected area. Impaired lung and thoracic development and chronic pulmonary compromise can be seen from radiation and/or chemotherapy. Pulmonary compromise is manifest as acute pneumonitis and pulmonary fibrosis. Dyspnea, dry cough, and low exercise tolerance are all signs of pulmonary fibrosis.

The heart may experience long-term effects from chemotherapy and/or radiation, which can be life-threatening. These treatments may cause irreversible damage to the heart. Anthracyclines are chemotherapeutic agents known to affect the heart by damaging cardiac myocytes. Chronic effects manifest as cardiomyopathy, pericarditis, or both. Cardiac toxicity from radiation alone may result in pericardial effusions or constrictive pericarditis. Decreased bone marrow function and immunosuppression may be long-term sequelae of cancer therapy and contribute to the increased risk of second malignancies. Bone marrow transplantation also places the child at greatest risk for hemtopoietic late effects.

The most devastating consequence of childhood cancer therapy is the development of a second malignancy. Approximately 3–12% of children treated for childhood cancer will develop a second malignancy within 20 years of the original cancer (Marina, 1997). The most common second malignancies are leukemia and soft tissue sarcomas. Long-term surveillance and the recognition of the potential for the development of these late effects allows the nurse, in the outpatient setting, to provide anticipatory guidance, supportive care, and interventions for symptom management. Long-term evaluations specific to the child's cancer therapy need to be done annually or more frequently, as needed. A long-term follow-up visit provides the opportunity to encourage clients to follow the recommendations for risk reduction and early detection. Those in the pediatric oncology field look forward to the day when late effects of therapy can be prevented; but in the meantime helping clients and their families anticipate and cope with late effects remains a critical element in the care of survivors of childhood cancer.

BOX 29-1 Camps for children with life-threatening illnesses

Around the country there are summer camps designed especially for children with life-threatening illnesses, cancer included. These camps offer these children a respite where they can get to know others that may struggle with the same emotions as they do and just be a kid. These camps offer activities that foster self-confidence. The activities (like swinging from a rope over a net) can be done with special equipment or with an adult so that every child can have the experience if they feel up to it.

Doctors, nurses, and other health care professionals often donate a week or two of their time to work at these camps. Thus, the campers always have medical care available to them to address their particular needs.

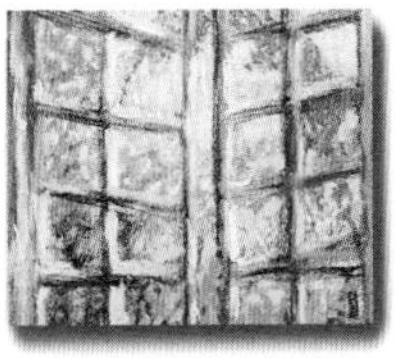

In the Real World

As a pediatric oncology nurse I am often asked, "Isn't it depressing to be around kids who are so sick and die? How can you go and work there everyday?" I respond that this is the most rewarding job I can ever imagine. Yes, there are sad days; when a child relapses or dies, the entire staff feels the family's pain, but oncology nursing is not depressing. Most children will have their cancer go into remission, and many will be cured. New advances in science improve the survival rates every year. Few other areas of nursing allow the nurse to get to know their clients and families so well. Pediatric oncology nursing is working on the cutting-edge of new scientific discoveries. I can counsel the caregiver and child, provide information, and offer comfort measures, whether it is pain medication or even rocking a child while reading him a book. The families whom I provide care to suffer great hardships, and I have the privilege to get to know them and be able to ease some of their burden.

Key Concepts

- Cancer is the leading cause of death from disease in children 1–14 years of age. Only accidents claim more lives.
- The primary treatment modalities for childhood cancer may include surgery, chemotherapy, radiation therapy, bone marrow transplantation (BMT), and biological response modifiers (BRMs).
- Colony stimulating factors are now widely used with children on chemotherapy to decrease the time the child is neutropenic and at risk for infection. Nurses are responsible for teaching the caregivers the administration of these agents in the home. Frequent monitoring of the CBC is needed to know when these agents can be stopped.
- The hematopoietic, gastrointestinal, hepatic, renal, integumentary, and reproductive systems are most commonly affected by side effects of chemotherapy. The nurse caring for the child undergoing chemotherapy is responsible for side effect management.
- Infection is the leading cause of death in the immunosuppressed child. Good handwashing and infection control measures are essential for the nurse to practice and teach the child and caregiver.
- Children with venous access devices are at increased risk of infection. Caregivers need to be taught the proper care of the devices and signs of infection.
- Bone marrow transplant is a treatment modality for leukemia, lymphomas, and certain solid tumors.
- The most common childhood malignancies are leukemia, brain tumors, and lymphomas.
- Children with leukemia commonly present with anemia, thrombocytopenia, and neutropenia, manifested as bleeding and fever. Pain is also a presenting symptom caused by bone destruction from leukemic infiltrates.
- Acute renal compromise can result from tumor lysis syndrome in children with leukemia and lymphoma. Nursing management includes IV hydration, alkalization of the child's urine with sodium bicarbonate, and the administration of allopurinol, prior to starting chemotherapy.
- Children with brain tumors may present with subtle neurological findings or signs of increased intracranial pressure.
- Children with neuroblastoma commonly present with advanced disease. Nursing care includes management of the presenting symptoms such as pain and, once chemotherapy has started, management of the side effects of therapy.
- Wilms' tumor is a malignancy of childhood that arises from the kidney. This tumor usually presents as an abdominal mass. Treatment is with surgery, chemotherapy, and sometimes radiation therapy.
- Limb-sparing surgery is commonly used for osteogenic sarcoma (bone tumors). Children with this type of cancer need to be prepared preoperatively both physically and emotionally. These individuals and their caregivers are to be informed of issues of body image and the expected amount of limb function prior to the procedure.
- Rhabdomyosarcoma and soft tissue sarcoma are the most common sarcomas of childhood. These children usually present with a hard, non-tender mass. Sarcomas are primarily treated with wide surgical excision, radiation therapy, and chemotherapy.
- Long-term effects of cancer therapy involve all major organs. Nurses in the outpatient settings need to assess for these specific side effects and provide prompt management and support.

Review Questions

1. List and describe the three most common childhood malignancies.
2. Describe how chemotherapy and radiation therapy are used in treating cancer.
3. List at least four common side effects of chemotherapy and describe how the nurse may manage these.
4. What are the client and family teaching needs of a child receiving a venous access device?
5. Describe the nursing interventions to use with a child who has recently been diagnosed with lymphoma to prevent tumor lysis syndrome.
6. Identify the nursing interventions in a child presenting with fever and neutropenia.
7. What is the single most important means of preventing infection?
8. How would you treat a child presenting with mucositis?
9. What would be included in a discharge care plan for the child recently diagnosed with a brain tumor?
10. Describe why the management of long-term effects of cancer therapy is important.

References

Abramovitz, L., & Senner, A. (1995). Pediatric bone marrow transplantation update. *Oncology Nursing Forum, 22*(1), 107–115.

American Brain Tumor Association. (1998). *A primer of brain tumors: A patient's reference manual,* Des Plaines, IL: Author.

American Cancer Society. (2000). *Cancer facts & figures: Childhood cancers.* [on-line]. Available: http:///www.cancer.org. Accessed: June 1, 2001.

Bernstein, L., Linet, M., Smith, M. A., & Olshan, A. F. (1999). Renal tumors. In L. A. G. Ries, M. A. Smith, J. G. Gurney, M. Linet, T. Tamra, J. L. Young, & G. R. Bunin (Eds.), *Cancer incidence and survival among children and adolescents: United States SEER Program 1975–1995,* National Cancer Institute, SEER Program. NIH Publication No. 99-4649. Bethesda, MD.

Brodeur, G. M., & Castleberry, R. P. (1997). Neuroblastoma. In P. A. Pizzo & D. G. Poplack (Eds.), *Principles and practice of pediatric oncology* (3rd ed., pp. 761–791). Philadelphia: Lippincott Raven Publishers.

Buschsel, P. C., Leum, E. W., & Randolph, S. R. (1996). Delayed complications of bone marrow transplantation: An update. *Oncology Nursing, 23*(8), 1267–1291.

Castiglia, P. T. (1995). Lymphomas in children. *Journal of Pediatric Health Care, 9*(5), 225–226.

De Vitta Jr., V. T., Hellman, S., & Rosenberg, S. A. (1997). *Cancer principles in oncology* (5th ed., pp. 2099–2103). Philadelphia: Lippincott Raven.

Dodd, M. J., Larson, P. J., Dibble, S. L., Miaskowski, C., Greespan, D., MacPhail, L., Hauck, W. W., Paul, S. M., Ignoffo, R., & Shiba, G. (1996). Randomized clinical trial of chlorhexidine versus placebo prevention of oral mucositis in patients receiving chemotherapy. *Oncology Nursing Forum, 23*(6), 921–927.

Friebert, S. E., & Shurin, S. B. (1998). ALL: Diagnosis and outlook. *Contemporary Pediatrics, 15*(2), 118–136.

Golub, T. R., Weinstein, H. J., & Grier, H. E. (1997). Acute myeloblastic leukemia. In P. A. Pizzo & D. G. Poplack (Eds.), *Principles and Practice of Pediatric Oncology* (3rd ed., pp. 317–384). Philadelphia: Lippincott Raven Publishers.

Goodman, M., & Riley, M. B. (1997). Chemotherapy: Principles of administration. In S. L. Groenwald, M. H. Frogge, & C. H. Yarbro (Eds.), *Cancer nursing principles and practice* (4th ed., pp. 317–384. Sudbury, MA: Jones and Bartlett Publishers.

Gurney, J. G., Smith, M. A., & Bunin, G. R. (1999). CNS and miscellaneous intracranial and intraspinal neoplasms. In L. A. G. Ries, M. A. Smith, J. G. Gurney, M. Linet, T. Tamra, J. L. Young, & G. R. Bunin (Eds.), *Cancer incidence and survival among children and adolescents: United States SEER Program 1975–1995,* National Cancer Institute, SEER Program. NIH Publication No. 99-4649. Bethesda, MD.

Gurney, J. G., Young, J. L., Roffiers, S. D., Smith, M. A., & Bunin, G. R. (1999). Soft tissue sarcomas. In L. A. G. Ries, M. A. Smith, J. G. Gurney, M. Linet, T. Tamra, J. L. Young, & G. R. Bunin (Eds.), *Cancer incidence and survival among children and adolescents: United States SEER Program 1975–1995,* National Cancer Institute, SEER Program. NIH Publication No. 99-4649. Bethesda, MD.

Heideman, R. L., Packer, R. J., Albright, L. A., Freeman, C. R., & Rorke, L. B. (1997). Central nervous system tumors of childhood. In P. A. Pizzo & D. G. Poplack (Eds.), *Principles and practice of pediatric oncology* (3rd ed., pp. 633–697). Philadelphia: Lippincott Raven Publishers.

Hobbie, W., Ruccione, K., Moore, I., & Truesdell, S. (1993). Late effects in long term survivors. In G. Foley, D. Fochtman, & K. H. Mooney (Eds.), *Nursing care of the child with cancer* (pp. 466–493). Philadelphia: W. B. Saunders.

Hudson, M. M., Tyc, V. L., Cremer, L. K., Luo, X., Rao, B. N., Meyer, W. H., Crom, D. B., & Pratt, C. B. (1998). Patient satisfaction after limb-sparing surgery and amputation for pediatric bone tumors. *Journal of Pediatric Oncology Nursing, 15*(2), 60–69.

Hudson, M. M., & Donaldson, S. S. (1997). Hodgkin's Disease. In P. A. Pizzo & D. G. Poplack (Eds.), *Principles and practice of pediatric oncology* (3rd ed., pp. 523–543). Philadelphia: J. B. Lippincott.

Lew, C. M., & La Vally, B. (1995). The role of stereotactic radiation therapy in the management of children with brain tumors. *The Journal of Pediatric Oncology Nursing, 12*(4), 212–222.

Margolin, J. F., & Poplack, D. G. (1997). Acute lymphocytic leukemia. In P. A. Pizzo & D. G. Poplack (Eds.), *Principles and practice of pediatric oncology* (3rd ed., pp. 409–462). Philadelphia: Lippincott Raven Publishers.

Marina, N. (1997). Long term survivors of childhood cancer. *Pediatric Clinics of North America, 44*(4), 1021–42.

Meyers, P. A., & Gorlick, R. (1997). Osteosarcoma. *Pediatric Clinics of North America, 44*(4), 973–989.

Moore, I. (1995). Central nervous system toxicity of cancer therapy. *Journal of Pediatric Oncology Nursing, 12*(4), 203–210.

Mosher, R. B., & McCarthy, B. J. (1998). Late effects in survivors of bone tumors. *Journal of Pediatric Oncology Nursing, 15*(2) 72–84.

Nemes, J., & Donahue, M. C. (1994). Solid tumors in children. *Nursing Clinics of North America, 29*(4), 585–598.

Nenstiel, R., White, G. L., & Aikens, T. (1997). Handwashing: A century of evidence ignored, *Clinician Reviews, 7*(1), 55–62.

Pearson, M. (1998). Historical perspective of the treatment of osteosarcoma: An interview with Dr. Norman Jaffe. *Journal of Pediatric Oncology Nursing 15*(2), 90–94.

Percy, C. L., Smith, M. A., Linet, M., Ries, L. A. G., & Friedman, D. L. (1999). Lymphomas and reticuloendothelial neoplasms. In L. A. G. Ries, M. A. Smith, J. G. Gurney, M. Linet, T. Tamra, J. L. Young, & G. R. Bunin (Eds.), *Cancer incidence and survival among children and adolescents: United States SEER Program 1975–1995,* National Cancer Institute, SEER Program. NIH Publication No. 99-4649. Bethesda, MD.

Pitler, L. R. (1996). Hematopoietic growth factors in clinical practice. *Seminars in Oncology Nursing, 12*(2), 115–129.

Potter, K. L., & Schafer, S. L. (1999). Nausea and vomiting. *American Journal of Nursing,* ONS Suppl. (April), 2–4.

Robinson, L. L. (1997). Principles of the epidemiology of childhood cancer. In P. A. Pizzo & D. G. Poplack (Eds.), *Principles and practice of pediatric oncology* (3rd ed., pp. 1–10). Philadelphia: Lippincott Raven Publishers.

Rust, D. M., Wood, L. S., & Battiato, L. A. (1999). Oprelvekin: An alternative for thrombocytopenia. *Clinical Journal of Oncology Nursing, 3*(2), 57–62.

Shad, A., & Magrath, I. (1997). Malignant non-Hodgkin's lymphomas in children. In P. A. Pizzo & D. G. Poplack (Eds.), *Principles and practice of pediatric oncology* (3rd ed., pp. 545–587). Philadelphia: J. B. Lippincott.

Shiminski-Maher, T., & Shields, M. (1995). Pediatric brain tumors: Diagnosis and management. *Journal of Pediatric Oncology Nursing, 12*(4), 188–198.

Shiminski-Maher, T., & Wisoff, J. H. (1995). Pediatric brain tumors. *Critical Care Nursing Clinics of North America, 7*(1), 159–169.

Smith, M. A., Ries, L. A. G., Gurney, J. G., & Ross, J. A. (1999). Leukemia. In L. A. G. Ries, M. A. Smith, J. G. Gurney, M. Linet, T. Tamra, J. L. Young, & G. R. Bunin (Eds.), *Cancer incidence and survival among children and adolescents: United States SEER Program 1975–1995,* National Cancer Institute, SEER Program. NIH Publication No. 99-4649. Bethesda, MD.

Stewart, S. K. (1995). *Bone marrow transplants; A book of basics for patients.* Highland Park, IL: Blood and Marrow Transplant Newsletter.

U.S. Department of Health and Human Services. (1998). *Clinician's handbook of preventive services: Put prevention into practice*, Washington, DC: U.S. Government Printing Office.

Woolery-Antill, M., & Colter, C. (1993). Biologic response modifiers. In G. Foley, D. Fochtman, & K. H. Mooney (Eds.), *Nursing care of the child with cancer* (pp. 179–207). Philadelphia: W. B. Saunders.

Yeaney, M. (1995). Care of the child requiring a bone marrow transplant. In L. Baker & B. Anderson (Eds.), *Inpatient pediatric nursing* (pp. 385–390). Albany, NY: Delmar Publishers.

Suggested Readings

Karian, V. E., Jankowski, S. M., & Beal, J. A. (1998). Exploring the lived-experience of childhood cancer survivors. *Journal of Pediatric Oncology Nursing, 15,* 153–162.

Keene, N. (1999). *Childhood leukemia: A guide for families, friends & caregivers.* Sebastopol, CA: O'Reilly Press.

Lehna, C. R. (1998). A childhood cancer sibling's oral history. *Journal of Pediatric Oncology Nursing, 15,* 163–171.

McCarthy, A. M., Williams, J., & Plumer, C. (1998). Evaluation of a school re-entry nursing intervention for children with cancer. *Journal of Pediatric Oncology Nursing, 15,* 143–152.

Nunez, A. M., & Leibman, M. C. (1999). Febrile neutropenia. *American Journal of Nursing,* ONS Suppl. (April), 9–12.

Resources

Organizations and Websites

American Brain Tumor Association
2720 River Road
Des Plaines, IL 60018
(847) 827-9910
www.abta.org

American Cancer Society
2200 Century Pkwy., Suite 950
Atlanta, GA 30345
(800) ACS-2345
www.cancer.org

Association of Pediatric Oncology Nurses
4700 W. Lake Avenue
Glenview, IL 60025
(847) 375-4724
www.apon.org

Candlelighters Childhood Cancer Foundation
3910 Warner St.
Kensington, MD 20895
(800) 366-2223
www.candlelighters.org

Childhood Brain Tumor Foundation
20312 Watkins Meadow Drive
Germantown, MD 20876
(301) 515-2900
www.childhoodbraintumor.org

Children's Oncology Group
Children's National Medical Center
Department of Hematology/Oncology
111 Michigan Ave., NW
Washington, DC 20010
childrensoncologygroup.org

The Leukemia & Lymphoma Society, Inc.
1311 Mamaroneck Ave.
White Plains, NY 10605
(800) 955-4572
www.leukemia.org/hm_lls

National Cancer Institute
Building 31, Room 10A31
31 Center Dr., MSC2580
Bethesda, MD 20892
(800) 4-CANCER (800-422-6237)
www.nci.nih.gov

National Childhood Cancer Foundation/Children's Oncology Group
440 Huntington Dr.
Arcadia, CA 91066
(800) 458-6223
www.nccf.org

National Marrow Donor Program
3433 Broadway St. NE, Suite 500
Minneapolis, MN 55413
(800) MARROW2 (800-627-7692)
www.marrow.org

Oncology Nursing Society
501 Holiday Drive
Pittsburgh, PA 15220
(412) 921-6565
www.ons.org

CHAPTER 30

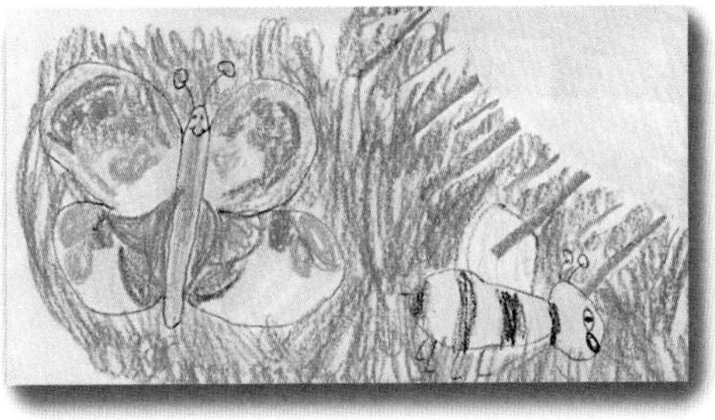

Jason started to develop eczema before he was 6 months old. His rash first appeared on his face and arms, and I could tell it made him uncomfortable. By the time he was a year old, the rash was on his lower legs as well. The rash was very itchy, and he would have raw, open areas from persistent scratching. We tried using many different lotions and creams on our own, but nothing really seemed to make a difference. Everyone seemed to have some well-meaning advice to offer. We tried to identify foods or activities that made the rash worse, but we couldn't find anything that increased the problem. By this time, it seemed he would scratch, almost out of habit, whether his skin had a rash or not. He became very irritable because we would tell him over and over not to scratch, and yet we knew he was uncomfortable. Over time, we came to learn more about eczema. We started giving him baths more frequently rather than less frequently and added baby oil to the bath water. We were careful to apply cream right after his bath and use steroid cream when the rash flared. Jason is now 9 years old, and he still has eczema. He still has times when he has flare-ups of the rash and will scratch. Overall, though, we have been able to help him take control of his eczema. It takes daily care, but his skin and his self-image are healthier for it.

INTEGUMENTARY ALTERATIONS

Linda S. Reig, PhD, RN
Phyllis Augspurger, PhD, RN
Lauri A. Linder, MS, RN

COMPETENCIES

Upon completion of this chapter, the reader will be able to:

- *Describe the impact of developmental and racial differences in caring for the skin of the pediatric client.*
- *Discuss the etiology, pathophysiology, clinical manifestations, and management of common integumentary disorders.*
- *Discuss nursing management and interventions appropriate for children with various integumentary disorders.*
- *Prepare a family centered plan of care for a child with a skin condition.*

The pediatric integumentary system plays a vital role in the child's health and well-being. From a physiological standpoint, it serves as a protective barrier against infective organisms and helps maintain the child's metabolic functioning. From a psychosocial perspective, the appearance of the skin influences others' perceptions of and reactions to the child. Alterations of the pediatric integumentary system can occur from many different causes including infectious and noninfectious sources. Although integumentary disorders are rarely life-threatening, they can have a major impact on the child's social functioning. This chapter begins with an overview of the major racial and developmental differences in the child's integument. A discussion of frequently seen pediatric integumentary disorders follows. They are grouped as infectious disorders, infestations, inflammatory disorders, bites and stings, and sunburn.

ANATOMY AND PHYSIOLOGY

The skin (integument) and its appendages (nails, hair, and certain glands) comprise the largest single organ of the body. It contains many types of cells that are crucial for health and survival. The three distinct layers of the skin are the epidermis, dermis, and subcutaneous tissue. Figure 30-1 illustrates the structures of the skin and epidermal and dermal layers. The outermost layer of the **epidermis,** the **stratum corneum,** is an effective barrier against the penetration of irritants, toxins, and organisms; it also holds in body fluids. **Melanocytes** within the epidermis are important for protection from the

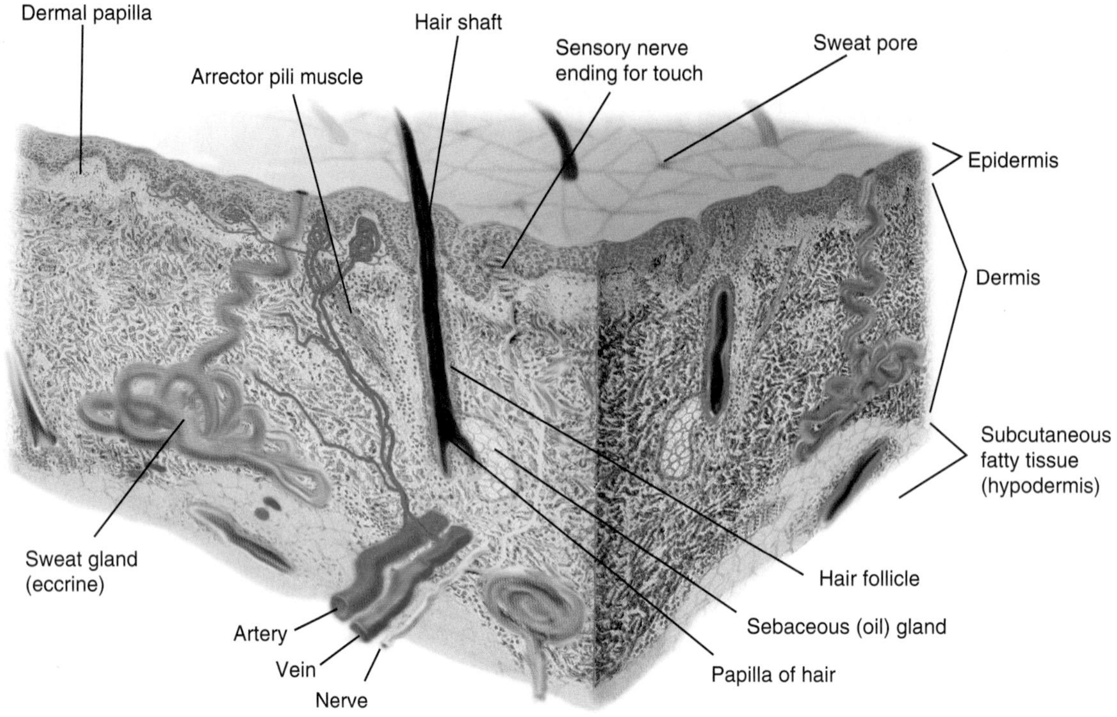

Figure 30-1 Structures of the Skin

harmful effects of ultraviolet light. These cells are also the major determinants of skin color (Wysocki, 1999).

The **dermis** consists largely of fibroblasts and collagen. It is a tough mechanical barrier against cuts, bites, and bruises. It provides nourishment to the epidermis and is essential for wound healing. Sebaceous glands, sweat glands, and hair follicles receive structural support by the collagenous matrix found in the dermis and subcutaneous tissue (Huether, 1998).

The integumentary system contributes to the protective, metabolic, and interactive functions of a person. The skin protects an individual from harmful external organisms, which may cause disease, as well as offers coverage to prevent leakage of vital bodily fluids. Linked to this protective function is the ability to warn of changes in stimuli, such as temperature, pressure, and pain, as well as provision of pleasure and comfort provided by touch (Wysocki, 1999; Huether, 1998). Storage and absorption are among the metabolic functions of the skin. Storage of water and fat in the subcutaneous tissues protects against mechanical forces and provides insulation and storage of nutrients. Absorption of ultraviolet (UV) light can be positive or harmful. Absorption is necessary for the conversion of substances to vitamin D; however, excessive UV exposure can lead to skin damage, the most serious being skin cancer. The skin also absorbs medications and chemicals applied topically, which can produce therapeutic or harmful effects (Wysocki, 1999; Huether, 1998).

The physical appearance of the skin may be perceived by the child and adolescent as its most important function. Much of young people's self-image and self-esteem comes from their body image; this includes how they appear to themselves as well as the reactions they receive from others, often as a result of their appearance. Health care providers can gain a wealth of information about a person from a brief survey of the integument. Clues such as pallor, cyanosis, jaundice, rashes, broken hair, **alopecia** (bald spots), signs of infestation, multiple bruises, and skin lesions are examples of indicators that require further evaluation. Often the integument serves as a window for observing a much broader view of the individual's overall health status.

Understanding the differences of the integument associated with developmental stages and various races is necessary to provide appropriate assessments and therapeutic interventions. Like most of the other body systems, the integumentary system is immature at birth. The newborn's skin is very thin and the epidermis is loosely bound to the dermis. Premature infants are susceptible to damage caused by friction with even minor handling. The neonate's thin epidermis results in increased absorption of medications and substances through the skin. They have limited subcutaneous fat, which limits their ability to adapt to environmental temperature changes. The pH of a newborn's skin is relatively alkaline during the first week of life, which renders the infant more susceptible to infection. Over time, the skin surface becomes more acidic. This lower pH discourages growth of microorganisms. The infant's **sebaceous glands** are active at birth because of the influence of maternal hormones. The sebaceous glands secrete **sebum,** which helps lubricate the skin. Sebaceous gland activity may result in the

Nursing Alert:

Topical Medications and Infants

Topical medications should be avoided, if possible, in infants less than 6 months of age. Young infants have an increased rate of absorption of topical medications, which may lead to toxicity.

appearance of neonatal acne. As sebaceous gland activity decreases, the skin may become more prone to drying and chapping requiring the use of moisturizing lotions.

The protective functions of the skin mature as the child reaches the preschool years. Secretory IgA is diminished until the child is about 2 to 5 years old. Until this time, the child has decreased mucosal resistance to organisms. Caregivers should be taught to monitor items the child places in his or her mouth to help reduce the risk of infection. **Eccrine glands** reach mature function by the time the child is 2 to 3 years old. Eccrine glands are distributed across the body and allow for perspiration. Maturation of these glands allows for more effective thermoregulation. Evaporation of eccrine sweat also decreases the skin's pH, providing increased resistance to microorganisms.

Apocrine glands become functional around 8 to 10 years of age. Apocrine glands are sweat glands concentrated in the axillae, scalp, face, abdomen, and genital area. Perspiration from appocrine glands begins a few years before puberty. Its appearance can indicate progress toward normal, pubertal development. Sebum secretion also occurs during the school-age years. In addition to providing lubrication to the skin, sebum functions to lower the skin's pH. Normal integumentary changes associated with adolescence include increased sebaceous gland activity under the influence of stimulation from normal androgen secretion. This contributes to the development of acne, which is a major concern for many adolescents. Axillary and pubic hair develops in both genders and facial hair develops in males under the influence of gonadal hormones.

Varied pigmentation is only one of the differences in the integumentary system among racial groups. Differences in hair texture and distribution, number of sweat glands, and cultural values regarding the integument may exist. For example, pallor or cyanosis may be difficult to assess in individuals of darker-skinned races such as African-American or Native American. Assessment of mucous membranes or nail beds provides a more reliable measure. Rashes also may be more difficult to discern in darker-skinned individuals. Rashes should be palpated to allow for more accurate assessment. Erythema may appear as a deep red or violet color. Table 30-1 provides a brief overview of the major variations in the integument of different races.

TABLE 30-1 Skin Variations by Race of Children

Race	Characteristics (and Implications for Care)
African-American	Skin
	Pallor best detected in nail beds or mucous membranes; cyanosis may appear deep blue/black on skin
	Varying degrees of pigmentation from very light to deep black; pigmentation increases similar to Asians. **Implications for care:** May need to palpate rashes because of difficulty visualizing; erythema often seen as deep red or violet.
	Apocrine sweat glands more numerous than Native Americans and Asians
	Increased cutaneous melanin; protects against sun damage
	Mongolian spots present in 90% of infants. **Implications for care:** Do not assume caregivers know what these are; explain that these spots are not uncommon in some races and tend to fade as the child gets older. Need to document because they can be misdiagnosed as bruises, common in child abuse.
	Other
	Pseudofolliculitis barbae: Papulopustules occur at hair follicles, caused by to hair reentering the skin. Seen almost exclusively in African-American males
	Hair
	Variety of textures; increased sebaceous secretions
	Hair may spontaneously knot; rubbing can have a wooling effect
	Nail Beds
	Diffuse pigmentation of nail, especially in darker clients

continues

TABLE 30-1 *Continued*

Race	Characteristics (and Implications for Care)
Asian	Skin
	Pallor is best detected in nail beds and mucous membranes
	Pigmentation varies from brown to pale yellow-tinged
	Pigmentation is very light at birth, darkens with age until 2 to 3 months old
	Apocrine sweat glands fewer than in Caucasians and African-Americans
	Mongolian spots (blue-black hyperpigmentation found in the lumbosacral area) present in 90% of infants. **Implications for care:** See African-American.
	Hair
	Sparse body hair; chest hair frequently absent in adolescent males
	Color very dark; usually deep brown to black
	Texture may be fine to coarse; generally straight but may be wavy
	Nail beds
	Darker pigmentation may be present
Caucasian	Skin
	Large variations in skin tones and degree of pigmentation
	More apocrine sweat glands than Asians and Native Americans
	Decreased melanin leads to high risk for sunburn, and skin damage leading to higher incidence of skin cancer than other races. **Implications for care:** Early skin cancer prevention education important for caregivers. Stress importance of routinely using sunscreen on children and infants older than six months.
	Freckles seen in fair-skinned school-aged children with frequent exposure to the sun
	Other
	Higher incidence of adolescent acne
	Hair
	Wide variation in hair color and texture
	Color ranges from blond to black; texture may be straight to very curly, thick to fine
	Nail Beds
	Pale to deep pink pigmentation
Hispanic American	Skin
	Pallor best detected in mucous membranes
	Varying degrees of pigmentation. Largest percentage have tan to dark brown skin
	Increases in pigmentation similar to Asians and African-Americans
	Mongolian spots present in 90% of infants. **Implications for care:** See African-American.
	Hair
	Varying textures: wavy, curly, straight; mostly black or dark brown
	Nail Beds
	Deep pigmentation may be present

continues

TABLE 30-1 *Continued*

Race	Characteristics (and Implications for Care)
Native American	Skin
	Pallor best detected in mucous membranes
	Varying degrees of pigmentation; increased pigmentation similar to Asians, African-Americans, and Hispanics
	Fewer apocrine sweat glands than in African-Americans and Caucasians
	Mongolian spots present in 90% of infants. **Implications for care:** See African-American.
	Hair
	Variations in texture may be coarse to fine; hair may be straight, wavy, or curly
	Nail Beds
	Deep pigmentation may be present

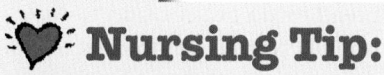

Nursing Tip:

Mongolian spots

Mongolian spots are areas of bluish-black hyperpigmentation that most frequently occur over the lumbosacral area of dark-skinned infants. These areas are normal skin variations and tend to fade as the child gets older. The presence of Mongolian spots should be included as a part of the child's documentation. Mongolian spots can be misdiagnosed as bruises, commonly found in child abuse.

BACTERIAL INFECTIONS

The skin of healthy infants and children is resistant to invasion by most bacteria because the cutaneous surface provides a dry mechanical barrier from which contaminating organisms are constantly removed by **desquamation,** or shedding of the outer layer of the epidermis. Intact skin and mucous membranes, in conjunction with both transient and resident flora, provide this protective barrier. Transient flora consist of almost all microorganisms that are deposited on the skin from the environment; they do not generally proliferate, and are easily removed by washing the affected area. Resident flora are fewer in number and can become established and multiply on the skin. These organisms are not easily dislodged and function as a defense against bacterial infection. Resident and transient bacteria can resist colonization by producing antibacterial substances or by competing for available nutrients. The combination of normal epidermal shedding, dryness of the cutaneous surface, integrity of the skin, virulence of the organisms, presence of normal flora and the host response determine if infections of the skin will occur (Wysocki, 1999). Children with compromised immune systems (such as infants, those with debilitating illnesses, immune deficiency disorders, or those taking immunosuppressive drug therapy) are at particular risk for developing bacterial skin infections. The bacterial infections, impetigo and cellulitis, are discussed.

Impetigo

Impetigo is a highly contagious superficial bacterial skin infection and is characterized by localized inflammation and infection in the epidermis. Two major disease forms exist: 1) impetigo contagiosa, which is characterized by crusted lesions, and 2) bullous impetigo, which is characterized by fragile bullae (Resnick, 2000).

Incidence and Etiology

Impetigo is more prevalent during mid to late summer and in hot, humid climates. Although the disease may affect any individual, it is most prevalent among infants and children. Poor sanitation and crowded living conditions place the child at increased risk for acquiring impetigo (Nicol & Huether, 1998). In most cases, minor trauma to the skin such as a scratch or insect bite is necessary to disrupt the skin barrier and allow introduction of bacteria, which are most commonly spread by direct contact with an infected individual. Individuals colonized with *Staphylococcus aureus*, however, may serve as their own source of infection (Resnick, 2000).

Pathophysiology

Both *Staphylococcus aureus* and group A beta-hemolytic streptococci can cause impetigo contagiosa. Bullous impetigo is almost always caused by *Staphylococcus aureus*. The development of the skin lesions occurs as a result of disruption of normal cellular adhesion. Both staphylococci and streptococci release exotoxins and enzymes that interfere with normal cellular function and allow destruction of connective tissue and exfoliation of the skin. The overall immune status of the affected individual also contributes to the extent and severity of the lesions.

Clinical Manifestations

The lesions of impetigo contagiosa begin as small red macules and progress to small, thin-roofed vesicles or pustules that rupture easily and expose weeping, denuded skin. Drainage from the lesions has a characteristic honey color and forms crusts. Lesions may enlarge to 1 to 2 centimeters in diameter, and smaller satellite lesions are common (Figure 30-2). Regional lymphadenopathy is often associated with impetigo contagiosa (Resnick, 2000; Nicol & Huether, 1998).

Bullous impetigo also begins as small red macules; however, these lesions rapidly progress to distinct vesicles, which may further enlarge to form fragile bullae. Ruptured bullae may result in shiny erosions of the skin or produce a honey-colored crust. Regional lymphadenopathy is uncommon with bullous impetigo.

Lesions of both forms of impetigo most often appear on the face, in particular, around the mouth and nares. Lesions originating on the extremities and buttocks may occur also. Lesions often cause mild discomfort and pruritus. Pruritus is associated with self-inoculation when the child scratches and then touches another area. Widespread involvement is possible and lesions may be present on any surface of the skin.

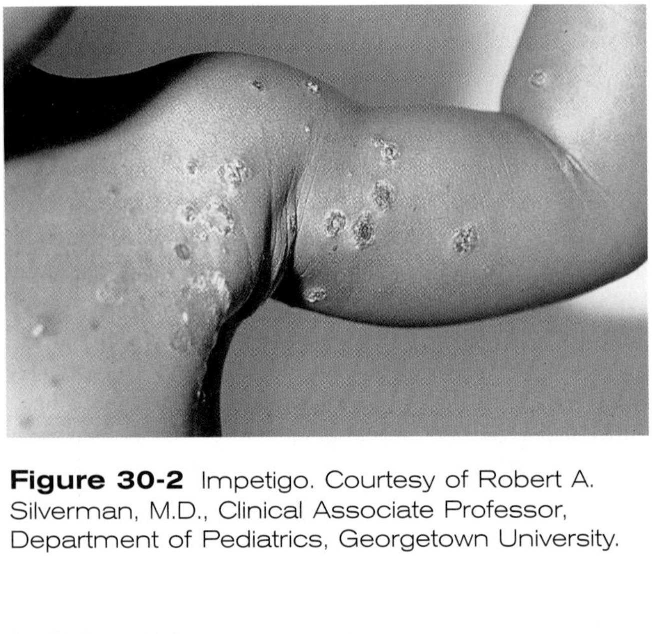

Figure 30-2 Impetigo. Courtesy of Robert A. Silverman, M.D., Clinical Associate Professor, Department of Pediatrics, Georgetown University.

Such involvement typically occurs in the presence of an underlying skin disorder such as atopic dermatitis.

Diagnosis

Diagnosis is based on clinical presentation. The presence of honey-colored crusts is considered the hallmark characteristic of impetigo. Of particular importance is the need to assess for underlying skin diseases such as atopic dermatitis, herpes simplex infections, or contact dermatitis that have become secondarily infected (Resnick, 2000).

Treatment

The treatment of impetigo is focused on eliminating the causative organism while utilizing comfort measures and preventing complications. Medical management consists of topical antibiotic therapy, which may be considered for initial therapy if only a few lesions are present and are limited to a small area of the skin. Mupirocin (Bactroban) is an example of a topical antibiotic that has been used. Studies have suggested that its effectiveness is equal to that of erythromycin or cephalexin (Resnick, 2000; Bass, et al., 1997).

If lesions are widespread or do not respond to topical therapy, administration of oral, systemic antibiotics is indicated. Neonates and children at high risk for widespread disease also should be managed with systemic antibiotics. Penicillinase-resistant penicillins such as dicloxacillin (Dynapen) or cephalosporins such as cephalexin (Keflex) are considered appropriate, cost-effective therapy for both forms of impetigo. Health care providers need to be aware of the local resistance patterns to certain antibiotics. For example, staphylococcal resistance to erythromycin may be as great as 50% in some geographic areas (Resnick, 2000; Nicol & Huether, 1998).

Nursing Management

Assessment

Nurses should discuss with the child and caregivers any previous exposure to anyone with similar lesions. Ask about the location and appearance of the first lesions and in what manner and how quickly they spread. Note the character and extent of lesions, the presence of vesicles, and crusting and drainage. As with any infection, nurses should observe for presence of elevated temperature, respiratory rate, and heart rate and ask about the child's comfort. Also, assess for the presence of regional lymphadenopathy and any underlying skin disorders such as atopic dermatitis.

Nursing Diagnosis

Nursing diagnoses for the infant or child with impetigo include:

1. Infection related to presence of infective organisms.
2. Impaired skin integrity related to presence of lesions.

3. Risk for secondary infection related to scratching or picking of lesions.
4. Deficient knowledge related to treatment and measures to control and prevent the spread of infection.

Outcome Identification

1. Child's infection will be resolved and lesions will heal without evidence of scarring.
2. Child's infection will not spread beyond the primary site of infection.
3. Caregivers will verbalize understanding of the treatment regimen and implement strategies to prevent spread of infection.

Planning/Implementation

The nursing management of children with impetigo focuses on resolution of the infection, comfort measures, and education for the caregivers related to preventing the spread of infection and prevention of complications. Careful handwashing before and after contact with the child is essential, along with wearing gloves during care. Although older children may understand instructions and attempt to keep from touching the lesions when awake, younger children will not. Comfort measures, such as gentle soaking and removal of crusts with warm soapy water and keeping the child's nails cut short, along with close supervision and distraction techniques are required for most children in order to contain the spread of infection.

Evaluation

The infection should be resolved by adherence to the antibiotic regimen, and lesions should not spread beyond the initial site of infection. Children and caregivers are able to utilize strategies to contain the infection and prevent spread to others.

Family Teaching

Strict adherence in taking the prescribed antibiotics as directed is essential. The nurse must emphasize the need to take the medications as instructed, even if the infection appears to be gone. The client and family members need to understand the contagious nature of impetigo and be instructed in principles about good hygiene including the need to use good handwashing with antibacterial soap. Towels and other personal items should not be shared. It is important to instruct caregivers to examine other individuals living in the home, particularly children, for signs of infection and to seek treatment if any lesions are found. Although the crusting lesions of impetigo may be distressful to the child and caregivers, they need to understand that simple uncomplicated ones will generally heal without scarring, if early treatment is initiated. The caregivers should notify the school of the diagnosis, and the child should remain out of school for 24–48 hours after the initiation of the systemic antibiotics. Instructions for seeking medical attention should be provided if the infection is not resolving.

Cellulitis

Cellulitis is a bacterial infection involving the dermis and subcutaneous tissue and is characterized by a painful area of erythema and swelling that may spread through the surrounding tissue. In contrast to impetigo, cellulitis is not considered contagious.

Incidence and Etiology

Cellulitis can occur in children of any age. The onset of symptoms typically occurs 1 to 2 days following minor trauma that disrupts the normal protective function of the skin. Infection can occur at any site on the body; however, the extremities and face, periorbital, and buccal areas are most commonly affected.

Streptococcus pyogenes and *Staphylococcus aureus* are the most common infective organisms (Darmstadt, 1997; 2000a). Children with cellulitis of the head and neck frequently have had an antecedent upper respiratory tract infection such as otitis media or sinusitis. *Haemophilus influenzae* was once a common causative agent of facial cellulitis in children from 3 months to 3–5 years; however, immunization with the *H. influenzae* type B (HIB) vaccine has resulted in significantly decreased numbers of cases (Givner, et al., 2000; Resnick, 2000). Immunocompromised children are at risk for acquiring cellulitis from opportunistic pathogens such as *Pseudomonas* species.

Pathophysiology

The symptoms of cellulitis result when the invading bacteria enter the skin, often following minor trauma. The subsequent inflammation and infection develop in the loose connective tissue. The infection also extends into the dermis, but most often spares the epidermis. Tissue necrosis does not occur with cellulitis.

Clinical Manifestations

The classic symptoms of cellulitis are those of an acute inflammatory process—erythema, swelling, warmth, and pain. The borders of the affected area are diffuse and will extend as the infection progresses (Figure 30-3). Lymphangitis, red streaks leading from the affected area to adjacent lymphatics, is often present as is lymphadenopathy. Systemic symptoms such as fever, chills, and malaise are common. Progressive infection may lead to abscess formation. Children with facial cellulitis caused by *Haemophilus influenzae* type B are at risk for developing meningitis.

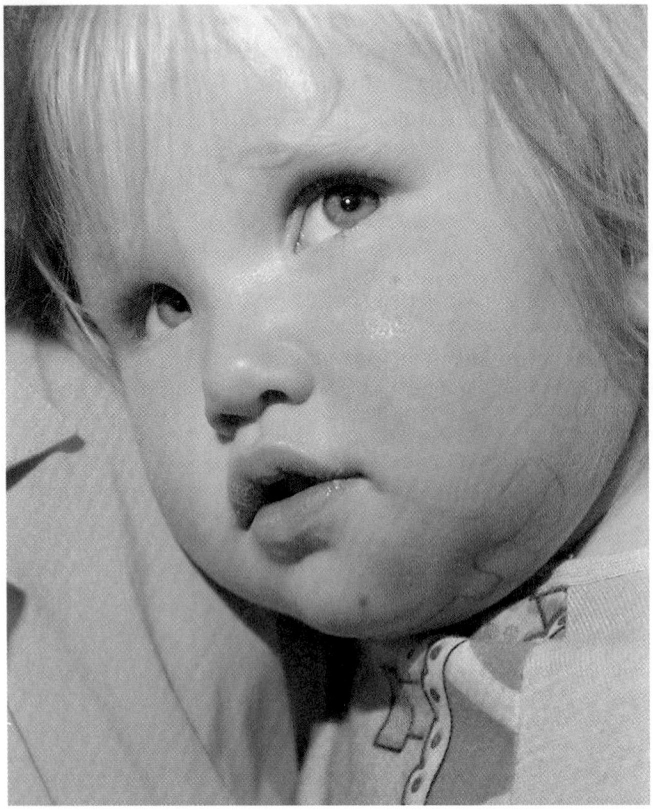

Figure 30-3 Cellulitis of the Face

Diagnosis

Diagnosis of cellulitis typically is based on history and clinical presentation. Identification of the specific pathogen in an immunocompetent host is difficult. Tissue aspirates, skin biopsies, and blood cultures often yield negative results and are not cost effective (Resnick, 2000; Sadow & Chamberlain, 1998).

Treatment

Prompt administration of systemic antibiotics is essential for treating cellulitis. Penicillinase resistant penicillins, cephalosporins, or erythromycin are appropriate agents for treatment (Rhody, 2000). If the child is febrile and acutely ill, hospitalization and administration of IV antibiotics are generally needed. The child with limited cellulitis can generally be managed on an outpatient basis with a regimen of oral antibiotics, warm compresses, immobilization and elevation of the extremity, and comfort measures (Resnick, 2000). Immobilization is recommended for comfort and to decrease edema. Warm compresses may be used to increase circulation to the area; however, cool compresses may be preferred to relieve discomfort. Acetaminophen and ibuprofen may be used to relieve pain and reduce fever. Close observation for early signs of potentially serious systemic infections is required.

Nursing Management and Family Teaching

Priorities for nursing management include eradication of the infection, promotion of the child's comfort, and prevention of complications. The assessment should include questioning the child or caregivers about a history of minor trauma to the affected area. The nurse also should ask about the development of symptoms related to the cellulitis and any associated systemic symptoms. Planning should emphasize teaching caregivers about the prescribed medical treatment and comfort measures. Children requiring IV antibiotic therapy will require coordination of home care services to provide the medication once the client's condition has been stabilized in the hospital. Caregivers should receive education regarding signs and symptoms of worsening infection.

FUNGAL INFECTIONS

Fungi are found throughout the environment including the soil, water, decaying vegetation, animals, rocks, and air. Although some fungal infections occur as an overgrowth of **commensal fungi,** most superficial ones result when fungi are introduced from the environment through the skin and mucous membranes. The body has several defense mechanisms, including general health, nutritional status, and various skin properties such as pH and rate of epithelial turnover that inhibit fungal infection. When these mechanisms are compromised in some way, fungal infections can occur. Fungal infections are also known as **mycoses.** The most common types of superficial mycoses are *Candida* and tinea infections.

Candidiasis

Candidiasis, or moniliasis, is a fungal infection caused by *Candida* species and is the most common type of fungal infection. *Candida albicans*, a commensal fungus of the mouth and gastrointestinal tract, is the most common causative organism. This infection exists in two forms: a yeast, or spore, which is relatively harmless, and a hyphal form. **Hyphae** are the branching outgrowths of a fungus that invade the tissue and establish an infection. The majority of *Candida* infections are superficial, although systemic infections may occur. In infants and young children, candidiasis is most often manifested as oropharyngeal candidiasis, or thrush, and as candidal diaper dermatitis.

Incidence and Etiology

The exact incidence of candidiasis is difficult to determine. The incidence of thrush in infants is approximately 2–4%. Bottle-fed infants are at greater risk than breastfed infants for developing thrush (Clayton, 2000; Hoppe, 1997).

Clinical evidence of infection occurs as a consequence of alterations in the host's immune system. Neonates are at risk for acquiring *Candida* intrapartally from the vaginal canal. They also may acquire *Candida* from the mother during nursing or from bottle nipples that are improperly sterilized. Neonates have increased susceptibility for infection as a consequence of an immature immune system and incomplete development of the normal flora. Other factors that place the child at risk for developing candidal infections include antibiotic therapy, immune compromised conditions, endocrine disease, immunosuppressive therapy, maceration of the mucous membranes, and iron-deficiency anemia.

Pathophysiology

In most cases, the source of *Candida* is the host's normal flora. Colonization with *Candida* begins with adherence of the organism to the mucosal cells. Adherence to the mucosal cells must occur to allow the spores to germinate. Under the appropriate host conditions, including temperature, pH, and other environmental factors, the yeast spores are able to transition to the hyphal phase. Organisms in the hyphal phase then penetrate the host tissue and establish an infection. Following infection, host neutrophils infiltrate the epithelium followed by dermal infiltration by lymphocytes and tissue macrophages (Clayton, 2000; Walpole, 1998).

Clinical Manifestations

Thrush is characterized by the development of creamy-white plaques on the buccal mucosa and lateral borders of the tongue. Lesions gradually become confluent and may cover the entire oral cavity (Figure 30-4). The plaques associated with thrush can by distinguished from residual milk curds by their inability to be removed from the buccal mucosa. Lesions may cause mild discomfort but generally do not interfere with sucking and swallowing. In children with immune compromised conditions, oropharyngeal candidiasis may progress to esophagitis or systemic disease.

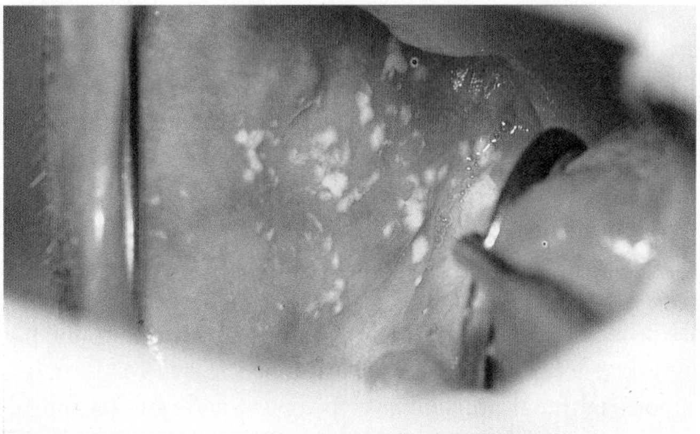

Figure 30-4 Candidiasis—Thrush. Courtesy of Dr. Joseph Konzelman, School of Dentistry, Medical College of Georgia.

Candidal diaper dermatitis is characterized by acute onset of erythematous papules beginning in the perianal area and progressing to cover the perineum. The papules coalesce to form a well-defined area of erythema with scalloped borders. Satellite vesico-pustular lesions are common. In African-American infants, the lesions may show depigmentation.

Candidiasis also may present as **intertrigo,** an erythematous skin eruption occurring on apposed skin surfaces. Apposed surfaces are those in direct contact such as the axillae and popliteal fossae. The presentation is similar to that of candidal diaper dermatitis with areas of well-defined erythema and satellite lesions (Figure 30-5). Common sites of occurrence are the axillae, interdigital spaces, and the gluteal cleft.

Diagnosis

Diagnosis commonly is based on the child's history and clinical presentation. Cytologic examination may be done to confirm the diagnosis. Smears from mucosal surfaces will reveal budding yeast cells with hyphae when examined using potassium hydroxide preparation or Gram stain. Diagnosis of the breastfeeding infant with thrush also should include evaluation of the mother for candidiasis of the nipple.

Treatment

Thrush usually responds quickly to oral nystatin suspension (100,000 U/ml) administered at intervals of 4 to 6 hours. Treatment should continue for 48 hours following resolution of symptoms (Clayton, 2000). Oral nystatin (Mycostatin) is poorly absorbed so it provides effective topical antifungal therapy. Nystatin lozenges or clotrimazole (Mycelex) troches provide an alternative means of delivering topical therapy to older children. Breastfeeding mothers with nipple candidiasis should apply nystatin cream to the nipples while treating the infant with oral nystatin (Bedinghaus, 1997). It should be wiped off prior to feeding.

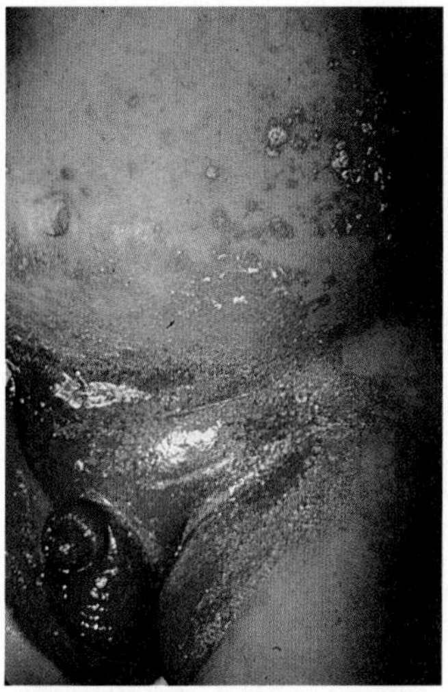

Figure 30-5 Candidiasis—Intertrigo. Courtesy of the Centers for Disease Control and Prevention.

Candidal diaper dermatitis and intertrigo most often are managed successfully with nystatin cream or ointment. A low-potency steroid such as 1% hydrocortisone cream may be used in addition to nystatin to manage diaper dermatitis (Clayton, 2000; Rex, et al., 2000). Additional supportive measures include keeping the affected area dry and exposed to air when feasible. Because of their increased risk of invasive candidiasis, children with neutropenia or those post solid organ or hematopoietic stem cell transplant often receive antifungal prophylaxis. Fluconazole (Diflucan) administered once daily is common therapy (Clayton, 2000; Rex, et al., 2000).

Nursing Management

Nursing care priorities for the child with candidiasis include resolution of the infection, promotion of the child's comfort, and continuation of breastfeeding. The nursing history should include prior antibiotic use in the child or mother and a history of yeast infections in the mother. Physical examination should note the pattern and distribution of lesions as well as nipple erythema and pain in the mother. Planning should include teaching about the prescribed medication and comfort measures for the child and mother. Because of the benefits to the infant, continued breastfeeding should be encouraged.

Family Teaching

Teaching should address proper use of the prescribed nystatin preparation. Because the medication is not absorbed systemically, it requires direct contact with the affected area to exert its antifungal activity. The suspension should be administered following a feeding to allow for prolonged contact. It should be administered in a manner that will allow for optimum contact with the lesions. Use of a toothette to swab the medication on the mucosal surfaces may be helpful. Nystatin ointment or cream should be applied to the diaper area four to six times a day following diaper changes. The skin should be thoroughly cleaned and dried prior to application. Diaper wipes should be avoided as they may irritate already inflamed skin. Exposing the skin to air when feasible may assist in promotion of healing. Teaching priorities for the breastfeeding mother include thorough handwashing before and after breastfeeding and following diaper changes. Breast pumps and pacifiers should be boiled for 20 minutes each day. Reinforcing proper positioning of the infant during feeding can prevent further nipple trauma to the mother. Expressed breast milk should be used immediately and not be frozen (Walpole, 1998).

Tinea Infections

The tinea infections are caused by **dermatophytes,** a group of closely related fungi that invade the outer keratin layer of the skin and its appendages, the hair and nails. Infection occurs when the fungus multiplies at a rate greater than the rate of keratin production. The five most commonly known tinea infections are distinct clinical entities, defined by the anatomic site of the infection and the fungus involved. They include tinea capitis (head ringworm), tinea corporis (body ringworm), tinea pedis (athlete's foot), tinea cruris (jock itch), and tinea unguium or onchomycosis (nail fungus). The clinical presentation of each infection as well as treatment are presented later in this section.

Incidence and Etiology

Tinea infections are the most common superficial fungal infections in children. Risk factors for acquiring an infection include close, prolonged contact with an infected individual, in particular a family member; exposure to an infected animal; and immunodeficiency (Honig, 1999; Rudy, 1999).

Tinea infections result from the transfer of dermatophytes to an uninfected individual. This transfer may be direct or through **fomites.** Fomites are inanimate objects on which disease-causing organisms may be conveyed and include such items as towels, shoes, or other objects shared by infected individuals. The household is the most common place for the spread of infection.

Pathophysiology

Tinea infections are caused by dermatophytes, keratin-loving fungi that are parasitic upon the skin. *Trichophyton*, *Micosporum*, and *Epidermophyton* species most often cause tinea infections. Infection occurs when dermatophytes invade and proliferate in the stratum corneum. Immune reactivity then develops and the T cell response produces a brief, intense inflammation and the process is terminated. The process of intense inflammation is shorter with reinfection. Clients who suffer from allergic reactions with strong familial tendencies (eczema, asthma, and seasonal allergies) tend to have chronic, recurring, and longer-lasting infections because they do not mount a sufficient T cell response in the skin.

Diagnosis

Diagnosis of tinea infections is based on the clinical presentation. Potassium hydroxide (KOH) examination is the most sensitive test for superficial fungal infections and provides a definitive diagnosis. The examination involves placing hair or scales from the leading border of a lesion on a microscope slide with a few drops of a potassium hydroxide (KOH) solution. The KOH solution helps dissolve the keratinous material for better visualization. Fungal cultures may be performed; however, this is often unnecessary because most superficial fungi are sensitive to topical and oral antifungal agents (Rupke, 2000). If indicated, scrapings for fungal cultures can be obtained by rubbing the edges of the lesions with the bristles of a clean toothbrush and transferring the specimen to the slides and culture media. A Wood's lamp examination often is not useful in establishing a diagnosis because the dermatophytes most commonly associated with tinea infections do not fluoresce (Rudy, 1999).

Treatment

Successful treatment of superficial fungal infections is achieved only when the antifungal agent can completely eradicate the causative fungal species and achieve a **mycologic cure** (defined as no fungal species present). A **clinical cure,** or resolution of all the clinical signs and symptoms of superficial fungal infection, is frequently achieved with less than the recommended course of treatment. Without a mycologic cure, determined by a negative microscopic KOH examination and negative cultures, the symptoms will recur.

A very different situation occurs with the treatment of onchomycosis, in which a mycologic cure is achieved before the clinical cure. This occurs because new nail growth must replace the infected nail before the clinical cure would be achieved; complete nail regrowth can take up to a year after the mycologic cure has been achieved.

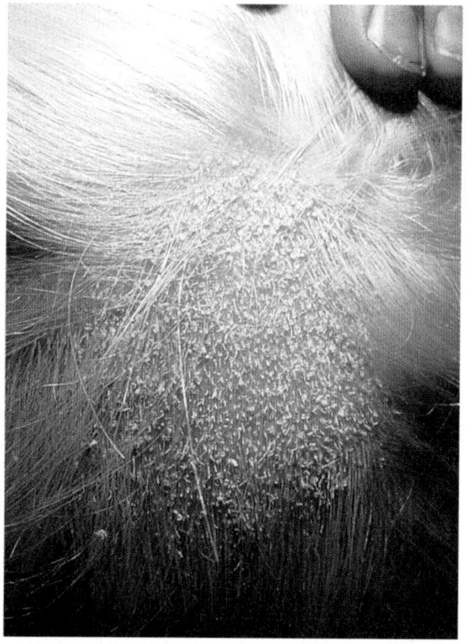

Figure 30-6 Tinea Capitis. Courtesy of Robert A. Silverman, M.D., Clinical Associate Professor, Department of Pediatrics, Georgetown University.

Tinea Capitis

Tinea capitis is the most common dermatophyte infection in children both in the United States and worldwide. *T. tonsurans* is the most common causative organism in the United States. Tinea capitis occurs most frequently in school-aged children, in particular, African-American children. Infection is transmitted more often from contact with fomites rather than direct contact. Factors associated with the development of tinea capitis include crowded living conditions, lower socioeconomic status, and large household size. Although transmission of infection most often occurs within the household, outbreaks of tinea capitis can occur in schools and day care centers where children's activities involve prolonged close contact.

Clinical Manifestations

The clinical presentation of tinea capitis varies. It presents most commonly as scalp scaling with or without alopecia (Figure 30-6). Areas of alopecia are well demarcated with or without erythema. Scale and black dots, resulting from broken hairs, may be present. Crusting, pustules, and lymphadenopathy may result as the infection progresses. Kerions, which are moist, boggy, scalp nodules, are associated with tinea capitis. These lesions may become secondarily infected with bacteria.

Treatment

Oral administration of griseofulvin (GrifulvinV, FulvicinP/G, Grisactin) remains the standard treatment for tinea capitis (Nesbitt, 2000). Treatment typically lasts for a minimum of 8 weeks. Terbinafine (Lamisil), a relatively new antifungal medication, may offer a more definitive cure with a shorter duration of treatment (Caceres-Rios, Rueda, Ballona, & Bustamante, 2000). Topical agents are ineffective in the management of tinea capitis because they are unable to penetrate the hair follicle. Shampoos containing 1% or 2.5% selenium sulfide or 2% ketoconazole have been found to be effective adjunctive therapies when used with griseofulvin in that they help to limit the spread of spores (Nesbitt, 2000; Howard & Frieden, 1999). In addition to medical therapy, clinical management must include identification and thorough cleaning of all objects that have come into contact with the infected child's hair.

Tinea Corporis

Tinea corporis, or "body ringworm," is a fungal infection occurring on nonterminal hair-bearing areas of the body. The dermatophytes most commonly associated with tinea corporis in the United States are *T. rubrum*, *T. mentagrophytes*, *M. canis*, and *T. tonsurans*. Tinea corporis can occur in children of any age and may be acquired from an infected domestic animal.

Clinical Manifestations

The classic presentation of tinea corporis is an annular, expanding lesion with a raised, erythematous border and a scaly, clearing center. The appearance of the lesion has led to the infection being commonly known as "ringworm." Lesions appear in an asymmetric pattern. When multiple lesions are present, their borders will overlap. Less common presentations of tinea corporis include clusterings of vesicles or pustules, widespread, scaly, polycystic lesions, or subcutaneous abscesses (Figure 30-7).

Treatment

Tinea corporis typically responds well to topical agents. Commonly used medications include miconazole (Micatin), and clotrimazole (Lotrimin) creams, which are applied twice daily for two to three weeks. Lesions should respond by the second week of therapy. If lesions are widespread or the client is immunocompromised, treatment with an oral agent such as itraconazole (Sporanox) or terbinafine may be indicated (Rupke, 2000; Howard & Frieden, 1999; Rudy, 1999).

Tinea Pedis

Tinea pedis is a dermatophyte infection of the feet. It is most commonly seen in adolescents. The organisms most often responsible for tinea pedis infections are *T. rubrum* and *T. mentagrophytes*. Tinea pedis is commonly called "athlete's foot" and is often acquired from contaminated showers or locker room floors.

Clinical Manifestations

Tinea pedis has three main clinical presentations. The interdigital form is the most common and consists of scaly, erythematous, pruritic lesions occurring between the toes (Figure 30-8). It may be complicated by fissuring and maceration. Contributing factors include warmth and tight-fitting shoes. The moccasin type consists of a dry, silvery scale covering the sole of the foot and tender, pink skin. The least common form of tinea pedis presents with vesicular or bullous lesions on the instep of one or both feet. All types of tinea pedis may be complicated by secondary bacterial infection, *Candida* infection, or spread of the infection to other areas of the body.

Treatment

Tinea pedis is treated with topical antifungal agents. Interdigital tinea pedis may be treated with clotrimazole, econazole (Spectazole), or sulconazole (Exelderm) cream. The cream should be applied twice daily for four to six weeks. If the infection involves areas with a thick keratin surface, oral agents such as itraconazole (Sporanox), fluconazole (Diflucan), or terbinafine (Lamisil) may be used (Boerio, Brooker, Freese, Phares, & Yazvec, 2000; Rupke, 2000; Rudy, 1999).

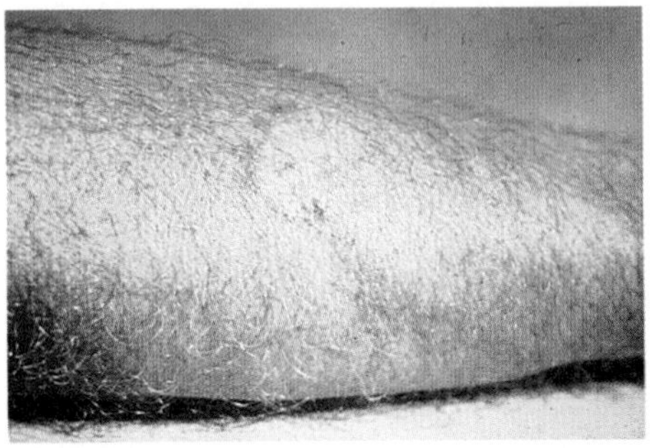

Figure 30-7 Tinea Corporis. Courtesy of the Centers for Disease Control and Prevention.

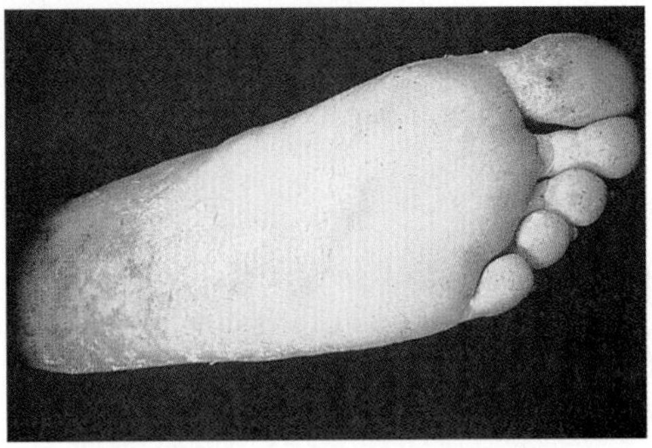

Figure 30-8 Tinea Pedis. Courtesy of the Centers for Disease Control and Prevention.

Tinea Cruris

Tinea cruris, commonly known as "jock itch," is a dermatophyte infection of the groin. It occurs most often in adolescent males although it can appear in infants. *E. floccosum*, *T. rubrum*, and *T. mentagrophytes* are common causative organisms. Factors associated with the development of tinea cruris are warmth, moisture, friction, obesity, and tight-fitting garments.

Clinical Manifestations

Tinea cruris typically presents bilaterally as an erythematous, scaly, red-brown eruption with defined borders. Central clearing and a vesiculopapular border may be present. Tinea cruris often causes intense pruritus.

Treatment

Tinea cruris is managed with topical antifungal medications. Miconazole (Micatin) and clotrimazole (Lotrimin) creams are commonly used and are applied twice daily for two to three weeks. The affected area also must be kept dry (Rupke, 2000; Rudy, 1999).

Tinea Unguium

Tinea unguium results from dermatophyte infection of the nail. It is relatively rare in children but may be associated with tinea pedis. Other associated conditions include immunocompromised states, Down syndrome, and tinea capitis. *T. rubrum* is most commonly associated with tinea unguium in children.

Clinical Manifestations

Tinea unguium occurs more frequently in toenails than fingernails. Distal-subungual infection, in which the infection begins at the underside of the distal nail and progresses to the proximal end, is most common in children. This form of infection presents as a yellow-brown discoloration of the nail plate, subungual hyperkeratosis, and breakdown of the nail.

Treatment

Tinea unguium is one of the most difficult tinea infections to resolve. Mycologic cures are difficult to achieve with the traditional antifungal agents because they only stop the growth of the fungus (fungistatic effect) and do not eradicate it (fungicidal effect). Standard treatment has consisted of oral griseofulvin for 6 to 9 months (Rudy, 1999). New oral antifungal agents that are both fungicidal and fungistatic include fluconazole, itraconazole, and terbinafine. These drugs have been highly effective for the treatment of tinea unguium (Huang & Paller, 2000).

Nursing Management of Tinea Infections

Careful handwashing before and after contact with the child is essential, along with wearing gloves during care. Nurses should ask the child and caregiver about the location of the lesions and when they first appeared and the manner in which the lesions spread. Identify previous exposure to anyone with similar lesions and any common precipitating factors. Note the character and extent of lesions, including the pattern and presence of scaling, vesicles, pustules, or crusting. The nurse should identify local lymphadenopathy, assess for pruritus, the child's level of comfort, and the presence of secondary skin conditions or infections.

The nursing management of children with tinea infections focuses on resolution of the infection, comfort measures, and education for the caregivers related to the treatment plan and preventing the spread of infection. Although many children and caregivers have heard of "ringworm," many mistakenly believe that they have worms, rather than a fungal infection. Resolution of the infection, as well as preventing spread to others, is easier if the child and caregivers understand the nature of the infection, how it is transmitted, and treatment issues. Nursing care also should include strategies to support the self-image of the affected child.

Family Teaching

Family education must address the importance of adherence to the prescribed medical therapy. Tinea capitis and unguium require long-term therapy, and non-adherence to the treatment plan may play a role in recurrence of infection. Tinea pedis, corporis, and cruris will usually respond well to the prescribed topical agents. Because resolution of clinical signs and symptoms of infection will occur with less than the recommended course of treatment, the caregiver will often mistakenly believe that the infection has been "cured" and stop using the medications. To prevent recurrence, application should continue for 5 to 7 days after signs of infection are gone. If the infection does not resolve, the child should receive further evaluation from a health care provider.

Griseofulvin, the agent most commonly used to treat tinea capitis is better absorbed in the presence of fatty foods. Caregivers should be taught to administer the medication with foods high in fat such as peanut butter or ice cream to enhance the drug's effectiveness. Children receiving griseofulvin for longer than three months should receive laboratory testing for leukopenia, anemia, and elevated liver enzymes.

Another important teaching point is thorough cleaning of fomites. Items such as combs, hair clips, hats, and towels should not be shared. Hair care products such as gels that have been used on infected hair should be discarded. Contamination of new containers may be avoided by removing the product with a spoon that does not come into contact with the infected hair. When treatment has been initiated, all items that may harbor shed spores such as pillows, linens, barrettes, and combs must be thoroughly washed and disinfected.

Children who are receiving therapy for tinea capitis do not need to be excluded from attending school. The most common place for prolonged contact leading to infection is the household, and shedding of spores will continue even after therapy is initiated. Haircuts, shaving of the head, or wearing of a cap during treatment are not necessary (American Academy of Pediatrics, 2000a). Caregivers and children should be taught to avoid factors that may precipitate the development of tinea infections. Maintaining dry and intact skin as well as avoiding tight-fitting shoes and clothing will help to decrease the development and spread of infection.

VIRAL INFECTIONS

Viral infections are responsible for many of the childhood communicable diseases, which are accompanied by characteristic rashes, such as rubella, roseola, or chickenpox (see Chapter 15). Verrucae (warts) and herpes simplex type I infections are common viral disorders of the skin seen in children and adolescents and will be discussed.

Verrucae

Verrucae, also known as cutaneous warts, are benign epidermal tumors caused by the human papilloma virus. Lesions are characterized by the formation of thick, hyperkeratotic lesions. Verrucae are classified according to their clinical presentation. Frequently occurring types include verrucae vulgaris (common warts), verrucae plantaris (plantar warts), and verrucae planus (flat warts).

Incidence and Etiology

Although individuals of any age may get warts, the highest incidence generally occurs during childhood and adolescence. An estimated 10% of children are affected with the greatest frequency occurring in children between 12 and 16 years of age (Plasencia, 2000; Silverberg, Lim, Paller, & Mancini, 2000; Verbov, 1999). Children with compromised immune systems are at increased risk for developing verrucae. Human papillomavirus (HPV) is responsible for the development of verrucae. Different types of the virus are responsible for the varying forms of verrucae. Infection occurs as a consequence of direct contact with HPV.

Pathophysiology

HPV infection occurs in the basal layer of keratinocytes. Often the virus is introduced into an area of broken skin. Transmission may occur through contact with the skin of an infected individual or via **autoinoculation,** that is, the transfer of infection from one site to another on the same individual. The exact incubation period is unknown, but is estimated to vary from several weeks to over a year (Benton, 2000; Plasencia, 2000). Once introduced, the virus causes proliferation of squamous cells resulting in the clinical manifestations of verrucae. In contrast to other skin infections, HPV does not incite the inflammatory response. This contributes to the extended period of time necessary for HPV infection to clear. The duration of the lesions varies from a few months to several years. Approximately two-thirds of affected individuals experience spontaneous clearing of lesions within 2 years (Plasencia, 2000). Deficiencies in cell-mediated immunity, in particular, contribute to extended infection. The ability of the affected individual to generate HPV-specific antibodies and increase expression of gamma-interferon have been associated with enhanced host immunity (Benton, 2000; Plasencia, 2000).

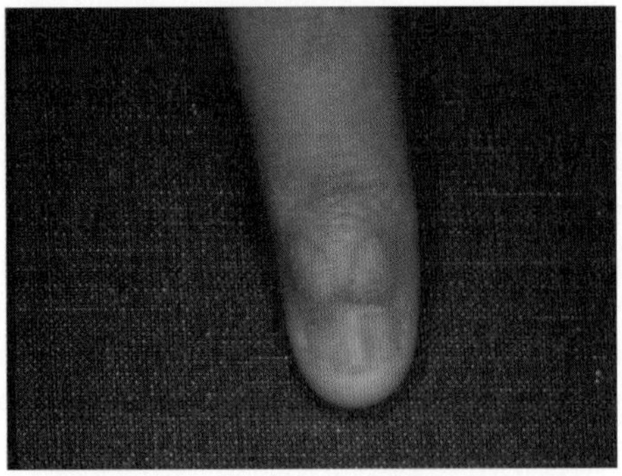

Figure 30-9 Verrucae Vulgaris on the Hand. Courtesy of Robert A. Silverman, M.D., Clinical Associate Professor, Department of Pediatrics, Georgetown University.

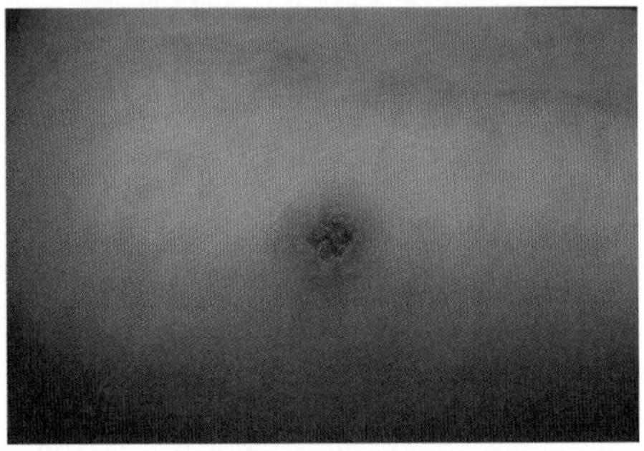

Figure 30-10 Verrucae Plantaris in an Adolescent. Courtesy of Robert A. Silverman, M.D., Clinical Associate Professor, Department of Pediatrics, Georgetown University.

Clinical Manifestations

The exact presentation of verrucae varies with the type of wart and the anatomic area affected. Verrucae vulgaris (common warts) are the most frequently occurring warts and account for approximately 70% of all warts (Plasencia, 2000). These warts appear predominantly on the dorsal surface of the hands or **periungual** (around the nail) regions; however, they may be present anywhere on the skin. Individuals may have a single lesion or multiple warts over the body. When these warts first appear, they are usually round, flesh-colored papules with well-defined borders. Over a period of a few weeks to months, they typically grow larger and may turn to yellowish tan, grayish, or brown papules or nodules (Figure 30-9). Verrucae vulgaris generally are not painful unless secondary lesions such as fissures develop.

Verrucae plantaris (plantar warts) develop on the plantar surfaces of the feet. They are most often located on weight bearing areas such as the heels or under the metatarsal heads. Lesions present as well-defined areas of compressed keratin surrounding a softer whitish substance (Figure 30-10). These lesions can become very painful as a consequence of the pressure and irritation of the lesion and deeper tissue when walking. Plantar warts are more common in adolescents and young adults. Factors such as increased perspiration and repeated microtrauma from athletic activities are believed to contribute to the increased incidence in these groups.

Verrucae plana (flat warts) are the least common cutaneous warts and represent only about 4% of warts (Plasencia, 2000). These warts most commonly occur on the face and dorsal surface of the hands. Lesions present as flat, flesh-colored papules and often measure less than 5 mm in diameter. These lesions tend to be less responsive to treatment.

Diagnosis

Diagnosis of verrucae typically is made based on clinical presentation. Because of the frequency of occurrence and easily distinguished clinical presentation, further evaluation is not likely to contribute to establishing the diagnosis (Young, Jolley, & Marks, 1998). If differential diagnosis is difficult, gentle paring or abrasion of lesions can be accomplished. This process will reveal small capillaries that can help distinguish the lesions from molluscum contagiosum or callus formation. In the latter two, capillaries will not be present (Verbov, 1999).

Treatment

No single recommended treatment for verrucae exists. Therapy must be based on the unique circumstances of each individual, including the age of the child and the degree to which the warts are a concern for him or her. Many children and caregivers will want warts removed because of cosmetic concerns and the associated embarrassment they often experience. Plantar warts are usually removed because of pain and difficulty walking. No matter what therapeutic approach is used, warts may be resistant to therapy, have a high recurrence rate, and may leave scars as a result of the treatment. Because verrucae rarely are a serious health problem and often spontaneously resolve over a period of time, no treatment must be considered as one option. A generally agreed upon principle of management is that the treatment should not be more unpleasant than the condition itself (Verbov, 1999).

Treatment of verrucae should include destruction of the wart by physical or chemical means as well as stimulation of an immune response to the virus. The treatment goal for warts is cytodestruction, which includes destroying the epidermal cells along with the virus. First-line therapies include application of topical agents. Salicylic acid solutions and plasters are the common chemical agents frequently used. Salicylic acid acts as a keratinolytic agent and also produces a local irritant effect. Preparations such as Duofilm, Occlusal, Duoplant, Trans-Plantar, and Mediplast are available without a prescription, can be applied at home with little pain, and are relatively inexpensive. The affected area is debrided with an emery board or pumice stone and then soaked in warm water to soften the keratin layer. The medication is applied, allowed to dry, and then reapplied as necessary to cover the entire wart. The solution may be applied once or twice daily until the wart has been removed. Often improvement is noted within one to two weeks of use; however, treatment may be indicated as long as 12 weeks. The estimated cure rate for verrucae vulgaris and verrucae plantaris is estimated to be approximately 70–80% with salicylic acid preparations (Benton, 2000; Plasencia, 2000). Other topical preparations that may be used in the management of verrucae include formalin, glutaraldehyde, and cantharidin. Guidelines for use are similar to those for salicylic acid.

Cryosurgery or "freezing" the wart is considered a second-line treatment for verrucae. Cryotherapy results in intracellular and extracellular ice formation, which causes disruption of the cellular membrane and results in cell death. The virus itself is not killed by cryotherapy, but it is released into the extracellular environment where an immune response is produced (Benton, 2000). Treatment involves pressing a liquid nitrogen (−195°C) cotton-tipped swab against the lesion. After a few days, a blister forms followed by sloughing of the lesion. Retreatment may be necessary to achieve complete destruction of the wart. This treatment must be performed by a health care provider and is more traumatic and expensive than over-the-counter remedies. Other treatment modalities have been investigated in the management of verrucae and usually are reserved for more severe cases. Surgical resection may be performed but may result in scarring or delayed healing. Laser therapy and squaric acid immunotherapy have been investigated and may offer benefit to children whose warts have been resistant to other conventional therapies (Jacobsen, McGraw, & McCagh, 1997; Silverberg, et al., 2000).

Nursing Management

Assessment

Ask the child and caregiver about the location of the lesions and when they first appeared. Note the character and distribution of lesions and determine whether the lesions have spread from the initial site. Identify the presence of pain in association with plantar warts. Assess for the presence of secondary skin conditions or infections. Identify whether an immune compromised condition is present.

Nursing Diagnosis

Nursing diagnoses appropriate for the child with verrucae include:

1. Body image disturbance related to lesions.
2. Pain related to pressure on lesions (plantar warts).
3. Deficient knowledge related to course of infection and treatment options.

Outcome Identification

1. Child and family will utilize positive coping mechanisms to manage body image changes.
2. Child will experience relief of pain associated with plantar warts.
3. Child and family will verbalize appropriate understanding of clinical management including medications and chronic nature of verrucae.

Planning/Implementation

The nursing care of children with verrucae should emphasize education of the child and caregivers and promotion

Nursing Alert:

Verrucae and Immune Function

Widespread warts may be present in children who have an underlying compromised immune system, for example, children with HIV infection or those receiving chemotherapy.

of the child's self-image. Children and caregivers need to understand the chronic nature of verrucae and to be reassured that warts frequently resolve spontaneously after several months. Because it is difficult to trace time and place of exposure to the virus, basic hygiene principles, such as handwashing, should be encouraged. Children should be instructed not to pick at lesions to avoid autoinoculation. Correct use of topical preparations should be demonstrated when possible. If treatments such as cryotherapy or surgical excision are to be used, the child and caregiver should receive appropriate preparation prior to the procedure.

Evaluation

The child and caregivers should understand that warts typically are not harmful and that, although bothersome, often resolve over a period of several months. Medications to be administered at home should be administered safely and for the indicated period of time. Follow-up care is indicated to evaluate the response of the lesions to treatment and to assess the need for further intervention.

Family Teaching

Appropriate teaching for the child and caregivers is an essential aspect of nursing care. Caregivers and children should be forewarned that treatment is sometimes slow, and that warts may recur. Treatment should be individualized for each child. Education should address the specific purpose for the treatment, what the child may expect during the treatment, and specific instructions following the treatment. If topical preparations are to be used, the child and caregivers should be taught to apply the medication only to the affected skin. Petroleum jelly may be applied to the skin surrounding the wart to avoid contact with the medication. Less concentrated preparations should be used for children to avoid potential toxicity. Typically side effects are minimal and are limited to contact dermatitis at the site of application. Children and caregivers should understand that cryotherapy is a painful procedure, and it may not be well tolerated by all children. Topical anesthetic creams applied before the procedure may provide some benefit. They should be instructed to avoid contact with the fluid inside the blister that forms following cryotherapy because further spread of the virus may occur.

Herpes Simplex Virus Type I

Herpes simplex virus type I (HSV-1) is a double-stranded DNA virus and one of 8 identified herpes viruses that may cause infection in humans. HSV-1 has the potential to cause infection on any area of the skin that comes into direct contact with the virus. In rare cases, HSV-1 may result in disseminated disease or encephalitis. This focus of this section will be oral–labial herpes caused by HSV-1.

Incidence and Etiology

Primary infection with HSV-1 occurs most commonly in children. Risk of exposure is greatest before age five, and an estimated 20–50% of children less than 5 years of age have HSV-1 antibodies. Children living in lower socioeconomic conditions are at increased risk of exposure and subsequent infection. Among these children, the incidence of HSV-1 antibodies may be as high as 90% (Goodyear, 2000; Riley, 1999). Neonates and children who are immunosuppressed are at increased risk for serious infection.

Primary infection with HSV-1 occurs as a consequence of direct contact with the virus, usually via saliva or respiratory secretions. Because HSV-1 can remain dormant in the dorsal root ganglia, reactivation of the virus is possible. Approximately 20–40% of those with primary HSV-1 infections will have recurrent infections, which may be precipitated by factors such as sunlight, wind, local injury, or emotional stress.

Pathophysiology

Primary infection occurs by direct contact with infected secretions. The virus must come into contact with abraded skin or mucous membranes to cause infection. The virus may be transmitted by an individual with active lesions or by an asymptomatic individual, someone who sheds the virus without clinical evidence of HSV-1 infection.

Once inside the cell, the virus replicates itself causing injury to the epidermal cells. Cellular damage results in the development of the papules and vesicles characteristic of HSV-1 infection. Following replication, the virus is transported to the dorsal root ganglia where it remains latent. During a recurrent infection, the virus is transported back down the sensory nerve and infects epithelial cells at the nerve root ending.

Clinical Manifestations

The clinical manifestations of primary HSV-1 infection vary greatly. Infections may consist of widespread lesions or be asymptomatic. In children, orolabial lesions, those occurring in the mouth and around the lips, are most common (Figure 30-11). Lesions may occur on any surface of the oropharynx, including the hard and soft palate, gingiva, buccal mucosa, tongue, and floor of the mouth. They also may extend away from the mouth. They classically present as small vesicles on an erythematous background. The vesicles progress to form ulcers with a yellow exudate that forms a crust. Lesions typically heal completely without scarring, tend to last 2 to 3 weeks, and often are painful. Underlying tissue may be swollen, erythematous, and susceptible to minor injury. Associated symptoms may include fever, malaise, cervical lymphadenopathy, and halitosis. A major complication is the spread of infection as a consequence of the child scratching the infected area and transferring the infection to other areas of the body.

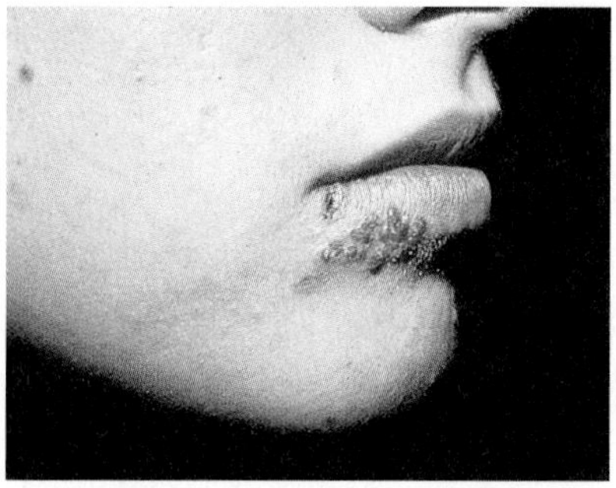

Figure 30-11 Herpes Simplex Type I. Courtesy of Robert A. Silverman, M.D., Clinical Associate Professor, Department of Pediatrics, Georgetown University.

Recurrent infections tend to occur on the lips and are commonly known as "cold sores." The most common site for recurrence is the mucocutaneous junction of the lips. Recurrent lesions tend to be fewer in number, less painful, and heal more rapidly. In approximately 80% of recurrences, only a single lesion is present (Goodyear, 2000). A prodrome sensation may be present within 6 hours of the appearance of a lesion. Irritation, numbness, tingling, or burning at the site may be present. Mood changes in young children also have been reported. Symptoms such as fever and malaise are uncommon.

Diagnosis

Although diagnosis may be made based on the appearance of clinical symptoms, viral cultures remain the "gold standard" for confirming diagnosis (Goodyear, 2000; Fitzpatrick & Schumann, 1999; Riley, 1999). Cultures are obtained by swabbing a lesion. When possible, the sample should be taken from the newest lesion—within 7 days of appearance and within 2 days of appearance for recurrent lesions. Swabs should be taken from the base of the lesion or from vesicular fluid where more virus is likely to be present. Culture results are available within 2 to 3 days following specimen collection. False negative results are possible. A false negative finding is one in which the testing process indicates that a condition is not present when, in fact, it is.

Treatment

Treatment priorities for HSV-1 infection are to relieve associated discomfort, promote healing of lesions, prevent complications, and decrease the duration of viral shedding. Mild, uncomplicated primary infections do not require specific treatment although supportive measures to provide analgesia, hygiene, and adequate hydration should be offered.

Oral acyclovir (Zovirax) may be used for more severe primary or recurrent infections or early in the course of infection. Acyclovir disrupts viral replication by interfering with DNA synthesis. It is most effective when initiated early in the infection when viral replication is greatest. Topical acyclovir cream may be used with recurrent infections. It is most useful when applied early in the prodrome phase.

Nursing Management

Nursing management priorities should include resolution of symptoms, prevention of the spread of lesions, promotion of the child's comfort, and prevention of complications. Assessment should include identification of the extent of the lesions and of the presence of any secondary infection such as impetigo. Additional areas for assessment should include the child's level of comfort and ability to maintain adequate oral fluid intake.

Planning should emphasize teaching caregivers about appropriate comfort measures including hygiene and mild analgesics. Caregivers also need to ensure that the child is receiving adequate oral fluids. If medications are indicated, appropriate education regarding the use of the medication should be provided.

Family Teaching

Caregivers need to understand the highly infectious nature of HSV-1. Good handwashing should be practiced by all household contacts to minimize spread of infection. Children with active lesions should be monitored to avoid picking at lesions and touching other unaffected areas of the body.

Caregivers and children should be reassured that lesions most often heal without scarring. Caregivers also should receive education regarding viral latency following initial infection and that recurrent infections can occur. Education should include factors that may trigger a recurrence and prodromal symptoms.

INFESTATIONS

Infestations from pediculosis and scabies are among the most prevalent communicable diseases that affect children. These highly contagious disorders may become epidemic, and the effects of these parasites often create discomfort and embarrassment for the child and caregivers.

Pediculosis

Pediculosis refers to infestation of an affected individual by lice. There are three types of pediculosis, each caused by a different species of louse. The following section will be limited to a presentation of pediculosis capitis, or head lice, which is caused by *Pediculosis humanus capitis*. Head lice are **ectoparasites,** that is, they live on the surface of the body. Lice require several meals of human blood each day, and they will die if they are away from a human host for more than two days. Although infestations are troublesome, the louse is not a vector of human disease.

Incidence and Etiology

Pediculosis capitis, or head lice, affects 6 to 12 million people in the United States each year (CDC, 2001). Infestations are most common among healthy children 3 to 10 years of age. Girls are at an increased risk, possibly because of increased head to head contact. All socioeconomic groups are affected; however, head lice are most common in Caucasian, school-aged females. In the United States, African-American children have fewer reported infestations. This is believed to be because of racial differences in hair texture and curl, which create difficulty for the louse to attach to the hair shaft. The classroom is considered the primary source of infestation.

Pathophysiology

Head lice are transmitted primarily through head to head contact. Fomites, such as hats, combs, bedding, and personal items also have been implicated in their transmission. Lice do not fly or jump, but they can crawl quickly on dry hair. The female louse lives on the scalp and lays approximately 4 to 10 eggs per day. The eggs are attached firmly to the proximal end of the hair shaft in egg casings (nits). A water-insoluble, glue-like substance holds the nits to the hair. Eggs are deposited most commonly in the posterior auricular and occipital areas where the warmth and moisture of the host's scalp allows the eggs to incubate. Nymphs emerge from the eggs within 7 to 10 days and mature into adults in another 7 to 14 days. The life span of the louse is approximately 30 days.

Clinical Manifestations

The most common presenting symptom of pediculosis capitis is persistent itching on the scalp. Initially, the pruritus may be localized in the occipital and postauricular areas and become particularly intense at night. The crawling insect and bites of the parasite along with the insect saliva create an allergic response of the skin causing the pruritus. Persistent scratching may result in excoriation and secondary bacterial infection. Mild fever, lymphadenopathy, and malaise may be present although most infestations are asymptomatic (Mazurek & Lee, 2000).

Individuals who are infested with head lice may have no more than 10 to 12 live lice at one time. The actual louse is about the size of a sesame seed, and it may be difficult to locate because of its small size, quick mobility, and brief life span. Nits are much more easily identifiable, and hundreds may be present at a time. Substances such as hairspray residue, dandruff, lint, and hair casts are often mistaken for nits. Closer examination reveals that these substances are easily removed from the hair and lack the characteristic shape of nits. Nits are oval in shape, approximately 0.8 mm by 0.03 mm) and are firmly attached to one side of the hair (Figure 30-12). Eggs that have hatched are white; newly formed nits are brown in color. Nits that are viable are often found within 6 mm of the scalp. The distance nits are from the scalp may be used as a measure of the duration of the infestation (CDC, 2001; Eichenfield & Colon-Fontanez, 1998).

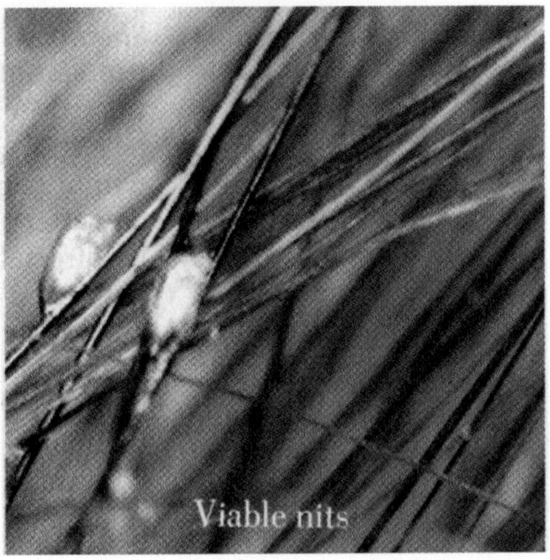

Figure 30-12 Louse Egg (Nit) Attached to a Hair Shaft. Courtesy of Hogil Pharmaceutical Corporation.

Diagnosis

Diagnosis of pediculosis capitis is confirmed by identification of a live louse in the hair on the scalp of the person. Numerous nits firmly attached to the base of the hair shafts within 6 mm of the scalp are highly indicative of an active infestation. Nits found only at distances greater than 6 mm from the scalp most likely indicate a previous infestation (CDC, 2001; Mazurek & Lee, 2000).

Treatment

Effective treatment of pediculosis capitis includes the use of pediculocides along with removal of nit cases. Many experts agree that treatment with pediculocides should be limited to those with live lice or unhatched nits. Prophylactic treatment of uninfested contacts is unnecessary. The Division of Parasitic Diseases of the CDC (2001) does not recommend use of pediculocides on children less than two years of age. Treatment for these children should consist of manual removal of nits and lice.

A solution of 1% Permethrin (Nix) is considered the treatment of choice for pediculosis capitis (Mazurek & Lee, 2000; Eichenfield & Colon-Fontanez, 1998) and is both pediculocidal and ovicidal. It has a residual pediculocidal activity, which lasts longer than two weeks. One application is often adequate for cure.

Other available products are less potent ovicidal agents. Lindane (Kwell, Scabene) requires re-treatment in one week to eliminate newly hatched lice. The most significant side effect is neurotoxicity, which generally results from misuse of

REFLECTIONS FROM FAMILIES

I was horrified when I found out that my 7-year-old daughter had head lice. I had no idea where she could have become infested. We always keep our home very clean, and I wash her hair several times a week. Nothing like this has ever happened to us before. I thought that only the "dirty" kids got head lice—certainly not my child. We eventually determined that she probably acquired the lice from a summer day camp where she and some of the other girls were sharing hats. It was a new experience for me to get the prescription for the lice shampoo and then to use it on her. The hardest part, though, was combing out her long blond hair. It was very tedious, but we decided to make a game of it and play "going to the beauty parlor." We then went through the house and cleaned all of the bedding, hairbrushes, hats, and hair clips and ribbons. Fortunately, no one else in our family got lice. This experience definitely made me more sympathetic to other families who have a child with head lice. It can happen to anyone.

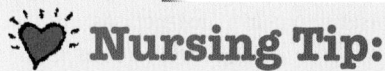

the product. Products such as RID and A-200 are natural pyrethrins and are not ovicidal nor do they have residual pediculocidal activity. Even after two applications, treatment may not be successful (Mazurek & Lee, 2000; Eichenfield & Colon-Fontanez, 1998).

Pediculocide resistance has become an increasing issue on a worldwide level (Chew, Bashir, & Maibach, 2000; Chosidow, 2000; Mazurek & Lee, 2000; Eichenfield & Colon-Fontanez, 1998). Presently, in the United States, most causes of treatment failure can be attributed to poor technique, noncompliance, or reinfestation. Oral trimethoprim/sulfamethoxazole (Bactrim, Septra) used in combination with 1% permethrin has been demonstrated to be effective therapy for children with multiple treatment failures or those with suspected lice-related resistance to traditional therapy (Hipolito, Mallorca, Zuniga-Macaraig, Apolinario, & Wheeler-Sherman, 2001).

Following application of an appropriate pediculocide the hair should be thoroughly combed to remove all nits and lice. A fine-toothed comb, often included in the pediculocide package, should be used. An application of 50% distilled white vinegar and 50% water or formic acid solution prior to combing may aid in loosening the nits from the hair shaft (Angel, Nigro, & Levy, 2000; Eichenfield & Colon-Fontanez, 1998).

Nursing Tip:

Treatment of the hair prior to use of pediculocide

Do not use a cream rinse or combination shampoo/conditioner before using the prescribed pediculocide. Do not rewash the hair for 1 to 2 days following treatment.

Treatment of the household includes identifying active infestations among household members. The Division of Parasitic Diseases of the CDC (2001) recommends checking household contacts every 2 to 3 days until all lice and nits are eradicated. Treatment of the environment is also essential to prevent reinfestation. Nits that are shed into the environment can survive in a warm environment and are capable of hatching for over a week.

Nursing Management

Careful handwashing before and after contact with the child is essential. If possible, hair should be wet to facilitate ease of identifying lice and nits. Conditioner should not be used prior to examination because the residual residue can create difficulty in identifying nits. The National Pediculosis Association (NPA) (2001a & b) does not recommend that gloves be worn during the examination. Instead, wooden tongue depressors, which are discarded following each examination, may be used to examine the child's hair. The examiner should separate small sections of hair at a time beginning at the posterior auricular and occipital areas because nits are most likely to be found in these areas. The presence of any lice or nits should be noted. If nits are present, the distribution and distance from the scalp are to be noted. Associated symptoms such as fever, lymphadenopathy, headache, and increased irritability should be identified as well. The examiner should assess for the presence of secondary skin lesions or infections. Household contacts of the affected child also should be examined.

The nursing management of children with pediculosis focuses on resolution of the infection, comfort measures, and education for the caregivers related to the treatment plan and preventing infestation. One of the most important messages for caregivers is reassurance that any child can get head lice. Early detection, treatment, and proper communication to the appropriate individuals, such as the school nurse or teacher is essential to prevent an epidemic in the community. Providing written information regarding the treatment plan may be useful to clarify instructions.

The effectiveness of the nursing interventions is measured by successful eradication of the pediculosis infestation. Monitoring follow-up care, treatment compliance, and effectiveness is an essential aspect of nursing care. The infestation should be eliminated by proper use of pediculocides, combing to remove nits, and treatment of the household. Children and caregivers should utilize strategies to prevent spread of the infestation or reinfestation.

Family Teaching

Teach the caregivers about the prescribed pediculocide. They need to understand the importance of following the directions that accompany the product. Hair should first be washed with regular shampoo. The pediculocide should be applied and left on the hair according to label instructions. Comb wet hair thoroughly to remove all nits following shampooing with pediculocide. The caregiver should work with small sections of hair at a time, working from the scalp outward. Hair should be recombed every two to three days until no nits are found.

Teach proper treatment of the household to prevent reinfestation. All potentially contaminated clothing, bedding, and linens should be washed in hot water (>120°F) or dry cleaned. Items that cannot be dry cleaned should be placed in a plastic bag and sealed for two weeks. Contaminated combs and brushes should be soaked in rubbing alcohol or immersed in boiling water. Floors and furniture should be vacuumed thoroughly. Use of fumigant sprays is unnecessary and may cause toxicity (CDC, 2001). Assess household contacts for presence of lice or nits every two to three days for two to three weeks and initiate treatment only if they are found. "Preventive" treatment is not beneficial.

Nursing Tip:

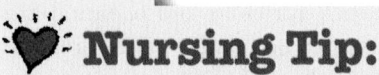

Psychological impact of pediculosis

The psychosocial impact of pediculosis can be more distressing for the affected child and family than the physiological aspects. Misconceptions regarding pediculosis and its transmission can have a significant impact on the affected child's self-esteem. If other children are aware of the condition, teasing may occur. The nurse can help the child and caregivers understand that pediculosis is an infestation that is common and is not associated with cleanliness or socioeconomic status. If the caregivers have a positive understanding about the infestation, they can provide appropriate support to their child.

Nursing Tip:

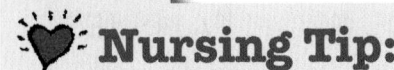

Obtaining cooperation during treatment

Children may have a difficult time cooperating with the treatment because the pediculocide must remain on the scalp for several minutes and the combing procedure can take 20 minutes or longer. The nurse or caregiver can prepare the child by providing developmentally appropriate activities or distraction techniques prior to starting the treatment. This preparation should include ways to prevent any medication from getting into the child's eyes such as playing beauty shop or wearing a colorful headband on the forehead.

Educate teachers and classmates about the usual modes of transmission. Children need to be cautioned about using each other's personal items and, if possible, hooks or lockers at school should be available that provide adequate individual space for coats and hats. Notify schools or day care centers where the affected child attended so that other children may be identified and treated. Identify the school's guidelines for returning to school following treatment. Many schools follow the educational programs available through the National Pediculosis Association, which advocates a "no nits" policy for treated children prior to reentry to school (NPA, 2001b). Advise caregivers to contact the National Pediculosis Association (www.headlice.org) for additional available educational programs and guidelines for management.

Scabies

Scabies is caused by the infestation of the scabies mite, *Sarcoptes scabiei*. Like pediculosis, the scabies mite is an ectoparasite and dependent on its human host for survival.

Incidence and Etiology

Scabies infestations are significant on a worldwide level with over 300 million cases occurring each year (Angel, Nigro, & Levy, 2000; Chosidow, 2000). The prevalence is greatest among individuals living in underdeveloped countries. Scabies is distributed across races, socioeconomic classes, and climates. It may affect people of any age, although children under two years of age are most commonly affected (Chosidow, 2000). Individuals with compromised immune systems are at increased risk for acquiring scabies.

Pathophysiology

Scabies is transmitted primarily by close person-to-person contact although fomite transfer may occur. The incubation period for scabies ranges from two to six weeks. During this time, the asymptomatic carrier may transmit the infestation to others.

Once on the human skin, mites burrow into the stratum corneum depositing feces. The impregnated female burrows under the skin to lay eggs at 2- to 3-day intervals. The eggs hatch after 3 to 8 days, and the immature mites emerge to the surface of the skin to **molt,** that is, to shed their exoskeleton to allow for growth. After molting, the mites burrow back into the skin; this process continues until the mites reach adult size. Adult mites are round, eyeless, and sac-like with females being 0.3 to 0.4 mm long and 0.25 to 0.35 mm wide. Males are slightly larger than one-half the size of females. The life span of the female mite is 2 months; males die shortly after mating.

Clinical Manifestations

Within a few weeks of infestation, an inflammatory response will occur anywhere the mite has traveled. Generalized pruritus, which increases at night, and a characteristic erythematous, papular, rash are considered the classic symptoms of scabies. The lesions are created as the impregnated female mite burrows into the stratum corneum of the epidermis to bury her eggs. Also characteristic of scabies are minute grayish-brown, threadlike, burrow tracks with a black dot at the end of the burrow.

The extent of lesions may range from a few erythematous papules, vesicles, and pustules to hundreds of excoriated lesions. The distribution of the rash is generally in **intertriginous** sites, that is, skin surfaces that are apposing or form folds such as the interdigital, axillary, cubital, popliteal, and inguinal areas (Figure 30-13). In infants, the face, head, neck, palms, and soles also may be involved. This presentation is often confusing and may result in a misdiagnosis or delayed diagnosis. Persistent scratching may lead to excoriation. Secondary bacterial infection may mask the initial infestation. Irritability and poor feeding may be associated with scabies in infants.

Diagnosis

A careful history and complete physical exam often are sufficient for a diagnosis of scabies. A microscopic examination of scrapings from a papule is useful in providing a definitive diagnosis. Mineral oil is placed on a scalpel blade, which is then used to scrape several skin lesions. The scrapings are then transferred to a glass slide that is observed under a microscope. Mites, eggs, or feces often are present; however, false negative findings may be obtained.

Treatment

Five percent permethrin cream (Elimite) is considered the treatment of choice for scabies (CDC, 2001; Chosidow, 2000). Permethrin is highly effective in eradicating scabies and has a low risk for toxicity. It has been used safely in infants as young as two months of age (Tanphaichitr & Brodell, 1999). A 1% lindane lotion (Kwell) also has been used in the successful management of scabies. Significant side effects associated with lindane include neurologic toxicity, including seizures. Typically one application of the prescribed scabicide is sufficient to eliminate the infestation. Because of the long incubation period associated with scabies, all household members and close physical contacts should be treated prophylactically. Although fomite transfer is less common, the household environment should be treated. Clothing, bedding, and linens used by the affected child in the two days prior to treatment should be washed in hot water and dried in a hot dryer.

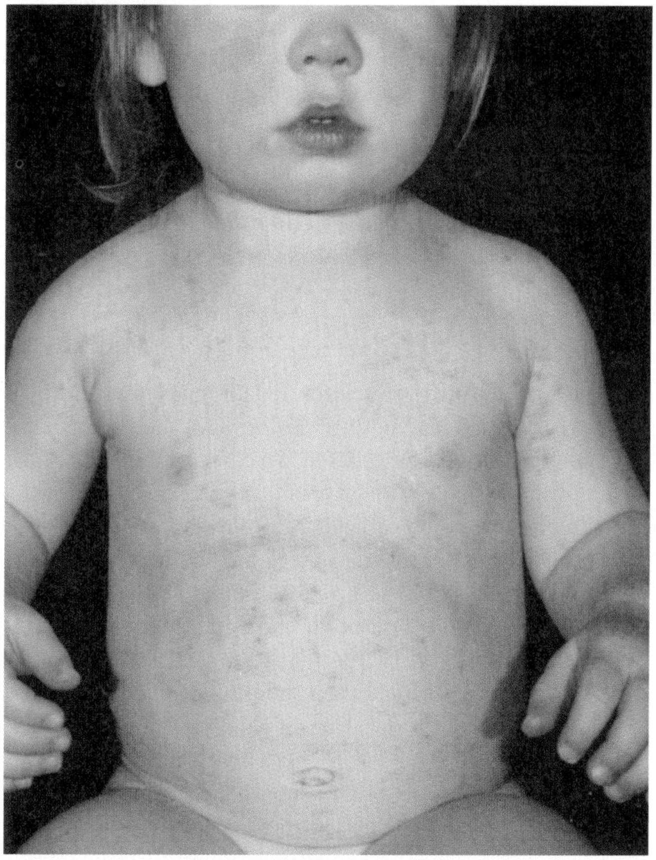

Figure 30-13 Diffuse Scabies in an Infant. Habif, T. P. (1996). *Clinical dermatology: A color guide to diagnosis and therapy* (3rd ed.). St. Louis: Mosby-Year Book, Inc. (p. 450, fig. 15-8).

Nursing Management

Priorities for nursing management include successful eradication of the infestation, promotion of the child's comfort, and prevention of complications such as secondary infection. Any complaints of severe itching or a skin rash should lead to further investigation to observe for the clinical signs of scabies. Until a definitive diagnosis is made the nurse should assume that the child might be contagious. Assessment also should include identification of secondary skin infections. Thorough handwashing should be implemented before and after client contact, and gloves should be worn during examination and care. The primary nursing responsibility is to provide teaching about the prescribed medical treatment and comfort measures. Caregivers should be taught to recognize clinical signs of scabies among other members of the household. Teaching also should address strategies to prevent reinfestation.

Family Teaching

As with pediculosis, education of caregivers is a priority aspect of the management of scabies. All members of the household need to be treated whether or not they have symptoms of scabies. Caregivers must be instructed to follow the directions for any scabicide carefully. Prior to application of the prescribed scabicide, the individual should bathe in tepid water. After the skin is dry, the scabicide should be applied to the entire body with particular attention given to the skin folds, fingernails, toenails, scalp, and posterior auricular areas. The individual then should put on clean clothes. After the prescribed duration of therapy, the scabicide is removed by bathing. If severe side effects such as redness or burning occur, the scabicide should be removed and the health care provider notified. Caregivers need to understand that one application is usually sufficient and that itching may persist for one to two weeks following treatment. If itching persists beyond that time, the child should be re-examined. Topical lubricants such as fragrance-free lotions and creams often are sufficient to manage pruritus following treatment. Children may return to the school or day care setting 24 hours after the completion of treatment. The school or day care should be notified of the child's condition so that peers and teachers may be monitored for signs and symptoms of infestation. Other individuals who have frequent close contact with the child should be notified and advised to seek prophylactic treatment.

INFLAMMATORY DISORDERS

Inflammatory skin disorders are among those skin conditions that are chronic in nature and challenging to manage. These disorders may occur in children of any age. With these disorders, the skin reacts with an inflammatory response to extrinsic or intrinsic factors. All responses include a visible component, either a rash or skin eruption, and frequently include a pruritic component. The appearance and discomfort of the associated skin lesions can impact the child's quality of life significantly. Attention to the psychosocial aspects of these conditions is essential to provide holistic care to these children and their families. The following inflammatory disorders are discussed: atopic, diaper, seborrheic and contact dermatitis, and acne.

Atopic Dermatitis

Atopic dermatitis has been described as "an itch that rashes." It is a chronic, relapsing inflammation of the dermis and epidermis resulting in itching, edema, papules, erythema, excoriation, serous discharge, and crusting. Although atopic dermatitis is commonly known as "eczema," it actually is one disease in a group of eczematous conditions.

Incidence and Etiology

The overall incidence of atopic dermatitis in the United States has increased significantly over the past 30 years. It is estimated that about 10% of the population has been affected by atopic dermatitis at some point in their lives compared with 2–5% in 1960 (Kristal & Klein, 2000; Nicol, 2000). Although it can occur at any time of life, it is most common in infants and young children. In the United States, 75% of cases appear by six months of age with three months being the common age of onset, 80–90% of cases present by 5 years of age. Approximately 40–75% of children "outgrow" atopic dermatitis by adolescence; however, many of them continue to experience dry skin that is easily irritated (Jaffe, 2000; Nicol & Boguniewicz, 1999).

The exact etiology of atopic dermatitis is unclear, although there appears to be a relationship to allergies. Children with atopic dermatitis are at increased risk for associated asthma or hayfever. A familial pattern is associated with the disorder.

Pathophysiology

The exact pathophysiology of atopic dermatitis is unknown. It is one of a group of atopic conditions, including asthma, allergic rhinitis, allergic conjunctivitis, and gastrointestinal allergy. These conditions may occur independently or in combination. The cause is believed to be multifactorial including familial, environmental, and infectious variables. The parallel increase in asthma over the past 30 years and the association of asthma with atopic dermatitis suggests a possible environmental trigger. The dry skin associated with atopic dermatitis is believed to result from changes in the epidermal barrier. One hypothesis is that essential fatty acid metabolism is altered resulting in changes in the lipid composition of the epidermal barrier. These changes may result in the initial pruritus and increased sensitivity to irritants (Bos, 2000).

Current research into the pathophysiological mechanisms involved in atopic dermatitis also suggests abnormalities in the child's immunoregulatory mechanisms. The skin lesions are believed to result from abnormal functioning of the immune system rather than the skin itself. Helper T lymphocytes, eosinophils, tissue macrophages, and Langerhans' cells have been identified as having a role in the immune response mechanisms associated with atopic dermatitis. Helper T cells that infiltrate the skin lesions often have skin-specific receptors. These cells also are involved in **cytokine** production. Cytokines are substances that participate in the immune response and are secreted by cells. Infiltration of skin lesions by eosinophils and deposition of granular proteins may be involved in further tissue injury. Tissue macrophages and Langerhans' cells have increased levels of immunoglobulin E (IgE), which may facilitate antigen processing and presentation to T cells (Nicol & Boguniewicz, 1999).

The pattern of cytokine production by T cells is believed to be specific to the acute and chronic phases of skin inflammation with different types of cytokines predominating each phase. Cytokine production also is involved in the "itch–scratch cycle." Children with atopic dermatitis often have a reduced threshold for pruritus, possibly because of changes in the lipid composition of the epidermal barrier and dermal nerve endings. Release of inflammatory cytokines promotes pruritus. Scratching results in further inflammation and tissue injury, promoting ongoing cytokine release (Nicol & Boguniewicz, 1999). The end result of these changes is impairment of the barrier function of the skin. Compromise of the skin's barrier function results in increased water loss, causing the skin to be dry and at increased risk for injury and irritation. These changes render the child susceptible to the chronic, ongoing cycle associated with atopic dermatitis.

Clinical Manifestations

The hallmark clinical manifestation of atopic dermatitis is persistent pruritus and scratching. The current hypothesis is that the "itch" causes the "rash," rather than the other way around because children will scratch at otherwise healthy, intact skin as well as affected skin. Itching often persists at night and results in lack of adequate sleep for the child. Over time the child's fingernails may take on a "polished" appearance as a consequence of constant rubbing and scratching. Areas of dryness and roughness on the young infant's skin may be the first clinical indications of atopic dermatitis. Pruritus, erythema, and papules develop after the skin has been irritated. The intense pruritus causes the child to rub or scratch the affected areas resulting in the erythema, excoriation, and subsequent serous discharge and crusting. African-Americans are more likely to have follicular and papular lesions. Lesions may be discrete and skin-colored or erythematous.

Lesions present in three stages: acute, subacute, and chronic. Acute lesions are characterized by extremely pruritic erythematous papules, which may occur with excoriation, erosion, serous exudate, and crusting. In the subacute stage, the papules are excoriated with fine scaling. Mild **lichenification,** or thickening of the skin with exaggeration of its normal markings, may be present. In the chronic phase, marked lichenification is present. Fibrotic papules and hyper- or hypopigmentation are present. The child with chronic disease may have acute and subacute lesions present as well (Nicol & Boguniewicz, 1999).

The distribution of skin lesions varies according to the child's age. During infancy, lesions occur primarily on the face, scalp, and **extensor surfaces** of the extremities (Figure 30-14). The extensor surfaces are those that do not come into contact when the extremity is flexed. The diaper area typically is not involved. Lesions tend to be of the acute stage and may be moist, oozing, or crusting. Drooling associated with teething may cause further irritation to affected skin. Chronic lesions with lichenification generally do not appear until the infant is capable of scratching. Young infants may "scratch" pruritic skin by rubbing their faces against bed linens or against the shoulder of someone holding them.

By the time the child is about two years of age, the pattern of distribution of lesions changes with appearance on the **flexural surfaces** of the body predominating. The flexural surfaces are the areas of an extremity that come into direct contact when the extremity is flexed. Areas most commonly affected include the antecubital and popliteal fossae, wrists, ankles, and neck. Lesions tend to consist of poorly defined erythematous, scaly patches although acute inflammatory areas may be present. Lesions occurring on the extensor surfaces in these children may indicate a poorer prognosis (Kristal & Klein, 2000).

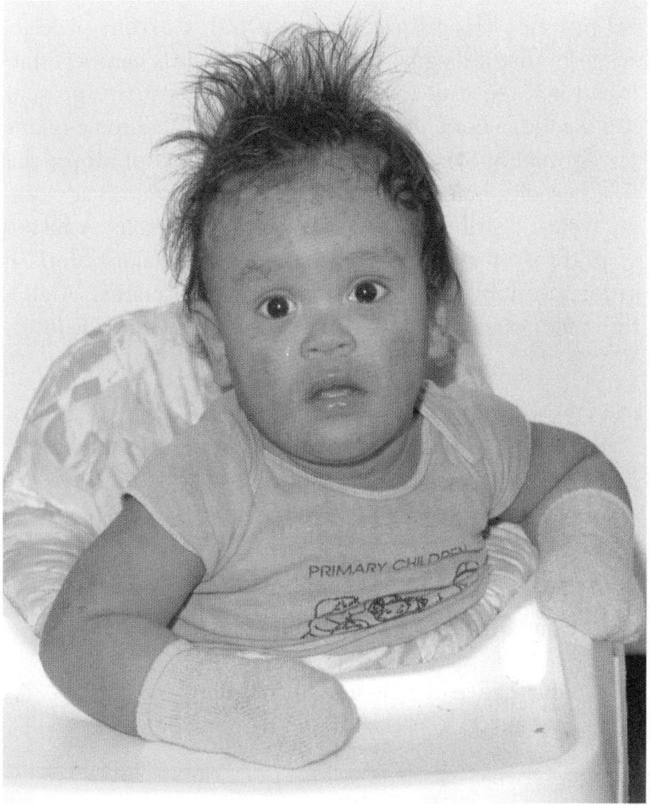

Figure 30-14 Generalized Atopic Dermatitis in a Toddler

Colonization of the skin by *Staphylococcus aureus* is present in approximately 90% of children with atopic dermatitis (Jaffe, 2000; Nicol, 2000). Superinfection may result as a complication of severely excoriated skin and may exacerbate eczematous lesions. Other complicating secondary infections include lesions from herpes simplex I and warts.

Exacerbations and remissions of lesions are common throughout the course of the condition. Although the majority of affected children experience relief of symptoms by adolescence, the exact clinical course of the disease for an individual child cannot be predicted. A number of factors have been associated with precipitating an exacerbation of atopic dermatitis. These are listed in Box 30-1. The significance of each factor in exacerbating atopic dermatitis is unique to each individual. Emotional stressors have a significant role in the course of atopic dermatitis, and affected children are more prone to respond to stressful stimuli by scratching. It is hypothesized that central nervous system stimulation may increase vasomotor and sweat responses of the skin, which contribute to the itch–scratch cycle (Nicol & Boguniewicz, 1999).

Diagnosis

No objective laboratory criteria exist for the diagnosis of atopic dermatitis. Diagnosis is made based on the child's history and clinical manifestations. Hanifin and Rajka proposed a set of diagnostic criteria based on major and minor characteristic features in 1980, which continues to be used in clinical practice (Hanifin & Rajka, 1980). Current practice suggests that a diagnosis of atopic dermatitis can be established if three major and three minor criteria are present. Among the major criteria are (1) pruritus; (2) chronic relapsing dermatitis; (3) a personal or family history of **atopy,** that is, a heredity predisposition to develop allergic disease; and (4) typical distribution and morphology of lesions. A history of pruritus must be present as one of the major criteria in order to establish a diagnosis of atopic dermatitis. Among the minor diagnostic criteria are elevated serum IgE levels, early age of onset, tendency toward cutaneous infections, orbital darkening, tendency toward nonspecific dermatitis of the hands or feet, food intolerances, and a clinical course influenced by environmental or emotional factors.

Laboratory tests may be useful in evaluating the child with atopic dermatitis. Although these tests may be associated with allergic or atopic disease, they are not necessarily specific for atopic dermatitis. Commonly performed tests include total serum IgE, specific IgE antibodies, and eosinophil counts. Results often indicate increased levels, which may correlate with the child's disease course (Jaffe, 2000; Kristal & Klein, 2000).

BOX 30-1 Factors associated with exacerbation of atopic dermatitis

- Dust mites
- Pets/animal dander
- Pollens
- Soaps/detergents
- Food allergies
- Changes in climate and temperature
- Sweating
- Infections
- Textiles
- Emotional stressors

Treatment

Presently, no cure for atopic dermatitis exists. Treatment focuses on control of symptoms by relief of itching, hydration of the skin, and minimization of inflammatory changes. Individualization of treatment for each child is a necessary aspect of effective management. Managing the intense pruritus and associated scratching is one of the most important goals of therapy, yet also one of the most challenging. Children's fingernails should be kept short to avoid trauma to the skin from scratching. Because very young children cannot understand "no scratching," distraction measures must be implemented. Care should be taken to avoid exposure to known irritants or triggers. Because heat may aggravate itching, an environment that avoids extremes in temperature should be maintained. Children should be dressed in light clothing that does not allow them to become overheated. Cornstarch or oatmeal baths may help provide relief of itching. Cool compresses and topical emollients also may provide benefit. Oral antihistamines such as diphenhydramine (Benadryl) and hydroxyzine (Vistaril, Atarax) may be necessary to control pruritus, especially at bedtime.

Because the skin's ability to retain water is decreased, care must be taken to promote adequate hydration of the skin. Previously, bathing had been thought to increase water loss and promote drying of the skin. Current practice recommends daily bathing in warm water followed by application of an occlusive product such as a cream or ointment to seal in moisture (Bingham, 2000; Nicol, 2000). Moisturizing emollients also should be applied liberally throughout the day. Products with a water-in-oil or lipid base are most effective in sealing moisture. Lotions have a higher water content; however, they promote drying of the skin because of an evaporative effect.

Topical corticosteroids are the most common prescribed treatment for atopic dermatitis and are used to reduce inflammation. The general principle is to use the least potent steroid that is effective in relieving the symptoms. Mild to moderate disease usually is managed successfully with 1% hydrocortisone cream or ointment. Higher-potency steroids should be avoided in infants and young children because of the risk of increased absorption and systemic side effects, in

Eye On:

Food Allergies and Atopic Dermatitis

Food allergies have been associated with atopic dermatitis although their exact role in the development of the disease is controversial. Food allergies may be an aggravating factor for 20% of children with severe disease. Common associated food allergens include eggs, milk, wheat, soy, seafood, and nuts. The practice of broad food restrictions has been questioned, and caregivers should be cautioned prior to eliminating foods from the child's diet. Unsupervised elimination of foods from the child's diet may result in malnutrition. Only if the food has been identified through testing should it be removed from the child's diet. The psychosocial implications of a severely restricted diet on both the child and the family should be taken into consideration.

particular, growth suppression (Bingham, 2000). High-potency steroids also should not be used on areas of extensive inflammation because of the risk of systemic side effects. As symptoms improve, steroids should be tapered to less potent preparations and finally to moisturizers.

Wet wrap therapy generally is reserved for clients with severe or persistent disease. Wet wrap dressings enhance penetration of topical corticosteroids and may help relieve pruritus. The prescribed agent is applied to the skin. Bandages or cotton-blend pajamas soaked in warm water are worn next to the skin. Dry pajamas are worn over the wet clothing. These dressings are best tolerated at night because of their cumbersome nature.

Development of new agents for management of atopic dermatitis has focused on immune regulation. Benefits from use of agents such as cyclosporine (Sandimmune, Neoral), tacrolimus (FK 506), azathioprine (Imuran), and interferon-gamma are being explored (Bingham, 2000; Kristal & Klein, 2000; Nicol, 2000). Failure to respond to traditional therapy does not necessarily imply that increased potency agents are indicated. Nonadherence has been identified as the most common cause of treatment failure. Health care professionals need to explore barriers to maintaining the prescribed treatment plan. Worsening of symptoms also may indicate a secondary infection or contact dermatitis.

Family Teaching

Education of caregivers is of great priority in the management of atopic dermatitis. Children should receive age-appropriate teaching and be involved in their own care. Caregivers and children need to understand the chronic nature of the disease as well as its course of unpredictable exacerbations followed by periods of relative remissions. They should be reassured that atopic dermatitis often resolves by adolescence. Teaching should emphasize avoidance of known irritants and strategies to relieve pruritus. Caregivers should be taught to maintain a thermoneutral environment in the home. When possible, the child should wear clothing that is loose fitting to allow air circulation over the skin. Light bed linens and loose-fitting pajamas will help prevent overheating and increased pruritus at night.

Efforts to promote adequate hydration of the skin should continue even when lesions are not present. Daily bathing in warm water is recommended, and the bath should not last longer than 15 to 20 minutes. Following the bath, the skin should be patted dry rather than rubbed to minimize further trauma to the skin. Moisturizers should be applied within three minutes of bathing to promote retention of water. Moisturizers also should be reapplied several times throughout the day. Box 30-2 provides an overview of the use and different types of emollients.

BOX 30-2 Use of emollients

In order to promote hydration of the skin, moisturizing creams and ointments must be applied within three minutes of the bath or shower. Agents should be applied thinly in smooth downward strokes in the direction of hair growth to minimize trapping heat and increasing the potential for pruritus.

Emollients are substances containing varying amounts of lipid and water and are used to promote hydration and softening of the skin. Application of emollients provides a thin film over the surface of the skin, trapping water and preventing further water loss.

A number of preparations of emollients are available for use. Selection of an emollient product should be individualized based on the child's condition. An appropriate understanding of available products and indications for use can assist the nurse in providing education to children and their caregivers.

Lotions contain the greatest proportion of water. Their consistency is lighter and less greasy. Their high water content may promote evaporative water loss. Lotions often contain fragrances that can be irritating to the skin. Caregivers should be instructed to select products that do not contain added fragrances.

Creams are heavier products than lotions and have a greater capacity to trap water under the skin. Creams are more readily absorbed than ointments.

Ointments are thicker, greasier, and contain the least water. Ointments have the greatest capacity to trap moisture but may not be practical because of their greasy consistency.

Bath oils provide benefit by allowing an emollient film to form on the skin during bathing.

Children with atopic dermatitis do not need to avoid swimming. The child's skin should be rinsed thoroughly after swimming, and a moisturizer should be applied. The amount of time spent swimming should be reduced if aggravation of symptoms occurs. Teaching should address safe use of steroids. Often caregivers express concerns related to side effects from misuse of high-potency steroids. They need to understand the strength of the topical steroid, potential side effects, and the correct amount to use. Topical steroids often are to be applied twice daily. When possible the nurse should demonstrate the correct amount to be applied to avoid over- or underuse of the medication. Box 30-3 provides guidelines for application of topical steroids on children of different ages. Caregivers need to understand the importance of follow-up care to evaluate the effectiveness of the current treatment plan.

Promotion of normal growth and development cannot be overemphasized. Caregivers often are concerned about the presence of a chronic disease and easily may become overprotective of the child, restricting his or her activity pattern and interactions with others. Children may feel "different" from their peers because of their appearance; however, they should be encouraged to participate in all developmentally appropriate activities. Teaching should address strategies for promoting the child's self-esteem.

BOX 30-3 Application of topical steroids in children

Questions often arise regarding the appropriate amount of steroid cream or ointment to apply to the child's skin. Overapplication may result in undesired systemic absorption. Underapplication does not provide adequate medication for relief of symptoms. In 1991, Long and Finlay developed the fingertip unit (FTU) technique for measuring the amount of cream or ointment. One fingertip unit is defined as the distance from the tip of an adult index finger down to the first joint. Guidelines for application of topical agents in children of different ages are as follows:

Location	6 months	1 year	5 years	10 years
Hand × 2	0.5	0.5	1	2
Arm × 2	0.5	1	2	3
Leg × 2	1	1.5	4	5
Foot × 2	0.5	0.5	2	2
Trunk (front)	1	1.5	3	4
Trunk (back)	1	1.5	3	4
Face and neck	0.25	0.5	0.5	1
Total FTU	4.75	7	15.5	21

Adapted from Long, C. C., & Finlay, A. Y. (1991). The finger tip unit–A new practical measure. *Clinical Experimental Dermatology, 16,* 444–447.

Diaper Dermatitis

Diaper dermatitis or "diaper rash" refers to an acute inflammatory process occurring in the diaper area. It most frequently appears as a consequence of primary irritant contact dermatitis, although rashes from other conditions, such as candidiasis, may appear in the diaper area.

Incidence and Etiology

Diaper dermatitis is the most common irritant contact dermatitis of childhood. Any child wearing diapers is at risk for the development of diaper dermatitis; however, peak incidence is between 9 and 12 months of age. This may be related to the transition from breastfeeding to bottle feeding and the introduction of solid foods. The prevalence of diaper dermatitis among infants in the United States is estimated to be 7–35%, and approximately 10% of these cases are referred for treatment (Kazaks & Lane, 2000; Ward, Fleischer, Jr., Feldman, & Krowchuck, 2000). The introduction of ultra-absorbent disposable diapers in developed countries has decreased the overall incidence of diaper dermatitis. The prevalence of diaper dermatitis in underdeveloped countries is less because of decreased use of diapers for infants.

At one time, diaper dermatitis was believed to result from the skin coming into contact with ammonia in the urine (Singleton, 1997). Although the exact etiology remains unknown, multiple factors are involved in its development. The environment created by wearing the diaper and diaper area hygiene are considered the primary factors that contribute to the development of diaper dermatitis. Factors involved in the environment include urine pH, stool consistency, frequency of urine and stool, the type of diaper used, and friction. Cloth diapers that are covered by tight-fitting plastic pants, in particular, reduce air circulation and create increased moisture within the diaper area. Factors related to hygiene that increase the incidence include infrequent diaper changes, inadequate cleaning and drying of the diaper area, and failure to use appropriate topical barriers to protect the skin (Bonifazi, 2000; Kazaks & Lane, 2000; Singleton, 1997). Other factors associated with an increased incidence include bottle feeding, prematurity, and intestinal carriage of *Candida albicans*. Children with atopic dermati-

Nursing Tip:

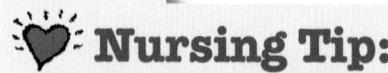

Infant feeding and diaper dermatitis

The pH of both the urine and stool of breastfed infants is lower than that of bottle-fed infants. This may explain the decreased incidence of diaper dermatitis in these infants.

Case Study/Care Plan

A Child with Rash and Itching

Rebecca is an 18-month-old Caucasian girl being seen by her primary care provider for a rash and itching of unknown etiology. The caregiver states that Rebecca has been crying, irritable, and not sleeping for the past week. She has a red rash on her legs, arms, and face. The rash includes macules and papules and in some spots is weeping a clear serous fluid. The caregiver states she has "tried everything" but Rebecca continues to scratch until her skin is bleeding.

Nursing Care Plan

Assessment The nursing assessment should begin with a detailed client history including the onset and distribution of the rash, whether this has changed since the rash first appeared, and any associated symptoms such as fever or recent illness. The nurse should determine what measures the caregiver has used to help relieve the symptoms and whether they have provided any relief. Specific questions should be directed toward exposure to infectious diseases or to any new substances or possible allergens in the child's environment such as foods, detergents, pets, plants, medications, and so forth. The nurse should ask whether any other members of the household have had similar symptoms and whether there is a family history of atopy.

The nursing assessment should note the type of lesion present, including primary and secondary lesions, and the distribution of the rash. The nurse should assess for evidence of superinfection.

Nursing Diagnosis #1

Impaired skin integrity related to the presence of lesions and scratching from pruritus.

Expected Outcomes

1. Child will exhibit signs of healing of lesions.
2. Child will exhibit decreased pruritus.

Interventions/*Rationales*

1. Provide moist environment–dressing or occlusive ointment for healing. *Wet environment provides moisture to the stratum corneum.*
2. Administer topical treatments and applications. *Topical ointments prevent transdermal water loss.*
3. Administer systemic medication if prescribed. *Systemic medicine such as corticosteroid may be needed to reduce the inflammation.*
4. Keep child away from irritant/allergen (if known). *Avoidance of exposure to the irritant, if known, is the best method of prevention.*
5. Avoid or reduce stimuli that exacerbate pruritus such as clothing, bed linen, and environmental allergens. *Reducing the stimuli for irritation will reduce the itching.*
6. Administer anti-pruritic medications. *Allergic reactions may be controlled with systemic medications such as antihistamines.*
7. Administer soothing baths–soaps may be drying, oils are hazardous with small children, baking soda and oatmeal baths do not decrease moisture in the skin. *Cool water relieves the itching; some additives may increase the effectiveness of the bath.*
8. Teach child and/or caregiver to pat skin dry rather than rub dry following a bath. *Rubbing the skin dry further traumatizes the skin and increases the itching.*

continues

continued

9. Apply occlusive emollient creams immediately after bathing. *Ointments or creams applied immediately after bathing help retain moisture in the skin and reduce the itching.*

Evaluation

The child exhibits healing of lesions as evident by decreased inflammation and excoriation of skin, decreased distribution of lesions, and absence of signs and symptoms of secondary infection. The child receives symptomatic relief of pruritus.

Nursing Diagnosis #2

Disturbed sleep pattern related to pruritus.

Expected Outcomes

Child will sleep undisturbed.

Interventions/*Rationales*

1. Administer soothing baths and apply creams prior to bedtime. *Baths will alleviate pruritus and help facilitate the child's sleeping.*

2. Administer mild anti-pruritic medication prior to bedtime. *Medication prior to bedtime will alleviate pruritus and increase the chance of restful sleep.*

3. Establish a bedtime routine that allows the child to wind down. *An established routine enables a child to be ready for sleep.*

Evaluation

Child sleeps undisturbed as evident by sleeping through the night with minimal waking and without scratching in his or her sleep. Child appears rested upon waking.

Nursing Diagnosis #3

Disturbed body image related to perception of appearance.

Expected Outcomes

Child will maintain a positive self-image as evident by normal age-appropriate behaviors.

Interventions/*Rationales*

1. Provide tactile stimulation of unaffected parts through caressing and touching. *Children need to be touched and held to feel accepted by caregivers and others.*

2. Hold child as often as possible. *Physical contact demonstrates acceptance of child rather than fear/disgust of the rash.*

3. Involve child in care activities when possible. *Participation in personal cares provides children with a sense of control of the situation.*

4. Encourage the child to continue normal age-appropriate activities. *Growth and development issues need to be addressed at all ages.*

5. Improve the appearance of the child using clothing and other appropriate measures. *The response of others is important in the formation of self-esteem and self-image.*

6. Give the child positive feedback for activities. *Praise for activities will enhance self-image.*

7. Allow the child to verbalize feelings about appearance. *Expression of emotions and acceptance by significant others will enhance self-image.*

Evaluation

Child maintains a positive self-image as evident by active participation in age-appropriate activities and expressing emotions regarding his or her condition. Child receives therapeutic tactile stimulation and support from caregivers and peers. Child utilizes appropriate coping skills to manage the psychosocial impact of the condition.

continues

continued

Nursing Diagnosis #4

Interrupted family processes related to having a child with a chronic skin condition.

Expected Outcomes

Caregiver will demonstrate positive coping skills.

Interventions/*Rationales*

1. Teach caregivers necessary skills to carry out treatments. *Competence in care giving activities will reduce stress.*

2. Teach caregivers about medications for child. *Knowledge of drugs and side effects is essential for competent care.*

3. Allow caregivers to express feelings of frustration, anger, and irritability. Emphasize that negative feelings are normal and expected, but that caregivers must find appropriate outlets for these feelings to remain healthy. *Expression of negative feelings and frustration by caregivers permits a positive venting of emotions.*

4. Praise caregivers for evidence of good care; provide reassurance that an exacerbation is not the caregivers' fault. *Praise for positive behaviors reinforces self-esteem and self-image.*

Evaluation

Caregivers exhibit positive coping skills as evident by discussing rationale for the child's treatment, expressing a sense of competence in the care, and expressing their emotions/concerns about the child's condition and care.

Nursing Diagnosis #5

Risk for infection (secondary) related to scratching of lesions.

Expected Outcomes

Child will have no evidence of secondary infection.

Interventions/*Rationales*

1. Keep child's fingernails short. *Contaminants under nails may harbor bacteria that can be introduced into open lesions by scratching.*

2. Cover child's hands with mittens or socks to prevent scratching. *Scratching can further damage skin, making it more susceptible to secondary infection.*

3. Dress child in clothing that is light, clean, and loose. *Tight clothing may cause more irritation and therefore more scratching. Clean clothing will prevent further infection.*

4. Wash hands or wear sterile gloves before changing dressings. *Exposure to bacteria should be kept at a minimum.*

5. Teach family hygienic methods to prevent infection such as use of antibacterial soap pumps for handwashing. *Exposure to bacteria should be kept at a minimum.*

Evaluation

Child is free of secondary infection as evident by skin that is clean and free of excoriation and secondary lesions and by absence of erythema or purulent drainage from lesions. The child is afebrile with vital signs within normal limits and free of associated systemic symptoms such as malaise and lymphadenopathy.

tis and those with biotin deficiencies also are at increased risk for developing diaper dermatitis.

Pathophysiology

Skin breakdown in the diaper area occurs as a consequence of prolonged contact with physical and chemical irritants. Increased wetness and warmth in the diaper area prevent evaporation of moisture and increases the damage caused by friction. The result is damage to the stratum corneum, which renders the skin more susceptible to irritating substances. An increased pH in the diaper environment causes further irritation to the damaged skin. Fecal enzymes and bile salts have an irritant effect on the skin, and their activity is increased by a higher pH. Urinary ammonia further elevates the pH of the diaper environment and causes increased irritation to the skin. If cloth diapers are used, residual detergent may cause additional irritation. The resulting injury to the skin places the infant at increased risk for overgrowth of microorganisms, including *Candida albicans* (Kazaks & Lane, 2000; Wahrman & Honig, 2000).

Clinical Manifestations

Primary irritant diaper dermatitis appears as a shiny erythema, which covers the convex surfaces of the diaper area. Because the rash affects skin that is in direct contact with the diaper, the skin folds commonly are spared. In more severe cases, vesicles, papules, and scaling may occur (Figure 30-15). This presentation distinguishes the rash from that caused by *Candida albicans* (Figure 30-16). The clinical manifestations of candidal diaper dermatitis are described under the section on candidiasis.

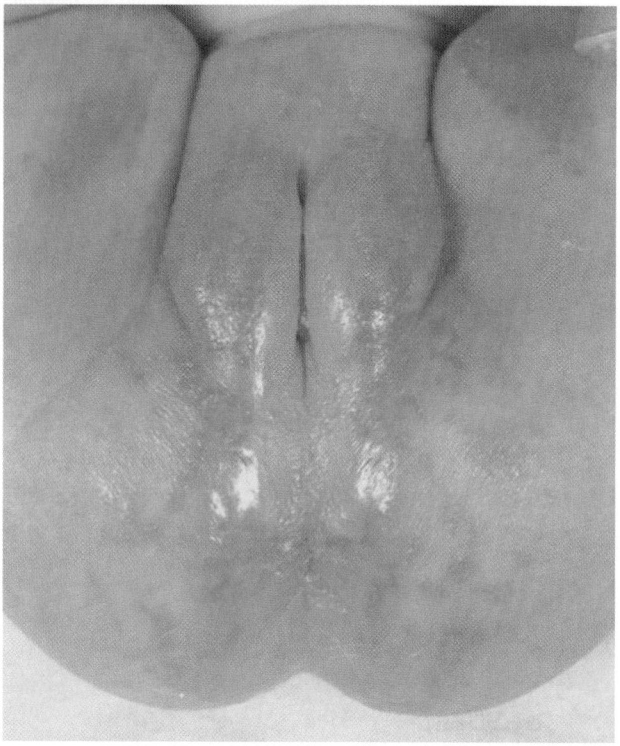

Figure 30-15 Severe Irritant Diaper Dermatitis. *Source:* Harper, J., Oranje, A. P., & Prose, N. (2000). *Textbook of pediatric dermatology.* Oxford: Blackwell Science, Ltd.

Diagnosis

Diagnosis is made from the characteristic rash in the diaper area. Because rashes originating from other sources, such as *Candida* or intertrigo, may occur in the diaper area, the examiner must note the specific appearance of the rash when making a diagnosis.

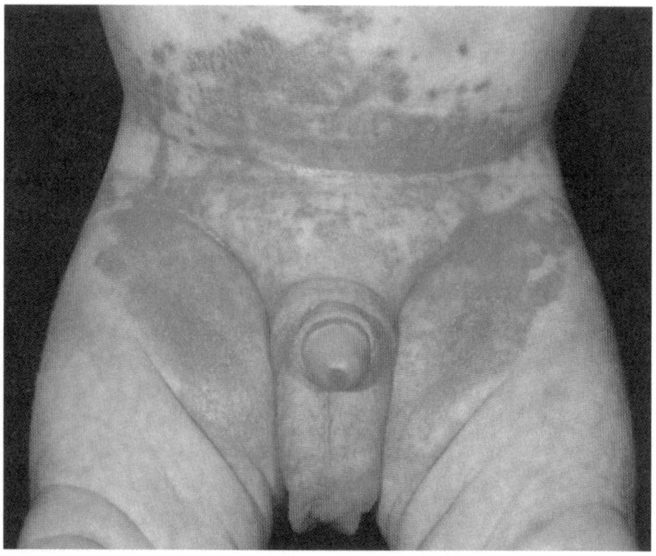

Figure 30-16 Candidal Diaper Dermatitis. *Source:* Habif, T. P. (1996). *Clinical dermatology: A color guide to diagnosis and therapy* (3rd ed.). St. Louis: Mosby-Year Book, Inc. (p. 398, fig. 13-51).

Treatment

Prevention is the best approach in the management of diaper dermatitis. Essential principles of management include keeping the skin dry, protected, and free of infection. Most cases are minor and respond quickly to this approach to care.

Increasing the frequency of diaper changes, along with good diaper hygiene, is considered the most important strategy to avoid prolonged skin contact with wetness. Superabsorbent disposable diapers, which move the moisture away from the skin and provide a pH control, are superior to cloth diapers; however, they are not a substitute for frequent diaper changes and good hygiene.

Barrier creams are useful to protect the skin from moisture and chemical irritants. White petrolatum products and zinc oxide are inexpensive products that are safe and soothing to irritated skin. Baby powder and over-the-counter products such as baking soda and boric acid should not be

Nursing Tip:

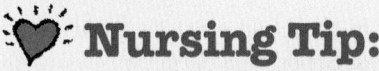

Baby wipes and diaper dermatitis
Baby wipes and lotions containing alcohol may exacerbate the rash. Mild soap and water are the best agents for cleansing.

used because of the risk for further irritation and toxicity. Baby powder also poses a risk for accidental inhalation and respiratory injury (Kazaks & Lane, 2000; Oranje; 2000).

Low-dose steroid creams such as 1% hydrocortisone may be beneficial to infants with severe inflammation. These products should not be used more than two weeks. Diaper dermatitis that occurs as a result of *Candida albicans* requires treatment with an antifungal agent, typically, nystatin (Mycostatin) cream or ointment. Combination products that contain both a corticosteroid and antifungal agent such as Lotrisone, which contains betamethasone 0.05% and clotrimazole 1%, should be avoided because of the high potency of the steroid and potential for systemic absorption (Singleton, 1997; Ward, et al., 2000).

Nursing Management

Nursing assessment of the infant with diaper dermatitis begins with a thorough history. Specific areas to cover with the history include the type of diaper used, frequency of diaper changes, presence and duration of diarrhea, and the use of any baby care products. The nurse also should ask the caregiver when the rash first appeared, what has been done to manage the rash, and what the results have been. When examining the infant, the nurse should note the distribution of the rash and the type of lesions present. The clinical appearance of the rash will assist the examiner in determining its etiology. For example, a primary irritant contact dermatitis typically will spare the skin folds and be shiny and erythematous in appearance. A rash caused by *Candida* will be a beefy red in appearance with satellite pustules.

Nursing management, like the treatments mentioned previously, is designed to remove the irritants and keep the diaper area dry. Changing diapers as soon as they are soiled and thoroughly cleaning the diaper area are the most important preventive and treatment measures. The nurse should identify the type of diaper used for the infant. When possible, super-absorbent disposable diapers should be used. If cloth diapers are used, plastic pants should be avoided. Interventions to promote healing of irritated skin include allowing the diaper area to dry thoroughly during diaper changes. When feasible, the diaper area may be exposed to air. Ointments and barrier creams that protect the skin from moisture and irritants may be used.

Critical Thinking

Diaper Dermatitis

What instructions about treatment would you give to caregivers of an infant with diaper dermatitis?

The rash should demonstrate initial improvement following increased frequency of diaper changes and application of barrier creams. Most cases of diaper dermatitis are relatively mild and show signs of improvement within one or two days. Cases that do not respond to initial intervention may require further evaluation.

Family Teaching

Most infants with diaper dermatitis are cared for in the home. Caregivers need to be taught factors that contribute to the development of diaper dermatitis and to recognize its early symptoms so that they can initiate interventions early. If cloth diapers are used, they should be rinsed thoroughly to avoid irritation from residual detergent. If the rash persists, the type of detergent may need to be changed. Mild soaps and lukewarm water should be used for cleansing the diaper area. Ointments and barrier creams, as described earlier, may be used. These products should be applied in a thick layer. They do not need to be removed completely with each diaper change. When the diaper is soiled, the top layer should be wiped away. More ointment or cream should be reapplied. Steroid creams should be applied to the affected area in a thin layer twice a day as indicated.

Seborrheic Dermatitis

Seborrheic dermatitis is a self-limiting inflammatory condition affecting infants and adolescents. Its exact etiology is unclear.

Incidence and Etiology

Seborrheic dermatitis is also known as "cradle cap" in infants. It most commonly presents within the first three months of life, often as early as the first 3 to 4 weeks of life, and resolves spontaneously by 8 to 12 months of age. In adolescents, seborrheic dermatitis develops following puberty. It has a prevalence of 2–5% and is more common in boys (Langtry, 2000). Seborrheic dermatitis occurring during adolescence has the potential to become chronic. An increased incidence is noted during the winter months.

The inflammatory changes are believed to result from dysfunction of the sebaceous glands and hormonal activity. Overgrowth of the yeast, *Pityrosporum ovale*, which normally is found on the scalp, also has been implicated in the development of seborrheic dermatitis in adolescents.

Pathophysiology

Increased activity of sebaceous glands is a normal occurrence of infancy and adolescence. Manifestations of seborrheic dermatitis are believed to occur as a consequence of a low-grade inflammatory process involving the sebaceous glands. Dysfunction of sebaceous glands may initiate the immune response resulting in symptoms of inflammation. Hormonal activity may influence increased sebum production. Circulating maternal hormones in the infant are believed to account for the onset of seborrheic dermatitis in early infancy and its resolution by the end of the first year of life when levels have decreased (Singleton, 1997).

Clinical Manifestations

Lesions typically are thick, adherent, whitish-yellowish, scaly, oily patches that may be mildly pruritic (Figure 30-17). **Spongiosis,** inflammation of the skin's spongy layer, also may be present. Seborrheic dermatitis can occur anywhere that sebaceous glands are plentiful. In infants, lesions most commonly are distributed on the scalp, although discrete lesions also may be present on the face, trunk, intertriginous skin folds, and flexural surfaces. During adolescence, lesions begin on the scalp and may involve the eyebrows, forehead, nasolabial folds, and retroauricular areas. Pustules may be present in the beard area.

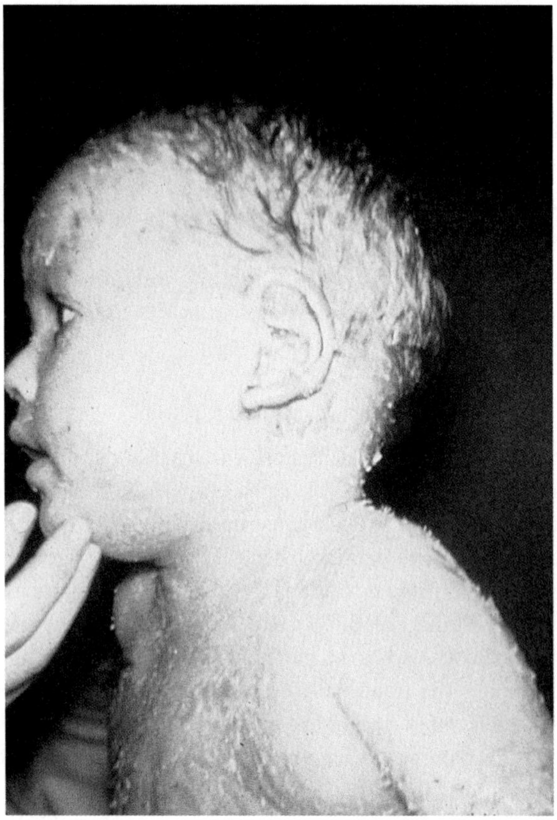

Figure 30-17 Seborrheic Dermatitis. Courtesy of the Centers for Disease Control and Prevention.

Diagnosis

Diagnosis is made from the characteristic location and appearance of the lesions. Seborrheic dermatitis can be distinguished from atopic dermatitis by its limited pruritus.

Treatment

Initial treatment of seborrheic dermatitis consists of removal of the crusts with good hygienic methods. Infants with mild symptoms often respond to daily shampooing with a mild, non-medicated shampoo or a baby shampoo. The shampoo should be left in place for a few hours to loosen the scales and then gently scrubbed while rinsing. Mineral oil or white petrolatum applied to the scalp and left overnight two to four weeks may aid in removing persistent scales. Low-potency topical corticosteroids can be used to manage generalized seborrheic dermatitis.

Treatment principles for adolescents are similar to those for infants although medicated shampoos may be used. Shampoos containing sulfur or salicylic acid may be used for lesions not responding to initial daily shampooing. Lesions that remain resistant to treatment are managed with topical corticosteroid lotion with or without 2–5% sulfur precipitate or salicylic acid applied to the scalp twice daily (Boerio, et al., 2000). Shampoos containing an antifungal agent such as ketoconazole are beneficial in suppressing growth of the *Pityrosporum* yeast (Langtry, 2000).

Nursing Management and Family Teaching

Priorities for nursing management include resolution of symptoms and education of the caregivers and adolescent. The nursing assessment should include a history of the onset of the lesions and any accompanying symptoms. The nurse should note the pattern and distribution of the lesions, including any accompanying pruritus. Teaching should include information about the nature of the condition. Caregivers of infants should be offered assurance that the condition may resolve within a few weeks and most often within 8 to 12 months. They may require assistance in shampooing because of fear of injury to the anterior fontanel. Teaching should address use of appropriate shampoos, appropriate time for leaving the shampoo in place, and the correct technique for removing scales. Caregivers should be assured that gentle scrubbing with a soft brush or toothbrush or the fingertips will not injure the fontanel. If topical corticosteroids are to be used, teaching should address correct use and application. Adolescents should be reassured that although the condition may require treatment for a long time, long-term prognosis is good.

Contact Dermatitis

Contact dermatitis occurs as a result of contact with an irritant or an allergen. Irritant contact dermatitis occurs as a local reaction to a sufficient amount of irritant, often as a consequence of prolonged contact. Allergic contact dermatitis is a cell-mediated response brought about by sensitization to an allergen.

Incidence and Etiology

The exact incidence of contact dermatitis in children is difficult to estimate. It is estimated that allergic contact dermatitis represents approximately 20% of all dermatitis occurring in children (Boerio, et al., 2000; Bruckner & Weston, 2001). Of children with dermatitis, approximately 15–66% are sensitized to contact allergens; however, the clinical significance has not been determined. Although sensitization to allergens was once believed to be less common in young children because of their less developed immune systems, sensitization can occur. Children who have frequent, repeated breaks in their skin are at increased risk for developing irritant and allergic contact dermatitis.

The development of irritant contact dermatitis depends on the ability of the skin to serve as an intact barrier, the type of irritant, and the duration of contact. Any process or substance that compromises skin integrity may function as an irritant. A common irritant for children is moisture such as that which occurs with repeated liplicking, increased drooling, and diaper dermatitis. Other irritants include latex, which also may contribute to allergic contact dermatitis, perfumes, and detergents (Boerio, et al., 2000).

Allergic contact dermatitis occurs in response to an antigen that elicits a hypersensitivity reaction. It requires an intact immune system that is capable of mounting a hypersensitivity response. The most common allergen in the United States is urushiol, which is the substance found in poison ivy, poison oak, and poison sumac. Others include nickel, which is common in jewelry and fasteners; neomycin, which is a topical antibiotic; potassium dichromate, which is used in leather tanning; and latex (Bruckner & Weston, 2001).

Pathophysiology

Irritant contact dermatitis occurs as a consequence of repeated insults to the skin from an irritating source. These repeated injuries to the skin cause it to lose its barrier function, leading to breakdown of the surrounding area. Factors that contribute to the severity of the dermatitis include the length of exposure, concentration of the irritant, and the integrity of the skin. Allergic contact dermatitis is a type IV hypersensitivity response. Two phases are required for a response to occur: first, a sensitization phase, and second, an elicitation phase.

The initial exposure to the antigen occurs during the **sensitization phase.** Most contact allergens have low molecular weights and readily penetrate the epidermis. Following the exposure, the antigen is processed by Langerhans' cells, which reside in the basal layer of the epidermis, and transported to T lymphocytes. The T lymphocytes then develop memory to the antigen and circulate throughout the body, including the skin. The clinical manifestations of the hypersensitivity response occur during the **elicitation phase.** Upon re-exposure to the antigen, the sensitized T lymphocytes proliferate and release inflammatory mediators that produce a localized dermatitis. The dermatitis most often occurs 12 to 24 hours following re-exposure (Weston & Bruckner, 2000).

BOX 30-4 Urushiol

Urushiol is the active allergen in plants belonging to the *Toxicodendron* genus. In the United States, these plants include poison ivy, poison oak, and poison sumac. Urushiol is widely distributed through the leaves, stems, and roots of *Toxicodendron* plants. It is a very potent resin that may cause an intense rash, blisters, and pruritus. Direct contact with the plant is the primary source of sensitization; however, the allergen can be carried on clothing, pets, tools, and toys and thus transferred to the sensitive individual. Even the smoke from burning the plants can cause irritation in the lungs of sensitive individuals. The peak age of sensitization is between 8–14 years of age. Sensitivity to urushiol is acquired and tends to run in families. Reactivity to urushiol is influenced by the degree of exposure, physical activity, and the affected individual's age and immune function.

Adapted from Tanner, T. L. (2000). Rhus (*Toxicodendron*) dermatitis. *Primary Care, 27,* 493–502.

Clinical Manifestations

Irritant contact dermatitis manifests as the injury occurs and most frequently presents as a localized area of erythema and dryness. Pruritus often is present. Repeated and intense exposure to the irritant may result in further fissuring and lichenification of the affected area. Severe injury may result in loss of function, in particular if the hands are involved (Shaw, 1996).

Because allergic contact dermatitis is a delayed hypersensitive response, symptoms do not appear until 12 to 24 hours following re-exposure to the antigen. The dermatitis will be fully developed in about 2 days and regress in about 3 to 4 weeks unless treated (Weston & Bruckner, 2000). Symptoms of allergic contact dermatitis include a pruritic rash occurring at the site of contact. The rash caused by potent allergens, such as poison ivy, is characterized by erythema, edema, and pruritus (Figure 30-18). Vesicles or bullae develop and may rupture, leaving a crust. As lesions rupture, the denuded skin is susceptible to secondary bacterial infection. Less potent allergens, such as nickel used in

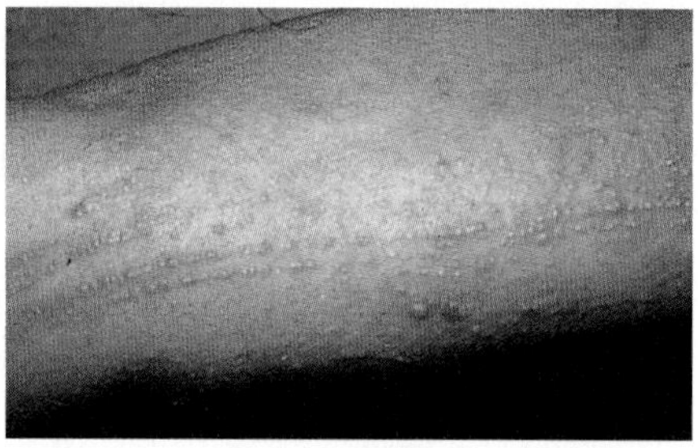

Figure 30-18 Allergic Contact Dermatitis from Poison Oak. Courtesy of the Centers for Disease Control and Prevention.

jewelry, result in a more chronic onset of dermatitis. Lesions are characterized by erythema, scaling, and lichenification. If allergic contact dermatitis is not treated, symptoms resolve over a period of 3 to 4 weeks. If exposure to the allergen is repeated, symptoms may become widespread. If the irritant allergen can be identified and avoided, long-term prognosis is excellent.

Diagnosis

Diagnosis is based on a history of exposure to the irritant and the appearance of the rash. For example, the rash associated with poison ivy exposure frequently appears as a linear distribution of vesicles. Areas of dryness and scaling on the earlobes are suggestive of nickel allergy associated with wearing earrings. If the diagnosis is not obvious, patch testing may be indicated to determine the specific allergen. Patch testing is used to determine a T lymphocyte response. It involves the placement of specific antigens on the skin for 48 hours and monitoring for evidence of a localized reaction. Patch testing should be performed by an experienced dermatologist to avoid error in interpreting findings.

Treatment

Prevention is the best treatment for contact dermatitis, which means avoidance of the irritant. Educating children and caregivers about potential sources of the allergen and to recognize known sources, such as poison ivy, is essential to avoid re-exposure (Box 30-5).

If a sensitive individual comes in contact with poison ivy, poison oak, or poison sumac, the area should be rinsed immediately (within 5 minutes) with water. Clothing should be removed and washed. Tools, toys, or other contaminated objects should be washed thoroughly to remove any residual resin. Corticosteroids are the mainstay of pharmacologic management of allergic contact dermatitis. If the dermatitis covers less than 10% of the skin surface, topical mild- to moderate-potency steroids are used. Typical treatment is twice daily application for two to three weeks. If the dermatitis covers more than 10% of the skin, oral steroids are used. The usual dose is 1 to 2 mg/kg/day given as a single dose for 7 to 10 days. The dose then is tapered over another 7 to 10 days. Whether topical or oral steroids are used, the treatment must be given for the prescribed two to three weeks to prevent recurrence of symptoms (Bruckner & Weston, 2001).

BOX 30-5 Plant identification

Toxicodendron plants are found throughout the United States: poison ivy is more common east of the Rocky Mountains, poison oak is found west of the Rocky Mountains, and poison sumac is usually found in the swamp regions of the Southeast. The appearance of the plants is varied according to the individual species and the season of year. Poison ivy grows either as a shrub or vine and is identified by clusters of three leaves ranging from 3 to 15 cm in length. Poison oak grows as a small bush-like plant or a climbing vine. Its leaves are 3 to 7 cm long and may grow in clusters of three, five, or seven. Poison sumac (also known as poison dogwood or poison elder) has smooth, pointed pale green leaves approximately 10 cm long. Seven to 13 leaves may be arranged on one stem.

Adapted from Tanner, T. L. (2000). Rhus (*Toxicodendron*) dermatitis. *Primary Care, 27,* 493–502.

Additional supportive care measures include the use of antihistamines such as diphenhydramine (Benadryl) or hydroxyzine (Vistaril) to relieve pruritus. Oral preparations should be used as opposed to topical agents. Topical antihistamines pose a potential risk of sensitization and further exacerbation of the condition (Tanner, 2000). Wet compresses, cool baths, and calamine lotion also may be used to relieve symptoms of itching and discomfort from the rash.

Nursing Management

Nursing management focuses on identification of the irritant, education of children and their caregivers to avoid contact with the irritant, prevention of secondary infections, and alleviation of the pruritus. The nursing history should address recent exposure to common environmental irritant allergens. Avoidance of the plant or other environmental irritants is the first line of management. When exposure to poison ivy, poison oak, or poison sumac is possible, long pants, shirts with long sleeves, and shoes with socks should be worn to avoid exposure. If exposure does occur, the exposed area should be rinsed with water immediately. The antigen penetrates the skin quickly and needs to be removed as soon after exposure as possible to avoid symptoms of allergic dermatitis. Children should be assisted to rinse their hands carefully to prevent spread of the reaction to sensitive areas of the body such as the face, mouth, and genitalia. Cotton balls or gauze soaked in rubbing alcohol can be used to remove plant sap from the skin. Clothing contaminated with the resin should be removed as soon after exposure as possible (Tanner, 2000). Regardless of the source of the allergen, meticulous hygiene of the skin is essential to avoid secondary bacterial infections. Efforts must be made to minimize symptoms of pruritus to avoid further damage to the skin.

Family Teaching

Teaching should emphasize measures to prevent re-exposure and management of the symptoms of the dermatitis. Caregivers and older children should be able to identify the offending plant or environmental irritant in order to avoid it. The adage, "Leaves of three, let it be," is useful to assist children in recognizing and avoiding contact with poison ivy. The various methods of transfer of urushiol on animals, clothing, toys, tools, and shoes should be stressed. Children who undergo patch testing will require education specific to the procedure. The patches will be in place for two days. Children should not bathe or engage in strenuous activity while wearing the patches to avoid interference with any localized reaction occurring at the patch site (Weston & Bruckner, 2000).

Acne

Acne vulgaris, commonly known as acne, is predominantly a skin disease of adolescence. It is considered a chronic condition and may persist into adulthood. In addition to the physical changes that occur as a consequence of the skin lesions, acne may result in considerable emotional distress for the adolescent (Aktan, Ozmen, & Sanli, 2000; Klassen, Newton, & Mallon, 2000). Successful management must address both physiological and psychosocial well-being.

Incidence and Etiology

It is estimated that 85% of adolescents and young adults between 12 and 25 years of age will develop acne. The highest incidence is in the late teens, 16–17 years of age for girls and 17–18 years of age for boys. Acne is more common in males than females (Krowchuk, 2000). The exact etiology is unknown but it has been associated with increased androgen and sebum production, which normally occurs during puberty. There is evidence of a familial tendency toward severe acne; however, other factors influence the actual course of the disease. Heat, humidity, increased friction, emotional stress, oil-based cosmetics, menstrual cycles, and steroid administration have all been associated with the development of acne. No evidence presently exists to suggest that any specific food has an influence on the development of acne (Krowchuk, 2000; Usatine & Quan, 2000).

Pathophysiology

Acne is a disease involving the **pilosebaceous follicles.** These units consist of a follicle, or pore, a sebaceous gland, and a tiny **vellus hair** (short, tiny, and often inconspicuous hairs distributed across the body). Pilosebaceous follicles are most abundant on the face, chest, and upper back. Acne is associated with an increased production of **sebum,** a complex lipid mixture that helps to maintain normal hydration of the skin. The sebaceous gland increases in size and production of sebum under the influence of the adrenal and gonadal hormones during the time of adrenocortical maturation (teen years). Sebum secretion peaks during adolescence and declines after age 20. In individuals with acne, the epithelial cells lining the follicle change and become more cohesive. This allows for the accumulation of sebum and keratinized material derived from the lining cells. The exact trigger for this process has not been determined. As a consequence of this obstruction the development of acne lesions occurs. *Propionibacterium acnes* (*P. acnes*) is a normally harmless anaerobic bacterium, which is part of the normal skin flora and often colonizes the pilosebaceous follicle. The bacteria use sebum as a nutrient for growth. *P. acnes* is believed to contribute to the development of acne by producing free fatty acids and enzymes that trigger the inflammatory response and damage the follicle wall.

> **Critical Thinking**
>
> **Pathophysiology of Acne**
>
> What are the four factors involved in the pathophysiology of acne?

Clinical Manifestations

A number of different classification systems exist for acne. The two common classification subtypes are 1) comedonal acne, which is obstructive and noninflammatory and 2) inflammatory acne, which is characterized by inflammatory papules, pustules, and nodules. Many individuals with acne have both types of lesions present. **Comedones** are the characteristic lesions of noninflammatory acne. Lesions may be closed or open. Closed lesions commonly are referred to as whiteheads. These lesions are slightly palpable nonerythematous papules with microscopic openings. They are approximately 1 to 3 millimeters in diameter and are whitish or flesh colored. Open lesions are known as blackheads. These lesions are follicles with widely dilated openings. The characteristic black color of these lesions is not dirt, but occurs as a consequence of oxidation of melanin.

Inflamed lesions result when the follicular wall ruptures, leaking sebum, hair, *P. acnes*, and cells into the dermis and causing the formation of papules, pustules, nodules, and cysts. Papules are erythematous lesions that range from 2 to 5 mm in diameter. Pustules are papules that contain purulent material. Nodules exceed 5 mm in diameter and are seated more deeply in the dermis than papules and pustules. The term cyst, when used with acne, is actually a misnomer. These lesions are nodules that have become filled with pus. Although nodules are most likely to result in scarring, any inflammatory lesion has the potential to produce scarring. Acne scars most frequently have the appearance of pits or depressions, although hypertrophic scars may result. Secondary infection, occurring as a consequence of picking at the lesions may result in further scarring.

The psychological aspects of acne should not be overlooked. The impact of acne is not necessarily related to the severity of the lesions, and girls are at greater risk for negative psychosocial effects (Aktan, Ozmen, & Sanli, 2000). Emotional sequelae may include low self-esteem, diminished self-confidence, social isolation, and depression.

Diagnosis

The diagnosis of acne is made based on the client's age and the appearance of lesions on the face, neck, and back. Evaluation of the adolescent is important to determine the appropriate course of treatment. The history should address factors associated with acne flares, activities that may aggravate the condition, and treatments that the adolescent used along with their effectiveness. Physical examination should include a "lesion count," noting the number of lesions present, their distribution, and type. Acne often is given a global grading of mild, moderate, or severe based on the presentation of lesions. The examiner also should note the psychosocial impact of the adolescent's acne. Acne appearing in prepubertal age children may be indicative of an underlying endocrine disorder and warrants further diagnostic evaluation.

Treatment

Although many treatments have been used, there is little evidence that any actually shorten the course of the disease. The objectives of the treatment are to promote the general health of the individual, improve appearance, decrease discomfort from inflamed lesions, prevent or minimize scar formation, and prevent adverse psychological outcomes. Medications for acne can be divided into topical and systemic agents. Topical medications include benzoyl peroxide, retinoids, adapalene, azelaic acid, and antibiotics. Oral agents include antibiotics, oral contraceptives, and isotretinoin.

Treatment should be individualized to the adolescent based on consideration of the type of lesions, severity of lesions, psychological impact of lesions, and the adolescent's personal preferences regarding treatment. Some treatment choices may be limited by health care reimbursement regulations. For example, some states do not allow Medicaid reimbursement for prescription topical acne medications. In addition, no single formula for treatment works for all adolescents. Regardless of the type of treatment used, improvement typically is not observed before 4 to 6 weeks.

Mild comedonal and inflammatory acne are managed with topical agents. A single agent is used initially, and, if no response is noted, additional medications may be substituted or added to the treatment regimen. Common agents used at the onset of treatment include benzoyl peroxide, tretinoin, or azelaic acid. Increased concentrations of topical agents are indicated for moderate comedonal acne. Oral antibiotics, such as tetracycline, often provide benefit to adolescents with inflammatory or mixed comedogenic and inflammatory acne. These agents reduce the activity of *P. acnes* and are taken over a period of several months. Topical tretinoin may continue to be used with oral antibiotic therapy.

Treatment with isotretinoin is limited to adolescents with severe inflammatory acne who have not responded to standard therapies. It is the only acne medication that can reverse the pathologic changes associated with acne. Its use is limited because of its high potency and potential side effects, and it should be prescribed only by a dermatologist or practitioner experienced in its use. Side effects include dry skin and mucous membranes, musculoskeletal symptoms, and premature epiphyseal closure. It is also highly tetratogenic, and strict contraceptive measures must be observed by females taking the medication. Isotretinoin therapy typically lasts for a period of 16 to 20 weeks. Adolescents who fail to respond to isotretinoin may be retreated 2 to 5 months after completion of the first course (Usatine & Quan, 2000).

Other adjunct therapies are available to the adolescent with acne. These include comedone extraction and steroid injections. Often referral to a dermatologist is required for treatment. Comedone extraction involves opening the comedone with a scalpel or 25 gauge needle followed by application of pressure with a comedone extractor to remove the contents of the lesion. Intralesional steroid injections are used to relieve the pain and inflammation associated with lesions and to reduce the potential for scarring. Approximately 0.05 to 0.3 ml of triamcinolone acetonide solution is injected into each lesion using a 30 gauge needle. Injections may be repeated after 3 weeks (Usatine & Quan, 2000).

Nursing Management

Nursing management focuses on reduction of the severity of the acne, supportive care, and education of the adolescent regarding the management of the acne. Because acne is a disease primarily of adolescence, interventions should be directed primarily toward the adolescent. The nurse should recognize that because benefit from treatment may take 6 to 8 weeks to become apparent, the adolescent may need support to follow the treatment regimen. A healthy support system also is helpful to the adolescent with decreased self-esteem and body image as a consequence of the acne.

Information about skin care, diet, and rest should be made available to the adolescent. Common myths associated with skin care need to be dispelled. For example, acne is not

Kids Want To Know

Are greasy foods making my acne worse?

I love chips, whether they are potato, cheese curls, or tortilla chips! Will I have to go cold turkey on eating chips to manage my pimples? The nurse should counsel that while scientific studies do not show a correlation between eating greasy items and acne, it is important to maintain a healthy balanced diet. If consumption of a particular food item seems to aggravate the condition, then discontinue eating it.

caused by dirt, and aggressive washing can damage the skin and limit the individual's ability to tolerate topical medications. No specific foods have been implicated as having a role in the development of acne. The adolescent should be discouraged from picking and squeezing the lesions. This can damage the skin and increase the possibility of secondary infection and scarring. Keeping the hair clean and off the forehead tends to lessen the severity of the lesions.

The adolescent should receive information specific to the treatment plan. Teaching should include the medication to be used, specific instructions for use, and significant side effects. Families should be encouraged to support the client to follow the treatments and to encourage the adolescent to stick with the regimen even if it does not seem instantly effective.

Family Teaching

Education is an important aspect in the management of acne vulgaris. As previously noted, adolescents may have many misconceptions regarding the development and management of acne that need clarification. The nurse should emphasize that acne is a chronic condition and will most likely have a waxing and waning course over several years. The adolescent should understand factors that may worsen acne. Cosmetics and moisturizers containing oils should be avoided; products labeled as "noncomedogenic" should be substituted. Picking at or squeezing lesions will result in further trauma and inflammation, which can delay healing and increase the potential for scarring. Acne flares may occur in young women prior to menstruation as a consequence of the androgenic effects of progesterone. Individuals who encounter environmental exposure to oils or grease, such as those working in auto-repair shops or fast-food restaurants, may experience aggravation of acne.

Appropriate use of over-the-counter and prescribed medications should be emphasized. The adolescent should be instructed to apply the topical medication to the entire area and not just the individual lesions. They should be warned that topical medications may cause erythema, peeling, itching, and burning with initial use. Assurance should be provided that these symptoms frequently improve with continued use of the medication.

Because the effectiveness of topical tretinoin is inhibited by exposure to ultraviolet light, it should be applied at night. Topical tretinoin also is oxidized by benzoyl peroxide, and these products should not be used simultaneously (Usatine & Quan, 2000). Several of the topical and oral medications cause photosensitivity. Adolescents taking these medications should be reminded to use sunscreen with an SPF rating of 15 or greater and wear protective clothing to reduce exposure to ultraviolet rays (Krowchuk, 2000; Usatine & Quan, 2000). Adolescent females receiving isotretinoin must receive thorough counseling of the necessity of observing strict contraceptive measures during and one month following therapy. Many providers require women of reproductive age to receive monthly pregnancy tests prior to beginning therapy and throughout therapy regardless of whether or not they claim to be sexually active. (Usatine & Quan, 2000).

BITES AND STINGS

Injuries to children from bites and stings have the potential to be life-threatening in young children. Each year, many children become seriously injured and disfigured as a consequence of animal bites. Because of their small size, children are less able to defend themselves from attacking animals and are more likely to receive fatal injuries. Bites and stings from arthropods, in particular insects and spiders, can be harmful to children because they receive a relative greater "dose" of venom than an adult does. Stings from insects such as bees and wasps have the potential to result in hypersensitivity reactions. Spider bites are more likely to cause systemic injury as a consequence of exposure to their venom.

Animal Bites

An estimated several million individuals in the United States are bitten by animals each year. Of those sustaining bites, fewer than one-fourth seek medical care for the bite (Weiss, Friedman, & Coben, 1998; Sacks, Kresnow, & Houston, 1996). Although the majority of injuries from animal bites are minor, severe trauma, infection, and even death may result.

Incidence and Etiology

Dogs and cats account for approximately 90% of all animal bites in the United States (Weiss, et al., 1998). Although occurring less frequently, the significance of bites from other mammals should not be overlooked. In 1999, bites from bats, foxes, raccoons, rodents, and skunks were documented in children in the United States (Litovitz, et al., 2000). Dog bites represent approximately 80% of animal bites in the United States (Garcia, 1997). National and regional reports indicate that bites from dogs occur more frequently in children and are more likely to result in severe injury (Bernardo, Gardner, O'Connor, & Amon, 2000; Gandhi, Liebman, Stafford, B., & Stafford, P., 1999; Patrick & O'Rourke, 1998; Weiss, et al., 1998). During 1997 and 1998, 27 dog bite related fatalities were recorded in the United States. Of these, 19 (70%) were children (Sacks, Sinclair, Gilchrist, Golab, & Lockwood, 2000).

The majority of reported dog bites involve large dogs such as pit bulls, German shepherds, rottweilers, and chows (Bernardo, et al., 2000; Gandhi, et al., 1999). These breeds of dogs also are most likely to cause fatal injuries (MMWR, 1997). Male, unneutered dogs tend to be more aggressive and have an increased frequency of reported attacks on children. Children are most likely to be bitten by a dog that is known to them, either owned by the child's family or someone familiar to the family. The majority of dog bites involve a single dog and occur in the afternoon. Approximately one-half of all bites are considered unprovoked although this is not always clearly reported. Boys tend to be bitten by dogs more frequently than are girls. Boys between 5 and 9 years of age are most frequently bitten. Children less than 5 years of age are at risk for the most debilitating injuries from dog bites. Their injuries are most likely to involve the head and neck (Bernardo, et al., 2000; Gandhi, et al., 1999; Patrick & O'Rourke, 1998).

Cat bites represent only about 10–15% of all animal bites in the United States. The majority of these bites are reported to be provoked. Cat bites are less likely to occur in children; however, they pose a greater risk of infection (Patrick & O'Rourke, 1998; Garcia, 1997).

Pathophysiology/Clinical Manifestations

The most common types of injuries resulting from animal bites include abrasions, punctures, and lacerations with or without **avulsion** (major tearing of tissue) (Ginsburg, 2000). The majority of injuries to children involve the face, in particular, the cheek, lips, and mouth (Bernardo, et al., 2000; Gandhi, et al., 1999). Facial injuries present the risk of permanent disfigurement. Attacks to the head and neck are particularly dangerous because of the risk of massive blood loss if a major blood vessel is punctured.

Infection is the most common complication resulting from animal bites. Wounds sustained as a consequence of dog and cat bites are at particular risk for contamination with *Pasturella* species. Clinical manifestations of *Pasturella* infection include intense inflammation accompanied by pain and swelling within 24 hours of the injury. Infection rates are significantly greater following cat bites than dog bites, and puncture wounds are more likely to become contaminated than lacerations (Garcia, 1997).

Diagnosis

Initial evaluation of bites should address the type of animal, whether the bite was provoked or unprovoked, the type of injury, the size and depth of the wound, the presence of foreign material in the wound, the integrity of underlying structures, and the duration of time that has elapsed since the injury. X rays should be obtained when there is a risk of fracture, such as in the case of an infant who has sustained injuries to the head and face (Ginsburg, 2000). Because of the risk for infection, cultures of the wound site should be considered. Dog bites that are treated within 8 hours have a less than 20% risk of infection. These bites are not considered to require culturing unless they are deep and extensive or are greater than 8 hours old.

In contrast, because cat bites have a much greater risk of infection, all wounds except those considered as trivial should be cultured. All wounds caused by bites from other animals should be routinely cultured (Ginsburg, 2000). An additional priority in the diagnosis of bites includes evaluation of the animal's rabies status. Although the overall incidence of human rabies in the United States has declined since the 1950s, rabies continues to remain a problem among wildlife (Adams, 2000; American Academy of Pediatrics [AAP], 2000b). Healthy, vaccinated domestic animals are held for 10 days of observation following the biting episode. Immediate rabies prophylaxis is necessary for individuals bitten by domestic animals suspected of being rabid and those bitten by wild animals such as bats, skunks, raccoons, and most wild carnivores. If at all possible, the animal should be captured and euthanized in a manner that will preserve its brain tissue for definitive diagnosis (AAP, 2000b).

Treatment

After the appropriate cultures have been obtained, the wound should be thoroughly irrigated with large amounts of sterile saline at pressures that will allow for adequate debridement yet will not cause further tissue damage (Ginsburg, 2000; Garcia, 1997). Local anesthesia may be necessary to accomplish adequate cleansing of the wound. Suturing and stapling are commonly performed procedures for wound management (Bernardo, et al., 2000). Disagreement exists over whether wounds should undergo **primary closure** (wound closure performed shortly after the injury in which the wound edges are approximated), **delayed primary closure** (wound closure performed 3–5 days after the injury), or be allowed to heal by **secondary intention** (Ginsburg, 2000). Secondary intention is the natural process of wound healing that occurs when the wound edges cannot be approximated because of extensive tissue loss. This process involves inflammation, reconstruction of epithelium, and scar formation without surgical intervention. Current recommendations are that a surgical consult be obtained for wounds that are deep and extensive, involve bones and joints, and that have become infected and require open drainage. Wounds to the face that are less than 5 hours old should undergo primary closure by a plastic surgeon (Ginsburg, 2000).

Guidelines for the use of prophylactic antibiotics are not well established. Considerations in determining antibiotic therapy include the depth and severity of the wound, the presence and degree of overt infection, and the immune status of the child (Ginsburg, 2000). Moderate to severe wounds, those to the face and hands, deep puncture wounds, cat bites, and individuals who are immune compromised are most likely to benefit from antibiotic therapy (Garcia, 1997). Extended spectrum penicillins are considered antibiotics of choice because of their activity against the majority of bacteria routinely cultured from bite wounds. Amoxicillin-clavulanate (Augmentin) is considered an effective oral antibiotic for prophylaxis and treatment of infection. Ticarcillin-clavulanate (Timentin) and ampicillin-sulbactam (Unasyn) are useful for intravenous management of bite-related infection. Appropriate tetanus prophylaxis should be administered to children who have not been immunized previously and who have not had a tetanus immunization in the past 10 years. Positive identification of the biting animal and evaluation of its rabies status should be made as soon after the injury as possible and, if indicated, appropriate rabies prophylaxis should be initiated (Box 30-6).

BOX 30-6 Rabies

Rabies remains a significant threat to those bitten by wild animals. Bats, raccoons, skunks, foxes, and other wild carnivores pose the greatest risk for transmitting the disease to humans. Unvaccinated domestic animals also are considered a risk to humans. If a human is bitten by one of these animals, rabies prophylaxis should be initiated immediately, and the case should be reported to appropriate public health authorities. The rabies virus is present in the saliva of the infected animal and is transmitted by biting. The average incubation period is 4 to 6 weeks although symptoms may appear within 5 days of exposure. Once symptoms appear, no specific treatment for rabies is available. The diagnosis of rabies is confirmed by demonstration of virus-specific fluorescent antigen in brain tissue. An animal that has bitten and is suspected of being rabid should be captured and euthanized so that the brain tissue is preserved. The head should be removed, refrigerated, and sent to a qualified laboratory for evaluation. Rabies prophylaxis consists of the administration of both passive and active immunoprophylaxis and should be initiated as soon as possible following exposure. Passive prophylaxis involves the intramuscular administration of human rabies vaccine (HRV) on the first day post-exposure followed by repeated doses on days 3, 7, 14, and 28 after the first dose. Active prophylaxis consists of administration of rabies immune globulin (RIG). The wound should be infiltrated with as much of the RIG as possible. The remainder of the dose is administered intramuscularly using a separate syringe and needle.

Adapted from Adams, W. G. (2000). Rabies. In R. E. Behrman, R. M. Kleigman, & H. B. Jenson (Eds.), *Nelson textbook of pediatrics* (16th ed., pp. 1014–1017). Philadelphia: W. B. Saunders; American Academy of Pediatrics. (2000b). Rabies. In L. K. Pickering (Ed.), *2000 Red book: Report on the committee on infectious diseases* (25th ed. pp. 475–482). Elk Grove, IL: Author.

Nursing Management

Prevention is the most important nursing consideration for animal bites. During routine well-child visits, nurses have the opportunity to ask the caregivers whether there is an animal in the home and to provide appropriate anticipatory guidance. Nurses also may develop educational programs to teach children in school and community settings about safe behavior around animals. A study of an educational program in Australia demonstrated that children who participated in an animal bite prevention program were more likely to display safe behaviors around dogs than children who did not participate in the program (Chapman, Cornwall, Righetti, & Sung, 2000). Nurses need to be aware of local and regional policies for reporting animal bites. Accurate reporting is essential to establish evidence for laws relating to animals such as leash laws and to receive funding for injury prevention programs.

Family Teaching

Teaching provided to children and caregivers should emphasize the child's safety and strategies for preventing injury. Children must be taught a healthy respect for animals, including safe behaviors around animals and actions to take if threatened. General dog bite prevention strategies for children are presented in Box 30-7. Children also should be taught to stay away from any wild animal.

Education of the caregiver should include selection of an appropriate animal for the family pet. The personalities of many animals are more adaptable to children than others; therefore, checking with a veterinarian about good pets is a major preventive measure. Exotic pets should be discouraged if young children are in the home. If the animal will not be used for breeding, neutering should be recommended to decrease aggressive behavior. Caregivers should be willing to make lifestyle and home environmental changes necessary to accommodate a pet. The importance of careful supervision of children and animals must be emphasized. Infants and young children never should be left alone with an animal. An increased incidence of animal bites occurring in the afternoon and early evening may be associated with decreased

BOX 30-7 Preventing dog bites in children

The following safety principles should be taught to children and reviewed regularly:

1. Never approach an unfamiliar dog.
2. Never run from a dog and scream.
3. Remain motionless when approached by an unfamiliar dog (e.g., "be still like a tree").
4. If knocked over by a dog, roll into a ball and lie still (e.g., "be still like a log").
5. Never play with a dog unless supervised by an adult.
6. Immediately report stray dogs or dogs displaying unusual behavior to an adult.
7. Avoid direct eye contact with a dog.
8. Do not disturb a dog that is sleeping, eating, or caring for puppies.
9. Do not pet a dog without allowing it to see and sniff you first.
10. If bitten, immediately report the bite to an adult.

Adapted from Sacks, J. J., Lockwood, R., Homreich, J., & Sattin, R. W. (1996). Fatal dog attacks, 1989–1994. *Pediatrics, 97,* 894. Reproduced with permission. Copyright 1996.

Reflective Thinking

Public Policy Concerning Specific Dog Breeds

Because of the greater incidence of specific dog breeds, namely pit bulls and rottweilers, involved in dog bite-related fatalities, many individuals support legislation to regulate these breeds. Do you think that this is an appropriate approach to reducing injury by these dogs? What legal responsibility should owners of these dogs be required to assume for their animals' actions?

adult supervision. Animal training and socialization programs may be helpful to promote appropriate behaviors around children (Bernardo, et al., 2000).

Insect Bites and Stings

Most bites and stings from insects produce only local skin reactions. Although relatively uncommon, life-threatening hypersensitivity reactions may occur. Bites and stings from insects involve separate, distinct mechanisms. Bites occur when the affected individual's skin is punctured by a sharp stylet on the insect's mouth. Stings occur when the skin is punctured by a stinger attached to the insect's abdomen.

Incidence and Etiology

Biting insects, mosquitoes, fleas, and flies, inflict their bites by penetrating the skin with a stylet covered with saliva. Warmth and moisture attracts the insects to humans. They are distributed throughout the world and have the potential to transmit diseases to humans. Mosquitoes are most prevalent among damp, marshy areas. In the United States, bites are most problematic during the summer months. Fleas are most commonly found on animals and in bedding and carpeting where the animal lies. Fleas are capable of jumping to attach to human hosts. Flies such as the deerfly, horsefly, and black fly are capable of producing painful bites. The common housefly does not cause bites. Although not insects, ticks and chiggers are other arthropods capable of producing disease or injury with their bites.

Although ticks and chiggers belong to the arachnid class of arthropods (as do spiders), they are often considered in discussions of insect bites. Ticks may grow as long as one centimeter and, like spiders, have four pairs of legs. They are vectors for a number of serious diseases. Ticks are found throughout the United States; however, specific species are more prevalent in specific geographic areas. Deer ticks are more common in the Northeast and are known for transmitting Lyme disease; in the West, Rocky Mountain spotted fever is transmitted by the Rocky Mountain wood tick.

Ticks often are found among tall grasses and bushes. When attached to a host, the tick's teeth penetrate the skin, and it becomes engorged by sucking blood. Tick bites are usually painless and may not be noticed for several hours when a pruritic wheal develops at the puncture site. If a bite occurs, the entire tick, including the mouth parts, should be removed carefully using a blunt forceps or tweezers. The tick should not be handled with bare hands to avoid contact with infective agents. Children should be checked carefully for ticks after activity in areas prone to them.

Harvest mites are more commonly known as chiggers. The six-legged larva is the only form of the chigger that is parasitic on humans. The larva does not ingest blood, but it must obtain a meal of epidermal and dermal tissue from a vertebrate host in order to mature into the adult form. After the larva has fed, it drops off into the soil. Chiggers often are found in areas with tall grass and underbrush. When attached to the human host with its claws, it produces digestive substances that liquefy the host's epithelium. This results in the appearance of intensely pruritic erythematous papules. Because chiggers prefer a warm environment, the intertriginous areas and those covered by clothing are most commonly affected. Typical treatment consists of measures to relieve pruritus such as oral antihistamines, cool compresses, and calamine lotion. Extensive bites may require treatment with oral corticosteriods. Yards may be treated with insecticides containing dursban and diazinon to control chiggers. (Angel, Nigro, & Levy, 2000; Habif, 1996a).

Insect stings are associated with insects of the Hymenoptera order, which includes apids (honeybees and bumblebees) and vespids (hornets, wasps, and yellow jackets), and ants. They inflict injury by penetrating the skin with a stinger attached to their abdomen, and their venom is responsible for hypersensitivity reactions. Reactions may range from mild, localized reactions to life-threatening systemic reactions. An estimated 0.15–3.3% of the general population will experience a systemic response to hymenopetera venom, and approximately 50 deaths each year in the United States are attributed to extreme hypersensitivity reactions (Maher, 1998; Novembre, et al., 1998). The exact prevalence of sensitization to hymenoptera venom among children is unknown. Yellow jackets and honeybees account for the majority of hymenoptera stings in the northern areas of the United States. In the Southeastern states and Gulf Coast area, fire ants and paper wasps are responsible for most stings (Maher, 1998). On a national level, yellow jackets, followed by honeybees and wasps, are most commonly associated with moderate to severe hypersensitivite reactions. The exact incidence of insect bites and stings among children is difficult to estimate because only rarely is medical attention required.

Pathophysiology

Antigens in the saliva of the biting insect cause the reaction in the host. Individual differences in sensitivity to the saliva result in the varied manifestations. Delayed reactions may occur; however, the rate of immediate reaction is increased in childhood (Habif, 1996a). Local reactions are most common, and anaphylactic reactions are very rare. The venom of hymenoptera species contains both antigens and pharmacologically active substances, including histamine and mast cell degranulating peptides (Burns, 2000). Both of these types of substances influence the individual's response to the venom, which may result in a hypersensitive or toxic response. Hypersensitive responses occur as a consequence of the release of endogenous cellular mediators in the affected individual. Toxic reactions are less common and result from poisonous effects of the venom itself (Maher, 1998).

Clinical Manifestations

Insect bites most commonly present as localized papules that are pruritic (Habif, 1996a). For most children there will be immediate discomfort, localized erythema, and edema. Individual reactions to insect bites depend on the degree of sensitivity to the saliva. An initial mosquito bite typically does not cause a reaction; however, with repeated bites, an immediate wheal develops and older bite sites may demonstrate flare-ups. Flea bites frequently appear as clusters of red papules located around the knees or ankles. These particular sites are common because fleas cannot jump higher than approximately 2 feet.

Stings from apids and vespids often are limited to a single lesion although multiple stings are possible if the stinger does not have barbs. The stinger may or may not be embedded in the skin. Eighty-five to 90% of individuals bitten by these insects will have local reactions only, which consist of pain, pruritus, erythema, and slight edema at the site. Typically, the symptoms resolve within 1 to 2 hours. Large local reactions also may occur. These reactions consist of more pronounced local symptoms and involve the side of the body on which the bite occurred. For example, if a child is stung on the hand, he or she may experience swelling of the entire arm. Symptoms of large local reactions often peak by 24 to 48 hours following the sting and may persist up to one week (Maher, 1998). Hypersensitivity, or systemic, reactions may range from generalized pruritus with a few hives to anaphylaxis. Most reactions in children consist of hives and are not associated with a recurrent reaction. Anaphylaxis is more common in adults although it may occur in children (Habif, 1996a). Symptoms most frequently occur within minutes of the sting and include generalized pruritus and hives, nausea, abdominal cramping, generalized edema, and shortness of breath and wheezing resulting from airway swelling. Such reactions may progress to shock and become life-threatening. Toxic reactions to apid and vespid stings are relatively rare because the individual must be stung repeatedly to receive sufficient venom to produce a response. The estimated lethal dose of venom is 19 honeybee stings per kilogram of body weight. A child would have to be stung approximately 500 times to receive this much venom (Maher, 1998). Ant stings are more likely to present as multiple lesions because the ants attack in numbers and a single ant may deliver multiple stings. Stings are initially painful and are followed by the development of a local wheal. Vesicles develop 8 to 24 hours later and progress to pustules that typically resolve within 10 days.

Diagnosis

Diagnosis is based on the individual's history of an insect bite or sting and the clinical presentation. Only about one-third of individuals who have been stung by Hymenoptera species can identify the insect correctly. A focused history regarding the child's activity at the time of the sting can aid in identifying the insect. A list of common activities and associated insects is presented in Box 30-8.

Diagnosis of allergy is based on the presentation of symptoms following a bite or sting. Individuals who have experienced a severe hypersensitivity reaction should receive further evaluation to determine the specific allergen. Cross-reactivity between venoms is uncommon; for example, the majority of people who are allergic to honeybee venom are not allergic to yellow jacket venom and vice versa.

BOX 30-8 Stinging insects and associated activities

Identifying the child's activity at the time of an insect sting can provide clues as to the insect most likely at fault.

Activity/Site	Insect
Walking barefoot in clover or grass	Bumblebee, honeybee, yellow jacket
Gardening near flowers	Bumblebee, honeybee, yellow jacket
Picnicking; picking apples; near garbage or a dumpster	Yellow jacket
Behind shutters; under electrical boxes or overhangs	Paper wasps
Under decks or roof overhangs; in trees or shrubs	Hornets

Adapted from Maher, L. (1998). Managing stinging insect allergies. *Patient Care Nurse Practitioner,* (June), 18–23.

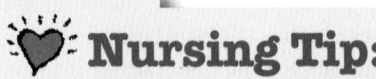

Nursing Tip:

Administration of oral corticosteroids

Oral corticosteroids require several hours to begin working. They should be given as soon after the sting as possible to promote their maximum effectiveness in limiting and reducing swelling.

Treatment

Prevention of insect bites and stings should receive priority consideration. Repellents containing diethyltoluamide (DEET) are highly effective against mosquito bites, flies, gnats, chiggers, and ticks, but do not offer protection against stinging insects (Habif, 1996a). Avoiding outside activity where biting and stinging insects are likely to be present should be emphasized to children and caregivers. Supportive care measures are sufficient to manage the majority of insect bites and stings. The stinger should be removed, if present, and cool, wet compresses should be applied to the site. Oral over-the-counter antihistamines such as diphenhydramine (Benadryl) may be used to alleviate pruritus and swelling. A mild analgesic such as acetaminophen is helpful to alleviate associated pain. Oral corticosteriods such as prednisone may be indicated for stings resulting in a large, local reaction. A paste made of 1 teaspoon of meat tenderizer mixed with 1 teaspoon of water may be applied to the site of a local reaction caused by an apid or vespid sting. In the case of fire ant stings, the paste should be made with baking soda (Habif, 1996a).

In the event of an anaphylactic reaction, emergency measures are required. Subcutaneous epinephrine often is the initial drug of choice. Antihistamines may be given as well. Limited hypersensitivity reactions may be managed with antihistamines alone. Individuals with a history of an anaphylactic reaction should have an emergency epinephrine kit (Epi-Pen, Ana-Kit) available for self-administration in the event of a sting (Maher, 1998).

Immunotherapy is indicated for those with a life-threatening anaphylactic reaction and a positive skin test to venom. Children under 16 years of age are less likely to be candidates for immunotherapy because of their lower rate of hypersensitivity reactions and decreased risk of recurrence. Immunotherapy requires a 3 to 5 year commitment for treatment and is considered 95–99% effective in eliminating future anaphylactic reactions to the specific venom (Burns, 2000; Maher, 1998; Habif, 1996a).

Nursing Management

Nursing management should emphasize prevention of insect bites and stings, initiation of supportive care measures, and education of the child and caregiver. Protecting the child from insect bites and stings is an important issue for caregivers.

If a child is stung, he or she should be closely monitored for the development of systemic symptoms. If anaphylactic symptoms develop, emergency services should be notified. If the individual has an emergency epinephrine kit available, a dose should be administered. Management of local reactions to bites and stings should consist of comfort measures such as removal of the stinger, application of cool compresses, and administration of antihistamines and analgesics.

Family Teaching

Priorities for family teaching include strategies to avoid insect bites and stings and appropriate management if they occur. Children and caregivers should be advised of common areas where biting and stinging insects are likely to be found.

Nursing Tip:

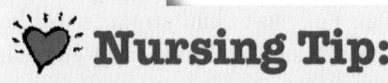

Application of insect repellents

Insect repellents should not be applied to children's hands because of the risk of injury if they rub their eyes.

Nursing Tip:

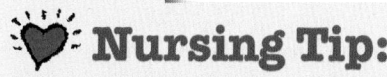

Expiration dates on epinephrine kits

Because of the infrequent use of emergency epinephrine kits, children and caregivers should be taught to check the expiration date routinely. Kits need to be replaced when the expiration date has passed.

When playing outside, children should avoid wearing clothing with bright, flowery prints because these may attract stinging insects. Fragrances such as those from perfumes, colognes, and scented soaps also should be avoided prior to outdoor play. Insect repellents provide one to several hours of protection. They should be reapplied after swimming, sweating, or exposure to rain. Products with high concentrations of DEET should be avoided in young children. The maximum recommended concentration is 10% (Hebert & Carlton, 1998). DEET is absorbed by the skin, and neurologic toxicities in children such as encephalopathy and seizures have been associated with products containing high concentrations.

Children who are allergic to insect venom should wear medical identification indicating their allergy. Caregivers and older children require instruction regarding correct administration of emergency epinephrine. Schoolteachers, babysitters, and others who are involved in the child's care should be informed of the individual's allergy and appropriate actions if a sting occurs. An extra emergency epinephrine kit should be kept at school or with other caregivers.

BOX 30-9 Spider Bites

Although most spiders in North America create relatively minor reactions, bites from the brown recluse spider and black widow spiders can have serious consequences. These spiders typically avoid humans and bite only if threatened. Counsel caregivers and children to stay away from areas where the spiders are likely to inhabit. These include warm, dry places, such as wood piles, basements (in bedding or clothing being stored). See Table 30-2 for symptoms and management. Figure 30-19 shows a brown recluse spider bite.

SUNBURN

Sun exposure is a major health concern for individuals of all ages. Although the long-term effects of sun exposure are not evident in children, the majority of skin damage in later life occurs as a consequence of sun exposure during childhood

TABLE 30-2 Symptoms and Treatment of Spider Bites

Spider	Clinical Manifestations	Treatment	Family Teaching
Brown Recluse	Mild stinging 2–3 hours after bite; mild erythematous, painful and puritic macule; fever, chills, malaise. Serious complications; edema and bullous formation; tissue necrosis.	Keep affected area below heart. Apply cool compress to affected area. Wound healing is slow. In the most severe bites, dapsone can be used. Surgical debridement may be necessary. If no bullae form, no further management is needed. Watch for secondary infection.	Avoid the areas that spiders inhabit; if bitten, seek medical attention. Keep affected area below heart. Apply cool compress to affected area.
Black Widow	Immediate pain, puncture marks and mild erythema may be present. Severe muscle cramping and spasm. Symptoms peak within 24 hours and may persist for 2–3 days; anxiety, diaphoreseis, parasthesias, and poor coordination. In young children, increased irritability and persistent crying. Severe symptoms include hypertension and shock.	Emergency treatment needed. Affected area should be kept lower than heart. Apply cool compress. Physiological stabilization is paramount due to possibility of cardiopulmonary collapse. Most common medical treatment is intravenous calcium gluconate. Antivenom can be used in severe cases not responding to calcium gluconate.	Avoid the areas that spiders inhabit; if bitten, seek medical attention. Keep affected area below heart. Apply cool compress to affected area.

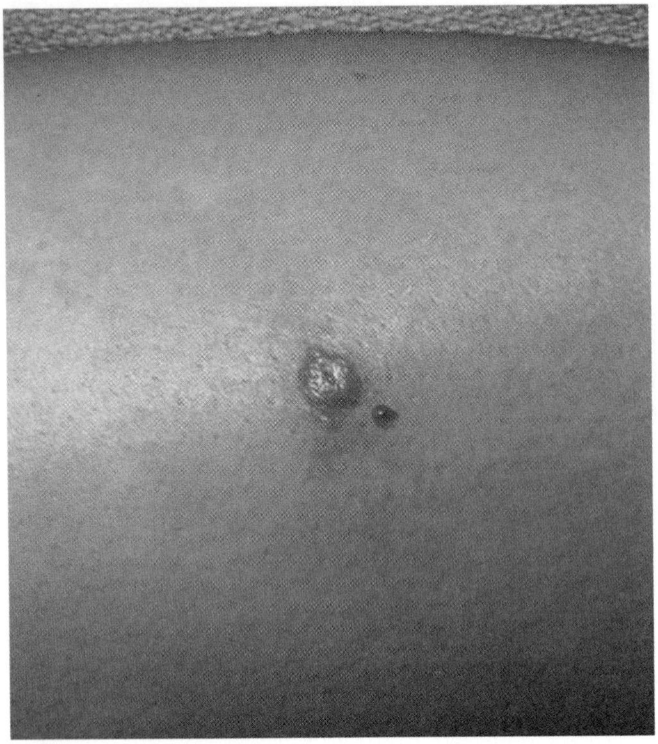

Figure 30-19 Brown Recluse Spider Bite.
Source: Habif, T. P. (1996a). *Clinical dermatology: A color guide to diagnosis and therapy* (3rd ed.). St. Louis: Mosby-Year Book, Inc. (p. 461, fig. 15-22).

and adolescence. Skin cancer represents approximately one-half of all cancers diagnosed each year in the United States. Sun exposure is deemed responsible for 90% of all skin cancers (Heffernan & O'Sullivan, 1998). Despite current awareness of the dangers of sun exposure, a significant proportion of children still do not receive adequate sun protection and sustain sunburns (Morris, McGee, & Bandaranayake, 1998; McGee, Williams, & Glasgow, 1997).

Incidence and Etiology

Sunburns are considered the most common photosensitive reaction seen in children (Darmstadt, 2000b). They are at increased risk for sunburns, in part, as a consequence of their daily activities. Current estimates suggest that individuals receive between 50% and 80% of their lifetime ultraviolet B radiation prior to age 20 years (Darmstadt, 2000b; Heffernan & O'Sullivan, 1998). Children spend more time outside than adults and receive approximately three times more annual ultraviolet B radiation (Robinson, Rigel, & Amonette, 2000). Much of the exposure occurs during the peak sun hours during the summer.

The most significant risk factor for sunburn is the child's genetics and racial background. A list of skin types and associated characteristics and sunburn risk is presented in Table 30-3. Those at greatest risk for sun-related damage include children with fair skin, fair hair, and a history of previous sunburn. Although darker skinned races tend to be less sensitive to damage from sun exposure, no individual is "immune" to the damaging effects of the sun.

Certain diseases such as atopic dermatitis and systemic lupus erythematosus increase the child's sensitivity to sunlight. A number of medications including sulfonamides, barbiturates, and retinoic acid also have been implicated in increased photosensitivity. Other risk factors associated with sunburn include the time of day, location, and geography. Ultraviolet B radiation is greatest between the hours of 9 AM and 6 PM during the summer months. Increases in altitude also increase the risk. Sun exposure is increased by 4% to 5% for every 1,000 feet of elevation (Heffernan & O'Sullivan, 1998). Up to 85% of ultraviolet rays are reflected on snow, sand, and concrete, creating an increased potential for sunburn. In addition, clouds and water do not provide protection against ultraviolet radiation. Approximately 80% of the sun's rays can penetrate clouds and approximately 50% can penetrate water (Heffernan & O'Sullivan, 1998) (Figure 30-20).

TABLE 30-3 Skin Types, Characteristics, and Sunburn Risk

Skin Type	Characteristics	Sunburn, Tanning HIstory
I	Red hair, freckles, Celtic origin.	Always burns easily, no tanning.
II	Fair skin, fair haired, blue-eyed, white.	Usually burns, minimal tanning.
III	Darker skinned white.	Sometimes burns, gradual light brown, tan.
IV	Mediterranean background.	Minimal to no burning, always tans.
V	Middle-eastern white, Mexican.	Rarely burns, tans profusely dark brown.
VI	Blacks	Never burns, pigmented black.

Adapted from: Darmstadt, G. L. (2000b). Photosensitivity. In R. E. Behrman, R. M. Kleigman, & H. B. Jenson (Eds.), Nelson textbook of pediatrics *(16th ed., pp. 1998–2001). Philadelphia: W. B. Saunders.*

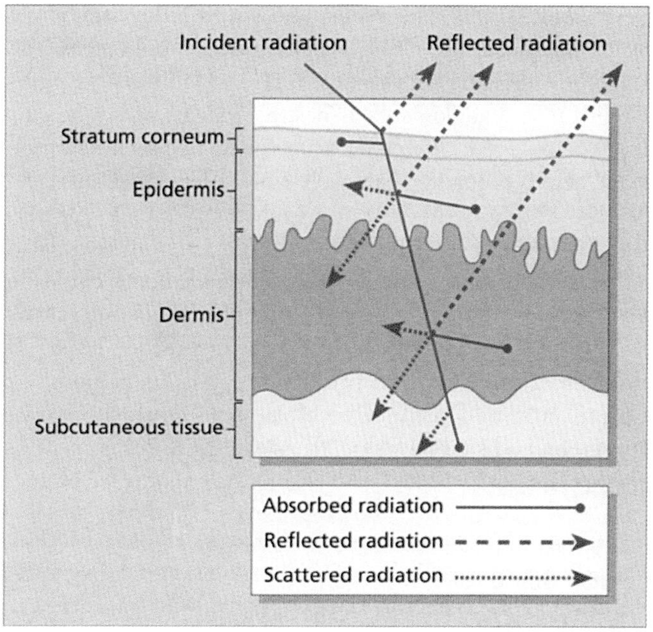

Figure 30-20 Effect of Ultraviolet Radiation on the Layers of the Skin. Source: Harper, J., Oranje, A. P., & Prose, N. (2000). *Textbook of pediatric dermatology.* Oxford: Blackwell Science, Ltd.

Nursing Alert:

Medications and Sunburn

Be certain to identify medications the child is receiving when obtaining a client history. Certain medications increase the child's sensitivity to sunlight and risk for sunburn.

Pathophysiology

Damage to the skin occurs as a consequence of exposure to ultraviolet radiation from the sun. The two types of ultraviolet rays responsible for damage to the skin are ultraviolet A (UVA) and ultraviolet B (UVB). Ultraviolet B rays make up only a short percentage of UV radiation; however, they are believed to be responsible for approximately 90% of sunburns (Heffernan & O'Sullivan, 1998). These rays are absorbed primarily in the epidermis although the dermis may be affected.

Ultraviolet A rays are able to penetrate the dermis and potentiate the effects of UVB radiation. They are responsible for "photoaging" by causing changes in collagen resulting in wrinkling, dryness, cracking, and freckling. These rays also are responsible for sunburns during winter recreational activities and the development of **photoallergies** associated with some medications. Photoallergies are delayed immune responses involving previous sensitization through exposure to a chemical substance, often a medication, and the appearance of a skin rash following exposure to UVA radiation. UVA rays are transmitted from fluorescent lights and are used in tanning booths (Heffernan & O'Sullivan, 1998; Morrison, 1997).

Clinical Manifestations

The development of the sunburn reaction occurs in two stages: immediate and delayed erythema. Immediate erythema appears within minutes following exposure and is caused by ultraviolet A radiation. Delayed erythema appears 6 to 12 hours following sun exposure and is a consequence of ultraviolet B radiation. Delayed erythema often reaches a peak in 24 hours and can persist for several days. With more severe sunburns, edema and vesicle formation occurs. This is followed by desquamation within a week of the sunburn (Darmstadt, 2000b; Habif, 1996b). Tanning refers to the delayed increased pigmentation of the skin following sun exposure. It is helps provide protection against further sun injury; however, it must be noted that it is a reparative response and indicates that the skin has been damaged (Morrison, 1997).

Diagnosis

Diagnosis of sunburn is based on the clinical presentation. The majority of sunburn cases do not require medical evaluation. Sunburn severity is classified according to color (pink to bright red) and the presence or absence of vesicles and bullae. Because sunburns do not scar, classifying sunburns according to guidelines developed for thermal burns is not useful (Morrison, 1997).

Treatment

Sunburns are most often managed with supportive measures. Cool compresses and topical corticosteroids aid in diminishing the inflammation and pain. Oral analgesics are beneficial in relieving associated pain. Ibuprofen, which is a prostaglandin inhibitor, offers the additional benefit of potentially decreasing associated erythema (Darmstadt, 2000b). Topical anesthetic preparations pose the risk of contact dermatitis and are not always effective. Fragrance-free emollients are beneficial during the desquamation phase of the sunburn.

Nursing Management

Assessment

Nurses should discuss with the child and caregivers the duration of sun exposure and the use of sun protective measures; ask about medications the child is receiving that may increase his or her susceptibility to sunburn; note the extent of the sunburn, including the development of vesicles; and assess for the presence of associated complications such as pain, edema, nausea, fever, and headache.

Nursing Diagnosis

Nursing diagnoses appropriate for the child with sunburn include:

1. Impaired skin integrity related to epidermal injury secondary to the sunburn.
2. Acute pain related to inflammation secondary to injury from the sunburn.
3. Risk for injury (sunburn) related to inappropriate use of sun protection.
4. Deficient knowledge related to inadequate understanding of factors, that increase the risk for sunburn and actions to decrease such risk.

Outcome Identification

1. Child will experience healing of injured skin.
2. Child will experience relief of pain.
3. Child and caregivers will utilize appropriate sun protection measures to avoid sunburn in the future.
4. Child and caregivers will discuss factors that increase the risk of sun-related damage to the skin and actions that will decrease the risk.

Planning/Implementation

The nursing management of children with sunburn focuses on promotion of healing of the injured skin, promotion of the child's comfort, and education for the child and caregivers regarding sun protection. Education also should include information regarding the long-term consequences of sun exposure in young children. Caregivers should understand principles of supportive care such as use of cool compresses, baths, and use of analgesics. Education regarding sun protection should take into consideration the child's developmental stage. Caregivers also should be encouraged to utilize appropriate personal sun protection. Children whose caregivers use sun protective measures such as wearing sunscreen or hats are more likely to be using those measures themselves (McGee, et al., 1997).

Evaluation

The injured skin should heal with use of supportive measures. Children and caregivers are able to utilize strategies to promote comfort and healing following the sunburn, to prevent further sunburn, and to articulate long-term consequences of sun exposure.

Family Teaching

Teaching for children and caregivers should emphasize both supportive measures to care for the sunburn and measures to prevent repeat sunburns. Because most children will not require a visit to their primary health care provider for a sunburn, teaching should be emphasized during well visits and should address general principles of sun protection, use of sun blocks and sunscreens, and specific developmental issues unique to the child. Teaching also should stress the long-term dangers of sun exposure and sunburn as many caregivers and adolescents associate a suntan with a healthy appearance. Even though a sunburn may not occur, damage to the skin is occurring with each "dose" of sun exposure.

Prevention is the best approach for avoiding sunburns and subsequent long-term sun injury. Current estimates indicate that approximately 80% of skin cancers could be avoided by regular use of sun protective measures (Robinson, et al., 2000; Heffernan & O'Sullivan, 1998). If children are outside, sun protection (sunscreen, sunblock agent, hats, and protective clothing) should be worn. Sunscreen and sunblock should have an SPF rating of 15 or greater (Boxes 30-10 and 30-11). Products that offer protec-

BOX 30-10 SPF ratings

The sun protection factor (SPF) is a measure of the estimated protection against sunburn offered by a sunscreen or sunblock. In theory, it can be considered a ratio of the time a sunburn would develop with or without protection. For example, if a child could remain in the sun for one hour without burning, he or she would be protected for 15 hours using a product with an SPF of 15. In practice, the SPF is diminished by factors such as sweating, swimming, and friction from clothes.

BOX 30-11 Sunscreens and sunblocks

Sunblocks and sunscreens are products that offer protection against the sun's radiation. Both are effective; however, each acts in a different manner. *Sunblocks* offer the greatest protection against the sun's rays. These products reflect and scatter ultraviolet rays and are opaque. They may be used as primary sun protection or only on frequently exposed areas such as the nose and face. Products marketed as sunblocks should have an SPF rating of 12 or greater. Common agents include zinc oxide, titanium dioxide, and red petrolatum. *Sunscreens* are products that absorb the sun's rays. Different types of sunscreens may offer protection against ultraviolet A and ultraviolet B radiation individually or against both. Products containing para-aminobenzoic acid (PABA) offer protection against ultraviolet B rays, and those containing benzophenones provide protection against both ultraviolet A and ultraviolet B radiation.

Adapted from Heffernan, A. E., & O'Sullivan, A. (1998). Pediatric sun exposure. *The Nurse Practitioner, 23* (7), 67–68, 71–72, 74–76, 78, 83–84, 86.

Research Highlight

Parents' Use of Sun Protection for Their Children

Study Purpose

Descriptive study to explore adults' use of summertime sun protection for their children. The study surveyed parents to identify the duration and time of their children's sun exposure, use of sun protection, and observed sunburning of their children.

Methods

Subjects were 503 parents of children less than 12 years of age. Potential subjects were identified via a random telephone calling procedure. Participants were asked to identify their child's age, gender, and skin type. Parents also were asked to determine the number of hours the child spent outside during the previous weekend, the types of sun protection used, and whether the child sustained a sunburn. They completed a survey regarding their beliefs and attitudes toward sun protection using a 4-point scale.

Findings

Use of all types of sun protection was positively associated with fair-skinned and Caucasian children and decreased with increasing age of the child. A sunscreen with an SPF of 15 or greater was the most frequently reported sun-protective behavior with 53% of participants reporting having used sunscreen on their child during the past week. Sunscreen use was significantly associated with sunny weather, a family history of skin cancer, previous sunburn in the child, fair skin, and higher family income. Twenty-six percent of respondents reported complimenting their child on the appearance of a tan. Factors associated with a perceived healthy appearance of a suntan included male gender of the reporting adult, older and darker skin-toned children, and lower educational levels. Thirteen percent of children in the sample were reported as having sustained a sunburn during the previous week.

Implications

Although the majority of adults in this study had used sunscreen on their children during the past week, the incidence of sunburns implies that the level of sun protection was inadequate. The findings of this study demonstrate the need for ongoing education regarding appropriate sun protection. Specific areas include proper use of sunscreen including application to all exposed body surfaces and reapplication during the day. Sunscreen should not be used as a means for prolonging sun exposure. Multiple methods of sun protection, including wearing wide brimmed hats, wearing long sleeves, and avoiding outdoor activity between 10 AM and 4 PM should be used to minimize the risk of sunburn.

Citation

Robinson, J. K., Rigel, D. S., & Amonette, R. A. (2000). Summertime sun protection used by adults for their children. *Journal of the American Academy of Dermatolotgy, 43* (5, Pt. I), 746–753.

tion against both ultraviolet A and ultraviolet B radiation need to be used and applied approximately 15 to 30 minutes prior to outside activity. They should be reapplied every 2 to 3 hours throughout the day, especially after swimming and sweating. Hats should have a wide brim (approximately 3 inches) to cover the face, neck, and ears appropriately. Long sleeves and long pants should be comfortable, lightweight, and tightly woven. Whenever possible, children should avoid outside activity between 10 AM and 2 PM.

Teaching also should address issues and considerations unique to the child's developmental level. An overview of teaching considerations for children of different ages is provided in Table 30-4. Infants and young children are dependent on their caregivers to provide them with adequate sun

TABLE 30-4 Developmental Considerations for Sun Protection

Developmental Stage	Teaching Considerations
Infant	Avoid sun exposure as much as possible. Infants less than 6 months of age may have small amounts of sunscreen applied to areas frequently exposed to the sun, (e.g., nose, neck, ears). Infants greater than 6 months of age should use a sunscreen with an SPF of 15 or greater. Use canopies or hoods on strollers and carriages. Wear wide-brimmed hats when exposed to the sun. Use window shades in vehicles.
Toddler/Preschool	Apply sunscreen with an SPF of 15 or greater liberally prior to outdoor activity. Limit outdoor activity during peak sun hours. Wear wide-brimmed hats when exposed to the sun. Wear protective clothing when outside. Supervise outdoor activity.
School-aged	Apply sunscreen of 15 or greater liberally prior to outdoor activity. Limit outdoor activity during peak sun hours. Wear hats and protective clothing. Avoid sheer clothing or bathing suits that allow penetration of the sun's rays. Teach appropriate sun protection measures and risks of sun exposure.
Adolescent	Apply sunscreen liberally prior to outdoor activity. Limit outdoor activity during peak sun hours. Wear hats and protective clothing. Avoid sunbathing or using tanning parlors. Avoid sheer clothing or bathing suits that allow penetration of the sun's rays. Teach appropriate sun protection measures and risks of sun exposure.

Nursing Tip:

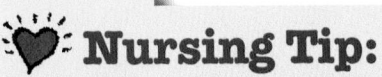

Selecting an appropriate SPF rating
Sun protection products on the market have SPF ratings varying from 2 to greater than 30. Products used for children should have an SPF rating of at least 15. Those with an SPF greater than 30 do not provide any greater benefit and may expose the child to greater concentrations of chemicals.

protection, and teaching should be aimed at the caregiver. Older children and adolescents are assuming greater self-care responsibilities, and education should be directed toward them as well as their caregivers. Promotion of sun protection among this age group is particularly challenging because although education efforts may increase knowledge and awareness, actual behaviors may not reflect appropriate sun protection (Hill & Dixon, 1999). Sunbathing, in particular, is popular among adolescents, and motivation for sun protective behaviors is largely influenced by peers.

Several educational programs have been initiated to teach children the dangers associated with sun exposure and safe sun protective behaviors. Younger school-aged children may be the most effective target group for such programs as they are beginning to assume greater personal responsibility for their actions. Evaluations of these programs have demonstrated an increase in both awareness of sun safety and actual sun protective behaviors (Glanz, Lew, Song, & Cook, 1999; Grant-Peterson, Dietrich, Sox, Winchell, & Stevens, 1999). Education efforts also should target those who work with children such as child care providers, schoolteachers, and scout leaders.

ADDITIONAL INTEGUMENTARY DISORDERS

The following disorders are uncommon in children; therefore, they are discussed only briefly.

Folliculitis

Folliculitis, an inflammation of the hair follicle, is caused by infection, irritation, or injury. It may occur in association with other inflammatory skin disorders. Coagulase-positive *Staphylococcus aureus* is the common causative agent (Rhody, 2000). Typical features include small, dome-shaped pustules occurring at the opening of the follicle. Deep folliculitis may involve the entire hair follicle. Lesions present as swollen, red pustules that may come to a point at the surface. Common sites for folliculitis include the scalp, the most common site in children, back, and extremities. Lesions can appear singly or in groups and may or may not be painful. Associated systemic symptoms are rare. Superficial folliculitis may resolve without treatment. Good hygiene and cleaning with antibacterial soap may be sufficient although topical 2% erythromycin solution may hasten clearing of lesions. Deep folliculitis usually requires treatment with oral antibiotics (Rhody, 2000). In both cases, treatment should include management of underlying skin disorders and teaching the child and family to avoid precipitating factors.

Furuncles and Carbuncles

Furuncles, known more commonly as abscesses or boils, are painful, firm, walled-off masses of granulation tissue and pus. Carbuncles are an aggregation of furuncles. Furuncles and carbuncles are most common after puberty, and the infective organism most often is *Staphylococcus aureus* (Rhody, 2000). Furuncles may occur at any site; however, they are most common in areas exposed to friction such as under a belt. A single lesion is most often present and is erythematous and painful. It may remain unchanged for several days before coming to a point and rupturing. Associated systemic symptoms are uncommon (Figure 30-21). Carbuncles most commonly occur where the dermis is thick, such as over the back and lateral thighs. They present as deep, erythematous, painful masses and form multiple points. Sloughing of the skin may result with severe infections. Symptoms such as malaise, fever, and chills are more common with carbuncles.

Treatment of furuncles and carbuncles involves the application of warm compresses to facilitate pointing of the lesions. When the covered skin has adequately thinned, the lesion may be incised to allow for drainage. If necessary, the wound may be packed to promote further healing and drainage. Culture of the lesions is not indicated (Rhody, 2000).

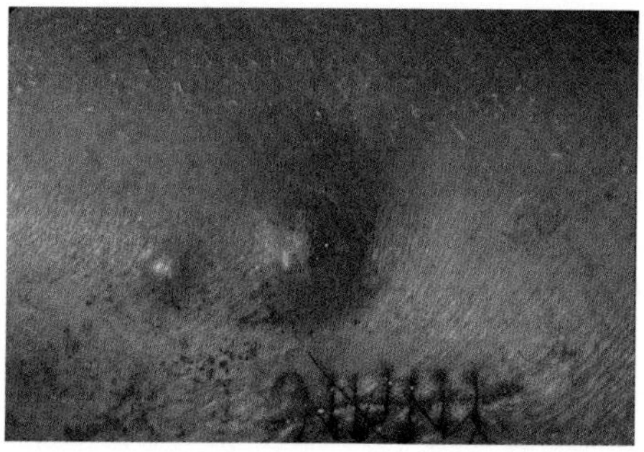

Figure 30-21 Furuncle. Courtesy of Robert A. Silverman, M.D., Clinical Associate Professor, Department of Pediatrics, Georgetown University.

Frostbite

Frostbite refers to the acute freezing of body tissues when exposed to temperatures below the freezing point of intact skin (Murphy, Banwell, Roberts, & McGrouther, 2000). The overall incidence of frostbite has increased over the past 20 years, most likely in conjunction with an increased participation in winter outdoor sports and activities. Children are less efficient at maintaining body heat because of their proportionately greater body surface area to body mass and, therefore, are at increased risk for the development of frostbite. Other risk factors include prolonged exposure to the cold, subfreezing temperatures, high humidity, and low wind chill factors (Kanzenbach & Dexter, 1999).

Injury from frostbite occurs as a result of direct cellular damage at the time of cold exposure and progressive dermal ischemia resulting in deterioration and necrosis of tissue. The extremities are most frequently affected, accounting for 90% of frostbite injuries. Other common sites include the ears, nose, and cheeks (Murphy, et al., 2000). The initial symptoms include numbness at the affected area. The skin may have a waxy or mottled appearance. Erythema, along with the formation of vesicles or bullae, develops within 6 to 24 hours. Severe, throbbing pain begins 48 to 72 hours following the injury and often requires narcotic analgesia. If the injury is severe, eschar develops within two weeks. Favorable outcomes are associated with sensation to a pinprick, healthy-appearing skin color, and no vesicles present (Kanzenbach & Dexter, 1999).

Prevention is the best measure to avoid frostbite. Children should be dressed in warm, layered clothing including hats, warm socks, mittens, and fitted neckwear. Prolonged exposure to the cold should be avoided. If the child's clothing becomes wet, it should be changed because wet clothing increases the child's vulnerability to cold injury. Drinking warm, nourishing liquids during outdoor activity may help to maintain body temperature. If frostbite is suspected, the child should be taken to an emergency department as quickly as possible. Any wet clothing should be removed, and the affected area should be splinted, elevated,

Nursing Alert:

Frostbite Outcomes in Children

Children with frostbite injury are at risk for destruction of the growth plates of the distal fingers and toes (Murphy, et al., 2000).

and covered with a dry dressing. The area should not be massaged as this may cause further tissue injury. Current initial medical treatment consists of rapid rewarming by immersing the affected area in water at a temperature of 40 degrees Celsius (Murphy, et al., 2000; Kanzenbach & Dexter, 1999). Appropriate tetanus and antibiotic prophylaxis should be implemented. Surgical resection may be indicated for severe cases but is usually delayed until the extent of injury has been determined.

In the Real World

"During nursing school, I was assigned to an inner city elementary school for my community clinical rotation. One of my often-performed responsibilities was to examine classrooms of children for head lice. On one particular morning, I was requested to examine the children in one of the fourth grade classes. I did identify numerous nits but no live lice in the hair of one of the girls. I then learned that the class was scheduled to leave for a field trip later that morning. I felt sorry that this little girl would have to miss an event she had been looking forward to for some time. I discussed the situation with the school's principal. She agreed that the child could attend the field trip and then be dismissed from school when she returned. When I contacted the girl's parents, they indicated that she had been treated with "lice shampoo," but that they had not removed all the nits from her hair. I explained the necessity of removing all the nits before she would be able to return to school and reviewed the procedure for treating the household. This situation helped me to feel good about my nursing care as a student because I was able to support this little girl's self-esteem and help her parents provide the treatment she needed for her condition."

Key Concepts

- The integumentary system provides for the protective, metabolic, and interactive functions of the child.
- A careful assessment of the integument can provide the health care provider with cues related to other disorders.
- Interventions to meet the needs of the child with an integumentary disorder are directed toward preventing infections, restoring altered skin integrity, and maintaining a positive self-image.
- Integumentary problems that alter children's appearances can affect their body image and self-esteem significantly.
- Impetigo is a highly infectious bacterial infection localized in the epidermis.
- Immunization for *Haemophilus influenzae* type B has reduced the incidence of this bacterium as a significant causative agent of cellulitis in young children.
- Thrush is characterized by creamy white patches on the buccal mucosa and tongue that cannot be scraped away.
- Fomite transfer within the household is a common source of tinea capitis infection.
- Primary infection with herpes simplex type I is greatest among young children, and recurrent infections may be triggered by sunlight, wind, local injury, or emotional stress.
- Treatment of the child with pediculosis consists of application of pediculocide followed by manual removal of nits and lice.
- Atopic dermatitis is a chronic skin condition believed to result from abnormal immune system function. Nursing care is directed toward teaching supportive measures to promote hydration of the skin and prevent further injury.
- Diaper dermatitis is most prevalent in infants 9 to 12 months of age. Increased attention to diaper hygiene and application of barrier creams and ointment often are adequate for effective treatment.
- Contact dermatitis may occur as a local reaction to prolonged contact with an irritant or as an allergic reaction following sensitization to a specific antigen. The most important treatment principle is avoidance of the known irritant.
- Nursing care for the adolescent with acne is directed toward reducing the severity of the condition, education regarding the prescribed treatment plan, and psychosocial support.
- Education of children and the community is a priority nursing consideration to reduce injury to children from dog bites.
- The majority of an individual's sun exposure occurs during childhood. Promotion of safe sun protective behaviors among children is an important nursing intervention to prevent skin cancer in adulthood.

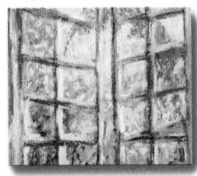

Review Questions

1. What are the three most important functions of the skin?
2. How do differences in the skin of children of different ages and races influence nursing care?
3. Discuss priority teaching principles for the caregivers of a child with impetigo.
4. Discuss treatment strategies for the infant with thrush and the breastfeeding mother.
5. Differentiate between clinical cure and mycologic cure in the management of tinea infections.
6. Explain the different treatment alternatives for verrucae. What factors are most important to consider related to treatment decisions?
7. Describe factors that may result in reactivation of herpes simplex type I infections.
8. How would you explain the management of pediculosis to the caregiver and child?
9. Compare primary irritant diaper dermatitis and diaper dermatitis caused by *Candida albicans*.
10. Describe appropriate teaching for the adolescent receiving systemic treatment for acne vulgaris.
11. How would you teach a child and caregivers to avoid injury from dog bites?
12. Discuss age-specific interventions for prevention of injury to the skin related to sun exposure.

References

Adams, W. G. (2000). Rabies. In R. E. Behrman, R. M. Kleigman, & H. B. Jenson (Eds.), *Nelson textbook of pediatrics* (16th ed., pp. 1014–1017). Philadelphia: W. B. Saunders.

Aktan, S., Ozmen, E., & Sanli, B. (2000). Anxiety, depression, and nature of acne vulgaris in adolescents. *International Journal of Dermatology, 39,* 354–357.

American Academy of Pediatrics. (2000a). Tinea capitis. In L. K. Pickering (Ed.), *2000 Red-book: Report on the committee on infectious diseases* (25th ed. pp. 569–570). Elk Grove, IL: American Academy of Pediatrics.

American Academy of Pediatrics. (2000b). Rabies. In L. K. Pickering (Ed.) *2000 Red-book: Report on the committee on infectious diseases* (25th ed. pp. 475–482). Elk Grove, IL: American Academy of Pediatrics.

Angel, T. A., Nigro, J., & Levy, M. L. (2000). Infestations in the pediatric patient. *Pediatric Clinics of North America, 47,* 921–935.

Bass, J. W., Chan, D. S., Creamer, K. M., Thompson, M. W., Malone, F. J., Becker, T. M., & Marks, S. N. (1997). Comparison of oral cephalexin, topical mupirocin and topical bacitracin for treatment of impetigo. *The Pediatric Infectious Disease Journal, 16,* 708–709.

Bedinghaus, J. M. (1997). Care of the breast and support of breastfeeding. *Primary Care, 24,* 147–160.

Benton, E. C. (2000). Human papillomavirus infection and molluscum contagiosum. In J. Harper, A. Oranje, & N. Prose (Eds.), *Textbook of pediatric dermatology* (pp. 307–320). London: Blackwell Science, Ltd.

Bernardo, L. M., Gardner, M. J., O'Connor, J., & Amon, N. (2000). Dog bites in children treated in a pediatric emergency department. *Journal of the Society of Pediatric Nurses, 5*(2), 87–95.

Bingham, E. A. (2000). Guidelines to management of atopic dermatitis. In J. Harper, A. Oranje, & N. Prose (Eds.), *Textbook of pediatric dermatology* (pp. 215–230). London: Blackwell Science, Ltd.

Boerio, M., Brooker, J., Freese, L., Phares, P., & Yazvec, S. (2000). Pediatric dermatology: That itchy scaly rash. *Nursing Clinics of North America, 35,* 147–157.

Bonifazi, E. (2000). Diaper dermatitis: Causative factors. In J. Harper, A. Oranje, & N. Prose (Eds.), *Textbook of pediatric dermatology* (pp. 140–142). London: Blackwell Science, Ltd.

Bos, J. D. (2000). Immunology of atopic dermatitis. In J. Harper, A. Oranje, & N. Prose (Eds.), *Textbook of pediatric dermatology* (pp. 178–185). London: Blackwell Science, Ltd.

Bruckner, A. L., & Weston, W. L. (2001). Beyond poison ivy: Understanding allergic contact dermatitis in children. *Pediatric Annals, 30,* 203–206.

Burns, D. A. (2000). Other noxious and venomous creatures. In J. Harper, A. Oranje, & N. Prose (Eds.), *Textbook of pediatric dermatology* (pp. 570–583). London: Blackwell Science, Ltd.

Caceres-Rios, H., Rueda, M., Ballona, R., & Bustamante, B. (2000). Comparison of terbinafine and griseofulvin in the treatment of tinea capitis. *Journal of the American Academy of Dermatology, 42,* 80–84.

Cacy, J., & Mold, J. W. (1999). The clinical characteristics of brown recluse spider bites treated by family physicians: An OKPRN study. *The Journal of Family Practice, 48,* 536–542.

Centers for Disease Control and Prevention. (2001). Parasites and health: Head lice. [On-line]. Available: www.dpd.cdc.gov/DPDx.html

Chapman, S., Cornwall, J., Righetti, J., & Sung, L. (2000). Preventing dog bites in children: Randomised controlled trial of an educational intervention. *British Medical Journal, 320,* 1512–1513.

Chew, A. L., Bashir, S. J., & Maibach, H. I. (2000). Treatment of head lice. *The Lancet, 356,* 523–524.

Chosidow, O. (2000). Scabies and pediculosis. *The Lancet, 355,* 819–825.

Clayton, Y. M. (2000). Candidosis (candidiasis). In J. Harper, A. Oranje, & N. Prose (Eds.), *Textbook of pediatric dermatology* (pp. 447–472). London: Blackwell Science, Ltd.

Darmstadt, G. (1997). A guide to superficial strep and staph skin infections. *Contemporary Pediatrics, 14,* 95–116.

Darmstadt, G. L. (2000a). Cutaneous bacterial infections. In R. E. Behrman, R. M. Kleigman, & H. B. Jenson (Eds.), *Nelson text-*

book of pediatrics (16th ed., pp. 2028–2036). Philadelphia: W. B. Saunders.

Darmstadt, G. L. (2000b). Photosensitivity. In R. E. Behrman, R. M. Kleigman, & H. B. Jenson (Eds.), *Nelson textbook of pediatrics* (16th ed., pp. 1998–2001). Philadelphia: W. B. Saunders.

Eichenfield, L. F., & Colon-Fontanez, F. (1998). Treatment of head lice. *Pediatric Infectious Disease Journal, 17,* 419–420.

Fitzpatrick, C. A., & Schumann, L. (1999). Herpes simplex infection. *Journal of the American Academy of Nurse Practitioners, 11,* 539–548.

Gandhi, R. R., Liebman, M. A., Stafford, B. L., & Stafford, P. W. (1999). Dog bite injuries in children: A preliminary study. *American Surgeon, 65,* 863–864.

Garcia, V. F. (1997). Animal bites and *Pasturella* infections. *Pediatrics in Review, 18,* 127–130.

Ginsburg, C. M. (2000). Animal and human bites. In R. E. Behrman, R. M. Kleigman, H. B. Jenson (Eds.), *Nelson textbook of pediatrics* (16th ed., pp. 790–793). Philadelphia: W. B. Saunders.

Givner, L. B., Mason Jr., E. O., Barson, W. J., Tan, T. Q., Wald, E. R., Schutze, G. E., Kim, K. S., Bradley, J. S., Yogev, R., & Kaplan, S. L. (2000). Pneumococcal facial cellulitis in children. *Pediatarics, 106*(5), e61.

Glanz, K., Lew, R. A., Song, V., & Cook, V. A. (1999). Factors associated with skin cancer prevention practices in a multiethnic population. *Health Education and Behavior, 26,* 344–359.

Goodyear, H. (2000). Herpes simplex virus infections. In J. Harper, A. Oranje, & N. Prose (Eds.), *Textbook of pediatric dermatology* (pp. 321–328). London: Blackwell Science, Ltd.

Grant-Peterson, J., Dietrich, A. J., Sox, C. H., Winchell, C. W., & Stevens, M. M. (1999). Promoting sun protection in elementary schools and child care settings: The SunSafe Project. *Journal of School Health, 69*(3), 100–106.

Habif, T. P. (1996a). Infestations and bites. In T. P. Habif, (Ed.), *Clinical dermatology: A color guide to diagnosis and therapy* (pp. 445–498). St. Louis: Mosby Year Book.

Habif, T. P. (1996b). Light-related diseases and disorders of pigmentation. In T. P. Habif, (Ed.), *Clinical dermatology: A color guide to diagnosis and therapy* (pp. 597–626). St. Louis: Mosby Year Book.

Hanifin, J. M., & Rajka, G. (1980). Diagnostic features of atopic dermatitis. *Acta Dermatovenerology, 92* (Suppl.), 44–47.

Hebert, A. A., & Carlton, S. (1998). Getting bugs to bug off: A review of insect repellents. *Contemporary Pediatrics, 15*(6), 85–95.

Heffernan, A. E., & O'Sullivan, A. (1998). Pediatric sun exposure. *The Nurse Practitioner, 23*(7), 67–68, 71–72, 74–76, 78, 83–84, 86.

Hill, D., & Dixon, H. (1999). Promoting sun protection in children: Rationale and challenges. *Health Education and Behavior, 26,* 409–417.

Hipolito, R. B., Mallorca, F. G., Zuniga-Macaraig, Z. O., Apolinario, P. C., & Wheeler-Sherman, J. (2001). Head lice infestation: Single drug versus combination therapy with one percent permethrin and trimethoprim/sulfamethoxazole. *Pediatrics, 107*(3), e30.

Honig, P. J. (1999). Tinea capitis: Recommendations for school attendance. *Pediatric Infectious Disease Journal, 18,* 211–214.

Hoppe, J. E. (1997) Treatment of oropharyngeal candidiasis and candidal diaper dermatitis in neonates and infants: Review and reappraisal. *Pediatric Infections Disease Journal, 16,* 885–894.

Howard, R. M., & Frieden, I. J. (1999). Dermatophyte infections in children. *Advances in Pediatric Infectious Diseases, 14,* 73–107.

Huang, P. H. & Paller, A. S. (2000). Itraconazole pulse therapy for dermatophyte onychomycosis in children. *Archives of Pediatric and Adolescent Medicine, 154,* 614–618.

Huether, S. E. (1998). Structure, function, and disorders of the integument. In K. L. McCance & S. E. Huether (Eds.), *Pathophysiology: The biologic basis for disease in adults and children* (3rd ed., pp. 1517–1554). St. Louis: Mosby.

Jacobsen, E., McGraw, R., & McCagh, S. (1997). Pulsed dye laser efficacy as initial therapy for warts and against recalcitrant verrucae. *Cutis, 59,* 206–208.

Jaffe, R. (2000). Atopic dermatitis. *Dermatology, 27,* 503–513.

Kanzenbach T. L., & Dexter, W. W. (1999). Cold injuries: Protecting your patients from the dangers of hypothermia and frostbite. *Postgraduate Medicine, 105,* 72–78.

Kazaks, E. L., & Lane, A. T. (2000). Diaper dermatitis. *Pediatric Clinics of North America, 47,* 909–919.

Klassen, A. F., Newton, J. N., & Mallon, E. (2000). Measuring quality of life in people referred for specialist care of acne: Comparing generic and disease specific measures. *Journal of the American Academy of Dermatology, 43* (2 Pt. 1), 229–233.

Kristal, L., & Klein, P. A. (2000). Atopic dermatitis in infants and children: An update. *Pediatric Clinics of North America, 47,* 877–895.

Krowchuk, D. P. (2000). Managing acne in adolescence. *Pediatric Clinics of North America, 47,* 841–857.

Langtry, J. A. A. (2000). Seborrhoeic dermatitis of adolescence. In J. Harper, A. Oranje, & N. Prose (Eds.), *Textbook of pediatric dermatology* (pp. 273–277). London: Blackwell Science, Ltd.

Litovitz, T. L., Klein-Schwartz, W., White, S., Cobaugh, D. J., Youniss, J., Drab, A., & Benson, B. E. (2000). 1999 Annual report of the American Association of Poison Control Centers Toxic Exposure Surveillance System. *American Journal of Emergency Medicine, 18,* 517–574.

Long, C. C. & Finlay, A. Y. (1991). The finger tip unit—A new practical measure. *Clinical Experimental Dermatology, 16,* 444–447.

Maher, L. (1998). Managing stinging insect allergies. *Patient Care Nurse Practitioner,* (June), 18–23.

Mazurek, C. M. & Lee, N. P. (2000). How to manage head lice. *Western Journal of Medicine, 172,* 34 –345.

McGee, R., Williams, S., & Glasgow, H. (1997). Sunburn and sun protection among young children. *Journal of Paediatric and Children's Health, 33,* 234–237.

Morbidity and Mortality Weekly Reports. (1997). Dog-bite-related fatalities—United States, 1995–1996. *Author, 46,* 463–467.

Morrison, W. L. (1997). Sunlight: An environmental toxin for humans. *Maryland Medical Journal, 46,* 227–230.

Morris, J., McGee, R., & Bandaranayake, M. (1998). Sun protection behaviors and the predictors of sunburn in young children. *Journal of Paediatric and Children's Health, 34,* 557–562.

Murphy, J. V., Banwell, P. E., Roberts, A. H. N., & McGrouther, D. A. (2000). Frostbite: Pathogenesis and treatment. *The Journal of Trauma: Injury, Infection, and Critical Care, 48,* 171–178.

National Pediculosis Association. (2001a). *Child care provider's guide to controlling head lice.* Newton, MA: Author. Retrieved February 15, 2001 from the World Wide Web: http://www.headlice.org/publications/ccguide.html

National Pediculosis Association. (2001b). *The no nit standard: A healthy standard for children and their families.* Newton, MA: Author. Retrieved February 15, 2001 from the World Wide Web: http://www.headlice.org/publications/nonitstandard.html

Nesbitt Jr., L. T. (2000). Treatment of tinea capitis. *International Journal of Dermatology, 39,* 261–262.

Nicol, N. H. (2000). Managing atopic dermatitis in children and adults. *The Nurse Practitioner, 25,* 58–79.

Nicol, N. H., & Boguniewicz, M. (1999). Understanding and treating atopic dermatitis. *Nurse Practitioner Forum, 10,* 48–55.

Nicol, N. H., & Huether, S. E. (1998). Alterations of the integument in children. In K. L. McCance & S. E. Huether (Eds.), *Pathophysiology: The biologic basis for disease in adults and children* (3rd ed., pp. 1555–1569). St. Louis: Mosby.

Novembre, E., Cianferoni, A., Bernardini, R., Veltroni, M., Ingargiola, A., Lombardi, E., & Vierucci, A. (1998). Epidemiology of insect venom sensitivity in children and its correlation to clinical and atopic features. *Clinical and Experimental Allergy, 28,* 834–838.

Oranje, A. P. (2000). Diaper dermatitis: Management. In J. Harper, A. Oranje, & N. Prose (Eds.), *Textbook of pediatric dermatology* (pp. 153–157). London: Blackwell Science, Ltd.

Patrick, G. R., & O'Rourke, K. M. (1998). Dog and cat bites: Epidemiologic analyses suggest different prevention strategies. *Public Health Reports, 113,* 252–257.

Plasencia, J. M. (2000). Cutaneous warts: Diagnosis and treatment. *Dermatology, 27,* 432–434.

Resnick, S. D. (2000). Staphylococcal and streptococcal skin infections: Pyodermas and toxin-mediated syndromes. In J. Harper, A. Oranje, & N. Prose (Eds.), *Textbook of pediatric dermatology* (pp. 369–383). London: Blackwell Science, Ltd.

Rex, J. H., Walsh, T. J., Sobel, J. D., Filler, S. G., Pappas, P. G., Dismukes, W. E., & Edwards, J. E. (2000). Practice guidelines for the treatment of candidiasis. *Clinical Infections Diseases, 30,* 662–678.

Rhody, C. (2000). Bacterial infections of the skin. *Primary Care, 27,* 459–473.

Riley, L. E. (1999). Herpes simplex virus. *Seminars in Perinatology, 22,* 284–292.

Robinson, J. K., Rigel, D. S., & Amonette, R. A. (2000). Summertime sun protection used by adults for their children. *Journal of the American Academy of Dermatology, 42,* 746–753.

Rudy, S. J. (1999). Superficial fungal infections in children and adolescents. *Nurse Practitioner Forum, 10,* 55–66.

Rupke, S. J. (2000). Fungal skin disorders. *Primary Care, 27,* 407–421.

Sacks, J. J., Lockwood, R., Homreich, J., & Sattin, R. W. (1996). Fatal dog attacks, 1989–1994. *Pediatrics, 97,* 891–895.

Sacks, J. J., Kresnow, M., & Houston, B. (1996). Dog bites: How big a problem? *Injury Prevention, 2,* 52–54.

Sacks, J. J., Sinclair, L., Gilchrist, J., Golab, G. C., & Lockwood, R. (2000). Breeds of dogs involved in fatal human attacks in the United States between 1979 and 1998. *Journal of the American Veterinary Medical Association, 217,* 836–840.

Sadow, K. B., & Chamberlain, J.M. (1998). Blood cultures in the evaluation of children with cellulitis. *Pediatrics, 101,* 461–462.

Shaw, S. (1996). Managing contact dermatitis. *Practitioner, 240,* 16–24.

Silverberg, N. B., Lim, J. K., Paller, A. S., & Mancini, A. J. (2000). Squaric acid immunotherapy for warts in children. *Journal of the American Academy of Dermatology, 42,* 803–808.

Singleton, J. K. (1997). Pediatric dermatoses: Three common skin disruptions in infancy. *The Nurse Practitioner, 22,* 32–37, 43–44, 49–50.

Tanner, T. L. (2000). Rhus (Toxicodendron) dermatitis. *Primary Care, 27,* 493–502.

Tanphaichitr, A., & Brodell, R. T. (1999). How to spot scabies in infants. *Postgraduate Medicine, 105,* 191–192.

Usatine, R. P., & Quan, M. A. (2000). Pearls in the management of acne: An advanced approach. *Primary Care, 27,* 289–308.

Verbov, J. (1999). How to manage warts. *Archives of Disease in Children, 80,* 97–99.

Wahrman, J. E., & Honig, P. J. (2000). Diaper dermatitis: Clinical features and differential diagnosis. In J. Harper, A. Oranje, & N. Prose (Eds.), *Textbook of pediatric dermatology* (pp. 143–152). London: Blackwell Science, Ltd.

Walpole, J. (1998). Oral candidiasis. *The Americal Journal for Nurse Practitioners, 2,* 37–43.

Ward, D. B., Fleischer, Jr., A. B. Feldman, S. R., & Krowchuck, D. P. (2000). Characterization of diaper dermatitis in the United States. *Archives of Pediatric and Adolescent Medicine, 154,* 943–946.

Watson, J., & Schumann, L. (1999). Spider bites: Assessment and management. *Journal of the American Academy of Nurse Practitioners, 11,* 215–223.

Weiss, H. B., Friedman, D. I., & Coben, J. H. (1998). Incidence of dog bite injuries treated in emergency departments. *Journal of the American Medical Association, 279,* 51–53.

Weston, W. L., & Bruckner, A. (2000). Allergic contact dermatitis. *Pediatric Dermatology, 47,* 897–907.

Wysocki, A. B. (1999). Skin anatomy, physiology, and pathophysiology. *Nursing Clinics of North America, 34,* 777–797.

Wright, S. W., Wrenn, K. D., Murray, L., & Seger, D. (1997). Clinical presentation and outcome of brown recluse spider bite. *Annals of Emergency Medicine, 30,* 28–32.

Young, R., Jolley, D., & Marks, R. (1998). Comparison of the use of standardized diagnostic criteria and intuitive clinical diagnosis in the diagnosis of common viral warts (Verrucae vulgaris). *Archives of Dermatology, 134,* 1586–1589.

Suggested Readings

Chamberlain, L. J. (2001). Permethrin should be first-line therapy for scabies, lice. *Infections Disease in Children, 14* (4), 46.

Howard, R. (2001). The appropriate use of topical antimicrobials and antiseptics in children. *Pediatric Annals, 30,* 219–224.

Kirsche, M. L. (2001). Tacrolimus ointment shows marked improvement in atopic dermatitis. *Infections Disease in Children, 14* (4), 44.

Knowell, K. A., & Greer, K. E. (1999). Atopic dermatitis. *Pediatrics in Review, 20,* 46–52.

Lewis-Jones, S. (2000). The psychological impact of skin disease. *NT Plus, 96*(27), 2–3.

Lovell, C., & Anderson, V. (2000). Skin reactions to toxic plants. *NT Plus, 96*(27), 7–9.

Lund, C. (1999). Prevention and management of infant skin breakdown. *Nursing Clinics of North America, 34,* 907–920.

Metry, D. W., & Herbert, A. A. (2000). Topical therapies and medications in the pediatric patient. *Pediatric Clinics of North America, 47,* 867–876.

Pomeranz, A. J., & Fairley, J. A. (1998). The systematic evaluation of the skin in children. *Pediatric Clinics of North America, 45,* 49–63.

Talan, D. A., Citron, D. M., Abrahamian, F. M., Moran, G. J., & Goldstein, E. J. C. (1999). Bacteriologic analysis of infected dog and cat bites. *New England Journal of Medicine, 340,* 85–92.

Spray, A., & Siegfried, E. (2001). Dermatologic toxicology in children. *Pediatric Annals, 30,* 197–202.

Winsor, A. (2000). Sampling techniques. *NT Plus, 96*(27), 12–13.

Resources

Organizations and Websites

American Academy of Dermatology
930 N. Meacham Road
P.O. Box 4014
Schaumburg, IL 60168-4014
(847) 330-0230
www.aad.org

American Association of Poison Control Centers
3201 New Mexico Avenue, Suite 310
Washington, DC 20016
(202) 362-7217
www.aapcc.org

Dermatology Online Atlas
Thibautstrasse 3
D-69115 Heidelberg
GERMANY
+49-(0)-6221-56-8751
Hartmannstrasse 14,
D-91052 Erlangen
GERMANY
+49-(0)-9131-85-33164
www.dermis.net/index.html
www.derma.med.uni-erlangen.de/index_e.htm

National Eczema Association for Science and Education
1221 SW Yamhill, Suite 303
Portland, OR 97205
(800) 818-7546
www.excema-assn.org

National Pediculosis Association
P.O. Box 610189
Newton, MA 02461
(781) 449-6487
www.headlice.org

Skin Cancer Foundation
245 Fifth Avenue, Suite 1403
New York, NY 10016
(800) SKIN-490
www.skincancer.org

The Society for Pediatric Dermatology
5422 North Bernard
Chicago, IL 60625
(773) 583-9780
www.spdnet.org

UNIT VII

Alterations in Sensorimotor Function

CHAPTER 31

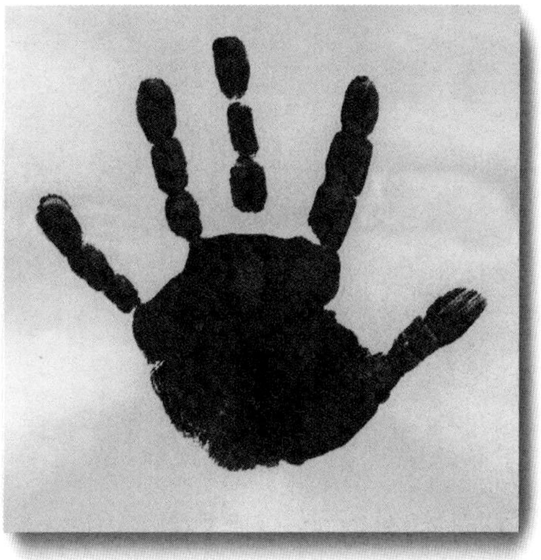

When I was 5 years old, I could hear sounds and spoken English only within a distance of about three feet. Even with the most powerful hearing aid, I had a difficult time understanding my friend's speech. Sometimes the other kids made fun of me because I couldn't hear; they thought I was stupid. When I was 8 years old I received a cochlear implant. My whole life has changed now because I can hear and understand my friends. Now my friends think I am smart. (Andrew, age 12)

SENSORY ALTERATIONS

Angela Ciolfi Murphy, PhD, RN

COMPETENCIES

Upon completion of this chapter, the reader will be able to:

- *Explain the eye and ear structures and how they differ between children and adults.*
- *Discuss normal language development.*
- *Describe the major types of language and speech disorders in children.*
- *Discuss normal hearing and vision development.*
- *Describe the common causes of hearing and visual impairment in children.*
- *Explain how hearing or visual impairments affect the child's development of speech and language.*
- *Discuss the nurse's role in early detection of sensory impairments.*
- *Describe the nurse's role in promoting optimal development of a child with a sensory impairment.*
- *Describe the nurse's role in preventing and treating traumatic injury to the sensory organs in children.*

Alterations in sensory function can have a profound effect on the child's ability to achieve normal growth and development. Children learn about themselves, their families, and the world through their senses and use of language and speech. Early identification of hearing, vision, and communication defects enables early intervention to assist the child and family to achieve optimal growth and development. This chapter focuses on the nurse's role in the care of children with impairment of language or speech, hearing, or vision, and in the prevention and treatment of traumatic injury to the sensory organs.

ANATOMY AND PHYSIOLOGY

The following discussion explains the anatomy of the ear and eye and discusses how structures differ between children and adults.

Ear

The ear has three main sections: the outer ear, the middle ear, and the inner ear (Figures 33-1A and B). The outer ear is composed of the auricle, the external auditory canal that directs sound to the tympanic membrane (eardrum). The tympanic membrane vibrates to conduct sound waves to the

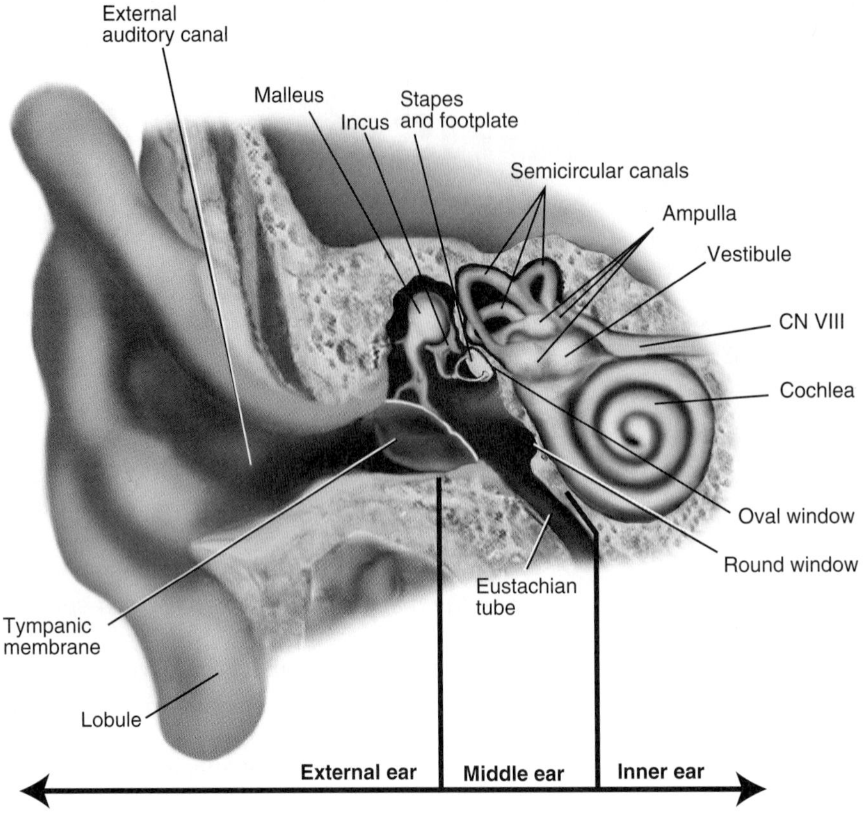

Figure 31-1A Cross-Section of the Ear (adult)

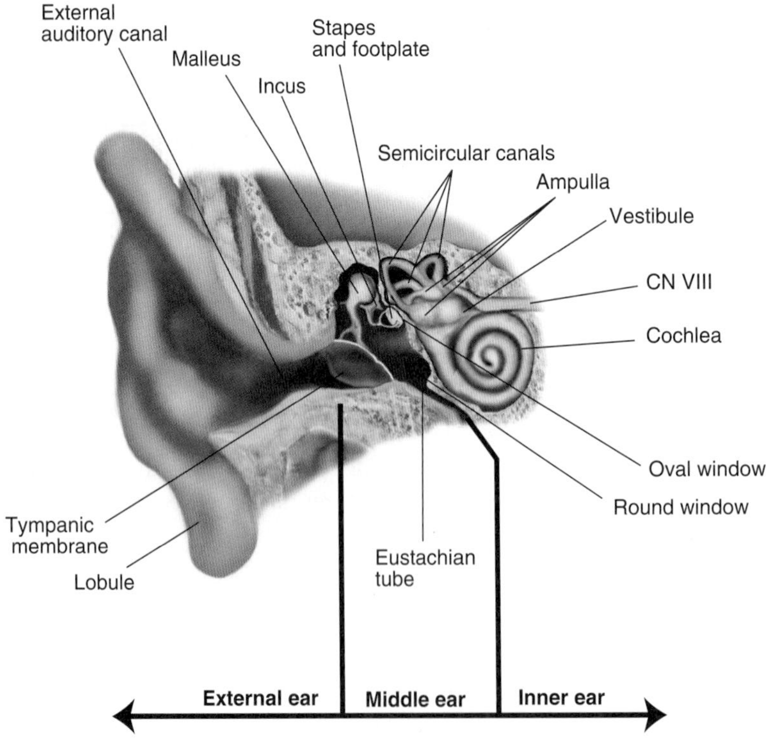

Figure 31-1B Cross-Section of the Ear (young child). Note shorter and flatter eustachian tube.

three bones [malleus (hammer), incus (anvil), and stapes (stirrup)] in the middle ear, which transmit sound to the nerve endings in the inner ear. The nerve endings are contained in the fluid-filled cochlea, which transmits the sound waves to the auditory nerve in the brain. The inner ear also contains the semicircular canal that maintains balance and body position. The eustachian tube connects the middle ear with the nasopharynx. It allows fluid to drain into the nasopharynx and equalizes pressure between the outer and middle ear. Infants and young children have shorter, more horizontal, and more flaccid eustachian tubes, predisposing them to middle ear infections.

Eye

The eye is composed of the external and internal eye (Figures 31-2 and 31-3). The external eye is composed of the eyelids, lacrimal glands, conjunctiva, and cornea. The internal eye is composed of the sclera, iris, pupil, lens, ciliary body, retina (containing rods and cones; the macula), and vitreous chamber. The eye is moved by six accessory muscles, and affected by cranial nerves II, III, IV, V, and VI. Light enters the eye through the cornea and moves through the lens, whose shape is changed by the ciliary muscles to focus light on the retina. The rods and cones and the macula transmit light impulses via the optic nerve (cranial nerve II) to the brain. Binocularity (ability to fixate on one visual field with both eyes) is established by 6 months of age. Visual acuity increases with age, reaching maturity by 5 years of age. Tears are not present until the lacrimal gland begins to function, usually at 1–3 months of age (Grover, 2000b).

SPEECH AND LANGUAGE

Speech involves the physical production of sound using the oral mechanism (tongue, teeth, oral cavity, larynx). **Language** refers to the meaningful use of words, phrases, and gestures to transmit meaning from one person to another.

Normal Language Development

Children are born with the capacity to learn the complex system of language and speech. A variety of theories have been proposed to explain how children acquire language. All theories agree optimal language development is influenced by cognitive ability, temperament, language environment, and intact auditory and visual senses. Communication is composed of speech and language. Speech has three characteristics: (1) *voice,* described in terms of the pitch, volume, or quality; (2) *articulation,* the ability to produce and sequence speech phonemes in an intelligible fashion; and (3) *fluency,* the rate, rhythm, and general flow of speech. Language

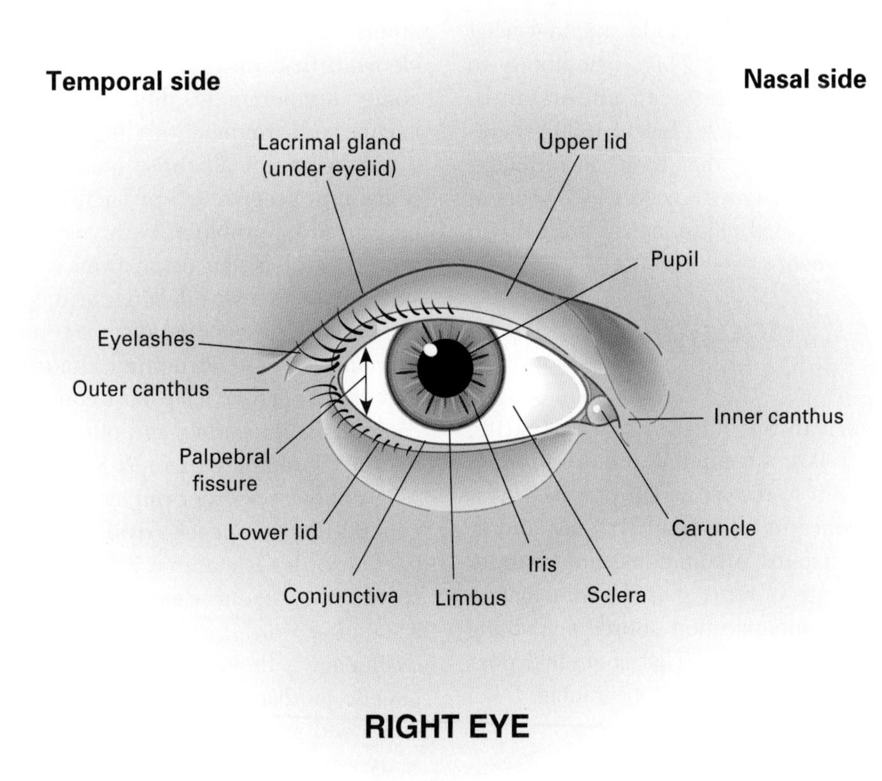

Figure 31-2 External View of the Eye

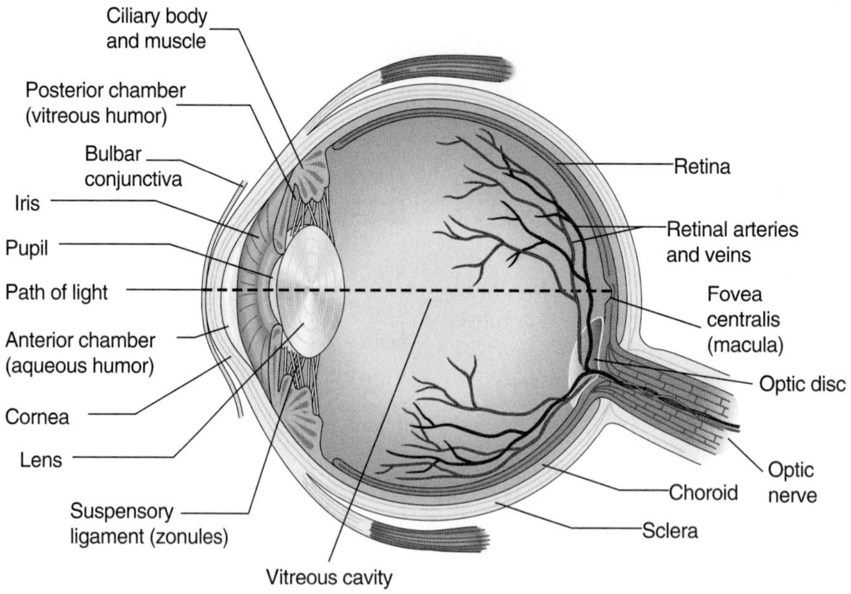

Figure 31-3 Lateral Cross-Section of the Interior Eye

involves three dimensions: *syntax* is the ordering or arrangement of words to communicate an idea; *semantics* is the acquisition of vocabulary and use of words to refer to objects, people, processes, actions, or conditions; and *pragmatics* involves the functional use of language as a social tool for communication, learning, and directing behavior (Coplan, 1995). Language development involves two interrelated processes: *receptive language* (understanding what others say to you) and *expressive language* (the ability to speak verbally in a way that others can understand). Children learn receptive language first (Taylor, 1999), therefore, children can understand more than they can verbalize. Approximately 80% of language growth occurs by 3 years of age. Table 31-1 outlines expected milestones in normal language and speech development.

Speech and Language Disorders

According to the American Speech-Language-Hearing Association (Goldstein, 1993), a communication disorder is any impairment in the ability to receive and/or process a symbol system, represent concepts or symbol systems, and/or transmit and use symbol systems. A communication disorder may involve speech, language, or hearing or any combination of these three functions. Communication disorders in young children are developmental in nature. That is, a child does not acquire language normally from the very beginning.

Incidence and Etiology

Between 5% and 10% of all children have language disorders (Grover, 2000a). Language disorders in children are either a receptive disorder (failure to comprehend), or an expressive disorder (deviation or delay in speech or qualitative aspects of language). **Receptive language** is the ability to understand spoken and written communication. Receptive disorders result from some type of central nervous system failure. **Expressive language** is the ability to use gestures, words, or written symbols to communicate with others. Expressive language disorders result when any of the elements that contribute to language development (cognitive ability, temperament, intact auditory or visual senses, and language environment) are impaired. Deviation or delay can occur in one or all three qualitative dimensions (syntax, semantics, pragmatics) of language. Speech disorders may be caused by problems with voice, articulation, or fluency. Voice disorders can result from vocal cord polyps, chronic shouting or excessive talking, or medical conditions, such as cleft palate. Articulation disorders may be caused by neuromuscular disease, structural abnormalities, immaturity, or may be idiopathic. The most common cause of articulation disorders is idiopathic, and often may disappear as children mature (Shriberg, Gruber, & Kwiatkowski, 1994).

A fluency disorder can include impaired rate, rhythm, or general flow of speech (**dysfluency**). An example of a fluency disorder is stammering or stuttering. **Stuttering** is a speech impairment where an individual involuntarily repeats a sound or word, resulting in loss of speech fluency. Speech dysfluency is thought to be caused by neurological damage, genetic predisposition, and anxiety. A persistent idea about childhood stuttering is that it is the consequence of a primary emotional disorder. However, research findings challenge this hypothesis. Stuttering is normal between the ages of two and four years. Persistence of speech dysfluency

TABLE 31-1 Normal Language/Speech Developmental Milestones

Age of Child	Speech	Receptive Language	Expressive Language
Birth to 6 months	• Makes vowel sounds	• Turns head to sound • Responds to name, "no," "bye-bye," "mama," "daddy" • Quiets when hears parent's voice	• Uses different cries to express hunger or discomfort • Coos or gurgles • Squeals when happy • Babbles
6 months to 12 months	• Utters one–two words with meaning	• Stops activity when "no" or name is said • Responds with gestures to words such as "up," "come," and so forth	• Babbles using two syllables • Imitates animal sounds • Imitates speech intonation • Uses "jargon"
12 months to 18 months	• Starts to combine two words • 18–22 words vocabulary	• Recognizes names of body parts • Identifies pictures of familiar objects when named	• Mixes real words with jargon and gestures • Says "ma-ma" and "da-da" • Uses words more than gestures • Announces familiar objects by name
18 months to 2 years	• Articulation lags behind • 270–300 words vocabulary	• Follows two consecutive related directions such as "pick up ball and bring it to me" • Understands more complex sentences	• Refers to self by name • Uses two- and three-word phrases
2 years to 3 years	• Uses consonants and pronouns • Begins to use word endings • 900 words vocabulary	• Learns concepts such as hot/cold, big/little, and so forth • Listens to and identifies sounds	• Begins combining words in short complete phrases • Inverts subject and verb such as "come lunch mommy" • Answers simple yes/no questions
3 years to 4 years	• Speaks clearly • 1,500 words vocabulary	• Can categorize objects • Carries out three-part command • Begins to identify colors, letters, or numbers in books	• Constantly asks questions • Uses complete sentences
4 years to 6 years	• Distorts s, z, sh, ch, and j. • 2,600+ words vocabulary	• Comprehends "if"	• Able to correctly use most grammatical forms • Appropriately uses pronouns and verbs

beyond five years of age is considered significant for early stuttering and will require therapeutic intervention (Dowling, 1994).

Clinical Manifestations

Signs of speech and language disorders can be subtle. Table 31-2 outlines the signs of problems in language and speech development. If a child displays any of these signs, a referral should be made immediately to a pediatrician and a speech-pathologist.

Diagnosis

School-aged children normally have well-developed communication systems; therefore, identification of a disorder in this population is a relatively simple task. However, language acquisition is a developmental process, so diagnosing irregularities

TABLE 31-2 Signs Suggesting Speech and Language Disorders

Communication	Signs
Language	6 mos: does not turn eyes and head to sound coming from behind or from side 10 mos: does not respond to own name 2 yrs: is not talking at all; does not respond to directions appropriately After 2 yrs: has excessive, inappropriate use of "jargon" 3 yrs: fails to use three or more word sentences; has speech that is not intelligible to strangers 5 yrs: exhibits noticeably impaired sentence structure
Articulation	After 3 yrs: uses vowels rather than consonants After 5 yrs: substitutes simpler sounds for difficult sounds According to developmental sequence, sounds appear more than a year late
Fluency	At 3 yrs: shows overt signs of tension when stuttering (i.e., grimacing, foot tapping) After 5 yrs: has dysfluent speech Has more than 10 speech dysfluencies per 100 words Excessive parental concern over the child's speech
Voice	Poor voice quality (monotone, loud, barely audible, or hoarse) Pitch is inappropriate for age

in speech and language in infants, toddlers, or preschoolers is not as simple. The link between hearing loss and poor communication has been well-documented. The evaluation of any child for speech or language dysfunction should begin with a thorough physical examination to ascertain whether hearing ability is normal. Parent reports of communication problems are the most reliable pieces of data for the pediatric health care provider (Hess, 1999). If no abnormalities are noted on the physical examination, then a language-screening test should be administered. Table 31-3 lists the name and the appropriate age for administration of the most common language-screening instruments. These screening tests are administered and interpreted by appropriate language specialists (Figure 31-4).

Treatment

Children with expressive language disorders should receive speech therapy. Some clinicians advocate a wait-and-see position with the belief that the problem is self-correcting for most children. Most researchers, however, hold the position that expressive disorders are not self-correcting, and therefore speech therapy should be instituted (Conture, 1996). Programs for stuttering utilize behavior modification of the child and education of parents as the treatment as language disorders have a major impact on development and learning. An effective communication system is essential for children to integrate the phenomenon in the world around them. Because the ability to communicate is critical to academic learning, children with expressive language deficits

TABLE 31-3 Language-Screening Instruments

Name	Appropriate Age
Denver Articulation Screening Examination (DASE)	$2^1/_2$ to 6 yrs
Early Language Milestone Scale (ELM)	2 to 3 yrs
Assessment of Children's Language Comprehension	3 to 6 yrs
Pre-School Language Scale	Birth to 3 yrs
Expressive One-Word Picture Vocabulary Test	2 to 12 yrs
Peabody Picture Vocabulary Test	$2^1/_2$ to 18 yrs
Rockford Infant Developmental Evaluation Scale	Birth to 4 yrs
SKI-HI Language Development Scale	Birth to 5 yrs

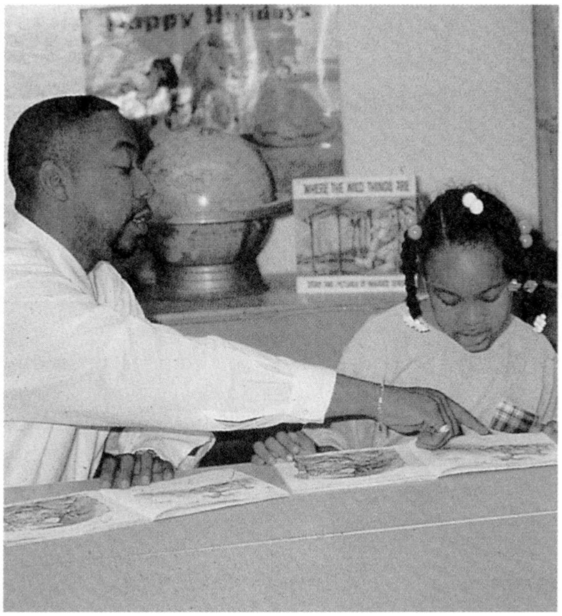

Figure 31-4 Speech therapists use a variety of techniques to help children with speech disorders, including having the child read aloud.

have difficulty in school and are usually academically delayed. The earlier correction is accomplished the less learning delay will occur (Rustin & Cook, 1995).

Nursing Management

The nurse's primary responsibilities when caring for children with communication impairments are assessment and family education. Assessment of abnormalities requires knowledge of normal language and speech development. Knowledge of normal milestones enables the nurse to distinguish when communication characteristics are normal and when there are deviations. During every well-child visit the nurse should assess the child's communication patterns and compare them to normal values for the age of the child. McGlothlin & Loera (1994) in *Speech-language Development in Bilingual Children: What to Look For* offers advice for the nurse on how to identify communication disorders in bilingual children. Box 31-1 suggests questions to ask the caregiver to assess the presence of communication impairment when there is a suspected problem.

Social interactions and the development of interpersonal relationships are impaired when communication is not optimal. The frustration of not being able to express needs and ideas, and the embarrassment of impaired communication, influence the child's developing self-image and self-esteem. A behavior disorder may coexist with a communication disorder. Therefore, the nurse must assess each child, and intervene by assisting the child and family to seek the appropriate professional resources to correct the communication disorder and thus diminish the impact on the child's development. Evaluation should be completed on each visit.

BOX 31-1 Questions to ask when taking a nursing history related to communication disorders

1. At what age did your child say his/her first words?
2. At what age did your child put two to three words together?
3. Does your child make mistakes in grammar? (For instance, "We goes home.")
4. Do directions need to be repeated?
5. Can your child follow two to three directions given at once? (For example, "Go upstairs, get your shirt, and put the shirt on.")
6. Can others understand your child's speech?
7. Does your child stutter?
8. Do you have any difficulty understanding your child's speech?
9. Has there been a recent change in your child's voice?

Nursing Alert:

Early Identification of Communication Disorder

Remember early identification and intervention of a child with a communication disorder can prevent long-term detrimental effects on learning and development. It is essential to conduct a thorough assessment and physical examination, make appropriate referrals, and encourage caregivers to follow through on therapy.

Prevention is one of the primary interventions for communication disorders, and involves early intervention in children who are at risk related to inadequate environmental stimuli, impaired vision or hearing, impaired cognition, or behavior problems (Gottwald & Starkweather, 1995). Nurses are in a pivotal position to recognize children at risk and initiate early intervention to prevent and/or diminish communication disorders. Caregivers must also be taught how to encourage language acquisition in their children (Wilkenfeld & Curlee, 1997). They should also be taught normal expectations of language for their child, and how to encourage language acquisition in the normal child, the child at risk, and the child with a diagnosed communication impairment. Caregivers should also be made aware of parental behavior outlined in Box 31-2 that can assist children acquire language.

Where stuttering has been diagnosed, the caregiver must be taught to interact with the child to decrease stress and, therefore, stuttering. Suggestions for behaviors that can decrease stuttering include: adopt a slow rate of speech (the child is likely to model the adult's rate of speech); positively reinforce periods of fluent speech; ask few direct questions and offer more open-ended comments; maintain eye contact

BOX 31-2 Family teaching: Guidelines to encourage language acquisition

- Talk to your child even when he or she cannot respond verbally; children learn through imitation.
- Use correct language; don't talk "baby talk."
- Describe daily activities as they occur.
- Build vocabulary by making new words part of the everyday activity.
- Do not respond to a child's gesture; encourage the child to say the word before fulfilling the request.
- Repeat the child's words using adult pronunciation.
- Look directly at the child's face when talking: 12 inches away from the newborn's face; increase the distance as the child grows.
- Initiate a play time each day when you talk to your child.
- Read to your child at a young age (under 12 months).
- Reinforce the child's attempt to use language with praise and affection.

Reflective Thinking

Caring for a Child who Stutters

To increase self-awareness about a child who stutters, ask yourself:

1. Do I believe stuttering is a result of a primary emotional disorder?
2. Do I believe the child who stutters is language impaired rather than cognitively impaired?
3. Do I believe the child cannot control the stuttering and can I convince his caregivers of this?
4. Do I have the patience to appear unhurried and take the time to listen to the child?
5. How can I foster the child's self-confidence?

Kids Want To Know

What can I do when other kids make fun of my stuttering?

- Ignore comments and continue as though nothing was said.
- Take a deep breath, relax, then repeat your thought slowly.
- Don't let comments keep you from talking to other kids.
- Practice speaking in your room and with your therapist to decrease incidence of stuttering.

and avoid appearing hurried; and finally, if possible, eliminate stressors associated with stuttering behavior.

A question may arise from bilingual caregivers in regard to when and how to teach more than one language to a child. According to Mills (1997), children can learn two (primary, secondary) languages simultaneously from birth. The essential process to avoid confusion is to keep the languages separate. For example, if the mother speaks Spanish, the father speaks French, and both speak English; then the mother should consistently speak to the child in Spanish, and the father should speak consistently to the child in French. The child will quickly learn which language to use with which parent in order to get needs met. A third language should be introduced only after the child has gained competence in the primary and secondary languages (Oller, Eilers, Urbano, & Cobo-Lewis, 1997).

HEARING IMPAIRMENT

Hearing impairment can range in severity from mild to profound. Deafness is defined as "a hearing impairment that is so severe that the child is impaired in processing linguistic information through hearing, with or without amplification" (National Information Center for Children and Youth with Disabilities [NICHCY], 1996).

Normal Hearing Development

Table 31-4 summarizes the normal development of hearing from birth through 24 months of age.

Hearing Loss

Being alert to the signs of hearing impairment early in the child's life enables the child to receive early intervention to prevent or reduce the effects of the disability on development.

Incidence and Etiology

The incidence of hearing loss in newborns is 1 in 1,000, and is one of the most common infant disabilities in the United States. Each year 4,000 children are born profoundly deaf, while 24,000 others have some degree of hearing loss (Ryan, 1997).

One to two additional children per 1,000 become deaf during childhood, and 16 to 30 per 1,000 children have an educationally significant hearing loss (limited ability to receive auditory information so that it interferes with learning). The U.S. Department of Education (1996) reports that

TABLE 31-4 Milestones of Normal Hearing Development

Age	Hearing
Birth to 3 months	Soothed by parent's voice Gives a startled response to loud sudden noises
3 to 6 months	Looks to see where sounds come from Becomes frightened by an angry voice Smiles when spoken to Wakes up when spoken to or when a loud noise is made nearby
6 to 12 months	Stops for a minute when someone says "no-no," "bye-bye," and own name Looks at objects or pictures when someone talks about them Enjoys rattle and similar toys for their sounds
12 to 18 months	Sings and hums spontaneously Discriminates between sounds such as doorbell, telephone, barking dog, and so forth "Dances" and makes sounds to music
18 to 24 months	Brings objects to others when asked Hears and identifies sounds coming from another room

during the 1994–95 school year, 5,568 students aged 6 to 21 received services for hearing impairment and deafness.

Hearing loss is caused by a number of prenatal and postnatal conditions that are related to congenital or acquired factors. Box 31-3 summarizes these etiologies. Environmental noise is an etiologic agent that is increasing in two distinct age groups, the neonate and the adolescent. The noise level in neonatal intensive care units is producing hearing loss in newborns, especially in premature low birth weight babies, by damaging the stereocilia of the cochlea directly and permanently. Sound levels over 80 decibels (dB) for a sustained amount of time have been shown to produce hearing loss in humans (Brogan, 1999). The average NICU environment produces low-frequency sounds at the 50–80 dB level. Peak decibel levels for some equipment in the NICU fall within this range (incubator motor [51–71 dB], IV pump alarm [76 dB], opening a plastic incubator sleeve [76 dB]). In the adolescent group, the practice of listening to loud music on earphones (80 dB) (Figure 31-5), or at a concert and in blaring speakers in cars (120 dB), puts this group at risk for permanent sensorineural deafness (Rajotte, 1997; Holmes, et al., 1997).

BOX 31-3 Etiology of childhood deafness

I. **Congenital**
   A. Genetic
   B. Nongenetic
      1. Perinatal infection–Maternal rubella, rubeola, cytomegalovirus, toxoplasmosis, herpes, syphilis, bacterial meningitis
      2. Metabolic disease
      3. Perinatal asphyxia
      4. Ototoxic drugs
      5. Rh incompatibility
      6. Radiation
      7. Anoxia and birth trauma
      8. Low birth weight

II. **Acquired**
   A. Infection–chickenpox, measles, mumps, otitis media, meningitis
   B. Ototoxic drugs
   C. Neoplastic disorders
   D. Trauma
   E. Metabolic disorders
   F. NICU noise
   G. Environmental noise

Pathophysiology–Classification

Four types of hearing loss have been identified. They include conductive, sensorineural, mixed, and central. **Conductive hearing loss** is a temporary or permanent hearing deficit resulting from any condition, such as fluids, that "affects the progress of sound into the ear canal or across the middle ear system" (NICHCY, 1996). The most common causes are damage, inflammation, obstruction, or malformation of the outer or middle ear. **Sensorineural hearing loss** results from damage or malformation of the middle ear and/or auditory nerve. The most common causes are congenital defects, infection, exposure to loud noises or ototoxic drugs, and prematurity. Sensorineural loss results in distortion of sound and

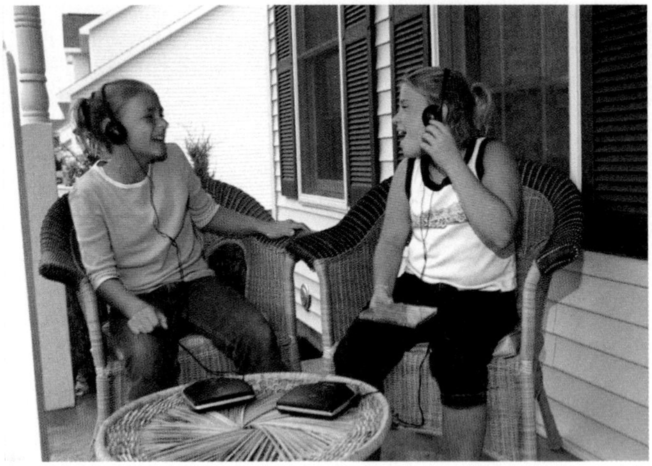

Figure 31-5 Listening to loud music through earphones has been attributed to hearing loss.

TABLE 31-5 Decibel Levels of Various Sounds

Decibel Level	Sound
0	Threshold of hearing
10	Heartbeat
45–55	Normal conversation
65	Telephone ringing
80	Loud music in earphones
120	Rock music concert, blaring car speakers
140	Jet airplane during departure
>140	Any sound at this level will cause pain and permanent damage

problems in discrimination and comprehension and is usually permanent. **Mixed conductive-sensorineural hearing loss** results from interference with transmission of sound in the middle ear and along neural pathways, which produces problems with sound distortion and a reduction in the child's ability to hear sounds below a certain decibel level or loudness. The conductive component is reparable; however, the sensorineural effect is irreversible. **Central hearing** loss is caused by damage that interrupts sound transmission between the brainstem and the cerebral cortex, resulting in difficulty in sound discrimination, auditory association of meaning to sound, auditory memory, and being able to differentiate sound from its background. Whether or not this is permanent depends upon the underlying cause.

Hearing impairment is described in terms of loudness (intensity) and pitch (frequency) of sounds. Loudness is described in terms of decibel units, and pitch is described in terms of Hertz (Hz) units. Table 31-5 describes decibel levels of various sounds. The softest sound the normal human ear can hear is 0 dB. Sustained listening to sound that is more than 140 dB will cause pain and permanent damage. Human beings can hear from a low pitch of 16 Hz to high pitch of 30,000 Hz. Normal speech tones generally fall between 45 and 55 dB and 500 and 2,000 Hz (Brogan, 1999). Hearing impairment can be classified according to decibel level (as measured by an audiometer) and the degree to which it affects one's ability to hear speech. Table 31-6 describes the degree of hearing loss and its effect on speech and language. Because approximately 80% of language growth occurs by 3 years of age, early detection of hearing impairment is critical.

Clinical Manifestations

Early recognition of hearing loss is essential to control the amount of developmental impact on the child. Children at risk, those with a family history of impairment, low birth weight, congenital prenatal infection, cranio-facial abnormalities, elevated bilirubin, asphyxia, low APGAR rating, meningitis, administration of ototoxic drugs, or being a member of the Asian race (Naeem & Newton, 1996) should be assessed very carefully. Children with hearing loss will show characteristic behavioral signs, described in Table 31-7 according to chronologic age. When any of these signs are present, a physical examination and tests of hearing function should be performed.

Diagnosis

Experts have known that congenital hearing loss causes major problems in a child's development. At least two major professional groups have recommended newborn screening to detect hearing loss and forestall developmental problems, the National Institute of Health in 1993, and the American Speech-Language-Hearing Association in 1994 (ASHA, 1994). Sixteen states currently screen all high-risk newborns. The major screening test for hearing is the Brainstem Auditory Evoked Response (BAER) (Ryan, 1997). The Otoacoustic Emission Test (OAE) has replaced the BAER as the major screening test of at-risk children because it is less expensive and easier to administer. The Crib-o-Gram can be used to follow at-risk infants; however, despite its low cost, it is not as definitive as the other two tests (Rouch & Matkin, 1994). See Box 31-4.

The OAE is used together with the BAER to obtain a complete picture of peripheral and brainstem functioning. These tests are performed by an audiologist to confirm suspected hearing impairment. Nurses must be alert to signs of hearing loss and able to explain how these tests are done to caregivers (Figures 31-6A and B).

Treatment

Treatment of hearing loss depends on the type of hearing impairment. Conductive loss can be improved with the use

TABLE 31-6 Hearing Loss: Effect on Speech and Language

Degree of Loss	Effect on Hearing	Effect on Speech and Language
Slight Loss 15–25 dB	No impairment	No significant speech and language delays
Mild Loss 26–40 dB	Difficulty hearing faint or distant speech May benefit from hearing aid	Usually will not have school difficulty
Moderate Loss 41–55 dB	Understands speaker face-to-face at 3–5 feet May need hearing aid	May miss 50% of class discussion if voices are faint or not within the line of sight May have problems pronouncing some speech sounds
Moderately Severe Loss 56–70 dB	To hear conversation needs to be louder than 70 dB Will need hearing aid	Has increasing difficulty in classroom activities Probably has difficulty pronouncing some speech sounds May have deficiencies in language comprehension and usage
Severe Loss 71–90 dB	May hear loud voices if at distance of one foot away from ear Can hear if using hearing aid	Speech and language development are delayed and will not develop spontaneously if loss present before two years of age
Deaf More than 90 dB	Deaf	Severe speech and language delay

TABLE 31-7 Behavioral Signs Associated with Hearing Loss

Age	Behavioral Signs
Birth to 6 months	• Does not startle, blink eyes, or change activity in response to a sudden loud noise • Is not soothed by mother's voice • Does not respond to voice • Does not imitate gurgling and cooing sounds or show response to noise-making toys • Does not turn eyes and head in direction of sound coming from the side or from behind
By 10 months	• Does not respond when name is called
By 12 months	• Does not respond to normal household sounds (dog barking, voice of a family member, etc.) • Engages in loud shrieking and sustained production of vowels • Tries to imitate speech sounds made by caregiver • Points to familiar objects when asked to
15 months to 4–5 years	• Watches a speaker's face intently • Follows simple spoken instructions • Frequently says "huh" and "what" when spoken to • Shows preference for high- or low-pitched sounds • Shows delayed acquisition of speech • Uses gestures rather than verbalization to get attention and objects

Research Highlight

Noise and Nursing Interventions in the NICU Environment

Study Purpose

To document the effects of loud noise and routine nursing procedures on the physiological and behavioral responses of premature infants in the NICU.

Methods

Fifty-five premature infants weighing from 480 to 1930 grams between the ages of 23 and 27 weeks gestation were assessed for the effects of loud noises (alarms, telephones, infant crying, loud speech) and nursing interventions [highly intrusive (suctioning, needle puncture), moderately intrusive (chest physiotherapy), minimally intrusive (administration of medications), and other activities (diaper changes, feeding)] on behavioral (sleep/wake states, amount of crying) and physiological (heart rate, respiratory rate, oxygen saturation) responses.

Findings

Noise and nursing interventions together resulted in oxygen saturation (SaO_2) dropping in 20% of infants. In addition, heart rate (HR) rose in 19% of infants and respiratory rate (RR) rose in 17% of infants. Noise alone caused drops in SaO_2 in 14% of infants, HR rose acutely in 16% of infants, and RR rose acutely in 13% of infants. Seventy-eight percent of infants changed their behavioral state in response to noise and nursing interventions. Most changes were from regular or irregular sleep to fussy and crying states. Forty-three percent of infants changed behavioral states from sleep to fussy/crying in response to noise alone.

Implications

Premature infants are susceptible to loud noises due to the immaturity of their organ of Corti and sensitive cochleas and may not be as able as full-term infants to shut out environmental stimuli. Nurses should take precautions to decrease the loudness of their conversations, radios, and telephones. Applying earmuffs to premature infants might also help decrease the effect of noise. Consolidating nursing interventions so only those essential for care are provided may also limit their effect on the premature infant.

Citation

Zahr, L., & Balian, S. (1995). Responses of premature infants to routine nursing interventions and noise in the NICU. *Nursing Research, 44*(3), 179–185.

of a hearing aid to amplify sound. Sensorineural hearing loss does not improve with amplification. However, a new technique of cochlear implantation has been helping children with sensorineural hearing loss. To assist communication in the hearing-impaired child a number of techniques are utilized—lip reading, sign language, cued speech, and speech therapy (Gatty, 1996). Hearing aid choice depends on the specific needs of the child. The four types of hearing aids commonly used for pediatric clients are behind the ear (postauricular), in the ear, body aid, and eyeglass aids. The most commonly used amplification aid in children is the postauricular aid (Seewald & Gagne, 1995). See Figure 31-7 for various types of hearing aids.

Cochlear implantation is a new technique that can benefit some deaf children. The device has two major components, an internal and an external component. The internal component consists of an electrode implanted into or on the cochlea and an internal receiver embedded into the temporal bone behind the auricle. The external components consist of a microphone, external transmitter, and signal processor. The signal processor transforms the sound stimulus received from the microphone and sends it to the external transmitter and then to the

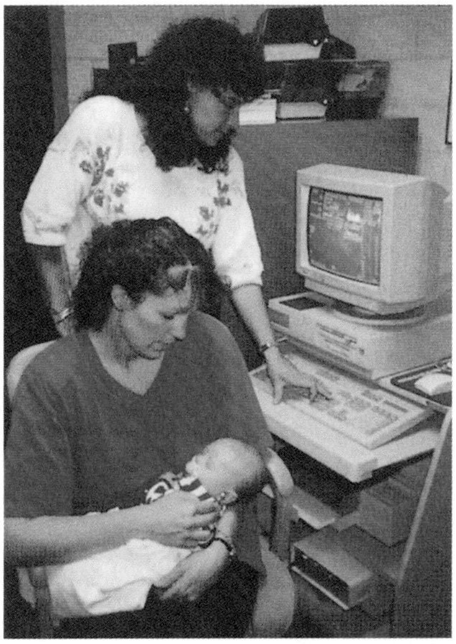

Figure 31-6A Infant Getting Hearing Tested. Courtesy of American Academy of Audiology.

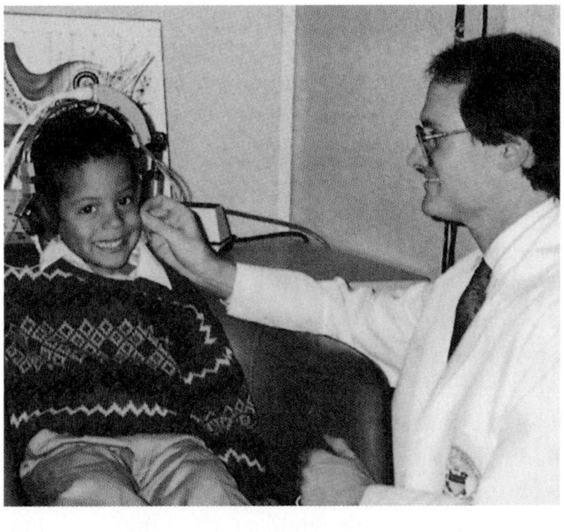

Figure 31-6B Preschooler Getting Hearing Tested. Courtesy of American Academy of Audiology.

BOX 31-4 Hearing tests

BAER = Electrodes placed on forehead and mastoid process. A stimulus is presented and brain wave responses are recorded. Requires sedation.

OAE = As sound moves through the cochlea, thousands of hair cells vibrate and send a signal to the eighth cranial nerve to the brain. If the cochlea is functioning normally, the hair cells simultaneously emit an echo of sound back to the middle ear where a small sensitive microphone records the sound.

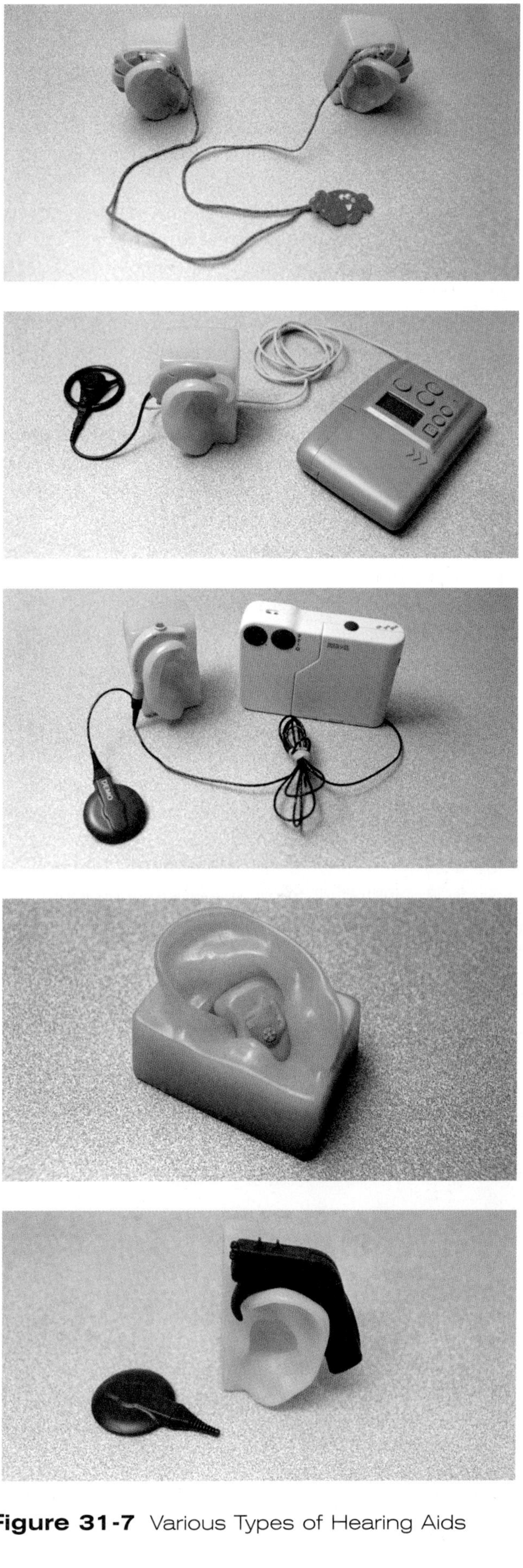

Figure 31-7 Various Types of Hearing Aids

internal receiver. The VIII cranial nerve is stimulated and the brain interprets the sound (Pronovost, 1999). To become a candidate for cochlear implantation a child must meet specific criteria, including being at least 2 years of age with normal IQ, having profound bilateral sensorineural deafness, having no other medical contraindications for surgery, and having strong family support (Rouch & Matkin, 1994).

Because cochlear implantation in children has only had FDA approval since 1990, long-term implications are unknown. A recent study (Tomblin, Spencer, Flock, Tyler, & Gantz, 1999) that compared language skills of children who used hearing aids and those with cochlear implants, found the children with cochlear implants had significantly better language skills than those who used hearing aids.

Vibrotactile aids are devices that present acoustic information decoded tactually on the skin's surface for the purpose of speech reception. The device can be attached to the wrist, forearm, stomach, back, leg, or sternum. An electrotactile signal is transmitted through the part of the body that is stimulated (usually the fingers or hands) to the language processing center in the brain for interpretation (Sarant, 1993). Other hearing assistive techniques such as lip reading, sign language, or cued speech are addressed under nursing management.

Nursing Management

Assessment

The nurse's most important role in caring for the child with hearing loss is careful assessment to detect impairment as early as possible. Assessment involves taking a careful nursing history to identify children who are at risk, screening all children during well-child visits, and observing the child's behavior. It is important to pay special attention if the caregiver reports behaviors indicating hearing loss described earlier in Table 31-7.

Nursing Diagnosis

Nursing diagnoses include:

1. Impaired verbal communication related to impaired hearing.
2. Impaired verbal communication related to anxiety.
3. Disturbed body image related to impaired hearing.
4. Delayed growth and development related to impaired hearing.
5. Interrupted family processes related to the diagnosis of deafness of a child.

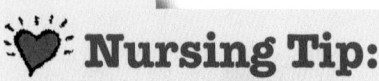

> **Nursing Tip:**
>
> **Detecting hearing loss**
>
> Remember, caregivers know their children well and notice subtle behaviors that may escape the attention of medical personnel. Listen to their comments carefully. If their input, together with a nursing assessment, indicates a possible hearing loss, the child must be referred to an audiologist and an ear, nose, and throat specialist for further evaluation.

Outcome Identification

1. The child will achieve optimum communication.
2. The child will experience optimal growth, development, and socialization.
3. The child and caregivers will understand measures to be taken to prevent further hearing impairment.
4. The child and caregivers will understand the impact of the hearing impairment and incorporate support interventions into their daily lives to enable positive psychological adjustment.

Planning/Implementation

Initial nursing interventions to accomplish the goal of promoting communication must first address the impact of the child's hearing impairment on caregivers as they may feel disappointed and need to be assisted to accept and adapt to the impairment. However, caregivers must go through the stages of a grieving process before they can adapt and begin to deal with the challenges of a hearing-impaired child. Depression and anger, especially toward medical staff, are normal stages in the grieving process. The nurse may refer caregivers to a support group for help.

The nurse should remember the family is an integrated system and therefore *all* are influenced by the birth of the hearing-impaired child. Siblings may experience the same feelings of sadness, anger, fear, and guilt that caregivers experience. Because much time and energy is devoted to the hearing-impaired child, the sibling may react to the inequity of attention by feeling jealousy and resentment. Each sibling's reaction will vary depending on age and developmental level, and often reflects the attitudes caregivers have expressed both by example and direct communication. Research, however, indicates siblings of children with disabilities appear to be much more positively, rather than negatively, affected by living with a child with a hearing loss (Weston, 1995).

Grandparents must also adapt to the child with hearing loss. Grandparents grieve for two reasons; they grieve the loss of the perfect grandchild, and they grieve because of their own child's pain (Simons, 1987). In the process of learning to accept this hearing-impaired child, the grandparents may reflect the parents' emotions. Parents can help grandparents adapt by encouraging them to spend time with the child and sharing information on how to help the child develop.

Nurses play a critical role in educating the public on how to prevent hearing loss. For families where impairment deviations that include hearing loss are common, genetic counseling should be encouraged. During pregnancy, steps should be taken to prevent the effects of any Rh incompatibility and birth trauma, and to avoid infection and ototoxic drugs. After birth, all infants and children should have ear infections treated promptly. Protection of the neonate in the NICU must be instituted to provide a quieter environment in order to protect against iatrogenic hearing loss. Preventive education must be undertaken with adolescents who expose themselves to loud music via earphones and car speakers to alert them to the potential damage to hearing ability.

How does the nurse communicate with the hearing-impaired child? The nurse must know what method (hearing aid, lip reading, sign language) the child uses to communicate, and make an effort to continue these methods in the health care setting. Box 31-5 lists practices enhancing the communication process between nurse and child.

Evaluation

The child and their family will have benefited from the nursing interventions including teaching, coping methods, and outside support.

Family Teaching

From birth, communication interchange is altered between caregiver and infant. Caregivers should be advised that deaf infants babble until approximately 6 months of age and then stop because of lack of auditory feedback (Lederberg & Everhart, 1998). Methods to enhance communication between child and caregivers should begin immediately upon detection of impairment. They must be taught how to use the various aids to hearing so they can manage and support the child's rehabilitation.

The nurse and caregivers must also learn to care for the hearing aid. All hearing aids must be fitted properly by the audiologist, and as the child grows, a new aid will be needed. For children under 4 years old, the aid must be changed every 3–6 months. After 4 years of age, the aid will need replacement yearly. All hearing aids have a volume control and an on/off switch. The ear mold is the only part that can be cleaned with pipe cleaners or toothbrushes. Heat and moisture damage the aid. Batteries that last 100–150 hours must be handled carefully, replaced when worn, and turned off when not in use to preserve battery life. Hearing aids amplify background noise as well as the speaker's voice, which can be annoying and confusing to a child. A whistling sound, termed **acoustic feedback,** is caused by improper fit into the ear or by too high a volume. To eliminate whistle, caregivers should be taught to clean the ear mold, reinsert the aid into the ear making sure no hair is caught between the ear mold and canal, and turn down the volume. Hearing aids should be removed before any medical procedures involving radiation because radiation damages the device.

There are two basic communication approaches the child can learn, lip reading or speech reading, and sign language. A third form that is less common is termed cued speech. When utilizing *lip reading or speech reading* only 40% of the spoken word is understood because during speaking, the tongue moves inside the mouth and is not visible. Therefore, the nurse or caregiver should speak clearly and slowly but without exaggeration, as exaggeration alters

BOX 31-5 Practices to enhance communication with the child who is hearing-impaired

1. Encourage use of hearing aid.
2. Look directly into child's face–be on same level as child–get child's attention before speaking.
3. Speak slowly with normal volume and simple sentence structure.
4. Eliminate background noise and visual distractions.
5. Use visual aids such as pictures, objects, hand gestures.
6. Utilize a sign language interpreter.
7. When talking, use normal body gestures and facial expressions.
8. Check comprehension by asking simple questions.
9. Write notes.
10. Avoid restraining child's hands.
11. Avoid darkened room; light should be on face rather than behind speaker's head.

Nursing Alert:

Battery Safety

Emphasize the importance of storing the batteries in a place where young children cannot reach for and swallow them. If this occurs, seek medical attention immediately.

Kids Want To Know

What do I say when other kids make fun of my hearing aid?

- Explain the hearing aid allows you to hear what they are saying to you.
- If they were listening to the radio and could not hear the music, they would turn up the volume. The hearing aid "turns up the volume" for you.
- Try to wear your aid so that it is not as obvious.

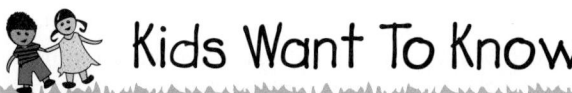

REFLECTIONS FROM FAMILIES

When I found out Spencer had impaired hearing, I was devastated! However, what hurt more, was trying to comfort my son when he was 7 years old and came home from school crying because the other kids had made fun of his hearing aid and his impaired speech. What can I say to improve Spencer's self-image and self-esteem? The nurse at his school encouraged me to help him see he is hearing challenged not hearing handicapped, and is challenged to learn and communicate more than the other kids in his school. The fact that Spencer is able to learn and communicate despite his diminished hearing makes him special rather than different.

Reflective Thinking

Self-induced Hearing Loss

In recent years there is increasing concern over sensorineural deafness induced by frequent exposure to loud music. Studies have discovered sound levels over 80 dB can produce hearing loss in adults. The sound from rock concerts, car stereos, and home speakers can easily exceed the 80 dB level. Availability of high-intensity speakers and personal earphones have put adolescents at risk because adolescents consider loud music part of their lifestyle. The absorption in loud music is an escape from daily living, and is consistent with the normal developmental task of adolescents of achieving independence and developing identity. What can the nurse do to change this behavior? What can caregivers do to change this behavior?

rhythm and decreases comprehension. Comprehension is further reduced if the speaker has a beard or an accent. The nurse or caregivers can refer to the suggestions in Box 31-5 to enhance comprehension.

Sign Language has three forms: American Sign Language (ASL), Signed Exact English (SEE), and British Sign Language (BSL). Sign language is a visual-gestural language that uses hand signals corresponding to words in the English language. The caregivers and child should learn sign language as an adjunct to lip reading. *Cued speech* is a method of communication that uses eight configurations and four positions of the hand to supplement lip reading when words look alike when formed by the lips (e.g., "sin," "tin"). Other aids for hearing are lights wired to flash when the telephone and doorbell ring, trained dogs to alert one to sounds, closed captioning on TV that provides subtitles to translate the audio portion of the program, or telecommunications devices for the deaf, such as a typewriter that transmits the typed message over telephone lines to a monitor so people with hearing impairment can communicate with each other.

Children with hearing loss can learn to communicate effectively if the proper training is instituted early. Nurses should teach caregivers that children learn with their eyes first, so stimulation is essential to development. Encouraging the child to speak by expecting speech and allowing time to try to speak no matter how the speech syllables sound is important. Caregivers should be reminded it is easy to spoil deaf children by giving them attention, overindulging their wishes, or overprotecting them. Techniques for handling behavior in hearing-impaired children are the same as for children with normal hearing. A feeling of adequacy and self-confidence is established in children if they learn to play with other children, especially hearing children. Educational opportunities for deaf children should be the same as for other children. Appropriate accommodations must be made in the educational setting for the hearing-impaired child.

Early Intervention Programs

The education that can take place in specialized or public school of the hearing-impaired child is essential to optimal development. The key element is that this education occurs as early as possible in the child's life, hence, early intervention program involvement. The Education for All Handicapped Children Act of 1975 (P.L. 94-142) was enacted to assure appropriate education to children with disabilities. In 1986, Public Law 99-457 reaffirmed P.L. 94-142 and amended it to include mandatory special education for children. It also funded Early Intervention Services for young children (birth to 3 years) with disabilities and changed the focus to include families. In 1990, P.L. 101-476 reauthorized the Education of the Handicapped Act (P.L. 94-142) and changed its name to the "Individuals with Disabilities Education Act" (IDEA). Revisions to Part H of P.L. 99-457 were made in P.L. 102-119 making the "case manager" a "family service coordinator" and also developing a system of services for infants and toddlers with developmental delay or disabilities. Under P.L. 94-142, the focus was on the individual with the IEP (Individual Education Plan). Under P.L. 102-119 the focus of services is on the family IFSP (Individual Family Service Plan).

This change in focus addresses the needs of the child within the dynamic of the family system. Nurses play a central position in delivering family centered care and are a piv-

Critical Thinking

Hearing Deficits

As a nurse in a pediatrician's office, you occasionally hear mothers mention that their infants do not seem to be aware that they have entered the room until they are seen and the infants will not awaken to a voice unless it is also accompanied by touch. Should you be concerned that these infants have a hearing deficit?

otal member of the early intervention team, which must learn to be cross-culturally competent in order to deliver appropriate care. Behaviors demonstrating cultural sensitivity include: respects individuals from other cultures, makes sincere attempts to understand the world from others' points of view, has a sense of humor, tolerates ambiguity well, and approaches others with a desire to learn. The delivery of services by the multidisciplinary team (including the nurse) coordinates the care and education of the child with a disability so optimal development occurs.

BOX 31-6 Color blindness

Color blindness (color deficiency or color vision deficit) occurs in about 8% of the general population and is seen more frequently in males than females. It tends to be inherited as a sex-linked disorder and affects the ability to distinguish red from green or blue from yellow colors. There is no cure for the condition and it is detected by use of the Ishihara color plates, which have numbers of a particular color hidden within them. Children who are color blind cannot see the numbers and just see colored dots. Children who are not color blind are able to see the numbers within the plates. Nursing care involves helping children and families learn other ways to discriminate colors, for example, learning the order of lights on traffic signals, or to be observant for warning signs that may have a flashing light associated with them (railroad crossing, school crossing walk). Other implications involve helping children match their clothes according to ways other than coloring, by organizing, labeling, purchasing clothes that can be worn together, or making sure teachers are aware of the condition, so children are not assigned color identification or discrimination tasks.

VISION IMPAIRMENT

Vision is also an important sense for normal child development. From the moment of birth, the child begins to bond with parents and learn about the world using sight. Through sight, the child learns to read, move about the environment, and interact with the world. Impaired vision requires early assessment and intervention to ensure the child's optimal development.

Normal Development

The eyes begin to develop at about 22 days of gestation. Development of the eye is not complete at birth. However, the newborn is able to focus on an object at a distance of 3 feet. Sensitivity to brightness develops rapidly in the first two months of life, and the infant displays the blink reflex. Tears begin to secrete within the first two weeks of birth. However, secretion in relation to emotion occurs between six and twelve weeks. By four to six months of age infants show preference for bright colors such as red and yellow, are able to reach for familiar objects, and have visual **accommodation** (the ability of the eye to focus clearly on objects at all distances) equal to an adult (see Box 31-6 for information about color blindness). **Binocularity** (fixation of two ocular images into one cerebral picture, i.e., fusion) is established by six months of age. **Visual acuity** (clearness or sharpness of the image) changes with age from 20/50 at 18 months to 20/20 at 4 years of age. At birth, the iris appears blue or light gray in color in light-skinned newborns, and brown in darker-skinned newborns. An indication of eventual color can be seen at 6 months of age. However, permanent eye color may not appear until one year of age.

Visual Impairment

Loss of vision is described in terms of its legal-medical, educational, and functional implications. The *legal-medical* definition emphasizes the clearness of vision at various distances (visual acuity). The *educational* definition emphasizes the extent to which vision can be used for reading and learning. The *functional* definition describes what a person actually can see. Box 31-7 summarizes these definitions.

Incidence, Etiology, and Pathophysiology

The three underlying reasons for visual impairment are: the eyeball may be proportioned incorrectly making it hard to focus on objects; there may be damage to one or more parts of the eye essential to vision that interferes with the way the eye receives or processes visual information; and the part of the brain processing visual information may not function properly, resulting in the brain not being able to analyze and interpret visual information (Holbrook, 1996). A visual impairment may be congenital (75%) or acquired (25%) (Espezel, 1994). Very low birth weight (VLBW) infants have

BOX 31-7 Definitions of vision impairments

The Legal-Medical Definitions

Blind = Visual activity of 210/200 or less in the better eye, with correction; a visual field which subtends to an angle of not greater than 20 degrees. (Federal Regulations, PL 94-142, 1975)

Sighted Partially = Visual activity between 20/200 and 20/70 in the better eye with correction (Federal Regulations, PL 94-142, 1975)

The Educational Definitions

Blind = Visual loss is severe enough so cannot read print

Partially Sighted = Residual vision is sufficient to allow child to read large print (for visually impaired) for educational purposes

The Functional Definitions

Blind = Vision allows only light perception

Low Vision = Can see if objects are a few inches to a maximum of two feet away

Limited Vision = Visual defects are correctable with lenses or surgery so child functions as a normally sighted person

BOX 31-8 Clinical manifestations of visual loss based on age

Infants:

Pupils do not react to light.
Does not gaze or stare at surroundings.
Does not follow a moving object with eyes.

Toddlers or Preschoolers:

Rubs eyes frequently.
Squints or tilts head to see.
Frequently bumps into objects.
Moves hesitantly or walks close to the wall.
Holds books or toys close to face.
Shows difficulty in identifying faces or numbers that designate rooms or floors.
Complains of headaches, dizziness, nausea/vomiting.

significantly increased incidence of ocular muscle weakness. Research is in process to determine if fluorescent lights are the cause of blindness observed in retinopathy of prematurity (ROP) in premature babies in the NICU (Gauzer, 1997). Partial vision (between 20/70 and 20/200) occurs in roughly 1 in 500 schoolchildren. 35,000 children in America have visual activity of 20/200 and total blindness (Behrman & Kliegman, 1998).

Clinical Manifestations

Total blindness can usually be identified during the first year of life. Partial vision loss often goes unnoticed until the child enters school and has functional difficulty. See Box 31-8 for a list of clinical manifestations based on age.

Diagnosis

The assessment of vision in the infant centers on evaluating fixation and following of each eye. An entirely satisfactory method of determining vision in the preverbal child has yet to be developed (Ryan, 1996). In early childhood or with developmentally delayed children, visual acuity can be tested with:

- Allen cards—seven black and white pictures of familiar objects (horse, house, etc.)—where the child is asked to name the objects
- Blackbird Preschool Vision Test—six cards, each with varying sizes of blackbirds—child indicates direction the bird is flying
- Snellen—child indicates which way the legs of the letter E point
- Denver Eye Screening Test (DEST)—a single E card—child indicates which way E is pointing
- STYCAR test—Chart with letters T, H, V, and O, and four individual cards with these same letters—child must match letter on chart with the appropriate letter on the card (American Academy of Pediatrics, 1996)

The Snellen Alphabet chart is used for older children who can identify letters (Figures 31-8 and 31-9). The numerical fraction, for example, 20/40, describes visual acuity. The numerator indicates the distance the child is from the chart. The denominator indicates the distance at which a person with normal vision can read the same letters.

Vision Disorders

A variety of disorders can affect a child's vision. The disorders can be classified into four groups: visual acuity (how clearly the child sees); muscular efficiency (how well the two eyes work together to focus on objects and to produce binocular vision); physical integrity (how intact and structurally normal are the physical mechanisms of the eye); and eye infections.

Impairment of Visual Acuity

Detection and correction of disorders that cause impaired visual acuity in children are important for two reasons: to prevent irreversible vision loss, and to eliminate any visual impairment diminishing the child's normal development.

Refractive Disorders

Refractive disorders include **myopia** (nearsightedness), **hyperopia** (farsightedness), and **astigmatism** (blurred vision). A discussion of the three disorders follows.

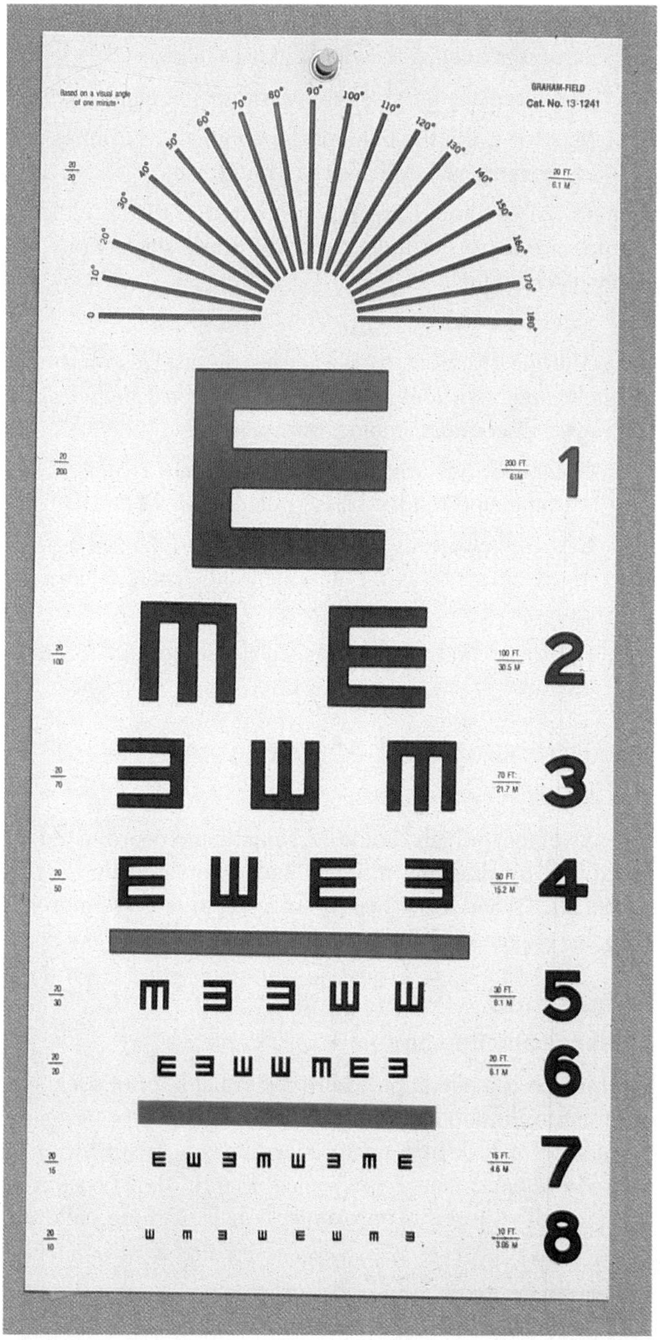

Figure 31-8 Snellen "E" or "Big E" Chart for Testing Distance Visual Acuity of Children

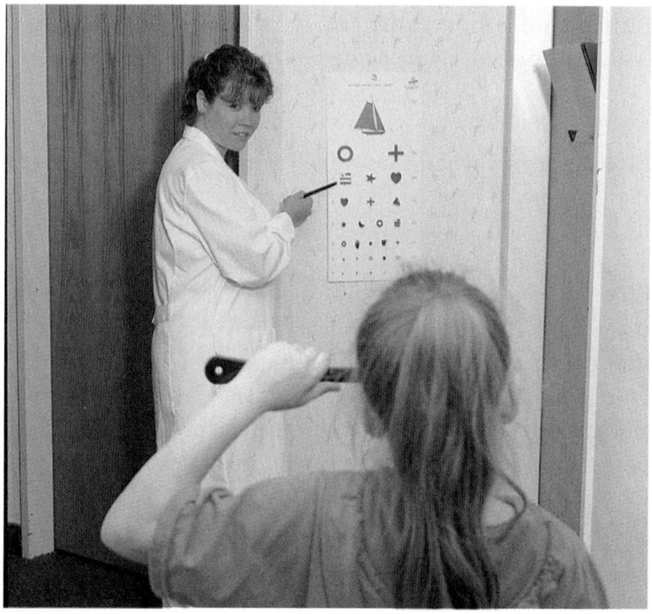

Figure 31-9 Measuring Distance Visual Acuity of a Child Using a Kindergarten Vision Screening Chart

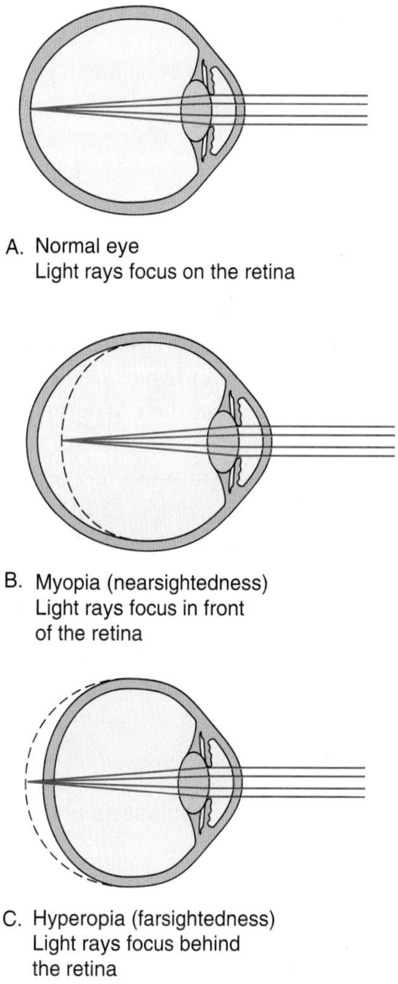

Figure 31-10 Eye Refraction

Incidence and Etiology

Refractive disorders are the most common type of visual disorders in children. **Refraction** refers to the process by which the cornea and lens of the eye bend light rays to focus on the retina. When the bending of the rays and the length of the eyeball are uncoordinated, the image does not fall on a single point on the retina. The three types of refractive disorders are illustrated in Figure 31-10. Theories on the etiology of myopia include it being inherited as a recessive gene, prolonged use of eyes on close work resulting in excessive tension on ciliary muscles, or vitamin deficiencies. Astigmatism is primarily caused by inheritance.

Pathophysiology

Myopia occurs when the eyeball is too long, causing light rays to focus in front of the retina resulting in difficulty with distance vision. Hyperopia occurs when the eyeball is too short, causing light to focus behind the retina resulting in difficulty with near vision. This is the most common refractive disorder in children. Astigmatism occurs when there is uneven curvature of the cornea or lens, preventing light rays from focusing correctly on the retina. Because normal refraction does not develop until the age of $4^1/_2$ years, diagnosis of refractive errors occurs after this age.

Clinical Manifestations

Each impairment results in poor visual acuity. Associated symptoms may include headache, irritated eyes, nausea, eyestrain, and irritability. Classic complaints of children are difficulty reading or seeing things at a distance, such as on the blackboard.

Diagnosis

Visual screening tests are routinely administered by nurses in various practice settings such as elementary schools, headstart centers, or well-child visits.

Treatment

Myopia is treated with biconcave lenses to improve distance vision. The child may need new lenses every year or two as he or she grows. A new treatment, photorefractive keratectomy laser surgery is used to correct myopia, but is not recommended for children yet (Wessel, 1997). Most young children need no correction for hyperopia because their ability to accommodate overcomes their hyperopia as they grow. Astigmatism is treated with special lenses to correct unequal curvatures. High astigmatism must be corrected early to avoid **amblyopia** (a reduction or loss of vision in one eye).

Nursing Management

Assessment is the primary nursing consideration. It is important to screen all children at well-child visits and listen carefully to the caregiver's history of the child's behavior. If vision impairment is detected, referral should be made to the appropriate professional.

Family Teaching—Care of Eyeglasses and Contact Lenses

Plastic or polycarbonate lenses are the safest lenses for children. Nurses should teach caregiver and/or child to:

- Prevent scratches, never lay glasses lens down
- Always remove glasses with both hands to prevent warping of the frame
- Avoid getting the elastic bands too tight when using harnesses to keep the child's glasses in place
- Never replace missing screws with paper clips or wires
- Monitor when the bend of the temple is in front of the ear because glasses have been outgrown

Contact lenses should not be prescribed until the child is able to care for them independently. Some suggestions for family teaching include:

- Safer for children engaged in active sports
- Allergic reactions to the lenses themselves or to the cleaning solutions may occur (symptoms include red eyes, discomfort, itching, burning)
- Complications are more likely to occur if lenses are worn on an extended basis (greater than 24 hours)
- Care and cleansing directions must be followed explicitly in order to avoid complications, such as corneal damage
- Improved body image—especially important for adolescents

Impairment of Muscular Efficiency

Eye movement, which should be smooth and coordinated, is controlled by six small muscles and innervated by cranial nerves III, IV, and VI. When the movement of these muscles becomes impaired, vision is compromised.

Strabismus

Incidence and Etiology

Strabismus is a condition where the visual lines of each eye do not simultaneously focus on the same object in space because of a lack of muscle coordination, resulting in a crossed-eye appearance. Strabismus (Figure 31-11) occurs in 2–3% of all children. Approximately half of these children

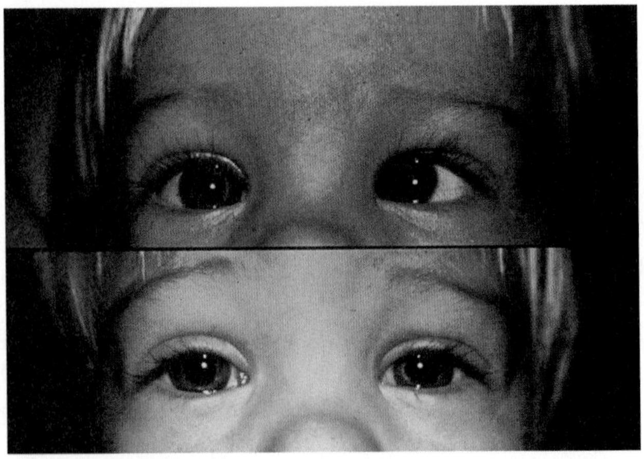

Figure 31-11 Child with Strabismus Before and After Corrective Treatment. Courtesy of the National Eye Institute.

have a positive family history for the defect. Pseudostrabismus is a condition that makes a child appear crossed-eyed because of prominent epicanthic folds and a flat nasal bridge. Pseudostrabismus disappears as the child grows, but true strabismus is not outgrown (Dreger, 1998).

Pathophysiology

When the extraocular muscles move the eyes in unison, the visual image falls on the fovea of each eye and the images fuse to form a single image. When one eye deviates (moves up, down, inward, or outward), the brain is unable to fuse the dissimilar images and double vision results. The brain will learn to suppress the image from the deviated eye (amblyopia) to allow clear sight in the straight eye. The earlier suppression begins and the longer it is allowed to continue, the more permanent the loss of vision (Huddleston, 1994).

Clinical Manifestations

Double vision in the older child causes the child to appear clumsy and to stumble or have difficulty picking up objects. The child may also squint to get a better image. Persistent crossing of the eyes is always abnormal regardless of the age of the client (Huddleston, 1994). Because of the potential loss of vision in the deviated eye, evaluation and treatment should begin as soon as possible, even as young as three months of age. If correction is not instituted before 6 years of age, reversal of the suppression of the image is difficult.

Diagnosis

Screening should begin at 3–6 months of age to prevent loss of vision from strabismus. There are two major screening tests to detect strabismus, the Hirschberg Corneal Light Reflex Test and the cover test. To perform the Hirschberg test, a light is held in front of the child's face as the child stares straight ahead. The light should reflect off the cornea symmetrically, just medially to the center of the pupil. The cover test is more sensitive than the light reflex test but requires the child's cooperation. As the child looks at a toy, the examiner covers one of the child's eyes. If the uncovered eye moves, then it can be assumed it was not fixed on the target simultaneously with the other eye, and, therefore, the child has strabismus. Strabismus is classified into three primary types as illustrated in Figure 31-12.

Esotropia (convergent) occurs when the eye turns toward the midline.

Exotropia (divergent) occurs when the eye turns outward or away from the midline.

Hypertropia occurs when the eyes are out of vertical alignment. One pupil appears higher than the other.

Treatment

The goal of treatment is to attain the best possible vision in each eye while also attaining binocular vision. The type of treatment varies with the age of the child and the type of strabismus. Treatment can be medical or surgical. The medical approach may utilize occlusion therapy (eye patching), glasses, pharmacologic therapy, or eye exercises. Surgical correction is typically utilized for infants less than 12–18 months of age when glasses and pharmocologic therapy do not work. Eye patching is used prior to surgery to stimulate the non-involved eye to function.

Patching the good eye is a common method of treatment. The stronger eye is covered to allow the weaker eye to work alone for all or part of each day, so it may become stronger. The duration of the therapy is determined by an ophthalmologist. Patching is most successful when done during the preschool years (American Academy of Ophthalmology, 1994). Eyeglasses with covered lenses are another method of occulsion. Pharmacologic therapy may utilize miotics (drugs that act on the ciliary muscle) to make accomodation easier. Another therapy is botulinum toxin (Botox, Oculinum), approved by the U.S. Food and Drug Administration in 1989 as an alternative to surgery. The toxin is injected into the eye muscle to produce temporary paralysis. This allows the muscles opposite the paralyzed muscle to straighten the eye. When the medication wears off in about two months the correction will be successful in 50% of clients. The most common side effect is a drooping eyelid, which resolves spontaneously (Dreger, 1998). Eye exercises may be prescribed in conjunction with patching and pharmacologic therapy.

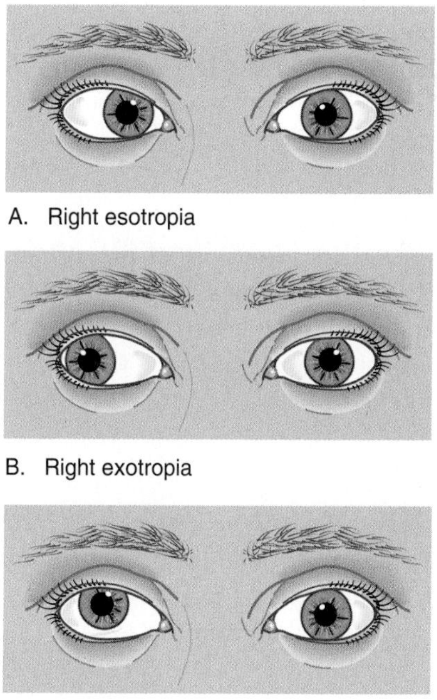

A. Right esotropia

B. Right exotropia

C. Hypertropia

Figure 31-12 (A) Right Esotropia, (B) Right Exotropia, (C) Hypertropia

Nursing Management

Assessment

The most important nursing responsibility is early identification of the child with strabismus. Children should be assessed during well-child visits and referred immediately if needed. The nurse must support the family in managing the prescribed therapy. If the child is in school, the treatment plan should be explained to the school nurse.

Nursing Diagnosis

1. Delayed growth and development related to impaired visual perception
2. Anxiety related to lack of knowledge about treatments used for strabismus.

Outcome Identification

1. The child will not experience any impairment of growth and development.
2. The child will wear patching as instructed.
3. Caregivers will report diminished anxiety related to the child's treatment.

Planning/Implementation

Education of the caregivers is essential if the prescribed therapy is to be successful as they must understand why patching or corrective lenses are necessary. The nurse must stress the importance of compliance in promoting normal visual development. Caregivers need help and support in order to ensure the child's compliance. If the child is going to have surgery, the nurse must prepare the family. Caregivers need to know surgery may correct alignment, but not vision. Families must also be prepared for the possibility that the surgery may not be successful and subsequent surgery may be necessary.

Evaluation

As a result of the consistent use of prescribed therapy the strabismus will resolve. If surgery is required, then the family will understand the potential outcomes of the surgery and incorporate postsurgical care into their daily lives until instructed otherwise.

Family Teaching

Children need to be taught how to take proper care of glasses. Caregivers and children must be provided with information about dressing changes, eyedrops, corrective lenses, eye patches, and restraints.

Amblyopia

Amblyopia is the chief cause of preventable visual loss in children. Early detection and referral to the ophthalmologist can avert permanent disability (Bacal & Hertle, 1998).

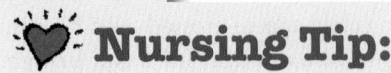

> **Nursing Tip:**
>
> **Care of eye patches**
>
> Suggest the following measures to maintain the treatment of eye patching:
>
> - Apply tincture of benzoin around the eye where the sticky part of the patch goes to improve adhesion.
> - If patch does not stay on, apply tape from the forehead to the cheek.
> - Another method to keep the patch on is to apply tincture of benzoin to the tape as well.
> - Wrap a bandage around the entire head and secure.
> - Encourage children to pretend they are pirates or monsters to encourage compliance.
> - When all else fails, restrict the child's ability to remove the patch by taping mittens on the hands of a young child. In older children, use cardboard tubes secured with gauze longitudinally around the elbows.
> - Remove the eye patch for 2 hours per day to minimize the risk of occlusion amblyopia in the good eye. Patches can be put on one hour after the child awakens and removed one hour before bedtime.
> - When child keeps patches on, use rewards, such as a trip to the park, to reinforce compliance.
> - If all methods to keep patch on fail, glasses with opaque lens may be utilized.

Incidence and Etiology

Amblyopia ("lazy eye") is a reduction or loss of vision in one eye unrelated to an organic cause. Approximately 2% to 3% of the population have amblyopia in the preschool years. The most common cause is strabismus, where the brain suppresses the vision in the deviated eye to avoid the double image it is receiving. Eventually, sight is lost from the deviated eye. Additional causes of amblyopia are congenital cataracts, corneal opacity, or prolonged patching of the eye to correct strabismus, and refractive amblyopia, which occurs when there is asymmetric refractive error in each eye. When both eyes are not equally hyperopic, the brain receives one clear image and one blurred image. Just as in strabismus, the image from the eye with the greater hyperopia will be suppressed (Bacal & Hertle, 1998).

Pathophysiology

During the first six months of life, the infant develops the ability to clearly perceive images seen through both eyes. The normal infant's brain merges the images from the two eyes, enabling binocular vision (i.e., two eyes seeing a single image). If the brain suppresses the vision in one eye, the lack of stimulation to the portion of the brain associated with the affected eye does not develop. The critical period for the visual center in the brain to develop is up until 6 to 7 years of age. The longer visual suppression is present, the less reversible it becomes. If detected after the age of 7 years, restoration of sight in the suppressed eye is unlikely (Kelsey, 1998).

Clinical Manifestations

Infants and young children with amblyopia often do not display any symptoms. However, they may occasionally develop a tendency to overreach for an object. Because of the lack of symptoms, and because amblyopia develops before the age of 7 years, tests for visual acuity should be part of routine health assessment for all young children.

Diagnosis

Unless strabismus with the obvious sign of crossed eyes is present to alert the professional, amblyopia is largely asymptomatic because the good eye assumes the burden of vision and the child is unaware there is a problem. Therefore, it is essential a child's eyes be examined periodically before the age of seven. If any difference in visual acuity between the two eyes is detected during routine screening, referral to an ophthalmologist for a detailed examination should be made as early detection is the key to treatment.

Treatment

The method of treatment is determined by the underlying cause. The underlying cause is always treated first, except when strabismus requires surgery, in which case the amblyopia is treated first (Kelsey, 1998). If cataracts are the cause, removal of cataracts and appropriate treatment are instituted. Refractive amblyopia is treated by correcting the refractive error with corrective lenses. The major treatment of amblyopia is occlusion of the good eye (occlusion therapy) to force vision in the "lazy eye."

Nursing Management

The screening of visual acuity to detect deficits during well-child visits in children younger than seven years of age is the primary nursing responsibility. The nurse should understand how to administer screening tests and be cognizant of physical signs and symptons of disorder.

Physical Integrity

Physical integrity problems occur when an alteration interferes with a child's vision. Cataracts and glaucoma are examples of such alterations.

Cataract

A **cataract** is an opacity (clouding) of the crystalline lens of the eye. Because light cannot pass through the opacity, vision is obscured.

Incidence and Etiology

Cataracts can be complete (entire lens is opaque) or incomplete (only part of the lens is opaque), bilateral or unilateral, or acquired or congenital. Acquired cataracts are caused by maternal infection during pregnancy, trauma, systemic disease, factors secondary to other eye malformations or diseases, or idiopathic factors. Congenital cataracts can be inherited as an autosomal dominant trait, caused by prenatal trauma, anoxia, or maternal systemic disease, or acquired through prenatal infection. The most frequent etiology of cataracts is congenital, which affects 1 out of 250 newborn infants (Behrman & Kliegman, 1998). The rubella virus was a primary cause of congenital cataracts in the past, but with widespread immunization, the incidence has decreased.

Pathophysiology

The lens capsule forms during the fourth and fifth weeks of fetal development. It is normally a clear membrane allowing light rays to enter the eye and refract the rays for a clear image on the retina. When an organism or other factors interfere with lens development, it becomes milky white and cloudy, obscuring light rays and thus vision. Figure 31-13 illustrates the appearance of a cataract.

Clinical Manifestations

The cloudiness of the lens is often visible to the naked eye. While checking pupils, an absent or abnormal reflex during a routine newborn examination is obtained. Caregivers might also notice their infant lacks visual attention to the environment or seems distressed in bright light. Nystagmus (oscillating movement of the eye) is a late sign.

Diagnosis

Infants with a family or prenatal history placing them at risk for cataracts should be assessed as soon after birth as possible. The cloudiness of the lens usually can be seen by the caregiver or the nurse with the naked eye, or when the nurse is checking pupils with a penlight and notices a white pupillary reflex and an absent or abnormal red reflex. Early identification is essential to prevent the suppression of development of the visual cortex in the brain, which occurs during the first two months of life.

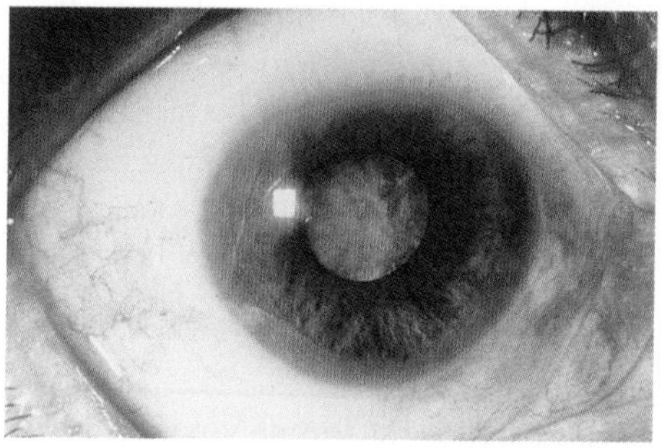

Figure 31-13 Cataract. Courtesy of the National Eye Institute.

Treatment

The definitive treatment is surgical removal of the cataract from the affected eye. Timing of surgery is crucial to prognosis. If cataracts are visually present at birth, surgery must take place before 8 weeks of age to prevent an irreversible lack of vision development. After removal of the lens, the infant is considered aphakic or without lens, and will need a corrective lens or contact lens to focus light on the retina. Intraocular lens implants have been used on some infants, but the long-term effects of permanent lens implants have not been established for infants. Because the developing eye will need frequent changes in corrective lenses, use of intraocular implants is not advised.

Nursing Management

Assessment

The nurse must assess the child and family's responses to the diagnosis and identified preoperative treatment. The nurse must also assess the caregiver's knowledge regarding the postoperative follow-up care (patching, eye medications, etc.) required.

Nursing Diagnosis

1. Anxiety related to the surgical procedure and the surgical outcome.
2. Deficient knowledge related to the postsurgical care.

Outcome Identification

1. Child will maintain a safe intraocular pressure.
2. Child will not develop an infection in the eyes.
3. Caregivers will be able to administer eye drops safely.
4. Caregiver will demonstrate aptitude in postsurgical care.

Planning/Implementation

In order to prevent an increase in intraocular pressure, the nurse must prevent the child from coughing, straining, or vomiting, with appropriate pain medication and comfort measures. The risk of infection can be minimized by using aseptic technique when handling dressings, and closely monitoring for signs of local or systemic infection. The nurse must instill the appropriate eye drops per the ordered schedule in order to prevent the complications of increased intraocular pressure, infection, and glaucoma. Care must be taken to not put pressure on the globe of the eye when instilling drops. To prevent edema and pressure on the eye, the nurse should not place the child with the affected eye in a dependent body position.

Family Teaching

Caregivers must be taught to safely perform the following postoperative care:

- Instillation of ordered eye drops
- Signs and symptoms of infection (drainage, redness, edema, itching)
- Signs and symptoms of increasing intraocular pressure (pain, bulging of eye)
- Care, purpose, and methods of maintaining eye patching

Glaucoma

Glaucoma is a rare but serious visual impairment that, if untreated, can potentially end in blindness.

Incidence and Etiology

Infantile (congenital) glaucoma occurs in children under 3 years of age, and although it can manifest itself in a child several months old, it is usually present at birth. Juvenile glaucoma affects children older than 3 years of age, and is usually secondary to some other disease process. The signs and symptoms are essentially the same for the two forms of glaucoma. Because juvenile glaucoma is similar to the adult form, the remainder of this discussion refers to infantile glaucoma. Infantile glaucoma occurs in 1 out of 10,000 live births, and is a disease where the intraocular fluid pressure of the eye is increased because of a defect in the drainage system of the eye (Grover, 2000a). This is usually caused by a developmental anomaly of the iridocorneal angle of the eye (also called trabeculodysgenesis).

Pathophysiology

Infantile glaucoma results from a defective development of the trabecular meshwork, which does not allow a sufficient amount of aqueous humor to drain out of the intraocular space. When the aqueous humor accumulates in the anterior chamber of the eye, increased intraocular pressure results. The pressure causes damage to the ganglion cells of the retina, leading to ischemia and necrosis of the optic disc, which may cause blindness (Grover, 2000b).

Clinical Manifestations

Clinical signs of glaucoma include excessive tearing (**epiphora**), involuntary closing of the eyelid, light sensitivity (**photophobia**), enlargement of the eyeball (**buphthalmos**), haziness or clouding of the cornea, and pain.

Diagnosis

Intraocular pressure of the eyes should be measured using tonometry. Normal intraocular pressure is 12 to 20 mm Hg. Measurement in the infant and young child often requires anesthesia. Assessment of corneal diameter and clarity, and an examination of the retina to assess for optic nerve cupping (damage reflecting pressure), should also be done.

Treatment

The definitive treatment is surgery (**goniotomy** or **trabeculotomy**) to open the outflow of the aqueous humor from the anterior chamber of the eye. It is essential to reduce the intraocular pressure as soon as possible (hours to days) in order to avoid cupping of the optic nerve. More than one surgical procedure is often necessary. Medications may temporarily improve the drainage pre- and postoperatively. However, topical anti-glaucoma drugs have been found to be generally ineffective in children.

Nursing Management and Family Teaching

The major postoperative nursing goals are management of intracoular pressure, management of pain, reducing fear and anxiety, and teaching the caregivers to manage care at home. Measures to prevent an increase in intraocular pressure are instituted (prevention of straining, crying, startling). Bilateral eye patches increase anxiety. Therefore, measures to decrease anxiety and encourage caregiver involvement are helpful. The nurse must teach the caregivers how to manage care at home after surgery. Elements to include are:

- Management of eye patches
- Signs of increasing intraocular pressure
- How to prevent increase in intraocular pressure
- How to instill eye drops
- Signs of infection
- Need for follow-up care and monitoring

Infections

Conjunctivitis

Conjunctivitis ("pinkeye") is an inflammation of the conjunctiva. Inflammation in and around the eye of infants and children is irritating to the child and can be frightening to the caregiver. This condition always requires attention and prompt treatment.

Incidence and Etiology

There are two types of conjunctivitis, neonatal conjunctivitis and childhood conjunctivitis. Neonatal conjunctivitis is caused by chemical irritation or infection. The incidence of neonatal conjunctivitis due to maternal chlamydial infection is 8:1000 live births (Grover, 2000c). Childhood conjunctivitis is caused by allergy or infection by bacterial or viral agents. The most common bacterial causes are *Haemophilus influenzae* and *Streptococcus pneumoniae* (Grover, 2000c).

Pathophysiology

In neonatal conjunctivitis, chlamydia and gonnococcus are spread to the newborn during passage through the birth canal. In childhood conjunctivitis, the child can be infected by either a bacteria or virus. Bacterial or viral conjunctivitis is highly contagious through contact with drainage from the eyes. Allergic conjunctivitis may arise in response to an allergen.

Clinical Manifestations

Signs and symptoms of conjunctivitis may include itching eyelids, burning, light sensitivity (photophobia), redness, edema, and discharge. The appearance of the discharge from the eye can assist in identifying the etiologic agent. When an allergy is the cause, the drainage is stringy. Bacterial drainage tends to be mucopurulent; viral drainage is watery (Grover, 2000c; Ruppert, 1996). Itching most often identifies the cause as an allergic response.

Diagnosis

Diagnosis is made primarily on the presentation of the clinical manifestations. A culture may be obtained on the drainage to confirm the diagnosis.

Treatment

In both neonatal or childhood conjunctivitis, identification of the etiologic agent is necessary to determine appropriate therapy. Antibiotic or antiviral eye drops or ointments are the common treatment of infectious conjunctivitis. Both are self-limiting conditions lasting approximately 1–2 weeks. In allergic conjunctivitis, treatment is symptomatic. Cool eye compresses, oral antihistamines, and Crolom ophthalmic solution will bring some comfort (Grover 2000c; Ruppert, 1996).

Nursing Management

If the conjunctivitis is allergic or viral in origin, the nursing management is primarily comfort measures, such as cold compresses on the eyes, reduced lighting, preventing rubbing of the eye, acetominophen for discomfort, and Crolom before allergy season (no effect on active inflammation). Conjunctivitis caused by bacterial agents is treated with appropriate antibiotic eye ointments applied from the inner to the outer canthus, the use of baby shampoo to soften and remove crusting, or the use of dark glasses for photophobia (Ruppert, 1996).

Family Teaching

Caregivers must be taught how to prevent transferring the extremely contagious drainage by following some simple steps:

- Use good handwashing after touching the eye.
- Use a separate towel, washcloth, sheets, and pillowcases.
- Don't allow the medicine dropper to touch the child's eyelid during medication administration.
- Use elbow restraints (infants or young children) to prevent rubbing of the eyes.
- Use Kleenex on each individual eye and discard after use.

- Discard old lenses and use new ones after the infection resolves.
- Discard old eye makeup, utilize new containers after the infection resolves.

The child will be excluded from school or day care until the infection is resolved, even though the child is not communicable after 24 to 48 hours of treatment.

Periorbital Cellulitis

Periorbital cellulitis is an infection of the eyelid and soft tissues of the orbit of the eye.

Etiology

Periorbital cellulitis can be caused by extension of infection from the sinuses or face, otitis media, upper respiratory infections, insect bites, or trauma.

Pathophysiology

Most often precipitated by organisms from wounds or infections elsewhere in the body (Powell, 1995), the most common causative organisms are *Staphylococcus aureus*, *Escherichia coli, group B streptococci, H. influenzae*, and *Staphylococcus pneumoniae* (Grover, 2000c).

Clinical Manifestations

Many of the same symptoms of conjunctivitis are exhibited in periorbital cellulitis, such as edema, warmth and tenderness of the eyelid. Other symptoms that may be present are malaise, fever, elevated WBC count, decreased vision, and painful and reduced movement of the eyeball.

Diagnosis

Diagnosis is made by close inspection and a culture of the drainage. Because sinusitis may be present, X rays of the paranasal sinuses are also recommended.

Treatment

Intravenous antibiotics are usually the treatment of choice. The antibiotic used depends on the causative organism. Broad-spectrum antibiotics such as Ceftriazone (Rocephin), or Naficillin (Nafcil) are utilized for a 10-day period. It is important to treat the cellulitis, because if untreated, the infection can spread to the optic nerve or the brain, causing meningitis. Analgesics may be given for the pain (Grover, 2000c).

Nursing Management

The nurse monitors the administration of the intravenous antibiotics and analgesics. Warm soaks to the eyes 3 to 4 times per day may increase comfort. The cellulitis usually resolves without complication after antibiotic therapy is completed.

Sensorineural Blindness

The inability of a child to see presents a great challenge in achieving normal growth and development milestones. An interdisciplinary team and early intervention are necessary to ensure a child attains his or her maximum potential.

Incidence and Etiology

A child is considered **blind** when other senses (hearing and touch) are relied upon as a chief means of task performance and learning (Holbrook, 1996). Legal blindness is defined as visual acuity of 20/200 or less with correction, or peripheral fields narrowed to an angle of 20 degrees or less. The legal definition must be verified by physical examination and determines eligibility for many rehabilitation programs. Approximately 5,000 cases of legal blindness are diagnosed in children younger than 20 years of age each year. Approximately 50% of the children who are visually impaired have concurrent disabilities. Blindness can result from any of the hereditary and acquired disorders noted in previous sections.

Pathophysiology

Damage to the optic nerve and/or the visual center of the brain prevent the child from using vision to explore the world.

Clinical Manifestations

Blind children have lost one of their most essential senses and must learn alternative ways to interact with their environment. Blindness may have an impact on every area of development, such as attachment, motor ability, mobility, language, learning, play, socialization, independence, self-concept, perception of space, and body image.

Diagnosis

Visual acuity tests, neurological tests and other diagnostic tests appropriate for specific etiologies are utilized to diagnose sensorineural blindness.

Treatment

The blind child will require the assistance of a multitude of specially trained individuals in order to develop normally. Specialized training and adaptation of the early environment are essential to alter the impact of blindness in all areas of development. Special technologies are now available to assist the blind child adapt to the environment. Technologies such as braille (a system of raised dots that represent numbers and letters) to assist in reading a message (Figure 31-14), and a braillewriter to write a message are useful. A tape recorder or a computer with a voice synthesizer can be used when the person being communicated with does not understand braille. The tape recorder can also be used for notetaking and listening to books on tape. With the visually-impaired child,

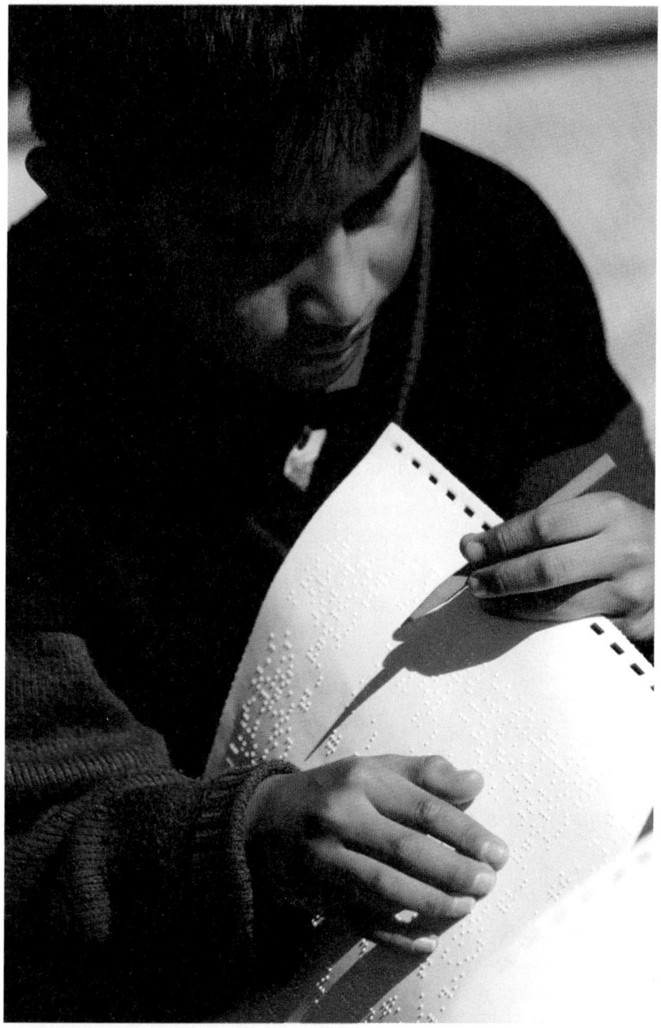

Figure 31-14 This young man takes a test in braille. Digital imagery © copyright 2001, PhotoDisc, Inc.

devices such as corrective lenses, magnifiers, large print books, magnified video projection systems, and tape recorders may also be helpful.

Families also need to understand the process of developing attachment to blind children and may require some adaptation in parenting behavior. When a child is blind, the usual facial interplay conveying emotion and communication between caregiver and child is impaired. The blind infant can develop attachment but usually does so more slowly (Moller, 1993). Fraiberg (1975) described a program that teaches caregivers to look for cues (other than visual) that suggest the infant is responding to them, for example, blinking of eyes, hand movements, and changes in activity level. Caregivers are also encouraged to show affection through nonvisual means, such as talking, cuddling, rocking, and so forth.

Self-initiated mobility is delayed about 4 months in blind infants (Espezel, 1994). Because the blind infant does not have the stimulus of reaching to encourage mobility, the child must be stimulated by the use of sound. Delay will still occur as sound is not as strong a stimulus as sight. Although the child is physically ready to be mobile, the functional delay causes frustration, which results in some children exhibiting physical signs of frustration termed "**blindisms,**" (for example, rocking and swaying) until the task is mastered. As a blind child becomes mobile, caregivers must make the environment safe as mobility is essential to later independence. Children are usually taught to walk by professionals known as orientation and mobility instructors. As the child becomes mobile, play takes on a new dimension. Blind children do not learn to play by imitation or active exploration, so they must be stimulated (especially by touch) and taught to play. Caregivers will need assistance in selecting toys and methods to teach the child how to play in order to develop their gross and fine motor skills. Socialization needs of blind children are the same as for other children.

Promoting independence in activities of daily living is also important so the child will develop a positive self-concept. Caregivers need to be patient and persistent when teaching activities of daily living, and focus on the child's abilities, not the child's disabilities. Guidelines for caregivers and nurses include:

- When describing the environment, use words that are familiar to the child.
- Call the child by name and identify yourself before touching child.
- Keep objects in the environment in the same location, that is furniture, toys, and so forth.
- Utilize natural environmental cues to orient the child to associated event—for example, keys = time to go for ride, water running = time for a bath.
- Do not overprotect the child; allow the child to gain self-confidence.
- A multidisciplinary team, together with the family, must collaborate to assist the child to gain optimum independence.

Eye Trauma

Children are more likely than adults to sustain eye trauma. Therefore, it is important to institute every possible measure to prevent injury that may cause transient or permanent loss of vision.

Incidence and Etiology

Trauma is the leading cause of blindness in children, with boys being twice as likely to sustain injury as girls. Boys between 11 and 15 years of age are the most vulnerable (McGrory, 1997). Injuries to the eyeball and adjacent structures are classified as *penetrating* and *nonpenetrating*. Penetrating injuries are usually the result of sharp objects such as scissors, forks, sticks, knives, screwdrivers, pencils, and BBs.

Case Study/Care Plan

Visual Impairment

Karl is a 5-year-old child with sensorineural blindness admitted to the hospital for a hernia repair. Karl is legally blind and has had specialized training to adapt to his visual limitation. His growth and development are delayed. The family reports they are having some difficulty assisting Karl integrate into the family and meet developmental tasks. You are the nurse admitting him to the pediatric unit. The nursing care plan is limited only to his visual impairment.

Nursing Care Plan

Assessment The nurse should identify what difficulties the family is having integrating Karl into the family and the feelings both Karl and his family have. Information as to where Karl is developmentally must also be obtained.

Nursing Diagnosis #1

Risk for injury related to visual perceptual alteration.

Expected Outcomes

1. Karl will move confidently within his environment.
2. Karl will not experience any injuries when ambulating independently.

Interventions/*Rationales*

1. Describe the environment in words familiar to Karl. *The child needs orientation to the layout of the room to navigate safely.*
2. Keep objects in the environment in the same location. *Enables child to move within room independently.*
3. Call Karl by name and identify yourself before touching. *This avoids frightening Karl and gives him a chance to control his own environment.*
4. Encourage the family to re-enroll Karl in special programs for the blind as soon as possible. *Enables Karl to learn skills to ambulate safely.*

Evaluation

Caregivers talk about their concern for Karl's safety and development. Karl moves confidently through his environment without injury.

Nursing Diagnosis #2

Delayed growth and development related to visual perceptual alteration.

Expected Outcomes

1. Karl will maintain or increase his level of development through play activities.
2. Karl will display acceptable behavior and tolerate frustration.

Interventions/*Rationales*

1. Explain the day's activities early in morning. *Enables Karl to anticipate which activities will require assistance and which can be managed independently.*
2. Offer Karl choices and ask for his help in arranging the day's schedule. *Allows Karl to have some control and promote self-reliance.*
3. Anticipate that all tasks will take more time for Karl. *Karl needs detailed description of how to perform new activities and must move slowly to remain safe.*
4. Guide the family to select play material and activities that are suitable for visually impaired children. *Select activities that stimulate motor development and stimulate the senses of hearing and touch.*

continues

continued

5. Discuss the importance of consistent limit-setting. *To assist learning acceptable behavior and tolerating frustration.*

6. Encourage Karl to play with other children on unit. *This will encourage socialization.*

Evaluation

Karl receives adequate stimulation to keep his growth and development moving in an acceptable direction.

Nursing Diagnosis #3

Interrupted family processes related to Karl's visual alteration.

Expected Outcomes

1. Caregivers will express their feelings regarding Karl's impaired vision.
2. Caregivers will express an understanding of Karl's unique abilities and special needs.
3. Karl will express feelings regarding his sight.
4. Caregiver and Karl will exhibit a positive relationship

Interventions/*Rationales*

1. Assist the family to gain a realistic concept of Karl's abilities. *Enables caregivers to encourage Karl to attain optimum level of development.*
2. Be available to the family for assistance. *Family will express problems and seek help when needed.*
3. Encourage and reinforce rehabilitation efforts for Karl. *Assists Karl to gain optimal level of independence.*
4. Demonstrate Karl's acceptance by example. *Assists the family to accept Karl in a positive manner.*
5. Encourage Karl and siblings to discuss their feelings regarding the disability. *Assists in positive reinforcement.*
6. Discuss the importance of grief and of chronic sorrow. *Helps them function in a healthier fashion.*

Evaluation

The family feels comfortable and confident in accepting Karl's blindness and fosters his confidence and positive self-esteem.

Nonpenetrating injuries are usually caused by foreign objects, such as blows from a blunt object (ball, fist, airbag), or thermal or chemical burns. A blow from the hand or foot of another child is the most frequent cause of traumatic injury to the eye. The baseball continues to be a common cause of sports-related eye injuries. **Hyphema,** a hemorrhage into the anterior chamber of the eye, is a major complication of a blow to the eye. Chemical burns of the cornea are among the most serious eye injuries; alkali burns are more destructive than acid burns because alkali damages cell membranes and allows continuing penetration of alkali into the eye (Hooper, 1997). Foreign bodies in the eye need to be removed carefully to avoid corneal abrasions and danger of an infection. Exposure to ultraviolet rays from the sun can cause solar retinopathy, cataracts, and age-related macular degeneration. Light-colored eyes are more sensitive than dark-colored eyes.

Emergency Treatment

All treatment is focused on preventing further damage to the eye as a complication of the traumatic injury. Immediate and appropriate treatment at the scene can make a critical difference in the extent and the permanence of the injury. Although the goal of treatment remains the same, once the child arrives at the hospital, the primary responsibility for care is in the hands of the ophthalmologist or eye surgeon. Nurses should understand and assist with treatment. See Box 31-9 and Box 31-10 for further information.

BOX 31-9 Care of penetrating eye injuries

At the Scene

Do not remove object.
Secure the object with tape to prevent movement.
Cover uninjured eye to limit eye movement.
Caution child against rubbing the eye.
Transport child to the emergency room.

At the Hospital

Sedate child.
Remove object using aseptic technique.
Observe for aqueous or vitreous leaks, hemorrhage, prolapsed iris (not perfectly circular), pupils (shape, equality, and reaction to light), intraocular pressure, emphysema (air within orbit).
Administer prophylactic antibiotics.
Place an eye patch over the eye.
Elevate head 30 degrees.
Check immunization status of child, give tetanus if necessary.

BOX 31-10 Care of nonpenetrating eye injuries

Foreign Body

At the Scene

Evert upper eyelid to look for foreign body; remove object with wet corner of a cotton swab.
Caution child against rubbing the eye.
If the eye irritation continues (continued blinking and tearing, pain, photophobia), take child to emergency room.

At the Hospital

Observe and treat hemorrhage or corneal abrasion (see below).

Corneal Abrasion

At the Scene

Attempt to remove foreign object from eye (as above).

At the Hospital

Carefully examine eye for any abrasion (scraping of the cornea), using a fluorescein dye and visualizing injury under a blue filtered light (Wood's lamp or slit lamp.)
If the abrasion is small, instillation of antibiotic ointment four times per day is sufficient. If the abrasion is large, patching the eye for 24 hours, followed by instillation of antibiotic drops will be necessary (Wingate, 1999).

Hyphema

At the Scene

Place eye patch over injured eye.
Caution child not to move the head.
Transport child to the emergency room.

At the Hospital

Determine amount of bleeding into the anterior chamber and intraocular pressure.
Both eyes should be patched and the child placed on bedrest in the hospital with the head elevated 30 degrees to reduce mobility. (This will control further bleeding into the eye and prevent increase in intraocular pressure.)
Cycloplegic (causing paralysis of the ciliary muscles of the eye) medications are administered to prevent movement of eye and to assist in reabsorption of blood.
Close monitoring of the child to ensure bleeding does not recur and intraocular pressure does not increase is essential.

continues

BOX 31-10 *Continued*

Chemical Burns

At the Scene

Irrigate eye with water or saline from the inner to outer canthus.

Transport immediately to the emergency room.

At the Hospital

Continue irrigation for 30 minutes if minor and 2 to 4 hours if severe.

If chemical is unknown, use pH paper to determine if is an acid or alkali. (pH paper also can be used after irrigation to check if it is normal.)

Administer cycloplegic drugs (will decrease eye movement and pain).

Patch eye (will decrease eye movement and pain).

Administer antibiotic drops.

Monitor for inflammatory response and intraocular pressure readings.

Ultraviolet Rays

At the Scene

If skin is burned, close and patch the eyes, secure eye patches with a bandage wrapped around the head.

Transport to the emergency room.

At the Hospital

Cold compresses can be applied to eyelids to decrease swelling.

Eyes must be examined to ascertain whether damage is more than just to the skin of eyelids.

Nursing Alert:

Eye Abrasions

Failure to treat an abrasion may result in corneal ulceration, infection, or permanent scarring and loss of visual acuity.

Topical anesthetics should never be used because they can retard healing and may mask painful symptoms of an infected abrasion.

Eye On:

Traditional Methods of Maintaining Health

A traditional Chinese practice is to prepare amulets (a charm with an idol or chinese character painted in red or black ink and written on a strip of yellow paper) to prevent evil spirits from causing them harm in the belief that children are kept safe with charms. Be sure whenever caring for a child who is wearing an amulet that you acknowledge its importance and integrate its use into practice.

Nursing Management

The primary goals after injury are to institute immediate treatment for an eye injury in order to prevent further damage to the eye (at the scene), to continually monitor the injured child to detect complications after initial treatment (at the hospital), to support the frightened child and family, and to teach management of injury and prevention of future injuries.

Eye injury statistics reveal a great need to educate caregivers, teachers, and coaches on the methods of prevention. Family and community education are a primary nursing role. As children grow and become mobile, the environment must be assessed for potential dangers and the child safeguarded. Chemicals such as cleaning and gardening products should be kept away from young children. Small objects that can be inserted into the nose, ear, and eye must be kept from the infant and toddler. If children play with sharp objects (such as scissors) and toys, they must be developmentally ready and supervised. Caregivers should be reminded of the dangers of glass (windows, doors, drinking) in the household.

In addition, many sports injuries can be avoided by the use of safety equipment. High-risk sports (those where no eye protection can be worn such as boxing, wrestling, martial arts), those using a rapidly moving ball or puck (baseball, basketball, hockey, racquet sports), or those involving aggressive body contact (football) are especially dangerous. The highest percentage of injuries occurs in the sports of baseball and basketball. To prevent some injuries, polycarbonate goggles should be worn in sports that do not require a helmet or face mask; goggles should be worn under helmets for the hockey goalie and the baseball batter.

Reflective Thinking

Prevention of Sports-related Injuries to the Eye

Although sports injuries occur in all age groups, far more children and adolescents incur eye injuries than adults. The greater number of children participating in high-risk sports, their athletic immaturity, and the practice of wearing inadequate or no eye protection, puts children and adolescents at greater risk for sports-related eye injuries. Although suitable eye protection exists for high-risk sports such as baseball, hockey, lacrosse, and racquet sports, children typically do not wear protective eyewear. Most of the traumatic eye injuries resulting in pain, decreased visual acuity, or permanent loss of vision could be prevented.

What do you think are the reasons these preventive measures are not taken?

What can you as a nurse or as a caregiver do to change this dangerous practice?

Can professional athletes, for example, Karem Abdul Jabbar, serve as role models for children?

Exposure to ultraviolet rays from the sun has caused solar retinopathy, cataracts, and age-related macular degeneration. Caregivers should be encouraged to have their children use sunglasses when exposed to the sun long enough to get a tan or a sunburn, or when in increased UV exposure situations such as beaches, snowfields, or high altitudes (Wagner, 1995). Some guidelines according to Wagner (1995) for selection of effective sunglasses are found in Box 31-11.

BOX 31-11 Sunglass guidelines

- Labeled with "99% UV protection" = "meets ANSI UV requirements"
- Labeled with "100% UV protection" = "absorption up to 400 nm"
- Polarization reduces glare but has no relation to UV absorption
- Darkness of lens has no relation to protective capacity

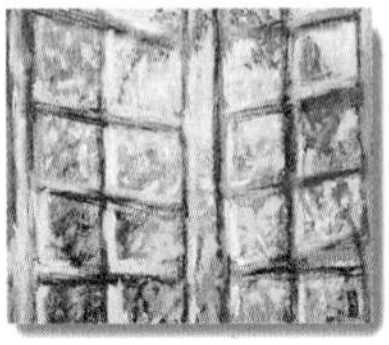

In the Real World

My experiences with Helen helped me to realize that each client requires critical thinking on my part to recognize his or her needs and individualize his or her care. Nurses must gather information about patient history, diagnosis, and present illness and then incorporate (organize, analyze) it into meaningful care. Because of her extensive medical experience, Lydia (mother) required far less general teaching and far more precise information. As nurses then, we need to adapt to schedules already established rather than trying to create our own for them. We need to be flexible and creative and help to make the hospital environment as normal as possible for the child and family. (Written in response to caring for a child diagnosed at an early age with sensorineural blindness and hearing loss who had been admitted to the hospital frequently for treatment and surgery.)

All sensory alterations have an impact on growth, development, and learning to some degree. The nurse can alter the degree of impact by accurate and timely assessment and appropriate referral to other disciplines for intervention that will enhance the child's and the family's adaptation and enable the attainment of optimal growth and development.

Key Concepts

- Any alteration in a child's sensory perception or communication will affect growth and development.
- Early identification and intervention can prevent some detrimental effects of sensory alterations.
- Optimal language development is influenced by cognitive ability, temperament, language, environment, and intact auditory and visual senses.
- Language disorders can be either receptive or expressive.
- Speech disorders may be caused by problems with voice, articulation, or fluency.
- Stuttering is the most common speech disorder. It may disappear as children mature.
- Hearing disorders may be classified as conductive, sensorineural, mixed, or central.
- Prevention of hearing loss includes genetic counseling, prenatal care, prompt treatment of infection, immunizations, cautious use of ototoxic drugs, auditory screening, and protection from excessive decibel levels.
- Refractive errors are the most common type of visual disorders in children.
- Strabismus is the most common cause of amblyopia.

- Cataracts must be surgically removed no later than 17 weeks of age to prevent an irreversible lack of vision development.
- It is essential to identify and reduce intraocular pressure immediately to avoid cupping of the optic nerve in a child with infantile glaucoma.
- Trauma is the leading cause of blindness in children.
- Nursing goals include early detection of impairment, assisting the child and family to adjust to the impairment, promoting parent-child attachment, referring to specialized training personnel, providing parent education and the opportunity for play and socialization, and fostering optimum development.

Review Questions

1. What is the difference between normal nonfluency and stuttering?
2. What would you include in a teaching plan to assist caregivers to enhance normal language acquisition?
3. What are the recommended practices encouraging bilingual language development in the young child?
4. What are the signs of visual and hearing impairment in children (infancy through adolescence)?
5. What are the leading causes of visual and hearing impairment in children?
6. What are the guidelines that caregivers and nurses can utilize to enhance independence in daily living for blind children?
7. What is the most important role of the nurse in relation to hearing and visual loss?

References

American Academy of Ophthalmology. (1994). Strabismus: Etiology, diagnosis, and treatment. *Journal of Opthalmic Nursing and Technology, 13*(3), 121–123.

American Academy of Pediatrics, Committee on Practice of Ambulatory Medicine, Section on Ophthalmology. (1996). Eye examination and vision screening in infants, children, and young adults. *Pediatrics, 98*(1), 153–157.

American Speech-Language-Hearing Association. (1994). Joint committee on infant hearing: 1994 Position statement. *American Speech-Language-Hearing Association Journal, 36*(12), 38–41.

Bacal, D., & Hertle, R. (1998). Don't be lazy about looking for amblyopia. *Contemporary Pediatrics, 15*(6), 99–100, 103–107.

Behrman, R., and Kliegman, R. (1998). *Nelson's Textbook of Pediatrics*, 3rd ed. Philadelphia: Saunders.

Brogan, J. (1999). Listen to this: Our noisy society is deafening us. *Providence Journal Bulletin*, M 1–2.

Conture, E. (1996). Treatment efficacy: Stuttering. *Journal of Speech and Hearing Research, 39*(5), 18–26.

Coplan, J. (1995). Normal speech and language development: An overview. *Pediatric Review, 16*(3), 91–100.

Dowling, C. (1994). Differentiating normal speech dysfluency from stuttering in children. *Nurse Practitioner, 19*(2), 30–35.

Dreger, V. (1998). Detection and treatment of strabismus. *Insight, 23*(3), 95–101.

Espezel, H. (1994). The visually impaired child. *Canadian Nurse, 90*(5), 1–7.

Fraiberg, S. (1975). Intervention in infancy: A program for blind infants. In B. Z. Friedlander, G. M. Sterritt, & G. E. Kirk (Eds.), *Exceptional infant, 3: Assessment and intervention* (pp. 40–62). New York: Brunner/Mazel.

Gatty, J. (1996). Early intervention and management of hearing in infants and toddlers. *Infants and Young Children, 9*(1), 1–15.

Gauzer, B. (1997, June 1). Can light be dangerous for babies? *The Providence Journal-Bulletin*, p.4, Parade Magazine.

Goldstein, B. (1993). Articulation disorders. *American Speech Language Hearing Association, 35*(11), 55–56.

Gottwald, S., & Starkweather, C. (1995). Fluency intervention for preschoolers and their families in the public schools. *Language, Speech and Hearing Services in Schools, 26*(2), 117–126.

Grover, G. (2000a). Language development: Speech and hearing assessment. In C. Berkowitz (Ed.), *Pediatrics: A primary care approach.* (2nd ed., pp. 54–58). Philadelphia: Saunders.

Grover, G. (2000b). Excessive Tearing. In C. Berkowitz (Ed.), *Pediatrics: A primary care approach.* (2nd ed. pp. 248–251). Philadelphia: Saunders.

Grover, G. (2000c). Infections of the eye. In C. Berkowitz (Ed.), *Pediatrics: A primary care approach.* (2nd ed., pp. 243–248). Philadelphia: Saunders.

Hess, L. (1999). Let's talk and play: A study of poverty mothers and toddler daughters. *Infant Toddler Intervention Transdisciplinary Journal, 9*(1), 1–16.

Holbrook, M. (Ed.). (1996). *Children with visual impairments: A parents' guide.* Bethesda, MD: Woodbine House, Inc.

Holmes, A., Kaplan, H., Phillips, R., Kemker, F., Weber, F., & Isart, F. (1997). Screening for hearing loss in adolescents. *Language Speech and Hearing Services in Schools, 28*(1), 70–76.

Hooper, M. (1997). Prompt treatment for chemical eye injuries. *Nursing Standard, 11*(36), 40–43.

Huddleston, K. (1994). Strabismus repair in the pediatric patient. *AORN Journal 60*(5), 754–755, 757–760.

Kelsey, A. (1998). Amblyopia: The condition, the challenge and the cure. *Journal of Ophthalmic Nursing and Technology, 17*(6), 227–229.

Lederberg, A., & Everhart, V. (1998). Communication between deaf children and their hearing mothers: The role of language, gesture and vocalization. *Journal of Speech, Language, and Hearing Research, 41*(4), 887–899.

McGlothlin, M., & Loera, B. (1994). Speech-language development in bilingual children: What to look for. *Texas Child Care, 18*(1), 2–7.

McGrory, A. (1997). Eye injuries: A review of the literature with nursing implications. *International Journal of Nursing Studies, 34*(2), 87–92.

Mills, B. (1997, May 22). Children are natural polyglots; Just be sure to keep the languages separate. *The Providence Journal-Bulletin*, p.13.

Moller, M. (1993). Working with visually impaired children and their families. *Pediatric Clinics of North America, 40*(4), 881–889.

Naeem, Z., & Newton, V. (1996). Prevalence of sensorineural hearing loss in Asian children. *British Journal of Audiology, 30*(5), 332–339.

National Information Center for Children and Youth with Disabilities. (1996). *Deafness and hearing loss.* (Special Education Programs Publication No. H030A30003) Washington, DC: U.S. Government Printing Office.

Oller, D., Eilers, R., Urbano, R., & Cobo-Lewis, A. (1997). Development of precursors to speech in infants exposed to two languages. *Journal of Child Language, 24*(2), 407–425.

Powell, K. (1995). Orbital and periorbital cellulitis. *Pediatrics in Review, 16*(5), 163–167.

Pronovost, A. (1999). From silence to sound. *Your Health*, Summer, 1999, p 14–15.

Rajotte, C. (1997). Protect those ears before it is your loss. *Kansas Nurse, 72* (7), 3–4.

Rouch, J., & Matkin, N. (Eds.) (1994). *Infants and toddlers with hearing loss.* Baltimore: York Press, Inc.

Ruppert, S. (1996). Differential diagnosis of pediatric conjunctivitis (red eye). *Nurse Practitioner, 21*(7), 12-26.

Rustin, L., & Cook, F. (1995). Parental involvement in the treatment of stuttering. *Language Speech Hearing Services in Schools, 26*(2), 127–137.

Ryan, J. (1996). Pediatric primary care vision examination. *Optometry Clinics, 5*(2), 1–34.

Ryan, M. (1997, July 20). A simple test to make sure baby can hear. *Parade Magazine*, p. 14.

Sarant, J. (1993). The effect of handedness in tactile speech perception. *Journal of Rehabilitation Research, 30*, 423–435.

Seewald, R., & Gagne, J. (1995). Approaches to hearing aid fitting in infants and young children. *Volta-Review, 97*(3), 161–173.

Shriberg, L., Gruber, F., & Kwiatkowski, J. (1994). Developmental phonological disorders: long-term speech-sound normalization. *Journal of Speech Hearing Research, 37*(5), 1151–1177.

Simons, R. (1987). *After the tears: Parents talk about raising a child with a disability*. New York: Harcourt, Brace, Jovanovich.

Taylor, C. (1999). An examination of the development of language in the normal child. *Journal of Child Health Care, 3*(1), 35–38.

Tomblin, J., Spencer, L., Flock, S., Tyler, R., & Gantz, B. (1999). A comparison of language achievement in children with cochlear implants and children using hearing aids. *Journal of Speech, Language, and Hearing Research, 42*(2), 497–511.

United States Department of Education. (1996). *Report on special services*. Washington, DC: Government Printing Office.

Wagner, R. (1995). Why children should wear sunglasses. *Patient Care, 29*, 178–182.

Wessel, H. (1997, July 23). Laser improves surgery for near-sighted. *The Providence Journal-Bulletin*, p. E3.

Weston, M. (1995). *What about me? A practicum addressing the needs of children who have a preschool sibling with impaired hearing*. Florida: Ed.D. Practicum, Nova Southeastern University.

Wilkenfeld, J., & Curlee, R. (1997). The relative effects of questions and comments on children's stuttering. *American Journal of Speech-Language Pathology, 6*(3), 79–89.

Wingate, S. (1999). Treating corneal abrasions. *Nurse Practitioner, 24*(6), 53–60.

Zahr, L., & Balian, S. (1995). Responses of premature infants to routine nursing interventions and noise in the NICU. *Nursing Research, 44*,(3), 179–185.

Suggested Readings

Castiglia, P.T. (1994). Strabismus. *Journal of Pediatric Health Care, 8*(5), 236–238.

Coplan, J. (1987). Deafness: Ever heard of it? Delayed recognition of permanent hearing loss. *Pediatrics, 79*(2), 206–212.

Friendly, D. (1993). Development of vision in infants and young children. *Pediatric Clinics of North America, 40*(4), 693-703.

Jones, G. (1998). Foreign bodies in the eye. *Accident and Emergency Nursing, 6*(2), 66–69.

Jurkus, J. (1996). Contact lenses for children. *Optometry Clinics, 5*(2), 91–104.

King, R.A. (1993). Common ocular signs and symptoms in childhood. *Pediatric Clinics of North America, 40*(4), 753–766.

Kutschke, P. (1994). Ocular trauma in children. *Journal of Ophthalmic Nursing & Technology, 13*(3), 117–120.

Lie, L., Runyan, C., Petridou, E., & Chang, A. (1994). American Public Health Association (American Academy of Pediatrics Injury Prevention Standards). *Pediatrics, 94*(6:2), 1046–1048.

Lieberth, A. (1988). *Degrees of hearing loss.* Boston: Communications Skill Builders, Inc.

National Institutes of Health (1993). Early identification of hearing impairment in infants and young children: Summary of the NIH consensus. *Pennsylvania Nurse, 48*(7), 14.

North American Nursing Diagnosis Association. (2001). Nursing diagnosis: Definitions and classifications 2001–2002). Philadelphia: Author.

Spires, R. (1995). Traumatic hyphema. *Journal of Ophthalmic Nursing and Technology, 14*(1), 21–4,40–1.

Stylianos, S., & Eichelberger, M. (1993). Pediatric trauma, prevention strategies. *Pediatric Clinics of North America, 40* (6), 1359–1367.

Trobe, J.D. (1993). *The physician's guide to eye care.* San Francisco: American Academy of Ophthalmology.

Resources

Organizations and Websites

Blindness

American Foundation for the Blind Information Center
11 Penn Plaza, Ste. 300
New York, NY 10001
(212) 502-7600
(800) AFB-LINE (800-232-5463)
E-mail: afbinfo@afb.net
www.afb.org

American Printing House for the Blind
P.O. Box 6085
Louisville, KY 40206-0085
(800) 223-1839
www.aph.org

The Blind Children's Center
4120 Marathon Street
Los Angeles, CA 90029
(323) 664-2153

The Foundation Fighting Blindness
11435 Cronhill Drive
Owings Mills, MD 21117-2220
(410) 785-1414
(888) 394-3937
TDD: (800) 683-5551
Local TDD: (410) 785-9687
www.blindness.org

National Association for Parents of Children with Visual Impairments
P.O. Box 317
Watertown, MA 02471
(800) 562-6265
(617) 972 7441
(617) 972-7444
www.spedex.com/napvi

National Eye Institute
2020 Vision Place
Bethesda, MD 20892-3655
(301) 496-5248
www.nei.nih.gov

National Federation of the Blind
1800 Johnson Street
Baltimore, MD 21230
(410) 659-9314
www.nfb.org

Hearing Impairment

Alexander Graham Bell Association of the Deaf & Hard of Hearing
2000 M Street, NW, Suite 740
Washington, DC 20036
(202) 337-5220
TTY: (202) 337-5221
E-mail: agbell2@aol.com

American Academy of Audiology
8300 Greensboro Dr., Ste. #750
McLean, VA 22102
800-AAA-2336
Fax (703) 790-8631
www.audiology.org

American Deafness Association
P.O. Box 555369
Little Rock, AR 72225

American Society for Deaf Children
P.O. Box 3355
Gettysburg, PA 17325
(800) 942-2732
TTY: (717) 334-7922
www.deafchildren.org

National Association for the Deaf
814 Thayer Avenue
Silver Spring, MD 20910-4500
(301) 587-1788
TTY: (301) 587-1789

National Deaf Education Network & Clearinghouse
Laurent Clerc Deaf Education Center
Gallaudet University
800 Florida Avenue N.E.
Washington, DC 20002-3695
(202) 651-5051
TTY: (202) 651-5052
www.clercenter.gallaudet.edu

National Institute on Deafness and Other Communication Disorders
Disorders Clearing House
31 Center Drive, MSC 2320
Bethesda, MD 20892-2320
(800) 241-1044
TTY: (800) 241-1055
www.nidcd.nih.gov

Self Help for Hard of Hearing People
7910 Woodmont Avenue, Ste. 1200
Bethesda, MD 20814
(301) 657-2248
TTY: (301) 657-2249
www.shhh.org

Speech and Language

American Speech-Language-Hearing Association
10801 Rockville Pike
Rockville, MD 20852
(800) 638-8255
www.asha.org

National Easter Seal Society
70 East Lake Street
Chicago, IL 60601
(800) 221-6827

Stuttering Foundation of America
P.O. Box 11749
Memphis, TN 38111-0749
(800) 992-9392
www.stuttersfa.org

CHAPTER 32

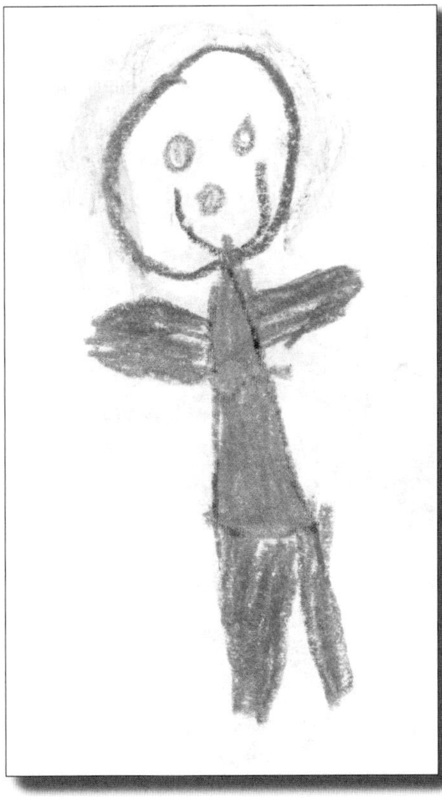

We love Luke so much! He is such a joy! Although he was born one and a half months early, and at one point we didn't know if he would make it, today at seven years of age, he is doing so well! He wears glasses because of his nystagmus and uses a cane to help him walk. He is in second grade now and able to read at the level of most of his friends. The doctors say that as he gets older his motor control may get better and his speech may improve. We just hope he will remain the happy-go-lucky child he is and be able to be independent as an adult.

—Sarah, mother of a child with cerebral palsy.

NEUROLOGICAL ALTERATIONS

Marcia C. Wellington, RNC, MS
Robert F. Wayner, MD
Barbara Mandleco RN, PhD

COMPETENCIES

Upon completion of this chapter, the reader will be able to:

- *Explain the anatomy and physiology of the nervous system and describe the differences in anatomy and physiology between children and adults.*
- *Describe the different types of seizures seen in children and demonstrate the appropriate nursing interventions.*
- *Discuss the etiology, signs and symptoms, and nursing management of hydrocephalus, craniosynostosis, and arteriovenous malformation.*
- *Describe the various types of neural tube defects and discuss appropriate pre- and post-operative nursing interventions.*
- *Discuss the etiology, signs, symptoms, and nursing care of a child with meningitis, encephalitis, or Reye's syndrome.*
- *Discuss the etiology, pathophysiology, and nursing care of a child with a head injury or a spinal cord injury.*
- *Explain the various types of drowning and the associated pathophysiology.*
- *Discuss the etiology, signs and symptoms, and nursing management of the various types of cerebral palsy.*
- *Describe interventions needed to help families cope with a child who has alterations in neurological functioning.*

Neurological alterations can be structural, infections, or caused by an injury. Most often, pediatric alterations can be classified as either acquired or congenital. In some instances, however, these delineations are not as clear. For example, seizures, hydrocephalus, or cerebral palsy may be present at birth or shortly thereafter, but also may occur later from infection, trauma, or neoplasm. This chapter describes and discusses a variety of alterations seen in infants, children, and adolescents.

ANATOMY AND PHYSIOLOGY

The nervous system consists of the brain, spinal cord, and nerves. A review of the anatomy and physiology of these components sets the stage for gaining an understanding of the alterations of the neurological system.

Head

The scalp is composed of five layers: the skin, the vascular subcutaneous tissue, the loose fitting galea or aponeurosis, the areolar tissue, and the periosteum. The skull is made up of the cranial vault and the calvarium or base. The outer surface of the skull is smooth, whereas the inner surface is rough and irregular, especially at the base. There are three membranes covering the brain called the **meninges** (Figure 32-1). The **dura mater** adheres to the inner surface of the skull, covering the meningeal arteries and veins. Below that is the thin, transparent **arachnoid mater** under which the cerebrospinal fluid flows. The third layer, the **pia mater,** is attached to the brain itself (Estes, 2002).

The **cerebrum** is the largest portion of the brain and consists of two hemispheres and several lobes. The frontal lobe controls personality, emotion, complex intellectual function, and voluntary movement. The parietal lobes, which are on the lateral and medial surfaces of the brain, are where sensory input such as pain, pressure, proprioception, and temperature are interpreted. Taste, smell, hearing, speech, and language are deciphered in the temporal lobes, whereas the vision center is in the occipital area, located at the back of the brain. The **cerebellum,** which is in the posterior fossa, controls motor coordination, posture, and equilibrium. The brain stem, which sits under the cerebellum, controls the vital centers. The **brain stem** is composed of three parts: the **midbrain,** which manages visual reflexes, tracking, and cranial nerves III and IV; the **pons,** which controls respiratory function and cranial nerves V, VI, VII, and VIII; and the **medulla oblongata,** which regulates the respiratory, cardiac, vasoconstrictor, sneeze, cough, and vomiting reflexes as well as cranial nerves IX, X, XI, and XII (Estes, 2002) (Figure 32-2).

Cerebrospinal Fluid

Cerebrospinal spinal fluid (CSF), which acts as a cushion to help protect the brain, is composed of **choroid plexus** secretions and interstitial brain fluid, and is produced at a rate of 100 (in neonates) to 500 (in adults) milliliters per day. Figure 32-3 illustrates the normal flow of CSF. This process works if the production rate of fluid is equal to the absorption rate and there is free flow within the ventricular system (Behrman & Kliegman, 1998).

Cerebral Blood Flow

Cerebral blood flow (CBF) must be maintained in order to meet the metabolic needs of the brain. In the adult and older child, flow is thought to be 45–50 milliliters per gram of brain tissue per minute; it is less than that in younger children, although exact parameters are unknown. When CBF falls below 18 to 20 milliliters per gram of brain tissue per minute, ischemia will occur. Cerebral blood flow, measured by monitoring systemic arterial pressure, should remain between 60 and 150 millimeters of mercury. Flow may be influenced by changes in systemic blood pressure, arterial blood gas levels, metabolic demands of the brain, and intracranial pressure (Walker, 1998).

Intracranial Pressure

Intracranial pressure (ICP), the force exerted by the brain, blood, and cerebrospinal fluid within the cranial vault, cannot accommodate any pressure increase without compromise. To compensate for increasing pressure in a rigid space, the body will first shunt cerebrospinal fluid through the subarachnoid space into the spinal canal, compress parenchymal tissue, and finally reduce blood flow to the brain, which

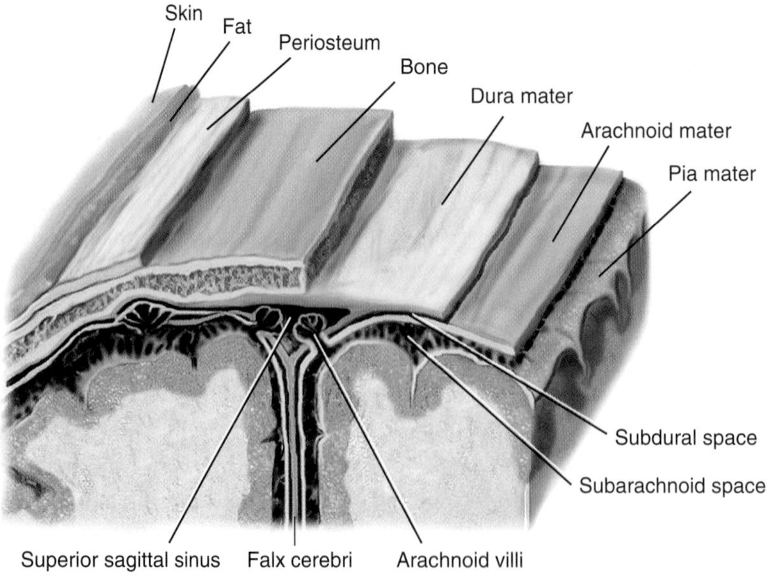

Figure 32-1 Brain coverings

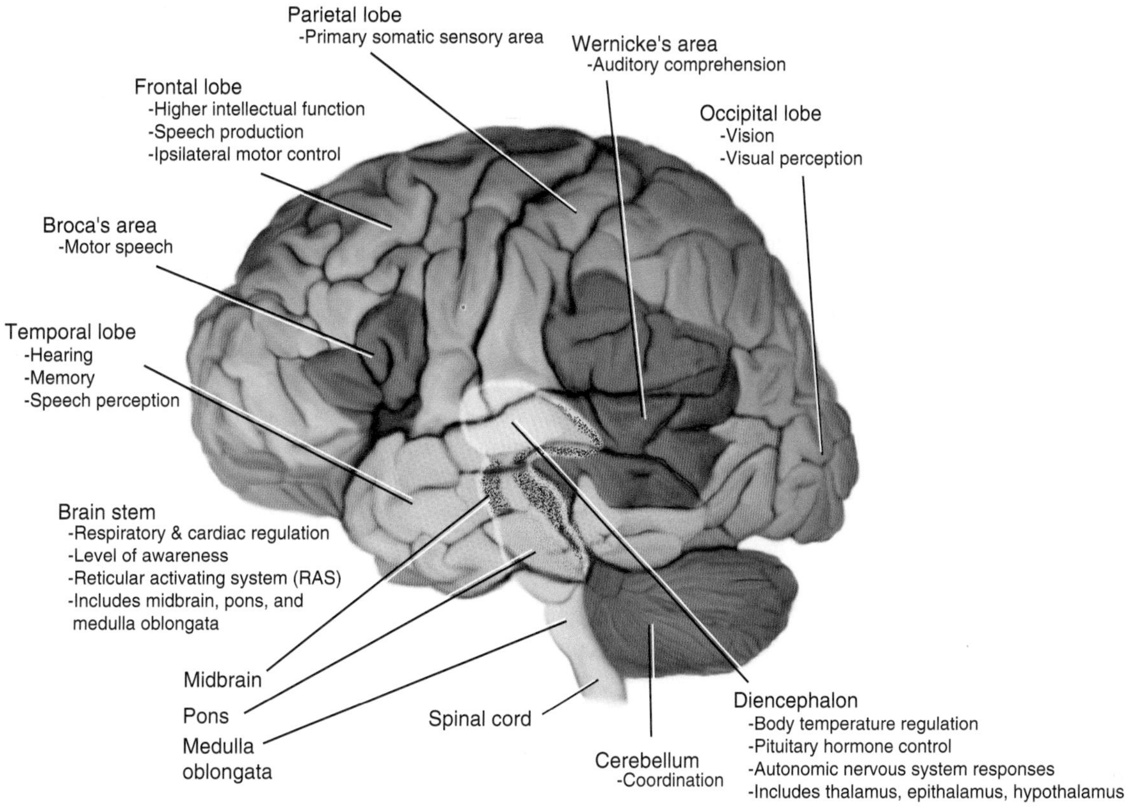

Figure 32-2 The locations and functions of the cerebral lobes, brain stem, and cerebellum.

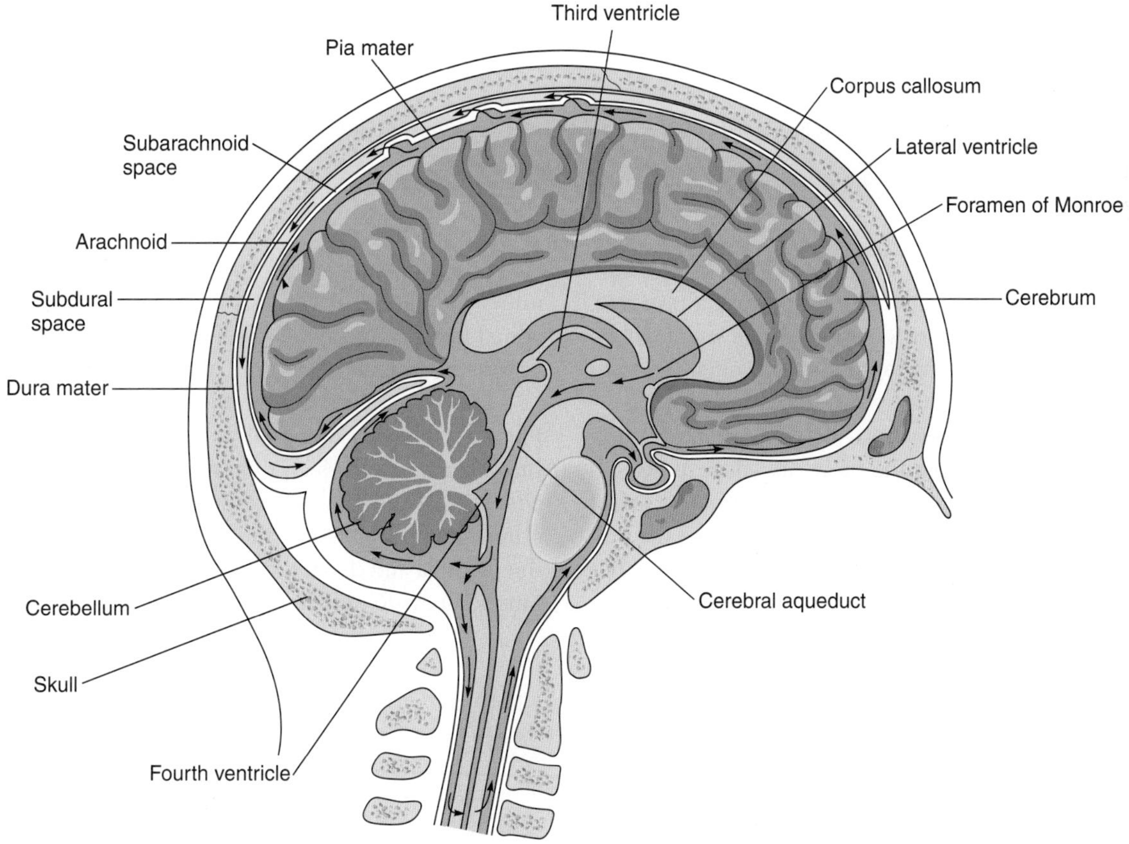

Figure 32-3 The flow pattern of the cerebrospinal fluid.

Research Highlight

Rethinking Physiologic Stability: Touch and Intracranial Pressure

Study Purpose

To examine the effect of nursing, medical, and caregiver touch not associated with a procedure on intracranial pressure in critically ill children.

Methods

Eight children between 7 months and 12 years who had intracranial hypertension from a variety of causes served as subjects. Nonprocedural touch was defined as touch by staff, family, or visitor that did not coincide with caregiving procedures (turning, suctioning, bathing). The change in ICP was evaluated by comparing the mean ICP obtained one minute prior to the touch and one minute after the touch.

Findings

Nonprocedural touch was often accompanied by talking, and usually did not cause a change in the level of ICP greater than the ICP variability for a particular child.

Implications

As nonprocedural touch had no harmful effects on ICP level, nurses should not avoid touching critically ill children. As caregiver touch had a stabilizing effect on the child's ICP level, caregivers need to be encouraged to touch and stroke their critically ill children.

Citation

Mitchell, P., & Habermann, B. (1999). Rethinking physiologic stability: Touch and intracranial pressure. *Biological Research for Nursing, 1*(1), 12–19.

affects cerebral blood flow and cerebral perfusion pressure. If increased intracranial pressure persists, brain tissue will be forced downward, past the tentorium, and through the foramen magnum (Behrman & Kliegman, 1998; Walker, 1998).

Normal intracranial pressure is between 0 and 12 millimeters of mercury, although the body can adapt to 20 millimeters of mercury without detrimental effects. The infant is better able to accommodate the rising pressure than an older child because the skull is more elastic, the fontanelles are not yet closed, and there is room inside the cranium for brain growth (Behrman & Kliegman, 1998).

The early and late signs and symptoms of increased intracranial pressure are found in Table 32-1.

Spinal Column and Cord

The spinal column is divided into several areas, each with a specific number of vertebrae: the cervical area has seven; the thoracic region, 12; the lumbar, five; the sacral, one; and the coccygeal, one. The spinal cord resides inside the spinal column, and there are 31 sets of nerves emerging from the spinal cord to enervate the body (Estes, 2002). Refer to Figure 32-4 for an illustration of the spine.

The spinal cord transmits nerve impulses to and from the brain. Sensory messages are sent via peripheral nerves to the spinal nerves, which then send the information to a specific area of the brain for response. Motor responses, on the other hand, originate in the cerebral cortex, travel through the medulla and down the cord to the anterior horn cells and muscle fibers to initiate movement (Estes, 2002).

Differences in Children and Adults

The anatomy and physiology of a child's nervous system is different from an adult. These differences are summarized in Box 32-1 and may explain why the child is more prone to specific structural defects, injuries, and other pathologic processes. On the other hand, these very distinctions also

TABLE 32-1 Signs and Symptoms of Increased Intracranial Pressure

Early Signs	Late Signs

• Headache
• Vomiting
• Slight change in vital signs
• Slight alteration in level of consciousness
• Pupils not as symmetrical or responsive
• Sunsetting eyes (sclera can be seen above the iris)
• Cranial nerve palsies (VI and VII)
• Generalized seizures
In addition, the infant will also display:
• High-pitched cry
• Bulging fontanelle
• Dilated scalp veins
• Wide sutures
• Irritability
	• Significant deterioration in level of consciousness
	• Respiratory distress including shallow breathing and Cheyne-Stokes respirations
	• Cushing's triad
	  • Bradycardia
	  • Wide pulse pressure
	  • Increased systolic blood pressure
	• One pupil fixed and dilated with extremities on the contralateral side either flaccid or spastic

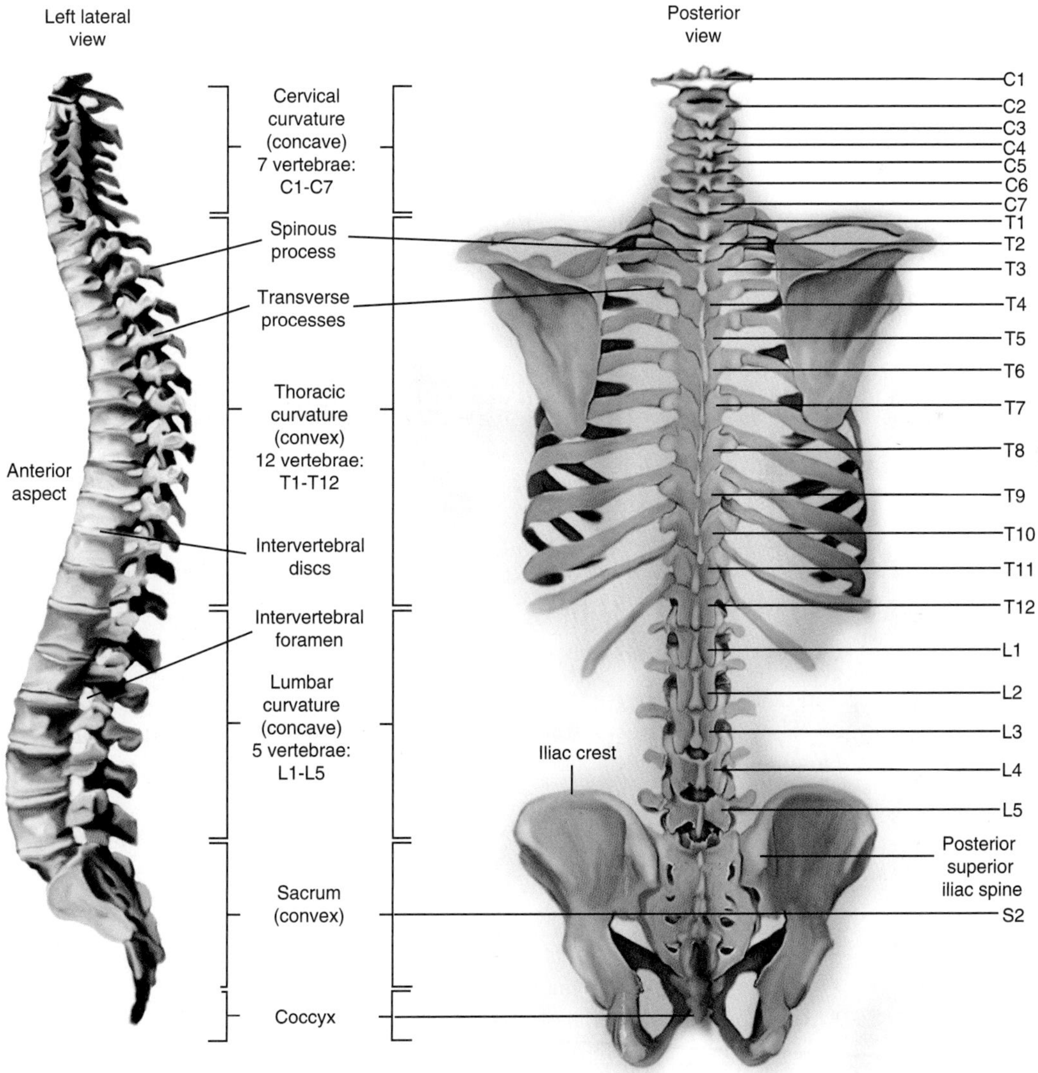

Figure 32-4 The Anatomy of the Spine

BOX 32-1 Anatomy and physiology differences between child and adult

- Normal infant head circumference = 34–35 cm, by 1 year = 47 cm.
- At birth, brain weight is 2/3 of an adult. By age 6, the brain weighs approximately 90% of adult brain.
- Cerebrospinal fluid is produced at a rate of 100 ml/day in infants as compared to 500 ml/day in adults.
- In the first year, the neurons become completely myelinated and primitive motor reflexes are replaced by purposeful movement. Myelinization occurs cephalocaudally and proximodistally.
- The infant has open fontanels; the posterior fontanel usually closes by 3 months of age; the anterior fontanel should close by 19 months of age with the average being between 12 and 18 months of age.

Adapted from Estes, M.E.Z. (2002). *Health Assessment and Physical Examination* (2nd ed.). Albany, NY: Delmar.

enable the child to recover more quickly and completely than the adult. Table 32-2 lists factors predisposing young children to alterations in neurological function.

CLINICAL MANIFESTATIONS AND ASSESSMENT OF ALTERED NEUROLOGICAL STATUS

Infants and children with neurological dysfunction display a wide variety of responses to neurological injuries or illnesses. Changes in levels of consciousness are common and can be manifested in varying degrees. The youngster, although alert, may demonstrate **confusion,** may be disoriented to time, place, and person, or unable to answer simple questions. The condition may deteriorate to **delirium,** where anxiety, fear, and agitation are seen. Level of consciousness may further diminish to **stupor** when the child is in an unresponsive state, reacts only to vigorous stimulation, and then returns to the original state once the insult is removed. **Coma,** the most severe form of depressed consciousness, is defined as no response to intense painful stimuli (Estes, 2002).

The child's level of consciousness may be evaluated several ways. "AVPU" is commonly utilized (refer to Box 32-2); however, it is necessary to state the exact stimulus and reaction elicited when used. For example, if assessing a painful response, the catalyst (pressure on a nail bed, a vigorous sternal rub) should be mentioned. The child's response should be specific; was the stimulus removed by request or did the child just moan or do nothing at all.

A second way to assess level of consciousness is a neurological assessment that includes the Glasgow Coma Scale

TABLE 32-2 Factors Predisposing Young Children for Alterations in Neurological Function

Level	Components
Developmental	• Poor judgment about dangerous situations • Unsteady gait • Immature immune system → increased susceptibility to infection
Cellular	• Fragile neurons • Nerve cells not completely myelinated

Structural	• Top-heavy: head large in relation to rest of the body
	• Neck muscles not very strong; may not be able to adequately support head
	• Cranium not well developed; thin and prone to fracture, especially temporal bones
	• Small subarachnoid space; decreases cerebrospinal fluid cushion
	• Dura: firmly attached to inner surface of skull, but can easily peel away with hemorrhage or hematoma
	• Brain: very vascular and prone to hemorrhage
	• Excessive spinal mobility caused by:
	  • Immature muscles, joints, and ligaments of the cervical spine
	  • Wedge-shaped cartilaginous vertebral bodies
	  • Incomplete ossification of vertebral bodies

Cognitive	• Has not yet learned hazards of the environment
Physical	• Fine or gross motor coordination not yet mastered

BOX 32-2 AVPU

A = **A**lert and **A**wake
V = Responsive to **V**erbal stimuli
P = Responsive to **P**ainful stimuli
U = **U**nresponsive

Nursing Tip:

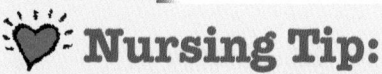

The child in an altered neurological status
Both verbalizations ("it hurts") or moans are positive responses to painful stimuli, but the level of stimulus and the child's response are vastly different. Therefore, in order to track neurological status, it is vital the stimuli used and client responses are documented in great detail.

(Table 32-3). However, the child's chronological age must be taken into account when using this scale. For example, a toddler may keep the eyes closed so what is happening in the environment will not be seen, whereas a five year old may not verbally respond to the nurse because caregivers have told the child never to talk to strangers.

TABLE 32-3 Glasgow Coma Scale Modified for Infants and Children

	Points
I. Eye opening	
a. Spontaneous	4
b. To command	3
c. With pain	2
d. No response	1
II. Verbal response	
a. Coos and babbles	5
b. Irritable cry	4
c. Cries to pain	3
d. Moans to pain	2
e. None	1
III. Motor response	
a. Normal spontaneous movement	6
b. Withdraws to touch	5
c. Withdraws to pain	4
d. Abnormal flexion	3
e. Abnormal extension	2
f. None	1
Maximum score	15

From Berkowitz, C. D. (2000). Pediatrics: A primary care approach *(2nd ed.). Philadelphia: W. B. Saunders.*

The presence or absence of posturing is another important indicator of level of consciousness (Figure 32-5). **Decorticate** or flexor posturing is associated with bilateral cerebral hemisphere injury. **Decerebrate** or rigid extensor posturing is secondary to trauma to the midbrain or pons; it is associated with poor prognosis (Estes, 2002). **Flaccid areflexia** or absence of response is indicative of severe brain stem injury and is evident most frequently in terminal coma.

DIAGNOSTICS

To determine the specific pathology of a neurological problem, definitive assessments are essential. Tests can include computed axial tomography (CT), magnetic resonance imagery (MRI), skull X rays, lumbar puncture, angiogram, and electroencephalogram (EEG). Before beginning the assessment, however, the nurse should explain the procedure to both the child and caregiver and allow time for discussion of feelings and anxieties concerning any and all diagnostic evaluations. In addition, any specific nursing actions needed before, during, and after the procedure should be taken to ensure the health, comfort, and safety of the child.

GENERAL NURSING ISSUES

The nurse caring for the child with alterations in neurological function must meet identified needs. This begins with a basic assessment of the child's physical condition using ABCDEs. Refer to Box 32-3 for the ABCDEs.

Once the nurse is assured the youngster's ABCDEs are stable, neurological status evaluation continues and should include:

- Level of consciousness, which can be assessed using AVPU or the Glasgow Coma Scale.
- Motor responses including strength, symmetry, spontaneity, and posturing.

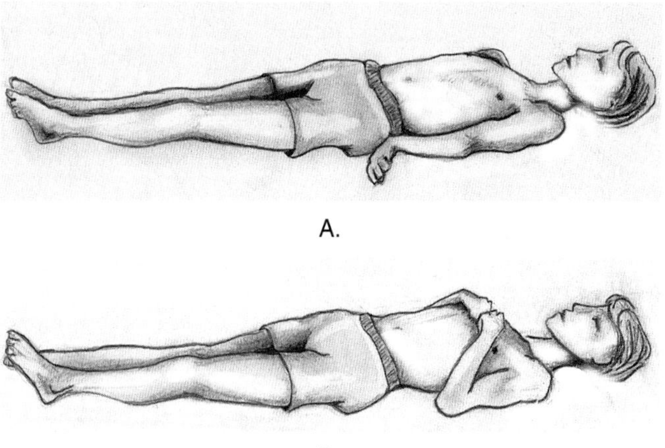

Figure 32-5 Motor System Dysfunction. A. Decerebrate Rigidity. B. Decorticate Rigidity

BOX 32-3 Assessment Using the ABCDEs

A = Airway
B = Breathing
C = Circulation
D = Disability or neurological status
E = Exposure of body

Evaluation always follows the ABCDE progression, only moving to the next step once the area assessed is determined to be stable. If not, appropriate interventions are initiated before moving on. For example, if an airway cannot be determined as patent, intubation should occur immediately. Once the airway is secure, the remaining assessment can be addressed.

- Sensory evaluation including responses to temperature (hot versus cold), pressure (mild, moderate, or severe), pain (sharp versus dull), and **proprioception** ("awareness of posture, movement, and changes in equilibrium and knowledge of position, weight, and resistance of objects in relation to the body," Taber's, 2001).
- Reflexes, noting presence, absence, symmetry, and strength of cranial nerves, as well as the Babinski, biceps, triceps, patellar, and ankle reflexes (refer to Table 32-4 for methods of assessing cranial nerves in an unconscious child).
- Physical abilities compromised by the illness or injury. In addition, any sequelae associated with immobility such as contractures or skin breakdown should be noted.

The nurse should then determine the care the child requires, including physical, intellectual, social, and emotional needs in order to encourage optimal development.

SEIZURES

Seizures are episodic, stereotypic behavioral syndromes that have an abrupt onset, generally are not provoked by external stimuli, and result in loss of responsiveness.

Incidence and Etiology

An estimated 0.5–1% of all children experience at least one afebrile seizure (Huff, 2000). Etiology can be caused by many factors (Table 32-5). Prognosis depends on the etiology, the type, and the age of initial onset.

Pathophysiology

Seizures are the result of a spontaneous electrical discharge of hyperexcited brain cells in an area called the **epileptogenic focus.** These cells can be triggered by either environmental or physiological stimuli such as emotional stress, anxiety, fatigue, infection, or metabolic disturbances. The exact location of the epileptogenic foci and the number involved determines the nature of the seizure. If a small area of the brain is affected, a focal (localized) seizure may occur. However, if the electrical discharge continues, it may become generalized. A generalized seizure will also occur if the epileptogenic focus is located in the brain stem, midbrain, or reticular formation.

The cause of seizures is often unknown, or idiopathic, although there may be genetic factors present predisposing

TABLE 32-4 Assessment of the Cranial Nerves in the Unconscious Child

Cranial Nerves	Reflex Evaluated	Evaluation
II and III	Pupillary	Shine light source directly into eye. ***Intact response:*** pupils will immediately constrict.
II, IV, and VI	Oculocephalic	Hold eyes open and turn head from side to side only *after* cervical spine has been cleared of injury. ***Intact response:*** eyes should be gazing upward.
III and VIII	Oculovestibular	*After* cervical spine has been cleared of injury and tympanic membrane has been determined to be intact, place head in midline with child's head elevated. Inject ice water into the ear canal. ***Intact response:*** eyes will deviate toward irrigated ear.
V and VII	Corneal	Gently swab cornea with sterile cotton tipped applicator. ***Intact response:*** Blink.
IX and X	Gag	Irritate pharynx with tongue depressor or cotton swab. ***Intact response:*** Gag.

TABLE 32-5 Common Seizure Etiologies

Type of Seizure	Common Etiologies
Partial	
Complex	• Intracranial lesions, tumors, cysts • Birth or other traumatic injury • Arteriovenous malformations • Prolonged febrile seizures
Simple	• Tumors or other lesions • Focal damage to the brain • Arteriovenous malformation • Brain abscess
Generalized	
Tonic/clonic	• Cerebral damage secondary to birth injury or trauma • Metabolic or neuromuscular degenerative disorders • Fever • Unknown
Absence	• Possible genetic link
Myoclonic	• Prenatal or perinatal encephalopathy • Tuberous sclerosis • Microcephaly
Myoclonic and akinetic	• Gray matter degenerative disorders • Subacute sclerosing panencephalitis • Unknown

children to particular types of seizures. **Febrile seizures** (seizures that occur with illness accompanied by fever) are an example of a type of seizure that has an unknown cause. Seizures can also be acquired, resulting from traumatic brain injury, central nervous system infection, hypoglycemia or other endocrine dysfunction, toxic ingestion or exposure, or intracranial lesion or vascular malformation. Typically, infants develop seizures because of birth injury, anoxic episodes, infection, intraventricular hemorrhage, or a congenital brain anomaly. Seizures in older children occur most often secondary to trauma or infection. In addition, changes in diet or hydration status, fatigue, or not taking prescribed medications may precipitate seizure activity. The various types of seizures as well as their etiology are found in Table 32-5.

Status epilepticus is a prolonged seizure or series of convulsions where loss of consciousness occurs for at least 30 minutes. **Refractory seizures** last more than 60 minutes. **Epilepsy** refers to a chronic seizure disorder that is often associated with central nervous system pathology.

Clinical Manifestations

Clinical manifestations depend on the specific type of seizure. **Partial seizures,** which arise from abnormal electrical activity in a small area of the brain, most often the temporal, frontal, or parietal lobes of the cerebral cortex, will have symptoms associated with the area of the brain that is affected. On the other hand, **generalized seizures,** secondary to diffuse electrical activity throughout the cortex and into the brain stem will cause the child to lose consciousness as well as demonstrate uncontrolled motor involvement with movements and spasms that are bilateral and symmetrical in nature (Huff, 2000).

Partial seizures are characterized by local motor, sensory, psychic, and somatic manifestations. There are two types of partial seizures, simple partial seizures and complex partial seizures. **Simple partial seizures** or focal seizures can be manifested at any age. There is no **aura** (a somatic, sensory, or psychic warning that the event will occur, which is often described as a strange sensation in the stomach that rises up to the throat) associated with these episodes and consciousness is generally not lost. Most often, the symptoms seen are motor or sensory in nature. Movements may involve one extremity, a part of that extremity, or the head and eyes will twist in the opposite direction of the extremities. The arm toward which the head is turned is abducted and extended with the fingers clenched. There may be numbness, tingling, or painful sensations as well that begins in one area of the body and spreads out to others. Alterations in sensory perception may also be present. The child may have visual hallucinations and report seeing images or light flashes. In addition, a buzzing sound may be heard, unusual odors identified, or an odd taste experienced. The child may also report feeling emotional or anxious (Behrman & Kliegman, 1998).

There are several specific types of simple partial seizures. **Jacksonian seizures** are motor episodes beginning with tonic contractions of either the fingers of one hand, toes of one foot, or one side of the face. The spasms progress into tonic/clonic movements that "march" up adjacent muscles of the affected extremity or side of the body (Encyclopedia Britannica, 2001). **Rolandic or sylvian seizures** are manifested as tonic/clonic movements of the face with increased salivation and arrested speech that occur commonly during sleep (Huff, 2000).

Complex partial seizures are also known as partial psychomotor or temporal lobe episodes. They can be manifested from age three years through adolescence. Just before the event, the child may have an aura. In addition, the youngster may have feelings of anxiety, fear, or deja vu, the sense that an event has occurred before, or complain of abdominal pain, having an unusual taste in the mouth, smelling an odd odor, or visual or auditory hallucinations.

Consciousness is not completely lost during complex partial seizures. Rather, the child will appear confused or dazed, especially at the onset. When the seizure begins, the child stops the activity involved in and begins purposeless behaviors such as staring into space or assuming an unusual posture. The child may also perform **automatisms,** or repeated nonpurposeful actions, such as lip smacking, chewing, sucking, or uttering the same word over and over, wander aimlessly, or remove clothing. Violent acts or rages are rare. A postictal period follows this type of seizure when the child will be drowsy, confused, aphasic, or display sensory and/or motor impairments. Children usually do not remember the behaviors displayed (Wertz, 2002).

Generalized seizures, arising from both cerebral hemispheres, can occur at any time and last from several seconds to hours. There is no aura, but always loss of consciousness. Generalized seizures appearing in children under four years of age are frequently associated with developmental delays, learning disabilities, and behavior disorders. There are four types of generalized seizures, tonic/clonic, absence, myoclonic, and akinetic.

Tonic/clonic seizures, often referred to as grand mal seizures, can occur at any age. Onset is usually abrupt and begins when the child loses consciousness and falls to the ground. The initial phase is tonic when there are intense muscle contractions. The jaw clenches shut; the abdomen and chest become rigid; and often the child emits a cry or grunt as exhaled air is forced through the taut diaphragm. Pallor or cyanosis may occur as oxygenation and ventilation are impaired. The airway is compromised because of increased salivation that the youngster cannot manage because of muscular contractions as well as the diminished mental status. The neck and legs are also extended while the arms are flexed or contracted. The eyes roll upward or deviate to one side, the pupils dilate, and there may also be bladder or bowel incontinence. The tonic phase of the seizure usually persists for 10 to 30 seconds. During the clonic phase, jerking movements are produced as a result of contraction and relaxation of the muscles. These spasms dissipate as the seizure ends, and can last from 30 seconds to 30 minutes after onset of the seizure (Wertz, 2002; Behrman & Kliegman, 1998).

A postictal or postconvulsive state follows a tonic/clonic seizure. Here, the child may be somnolent or if awake, confused or combative; there may be no memory of the event, hypertension, and diaphoresis. Headache, nausea, vomiting, poor coordination, slurred speech, and/or visual disturbances may follow.

Absence seizures, which used to be called petit mal seizures, appear around the fourth birthday and generally disappear near adolescence. They are characterized by a transient loss of consciousness, which may appear as cessation of current activity. The child seems to stare into space or the eyes may roll upward with ptosis or fluttering of the lids. There also may be lip smacking or a loss of muscle tone causing the head to droop or any objects in the hands to be dropped. These events usually last from five to ten seconds and can occur as often as 20 or more times per day. Children with this type of seizure are often accused of daydreaming and being inattentive in school (Huff, 2000; Wertz, 2002; Behrman & Kliegman, 1998).

BOX 32-4 Febrile seizures

Febrile seizures are a type of tonic/clonic seizure usually associated with rapid rise in temperature that reaches a minimum of 39° (102.2°F) centigrade. These episodes usually occur in children between six months and five years of age. There is often a positive family history of febrile seizures and they frequently accompany infectious processes such as upper respiratory infections, pneumonia, pharyngitis, shigella, urinary tract infections, otitis media, roseola, and meningitis. The seizures are often self-limiting and with a postictal period lasting for less than 15 minutes (Behrman & Kliegman, 1998).

REFLECTIONS FROM FAMILIES

Chad just had a cold and fever. All of a sudden, I heard a cry and I ran in to see him shaking all over. His face was pale and his eyes rolled back into his head. This seemed to last forever. I called 911 and by the time the paramedics got there, the shaking stopped and Chad just slept. I was never so scared in my life. What was it caused by? Will it happen again?

BOX 32-5 Infantile spasms

Infantile spasms, also referred to as salaam seizures, begin at three months of age. Many children with this disorder suffered from gestational difficulties, are developmentally delayed, or have other neurological abnormalities. Twice as many males as females are affected. During the seizure, this infant's head may suddenly drop forward while both arms and legs are flexed. The eyes may roll upward or downward, and the infant may cry out and turn pale, cyanotic, or flushed. There may be a loss of consciousness or awareness (Behrman & Kliegman, 1998; Wertz, 2002).

Myoclonic seizures are sudden repeated contractures of the muscles of the head, extremities, or torso. The child, who can be as young as two years but is usually school-aged or an adolescent, recovers quickly. These seizures occur when the child is drowsy and just falling asleep, or just waking up. There is usually no loss of consciousness nor is there any postictal period (Wertz, 2002).

Atonic or astatic-akinetic seizures (drop attacks) occur between ages two and five years, and are manifested by sudden loss of muscle tone with the head dropping forward for a few seconds. More significant events occur when the youngster loses consciousness and falls to the ground, most often face down. In either case, amnesia follows. These seizures often cause repetitive head injuries if the child is not protected by wearing a football or hockey helmet. Many have underlying brain abnormalities and are mentally retarded (Behrman & Kliegman, 1998; Wertz, 2002).

Akinetic seizures are manifested by total lack of movement as the child appears frozen in a position. Mental status during the event is diminished.

Diagnosis

The objectives of diagnosis are threefold: to ascertain whether or not the child truly had a seizure, to determine the cause of the episode, and to classify the type of seizure. This process begins with obtaining a thorough history from the caregivers and/or witnesses. In addition, a complete medical history must be obtained, noting any illnesses, medications, hospitalizations, or toxic exposures the child may have had as well as if previous episodes occurred. Family history is also important because of genetic predisposition to some types of seizures (Behrman & Kliegman, 1998; Huff, 2000).

Nursing Tip:

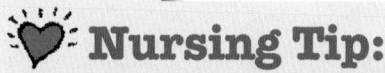

Obtain the following information if a seizure is suspected:

- Suffered a loss of consciousness or awareness?
- Became pale, cyanotic, or flushed?
- Displayed any unusual movements, especially tonic/clonic actions, repeated muscle spasms, or head drops?
- Had dilated pupils and/or eyes rolled upward or deviated to one side?
- Was incontinent of urine or stool?
- What happened after the episode? Was there a postictal period? If so, describe it.
- How soon after the event did the child's behavior returned to normal?

Eye On:

Neurological Tests and Procedures

In many Asian cultures, the head is sacred and considered to be the carrier of the soul. Therefore, when teaching family members about a CT scan and the child's need for the examination, nurses should be careful not to touch the child's head. It would be better for the nurse to use a drawing of a child's head, or point to her own head instead.

A detailed account of the event must be explored, and an assessment made of whether or not the child suffered any trauma, had been ill or febrile, ingested any toxin or poison, or was exposed to dangerous chemicals. It is also important to determine if the youngster had an aura just before the event.

Once the history is obtained, a complete physical examination must be performed. A complete blood count can determine the presence or absence of infection such as meningitis or encephalitis, and serum electrolytes should be analyzed to rule out metabolic disturbances, particularly hypoglycemia. A lumbar puncture may also be performed to investigate for infectious processes or bloody cerebrospinal fluid. If a toxic ingestion is suspected, both urine and blood can be checked for its presence (Huff, 2000).

A complete neurological evaluation should follow, including checking the level of consciousness, reflexes, and sensory and motor responses. Radiologic imaging such as CT or MRI may be performed to note any structural abnormality while angiography would pinpoint vascular irregularities. In addition, an electroencephalogram (EEG) might be indicated to assess the brain's electrical activity while the child is asleep, awake, or receiving noxious stimuli, and a positron emission tomography (PET) scan done to highlight areas of brain abnormality (Huff, 2000).

Treatment

The child with tonic/clonic seizures must be managed quickly. The airway must be assured; a short-term method is to perform the jaw thrust. Nothing, including a tongue blade, should ever be placed in the child's mouth. The child may then be placed on the side if the airway is patent to help prevent secretions from pooling in the mouth, and suction should be readily available. Because of thoracic and diaphragmatic muscle rigidity, air exchange is impaired and hypoxia may result. Therefore, children having tonic/clonic seizures should receive oxygen during the event either by face mask or assisted ventilations. Many seizures are self-limiting and last less than five minutes; these require no further management other than the jaw thrust and oxygen administration (Behrman & Kliegman, 1998).

On the other hand, the child in status epilepticus will need intravenous medications. The benzodiazepines (diazepam [Valium] or lorazepam [Atavan]) are usually administered first, and if seizures continue, phenytoin (Dilantin) or fosphenytoin (Cerebyx) are administered next. Phenobarbital (Luminal) may also be given, but it takes 30 minutes before onset. It is important to place the child on a cardiorespiratory monitor during medication administration as an apneic response may follow administration of the benzodiazepines. There is also the risk of hypotension or cardiac dysrhythmias when phenytoin is administered. Once the seizure is over, the child should be closely monitored during the postictal period. If the episode is a first time event, diagnostics should begin after recovery (Behrman & Kliegman, 1998; Wertz, 2002).

Once the diagnosis and the type and cause of the seizure is identified, more definite treatment can begin. If the cause was infectious, a toxic exposure, metabolic abnormality, an intracranial lesion, or a vascular malformation, that particular cause would be treated. For the child with convulsions caused by nonstructural pathology, anticonvulsant medications would be prescribed, and the child followed by neurologists who would carefully monitor drug serum levels to ensure they remained within therapeutic ranges. If episodes continued, medications could be changed or added to the youngster's current regimen. Refer to Table 32-6 for drugs used to treat seizures.

Over the last ten years, the Ketogenic Diet has gained popularity in treating absence, akinetic, and myoclonic seizures. The diet severely limits the intake of proteins and carbohydrates thereby forcing the body to use ketones for fuel. The amount of protein in the diet is regulated so that 90% of the calories are derived from fat, and the fat to carbohydrate ratio is 4:1. The reason ketones have an effect on seizures is not well understood, but theoretically to (1) change lipid concentrations, (2) change fluid and electrolyte balances, (3) modify the seizure threshold, or (4) stabilize the central nervous system (Le Fevre & Aronson, 2000).

TABLE 32-6 Drugs Useful for Treating Seizures

Seizure Type	Toxic Symptoms
Absence Seizures	
Ethosuximide (Zarontin)	Nausea, hiccups
Valproic acid (Depokene)	Tremors, sedation
Generalized Seizures	
Valproic acid	Tremors, sedation
Felbamate (Felbatol)	Insomnia, anorexia
Topiramate (Topamax)	Weight loss, speech disturbance
Infantile spasms	
Adrenocorticotropic hormone	Increased appetite, acne
Valproic acid	Tremors, sedation
Vigabatrin	Drowsiness, behavioral disturbances
Myoclonic seizures	
Clonazepam (Klonopin)	Drowsiness, ataxia
Neonatal seizures	
Phenobarbital (Luminal)	Lethargy, irritability
Partial seizures	
Carbamazepine (Tetrazol)	Gastrointestinal distress, headache
Phenytoin (Dilantin)	Ataxia, nystagmus
Primidone (Mysoline)	Drowsiness, ataxia
Newer medications	
Lamotrigine (Lamictal)	Dizziness, sedation
Gabapentin (Neurontin)	Somnolence, ataxia
Vigabatrin	Drowsiness, behavioral disturbances
Topiramate	Weight loss, speech disturbances

Adapted from Berkowitz, C. D. (2000). Pediatrics: A primary care approach *(2nd ed.). Philadelphia: W. B. Saunders.*

For the child with intractable seizures, surgery may be the last hope for control. The epileptogenic focus may be removed if there are no critical structures involved. Temporal lobectomy or a hemispherectomy could be performed on the client with unrelenting partial seizures with widespread hemispheric origin. Oftentimes, these youngsters will also display preexisting motor, cognitive, and sensory deficits. The goal of surgery is not only to decrease seizure activity, but also to improve the child's behavior and intellectual status.

Nursing Management

The nurse caring for the child with seizures has multiple responsibilities. If the child is actively convulsing, a patent airway and adequate oxygenation must be assured. Prescribed medications need to be administered in a safe and efficient manner, noting the specific rates of delivery, need for cardiorespiratory monitoring, and watching for potential adverse reactions. Once the episode is controlled, the nurse must document the event in detail, including the onset of any aura to resolution.

Nurses should provide a safe environment for the child with seizures to ensure injury will not occur. Suction and oxygen should be at hand and bed rails padded. If the event occurs when the child is in a chair or standing, the child should gently be helped to the ground and placed on one side and any nearby objects moved out of the way. Children with recurrent seizures may wear helmets to protect their heads during falls.

The nurse must also care for the emotional needs of the child and family as seizures can often have a negative stigma, making the victim as well as caregivers and siblings uncomfortable or ashamed. The child may resent feeling different from peers and taking medications several times per day, or fear having a seizure in front of friends. The nurse should encourage the child to talk about these feelings and provide help so the condition can be accepted.

Family Teaching

The nurse must work with the family as well. Some caregivers feel guilty, especially if the episodes are a result of trauma or genetic predisposition. The nurse should allow these family members to express their feelings and frustrations. Caregivers may also worry about the financial aspects of having a youngster with a chronic condition, requiring daily medications, visits to the neurologist, and frequent drug serum monitoring. The nurse can arrange for caregivers to speak with social services for assistance in working out these issues.

Caregivers must also be taught how to give medications, and the importance of not missing doses. They also need to know drug serum levels should be checked periodically as the child grows. School-aged children should be encouraged to accept responsibility for taking their own medications as this gives them feelings of control over their illness.

Safety is another issue to discuss with the child, caregivers, teachers, baby-sitters, and family members. All should know what do to when a seizure occurs, and when to call emergency medical services. The child should wear a Medic Alert bracelet or necklace, and people caring for this youngster should be aware of activities that can and should not be encouraged. While most play is acceptable, contact sports are ill-advised. In addition, the child with a seizure disorder must be carefully watched at all times during a bath or if involved in any water activities such as swimming or boating. Instruct what to do if child seizes and when to call

Case Study/Care Plan

Idiopathic Seizure Disorder

Ryan, a three year old, was in apparent good health until one afternoon when he was playing with his siblings, he suddenly cried out, fell to the floor, and began shaking violently. In a panic state, Helen, his mother, who witnessed the event, grabbed him, put him in the car, and drove him to the hospital just a few blocks away.

When they got to the emergency department, Ryan was having tonic/clonic movements. His skin was pale; his eyes rolled upward. Helen told the staff that the episode began about 15 minutes before her arrival. She denied trauma, infection, fever, toxic exposure, or family history. This was the first such episode Ryan had exhibited.

The nurse performed a jaw thrust to keep Ryan's airway patent. She administered oxygen via face mask. An intravenous line was started and diazepam administered slowly. The convulsive activity ceased; however,

continues

continued

within five minutes, they began again. A second dose of diazepam was given with only short-term resolution. Next, phenytoin was pushed through the intravenous catheter and the seizure finally dissipated. Ryan then slept for over an hour. When he awoke, he said his head, arms, and legs hurt; he did not remember what happened. A complete physical assessment was done in the emergency department. No pathology consistent with seizures was discovered, and Ryan was referred to a neurologist for follow-up.

The neurologist saw Ryan the next day and ordered more extensive evaluations that would require a hospital admission.

Nursing Care Plan

Assessment Ryan has been admitted to the inpatient medical unit with a diagnosis of seizures of unknown etiology. He is accompanied by his mother. Ryan currently is receiving phenobarbital and dilantin. Because his seizures are newly diagnosed and may not be fully controlled, his caregiver will need information about his diagnosis, treatments to be experienced in the hospital, medication regimen, and what to do if he seizes. Seizure precautions will need to be implemented for his hospital stay as well, since he seized right after the initial assessment.

Nursing Diagnosis #1

Ineffective breathing patterns related to tonic/clonic motions.

Expected Outcomes

Child's breathing patterns will not be compromised.

Interventions/*Rationales*

1. Perform jaw thrust as needed; administer oxygen either by face mask or assisted ventilations. *The positioning will help to maintain a patent airway during the seizure. Oxygen is administered to any client with tonic/clonic seizure activity for two reasons: first, the rigidity of the diaphragm as well as thoracic and abdominal muscles impede adequate air exchange; and second, the convulsing elevates body metabolism, thus increasing oxygen demand to the tissues.*

2. Suction as necessary. *Clients who are experiencing generalized seizures often have increased secretions, which they cannot manage because of their diminished level of consciousness. These secretions may pool in the hypopharynx and occlude the airway or pose a risk for aspiration.*

3. Time the event. *Most seizures are self-limiting and last less than five minutes. If they are longer, however, interventions will need to be instituted to curtail the activity. Medications may be delivered, starting with benzodiazepins and followed by anticonvulsants as indicated.*

4. Assist with intubation for prolonged convulsive activity. *The child who is having a prolonged seizure will need to have his airway protected; therefore, intubation will be necessary.*

Evaluation

Ryan's airway will be protected throughout the event; hypoxia or hypercapnia will not occur.

Nursing Diagnosis #2

High risk for injury related to tonic/clonic movements as well as diminished level of consciousness.

Expected Outcomes

Ryan will not sustain injury during the seizure.

continues

continued

Interventions/*Rationales*

1. Pad bed side rails and ensure no objects in the bed can cause harm if Ryan has a seizure again. *The child having tonic/clonic convulsions must have a safe environment in which to move during the episode.*

2. Have seizure precaution equipment at the bedside. *Suction and a ventilation bag and mask may be needed for prolonged activity. It is more prudent to have them at hand than to find them during an emergent situation.*

3. If Ryan begins to convulse when standing or sitting, gently ease him to the ground and remove any furniture or objects nearby that may be hazardous. *Helping to ease the child down prevents falls and possible trauma. The floor is a safe place for the youngster as long as there is nothing in the area on which he can be injured.*

4. Place Ryan on his side during the event. *Prevents aspiration of secretions and emesis if child vomits.*

Evaluation

Ryan will not be injured during the tonic/clonic event.

Nursing Diagnosis #3

High risk for injury related to medication administration during the acute episode.

Expected Outcomes

Ryan will have no adverse reactions to medications.

Interventions/*Rationales*

1. Administer benzodiazepines slowly; place Ryan on a monitor while giving them. *Respiratory depression or apnea may occur if these medications are delivered too quickly.*

2. Administer phenytoin very slowly using only normal saline as the fluid to flush the line. Place Ryan on cardiac monitor with rhythm recording capabilities. Also measure blood pressure frequently. Check intravenous catheter site often. *Phenytoin is an alkalotic compound, incompatible with all intravenous solutions except normal saline; others will cause it to precipitate. This drug must be administered at a rate no greater than 0.5 to 1 milligram per kilogram per minute. Cardiac dysrhythmias and/or hypotension are not uncommon during delivery. In addition, the site may become red or extravasated.*

Evaluation

Ryan will experience no adverse reactions to the medications.

Nursing Diagnosis #4

High risk for continued seizure activity related to seizures of unknown origin.

Expected Outcomes

Ryan will have decreased seizure activity related to seizures of unknown origin.

Interventions/*Rationales*

1. Provide information to the family about how to handle seizures at home. *Decreases anxiety and allows them to ensure the safety of the child.*

2. Teach caregivers about the importance of giving all medications as ordered by the physician and the need for periodic drug serum level testing. *Missing doses may precipitate a seizure; as child gets older or grows in size, medication dosages may need to be adjusted.*

continues

continued

3. Ensure the caregivers are aware of the side effects of the oral preparations Ryan will take at home. *Family will be prepared to handle any reactions that may occur.*

Evaluation

Ryan will experience reduced seizure activity; caregivers will better understand Ryan's special needs.

Nursing Diagnosis #5

Interrupted family dynamics related to caring for a child with a chronic condition.

Expected Outcomes

Ryan's chronic condition will demonstrate minimal effects on family dynamics.

Interventions/*Rationales*

1. Work with the family on accepting the diagnosis. *Giving the family control of their child's well-being will empower them and make them less angry and frustrated by their child's condition.*

2. Stress the actions and activities Ryan can participate in rather than dwelling on what cannot or should not be done. *Be positive with the family and encourage them to treat Ryan as normally as possible. Also, encourage them not to make Ryan their "special" child at the expense of the other siblings.*

Evaluation

The family will be able to accept the child's special needs.

Nursing Diagnosis #6

Deficient caregiver knowledge related to seizures and treatment.

Expected Outcomes

Helen will learn information about seizures.

Interventions/*Rationales*

1. Explain what the seizure may be caused by. *Will help Helen unravel the mystery of seizure.*

2. Explain medication treatment and how the medication works. *Medication compliance will be enhanced when Helen understands why the medication is needed to control seizures.*

3. Explain safety measures. *Helen will feel more comfortable with understanding what she can do to minimize injury to Ryan during a seizure.*

Evaluation

Helen will feel comfortable in caring for Ryan.

911 for help. It will be also helpful to teach them CPR. Provide teachers, classroom assistants, school nurses or health aides, and administrative staff with information on what to do if the child has a seizure in school. If the school nurse or health aide must give a medication during the day, provide information about the drug. If the child and caregiver agree, talk to the children in the class at school about the child's condition as well as what a seizure is and what it looks like in order to reduce fears and anxieties about their classmate. Refer the family and child to groups offering support to families whose child has a seizure disorder.

STRUCTURAL ABNORMALITIES

Structural abnormalities discussed include hydrocephalus, spina bifida, craniosynostosis, and arteriovenous malformation.

Hydrocephalus

Hydrocephalus is caused by increased production, impaired absorption, or a block in the flow of CSF that results in an excessive amount of cerebral spinal fluid within the cerebral ventricles (Behrman & Kligeman, 1998).

Incidence

The incidence is 3–4 per 1,000 births (Pillitteri, 1999).

Etiology and Pathophysiology

Hydrocephalus may be an acquired congenital disorder or of unknown etiology. There are two types of hydrocephalus: communicating and noncommunicating. In **communicating hydrocephalus,** there is an obstruction outside the ventricular system causing decreased absorption of cerebrospinal fluid in the subarachnoid space at the subarachnoid villi.

Noncommunicating or obstructive hydrocephalus, which is responsible for 99% of all occurrences in children (Wellington & Wayner, 1995), is caused by an impediment of cerebrospinal fluid flow within the ventricular system. Most often, this is secondary to congenital malformation such as **aqueductal stenosis,** a sex-linked hereditary deformity (Johnson & Oski, 1997), **meningomyelocele** (MMC) (where the meninges protrude through an opening of the skull or spinal column), **Dandy-Walker syndrome** (an obstruction in the foramina of Luschka and Magendie) usually evident by age two years, or **Arnold-Chiari malformation** (ACM), a brain defect in the posterior fossa where there is herniation of the cerebellum, medulla, pons, and fourth ventricle into the cervical spinal canal through an enlarged foramen magnum (Behrman & Kliegman, 1998).

During the neonatal period and early infancy, hydrocephalus is regarded as a primary dysfunction caused by either intraventricular hemorrhage associated with prematurity, gram negative meningitis, or a structural defect such as aqueductal stenosis, ACM, or meningomyelocele (Page, 1992). The child and adolescent, however, develop hydrocephalus most often from intracranial tumors such as medulloblastoma, craniopharyngioma, ependymoma, or astrocytoma (Page, 1992); infection such as meningitis; or head injury.

Prognosis depends on the cause of the obstruction. If the child has a neoplasm, the outcome will be based on the state and dissemination of the tumor. On the other hand, if the disorder is secondary to trauma, infection, or hemorrhage, the prognosis is based on the amount of brain damage incurred before treatment. Children who have shunts placed soon after diagnosis have a better survival rate, although some will display ataxia, decreased fine motor coordination, spasticity, diplegia, and/or perceptual deficits. Clients with additional complications, such as meningomyelocele, have more complications and disabilities (Johnson & Oski, 1997).

Clinical Manifestations

The signs and symptoms of hydrocephalus are generally caused by large ventricles (Figure 32-6) resulting from the trapped cerebrospinal fluid leading to compression of the brain parenchyma against the inner table of the skull and increased intracranial pressure.

During the neonatal period, hydrocephalus is common with a meningomyelocele at the thoracolumbar junction or above. If a structural defect is not immediately apparent, however, the only sign of the disorder may be a rapidly

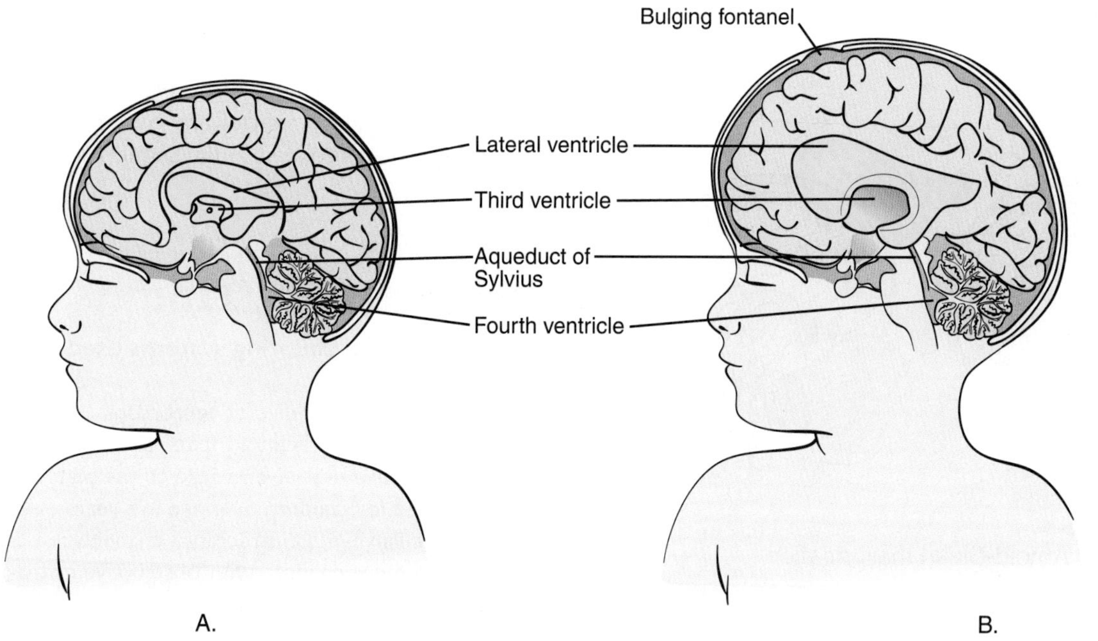

Figure 32-6 Comparison of A. Normal Size Ventricles and B. Enlarged Ventricles Associated with Hydrocephalus

increasing head circumference. In fact, within the first two to four weeks of life, the measurement may be as much as one to two standard deviations above normal.

The head of the infant with hydrocephalus will be disproportionately large when compared to the face. In addition, there will be protrusion of the frontal region, translucent skin covering the forehead, prominent scalp veins, and wide palpable suture lines. The eyes may have a wide bridge between them and visible sclera above the iris (sunsetting sign). The anterior fontanelle may be bulging and/or tense (Johnson & Oski, 1997). Other anatomic and physiologic abnormalities include a thin cerebral cortex; less dense cranium; and a positive **Macewen's sign** (a hollow or "cracked-pot" sound produced on percussion of the skull). Neurologically, the infant may be fussy, restless, irritable, apathetic, or have an altered or diminished level of consciousness accompanied by sluggish pupillary response to light, posturing, atypical reflex reaction, and lower extremity spasticity. In addition, the infant may feed poorly because of difficulties in proper positioning and/or swallowing, and the cry may be high-pitched and cat-like. In extreme cases, cardiopulmonary depression may occur (Wellington & Wayner, 1995).

The infant with Arnold-Chiari malformation displays cranial nerve dysfunction caused by brain stem compression. In addition, there may be difficulties swallowing, stridor, apnea, respiratory distress, diminished or absent gag reflex, and upper extremity weakness or spasticity. Refer to Figure 32-7 for an illustration of Arnold-Chiari malformation.

With Dandy-Walker syndrome, the posterior fossa of the baby's head will be prominent with bossing below the tentorium; the face will appear small as compared to the head, and nystagmus, cranial nerve palsies, and ataxia will be present.

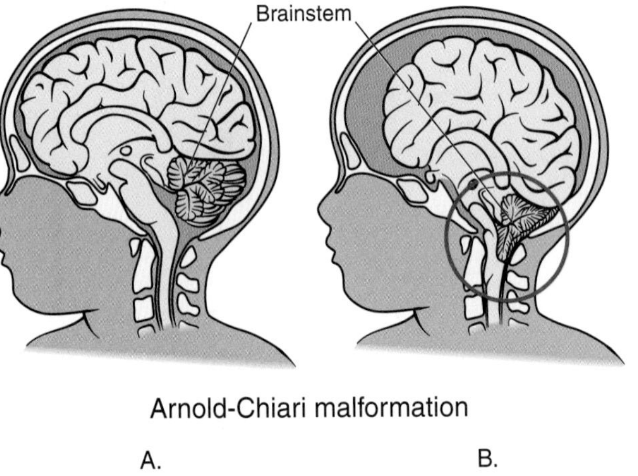

Figure 32-7 A. Brain in child without spina bifida. B. Brain with Arnold-Chiari malformation.

The hydrocephalic older child and adolescent display no enlargement of the head. Instead, most signs and symptoms are consistent with those of increased intracranial pressure. Upon awakening in the morning, the child may have a headache, often accompanied by nausea and vomiting. In addition, irritability, lethargy, apathy, or confusion may be reported. Judgment and reasoning skills may be impaired, and the child may become incoherent. There will also be change in motor abilities (ataxia, spasticity). Further examination may reveal papilledema, strabismus, and/or decrease in visual acuity secondary to compression of the optic nerve. Other manifestations will be focal in nature resulting from the location of the space-occupying lesion (Behrman & Kliegman, 1998; Johnson & Oski, 1997).

Diagnosis

Rapid head enlargement is the first indication of hydrocephalus; therefore, daily measurement of cranial circumference is critical. Awareness of the clinical manifestations displayed by all age groups will also help in diagnosis. Most often, CT scans and MRIs are used to confirm the diagnosis and ventricular dilatation or enlargement, as well as the structural defect or lesion responsible for the obstruction may be observed.

Other radiologic and imaging examinations may also be utilized. Ultrasound or echoencephalography, used exclusively in the neonate because of the open fontanelle, will show disproportionately large lateral and third ventricles. Plain skulls X rays may also be taken, and in the infant, macrocranium with wide cranial sutures will be evident. The films of the adolescent, however, will display a splitting of the sutures with a "beaten silver" look to the skull bones (Page, 1992).

Treatment

Treatment is directed toward relief of the hydrocephalus, prevention or management of any complications, and handling any problems related to the sequela of the underlying

Nursing Tip:

Other types of shunting systems used for children:

- Lumboperitoneal: diverts cerebrospinal fluid from the lumbar subarachnoid space to the peritoneum
- Ventricular plural: diverts fluid to the pleural cavity; it is used for children over age five years
- Ventricular bypass: intracranial channels are created in older children with obstructive hydrocephalus secondary to aqueductal stenosis or posterior fossa mass

pathology. With few exceptions, treatment is surgical: the removal of any space occupying lesion and the insertion of a shunt. The shunt system, made of radio-opaque plastic material, has a ventricular catheter, a unidirectional pressure valve and pumping chamber, and a distal catheter that work together to direct the flow of cerebrospinal fluid from the ventricles to other areas of the body for absorption. In pediatrics, shunts are placed to manage progressive ventricular enlargement and increased intracranial pressure in the presence of the large ventricles. Most often, they are ventriculoperitoneal, from the ventricle to the peritoneum (Figure 32-8), or ventriculoatrial (from the ventricle to the left atrium). The first is more commonly used in infants and children as the peritoneal cavity provides both an adequate blood supply to ensure cerebrospinal fluid reabsorption and a large space to accommodate the coiled catheter tubing.

In clients with congenital hydrocephalus, shunts are typically placed as soon as the diagnosis is made, and modifications to handle physical growth are planned at regular intervals. Unexpected revisions, however, may occur at any

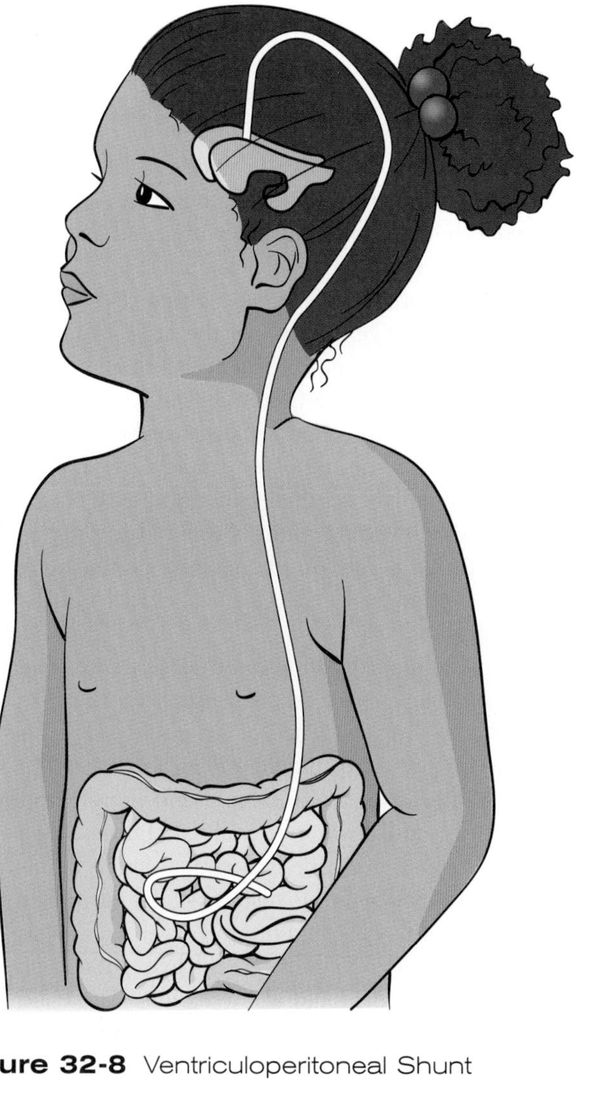

Figure 32-8 Ventriculoperitoneal Shunt

Nursing Alert:

Signs of a Shunt Infection:

- *Ventriculitis with a low-grade fever, malaise, nausea, and headache.*
- *Blood cultures may be negative, although there will be an increase in serum leukocytes.*
- *Cerebrospinal fluid will have an increase in white blood cell count and protein, a decrease in glucose, and the pathogen seen in cultures or Gram stain.*
- *Sepsis with a modest fever and weakness; laboratory tests reveal positive blood and cerebrospinal fluid cultures, leukocytosis, and anemia.*

Nursing Alert:

Signs and Symptoms of Over-draining Ventricles When Using an External Drainage Device

- *Change in blood pressure*
- *Decreased heart rate*
- *Apnea or change in respiratory pattern*
- *Severe headache*
- *Nausea and vomiting*
- *Lethargy, drowsiness, and/or irritability*
- *Seizures*

REFLECTIONS FROM FAMILIES

My son Carl is 10 years old and had his first V-P shunt placed just a week after birth. Over the years, we had some problems with malfunctions and once he even had an infection. Usually, when there are mechanical problems with the shunt, I know about them. His behavior changes just a little—this is so subtle that only his Dad and I are aware of it. I wish that when we went to the clinic and voiced our concerns the doctors and nurses would listen to us. Last time, we made three trips before they even ordered a CT scan. By then, Carl's ICP started to build up and he had to be literally rushed to the operating room.

My plea is simple: Please pay attention to parents and what they are telling you. You do not know my son, I do. When something is "not right" I can tell immediately. Perhaps, next time, we can avoid the dramatic rush to fix something that could have been taken care of quite simply.

time. The most serious complication associated with shunt placement is infection. It occurs in about 30% of the cases (Scheinblum & Hammond, 1990), most often within two months of the surgery. The causative agents are usually *Staph epidermidis* and *Staph aureus*. Children under three months of age and those infants who have had an intraventricular hemorrhage or central nervous system infection are at particular risk for shunt infection (Dallacasa, et al., 1995).

Conservative treatment for shunt infection is administration of antibiotics. The medication used, however, will depend on the pathogen as well as the ability of the drug to cross the blood-brain barrier. After 48 hours of therapy, repeat cultures are taken. If there is still evidence of infection, an external ventricular drainage (EVD) device may be necessary.

Shunt malfunction, the other major complication, is caused by mechanical problems such as kinking, plugging, migrating, or separating of the tubing. Signs and symptoms mimic those of increased intracranial pressure as the CSF fluid is not draining effectively from the ventricles. Most often, surgical repair is needed.

Nursing Management

Assessment

Preoperatively, the nurse must assess the child carefully by measuring head circumference daily, watching for signs and symptoms of increased intracranial pressure, assessing respiratory status, measuring intake and output, and monitoring nutritional status. Postoperatively, the nurse must assess vital signs and perform neurological checks every two hours. Baseline behaviors should be used to evaluate interactions with people and the environment, sleep patterns, and developmental capabilities. Intake and output, skin integrity, bowel sounds, and signs of infection should be monitored. The nurse must also watch for evidence of increased intracranial pressure.

Nursing Diagnosis

Preoperatively:

1. Risk for injury to neck muscles related to enlarged head and large, heavy cranial vault.
2. Risk for impaired skin integrity related to thin skin.
3. Imbalanced nutrition: less than body requirements related to potential for vomiting and need for proper positioning when feeding.
4. Excess fluid volume related to alteration in CSF flow.
5. Decrease intracranial adaptive capacity related to alteration in CSF flow.

Postoperatively:

1. Risk for imbalanced fluid volume related to cerebrospinal fluid draining too quickly.
2. Risk for excess fluid volume related to surgery.
3. Risk for impaired skin integrity related to thin skin.
4. Risk for infection related to surgical site.
5. Decrease intracranial adaptive capacity related to alteration in CSF flow prior to surgery.

Outcome identification

Preoperatively:

1. The child's neck muscles will not show signs of strain.
2. The child will not show signs of skin breakdown.
3. The child will have proper intake of nutrition and exhibit normal weight gain.
4. The child will not have increased fluid volume prior to operation.

Postoperatively:

1. The child will not suffer from CSF drainage and pressure on valves.
2. The child will not show signs of intracranial pressure.
3. The child will not show signs of skin breakdown.
4. The child will not develop an infection.

Planning and Implementation

Preoperatively, the nurse must take particular care when positioning the child, assuring the neck muscles are well supported and not stretched as they try to accommodate the large, heavy cranial vault. As the skin is so thin, there is an increased chance for breakdown; therefore, sheepskin or lamb's wool should be placed under the head, and the position changed frequently. Special attention must be paid to the nutritional status of the infant as well. Holding to feed may prove a challenge because of the large head. Because the infant is prone to vomiting, the nurse should offer small, frequent feedings with intermittent burping.

Postoperatively, the child will be placed in a flat position on the unoperated side to prevent rapid CSF drainage and pressure on the valves. Gradually, the head of the bed will be elevated. If cerebrospinal fluid is drained too quickly, the child is at risk for a subdural hematoma caused by tears in the vessels secondary to the cerebral cortex pulling away from the dura.

The child should be monitored closely with vital signs and neurological checks taken frequently. Level of consciousness as well as evidence of irritability or restlessness should also be evaluated. Baseline behaviors should be used to evaluate interactions with people and the environment, sleep patterns, and developmental capabilities. Head circumference must be measured as should intake and output, especially as fluids may be restricted during the first 24 hours postoperatively. In addition, bowel sounds must be evaluated and reappear before oral hydration is started. Meticulous skin care should also continue. The child must be observed for signs of infection, such as fever, increased heart and respiratory rates, poor feeding or vomiting, altered mental status, seizures, and focal symptoms such as redness or cerebrospinal fluid leakage at the surgical site or erythema along the shunt tract. The nurse must also watch for evidence of increased intracranial pressure.

Evaluation

The child will not show signs of strained neck muscles or skin breakdown. The child will take normal amount of nutrition and will maintain current levels of fluid retention prior to the operation. Postoperatively, the child will experience proper CSF drainage. The child will exhibit normal vital signs, bowel sounds will be heard, skin integrity will be maintained, and the child will not exhibit signs of infection or increased intracranial pressure.

Family Teaching

The child's caregivers need support. If the disorder is diagnosed in the neonatal period or early infancy, the family will fear the obstruction sequelae or the surgical procedure itself. They are most often afraid of brain damage, mental retardation, or other developmental difficulties. On the other hand, if the hydrocephalus is secondary to neoplasm, the caregivers' anxieties are compounded by their child's potentially life-threatening illness. In either case, it is prudent to provide support and allow them to ventilate.

The caregivers will also need explanations about the anatomy and physiology of hydrocephalus, how it affects the child, surgical procedures, and nursing care. As much of the information may seem confusing or overwhelming, it is helpful to use photographs and illustrations. Once there is a clear understanding of what will initially happen, the nurse should begin teaching the caregivers how to care for their child. This will foster feelings of control and mastery of the situation, and help them become members of the health care team.

Before discharge, the nurse should speak with the family about caring for the child with a shunt. They will need to know this is a lifelong condition requiring frequent follow-up consultation, and taught the signs and symptoms of shunt infection and failure as well as what to do if they suspect either is present.

Most children with shunts lead normal lives. They go to school, interact with peers, should not be overprotected, but should avoid contact sports, and in general, be allowed to grow and develop as typically as their friends.

Neural Tube Defects

Spina bifida is a neural tube defect where there is an incomplete closure of the vertebrae and neural tube.

Incidence

Spina bifida develops during the first 28 days of gestation. It is a common developmental anomaly of the central nervous system, occurring in approximately 0.4–1 birth per 1,000 in the United States each year. Incidence is higher in families with English and Irish ancestry and in females. If other family members are affected the chance of another infant having the defect is higher (Wallace, et al., 1997).

Etiology and Pathophysiology

Spina bifida, which can occur anywhere along the spine, may be due to failure of the neural tube to close completely during the fourth week of gestation, or to a fissure resulting from increased cerebrospinal fluid pressure.

Currently, the cause remains unknown. Environmental factors such as exposure to chemicals and medications and maternal nutrition may also play an important role, especially the mother's intake of folic acid, as low levels in the mother have been associated with spina bifida in their children. In 1993, the American Academy of Pediatrics recommended all women take 0.4 milligrams of folic acid per day at least one month before conception, a dose found in most vitamin preparations. For those women with a family history of spina bifida, the dosage is raised to four milligrams of folic acid each day beginning at least one month before conception and continuing through the first trimester (AAP, 1999). Prognosis depends on the type and level of the defect, the presence of other congenital anomalies, and whether or not there are additional complicating factors, such as hydrocephalus.

Clinical Manifestations

Spina bifida can occur anywhere along the spinal cord with varying pathologies. The most common defects include:

- **Ancephaly:** absence of the cranial vault with cerebral hemispheres either completely missing or greatly reduced in size. At times, the brain stem will be intact and vital functions can be maintained for weeks or even months. Death is usually caused by respiratory failure.
- **Cranioschisis:** a skull defect through which neural tissue protrudes.
- **Exancephaly**: a malformation where the brain is totally exposed or herniated through a skull defect.
- **Encephalocele** (Figure 32-9): a protrusion of the brain and meninges into a fluid-filled sac through a skull defect.
- **Spina bifida occulta:** failure of the posterior vertebral arches to fuse, most often at the fifth lumbar or first sacral vertebrae; there is no herniation of the spinal cord or meninges. This defect is not usually visible externally, although a dimple or small depression may be noted. It can, however, be seen on X ray. Initial suspicion that a problem may be present is not usually detected until toddlerhood. When the child begins to walk, there may be an abnormal gait with foot weakness or deformity. Later on, when toilet training is

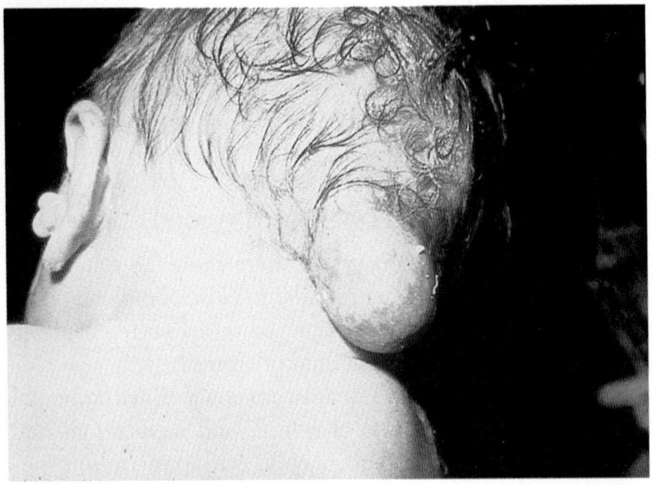

Figure 32-9 Encephalocele

attempted, there may be disturbances in controlling either or both the bladder or bowel.

- **Rachischisis:** fissure in the vertebral column exposing the meninges and spinal cord.
- **Spina bifida cystica:** a defect in the closure of the posterior vertebral arch resulting in one of the following two anomalies:
  - **Meningocele:** a sac-like herniation through the bony malformation containing the meninges and cerebrospinal fluid. The sac covering may be thin and translucent or membranous (Figure 32-10).
  - **Meningomyelocele:** a sac-like extrusion through the bony defect containing the meninges, cerebrospinal fluid, and a portion of the spinal cord and/or nerve roots. This lesion is poorly covered so there may be cerebrospinal fluid leakage at the site. It occurs most often at the lumbar or lumbosacral areas of the vertebrae (Figure 32-11).

Spina bifida, the generic term used to describe meningomyelocele, is noted at birth with the sac-like protrusion or the neonate's back. The clinical manifestations depend on the location of the lesion: the higher the deformity, the more neurological deficits will be present. The lower extremities may be partially or completely paralyzed and the bowel and bladder may or may not be affected. In addition, there may be renal impairment secondary to faulty kidney innervation. Orthopedic complications such as flexion or extension contractures, talipes valgus, or varus contractures may also be present at birth. Hydrocephalus is extremely common in infants with neural tube deformities and the higher the defect, the more likely it is that the child will have hydrocephalus (Pillitteri, 1999).

Infants and children with spina bifida may develop signs and symptoms of complications associated with the defect, the most common being urinary tract infections. Orthopedic problems are also seen in children with spina bifida. Although only 10% of the children with thoracic lesions are

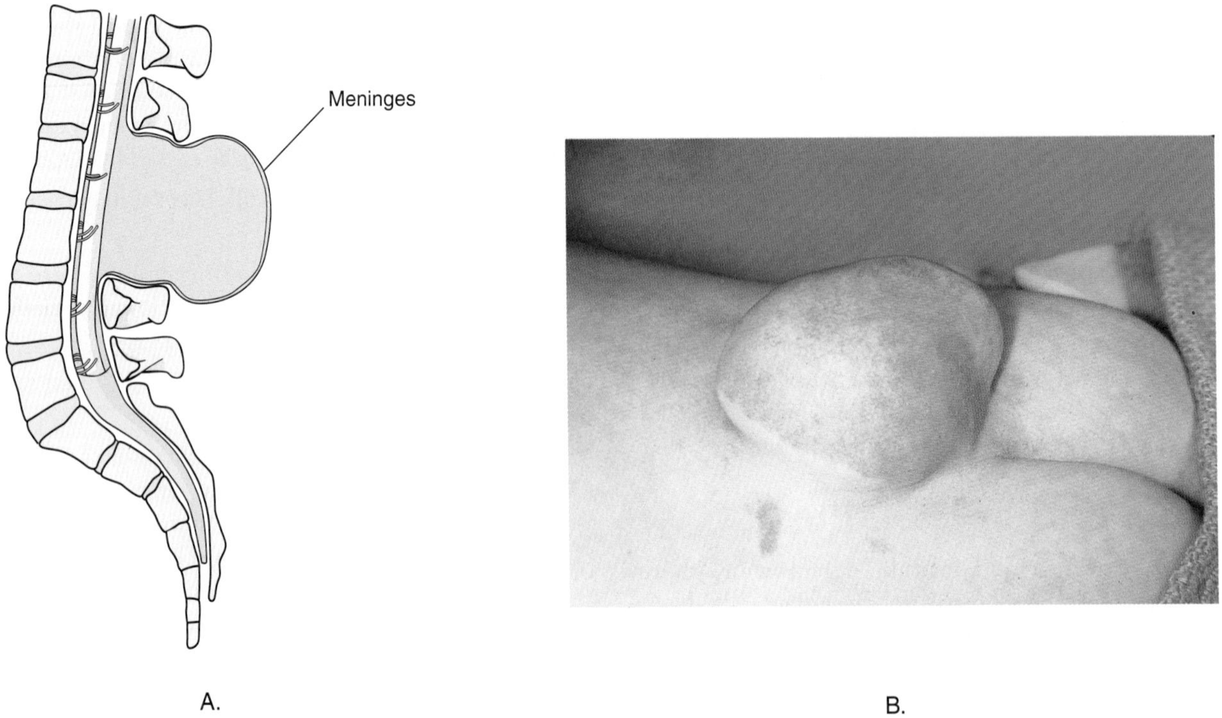

Figure 32-10 A. Illustration of Meningocele. B. Meningocele

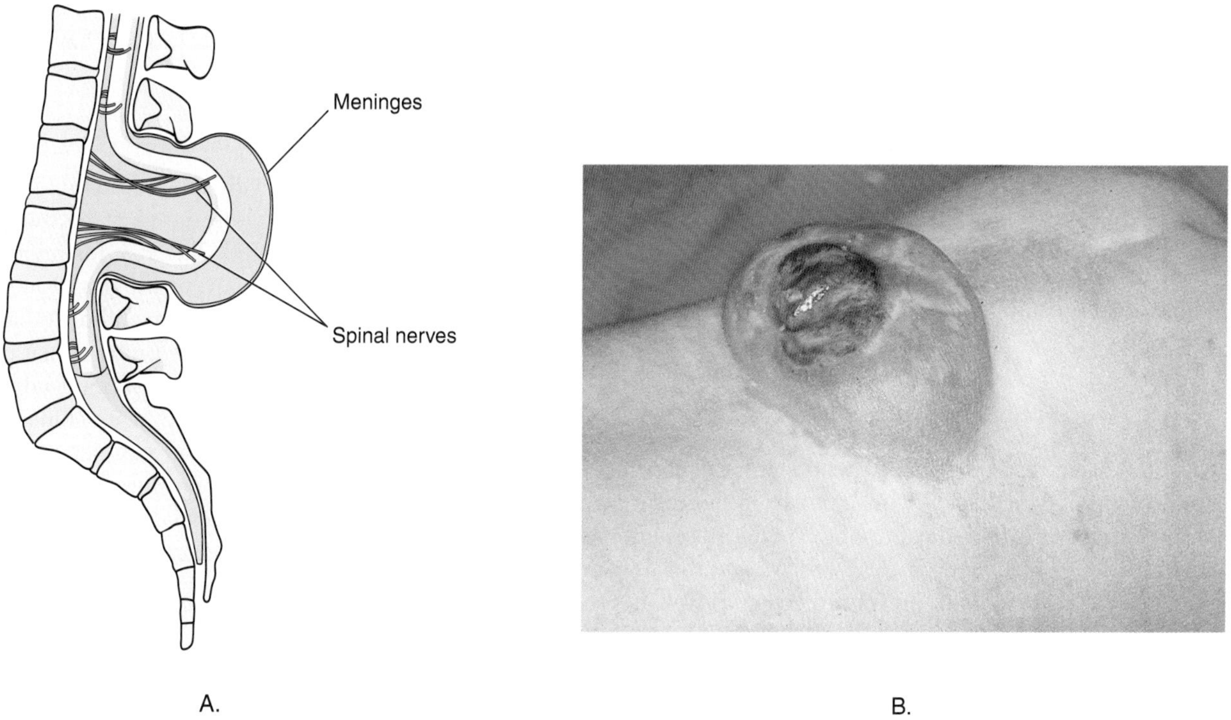

Figure 32-11 A. Illustration of Meningomyelocele, B. Meningomyelocele

Kids Want To Know

A Brother with Meningomyelocele

What's wrong with Ronnie? (newborn brother) Will he ever be normal? Can he run and play like other kids?

Answer: Ronnie has a defect in his back called a meningomyelocele. At this point we do not know if he will be able to walk independently, but he may be able to use a brace, crutches, or a cane. He should develop normally and will be able to play with you.

born with **kyphosis,** an abnormal curvature of the spine occurring in the thoracic region, by adolescence, the rate increases to 35% (Wellington & Wayner, 1995). This deformity is not merely a cosmetic problem as it can lead to back pain, respiratory distress, recurrent skin breakdown, and difficulty ambulating. Scoliosis is also frequently seen, especially in adolescents, but lordosis (forward curvature of the spine) occurs less frequently. Tethering (abnormal adhesion to a bony structure causing traction) of the spinal cord because of adhesions may cause difficulties in older children and adolescents as well, resulting in back pain, increased spasticity, and decreased urinary control.

Because loss of sensation is secondary to interrupted nerve pathways, trauma to the lower extremities may occur without the infant or child's knowledge and skin breakdown frequently is seen over bony prominences. In addition, these children are more susceptible to burns from both water and the sun as well as idiopathic fracture because their bones are brittle. Finally, infants and children who have had shunts placed may develop shunt failure or infection.

Diagnosis

Some neural tube defects may be diagnosed prenatally by ultrasound. In addition, an amniocentesis test may reveal an increase in alpha-fetoprotein, a fetal specific gamma-1 globulin in the amniotic fluid that indicates the presence of meningomyelocele, just before these protein levels normally diminish.

Diagnosis after birth is made during the neonatal examination. If a lesion is noted, it can be evaluated using several techniques. **Transillumination** (shining a light through the sac) may be utilized to determine the structures in the sac. If the sac becomes translucent when the light source is held to it, it is a meningocele; if the sac does not become translucent, it is a meningomyelocele. Radiologic studies may also be performed. CT scans and MRIs as well as flat-plate films of the spinal column may be used to determine bony deformities and tissue herniation. In addition, neuroimaging may be used to determine the presence of other structural defects such as hydrocephalus or Arnold-Chiari malformation. As the child gets older, radiologic studies are used to evaluate the onset of hydrocephalus or shunt failure, orthopedic complications, or renal and/or urinary dysfunction.

Neurological examination of the extremities must also be performed. Motor response and strength, sensory reaction to specific stimuli, and reflexes should be evaluated on an ongoing basis. In addition, routine developmental assessments are necessary to note delays. If milestones are not reached at the appropriate time, additional therapies may be added to the established regimen to encourage optimal development.

Treatment

Once the diagnosis is confirmed, treatment is begun using a multidisciplinary approach with input from neurosurgery, plastic surgery, orthopedics, urology, pediatric medicine, nursing, occupational and physical therapy, and social work. The goal of this team is to prevent infection as well as preserve or enhance whatever neurological and urologic function is present. Surgical intervention is the first method used to achieve that end.

Before surgery to close the defect, the infant is placed in a prone position with a sterile dressing moistened with normal saline covering the area. The prone position also keeps the urine and feces away from the defect. The child my be kept in an isolette to maintain temperature. A towel roll, placed between the knees with the hips slightly flexed and legs abducted, can be used to maintain hip alignment and decrease pressure on the sac. Meticulous skin care must be provided as well; sheepskin, a lamb's wool sheet, or an egg-crate mattress pad should be placed under the infant.

After surgery, the infant is again placed in the prone position for several days until the incision has healed. The infant will also receive antibiotics, and must be watched closely for signs of infection and hydrocephalus. In addition, bowel and bladder dysfunction must be noted as incontinence may contaminate the operative site.

Neurological assessments of the extremities assist in planning the therapeutic regimen, as management of any orthopedic malformations often begins just after birth. Positioning, casting, splinting, bracing, traction, and surgeries are performed as soon as possible to enhance the chance for ambulation and decrease the risk of complications. Walkers, crutches, canes, and lightweight braces may be used with lesions at L-2 to L-5 while customized wheelchairs can be used with a high-level deformity, usually at L-2 or above.

Infants and children with neural tube defects often have neurogenic bladder and, therefore, are prone to urinary retention and frequent infection. Intermittent catheterization along with medications to enhance bladder storage and continence are utilized to help manage this problem. A vesicostomy where a stoma is created by bringing the anterior wall of the bladder to the abdominal wall is a surgical option for some children (Wertz, 2002). To maintain bowel control, stool softeners and diets high in fiber have proven to be valuable.

Nursing Management

The neonate diagnosed with spina bifida must be carefully observed. Preoperatively, the sac must be watched closely and its integrity maintained. The risk for infection is high and the nurse must be aware of the symptoms associated with it, including fever, irritability and/or lethargy, nuchal rigidity, and the signs of increased intracranial pressure. In addition, as hydrocephalus is a common adjunct to the deformity, nurses must be aware of its clinical manifestations. In both cases, the neurosurgery department must be notified as soon as possible when these conditions appear as immediate intervention is indicated.

Because providing comfort may be difficult, tactile stimulation such as touching, rubbing, and stroking are important. If held, the infant should be placed prone on a pillow on the nurse or caregiver's lap. Feeding in the prone position can be challenging. Therefore, the infant should be fed with the head turned to one side. Because breastfeeding may be

Nursing Alert:

Latex Allergy

Infants, children, and adolescents with spina bifida are 41% more likely to have latex allergy than the general public. The nurse must be aware of the signs and symptoms:

- *Urticaria*
- *Wheezing*
- *Watery eyes*
- *Rash*
- *Anaphylaxis, in extreme cases*

Equipment such as tourniquets, intravenous tubing, urinary and intravenous catheters, and tapes are now available latex free; therefore, the nurse must ensure that all products be checked before they are brought into client rooms, and not used if they contain latex.

Nursing Tip:

Monitor height

Many children with spina bifida do not reach normal heights. Recombinant human growth hormone has been administered to some children with success as it improves both their growth rate and length. The effect on the adult stature, however, is unknown at this time (Rothstein & Reigel, 1996).

Reflective Thinking

Mom's Have Special Needs, Too

It is important to remember that during the neonatal period, the mother has special needs. Not only is she dealing with the grief associated with not having a "normal" child and the medical, social, and intellectual implications associated with spina bifida, but she is going through the postpartum period and may be extremely emotional and vulnerable. Put yourself in her shoes. Can you imagine what your responses would be?

contraindicated before surgery, mothers should be encouraged to pump their breasts and begin breastfeeding later.

Before surgery, a neurological assessment should be performed. Absence or presence of extremity movement must be observed as should any evidence of flaccidity or spasticity. In addition, dribbling urine or continuous stooling should be noted.

Postoperatively, the neonate should be monitored carefully and vital signs taken frequently. In addition, the infant must be observed for any signs of local or systemic infection, meningitis, hydrocephalus, or increased intracranial pressure. Also, the surgical site must be watched for cerebrospinal fluid leakage. The neonate's position now can be prone, side-lying, or upright while leaning against someone's chest. After the incision has healed, the infant may be held

Research Highlight

Mother's Experiences of "Living Worried" When Parenting Children with Spina Bifida

Study Purpose

To gain a better understanding of the day-to-day experience of mothers raising a child with spina bifida so nurses and other health care providers might improve their practice.

Methods

A convenience sample of 13 mothers between 34 and 54 years of age raising children with spina bifida who were between 12 and 18 years of age participated in this phenomenological study. Mothers were asked to describe day-to-day experiences they had while raising their children. Interviews were audiotaped and analyzed using appropriate Heideggerian hermeneutic interpretation.

Findings

The major theme identified was "living worried," which began at the child's birth and was always present. The worry involved concern about the child's future, health and school problems, and the fact that the child might not "fit in" with their peer group. The worry also involved "staying with the struggle." This meant the mothers worked hard not to give up and keep open the possibility of the child having a meaningful future.

Implications

Parenting a child with a disability is a challenge. Nurses need to be aware of the impact this disability has on a mother's life and provide help and support for these parents. Nurses also need to integrate this information into their daily practice in order to help families learn from one another and cope with the challenges and worries of raising a child with spina bifida.

Citations

Monsen, R. (1999). Mother's experiences of living worried when parenting children with spina bifida. *Journal of Pediatric Nursing, 14*(3), 157–163.

Reflective Thinking

High Neural Tube Defects

Neonates and infants with ancephaly are most often provided with comfort measures and palliative care. There is the ethical dilemma, however, about providing aggressive management of respiratory failure of these infants and the need for resuscitation following an arrest.

At least one case went to court where the mother of such an infant demanded that her child receive the maximum care and most aggressive treatments available, while the hospital medical staff argued that that was a futile and painful effort for a child with no chance for long-term survival. The court decided in favor of the mother.

Think about how you would feel if you had to work with this mother when your personal feelings differed from hers.

in a normal fashion for feeding either from the breast or bottle.

Because most problems associated with spina bifida are related to motor and/or sensory impairments, skin integrity must be maintained. To reduce the chance of breakdown, bony prominences should be protected, gentle massage provided, and linen changed frequently.

Orthopedic sequelae are common as well. For most children, range of motion exercises and other physical therapy maneuvers should be initiated early to prevent muscle atrophy and contractures.

Because urinary and bowel sequelae occur, the nurse should watch for retention difficulties or infection. In addition, hydrocephalus may emerge at any time, so any change in neurological status must be investigated.

The child with spina bifida has needs beyond those of the neonate and infant. Development must be assessed carefully, and it is critical the child be treated according to cognitive rather than motor capabilities. Independence should be encouraged and opportunities for choices provided. The physical, emotional, and intellectual environment must be stimulating, yet not frustrating. Because the adolescent may have concerns about physical disabilities (how they affect peer relations, sexual identity, career), sensitivity, respect, and referral to appropriate staff may be necessary.

At the time of diagnosis, the family has tremendous needs coping with a child who will have lifelong challenges and needs. The initial facts are usually overwhelming, especially as they make decisions relative to surgeries and treatments. The nurse might become the central figure to help caregivers sort out their feelings and learn about useful resources. Clergy or social workers might also be helpful in answering nonmedical questions such as how bills will be paid and in arranging for care of the other children at home.

Before the infant is discharged, the nurse should help the family contact needed community resources. In addition, home care services should be arranged so all clinic appointments, therapy sessions, and in-hospital teaching can be reinforced and coordinated. Also, any special equipment must be ordered and in place before the infant goes home.

Family Teaching

The infant will have special needs in terms of positioning, feeding techniques, skin care, intermittent catheterization, exercises, and special equipment such as braces or splints. Physical therapists, nutrition specialists, and nurses should teach caregivers how to care for the infant at home. In addition, caregivers need to realize the importance of follow-up care by the many specialists working with the child.

The family must not only learn the signs of hydrocephalus, idiopathic fractures, and urinary dysfunction and/or infection; but also what to do if these manifestations appear. They also need to understand that while some symptoms are not life-threatening, others, such as shunt failure, are, and require immediate medical attention.

Craniosynostosis

Craniosynostosis is the premature closing of the cranial sutures (Figure 32-12).

Incidence

Although rare, occurring in approximately 0.4 per 1,000 births, craniosynostosis is often a complex problem. There does not appear to be a racial predilection. Premature fusion of the sagittal sutures is the most common type (55% of all cases) with boys being more commonly affected (4:1). Twenty to twenty-five percent of cases are unilateral or bilateral coronal synostosia, which is seen more commonly in females (Johnson & Oski, 1997). In as many as 10–20% of the cases, it presents itself concurrently with inherited syndromes such as Apert's or Crouzon's. Most children with this abnormality, however, have no family history of the disorder.

Etiology and Pathophysiology

The cause of craniosynostosis is unknown. Usually, bone growth occurs perpendicular to the suture lines, and normal suture closure occurs at predetermined times during infancy and early childhood. If the sutures close prematurely, bone growth will continue but in a direction that is parallel to the suture line, leading to compensatory overgrowth at the normal suture lines and skull deformity.

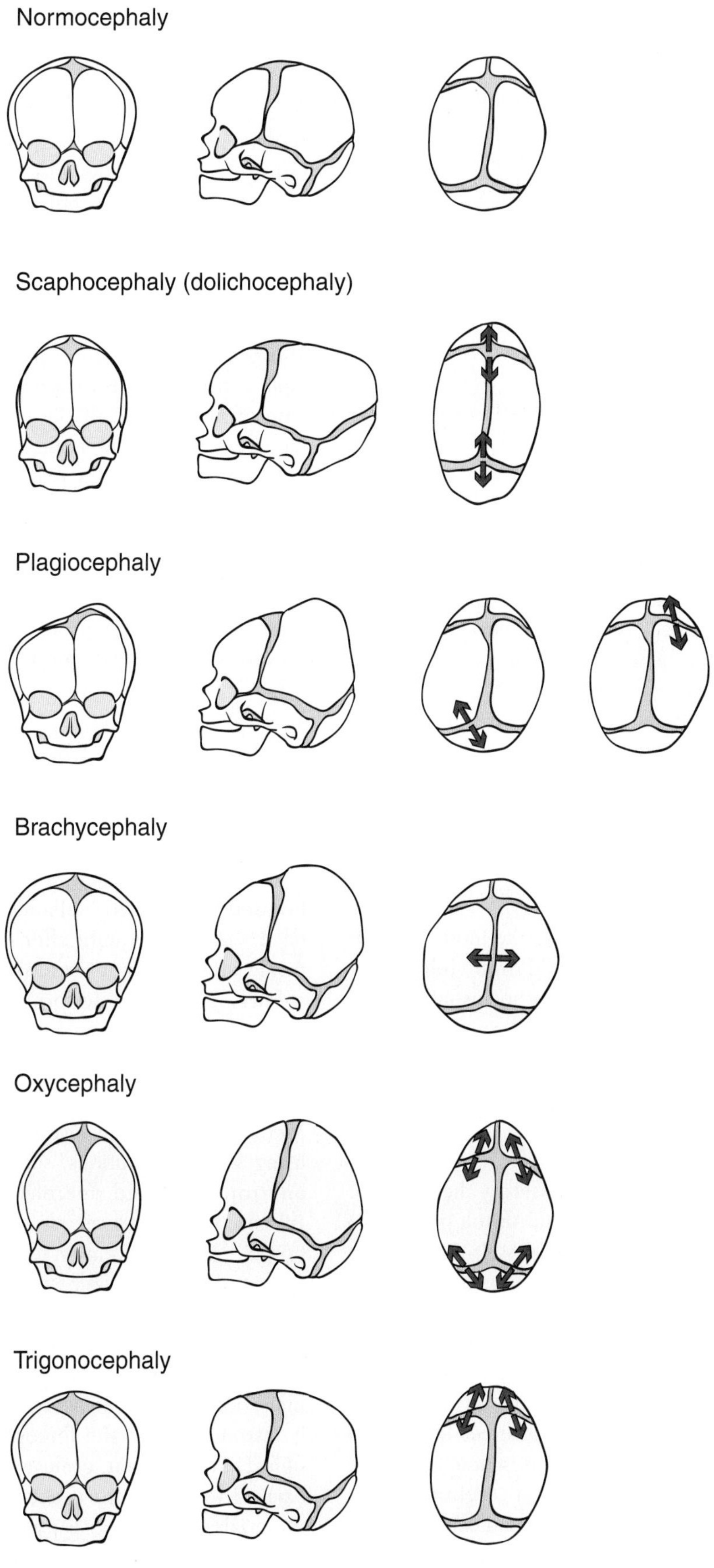

Figure 32-12 Craniosynostosis

Clinical Manifestations and Diagnosis

The predominant feature is skull deformity, but the clinical picture depends on the sutures affected. In addition to the structural defect, the small or misshapen skull may cause problems with brain growth. Therefore, signs of increased intracranial pressure may be evident. Papilledema may also occur, and if left untreated may lead to blindness caused by atrophy of the optic nerve. Diagnosis is made by clinical appearance, skull X rays, CT, and MRI.

Treatment

Surgical intervention is the most common form of treatment. The procedure is usually a linear craniotomy parallel to the fused sutures. Polyethylene film is inserted over the cut bony surface to delay closure (Johnson & Oski, 1997).

Nursing Management

The nurse must support the family, as the appearance of their child can be a concern. Referral to social workers or peer groups can often be beneficial. The nurse should also be able to manage the postoperative course of treatment for the child, including watching for signs and symptoms of increased intracranial pressure, infection, bleeding, and the effects of immobility associated with any intracranial surgery.

Arteriovenous Malformation

Incidence

Arteriovenous malformations (AVMs) are the most common cause of intracranial hemorrhage in children (Johnson & Oski, 1997). Clinical presentation does not usually occur before the age of 10; oftentimes, the malformation is only noted when the child has a head CT or MRI for other reasons such as trauma.

Etiology and Pathophysiology

An **arteriovenous malformation** is caused by the failure of cerebral capillaries to form during fetal development. To compensate for this, a web-like tangle of vessels is created to provide a network between the arteries and veins. The vessels in the malformation are dilated and thin-walled, resulting in decreased resistance that causes increased blood volume at high pressure as blood moves from the artery involved to the vein. Initially, blood is shunted toward the malformation because of the low resistance, leading to "stealing" of cerebral blood with resulting ischemia in other areas of the parenchyma. This increased cerebral venous return can lead to congestive heart failure and cardiomegaly, especially in neonates whose cardiovascular status is exquisitely sensitive to change in fluid status. The vessels themselves may also become compromised and rupture causing intracranial hemorrhage. Aneurysms can also form because of the incredibly high flow (Behrman & Kliegman, 1998; Johnson & Oski, 1997).

Clinical Manifestations

In neonates, the initial signs of an AVM are congestive heart failure, cardiomegaly, and a cerebral bruit. In addition, hydrocephalus may occur because of aqueductal stenosis secondary to congestion of the dilated vein of Galen. In children, a seizure is often the first sign of neurological problem. The convulsion may be focal, Jacksonian (localized motor), or generalized. Headache may also occur, usually described as migraine-like in nature. In fact, if a child complains of this type of pain and has a seizure, there should be high suspicion of an AVM. Half the children have a remote, silent bleed before hospital admission. When hemorrhage occurs, there may be signs of increased intracranial pressure or cerebral edema, syncope, fainting, vertigo, dizziness, sensory deficits, tingling of extremities or motor weakness, aphasia, dysarthria, visual impairments such as hemianopia (blindness in half of the normal visual field), and confusion. In severe cases, there may be a profound decrease in the level of consciousness or coma (Johnson & Oski, 1997).

Diagnosis

Cerebral angiography is used in diagnosis as the defect can be well visualized. In addition, CT with contrast, MRI, and skull films may be used. An EEG may be done; however, abnormal waves might be a reflection of brain ischemia rather than the vascular deformity. A lumbar puncture may be used to assess for subarachnoid bleeding, but it should not be performed until after CT has ruled out other structural pathology or intracranial shifts. Cerebral blood flow studies may also be performed, and chest X-ray may reveal cardiomegaly.

Treatment

Medical management involves close observation of the child using "AVM precautions" such as bed rest, sedation, a quiet environment, and decreased activity and stimulation. Invasive techniques can also be used to treat the malformation. Surgical intervention to excise the web is the ideal therapy but often impossible because of its location. When this is deemed the treatment of choice, the child must be medically stable for at least two to three weeks post initial bleed.

Flow-directed embolization is also used, especially with malformations in critical areas of the brain. Here, a catheter is introduced into the femoral artery and advanced to the defect. At that point, occlusive materials are introduced and carried to the malformation by direct blood flow. These materials, in essence, cause an occlusion to the deformity and divert blood flow through more normal channels (Behrman & Kliegman, 1998; Johnson & Oski, 1997).

For those children where surgery or embolization is not an option, radiotherapy using stereotaxic techniques may be utilized. The major disadvantage to this therapy is time as it may take up to two years before the treatment is completed.

Nursing Management

The nurse should manage the child with an AVM as any other client with a fragile neurological status. The ABCDEs, vital signs, and intracranial pressure should be closely monitored. Pupils should be checked and the Glasgow Coma Score calculated. "AVM precautions" must be strictly adhered to in order to maximize the child's recovery.

In addition, the nurse should watch for the sequelae of the treatment protocol chosen for the child whether it be surgical or radiological. The child who undergoes a craniotomy must be treated as all clients with intracranial surgery. On the other hand, the child who has embolization needs to be kept immobilized with pressure on the groin area to prevent arterial bleeding, and pedal pulses routinely checked. Families need information about the deformity and management options. The nurse should explain procedures as well as the post-treatment course for the child.

INFECTIONS

Infections of the neurological system that are discussed include meningitis (bacterial and viral), Reye's syndrome, and encephalitis.

Meningitis

Meningitis is an inflammation of the meninges that develops as a result of infection from either bacterial or viral agents. The causative organism is often age dependent. Neonates develop meningitis as a result of *Escherichia coli*; *Haemophilus influenzae*, type B; Group B *Streptococcus*; *Neisseria meningitidis*; *Streptococcus pneumoniae*; and *herpes*. Infants and children are susceptible to *Haemophilus influenzae*, type B; *Neisseria meningitidis*; *Streptococcus pneumoniae*; enterovirus; adenovirus; and the mumps virus. On the other hand, adolescents are at risk from exposure to *Neisseria meningitidis*; *Streptococcus pneumoniae*; *herpes*; adenovirus; and arbovirus (Behrman & Kliegman, 1998; Johnson & Oski, 1997; Wertz; 2002).

Bacterial Meningitis

Incidence and Etiology

Bacterial or pyogenic meningitis affects many infants, children, and teenagers in the United States each year; 90% of all cases are in children under five years of age (Wertz, 2002). The mortality rate is significant, even with appropriate antibiotic therapy (8% *H. influenzae*; 15% meningococcal; 25% pneumococcal). The infant and young child are at great risk for bacterial infection with males being affected more often than females (Behrman & Kliegman, 1998). The most common pathogens have a seasonal pattern: *Haemophilus influenzae*, type B, occurs most frequently in the autumn and early winter although with the administration of the Hib vaccine, the rate of infection has fallen. *Neisseria meningitidis* and *Streptococcus pneumoniae* are prevalent in the later winter and early spring. Meningitis can also follow penetrating trauma or neurosurgical intervention, but it is usually a secondary response to a primary infection such as otitis media, sinusitis, pharyngitis, cellulitis, pneumonia, septic arthritis, or dental caries.

Pathophysiology

The bacteria enter the blood supply and are disseminated throughout the body, including the meninges. There, they are seeded into the cerebrospinal fluid and spread throughout the subarachnoid space. An inflammatory response follows, and white blood cells accumulate over the surface of the brain with a thick, purulent exudate. *Neisseria meningitidis* tends to cover the parietal, occipital, and cerebellar regions of the brain while *Streptococcus pneumoniae* spreads over the anterior lobes. In either case, the brain becomes hyperemic and edematous resulting in increased intracranial pressure. Hydrocephalus may occur if the ventricles become infected and obstructed, or if the flow of cerebrospinal fluid within the subarachnoid space is impeded.

Prognosis depends on age, the organism, how quickly antibiotics and other medical interventions are initiated, and if there are complicating factors such as hydrocephalus, cerebritis, or disseminated intravascular coagulopathy. Sequelae such as hearing loss, blindness, paresis of facial muscles, and intellectual impairments are not uncommon (Behrman & Kliegman, 1998).

Clinical Manifestations

Manifestations depend on age and the pathogen. The infant less than three months of age may have subtle signs and symptoms, including being lethargic, fussy, irritable, or displaying paradoxic irritability, a state in which activities that normally soothe a baby, such as rocking or cuddling, aggravate the infant further. Fever may or may not be present; hypothermia is a possibility. In addition, alterations in feeding or sleep patterns and/or vomiting or diarrhea with or without weight loss may be seen. The infant will usually have a bulging anterior fontanelle unless dehydration is present. The infant who is further compromised may seize, show diminished level of consciousness, and have a depressed respiratory state where apneic episodes are not uncommon (Behrman & Kliegman, 1998; Johnson & Oski, 1997).

The infant over three months of age and the toddler will show many of the same manifestations, with usually a gradual onset of symptoms and change in activity level, fever, or irritability. The child over age two years may have gastrointestinal upset and cold-like prodromal signs. Later, chills and fever will develop. The extent of the inflammatory process determines many other symptoms. When there is cortical involvement, the child may become irritable, agitated, confused, delirious, or lethargic and somnolent. In addition, there may be nausea and projectile vomiting. If the cranial nerves are involved, the youngster will suffer from photophobia (extreme light sensitivity), diplopia (double vision), and tinnitus. If the cervical nerves are irritated, the child will have nuchal rigidity. If this is the case, an **opisthotonic** position may be assumed, whereby the head and neck are hyperextended (Figure 32-13). This child may also complain of headache, most often frontal; myalgias; joint pain; and malaise.

If the child is seriously compromised, there may be signs of shock including poor perfusion with delayed capillary refill time, elevated heart rate, normal or low blood pressure, cool and pale extremities, and diminished level of consciousness. In addition, signs of increased intracranial pressure may be noted. A rash may also be present; if it is petechial, purpura-like, or ecchymotic, the child may have meningococcemia and need immediate medical intervention.

On further examination, the child with meningitis may have hyper-reactive reflexes. In addition, positive Kernig and Brudzinski's responses may be seen (Behrman & Kliegman, 1998). **Kernig's** sign (Figure 32-14) is tested by having the child lie supine with hips flexed. If meningitis is present, the child will either resist the examiner's attempts to extend the leg or complain about pain on extension. **Brudzinski's** sign (Figure 32-15) is evoked when the youngster is supine. If there is meningeal irritation when the child's head is flexed forward, the child will automatically flex the hips and knees.

The meningitic infant or child is at risk for numerous complications including sepsis, seizures, subdural effusions, brain abscess, and/or hydrocephalus, all of which will increase intracranial pressure or septic arthritis. This child is also at risk for developing syndrome of idiopathic antidiuretic hormone secretion (SIADH) as well as disseminated intravascular coagulopathy (DIC). Refer to Chapter 26 for information about DIC and Chapter 28 for information about SIADH.

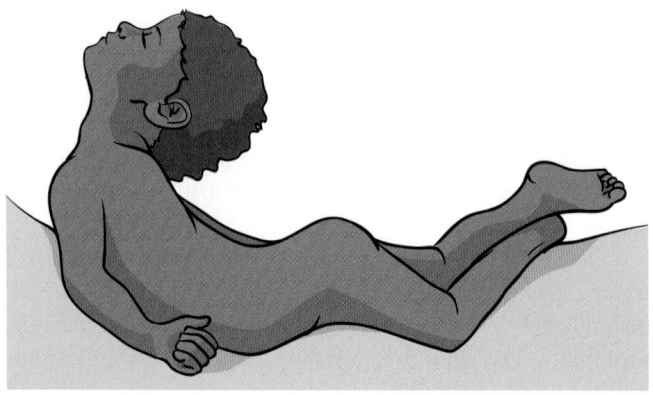

Figure 32-13 Opisthotonic Position

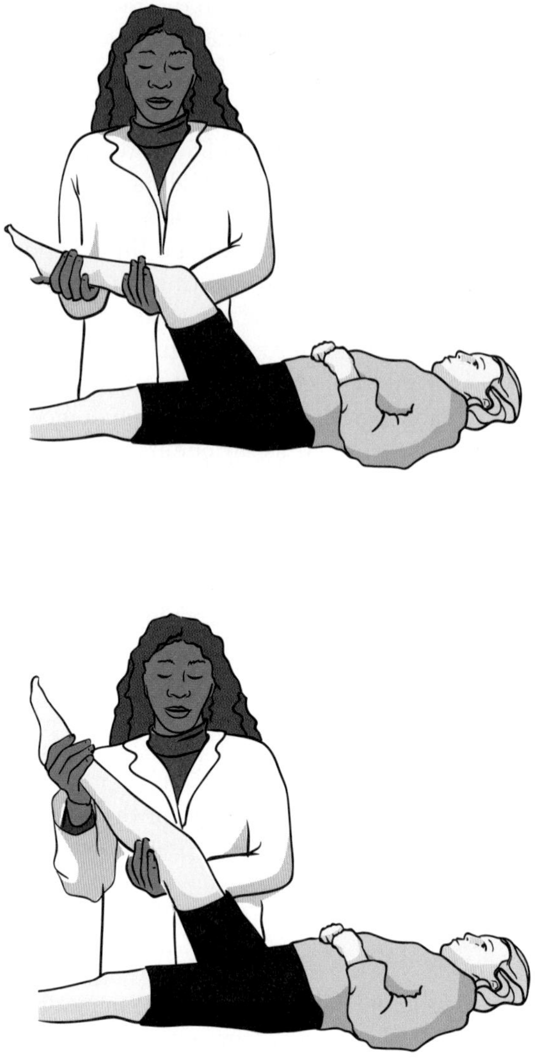

Figure 32-14 Kernig's Sign

Diagnosis

A detailed history is important, especially regarding the child's contact with other ill individuals, the duration of those illnesses, and their symptoms. The caregivers should also be asked if the youngster has developed a rash, had a seizure, or appears pale. In addition, they should be questioned about any changes in behavior, feeding, or sleeping patterns.

Laboratory tests include microscopic examination of blood, cerebrospinal fluid, and urine. A complete blood count will indicate if infection is present and whether or not it is bacterial. A culture of the CSF will identify the pathogen. Serum electrolytes and osmolarity should be checked to monitor hydration and note any signs of SIADH (headache, drowsiness, lethargy, confusion, diminished reflex response, hyponatremia, increased urine sodium, or urine specific gravity). In addition, clotting studies should be performed to determine if DIC is present.

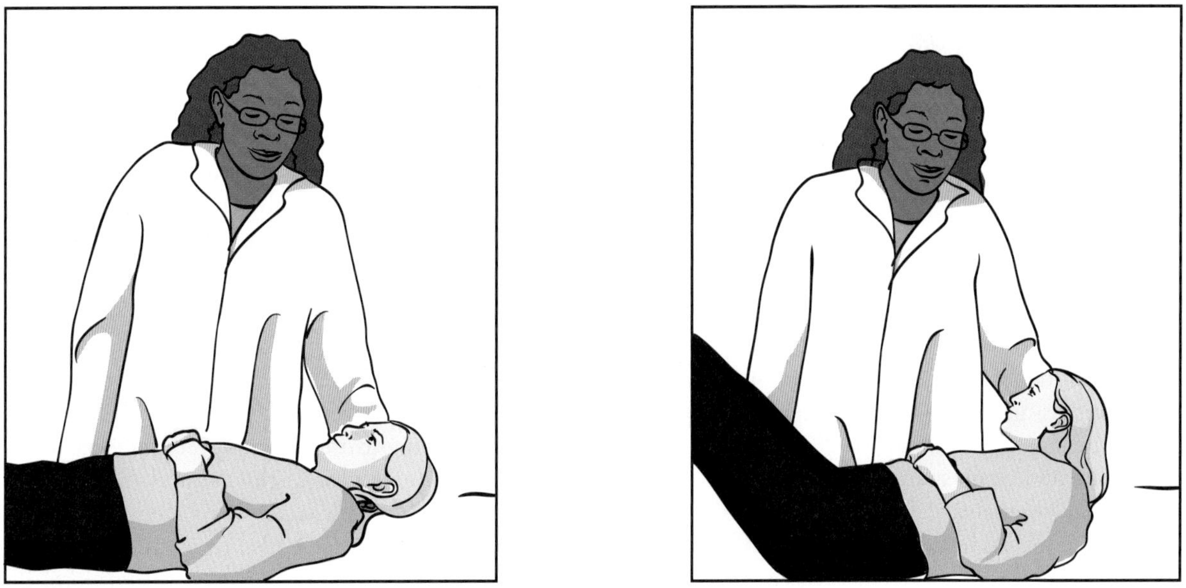

Figure 32-15 Brudzinski's Sign

Nursing Alert:

Meningococcemia

Meningitis caused by Neisseria meningitidis is a particularly virulent form of the disease that occurs concurrently with sepsis. It is spread by droplet and extremely contagious, especially in school or military settings.

The early signs are flu-like in nature: headache, fever, dizziness, malaise, and myalgia. Within hours, the child becomes significantly more ill with either sudden high rise in temperature or hypothermia. Behavior changes as well as delirium, apprehension, or a diminished level of consciousness may also be seen. Within 12 hours, the classic petechial to ecchymotic rash appears. This is caused by endotoxin release from the bacteria and indicates the onset of disseminated intravascular coagulopathy. In addition, signs of septic shock with alteration in vital signs, cyanosis, oliguria, and further depression of mental status may be seen. ***Waterhouse-Friedrichsen syndrome*** *is fulminating meningococcemia; the child is in septic shock, with disseminated intravascular coagulopathy and bilateral adrenal hemorrhage.*

Immediate medical interventions are needed. The airway must be protected by intubation. Poor perfusion is treated with fluid bolus administration as well as inotropic support. Antibiotics are given as soon as possible; however, further deterioration may occur as antibiotic lysis releases an overwhelming amount of endotoxin, further compromising the client and possibly causing death. Family members as well as others who come into close contact with children who have meningococcemia must be treated prophylactically with rifampin (Behrman & Kliegman, 1998).

Critical Thinking

Signs and Symptoms of Meningitis

There are numerous signs and symptoms of meningitis that are neurological in nature: bulging fontanelle, irritability, photophobia, nuchal rigidity, opisthotonic position, nausea, and vomiting. Discuss why these manifestations occur.

Lumbar punctures should be performed on all children suspected of having bacterial meningitis, except in the presence (other than a bulging fontanel) of increased intracranial pressure (Behrman & Kliegman, 1998). This assessment not only provides fluid samples, but also opening pressure measurements as well. The normal opening pressure value for the infant who is not crying is 50 millimeters of water; for the child, 85 millimeters of water. If the value exceeds 180 millimeters of water, meningitis should be suspected. Cerebrospinal fluid must also be examined microscopically, and the presence of white blood cells greater than 100 per cubic millimeter indicates meningitis. Fluid will appear

Nursing Alert:

Contraindications to a Lumbar Puncture

- *Evidence of airway instability*
- *Risk of apnea or respiratory arrest during the procedure secondary to positioning*
- *Shock (either hypovolemic or septic)*
- *Evidence of coagulopathy*
- *Any possibility of increased intracranial pressure*

cloudy to purulent depending on the number of neutrophils, and with meningitis, glucose will be decreased and protein increased (Behrman & Kliegman, 1998). To identify the pathogen, culture and Gram stain should be performed.

Urine should be analyzed for culture, specific gravity, and osmolarity. Latex agglutination should also be done to rapidly identify the bacterial antigen. Chest X-ray is usually performed in conjunction with the septic work-up as a silent pneumonia may be present. In addition, a CT or MRI may be needed to confirm a subdural effusion, cerebral edema, or hydrocephalus.

Treatment

The child with meningitis may be critically ill. Although intubation may not be needed, the child should be placed on a cardiorespiratory monitor until stable. In addition, this client may need supplemental oxygen as the illness will increase metabolism, thus raising oxygen consumption. It is not uncommon for infants and children with meningitis to be poorly perfused during the initial stages of this illness as vomiting and anorexia are often present. If signs of shock appear, the child may need fluid boluses or inotropic support. Signs of petechiae or purpura may indicate meningococcemia, DIC, or both, which need emergent management including intubation, fluid boluses, inotrope administration, blood or blood product infusions, and measures to control bleeding.

Seizure activity, generalized or focal, may also be present. If the episode is self-limiting or lasts less than five minutes, a jaw thrust and oxygen administration will be the only interventions necessary. On the other hand, if status epilepticus is evident, benzodiazepine will be given as the first drug of choice; phenytoin may be needed as well if seizure activity remains uncontrolled. Generally speaking, seizures do not continue past the acute phase of the illness unless there is accompanying parenchymal damage.

Antibiotics should be ordered immediately and continued for a total of seven to ten days, depending on the bacteria and the child's clinical response. Dexamethasone may be administered as an adjunct with the first dose and may continue for the first four days of treatment to help decrease the inflammatory response to lysis of the bacterial cell walls (Behrman & Kliegman, 1998). The antibiotics are usually given intravenously, the dosages are generally quite high, and peak and trough serum blood levels of the antibiotic are frequently obtained.

Complications must be quickly managed. Serum electrolytes and urine osmolarity should be checked daily during the acute phase to monitor trends toward SIADH. In addition, if septic joints appear, they should be treated vigorously with antibiotics. Subdural effusions or hydrocephalus should be treated in consultation with neurosurgery. Hearing loss or other sensory or motor deficits must be handled using a multidisciplinary approach.

Nursing Management

Before entering the room, the nurse caring for the child with bacterial meningitis must don appropriate protective attire, which includes a gown, gloves, and mask. These items should be used for at least 24 hours after the antibiotics have been started. The nurse is also responsible for ensuring visitors adhere to these precautions. Furthermore, the family members or other individuals who have had recent close contact with the child should be encouraged to speak with the health care provider to assess their need for prophylactic antibiotics.

The nurse should check vital signs frequently. Tachycardia may be a sign associated with fever or septic shock. The child's blood pressure and capillary refill time should also be monitored, and the skin evaluated carefully for signs of petechiae or purpura. A neurological evaluation should be performed. Although it is common for this child to be fussy or irritable, level of consciousness should be assessed frequently as alteration in mental state may be caused by a myriad of potential complications associated with the disease such as subdural effusion, cerebral edema, or increased intracranial pressure. The infant's fontanelle must be frequently palpated for bulging (common in meningitis) or depression (a result of dehydration), and head circumference measured daily as rapid enlargement may be secondary to development of hydrocephalus. The nurse should also observe for any seizure activity and notify the health care provider at once if it appears.

Antibiotics should be administered as prescribed. The nurse must try to maintain normothermia as elevated fever will increase metabolism and oxygen consumption. Either acetaminophen or ibuprofen can be administered to reduce fever, but if it persists, a hypothermia blanket may be utilized. In addition, the nurse should measure input and output along with urine specific gravity to watch for the signs associated with the SIADH.

Comfort measures include keeping the environment quiet and dark (the child may have photophobia), and allowing the child to assume a comfortable position. Pain should be managed using acetaminophen or a non-steroidal anti-inflammatory preparation. Furthermore, the nurse caring for the child with meningitis should be on the alert for sequelae that may appear at any time. Changes in neurological status or urine output may become evident, and a warm, red, swollen joint may indicate the bacteria has spread, creating a septic arthritis.

The nurse should also address developmental and social needs. Family members should be encouraged to visit and bring toys or music from home to make the hospital a more familiar and less frightening environment. Once the child's condition is stable, the nurse should enlist the assistance of the youngster's primary caregivers in helping with bathing, feeding, and dressing. This activity not only makes the client feel more comfortable and secure, it also empowers the family members as they are providing care their child needs to become healthy again.

The child with meningitis may have deficits as a result of the infection such as cognitive changes or hearing impairment. Therefore, the nurse should enlist the assistance of the rehabilitation team within the hospital to begin working with the child and family and begin discharge planning with community resources if these complications occur.

Family Teaching

The family should first be educated about the Hib vaccine to ensure this child and other children in the home are not at risk for *Haemophilus influenzae*, type B. A copy of the immunization protocol for children should be provided and referrals made to a clinic or health care provider for follow-up testing and treatment of any sequelae. If the child has sequelae, the caregivers will need to learn how to manage the problems at home. If the child has seizures or hydrocephalus, extensive teaching will be required. Learning or hearing difficulties will need special education, speech therapy, hearing aids, or classes in sign language or lip reading. The nurse may initiate treatment and education, and arrange for community support.

Viral (Aseptic) Meningitis

Incidence and Etiology

Aseptic or viral meningitis is an inflammatory response of the leptomeninges. Eighty-five percent of the cases are caused by the non-polio enterovirus. Most cases occur in the summer or fall, and many are the result of inappropriately or partially treated bacterial disease (Behrman & Kliegman, 1998).

Pathophysiology

Although many pathogens are not identified, adolescents are usually more at risk for viral meningitis than infants and toddlers. The pathogens include herpes, adenovirus, and arbovirus. Some cases may also be caused by mycoplasma, chlamydia, various protozoa, and fungi.

Clinical Manifestations

The child with aseptic meningitis does not appear to be as ill as the child with bacterial infection. The onset may be gradual or abrupt, and the youngster irritable or lethargic. General malaise compounded by myalgia; headache; photophobia; anorexia, nausea, and/or vomiting; upper respiratory symptoms such as sore throat or chest pain; and a maculopapular rash may be seen. In addition, signs associated with meningeal irritation: nuchal rigidity, back pain, and positive Kernig's and Brudzinski's reflexes may occur. Fever is usually present, but rarely over 40° centigrade (104°F). If seizures occur, they are associated with hyperthermia rather than the meningitis. Signs and symptoms subside within three to ten days (Behrman & Kliegman, 1998).

Diagnosis

A septic work-up is needed, as meningitis must be confirmed as either bacterial or viral in nature. Analysis of cerebrospinal fluid will confirm the diagnosis: there will be less than 500 white blood cells per cubic millimeter; most will be leukocytes. Glucose will be greater than 40 milligrams per deciliter and protein decreased. Gram stain and culture will be negative. Initially, it may be difficult to distinguish between bacterial and viral meningitis as the signs and symptoms are similar. Therefore, a second spinal tap should be performed within six to eight hours for re-examination of the fluid.

Treatment

Until aseptic meningitis is verified, the child is treated as if the cause is bacterial, and antibiotics started. Once the diagnosis is determined to be viral, management usually becomes more palliative and supportive in nature.

Nursing Management

The nurse caring for this child should concentrate on comfort measures. The room should be kept quiet with the lights dim, fluids given intravenously and/or orally, and medications administered to control fever, headache, and myalgias.

Family Teaching

The nurse should help the caregivers prepare for managing their child at home as hospitalization will be brief, and provide the name of community resources for follow-up appointments and evaluations. Although viral meningitis is generally considered a benign disease where most children recover quickly and without incident, there may be sequelae. Many children complain of fatigue, weakness, irritability, incoordination, and/or muscle pain or spasms for several weeks postinfection. In addition, they are at risk for hearing loss, altered language development, or other learning deficits. Caregivers should be taught comfort measures and fever control as well as signs of any complications that need immediate medical attention such as change in mental status or development of seizures.

Reye's Syndrome

Reye's syndrome, first described in 1963, is an acute life-threatening encephalopathy with accompanying microvascular fatty deposits in the liver and kidney (Behrman & Kliegman, 1998; Johnson & Oski, 1997).

Incidence and Etiology

The incidence of Reye's syndrome in the United States has been steadily falling since its peak in 1980. The most vulnerable children are European American under five years of age who live in urban and suburban areas.

The etiology of Reye's is unclear although there is consensus that it follows a mild viral illness such as varicella, influenza B, influenza A, Epstein-Barr, adenovirus, or coxsackievirus. Links between aspirin use with the original illness and Reye's have been suspected for some time, even though no definitive data have ever been produced to either confirm or deny this hypothesis. However, since caregivers have been advised to use acetaminophen rather than salicylates (aspirin) for their children, incidence rates of Reye's syndrome have declined (Johnson & Oski, 1997).

Even though mortality from Reye's has dropped dramatically in the last few years, many children do suffer from residual effects such as attention disorders, speech and language delays, fine and/or gross motor impairments, diminished visual acuity or coordination, and intellectual deficits.

Pathophysiology

The liver becomes enlarged and assumes a yellow hue caused by fatty deposits in its microvasculature, which precipitate depletion of glucose stores, reduction in enzymes to convert ammonia to urea, and abnormalities in liver enzymes. At the same time cerebral edema with accompanying increased intracranial pressure becomes evident (Behrman & Kliegman, 1998; Johnson & Oski, 1997).

Clinical Manifestations

Initially, the child has symptoms of a mild viral infection, and signs of recovery may be noted; however, within 24 to 48 hours, the child's condition worsens. Vomiting with or without fever may be present, and when vomiting diminishes, there will be a marked change in the child's behavior, with confusion, fear, irritability, anxiety, or a flat affect apparent. Speech patterns may change and the level of consciousness deteriorates into a coma-like state, interrupted by periods of screaming, ranting, and raving. Either pupil will be dilated and exquisitely sensitive to light, or the child may lose vision entirely. Within 24 hours, the child slips into a deeper coma and demonstrates either decorticate or decerebrate posturing. Cranial nerve reflexes may be lost. Death from Reye's usually occurs within two to three days of onset, although the downward progression of the illness may stop abruptly at any time (Johnson & Oski, 1997).

Diagnosis

A complete blood count, chemistries, blood/urea/nitrogen, amylase, liver function tests, clotting times, and urine analysis should be done. Arterial blood should also be sampled to evaluate pH as well as for signs of acidosis, alkalosis, and respiratory sufficiency. Cerebrospinal fluid should be examined; if less than eight leukocytes per cubic millimeter with normal glucose and protein concentrations are found, Reye's is the diagnosis. The lumbar puncture, however, may not be a safe procedure to perform during the acute phase of the illness as the increased intracranial pressure associated with cerebral edema may precipitate brain herniation. CT may be done to confirm the presence of cerebral edema. A liver biopsy will also be done as it is the only test that can confirm Reye's (Behrman & Kliegman, 1998).

Treatment

Because children are acutely ill and at risk for rapid deterioration, they should be placed in an intensive care unit and intubated. Neuromuscular blocking agents, sedatives, and analgesics are administered to protect the airway, provide for adequate ventilation, correct any respiratory acidosis or alkalosis, and decrease intracranial pressure. As blood gases and other serum assessments are frequently measured, an arterial catheter is inserted. Electrolytes and glucose levels should be monitored often with replacements administered intravenously as needed. If clotting times are abnormal, vitamin K or fresh frozen plasma may be given (Johnson & Oski, 1997). To correct elevated ammonia levels, neomycin may be provided through a nasogastric tube. Once prothrombin levels are normal, neurosurgeons may place an intraventricular catheter to monitor intracranial pressure. If pressures remain elevated despite ventilatory interventions, mannitol, a hyperosmotic diuretic, may be administered to decrease the edema. Although fluid restriction is no longer recommended, strict measurement of intake and output is warranted; therefore, an indwelling urinary catheter should be placed. Seizures should be controlled with benzodiazepines and phenytoin.

Nursing Alert:

Over-the-Counter Medications Containing Aspirin

- *Alka-Seltzer*
- *Anacin*
- *Anacin Maximum Strength*
- *Aspergum*
- *Bufferin*
- *Bufferin Extra-Strength*
- *Coricidin*
- *Coricidin Demilets*
- *Dristan Tablets*
- *Excedrin*
- *4-Way Cold Tablets*
- *Medilets*
- *Pepto Bismol*
- *Triaminicin*

Nursing Management

The child requires intensive care by the nurse including frequent monitoring of vital signs, respiratory effort, neurological status, and laboratory values. The nurse also needs to observe for responses to the interventions performed and medications administered. Once the child is past the acute phase, emotional support, appropriate play activities, and interactions with others should be provided.

Family Teaching

The family needs to be prepared for the sequelae associated with Reye's, and the nurse should work with them and community resources to ensure special needs are met upon discharge. In addition, the nurse must educate the family about the use of salicylates in children with viral illnesses, given a list of over-the-counter medicines to avoid, and shown where to find ingredients on all over-the-counter preparations, thereby avoiding any exposure.

Encephalitis

Encephalitis is an inflammation of the brain that can be diffuse or localized.

Incidence and Etiology

Encepalitis can be caused by bacteria, viruses, fungi, or protozoa, although most are caused by viruses. Table 32-7 lists the causes of encephalitis. The most common cause beyond the neonatal period is herpes type I, *herpes simplex*. The arboviruses, caused by arthropod bites to humans, are usually endemic to specific regional areas. Some children will develop encephalitis following vaccines for tetanus, measles, rubella, diphtheria, or pertussis; however, these cases are rare. More commonly though, cases of encephalitis occur in immunosuppressed children, especially those with AIDS (Behrman & Kliegman, 1998).

Pathophysiology

Primary encephalitis is a result of the invasion of the pathogen into the central nervous system resulting in cerebral or cerebellar dysfunction. Postinfectious or parainfectious encephalitis occurs with other illnesses or following the administration of a vaccine or other substance. During the initial or non-neural stage, the child suffers from an acute febrile illness secondary to ingestion or vector bite. The neuronal phase occurs when the infection is seeded from the point of origin to the central nervous system.

Clinical Manifestations

The manifestations depend on the invading organism as well as the location of the infection within the brain. The disease has an acute onset with a strong neurological component. At first, the child may have an intense headache, signs of respiratory infection, nausea, or vomiting. Meningeal irritation (nuchal rigidity, photophobia, positive Kernig's and Brudzinski's signs), disorientation, confusion, personality and

TABLE 32-7 Causes of Encephalitis

Viruses	Enteroviruses: Poliovirus, Echovirus, Coxsackievirus Adenoviruses/Herpesviruses: Herpes Type I, Herpes Type II, Varicella, Herpes Zoster, Epstein-Barr, Cytomegalovirus Arboviruses: California Virus, Western Equine, St. Louis, Colorado Tick Measles Mumps Rubella Rabies Hepatitis B
Bacteria	*Haemophilus influenzae* *Neisseria meningitidis* *Streptococcus pneumoniae* Cat Scratch Fever
Other	*Chlamydia pneumoniae* Rickettsial Infections Rocky Mountain Spotted Fever Lyme Disease Fungi Protozoa Drugs: Trimethoprim

behavior changes, hemiplegia, ataxia, weakness, or slurred speech may also be seen. Alterations in cranial nerve and other reflex responses may be present as well as generalized or focal seizure activity with intermittent periods of screaming, hallucinating, or moving in bizarre fashions. Lastly, the child's level of consciousness may deteriorate from stupor to coma (Johnson & Oski, 1997).

Generally speaking, the younger the patient, the more devastating the sequelae. Although some children will recover completely, many have motor, intellectual, visual, and auditory deficits. The cardiovascular system, liver, and lungs may also be adversely affected by the pathogen.

Diagnosis

Diagnosis of encephalitis occurs when other pathologies such as mass lesions, metabolic disturbances, and other infectious processes have been ruled out. To confirm encephalitis, several procedures must be performed, including a complete history and physical examination. Laboratory analysis of blood, cerebrospinal fluid, and urine should be obtained. Initially, the CSF values may be within normal limits, but within two days, there is an increase in the number of leukocytes (most often monocytes). There also may be an elevation in protein. Stool and nasopharyngeal swabs should be taken to check for the presence of enteroviruses. Serologic assays can be done to detect Epstein-Barr virus. Brain biopsy is the only way to confirm *herpes simplex*. Noninvasive measures (CT, MRI) can be utilized to assess for cerebral edema, ventricular compression, or temporal lobe necrosis associated with herpes simplex. Electroencephalography may show slight diffuse slowing.

Treatment

Supportive care is needed and antibiotics are administered to all children until bacterial infection is ruled out. Youngsters with viral infections should be given anti-viral agents. There is an increased risk for seizures, respiratory failure, and increased intracranial pressure; therefore, during the acute phase of illness, close monitoring in intensive care units is important as the children may need to be intubated, mechanically ventilated, oxygenated, and treated for cerebral edema. Nutrition is supported either through intravenous supplementation or gastric tube placement. Meticulous skin care must occur if the child is in a coma (Behrman & Kliegman, 1998).

Nursing Management

Continual assessment of vital signs and paying special attention to the airway and respiratory function is critical. A complete neurological assessment should include pupil checks and Glasgow Coma Score evaluations to note possible increases in intracranial pressure. Being aware of seizure activity, and completing passive range of motion exercises, maintaining good skin integrity, and providing for adequate nutrition are other areas of nursing intervention. Caregivers should be involved in the child's care as appropriate.

Family Teaching

The family should always receive education about the causes of encephalitis, as well as procedures the child will undergo and any treatment needed. If the child has sequelae, caregivers will need to learn how to manage the problems at home. Sequelae involving any learning or hearing difficulties will require special education, speech therapy, hearing aids, or classes in sign language or lip reading. Caregivers will also need to become aware of governmental and private community agencies that can be helpful if their child has any residual problem.

NEUROLOGICAL INJURIES

Injuries discussed in this section include head trauma, spinal cord injury, and submersion (drowning).

Head Trauma

Head trauma or injury, defined as any pathologic process occurring to the scalp, skull, or brain parenchyma resulting from mechanical force, is a major cause of pediatric mortality.

Incidence and Etiology

It is estimated that 60–70% of all children with multiple trauma suffer from head injury, and these injuries account for up to 70% of all trauma deaths (Bruce, 1993). Of the nearly 5 million children sustaining a head injury every year, around 200,000 are hospitalized. More frequent in males than females, the causes may be varied: falls, bicycling, abuse, competitive sports, or motor vehicle accidents (Johnson & Oski, 1997). Traumatic brain injury (TBI) is the largest source of intellectual impairment, seizures, and physical disability in children.

Children are prone to head injury because of their physical immaturity (refer back to Table 32-2), as well as their high activity level, immature developmental skills, and increased head to body mass ratio (Palmer, 2000). In addition, developmentally they are at great risk for trauma, as infants, toddlers, and preschoolers are not aware of the dangers in their environments and cannot take precautions to avoid them. Once faced with a dilemma, young children do not have the experience or cognitive ability to quickly problem solve.

Age determines the type of head trauma seen in children. Infants who are not carefully attended often fall from high surfaces such as dressing tables, bed, sofas, and stairways. However, child abuse is the most prevalent cause of head injury in this age group. Shaken baby syndrome occurs when the infant is shaken violently or hit against a hard surface such as a wall or mattress. Refer to Chapter 36 for more information about shaken baby syndrome.

Toddlers and school-aged children are often injured in motor vehicle crashes (MVCs) either as passengers, pedestrians, bike-riders, or skateboarders. According to the American Automobile Association, in 1995, car crashes killed 195 pedestrians younger than five years and 272 pedestrians between ages five and nine years (Washington Post, 1997). The adolescent, on the other hand, is typically involved in a vehicle crash as either a passenger or driver or injured during sports activities. Furthermore, in our violent society, more and more teens fall victim to penetrating trauma from firearms or sharp weapons. Children are also prone to particular types of head injuries. Skull fractures, which are often accompanied by underlying hematomas and brain injury, are common. Furthermore, the secondary effects of trauma including cerebral edema, increased intracranial pressure or cerebral hypertension, and malignant brain edema (hyperemia) may occur.

Pathophysiology

Head injuries are categorized as either primary or secondary in nature (Wertz, 2002). Primary injury, which occurs at the moment of impact, is when initial cellular damage occurs. The mechanism of injury (Figure 32-16), or external force to the head and/or neck, may be a result of a direct blow to the head (such as being hit with a baseball bat) producing a coup injury. On the other hand, acceleration/deceleration movement of the brain within the skull causes a coup-contrecoup injury in which there are two points of trauma within the cranial vault (such as hitting the head on the windshield of a car when hit from behind). One is at the initial or coup site while the other is a result of the moving brain hitting the opposite side of the cranium. In this case, there may be shearing of the small veins and arteries that travel from the cerebral surface to the dural sinuses as well as diffuse axial injury. Regardless of the mechanism, at the time of impact, there is an increase both in arterial and intracranial pressures, bradycardia, hypertension, and alteration in level of consciousness. Table 32-8 presents information relative to the various forms of head trauma related to the specific type of injury received. Figures 32-17 and 32-18 provide illustrations of epidural and subdural hematomas which can occur due to head trauma.

Secondary injury involves both the brain and the body's response to the trauma, and is evident immediately after impact or several minutes, hours, days, weeks, or months later. Usually it is a result of brain tissue destruction secondary to hypoxia, hemorrhage, space occupying lesions, hypotension, edema, or change in the blood-brain barrier.

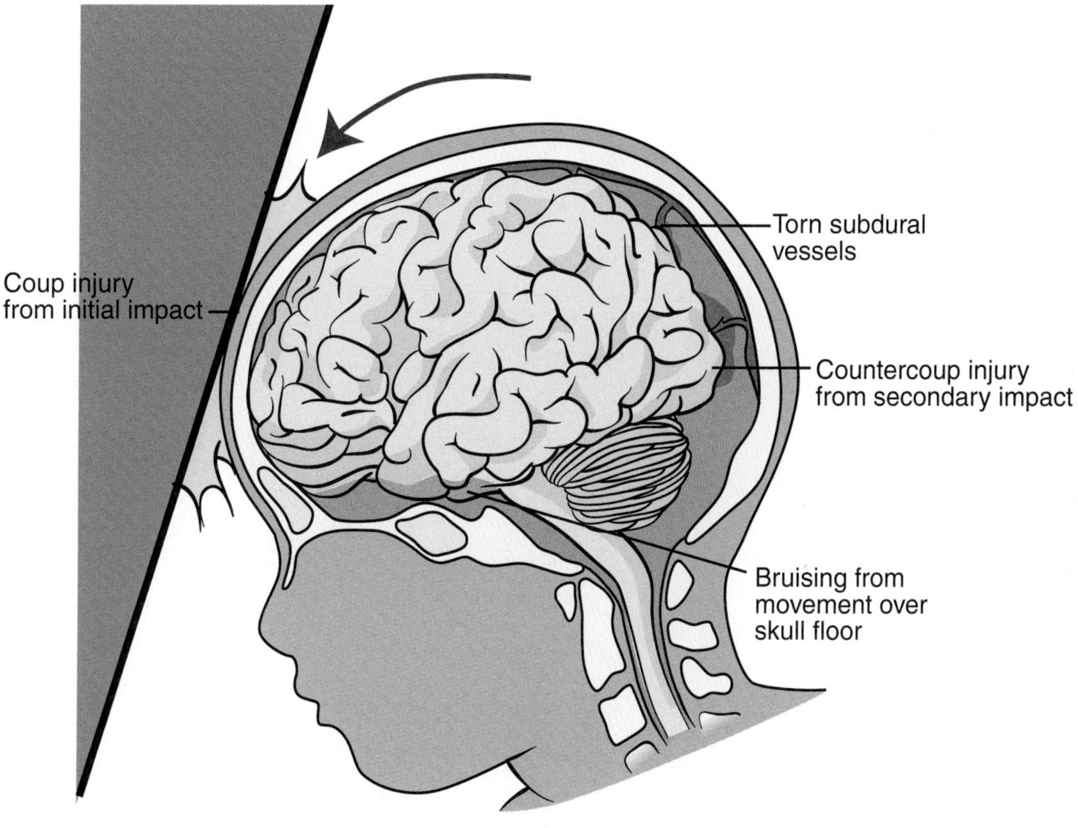

Figure 32-16 Coup/Contrecoup Injury

TABLE 32-8 Forms of Head Trauma, Pathology, Manifestation, Treatment, and Nursing Issues

Injury	Pathology	Clinical Manifestations	Treatment	Nursing Issues
Scalp Injury	• Laceration to scalp which can be very vascular	• Copious bleeding at site • Hypovolemia if large vessel or small infant	• Irrigation with normal saline • Sutures	• Provide comfort to child during procedure
Concussive Injuries *Concussion*	• Usually secondary to blunt injury • Caused by the stretching, compression, or tearing of nerve fibers near the brain stem without accompanying gross structural damage	• Transient alteration in mental status with loss of awareness or responsiveness • Soft neurological signs such as headache, nausea with or without vomiting, vertigo or dizziness, amnesia	• Palliative	• Observe closely for several hours as clinical manifestations seen mimic those of more serious injury
Pediatric Concussive Syndrome	• Results from insult to brain stem • Occurs most often in children under three years of age	• At time of injury, appears stunned • Later on, clammy, pale, lethargic, frequent episodes of vomiting	• IV hydration	• Observe closely for signs of more serious injury

Skull Fractures
Linear
	• Account for 75% of cranial trauma
	• Results from impact to large area of the skull
	• Most benign unless middle meningeal artery is nicked, then epidural hematoma is formed
		• No focal signs
		• Headache and tenderness at site
			• Palliative	• Watch for signs of complications:
				  • Subgaleal hematoma, a soft boggy mass at the site, which may be seen 2 to 3 days post-injury
				  • Growing fracture in which the dura is trapped in the healing fracture line forming a leptomeningeal cyst

Depressed	• Rare in children under 3 years as skull bones are soft; instead an indentation forms in the cranium at the point of impact causing a "ping-pong" appearance • Break in the integrity of the skull, shattering it into fragments that may be depressed into the brain tissue with a hematoma forming on top	• Pain and tenderness at the site • Visible or palpated depression of the skull • Seizures	• Surgical elevation of any bony fragment depressed more than the thickness of the skull or 5 millimeters • Antibiotics and tetanus prophylaxis	• Observe for signs of seizure activity and infection

TABLE 32-8 *Continued*

Compound	• Combination of a scalp laceration and depressed skull fracture	• Same as above	• Same as above	• Same as above
Basilar	• Occurs in the inferior, posterior portion of the skull and involves the frontal, ethmoid, sphenoid, temporal, or occipital bones with or without dural tear	• CSF leakage from the nose or ears • Periorbital ecchymosis and Battle's sign/mastoid bruising	• Palliative • Dural repair for persistent CSF leak	• Check for presence of CSF in draining fluid • Test fluid present for glucose • Assure an NG tube is *never* placed as it may migrate through the fracture site into the cranial vault and into the brain itself • Watch for signs of cranial nerve injury, a common sequela, involving nerves I, II. III,VII, or VIII
Diastatic	• Separation of the sutures of the skull secondary to trauma • Most common site: lambdoid • Occur most often in children under 4 years of age	• Pain at the site	• Palliative	
Diffuse Brain Injury	• Results from tearing of the anterior bridging veins, petechial hemorrhage of white matter, shearing of myelin and axons, and/or contusion of the corpus callosum • May be secondary to increased ICP or subarachnoid hemorrhage • In infants, secondary to abuse; in older children, associated with other trauma such as cerebral contusion or laceration, cerebral edema, cortical trauma, or scattered intracranial hemorrhage	• No external signs of injury • Deep coma with decorticate posturing or flaccid areflexia • Fixed and dilated pupils • May be periods of apnea and bradycardia	• Dependent on concurrent trauma • Airway and ventilatory support as indicated	• Watch for change in neurological status • Observe for alterations in respiratory or cardiovascular systems

continues

TABLE 32-8 *Continued*

Injury	Pathology	Clinical Manifestations	Treatment	Nursing Issues
Cerebral Contusion or Laceration	• Bruising or pulping of brain tissue along with tears to vessels and petechial hemorrhage • Parenchymal and vessel injury causes brain necrosis and infarction	• Focal signs based on the area of the brain injured • Level of consciousness can range from confusion to deep and prolonged diminished mental state • Signs of increased ICP	• Rarely surgical • Management of any rise in ICP • Palliative	• Observe for change in neurological status

Intracranial Hematomas and Hemorrhages
Epidural
	• Rare in children, but may occur with linear skull fractures
	• Temporal and parietal areas most common site
	• After trauma, blood accumulates between the dura and skull (epidural hematoma, see Figure 32-17) forcing tissue downward and inward, as hematoma forms and expands, displacing brain parenchyma under tentorium, and precipitating herniation through foramen magnum
	• Pressure placed on cranial nerves and vessels
	• May be either arterial (rapid onset of symptoms) or venous in nature
		• Diminished level of consciousness
		• Cushing's triad with wide pulse pressure, increased systolic blood pressure and bradycardia
		• Increased ICP
		• Respiratory depression
		• Fixed and dilated pupil with contralateral extremity spasticity or flaccidity
		• Paresis of cranial nerves III and VI
		• Papilledema
			• Management of increased ICP
			• Surgical evacuation of hematoma
				• Be aware pediatric presentation is different from adult:
				  • Adults: period of unconsciousness caused by primary injury, then lucid period as concussive effects diminish, then degeneration of consciousness caused by expanding hematoma
				  • Children: 1/3 present like adults, 1/3 have no initial loss of consciousness, 1/3 have immediate loss of consciousness not followed by lucid period

Subdural	• Occur most frequently under six months of age as a result of shaken baby syndrome • Results from damage to bridging veins, and spreads over both hemispheres (subdural hematoma, see Figure 32-18) until it reaches the tentorium and solidifies into	• Altered mental status ranging from confusion and agitation to lethargy to stupor • Increased ICP • Retinal hemorrhage • Papilledema • General: vomiting, fever, seizures, irritability • Infant also: full fontanelle, increase in head circumference	• Surgical evacuation of hematoma if large and causing neurological or systemic compromise • Subdural taps in infant in which CSF is removed through a catheter placed into the ventricles	• Watch for change in neurological status • Help family accept child's changed state as many have neurological sequelae such as seizures and developmental regression

TABLE 32-8 ***Continued***

	a hematoma placing wide-spread pressure on the brain • May occur with and without skull fracture • May be acute with signs and symptoms appearing within 72 hours post-injury or chronic in which manifestations are not seen for weeks or months	• Older child: headache with nausea, unsteady gait		
Subarachnoid	• Associated with severe head trauma and often accompany other intracranial injuries	• Those associated with concurrent injury • Signs of meningeal irritation from bloody CSF such as nuchal rigidity, diplopia, photophobia, and headache	• Manage concurrent trauma • Manage increased ICP • Palliative for meningeal irritation	• Observe for signs of severe concurrent injury • Comfort measures
Intracerebral	• Deep contusion or laceration of brain tissue most often as a result of penetrating injury • Result in diffuse bleeding within the parenchyma and formation of hematoma associated with the many, small hemorrhages	• Focal signs dependent upon area of the brain injured • Increased ICP	• Manage increased ICP • Usually surgery not indicated because of diffuse nature of injury	• Monitor neurological status
Penetrating Injury *Impalement*	• Foreign body traumatically entering the skull and brain	• Hemorrhage at site • Focal signs dependent upon area injured	• Removal of object in the operating room • Antibiotics and tetanus prophylaxis	• *Never* remove object, but stabilize until child gets to the operating room
Gun Shot Wounds	• Low velocity bullets enter the skull and ricochet within it causing multiple tracks of destruction of parenchyma and vessels • High velocity bullets create immediate shattering of bone, tissue, and vessels	• Immediate loss of consciousness • Hemorrhage • Focal signs dependent upon area injured	• Surgical debridement of the track as well as removal of bony and bullet fragments	• Prepare family as children who survive often have seizures and multiple focal deficits

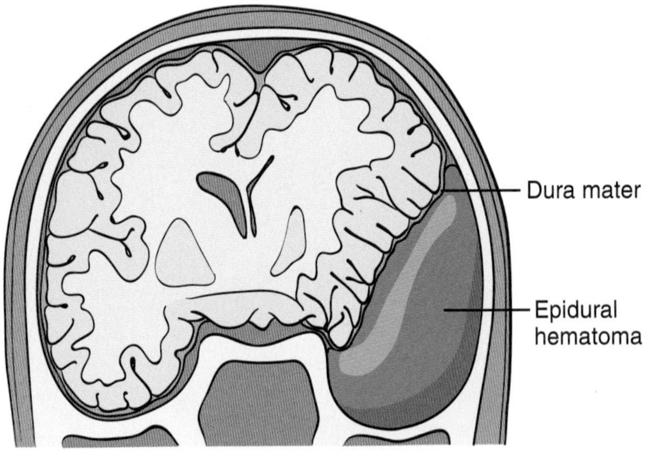

Figure 32-17 Epidural Hematoma

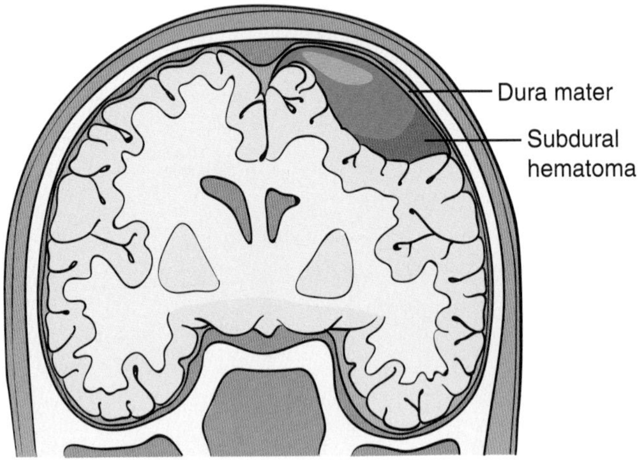

Figure 32-18 Subdural Hematoma

Whatever the cause, however, the end result is increased intracranial pressure, which if left unresolved will lead to irreversible brain damage and death.

Two forms of secondary injury (cerebral edema and malignant brain edema) are particularly devastating to children. **Cerebral edema,** defined as an increase in intracellular fluid in the brain resulting from anoxia, vasodilation, vessel damage, and/or vascular stasis (Behrman & Kliegman, 1998), may not be seen for the first day or two post-injury. Cerebral edema leads to an increased extravascular volume which in turns precipitates a rise in intracranial pressure. As autoregulation becomes impaired, edema continues to build and pressure rises further, causing compression of the ventricles, small cisterns, and a midline shift.

Malignant brain edema or cerebral hyperemia, is unique to children. Rather than an edematous response to trauma, there is a hyperemic or vascular reaction because of the disruption in the blood-brain barrier. In addition, the mechanism to control cerebrospinal fluid absorption is impaired.

Clinical Manifestations

Children with head injuries display a variety of symptoms depending on the specific pathology as well as its severity. The child with a mild injury or concussion may have no loss of consciousness or a very short episode (less than two minutes), and may or may not have amnesia of the event. In addition, headaches, nausea, or vomiting may occur. Behavior initially is within normal limits, and the child discharged from the emergency department or urgent care center to home after a period of observation.

With a moderate injury, the child will have loss of consciousness in the field; by the time the emergency room is reached, the level of consciousness may improve. The infant with moderate injury may be lethargic, vomit, or have a post-traumatic seizure. The child, on the other hand, may complain of headache, nausea, vertigo (which may be caused by compression of the eighth cranial nerve), and fatigue, and may vomit, seize, become irritable, and/or be amnesic of the event. If the trauma is to the frontal area, aggressiveness and combativeness may also be seen. In either case, it is important to remember diminished mental status may be caused by a postictal period rather than the head injury itself. Generally, children with this type of trauma are admitted to the hospital for observation and close evaluation as their injuries have similar signs and symptoms of more severe trauma.

The child with severe injury will demonstrate symptoms consistent with increased intracranial pressure, and will have a long period of seriously diminished mental status or unconscsiousness. Most often, these children will remain in a coma for a maximum of two weeks; beyond that time, they will either begin to show subtle signs of improvement or deteriorate further and be declared brain dead (Bruce, 1993).

The child's vital signs will reflect the seriousness of the injury. Changes in respiratory effort or periods of apnea can occur because of hypovolemic shock, injury to the spinal cord above C-4, metabolic disturbances, and/or damage to or pressure on the medulla. In addition, the increased intracranial pressure will produce a pattern where respiratory rate is increased, decreased, again increased, and then becomes Cheyne-Stokes in nature. Heart rate is an index of brain stem function. Bradycardia is frequently associated with increased intracranial pressure. However, tachycardia (sign of blood or fluid loss, hypovolemic shock, hypoxia, anxiety, or pain) following bradycardia is a grave, preterminal sign in the head-injured child. Blood pressure also reflects the seriousness of injury. Hypotension is rare with isolated injury except as a terminal event; therefore, the child with low pressure should be evaluated for concurrent trauma and shock. Increased systolic pressure with a wide pulse pressure are classic signs of increased intracranial pressure. Hypertension alone may indicate pain, anxiety, or a preexisting condition.

Pathologic neurological changes may also be seen in the severely injured child, with signs of either extreme irritability or restlessness. Both can be attributed to increased intracranial pressure, an enlarging intracranial mass, cerebral edema, malignant brain edema, or hypoxia. Reflexes may become either hyporesponsive, hyperresponsive, or nonexistent, and motor responses may deteriorate. In addition, the child might assume either a decorticate, decerebrate, or flaccid posture. Pupils may be sluggish in reacting to light and/or unequal in size. The child with one dilated pupil and contralateral spasticity or flaccidity displays the classic signs of intensely high intracranial pressure and is at risk for brain herniation if measures to mediate the pressure are not initiated immediately (Behrman & Kliegman, 1998; Johnson & Oski, 1997).

Box 32-6 Classification of head injury based on GCS

Total Glasgow score from 13 to 15 or motor score of 6: mild head injury

Total Glasgow score from 9 to 12 or motor score from 4 to 5: moderate head injury

Total Glasgow score less than 7 or motor score of 1, 2, or 3: severe head injury

Diagnosis

Identification of the type and severity of head injury involves obtaining a history of the trauma, past medical history, observation, assessment, and evaluation. The first issue is to ascertain exactly what happened, the victim's initial response to the trauma, and how the status has changed. A thorough medical history must also be obtained to learn if the child has any congenital or acquired conditions that might have an impact on the head trauma or the response to it, such as previous head trauma, seizures, hydrocephalus, cranial surgery, or hemophilia. Furthermore, the child's baseline abilities and behavior should be ascertained, as intellectual or motor deficiencies, attention deficit disorder, or autistic or pervasive developmental disorder traits. Also, information should be obtained from caregivers relative to the child's reactions to stressful situations, especially with strangers, as what might be called abusive or combative behavior in one child might be considered normal in another.

Neurological evaluation, rather than a single assessment, is a continual series of observations and examinations that indicate the child's clinical improvement or deterioration. Generally speaking, maximum depression should occur just after the incident with some improvement beginning to show shortly thereafter. If this does not occur, serious brain injury may be diagnosed.

Two common tools for evaluation of neurological status are the Glasgow Coma Scale (GCS) and AVPU. Refer back to Box 32-2 for AVPU and Table 32-3 for GCS information. For them to be meaningful, however, they must be used frequently with results compared so trends in improvement or deterioration can be noted. Generally speaking, Glasgow scores can be used to help in the classification of head injury (Box 32-6).

Cranial nerves should also be assessed. The conscious child is asked to perform a variety of activities such as opening and closing the eyes, moving the mouth, and sticking out the tongue to evaluate nerves. In the unconscious child, however, other methods must be employed. Refer back to Table 32-4 for methods of assessing the cranial nerves in an unconscious child.

Pupils must also be assessed frequently. A unilateral fixed and dilated pupil implies pressure on the third cranial nerve, usually resulting from increased intracranial pressure, one of the classic signs of impending herniation. The eyes should also be carefully evaluated. It is crucial retinal hemorrhage be identified as it is frequently associated with subdural hematoma, an injury that is most often secondary to abuse. In addition, papilledema, a late sign of increased intracranial pressure, may be present.

Examination of the head is critical. The face and scalp should be inspected for hematomas, abrasions, or lacerations. If the latter are present, the wound should be checked for debris as well as a dural tear or bony fragments. The cranium should be palpated for depressions or signs of crepitus. In addition, the ears and nose should be evaluated for blood or cerebrospinal fluid leakage.

Radiologic examinations are performed to determine specific pathologies. Most often, the first X ray is the lateral cervical spine. Most victims of head injury are multiply-injured; therefore, this assessment must be done to rule out spinal trauma. Other plain films may be done to confirm simple skull fractures. The most widely used tool in the diagnosis of head injury is computerized axial tomography (CT), which is performed on all infants and children with altered level of consciousness, suspected basilar or depressed skull fracture, penetrating injury, or neurological or focal deficits. Structural injuries such as hematomas, hemorrhages, contusions, or fractures can usually be visualized clearly. There may be times, however, when a CT appears normal despite a severely depressed sensorium. If the child shows signs of improvement after a short period of time, the injury may have been concussive in nature; however, if there is no change in client status or if deterioration begins, another series of films should be obtained to determine if venous hemorrhage has occurred. Magnetic resonance imaging (MRI) is an excellent adjunct to CT as subtle injury can be clearly detected. It is nearly impossible for this equipment to be used with the unstable child, however, as the process is slow, sometimes lasting 45 minutes.

Laboratory tests for the child with head injury involve complete blood count, chemistries, urine assays, and clotting times. If the child is intubated and/or hyperventilated, arterial blood gases will need to be checked frequently to ensure paO_2 is kept at 100 while $paCO_2$ is between 30 and 32. An electroencephalogram may be performed if the child seizes to determine the area of the brain involved and the type of convulsion occurring.

Treatment

The primary goals of care are to maintain ventilation, oxygenation, and perfusion while achieving an intracranial pressure that is safe; and prevent secondary injuries. To provide this, severely injured children should be in pediatric intensive care units with both invasive and noninvasive monitoring of their vital signs and pressures.

The child with a diminished level of consciousness or Glasgow Coma Score less than eight must be intubated, and arterial blood gases and pulse oximetry frequently monitored. To help control intracranial pressure, most intubated, head-injured children are sedated and chemically paralyzed, and oxygen and carbon dioxide levels frequently monitored. By keeping the paO_2 near 100 and the CO_2 between 30 and 32, cerebral blood flow can be reduced by 50% without compromising oxygen or nutrient requirements (Silverman, 1992). The child who is not intubated must also be observed carefully for changes in respiratory status (apnea, Cheyne-Stokes), which might indicate neurological deterioration and the need to receive manual ventilation.

Perfusion must be maintained to ensure adequate cerebral perfusion pressure, and signs of hypovolemia aggressively treated with crystalloids. Response to fluid administration can be assessed by evaluating heart rate, blood pressure, capillary refill time, and the level of consciousness. Urine output can be measured by an indwelling catheter. If perfusion is not adequate despite aggressive fluid resuscitation or if signs of cerebral edema appear, inotropes such as dopamine or dobutamine will need to be administered. Until adequate cerebral perfusion pressure is ensured, the bed should be kept flat to promote blood flow to the head.

Increased intracranial pressure must be treated. Only during the initial phase is hyperventilation performed. Mannitol, a potent diuretic, may also be administered to shrink brain volume. It should be given slowly while watching for signs of tachycardia and low blood pressure. In some children, there may be a rebound effect with mannitol as it may increase cerebral blood flow. If that occurs, the signs of increased intracranial pressure will reappear with more intensity than originally noted, and the neurosurgery department must be called at once so other modalities to control the pressure can be initiated. Neurological status is difficult, if not impossible, to assess during this time. Therefore, intracranial monitoring will be needed. Steroids do not have a place in the acute management of head trauma.

BOX 32-7 Measuring brain oxygenization

The Licox tissue probe measures oxygen levels of the brain tissue itself near the site of injury to ensure that the brain tissue is not infarcting. ICP monitoring is also in place. To ensure oxygen above levels of 20, propofal (Diprivan), increased FiO_2, increased pCO_2, mannitol, and blood products are utilized. For children older than 8 years of age, SiO_2 monitors are used to keep track of brain oxygenization. (Personal communication, M. Wellington, June 2001)

Managing the environment may help keep intracranial pressure under control. The room should be kept quiet and minimal invasive procedures performed. If suctioning needs to be done, administering lidocaine may help block the gag and cough reflexes, which intensify intracranial pressure. In addition, once cerebral perfusion pressure is adequate, the head of the bed should be elevated about 30 degrees. The child's head should be kept in the midline to promote venous drainage and the hips and knees should not be hyperflexed. Pain should initially be managed with acetaminophen, and if this is not effective, narcotics should be given and neurological assessments made with invasive ICP monitoring equipment. The room temperature should be kept comfortable; if the room is too hot, cerebral metabolism will increase; if the room is too cold, the child will shiver, and again raise cerebral metabolism.

Intracranial monitoring catheters may be placed in the epidural or subdural spaces; however, the standard at this time is the intraventricular probe. This equipment has several advantages: it measures intracranial pressure and it also allows for withdrawal of fluid. In children, removing just 30 milliliters of cerebrospinal fluid may create enough room inside the skull to mediate the high pressure inside. There will be times when increased intracranial pressure will need

Kids Want To Know

When can I go back to school?

Ten-year-old Barbara was hit by a car and suffers from right-sided hemiplegia. There are no other neurological problems. She wonders when she can return to school.

Explain that she needs to finish up rehab, but will return to school. In the meantime, encourage visits from schoolmates while Barbara is in the rehab unit. Reassure her that if she needs any special help while at school, it will be provided.

to be managed surgically. Burr holes or craniotomies may be needed to remove hematomas, bony fragments, or foreign bodies. Some studies have even indicated that a bony window be removed from the skull to allow more space for brain expansion and when the pressure is down, the flap replaced.

Complications of head trauma are listed in Table 32-9. Some complications must be treated aggressively and quickly while others may be handled through rehabilitation.

Nursing Management

Nursing management begins with assessing the head-injured client using the ABCDE approach. The nurse also evaluates the child's physical, developmental, and social needs and plans actions accordingly. Working with these children, however, requires a team approach with nursing, medicine, neurosurgery, rehabilitation experts, and social services collaborating to meet the needs of the child and family, because if the trauma is severe, their life will be different.

The nurse must assess the airway of the child and check endotracheal placement frequently. Arterial blood gases and pulse oximetry should be monitored, and if intubated, the child positioned comfortably and assessed for signs of pain or need for sedation.

The child's respiratory status must be evaluated whether intubated or not because of being at risk for deterioration from the unstable neurological condition. Perfusion must also be assessed frequently, and if inotropes such as dopamine or dobutamine are administered, the nurse must be aware of the side effects (tachycardia, increased blood pressure, cardiac dysrhythmias). Frequent monitoring for signs of increased intracranial pressure and being aware of the modalities used to treat increased ICP are also important.

If neurological sequelae are present, the nurse must work with the child in accepting the disability. The older child and adolescent can be challenging if they feel they have lost control of their lives and bodies and are different from their peers. The nurse can work with these children by encouraging venting frustrations, providing positive feedback,

Nursing Tip:

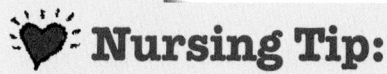

Assessing for pain in the chemically paralyzed child

- Tachycardia
- Increased blood pressure
- Tears

TABLE 32-9 Common Complications of Head Injury

Complication	Management
Seizures • Immediate: usually occur within seconds of injury; not precursor of long-term epilepsy • Early: occur within first week post-injury, but most often within first 24 hours; are associated with minor trauma or focal injury	• Assure patent airway and provide oxygen • If occur 30 after minutes injury, may administer benzodiazepines • If still seizing after benzodiazepins, may give phenytoin
• Late: occur one week after trauma; secondary to cortical scarring	• Give benzodiazepins and phenytoin initially • Since there is a high incidence of recurrent or permanent epilepsy, may be placed on oral anticonvulsants and then weaned off medication after six seizure-free months
Alterations in fluid homeostasis: either SIADH or diabetes insipidus (DI)	• Monitor electrolytes and fluid status • For DI, administer medications such as DDAVP
Post-concussive syndrome: may occur any time after the event; signs and symptoms include dizziness, vertigo, nausea, vomiting, photophobia, headache, trouble concentrating, changes in memory, and alterations in behavior such as aggression, regression, withdrawal, and emotional lability	• Provide palliative treatment • Refer to special education, rehabilitation, counseling for child as well as caregivers
Intellectual impairment, focal deficits, sensory disturbances, communication dysfunctions, motor abnormalities, or chronic alteration in mental status	• Refer to special education, rehabilitation, counseling for child as well as caregivers

and working with families and peers to ensure needed support is available.

Physical, occupational, and speech therapists should begin working with traumatic brain injured children as soon as possible. The nurse, even in the intensive care unit, should reinforce the regimens and encourage family members to participate in therapeutic exercises as well.

If the child's injuries lead to a diminished level of consciousness or a vegetative state, the nurse should work with the family in collaboration with social workers, psychologists, and clergy. Caregivers should be encouraged to bring in favorite toys and tapes of music or the family speak so the child can hear the familiar voices often during the day. When performing the daily assessments, all lacerations, abrasions, and hematomas should be examined to evaluate how well they are healing. Dressings, surgical incisions, and the child's temperature should also be assessed to determine their status.

Discharge planning needs to begin as soon as the child enters the hospital. The rehabilitation unit and social workers should help determine the services needed and how the family can arrange for them. Planning might include transfer to another center for therapy, making physical adjustments to the family home to accommodate a hospital bed or wheelchair, and/or securing appliances such as walkers or braces. The nurse should also arrange for follow-up with the multidisciplinary team members caring for the child during the acute phase of his recovery.

Family Teaching

Families with head-injured children have had their lives changed in seconds, and often come into emergency departments fearing the worst and hoping for the best, not really knowing what lies ahead. Most caregivers are ill-prepared for dealing with intensive care stays, surgical interventions, and long-term therapies including acute care hospitalizations as well as rehabilitation in inpatient and ambulatory settings. They usually go through highs and lows emotionally as their child improves, plateaus, and deteriorates. The nurse can help by supporting and educating caregivers about the recovery process of brain injury, and enlist the help of other professionals as well as encourage the family to seek out peer groups and national foundations.

Furthermore, the nurse should act as liaison for the child, the family, and the resources needed for rehabilitation. This can begin in the hospital setting when caregivers can be taught various therapeutic techniques to perform. In addition, family members should be encouraged to bring in toys and books based on the child's new level of functioning. Finally, the nurse must be an advocate for injury prevention. It is important to talk with families about safety issues emphasizing that bike helmets can avert as many as 85% of brain injuries while proper utilization of car seats and seatbelts can eliminate between 65% and 75% of head trauma (Chameides & Hazinski, 1994).

Spinal Cord Injury

Spinal cord injury includes damage to the cervical, thoracolumbar, and lumbar regions.

Incidence and Etiology

Vertebral injuries account for 2% to 3% of all childhood traumas (Scully & Luerrsen, 1995). Children under ten years of age have the lowest incidence. The number of young adults (ages 20 to 24 years) injured is four times greater than children and adolescents together. As with most trauma, males predominate over females with a 2:1 ratio (Dickman & Rekate, 1993).

Most spinal injuries are the result of motor vehicle crashes. In young children, the mechanism is either pedestrian-vehicle, bike-vehicle, or passenger-related, whereas in adolescence, passenger- and driver-related injuries account for most cord trauma. Mortality rate for cord trauma is exceedingly high in children, and over half the victims will die within the first hour following injury. Another 20% will succumb within the first three months (Dickman & Rekate, 1993).

Pathophysiology

Children suffer from different types of injury than adults because of their physical and developmental immaturity. Because of these characteristics, 75% of all spinal injuries of

Nursing Alert:

Lap-Belt Syndrome

"Lap-belt syndrome" is often seen in children under age 13 years who are passengers in motor vehicle crashes and wearing two- or three-point restraints. However, because of their anatomic immaturity, these belts do not protect children from injury. The seat belts, which normally sit on the pelvic girdle of adult passengers, lie on the abdomen of the child. When a crash occurs, the child is extremely hyperflexed over the belt, which acts as a fulcrum, and then snaps back upright. This impact directly hits the abdominal area with the force continuing posteriorly to the spinal column and cord.

Signs and symptoms include bruising across the pelvis and hematuria.

Injuries include:

- *Lumbar/sacral fracture or subluxation, most commonly at L-1 or L-2*
- *Lumbar/sacral cord injury, either complete or incomplete, most commonly at L-1 or L-2*
- *Abdominal injury to hollow and/or solid organs*
- *Perforated intestinal viscera*
- *Bladder hematoma/rupture*
- *Mild to moderate head injury*

children under age eight years are in the cervical area, with the highest incidence at the C-3 segment. The second most common area is the thoracolumbar region, probably because of improperly placed seat belts (Sivit & Bulas, 1993). Between ages eight and 14 years, 60% of injury is cervical, 20% thoracolumbar, and the remaining solely lumbar.

Most spinal cord injuries resulting in permanent loss of movement or sensation are not caused by complete transection, but rather by contusion, compression, vascular damage, and/or hemorrhage.

Clinical Manifestations

The clinical manifestations depend on whether or not concurrent injuries are present, the level of the trauma, and if the lesion is complete or incomplete. As the child is usually a victim of multiple trauma, the presenting picture is complex. Refer to Table 32-10 for manifestations of neurogenic and spinal shock and Table 32-11 for the symptoms according to the level of injury.

Diagnosis

All children with multisystem injury must be treated as if spinal cord injury is present until it has definitively been ruled out. Diagnosis of injury can be made either clinically and/or radiologically.

Treatment

The goals of the initial phase of managing the child with a spinal cord injury are to do no further harm and prevent further damage. Airway patency must be assured. Breathing will need to be evaluated and if high injury is present, the child must be intubated. If mechanical ventilation is a long-term possibility (clients with trauma above C-4), a tracheostomy should be performed. Proper perfusion and hydration must be ensured. Heart rate and blood pressure should be monitored by using electronic equipment, and any pathologic changes need to be treated quickly. The injuries to the vertebral column or spinal cord must be managed aggressively. Immobilization, the first step, is started where the trauma occurred by the prehospital providers and carried through to the hospital. Surgical management may be necessary to prevent further injury and promote healing. Debridement and decompression should take place as soon as possible after the injury; eight hours should be the maximum delay time. To stabilize the vertebrae, a spinal fusion may be performed using bone from other areas of the body. After this type of surgery, a body brace or shell is usually worn for six weeks for protection and alignment. If extensive trauma to the column has occurred, internal fixation devices may be required. To decrease the neurological sequelae associated with cord damage, methylprednisolone is administered to those clients with motor deficits. It *must* be started within eight hours of the injury, although it is prudent to begin the infusion as soon as possible (Bracken, et al., 1990).

Rehabilitation should begin early in the treatment regimen. Simple range of motion and other passive exercises may prevent contractures and muscle wasting as well as promote healing. Basic equipment such as footboards and

TABLE 32-10 Comparison of Neurogenic and Spinal Shock

Neurogenic Shock	Spinal Shock

Neurogenic shock is a form of distributive shock that accompanies complete high spinal cord injury. It is caused by interruption of sympathetic impulses from the spinal cord in the cervical/thoracic region.
 	
The hallmark signs include:
• Vasodilation
• Hypotension
• Bradycardia
• Warm flushed skin
• Inability to perspire
• Hypothermia
	Spinal shock is the complete loss of all reflex activity after spinal cord injury. This is a transient event that often occurs shortly after the trauma and can persist for as long as seven to 10 days.
	
	Signs include:
	• Below the level of the lesion
	  • Flaccid, areflexic extremities
	  • Loss of deep tendon reflexes
	  • No sensory response
	• Autonomic dysfunction
	  • Hypotension
	  • Bradycardia
	  • Decreased peripheral vascular resistance
	  • Impaired temperature control
	  • Warm, flushed, dry skin
	• Loss of sphincter control with urinary retention
	• Priapism

TABLE 32-11 Deficits Displayed Secondary to Level of Lesion

Level	Deficits
C-1 to C-2	• Quadriplegia with total loss of respiratory function • Flaccid paralysis
C-2 to C-4	• Quadriplegia with loss of phrenic innervation to diaphragm
C-4 to C-5	• Quadriplegia with possible phrenic nerve involvement caused by edema resulting in loss of respiratory function
C-5 to C-6	• Quadriplegia but with gross arm movements • Diaphragmatic breathing • No intercostal respirations
C-6 to C-7	• Quadriplegia but with biceps intact • Diaphragmatic breathing • Complete loss of shoulder movement
C-7 to C-8	• Quadriplegia with biceps and triceps intact • Diaphragmatic breathing • No function of intrinsic hand muscles
T-1 to T-2	• Paraplegia with loss of leg, bowel, bladder, and sexual function • Some loss of intercostal muscles • Arm function intact
T-2 to L-2	• Paraplegia with loss of varying degrees of intercostal and abdominal muscles
Below L-2 Cauda Equina	• Varying amounts of motor and sensory loss • Bowel and bladder dysfunction

Nursing Alert:

Autonomic Dysreflexia

After spinal shock has resolved and reflex activity has returned, children with high cervical or thoracic lesions may react to a noxious stimulus such as a distended bladder, constipation, or fecal impaction with a potential life-threatening sympathetic nervous system response. Spasms of the pelvic viscera and arterioles produce vasoconstriction below the lesion resulting in hypertension and superficial vasodilation, flushing, piloerection, and perfuse perspiration above the injury. To compensate for the increased blood pressure, the heart rate is slowed via vagal stimulation; however because of the trauma to the cord, this impulse cannot be sent to areas below the damage. Without rapid reversal of these symptoms, which is usually just removal of the stimulant, the victim may stroke, seize, or die.

splints should also be used in the initial stages of recovery. Later on, the physical and occupational therapists will work with the child in adaptive behaviors and use of equipment such as braces, crutches, walkers, or wheelchairs. In addition, if the youngster is mechanically ventilated, team members from respiratory and pulmonary will be able to assist in ensuring portable ventilators are available.

The emotional needs of the client must also be addressed, and opportunities provided to express anger, frustrations, and expectations. Working with psychologists, psychiatrists, social workers, and/or clergy may prove very beneficial.

Nursing Management

The nurse's primary responsibility is to ensure adequate oxygenation, ventilation, and perfusion by carefully monitoring vital signs and respiratory status. Bony prominences must be checked often for breakdown although skin integrity can be maintained with proper alignment, positioning, and use of lotions, egg crates, or sheepskin. If external devices are used to maintain immobility, pin or screw care is important, and all surgical sites should be watched carefully for signs of leakage, inflammation, or infection.

Providing adequate nutrition can be challenging. The child with a lower lesion can eat regular food without problem; however, the youngster who is quadriplegic may need gastrostomy tube placement. If this occurs, skin care must be provided.

Nursing Alert:

SCIWORA

SCIWORA, spinal cord injury without radiologic abnormality, accounts for as much as one-quarter of all pediatric spinal cord trauma. The child may initially experience brief sensory or motor deficits; however, these symptoms are usually gone by the time the victim reaches the emergency room and are often not reported. Initial X rays or CT show no bony abnormality. Therefore, based on the clinical and radiologic evidence, it is determined that the youngster has no spinal cord injury.

Onset of neurological symptoms can appear as late as four days post-trauma. Usually, signs of neurological deterioration are noted along with characteristics of either complete transection or partial cord syndromes.

Approximately two-thirds of the victims are under age eight years. Half the injuries are complete and thoracic in nature while the remaining 50% are incomplete and involve the cervical and lumbar regions.

This injury occurs as a result of the spinal column's cartilaginous structure and flexibility. It can withstand up to two inches of stretch without disruption. The cord, on the other hand, can rupture with only a quarter-inch elongation. Thus, on traditional X ray, the vertebrae will appear normal. MRI will be needed to appreciate the cord injury.

Bowel and bladder control may be difficult to achieve. The child may have an indwelling urinary catheter early in the course of recovery; but later on, training can begin with intermittent catheterization as the goal. Credé's method, where pressure is placed over the symphysis pubis to expel the urine, is not advised if the bladder is full as it may rupture with pressure. Bowel training involves a diet high in fiber and use of stool softeners. The nurse should work with the rehabilitation specialists and reinforce all the exercises and skills learned during the sessions, and utilize any equipment specially adapted to the child's needs.

Perhaps the most difficult issue for the nurse working with these children is the emotional aspect of care. The lives of these youngsters change in an instant, and the nurse must provide the support needed in adapting to their different body function and image. It is important to avoid being too solicitous or overprotective, yet at the same time encourage the children to meet small, short-term goals that will offer them as much independence as possible. The nurse should also provide an environment where the child is able to speak freely about frustrations, anxieties, and fears. Finally, as much normal activity as possible should be provided, while at the same time not presenting challenges that are too difficult to meet. In-house school or tutors may help meet educational needs and allow the school-aged child and adolescent to keep up with classmates.

Family Teaching

The family of the child with a cord injury often goes from a state of shock and disbelief to one of unresolved grief, and may need professional help. The family needs to be involved with the multidisciplinary team and learn how to work with their youngster in the normal activities of living such as dressing, feeding, and mobility. They will also need to learn exercises and various therapeutic techniques. Once these skills are mastered family members will feel they have gained some control over their lives.

Discharge planning should begin early, and most often a rehabilitation center is the next step for these children as it helps them achieve their maximum potential physically, emotionally, and intellectually. The family will decide if the child is treated as an inpatient or as an outpatient. The financial burdens associated with having a spinal cord injured child are phenomenal. Social workers can be helpful in securing funds for training, special appliances, and alterations that may need to be made to the home.

Drowning

Drowning is defined as death from a submersion incident in a liquid medium within the first 24 hours post-injury. **Near-drowning** refers to survival for more than 24 hours regardless of the final outcome. **Secondary drowning** refers to the rapid deterioration of respiratory function from several hours to days after successful resuscitation.

Incidence and Etiology

Drowning is one of the most preventable causes of childhood morbidity and mortality. Claiming around 2,000 victims per year, it is second only to transportation injuries as the most common cause of unintentional injury in the pediatric population. Almost half the children are under four years of age, with the peak incidence between one and two years of age, and then again during adolescence. The annual rate for boys to suffer from submersion injuries is almost 10 times higher than for girls (Behrman & Kliegman, 1998).

Over 90% of all submersion injuries occur in fresh water; 50% of those are in swimming pools. Ninety percent are residential pools. Drownings most often occur between 4:00 PM and 6:00 PM when family members are busy preparing dinner. Caregivers suspect something is wrong when the child is missing, usually for less than five minutes. Interestingly, splashes, screams, or cries for help, are rarely heard.

Bathtubs account for about 7% of all drownings; most often from either poor supervision or intentional trauma. Hot tubs and spas cause 10% of the drowning deaths of toddlers between ages 10 and 23 months by entrapping their hair or extremities in the mechanical suction devices. As these tubs and spas are filled with warm or hot water that is often laden with *Pseudomonas aeruginosa*, survivors of this type of submersion have a recovery complicated by infection. Three- to five-gallon buckets can also be hazardous, especially to toddlers as they are too top-heavy and uncoordinated to lift themselves out of the pail if they fall in head first. Only a very small number of submersion injuries are a result of boating or diving mishaps.

Children with convulsive disorders are high risk for submersion. Although swimming and water activities are not ill-advised for these youngsters, they must be carefully supervised in pools, tubs, or boats at all times.

Pathophysiology

There are two types of drowning. **Wet drowning** is caused by the aspiration of fluid into the lungs; it is the most common form especially for infants and toddlers. **Dry drowning,** which only occurs 10–15% of the time, is secondary to hypoxemia resulting from intense laryngospasm. In these cases, fluid has not entered the lungs.

Cold water victims have a better chance of recovery than warm water victims because either the reduced body temperature slows cerebral metabolism enough to protect the brain and heart, or the child undergoes a diver's reflex where blood is diverted to the vital organs. Most often, children whose body temperatures are lower than 28° centigrade have the best survival rates and outcomes.

The sequences occurring with drowning are that first, the child who is trapped in the water panics, struggles, and attempts to move using swimming-like motions. The breath is then held before some water is swallowed. Vomiting, and then aspiration of the vomit, and laryngospams, lasting less than two minutes, follow. The child then panics, and hypoxia follows, then the child swallows even more fluid. If this is a dry drowning, profound laryngospams then occur, and the child becomes severely hypoxic, seizes, and dies. If it is a wet drowning, the child will become unconscious. Laryngospams lessen as reflexes are lost and large amounts of fluid passively enter the airway and stomach.

The major insult associated with submersion is hypoxemia, and, initially, the body will try to compensate for this by shunting blood to the lungs to increase circulating oxygen. This fluid shift results in pulmonary edema, which when combined with the aspirated liquid causes decreased lung compliance. This is further complicated by the inactivation of pulmonary surfactant.

Hypoxia and acidosis lead to the complications associated with submersion. Cardiac dysrhythmias such as asystole, bradycardia, and ventricular fibrillation are frequently manifested. Other common pathologies seen include neurological dysfunction and renal failure. Hypothermia may also occur with submersion as youngsters tend to lose heat rapidly as their surface area is large and their fat stores do not provide enough insulation. Although extreme hypothermia may prove advantageous, a milder form may precipitate decreased coordination, increased muscle rigidity, decreased breath holding time, and deterioration in the level of consciousness.

Clinical Manifestations

The clinical presentation depends on the length of time underwater, the temperature of the fluid, the child's response to the event, and the initial maneuvers or treatments done at the scene, first by bystanders and then by the prehospital providers. Refer to Table 32-12 for the signs and symptoms.

The child submerged for a short period of time and those needing no immediate interventions will present with the least symptomatology, and may show few, if any, signs of neurological dysfunction; display minimal respiratory distress; have normal or almost normal blood gases and chest X rays; and be mildly hypothermic. Most often, there are no concurrent injuries. This child usually recovers without complication. However, the child with a longer submersion will display more pathology; if cardiopulmonary resuscitation was required at the scene, symptoms will be more devastating. There will be a diminished level of consciousness, ranging from stupor to coma, and there may or may not be appropriate reactions to painful stimuli. Reflex responses may or may not be intact, and decorticate, decerebrate, or areflexive posturing may be present. If the victim was also hypothermic, cardiac dysrhythmias commonly associated with hypoxia and acidosis may be exacerbated.

The child's clinical picture may change within the first 24 hours after the event. Cerebral edema may occur, leading to the classic signs of increased intracranial pressure as well as seizures. Respiratory function may also be affected as pulmonary edema, bronchospasm, and irregularities in breathing pattern such as Cheyne-Stokes, periodic breathing, or apnea may occur. In addition, chest X-ray may show marked abnormalities. Signs and symptoms of concurrent injuries may be manifested at this time as well, and the child may be hypovolemic, neurogenic, or exhibit spinal shock. Furthermore, the victim of a wet drowning may be a prime candidate for pneumonia. Other complications such as clotting abnormalities, electrolyte imbalances, and renal disturbances may also be seen.

Recovery from a submersion incident is painfully slow. Some children will survive intact, while others will have neurological sequelae such as cerebral palsy, intellectual deficits, and emotional lability. Still other victims will remain in a chronic vegetative state.

Diagnosis

The first step in making the diagnosis of drowning or near-drowning is getting an accurate history from any witnesses at the scene as well as the prehospital providers. It is vital to ascertain the following information:

- Amount of time the child was submerged
- Temperature of the fluid

TABLE 32-12 Manifestations of Near-Drowning by Category

Category	Signs and Symptoms
A	• Awake, alert, and oriented with Glasgow Coma Score of 14 to 15 • Minimal, if any, concurrent injury • Mild, if any, hypothermia • Minimal, if any, changes on chest X-ray • Slight signs of acidosis on arterial blood gas • May develop characteristics of neurological or pulmonary deterioration in 24 hours
B	• Alteration in neurological status ranging from stupor to coma with Glasgow Coma Score between 8 and 13; intact pupil and pain responses • Moderate concurrent injury • Mild to moderate hypothermia • Alteration in respiratory pattern • Abnormal chest X-ray and arterial blood gas
C	• Comatose with nonpurposeful response to pain and reflex responses, which may or may not be intact • Seizures • Compromised cardiovascular system with dysrhythmias, signs of shock, and DIC • Alteration in pulmonary function ranging from slight respiratory distress to failure • Abnormal chest X-ray • Arterial blood gas with a metabolic acidosis • Electrolyte imbalance such as hyperkalemia and hyperglycemia
C-1	As in "C" plus • Decorticate posturing • Cheyne-Stokes respirations
C-2	As in "C" plus • Decerebrate posturing • Central hyperventilation
C-3	As in "C" plus • Flaccid posturing • Apneustic breathing
C-4	As in "C" plus • Flaccid posturing • Apneic • No detectable circulation

Adapted from Wellington, M. C., & Wayner, R. F. (1995). Alterations in neurologic function. In J. Ball & R. Bindler (Eds.). Pediatric nursing: Caring for children. *Norwalk, CT: Appleton and Lange.*

- What the fluid was: salt or fresh water, from a hot tub or spa, or a cleaning solution in a bucket
- If the mechanism (inability to swim versus diving into a shallow pool) was conducive to causing other trauma such as head or spinal cord injury
- Victim's initial response after the rescue:
  - If there were spontaneous respirations or heart beats
  - If the child was awake, semi-conscious, or totally unresponsive
- Actions taken by the bystanders, including CPR, and the child's response to them
- Time the prehospital providers arrived
- Interventions performed by the paramedics and the victim's reaction
- Child's status during transport to the hospital

The child must have a thorough physical assessment with evaluation of the airway, ventilatory status, and circulation occurring immediately. If signs of shock are present, causes should be quickly determined as either from hypovolemia or neurological injury. Temperature must be monitored to rule out hypothermia. In addition, level of consciousness should be measured and pupils checked for both size and reaction to light. Arterial blood gases should be drawn to note pathologic changes in carbon dioxide and/or oxygen levels; pulse oximetry may not be a useful tool initially because of poor perfusion and/or hypothermia. Other laboratory assessments should include serum chemistries, blood/urea/nitrogen, creatinine, and clotting factors as well as cultures of blood, urine, and tracheal aspirate if the drowning occurred in a pond, spa, hot tub, or other source of potential infection. The radiologic examinations performed are chest X-ray to note the presence of an infiltrate, and a head CT to observe for intracranial or skull injury and/or cerebral edema. If concurrent injury is suspected, other films such as lateral cervical spine and pelvis are also taken.

Treatment

Treatment of the submersion victim must begin at the scene with immediate initiation of ventilations, compressions, and rewarming as indicated. If the airway is unstable, gas exchange poor, breathing effort minimal at best, and level of consciousness diminished (Glasgow Coma Score of 8 or less), the child must be intubated. A nasogastric or orogastric tube should then be placed both to empty the stomach to prevent emesis and the threat of aspiration as well as to relieve gastric distention and enhance ventilation. Furthermore, if the respiratory status is compromised by pulmonary edema and aspiration, positive end expiratory pressure will need to be delivered. If the victim has a stable airway and normal ventilation, he should receive oxygen by mask. In either case, bronchodilators may be delivered by either intravenous route or aerosol to control bronchospasm.

Circulation and perfusion must be maintained. Fluid boluses should be given in the amount of 20 milliliters per kilogram for signs of hypovolemic shock. If the condition does not improve after two infusions or if signs of pulmonary edema occur, inotropic support should be initiated. Cardiac rhythms must be closely monitored. If severe hypothermia is present; that is, the child's core body temperature is less than 28° centigrade, rewarming must be accomplished before treatments are initiated as they are ineffective in the cold victim.

Hypothermia accompanies many submersion injuries. Warming should begin at the scene by removing wet clothing and covering the victim with blankets and heat packs. In the hospital, it is vital to begin rewarming. Body surfaces can be warmed using heat lamps or warm blankets. However, internal methods such as providing humidified oxygen at a temperature between 42° and 46° centigrade through the endotracheal tube; administering intravenous fluids and blood warmed to 43°centigrade; performing peritoneal or gastric lavage with fluids heated to 43° centigrade; and/or utilizing extracorporeal rewarming technologies are far more successful. These modalities begin in the emergency department and may need to be continued after admission to the intensive care unit. It is important to remember that a drowning victim cannot be pronounced dead if extremely hypothermic; rewarming must take place first, even if the outcome is certain (Ochsenschlager,1992).

Neurological dysfunction will be managed after the victim's airway, breathing, and circulation have been stabilized, and may range from not being affected at all to being severely obtunded and in coma. If signs of increased intracranial pressure are evident just after the event, head injury should be suspected as cerebral edema usually does not manifest itself until 24 hours later. Signs and symptoms must be quickly recognized as interventions should begin at once. First, the child should be hyperventilated to achieve a $paCO_2$ level between 30 and 32, by intubation, sedation, and chemical paralysis. If there is no clinical or radiologic indication of spinal injury, the head of the bed should be elevated at least 30° keeping the child's head in the midline. If there is still no response, administration of mannitol should be considered. Any seizure activity should be controlled initially giving benzodiazepines. If, however, convulsions continue, anticonvulsants such as phenytoin or phenobarbital should be administered. If despite aggressive measures, intracranial pressure is still not reduced to below 30 millimeters of mercury and cerebral perfusion pressures remain below the normal 50 to 60, the prognosis for the child's survival is dismal. If the victim shows any signs of infection, aggressive treatment with antibiotics is essential.

Nursing Management

Assessment

The nursing management of the near-drowining victim depends of the level of injury. Assessment and monitoring of the minimally involved child is important as well as close observation for late developing sequelae. The more impaired child, on the other hand, will need intensive care for continual monitoring of respiratory, cardiac, and neurological status. In addition the nurse will need to monitor for increased intracranial pressure, cardiac dysrhythmias, electrolyte imbalances, clotting abnormalities, and closely watch for changes in laboratory values.

Nursing Diagnosis

1. Impaired communication related to altered state of consciousness.
2. Impaired mobility related to altered state of consciousness.
3. Decreased cardiac output related to near-drowning sequelae.
4. Decreased intracranial adaptive capacity related to brain anoxia.
5. Impaired skin integrity related to inability to control movements.
6. Compromised family coping related to feeling of guilt.
7. Interrupted family processes related to hospital stay and subsequent sequelae.

Outcome Identification

1. The child will feel comfort and less isolated through touch and listening to the nurse and family members.
2. The child will not suffer from contractures and muscle atrophy.
3. The child will maintain acceptable cardiac output.
4. The child will maintain acceptable intracranial pressure.
5. The child will not exhibit signs of skin breakdown.
6. The family will work through feelings of guilt.
7. The family will adapt to their child's disabilities.

Planning and Implementation

Care for the child with a severely diminished level of consciousness means providing a safe, comfortable environment where attention is paid to skin care, positioning, and communication. Furthermore, arrangements should be made for occupational and physical therapies to begin to prevent contractures and muscle atrophy that may occur from immobility. Ideally, plans for and initiation of rehabilitation must begin in the intensive care unit just after admission.

The nurse must work with the family. Often, they are tormented by feelings of guilt; therefore, the nurse should provide a non-threatening, non-judgmental environment where they can vent frustrations, anxieties, and fears. Most often, caregivers of a near-drowning victim are faced with an unknown prognosis; but most have hope of recovery. At other times, however, when family members realize the outcome for their child is dismal, they may wish for the end of suffering and death. In either case, the nurse should support the caregivers through the crisis with the assistance of social work, clergy, friends, or other family members. It is also important to remember the siblings and ensure their emotional needs are met.

Evaluation

The hope is that the child will fully recover and receive appropriate care, and the family who loses a child will effectively recover from their loss.

Family Teaching

If the child survives with minor deficits, home care and special education can be arranged before discharge. Follow-up visits with physicians at the hospital or in the community can also be scheduled. The child who is more impaired may also be discharged home. Those children with severe hypoxic responses may need special appliances such as wheelchairs. Even children in a coma can be managed in their residences with home care nurses assisting family members. Caregivers of these children will need to learn how to work with any equipment, handle their child, and meet special needs. They should also be informed about caregiver support groups as well as government or private facilities that may be helpful.

Prevention is the best education for these families. It is up to the nurse to make all families aware children must be carefully supervised when near any body of water, including bath tubs, hot tubs, and spas; residential pools must be surrounded by a four-sided, locked barrier; and large buckets of water emptied. In addition, the nurse should advise families that the American Academy of Pediatrics states children under the age of three years are too young to learn to swim. Therefore, caregivers of toddlers who have attended swimming lessons should not allow their children to be near water without an adult close by. Furthermore, life jackets on boats and watercraft must be the correct size; if not, children will come out of them when in the water. Finally, the nurse should emphasize learning CPR so, if tragedy occurs despite all these efforts, interventions can begin immediately to enhance the child's chance of survival.

CEREBRAL PALSY

Cerebral palsy (CP) is defined as non-progressive motor dysfunction caused by damage to the motor areas of the brain.

Incidence and Etiology

The incidence is estimated to be 7 per 1,000 live births per year (Behrman & Kliegman, 1998). Many persons with CP have accompanying disabilities such as cognitive and language delays, which range from mild to severe. The most common cause of cerebral palsy is premature birth or very low birth weight. Neonates are at especially high risk because of central nervous system immaturity.

Pathophysiology

Congenital malformation of or injury to the brain, or anoxia of the brain, at any time before, during, or after birth may contribute to the development of CP (Behrman & Kliegman, 1998; Johnson & Oski 1997). Table 32-13 lists the various factors contributing to cerebral palsy.

Prognosis for infants and children diagnosed with CP depends on the level of physical involvement as well as concurrent medical problems. Many children with hemiplegia and ataxia show improvement with therapy and are eventually able to ambulate independently. However, if a toddler does not sit alone by two years of age, there is almost no chance of walking, even with intense therapy and the use of braces, crutches, or a walker.

Clinical Manifestations

Cerebral palsy is an abnormality of muscle tone and movement. Tables 32-14 and 32-15 present the characteristics of cerebral palsy according to the muscle response seen and the area of the body involved.

TABLE 32-13 Factors Contributing to Cerebral Palsy

Time Period	Factors
Prenatal	• Genetic or chromosomal abnormalities • Brain malformation • Exposure to teratogens • Multiple fetuses • Intrauterine infection • Ineffective placenta causing insufficient nutrition and oxygen delivery to fetus
Birth	• Preeclampsia • Complicated labor and delivery • Birth injury caused by direct head trauma • Asphyxia secondary to cord collapse or strangulation
Perinatal	• Central nervous system infection and/or sepsis • Kernicterus
Childhood	• Head trauma • Meningitis • Toxic ingestion or inhalation

TABLE 32-14 Characteristics of CP According to Muscle Response

Descriptor	Characteristics
Hypotonia	• Floppiness • Increased range of motion of the joints • Diminished reflex responses
Hypertonia	• Rigidity; muscles are extremely tense or tight • Spasticity; movements are uncoordinated, awkward, and stiff • Scissoring or crossing of the lower extremities • Reflex reactions (Babinski, deep tendon) are exaggerated
Athetosis	• Constant involuntary writhing motions; affect entire body but more severe distally
Ataxia	• Irregularity in muscle action or coordination • Wide-based gait

Infants and children with cerebral palsy display a wide range of clinical manifestations. Alterations in muscle tone such as abnormal posturing and movements, and continued primitive reflex responses make reaching normal developmental milestones almost unattainable. There is usually delay in gross motor skills such as sitting, crawling, cruising, or walking. In addition, fine motor coordination may be affected, hampering the ability to perform activities of daily living including self-feeding and dressing. Furthermore, many infants and children have other deficits such as poor vision, strabismus or nystagmus, hearing loss, cognitive impairments, speech or language delays, and seizures.

Diagnosis

Diagnosis is based on clinical findings. However, a definitive diagnosis may not be possible until the child is between 18 months and two years of age as many infants displaying delayed development may improve with maturation. Table 32-16 presents the early warning signs of cerebral palsy.

Infants and children suspected of having cerebral palsy must be carefully and continually evaluated to determine if and when specific motor milestones are met, such as holding onto an object or sitting without support. In addition, if primitive postures or reflexes are present or last beyond normal parameters, if feeding or swallowing difficulties

TABLE 32-15 Characteristics of CP According to the Body's Topographic Response

Type of CP	Characteristics
Hemiplegia	• Involvement of one side of the body with the upper extremities more dysfunctional than lower extremeties • Sensory deficits • Asymmetric postures or positions • Atypical reflex responses on affected side • Alteration in muscle tone, most often spastic
Diplegia	• Involvement of similar parts of both sides of the body, such as the arms or legs • Lower extremity dysfunction greater than upper extremity function • Alteration in muscle tone (hypertonicity or spasticity) • Delay in meeting gross motor developmental milestones such as sitting, standing, or walking • Achievement of fine motor hand skills usually at normal pace
Quadriplegia	• Involvement of all four extremities with equal involvement although arms are usually flexed while legs are extended • Delay in attaining developmental milestones dependent on motor ability • Speech dysfunction; swallowing may be impaired • Emotional lability not uncommon

TABLE 32-16 Early Warning Signs of Cerebral Palsy

Age	Warning Signs
Neonate	• Weak or absent sucking or swallowing difficulties • Periods of apnea or bradycardia • Encephalopathic cry (high pitched) • Extreme fussiness and irritability • Poor tone • Twitching of an arm or leg • Not moving extremities normally • Absent or weak primitive reflex responses
3 months	• Feeding difficulties, may be caused by tongue thrust and/or poor swallowing • Irritability and/or listlessness • Hypotonia, but may have head control in prone position • One or both hands in fisted position • Strabismus • Presence of primitive reflexes • Brisk tendon reflex response
6 months	• Delay in reaching developmental milestones (motor, speech) • Continued primitive reflexes • Hands remain clenched; one hand becomes dominant • Hypertonia • Arching and/or tendency to stand when held up • Lack of interest in people or toys • Unaware of or indifferent to stimuli in environment • Little if any spontaneous actions
9 months	• Persistent delay in motor milestones • Reach may be atypical as fingers are extended and arms tremble with purposeful movement • Arms flexed

continues

TABLE 32-16 *Continued*

Age	Warning Signs
12 months	• Inability to sit alone • Scissoring of lower extremities • Toe walking while held, but unable to stand alone • Crawl, if present, may be abnormal as only arms may be used • Athetoid (irregular, twisting) movement • Poor articulation or lack of speech

remain, if other central nervous system dysfunctions are present, or if the neurologic abnormalities seem static or are progressively worse, the child should be referred for further evaluation.

Treatment

There is no cure for cerebral palsy. Therefore, interventions enable the infant or child to achieve the best movement, locomotion, and communication skills possible as well as encourage as much self-sufficiency as he or she is able to achieve.

Many toddlers and children are fitted with technical aids such as braces and walkers, enabling them to ambulate independently. Others must use customized wheelchairs powered either manually or with special electronic devices. Physical and occupational therapies are provided to enhance the child's motor potential and prevent contractures or other complications associated with immobility. Speech therapy is also available to help with feeding as well as language and communication skills. For those unable to verbalize clearly, computers and voice synthesizers may be utilized.

Some children, especially those with spastic CP, may need surgical interventions to reduce the effects of hypertonic muscles. The Achilles tendon may be lengthened to increase the range of motion of the ankle and allow the heel to touch the floor. Hamstrings can be released to correct knee flexion. Other procedures may be needed to prevent hip contractures or adduction, or improve the foot positioning. To reduce muscle spasms or improve muscle tone, a **rhizotomy,** a procedure in which a small section of the spinal cord is cut, may be performed (Krach, 2000).

Medication administration is usually reserved for the older child or adolescent. Muscle relaxers may be used to decrease contractures, and can be given orally, intravenously, or intrathecally. Antianxiety drugs may reduce the excessive motions associated with athetosis.

Nursing Tip:

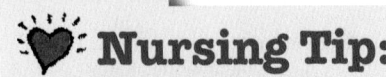

Use of botulinum toxin
A new and relatively innovative therapeutic intervention for children with cerebral palsy is to use botolinum toxin A to manage their spasticity. Children receiving this therapy have had significant improvement in muscle tone, range of motion, and functional motor status (Shaw, 1997).

Nursing Management

The nurse should ensure the infant's or child's body is in the best possible alignment, using pillows and bolsters as supports. Special care should be taken to protect bony prominences as they are prone to breakdown. Handling and moving the child can be challenging. For example, the floppy infant will need extra head and body support, the spastic child's extended legs may scissor when lifted, and the athetoid patient will writhe constantly. Caregivers as well as therapists may assist the nurse determine the best way to handle and move these children. Feeding may prove challenging as chewing and swallowing problems are commonplace. Techniques such as stroking the throat may help; however, the nurse should turn again to the family for guidance.

If the infant or child is hospitalized, the at-home regime should be followed as much as possible, and physical, occupational, and speech therapy departments should be contacted so therapy sessions can be scheduled. Care for the older child or adolescent can be challenging since many are mentally competent but physically limited. Therefore, respect and dignity need to be integrated into all interventions.

Family Teaching

Nurses must work with the families, providing them with support and resources to meet their child's needs. As soon as a diagnosis is confirmed, caregivers should be referred to a developmental clinic or center. These agencies will often have peer support groups for family members including siblings, as well as financial advisors.

Because the child will need a wide range of therapeutic services, family members will have to learn how to do the exercises and follow the techniques used by the rehabilitation specialists so their child receives consistent therapy at home. They may also need to learn about braces or walkers, and purchase adaptive feeding equipment.

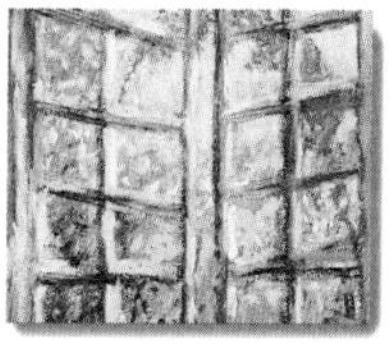

In the Real World

As a student nurse I wondered how I would care for a child who suffered from severe neurological injuries. When youngsters get sick, I think that is something out of their control, but serious neurological injuries can often be prevented. It makes me angry that parents do not put their children in car seats or use bike helmets. I spoke with some of the nurses on the floor and in the emergency department about this. They advised me to concentrate on the child's needs; care should be my first priority. When I questioned how to approach "negligent" parents, they told me mothers and fathers sometimes just do not have the correct or up-to-date information to make informed decisions about their child's care (such as the recommendations not to use walkers) and I should be nonjudgmental when dealing with them. If they do have all the information, however, and choose the path of least resistance (such as not using a car seat because the restraints make the child cry), they will probably feel extremely guilty about the incident and I should allow them to vent those feelings. In addition, when the time seems right, I should present information to them on injury prevention.

Key Concepts

- Differences in the anatomy and physiology of the nervous system from infant to adult include head circumferences, brain weight, cerebrospinal fluid production, myelinization of neurons, and open/closed fontanelles.
- Different types of seizures include partial: complex and simple; generalized: tonic/clonic, absence, myoclonic, and akinetic.
- Management of seizure activity includes maintaining a patent airway and oxygenation, providing a safe environment, and medication administration as indicated.
- Hydrocephalus, an increased amount CSF within the ventricles, is most often treated with a shunt. Nurses must be aware of the signs and symptoms of shunt infection or failure.
- Neural tube defects range in severity from simple spina bifida occulta to complex meningomyelocele. The defect's type and location determine the level of dysfunction, treatment, and care required.
- Initial signs of arteriovenous malformation include congestive heart failure, cardiomegaly, and a cerebral bruit.
- Meningitis can have a viral or bacterial cause. Signs and symptoms include change in level of consciousness or feeding, irritability, bulging fontanelle (infants), or headache, nuchal rigidity, photophobia, and malaise (child).
- Reye's syndrome usually follows a viral illness, and even though there is a rapid deterioration in patient condition, many survive because of prompt ventilatory and circulatory support in intensive care settings.
- Head injury is a common cause of childhood morbidity and mortality. Management depends on the particular trauma as well as the child's response.
- The major insult associated with near-drowning is hypoxemia.
- Cerebral palsy is a non-progressive motor dysfunction caused by damage in the motor areas of the brain. It is most commonly associated with prematurity but it can be caused by other kinds of neurologic trauma as well. Rehabilitation should begin as soon as diagnosis is made, as early therapy promotes improvement in both fine and gross motor skills.
- Families must be closely involved in the planning and management of their neurologically impaired child.

Review Questions

1. Describe a neurologic assessment based on a child's developmental age.
2. Define increased intracranial pressure. List the signs and symptoms associated with it.
3. Differentiate between partial and generalized seizures. Identify the characteristics of each.
4. Explain how the signs and symptoms of hydrocephalus are related to its pathology.
5. Describe the preoperative and postoperative care of the infant with spina bifida.
6. Describe the nursing assessments and interventions for an infant with bacterial meningitis.
7. Discuss the early signs and symptoms of Reye's syndrome.
8. Describe the ABCDE assessment of a neurologically injured child.
9. Explain the initial management of a child with a severely diminished level of consciousness secondary to head trauma.
10. Describe the difference between incomplete and complete spinal cord lesions.
11. Identify the signs and symptoms of a child with a cervical, thoracic, or lumbar cord lesion.
12. Explain the difference between drowning and near-drowning.
13. Describe the processes of both wet and dry drowning.
14. Discuss several characteristics displayed by infants who should be assessed for cerebral palsy.
15. Describe how neurologic pathology may have been averted by using preventive techniques.

References

American Academy of Pediatrics Committee on Genetics. (1999). Folic acid for the prevention of neural tube defect (RE9834). *Pediatrics, 104*(2), 325–327.

Behrman, R., & Kliegman, R. (1998). *Nelson; Essentials of pediatrics* (3rd ed.). Philadelphia: W. B. Saunders.

Berkowitz, C. D. (2000). *Pediatrics: A primary care approach* (2nd ed.). Philadelphia: W. B. Saunders.

Bracken, M., Shepard, M., Collins, W., Holford, T., Young, W., Baskin, D., Eisenberg, H., Flamm, E., Leo-Summers, L., Maroon, J., Marshall, L., Perot, P., Piepmeier, J., Sonntag, V., Wagner, F., Wilberger, J., & Winn, H. (1990). A randomized, controlled trial of methylprednisolone or naloxone in the treatment of acute spinal-cord injury. *The New England Journal of Medicine, 322*, 1404–1411.

Bruce, D. (1993). Head trauma. In M. Eichelberger (Ed.), *Pediatric trauma: Prevention, acute care, rehabilitation*. St. Louis: Mosby Year Book.

Chameides, L., & Hazinski, M. F. (1994). *Textbook of pediatric advanced life support*. Dallas: American Heart Association and American Academy of Pediatrics.

Dallacasa, P., Dappozzo, A., Galassi, E., Sandri, F., Cocchi, G., & Masi, M. (1995). Cerebrospinal fluid shunt infections in infants. *Child's Nervous System, 11*, 643–648.

Dickman, C., & Rekate, H. (1993). Spinal trauma. In M. Eichelberger (Ed.), *Pediatric trauma: prevention, acute care, rehabilitation*. St. Louis: Mosby Year Book.

Encyclopedia Britannica. (2001). [On-line]. Available: www.britannica.com/seo/f/focal-seizure/htm.

Estes, M. (2002). *Health assessment and physical examination* (2nd ed.). Albany, NY: Delmar.

Huff, K. (2000). Seizures and epilepsy. In C. Berkowitz (Ed.), *Pediatrics: A primary care approach* (2nd ed., pp. 559–565). Philadelphia: W. B. Saunders.

Johnson, K., & Oski, F. (1997). *Oski's essential pediatrics*. Philadelphia: Lippencott Raven.

Krach, L. (2000). Selective dorsal rhizotomy in the treatment of cerebral palsy. *Physical Medicine and Rehabilitation: State of the Art Reviews*. 14(2), 263–274.

Le Fevre, F., & Aronson, N. (2000). Ketogenic diet for the treatment of refractory epilepsy in children: A systematic review of efficacy, *Pediatrics 105*(4) p 46.

Mitchell, P., & Habermann, B. (1999). Rethinking physiologic stability: Touch and intracranial pressure. *Biological Research for Nursing, 1*(1) 12–19.

Monsen, R. (1999). Mother's experiences of living worried when parenting children with spina bifida. *Journal of Pediatric Nursing, 14*(3) 157–163.

Ochsenschlager D. (1992). Drowning and near drowning. In R. Barkin (Ed.), *Pediatric emergency medicine and concepts and clinical practice*. St. Louis: Mosby Year Book.

Page, R. (1992). Hydrocephalus. In R. Hoeckleman (Ed.), *Primary Pediatric Care* (2nd ed.). St. Louis: Mosby Year Book.

Palmer, J. (2000). Management of raised intracranial pressure in children. *Intensive and Critical Care Nursing. 16*(5), 319–127.

Pillitteri, A. (1999). *Child health nursing: Care of the child and family*. Philadelphia: Lippencott.

Rothstein, D., & Reigel, D. H. (1996). Growth hormone treatment of children with neural defects: Results from 6 months to 6 years. *Journal of Pediatrics, 128*, 184–189.

Scheinblum, S., & Hammond, M. (1990). The treatment of children with shunt infections: Extraventricular drainage system care. *Pediatric Nursing, 16*, 139–143.

Scully, T., & Luerrsen, T. (1995). Spinal cord injuries. In W. Buntain (Ed.), *Management of pediatric trauma*. Philadelphia: W. B. Saunders.

Shaw, M. (1997). Botulism toxin in the treatment of spasticity in children with cerebral palsy. *Physical and Occupational Therapy in Pediatrics,17* (4) 65–75.

Silverman, B, (Ed.). (1992). *APLS: The pediatric emergency medicine course* (2nd ed.). Chicago: American Academy of Pediatrics and the American College of Emergency Physicians.

Sivit, C., & Bulas, D. (1993). Diagnostic imaging. In M. Eichelberger (Ed.), *Pediatric trauma: Prevention, acute care, rehabilitation*. St. Louis: Mosby Year Book.

Taber's Cyclopedic Medical Dictionary, 19th ed. (2001). Philadelphia: FA Davis.

Walker, F. (1998). Internal pressure and cerebral blood flow. *Phonology, 8* [On-line]. Available: www.nda.ox.ac.uk/wfsa/html/u08/u08_013.htm.

Wallace, H., Biehl, R., MacQueen, J., & Blackman, J. (1997). *Mosby's resource guide to children with disabilities and chronic illness*. St Louis: Mosby Yearbook.

Washington Post. (1997). Child killed by mother's car. January 1, B1.

Wellington, M. C., & Wayner, R. F. (1995). Alterations in neurologic function. In J. Ball & R. Bindler (Eds.), *Pediatric nursing: Caring for children.* Norwalk, CT: Appleton and Lange.

Wertz, E. (2002). *Emerging care for children.* Albany, NY: Delmar.

Suggested Readings

Altumier, L. (1992). Pediatric central neurologic trauma: Issues for special patients. *American Association of Critical Care Nurses, 3,* 31–43.

American Academy of Pediatrics. (1990). Decline in *Haemophilus influenzae* type b meningitis—Seattle—King County, Washington, 1984–1989. aap.org

American Academy of Pediatrics. (1993). Shaken baby syndrome: Inflicted cerebral trauma. *Pediatrics, 92,* 872–875.

American Academy of Pediatrics. (1998). Recommended Childhood Immunization Schedule, United States, January 1998–December 1998. aap.org

American Liver Foundation. (1997, January). *Reye's syndrome information sheet.* Cedar Grove, NJ: author. [Online] Available: www.liverfoundation.org/html/livheal.20010118.dir/lhimdox.dir/iml3dox.fol/onlmats.dir/_lpe001.htm

Apple, D., Anson, C., Hunter, J., & Bell, R. (1995). Spinal cord injury in youth. *Clinical Pediatrics, 34,* 90–95.

Ashwal, S., Tomasi, L., Schneider, S., Perkin, R., & Thompson, J. (1992). Bacterial meningitis in children: Pathophysiology and treatment. *Neurology. 42,* 739–746.

Athey R. (1991). A 3 year old with spinal cord injury without radiologic abnormality (SCIWORA). *Journal of Emergency Nursing, 17,* 380–385.

Barkin, R. (1990). *Emergency pediatrics: A guide to ambulatory care.* St. Louis: Mosby.

Blarney, S. F. (1995). Arterio-venous malformation hemorrhage in children: the importance of nursing neurological assessment during the acute and early recovery. *Axon, 17,* 36–41.

Blasco, P. A. (1994). Primitive reflexes: Their contribution to the early detection of cerebral palsy. *Clinical Pediatrics, 33,* 388–397.

Brookshire, B. L., Fletcher, J. M., Bohan, T. P., Landry, S. H., Davidson, K. C., & Francis, D. J. (1995). Verbal and nonverbal skill discrepancies in children with hydrocephalus: A five year longitudinal follow-up. *Journal of Pediatric Psychology, 20,* 785–800.

Bruce, D. (1990). Head injuries in the pediatric population. *Current Problems in Pediatrics,* February, 61–107.

Calderon-Gonzales, R., Calderon-Sepulveda, R., Rincon-Reyes, M., Garcia-Ramirez, J., & Mino-Arango, E. (1994). Botulism toxin A in management of cerebral palsy. *Pediatric Neurology, 10,* 284–288.

Case-Smith, J. (1996). Fine motor outcomes in preschool children who receive occupational therapy services. *American Journal of Occupational Therapy, 50,* 52–61.

Centers for Disease Control and Prevention. (1995). Summary of notifiable diseases, United States, 1994. *Mortality and Morbidity Weekly Reports, 43,* 71.

Cherry, J. (1992). Aseptic meningitis and viral meningitis. In R. Feigin & J. Cherry (Eds.), *Textbook of Pediatric Infectious Diseases* (3rd ed.). Philadelphia: W.B. Saunders.

Choudhury, A. R. (1995). Infantile hydrocephalus: Management using CT assessment. *Child's Nervous System, 11,* 220–226.

Christoph, C. L., Poole, C. A., & Kochan, P. S. (1995). Operative gastric perforation: A rare complication of VP shunts. *Pediatric Radiology, 1,* 5173–5174.

Denislic, M., & Meh, D. (1995). Botulism toxin in the treatment of cerebral palsy. *Neuropediatrics, 26,* 249–52.

Eichelberger, M. (Ed.). (1993). *Pediatric trauma: prevention, acute care, rehabilitation.* St. Louis: Mosby Year Book.

Feigin, R., & Cherry, J. (Eds.). (1992). *Textbook of Pediatric Infectious Diseases* (3rd ed.). Philadelphia: W. B. Saunders.

Fields, A. (1993). Near drowning. In M. Eichelberger (Ed.), *Pediatric trauma: prevention, acute care, rehabilitation.* St. Louis: Mosby Year Book.

Freeman, J., (1992). What have we learned from febrile seizures? *Pediatric Annals, 21,* 355–361.

Ghajar, J., & Hairi, R. (1992). Management of pediatric head injury. *Pediatric Clinics of North America, 5,* 1090–1125.

Givens, T., Polley, K., Smith, G., & Hardin, W. (1996). Pediatric cervical spine injury: A three-year experience. *The Journal of Trauma, Injury, Infection, and Critical Care, 41,* 310–314.

Glaze D. (1992). Guillian-Barre syndrome. In R. Feigin & J. Cherry (Eds.), *Textbook of Pediatric Infectious Diseases* (3rd ed.). Philadelphia: W. B. Saunders.

Goldstein, B., & Powers, K. (1994). Head trauma in children. *Pediatrics in Review, 15,* 213–219.

Graf, W. D., Cumings, P., Quan, L., & Brutocao, D. (1995). Predicting outcome in pediatric submersion victims. *Annals of Emergency Medicine, 26,* 312–319.

Hazinski, M. F. (1992). *Nursing care of the critically ill child.* St. Louis, Mosby Year Book.

Hendricks, M. (1995). High fat and seizure free. *Johns Hopkins Magazine, XLVII,* 14–20.

Hoeckleman, R., (Ed.). (1992). *Primary Pediatric Care* (2nd ed.) St. Louis: Mosby Year Book.

Keating, J. (1992). Reye syndrome. In R. Feigin & J. Cherry (Eds.), *Textbook of pediatric infectious diseases,* (3rd ed.). Philadelphia: W.B. Saunders.

Key, C. B., Rothrock, S. G., & Falk, J. L. (1995). Cerebrospinal fluid shunt complications: An emergency medicine perspective. *Pediatric Emergency Care, 11*, 265–273.

Kloss, D. (1996). Caring for the patient with meningococcal meningitis. *American Journal of Nursing, 96*, 16F–16L.

Koman, L. A., Mooney, J. F., & Smith, B. P. (1994). Management of spasticity in cerebral palsy with botulinum-A toxin: Report of a preliminary, randomized, double-blind trial. *Journal of Pediatric Orthopedics, 14*, 299–303.

Kyriacou, D. N., Arcinue, E. L., Peek, C., & Kraus, J. F. (1994). Effect of immediate resuscitation on children with submersion injury. *Pediatrics, 94*, 13–142.

Lang, S., & Bernardo, L. (1993). SCIWORA syndrome: Nursing assessment. *Dimensions of Critical Care Nursing, 12*, 247–254.

Lazareff, J., & Becker, D. (1994). Acute neurosurgical conditions. *Pediatric Annals, 23*, 258–262.

Liptak, G. (1987). Spina bifida. In R. Hoeckleman (Ed.), *Primary pediatric care*. St. Louis: Mosby Year Book.

Lipton, J. (1993). Evolving concepts in pediatric bacterial meningitis—Part I: Pathophysiology and diagnosis. *Annals of Emergency Medicine, 22*, 1602–1615.

Lipton, J. (1993). Evolving concepts in pediatric bacterial meningitis—Part II: Current management and therapeutic research. *Annals of Emergency Medicine, 22*, 1616–1629.

Luerrsen, T. (1993). General characteristics of neurologic injury. In M. Eichelberger (Ed.), *Pediatric trauma: prevention, acute care, rehabilitation*. St. Louis: Mosby Year Book.

Lumenta, C. B., & Skotarczak, U. (1995). Long-term follow-up in 233 patients with congenital hydrocephalus. *Child's Nervous System, 11*, 173–175.

Mann, D., & Dodds, J. (1993). Spinal injuries in 57 patients 17 years or younger. *Orthopedics, 16*, 159–164.

McCracken, G. (1992). Current management of bacterial meningitis in infants and children. *The Pediatric Infectious Disease Journal, 11*, 169–174.

Mee, C. L. (1996). Hypothermia. *Nursing96, 26*, 33.

Michaud, L., Duhaime, A. C., & Batshaw, M. (1993). Traumatic brain injury in children. *Pediatric Clinics of North America, 40*, 553–565.

Monsen, R. (1992). Autonomy, coping, and self-care agency in healthy adolescents and in adolescents with spina bifida. *Journal of Pediatric Nursing, 7*, 9–13.

Morgan, S. (1991). A passage through paralysis. *American Journal of Nursing. 91*, 70–74.

Mori, K., Shimada, J., Kurisaka, M., Kurisaka, M., Sato, K., & Watanabe, K. (1995). Classification of hydrocephalus and outcome of treatment. *Brain and Development, 17*, 338–348.

Mulhauser, L. (1993). Spina bifida: An overview. *Ethiscope*, Winter Edition.

Nichols, D., Yaster, M., Lappe, D., & Buck, J. (Eds.). (1991). *Golden hour: The handbook of advanced pediatric life support*. St. Louis: Mosby Year Book.

Noah, Z., Hahn, Y., Rubenstein, J., & Aronyk, K. (1992). Management of the child with severe brain injury. *Critical Care Clinics, 8*, 59–77.

North American Nursing Diagnoses Association, (2001). Nursing diagnoses: Definitions and classifications 2001–2002. Philadelphia: Author.

O'Neill, M. (1994). Delayed-onset paraplegia from improper seat belt use. *Annals of Emergency Medicine, 23*, 1123–1125.

Patterson, R., Brown, G., Salassi-Scotter, M., & Middaugh, D. (1992). Head injury in the conscious child. *American Journal of Nursing, 84*, 22–30.

Peterson, P. (1992). Spina bifida—nursing challenge. *RN, 55*, 40–47.

Quam, D. A. (1994). Recognizing a case of Reye's syndrome. *American Family Physician, 50*, 1491–1496.

Quillen, T. (1996). ... About Reye's syndrome. *Nursing96, 26*, 17.

Rahman, S., Teo, C., Morris, W., Lao, D., & Boop, P. A. (1995). Ventriculosubgaleal shunt: a treatment option for progressive post-hemorrhagic hydrocephalus. *Child's Nervous System, 11*, 650–654.

Reynolds, E. (1992). Controversies in caring for the child with a head injury. *American Journal of Maternal/Child Nursing (MCN), 17*, 245–251.

Rogers, M., (Ed.). (1992). *Textbook of pediatric intensive care*. Baltimore: Williams & Wilkens.

Roos, K. (1992). Management of bacterial meningitis in children and adults. *Seminars in Neurology, 12*, 155–164.

Rutkowski, K. (1990). Grid implantation in seizure patients. *AORN Journal, 52*, 953–975.

Ryan, J. A., & Shiminski-Maher, T. (1995) Hydrocephalus and shunts in children with brain tumors. *Journal of Pediatric Oncology Nursing, 12*, 223–229.

Scipien, G., Chard, M., Howe, J., & Barnard, M. (1990). *Pediatric Nursing Care*. St. Louis: Mosby.

Seigler, R. (1990). The administration of rectal diazepam for acute management of seizures. *The Journal of Emergency Medicine, 8*, 155–159.

Shantz, D., & Spitz, M. (1993). What you need to know about seizures. *Nursing93, 23*, 34–40.

Slater, J. (1989). Rubber anaphylaxis. *The New England Journal of Medicine, 320*, 1126–1130.

Slater, J., Mostello, L., & Shaer, C. (1991). Rubber-specific IgE in children with spina bifida. *The Journal of Urology, 146*, 578–579.

Slater, J., Mostello, L., Shaer, C., & Honsinger, R. (1990). Type I hypersensitivity to rubber. *Annals of Allergy, 65*, 411–414.

Stewart, K. (1994). Tetanus. *Nursing94, 24*, 51.

Taft, L. (1987). Cerebral palsy. In R. Hoeckleman (Ed.), *Primary Pediatric Care*. St. Louis: MosbyYear Book.

Thompson, J., McFarland, G., Hirsch, J., Tucker, S., & Bowers, A. (1989). *Mosby's manual of clinical nursing*. St. Louis: Mosby.

Tunik, M., & Young, G. (1992). Status epilepticus in children: The acute management. *Pediatric Clinics of North America, 39*, 1007–1029.

Vernon-Levett, P. (1991). Head injuries in children. *Critical Care Nursing Clinics of North America, 3*, 411–421.

Wald, E., Kaplan, S., Mason, E., Sabo, D., Ross, L., Arditi, M., Wiederman, B., Barson, W., Kim, K., Yogev, R., & Hofkosh D. for the Meningitis Study Group. (1995). Dexamethasone therapy for children with bacterial meningitis. *Pediatrics, 5*, 21–28.

Wallech, C. (1994). Neurotrauma: Spinal cord injury. In E. Barker (Ed.), *Neuroscience Nursing*. St. Louis: Mosby Year Book.

Walsh, E. A. (1994). Childhood near-drowning: Nursing care and primary prevention. *Pediatric Nursing, 20*, 265–269.

Waugh, J. H., O'Callaghan, M. J., & Pitt, W. R. (1994). Prognostic factors and long-term outcomes for children who have nearly drowned. *Medical Journal of Australia, 161*, 598–599.

Weinstein, L. (1992). Tetanus. In R. Feigin & J. Cherry (Eds.), *Textbook of pediatric infectious diseases* (3rd ed.). Philadelphia: W. B. Saunders.

Zamula, P. (1990). Reye syndrome: The decline of a disease. *Consumer*, November, p. 20–24.

Resources

Organizations and Websites

American Liver Foundation
75 Maiden Lane, Suite 603
New York, NY 10038
(800) 465-4837
www.liverfoundation.org

Epilepsy Foundation
4351 Garden City Drive
Landover, MD 20785-7223
(800) 332-1000
www.efa.org

Meningitis Foundation of America
7155 Shadeland Station, Suite 190
Indianapolis, IN 46256-3922
(800) 668-1129
www.musa.org

Spina Bifida Association of America
4590 MacArthur Blvd. NW, Suite 250
Washington, DC 20007
(800) 621-3141
www.sbaa.org

United Cerebral Palsy
1660 L Street, NW, Suite 700
Washington, DC 20036
(800) 872-5827
www.ucp.org

CHAPTER 33

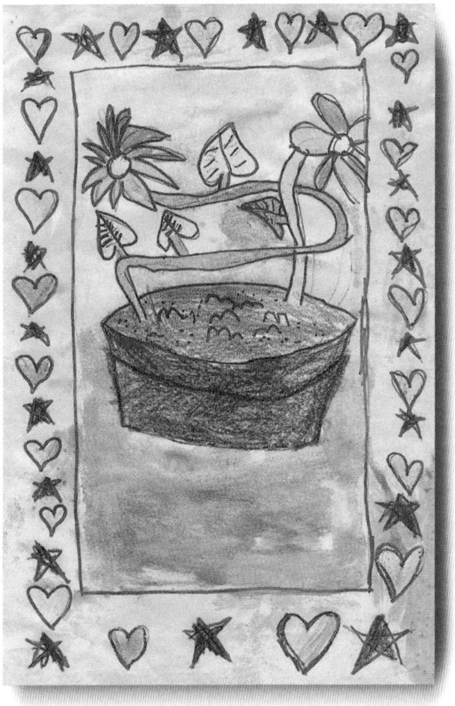

Once you have children your lives will never be the same. How little did my husband and I realize the impact of that statement 18 years ago! Our son Phillip, the oldest of our three children, was diagnosed with autism. A life altering diagnosis! Parents must rethink hopes, dreams, and goals. All sorts of things go through your mind in this moment: What happened? What did I do? Is this some family thing no one told us about! Without answers to these questions other than "these things happen" and "life goes on," we continued down the path rejoicing at triumphs and milestones that Phillip achieved. It took a great amount of work to get even the smallest of skills accomplished. His first step was at 18 months, his first word at three years. He was completely toilet trained at age 10 and his first reasonable night of full sleep at are 17, which meant the entire family slept a full uninterrupted night also. We felt like we had finally joined the real world! There is not a cure for autism; however, many of these individuals lead full, fun and very productive lives, and thankfully Phillip can be counted among these.

COGNITIVE ALTERATIONS

Suzanne Sutherland, RN, PhD

COMPETENCIES

Upon completion of this chapter, the reader will be able to:

- *Discuss the various causes of mental retardation.*
- *Describe the characteristics of a child with mental retardation.*
- *Discuss at least three commonly used tests for evaluating the presence and extent of mental retardation.*
- *Describe the appearance and behaviors of a child with Down syndrome, a child with fragile X syndrome, and a child with autism.*
- *Discuss the family's reaction to having a child with a cognitive alteration and the anticipated grieving process.*
- *Formulate a plan of care for the family and the child with a cognitive alteration.*

A child's cognitive alteration or impairment has an impact on the child, the family, and the community. The nature and severity of a specific impairment represent a given set of facts, embodying the raw material with which the family must work in order to craft an adult who can be, at least to a degree, communicating and self-sustaining. The environments of home and school then become the variables, the factors that can be altered in order to maximize the child's ability to eventually function in the adult world.

This chapter presents an overview of mental retardation, the manner in which it is identified and quantified in children. The two most prevalent syndromes associated with mental retardation, Down syndrome and fragile X syndrome, are presented. The symptom cluster autism is described, with its probable causation and most prevalent treatment modality.

MENTAL RETARDATION

Mental retardation (MR) is defined as significantly subaverage general intellectual functioning manifested before age 18, with limited adaptive skills in at least two or more areas of functioning: communication, self-care, social skills, community use, self-direction, health and safety, academics, and work. It is, at this point in time, an unalterable condition. Despite the irreversible nature of the condition, the abilities of children with MR can be maximized, primarily through caregiver excellence and educational and training programs in the schools and in the community.

Reflective Thinking

Valuing Cognitively Impaired Children

Cognitive alterations in children produce effects upon the child, the family, and the whole of society. Humans revel in their ability to conceptualize. Some of their richest delight is grounded in their own cleverness. Like peacocks, they are possessed of an array of gifts that they confidently flaunt for purposes of befriending, courtship, or dominance. Unlike peacocks, whose brains are a disappointing contrast to their stunning green and blue tail feathers, humans are, at turns, witty, creative, amusing, cynical, or profound. They draw others to them, using their scintillating mental attributes as coin.

How then do humans as a society value a person with a cognitive alteration? How can we bright and educated humans reevaluate our self-serving stance of "brighter is better" to embrace humans on a multifaceted basis of worth that is grounded in philosophical and spiritual beliefs, as well as in the egotism of our own cognitive endowments? How can you value the child who is cognitively impaired and transmit wholly and sincerely to the caregivers that the child is indeed respected and unique, and of inestimable worth?

TABLE 33-1 Categories and Examples of Causes of Mental Retardation

Cause	Example
Genetic	
Entirely genetic	Down syndrome
Combination of genetic and environmental	Anencephaly
Prenatal	
Environmental	Profound maternal acid-base balance disorder
Chemical	Maternal ingestion of drugs and alcohol
Infectious	Maternal rubella
Perinatal	
Environmental	Maternal exposure to a powerful toxin; low birth weight; prematurity
Perfusion-related	Premature placental separation
	Umbilical cord kinking
Oxygen-related	Maternal asphyxia
Chemical	Maternal overdose
Traumatic	Intrapartal brain injury
Infectious	Maternal cytomegalovirus
Postnatal	
Perfusion-related	Severe shock
Oxygen-related	Aspiration of a foreign object
	Drowning
Chemical	Poisoning
Traumatic	Cranial injury, especially motor vehicle accidents and child abuse
Infectious	Meningitis, encephalitis

Incidence and Etiology

The incidence of MR is estimated to be about 2–3% of the general population and 3% in the school-aged population (Goldson, 1999). It may exist in isolation or in a **syndrome** (a named condition characterized by a group of findings or attributes), such as Down syndrome or fetal alcohol syndrome. There are many causes of MR that can be categorized as genetic, prenatal, perinatal, or postnatal. Genetic causes may be purely genetic or a combination of genetic and environmental. Prenatal causes may be environmental, chemical, or infectious. Perinatal causes may be environmental, perfusion-related, oxygen-related, chemical, traumatic, or infectious. Postnatal causes may be perfusion-related, oxygen-related, chemical, traumatic, or infectious. Table 33-1 lists categories and examples of etiologies of MR.

Pathophysiology

In general, MR is associated either with syndromes in which genetic or structural differences in the brain affect its physiology, or with damaged or absent cerebral structures. The former case is found in infants who are born with genetic alterations or intracranial lesions. The latter case is typical of children who have suffered hypoxic brain damage resulting from perinatal mishap or from accidents in the developmental years.

Plasticity refers to the ability of neural cells in a certain area of the brain to assume the functions of a different area, or to the ability of the brain to act as a computer does in rerouting signals around a nonfunctioning piece of circuitry (Carpenter, 1996). Because the brain of the neonate displays considerable anatomic plasticity, an infant may be able to reassign portions of the brain to replace those lost through an hypoxic incident (Kostovic & Judas, 1998). The older child's brain relies most heavily upon rerouting around

Kids Want To Know

Will my kids be mentally retarded?

I'm Kenny. My sister Joellen is mentally retarded. I'm 18 and my girlfriend Carrie and I are getting married some day. I want to know if we'll have retarded children, or if we should just skip having children. Answer: Kenny, we all dream about our futures, and we need to do this. Of course you're wondering what life with Carrie would be like. You need to find out more about why your sister Joellen is mentally retarded. A few causes of mental retardation run in families but most do not. If you can talk to your parents, you can let them know this is worrying you. Your family physician or nurse practitioner, or a geneticist recommended by them, will be able to explain Joellen's type of mental retardation and what are the chances that you and Carrie could have a normal baby.

Nursing Tip:

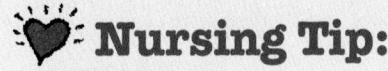

Sibling sensitivity

Sisters and brothers of a child with MR are aware that their sibling is different and are changed by the experience. Perhaps as early as the preschool years, but certainly by school-age, they experience both protective affection and resentment of the sibling. They begin to feel different from their peers and sometimes even isolated, especially during late school-age and adolescence. They may feel reluctant to let new friends and acquaintances know about their sibling. When they meet new people, they often don't know how to bring the subject up. Teenagers can feel very embarrassed by even an average-intelligence sibling's "uncool" mannerisms or appearance: imagine how much greater this can be for the siblings of a child with MR. The nurse should take opportunities to allow the siblings to discuss their feelings.

injured areas, producing substantial rehabilitation but not to the degree seen in infants.

Clinical Manifestations

The clinical manifestations vary according to the severity of MR, which can be classified as mild, moderate, severe, and profound (American Psychiatric Association [APA], 1994). Mild MR is the most common type. Infants with mild degrees of mental retardation are often not noticed as mentally retarded to observers. However, during infancy and early childhood, the caregiver may note **developmental delays** (achievement of developmental milestones later than expected) in language acquisition, social development, and motor skills. These children may be undiagnosed until primary grades, when they manifest delays in reading or arithmetic or both. Eventually with special education, they can acquire these skills to the 3rd to 6th grade level, and can be guided toward social appropriateness.

Children with moderate MR display obvious delays in motor development and speech; yet, they can learn self-help activities. During the school-age years, they can learn simple methods to communicate, basic health and safety habits, and simple manual skills. They may benefit from vocational training, but seldom progress academically beyond the 2nd grade level. Peer relationships often deteriorate during adolescence because of problems in recognizing socially correct interactions.

With severe MR, children typically acquire little if any communicative speech during early childhood but may learn to talk and develop elementary self-care skills (e.g., feeding self) in the school-age period. They usually walk if no other disability is present. Some understanding of speech eventually develops, and they may profit from learning to sight read some "survival" words such as restroom, stop, no walking.

Most children with profound retardation also have an identified neurological condition causing their retardation. They have minimal capacity for functioning in sensorimotor areas and require a highly structured setting with constant monitoring and supervision. Delays are obvious in all developmental areas. The child with profound retardation may display basic emotional responses and respond to training in using their legs, hands, and jaws.

Diagnosis

The diagnosis of mental retardation is based on the following: (1) a thorough physical examination and history; (2) routine developmental assessments; and (3) standardized tests of intellectual and adaptive functioning. Table 33-2 identifies commonly used instruments in the diagnosis of MR. One of the frequently used developmental test is the *Denver Developmental Screening Test II* (DDST-II) (Frankenburg, Dodds, Archer, Shapiro, & Bresnick, 1992) (Chapter 14 and Appendix E). The *Denver II*, designed for screening the child from birth through 6 years, identifies a broad range of ages at which achievement of certain verbal, motor, and social skills is expected. Failure to meet these milestones by the designated age range is labeled a delay. A child who is delayed is screened again in a week or two. If the delay persists, referrals are initiated.

General intellectual functioning is assessed with a standardized test of intelligence quotient (IQ), such as the *Stanford-Binet Intelligence Scale* (Terman & Merrill, 1973).

TABLE 33-2 Common Tests for the Diagnosis of Mental Retardation

Test	Age Range	Special Considerations
Denver II	Birth to 6 years	Identifies delay but does not quantify intelligence
Bayley Scales of Infant Development (Bayley, 1969)	1 month to 30 months	Provides scores with a mean of 100
Stanford-Binet Intelligence Scale (4th ed.)	2 years to adulthood	Provides scores with a mean of 100
Wechsler Preschool and Primary Scale of Intelligence–Revised (WPPSI-R)	3 years to 7 years	Provides scores with a mean of 100
Wechsler Intelligence Scale for Children (3rd ed.) (WISC-III)	6 years to 16 years, 11 months	Same as WPPSI-R—scores on this are quite close to scores children obtain years earlier on the WPPSI-R
Peabody Picture Vocabulary Test–Revised	2.5 through 18 years	Designed for the physically or language handicapped—Gives scores with mean of 100
Leiter International Performance Scale–Revised	2 years to 20 years	For hearing-impaired children—Provides scores with a mean of 100
Vineland Adaptive Behavior Scales	Birth to 18 years also delayed adults	Provides checklist information related to behavior and self-care skills
AAMR Adaptive Behavior Scale	Any age	Provides checklist information related to behavior and self-care skills

The **intelligence quotient** is the child's functional age on the intelligence test divided by the chronological age and then multiplied by 100. All this gives is a number. A child with a measured IQ that is confirmed as less than 70 on the *Stanford-Binet*, corroborated by other tests as necessary, is classified as mentally retarded (APA, 1994). Examples of tests that assess adaptive skills are the American Association on Mental Retardation's (AAMR) *Adaptive Behavior Scale* (Nihira, Foster, Shellhaas, & Leland, 1975) and the *Vineland Behavior Scale* (Sparrow, Balla, & Cicchette, 1984). Children's performance on these tests can fluctuate according to mood, sleep, wellness, attention level, arousal, and many other factors. Because of this, and because the diagnosis of MR is so traumatic for a family, repeat testing before definitive diagnosis is mandatory.

Critical Thinking

How to Help Caregivers Accept the Diagnosis of MR

How might the nurse assist the caregivers in accepting the fact that their child has just been diagnosed with severe mental retardation?

Treatment

There is no standard medical treatment of mental retardation; however, an interdisciplinary approach is frequently used. Management is directed toward maintaining the child's health and early intervention to improve the degree of adaptive functioning. Specialized educational and therapeutic services are central elements in the treatment of children with MR. Functionally speaking, however, the child will need more than an average child—extra attention in school, extra time to master some concepts, extra vigilance by caregivers, and extra options by society in order to learn safely how to survive and to reach one's maximum potential. Educationally, this may include infant stimulation programs, preschools with a low teacher-to-pupil ratio, special education programs in school years, and special work-training programs in secondary and post-secondary education.

Family Teaching

A vital part of planning and implementation is that of teaching. Although this can take the form of teaching actual psy-

REFLECTIONS FROM FAMILIES

Paul is severely mentally retarded. His brother Vernon is not. In fact, Vern was tested as very mentally gifted at the age of 5, with an IQ of 160, as were his sister and other brother. One day Vern asked me, "Mom, if all three of us gave Paul our extra brains, we'd still be smart enough. Would it be enough to make him normal?" I was so touched by his generosity and by his graciously and magically creative notion that brains, like water to the thirsty, might be siphoned among all the children of the family, for the common good.

chomotor skills to caregivers, the nurse functions just as often as interpreter, clarifying for them information from professionals of the interdisciplinary team. The child with MR may not differ at all from an average child, except in delay of developmental milestones. Caregivers may need assistance in teaching the child self-care skills such as self-feeding. If a physical impairment prevents the child from using cups, plates, and utensils, specially designed ones can be obtained (Figure 33-1).

It is important to remember, though, that the caregiver is also a solace person and comforter, not a therapist. The tendency for a caregiver to work at skills for all the child's waking hours should be discouraged. A well-rounded child, whatever his or her IQ, requires singing, cuddling, field trips to malls or zoos, tickling, pretending, visits to playgrounds, laughing, water play, games, and silliness. These activities may seem almost as important for caregivers as for children.

Case Study/Care Plan

The Child with Mental Retardation

Amanda became mentally retarded as a result of a bout with meningitis. Her parents have come to you to help guide them in a positive direction.

Nursing Care Plan

Assessment

Nurses can be instrumental in identifying the child who is mentally retarded through history taking, developmental screening, and observation. The family history should be obtained and hereditary disorders in which MR is a feature (e.g., fragile X syndrome) should be investigated. A pregnancy and birth history can provide important information, that is, prenatal maternal infection, alcohol or drug consumption; prenatal, perinatal, or postnatal trauma or physical injury. Infancy and early childhood developmental screening is of primary importance in finding children at risk for MR. The nurse's observational skills in noting gross and fine motor movements, visual and auditory acuity, and emotional responses provide significant data in making the diagnosis. It is important to determine whether physical factors such as hearing, vision, or motor deficits are the cause of or contributing to the child's developmental delays. Assessment by the nurse can identify early infant behavior that may indicate MR such as non-responsiveness to contact, poor eye contact during feeding, diminished spontaneous activity, decreased responsiveness to the surroundings, and decreased alertness to voices or movements. A complete physical, especially neurological, examination should be performed.

A family assessment is vital to obtaining information for planning care. It should include the effect of the child's behavior on the family members, the degree of independence encouraged at home, and the stability of the family unit. Assessment of the family's progress through the grieving process should also be made.

continues

continued

Nursing Diagnosis #1

Self-care deficit related to impaired cognitive and motor functioning.

Expected Outcome

Child will be able to participate in aspects of self-care.

Interventions/*Rationales*

1. Help family determine child's readiness to learn self-care activities and skills. Encourage caregivers to teach these skills as soon as child achieves readiness. *Readiness may not be easily recognized by the family. To facilitate optimum development.*

2. Encourage independence and for caregivers to avoid "taking over" a task but intervene when child is unable to perform. *To provide child a sense of accomplishment.*

3. Offer positive feedback for performance of self-care activities. *Positive reinforcement enhances self-esteem and encourages repetition of desirable behaviors.*

Evaluation

The child performs activities of daily living at optimum capacity and is able to fulfill some self-care needs independently.

Nursing Diagnosis #2

Impaired social interaction related to difficulty in learning appropriate social behaviors and skills.

Expected Outcome

Child will achieve optimum socialization.

Interventions/*Rationales*

1. Encourage caregivers to teach child some socially appropriate behaviors such as saying "hello" and "thank you" and waving good-bye. *Performance of such behaviors encourages acceptance by others.*

2. Encourage caregivers to remain with the child during initial interactions with others. *Presence of a trusted individual provides a feeling of security.*

3. Provide caregivers with information about programs that promote peer relationships such as Boy/Girl Scouts, Special Olympics, and camps for children with similar conditions. *To expose child to other children and to group situations in order to accommodate to social demands and expectations.*

Evaluation

The child demonstrates acceptable social behaviors. The child has peer relationships and is not socially isolated.

Nursing Diagnosis #3

Interrupted family processes related to raising a child with MR.

Expected Outcome

The family will receive adequate information about MR and emotional support.

Interventions/*Rationales*

1. Encourage family members to express fears, ambivalent feelings, frustrations, hopes, and aspirations about having a child with MR. *Allows them to express feelings and concerns about child's chronic condition and dependency on them. This process may help them to better cope with frustrations involved in raising a child with MR.*

continues

continued

2. Introduce caregivers to other families with a child with MR. Assist them to connect with support groups. *To avoid isolation of family that frequently occurs.*

3. Provide referrals to community resources that can offer educational information about MR, availability of early intervention programs, special education schools, and recreational programs for the child. *Early involvement in stimulation and educational programs results in the best outcomes for the child.*

4. Discuss the availability of respite care for caregivers. *Caregivers may not be aware of or willing to admit their need for assistance in care taking.*

5. Role model acceptance of the child through own behavior. *The nurse's validation of the child's inherent worth sets a tone for all concerned.*

Evaluation

Caregivers express feelings and concerns about raising a child with MR. They contact and use community resources. All family members receive adequate support and demonstrate acceptance of the child.

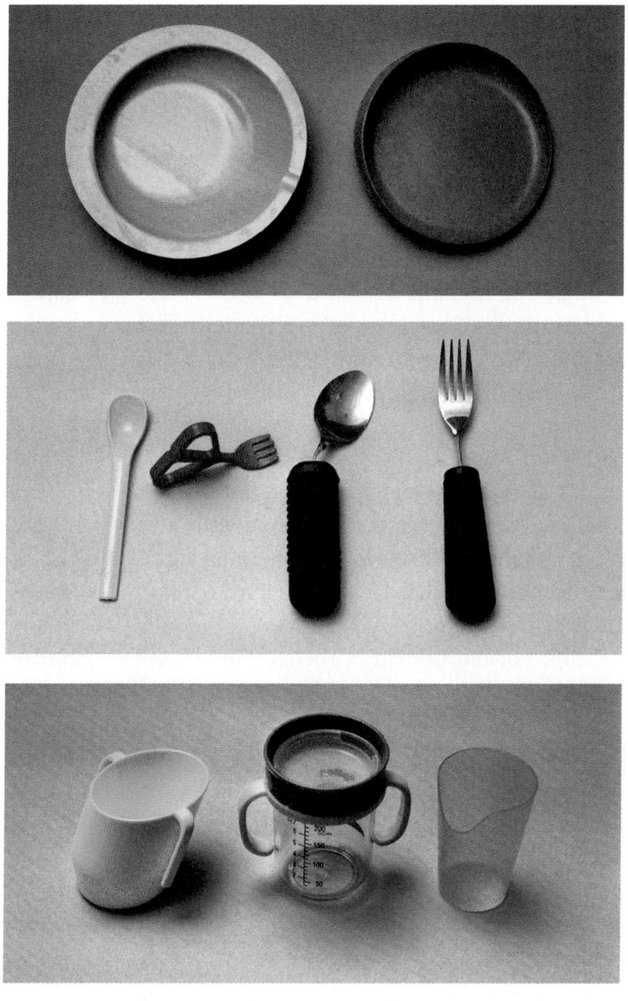

Figure 33-1 Several self-care aids are available commercially for the child with MR to promote optimum independence.

The nurse needs to decide what bits of knowledge are essential and which are optional. Then the individual must communicate this real-world knowledge to the caregiver. Sometimes all they can do is try to get through the next day without mishaps. The nurse has a responsibility to ask whether the caregiver would like to know something and then to prioritize teaching intelligently. Parents of a child who is mentally retarded may seek genetic counseling in order to make decisions about having subsequent children. (This is more commonly performed when MR exists within an identifiable syndrome or when the child has physical impairments in addition to MR.) The nurse can be enormously helpful to them both as moral support before counseling and as a person able to remember, clarify, and define medical terms after the process.

The Family's Response to Having a Child with MR

Imagine for a moment what it is like for caregivers to learn their child will be mentally retarded, developmental milestones will be achieved later than they expected, and they will have to worry about keeping her/him safe in a world filled with taunts and exclusions. They will have to endure stares and questions. They will put on their "public face" when they take the child out in the world, uncertain of the degree of warmth or rejection they will encounter. Words like "retard" and "dummy" will burn their ears. Goldson's (1999) observation that "the diagnosis of mental retardation is an event for which few families are prepared" is an understatement.

Many caregivers' react with significant grief when they learn that their child is mentally retarded. Moses (1988) has

REFLECTIONS FROM FAMILIES

Mrs. Anderson used to work in the neonatal intensive care unit, years ago when my youngest son was born. Peter arrived on the planet, far tinier than my other children, with a complete bilateral cleft lip and palate and hypotonia. He was a very difficult feeder and spent twelve days in the hospital. He would grow up to be deaf, mentally retarded, and autistic, with slight cerebral palsy. But when Peter was an infant, thirty years ago, I didn't know that. In fact, I didn't even know what hypotonia was. I just knew he wasn't as strong as my other children.

Mrs. Anderson took care of him all the days that she worked. She held him carefully. She held my concerns and my heart just as carefully, as she taught me how to feed my little baby with a cross-cut preemie nipple and how to keep him safe. She smiled at him. She beamed at him. She told me, without a word, that he was precious, and decent, and just as lovable as any baby in her nursery. She sent us home and told me to bring him back to see her and she meant it.

For about a year after he was born, every month or so, I would drive over to the hospital and bring Peter to see Mrs. Anderson. I would call up to the nursery and she would come down to see him. She would smile at him, laughing when he finally learned to smile back. She would comment on how big he was getting. After his repair surgeries for the clefts, she would remark on what a good repair he had had. Her approval set the stage for me to value him. Her approval of me made me proud of the good job I did.

BOX 33-1 The grieving process for caregivers of a child with an impairment

Denial–denial of reality or of one of its aspects; denial of the importance of the reality in one's child's life or in one's own.
Anxiety–a state of chronic uneasiness, often accompanied by physiological symptoms such as hyperventilation, nervousness, or hyperactivity.
Fear–a state of dread, apprehension, or trepidation, related to the future.
Depression–overwhelming, heavy, deep sadness or sorrow; a lack of ability to see a clear and positive future.
Guilt–the taking upon oneself of responsibility for a past event.
Anger–rage, indignation, or hostility, born of pain and injury.

described caregivers' journeys of adaptation after the birth of a child with an impairment of any kind, for instance mental retardation, club foot, or missing fingers. The grieving process is composed of six principal stages: denial, anxiety, fear, depression, guilt, and anger (Moses & Kearney, 1995) (Box 33-1).

Denial serves the purpose of buying time, delaying the impact of the purported diagnosis until the caregivers can brace themselves and gather strength. Denial can be total denial: denial of the impact upon one's own life, denial of the permanency of the impairment, denial of its extent or seriousness, or denial of the steps one must take in order to create possibilities for oneself and the child (Moses, 1988). Anxiety serves the purpose of alerting one's family and friends that there is something amiss (Moses, 1987). It also has the added benefit of contributing energy to the equation. It is almost as if one's unconscious mind declares, "There's an appalling amount of work to do here and I'm going to have to do it!" Caregivers have experienced the worst thing that they can know: loss of their dream of a healthy, perfect child. They are bound to be fearful of what else is in store for them. They may feel depressed and guilty, as they search for reasons, because any cause is better than no identifiable one for such a life-changing event. They feel anger because they have done their best to be healthy during the pregnancy, to diminish risks, to seek prenatal care, and what happened? Despite all their efforts, their dream was crushed, and it just isn't fair.

The normal grieving process runs its course, and new dreams are generated in the process. Ideally, a mentally retarded baby's smile and sunny disposition become an unforeseen joy. The caregivers come to see the child as unique, important, and irreplaceable. And hopes for the future, new dreams, are crafted by them. Counseling may be helpful for some families so that they can be reassured that their feelings are normal. It may also help families who are immobilized in one stage or another to work through subsequent stages. However, with or without counseling, they will eventually progress toward some resolution of their grief.

Nurses can act as sounding boards for families who are grieving. During all phases of grieving over a child's impair-

Reflective Thinking

Placement When Caregivers Can No Longer Care for Their Child

Ephraim Smith is mentally retarded. He lives at home with his caregivers, is 18 years old, goes to work at a fast-food restaurant four days a week for five hours each day, eats lunch there, and then goes to a group day care facility. In the evenings he goes home. His life is routine, predictable, and happy. He talks about the events of his day to his caregivers every evening, looks forward to trips and family outings, and is proud to have a job. He collects little plastic animals; teddy bears are his favorite. He has forty-one little plastic teddy bears, which are arranged on display stands along the west wall of his room.

Ephraim has an older brother Lee, who has been married and divorced a number of times. He is a very successful attorney, and despite alimony and child care payments, is extremely wealthy. He is in his forties, is a chronic alcoholic, with a tendency to overuse sedatives, and has attempted suicide twice in the past three years. He lives in the same town as does Ephraim. Lee wants their parents to make a will stating Ephraim will live with him in case anything happens to them. They are in excellent health now, but are in their late sixties. Lee assures them Ephraim will have everything he wants. The brothers love each other and seem to enjoy one another's company. There are also three sisters; none of them thinks she would be able to take Ephraim at such a time, although they are open to the possibility later when their own children are older. What should Ephraim's caregivers do? Should they make a will? Can they trust Lee? What is your opinion about Ephraim's future?

ment, they can benefit by telling their story, with its feeling and emotion, to someone who listens and cares. For example, caregivers may be in denial, but they can hear themselves talking about the very issues they are denying when a nurse takes the time to listen. They can, little by little, summon their inner resources and get close enough to the end of their denial to ask, "What if my daughter really is mentally retarded? What will I do then? What can I do then? How will I act? What can I do for her?" Nurses frequently interact with individuals with MR, on the job and during social times. The tone that they set in acceptance, in daily living as well as on the job, serves as a role model for members of the community and the health care profession. Nurses have the responsibility and the privilege of being central figures in the growing emancipation and acceptance of individuals with MR and other cognitive alterations.

Institutionalization and Out-of-Home Placement

Caregivers make the difficult decision about whether or not their child with MR will live with them, in their home, not once but many times. Most attempt to raise their children in their homes or nearby, visiting with them when they are able. Those who raise their children at home may do so because it is easier or because they experience less guilt with this arrangement. They make such choices based on what they were taught in their formative years, what their families and friends believe, how their extended families feel, what other children they have in the home desire, the availability of safe out-of-home placement, the number of other caregivers who are able to share raising of the child, and many other variables about which they are not even aware. Not all caregivers can bear the scenario of trusting their dependent child to others. For them, institutionalization and out-of-home placement are to be avoided at all costs. When placement becomes inevitable, it must be complete, because every brief visit with the child brings back the pain of the original decision.

It is never the nurse's responsibility to make the decision regarding placement. It is, however, the nurse's responsibility to offer information about options. Information about out-of-home placement is usually provided when the caregiver requests it, but it is not inappropriate to broach the subject when the child has achieved certain developmental milestones, such as the end of high school. Caregivers will invariably have thought about placement on their own, and their first reply will be that they are not interested. A wise nurse replies, "Of course you're not. But if you are interested, some day, I will be happy to tell you more."

Special Olympics

The Special Olympics organization provides both training and formal athletic events for children and adults with MR. The Special Olympics effort is truly international; the organization has officially sanctioned programs in more than 100 countries. Within the United States and many other countries, schools serve as centers of the athletic programs that lead to the Special Olympics competition. The object is to allow participation and competition with people of similar age and ability. Each participant is welcomed as he or she completes an event by a person designated to recognize the effort. These designees bestow a handshake or a hug, sometimes both, upon the contestant. Competitions in the United States and elsewhere boast an array of well-known celebrity, sports, and entertainment figures. The Special Olympics oath further underscores the importance of competition: Let me win. But if I cannot win, let me be brave in the attempt.

DOWN SYNDROME

Down syndrome (DS) is a congenital chromosomal disorder and is characterized by varying degrees of mental retardation and a characteristic appearance. Years ago, children with DS were called mongoloids (or, worse, mongoloid idiots) because their eyes have the epicanthic fold seen in Asian racial groups.

Incidence and Etiology

Down syndrome is the most common chromosomal disorder caused by the presence of an extra chromosome 21 (resulting in three instead of two), hence the name trisomy 21. It occurs in 1 in every 1,000 live births (Bachman, 1998). The incidence has increased somewhat in the United States within the past half century, as more women are postponing childbearing until after 35 years of age. The exact cause of DS is not known; however, the incidence increases as the mother's age increases. The incidence of DS for women over 30 years of age is 1 in 1,500, and it increases in women over 40 years to 1 in 100 live births.

Pathophysiology

In most children with DS, every cell of the body contains extra chromosomal material. An extra chromosome in each cell causes the dozens of changes associated with the syndrome. Many of these changes affect musculature or connective tissue. Several changes represent pathophysiological conditions. For example, defects that involve valves or chambers of the heart are common, with 30% to 40% of children with DS having congenital heart disease (Burns, 2000).

By microscopic examination during chromosome analysis, about 4% of individuals with DS appear to have 46 chromosomes (Hall, 1996); however, upon closer scrutiny, the genetic material for an extra cell is found attached or translocated onto another chromosome. Rarer still, about 1% of children have some cells with 46 chromosomes and some with 47. Like people with one blue eye and one brown one, or like calico cats, they possess two different genetic strains. The presence of two different cell lines in an individual or an organism is called **mosaicism** (Hall, 1996). Children with DS who have this cellular mosaicism are less severely affected than are children in whom all the cells have 47 chromosomes.

> **Nursing Alert:**
>
> **Cardiac Defects in Neonates with Down syndrome**
>
> *Early detection of cardiac defects in neonates with DS can vastly improve both the duration and the quality of their lives. Defects that produce cyanosis and a heart murmur are almost always detected. However, many heart murmurs are difficult to hear in a newborn, and some cardiac defects do not produce cyanosis. Consequently, major medical centers routinely perform echocardiograms for neonates with DS. If an infant with DS in your care has not received an echocardiogram, be sure to obtain an order for this noninvasive screening procedure.*

Clinical Manifestations

Common features of Down syndrome include:

- Epicanthic folds (small skin folds on the inner corners of the eyes)
- Square hands with a simian (single transverse) crease across the palm of the hand
- A large tongue in a small mouth
- A high arched palate
- Muscle weakness and hypotonia
- Oblique palpebral fissures, an upward slant to the eyes
- Small nose and depressed nasal bridge
- Wide space between the big and second toe

Some children may have only a few of these distinguishing features while others may have many (Figures 33-2 and 33-3 A and B). There are numerous physical conditions associated with DS. Congenital heart defects (septal defects) are common. Respiratory tract infections and chronic otitis media occur with greater frequency among children with DS because of hyopotonicity of the chest and abdominal muscles, altered immune system, and anatomical differences of

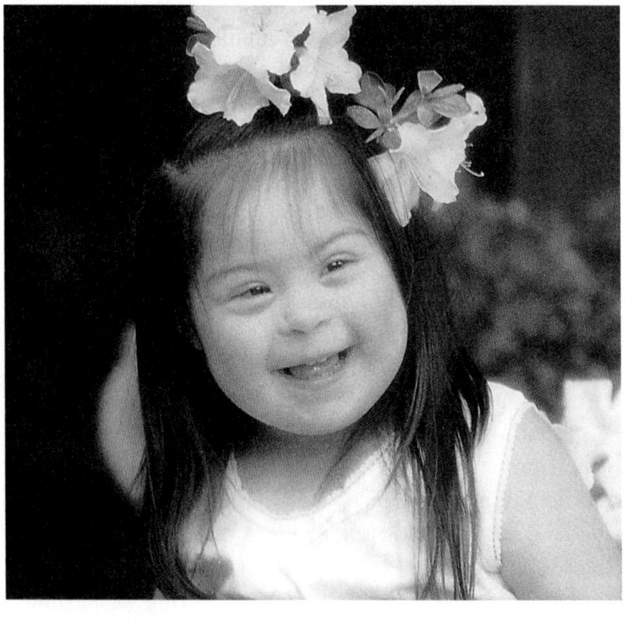

Figure 33-2 Young Girl with Down Syndrome. From Down Right Beautiful 1996 calendar, © Marijane Scott, Marijane's Designer Portraits.

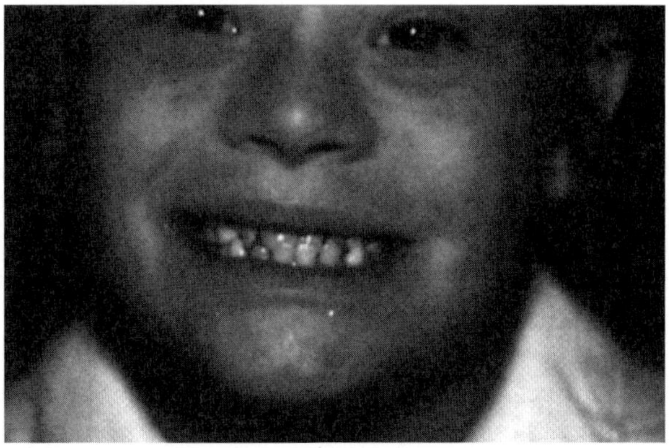

Figure 33-3A Spacing Abnormality of the Teeth in a Client with Down Syndrome

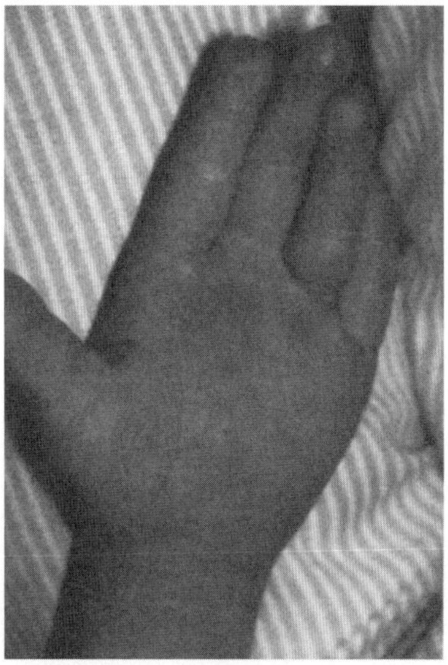

Figure 33-3B A Transverse Palmar Crease, Often Called a Simian Crease, in a Client with Down Syndrome

REFLECTIONS FROM FAMILIES

As I look back on it now, my first recollection of our Theodore, kind of like a snapshot, was when he was just seconds old. The nurse midwife held him up so I could see him and touch him. I wasn't allowed to hold him for the first few minutes, though, because he was pale and blotchy, and a little blue. The nurse rubbed him with a towel and put him under a warmer. I saw that he was pretty floppy, compared with our older girls. Right after birth, their bodies had tended to go back into that egg-shaped newborn roundedness, curling up like Alice's hedgehog. The nurse midwife told me what a beautiful baby boy he was, but then she said she wanted a pediatrician to look at him right away because she was concerned. So then, of course, I was concerned, too. Really, those first hours were like an overcast day, with skies the color of uncertainty. The pediatrician confirmed the nurse midwife's suspicions—here was a little fellow who had a heart defect and who probably had Down syndrome. The pediatrician was honest with me, uncovering Theodore for a more complete physical exam—his skin became even more blotchy when he was chilly. After the exam, I bundled him up. He was very floppy, with noodle-like muscles. Yet all the time we were fussing over him, he never cried but looked placidly at me with his lovely almond eyes.

the ears (narrow and short eustachian tube). Other problems include gastrointestinal conditions (Hirschsprung's megacolon, tracheoesophageal fistula), hypothyroidism, ocular cataract, **atlantoaxial deformity** (a spinal deformity resulting in instability of the upper cervical spine), leukemia, and Alzheimer's disease after the age of thirty (Hales, Yudofsky, & Talbott, 1999). The teeth are abnormally aligned and eruption is delayed.

Diagnosis

The diagnosis of DS is usually based on the characteristic features alone. Definitive diagnosis is based on **karyotyping,** or identification of the chromosomes' appearance, performed by growing cells from a blood or tissue sample, staining them during the metaphase stage of replication, and scanning them with a microscope. Chromosomes are examined, revealing extra genetic material.

Treatment

There is no cure for DS. However, several physical problems may be present that must be addressed in order to make these children as healthy as possible. The visible stigmata of DS, the uptilting almond-shaped eyes, enlarged tongue, flat bridge of the nose, can be altered with plastic surgery. However, this is a highly personal choice and is controversial. Early intervention programs include enrichment during the infant, toddler, and preschool years, either within an infant-stimulation or preschool-stimulation program, and/or with one-on-one time in the home. Modern wisdom stresses the importance of early enrichment programs because of the belief that transneuronal attachments in all babies are profuse but that they extinguish with disuse (Gordon, 1998). Some communities may school children with DS exclusively in the "mainstream" setting of the public school system. Others maintain special needs schools, in which children have academic and social education. Caregivers' beliefs and attitudes, the child's aptitudes, and the community's resources all contribute to the decision about which educational services the family chooses.

Treatment also includes monitoring of growth and development; special growth charts developed for the child with DS, who tend to be shorter than the average child, can be used. These growth charts are available at http://www.growthcharts.com. In the neonatal period, assessment of cardiac structural integrity is imperative, as are tests of thyroid function, assessment for ocular cataract, and screening of vision and hearing. Symptoms of Hirschsprung's megacolon should be evaluated. Constipation should be addressed with stool softeners and the possibility of Hirschsprung's reevaluated if problems persist. Failure to thrive is a distinct possibility, especially if a heart defect is present. Recurrent otitis media should be referred to an otorhinolaryngologist. The child or adolescent should have a thyroid function test at yearly intervals. Atlantoaxial instability should be frequently assessed.

Nursing Management

The nurse's role in the care of a child with DS is much the same as that discussed in the section on MR. However, it also includes follow-up to confirm that periodic screening is performed for the specific anomalies and malfunctions that are found more commonly in these children. Caregivers of infants need to be aware of the increased likelihood of respiratory infection. If a cardiac defect is present, they must learn about its medical or surgical treatment. If hypothyroidism is present, they need to know how to administer thyroid replacement hormone.

Parents of children with DS routinely receive genetic counseling and are informed of their relative risk of having subsequent children who also have DS. But before genetic counseling can be initiated, the family suffers the huge jolt of learning that their infant has a chromosomal disorder. The initial impact upon a family may be immense. Prenatal tests are available to detect DS and include amniocentesis, chorionic villus sampling (CVS), and measurement of various substances in maternal serum (alpha-fetoprotein, human chorionic gonadotropin, and unconjugated estriol and inhibin). Screening tests have proceeded from mid second trimester to very early second trimester. Initially, amniocentesis was performed at 16 weeks or greater gestation and followed by a three-week period during which cells were grown in culture and then analyzed. Failed cell growth occasionally resulted in a second waiting period of three more weeks. However, with modern gene marker techniques, a one-day result can be obtained, followed by confirmation with cell analysis (Verma, MacDonald, & Leedham, 1998). **Chorionic villus sampling** is a procedure for obtaining prenatal evaluation data in early pregnancy by withdrawing a chorionic villi sample from fetal membranes. Another method of first trimester screening examines alpha-fetoprotein, human chorionic gonadotropin, and unconjugated estriol and inhibin levels in maternal serum. Although amniocentesis was seen as the gold standard of decision-making, maternal blood testing is becoming more refined and has lower incidences of both false positives and false negatives in diagnosis (Haddow, 1998). A new technique involving ultrasound in late first trimester is being developed that may be even more effective than maternal blood testing (Lancet, 1998). Even after a woman is confirmed as carrying a child with DS, she must then choose whether or not to have an abortion. This is a highly personal choice based on religious and personal beliefs, personal experience, duration of pregnancy, and individual circumstances. The sensitive nurse can provide accurate information and support. The decision must rest with the woman herself, since she will be affected for the rest of her life, regardless of what course she follows.

Society's Response to Children with Down Syndrome

With all its cleverness and research and innovation, society has not yet devised a way to perform microsurgery on every

Family Teaching

Respiratory Infections in Children with Down Syndrome

The following topics are important to teach:

- The increased incidence and severity of both upper and lower respiratory infections.
- Symptoms of a respiratory illness, such as elevated temperature, foul-smelling nasal discharge, or a rattling, frequent cough, which should be reported to the health care provider.
- Minimal exposure to cigarette smoke.
- Importance of school personnel notifying caregivers if symptoms of a respiratory illness are observed in the child.
- Coordination of administration of medications with the school.
- Referral to an allergist, pulmonologist, or otorhinolaryngologist if respiratory infections are severe.

cell in the body of a child with DS, thus altering such societally important variables as intelligence, independent living capability, earning capacity, and ability to create and raise children. Consequently, based on the values of the nineteenth and early twentieth centuries, society's efforts toward DS have been either eugenic or compensatory in nature: either abort the fetus based on prenatal diagnosis, or attempt to improve intelligence, independent living capability, and earning capacity.

Since the middle of the century, a peculiar tendency has been noted. The measured intelligence quotient and the expected life span for people with DS in the United States have both increased markedly. Concurrently, there are more school-aged children with DS today than there were 50 years ago. Actually, there are at least two reasons for the changes. In the 1940s, many considered the child with DS as "hardly human" (Spock, 1949). Since the 1960s, social patterns have changed. In the first half of the century, DS neonates and other babies with birth anomalies were often relegated to the back rows of the hospital nursery in bassinets with signs that read, "Do not feed!" They were kept warm, bundled in blankets but were allowed to die from dehydration. In 1975, 77% of pediatric surgeons in this country favored withholding food and medical treatment from newborns with DS (Colson & Pearcey, 1997). Others were placed in institutions or in foster homes from birth. Mothers were told of a child who would not be able to learn and might not even be able to speak. Families were told that the children would surely need institutionalization in a few years and that it was easier on the caregivers, the siblings, and the infant to place him/her in an institution at birth. A generation ago life expectancy for infants with DS who were raised in institutions was only 9 years (Riccitiello & Adler, 1997).

In the 1960s there was a growing consciousness of developmental slowness as a normal variant of the human race and not a shameful condition. In the same time period legal mandates were enacted that protected infants and children from lack of medical intervention based solely upon their impairments. Additionally, it became more socially acceptable for families to keep their mentally retarded children at home for an extended period of time instead of institutionalizing them at birth. Individuals with DS live longer and experience better health than their cohorts did half a century ago. With adequate care, it turns out that life expectancy now is 58 years and rising (Riccitiello & Adler, 1997).

AUTISM

Autism is a genetic developmental disorder, characterized by extreme difficulty communicating with and relating to the environment. It is manifested by bizarre behavior, delayed language acquisition, poor social relations, impairment of self-care skills, and altered sensory responses. Kanner (1943), a psychiatrist at Johns Hopkins University, initially described autism in children exhibiting relationship impairment before age 30 months, language impairment, and a combination of ritualism and obsessiveness. These children were self-absorbed, aloof, and indifferent to others. They made little eye contact and demonstrated lack of imaginative or pretend play (American Academy of Pediatrics, Committee on Children with Disabilities, 2001a). Autism was first classified as a type of schizophrenia (Creak, 1961). "Infantile autism" first appeared as a diagnostic label in the *Diagnostic and Statistical Manual of Mental Disorders, Third Edition* (DSM-III) (American Psychiatric Association, 1980).

Incidence and Etiology

The incidence of autism has been reported to be 1 in 1,000 children (Fombonne, 1999). Boys are affected more often than are girls, by a ratio of three or four to one. It is also more common in siblings of affected children. The exact cause of autism is unknown; however, like most other behavioral syndromes, it seems multifactorial. Hypotheses regarding the cause of autism range from a genetic link to environmental events (Juul-Dam, Townsend, & Courchesne, 2001). Genetic studies indicate a greater likelihood that two monozygotic (i.e., identical) twins will have autism than two dizygotic (i.e., fraternal) twins.

Autism is sometimes associated with other syndromes or diseases. Between 2% and 5% of autistic children test positive for fragile X syndrome (Hales, Yudofsky, & Talbott, 1999). Tourette's syndrome is present in as many as 8% of autistic children (Baron-Cohen, Mortimore, Moriarty, Izaguirre, & Robertson, 1999). Some children with chromosomal disorders also exhibit autism, as do a few blind, hearing impaired, and mentally retarded children. Some autistics are mentally retarded. An association between unfavorable events in pregnancy, delivery, and the neonatal phase and autism has also been reported. Examples of these factors or events include uterine bleeding, induced labor, prolonged or precipitous labor, oxygen deficit at birth, and hyperbilirubinemia (Juul-Dam, et al., 2001).

Historically, autism was described as a result of altered mothering, and mothers were described as cold and unloving (the "refrigerator mother theory") (Bettelheim, 1967). Autistic children's mothers were observed to touch and interact socially with their children in a different way than did those of children without autism. Then it was realized that the child-caregiver dyad is a complex feedback system. A caregiver responds to a child's cues; a child responds to a caregiver's cues. A child who responds in a negative way to traditional cues stimulates different behavior in the caregiver: For instance, if a child does not present a positive response when smiled at, the caregiver will show approval or affection in different ways. This pattern was initially confusing to the observers of autistic children and their mothers. It was later noted that autistic children commonly developed seizure disorders often in adolescence (Rutter, 1970). The occurrence of seizures, as high as 75%, in some children with autism indicated that the disorder was rooted in abnormalities of the brain chemistry. Therefore, it was a neurodevelopmental disorder, and not a result of abnormal parenting.

Pathophysiology

Although the etiology of autism remains unclear, there is strong support for a genetic model of inheritance (Rutter, Bailey, Simonoff, & Pickles, 1997). There is an occurrence rate of 2% to 8% in siblings of autistic children (Fombonne, 1998; Mesibov, Adams, & Klinger, 1997). Identical twins demonstrate a concordance rate of 36% to 91%, whereas fraternal twins' concordance rate is about 5%, the same as for non-twin siblings (Mesibov, et al., 1997). Currently research has focused on locating the gene(s) associated with autism. One of the genes may be located on the seventh chromosome. Others on the second, fifteenth, sixteenth, and nineteenth chromosomes have been identified as potentially significant in autism inheritance (International Molecular Genetics Study of Autism Consortium, 1998; Philippe, et al., 1999).

There is indirect evidence to support a genetic model, acted upon by an environmental trigger. Historically, in studies of identical twins, the one with autism had the more difficult delivery (Folstein & Rutter, 1977). However, abnormalities of the affected twin could account for the difficulty during the delivery process. Presumably, differences in brain chemistry and in the stress response could precipitate changes in measurements of vital signs, tone, and neonatal responses. Caregivers of an autistic child with documented allergies often refuse routine immunizations for their subsequent children, especially the MMR, believing that it could represent the trigger if genes for autism are present (Waterhouse, 2000).

Clinical Manifestations

Aberrant social skill development is a hallmark for autistic disorder (American Academy of Pediatrics [AAP]), Committee on Children with Disabilities, 2001b). These children have poor communication, unusual forms of play, bizarre body movements, repetitive actions, withdrawal, absent eye contact, an aversion to some or all physical contact, unusual hand movements, sensitivity to tactile stimuli,

REFLECTIONS FROM FAMILIES

Thinking back on it, four years later, the most awful thing about that first couple of years was the exhaustion. Babies are supposed to be asleep most of the time, right? Here we were with this new baby, our first, and even though we weren't experienced at this sort of thing, it seemed suspiciously as if this was that dreaded entity we'd read about called The Difficult Child pattern. Matthew never slept. Never.

OK, so he slept, but it wasn't enough, and it wasn't nearly enough for my wife Martha. At a year, Matt was sleeping for an hour or two every afternoon and about six hours at night. That was it. Martha was so tired that all she had to do was sit down and she'd nod off. I have pictures (and he displays a picture of a very tired-looking woman sprawled in an easy chair), and the lack of sleep wasn't all of it. Matt insisted on breastfeeding, making Martha even more tired. Matt was never still. He walked well before a year, he was into everything. He was exploring, but in a way that wasn't like other kids. He was relentless in checking out one thing and then moving on to something else, climbing, reaching, climbing, checking doors, opening cupboards. He seemed to be on a mission from God. Supervising him was a full-time stand-up job, and injury—he was absolutely fearless. You know how other children are timid about this and that, how they won't go near the furnace because it makes a loud noise? He had no fear. He didn't climb the furniture—he swarmed up it, absolutely swarmed. He had no rubber band. (What's a rubber band?) That's the invisible cord that goes between a toddler and his mother—the kid gets just so far and then is uncomfortable with the amount of physical distance between them. Matt didn't have one. Consequently, all our doors have two-handed locks up by the ceiling, but it's just a matter of time before he figures that out, too. He can already scale six-foot fences. At four, he has finally begun to sleep—to sleep at predictable times and to stay asleep. We used to have to tiptoe but he'd wake too often anyhow. Thank Heaven he's sleeping. After a few years, I wasn't sure whether we'd all make it through as a family, whether we'd all be living together, whether we'd all be left standing. That's the thing that causes institutionalization faster than anything else, you know, the inability to survive the sleeplessness.

unresponsiveness to auditory stimuli, altered responses to pain, and a resistance to normal teaching and learning methods. The play, or behaviors, of an autistic child will typically involve solitary activities. These are repeated, apparently meaningless activities that the child finds essentially important and seems compelled to repeat in sequence (Waterhouse, 2000). One or more objects or toys are of great importance in these behavioristic rituals or play activities (American Psychiatric Association, 1994; Gray, 1998). Obsessive behaviors concerning eating, dressing, moving, and the physical environment, including the people in it, are often present.

Some of the bizarre body movements seen in autistic children are stiff gestures, awkward gait, rocking, and waving or flipping the hands back and forth. If repeated, these body movements are often accompanied by repetitious sounds. Sensitivity to tactile stimulation is most often seen as aversion to being touched. It can also include seeking contact with the hands or head by slapping an object or banging the head into it, or as extreme delight in touching or holding certain objects. Autistic children's altered response to pain usually takes the form of impassivity to mild or moderate pain, but can also be observed as loud howling in response to insignificant injuries.

The root of these odd behaviors seems to be the impaired ability of autistic children to assign meaning to the same objects and events that others find meaningful. Their behaviors may also reflect their compulsion for sameness and ritual in objects and events that others fail to grasp (Mesibov, et al., 1997). The child who is autistic may begin life as a normal infant or may display abnormal signs in infancy including an unusual response to auditory stimuli, a severe sleep disorder, a feeding disorder, lack of normal eye contact, and a lack of interaction (Mesibov, et al., 1997). The classic picture is the toddler who has apparently begun to use language and then loses most or all of it. Subsequently, the child develops abnormal behaviors, hyperfocusing on some objects and ignoring others. An autistic child typically is hyperfearful of some situations, does not indicate wants by pointing, seems to have a hearing deficit, does not exhibit "pretend" activities, does not interact voluntarily with others. He, for most autistic children are boys, may show extreme food preferences, exaggerated attachments to key possessions, complete lack of stranger anxiety, no desire when in strange environments to maintain closeness to caregivers, lack of spontaneous language, **echolalia** (repeating the last word or words heard, sometimes initially mistaken for real speech), and extreme difficulty in toilet training.

Reflective Thinking

I'm the Child's Parent. Why Won't You Believe Me?

Your 14-month-old child babbled and said about four words at 1 year of age. Now he says only one word, and that is infrequent. You know something is wrong. Your heart is cold with fear because you used to live next door to a little boy who was autistic, and you are beginning to see commonalties, one by one, week by frightening week. This loss of speech in your child is the saddest and cruelest thing you have known. You make an appointment and take him to the pediatrician. You tell the physician that you think your child is autistic. He tells you that many children are late to talk and that you shouldn't worry. You ask for a referral for hearing evaluation. The pediatrician is reluctant to make one because you had told him previously that the child was a light sleeper and woke to every little noise. You insist and get your referral. The physician tells you that your child looks fine to him. It seems as if you are being patronized. How would you feel about this whole experience?

Diagnosis

The diagnosis of autism is based mainly on the clinical manifestations and begins by ruling out other disorders such as deafness. Interviews, observations, and autism-specific assessment instruments are used in formulating the diagnosis. Correct diagnosis depends on an accurate developmental history focused on types of behavior typical of autism and on an evaluation of current social skills. A developmental history can determine if there is coexisting mental retardation and if the child's social skills are significantly below her or his global level of functioning. Social skills which are significantly delayed relative to overall developmental functioning is one of the most important criteria for the diagnosis of autism (AAP, 2001a).

Standardized autism-specific assessment instruments exist to aid in making the diagnosis of autism. A widely used one is the *Childhood Autism Rating Scale* (CARS) (Schopler, Reichler, & Renner, 1988). With this instrument, the child is evaluated in fourteen areas of behavior such as listening response, verbal communication, activity level, relating to people, object use, and imitation. The examiner provides an overall impression of whether the behavior in general seems autistic. The scale was designed for use with children 2 years and older and requires training in order to administer. The reliability of the diagnosis of autism in children under 3 years of age has been supported (Adrien, et al., 1992; Baron-Cohen, et al., 1996; Stone, Ousley, Yoder, Hogan, & Hepburn, 1997), and early diagnosis is best for both child and caregivers, for reasons of intervention.

Treatment

Although there is no cure for autism, various treatment modalities have been used. There is a growing body of evidence that intensive early intervention services for children diagnosed with autism before the age of 5 years may lead to better overall outcomes (Hurth, Shaw, Izeman, Whaley, & Rogers, 1999). However, the only controlled study of early intensive interventions with young children was conducted by Ivar Lovaas (Lovaas, 1987). This study has received significant attention because of its remarkable results. Children in the experimental group were treated with an intensive program of behavioral training on a one-to-one basis for 40 hours per week for 2 years. The program focused on acquisition of language, compliance behavior, imitation activities, and integration with peers. Caregivers adhered to the same treatment regimen during the remainder of the child's waking hours. After 2 years of therapy almost 50% of the children were functioning typically for their age in intellectual and academic areas. Yet, classically designed confirmatory studies in this area are lacking at present, and there are a number of methodological concerns regarding Lovaas's original study (Sheinkopf & Siegel, 1998).

Various developmental, behavioral, and educational strategies have been developed for the treatment of autism during the last 20 years; however, there is no consensus about which strategy is most effective (AAP, 2001a). It is generally agreed that early and intensive educational services (including special education) and behavior management are the most important intervention in autism (Rapin, 1997). Generally, the goals of treatment are to improve the overall functional status of the child by teaching communication, social, adaptive, and academic skills; decreasing unacceptable behaviors through behavioral interventions; and helping the family manage the stress associated with raising a child with autism.

Providing a highly structured environment with as much one-on-one instruction as possible is very important in the management of autism. These interventions are designed to stimulate the child's communication skills, stressing expressive and receptive speech, and to promote development of other developmental tasks including eye contact, play skills, repetitive pattern recognition, and social interactions. Because negative behavior patterns can emerge and become ingrained in a very short time, common undesired behaviors that are developmentally normal, such as hitting or biting, are predicted, immediately identified, and redirected by use of supervision, vigilance, and consistent response. The caregivers are partners in the treatment plan and are educated in the delivery of behavioral reinforcers and systematic responses to the child's behavior so that desired behaviors can be reinforced at all times of day.

Several comprehensive educational curricula have been developed specifically for children with autism including the most well known, *Treatment and Education of Autistic and Communication Handicapped Children* (TEACCH) (Schopler, 1997). In such programs, the educational approach is tailored to the child's particular preferences, the caregivers' ability to be personally and financially involved, and the child's functional level (Rutter, 1999). The basic elements of the TEACCH philosophy include the following (Schopler, 1997):

1. Collaboration between caregiver and professional.
2. Individualized treatments based on comprehensive assessments of the child.
3. Highly structured and holistic teaching.
4. Improved adaptation by teaching new skills and environmental accommodations.
5. Lifelong and community-based services.

Kids Want To Know

How should I feel about my autistic brother?

"My brother Joe is 4 and he's autistic. I'm 7 and I think he's really a pest. He gets into my dolls and my play horses and my games. He makes a mess of everything that isn't locked up, and sometimes I forget to lock my room door. It's like being a prisoner in my own house. What I want to know is this—Joe's my brother and all, but do I have to like him?"

The nurse can reply: "How frustrating for you to have to be so careful every time you leave your room. Having a little brother who is autistic is almost always harder than having a little brother who is not. You have to take special care to protect your toys and treasures, because Joe isn't good at following directions and staying in the rooms he's supposed to be in. What is really sad is that he may not ever learn this, so locking your room might be something you always have to do. He's probably pretty crafty at getting into your room quickly before your mom even knows he's in there. It sounds as if Joe would be hard for any big sister to like, and it's especially hard for you when he bothers your possessions. While we are supposed to love and respect our family members, there's nothing that says that we have to like them all the time. The way you feel is the way you feel, and it's OK to love him and at the same time not like him much when he doesn't behave."

Nursing Management

Assessment

When a child with autism is hospitalized, it is important for the nurse to obtain information from the caregivers about

Eye On:

Alternative Therapies for Children with Autism

Because autism is a chronic, lifelong condition for which there is no cure, it has become the focus of several nontraditional, alternative treatments. Several nutritional supplements have been used such as high-dose pyroxine (vitamin B_6) and magnesium (Findling, et al., 1997), ascorbic acid (vitamin C), and dimethylglycine (DMG) (Bolman & Richmond, 1999). Food allergies and intolerance are beginning to receive much attention as possible contributors to autistic behaviors. It is proposed that the body is unable to break down certain ingested proteins into amino acids (Lucarelli, Frediani, & Zingoni, 1995). Therefore, families have eliminated certain foods from their child's diet such as those containing gluten (e.g., wheat and barley) and casein (found in milk). Another controversial alternative therapy for children with autism is the administration of the synthetic human secretin hormone. However, one recent study failed to demonstrate significant improvement in autistic behaviors (Sandler, et al., 1999). Controversial, nontraditional therapies will continue to gain local and national attention because of the caregivers' desire to pursue anything that might help their child and their hope for a cure. Some treatments are detailed in journals, others on the Internet, and caregivers often have accessed and used them. Therefore, health care providers should become familiar with the more popular alternative therapies and approach the issue objectively and compassionately (Hyman & Levy, 2000).

the child's routines, likes and dislikes, and rituals. The nurse needs to evaluate as well as ask the caregivers about the child's skills and abilities regarding self-care, such as feeding, dressing, bathing, and toileting. Assessment should also include the child's communication skills, interactive patterns, and response to others. The nurse should inquire about the method the caregivers use to give the child medications, as well as ask about the family's support system.

Nursing Diagnosis

Nursing diagnoses that may be appropriate for the child and family include:

1. Risk for injury related to the potential for self-mutilation and sensory deficits.
2. Impaired verbal communication related to limited language skills.
3. Impaired social interaction related to inability to develop and maintain social relationships and lack of social or emotional reciprocity.
4. Caregiver role strain related to child's need for constant care and/or supervision, limited ability to relate to caregivers, and increased stress.

Outcome Identification

1. The child will not harm self.
2. The child will develop a means of communicating needs and wants to others.
3. The child will acknowledge others in the environment and attempt to initiate interaction with them.
4. The caregivers will discuss their need for respite care and their feelings related to the frustrations and stress of having a child with autism.

Planning/Implementation

Children with autism lack organic disturbances that would bring them into contact with health care providers more frequently than the average child, yet nurses will occasionally encounter them in the health care setting, either for wellness care or for treatment of childhood illnesses. Each autistic child is an individual, often with strong, even violent, preferences and aversions. Incorporation of the caregivers in the care of these children is absolutely essential. In the school setting, roles of teachers and nurses may overlap, especially around problem issues such as nutrition, communication, and undesirable behaviors. Nurses, as well as educators, bring specialized background knowledge related to normal nutritional needs, the range of communication patterns in the growing child, and limit-setting. The specialized role of the nurse as the child's advocate is of utmost importance throughout planning meetings and daily work with the individual. Additionally, the nurse may be called upon to administer medication during the school day. This should not be attempted until the caregivers have clarified their at home strategies and a cooperative plan has been devised. It is important to maintain consistency for medication administration, especially for children who are orally aversive.

Everything the caregivers know about the child may be helpful to the nurse who is planning care. This is especially true in the hospital setting, especially if the caregivers have other responsibilities and must leave the child for a period of time. Regardless of the hospital policies on visitation, caregivers need to have 24-hour access to the autistic child or, more important, vice versa. Caregivers can be extremely valuable in calming the child, explaining the environment, supervising the child in areas that would not present hazard to an average child, and assisting with procedures. They need to be acknowledged by nursing staff as the experts. Caregivers' detailed knowledge about their autistic child is golden.

However, caregivers do not come by this expert knowledge of their autistic child benignly. Often their lives are a symphony of sleep deprivation, misinformation, cognitive dissonance, and lulls in motivation. The misinformation that they accrue from various sources ranges from laughable to discriminatory. It includes a stereotypic view of all autistic children ("Oh, he's just like the Rain Man!"), the assumption that autistic children are all savants, the expectation that autistic adults can never survive independently, a lingering perception by some that autistics are created, not born, and a reluctance of funding agencies to support what they consider excessively expensive experimental behavioral programs.

The cognitive dissonance that caregivers of autistic children experience emanates from the gap between their own knowledge and the expectations of the health care community, the school system, and society in general. On one hand, the health care community sets itself up as expert in matters of medication; however, the caregivers of an autistic child may be told only to administer a medication to their orally aversive toddler, not *how* to administer it. School systems, the experts on children's education, may offer no publicly funded toddler or preschool programs for autistic children, despite the knowledge that intervention is best instituted early. Programs that do exist can be expensive, inadequately staffed, or of inadequate duration to produce behavioral change.

Lulls in motivation are experienced by all caregivers, regardless of whether their children are average or have special needs. However, caregivers of autistic children experience motivational dips because of three unrelated factors: first, the gap between their own instinctive and self-acquired knowledge and the world's knowledge, second, their enormous time and energy expenditure between the initiation of the intervention program and any lasting behavioral change, and third, their chronic sleep deprivation. It is very difficult to feel optimistic implementing a program that experts consider experimental, when there is no end in sight and no real improvement in any behavior for months at a time.

In the community setting, the nurse may encounter children with mild rather than severe forms of autism in the public school system or in special needs classrooms within larger schools. However, siblings of autistic children attend public schools and the nurse may be called upon to provide information and referrals. It is important to recognize the large extent to which these siblings are expected to be responsible for themselves, physically, socially, and emotionally, because of their caregiver's expenditure of time with the affected sibling. The nurse's role here includes provision of support as well as formal teaching. Caregivers can be experts in autism and yet have difficulty perceiving the effects it has on their families.

Evaluation

Questions for evaluating nursing interventions may include:

- Have the interventions directed toward preventing destructive behaviors been effective in protecting the child from injury?
- Has the child established a way to communicate needs and wants?
- Have all self-care needs been met?
- Has the child acknowledged others in the environment and attempted to interact with them?
- Has eye contact improved?
- Have the caregivers expressed their feelings and needs with the nurse?

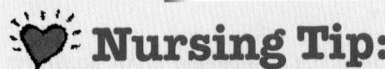

> **Nursing Tip:**
>
> **Ideas for medicating an autistic child**
>
> It is almost impossible to administer a disagreeable oral medication to an autistic child. If a health care provider orders a new medication for an autistic child, the nurse should perform the following actions:
>
> - Urge the provider to talk with the caregivers before selecting the medication, the route, and the amount.
> - Suggest prescribing double-doses if the child is likely to spit the medication.
> - Inform the caregivers of a child who is intensely oral-aversive that acetaminophen, for example, is available in rectal suppositories, which may be accepted better than the oral form.
> - Clarify alternatives for the caregivers.

Family Teaching

Teaching the family of a child who is autistic is a delicate matter. The typical caregiver raising a child with autism is far more knowledgeable about the care of that child than is the average nurse. Consequently, the critical cluster of things for the nurse to remember is to listen, to learn, to respect, and to remember. The nurse needs to understand each particular caregiver's knowledge base and beliefs about autism, its cause, its treatment, its prognosis and, most important, the individual hopes and concerns the caregiver holds for this child. Will the caregiver be able to keep him at home, at least for his childhood? Will he speak? Will he be able to coexist peacefully with siblings he may have? Will he learn to read? Will he be able to live independently?

In general, the school nurse will be the person who is close enough to the caregiver to be entrusted with specific hopes for the child's future. Alternatively, a nurse or nurse practitioner in a primary care setting might develop such a relationship with the caregiver over time. Occasionally, a community health nurse would be in this privileged position of trust with a caregiver. Then, within the framework of caregiver beliefs and hopes, the nurse can proceed with teaching. The first foci is routine health care. This caregiver needs to know about healthy practices that encompass all children. For instance, a nurse may have information about a strategy or product that may improve general safety, such as a new brand of childproof doorknob covers, or be able to suggest an unusual but especially nutritious food or food product, such as tofu, that other children with strong food preferences have tolerated. Caregivers of autistic children may be so busy with other issues that they forget simple routines, such as initiating dental visits during toddlerhood.

Research Highlight

Siblings of Special Needs Children

Study Purpose

The purpose of this correlational study was to investigate connections between parental and school-aged sibling's functioning in families where there is a younger child with special needs, and then compare these parents and children to another group of parents and children where there are younger well siblings.

Methods

The first group consisted of 39 parent pairs and their well school-aged children from families where there was a younger child with special needs. The second group was a sample of 39 parent pairs and children from families with younger well children. The two groups were matched by age and gender of the well sibling. Teachers who had known the children for at least six months evaluated the children's social skills. Both parents independently completed instruments measuring depression, marital conflict, and family conflict.

Findings

Results indicated there were no differences in groups in the school-aged children's problem behaviors. However, siblings of children with special needs scored higher than siblings of well children in cooperation and self-control. Both parents of children with special needs scored higher on the depression scale than parents of well children. In families with special needs children, maternal depression was related to sibling internalizing behavior. In families with well children, maternal depression was related to internalizing behavior and paternal depression was related to cooperation. There were no differences between groups relative to marital conflict or family conflict. However, in families with a child with special needs, marital conflict was positively related to internalizing and externalizing problem behaviors and negatively related to self-control. In families with well children, marital conflict was negatively correlated with cooperative behavior. Family conflict scores were related to teacher ratings of sibling problem behaviors in families with a child with a special need; in families with a well sibling, family conflict scores were linked to externalizing behaviors and self-control.

Implications

This information will assist nurses develop programs for all family members raising a child with special needs. It will also encourage family practitioners to enhance well-child and parent competence by providing needed support as they cope and adjust to the stresses and challenges of having a sibling with special needs.

Citation

Mandleco, B., Olsen, S., Robinson, C., Marshall, E., & McNeilly-Choque, M. (1998). Children's sibling and peer relationships in families with a disabled child. In P. Slee & K. Rigby (Eds.), *Children's peer relations: Current issues and future directions (pp.106-120).* London: Routledge.

Another teaching foci is caregiver emotional health. This again is individualized. Because many children with autism have sleep disturbances, caregivers may be too exhausted to cognitively realize that they are tired. Initiating a referral for respite care, so the caregiver can get some much needed sleep, may be the most important thing the nurse can offer. Caregivers may be deep within the grieving process and have a wealth of anger displayed inappropriately, or they may be very depressed and in need of someone to hear about how they feel. If caregivers will accept a referral for supportive counseling, that can be initiated. However, most caregivers realize this is not a "fix-it" problem, and their time is very much at a premium. Consequently, the nurse must be familiar with the grieving process and prepared to listen empathetically to caregivers' stories (Moses & Kearney, 1995).

Parents who originally planned to have other children may seek genetic counseling when their toddler is diagnosed as autistic. At present, although a genetic contribution is suspected, and although the incidence of autism is higher in families where other autistic individuals are found (Sigman & Capps, 1997), no genes causing autism have been positively identified. Siblings are certainly affected by having to adapt to living with someone who is autistic, and their feelings must also be expressed and heard. Caregivers may consciously or unconsciously treat the siblings of the autistic child as co-caregivers, as small adults sharing a common task. Caregivers need to be encouraged to see the siblings' achievements, tasks, sorrows, and needs, and to acknowledge important milestones in their lives. An autistic child is reared predominantly for a protected, circumscribed, and sheltered adulthood; the siblings need to be raised for full inclusion in the wide world that is both their heritage and their burden.

FRAGILE X SYNDROME

Fragile X syndrome is a commonly inherited cause of mental retardation (Hall, 1996). In 1991, the genetic code of the fragile X mental retardation 1 gene (FMR1) located on the X chromosome was discovered (Sherman, 1991).

Incidence and Etiology

Fragile X syndrome, occurs once in 1,000 to 2,500 births (Hagerman, 1997). The rate in males is about 1 in 1,000 to 1 in 1,500 (Giangreco, Steele, Aston, Cummins, & Wenger, 1996; Hales, et al., 1999). The occurrence in females is 1 to 3 per 10,000, and they are less severely affected than males (Hagerman, 1997). Approximately 7% of mild mental retardation in females is caused by fragile X. About 30% of families with an X-linked pattern of inheritance of mental retardation are those with fragile X syndrome (Hagerman, 1997). It has been described in all races and ethnic groups.

Pathophysiology

The gene mutation in fragile X syndrome is a nucleic acid repeat on the X chromosome. When this nucleic acid occurs more than 200 times, an individual is said to have the "full mutation" and fragile X syndrome. If the nucleic acid repetition occurs fewer than 200 times, the individual is unaffected or less severely affected. This is said to be the premutation, and the individual is identified as a carrier (Giangreco, et al., 1996). The disorder transmits from a mother with the premutation to a son with either the premutation or the full mutation, and occasionally from a father with the premutation or the full mutation to a daughter. Because of shortening of the nucleic acid repeat in gamete production, affected individuals can produce children with the premutation.

Clinical Manifestations

The manifestations of fragile X syndrome are seen very infrequently in girls. However, boys with fragile X syndrome have large ears, cupping of the ears, velvet-like skin, a slim build, broad and somewhat squinting eyes, large testes, and mental retardation (Figure 33-4) (Hagerman, 1996b, 1997).

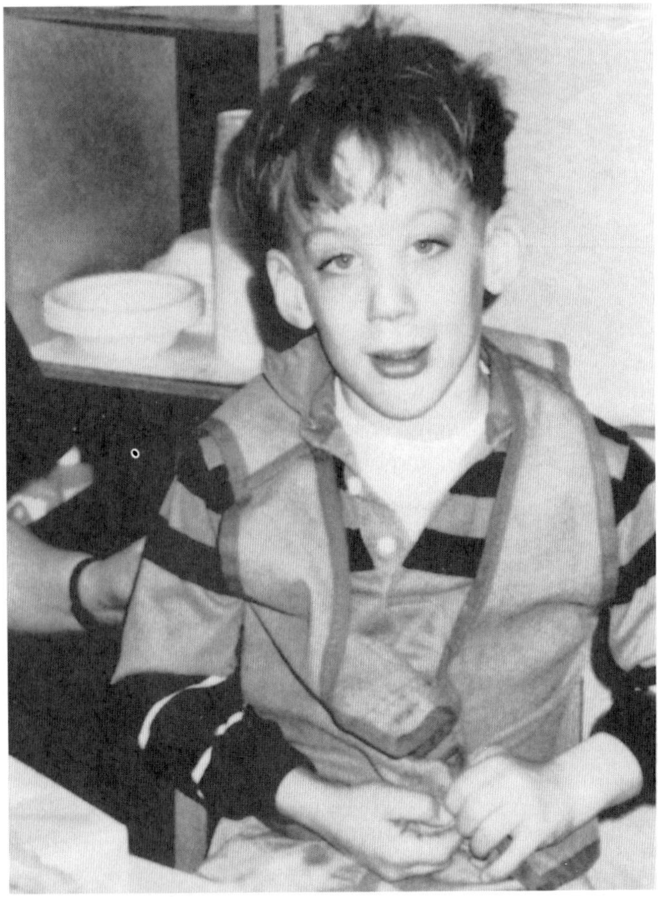

Figure 33-4 Young Boy with Fragile X Syndrome

Research Highlight

Screening for Fragile X

Study Purpose

Because screening by Southern blot analysis for fragile X is expensive, with many children testing negative, a prescreening checklist was sought that would eliminate the negatives without missing any positive cases.

Methods

Three hundred thirty-five cases previously screened by Southern blot for fragile X syndrome were compared with various physical and behavioral characteristics. Correlations between positive findings and characteristics were sought.

Findings

A correlation of positive fragile X diagnosis was found with six of the nine known characteristics of the disorder: mental retardation, a family history of mental retardation, an elongated face, large ears, attention deficit hyperactivity disorder (ADHD), and autistic-like behavior. A retrospective scoring of these six factors, on a scale from 0 to 2, yielded the information that a total score of five to twelve was obtained when 12 known fragile X children were scored, whereas a total score from 0 to 10 was found when 323 children who had tested negative for fragile X were scored. In a separate scoring, another 6 children positive for fragile X were found to have total scores of 5 and above, as well, validating the original findings.

Implications

The implications for cost containment are that children with scores of 4 or less need not have been screened for fragile X, eliminating approximately 60% of those in the original population. A second implication is that careful observation and history-taking may enable the nurse to request a genetic workup for fragile X for children who possess the characteristics of interest.

Citation

Giangreco, C. A., Steele, M. W., Aston, C. E., Cummins, J. H., & Wenger, S. L. (1996). A simplified six-item checklist for screening for fragile X syndrome in the pediatric population. *Journal of Pediatrics, 129*(4), 611–614.

The degree of mental retardation is in the moderate to severe range, with IQ scores of about 20 to 50. Many are autistic, with a 20% to 40% occurrence rate (Hales, et al., 1999). They also may have a high, arched palate, flat feet, large heads, a transverse palmar crease, and prominent ears. In adulthood, a defined jaw line develops and the face becomes longer. They are often shy and hyperactive, have a short attention span, exhibit hand-biting and hand-flapping, but have a fairly good ability to relate to other people (Hagerman, 1996a, 1997). Speech is typically delayed in both acquisition of language and complexity of sentence structure. In the school years, children with fragile X syndrome have problems with mathematics. They have poor auditory memory skills but good visual memory (Hagerman, 1996b). Behaviorally, children may also display mood instability, poor eye contact, and a tendency to chew on their clothes (Hagerman, 1997). A very good example of some of the behaviors of a teenaged boy with fragile X syndrome is in the movie *What's Eating Gilbert Grape?* Although the movie is not a presentation of mental retardation, it provides a good example of some of the stressors the sibling of an adolescent with fragile X experiences.

There appears to be a "developmental decline" in IQ, a decrease as boys with fragile X pass from preschool years to adulthood (Bennetto & Pennington, 1996; Hagerman, 1996b). Although preschool-aged boys display normal or borderline IQ 44% of the time, studies of adults reflect a deterioration in IQ, with only 13% of men high-functioning (Freund, Peebles, Aylward, & Reiss, 1995). As is true in Down syndrome, children who are mosaics display higher levels of functioning (Bennetto & Pennington, 1996). In families in which fragile X syndrome occurs over subsequent generations, there seems to be increased severity with each generation (Hagerman, 1996b).

Diagnosis

Diagnosis of fragile X syndrome is made by karyotyping. Although prenatal diagnosis through amniocentesis is possible, testing for fragile X syndrome is not routinely performed, unless there is a positive family history. As with Down syndrome, amniocentesis can be performed promptly in order to allow an early second trimester abortion, should the mother decide upon this course.

Treatment

Most persons with fragile X syndrome need special education and therapeutic services. Unfortunately little research has systematically examined the effectiveness of various treatments or interventions. Generally treatment resembles that for other developmentally delayed children. Suggestions include providing a structured, predictable environment, eliminating distractions, and clear communication of expectations and feedback. Diagnosis is often not made until the child is past toddler age. At that time, enrollment in a preschool is valuable for the acquisition of social skills and for caregiver support and respite. The majority of children with fragile X syndrome manifest hyperactivity, which may be treated with a combination of medication and behavior modification. Medically, children with fragile X syndrome are prone to otitis media from early childhood and are also are at risk for mitral valve prolapse and for gastroesophageal reflux (Hagerman, 1996a, 1996b).

Nursing Management

It is rare for a child with fragile X syndrome to be identified in the first year of life. Occasionally children with fragile X syndrome will be hospitalized for reasons unrelated to this diagnosis. Nurses involved in wellness care of children with fragile X syndrome need to be aware of their more frequent health complications. Aside from mitral valve prolapse, gastroesophageal reflux, and otitis media, there appears to be an increased incidence of visual problems, sinus problems, seizure disorders, and hearing loss associated with otitis. Special precautions in caring for the child with fragile X syndrome are related to these deficits.

Caregivers can be extremely helpful providing information as to preferences, level of supervision required, and aversive stimuli. They will need information about the nature of the genetic impairment and their child's expected development. Genetic counseling is advised if other children are planned. Although the syndrome can be identified through amniocentesis, counseling is also required in order to inform caregivers about the differing manifestations of the full mutation in boys and girls. Siblings may have the same difficulties as those of any mentally retarded child. If autism is also present, siblings may also encounter the stresses of living with an autistic brother or sister.

ADDITIONAL COGNITIVE ALTERATIONS

Fetal Alcohol Syndrome

Fetal alcohol syndrome (FAS) is a cluster of physical, behavioral, and cognitive abnormalities associated with a history of maternal alcohol exposure, which is defined as substantial regular intake or heavy episodic drinking (American Academy of Pediatrics, Committee on Substance Abuse and Committee on Children with Disabilities, 2000). FAS occurs in 0.5 per 1,000 live births (Abel, 1998). Higher rates are reported for selected subgroups such as Native Americans. The exact amount of maternal alcohol ingestion that causes FAS is not known; however, the harm to the fetus is greater with large amounts of maternal alcohol intake compared with smaller amounts.

Clinical Manifestations

A triad of characteristic features is seen in the infant with FAS: growth retardation, central nervous system abnormalities, and craniofacial abnormalities.

- Prenatal and/or postnatal growth retardation—height, weight, and head circumference below the 10th percentile; decreased adipose tissue. Weight is affected more than height.
- Central nervous system neurodevelopmental abnormalities—developmental delay, intellectual impairment, mental retardation, abnormal cognitive functioning (learning and attention difficulties), behavioral problems (infant irritability, child hyperactivity, oppositional behavior)
- Craniofacial abnormalities—microcephaly, abnormally small eyes, short palpebral fissures, poorly developed philtrum, thin upper lip, and flattened or absent maxillary area (Figures 33-5 and 33-6)
- Other abnormalities such as cardiac, skeletal, or ocular defects and renal anomalies

Treatment

FAS is permanent and irreversible but not degenerative. Treatment is mainly supportive during the neonatal period. Because poor feeding is common with these infants, nutritional intervention is necessary. Strategies include monitor-

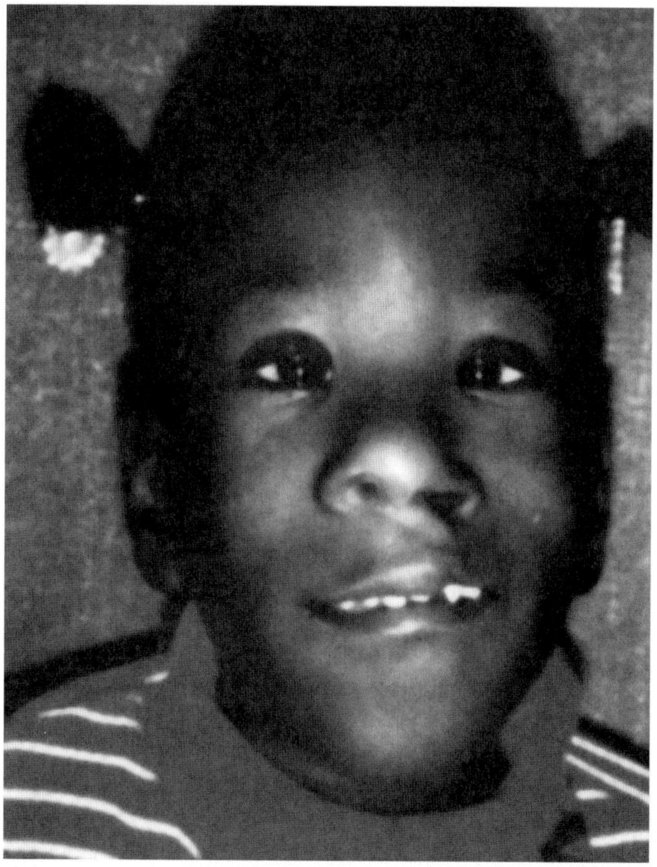

Figure 33-5 Young Girl with Fetal Alcohol Syndrome. In this case, the mother drank heavily from the onset of conception.

ing weight gain, optimizing caloric intake, and promoting suck and swallow patterns. Infants and children who are suspected to have FAS should be evaluated at an early age. For those with the disorder, referral to early intervention and education agencies should be made. Caregivers, especially the mother, should receive support services such as alcohol treatment so similar problems are prevented in the future. Because there is no known "safe" amount of alcohol consumption during pregnancy, health care providers should caution pregnant women and those planning pregnancy to abstain from all alcohol use.

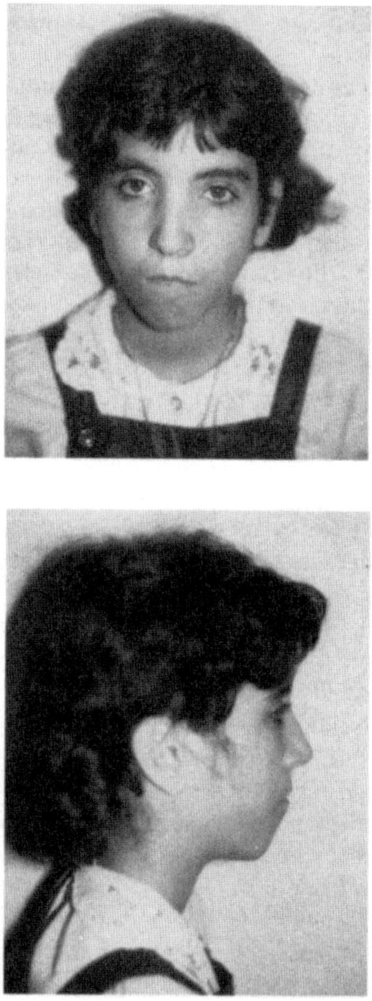

Figure 33-6 Young Girl with Fetal Alcohol Effects Whose Mother Drank Heavily Only During the Last Trimester

In the Real World

When I was between college semesters, I spent some time volunteering at various agencies. The volunteer coordinator scheduled me for two days at a school for mentally retarded preschoolers and primary grade children. I told her I just wanted to do one day but, no, she insisted that I would do a Friday and a Monday. She told me that volunteers tended not to want to go back unless they had two days at the school, because it took some desensitization. I did my two days and subsequently did many more. After that first Friday, though, I remember thinking that if I hadn't promised to go back on Monday I wouldn't have done it. Now I teach pediatric nursing. I schedule some of my students into school experiences with mentally retarded children. At first I scheduled them for two half-days. This semester, I acceded to their requests for longer experiences and less travel, and scheduled some of them for a whole school day, expecting negative reactions. Maybe times have changed in the intervening years. Maybe our young adults have been introduced to mentally retarded people all their lives and are less squeamish. However, my nursing students are so mature, so less apt to shrink from children with deficits than I was. Almost all enjoyed their school day, learning something about remedial reading or language development or special equipment or physical therapy or the role of the school nurse. In fact, one nursing student, a young man, had to schedule a two-hour experience to make up for short hours. Faced with many choices, he asked, "Can't I just go back to that school that has the mentally retarded children? There was a kid there named Arthur who asked me at the end of my day, 'Are you coming back to play with me tomorrow?' and it just broke my heart to say no."

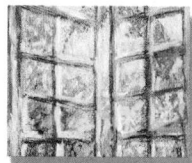

Key Concepts

- Two to three percent of the human population is mentally retarded. There is no treatment or cure.
- A mentally retarded person has subaverage general intellectual functioning existing concurrently with deficits in adaptive behavior.
- Diagnosis of mental retardation is made on the basis of history and physical examination, developmental assessments, and tests of intellectual and adaptive functioning.
- Siblings of mentally retarded children may have to expend extra patience and assume added responsibility. This may affect their lives both positively and adversely.
- Caregivers, and siblings, of mentally retarded children undergo a grieving process related to their separation from a significant dream.
- Down syndrome is the most frequent and most widely recognized chromosome disorder of humans.
- Health problems associated with Down syndrome include cardiac defects, hypothyroidism, ocular cataract, atlantoaxial deformities, frequent respiratory infections ranging from pneumonia to chronic sinusitis, hearing deficit, and Down-associated Alzheimer's syndrome after the age of thirty.
- Autism is a genetic developmental disorder, characterized by extreme difficulty communicating with and relating to the environment, and manifested by bizarre behavior, delayed language acquisition, poor social relations, impairment of self-care skills, and altered sensory responses.
- Because of behavior disturbances and disordered sleep patterns, caregivers of autistic children experience substantial stress.
- Individuals with fragile X syndrome have large ears, velvet-like skin, a slim build, broad and somewhat squinting eyes, large testes, and mental retardation. Some are autistic.

Review Questions

1. By percentage, how many children are mentally retarded?
2. Describe the appearance of a child with Down syndrome.
3. Explain the importance of knowing whether or not an echocardiogram was performed for a neonate with Down syndrome.
4. Give two reasons why the age span of Down syndrome children has increased over the past fifty years.
5. List the behavioral manifestations of an autistic child.
6. Explain why the care plan for the autistic child should include the diagnosis potential for injury.
7. Explain why genetic counseling may or may not be important for the parents of an autistic child if they are planning on subsequent children.
8. Describe the appearance of a boy with fragile X syndrome.

References

Abel, E. (1998). Fetal alcohol syndrome: The American paradox. *Alcohol and Alcoholism, 33,* 195–201.

Adrien, J. L., Barthelemy, C., Perrot, A., Roux, S., Lenoir, P., Hameury, L., & Sauvage, D. (1992). Validity and reliability of the Infant Behavioral Summarized Evaluation (IBSE): A rating scale for the assessment of young children with autism and developmental disorders. *Journal of Autism and Developmental Disorders, 22,* 375–394.

American Academy of Pediatrics, Committee on Children with Disabilities. (2001a). Technical report: The pediatrician's role in the diagnosis and management of autistic spectrum disorder in children. *Pediatrics, 107*(5), e85.

American Academy of Pediatrics, Committee on Children with Disabilities. (2001b). The pediatrician's role in the diagnosis and management of autistic spectrum disorder in children. *Pediatrics, 107*(5), 1221–1226.

American Academy of Pediatrics, Committee on Substance Abuse and Committee on Children with Disabilities. (2000). Fetal alcohol syndrome and alcohol-related neurodevelopmental disorders. *Pediatrics, 106*(2), 358–361.

American Psychiatric Association. (1980). *Diagnostic and statistical manual of mental disorders* (3rd ed., DSM-III). Washington, DC: Author.

American Psychiatric Association. (1994). *Diagnostic and statistical manual of mental disorders* (4th ed., DSM-IV). Washington, DC: Author.

Bachman, J. W. (1998). Genetic disorders. In R. B. Taylor (Ed.), *Family medicine principles and practice* (5th ed.). New York: Springer Verlag.

Baron-Cohen, S., Cox., A., Baird, G., Sweettenham, J., Nightingale, N., Morgan, K., Drew, A., & Charman, T. (1996). Psychological markers in the detection of autism in infancy in a large population. *British Journal of Psychiatry, 168,* 1–6.

Baron-Cohen, S., Mortimore, C., Moriarty, J., Izaguirre, J., & Robertson, M. (1999). The prevalence of Gilles de la Tourette's Syndrome in children and adolescents with autism. *The Journal of Child Psychiatry and Psychology, 40*(2), 213–218.

Bayley, N. (1969). *Bayley scales of infant development.* New York: Psychological Corporation.

Bennetto, L., & Pennington, B. F. (1996). The neuropsychology of fragile X syndrome. In R. J. Hagerman & A. Cronister (Eds.), *Fragile X syndrome: Diagnosis, treatment and research* (2nd ed., pp. 210–248). Baltimore: The Johns Hopkins University Press.

Bettelheim, B. (1967). The empty fortress: *Infantile autism and the birth of self.* New York: Free Press.

Bolman, W., & Richmond, J. (1999). A double-blind, placebo-controlled, crossover pilot trial of low dose dimethylglycine in patients with autistic disorder. *Journal of Autism and Developmental Disorders, 29,* 191–194.

Burns, C. (2000). Genetic disorders. In C. Burns, M. Brady, A. Dunn, & N. Starr (Eds.), *Pediatric primary care: A handbook for nurse practitioners.* (2nd ed., pp. 1260–1282). Philadelphia: W. B. Saunders.

Carpenter, R. H. S. (1996). Neurophysiology (3rd ed.). New York: Oxford University Press.

Colson, C., & Pearcey, N. (1997). Why Max deserves a life. *Christianity Today, 41*(7), 80.

Creak, M. (1961). Schizophrenic syndrome in childhood: Progress report of a working party. *Cerebral Palsy Bulletin, 3,* 501–504.

Findling, R., Maxwell, K., Scotese-Wojtila, L., Huang, J., Yamashita, T., & Wiznitzer, M. (1997). High-dose pyridoxine and magnesium administration in children with autistic disorder: An absence of salutary effects in a double-blind, placebo-controlled study. *Journal of Autism and Developmental Disorders, 27,* 467–478.

Folstein, S., & Rutter, M. (1977). Infantile autism: A genetic study of 21 twin pairs. *Journal of Child Psychology and Psychiatry, 18,* 297–321.

Fombonne, E. (1998). Epidemiological studies of infantile autism. In F. Volkmar (Ed.), *Autism and developmental disorders* (pp. 32–62). New York: Cambridge University Press.

Fombonne, E. (1999). The epidemiology of autism: A review. *Psychological Medicine, 29,* 769–786.

Frankenburg, W. K., Dodds, J. B., Archer, P., Shapiro, H., & Bresnick, B. (1992). The Denver II: A major revision and restandardization of the Denver Developmental Screening Test. *Pediatrics, 89*(1), 91–97.

Freund, L., Peebles, C.A., Aylward, E., & Reiss, A.L. (1995). Preliminary report of cognitive and adaptive behaviors of preschool-aged males with fragile X. *Developmental Brain Dysfunction, 8,* 242–261.

Giangreco, C. A., Steele, M. W., Aston, C. E., Cummins, J. H., & Wenger, S. L. (1996). A simplified six-item checklist for screening for fragile X syndrome in the pediatric population. *Journal of Pediatrics, 129*(4), 611–614.

Goldson, E. (1999). Mental retardation. In W. W. Hay, A. R. Hayward, M. J. Levin, & J. M. Sondheimer (Eds.), *Current pediatric diagnosis and treatment.* Stamford, CT: Appleton & Lange.

Gordon, N. (1998). Some influences on cognition in early life: A short review of recent opinions. *European Journal of Paediatric Neurology, 2*(1), 1–5.

Gray, D. E. (1998). *Autism and the family: Problems, prospects, and coping with the disorder.* Springfield, IL: Charles C. Thomas Publisher, Ltd.

Haddow, J. E. (1998) Antenatal screening for Down syndrome: Where are we and where next? *Lancet, 352*(124), 336.

Hagerman, R. J. (1996a). Physical and behavioral phenotype. In R. J. Hagerman & A. Cronister (Eds.), *Fragile X syndrome: Diagnosis, treatment and research* (2nd ed., pp. 3–87). Baltimore: Johns Hopkins University Press.

Hagerman, R. J. (1996b). Biomedical advances in developmental psychology: The case of fragile X syndrome. *Developmental Psychology, 32*(3), 416–424.

Hagerman, R. J. (1997). Meeting the challenge of fragile X syndrome. *Patient Care, 31*(14), 146–156.

Hales, R. E., Yudofsky, S. C., & Talbott, J. A. (1999). *The American psychiatric press textbook of psychiatry.* Washington, DC: American Psychiatric Press, Inc.

Hall, J. G. (1996). Chromosomal clinical abnormalities. In R. E. Behrman, R. M. Kliegman, & A. M. Arvin (Eds.), *Nelson textbook of pediatrics* (15th ed., pp. 312–321). Philadelphia: W. B. Saunders.

Hurth, J., Shaw, E., Izeman, S., Whaley, K., & Rogers, S. (1999). Areas of agreement about effective practices among programs serving young children with autism spectrum disorders. *Infants and Young Child, 12,* 17–26.

Hyman, S., & Levy, S. (2000). Autistic spectrum disorders: When traditional medicine is not enough. *Contemporary Pediatrics, 17,* 101–116.

International Molecular Genetics Study of Autism Consortium (1998). A full genome screen for autism with evidence for linkage to a region on chromosome 7q. *Human Molecular Genetics, 7,* 571–578.

Juul-Dam, N., Townsend, J., & Courchesne, E. (2001). Prenatal, perinatal, and neonatal factors in autism, pervasive developmental disorder—not otherwise specified, and the general population. *Pediatrics, 107*(4), e63.

Kanner, L. (1943). Autistic disturbances of affective contact. *Nervous Child, 2,* 217–250.

Kostovic, I., & Judas, M. (1998). Transient patterns of organization of the human fetal brain. *Croatian Medical Journal, 39*(2), 107–114.

Lancet, R. (1998). UK multicentre project on assessment of risk of trisomy 21 by maternal age and fetal nuchal-translucency thickness at 10–14 weeks of gestation. *Lancet 352*(9124), 343.

Lovaas, M. (1987). Behavioral treatment and normal educational and intellectual functioning in young autistic children. *Journal of Consulting and Clinical Psychology, 55,* 3–9.

Lucarelli, S., Frediani, T., & Zingoni, A. (1995). Food allergy and infantile autism. *Panminerva Medicine, 37,* 137–141.

Mandleco, B., Olsen, S., Robinson, C., Marshall, E., & McNeilly-Choque, M. (1998). Children's sibling and peer relationships in families with a disabled child. In P. Slee & K. Rigby (Eds.), *Children's peer relations: Current issues and future directions* (pp. 106–120). London: Routledge.

Mesibov, G. B., Adams, L. W., & Klinger, L. G. (1997). *Autism: Understanding the disorder.* New York: Plenum Press.

Moses, K. (1987). *The impact of childhood disability: The parent's struggle. Ways Magazine,* (Spring). Evanston, IL: First Publications.

Moses, K. (1988). *Lost dreams and growth : Children with disability; parent issues* (videorecording). Evanston, IL: Resource Networks, Inc.

Moses, K., & Kearney, R. (1995). *Transition therapy: An existential approach to facilitating growth in the light of loss.* Evanston, IL: Resource Networks, Inc.

Nihira, K., Foster, R., Shellhaas, M., & Leland, H. (1975). *AAMD Adaptive Behavior Scale.* Washington, DC: American Association on Mental Deficiency.

Philippe, A., Martinez, M., Guilloud-Bataille, M., Gillberg, C., Råstam, M., Sponh, E., Coleman, M., Zappella, M., Aschauer, H., van Malldergerme, L., Peret, C., Feingold, J., Brice, A., & Leboyer, M. (1999). Genome-wide scan for autism susceptibility genes. Paris Autism Research International sibpair study. *Human Molecular Genetics, 8*(5), 805–812.

Rapin, I. (1997). Autism. *New England Journal of Medicine, 337,* 97–104.

Riccitiello, R., & Adler, J. (1997). Your baby has a problem. *Newsweek, 129,* 46–48.

Rutter, M. (1970). Autistic children: Infancy to adulthood. *Seminars in Psychiatry, 2,* 435–450.

Rutter, M. (1999). The Emmanuel Miller Memorial Lecture 1998. Autism: Two-way interplay between research and clinical work. *Journal of Child Psychology and Psychiatry, 40*(2), 169–188.

Rutter, M., Bailey, A., Simonoff, E., & Pickles, A. (1997). Genetic influences and autism. In D. J. Cohen & F. R. Volkmar (Eds.), *Handbook of autism and pervasive developmental disorders* (2nd ed., pp. 370–387). New York: John Wiley.

Sandler, A. D., Sutton, K., DeWeese, L., Girardi, M., Sheppard, V., & Bodfish, J. (1999). Lack of benefit of a single dose of synthetic human secretin in the treatment of autism and pervasive developmental disorder. *New England Journal of Medicine, 341,* 1801–1806.

Schopler, E. (1997). Implementation of TEACCH philosophy. In D. J. Cohen & F. R. Volkmar (Eds.), *Handbook of autism and pervasive developmental disorders* (2nd ed., pp. 767–795). New York: Wiley & Sons.

Schopler, E., Reichler, R. J., & Renner, B. R. (1988). *The Childhood Autism Rating Scale.* Los Angeles: Western Psychological Services.

Sheinkopf, S. J., & Siegel, B. (1998). Home-based behavioral treatment of young children with autism. *Journal of Autism and Developmental Disorders, 28*(1), 15–23.

Sherman, S. (1991). Epidemiology. In R. J. Hagerman & A. Cronister (Eds.), *Fragile X syndrome: Diagnosis, treatment and research* (2nd ed., pp. 69–86). Baltimore: The Johns Hopkins University Press.

Sigman, M., & Capps, L. (1997). *Children with autism: A developmental perspective.* Cambridge, MA: Harvard University Press.

Sparrow, S. S., Balla, D. A., & Cicchette, D. V. (1984). *Vineland Adaptive Behavior Scales.* Circle Pines, MN: American Guidance Service.

Spock, B. (1949). *The pocket book of baby and child care.* New York: Pocket Books.

Stone, W. L., Ousley, O. Y., Yoder, P. J., Hogan, K. L., & Hepburn, S. L. (1997). Nonverbal communication in two- and three-year-old children with autism. *Journal of Autism and Developmental Disorders, 27*(6), 677–696.

Terman, L., & Merrill, M. (1973). *Stanford-Binet Intelligence Scale.* Boston: Houghton Mifflin.

Verma, L., MacDonald, F., & Leedham, P. (1998). Rapid and simple prenatal DNA diagnosis of Down syndrome. *Lancet 351*(9121), 9.

Waterhouse, S. (2000). *A positive approach to autism.* London: Jessica Kingsley Publishers.

Suggested Readings

Catalano, R. (1998). *When autism strikes: Families cope with childhood disintegrative disorder.* New York: Plenum Press.

Department of Developmental Services. (1999). *Changes in the population of persons with autism and pervasive developmental disorders in California's Developmental Services System: 1987 –1998. Report to the Legislature, March 1, 1999.* Sacramento, California: State of California, Department of Developmental Services. Available at: http://www.dds.ca.gov.

Gillberg, C., & Wing, L. (1999). Autism: Not an extremely rare disorder. *Acta Psychiatrica Scandinavica, 99*(6), 399–406.

Neuwirth, S. (1997). *Autism: Decade of the Brain.* Bethesda, MD: National Institute of Mental Health, Information Resources and Inquiries Branch.

Penn, A. A., & Shatz, C. J. (1999). Brainwaves and brain wiring: The role of endogenous and sensory-driven neural activity in development. *Pediatric Research, 45,* 447–458.

Resources

Organizations and Websites

ARC of the United States (mentally retarded persons)
1010 Wayne Ave., Suite 650
Silver Spring, MD 20910
(301) 565-3842
www.thearc.org

Association for Children with Down Syndrome
4 Fern Place
Plainview, NY 11803
(516) 933-4700
(800) LUV-ACDS
www.acds.org

Autism Society of America
7910 Woodmont Ave., Suite 300
Bethesda, MD 20814
(800) 328-8476
www.autism-society.org

California Department of Developmental Services
www.dds.ca.gov/Autism/main/AutismReport.cfm
This site offers a twelve-year overview of population changes in persons with autism, as compared with cerebral palsy, mental retardation, and seizure disorders.

Center for the Study of Autism
P.O. Box 4538
Salem, OR 97302
www.autism.org

Families for Early Autism Treatment
P.O. Box 255722
Sacramento, CA 95865
(916) 843-1536
www.feat.org

FRAXA Research Foundation
45 Pleasant Street
Newburyport, MA 01950
(978) 462-1866
www.fraxa.org

Growth Charts for Children with Down Syndrome
www.growthcharts.com

National Association for Down Syndrome
P.O. Box 4542
Oak Brook, IL 60522
(630) 325-9112
www.nads.org

National Down Syndrome Congress
7000 Peachtree-Dunwoody Rd. NE
Lakeridge 400 Office Park
Building #5, Suite 100
Atlanta, GA 30328
(770) 604-9500
(800) 232-NDSC
E-mail: NDSCcenter@aol.com
www.ndsccenter.org

National Fragile X Foundation
P.O. Box 190488
San Francisco, CA 94119
(510) 763-6030
(800) 688-8765
www.fragilex.org

New York Families for Autistic Children
95-16 Pitkin Ave.
Ozone Park, NY 11417
(718) 641-3441
www.nyfac.org

Special Olympics
1325 G St. NW, Suite 500
Washington, DC 20005-3104
(202) 628-3630
www.specialolympics.org

CHAPTER 34

MUSCULOSKELETAL ALTERATIONS

Jo Trilling, RNC, MS
Nicki Potts, PhD, RN

A special acknowledgment to Helene Harris, MSN, RN

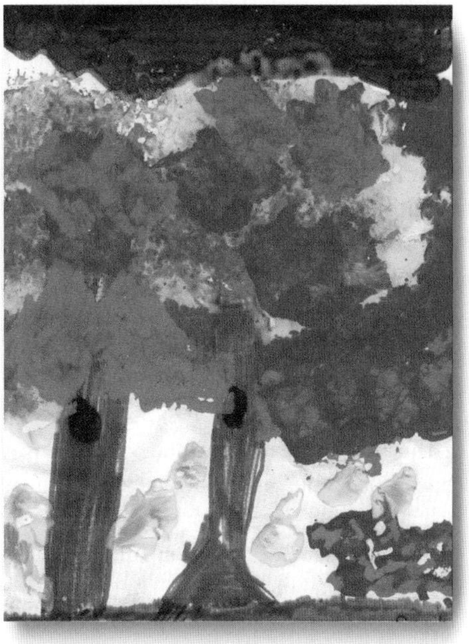

My pregnancy was uneventful. I had the usual morning sickness and food cravings, but I felt well. My ultrasounds were all normal and my husband and I were so looking forward to the birth of our son. We had so many wonderful plans for him. My husband was going to teach him to play football, ride a bike, all those things parents do for their children. Justin was born and was a very happy child. He never cried much except when he was hungry or wanted attention. We were never really worried when at 12 months he wasn't walking yet. Justin was just slow in walking, but when he did walk, he would walk on his toes. He had difficulty standing up. He would get in a position like he was going to crawl, pull his hands in close to his feet, and raise himself up by placing his hands on his knees and thighs. When Justin was about 2$\frac{1}{2}$ years old, we enrolled him in a day care center so I could go back to work. It was there that the problems really began. Justin had problems in the day care center keeping up physically with the other children.

Justin could not walk up the three steps to the slide during playtime. The teacher became concerned when Justin kept falling down all the time and called my husband and me to express her concerns. We took Justin to the pediatrician. The doctor did a range of tests on him. After 3 weeks we were given the news, Justin has Duchenne muscular dystrophy. If we're lucky he'll live to be 20 years old, but he will be confined to a wheelchair. Our only hope is that a cure is found. Maybe then my Justin will have a chance at a semi-normal life.

COMPETENCIES

Upon completion of this chapter, the reader will be able to:

- *Describe the anatomy and physiology of, and differences between, the musculoskeletal systems of the developing child and an adult.*
- *Describe various acute musculoskeletal injuries that may occur in children, including sprains, strains, contusions, dislocations, and fractures.*
- *List and identify different types of fractures. Explain the use of casts and types of fractures.*
- *Discuss the importance of identifying an injury of the epiphyseal growth plate.*
- *Identify the inflammatory and infectious disorders that can affect the pediatric musculoskeletal system.*
- *Describe congenital musculoskeletal disorders common to children and adolescents.*
- *Describe the nursing management associated with various musculoskeletal disorders.*
- *Identify the education needs of the families of children with musculoskeletal alterations.*

Disorders of the musculoskeletal system affect a child's movement and normal physical activity, thus influencing the ability to achieve developmental milestones. Alterations may be congenital or acquired during childhood from trauma, infection, or disease. Children and their caregivers may struggle with limitations of mobility and the discomfort associated with treatment of musculoskeletal disorders. This chapter highlights the common musculoskeletal alterations experienced during childhood and is organized into the following categories: (1) injuries, (2) inflammatory and infectious disorders, (3) congenital disorders, and (4) disorders related to growth. This chapter also focuses on the nurse's role in supporting children and their caregivers during assessment, diagnosis, treatment, and evaluation of musculoskeletal alterations.

ANATOMY AND PHYSIOLOGY

The musculoskeletal system is composed of bones, muscles, joints, and tendons that maintain form and perform specific functions of the body. This system provides protection for the internal organs and allows for movement. The skeletal system manufactures erythrocytes in the bone marrow and provides storage for minerals such as calcium and phosphorus. Bone is unique as a tissue and an organ because it is a rigid and variable structure, and it can heal and replace itself with normal tissue without scarring. There are many differences in the musculoskeletal system of a child in comparison to an adult. The bones of children contain large amounts of cartilage making them more flexible and more porous, thus, allowing them to bend and buckle rather than break. The periosteum is also stronger and tougher. These qualities account for children's bones being able to absorb more energy before breaking and healing more quickly. Another major difference is that children have an epiphyseal growth plate at the end of the long bones. A fracture that disrupts or transects this plate may interfere with the growth of the bone and lead to serious complications such as limb length discrepancy or cessation of growth in height. Musculoskeletal injuries in children also differ significantly from those of adults. Because soft tissue attachments are stronger in children, bony injury especially at the growth plate is more common than sprains, which are frequently seen in adolescents and adults. The tissues also heal at a much faster rate, allowing quicker resumption of activity.

As shown in Figure 34-1 each bone consists of a diaphysis, epiphysis, and the metaphysis. The **diaphysis** is the shaft of the long bone; the **epiphysis** is the proximal and distal ends of the long bone. The epiphysis is considered the ossification center of the bone. Muscles are attached to the proximal and distal epiphysis. The **metaphysis,** a section of the long bone in which the diaphysis and epiphysis converge, is responsible for growth until the child's adult height is

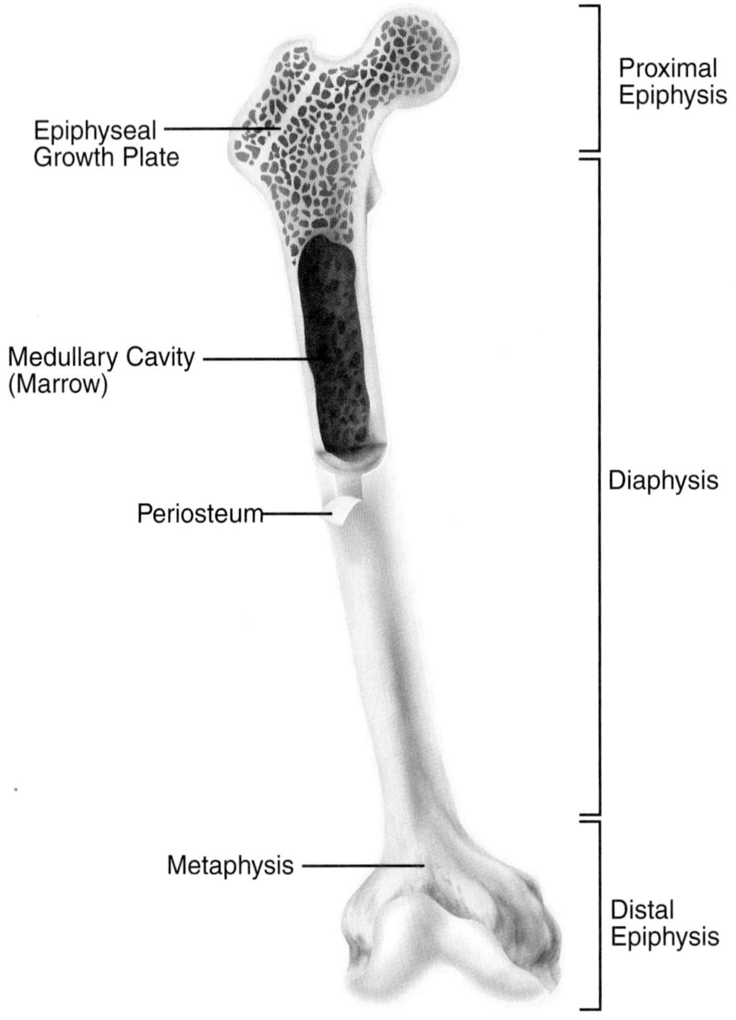

Figure 34-1 Structure of a Long Bone

attained. The metaphysis contains cartilage and produces bone. The medullary cavity is the interior of the bone, which contains red and yellow marrow. Hematopoiesis (production of blood cells) occurs in the red marrow. The yellow marrow is the site for fat storage.

Bone formation begins in the second month of life and ossification is nearly complete at birth. Bone growth occurs in two ways: **osteoblastic** activity (bone formation by osteoblasts), and **osteoclastic** activity (resorption of old bony tissue by osteoclasts). The **epiphyseal growth plate** is a thin layer of cartilage located between the metaphysis and the epiphysis at the end of the long bones. This growth plate controls long bone growth and is a vascular area of active cell division. New cartilage is laid down on the epiphyseal end of the plate. It is converted to bone at the metaphyseal end of the growth plate. The growing cells of the epiphysis are sensitive to nutrition and hormonal changes. Growth hormone, secreted by the anterior lobe of the pituitary gland, is responsible for increasing bone length. Maturation and bone shaping continues until 21 years of age. The skull is not rigid during infancy and fusing of the posterior fontanel occurs at 2 to 3 months of age. The anterior fontanel closes at approximately 16 to 18 months of age. This allows for growth of the brain and skull. Increased intracranial pressure prior to fontanel closure leads to separation of the sutures causing the infant's head to enlarge.

All muscles are present at birth, and as the child grows, the length and circumference increases. Muscle tissue is of two types, striated and smooth. Striated muscle is the predominant type, which provides movement, maintains the body's posture, and accounts for about half the body's weight. Smooth muscle is responsible for, among other things, gastrointestinal peristalsis. Muscle actions are controlled through sensory mechanisms, reflexes, and the nervous system.

MUSCULOSKELETAL INJURIES

Although all children old enough to walk can suffer musculoskeletal injuries, older preadolescents and adolescents are most at risk because of their higher level of athletic activity and greater body mass. Accidents and injuries may be caused by immature cognitive development, increased mobility, and immature or underdeveloped motor skills. They often occur during play and during participation in sports and recreation activities. Trauma is a frequent cause of injuries, especially fractures.

An understanding of growth and development is helpful whether assessing, planning interventions, or evaluating care of the child with injuries. Nurses can teach children and caregivers preventive and safety measures, not only in health care settings, but also in schools and after-school activities, such as scouting, and in the community. Common musculoskeletal injuries that are discussed include sports injuries, sprains, strains, contusions, dislocations, and fractures.

Sports Injuries

Every year at least 3 million school-aged children and adolescents in the United States experience injuries related to sports and recreation, which account for substantial morbidity and cost (Landry, Lilligard, & Rice, 1998; Hergenroeder, 1998). Most injuries in organized sports occur in ice hockey, wrestling, and football. Nonorganized sports and activities such as Rollerblading and skateboarding also contribute large numbers of injuries every year (Mankin & Zimbler, 1996). In 2000, with the increased popularity of scooters, there was a sharp increase in scooter-related injuries. Sports injuries in young children are predominately caused by fractures, contusions, and overuse. However, in adolescents sports-related injuries become more similar to those of adults, and ligament injuries, especially about the knee, are common. Sports injuries are classified as acute or overuse injuries. Acute injuries are caused by direct and forceful impact on the bones, joints, tendons, or ligaments. They may be caused by a blow, twisting, or overstretching that results in sudden stress to the tissue. Acute injuries occur most frequently with contact sports such as football. Overuse injuries are the result of chronic repetitive microtrauma to tissue that is not given sufficient time to heal (Mills & Muscari, 1998).

Of all the acute injuries, those that have the potential to be the most devastating are of the neck and head. Neck injuries are estimated to account for 10–15% of the reported injuries in recreational and organized sports. Approximately 30–50% of cervical spinal cord injuries result in quadriplegia (Luke & Micheli, 1999). However, spinal cord injury is rare among children younger than 11 years of age. Yet, the rate of neck injuries increases between 15 and 18 years of age. The sports that have the highest risk of spine injury are football, gymnastics, ice hockey, and wrestling. Diving is the most common source of recreational sport associated with cervical spine injury. Head injury should be considered in any athlete in whom contact involving the head results in disorientation or confusion. Almost 50% of all head injuries in sports are caused by bicycle riding, skating, and skateboarding accidents. Other sports associated with head injuries are football, baseball, martial arts, diving, and hockey (Luke & Micheli, 1999).

Common overuse injuries are seen in running sports such as soccer and basketball and in sports involving potential injury to the shoulder, elbow, or knee, that is, swimming and tennis. The major symptom is typically activity-related pain that is relieved by rest. Training factors, especially training abuses, are the most common source of overuse injuries (Thompson & Scoles, 1996). Overuse injuries can also produce stress fractures, which occur when soft tissue does not protect bone from repeated stress.

Prevention of sports injuries involves understanding risk factors, knowledgeable coaching and supervision, use of protective equipment when appropriate, and safe playing conditions. Risk factors are related to the type of sport and level of training intensity. Individual activities with continual and repetitive training, such as skating or dancing, have a greater risk for overuse injury. While team sports are generally considered safer, sports involving running, blocking, or cutting increase the risks of acute injures. Inadequate conditioning is a major factor in both types of injuries as muscles are tighter and susceptible to injury without warm-up periods.

Readiness to participate in sports is related not only to chronological age but the individual's physical and emotional readiness. The smaller child who is placed on a team with bigger, more skeletally mature children is at greater risk for injury. Children of the same chronological age may have different levels of cognitive maturity, and their understanding of the concepts of position or a role on a team may be different. Placing children on a team is best determined by several factors including age, size, and emotional, social, and cognitive maturity.

Warm-ups and cool-downs help, and the use of proper protective equipment protects against and prevents some sprains and strains. Conditioning before beginning an intensive sports season is also critical. All equipment should be well-fitting and specific to the sport. Helmets, protective eye gear, footwear, chest protection, and facemasks are types of protective gear available for different sports.

Many youths are injured in unsafe sports settings, for example, poor field conditions or unsafe locations, suggesting a need for and use of available and safe locations for recreation (Cheng, et al., 2000). The health professional's role is directed toward prevention, treatment, and rehabilitation of injuries as well as education about safety, use of protective equipment, and risks associated with different types of sports. Environmental safety, availability of first aid, and medical services may be the school nurse's responsibility. Education about the risks involved in the use of anabolic steroids and additional nutrition needs of the young athlete are additional concerns that the school nurse may address (Patterson, 1999).

Soft Tissue Injuries

Most sports injuries in older children and adolescents are not skeletal (fractures) but rather are injuries to soft tissues, including sprains, strains, and muscle contusions. In young children sprains and strains are very uncommon because the growth plates or physes are weaker than the ligaments and will usually separate before a ligament will tear.

A **sprain** is the stretching or tearing of a ligament from injury to a joint. A **strain** is the stretching or tearing of either a muscle or a tendon from overuse, overstretching, or misuse. A **contusion** occurs when there is damage to soft tissues, subcutaneous structures, small vessels, and muscles, yet, the integrity of the skin is not disrupted. Contusions are the most common of all sports injuries.

Incidence and Etiology

Sprains usually occur during forceful sports activities such as football, wrestling, or from a fall. Common sites include the knee, ankle, wrist, shoulder, and elbow. Strains are related to excessive physical activity or effort such as high action sports or from lifting heavy objects. Muscle contusions are common in contact and collision-type sports such as football and are caused by a blow to the body. The quadriceps muscle is the most common site of a contusion.

Pathophysiology and Clinical Manifestations

A sprain is the result of a twisting or turning injury to a joint in which the ligaments are stretched or torn. Strains are caused by excessive stretching of a muscle-tendon unit from an antagonist muscle group, an external object, or active muscle contraction. Sprains and strains are graded according to the severity of the injury. With a mild sprain there is microscopic tearing of the ligament with local tenderness and minimal swelling with no instability of the affected joint. A moderate sprain involves partial tearing of the ligament, partial joint instability, immediate pain, a moderate amount of swelling, and **ecchymosis** (black and blue discoloration of an area of skin caused by extravasation of blood into subcutaneous tissue as a result of trauma). A severe sprain is associated with less pain than a moderate one because the pain fibers are not being stretched. However, other manifestations of a severe sprain are markedly diffuse swelling, severe ecchymosis that develops rapidly, complete tearing of a ligament, joint instability, and loss of function.

The clinical manifestations of strains vary depending on whether the muscle or tendon is injured and the severity of the injury. Mild muscle strains are associated with microscopic tears in the muscle, local tenderness, and minimal swelling and ecchymosis. With a moderate strain a larger number of muscle fibers are torn, a "pop" is felt by the individual, and a small defect can be palpated. In severe muscle strains there is a popping or snapping sound complete with rupture of the muscle, severe pain, marked ecchymosis, and loss of function. Because tendons are relatively avascular, injuries involving them swell and are painful but do not bleed.

In a contusion, tearing of the soft tissues and small blood vessels occurs, leading to an inflammatory response. Hemorrhaging into the damaged tissues results in ecchymosis. The injured body part is painful to move.

Diagnosis

Soft tissue injuries are diagnosed based on the clinical manifestations. Radiographic studies may be obtained to rule out a fracture; however, they are routinely negative if the injury resulted in a sprain, strain, or contusion.

Treatment

Initial treatment of sprains, strains, and contusions includes rest, ice, compression, and elevation. The acronym RICE is used to describe this treatment plan. The RICE method is used for the first 24 hours followed by 48 hours of heat (Salmond, Mooney, & Verdisco, 1996). The first six to twelve hours are the most critical for controlling swelling and reducing muscle damage. Box 34-1 includes a description of the acronym RICE.

Analgesics, such as acetaminophen (Tylenol) or ibuprofen (Advil), are usually adequate to achieve pain control. Further treatment for mild sprains includes supporting the injured area with elastic bandages or splints. For moderate and severe sprains in which ligaments are torn, casting or bracing for several weeks is usually required. Severe sprains with complete tearing of ligaments may also be treated surgically. Healing time is determined by the extent of the injury. As the pain decreases, weight bearing is increased, moving from partial weight bearing to full weight bearing as tolerated. Stretching and strengthening exercises may be helpful when resuming weight bearing. Physical therapy referrals may be necessary if the exercise regimen is long-term or complex.

Nursing Management

Determining the severity of a soft tissue injury as well as the presence of fractures is the major function of the nurse's assessment. Range of motion, neurovascular involvement, localized tenderness of the joint, and limited joint movement are also considered. Goals for management include keeping the child as pain free as possible and helping the individual to return to normal activity level as the soft tissue injury heals. Nursing interventions include monitoring the neurovascular status of the child. Skin color should be pink with brisk capillary refill; skin temperature should be warm, and motion and pulses of the distal extremity should be present. Elevation of the affected limb will reduce swelling. If elastic wraps are used they should not be wrapped too tightly as this may impair neurovascular status. Activity restriction may be necessary in the effective management of the child's pain.

BOX 34-1 Treatment for soft tissue injuries (RICE)

Rest–Staying off the injury for several hours to several days depending on the severity.

Ice–On for 30 minutes, off for 15 minutes.

Compression–Use of an elastic wrap.

Elevation–Elevation of the injured part level with or above the level of the heart.

Family Teaching

Family teaching focuses on the need for rest, elevation of the affected extremity, and the use of ice or heat. Teaching crutch-walking principles is necessary if the child requires the use of crutches. Activity restrictions pose a challenge for caregivers if the child has been active in sports, therefore stressing the importance of maintaining restrictions is essential. Follow-up appointments and further sports restrictions need to be adhered to until the injury is fully healed.

Dislocations

A **dislocation** is a displacement of two bone ends or of a bone from its articulation with a joint. **Subluxation** is an incomplete or partial dislocation of the articular surfaces of a joint.

Incidence and Etiology

Areas of dislocation commonly seen in children are the fingers and elbows. Dislocation of the elbow, known as **nursemaid's elbow** or subluxation of the radial head, typically occurs in children younger than 5 years of age. This type of injury results when a child's hand is suddenly jerked by an adult to prevent a fall or when a child is forcibly lifted by the hand. Dislocation of the shoulder is uncommon in children but increases in frequency during adolescence as a result of participation in sports. Dislocation occurs when the force of stress on the ligament is so great as to displace a bone from its normal articulation within a joint.

Pathophysiology and Clinical Manifestations

A dislocation is associated with severe damage to the ligaments and joint capsule. Typical manifestations include pain, immobility, and change in the normal contour of the joint or length of the extremity.

Diagnosis

Observation and physical assessment also are used to determine the presence of a dislocation. Radiographs are used to diagnose the dislocation. They frequently reveal an associated fracture.

Treatment

Dislocations are treated with closed manual reduction with the child under conscious sedation or general anesthesia. Following reduction the joint is immobilized with a splint, sling, or cast for at least 3 weeks. Mobilization of the joint with active range of motion should begin after the immobilization period.

Nursing Management and Family Teaching

Nursing interventions include pain management and assessment of neurovascular status. The family needs to be instructed on caring for equipment such as slings or support devices and prevention of reinjury. The nurse also needs to provide information for appropriate school personnel about resumption of activity and participation in sports.

Fractures

Fractures of the bones are common injuries during childhood because children have many falls and mishaps. A fracture is a break or disruption in the structure of the bone when more stress is placed on the bone than it can absorb. Fractures can lead to serious and life-threatening complications; therefore, early diagnosis and appropriate treatment and nursing management are essential.

Incidence and Etiology

Fractures are one of the most common musculoskeletal injuries of childhood. The incidence peaks in both males and females between the ages of 6 and 16 (Maher, Salmond, & Pellino, 1998). Age and developmental level place children at a high risk for fractures that may result from direct trauma to the bone, for example, falls, motor vehicle accidents, sports injuries, or child abuse. Fractures are frequent in early childhood because of the porous nature of immature bones.

Pathophysiology

Fractures are described as simple (closed) or compound (open). In a simple or closed fracture, the skin surface over the broken bone remains intact. In a compound or open fracture, the broken bone protrudes through the skin causing an external wound and the potential for infection and significant blood loss. Figure 34-2 illustrates the most common types of fractures seen in children. They can also be classified by the description of the type of break as:

- Transverse—the fracture line is at right angles to the long axis of the bone; occurs on the shaft of the bone; often results from a sharp, direct blow or from stress as during prolonged running.
- Oblique—the fracture line is slanting or diagonal across the bone.
- Spiral—the fracture line is circular and twists around the bone shaft; produced by a twisting force; commonly seen in child abuse.
- Greenstick—a break through the periosteum and bone on one side while the other side only bends resulting in an incomplete fracture; similar to a green stick when it is broken; frequently seen in children.

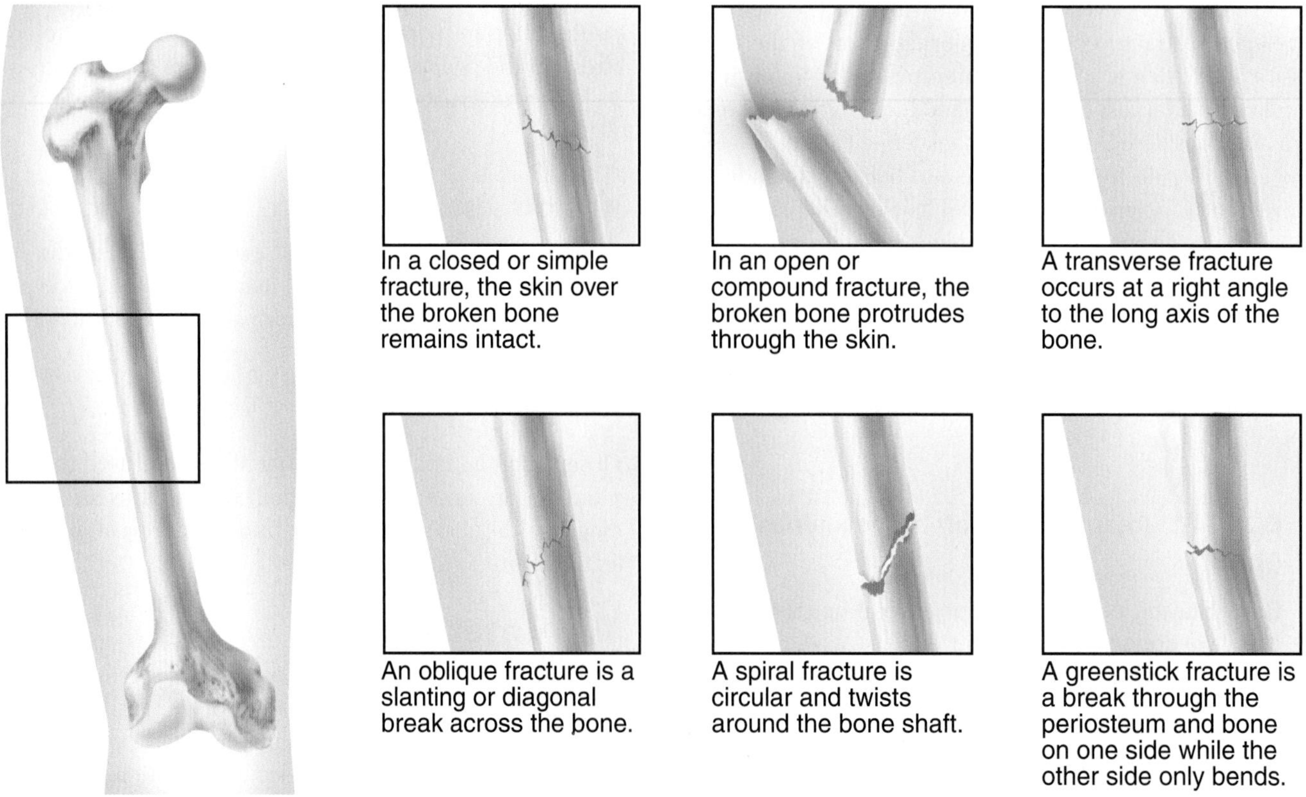

In a closed or simple fracture, the skin over the broken bone remains intact.
In an open or compound fracture, the broken bone protrudes through the skin.
A transverse fracture occurs at a right angle to the long axis of the bone.
An oblique fracture is a slanting or diagonal break across the bone.
A spiral fracture is circular and twists around the bone shaft.
A greenstick fracture is a break through the periosteum and bone on one side while the other side only bends.

Figure 34-2 Common Childhood Fractures

Another type of injury seen in children occurs at the epiphyseal growth plate, which is vulnerable because it is the weakest part of the long bone. These injuries can be serious because they can cause growth disruption, arrest, or uneven growth. Injuries of the growth plate can be classified with the Salter-Harris system (Figure 34-3). Salter I and II injuries generally have the best prognosis for normal growth.

The healing process that repairs the fracture is divided into several stages:

- Inflammatory stage: Immediately following the fracture a hematoma forms at the site of the break caused by ruptured blood vessels from injury to surrounding tissues. Blood begins to clot at the site and provides a fibrin network for cellular invasion. Granulation tissue begins to invade the area.
- Reparative stage: **Osteoblasts** (cells of mesodermal origin concerned with formation of bone) are produced and migrate to the fracture site. These cells form a new bone matrix between the bone fragments. This is followed by calcium salts being deposited and forming new tissue known as a **callus** (osseous material woven between the ends of a fractured bone that is

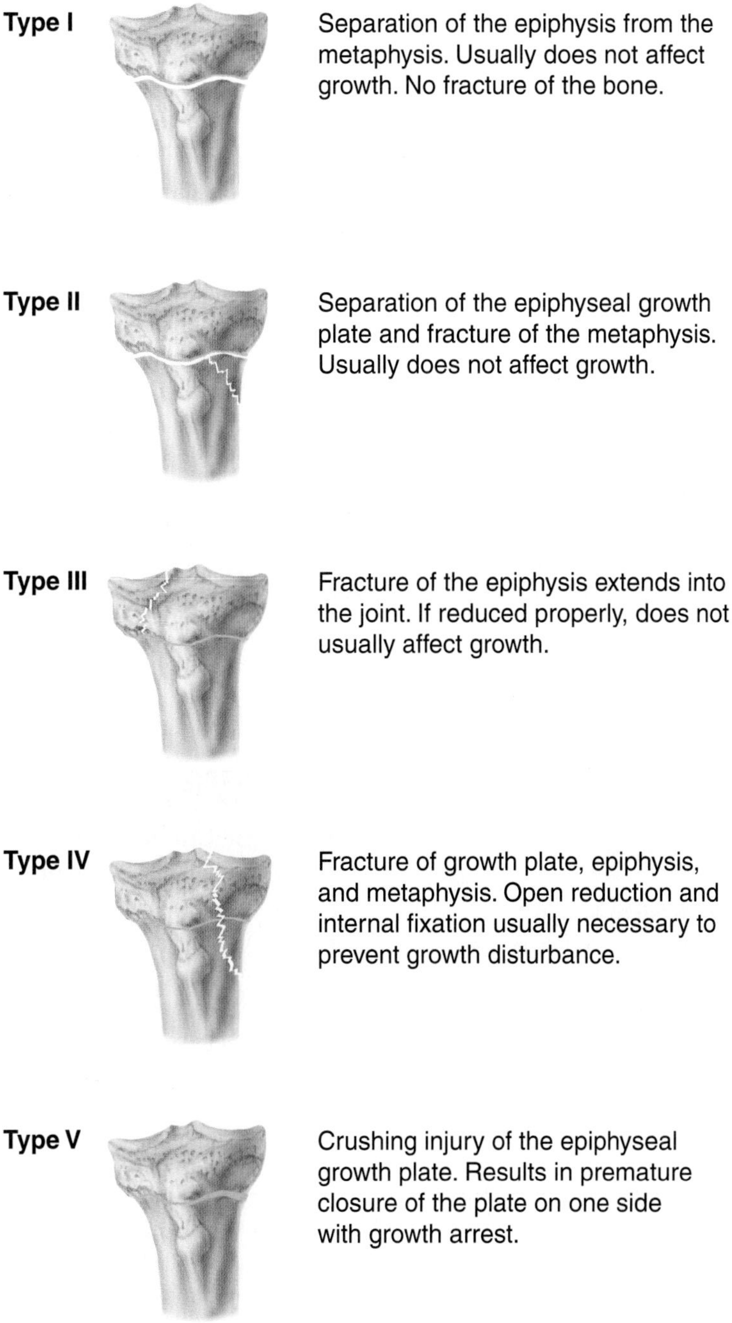
Type I
Separation of the epiphysis from the metaphysis. Usually does not affect growth. No fracture of the bone.
Type II
Separation of the epiphyseal growth plate and fracture of the metaphysis. Usually does not affect growth.
Type III
Fracture of the epiphysis extends into the joint. If reduced properly, does not usually affect growth.
Type IV
Fracture of growth plate, epiphysis, and metaphysis. Open reduction and internal fixation usually necessary to prevent growth disturbance.
Type V
Crushing injury of the epiphyseal growth plate. Results in premature closure of the plate on one side with growth arrest.

Figure 34-3 Salter-Harris Classification of Epiphyseal Injuries

Nursing Alert:

Damage to the Epiphyseal Growth Plate

Damage to the epiphyseal growth plate disrupts the growth process of the child who has not reached skeletal maturity and is still growing. Preserving normal growth is essential; therefore, injuries to this area should be evaluated as soon as possible.

ultimately replaced by new bone). The callus becomes firm enough so that no movement occurs at the fracture site, and there is a gradual increase in the stability of the fracture.

- Ossification stage: The callus turns into bone, the gap in the bone is bridged, and union occurs. Bony union has occurred at this point.
- Remodeling stage: Complete healing occurs when mature bone cells have replaced all temporary callus formation. The bone has now regained its normal shape and contour. This stage is usually complete within a year (Maher, et al., 1998; Morrissy & Weinstein, 1996).

Clinical Manifestations

Signs and symptoms of a fracture vary depending on type, location, and cause. The usual clinical manifestations include pain or tenderness, edema, and decreased range of motion. Others that may occur are obvious deformity of the extremity, bruising, muscle spasms, and **crepitus** (grating sound heard on movement of the ends of a broken bone). The functional use of the fractured bone is decreased. If the periosteum is intact, the fracture may remain stable, and the child may be able to use the affected extremity. Most frequently observed sites of fractures in children include the forearm, elbow, femur, knee, clavicle, and long bones in the leg.

Nursing Alert:

Is the Fracture the Result of Physical Abuse?

Some fractures in childhood are caused by child abuse. Factors strongly suggestive of abuse include:

- *Fracture is inconsistent with the history of the injury*
- *Fracture is inconsistent with the developmental stage of the child (Can an infant of three months "fall down"?)*
- *Multiple fractures, especially in various stages of healing*
- *Spiral fractures of the femur or tibia in a child who is not walking*
- *Spiral fracture of the humerus*
- *Multiple or depressed skull fractures (Bachman & Santora, 1993)*

Diagnosis

The diagnosis of a fracture is based on the child's signs and symptoms, history of the injury, physical examination, and radiographs. It is often difficult to obtain a history of the trauma from a young child. The caregivers may be able to provide information if they were present; however, the best informant is usually someone who witnessed the events leading to the injury. Radiographs are the most reliable method of determining if a bone is fractured as well as the type of fracture.

Treatment

The goals of treatment are to promote bone healing, restore function and appearance, and return the child to his or her normal lifestyle as soon as possible. For bone union to occur the fragments should be in approximation and alignment and must be held relatively immobile during the period of healing. Closed or open reduction and casting are the usual treatment methods. **Closed reduction** is the alignment of the bone by manual manipulation or traction. **Open reduction** is surgical alignment of the bone using wires, pins, bone screws, or plates. The majority of fractures in children can be managed by closed reduction. Immobilization following reduction is necessary to reduce pain, to prevent rotation at the fracture site, to maintain the position by preventing displacement or angulation until bony union occurs, and to allow free movement of uninvolved joints.

Casts

Casts hold bones immobile and offer protection after reduction of a fracture or may be used to correct a deformity

Eye On:

Need for Calcium in African-American Children with a Fracture

Foods high in calcium are important for children for the growth of bones. When a child sustains a fracture, the need for calcium may be increased. A major source of calcium is dairy products. Many African-Americans have a lactose intolerance in which they are unable to digest lactose, and ingestion of dairy foods causes abdominal bloating, diarrhea, and excessive flatus. Therefore, when they experience a fracture, they may need to obtain calcium from other food sources such as green leafy vegetables, broccoli, cauliflower, and cabbage. If they do consume dairy products, they may need to take a commercially available lactose preparation such as Lact-Aid or Dairy-Ease.

(Figures 34-4 and 34-5). Immobilization casts are most often made of plaster or a synthetic material such as fiberglass. Plaster conforms more readily to the body part but deteriorates when wet and is relatively heavy. Synthetic casts are lightweight, water resistant, available in colors, and dry quickly (15 minutes); yet, they are more expensive than plaster. Synthetic casts do not mold as well as plaster casts and, therefore, are not recommended for young children or those with serious fractures (Adkins, 1997). Most casts are applied on an outpatient basis, and hospitalization is not required. The nurse needs to educate the caregivers about caring for the child with a cast at home (see Box 34-2).

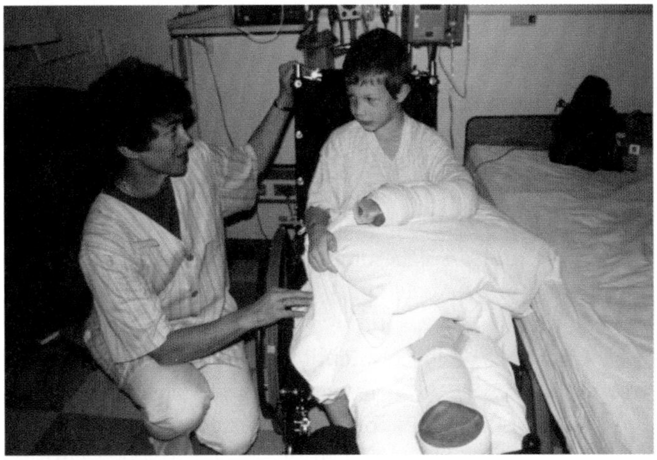

Figure 34-4 This child has a short leg cast for a fracture of the distal tibia and an arm cylinder cast for a dislocated elbow.

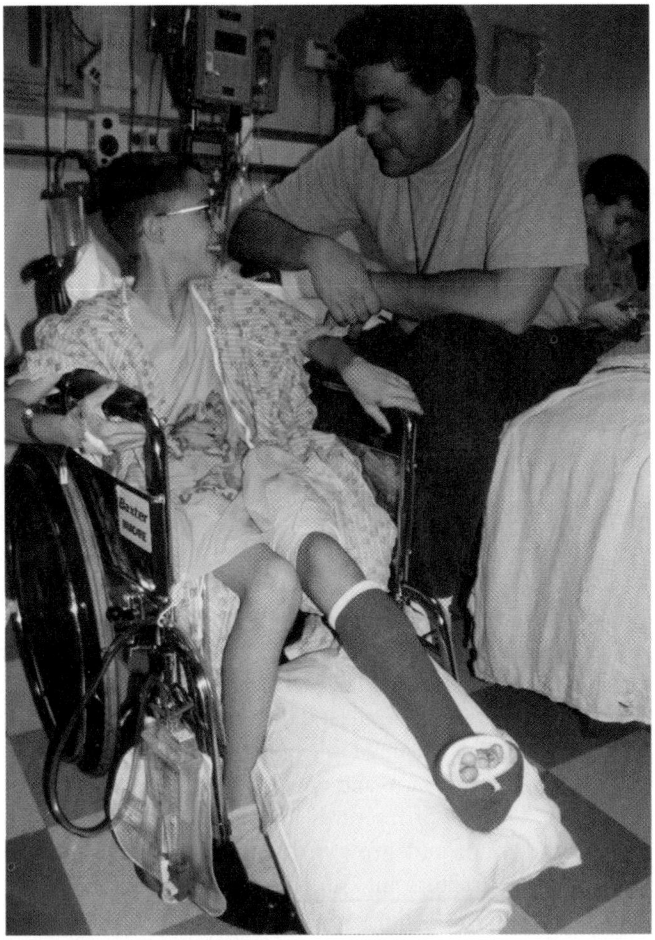

Figure 34-5 A Short Leg Fiberglass Cast. Advantages of fiberglass casts include the availability of a wide variety of colors, fast drying time, and their light weight.

Traction

Traction is the application of pulling force to a body part against a countertraction pull exerted in the opposite direc-

BOX 34-2 Home care for the child with a cast

1. After application of a plaster cast, let it dry thoroughly. This will take from 24 to 48 hours. Handle the cast gently. Use the palms of the hands to pick up the cast to prevent dents. Use of a fan or cool-air hair dryer will facilitate drying.
2. Elevate the cast on a pillow above the level of the heart to reduce swelling and improve circulation.
3. Do not hit or bang the cast as this may damage the cast or cause reinjury.
4. Avoid getting plaster casts wet. Plastic wrap or a plastic bag can be used to protect the cast from moisture during bathing.
5. "Petal" the edges with moleskin or adhesive tape to protect the child's skin from rough and irritating edges. The edges are rounded with scissors, and each of these "petals" is placed over the edge of the cast, with each slightly overlapping the previous one to form a smooth, finished edge. "Petaling" the cast around the edges, especially the groin and perineum, will protect it from urine and stool.
6. Do not allow the child to push small or sharp objects under the cast, such as a pencil, pen, or small game piece, as these may injure the skin.
7. Assess neurovascular status frequently on the extremity distal to the cast.
8. For itching, a hair dryer set on a cool setting can be used to blow air into the cast. An antihistamine can be used if the itching is bothersome.
9. Report any foul smelling odors, excessive swelling, bleeding, or excessive pain to the health care provider. The odor may indicate infection or skin breakdown. Bleeding, excessive pain, or swelling indicate problems and are not to be ignored.
10. Report any slippage, cracking, softness, or looseness of cast to the health care provider.

tion. The process is used to treat a variety of injuries such as of the spine, long bones of the upper and lower extremities, and pelvis. In straight traction the child's body weight serves as the countertraction. In balanced or suspended traction the body part is suspended by a sling, and the countertraction as well as the primary pull is accomplished by pulleys and weights. The angle of the involved joint and the angle formed by placement of the pulley on the bed determine the direction of the pull or force. The primary purposes of traction are to immobilize the fracture, realign the proximal and distal ends of the bone while healing takes place, decrease muscle spasms, and prevent further soft tissue damage. The two types of traction are skin and skeletal.

Skin Traction

Skin traction is applied directly to the skin and exerts force on the body surface. It is easy to use, noninvasive, and does not require anesthesia. A variety of materials such as ace bandages, boots, or belts are secured around a body part and attached to weights. The amount of weight used as a pulling force is limited to prevent injury to the skin. Skin traction should not be used if the child has a skin infection or breakdown, open wound, or extensive tissue damage. Several types of skin traction are discussed and are illustrated in Figure 34-6.

Buck Extension. A boot or circular wrap is applied to the skin. Traction is applied to the boot or the wrap, and countertraction is provided by the child's body. It is used for short-term immobilization such as preoperatively for a dislocated hip and to treat contractures and muscle spasm. It is important to keep the ropes and pulleys hanging freely for this type of traction to be effective.

Bryant Traction. The child is in a supine position with both legs flexed slightly less than 90 degrees. The child's buttocks should be off the mattress. It is used to treat developmental hip dysplasia and fractured femurs in children younger than 2–3 years of age or weighing less than 30 pounds. Countertraction is provided by the child's weight; therefore, the child needs to remain in the supine position. Both legs are always suspended, even if just one is broken. This type of traction must be used with caution as it is possible to create a tourniquet effect with the bandages and traction leading to vasospasms and avascular necrosis.

Russell Traction. Russell traction is similar to Buck's except a sling under the knee suspends the affected leg. The traction pulls from two directions, from the knee sling and from the foot. Elevating the foot of the bed provides countertraction. It is used to treat fractured femurs. Sling placement needs to be checked frequently to maintain the desired amount of flexion and to prevent damage to the nerve under the knee, thus preventing footdrop.

Cervical Traction. Cervical traction provides traction to the cervical spine and uses a head halter and weight to maintain the head in extension. A front strap fits under the chin and a rear strap rests at the base of the skull. It is used to treat injuries to the cervical muscles. The head of the bed is elevated 20 to 30 degrees for proper alignment.

Skeletal Traction

Skeletal traction uses pins, wires, tongs, or other special apparatus that have been surgically placed through the distal end of the bone to apply direct pull to the bone. This allows the use of longer traction time and heavier weights. It is used to ensure correct alignment of the bony fragments and proper healing. Without traction, muscle contractions cause overriding and displacement of bone fragments and may result in improper healing. A discussion of several types of skeletal traction follows; these are illustrated in Figure 34-7.

Crutchfield Tong. Crutchfield Tong is used to stabilize fractures or displaced vertebrae in the cervical and high thoracic areas of the spine. Tongs are inserted into either side of the scalp through burr holes in the skull. The head must be maintained in proper alignment, and the tongs should be checked frequently for displacement or looseness.

Balanced Suspension. Balanced suspension may be used with skeletal or skin traction for fractures of the femur, hip, and tibia. The Thomas ring splint fits around the upper leg and provides support of the hip. The Pearson attachment is connected with the ring at the knee and supports and provides flexion of the lower leg. Canvas slings may be used to further support the lower leg. The child is able to move, and the suspension apparatus adjusts without disturbing the traction pull. A footplate is used to prevent foot drop. The bed should be maintained in a flat position to reduce flexion contracture of the hip. This type of traction may be used with an older, heavier child, especially if much lifting is anticipated in the child's care.

90/90 Femoral Traction. This type of traction is the most commonly used traction for complicated fractures of the femur. The lower part of the leg is in a boot cast, and a skeletal Steinmann pin or Kirschner wire is placed in the distal fragment of the femur. Traction ropes are applied on the boot cast and at the pin site to maintain a 90 degree flexion of the hip and knee.

Dunlop or Sidearm Traction. Dunlop traction can use either skeletal or skin traction for supracondylar fractures of the humerus (fractured elbow). The upper arm is abducted and the forearm is placed in a 90 degree angle from the plane of the child. Pull is obtained in two directions, one in line with the upper part of the arm and one in line with the lower part.

Complications of fractures include malunion, compartment syndrome, and growth disturbances. Malunion or growth of the fracture into an incomplete or faulty position may occur even with the use of traction or casting. If malunion is severe, surgical repair may be necessary. **Compartment syndrome** is a serious condition in which increased pressure within one or more compartments leads to massive impairment of circulation to the area.

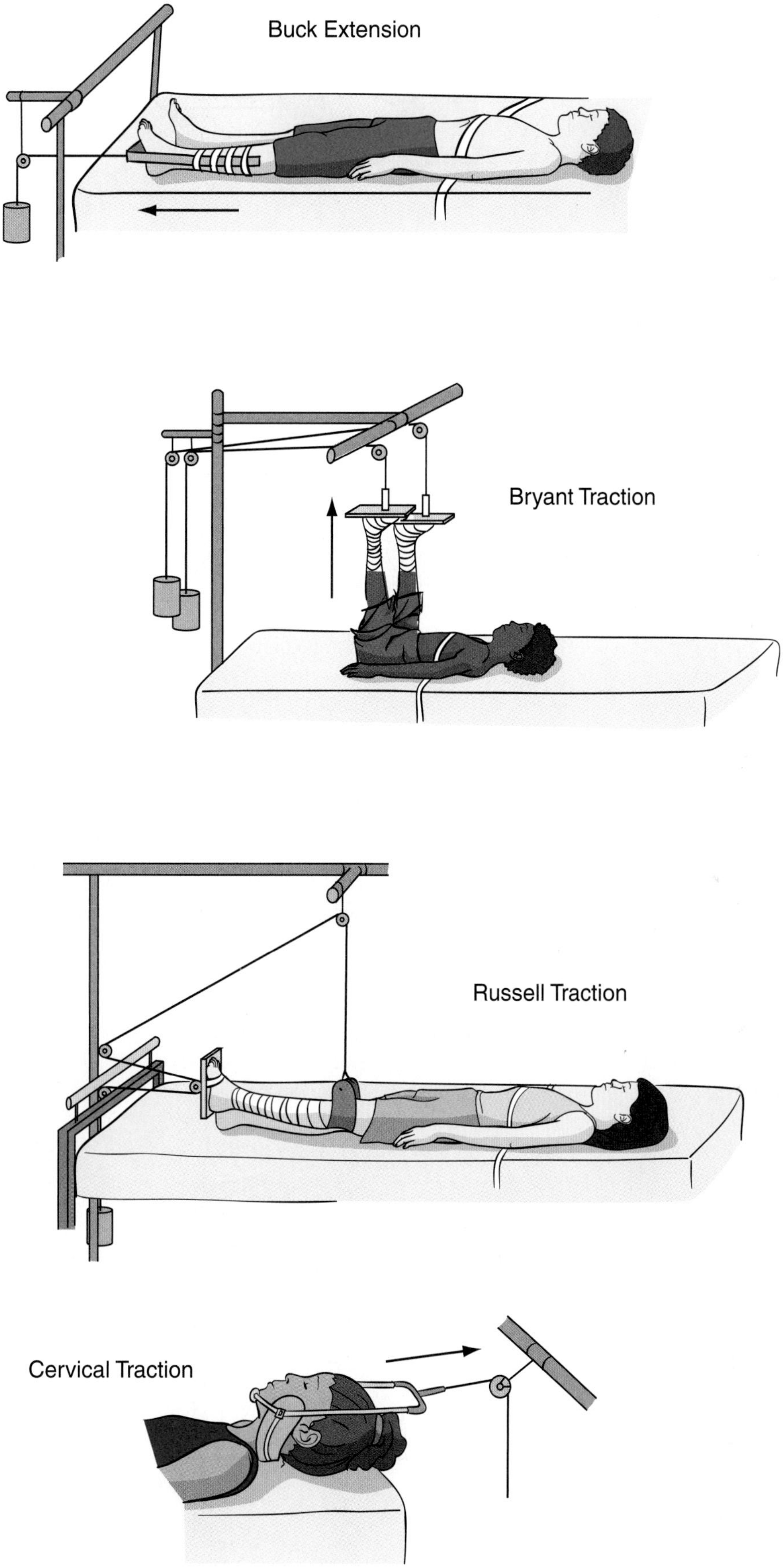

Figure 34-6 Types of Skin Traction

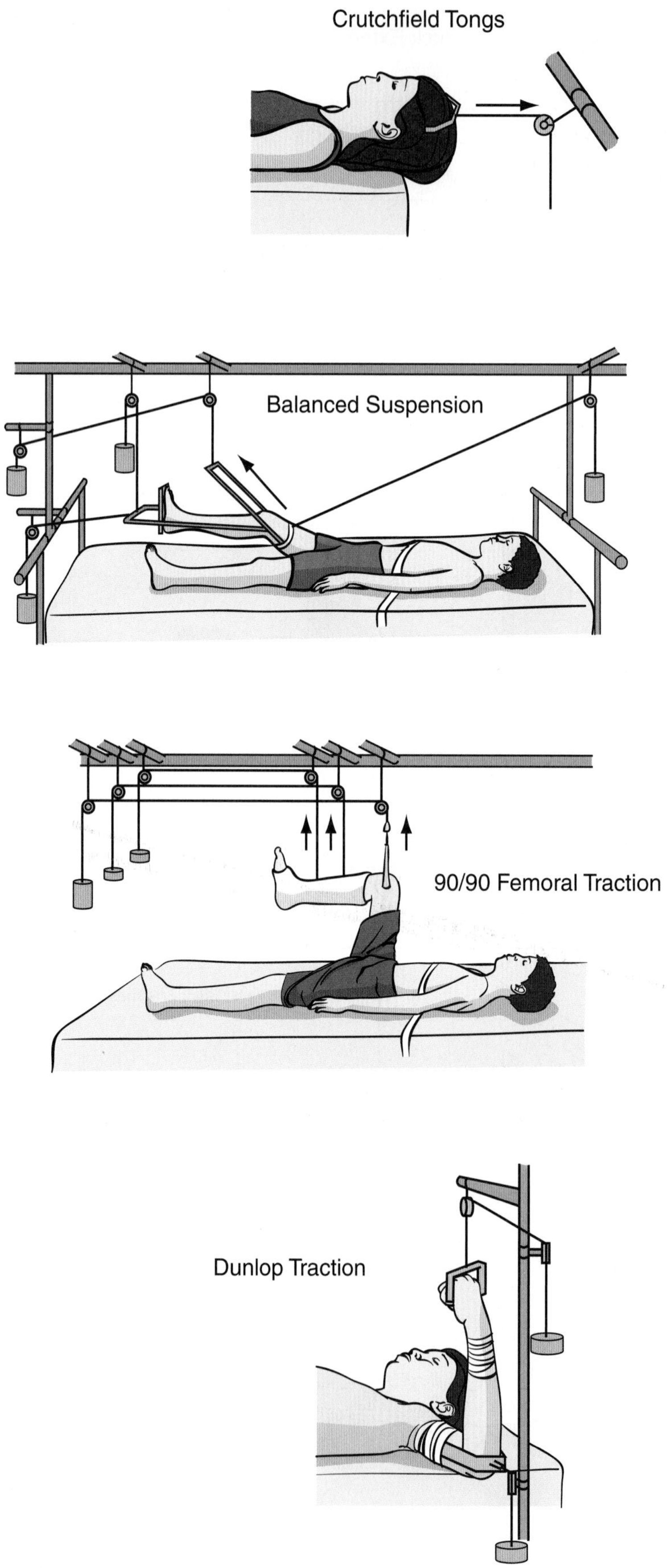

Figure 34-7 Types of Skeletal Traction

Compartments are sheaths of inelastic fascia that support and partition muscles, blood vessels, and nerves. Compartment syndrome occurs when the inelastic fascia fails to expand enough to compensate for the bleeding or swelling from the damaged tissues or the pressure from splints, casts, or tight bulky dressings (Monk, 1993). This lack of expansion results in impairment of blood perfusion to the muscle and tissue within the compartment producing severe ischemia, paralysis, or necrosis. The compartments involved are usually the forearm and the lower leg. The child complains of severe, unrelenting pain distal to the injury site that is unrelieved by analgesics. Severe swelling and **paresthesia** (numbness or tingling sensation) are noted of the digits below the affected compartment. Treatment involves immediate relief of the pressure, by splitting of the cast if present. In some cases, surgical intervention is required. The surgical procedure is a fasciotomy in which an incision is made along the outside of the compartment, thus relieving the pressure and allowing for adequate perfusion. Growth disturbances, another complication of fractures, are a result of shortening of a fractured extremity as a result of injury to the growth plate.

Nursing Management

Immediately following a musculoskeletal injury, immobilization with splints or sandbags may be necessary to avoid further trauma and reduce pain. Assessment of neurovascular status is performed to monitor for injury to the blood vessels and nerves after application of an immobilization device (cast, traction) and after surgery. Swelling or compression can interfere with blood flow, damage nerves beyond repair, and cause permanent disability or loss of limb. A neurovascular assessment includes evaluation of the following seven areas: pain, skin color, pulses, sensation, motion, skin temperature, and capillary refill (Table 34-1). The affected extremity should be

TABLE 34-1 Assessment of Neurovascular Status

Technique	Normal	Abnormal
Pain Assess using behavioral and physiological cues and age-appropriate rating scales	Some pain is normal after an injury or surgery	Excessive or increasing pain especially with passive motion or unrelieved with analgesia may indicate neurovascular compromise
Skin Color Inspect area distal to the injury	No change in color compared with unaffected extremity	Pallor, cyanotic, or dusky
Pulses Palpate pulses distal to the injury or immobilizing device if possible	Pulses are strong; no difference in affected and unaffected extremity	Weak or absent pulse (pulselessness)
Sensation Ask child if numbness or tingling is present Touch fingers or toes of affected and unaffected extremity, especially the web space between thumb and index finger and between first and second toes	No difference in sensation in both extremities	Numbness or tingling (paresthesia); decreased sensation
Motion Ask child to move fingers or toes of affected extremity	Able to move fingers or toes of affected extremity	Unable to move fingers or toes of affected extremity; paralysis
Skin Temperature Palpate extremity (the back of the hand is most sensitive to temperature)	Skin is warm or comparable to unaffected extremity	Cool or cold (may be caused by cool environment; if so, apply blanket to extremity, then reassess)
Capillary Refill Press each nail bed and note the time until color returns	Returns to usual color in less than 3 seconds	Returns to usual color in more than 3 seconds

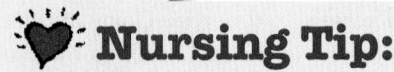

Nursing Alert:

Compartment Syndrome

Compartment syndrome is a limb-threatening emergency. If treatment does not occur within 4–6 hours after the onset, neuromuscular damage is irreversible. The outcome may be permanent disability to the extremity (Fecht-Gramley, 1994).

compared with the unaffected extremity. A general rule for frequency is to assess neurovascular status (NVS) every hour for the first 24 hours and then every 4 to 8 hours. Variations depend on the diagnosis and severity of the injury (Dykes, 1993).

Musculoskeletal pain associated with soft tissue damage, fractures, muscle spasms, surgical procedures, and immobilization devices is one of the most severe types of pain that can be experienced (refer to Chapter 18). The child often has pain for a prolonged period of time, making management and control difficult. It is important to remember that an initial sign of compartment syndrome is often sudden inability of the medications to relieve pain.

Immobilization is the usual method for treating musculoskeletal disorders, yet, it can cause physiological and psychosocial complications. No body system is immune from the effects of immobility. The greater the extent and longer the duration of immobility, the more pronounced the consequences. Table 34-2 presents the physiological effects of immobilization and nursing interventions.

The nurse caring for a child who is immobile needs to recognize that a variety of psychological responses are possible. The child may become angry, uncooperative, or engage in aggressive behaviors (especially towards caregivers), or may become withdrawn, passive, and submissive. It is important to reassure caregivers that if their child lashes out at them, they should not take it personally. The child is displacing anger about the loss of physical mobility, and they are safer "targets" than the nurses and other health care providers. Immobilizing a young child for an extended period of time may result in regressive behaviors. For exam-

Critical Thinking

Child in Skeletal Traction

Four-year-old Juan was hit by a car while riding his bicycle and sustained a fractured left femur. He has been in skeletal traction for 3 weeks. His mother tells you he has been impatient and demanding with her. She says Juan is always on the go, never sits still, and is bored and frustrated with being in bed for so long. How would you respond to her concerns? What suggestions would you make to help alleviate his boredom and frustration?

Nursing Tip:

Cast removal

Cast removal is very frightening for most children. The cast cutter creates vibrations and generates heat and a "tickling" feeling on the skin. Removing the cast is noisy, and many children are afraid that their skin will be cut. Demonstration of how the cast cutter works may relieve some of the child's fears. Therapeutic play, such as allowing the child to hold the cast cutter, even remove a cast from a doll with supervision, can be helpful. Caregivers should be allowed to stay with the child during the procedure. After removal of the cast, good skin care is essential as the skin under the cast may be flaky and yellow or brown because of the accumulation of dead skin. Some muscle atrophy may have occurred if the extremity has been immobile for a period of time. The extremity may also be stiff. Reassure the child and caregivers that muscle mass will return soon with normal use and movement.

Critical Thinking

Care of the Child with an Orthopedic Problem

Caitlin, age 8, is admitted to your unit at 8:30 PM after a softball injury. Her diagnosis is a fractured right fibula. She is currently in a long leg cast until an open reduction and internal fixation will be performed the next day. Caitlin arrives on your unit crying in pain. Her mother asks if you can give her something for pain. You check the orders and find one for Demerol 10–15 mg IV PRN every 3–4 hours. According to the nurses' notes, Caitlin was last given 15 mg of Demerol IM at 6:30 PM in the emergency room. Caitlin is also complaining of tingling in her right foot.

1. What would you include in your initial assessment of Caitlin?
2. What areas are assessed in a neurovascular assessment?
3. What would you do regarding Caitlin's pain status, as it is too soon to administer the pain medication?

TABLE 34-2 Physiological Effects of Immobilization and Nursing Interventions

Body System	Clinical Manifestations	Nursing Interventions
Respiratory	• Decreased lung expansion • Weakness of respiratory muscles • Stasis of secretions • Increased potential for pneumonia and atelectasis	• Frequent repositioning • Turn, cough, and deep breathing • Incentive spirometer
Cardiovascular	• Increased venous stasis • Decreased cardiac output and circulatory fluid volume • Formation of thrombus • Potential for pulmonary emboli	• Passive and active range of motion exercises • Antiembolism stockings • Mobilize child as soon as possible
Musculoskeletal	• Decreased muscle strength and mass • Atrophy of muscle • Decreased bone density • Joint contractures • Foot drop	• Passive and active range of motion exercises • Foot support
Gastrointestinal	• Constipation • Anorexia	• Increased intake of fiber and fluids • Stool softeners and rectal suppositories as ordered • Small frequent meals • Encourage family to bring child's favorite foods
Urinary	• Decreased urine output • Increased urine concentration • Retention of urine • Renal calculi • Urinary tract infection	• Increased fluid intake • Maintain acidic urine with cranberry juice • Monitor intake and output • Monitor urine concentration
Integumentary	• Skin breakdown • Pressure ulcers	• Frequent repositioning • Keep skin clean and dry • Use pressure reducing devices, such as sheepskin

Nursing Alert:

Calcium Loss Caused by Immobility

Loss of calcium is a response to immobility and indicates an imbalance between bone formation and breakdown. The lack of pressure (e.g., weight-bearing) on bones triggers calcium loss. Bone demineralization occurs as early as 2–3 days after the onset of immobility; therefore, the nurse needs to perform or encourage passive and active range of motion exercises for the child.

ple, a toddler who was drinking from a cup and feeding him/herself may demand a bottle and to be fed by the caregiver or nurse. Again caregivers need to be told that disruptions in development (regression) are temporary. The immobilized toddler who is striving for autonomy and independence may feel angry about losing autonomy and enforced dependence. To encourage a sense of autonomy allow the child to make choices (e.g., food, daily schedule, clothes, activities). If the child is school-aged, it is important to continue with schoolwork via tutoring. This allows the child to participate in age-appropriate activities and alleviates some of the social isolation.

Additionally, children whose mobility is restricted and who are confined in a hospital room often experience sensory deprivation and social isolation. Promoting mobility as soon as allowed by the health care provider's orders and the child's recovery will ameliorate some of these effects. Use of crutches, walkers, beds, wheelchairs, wagons, and carts provide means of transporting children out of their rooms and increasing their environmental stimulation. The nurse needs to encourage the child and family members to invite peers and relatives to visit. Caregiver participation helps to channel energies in positive directions and provides the child with a measure of security and safety.

Family Teaching

Initially, family teaching focuses on the hospital routine, casts, traction devices, and mobility restrictions. Before discharge the nurse must teach caregivers cast care and review restrictions on mobility and activities of daily living. Nurses should help caregivers identify any modifications they need to make

Case Study/Care Plan

The Child in Skeletal Traction

Jamel, age 6, fractured his femur and his elbow in a bicycle accident. He will be in skeletal traction for approximately a month. His father will care for him after he is discharged from the hospital.

Nursing Care Plan

Assessment Nursing assessment includes both the history of the injury and physical assessment. Careful history taking is important to determine how the child was injured. The child, caregivers, family members, and anyone present at the time may be able to share important details. Assessment should be made regarding the consistency of the history of the injury among those providing information. The nurse must be aware of the possibility of inflicted injury. Child abuse needs to be ruled out with all accidents.

Nursing Diagnosis #1

Risk for injury related to peripheral neurovascular compromise, trauma, and traction apparatus.

Expected Outcomes

1. Jamel will maintain neurovascular function.
2. Jamel will maintain adequate peripheral tissue perfusion.

Interventions/*Rationales*

1. Assess neurovascular status (NVS) to establish baseline for future assessments. Continue to monitor every 2 hours (or standards of care established within individual health care facilities). *Changes in NVS indicate circulatory compromise, nerve injury, vascular compromise, or pressure from traction.*
2. Assess for sensation in the toes of the affected extremity. Do not allow the child to see which area is being touched. *Verbalization of decreased sensation indicates neurovascular compromise.*
3. Encourage the child to tell the nurse if there is an increase in pain, tingling, or numbness. Increased irritability may be the only sign present in the nonverbal child. *Increasing pain, tingling, or numbness indicates circulatory compromise, nerve injury, or compartment syndrome.*
4. Maintain traction in proper alignment. Inspect apparatus frequently for correct position and functioning of ropes, pulleys, amount of weights. *Maintains effectiveness of traction and alignment during healing.*
5. Assess for pressure areas over major blood vessels and nerves by traction device. *Excessive pressure can cause neurovascular impairment.*

Evaluation

Jamel maintains neurovascular integrity as evident by:

- Strong and equal pulses in both extremities
- Absence of severe pain
- Skin color and temperature equal in both extremities

continues

continued

- Capillary refill time < 3 seconds
- Ability to move affected extremity
- Normal sensation in both extremities

Maximum effectiveness of the traction is maintained. Jamel is free from injuries.

Nursing Diagnosis #2

Risk for impaired skin integrity related to immobilization and traction.

Expected Outcomes

1. Jamel's skin will remain intact with no evidence of irritation or breakdown.
2. By time of discharge Jamel's skin integrity will return to prehospitalization level.

Interventions/*Rationales*

1. Assess for changes in the skin at the beginning and the end of each shift. Document all findings. *Careful assessment and documentation provide the nurse with base-line data and serve as a guide for future nursing interventions.*
2. Wash skin surfaces with a mild soap, dry thoroughly. *Mild soap will prevent skin irritation. Thorough drying prevents skin breakdown.*
3. Change position frequently. *Prevents skin breakdown and reduces pressure on bony prominence.*
4. Provide a sheepskin, mattress overlay or alternating pressure mattress for long-term immobilization. *Reduces skin abrasions and pressure on skin surfaces.*
5. Clean pin sites per the health care provider's orders or agency protocol. *Decreases the risk of infection.*
6. Observe pin sites for redness and purulent drainage. *Signs of infection should be reported to the health care provider.*

Evaluation

Jamel's skin shows no signs of irritation or breakdown. Pin sites remain clean, dry, and show no evidence of redness, swelling, or drainage.

Nursing Diagnosis # 3

Impaired mobility related to pain of injury or traction, immobilization, or presence of traction.

Expected Outcomes

1. Jamel will maintain optimal age-appropriate physical mobility within the limits of treatment.
2. Jamel will maintain full range of motion within the limits of treatment.

Interventions/*Rationales*

1. Assess and document mobility before application of traction, if possible. *Assists the nurse in providing appropriate care after the traction is in place.*
2. Encourage the child to move the affected extremity demonstrating flexion and extension to the child's fullest ability. *Maintains muscle tone and improves cardiovascular circulation.*
3. Provide range of motion exercises and other opportunities for movement. *Maintains strength of unaffected muscles and preserves joint function.*
4. Use age-appropriate play activities. *Encourages muscle movement, provides exercise for uninvolved muscles and joints, and reduces boredom.*

continues

continued

Evaluation

Jamel experiences minimal complications of immobility. He maintains full range of motion of unaffected extremity.

Nursing Diagnosis # 4

Imbalanced nutrition: less than body requirements related to loss of appetite secondary to pain and immobility.

Expected Outcomes

1. Jamel will maintain normal growth.
2. Jamel will consume an adequate amount of calories throughout hospitalization.
3. Jamel will maintain normal bowel elimination.

Interventions/*Rationales*

1. Ask Jamel or the caregivers what his favorite foods are. Encourage them to bring these foods to the hospital. Encourage a well-balanced diet, high in calcium. *The child is more inclined to eat foods he likes. At least 2,000 calories daily including calcium are needed to promote bone healing.*
2. Assess bowel movements for frequency and consistency. *Monitoring bowel movements helps in determining the need for intervention.*
3. Encourage fluids and high-fiber foods. *Promotes bowel elimination.*
4. Administer stool softeners, as ordered. *Enables water to penetrate fecal material, which allows for easy passage.*

Evaluation

Jamel maintains adequate nutritional status as evident by adequate caloric intake and maintenance of pre-injury weight. He maintains normal bowel elimination as evident by normal bowel movements and passing softer stools.

in the home or school environment, and refer them to social services and physical therapy for special services and equipment that may be needed in the home, school, or community. Child and caregiver education may be necessary about the use of safety equipment during sports activities. All equipment should be well-fitting and in good repair.

INFECTIOUS DISORDERS

Infections of the bones (osteomyelitis) and joints (septic arthritis) usually are caused by bacterial pathogens. If infections of the bones and joints are not diagnosed and treated quickly and adequately, permanent damage as well as alterations in growth may result.

Osteomyelitis

Osteomyelitis is an infection of the bone and is caused by a microorganism, which is usually bacterial but may be viral or fungal, and involves the entire bone (periosteum, cortex, and marrow).

Incidence and Etiology

Osteomyelitis occurs at any age but is more common in children between the ages of 3 and 12 years. Males are affected 2 to 4 times as often as females. Osteomyelitis may occur through the bloodstream from an infection in another part of the body (**hematogenous** spread), or direct introduction of the organism from the outside through a penetrating wound or open fracture. Infection through the bloodstream (hematogenous) is the most common form of osteomyelitis in children and usually occurs in the metaphyses or long bones, especially of the lower extremities (Mandell, 1996).

Common sources of infection include acute otitis media, impetigo, upper respiratory infection, abscessed teeth, and burn infections. Trauma to a bone may also predispose to osteomyelitis. The most common causative organisms are

Staphylococci aureus, which account for 80–90% of all cases. *Haemophilus influenzae*, *Streptococcus pneumoniae*, *Escherichia coli*, group B streptococci, (in neonates) gram-negative enteric bacilli, and anaerobic bacteria are other causative agents (Morrissy & Weinstein, 1996).

Pathophysiology

Pathogenic organisms from the local site of infection travel to the small end arteries in the bone metaphysis, where inflammation with hyperemia and edema occur. The infectious process leads to local bone destruction and abscess formation. Edema, pus, and vascular congestion are the result of the body's inflammatory response to the infection. Pressure increases as the pus collects and is confined within the rigid bone, contributing to vascular occlusion, ischemia, and eventually bone necrosis.

Clinical Manifestations

In infants, the manifestations may be quite subtle, presenting as irritability, diarrhea, or poor feeding. The temperature may be normal or slightly below normal. In older children the manifestations are more striking, with bone pain that is constant, localized, and increases with movement. There may also be restricted movement, swelling, heat, erythema, and fever, with the temperature usually above 101 degrees F. Further assessment may reveal a systemic infection.

Diagnosis

Laboratory tests include complete blood count, C-reactive protein test (CRP), erythrocyte sedimentation rate (ESR), and aerobic and anaerobic cultures. C-reactive protein and ESR are usually elevated, which indicates the presence of an inflammatory process. The white blood cell count (WBC) may be elevated. Before the initiation of antibiotic therapy, blood cultures are obtained. Cultures of pus, bone, and other tissues may be obtained to further delineate the causative organism. Displacement of the soft tissue adjacent to the bone secondary to an elevated periosteum or bone necrosis is visible on radiograph. Bone necrosis appears between the tenth and fourteenth days following the onset of osteomyelitis and is visible on radiograph.

Treatment

A broad-spectrum antibiotic is administered intravenously once cultures have been obtained. When the causative organism has been identified, the antibiotic may be changed. The initial response is determined by resolution of systemic signs of infection: a decrease in CRP, ESR, and WBC. CRP increases sooner than ESR or WBC and decreases significantly faster, reflecting the effectiveness of the therapy more sensitively than ESR or WBC (Unkila-Kallio, Kallio, Eskola, & Peltola, 1994). Although the length of antibiotic therapy is not well established, 3 to 4 weeks is recommended for most cases (Nelson, 1997).

Initially, antibiotics are always given intravenously in order to obtain and maintain high concentrations of the drug in the serum. If the initial treatment is positive, antibiotics are changed from the intravenous to the oral route. Splinting of the limb minimizes pain and decreases the speed of infection by lymph channels. The splint should be removed periodically to allow movement and to prevent stiffening and muscle atrophy. Surgery may be necessary if the infection fails to respond to antibiotics or an abscess is present. Drainage and surgical debridement cleans and removes dead bone and soft tissue and improves blood supply to the underlying bone.

Nursing Management

Health history and assessment are necessary to establish the onset of pain, restricted movement, or loss of mobility. Information from the caregivers helps to determine the source of infection; therefore, the nurse asks if the site was traumatized, or if the child had a recent infection. Soft tissue swelling at the site may indicate elevation of the loosely attached overlying periosteum by purulent effusion within the subperiosteum. The nurse administers analgesics as prescribed and monitors their effectiveness. Splints or traction may be ordered for comfort. The nurse should help the client maintain proper alignment and move the limb cautiously to avoid further injury to the bone. As the child is able to bear weight, participation in activities of daily living will increase. Crutches, wheelchair, or walker may be necessary for a short while. Because multiple antibiotics are frequently used thorough knowledge of side effects, therapeutic blood levels, and incompatibility problems is necessary. Maintaining adequate blood level of antibiotics is a critical component of successful therapy. Neurovascular and skin assessments are performed at least once every shift.

Family Teaching

Because antibiotics are continued at home, family teaching relevant to administration of oral or intravenous medications is necessary. Since many of the antibiotics used in treating osteomyelitis have adverse audiologic side effects, caregivers need to be taught to watch for hearing loss, and to report this to their health care provider. The family should be instructed in the importance of administering all of the medication prescribed.

Septic Arthritis

Septic arthritis is an infection of the joint that usually develops through the hematogenous route (bloodstream) from another site of infection.

Incidence and Etiology

The hip and the knee are the most common sites, and children 1 to 2 years of age are most often affected (Morrissy &

Weinstein, 1996). The incidence of joint infection in infancy is equal between male and females, but in adolescence it occurs predominantly in males. *Haemophilus influenzae* type b is a common pathogen accounting for 20–50% of cases in children ages 2 months to 5 years. *Staphylococcus aureus* is the most common organism in neonates and in children older than 5 years of age. Other organisms include pyrogenic *Streptococcus* and *Streptococcus pneumonia*.

Pathophysiology

Inflammation begins in the synovial membrane, and as pus forms, the synovial fluid thickens. The purulent effusion destroys the articular cartilage within hours after the bacteria enter the joint. Cartilage disintegration may be followed by osteomyelitis in the underlying bone. Scar tissue replaces the cartilage and eventually the mobility of the joint is impaired.

Clinical Manifestations

Pain, localized inflammation, restricted motion, fever, and swelling of the joint are present. An elevated white blood cell count is present and helps to differentiate septic arthritis from synovitis. **Synovitis** is an acute, nonpurulent inflammation of the synovial membrane of a joint, and occurs most commonly in the hip joint.

Diagnosis

Leukocytosis and an elevated ESR are common. The test of choice for rapid diagnosis of septic arthritis is aspiration of the joint fluid. Normal synovial fluid is clear, colorless, or straw colored. Purulent, cloudy fluid indicates the presence of an infection. The aspirated fluid is cultured to identify the causative organism. Plain radiography, ultrasound, and bone scan aid in the diagnosis.

Treatment

Treatment for septic arthritis is the same as for osteomyelitis. Initial treatment includes needle aspiration or open surgical drainage of the joint, administration of intravenous antibiotics after wound cultures have been obtained, immobilization of the joint, and pain relief. The length of antibiotic therapy is based on the type of causative organism; however, usually 4 to 6 weeks is required. Intravenous antibiotic therapy is administered initially, followed by oral medications.

Nursing Management

The nurse focuses on maintaining comfort, administering antibiotics, and avoiding complications of impaired mobility. (See nursing management for the child with osteomyelitis.)

Family Teaching

Education for the family and child is similar to that of the child with osteomyelitis. If the infection is in a superficial joint, it may be swollen and intensely painful; therefore, extreme care must be used when moving or handling it. Caregiver reliability in oral antibiotic administration is important because the usual course of therapy is several weeks long. Caregivers need to notify the health care provider if the child vomits or has diarrhea while on the antibiotics. If bedrest is necessary because of a painful joint, caregivers need to support and enforce this restriction.

CONGENITAL DISORDERS

Congenital disorders include clubfoot, developmental dysplasia of the hip, and muscular dystrophy.

Clubfoot

Clubfoot, also known as talipes equinovarus, is a congenital anomaly of the foot and the entire lower leg involving abnormalities of bony architecture and soft tissue Although not life-threatening, the birth of a child with a clubfoot has a significant impact on the family (Figure 34-8).

Incidence and Etiology

The incidence of clubfoot is 1.5 per 1,000 live births. Males are affected twice as often as females (Kyzer & Stark, 1995). The exact cause of clubfoot is unknown; however, several theories have been postulated. It may be caused by arrested fetal development in utero during the first trimester when the foot is formed or by neuromuscular abnormalities. There is a genetic predisposition for clubfoot as seen in the increased incidence in first-degree relatives (parents, sib-

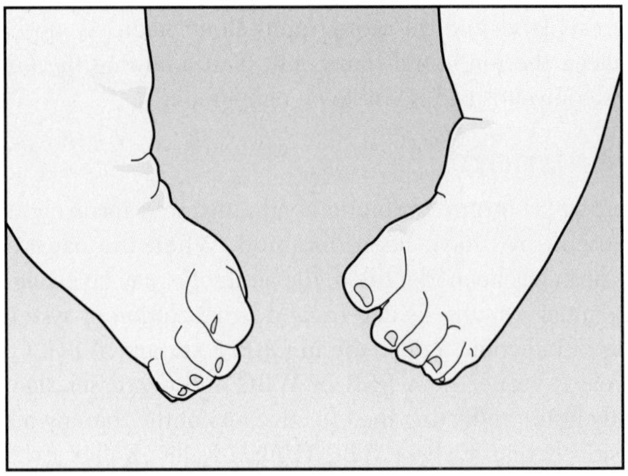

Figure 34-8 Bilateral Clubfoot

Eye On:

Incidence of Clubfoot

The incidence of clubfoot varies among ethnic populations, with Caucasians and Asians having the lowest. The incidence is higher in Mexican and South African groups; the condition is most commonly found in Hawaiian Polynesians.

lings). Clubfoot deformities are also seen in conjunction with congenital abnormalities such as cerebral palsy.

Pathophysiology and Clinical Manifestations

Clubfoot can be unilateral or bilateral and has three components of deformity: 1) the foot points downward (equinus), 2) the forefoot turns inward (adductus), and 3) the sole of the foot turns inward (inversion, suppination, or varus) (Kyzer & Stark, 1995). The affected foot is rigid, fixed, and difficult to move. The Achilles tendon is always shortened, the calf muscle is thin and atrophic, and the foot is small.

Diagnosis

Diagnosis is made at birth on the basis of visual inspection. Radiographs are used to confirm the degree and severity of the deformity. Magnetic resonance imaging (MRI) may be used in further diagnosis.

Treatment

Treatment is begun as soon as possible after birth. Serial casting, the major method of nonsurgical treatment, consists of manipulation of the foot into the correct anatomic position and application of a series of casts. The cast is changed every 1–2 weeks until complete correction has occurred, usually requiring 3 months. If casting does not achieve correction, surgical intervention is considered. The most common surgical approach is cutting the joint and tendons and restoring the bones to their normal positions. Realigned bones are held in place by pins. The surgery is followed by 2 to 3 months of casting. After the casts are removed, braces may be used to maintain the correction.

Nursing Management

Nursing assessment begins at birth. Visual inspection and straightening the newborn's feet to the midline is part of the initial assessment to detect this defect. The nurse obtains a history that includes information about the birth and any genetic defects in other members of the family. Providing support and education for the caregivers about care of the infant with a cast is an important aspect of nursing. If surgery is required, postsurgical care includes neurovascular status checks, assessment for edema, and drainage. Ice bags applied to the casted area and elevation of the foot with a pillow help reduce swelling. Analgesia is administered as needed.

Emotional support for the family allows them the opportunity to explore and verbalize their feelings regarding their child with a physical deformity. Caregivers should participate in all aspects of the child's care, as this allows them to carry out the normal activities of parenting and reinforces their role as important. Promoting a healthy body image is essential as the prognosis for clubfoot is for the child's foot to become fully functional. The calf muscle on the affected side will remain slightly underdeveloped, and the corrected foot will be smaller for the child's entire life; yet many children with surgical intervention are able to run, play, and walk without a limp (Hoffinger, 1996). Follow-up is required until the child reaches skeletal maturity because a major long-term problem is the tendency for the deformity to recur (Kyzer & Stark, 1995).

REFLECTIONS FROM FAMILIES

I was 35 years old when Juan was born. I had put off marriage until my career as an attorney was well established. I had two miscarriages before I became pregnant with Juan. My husband and I were so excited when this pregnancy did not end in a miscarriage. We both wanted a child so much. When Juan was born, he had bilateral clubfoot. We were so disappointed because we had waited so long for this event. Then our thoughts turned to the baby. We wondered if he would ever walk and run or if his feet would ever look like a normal child's.

Family Teaching

Bathing, skin care, dressing, and safety are areas for the nurse to address with the caregivers. Since tub baths are not allowed while the child is in a cast, nurses should teach the caregivers how to give a sponge bath. Teaching should include checking the skin around the cast edges for redness or irritation and assessing the neurovascular status of the foot. Other important areas to be covered include precautions for fresh casts and signs of infection. Clothing will need to be selected or adapted so it will fit over the cast. The nurse needs to discuss potential safety hazards when using various equipment. Caregivers need to check car seats, swings, and infant carriers to make sure the cast allows the safety belt, pads, and so forth to operate correctly. When using an infant seat on the floor or in a grocery cart, they need to make sure the additional weight of the cast does not overbalance it.

Developmental Dysplasia of the Hip

Developmental dysplasia of the hip (DDH) is a term used to describe the condition in which the femoral head has an abnormal relationship to the acetabulum (hip socket). Congenital dysplasia of the hip and congenital dislocated hip are other names commonly used for this group of hip disorders; however, the term developmental dysplasia of the hip is more accurate because many of the findings may not be present at birth (American Academy of Pediatrics [AAP], 2000). While hip dysplasia is commonly diagnosed in the newborn, it is also noted later in infancy. DDH may be found in older children, especially those with neuromuscular disorders such as spina bifida or cerebral palsy.

Incidence and Etiology

Developmental dislocated hip occurs in 1 to 1.5 in 1,000 births and affects females more frequently than males (6:1 ratio). DDH occurs in 1 in 300 females versus an incidence of 1 in 2,000 in boys (Novacheck, 1996). The left hip is involved 3 times as commonly as the right (AAP, 2000). The cause of DDH remains unknown, yet environmental and genetic factors have been clearly demonstrated to play a role in its development. Up to one-third of those affected may have a positive family history for DDH. Identical twins have a 36% increased chance of both twins having the syndrome. Prenatal factors include breech presentation associated with knee extension, ligamentous laxity associated with high levels of estrogen when the infant is female, and small uterine size. Postnatal positioning such as swaddling, strapping the infant to a cradle board, or carrying the infant with legs extended and adducted (pulled toward the midline of the body) have been associated with developmental dysplasia of the hip (Novacheck, 1996).

Pathophysiology

DDH includes **luxation** (complete dislocation of a joint, with no contact between articular surfaces of the joint), subluxation (incomplete or partial dislocation of the articular surfaces of a joint), and instability. Frank dislocation is characterized by complete loss of contact of the femoral head with the acetabulum; therefore, the femoral head lies completely out of the acetabulum. A dislocatable hip is one that can be manually displaced with stress, but returns to the acetabulum when the stress is removed. A subluxated hip is one in which the femoral head remains in contact with the acetabulum; however, an abnormal relationship exists between the two. A hip is unstable when the tight fit between the femoral head and acetabulum is lost, and the femoral head is able to be subluxated (partially dislocated) or dislocated by manipulation.

Clinical Manifestations

Unequal leg length, asymmetry of the thigh and gluteal folds, and limited abduction are usually the first signs of DDH (Figure 34-9). If the dysplasia is present bilaterally, clinical manifestations are difficult to detect because symmetry is maintained. In the older child the physical signs are more obvious. Gait abnormalities such as toe walking or limping

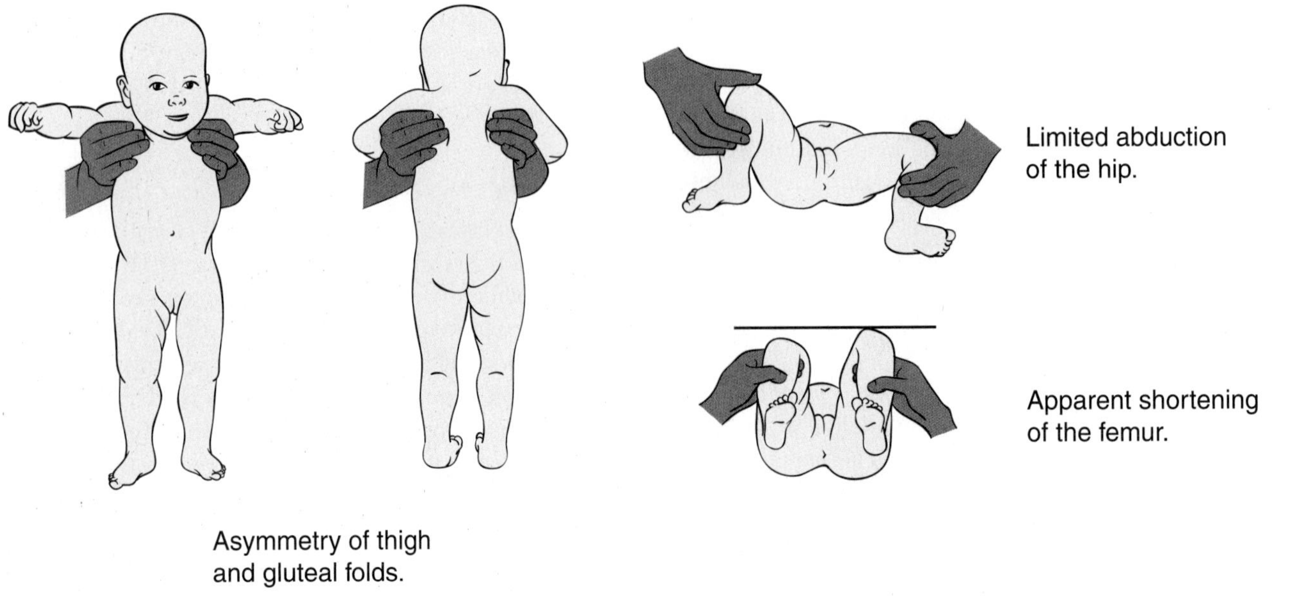

Figure 34-9 Signs of Developmental Dysplasia of the Hip

may be present, or the level of the pelvis may be unequal. The longer the disorder goes undiagnosed, and therefore untreated, the more severe the clinical manifestations.

Diagnosis

Diagnosis is made using Barlow or Ortolani test. In the Barlow maneuver, the examiner pushes an unstable femoral head out of the acetabulum by use of gentle lateral pressure of the lower trochanter. In the Ortolani maneuver, the examiner reduces the dislocated femoral head into the acetabulum by gentle abduction and external rotation. A "clunk" is heard and felt as the dislocated femoral head reduces into the acetabulum. Refer to Chapter 14 for further explanation of Ortolani maneuver. The disorder is usually, but not always, diagnosed at birth. Therefore examination of the hip is carried out at each well-child visit to detect late-onset dislocation. Radiographic examination is used to confirm the diagnosis, but is not reliable in early infancy because ossification of the femoral head does not normally take place until the third to sixth month of life.

Treatment

The treatment plan varies depending on the age of the child. For infants younger than 3 months an abduction device is the preferred method. The Pavlik harness is a commonly used device that seats the head of the femur in the acetabulum by keeping the knees and hips flexed and the hips abducted (Figure 34-10). It is worn 24 hours a day for 3 to 4 months. After this period the child is examined for a decreased laxity. Radiographs and ultrasounds will confirm improvement in position. Skin traction and/or surgery is used if the abduction device is not successful or if the child is older than 3 months. Traction stretches the soft tissue and moves the femoral head down to the level of the acetabulum. Achieving closed reduction without disruption of the blood supply to the femoral head is the goal. Surgery may be performed to reduce the dislocated hip. This procedure is followed by application of a hip spica cast (Figure 34-11).

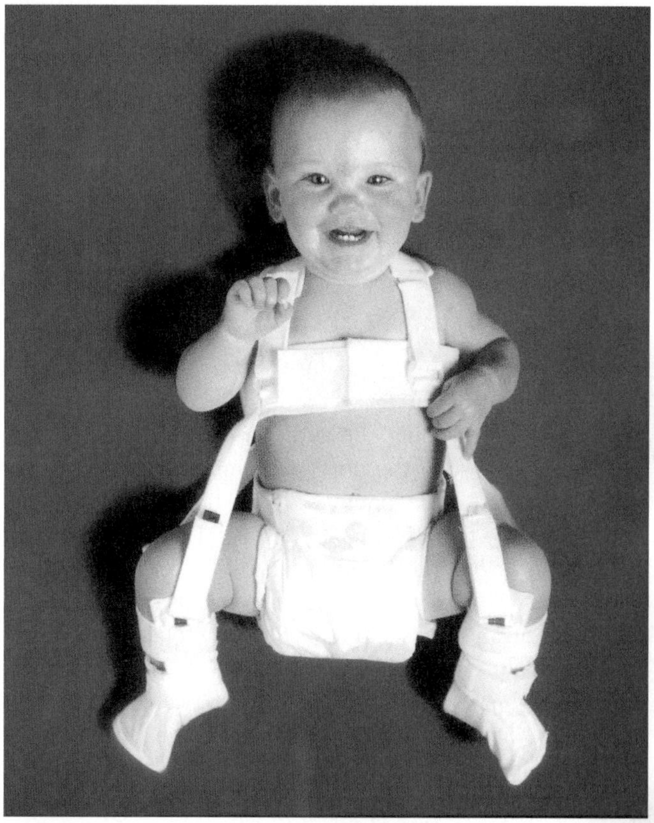

Figure 34-10 Infant with Developmental Dysplasia of the Hip in a Pavlik Harness. Courtesy of the Wheaton Brace Co., Carol Stream, IL.

Nursing Management

Nurses are in a position to detect DDH in the newborn. During routine assessments, bathing, and diaper changes the hips can be inspected for any deviations from normal.

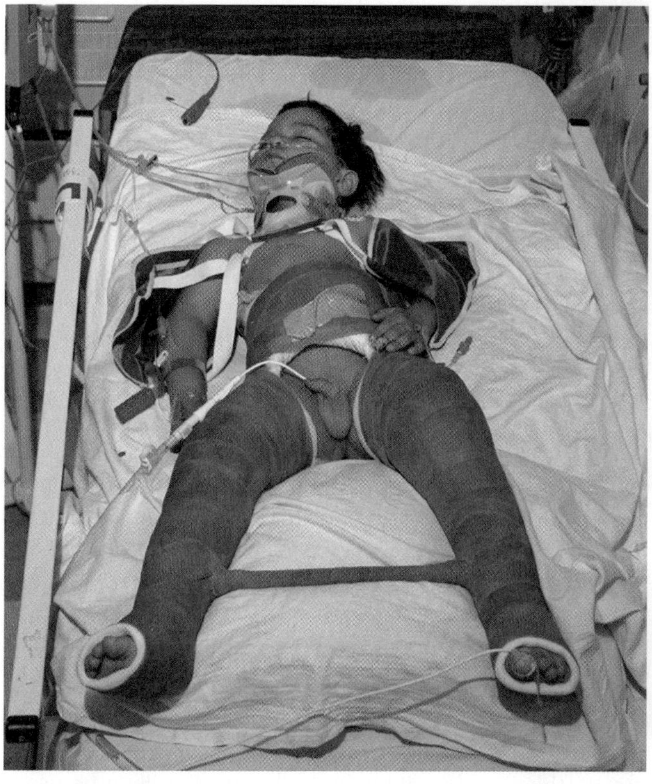

Figure 34-11 Boy in a Hip Spica Cast

Reflective Thinking

DDH

Suppose your child was born with DDH. What feelings would you expect to have? How would you channel any negative feelings into positive ones?

Nursing Alert:

Triple Diapering

The use of triple diapers in the treatment of DDH in the newborn is not recommended because it promotes hip extension and delays the initiation of more appropriate treatment such as the Pavlik harness (AAP, 2000).

Nursing management considers the normal growth and development of the infant or toddler. Reaching and pulling at toys or mobiles hung above the crib provide distraction and encourage use of the upper extremities for infants who are immobilized. Development of fine motor skills may be rapid while the child is immobilized, while development of gross motor skills may be delayed until after treatment is completed when the rate will return to normal. The child will use her or his arms and uncasted limb to aid in mobility. Nurses should reassure family members that the child will learn to maximize mobility in the cast or brace.

Immobility from traction, casts, or braces may lead to alterations in physiological functions. Use of bulk and bran in the child's diet will help maintain good bowel function and prevent constipation. Another complication of immobility is pressure on bony prominences and skin breakdown. Use of adequate padding, skin wrapping, and position changes every two hours will prevent skin breakdown and pressure sores. Pillows and blankets or even the floor may be used to allow for changes in position and diversion.

The principles of cast care were outlined in Box 34-2. For the infant in a spica cast the coarse, rough edges of the cast cause irritation and need to be trimmed. All edges should be covered with moleskin or waterproof tape to form a waterproof barrier between the diaper and skin. Irritation of the lower torso and legs can be avoided by tucking a disposable diaper up into the cast edges so that the plastic is between the baby and the cast. Change diapers frequently and use a folded cloth diaper or sanitary napkin to increase diaper absorbency.

Family Teaching

Care of the child in traction or a cast presents significant change in the caregivers' routine. Instructions and support are essential to ensure compliance. They need adequate time to practice and demonstrate skills with equipment and procedures (toileting, etc.) and to adjust daily routines to accommodate the child's special needs. They should be encouraged to verbalize fears and concerns about the impact of treatment on the family's life.

Family members will need to be informed about cast care including issues related to urinary and bowel elimination, bathing, and positioning. If skin traction is to be used, additional instructions will be required for skin care and traction application. Planning for nutritional requirements for the growing infant or toddler with restricted movement is necessary. An understanding of the age-appropriate developmental milestones will help the family members plan activities that will promote normal growth and development.

Caregivers need time to practice and demonstrate proper application of the Pavlik harness if used. They need to be taught how to diaper the child without removing the harness. Feeding is done in the upright position to maintain abduction of the hips. Wearing a cotton undershirt and cotton socks protects the skin by absorbing perspiration in warm weather and providing warmth in cold weather. Lotions, oils, or powder should not be used under the straps. Soothing and pacifying the infant or child may be a challenge. Caregivers need to be encouraged to hold the child despite a bulky harness or cast. They should bring experiences to the child because the child is unable to crawl or walk toward new and interesting objects in their surroundings.

Muscular Dystrophy

Muscular dystrophy (MD) refers to a group of progressive degenerative inherited diseases causing wasting of the muscles. The word dystrophy, with Latin and Greek roots, means "faulty nutrition." Muscles waste away in this disease, and it was theorized that persons with muscular dystrophy were not being properly nourished. This has proven unfounded. There are various patterns of inheritance and age of onset. The most common type of muscular dystrophy of childhood is Duchenne muscular dystrophy (DMD); therefore, the following discussion relates to DMD. Table 34-3 describes the common types of MD seen in children and adolescents.

Incidence and Etiology

DMD has an incidence of 0.3 in 1,000 live male births and affects all races and ethnic groups (Janas, 1996). It is inherited as an X-linked recessive disease; therefore, it affects males almost exclusively. Females may be carriers and pass the defect to their male children. Although DMD is genetically transmitted, as many as one-third of affected children have no family history of the disease.

Pathophysiology

In DMD there is an absence of the muscle protein dystrophin, which appears to play a role in supporting the structure of muscle fibers. The absence of dystrophin results in degeneration of skeletal or voluntary muscles that control movement. Fat and connective tissue replace the degenerated muscle fibers.

Clinical Manifestations

Early motor development in DMD is usually normal or just minimally delayed; however, between 2 and 4 years of age, the pelvic muscles begin to weaken. Children have difficulty

TABLE 34-3 Common Childhood Muscular Dystrophies

Type	Onset/Progression	Inheritance/Incidence	Clinical Manifestations
Duchenne	Onset: 2–6 yr. Progression: Rapid	X-linked/males Most common childhood form Affects all races Incidence: 0.3 per 1,000 live births	Affects upper arms and legs and trunk muscles first; calves enlarged due to fatty infiltrates; child has difficulty getting up from a sitting or lying position; waddling gait; mental retardation in some cases; life expectancy: adolescence–early 20s
Becker	Onset: 2–16 yr. Progression: slow	X-linked/males Incidence: 0.05 per 1,000 live births	Similar to Duchenne but appears later and progresses more slowly; child is mobile until late adolescence; normal intelligence; longer life expectancy than Duchenne
Limb-Girdle (LCMD)	Onset: Adolescence to early adulthood Progression: Usually slow	Autosomal recessive and dominant forms/males and females	Weakness begins in hips and moves to shoulders; progresses to include arms and legs
Facioscapulohumeral	Onset: Adolescence to early adulthood Progression: Slow, with long periods of stability interspersed with shorter periods of rapid muscle weakness	Autosomal dominant/ males and females	Muscles of face and shoulder area are affected first; forward sloping shoulders, difficulty closing eyes, and lifting arms above head; progresses in following order: abdomen, feet, upper arms, pelvic area, and lower arms; half are able to walk for their entire life

climbing stairs, running, and riding a bicycle. They develop a waddling gait and fall often. By 5 to 6 years of age, in order for the child to rise from a sitting to a standing position he must use a series of maneuvers and walks his hands up his legs. This is known as Gower's sign, and the maneuver is necessary because of weakness of the pelvic and trunk muscles (Figure 34-12).

Involvement of the shoulder girdle muscles usually occurs within 3 to 5 years after the onset of the disease, and the arms become weak. As muscles of the trunk atrophy, scoliosis often occurs. Enlargement of the calves and wasting of the thigh muscles are classic features. The calves appear large and strong, but they are weak because of infiltration of the muscles with fat and connective tissue. This abnormal enlargement of the muscles caused by an overgrowth of fatty and fibrous tissues is referred to as **pseudohypertrophy.** As the disease progresses, contractures develop usually in the ankles, knees, hips, and elbows. Between the ages of 9 and 12 years walking becomes impossible. In the later stages of the disease the auxiliary muscles of breathing and the diaphragm weaken, and respiratory function is poor. Respiratory infections become more common. The myocardium of the heart deteriorates and weakens resulting in cardiomyopathy. Eventually death results from respiratory infections or cardiac failure in the child's late teens or early twenties.

Diagnosis

The diagnosis is made by observation of clinical manifestations during physical examination and several tests. The most common diagnostic tests are muscle biopsy, electromyogram (EMG), nerve conduction velocity (NCV), and blood enzymes tests. With a muscle biopsy a small piece of muscle tissue is taken from an individual. If muscular dystrophy is present, the biopsy will reveal a replacement of normal muscle with connective and fatty tissue. An EMG involves placing a small electrode into the muscle to measure the electrical impulses, which are decreased in DMD. NCV involves sending electrical impulses down the nerves of the arms and legs. The speed of these impulses is measured with electrodes to determine whether the nerves are functioning normally. Because EMG and NCV are uncomfortable for most children, they will need adequate support during these tests. Blood enzyme tests are used to determine levels of the enzyme creatine kinase (CK). The CK level is

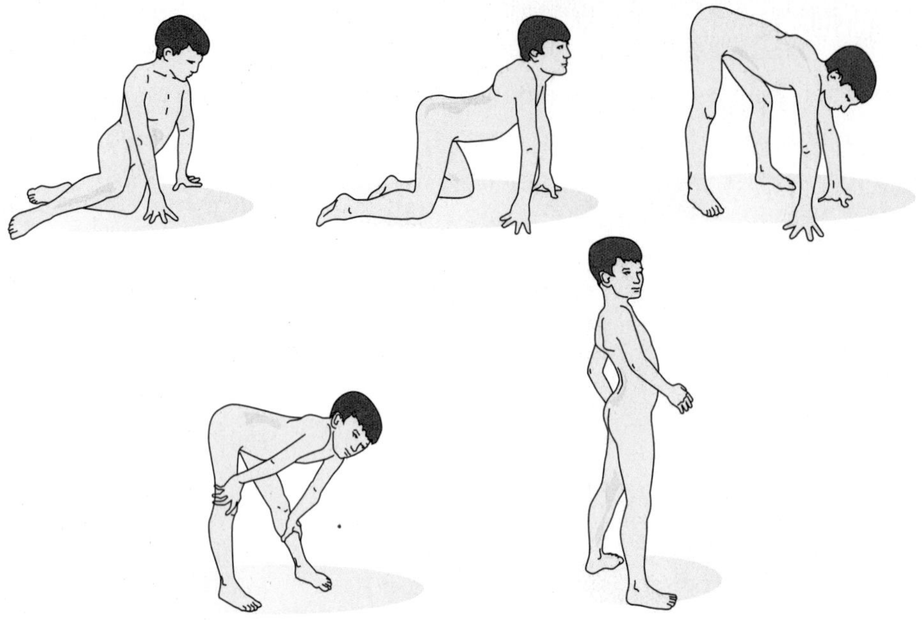

Figure 34-12 Gower's Sign. Because of the weakness of the pelvic and trunk muscles, the child with muscular dystrophy must use a series of maneuvers to rise from a sitting or lying position.

elevated in many forms of muscular dystrophy because these enzymes leak from degenerating muscles.

Treatment

Treatment is supportive, as there is no cure for muscular dystrophy. A team approach including the caregivers, health care provider, nurse, physical and occupational therapists, nutritionist, and social worker is necessary. The goal of management is to provide support and prevent complications. Physical and occupational therapies help children achieve their maximum level of functioning and independence. Physical therapy helps the individual maintain strength and maximize range of motion, posture, and comfort. Muscle weakness can lead to contracture and shortening of muscle tissue. A child with DMD typically walks on the tips of the toes as the tendon shortens, which is the result of the muscle breakdown and fibrosis in calf muscles. A daily routine of stretching these muscles delays the deformities caused by the contracture. Physical therapies help the individual and the family members develop an individualized exercise program that include the type and amount of activity best for each child. The goal of occupational therapy is to help the child compensate for physical limitations and learn to adapt to a new level of achievement in the activities of daily living at home and school. Adaptation of wheelchairs, seating systems, and computers to aid with writing are a few of the possibilities.

Surgery may be performed as contractures progress. One of the common procedures is a release of the heel cord, which relieves developing contractures and improves mobility. Surgery is performed on the hips and knees as they become contracted, thus allowing the child to sit in a wheelchair with an increased level of comfort.

Nursing Management

The care of the child with DMD is complex and requires cooperation among many health care providers and the child's caregivers. Monitoring of respiratory and cardiac status needs to be performed regularly. Proper nutrition and avoiding obesity are ongoing concerns. Activities such as swimming or water exercises are often recommended as a way to keep muscles toned and to promote mobility without causing undue stress on the muscles. As the child's stamina decreases, activities that involve less expenditure of energy can be suggested.

Members of the interdisciplinary team may need to meet with teachers and caregivers to evaluate the child's learning needs and functioning in the classroom. Reading books to the child, listening to tapes, and using the computer offer the child stimulation and promote normal development. It is important to provide good back support and posture by keeping the child's body in alignment when confined to a wheelchair.

In the later stages of DMD the child is unable to move himself and needs to be turned frequently to prevent skin breakdown. Adequate amounts of fluids must be encouraged to prevent urinary stasis. The combination of weak abdominal muscles and immobility can lead to severe constipation; therefore, the child's diet should be high in fluid, fiber, and fresh fruits and vegetables. A bowel regime including stool softeners and laxatives may be necessary to prevent stool retention and constipation. Respiratory therapy is needed to maintain pulmonary function for as long as possible. Modifications of the home to accommodate a wheelchair may be necessary. Supportive devices and lifts may be necessary to get the child in and out the bathtub without undue strain on the caregivers.

Genetic counseling and testing are recommended for females in the family of the affected child to determine if they are carriers of DMD. Accurate protein and DNA-based carrier detection tests are available. As gene and protein defects are identified, better diagnostic tests and understanding of the biological basis of a disease may lead to more effective treatment. Genetic counseling provides families with valuable information about current genetic testing methods.

Family Teaching

Mothers may deal with feelings of guilt since they are the carriers of DMD and pass the defective gene to their child. Nurses should encourage the family to discuss their feelings about the genetic aspect of the disease, the eventual fatal outcome, and how the disease is affecting all members and their lifestyle. Feelings of hopelessness are common as the child's disease progresses and he requires total care. Caregivers need to be taught how to assist with basic activities of daily living. Attention to the needs of siblings is important, as they may feel neglected because the child with DMD receives so much attention. If the child with muscular dystrophy needs a special diet, it is important to make mealtimes a family affair and to include that child despite his special diet. Use of an electric wheelchair, cellular phones, and other assistive devices decrease the risk for social isolation. Resources, such as the Muscular Dystrophy Association of America, can provide emotional support and arrange for special assistance as family energies are depleted.

GROWTH RELATED DISORDERS

Growth related disorders occur during periods of rapid growth of the musculoskeletal system before skeletal maturity is reached. The disorders discussed in this section include scoliosis, kyphosis, lordosis, and Legg-Calve-Perthes disease. Scoliosis, kyphosis, and lordosis are deformities that affect the spine (Figure 34-13).

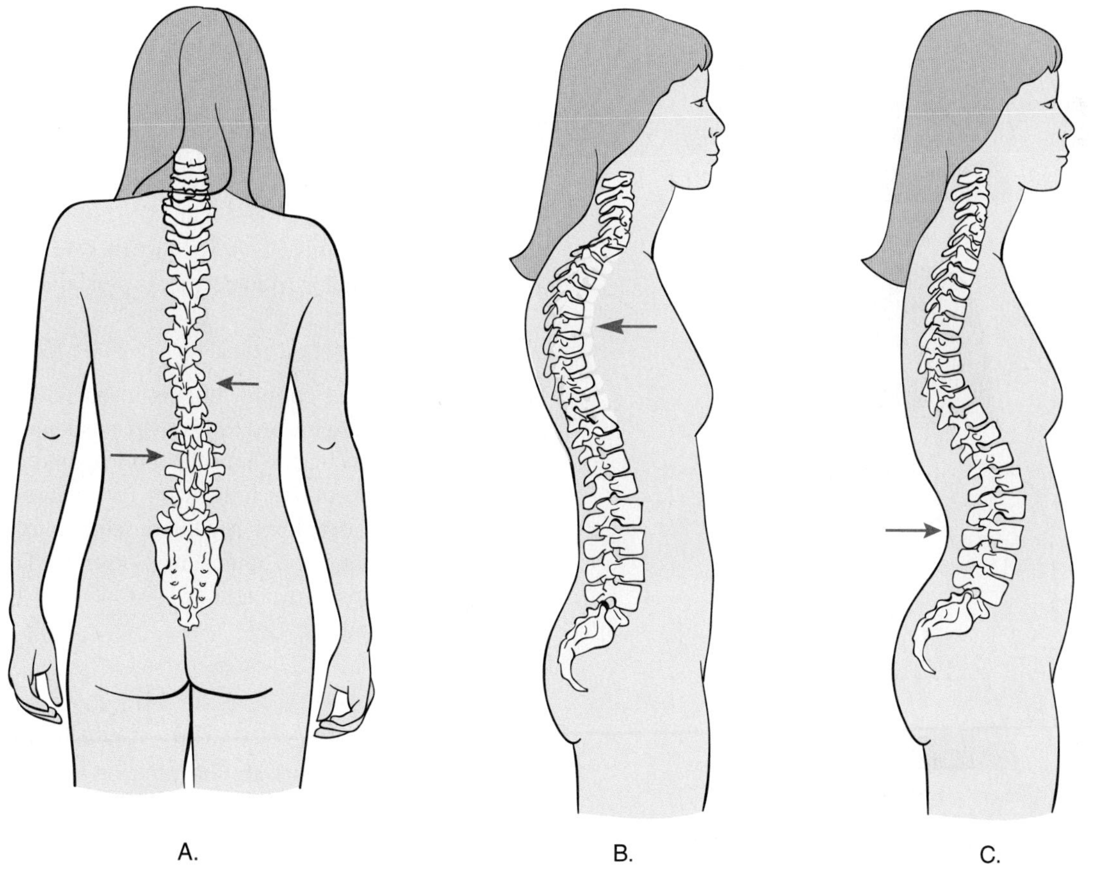

Figure 34-13 Spinal Deformities: (A) Scoliosis (B) Kyphosis (C) Lordosis

Scoliosis

Scoliosis is the lateral curvature of the spine with vertebral body rotation. As the spine curves, the vertebra column rotates around its long axis, pulling the ribs in the thoracic region along and causing them to become prominent on the convex side. The disorder can be structural, a primary deformity, or functional, a curve caused by a secondary problem. Figures 34-14A and B illustrate an adolescent girl with scoliosis.

REFLECTIONS FROM FAMILIES

When I was 15 years old, I was diagnosed with scoliosis and was told I would have to wear a Milwaukee brace for at least one year. When I saw pictures of the brace, I thought it was ugly, like something out of the Dark Ages. I was a sophomore in high school and was just beginning to like the attention I was receiving from boys. I was so angry about having to wear this awful brace. Even wearing blouses and shirts in bigger sizes couldn't conceal the head and chin rests. I was so worried that all the kids would stare at me. I didn't even want to go to school.

Incidence and Etiology

The incidence of scoliosis is 100 out of 1,000 children; however, only 2 per 1,000 require treatment. The child is usually healthy and has a normal spine at birth. The curvature develops between 9 and 12 years old. The incidence is slightly greater in males, but females have a greater tendency than males for progression of the curve to the point at which treatment is required. In some cases other family members are also affected; thus, a family history is valuable in detecting the problem in siblings (Morrissy & Weinstein, 1996).

The etiology of scoliosis is unknown, but several theories have been postulated. These include malfunctioning of the vestibular balancing system, genetic patterns, muscular weakness, and collagen metabolism. In the majority of cases the cause is unknown, called idiopathic scoliosis. This type is further divided into three classes: infantile, juvenile, and adolescent. The age of the child at the time of the diagnosis determines the classification. The most common of all types of scoliosis is adolescent idiopathic. Other conditions known to cause spinal deformity are congenital spinal column abnormalities, neuromuscular disorders (muscular dystrophy, cerebral palsy, spina bifida), and radiation therapy. Radiation often produces asymmetric growth in adjacent growth plates and soft tissues, leading to subsequent spinal deformity.

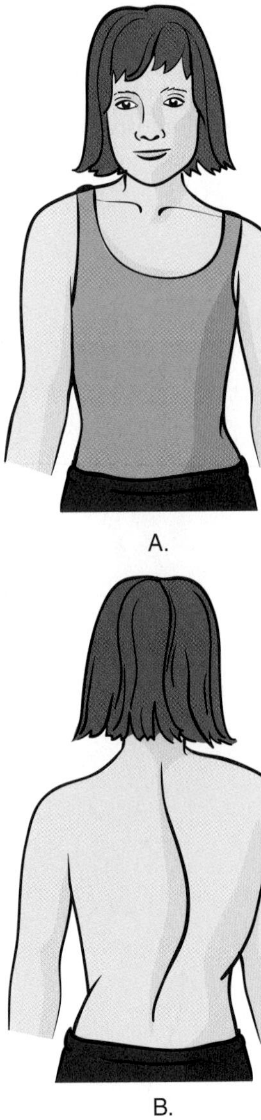

Figure 34-14 Adolescent Girl with Scoliosis: (A) Frontal View (B) Posterior View

Pathophysiology

When the vertebral column begins to curve laterally, the spine and ribs rotate toward the convex portion of the curve. On the concave side, the muscles and ligaments are contracted and thickened, whereas on the convex side they become thin and atrophied. A compensatory curve results as the child attempts to maintain erect posture. The thoracic cavity also changes and becomes asymmetrical resulting in respiratory problems.

Clinical Manifestations

In adolescent idiopathic scoliosis the time of highest risk for curve progression occurs around puberty when the growth rate is the fastest. The individuals may have unequal shoulder and hip level, prominence of one scapula or a curved spinal column, and truncal asymmetry. In normal children the elbow level falls above the iliac crest; in those with scoliosis one elbow will be closer to the iliac crest than the other. When the child bends over the rotation of the spine becomes more prominent. The scapula on one side becomes prominent, and the other side is hollow. Scoliosis curves occur in the thoracic, lumbar, or thoracolumbar sections of the spine, with the thoracic being the most common. Pain is uncommon until the deformity is well established.

Diagnosis

Scoliosis is frequently detected initially during routine physical examinations or school screenings. Box 34-3 describes a procedure for a school screening. Radiographs confirm the diagnosis of scoliosis.

Treatment

The treatment of adolescent idiopathic scoliosis is determined by a complex equation that includes the adolescent's physiologic, not chronologic, age; magnitude, location, and potential for progression of the curve. Thoracic curves, the most common, are at greater risk for progression than thoracolumbar or lumbar ones. Treatment includes observation, bracing, and/or surgery. Periodic reevaluation, often including radiographs, is recommended for the skeletally immature child with a curve less than 25 degrees and for the more skeletally mature with a curve less than 45 degrees.

For children who are skeletally immature with significant growth remaining and a curve between 25 and 40 degrees appropriate treatment is bracing (orthotics). The goal of a brace is to stop progression of the curve, not necessarily curve correction. The decision to begin a bracing program is often difficult. Although there are guidelines to help predict that a curve may progress, the health care provider must consider the child's willingness to participate. The emotional and monetary expense of bracing is high; therefore, the decision is made on an individual basis. The most common braces used are the Boston brace, the TLSO custom molded jacket, and the Milwaukee brace. The Boston brace, an underarm prefabricated plastic shell, is used for curves of the low thoracolumbar and lumbar spine. This brace is more socially acceptable because it can be concealed by loose-fitting clothing (Figure 34-16). The TLSO, used for thoracolumbar curves, is molded to the individual's body and built like a jacket. The Milwaukee brace is used for high thoracic curves and consists of plastic and metal with a chin extension. Curves between 20 and 40 degrees are of the optimal range for use of this brace (Maher, et al., 1998) (Figure 34-17). The

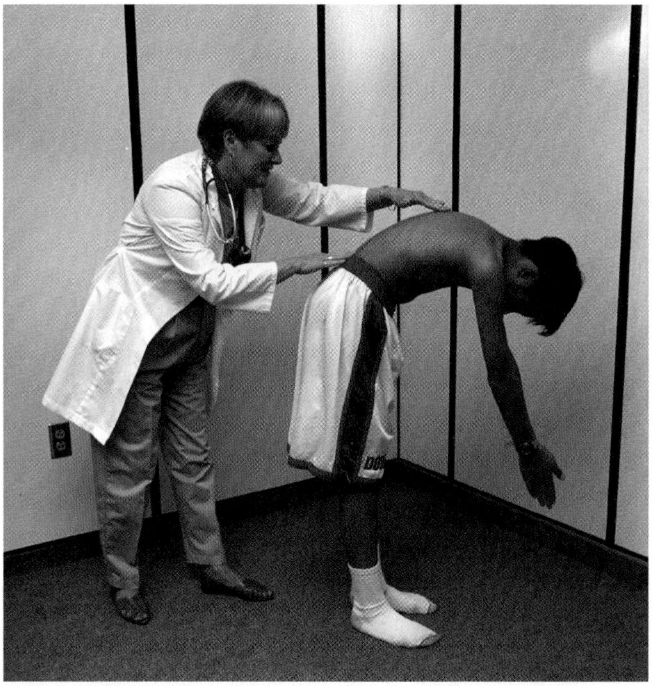

Figure 34-15 School Nurse Performing Scoliosis Screening

BOX 34-3 Scoliosis screening procedure (Figure 34-15)

1. Remove the blouse or shirt so the back is visible.
2. Explain the procedure so the child is at ease.
3. Pull back shoulder length hair with a barrette or rubber band. The child cannot hold the hair up or the screening will be inaccurate.
4. Screen boys and girls separately to reduce embarrassment.
5. Have the child stand upright with the feet together.
6. Stand behind the child and stabilize the pelvis by holding both hips at the iliac crest level.
7. Instruct the child to flex forward from the waist, allowing the arms and head to hang loosely.
8. Palpate the spinous process and place a dot on each with a felt-tip pen.
9. Draw an imaginary line through the dots with the child in a flexed position and then in an upright position. The line through the dots should be straight in both the upright and flexed positions.
10. Evaluate symmetry of the shoulders, scapula, and waist creases as well as arm lengths.
11. Observe the child from the front, looking for anterior chest deformity and asymmetry.
12. Look for symmetry of the shoulders, breasts, anterior rib cage, waist creases, and arm lengths.
13. Observe the child from the side in both the standing and bending positions to visualize increased kyphosis and lordosis.
14. Rescreen or refer the child with positive findings to a pediatrician or family physician for further evaluation (Maher, et al., 1998).

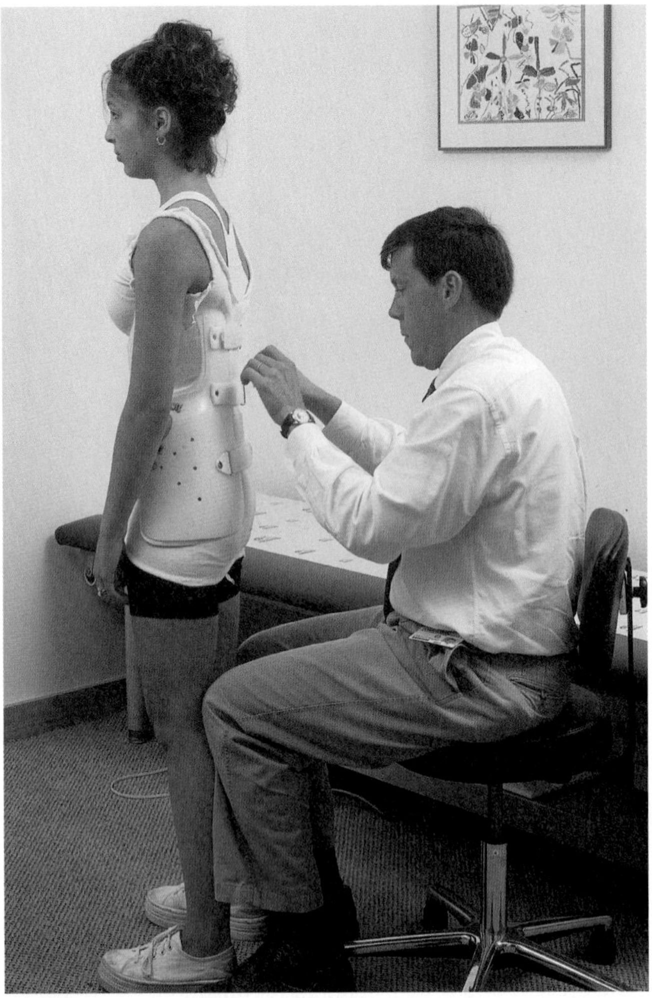

Figure 34-16 Boston Brace for Scoliosis. Courtesy of Boston Brace International.

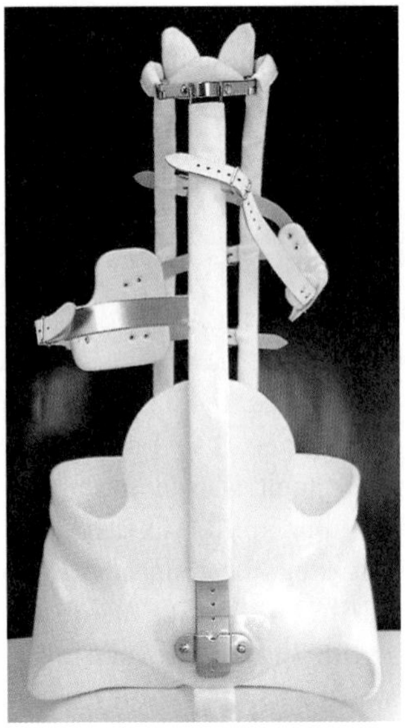

Figure 34-17 The Milwaukee brace is used for high thoracic scoliosis curves. Courtesy of Bertil Holmbert, MD, Malmoe, Sweden.

type of brace chosen and the number of hours it must be worn (usually between 16 and 23 hours a day) are based on the degree and location of the curve, age of the child, and the health care provider's recommendation.

In some cases, when the curve is 40 degrees or more in either the previously untreated child or in one in whom bracing was ineffective, surgery is suggested. There are two goals of surgery: to prevent progression of the curve and to diminish spinal deformity. The approach to the spine may be either anterior, posterior, or a combination of both. The most common surgical procedure used to correct idiopathic adolescent scoliosis is a posterior spinal fusion with instrumentation and bone grafting. This is achieved by the fusion of one vertebra to an adjacent one, which prevents motion between them. Instrumentation is used to stabilize the spine and obtain some correction of the deformity. The type of instrumentation used depends on the surgeon's preference, the approach to the spine, and the location of the curve. Examples of instrumentation are the Texas Scottish Rite Hospital, Luque, Cotrel-Dubousset, Dwyer, and Harrington. The first three types allow the child to be up without a cast or brace shortly after surgery and to be discharged from the hospital within 7–10 days. There is progressive resumption of routine daily activities including returning to school. An **autogenous** (originating within the child's body) bone graft taken from the iliac crest, fibula, tibia, or rib is used to augment the fusion (Puno, Mehta, & Byrd, 1994).

Kids Want To Know

Do I really have to wear this Milwaukee brace when I go to school? I'll look like a freak!

I understand you're concerned about the appearance of the brace, but wearing loose, colorful shirts, blouses, sweaters, or sweatshirts will help. You'll also feel better about how you look if you continue using your makeup and keep your hair clean and stylish. Instead of waiting for others to ask about the brace, a better approach is for you to mention it first and explain why you're wearing it. I know many kids think not wearing the brace now is more important than preventing progression of the curve in the future. However, the curve will get worse and may cause you considerable pain and difficulty breathing. I can get you in touch with another girl your age who also has a Milwaukee brace so you can share your feelings and concerns. Would you like that?

Nursing Alert:

Spinal Cord Injury after Surgery for Scoliosis

During surgical intervention for scoliosis, spinal cord injury is a potential complication caused by compression or trauma. Therefore, all clients who will be undergoing surgery should be assessed for neurological impairment. Assessment includes numbness, sensation, motion, paresthesia in all extremities, and bowel and bladder function.

Kyphosis

Kyphosis (humpback or round back deformity) is an excessive convex curvature at the thoracic level of the spine. A certain degree of kyphosis is normal but curvature greater than 45 degrees is generally considered excessive.

Incidence and Etiology

Kyphosis may be congenital, postural, or secondary to other diseases. Congenital kyphosis is the result of a failure of formation or segmentation of the vertebral structures in utero.

Case Study/Care Plan

The Child Undergoing Surgery for Scoliosis

Clara, 14 years of age, has been followed for three years in the scoliosis clinic. Her spinal curve has progressed significantly over the past year. She has worn a Milwaukee brace for one year. Her older sister also had scoliosis and wore the same brace during her adolescence. Asymmetry of the shoulder, scapular prominence and increase in pain are present. Radiographs, including anterior, posterior, and lateral, indicate a spinal curve of 50 degrees. Clara has no other health-related problems. Spinal fusion with Cotrel-Dubousset instrumentation is planned. Both an anterior and posterior approach will be used. Removal of the lower ribs is planned to allow better respiratory function. Rib bone will be used for autogenous graft for the spinal fusion.

Nursing Care Plan

Assessment Preoperatively, the nurse should assess the child's and family's understanding of the diagnosis of scoliosis and ask about what treatments, if any, have been used in the past. It is also important to determine their understanding of the treatment plan, specifically bracing, which must be explained so they know the anticipated results. Education is essential to promote compliance with bracing. If noncompliance is detected early, other approaches to treatment can be considered before spinal curvature has time to worsen. The nurse must also assess the child's concerns about body image. Before surgery, an assessment of the child's and family's understanding of the surgical procedure and postoperative care is performed. Significant information to obtain includes plans to continue schoolwork and expectations for the recovery period at home. Postoperatively, it is important for the nurse to monitor for complications such as respiratory alterations, altered neurovascular status, hemorrhage, fluid imbalances, altered cardiac status, pain, and paralytic ileus.

Preoperative

Nursing Diagnosis #1

Risk for impaired skin integrity related to bracing and other corrective therapies.

Expected Outcomes

1. Clara will not experience skin irritation or breakdown.
2. Clara's brace will fit appropriately without skin irritation.

continues

continued

Interventions/*Rationales*

1. Gradually increase orthosis wearing time as comfort allows. *Protects the skin from breakdown or irritation.*

2. Develop goals with Clara to achieve optimal orthosis wearing time. *The likelihood of compliance improves if the individual is allowed to participate in planning increased orthosis wearing time.*

3. Assess skin for breakdown or irritation. *Orthosis wearing time is uninterrupted if skin irritation or breakdown is avoided. Decreases the risk of infection, and comfort is maintained.*

4. Assess orthosis for proper fit. *An improperly fitting brace can result in skin breakdown and pressure sores.*

Evaluation

Clara's brace is properly fitted, and she wears it as prescribed. Her skin remains intact with no evidence of redness, irritation, or breakdown.

Nursing Diagnosis #2

Disturbed body image related to curvature of the spine, presence of brace, and scar after surgery.

Expected Outcomes

1. Clara will verbalize feelings about how the disorder and treatments affect her body image and self-esteem.

2. Clara will demonstrate a positive self-image and involvement with activities and support groups.

Interventions/*Rationales*

1. Assess and encourage verbalization of feelings about bracing, surgery, casting, and other procedures related to spinal deformity. *Assessment of her feelings and perceptions provides information to use in planning care. Verbalization provides an outlet for possible anger and resentment about disorder and its treatment.*

2. Encourage participation in activities of daily living as limitations allow (e.g., hair washing, grooming, and dressing in own clothing). *Promotes a positive self-image.*

3. Provide contact with other adolescents who have undergone treatment for scoliosis. *Support from others who have experienced the same treatments is often therapeutic.*

Evaluation

Clara's grooming demonstrates that she feels positive about herself. She is able to emphasize her strengths. She becomes involved with others who have scoliosis.

Nursing Diagnosis #3

Deficient knowledge regarding condition, treatment, brace care, and surgical procedure related to lack of prior experience.

Expected Outcomes

1. Clara and her family will verbalize an understanding of scoliosis, treatment aims, and surgery.

2. Clara and her family will ask appropriate questions about postoperative care.

Interventions/*Rationales*

1. Teach the adolescent and family about scoliosis, its nonsurgical and surgical treatment, anticipated outcomes of both types of treatment, and follow-up care. *Education and knowledge increase comfort level and compliance with treatment, and decrease fears.*

continues

continued

2. Explain preoperative tests and routines to Clara and family members. *Understanding of procedures and tests increases compliance and decreases anxiety.*

3. Encourage questions and provide honest answers. *Adolescent and family may be hesitant to ask questions. An honest approach establishes a trusting relationship with the nurse.*

4. Provide explanations and rationale for surgical procedure and postoperative care. *Information about upcoming surgery decreases anxiety, and an understanding of the reasons for postoperative routines may increase client cooperation.*

Evaluation

Clara and her caregivers express an understanding of the disorder, treatment plan, preoperative and postoperative care, and comply with treatment plan.

Postoperative

Nursing Diagnosis #1

Ineffective breathing pattern related to bedrest, anesthesia, and immobility.

Expected Outcomes

Clara will maintain effective breathing pattern and avoid pulmonary complications (pneumonia, atelectasis).

Interventions/*Rationales*

1. Reposition Clara every 2 hours. *Frequent position changes prevent pooling of secretions.*

2. Administer oxygen as needed. *Increases peripheral oxygen saturation.*

3. Provide respiratory care: coughing, deep breathing, and use of incentive spirometer every 2 hours for first 24 hours, then every 4 hours until ambulatory. *Promotes adequate pulmonary hygiene. Spirometry increases lung expansion and aeration of alveoli, prevents pooling of secretions and atelectasis.*

4. Monitor intake and output. Provide approximately 2,000–3,000 ml of fluid per 24 hours. *Ensures adequate hydration of the client, which helps to loosen lung secretions.*

Evaluation

Clara achieves adequate ventilation and remains free of respiratory distress or infections. Lung sounds are clear bilaterally with no adventitious sounds.

Nursing Diagnosis #2

Pain related to surgery, incision, donor site, and muscle stretching.

Expected Outcomes

Clara will demonstrate diminished pain.

Interventions/*Rationales*

1. Assess physiological, behavioral, and verbal indicators of pain. *Physiological manifestations and behavior provide clues to pain experience. Children and adolescents may be unwilling to express pain and to request medication because of fear of an injection.*

2. Use a pain assessment scale appropriate for developmental level to determine severity of pain. *A pain scale provides objective data about pain.*

3. Administer prescribed analgesics by patient controlled analgesia (PCA), epidural, or intermittent IV "around the clock." *Optimal pain management allows client to be more cooperative with postoperative respiratory regimen and promotes faster healing and recovery. Postoperative pain is intense for 72 hours after a spinal fusion.*

continues

continued

4. Encourage use of nonpharmacological methods to manage pain such as therapeutic touch, music, relaxation, and guided imagery. *These techniques can be an effective adjunct to medication.*

Evaluation

Clara experiences effective pain relief early in the postoperative period. She has no verbal complaints of pain and participates in conversations and diversional activities.

Nursing Diagnosis #3

Impaired physical mobility related to postsurgical restrictions.

Expected Outcomes

Clara will progress with physical activity as prescribed.

Interventions/*Rationales*

1. Reposition the child every 2 hours using the logrolling technique. Support the head and legs by using pillows. *Promotes circulation, increases comfort, and prevents skin breakdown. Proper positioning prevents injury to the spine.*
2. Perform passive and active range of motion exercises. *Exercises help maintain circulation, muscle tone, and strength, and prevent muscle atrophy.*
3. Dangle on the side of the bed when allowed per health care provider's order and gradually progress to unassisted ambulation. *Early mobilization decreases risk of thrombophlebitis and pulmonary emboli.*
4. Assist client with a return to normal activities and self-care as ordered and as client's condition allows. *Maintains circulation, muscle tone, and strength.*

Evaluation

Clara resumes full ambulation without adverse complications.

Nursing Diagnosis #4

Risk for injury related to altered neurovascular status secondary to circulatory or nerve damage during surgical instrumentation.

Expected Outcomes

Clara will not experience neurovascular injury as evident by intact sensation/motion of extremities, voluntary control over voiding and bowel evacuation, warm extremities, and capillary refill < 3 sec.

Interventions/*Rationales*

1. Assess circulatory and nerve status of all extremities every 2 hours for the first 24 hours, then every 4 hours for the next 48 hours. *Altered neurovascular status, paralysis, and thrombus formation are complications of surgery for scoliosis secondary to injury and compression of the spine.*
2. Monitor intake and output and assess for bladder distention or bowel incontinence. *Loss of bowel and bladder control may indicate spinal cord injury.*
3. Maintain flat position if prescribed. Logroll every 2 hours. *Maintaining proper alignment prevents injury to the spine. Logrolling is necessary to prevent nerve damage.*

Evaluation

Clara is free of neurovascular impairment and has full range of motion and sensation in lower extremities.

Family Teaching

The Child after Spinal Fusion for Scoliosis

- Instruct and demonstrate the correct technique for wound care.
- Instruct the child to avoid any extremes of bending, twisting, stooping, or lifting of heavy objects.
- Encourage caregivers to administer an iron supplement if the child is anemic because of blood loss during surgery.
- Explain that the diet should be well-balanced, especially with adequate protein, vitamin C, and calcium to promote healing.
- Discuss the potential for constipation caused by decreased motility and pain medication. Encourage increased fluid and fiber intake for prevention.
- Teach caregivers about appropriate medications for constipation, such as stool softeners.
- Make arrangements for child to contact someone who has undergone similar treatment for scoliosis as a support.
- Assist caregivers in obtaining home tutor until child returns to school, usually within 4–6 weeks after surgery.
- Provide appropriate school personnel (teachers, coaches, etc.) with instructions about activity restrictions, such as playing contact sports, diving in a pool, gymnastics, bicycle riding, ice skating, and horseback riding.
- Refer family to the National Scoliosis Foundation, for educational support materials and support groups.
- Provide referral to appropriate community agency for special equipment if needed such as a raised toilet seat, straight backed chair, and so forth.

Postural kyphosis tends to occur in pre-adolescent years, especially among girls who are self-conscious about breast development and increasing height. Kyphosis may be associated with diseases or disorders, such as cerebral palsy, tuberculosis, spinal muscle atrophy, muscular dystrophy, and metabolic disorders. Radiation and tumor removal from the spinal cord are other conditions that may cause kyphosis.

Pathophysiology

With congenital kyphosis one side of the vertebrae either incompletely develop or fail to grow resulting in narrowing of the vertebrae and the disks. The affected vertebrae rotate and cause physical changes in the spine. Spinal curvature occurs in postural kyphosis; however, there are no changes in the vertebrae. Kyphosis secondary to neuromuscular disorders results from an imbalance of the pull of muscles on either side of the spine.

Clinical Manifestations

Children with kyphosis have a hunchback or rounded appearance to their spine. Lumbar lordosis usually develops as a compensatory curve in children with postural kyphosis. Some children complain of mild pain in the back or shoulders.

Diagnosis

The diagnosis is made by visualizing the spine and scapular area from the side with the child bending 90 degrees at the waist. A comprehensive orthopedic and neurologic evaluation may be performed to determine if the kyphosis is associated with other diseases or conditions.

Treatment

Treatment for kyphosis depends on the age of the child, the degree of curvature, and the presence or absence of pain. Treatment options are: no treatment if the curvature is less than 40 degrees; exercises for curvature between 40 and 50 degrees; bracing and exercise for curvature between 50 and 70 degrees; and surgical intervention for curvature greater than 70 degrees (Maher, et al., 1998). Most cases of kyphosis can be corrected without surgical intervention (see Figure 34-18).

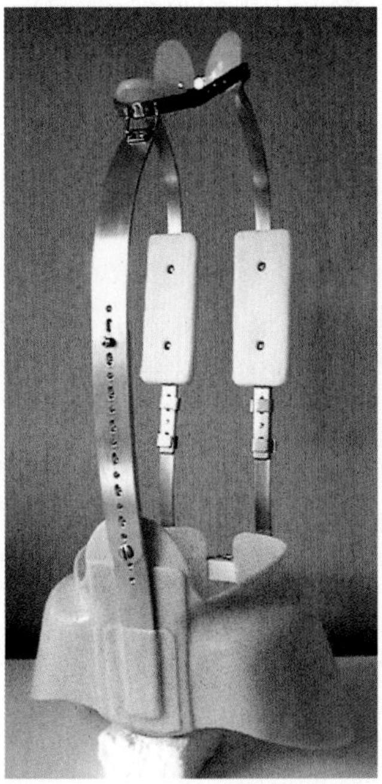

Figure 34-18 This brace is used in the treatment of kyphosis. Courtesy of Bertil Holmbert, MD, Malmoe, Sweden.

However, it is indicated for those who have completed skeletal growth, a significant degree of curvature, and chronic pain. The treatment involves fusion of the spine with some type of instrumentation. Nursing management is similar to that discussed in the section on scoliosis.

Lordosis

Lordosis is an excessive concave curvature of the lumbar spine. In the normal spine a mild concave curve exists in the lumbar region. Lordosis is an exaggeration of that normal curve.

Incidence and Etiology

Lordosis is a normal finding in toddlers that should disappear as the child grows in height, usually by school-age. It is often observed in adolescents, especially girls, during the growth spurt. However, in other children it may be associated with conditions such as obesity, flexion contractures of the hip, developmental dysplasia of the hip, and slipped femoral capital epiphysis.

Pathophysiology

With lordosis the muscles of the spine are unable to support an erect position. This results in straining of the ligaments, which causes lower back pain and fatigue.

Clinical Manifestations

The child with lordosis presents with a swayback and may exhibit a protruding chest and abdomen. Other clinical manifestations include complaints of lower back pain, hip pain, and fatigue.

Diagnosis

Lumbar lordosis is diagnosed by visualization of the spine and radiographs.

Treatment

One aspect of treatment is managing or correcting the associated etiological factor. Postural exercises are the usual form of treatment once the associated condition has been dealt with. Bracing and surgery are rarely needed. Nursing management is similar to that discussed in the section on scoliosis.

Legg-Calve-Perthes Disease

Legg-Calve-Perthes (LCP) disease, also known as osteochondrosis of the femoral head, coxa plana, osteochondritis deformans, and coxa juvenile, is characterized by avascular necrosis of the femoral head with collapse and subsequent regeneration. It is a self-limiting disease.

Incidence and Etiology

LCP disease occurs between the ages of 2 and 12 years, most frequently from 4 to 8 years of age. The incidence is 0.15 in 1,000, and males are four times more likely than females to be affected. It is more common among first-born children and those with low birth weight. The cause is unknown but proposed theories indicate heredity, metabolic, chemical, and mechanical dysfunction. Hereditary factors seem to be implicated as the risk is 20% greater in families with a history of the disease than in the general population. In some cases the onset of the disease is preceded by a traumatic injury, which may cause a subchondral fracture.

Pathophysiology

LCP occurs as a result of the temporary loss of blood supply to the femoral capital epiphysis resulting in avascular necrosis of the femoral head. Four stages occur over approximately a 36-month period. Stage one is the incipient or synovitis stage and is characterized by soft tissue changes with swelling of the synovial membrane and joint capsule. Stage two is aseptic necrosis, with opacity of the epiphysis. During this stage radiographs demonstrate a characteristic opacity of the femoral epiphysis and widening of the medial joint space. Stage three is revascularization; the epiphysis is mottled and fragmented. During this stage healing occurs as new bone forms and the necrotic bone is absorbed. It is at this point that the hip becomes painful with effusion, and movement is decreased. This is a critical period and if LCP is not treated, progressive deformity may occur. Stage four is the reossification with gradual reformation of the femoral head (Maher et. al., 1998).

Clinical Manifestations

The onset of LCP disease is insidious with a prolonged course of symptoms. Pain, present in the hip or only in the knee or groin, may be worse with activity and relieved with rest. In some children a limp is present with or without pain. The child presents with an abnormal gait and limitations of hip range of motion, especially abduction and internal rotation. Inspection of the affected leg may show atrophy of the thigh muscles.

Diagnosis

LCP disease is diagnosed and classified with use of radiograph. Occasionally a bone scan may be used to differentiate LCP from toxic synovitis of the hip, septic hip joint, or osteomyelitis.

Treatment

Permanent deformity of the bone may occur without treatment. The goals of treatment are to keep the femoral head in the acetabulum and as round as possible and to prevent deformity during the healing process with traction, casting, brace wearing, and/or surgery. Bed rest and the use of abduction traction will reduce pain and improve range of motion. A non-weight-bearing brace device or harness may be used. Performing non-weight-bearing exercises prevents atrophy of the extremity during this time. Another approach is to allow weight bearing as long as the femoral head remains in the acetabulum; therefore, treatment may consist of a long leg cast with an abduction bar. Surgery is necessary in some cases to maintain the femoral head within the acetabulum.

Nursing Management

To prevent injury and complications it is necessary to assess and plan interventions to maintain neurovascular integrity. Ongoing assessment of the neurovascular system is important during therapy with traction or surgery throughout the course of treatment. Meticulous skin care is important to reduce friction between the skin and traction equipment, cast, or brace. Teaching the child to crutch walk during hospitalization reduces the risk of falls after discharge as well as instructing caregivers to make the home environment safe. Rearranging furniture and removing loose rugs promote safe space for ambulating with either a brace or crutches.

Deficient knowledge related to home care is addressed early in the course of treatment. The child is usually in the hospital during the initial stages of treatment. During this time the nurse is able to work with the child and family to increase their understanding of the rationale for treatment and the correct use of the equipment. Other teaching includes the assessment of the skin and neurovascular status, signs of muscular atrophy, appropriate activities of daily living, and safety measures to be initiated in the home or school.

Family Teaching

Family teaching includes assessment skills of the skin and neurovascular system. The emphasis on safety and promoting a positive self-image of the child are two issues that involve ongoing recognition and support from the hospital and follow-up clinic staff. The child, between the ages of 4 and 8, is likely to associate disease and its accompanying restrictions with punishment; therefore, raising the caregivers' awareness of this developmental issue is critical. They are then better able to provide positive reinforcement for the child. It may be necessary to work with school personnel about adaptations to accommodate the child's limitations, such as safe hallways or an elevator for going up and down stairs.

ADDITIONAL MUSCULOSKELETAL DISORDERS

The following disorders are rare in children; therefore, they are discussed only briefly.

Osteogenesis Imperfecta

Osteogenesis imperfecta (OI), known as brittle bone disease, is a connective tissue disorder and is characterized by disturbed formation of periosteal bone. Children with OI have fragile bones that fracture easily. It is an inherited disease, usually in an autosomal dominant pattern. A ribbonlike or mosaic pattern is seen in the bones on X ray.

Clinical Manifestations

The major clinical manifestation is severe bone fragility with multiple fractures caused by poor collagen formation. Some children's bones are so fragile that fractures result not only from trauma, but also from normal activities of life such as walking. Other manifestations include associated deafness, dental deformities, blue sclera, hyperlaxity of ligaments, and short stature. The child may develop kyphosis or scoliosis if the vertebral bones are involved. Multiple fractures throughout childhood tend to cause limb and spinal column deformities that interfere with growth and bone aliment. Usually there is little pain at the site of the fracture; however, the older child may report tenderness. Soft tissue damage may be minimal secondary to bone fragility. The child bruises easily and there is a tendency for frequent epistaxis. Dentition may be immature, and the teeth may break easily.

Treatment

Treatment consists of early intervention of fractures and prevention of deformities using splints, braces, casts, and surgery. Insertion of rods into the long bones may prevent future fractures. Healing usually requires long periods of time to promote remineralization of the bones. Adequate nutrition with supplements of calcium, magnesium, and vitamins are used to strengthen the bony structure. Because of the multiple fractures and bruising, caregivers of children with OI are often accused of child abuse until the disorder is diagnosed. A supportive, nonjudgmental approach is important for these families. Education of caregivers should include information about promoting normal development within the child's limitations and methods to protect the individual from injury.

Slipped Capital Femoral Epiphysis

Slipped capital femoral epiphysis (SCFE), the most common adolescent hip disorder, is the displacement of the femoral head from the femoral neck occurring through an open femoral capital physis (growth plate). The femoral head remains seated in the acetabulum, and the femoral neck moves upward and outward. The incidence of SCFE is 0.01 in 1,000 children and varies greatly with race, sex, and geographic location. Males are affected two to five times more than females. African-Americans have an increased incidence.

This disorder typically occurs during the adolescent growth spurt, and the left hip is affected more often than the right.

While the etiology of SCFE is unknown, an endocrine basis has been suggested because it is frequently accompanied by growth disturbances. Slippage most often occurs in obese and skeletally immature children, indicating a decrease in sex hormones, or in tall, thin individuals who have had a recent growth spurt, indicating an excess of growth hormone. Trauma is also a factor in its development and may cause an abrupt slip of the weakened growth plate.

Clinical Manifestations

Walking with a limp and pain are frequent findings in children with SCFE. The pain may be in the hip or groin or referred to the thigh or knee. Hip range of motion demonstrates limitation with internal rotation, abduction, and flexion. The child tends to walk with the leg externally rotated.

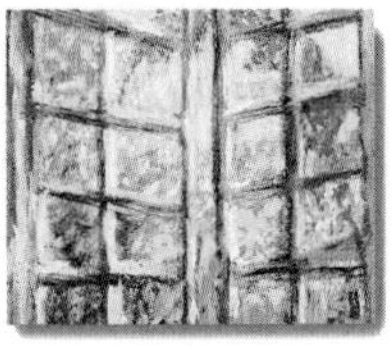

In the Real World

I began working with a boy born with clubfeet. The degree of severity was significant. Over the years this child has endured countless casts and surgeries. He has spent many days in a wheelchair and had to ride the special bus to school, not easy things when one is growing up. At 13, he has visible scars on his feet and ankles, heels that need to be aligned, and abnormally thin calves. In some people these issues would be devastating. However, this child is a bright, energetic, wonderful young man. I credit his parents for his positive adjustment to the clubfeet. They never held him back from doing anything, promoted his self-esteem, and allowed him to voice his feelings. I am buoyed by the physical and mental outcome of this young man. When I asked him how he is doing, he replied, "I am great! Happy to be walking around on my own two feet." I often think of this statement as I work with families in similar situations. It encourages me to really emphasize the client-teaching part of my job. I know that my teachings can have a positive effect.

Treatment

The goal of treatment is to prevent further slippage and complications and involves surgery. For mild to moderate SCFE the surgical procedure is percutaneous placement of pins across the growth plate into the femoral head to hold the head in place until closure of the femoral physis is attained. A small incision is made, and the child is able to ambulate with crutches shortly after surgery. Open correction (**osteotomy**) may be performed for chronic cases of SCFE or severe degrees of displacement. In this procedure the bone is redesigned surgically to alter the alignment or weight-bearing stress areas. Since there is an increased likelihood of SCFE to occur in the opposite hip, nurses should make sure the child and family are aware of symptoms such as pain or decrease in range of motion.

Key Concepts

- The differences in the musculoskeletal system of children as compared to adults' includes the child having a large amount of cartilage, the periosteum being stronger and tougher, and the growth plates being not yet closed.
- A significant number of school-aged children and adolescents experience musculoskeletal injuries related to sports and recreation, which account for substantial morbidity and cost.
- Most sports injuries in older children and adolescents affect the soft tissues rather than the bones. Examples of soft tissue injuries include sprains, strains, and muscle contusions.
- Types of fractures include transverse, oblique, spiral, and greenstick.
- Casting and traction are common fracture treatments.
- Injury to the epiphyseal growth plates is very serious in skeletally immature children because they can cause growth disruption, arrest, or uneven growth.
- Many musculoskeletal injuries and treatment methods can result in neurovascular compromise. Therefore, continuous assessment of neurovascular status is a key nursing responsibility.
- Oral antibiotic treatment for osteomyelitis and septic arthritis is effective only if the caregivers are compliant with the treatment protocol.
- Clubfoot is treated with serial casting. Surgery is necessary if casting is not effective.
- Treatment for developmental dysplasia of the hip includes an external abduction device such as a Pavlik harness, which maintains the head of the femur in the acetabulum.
- Instructing caregivers in the general care, skin care, and handling and positioning methods for the infant in a Pavlik harness ensures infant safety and the benefits of maintaining the hips in flexion and abduction.

- Duchenne muscular dystrophy is the most common type of muscular dystrophy in childhood. It is rapidly progressive resulting in loss of the ability to walk between 9 and 12 years of age and death by the early 20s.
- Scoliosis is treated with bracing and/or surgery, that is, spinal fusion with instrumentation.
- Legg-Calve-Perthes disease is characterized by avascular necrosis of the femoral head. The goal of treatment is to keep the femoral head in the acetabulum during the healing process with traction, casting, bracing, and/or surgery.

Review Questions

1. Discuss the nurse's role in preventing sports injuries.
2. Describe the differences between a sprain and a strain.
3. Discuss the treatment for a sprain.
4. What would be included in teaching caregivers about cast care?
5. List the different types of traction and explain each.
6. What important principles will the nurse use when caring for the child in traction?
7. What should be included in the assessment of the neurovascular status of a child who is immobilized?
8. List the clinical manifestations associated with osteomyelitis.
9. How would the nurse plan for caregiver involvement following surgery on the child with a clubfoot?
10. How would the nurse prepare the caregivers for the child going home in a Pavlik harness?
11. How would the nurse provide emotional support for the child with Duchenne muscular dystrophy and for the family?
12. What initial and ongoing assessments would the nurse make for an adolescent after spinal surgery?
13. Describe the treatment for the child with Legg-Calve-Perthes disease.
14. Why would the nurse advise parents of genetic testing if their child was born with osteogenesis imperfecta?

References

Adkins, L. (1997). Cast changes: Synthetic versus plaster. *Pediatric Nursing, 23*(4), 422–427.

American Academy of Pediatrics. (2000). Clinical practice guideline: Early detection of developmental dysplasia of the hip. *Pediatrics, 105*(4), 896–905.

Bachman, D., & Santora, S. (1993). Orthopedic trauma. In G. Fleisher & S. Ludwig (Eds.), *Textbook pediatric emergency medicine* (3rd ed.). Baltimore, MD: Williams & Wilkins.

Cheng, T., Fields, C., Brenner, R., Wright, J., Lomax, T., & Scheidt, P. (2000). Sports injuries: An important cause of morbidity in urban youth. *Pediatrics, 105*(3), e32.

Dykes, P. C. (1993). Minding the 5 P's of neurovascular assessment. *American Journal of Nursing, 93*(6), 38–39.

Fecht-Gramley, M. E. (1994). Emergency: Recognizing compartment syndrome. *American Journal of Nursing, 94*(10), 41.

Hergenroeder, A. (1998). Prevention of sports injuries. *Pediatrics, 101,* 1057–1063.

Hoffinger, S. (1996). Evaluation and management of pediatric foot deformities. *Pediatric Clinics of North America, 43*(5), 1091–1111.

Janas, J. (1996). Muscular dystrophy. *Nurse Practitioner Forum, 7*(4), 167–173.

Kyzer, S. P., & Stark, S. L. (1995). Congenital idiopathic clubfoot deformities. *Association of Operating Room Nurses, 61*(3), 492–503.

Landry, G. L., Lillegard, W. A., & Rice, S. G. (1998). Preventing sport injuries in kids. *Patient Care for the Nurse Practitioner, 1*(4), 24–35.

Luke, A., & Micheli, L. (1999). Sports injuries: Emergency assessment and field-side care. *Pediatrics in Review, 20*(9), 291–301.

Maher, A. B., Salmond, S. W., & Pellino, T. A. (1998). *Orthopaedic nursing* (2nd ed.). Philadelphia: W.B. Saunders.

Mandell, G. A. (1996). Imaging in the diagnosis of musculoskeletal infections in children. *Current Problems in Pediatrics, 26*(17), 218–237.

Mankin, K., & Zimbler, S. (1996). Foot and ankle injuries: Solving the diagnostic dilemmas. *Contemporary Pediatrics, 13*(3), 25–45.

Mills, D., & Muscari, M. (1998). Preventing sports injuries. *American Journal of Nursing, 98*(7), 58–60.

Monk, H. (1993). Fractures are never simple. *RN, 56*(4), 30–35.

Morrissy, R. T., & Weinstein, S. L. (Eds.). (1996). *Pediatric orthopaedics* (4th ed.). Philadelphia: Lippincott-Raven.

Nelson, J. (1997). Toward simple but safe management of osteomyelitis. *Pediatrics, 99*(6), 883–884.

Novacheck, T. F. (1996). Developmental dysplasia of the hip. *Pediatric Clinics of North America, 43*(4), 829–848.

Patterson, M. (1999). Prevention: The only care for pediatric trauma. *Orthopaedic Nursing, 18*(4), 16–20.

Puno, R., Mehta, S., & Byrd, J. (1994). Surgical treatment of idiopathic thoracolumbar and lumbar scoliosis in adolescent patients. *Orthopaedic Clinics of North America, 25*(2), 275–286.

Salmond, S. W., Mooney, N. E., & Verdisco, L. A. (Eds.). (1996). *National Association of Orthopedic Nurses (NAON): Core curriculum for nursing.* Pitman, New Jersey: Anthony J. Jannett.

Thompson, G., & Scoles, P. V. (1996). Sports medicine. In R. Behrman, R. Kliegman, & A. Arvin (Eds.), *Nelson textbook of pediatrics* (15th ed., pp.1958–1964), Philadelphia: W. B. Saunders.

Unkila-Kallio, L., Kallio, M., Eskola, J., & Peltola, H. (1994). Serum C-reactive protein, erythrocyte sedimentation rate, and white blood cell count in acute hematogenous osteomyelitis in children. *Pediatrics, 93*(1), 59–62.

Suggested Readings

Bialik, V., Bialik, G., Blazer, S., Sujov, P., Wiener, F., & Berant, M. (1999). Developmental dysplasia of the hip: A new approach to incidence. *Pediatrics, 103*(1), 93–99.

DeBoisblanc, B. (1997). The science of turning. *Critical Care Medicine, 25*(9), 1457–1645.

Goldberg, M. (2001). Early detection of developmental hip dysplasia: Synopsis of the AAP clinical practice guideline. *Pediatrics in Review, 22,* 131–134.

Gram, M., & Hasan, Z. (1999). The spinal curve in standing and sitting postures in children with idiopathic scoliosis. *Spine, 24*(2), 169–177.

Harcke, H. (1999). Developmental dysplasia of the hip: A spectrum of abnormality. *Pediatrics, 103*(1), 152–153.

Loder, R. (1998). Slipped capital femoral epiphysis. *American Family Physician, 59*(9), 2135–2142.

Peltola, H., Kallio, M., & Unkila-Kallio, L. (1998). Reduced incidence of septic arthritis in children by *Haemophilus influenzae* type B vaccination. *Journal of Bone and Joint Surgery, 80B,* 471–473.

Staheli, I. (1998). *Fundamentals of Pediatric Orthopedics* (2nd ed.). Philadelphia: Lippincott-Raven.

Theophilopoulos, E., & Barrett, D. (1998). Get a grip on the pediatric hip. *Contemporary Pediatrics, 15*(11), 43, 45, 49–50.

Resources

Organizations and Websites

Muscular Dystrophy Association of America
3300 East Sunrise Drive
Tucson, AZ 85718
(800) 572-1717
www.mdausa.org

Muscular Dystrophy Family Foundation, Inc.
2330 North Meridian Street
Indianapolis, IN 46208
(317) 632-8255
(800) 544-1213
www.mdff.org

National Scoliosis Foundation
5 Cabot Place
Stoughton, MA 02072
(781) 341-6333
(800) 673-6922
www.scoliosis.org

Osteogenesis Imperfecta Foundation, Inc.
804 West Diamond Avenue, Suite 210
Gaithersburg, MD 20878
(301) 947-0083
(800) 981-2663
www.oif.org

Scoliosis Association, Inc.
P.O. Box 811705
Boca Raton, FL 33481-1705
(800) 800-0669

Scoliosis Research Society
6300 N. River Road, Suite 727
Rosemont, IL 60018-4226
(847) 698-1627
www.srs.org

UNIT VIII

Other Alterations to Children's Health

CHAPTER 35

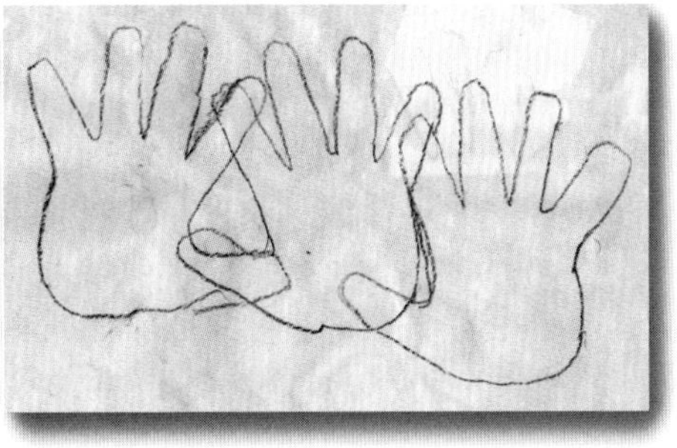

Even as a little boy, only 4 years old, Carson was unable to sit still. His attention span was very short, and he was disruptive in preschool. He would run around the library and pull all the books off the shelves. The librarian would walk over and ask him to help pick up the books, and he would shout, "I don't want to! I don't have to!" When he started school, the problems continued. Carson was getting bad grades, and his teachers were always sending home notes about his inability to complete tasks, blurting out answers before they could even finish asking questions, and forgetfulness. I knew he could do better. By the time he was 8 years old, I took him to our pediatrician. We went to several doctors before he was diagnosed with attention-deficit hyperactivity disorder. After much discussion and research, he began taking Ritalin at the age of $8^1/_2$. After a month, Carson was so happy with how much better his grades were and how many more friends he had. That was about 4 years ago. If Carson takes the medicine every day, he gets along so much better with me, his father, his brother, Sammy, and his friends, and he gets good grades.

PSYCHOSOCIAL ALTERATIONS

Jo Trilling, RNC, MS
Nicki L. Potts, PhD, RN

COMPETENCIES

Upon completion of this chapter, the reader will be able to:

- *Discuss various treatment modalities for children and adolescents with psychosocial alterations.*
- *Identify the primary clinical manifestations of attention-deficit hyperactivity disorder (ADHD).*
- *Develop a nursing care plan for a child with ADHD and the family.*
- *Differentiate between major depressive disorder and dysthymic disorder.*
- *Explain the conditions and circumstances that make an individual at high risk for suicide.*
- *Describe a means for assessing suicide potential in a child or adolescent.*
- *Define and describe the major anxiety disorders of childhood (separation anxiety disorder, school phobia or refusal, generalized anxiety disorder, social phobia, and post-traumatic stress disorder).*
- *List the types of substances subject to abuse by children and adolescents.*
- *Plan nursing care for individuals with eating disorders, including nutritional rehabilitation and psychotherapy.*

The number of children and adolescents in the United States who suffer from mental health disorders is staggering and has long-term implications, affecting their family and peer relationships, academic performance, future career and job potential, and economic self-sufficiency. However, children with mental health problems are one of the most underserved populations in the health care system. Inadequate distribution of services continues to compound the lack of availability of mental health services for children in rural and some urban areas.

Children and adolescents with psychosocial alterations or disorders are primarily treated in ambulatory and community settings. The nurse's role focuses on assessment, identification, referral, education, and support of the child and family, and working collaboratively with other disciplines in their therapy programs. The alterations included in this chapter include attention-deficit hyperactivity disorder, mood or depressive disorders, suicide, anxiety disorders, substance abuse, eating disorders, and failure to thrive.

Reflective Thinking

The Politically Active Nurse

A large percentage of children require mental health services. Even children with serious emotional disturbances appear to be greatly underserved. There is a need for effective systems of care in which agencies work collaboratively, and in which service delivery and financing are viewed comprehensively. The current political climate does not bode well for an increase in funds for services that are under considerable stress from high utilization. A proactive voice from professionals will be necessary to improve the availability of mental health services for children. How can you become politically active as a proponent of improved availability, access, and funding of mental health services for children and adolescents?

TREATMENT MODALITIES

Through therapy, improved communication skills, and self-knowledge children and their families gain hope and the ability to see their current situation in a new light, focusing on their strengths and abilities. They may be able to develop new patterns of behavior and more effective methods of coping with problems and concerns. The modalities and types of interventions used are based on the child's specific diagnosis, age, and developmental stage and are provided in the context of individual, family, or group therapy. Several modalities commonly used with children are discussed in the following sections.

Individual Therapy

Individual therapy involves the child or adolescent and a therapist and is usually used in conjunction with other treatment modalities. The focus is on the child's behavioral, developmental, and psychological issues and problems. The age, developmental level, and psychosocial alteration of the child determine the therapeutic interventions used. Caregivers are not in the session during individual therapy, but they are an important part of a comprehensive treatment program. The therapist and the child determine what will be shared with the caregivers. Older children may request that caregivers be denied access to their records.

Family Therapy

The focus of **family therapy** is the relationships and communication patterns among family members. The therapist looks at the child's symptoms or problems as a reflection of the family's problems. Family therapy may include the child, the primary caregivers, siblings, and other people from the extended family, for example, grandparents, ex-partners, and step siblings. The goal of therapy is to change family interactions, improve communication, and help each member achieve autonomy, independence, and self-effectiveness.

Group Therapy

Group therapy involves a group of children or adolescents, usually 6 to 10, with a focus on interpersonal relationships. Socialization process occurs among group members, and feedback and support come from peers rather than the therapist alone. This treatment modality is powerful and effective for the school-aged child and the adolescent because of the importance of peers for these age groups. Children learn to improve their social and communication skills through role modeling, group socialization, reality testing, feedback, and practice (Johnson, 1995).

Play Therapy

Play is the child's means of expression and often is called the work of childhood. As the child moves through each developmental stage, he or she learns to explore and communicate feelings and needs through play. One of the ways the child is prepared for more complex cognitive tasks of problem solving and abstract thought is through play. A child can also learn self-control and self-mastery, thereby increasing self-esteem. The focus of **play therapy** is to help the child reveal emotions, feelings, and problems. Toys, dolls, blocks, cars, or other play objects are used in the sessions. The process of being with the therapist, toy selection, and interaction during the therapy session are part of the therapeutic process. Anger, sadness, fear, and stress may be revealed, consciously or unconsciously, through play. The therapist is available to help the child understand her or his emotions and response to these emotions. Play therapy is usually individual but may be conducted in a group setting.

The initial stage of this type of therapy allows the therapist to assess the child and build a therapeutic relationship. In the middle stage, the child attempts to resolve conflicts and problems and work toward healthy personality change. During the termination, feelings of separation and rejection are worked through, and the therapist summarizes what changes have occurred for the child.

Art Therapy

In **art therapy** drawings and other art objects are used to help the therapist gain information about the child, her or his behaviors, concerns, and problems. The child is encouraged to use drawing as means to express feelings and issues that are difficult to verbalize. Drawings provide information about relevant situations and problems that are complex and remain hidden from the child's immediate level of consciousness.

Nursing Alert:

Using Drawing to Diagnose

Drawings should never be used solely to form a definitive diagnosis. They are used in conjunction with the history, assessment data, and other information.

ATTENTION-DEFICIT HYPERACTIVITY DISORDER

Attention-deficit hyperactivity disorder (ADHD) is characterized by inattention, hyperactivity, and impulsivity. It is the most commonly encountered neurobehavioral disorder of childhood (Brown, et al., 2001) and among the most prevalent chronic health conditions of school-aged children (American Academy of Pediatrics [AAP] Committee on Quality Improvement, Subcommittee on Attention-Deficit/Hyperactivity Disorder, 2000). The basic impairment in ADHD is a deficit with inhibiting behavior that interferes with the process of learning self-regulation behaviors. This deficiency of internal self-regulation typically results in school difficulties, academic underachievement, low self-esteem, and difficulties with family and social relationships. ADHD is now seen as a chronic disorder that may persist into adulthood. There are three subtypes: (1) ADHD primarily of inattentive type, (2) ADHD primarily of hyperactive-impulsive type, and (3) a combination of subtypes 1 and 2 (American Psychiatric Association [APA], 1994).

Incidence, Etiology, and Pathophysiology

Incidence rates generally range from 4% to 12% in school-aged children, ages 6 to 12 years (Brown, et al., 2001). Boys are four times more likely to be diagnosed with ADHD than girls (Scahill & Schwab-Stone, 2000). Girls are less likely than boys to exhibit disruptive and hyperactive behaviors, but tend to display more inattentive behaviors. The disorder is found in all cultures, although incidences differ. Whether these differences reflect real biological and psychological variation or merely variable diagnostic criteria is unclear. ADHD is frequently associated with the development of other disruptive disorders, particularly conduct disorder and oppositional-defiant disorder. Some experts think that the impulsivity and attention deficits associated with ADHD interfere with social learning or with attachment to caregivers in a way that predisposes to the development of behavior disorders (Barkley, 1998).

Etiology of ADHD is unknown, but the following factors have been suggested: genetic, neurophysiological, dietary, and environmental. The disorder is more common in first-degree relatives of the affected child than in the general population. Between 10% and 35% of these children have a first-degree relative with past or present ADHD (Swanson, et al., 2001). In fact, many of the parents of these children go through childhood and early adulthood with undiagnosed ADHD only to discover their own diagnosis when their child's symptoms bring her or him to clinical attention (Faraone & Doyle, 2000). Twin studies have shown that when ADHD is present in one twin, it is significantly more likely to occur in the other twin if the relationship is identical (monozygotic) rather than fraternal (dizygotic).

A deficiency in the neurotransmitter dopamine has also been implicated in ADHD. Dopamine plays a key role in initiating purposive movement, increasing alertness and motivation, reducing appetite, and inducing insomnia.

Dietary hypotheses have focused on food additives and refined sugar in children's diets. Although food coloring, additives, aspartame, and sugar may cause behavioral problems and hyperactivity in some children, well-controlled studies have demonstrated food additives and sugar have no adverse effects on children's cognitive functioning or behavior (Borowsky, 2000). Environmental factors that have been suggested as a cause of ADHD are maternal cigarette smoking (Milberger, Biederman, Faraone, & Jones, 1998), ingestion of alcohol or drugs, and elevated lead levels during pregnancy.

Clinical Manifestations

The primary clinical manifestations of ADHD are dependent on the subtype and include inattention, hyperactivity, and impulsivity. Inattention is the inability to sustain concentration for an appropriate period of time, and to disregard attending to external stimuli. Children with the symptom of inattention have difficulties with paying attention, excessive shifting of attention, distractibility, and screening out unimportant information. As a result they almost always have problems in school and are often mistakenly thought by teachers and caregivers to ignore instructions or assigned tasks or chores purposefully. Inattentive children have problems keeping their concentration on one idea; therefore, they may not listen, remember, or complete tasks. Because of these behaviors, they may underachieve in school and become frustrated or even depressed.

Hyperactive or overactive children tend to fidget or squirm, are disruptive in the classroom by frequently getting out of their seat, and interfere with teaching activities for other students. These behaviors often result in negative social consequences for the child with ADHD and interfere with peer relationships. Children exhibiting impulsivity may appear socially immature because they tend to interrupt and have difficulty delaying responses such as volunteering answers to class questions without being called on by the teacher. These behaviors are unpopular not only with fellow students but also with teachers. Impulsive children act before they think and are impatient.

Nursing Tip:

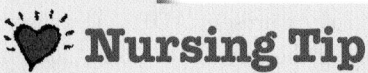

Conditions producing behaviors similar to ADHD

Children with other conditions can exhibit behaviors similar to those seen with ADHD:

- Underachievement at school because of a learning disability
- Attention lapses caused by absence seizures
- Intermittent hearing problems caused by otitis media
- Disruptive or unresponsive behavior caused by anxiety or depression

Diagnosis

Distinguishing between normal and ADHD behaviors is often difficult in the young child because developmental changes occur rapidly. Caregivers often wonder whether the child is just going through a stage, such as the "terrible twos," or whether the behaviors are early signs of ADHD (Lobar & Phillips, 1995). No one test or instrument is able to diagnose a child as having ADHD. Multiple data sources are used over a period of time to make the diagnosis and include: a complete health history; physical examination; behavior rating scales completed by teachers and caregivers; psychoeducational tests to identify learning disabilities, cognitive, language, and visual-spatial-motor problems; and the DSM-IV criteria.

In order to be diagnosed with ADHD the child must have six or more of the following symptoms of *inattention:* (1) fails to attend to details or makes careless mistakes in schoolwork, work, or other activities; (2) has difficulty sustaining attention with tasks or play activities; (3) is easily distracted; (4) does not follow instructions and complete what is started; (5) has difficulty with organization; (6) avoids or is reluctant to perform tasks that require sustained mental effort; (7) loses things needed for schoolwork or play activities; (8) does not seem to listen; and (9) is often forgetful. Additionally, six or more of the following symptoms of *hyperactivity/impulsivity* must also be present: (1) fidgets with hands or feet and squirms in seat; (2) leaves seat when remaining seated is expected; (3) talks excessively; (4) has difficulty playing quiet leisure activities; (5) runs or climbs excessively in situations where it is inappropriate; (6) is often characterized as "on the go" or "driven"; (7) interrupts with answers before the question is completed; (8) has difficulty taking turns; and (9) interrupts or intrudes in others' activities. The symptoms must have been present before the age of 7; occurred in two or more settings (home, school, or work); persisted for 6 or more months; and adversely affected functioning in school, work, or social situations (APA, 1994).

Treatment

Treatment includes pharmacotherapy, behavior management, educational interventions, and family education. Stimulant medications including methylphenidate (Ritalin), dextroamphetamine (Dexedrine), pemoline (Cylert), and a mixture of amphetamine salts (Adderall) consistently improve the symptoms of ADHD in the majority of children (Shaywitz, Fletcher, & Shaywitz, 2001). These drugs increase the availability of dopamine and norepinephrine in the neural synapses, thus improving concentration and attention, and reducing the child's activity level. Common side effects of these medications include anorexia, weight loss, abdominal pain, headache, insomnia, tachycardia, and hypertension or hypotension. If stimulants are ineffective or produce adverse side effects that are unacceptable to the child or caregivers, other medications may be used. Tricyclic antidepressants such as desipramine (Norpramin) and bupropion (Wellbutrin) have been used effectively.

Behavior management includes assisting the child to follow rules, complete tasks, and improve self-control, and providing positive feedback for appropriate behavior. Other techniques are clearly defining acceptable and unacceptable behaviors and the accompanying consequences and rewards, and periodically changing or varying them to motivate the child.

ADHD is regarded as a developmental disability; therefore, according to the federal law The Education for All Handicapped Children Act (Public Law 94-142), these children must receive free public education in the least restrictive environment. For this reason, many children with ADHD are "mainstreamed" in regular classrooms with their peers. When disruptive behavior is severe, special education or resource placement where the setting is smaller and more controlled may be recommended. Children with ADHD are often placed in classes with individuals who have serious psychiatric morbidity. Many caregivers are hesitant to agree to such placements out of concern for their child's emotional development and safety. Family education should provide information about the disorder, address concerns, and emphasize the child's and family's strengths. Caregivers should be reminded that they are not at fault for their child's situation and should be referred to and encouraged to seek ADHD support groups (Borowsky, 2000).

Many controversial treatments for ADHD have been proposed and used by caregivers who are eager to help their child. These alternative methods have been successful for some children but are not standard therapeutic treatments. There is no scientific evidence of improved behavioral or cognitive symptoms. Some of these controversial therapies include restricted diets, EEG biofeedback, megavitamins and mineral supplements, and chiropractic adjustment and bone re-alignment.

Nursing Management

Assessment

Assessment incorporates information from the child, caregivers, and teachers. The nurse may interview the child to gain information from his or her perspective. Direct observations of the child within the home and school will provide valuable data to assess the degree of inattention, impulsivity, motor hyperactivity, and behavioral problems.

Caregivers are an essential part of the assessment interview as their perceptions of the child's behaviors help determine the diagnosis. They can provide a detailed family and developmental history. They are also able to share information about the child's hyperactivity, attention deficits, and moods in the home. Standardized behavior rating scales are available for them to complete as part of the assessment process. Teachers' reports are also a part of the clinical assessment. Developmental age, language, and conceptual ability must be assessed to ensure an appropriate treatment plan is instituted. A physical examination should be performed to rule out any medical problems.

Nursing Diagnosis

The following diagnoses are relevant for the child with ADHD:

1. Impaired social interaction related to poor impulse control, short attention span, and aggressive behavior.
2. Risk for injury related to impulsivity and inability to perceive harm.
3. Chronic low self-esteem related to lack of satisfactory peer relationships and positive feedback, and academic underachievement.
4. Compromised family coping related to the child's disruptive and intrusive behaviors, hyperactivity, and inability to heed directions.

Outcome Identification

1. The child will demonstrate acceptable social skills and improved ability to interact with peers.
2. The child will be free of injury and/or unnecessary risks.
3. The child will demonstrate increased feelings of self-worth by verbalizing positive statements about himself or herself.
4. The family will identify coping strategies for managing disruptive and intrusive behaviors.
5. The caregivers will set appropriate limits and structure the environment to facilitate the child's developing increased control over own behavior.

Planning/Implementation

Because pharmacotherapy is a major aspect of the treatment for the child with ADHD, education of the caregivers about the medication regimen is vital. The nurse teaches them about the importance of the regimen and about the side effects. The nurse works with the family to encourage compliance and explores their feelings and concerns that might impede this. Do they fear they are "drugging" their child by giving the medication? Are they concerned that giving their child a stimulant medication will lead to drug addiction later in life? Weight, height, and blood pressure are frequently monitored if the child is taking stimulant medication. Growth rate may be decreased, and weight loss is common during the first few months of treatment and with long-term use because of appetite suppression. "Drug holidays" may be used every few months to determine if therapy is still necessary.

Caregivers need to be well educated about ADHD because of their involvement in the treatment, that is, implementing a behavioral management program at home. They often have to educate others, such as school personnel, about the needs of their child. The nurse should provide them with information about strategies for implementing the treatment regimen at home (see Box 35-1 and Box 35-2).

BOX 35-1 Home interventions for the child with ADHD

1. Develop specific time periods for waking, bedtime, chores, homework, playtime, TV, and meals. Maintain consistency in the child's routine. Explain any changes in routine ahead of time so that the child understands and can anticipate the changes.
2. Establish clear and concise rules of acceptable and appropriate behavior for the child. Rules, as well as consequences and rewards for appropriate behavior, can be written down and posted in a prominent place.
3. Give instructions as simply and clearly as possible, demonstrating if necessary. Ask the child to repeat them back to you. Then praise the individual when responding correctly.
4. Do not give more than one or two instructions at a time. If a task is difficult, break it into smaller parts and teach each separately.
5. Provide the child time with his or her own "special" quiet spot without distractions in which to do school work.
6. Allow the child choices within the limits you have set.
7. Help the child find avenues of self-expression that will help him or her express wants in acceptable, useful ways.
8. Provide positive feedback and praise for appropriate behaviors and tasks completed.

BOX 35-2 Controversy regarding Ritalin

There has been concern from the public regarding the overdiagnosis of ADHD and the overprescribed use of Ritalin (AAP, 2000). There are many opinions circulating. It is important for the caregivers to understand that they are just opinions. What is right for their child can only come from consultation with qualified individuals and thorough diagnostic testing.

Family support is necessary initially to help caregivers understand the complexity of the disorder and to deal with their feelings of possible guilt and shock. Support groups for families are helpful and may offer understanding and expertise in managing daily problems of living with the child with ADHD.

Evaluation

The nurse acts as a liaison between health care providers, the home, and school to coordinate referrals and to promote ongoing evaluation of intervention strategies. Indications that the interventions are effective include an increase in the child's ability to concentrate, fewer disruptive and intrusive behaviors, improvement in academic performance, and more positive social relationships. An evaluation of the interventions for the caregivers and other family members focuses on their acceptance of the diagnosis, understanding of the disorder and treatment regimen, compliance with the medication administration, and provision of a safe and supportive home environment.

Family Teaching

Caregivers will monitor medication administration for the younger child; therefore, awareness of side effects is essential. Education for the caregivers, child, and siblings regarding characteristics and interventions for ADHD is essential. Children with ADHD need to understand that they have a manageable illness, and that there are many resources such as support groups, medication therapy, and organizational strategies available to help them.

MOOD DISORDERS

Mood disorders, also referred to as depressive disorders, are common among children and adolescents, but are frequently unrecognized. Only recently have mood disorders come to be recognized and treated in this population. In the past it was believed that this age group lacked the psychological and cognitive structure necessary to experience these problems. Previously children could spend years in severe depression without their symptoms being recognized, diagnosed, or treated. However, a growing body of evidence has confirmed that they not only experience the whole spectrum of mood disorders, but also suffer from the significant morbidity and mortality (from suicide) associated with them (Son & Kirchner, 2000).

There are two types of mood disorders: bipolar disorder and depressive disorder, which has two subtypes, major depressive disorder (MDD) and dysthymic disorder (DD). Bipolar disorder is characterized by episodes of depression alternating with episodes of mania. MDD is marked by a single episode or recurrent episodes of depression, whereas DD involves a chronic disturbance of mood.

Incidence, Etiology, and Pathophysiology

The incidence of MDD is estimated to be approximately 1% in preschoolers, 2% in school-aged children, and 5–8% in adolescents (Birmaher, Brent, & Benson, 1998; Jellinek & Snyder, 1998). The ratio of boys and girls is equal in prepubertal children but increases to a 2:1 female-to-male ratio in adolescents. The incidence of depression appears to be increasing with each successive generation, and depressive disorders are being recognized at a younger age (Birmaher, et al., 1998). DD has an incidence of 0.6%–1.7% in prepubertal children and 1.6%–8% in adolescents (Birmaher, et al., 1996).

Many theories about the etiology of depression have been proposed, such as genetic, biological, and psychosocial ones; however, the exact cause is not known, partly because less research has been conducted with children. Children with at least one depressed parent are more than three times as likely to have a lifetime episode of MDD than children with non-depressed parents (Birmaher, et al., 1996). Biological theory proposes that the lack or excess of one or more neurotransmitters, specifically, serotonin, and endocrine dysfunction may contribute to the development of depression (Laraia, 1996).

Psychosocial factors include family dysfunction, personality dynamics, and exposure to negative or adverse life events. Family interactions characterized by conflict, child maltreatment, rejection, and lack of expression of affection and support may be risk factors. Caregivers of depressed children have high rates of psychiatric disorders, including anxiety, substance abuse, and personality (antisocial) disorders (Kovacs, Obrosky, Gatsonis, & Richards, 1997). Personality dynamics such as unrealistic, overly harsh, internal judgment of the child's own impulses, thoughts, and mood may contribute to the development of depression. These dynamics contribute to low self-esteem, self-blame, and shame, which are prominent in MDD. Depressed children report having experienced significantly more adverse or negative life events in areas of school, relationships with friends or caregivers, health, and work than their non-depressed counterparts. Exposure to the loss of a caregiver through death, separation, or divorce also raises the risk (Birmaher, et al., 1996).

Clinical Manifestations

The clinical manifestations of MDD in children and adolescents are similar to those seen in adults and include one or more major depressive episodes lasting on average from 7 to 9 months (Birmaher, et al., 1996). In order to be diagnosed with MDD, the child must experience five or more of the following symptoms: (1) depressed or irritable mood; (2) markedly diminished interest or pleasure in previously enjoyed activities (**anhedonia**); (3) changes in eating habits indicated by weight loss or gain; (4) psychomotor agitation or retardation; (5) feelings of worthlessness or inappropriate guilt; (6) diminished ability to think or concentrate; (7) fatigue or energy loss; (8) insomnia or hypersomnia; and (9) recurrent thoughts of death and suicidal ideation. The symptoms must cause clinically significant distress or impairment in social, school, or other important areas of functioning (APA, 1994). The distinction between the depressed child and the unhappy child is made by determining the duration of the sad mood. A child with MDD experiences a depressed mood that persists for most of the day, nearly every day for least 2 consecutive weeks (APA, 1994) (Figure 35-1).

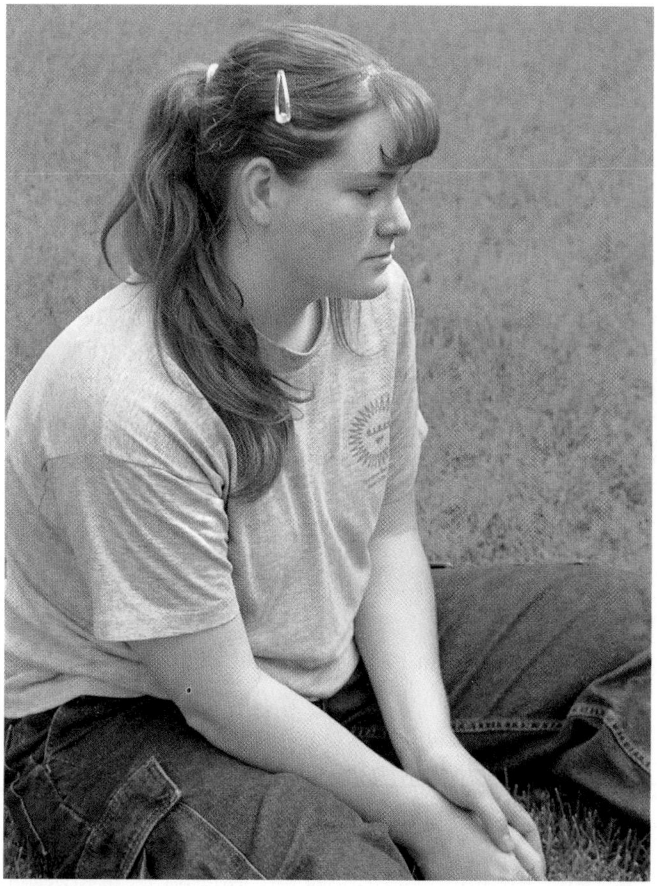

Figure 35-1 Loneliness and depression may be seen in some adolescents.

Nursing Alert:

Irritability in Children with Depressive Disorders
Children with depressive disorders often exhibit irritability as a manifestation of depression. This irritable mood may lead to aggression.

Compared to adults, depressed children are often irritable, are more likely to express symptoms of anxiety (such as school or social phobia), and have more somatic complaints, such as stomachaches and headaches. The presentation of MDD in adolescents is manifested by more impairments in functioning than younger children, but more behavioral problems than adults. Forty to 70% of children and adolescents with MDD also have other psychiatric disorders including anxiety disorders, disruptive disorders (conduct disorder, ADHD), substance abuse, and personality disorders (Son & Kirchner, 2000).

DD consists of a persistent long-term depressed mood that is less intense but more chaotic than in MDD. The affected child has a depressed or irritable mood for most of the day, on most days, for a period of one year (Kovacs, et al., 1997). Other manifestations of DD are poor appetite or overeating, low energy or fatigue, poor concentration, difficulty making decisions, and feelings of hopelessness (Son & Kirchner, 2000). Because the development of DD is one of the major pathways to recurrent depressive disorders, early identification and treatment are critical (Cicchetti & Toth, 1998).

Diagnosis

The most useful tool in diagnosing depressive disorders is a comprehensive evaluation, including interviews with the child, caregivers, teachers, and social services professionals if appropriate. Clinician-completed rating scales and self-report instruments may also be used. The following instruments are used in pediatrics: (1) Children's Depression Inventory, (2) Beck Depression Inventory, (3) Zung Self-Rating Depression Scale (Kowath, Emslie, & Kennard, 1996). A thorough physical evaluation is necessary as a number of medical disorders can mimic depression, such as mononucleosis, seizure disorder, hypo- and hyperthyroidism, drug abuse and withdrawal, and other psychiatric disorders. Lastly, a developmental history, a family history of psychiatric disorders, and an assessment of home and school environments, and potential stressors are obtained (Cassidy & Jellinek, 1998). The history and physical examination can help determine which laboratory tests may be appropriate.

Treatment

Treatment is usually psychotherapy and psychotropic medication. Psychotherapy encompasses a multitude of approaches including play therapy; individual, family, and

Nursing Tip:

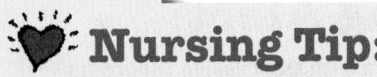

Ethnic and cultural factors and depression

It is imperative for the health care provider to be alert to ethnic and cultural factors that may influence the assessment of depressive disorder. Children from many cultures or ethnic groups are encouraged to be silent and to avoid direct eye contact when in the presence of authority figures. These behaviors easily can be misinterpreted as indicators of depression, and the child may be misdiagnosed with MDD or DD.

Eye On:

Complementary Alternative Therapy for the Child with Depression

Complementary alternative medicine (CAM) may be used in the treatment of depression. St. John's wort and many other herbal remedies have been effective for some individuals. Knowledge about the side effects and efficacy of CAM for treating depression is important, but research with herbs is limited in children. The research that has been performed has used adults as subjects. The nurse should query caregivers and the child as to herbal use.

group therapy; and **cognitive behavioral therapy** (CBT). CBT is a behavioral modification using stimulus and response to alter inappropriate behavior. Appropriate behavior is reinforced while inappropriate behavior is extinguished and replaced with a more desirable one. CBT is based on the premise that individuals with depression have cognitive distortions in how they view themselves, the world, and the future that contribute to their depression. CBT teaches them to identify and change these cognitions. It is important to determine the child's developmental and cognitive level in deciding the most appropriate approach. For example, play therapy would be appropriate for the preschool-aged child with depression, while individual, group, and CBT would be more appropriate for older children and adolescents (Son & Kirchner, 2000). Group therapy is effective for adolescents because of the importance of the peer group and is most effective if individuals in the group have a variety of diagnoses, as the depressed adolescent is often quiet, withdrawn, and non-interactive. Within the group the adolescent learns interpersonal and communication skills and expression of affect. Role playing and social interaction skills are used in the group setting (Pearson, 1995).

Antidepressants may be prescribed. Research in children and adolescents has failed to demonstrate the effectiveness of tricyclic antidepressants, including imipramine (Tofranil) and amitriptyline (Elavil). However, the selective serotonin reuptake inhibitors (SSRIs) such as fluoxetine (Prozac), sertraline hydrochloride (Zoloft), and paroxetine (Paxil) appear to have efficacy and safety (Kutcher, 1998; Emslie, et al., 1997; Strober, et al., 1999). The SSRIs dominate the pharmocotherapy of depression because of their relatively safe side effect profile, very low lethality after overdose, and easy administration (once a day).

Hospitalization is based on the seriousness of the mood disorder as determined by assessment and observation of the child. The hospital provides a safe and controlled environment and has strategies for protecting the child with suicidal behaviors or ideation. These measures include restrictions or precaution status that limit the child's movements and activities in the hospital setting (Pearson, 1995).

Nursing Management

Assessment

A thorough history from the child and caregivers is important in the nurse's assessment. When asking children about the feelings of depression, a variety of words such as sad, depressed, blue, down, and very unhappy should be used. Depending on the child's developmental and cognitive level, information about sleep problems, somatic complaints, worries and stressors, feelings of worthlessness, and suicide ideation should be obtained. Caregivers can provide information about the duration of depressed mood, observable behaviors, sleep disturbances, somatic complaints, self-deprecatory remarks, and recent family stressful events (moving, death of family member or pet, loss of a job). Teachers need to be asked about changes in the child's academic performance and grades and peer relationships.

Nursing Diagnosis

Nursing diagnoses for a child with depression may include the following:

1. Low self-esteem related to cognitive distortions, negative view of self, feelings of worthlessness.
2. Impaired social interaction related to low self-esteem, withdrawn behavior, and feelings of worthlessness.
3. Disturbed sleep pattern related to biochemical alterations (decreased serotonin), lack of activity, and anxiety.
4. Risk for injury: self-directed, related to depressed mood, feelings of worthlessness and hopelessness, and verbalization of suicidal ideation or plan.

Outcome Identification

1. The child will express positive feelings about self and will display more self-confidence.
2. The child will interact appropriately with others.
3. The child will demonstrate less withdrawn behavior and will be less socially isolated.
4. The child will verbalize improved sleep patterns and will be free of signs of sleep deprivation (irritability, lethargy).
5. The child will remain safe and free from self-inflicted harm.

Planning/Implementation

A major focus for nursing intervention is education of the child and family about the disorder and treatment. This not only enhances their understanding but can also improve compliance with therapy. Because of the high incidence of depressive disorders in first-degree relatives of the child with MDD, family education can be an integral component of improving the individual's environment and support structure by allowing for the treatment of the whole family. This education should occur within the child's community as well, especially the school, to provide improved support in all settings.

Caregivers need to know that SSRIs usually take several weeks before the child will feel less depressed. The nurse instructs the child and caregivers about the possible side effects such as agitation, nausea, increased anxiety, insomnia, and changes in appetite. Depression in children and adolescents is often unrecognized and unnoticed; therefore, an important nursing function is the recognition of depression and suicidal ideation. Because mood disorders do increase the risk of suicide, any suicidal ideation or behavior should be taken seriously and appropriate action taken.

Evaluation

Evaluation of nursing interventions for the depressed child may be facilitated by gathering information using the following types of questions: Is the child able to express being less sad? Does the child express positive aspects of self and feelings of worthiness? Does the child resume normal sleeping patterns? Does the child seem interested in others? Is the child seeking out interaction with others? Has self-harm to the child been avoided?

Family Teaching

Family dysfunction is a risk factor for depression; therefore, the nurse works with the family to improve their overall functioning. Interventions with the family focus on their willingness to participate in therapy and the importance of following planned interventions in the home. The family needs to be able to assess the child's risk to himself or herself.

SUICIDE

Suicide is the intentional or purposeful taking of one's own life. It is the ultimate act of self-destruction. Suicide may be completed, attempted, or **suicidal ideation** (thoughts about killing oneself). Because mood disorders increase the risk of suicide, any suicidal behavior is a matter of serious concern.

Incidence, Etiology, and Pathophysiology

While completed suicide is relatively rare in children, the incidence of suicide attempts reaches a peak during mid-adolescent years. Mortality from suicide, which increases steadily through the teens, is the third leading cause of death in 15 to 19 year olds. The number of adolescents committing suicide in the United States has increased dramatically over the last few decades. The actual incidence from suicide is estimated to be 0.11 per 1,000 (AAP Committee on Adolescence, 2000). From 1950 to 1990, the suicide rate for the 15 to 19-year-old group increased by 300%. The National Youth Risk Behavior Survey of students in high school indicated that nearly one-fourth (24%) had seriously considered suicide; 17.7% had made a specific plan; and 8.7% had attempted suicide during the 12 months preceding the study (CDC, 1996).

Suicide affects adolescents of all races and socioeconomic groups, yet some groups have higher rates than others. Native American males have the highest rates; African-American females have the lowest. Gay and bisexual individuals have rates of attempting suicide three times higher than other adolescents. Females are three times as likely to attempt suicide, whereas males are three times as likely to succeed in their attempts. Firearms are the leading cause of death for males and females committing suicide and are used in more than 67% of all suicides. Ingestion of pills is the most common method used among those who attempt suicide (AAP Committee on Adolescence, 2000).

Stresses related to psychosocial, psychosexual, and physiological issues have been identified as causes for the increasing number of suicides (Murray & Zentner, 2001). Children and adolescents at higher risk for suicide typically have a history of depression, have previous suicide attempts, a family history of psychiatric disorders (depression and suicidal behavior), family disruption, alcohol use and abuse, a chronic or debilitating physical disorder, history of physical or sexual abuse, and a recent relationship breakup (Borowsky, Ireland, & Resnick, 2001).

Diagnosis

The suicide-risk diagnosis is made when certain warning signs are present (Box 35-3) (Fritz & Barbie, 1993). Many suicidal children and adolescents have experienced the warning signs for at least a month before the suicide or

BOX 35-3 Warning signs of suicide

- Major life changes such as death of a family member or friend (especially by suicide), separation or divorce, and loss of financial security
- Suicidal clues (giving away possessions, writing or talking about death, suicide, or self-harm)
- Decreased performance in school or work
- Accident proneness
- Mood swings
- Withdrawal from family and friends
- Increase in alcohol or drug use
- Change in appetite
- Loss of interest in personal appearance

Nursing Alert:

The Decision to Commit Suicide

A sudden change in affect for the better or a dramatic lifting of depression may be an indication that the individual has resolved the ambivalence about living or dying and has made the decision to commit suicide. Increased energy and the ability to concentrate and plan facilitate the suicidal actions.

attempt. Days or weeks of loneliness usually precede the attempt due to the loss of the few remaining relationships.

Treatment

Children and adolescents who are at high risk for suicide have a well-thought-out plan that includes the method, place, time, clear intent, and no rescue plan. The degree of intent is related to the lethality of the method. Use of a firearm has a high degree of lethality, whereas taking pills in the presence of friends is considered a low risk because there is a good chance of rescue (Jellinek & Snyder, 1998). For those who are at high risk or have previously attempted suicide, evaluation by a mental health professional should be performed immediately. This can be obtained in a hospital, an emergency department, or via an appointment the same day with a professional. The safest course of action is hospitalization in which a safe, protected environment can be provided. The individual can have a thorough medical and psychiatric evaluation, and therapy can be initiated. Those who are not at high risk should be followed up closely and/or referred for a psychological or mental health evaluation.

Nursing Management

Assessment of clients at risk for suicide includes gathering information about individual and family history of depression and suicide attempts, mood changes, cognitive changes including suicidal ideation, expression of feelings of despondency and hopelessness, and behavioral or social changes. Obtaining information from caregivers and significant others in the child's social and support systems is essential. Physical assessment for health problems and changes in sleeping and eating patterns is also part of the assessment. Children and adolescents with high risk behaviors and high risk factors should be asked about suicide. Inquiring about suicide does not precipitate the behavior, as is commonly believed. In fact, most individuals are relieved that someone has heard and recognized their cry for help. One approach to this process is to ask a general question such as "Have you ever been so depressed or sad that you thought about killing yourself or wished you were dead?" (AAP Committee on Adolescence, 2000). If the answer is yes, the nurse should ask about the suicide plan (method, time, place), availability of the means (gun, rope, medication), lethality of the means, the individual's support system, and coping resources.

Nursing management focuses on the safety of the child and all family members. Threats or gestures to hurt oneself are always taken seriously regardless of the child's developmental age (Figure 35-2). Interventions are on the primary, secondary, or tertiary level. The focus of the interventions is to keep the child safe and provide the least restrictive setting possible (Pearson, 1995).

Primary interventions include activities that provide support, information, and education. At the primary level the nurse can offer educational programs for children and their caregivers that focus on parenting, development of coping skills, normal growth and development, and risk factors. Caregivers need to be taught to identify risk factors and symptoms of depression. The school nurse and counselor can

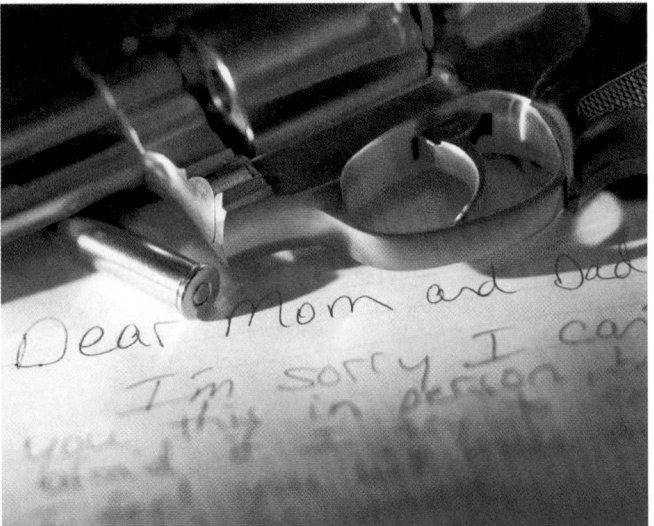

Figure 35-2 The nurse must raise awareness of the warning signs of suicide risk. Copyright ©2001 PhotoDisc, Inc.

Research Highlight

Suicide and Access to Firearms

Study Purpose

To determine whether there was a difference in an adolescent's household access to firearms between those who did commit suicide and those who did not.

Methods

A case-control design was used to compare 36 adolescents who committed suicide using firearms with an equal number of adolescents matched for age and sex. Controls were randomly selected from the same schools attended by the adolescents who committed suicide. Study participants were an average of 15 years of age, and 75% were males. Data were collected by telephone interview with caregivers of both groups.

Findings

The majority (67%) of those who committed suicide used a gun (handgun = 42%; rifle = 46%) obtained from their homes. The majority of these guns were not in locked storage. Those who committed suicide were significantly more likely than controls not to attend school and to be the only child in the family. Past mental health problems and conduct disorder were found as independent risk factors associated with those who committed suicide with guns.

Implications

Findings from this research suggest that public health interventions should be instituted to limit household access to firearms and to identify those at risk for this type of suicide. Although previous suicide attempts were not measured in this study, it is important for nurses and health care providers working in emergency departments to discuss access to firearms with caregivers of any adolescent who is treated for attempted suicide. It is also important for school nurses to follow up by implementing suicide prevention with adolescents who have a history of mental health problems or conduct disorder.

Citation

Shah, S., Hoffman, W., & Marine, W. (2000). Adolescent suicide and household access to firearms in Colorado: Results of a case-control study. *Journal of Adolescent Health, 26,* 157–163.

be instrumental in the development of programs that focus on strengthening children's awareness of their feelings, building self-esteem, and enhancing coping skills (Pearson, 1995). Secondary interventions involve the treatment of the actual suicidal crisis. Key elements in the success of any treatment modality include: establishing a personal relationship with the suicidal child or adolescent; encouraging more realistic problem solving behavior; and reaffirming hope for the individual.

Tertiary interventions are provided for the child or adolescent after a suicide attempt or for the family and friends of a person who has committed suicide. Self-help groups have been beneficial for the survivors of the youth who has committed suicide. Nurses working with clients who successfully commit suicide need the opportunity to work through their own feelings of self-blame, grief, and guilt. Debriefing sessions and support groups may be a routine part of work environments to support nurses after a client successfully commits suicide (Workman & Prior, 1997).

Family Teaching

Caregivers' ability to identify behaviors associated with depression and anxiety disorders decreases the risk of a successful suicide for the child. Therefore, educational programs focusing on suicide and risk factors can be part of family educational programs offered by community-based nurses.

Family dysfunction is correlated with depression and suicide. Social service programs that improve family functioning for the at-risk family will improve the outlook for the at-risk child.

ANXIETY DISORDERS

The child growing up in today's world deals with complex and rapidly changing norms. Anxiety is unavoidable and can be useful in promoting growth and helping the child adapt to new experiences. However, if anxiety is overwhelming, it can result in psychosocial alterations. Anxiety is a sense of apprehension or uneasiness caused by uncertain, nonspecific danger or threat. The child may cope with anxiety or fear by becoming overly dependent, avoiding problems, or withdrawing. Anxiety disorders are one of the prevalent categories of child and adolescent psychopathology (American Academy of Child and Adolescent Psychiatry [AACAP], 1997a). Included in the category of anxiety disorders are separation anxiety disorder, school phobia or refusal, generalized anxiety disorder, and social phobia.

The essential characteristic of separation anxiety disorder (SAD) is marked anxiety about separation from major attachment figures, home, or familiar surroundings, which is beyond that expected for the child's developmental level (APA, 1994). At the time of separation, the child's anxiety may approach panic level. Separation anxiety is a part of normal development from the age of 7 months through preschool years (Dashiff, 1995). Separation anxiety that occurs in older children, persists for more than 1 month, and causes difficulty in functioning (e.g., refuses to leave the caregiver and house to play with peers) is considered SAD (APA, 1994).

A form of separation anxiety is school phobia or refusal, which is defined as difficulty attending or remaining in school for an entire day, associated with emotional distress, especially anxiety and depression (King & Bernstein, 2001). Children who refuse to attend school are generally suffering from separation anxiety rather than a true phobia. The caregivers often have ambivalent feelings about their child's attendance, which contributes to their ineffectiveness in helping to return the child to school.

Generalized anxiety disorder (GAD), previously called overanxious disorder, is characterized by excessive worry and anxiety about future events, such as academic or athletic performance, being on time, or natural disasters (hurricanes, earthquakes). These children and adolescents worry even when school and social successes demonstrate that they have nothing substantive to be concerned about. They are often labeled as "worriers."

Children with social phobia either avoid or endure with significant distress social or performance situations in which they anticipate scrutiny by others, embarrassment, and humiliation (Compton, Nelson, & March, 2000). For some children anxiety can be provoked by nonjudgmental situations such as simple conversation or even eating in public.

Incidence, Etiology, and Pathophysiology

The incidence of SAD ranges from 3.5% to 5.4% (Compton, et al., 2000) and the disorder manifests at anytime from 5 to 16 years of age, with a mean age of 9 years. The incidence decreases with age. School refusal occurs in approximately 5% of all school-aged children, tends to be equally common in boys and girls, and can occur throughout the entire range of school years. However, the disorder peaks at certain ages (between 5–6 years and 10–11 years) and certain transition points in the child's life. The incidence of generalized anxiety disorder is relatively stable for girls from 10 to 20 years of age at 14% to 15%. For boys the rate declines with age from 13% in 10 to 13 year olds, to 5% thereafter (Cohen, Cohen, & Brook, 1993). The onset of social phobia most commonly occurs in early to mid-adolescence, and similar numbers of males and females develop the disorder (Bernstein, Borchardt, & Perwien, 1996). Individuals with social phobia have a high incidence of concurrent anxiety and mood disorders. Social phobia is more prevalent in girls than boys and in Caucasian children from middle- and upper-class families.

The cause of anxiety disorders is not known. Environmental as well as biological factors have been suggested. More research is needed to determine the exact cause. Some researchers have suggested that between the ages of 6 and 8 children should be watched for signs of anxiety disorders because at this age they are usually less fearful of the dark and imaginary images, but may become fearful of school, social situations, and relationships.

Clinical Manifestations

A child with separation anxiety disorder may exhibit complaints of stomachaches, headaches, nausea, vomiting, and low-grade fevers that occur without any underlying physiologic cause. Older children experience symptoms such as vertigo, palpitations, and faintness. These symptoms usually improve gradually as the day progresses.

School refusal behavior is a serious problem because it is often associated with significant short- and long-term consequences. Short-term problems include poor academic performance, family difficulties, and peer relationship problems. Long-term sequelae may include fewer opportunities to attend institutions of higher learning, employment problems, social difficulties, and increased risk for later psychiatric illnesses (Kearney & Albano, 2000). Clinical manifestations may also include frequent somatic complaints in the absence of a physical condition (stomachache, headache, dizziness, fatigue), sleep difficulties, morning tantrums, and marked distress on school days (King & Bernstein, 2001).

In addition to excessive worry and anxiety about future events, the clinical manifestations of generalized anxiety disorder include:

- Restlessness
- Fatigue
- Difficulty concentrating
- Irritability
- Sleep disturbances
- Muscle tension

Children with social phobia experience feelings of anxiety, which can often produce physical reactions such as tremors, palpitations, sweating, diarrhea, and blushing.

Diagnosis

The diagnosis is made if excessive anxiety or worry predominates the child's thoughts and begins to interfere with the ability to function and perform regular activities. Inquiry about anxiety symptoms should be a standard part of a diagnostic interview regardless of the presenting problem. Often these symptoms will not be elicited unless specifically asked about. Caregivers should be asked about the child's verbal expressions of fear or worry and signs of anxiety such as sweating, hyperventilation, and somatic complaints. A family history of anxiety and mood disorders and other psychiatric conditions should be obtained. The developmental and social history needs to be detailed enough to give the examiner a sense of the child's usual style of coping with stress in general and anxiety provoking situations in particular. The caregivers' coping styles should also be asked about.

Treatment

The broad goals of treatment are (1) to reduce the symptoms and relieve distress, (2) to minimize the disability associated with the disorder, and (3) to enhance the developmental potential of the child or adolescent. Although anxiety disorders are relatively common in children and adolescents, there has been little definitive research on the efficacy of psychotherapy (Kendall, et al., 1997). The treatment usually involves a variety of approaches including education of the individual and caregivers about the disorder, consultation with school personnel, cognitive behavioral interventions, individual and family psychotherapy, and pharmacological therapy. Treatment approaches are individualized for the child and the specific disorder. Family therapy allows the family to gain insight into the dynamics of the disorder. Cognitive, supportive, and behavioral psychotherapy have been used with varying degrees of success. Individual therapy is used to address the specific problems the child or adolescent experiences. For the child with school refusal the goal of therapy is to return the child to school as soon as possible. Cognitive techniques such as desensitization and operant conditioning are treatment methods used for this purpose (Martini, 1995).

Psychotropic drugs should not be used as a sole intervention, but as an adjunct to psychotherapeutic interventions. Commonly used medications include the antidepressants (tricyclics and SSRIs) and the benzodiazepines or anti-anxiety drugs. The benzodiazepines such as lorazepam (Atavan) or diazepam (Valium) may be used on a short-term basis for the anxiety symptoms and/or sleep disturbances.

Nursing Management

Assessment

A school nurse may be the person who identifies patterns of absenteeism or tardiness in attendance. Calling caregivers to inform them and discuss the patterns may give them an opportunity to discuss their concerns about the child's fear of school. A child with school phobia or refusal will present with frequent complaints of illness especially of stomachaches early in the morning, which go away as the day progresses. Well-child visits to the care providers are another avenue where the nurse may be available to listen to a caregiver's concerns about the child's anxiety about school or other anxious situations.

Nursing Diagnosis

Nursing diagnoses for children experiencing anxiety disorders may include the following:

1. Fear related to separation from caregiver and social or performance situations.
2. Impaired social interaction related to inability to interact with unfamiliar people and insufficient contact with peers.
3. Ineffective individual coping related to perception of the situation and changes in personal and family life.

Outcome Identification

1. The child will be able to experience normal developmental situations (staying overnight at a friend's house, attending camp) with minimal anxiety.
2. The child will attend school and experience minimal or no anxiety.
3. The child will initiate social interactions with peers.
4. The child will cope effectively with anxiety.
5. The child will use relaxation, deep breathing techniques, and self-talk to control anxiety.

Planning/Implementation

The family of the child with an anxiety disorder should be included in every aspect of the care. Caregivers provide important historical information about the child and give insight into the working of the family unit. They are involved in the implementation of the treatment plan; therefore, compliance depends on their cooperation (Martini, 1995). The nurse can assist the child in identifying sources of anxiety and tensions, and environmental factors that create a feeling of anxiety. Nurses should teach caregivers to recognize that a change in school performance may indicate anxiety. The child should be helped to identify alternative outlets for anxiety such as sports, running, climbing, and group games. The nurse can assist caregivers in exploring ways in which they reinforce dependent behavior in the child and in adopting alternative patterns of behavior. Teaching the child and caregivers to monitor the effectiveness and side effects of psychotropic drugs is also an important part of the nurse's role.

Evaluation

Is the child able to attend school? Does the child participate in social activities, such as visits to a friend's home, "sleep-overs," and camp? Is the child able to recognize feelings of anxiety and use techniques that help control the feelings? Are caregivers knowledgeable about normal developmental milestones and are their expectations of the child realistic?

Family Teaching

Changing family structure and contemporary culture contribute to the stress of childhood, and caregivers serve as protectors and teachers for their children. Parenting skills that reinforce adaptive behaviors and provide positive role models for children are critical. Limit-setting skills are complex, and even the most skilled caregivers need guidance. They also need to learn functional coping behaviors if they hope to guide and influence their children positively.

POST-TRAUMATIC STRESS DISORDER

Post-traumatic stress disorder (PTSD) is an anxiety disorder characterized by a constellation of symptoms and psychological reactions that follows an extreme and/or life-threatening traumatic event. The trauma can be the result of a single event that is abrupt, often lasting a few minutes and as long as a few hours, or chronic, repeated, and ongoing events such as physical and sexual child abuse.

Incidence and Etiology

The incidence rates of PTSD for children are reported as 1% (APA, 1994). Traumatic events capable of causing PTSD fall into three categories:

1. Natural disasters—tornadoes, floods, hurricanes, earthquakes
2. Accidental disasters—automobile, train, and airplane accidents, fires, explosions, nuclear plant accidents
3. Intentional human-made disasters—combat, bombings, rape, armed robbery, assault, physical and sexual abuse (Terr, 1991)

Clinical Manifestations

The hallmark symptoms of PTSD are re-experiencing the trauma, avoidance of stimuli associated with the event and numbing of general responsiveness, and increased states of arousal. Re-experiencing symptoms include recurrent, intrusive, unwanted thoughts and dreams related to the traumatic experience. In young children this symptom may be manifested by repetitive play in which the traumatic themes occur. Avoidance symptoms involve physical avoidance of situations that resemble the traumatic event, efforts to avoid thoughts, feelings, or conversations associated with the trauma, and numbing of responsiveness to the outside world (diminished interest in normal activities, restriction of emotions). Increased arousal states are exemplified by hypervigilance, an exaggerated startle response, sleep difficulties, and irritable or angry outbursts. These symptoms must be present for more than one month and cause significant impairment in daily functioning (Cohen, 1998).

Diagnosis

A comprehensive clinical interview with the child and caregivers is a primary assessment tool in the evaluation of PTSD. Both the child and caregivers should be asked directly about the traumatic event and re-experiencing, avoidant, and hyperarousal symptoms. Teachers should also be questioned about behavior changes in the child and the time these changes began. Although there are several questionnaires and semi-structured interviews that purport to measure this disorder, there is no single instrument accepted as a "gold standard" in making the diagnosis.

Treatment

The cornerstone of treatment for PTSD is the education of the child and family regarding the nature of the disorder so that the child's symptoms are not mistakenly viewed as "crazy" or "manipulative" (Clark, 1995). Essential components of treatment include (1) direct exploration of the trauma, (2) use of stress management techniques, (3) exploration and correction of inaccurate attributions regarding the event, and (4) inclusion of caregivers. Direct exploration of the traumatic experience and its meaning to and impact on the child is crucial. Stress management techniques such as muscle relaxation, positive imagery, and deep breathing frequently are used in conjunction with direct discussion of the event. This intervention enables the child to gain a sense of control over thoughts and feelings instead of being overwhelmed by them. The child can then directly discuss the trauma with diminished hyperarousal and negative feelings states through relaxation and desensitization procedures. The third element of treatment is exploration of attributional distortions such as "It was my fault," or "Nothing is safe anymore." These attributions should be challenged by step-by-step logical analysis of the child's cognitive distortions during therapy. Caregivers should be included in treatment because they can provide support, monitor the child's symptoms, and learn appropriate behavioral management techniques.

Despite a lack of systematic research of pharmacologic therapy for children with PTSD, clinicians have prescribed a variety of medications. However, medications should be considered as an adjunct to treatment, not the sole mode of therapy. Clonidine (Catapres) has been shown to reduce hyperarousal symptoms. Propranolol (Inderal) appears to regulate anxiety and panic symptoms. Tricyclic antidepressants and SSRIs may be used to treat re-experiencing of traumatic symptoms and depression (Vargas & Davidson, 1993).

Nursing Management

It is important for the nurse to establish a trusting relationship with the child, to offer reassurance of safety and security, and to explain that the symptoms are not uncommon following a trauma of the magnitude she or he has experienced. Resolution of the post-trauma response is largely dependent on the effectiveness of the coping strategies employed. Therefore, the nurse should discuss with the child coping strategies used in response to the trauma, as well as those used during stressful situations in the past, and together determine the most helpful. Guilt at having survived a trauma in which others have died is common. The child needs to discuss these feelings and recognize that he or she is not responsible for what happened. It is important to assess the impact of the trauma on the child's ability to resume activities of daily living. The child should be assessed for self-destructive ideas and behavior as the trauma may result in feelings of hopelessness and worthlessness, leading to high risk for suicide. The child and family may need to be referred to community resources such as support groups for victims of trauma during the recovery process.

SUBSTANCE ABUSE

Substance use is a precursor to dependence or abuse, and regular use increases the risk of developing a substance use disorder (SUD) (AACAP, 1997b). SUD encompasses both substance abuse and sunstance dependence. **Substance abuse** is a maladaptive pattern of substance use leading to significant distress or impairment (APA, 1994). In children and adolescents the impairment is usually in psychosocial and academic functioning. Substance abuse is further manifested by recurrent substance use in situations in which it is physically hazardous (driving an automobile while impaired); recurrent substance-related legal problems; and continued substance use although the individual is having persistent social or interpersonal problems. **Substance dependence** involves a substantial degree of involvement with a substance, including withdrawal (adverse physical symptoms due to cessation of or reduction in prolonged and heavy substance use); tolerance (a need for increased amounts of the substance to achieve the desired effect); and loss of control over use (efforts to cut down use are unsuccessful) (APA, 1994). Substances that are used and abused by pre-adolescents and adolescents include alcohol, tobacco, marijuana, opiates, cocaine, amphetamines, barbiturates, hallucinogens, and inhalants (AAP Committee on Substance Abuse, 1998) (See Box 35-4).

Incidence and Etiology

From 1991 through 1996 there has been a steady increase in the use and abuse of substances among students in 8th through 12th grades (AAP Committee on Substance Abuse, 1998). The use of a variety of psychoactive substances is common among adolescents; yet, alcohol is the drug most often used and abused. In 1999, 80% of high school seniors and 52% of 8th grade students reported using alcohol (AAP Committee on Substance Abuse, 2001). By the end of high school, 90% of high school students have tried alcohol, and more than 40% have tried an illicit drug, mostly marijuana. More boys than girls are involved in alcohol and other drugs (Tweed, 1998). For both boys and girls abuse of substances is minimal from 10 to 13 years of age, but doubles between mid-adolescence (12 to 16 years) and late adolescence (17 to 20 years) (Cohen, et al., 1993). Substance abuse occurs in children from all socioeconomic levels, family types, and academic abilities.

BOX 35-4 Ecstasy

Methylenedioxymethamphetamine (MDMA) is the drug known as Ecstasy, also referred to as *XTC, Adam, the love drug*. MDMA is both a CNS stimulant and hallucinogenic. According to users, MDMA replaces anxiety and depression with feelings of pleasure. According to the Partnership for a Drug-Free America, MDMA use has doubled among the teenage population since 1995, and one in 10 adolescents has experimented with the drug. It is often used in combination with LSD. The rate of emergency room visits for complications of use and overdose of this drug are on the rise.

Adapted from Reiss, B., Evans, M., & Broyles, B. (2001). *Pharmacological aspects of nursing care* (6th ed.). Albany, NY: Delmar.

There are multiple theories concerning causes of substance abuse and SUD that include (AAP Committee on Substance Abuse, 2001; Berman, 1995; AACAP, 1997b):

- Genetic factors—twin and adoption studies point to the probable contribution of genetic or constitutional factors to the risk for SUDs.
- Family factors—caregiver substance use; their beliefs, attitudes, and tolerance of substance use; dysfunctional family relationships (e.g., lack of closeness, neglect, lack of supervision); poor parenting skills.
- Peer influence—peer network substance use; peer pressure; peer attitudes; desire to be "in the mainstream"; feeling inadequate because of social or cultural group.
- Individual factors—early anti-social behavior; poor academic performance and school failure; ineffective coping skills; psychiatric conditions (e.g., ADHD, depression, conduct disorder); low self-esteem.
- Community or neighborhood factors—low socioeconomic status; high crime; high population density.
- Media factors—advertising that links drinking and drug use with highly valued personal attributes.

Clinical Manifestations and Pathophysiology

Generally all drugs involve alterations in sensorium as well as other physiological and psychological alterations that become more significant as the amount and frequency of usage increases. Clinical manifestations will vary depending on the type of substance used and the age and weight of the child. Central nervous system depressants such as alcohol, barbiturates, and nonbarbiturate sedatives produce states that range from calmness and drowsiness to delirium and coma. Physiological alterations include cardiac and respiratory depression, hyperthermia, coma, and death. Alcohol decreases inhibitions and causes relaxation and slurred speech. Toxicity leads to lack of coordination, impaired judgment, accidents, respiratory depression, coma, and death. Opiates create a feeling of euphoria or analgesia. Toxicity leads to respiratory depression, cerebral edema, and death.

Central nervous system stimulants such as amphetamines create a feeling of well-being or euphoria. Toxicity leads to hypertension, hyperthermia, convulsions, cardiovascular shock, and death. Hallucinogens alter perceptions, thoughts, and feeling. Side effects include convulsions and cardiovascular collapse. Suicide, fatal accidents, and homicide often occur secondary to paranoid delusions, hallucinations, psychosis, and flashbacks. Effects of marijuana include feeling of unreality, distorted sense of time, and perceptual distortions. Side effects range from hallucinations to tachycardia, decreased motor skills, impaired memory, and chronic bronchitis. Inhalants create feelings of euphoria and excitement. Side effects include ataxia, stupor, seizures, and cardiac and respiratory arrest (Woodard, 1995).

Kids Want To Know

How intoxicating are different types of alcohol?

I overheard my older brother and his friends talking about alcohol yesterday. By the way, he is in college. They were saying that beer has less alcohol than wine or "hard" liquor like vodka or bourbon, so you can drink more of it before you get "drunk." Is this true?

The nurse should explain that this is not true. A 12-ounce can or bottle of beer, an 8-ounce glass of wine, and a 1.5-ounce glass of liquor all have about the same alcohol content. When a person drinks one of any of these, it is enough to impair judgment and reflexes and interfere with driving.

Treatment

Treatment varies depending on the substance being abused, the willingness of the child and family to cooperate with treatment, the age of the client, and the availability of treatment modalities. Broad treatment goals include the elimination of substance abuse and any accompanying undesirable behaviors and restoration of the child to a healthy functional status. Individuals with substance abuse should be treated in the least restrictive setting that is safe and effective. Treatment settings can range from inpatient (hospital-based or free-standing rehabilitation center); residential; partial-hospitalization or day treatment; and outpatient. Children who require inpatient treatment include (1) those with severe psychiatric disorders, symptoms, or behaviors (acute psychosis, suicidal, homicidal, or other acutely dangerous behavior); (2) those with a history of treatment failure in less restrictive programs; and (3) those at risk for substance use withdrawal or with a history of withdrawal problems (AACAP, 1997b). Because family dysfunction is frequently a factor in the etiology of the problem, family-based treatment programs and family participation are essential.

Pharmacotherapy may also be used for treating withdrawal effects and other psychiatric disorders. Although significant symptoms of withdrawal from substances are rare in children, the treatment should proceed as for adults. Initially, short-term attempts to treat psychiatric symptoms, such as anxiety and depression, should consist of abstinence from psychoactive substances and psychosocial interventions. If symptoms persist beyond several weeks, pharmacotherapy may be necessary (AACAP, 1997b).

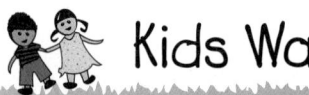

Self-help or peer-support groups such as Alcoholics Anonymous (AA) and Narcotics Anonymous (NA) are important adjuncts to the treatment program. These groups are thought to be an essential element in the recovery process and help prevent relapse. Members meet and support each other in dealing with their substance abuse problems. The programs offer suggestions for a way of living without the use of substances. Both AA and NA are nonprofessional, multicultural, nondenominational, and apolitical and are located in communities throughout the world. Several reports conclude that AA or NA have a high success rate secondary to group support and one-on-one interactions between the sponsor and the affected individual (Woodard, 1995).

Diagnosis

The first goal of assessment for suspected substance abuse is to determine whether a problem of using substances exists. A physical examination is performed to identify signs and symptoms that may indicate a substance use problem, such as bloodshot eyes, weight loss, nasal irritation, slurred speech, abnormal pupil constriction or dilation, and increase in accidents and injuries. Because of the covert nature of substance abuse, information should be gathered from a variety of sources, such as the child or adolescent, caregivers, other family members, peers, and school personnel. A comprehensive developmental, social, and medical history is part of a complete assessment. Information is gathered about the child or adolescent's substance use behavior. The health care provider needs to determine the effect of the substance use on various areas of the individual's life and psychosocial functioning. It is also essential to ascertain if associated problems, such as mood disorders or antisocial behavior, are present and what family and environmental stressors exist. Substance abuse is differentiated from social drinking or non-pathological substance use by the presence of compulsive use, craving, or substance related problems (AACAP, 1997b).

Nursing Management

Assessment of risk factors is important in identifying individuals who may be using and/or abusing substances. Nurses may suspect substance abuse when they observe irrational behavior; preoccupation with the occult; frequent absences from school and decline in academic performance; disinhibition, lethargy, hyperactivity or agitation, and hypervigilance; changes in personality, friends, activities, or appearance; difficulty communicating; rebelliousness; mental or physiological deterioration; unexplained loss of money; and actual substances or paraphernalia.

Children with low self-esteem, family history of substance abuse, and peer pressure often use drugs to "be cool" or to cope with social pressures; therefore nursing management focuses on the causes of the substance abuse (Figure 35-3). Long-term counseling may be necessary to support changes in lifestyle and behaviors and address and resolve underlying issues of self-esteem and family history of abuse. The nurse must identify the precipitating problems and plan interventions to help the child or adolescent cope with these. The nurse focuses on social skills such as problem solving, self-esteem building, and values clarification.

Another important role for nurses is prevention of substance abuse, which focuses on drug education, self-awareness, decision-making abilities, and clarification of values and beliefs about substances. Prevention programs may begin as early as elementary school and include education and family involvement. Children are taught to make knowledgeable and value-based choices, ways to resist social and peer pressure, methods of improving communication with caregivers,

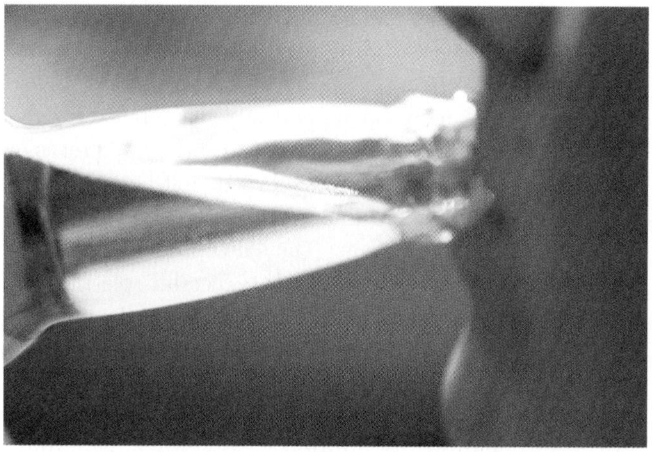

Figure 35-3 Some adolescents engage in risky behavior they later regret. Copyright ©2001 PhotoDisc, Inc.

REFLECTIONS FROM FAMILIES

January: My family. On the outside we seem perfect. Big house, nice cars, best schools, vacations every year. On the inside, that is a different story. My mom drinks through the day, my dad avoids her at all cost and spends most of his time at work. Me? I drink alcohol and do drugs. The release I feel from my problems is tremendous. After snorting some cocaine, I feel invincible. Ecstasy helps me dance the night away.

January, one year later: My family. My mom still drinks. I am not sure what Dad does. Me? I am in jail pending conviction of running a child over while DWI. How I wish I could bring that child back. How I wish I could rewind my life and get the counseling I needed to stop my drug abuse.

and alternative ways to feel good about oneself without using substances. Strategies can be small group discussions and role-playing.

Interventions focus on support and reassurance for the child and the family. Changes in lifestyle and new patterns of coping with stress need to be reinforced. Self-help and support groups encourage abstinence through a framework for lifestyle and personal change. They also provide a place to learn social skills and interact with successful role models. Other nursing interventions include individual, family, and group therapy. After a short time in individual therapy, the older child is often moved to a group therapy setting because this is an excellent place to learn new behaviors and interact with others who are struggling with similar problems. Substance abuse is often a coping mechanism for living in a dysfunctional family; therefore, the interventions must focus on resolving the family problems or treatment for the substance abuse will not be successful.

Critical Thinking

Cultural Trends and Eating Disorders

Cultural ideals of beauty have always been reflected in fashion for women. The trend in fashion since the 1960s has been increasingly toward thinness. With the media as the vehicle, adolescents are bombarded with images of the thin, fit, "perfect" woman, an ideal unattainable for most of them. Very few women have a natural body type that matches the ideal, leading most to believe that their normal, healthy shape is too fat. Many resort to excessive and unhealthy dieting to achieve this ideal body, which may lead to an eating disorder in some individuals. As a school nurse in a junior high school, what can you do to prevent adolescents from developing an eating disorder?

EATING DISORDERS

Eating disorders such as anorexia nervosa (AN) and bulimia nervosa (BN) are common disorders encountered in children, especially adolescents. These disorders are affecting adolescents with increasing frequency and continue to be associated with serious physical complications and significant morbidity and mortality. The mortality rate associated with eating disorders is the highest of any major psychiatric disorder (Panagiotopoulos, McCrindle, Hick, & Katzman, 2000).

Anorexia Nervosa

AN is characterized by voluntary refusal to eat, significant weight loss, an intense fear of becoming overweight, and a pronounced disturbance of body image. The individual with AN may exclusively restrict dietary intake (restrictive subtype), or may regularly engage in binge eating or purging behaviors (i.e., self-induced vomiting or misuse of laxatives, diuretics, or enemas) (binge eating/purging subtype) (APA, 1994).

Incidence and Etiology

The incidence of AN is approximately 0.5% to 1.0% of adolescents (Seidenfeld & Rickert, 2001). The highest incidence is for females aged 10 through 19 years, thus, the first occurrence takes place almost exclusively during adolescence (Lewinsohn, Striegel-Moore, & Seeley, 2000). Although AN is predominately a disorder of females, it does occur in males at a 1:9 ratio.

While the exact etiology of AN is unknown several theories offer insight into the complex nature of the disorder. Biological theory suggests that anorexic individuals suffer a disturbance in levels of neurotransmitters in the brain. Norepinephrine and its metabolites have been found to be low, but they increase to normal levels as weight is restored. However, it is not clear whether these biochemical changes are the cause or the effect of the disorder (Woodside, 1995).

The psychodynamic theory suggests that deficits in ego development may predispose the young woman to AN. Appropriate ego development is necessary for the child to function separately from the family. Without encouragement for independence during the individuation-separation phase, the child does not develop autonomy and the ability to make decisions (Bruch, 1982).

Family systems theory suggests that AN is caused by intrafamilial conflicts and dysfunctional family patterns. The adolescent's eating behavior allows the family to focus on the problem of the sick child, rather than on the conflicts among the adult partners and other family members. Alliances are formed, and the child is encouraged to side with one caregiver against the other. Subsequently, this behavior allows the child some degree of control in the family.

Clinical Manifestations and Pathophysiology

The clinical manifestations of AN include the following:

- Extreme weight loss
- Refusal to maintain body weight at or above the minimum recommended weight for age and height (weight less than 85% of that expected)
- Intense and irrational fear of gaining weight or becoming fat, although underweight
- Denial of the seriousness of the current low weight
- Distorted body image, weight, or shape, that is, seeing oneself as fat when emaciated

- Physical manifestations (amenorrhea or absence of at least three consecutive menstrual cycles, hypothermia, muscle wasting, growth of lanugo, cardiac dysrhythmias, and osteoporosis)

Diagnosis

Criteria for the diagnosis of AN includes: refusal to maintain body weight at or above a minimally normal weight for age and height; weight loss leading to maintenance of body weight at less than 85% of expected weight; intense fear of gaining weight; in the postmenarcheal female absence of at least three consecutive menstrual cycles; altered perceptions of how the body looks; and denial of the seriousness of the current body weight (APA, 1994).

Treatment

The initial goals for managing the individual with AN are overall improvement of body weight, normalization of eating patterns, and the restoration of physical health through weight gain. Until this goal is achieved, disordered thinking caused by malnutrition may inhibit the success of other therapies (Seidenfeld & Rickert, 2001). Because the real issue is not food, but rather issues such as poor self-esteem, a need to be in control, a need for perfection, and a belief in the myth of thinness and dieting, effective treatment is complex and long-term. Other goals for treatment include correction of medical complications such as fluid, electrolyte, and nutritional imbalances; improvement in personal and social functioning; improvement of family dynamics; and treatment of additional conditions (e.g. depression) (Joffe, 1995).

Currently, hospitalization is limited to brief, acute weight restoration and refeeding for severe cases. Weight should not be regained too quickly as it is medically unsafe and may lead to cardiac overload and death. An appropriate target goal weight should be within 10% of the individual's ideal body weight (Fisher, 1997). Referral to a dietitian, education related to healthy eating habits, and a balanced diet with sufficient calories to allow weight gain are all part of the treatment plan.

Numerous medications have been studied for treatment of AN: antidepressants, hormones, antipsychotics, and gastric motility enhancers. Most have shown inconsistent benfits. However, the antidepressants, selective serotonin reuptake inhibitors, have been effective in the treatment of AN. Individual and family therapy are also used in the treatment of AN, often for years.

Nursing Management

During the nutritional rehabilitation phase the priority is to establish nutrition adequate to stop and reverse the malnutrition and starvation. The nurse may need to promote the individual's physical well-being by monitoring food intake and weight gain. Once an appropriate eating pattern is established, the adolescent should focus on psychotherapy. Most anorectics experience a significant amount of fear and anxiety as they begin to gain weight. The nurse needs to adopt a kind, nurturing yet firm manner in managing the care of the individual. Interventions that increase self-esteem and self-worth are helpful as the individual learns to like herself, learns to trust, and develops an identity beyond her thin body.

Bulimia Nervosa

Whereas the prominent features of AN are the caloric restriction and resulting weight loss, the major elements of BN are episodes of binge eating (large amounts of food with a lack of control) followed by various compensatory behaviors (e.g., self-induced vomiting) to control weight gain. The individual usually suffers painful guilt and remorse after such behaviors but is unable to control the impulse to repeat the cycle of binge-purge.

Incidence and Etiology

Incidence of BN is higher than AN and occurs in about 1% to 1.5% of females with lower rates in males. The client with BN is typically between the ages of 15 and 30 with a peak in later adolescence, at about 18 to 19 years of age (Dunn, 2000). BN is found in all socioeconomic and ethnic groups. Individuals most at risk for developing this disorder are those who are involved in a career or sport requiring low body weight or frequent "weigh-ins" (e.g., ballet, wrestling); who have been sexually abused; and who have a family history of depressive disorders, substance abuse, and eating disorders (Muscari, 1996).

Clinical Manifestations and Pathophysiology

The individual with bulimia may be unable to express feelings accurately. Low self-esteem, feelings of ineffectiveness, depression, and substance abuse are frequently seen. The bulimic typically has an intense fear of getting fat, is very sensitive to weight gain, and fears she is constantly at risk for getting fat because she lacks impulse control.

Binge eating usually occurs in secret and stops when the individual experiences abdominal discomfort. During a binge high-carbohydrate, high-fat, high-calorie foods such as sweets, ice cream, and pastries are usually consumed. Insulin production is increased during the binge. When vomiting occurs, the extra insulin stimulates hunger and eating, and the binge-purge cycle begins again. Following the binge the adolescent feels out of control, depressed, guilty, and anxious. Purging behaviors, commonly self-induced vomiting and laxative abuse, decrease the anxiety, abdominal discomfort, and bloating. The binge-purge cycle is practiced many times a day, and the bulimic loses the ability to respond to normal cues of hunger and satiety. Vomiting and laxative misuse result in complications such as dehydration, abdominal distension, fluid and electrolyte imbalances, esophagitis, and esophageal lacerations. Erosion of tooth enamel, increased dental caries, and tooth discoloration are present secondary to regurgitation of gastric acids. Frequent vomiting also may result in parotid gland enlargement. Cardiovascular symptoms may include hypotension, arrhythmias, and cardiomyopathy.

Diagnosis

Criteria for the diagnosis of BN include the following: recurrent episodes of binge-eating; a sense of lack of control over eating; recurrent inappropriate compensatory behavior to prevent weight gain, such as self-induced vomiting, misuse of laxatives, diuretics, or other medications; fasting; or excessive exercise (APA, 1994).

Treatment

Therapeutic interventions for the person with BN include individual, family and group therapy, and pharmacologic interventions. Behavioral modification is used to control the binge eating and purging. Cognitive therapy may be used after the client's weight has stabilized. Most individuals with BN, as well

Case Study/Care Plan

An Adolescent with Bulimia Nervosa

Cara is a 16-year-old eleventh grader diagnosed with bulimia nervosa. She is 5 feet 5 inches tall and weighs 95 pounds. Her mother and father are divorced. She now lives with her mother and stepfather. Her stepfather is a minister and her mother is a physical therapist. Cara describes her family as close but says her mother and stepfather are involved in their careers and busy. Her grades in school had been above average until 10th grade but have been below average in the last year. During the past year Cara has lost 35 pounds (from 130 to 95 pounds). A friend went to the school counselor and told him that Cara was vomiting every day and had been doing so for over a year. She has also been running 5 miles a day to lose weight. The counselor notified Cara's mother.

Nursing Care Plan

Assessment Assessment data includes: Cara states she felt "really good" when she began to lose weight. Cara has little motivation for working hard and doing well in school. Social interactions consist of watching television, talking on the phone, and shopping. She does not have an after-school job. Her mother's history includes lifelong dieting and sexual abuse as a child. Her father's history includes substance abuse and suicide in his family of origin. Cara's own history includes experimentation with alcohol and marijuana and shoplifting. Cara was encouraged to take ballet and modeling lessons as a young girl.

Nursing Diagnosis #1

Imbalanced nutrition, less than body requirement related to purging and inadequate food intake.

Expected Outcomes

1. Cara will regain weight within normal range for height and age.
2. Cara will demonstrate nutritionally adequate eating pattern without binging or purging.
3. Cara will verbalize an understanding of her nutritional needs.
4. Cara will reduce energy expenditure.

Interventions/*Rationales*

1. Implement nutritionally balanced diet as prescribed. *To allow gradual weight gain. Malnutrition is a mood altering condition affecting cognitive functioning and decision making. Improving nutrition enhances thinking ability and therapeutic work can begin.*

continues

continued

2. With a nutritionist, Cara, and her caregivers, select a balanced diet with gradual increase in calories and allowing Cara choices as much as possible. *Allows client to have some control over diet plan, encourages compliance, and avoids cardiac overload from rapid weight gain.*

3. Provide supervision of Cara after meals and snacks to prevent purging. *As weight is gained, the bulimic experiences severe anxiety and fear and may resort to purging.*

4. Supervise selection and performance of activity. Watch for secretive exercising. *Client may use excessive exercising as weight loss strategy.*

Evaluation

Cara will be within 10% of ideal body weight. She will understand and demonstrate positive eating habits and engage in normal levels of exercise activity.

Nursing Diagnosis #2

Disturbed body image related to inaccurate perception of body size and shape.

Expected Outcomes

1. Cara will develop realistic attitudes and perception of body size and shape.
2. Cara will display evidence of developing a positive self-image.
3. Cara will express feelings and concerns.

Interventions/*Rationales*

1. Discuss misconceptions of body image. *Provides opportunity to discuss client's perception of self/body image and realities of her own body.*

2. Encourage identification and expression of feelings. *Learning to express feelings and having a sense of internal control helps the client deal with emotions in ways other than binging and purging. Bulimics are often not aware of unpleasant or unacceptable feelings such as anger and resort to binge eating to control anxiety associated with such feelings.*

3. Provide positive support and encouragement for accurate perceptions of body. *To reinforce new and appropriate behaviors.*

4. Teach assertion skills and identify strengths. *Lack of control and feeling ineffective are common problems for the bulimic. Enables client to focus on inner strengths rather than physical appearance.*

Evaluation

Does Cara have a realistic view of normal body size and shape? Does she seem to project a positive self-image? Does she express worries and concerns and seek assistance?

Nursing Diagnosis #3

Compromised family coping related to issues of control and dysfunctional dynamics.

Expected Outcomes

1. Family members will learn about dysfunctional family dynamics that contribute to eating disorders.
2. Family members will establish boundaries that are clearly defined.
3. Family members will demonstrates effective communication patterns.

continues

continued

Interventions/*Rationales*

1. Educate the family about healthy boundaries and normal separation and individuation versus overprotection and family enmeshment. Interact with family members to help increase their awareness of dysfunctional patterns of interaction. *An enmeshed or overprotective family often is not aware of the dysfunctional dynamics. To help the family relinquish unnecessary controls. To promote mutually satisfying interpersonal relationships among family members.*

2. Encourage caregivers to recognize the importance of their relationship as a couple. *Caregivers need to improve their relationship and restore balance in their lives, thus moving the focus off the bulimic's illness. Attention directed toward the bulimic often serves to protect the caregivers from dealing with their own issues.*

3. Help arrange referrals for family therapy. *Family therapy is directed toward redirection of malfunctioning process in the family.*

Evaluation

Have family members begun to alter interaction patterns and improve dynamics of the family? Does every family member communicate in a healthy manner?

as AN, demonstrate distorted thoughts and beliefs related to food, weight, body image, and self-concept. The goals of cognitive therapy include: developing an initial sense of self and an understanding of the underlying conflicts; developing a realistic perception of one's body; and enhancing self-esteem and self-concept. Other interventions are psychoeducational groups, dietary counseling, and psychotropic drugs. SSRIs have been effective in reducing the urge to binge and in treating depression (Woodside, 1995). Hospitalization may be necessary for an individual with severe symptoms such as dehydration and fluid and electrolyte imbalances.

FAILURE TO THRIVE

Failure to thrive (FTT) is a term used to describe a child with inadequate growth, usually weight, on standardized growth charts. There is no clear consensus regarding the definition of FTT; however, the term usually describes a child whose weight is below the 3rd to 5th percentile or falls more than 2 major percentile groups (i.e., from above the 75th percentile to below the 25th).

Incidence and Etiology

The incidence of FTT has been reported as 1–5% of hospitalized children under 1 year of age (Maggioni & Lifchitz, 1995). The causes of FTT can be classified as organic (OFTT), caused by a physical problem, or non-organic (NOFTT), caused by psychosocial factors, or mixed failure, caused by a combination of organic and non-organic factors. Most cases of FTT are non-organic in origin. Organic causes vary widely, with the most common being gastrointestinal, such as gastroesophageal reflux, celiac disease, and pyloric stenosis. Other causes of OFTT are increased metabolic demands (e.g., congenital heart disease, chronic infections, very low birth weight), central nervous system abnormalities, and endocrine disorders (e.g., diabetes mellitus, growth hormone deficiency). Several environmental and psychological factors have been identified as the cause of NOFTT (Chatoor, Ganiban, Colin, Plummer, & Harmon, 1998). These include:

- Poverty
- Insufficient social support
- Family stress
- Inadequate caregiver nutritional information
- Errors in formula preparation
- Inadequate breast milk
- Difficulties in the maternal-child attachment
- Maternal psychopathology (affective, anxiety, psychotic, and substance abuse disorders)

Clinical Manifestations and Pathophysiology

The clinical manifestations of FTT include:

- Growth failure—weight/or weight and height below the 3rd to 5th percentile

- Failure to maintain previously established growth trajectory
- Loss of subcutaneous fat
- Reduced muscle mass
- Developmental delays
- Apathy and listlessness
- Flattened occiput from lying in one position
- Infrequent and scanty stools
- Signs of neglect: poor hygiene such as dirty body, clothes, fingernails, and extensive diaper rash
- Avoidance of eye contact
- Expressionless face

Long-term effects of failure to thrive include developmental delays, secondary immune dysfunction, and growth delays.

Diagnosis

To rule out an organic cause of FTT, dietary interventions including provision of nutrients and nurturing should be implemented. If the infant/child gains the expected amount of weight, a diagnosis of NOFTT is appropriate. The history should include past and present medical histories of the child and family members, a social history to obtain information about economic resources and social supports of the family, and a detailed dietary and feeding assessment. The dietary history can be used to determine whether the child's diet is appropriate for age (MacPhee, 1996). The caregiver-child feeding interaction observation is another essential aspect of the FTT assessment. Other diagnostic tests are used only to rule out organic problems.

Treatment

The primary goal of treatment is to provide sufficient calories and nutrition for the child to attain **"catch-up" growth** (a rate of growth greater than the expected rate for age). Additionally, other medical and psychosocial problems must be addressed. One critical factor contributing to success with management of FTT is to use a multidisciplinary team approach (nurse, health care provider, dietitian, social worker, occupational/physical therapist, mental health professional) as the problems are complex. Any underlying organic conditions should also be treated.

Nursing Management

Nursing care focuses on observation of the caregiver-child interactions during feeding and when not feeding. A feeding schedule should be developed and taught to the caregivers. Education is provided about appropriate feeding techniques, for example, how to hold the infant, the importance of eye contact, cues from the infant about satiety, and desire to feed more. The nurse monitors weight gain, intake, and plots weights and lengths/heights on grids to monitor growth. It is important for the nurse to role model appropriate caregiver-child interactions. The nurse can role model feeding behaviors, can talk to the infant or child, and initiate playful interactions. Caregivers may need to see that the nurse views it as appropriate to talk to an infant or young child and that the child can respond.

Success in this educational process depends on building a trusting relationship between the family and the professionals. A supportive, nonblaming approach is essential. By adopting the attitude that the caregivers have not had the opportunity to learn healthy parenting behaviors rather than assuming their behavior is willful, a trusting relationship can be established. Another nursing intervention is providing emotional support for the caregivers. The nurse can help them increase their self-esteem through positive parenting skills. The nurse should praise and encourage them for displaying any such skills, and encourage as much caregiver participation in care as is practical. Another significant nursing role is to emphasize the importance of frequent health visits to monitor weight gain and developmental progress. A home health referral may be appropriate in some situations so these parameters can be assessed on a regular basis.

Reflective Thinking

Failure to Thrive

You have been assigned to work with a caregiver whose child is suffering from non-organic failure to thrive. Assuming you have not met with the child and caregiver yet, what are your initial feelings toward this caregiver?

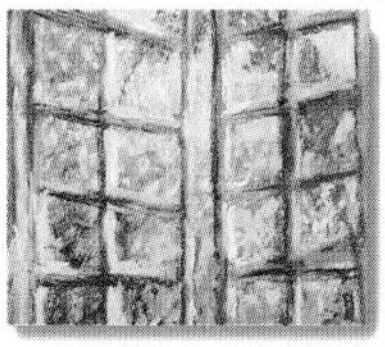

In The Real World

Her mother cried, "If I only knew the signs!" Her father said through tears, "Why didn't we see?" Her grandmother was too distraught for words. Her brother said, "What could have been so bad?" These are words or feelings expressed in the hospital emergency room reacting to news that 15-year-old Elizabeth had committed suicide.

As a nurse who has had opportunities to counsel children who have tried to commit suicide and their families, the suicide risk signs are almost always apparent. It just doesn't happen out of the blue. We must as nurses strive to observe for these signs in our clients and to encourage caregivers, school officials and teachers, coaches, and the general public to take notice of these signs and be proactive. Working together we might just save a life.

Key Concepts

- Individual, family, group, play, and art therapy are the various types of therapy used to treat the pediatric client with psychosocial alterations. The modalities and types of interventions are based on a child's diagnosis, age, and developmental stage.
- Children with attention-deficit hyperactivity disorder have difficulty inhibiting behavior, which interferes with the process of learning self-regulation behaviors.
- Nursing management of attention-deficit hyperactivity disorder includes pharmacological education, providing family support, and acting as a liaison with health care providers, caregivers, school, and other members of the interdisciplinary team.
- Nursing management of mood disorders includes assessing the child physically; talking with the child and family about their feelings and concerns; and educating the family about the disorder and treatment. The nurse should work with the family to improve intrafamily communication and resolution of dysfunctional family patterns.
- The incidence of suicide is rising in the adolescent age group. The nurse should be active in promoting the signs of suicide risk including identification of potential stressors.
- Nursing interventions for attempted suicide include primary, secondary, and tertiary levels of intervention.
- Anxiety disorders include separation anxiety disorder, school phobia or refusal, generalized anxiety disorder, and social phobia.
- Nurse interventions for anxiety disorders include pharmacologic teaching, encouraging identification of sources of anxiety, teaching caregivers to recognize signs of anxiety, and methods for diffusing the anxiety.
- Nursing interventions for substance abuse include support and reassurance for the client and family, encouraging positive changes in lifestyle, and referral to support groups.
- The mortality rate for anorexia nervosa and bulimia nervosa are the highest of any of the major psychiatric disorders.
- Causes of non-organic failure to thrive include poverty, insufficient social support, family stress, inadequate caregiver information, difficulty in maternal/child attachment, and maternal psychopathology.

Review Questions

1. Explain why you would use play therapy for one child and art therapy for another.
2. What are the clinical manifestations of ADHD?
3. Explain the difference between major depressive disorder and dysthymic disorder.
4. What interventions would you include in a primary prevention education program related to suicide?
5. What are the goals for the caregivers of a child with school refusal?
6. Compare anorexia nervosa symptoms and nursing interventions with those of bulimia nervosa.
7. What information would you include in a class you planned to teach junior high-school-age students about substance abuse?
8. List 3–5 risk factors for the development of substance abuse and substance abuse disorder.
9. List 3 factors identified as causes of non-organic failure to thrive.

References

American Academy of Child and Adolescent Psychiatry. (1997a). Practice parameters for the assessment and treatment of children and adolescents with anxiety disorders. *Journal of the American Academy of Child and Adolescent Psychiatry, 36*(Suppl. 10), 69S–84S.

American Academy of Child and Adolescent Psychiatry. (1997b). Practice parameters for the assessment and treatment of children and adolescents with substance use disorders. *Journal of the American Academy of Child and Adolescent Psychiatry, 36*(Suppl. 10), 140S–156S.

American Academy of Pediatrics Committee on Adolescence. (2000). Suicide and suicide attempts in adolescents. *Pediatrics, 105*(4), 871–874.

American Academy of Pediatrics Committee on Quality Improvement, Subcommittee on Attention-Deficit/Hyperactivity Disorder. (2000). Clinical practice guideline: Diagnosis and evaluation of the child with attention-deficit/hyperactivity disorder. *Pediatrics, 105*(5), 1158–1170.

American Academy of Pediatrics Committee on Substance Abuse. (1998). Tobacco, alcohol, and other drugs: The role of the pediatrician in prevention and management of substance abuse. *Pediatrics, 101*(1), 125–128.

American Academy of Pediatrics Committee on Substance Abuse. (2001). Alcohol use and abuse: A pediatric concern. *Pediatrics, 108*(1), 185–191.

American Psychiatric Association. (1994). *Diagnostic and statistical manual of mental disorders* (4th ed.). Washington, DC: Author.

Barkley, R. (1998). Attention-deficit/hyperactivity disorder. *Scientific American, 279*(3), 66–71.

Berman D. S. (1995). Risk factors leading to adolescent substance abuse. *Adolescence, 30*(117), 201–208.

Bernstein, G., Borchardt, C., & Perwien, A. (1996). Anxiety disorders in children and adolescents: A review of the past 10 years. *Journal of the American Academy of Child and Adolescent Psychiatry, 35,* 1110–1119.

Birmaher, B., Brent, D. A., & Benson, R. S. (1998). Summary of the practice parameters for the assessment and treatment of children and adolescents with depressive disorders. *Journal of the American Academy of Child and Adolescent Psychiatry, 37*(1), 1234–1238.

Birmaher, B., Ryan, N., Williamson, C., Brent, D., Kaufman, J., Dahl, R., Perel, J., & Nelson, B. (1996). Childhood and adolescent depression: A review of the past 10 years. Part I. *Journal of the American Academy of Child and Adolescent Psychiatry, 35,* 1427–1439.

Borowsky, I. (2000). Attention-deficit/hyperactivity disorder. In C. Berkowitz (Ed.), *Pediatrics: A primary care approach* (2nd ed., pp. 469–473). Philadelphia: W. B. Saunders.

Borowsky, I., Ireland, M., & Resnick, M. (2001). Adolescent suicide attempts: Risks and protectors. *Pediatrics, 107*(3), 485–493.

Brown, R., Freeman, W., Perrin, J., Stein, M., Amler, R., Feldman, H., Pierce, K., & Wolraich, M. (2001). Prevalence and assessment of attention-deficit/hyperactivity disorder in primary care settings. *Pediatrics, 107*(3), e43.

Bruch, H. (1982). *The golden cage: The enigma of anorexia nervosa.* Cambridge, MA: Harvard University Press.

Cassidy, L., & Jellinek, M. (1998). Approaches to recognition and management of childhood psychiatric disorders in pediatric primary care. *Pediatric Clinics of North America, 45,* 1037–1052.

Centers for Disease Control and Prevention (CDC). (1996). Youth risk behavior surveillance: United States, 1995. *Morbidity and mortality weekly reports CDC surveillance summary, 45*(ss-4), 1–84.

Chatoor, I., Ganiban, J., Colin, V., Plummer, N., & Harmon, R. (1998). Attachment and feeding problems: A reexamination of nonorganic failure to thrive and attachment insecurity. *Journal of the American Academy of Child and Adolescent Psychiatry, 37,* 1217–1224.

Cicchetti, D., & Toth, S. (1998). The development of depression in children and adolescents. *American Psychologist, 53*(2), 221–241.

Clark, R. B. (1995). Psychosocial aspects of pediatrics and psychiatric disorders. In W. Hay, J. Groothuis, A. Hayward, & Levin, M. (Eds.), *Current pediatric diagnosis and treatment* (12th ed., pp. 154–194). Norwalk, CT: Appleton & Lange.

Cohen, J. (1998). Summary of the practice parameters for the assessment and treatment of children and adolescents with post-traumatic stress disorder. *Journal of the American Academy of Child and Adolescent Psychiatry, 37*(9), 9897–1011.

Cohen, P., Cohen, J., & Brook, J. (1993). An epidemiological study of disorders in late childhood and adolescence—II: Persistence of disorders. *Journal of Child Psychology and Psychiatry, 34,* 869–877.

Compton, S., Nelson, A., & March, J. (2000). Social phobia and separation anxiety symptoms in community and clinical samples of children and adolescents. *Journal of the American Academy of Child and Adolescent Psychiatry, 39,* 1040–1046.

Dashiff, C. (1995). Understanding separation anxiety disorder. *Journal of Child and Adolescent Psychiatric Nursing, 8,* 27–38.

Dunn, A. (2000). Nutrition. In C. Burns, M. Brady, A. Dunn, & N. Starr (Eds.), *Pediatric primary care: A handbook for nurse practitioners* (2nd ed., pp. 243–302). Philadelphia: W. B. Saunders.

Emslie, G., Weinberg, W., Kowatch, R., Hughes, C., Carmody, T., & Rush, A. (1997). Fluoxetine treatment of depressed children and adolescents. *Archives of General Psychiatry, 54,* 1031–1037.

Faraone, S., & Doyle, A. (2000). Genetic influences on attention deficit hyperactivity disorder. *Current Psychiatry Report, 2*(2), 143–146.

Fisher, M. (1997). Anorexia and bulimia nervosa. In R. Hoekelman (Ed.), *Primary pediatric care* (3rd ed.). St. Louis: Mosby.

Fritz, T., & Barbie, M. (1993). What are the warning signs for suicidal adolescents? *Journal of Psychosocial Nursing, 32*(2), 37–40.

Jellinek, M., & Snyder, J. (1998). Depression and suicide in children and adolescents. *Pediatrics in Review, 19,* 255–264.

Joffe, A. (1995). Anorexia nervosa and bulimia. In S. Parker & B. Zuckerman (Eds.), *Behavioral and developmental pediatrics* (2nd ed., pp. 63–69). Boston: Little, Brown, and Co.

Johnson, B. S. (1995). *Adolescent and family psychiatric nursing.* Philadelphia: J. B. Lippincott.

Kearney, C., & Albano, A. (2000). *When children refuse school: A cognitive-behavioral therapy approach—therapist guide.* San Antonio, TX: Psychological Corporation.

Kendall, P., Flannery-Schroeder, E., Panichelli-Mindel, S., Southam-Gerow, M., Henin, A., & Warman, M. (1997). Therapy for youths with anxiety disorders: A second randomized clinical trial. *Journal of Consulting and Clinical Psychology, 65,* 366–380.

King, N., & Bernstein, G. (2001). School refusal in children and adolescents: A review of the past 10 years. *Journal of the American Academy of Child and Adolescent Psychiatry, 40,* 197–205.

Kovacs, M., Obrosky, D., Gatsonis, C., & Richards, C. (1997). First-episode major depressive and dysthymic disorder in childhood: Clinical and sociodemographic factors in recovery. *Journal of the American Academy of Child and Adolescent Psychiatry, 36,* 777–784.

Kowatch, R., Emslie, G., & Kennedy, B. (1996). Mood disorders. In D. X. Parmelee (Ed.), *Child and adolescent psychiatry.* St. Louis: Mosby Year Book.

Kutcher, S. (1998). Affective disorders in children and adolescents: A critical clinically relevant review. In B. T. Walsh (Ed.), *Child psychopharmacology* (pp. 91–109). Washington, DC: American Psychiatric Association Press.

Laraia, M. (1996). Current approaches to the psychopharmacologic treatment of depression in children and adolescents. *Journal of Child and Adolescent Psychiatric Nursing, 4,* 15–26.

Lewinsohn, P., Striegel-Moore, R., & Seeley, J. (2000). Epidemiology and natural course of eating disorders in young women from adolescence to young adulthood. *Journal of the American Academy of Child and Adolescent Psychiatry, 39,* 1284–1292.

Lobar, S. L., & Phillips, S. (1995). Developmental conflicts for families dealing with the child who has attention deficit hyperactivity disorder. *Journal of Pediatric Heath Care, 9*(3), 115–122.

MacPhee, M. (1996). Failure to thrive. *Journal of the Society of Pediatric Nurses, 1*(3), 139–142.

Maggioni, A., & Lifchitz, F. (1995). Nutritional management of failure to thrive. *Pediatric Clinics of North America, 42*(4), 791–810.

Martini, D. R. (1995). Common anxiety disorders in children and adolescents. *Current Problems in Pediatrics 25*(9), 271–279.

Milberger, S., Biederman, J., Faraone, S., & Jones, J. (1998). Further evidence of an association between maternal smoking during pregnancy and attention deficit hyperactivity disorder: Findings from a high-risk sample of siblings. *Journal of Clinical Child Psychology, 27*(3), 352–358.

Murray, M., & Zentner, J. (2001). *Health assessment and promotion strategies throughout the lifespan.* (7th ed.). Stamford, CT: Appleton & Lange.

Muscari, M. (1996). Primary care of adolescents with bulimia nervosa. *Journal of Pediatric Health Care, 10,* 17–25.

Panagiotopoulos, C., McCrindle, B., Hick, K., & Katzman, D. (2000). Electrocardiographic findings in adolescents with eating disorders. *Pediatrics, 105*(5), 1100–1105.

Pearson, G.S. (1995). Mood disorders. In B. S. Johnson (Ed.), *Child adolescent psychiatric mental health nursing* (pp. 253–269). Philadelphia: J. B. Lippincott.

Reiss, B., Evans, M., & Broyles, B. (2001). *Pharmacological aspects of nursing care* (6th ed.). Albany, NY: Delmar.

Scahill, L., & Schwab-Stone, M. (2000). Epidemiology of ADHD in school-age children. *Child and Adolescent Psychiatric Clinics of North America, 9*(3), 541–555.

Seidenfeld, M., & Rickert, V. (2001). Impact of anorexia, bulimia and obesity on the gynecologic health of adolescents. *American Family Physician, 64*(4), 445–454.

Shah, S., Hoffman, W., & Marine, W. (2000). Adolescent suicide and household access to firearms in Colorado: Results of a case-control study. *Journal of Adolescent Health, 26,* 157–163.

Shaywitz, B., Fletcher, J., & Shaywitz, S. (2001). Attention-deficit hyperactivity disorder. *Current Treatment Options in Neurology, 3,* 229–236.

Son, S., & Kirchner, J. (2000). Depression in children and adolescents. *American Family Physician, 62*(10), 2297–2310.

Strober, M., DeAntonio, M., Schmidt-Lackner, S., Pataki, C., Freeman, R., Rigali, J., & Rao, U. (1999). The pharmacotherapy of depressive illness in adolescents; An open-label comparison of fluoxetine with imipramine-treated historical controls. *Journal of Clinical Psychiatry, 60*(3), 164–169.

Swanson, J., Posne, M., Fusella, J., Wasdell, M., Sommer, T., & Fan, J. (2001). Genes and attention-deficit hyperactivity disorder. *Current Psychiatry Report, 3*(2), 92 –100.

Terr, L. (1991). Childhood trauma: An outline and review. *American Journal of Psychiatry, 148*(1), 10–20.

Tweed, S., (1998). Intervening in adolescent substance abuse. *Nursing Clinics of North America, 33,* 29–45.

Vargas, M., & Davidson, J. (1993). Post-traumatic stress disorder. *Psychopharmacology, 16,* 737–748.

Woodard, V. A. (1995). Chemical dependency. In B. S. Johnson (Ed.), *Child, adolescent and family psychiatric nursing* (pp. 315–331). Philadelphia: J. B. Lippincott.

Woodside, D. B. (1995). A review of anorexia nervosa and bulimia nervosa. *Current Problems in Pediatrics, 25*(2), 67–87.

Workman, C. G., & Prior, M. (1997). Depression and suicide in young children. *Issues of Comprehensive Pediatric Nursing, 20,* 125–132.

Suggested Readings

Estok, P. J., & Rudy, E. B. (1996). The relationship between eating disorders and running in woman. *Research in Nursing & Health, 19*(5), 377–387.

Johnston, L., O'Malley, P., & Bachman. J. (1996). *National survey results on drug use from the Monitoring the Future Study, 1973–1995; Volume I: Secondary school students.* Rockville, MD: National Institute on Drug Abuse.

O'Connell, K. (1996). Attention deficit hyperactivity disorder. *Pediatric Nursing, 22*(1), 30–33.

Stein, K. F. (1996). The self-schema model: Theoretical approach to the self-concept in eating disorders. *Archives of Psychiatric Nursing,19*(2), 96–109.

Stein, K. F., & Hedger, K. M. (1997). Body weights and shape self-cognitions, emotional distress, and disordered eating in middle adolescent girls. *Archives of Psychiatric Nursing, 11*(5), 264–275.

Wright, C. (2000). Identification and management of failure to thrive: A community perspective. *Archives of Diseases in Childhood, 82,* 5–9.

Resources

Organizations and Websites

Al-Anon and Alateen
Al-Anon Family Group Headquarters, Inc.
1600 Corporate Landing Parkway
Virginia Beach, VA 23454
(757) 563-1600
(888) 4AL-ANON

Alcoholics Anonymous
A.A. World Services, Inc.
P.O. Box 459
New York, NY 10163
(212) 870-3400
www.aa.org

American Academy of Child and Adolescent Psychiatry
3615 Wisconsin Ave., NW
Washington, DC 20016-3007
(202) 966-7300
www.aacap.org

American Association of Suicidology
4201 Connecticut Avenue, NW, Suite 408
Washington, DC 20008
(800) SUICIDE (24 hours a day, 7 days a week)
(202) 237-2280
www.suicidology.org

Children and Adults with Attention-Deficit/Hyperactivity Disorder
8181 Professional Place, Suite 201
Landover, MD 20785
(800) 233-4050
www.chadd.org

Mothers Against Drunk Driving (MADD)
P.O. Box 541688
Dallas, TX 75354
(800) GET-MADD
www.madd.org

National Association of Anorexia Nervosa and Associated Disorders
Box 7
Highland Park, IL 60035
(847) 831-3438
www.anad.org

National Attention Deficit Disorder Association
1788 Second St., Suite 200
Highland Park, IL 60035
(847) 432-ADDA
www.add.org

National Clearinghouse for Alcohol and Drug Information
P.O. Box 2345
Rockville, MD 20847
(800) 729-6686
www.health.org

National Mental Health Association
1021 Prince Street
Alexandria, VA 22314
(703) 684-7722
www.nmha.org

Students Against Drunk Driving (SADD)
P. O. Box 800
Marlboro, MA 01752
(877) SADDINC
www.saddonline.org

Substance Abuse and Mental Health Services Administration (SAMHSA)
U.S. Department of Health and Human Services
5600 Fishers Lane
Rockville, MD 20857
(301) 443-8956
www.samhsa.gov

CHAPTER 36

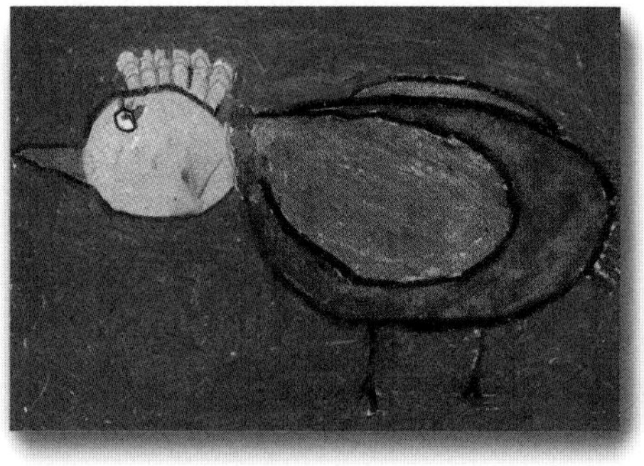

A Child's Thought
"I AM A PERSON
I AM SPECIAL
I AM IMPORTANT
NOT BECAUSE OF THINGS I DO,
NOT BECAUSE OF WHAT I LOOK LIKE,
NOT BECAUSE OF WHAT I HAVE
JUST BECAUSE I AM"

Excerpt: Just because I am: A child's book of affirmations *by Lauren Murphy Payne & Claudia Rohling, 1994, Free Spirit Publishing Inc., Minneapolis, MN.*

CHILD ABUSE AND NEGLECT

Barbara Caldwell, RN, PhD, CNS-C

COMPETENCIES

Upon completion of this chapter, the reader will be able to:

- *Compare child abuse and child neglect.*
- *Describe the incidence and prevalence of child abuse and neglect in the United States.*
- *Explain the theoretical origins of family violence in the United States.*
- *Describe components of a nursing assessment for a child who has been abused and/or neglected.*
- *Describe the clinical manifestations of physical, psychological, and sexual abuse.*
- *Identify nursing interventions related to child abuse and neglect.*
- *Understand and explain the nurses' legal and ethical roles and responsibilities in assessing child abuse and neglect.*

The United States, currently involved in a war on violence, is considered the most violent country in the industrialized world (Osofsky, 1997). Bentovin (1992) describes the family as a violent institution in our country that teaches hurtful and harmful behaviors. The family clearly provides part of the intergenerational transmission of violence as some children witness the abuse of their mother, father, or caregiver. These experiences influence how individuals resolve problems and cope with difficult situations. Nurses have an integral role in preventing child abuse and family violence through educating the public and in national, state, and community health policy and advocacy efforts supporting family health and mental health initiatives.

Child abuse and neglect include physical, emotional, and sexual abuse. Children of any age, race, gender, religion, and socioeconomic group can be victims (Figure 36-1). Therefore, it is imperative the nurse utilize skills, knowledge, and intuition to ensure a child is safe and not in an abusive environment. The following pages not only define and discuss child abuse and neglect, but also provide information regarding the nursing care of these children.

Several terms are used when discussing child abuse. **Child maltreatment** is the intentional injury of a child. **Child neglect** is harmful, malicious, or ignorant withholding of physical, nutrition and health care, or emotional and educational necessities that provide a foundation for healthy childhood development. **Child abuse** includes a range of intentional behaviors by a parent or caregiver that can involve neglect, or physical, emotional, and/or sexual abuse. **Physical abuse,** the most commonly

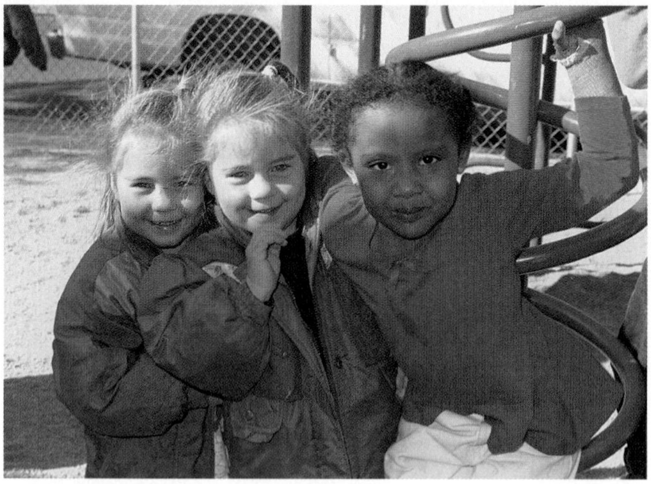

Figure 36-1 Child abuse occurs in any family regardless of race, class, income bracket, religious background, neighborhood, or sexual orientation.

reported type of abuse, represents bodily injury to a child that appears to have been inflicted by other than accidental means. The type of physical injuries a child receives may include damage to skin, as bruises, burns, bite marks, and lacerations; damage to the head including scalp hematomas, lacerations, bruises, brain injuries, or shaken baby syndrome; damage to the internal organs (chest, abdomen, liver, pancreas, spleen, kidney, bladder); or damage to the skeleton (fractures). **Psychological** or **emotional abuse** results from habitual lack of attention to the child's needs, and includes lack of affection, emotional support, or supervision. Emotional abuse may also occur when a caregiver refuses to accept recommended treatment or services by school officials or medical personnel.

All types of abuse have profound implications on a child's growth and development; some effects are short lived, and others are lifelong. Therefore, understanding the incidence, etiology, clinical manifestations, and nursing management of child abuse is important and can affect the course of the child's developmental trajectories.

In 1997 an estimated 3 million children were reported to state Child Protective Service (CPS) agencies as suspected victims of abuse and neglect, and approximately 984,000 were confirmed victims of maltreatment (physical abuse, neglect, sexual abuse, medical neglect, psychological abuse, other abuses). Three-fourths of the perpetrators were caregivers, and an additional one-tenth were relatives. However, only about one-half of the child abuse and neglect reports are investigated nationally, and on average only about one-third of the investigations find evidence of child abuse and/or neglect. Of those who are abused and neglected, only about half receive post-investigation services. Fifty-five percent of child victims are neglected, 25% are physically abused, 12% are sexually abused, and 6% are emotionally abused. Young children are most at risk for being abused/neglected, and 40% of the victims are under the age of 6. Both domestic violence and child maltreatment occur in 30% to 60% of families experiencing some form of family violence, and it is estimated millions of children witness family violence. African-American and Native American children are overrepresented in these statistics at twice their proportion to the general population. Children whose caregivers abuse substances are 3 times more likely to be abused and more than 4 times more likely to be neglected than children of caregivers who do not abuse drugs or alcohol (Reid, Machetto, & Foster, 1999).

The Third National Incidence Study of Child Abuse and Neglect (NIS-3; Sedlak & Broadhurst, 1996), estimates that 20% to 35% of children identified as maltreated suffered serious injury, defined as "long-term impairment of physical, mental or emotional capacities requiring professional treatment aimed at preventing such long-term impairment." In 1995, an estimated 1,500 fatalities related to child abuse and neglect were confirmed by CPS agencies (National Center on Child Abuse and Neglect, 1996). Based on these numbers, more than 3 children die each day as a result of abuse and neglect (Lung & Daro, 1996).

THEORETICAL APPROACHES TO CHILD ABUSE AND NEGLECT

Three theoretical models can be used to explain the phenomena of child abuse and neglect. These models include the sociological model, the social-interactional systemic perspective model, and the attachment model.

Sociological Model

The sociological model of family violence helps the professional understand how social structures affect people and their behavior (Straus & Gelles, 1989). Here, child abuse and neglect are seen as isolated events in a family system, and family violence is a pattern of behavior that is passed from generation to generation. Although the form of abuse may change, the pattern continues, as, for example, physical abuse in one generation changing to sexual abuse in the next generation.

Gelles (1987) described nine risk factors that make families less nurturing and more prone to hurtful, violent behavior. They are found in Table 36-1.

Social-Interactional Systemic Perspective Model

The social-interactional systemic perspective suggests society contains the attitudes, values, and beliefs that legitimize violence in the family (Bentovin, 1992). For example, violent

TABLE 36-1 Risk Factors for Abuse

Factors	Rationale	Example
Stress	Families who spend increased time together under stressful conditions may not have appropriate social supports.	Poor environment, poverty, unemployment, lower educational level.
Intolerance for normal development	Caregivers may not know normal development and have inappropriate expectations.	Hostility toward the very young child who asks many questions or is very active.
Intensity of involvement	Communication patterns expose mutual antagonism, higher levels of criticism, threatening behaviors or conflict.	Belittling adolescent for attempting to dress differently; criticizing a school-aged child for failing to make a goal at a soccer game.
Coercive actions	Deficient parenting skills related to age-appropriate discipline techniques, and use of coercive tactics and physical punishment to maintain control of family members.	Physically punishing a child rather than using time-out strategies or a behavioral chart.
Right to influence	Abusive caregivers are either very authoritarian and punitive to the child's developmental needs or neglectful of emotional needs. The child has little power to negotiate or claim a safe space in such a family system.	The caregiver directs and supervises clothes shopping for a 17-year-old daughter, or on the other hand, punishes the daughter when she interacts with peers in after-school activities.
Gender and age differentials	More than 80% of all perpetrators of child abuse and neglect are under 40 years of age and two-thirds are female (U.S. Dept of Health and Human Services, 1998).	Family violence occurring within patriarchal and matriarchal dominated systems.
Patterns of abuse	Intergenerational patterns of violence are passed down from generation to generation.	Caregivers will construct similar abusive relationships with their own children based on their own experiences of having violent caregivers. Mothers and fathers abused as children sometimes do not know any other method of disciplining than what they experienced as children.
Privacy of the home	Rules for appropriate punishment and discipline can grow and become extreme in a family system that has little contact with community groups such as school, church, or recreational programs. These rules may give rise to abnormal, inappropriate, harmful, and secretive practices that can destroy the self-worth of a child or family member.	Children are not involved in after-school programs or activities, or not allowed to play with other neighborhood children.
Difficult transitions	Family transition periods (births, deaths, separations, loss, unemployment, illness) create stressful conditions, and when abuse is present, these transitions can be particularly problematic and sources of violent and hurtful acts.	Alcohol use may increase during stressful periods for at-risk families and can precipitate violent behaviors.

Adapted from Gelles, R. J. (1987). Family violence *(2nd ed.). London: Sage.*

acts, interactions, and roles are part of society, and television programs, movies, and videos demonstrate and illustrate the value society places on violence. In this model then, the family selects behaviors that maintain, escalate, or reduce the level of violence tolerated by its members. The behaviors selected by family members best suit the psychological disposition, cultural background, and coping strategies used to resolve conflict within the family. Unfortunately, social norms also expose individuals to violent methods of resolving problems, resulting in impulsive and violent acts toward family members.

According to this perspective, four factors place family members at risk for abuse. These risk factors include the family itself, the caregiver, the child, and the presence of a family crisis. Sources of family violence include physical abuse the caregivers either experienced or witnessed in their past (Straus & Gelles, 1989). Poor impulse control, anger management, conflict, and problems solved by blaming or hurting others also contribute to family violence (Youngblade & Belsky, 1990). Caregivers who have a history of domestic violence are also at risk for harming their children (McCloskey, Figueredo, & Koss, 1995), as are children who are born into family systems that lack the financial or psychological resources to create healthy nurturing environments for their individual personalities.

Caregivers who abuse their children tend to be young. Many are single mothers struggling with poverty, role strain, lack of education, and limited personal resources (Gelles, 1992). Many are unprepared for their role in childrearing, immature, impulsive, and have low self-esteem (Widner-Kolberg, 1997). Caregivers who are physically abusive may not only have been abused as children, but also have poor role models and weak social supports.

Another characteristic of caregivers at risk for abusing children is a lack of knowledge, skills, and emotional maturity in understanding and meeting the needs of their child in developmentally appropriate ways as well as inappropriate expectations for their children's behavior. In this situation, the child also often assumes a caregiver role toward the caregiver, as when a five-year-old consoles the unemployed parent. Termed "role-reversal," this commonly occurs in abusive families.

A depressed caregiver is also at risk for physically or emotionally abusing children (Radke-Yarrow, et al., 1995). Such an individual may be irritable or withdrawn from family members, not have the emotional energy to manage the demanding developmental needs of a child, or become provoked and use harsher punishment than necessary or appropriate. Finally, caregivers who abuse substances are more likely to utilize severe punishment and be unable to tolerate a child's normal developmental behaviors (Murphy, Orkow, & Nicola, 1985).

Some infants are born with "fussy" or difficult temperaments, and not easily soothed or calmed. One caregiver may become frustrated and short tempered with such an infant, whereas another caregiver may have the skills or patience to comfort the infant. Fussy, overactive, and unsoothable infants are also more likely to resist a caregiver's attempt at comforting, placing them at greater risk for abuse. Prolonged hospitalization by either the child or caregiver can also interfere with establishing a nurturing bond or appropriate attachment behaviors. Weak attachment bonds from chronic hospitalization can result in a caregiver viewing the child as an "imperfect child" (Brayden, Altemeier, Tucker, Dietrich, & Vietze, 1992; Kotch, et al., 1995), and place her or him more at risk for abuse.

Finally, the child's age, gender, and health status may effect caregiver abuse. Premature infants, a history of low birth weight, children under 3 years of age, and young children with hyperactivity, cerebral palsy and mental retardation are at an elevated risk. Unwanted pregnancies, illegitimacy, and negative attitudes toward a pregnancy also place the child at risk for abuse (Widner-Kolberg, 1997).

Family members are often in situational crises (sudden or prolonged unemployment, illness of family members, residential changes, a caregiver's separation or possible divorce) that precipitate child abuse. Here minor misbehavior can precipitate an abusive interaction, especially when caregivers have exhausted their ability to cope effectively with everyday hassles. In addition, families experiencing constant and chronic stress (financial, physical, mental health problems) are more susceptible to being physically and/or emotionally abusive (Kotch, et al., 1995). Finally, extra-marital affairs, which can create situations where the caregiver is angry and burdened with additional childrearing responsibilities, may result in child abuse and neglect (Brayden, et al., 1992).

Attachment Model

James (1994) defined **attachment** as a reciprocal, enduring, emotional and physical affiliation between a child and a caregiver. Bowlby (1969) considered attachment behavior a preprogrammed set of behavior patterns designed to keep the mother/caregiver close to the infant. Four attachment styles (Florsheim, Henry, & Benjamin, 1996; Main, 1996) assist in understanding how infants and children are emotionally connected to their caregiver. These attachment patterns are listed in Box 36-1.

Children demonstrating avoidant, ambivalent, and disorganized attachment are at risk for being abused.

TYPES OF CHILD ABUSE

Child abuse includes physical abuse, abandonment and neglect, psychological abuse, and sexual abuse. Each is discussed.

Physical Abuse

Physical abuse should always be suspected when there is an injury that cannot be explained, or when the history pro-

BOX 36-1 Patterns of attachment

Secure Attachment: The caregiver meets physical, developmental, and psychological needs, and the infant is able to balance proximity to the caregiver with exploration prior to separation. When an infant is distressed during separation, contact with the caregiver is sought, who then soothes the infant.

Avoidant Attachment: Infant realizes the caregiver will not always be available to provide comfort. The infant exhibits "independent" behavior without acknowledging the caregiver prior to separation, exhibits minimal distress during separation, and avoids emotional support offered by the caregiver upon reunion.

Ambivalent Attachment: The infant understands the caregiver is not reliable in meeting physiological and psychological needs and remains close before separation, is distressed during separation, demonstrates a combination of contact-seeking behaviors with temper tantrums during reunion, and may display indifference when comforted by the caregiver.

Disorganized Attachment: The infant is confused and cannot understand how to get physiological and psychological needs met by the caregiver. This infant may be rejected and/or comforted by the caregiver. Children with this type of attachment display no organized strategy toward the attachment figure.

Adapted from Florsheim, P., Henry, W, & Benjamin, S. (1996). *Integrating individual and interpersonal approaches to diagnosis: The structural analysis of social behavior and attachment theory.* In F. Kaslow (Ed.), *Handbook of relational diagnosis.* New York: John Wiley & Sons; Main, M. (1996). Introduction to the special section on attachment and psychopathology: Overview of the field attachment. *Journal of Consulting and Clinical Psychology, 64*(2), 237–243.

vided is incongruous with the physical findings or the child's developmental level. Suspicion should also be aroused when the caregiver claims the injury was self-inflicted, inflicted by a sibling, or when there is a delay in seeking medical services. However, the cultural background of the family must be considered as well because some folk medicine practices resemble abuse. For instance, **cao gao** practiced by Southeast Asians to treat minor ailments, involves rubbing a coin or a spoon heated in oil on an ill child's neck, spine, and ribs (Monteleone, 1996), may create a burn or abrasion (Figure 36-2). **Cupping** (Ventosos) practiced by Latin American and Russian cultures to treat headaches or abdominal pain, occurs by creating a vacuum under a cup or glass when a small amount of burning material is placed on the skin. The child may then present with first or second-degree burns (Monteleone, 1996).

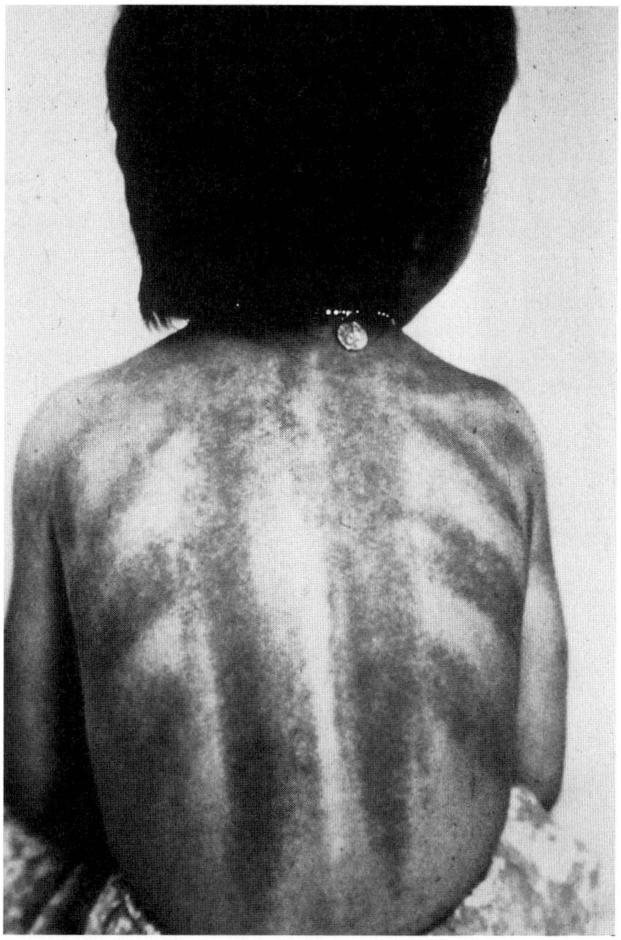

Figure 36-2 Coining, or cao gao, is a folk practice where hot coins are rubbed over a child's back or chest to cure fever. (Used with permission of the American Academy of Pediatrics.)

Clinical Manifestations: Physical

Physical abuse indicators include unexplained bruises, scars, or welts that appear to be in various stages of healing; bruises on the mouth, lips, or eyes; an unexplained swollen extremity; bite marks, especially around the genitals or buttocks; bruises that are the shape of recognizable objects (hand, belt, electric cord), or injuries in locations that a child cannot reach. Burns may be visible on the face, hands, legs, and/or feet; or appear as hot water scalding marks (an even line across the skin, usually on the legs or buttocks). Limited range of motion and complaints of tenderness may suggest skeletal injuries that are the result of direct blows, twisting forces, shaking, or squeezing. Figures 36-3 and 36-4 show marks and burns caused by commonly used objects. Figure 36-5 provides five examples of physical abuse.

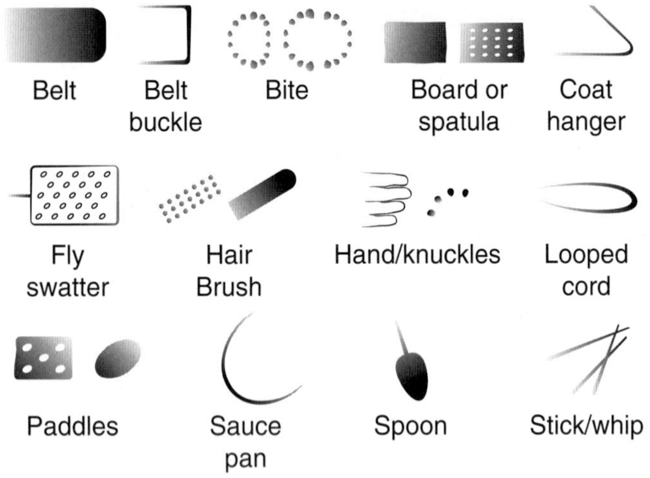

A.

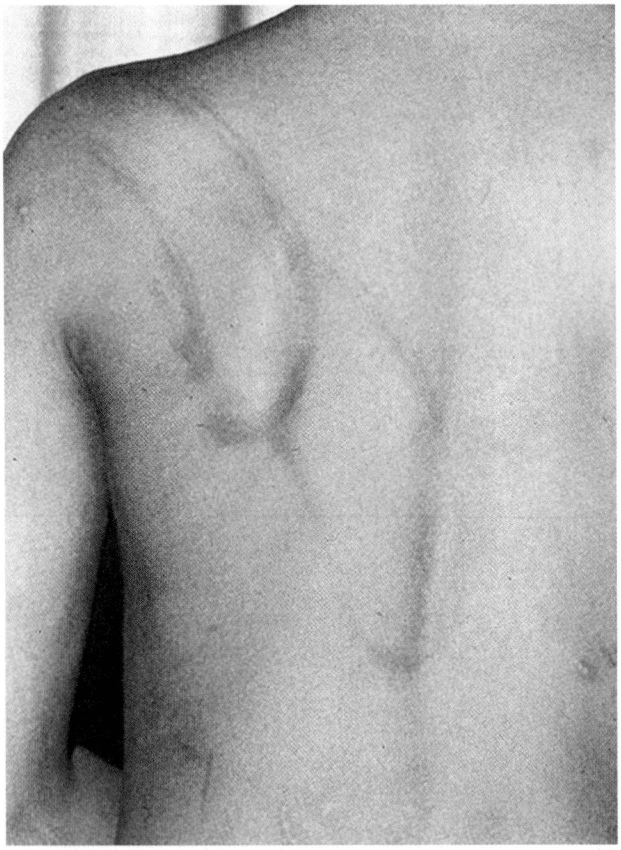

B.

Figure 36-3 (A) Marks on Skin Left by Objects. (B) Bruising in specific patterns such as the loop of a strap often is an indicator of child abuse. Photo courtesy of Emergency Medical Services for Children, NERA, Torrance, CA.

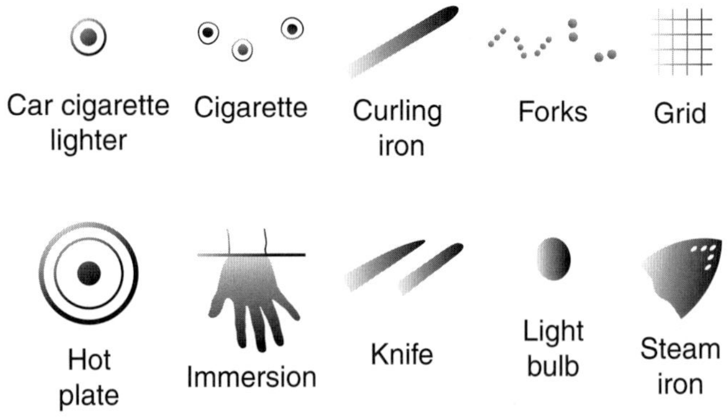

Figure 36-4 Burns on Skin Left by Common Objects

Nursing Alert:

Signs of Abuse

- *Unusual ecchymotic areas such as at the base of the skull or the face, buttocks, breasts, or abdomen should warrant a high index of suspicion of abuse.*
- *Burns, belt marks, or whip marks should always be investigated.*
- *The explanation of the injury doesn't seem consistent with the injury.*

Critical Thinking

Suspecting Child Abuse

Mary, a young mother of five children brings her 2-year-old, Helen, into the emergency department. The child has been vomiting for the past 24 hours, and appears dehydrated, weak, and smells of urine and feces. Upon examination, you notice 6 circular 3 mm areas on the lower back thigh areas that appear to be healing burns. There is erythema and tissue damage surrounding each of the borders. Mary appears angry at having to be in the emergency department and curses at Helen several times. Helen is lying on the stretcher in a fetal position with no eye contact and a sad and withdrawn affect.

1. How does a child receive this type of injury to the back of the legs?
2. How would you proceed with the assessment process? What are the questions that you need to focus on with the mother?

Bruises are injuries to the surface of the skin resulting from accidental falls or bumps. The skin may or may not be broken, and will be discolored. Table 36-2 provides a guide for assessing the characteristics and timeframe for bruising in children. Because young children may have a number of bruises as a result their normal activities, nurses must be able to talk with children and caregivers about the origins of the bruises.

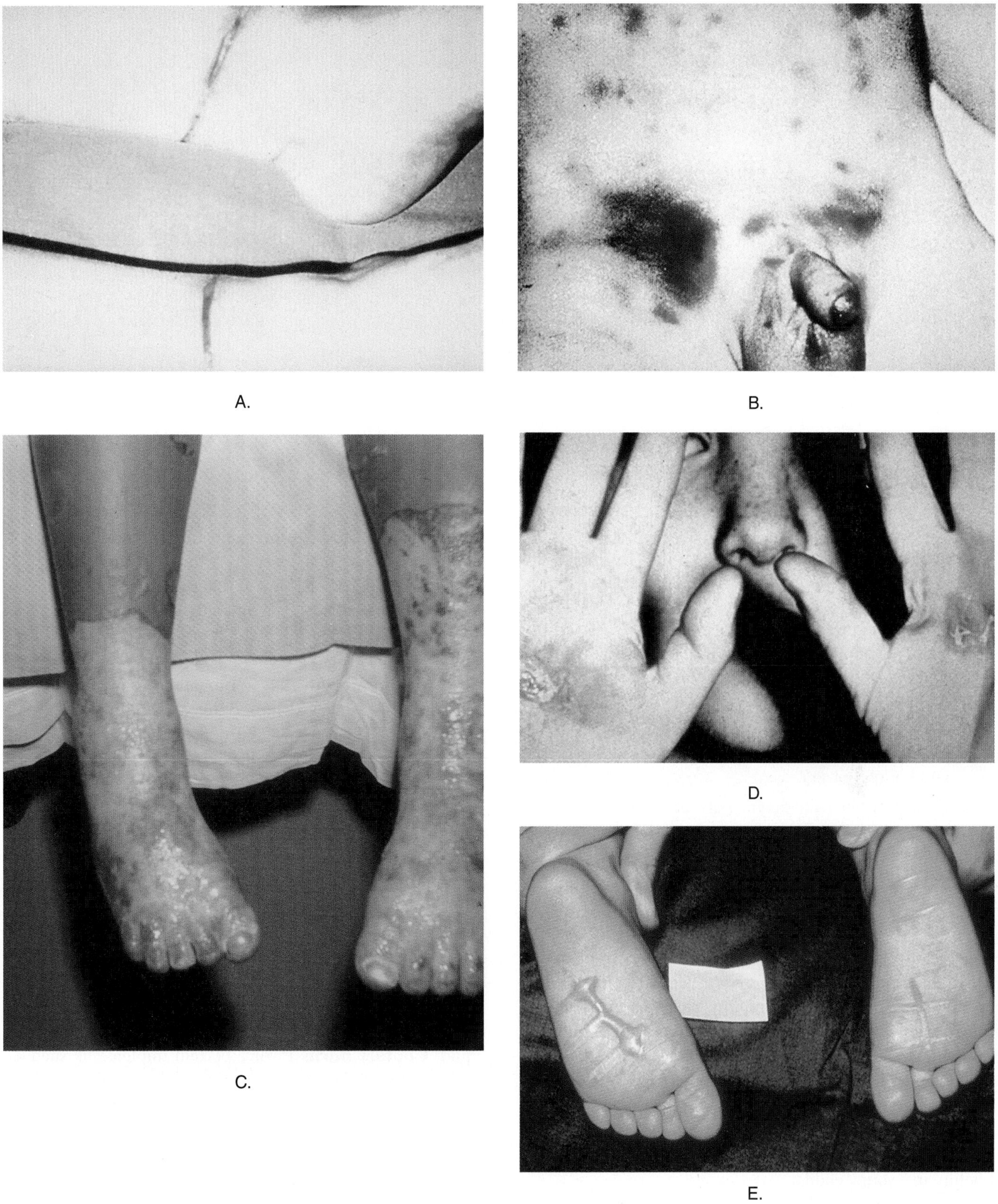

Figure 36-5 Photos of Child Abuse. (A) Bruises that encircle the extremities may indicate the child has been bound. (B) Bruises in various stages of healing may indicate a child is being abused. (C) Circumferential burns (stocking or glove burns) to the extremities may indicate the child was intentionally held in scalding water. (D) Cigarette Burns. (E) Burns that have specific shapes and patterns, called branding, may be an indicator of abuse. All photos courtesy of Emergency Medical Services for Children, NERA, Torrance, CA.

TABLE 36-2 Date Estimation of Bruising in the Abused Child

Time Elapsed	Characteristics
Less than one day	Reddish-blue to purple with margins
1 to 2 days	Bluish-brown to dark purple
3 to 5 days	Yellowish-green to brown
5 to 7 days	Yellow-fading
Past one week	Yellow- brown-fading

Reflective Thinking

Physical Abuse

As a new pediatric intensive care unit nurse, you are assigned to care for a child with second-degree burns on her buttocks and legs. According to Tena, her mother, Emily had been placed in a tub of scalding water by accident. Now Emily requires twenty-four hour intensive care but each time care is provided, one had to wonder how such an "accident" could have occurred. The family was referred to Child Protective Services.

1. How does your attitude influence the care you provide an abused and neglected child like Emily, and her caregiver?
2. What responsibility do you have to ensure the care provided to Tena is nonjudgmental and still professional?

Because the skeletal system is commonly traumatized when children are physically abused, all extremities should be examined for swelling, crepitus, or hematomas. Pulse, color, sensitivity, and function of all limbs are also part of the assessment. Suspicious fractures include chip fractures of the metaphysis, spiral fractures resulting from twisting of the limb, epiphysis separations, and fractures in unusual places such as the ribs, vertebrae, scapula, sternum, or metacarpal bones (Widner-Kolberg, 1997). Figure 36-6 depicts spiral fracture in a young child.

Children between one and five years of age are at risk for burn injuries because their skin is thinner and more sensitive than an adult's. Serious burning also occurs more rapidly and at lower water temperatures. Abusive burns include scald burns, immersion burns, splash burns, flexion burns, and contact burns. **Scald burns** are skin injuries caused by hot water from the tap, coffee, tea, or hot cooking grease from the stove. **Immersion burns** to the buttocks or genitals are sometimes used as a form of punishment for soiling or problem behaviors in toilet training, and create an even line across the legs, buttocks, or hands. They are caused either by an accidental fall into hot bath water or by purposefully placing the child in a tub of hot water.

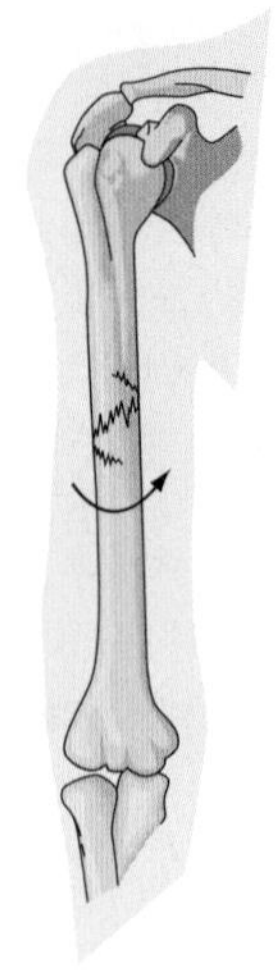

Figure 36-6 Spiral fractures of long bones are caused by twisting forces.

"Stocking or glove" type **burns** represent attempts by the child to prevent and protect him or herself from being immersed in hot scalding tub water; the burn has the appearance of a glove or stocking with an even edge (Monteleone, 1996). **Splash burns** occur when the caregiver pours hot liquid on the child, and usually involve the back, lateral side of the face, or shoulder. The direction the hot liquid flows down the child's body assists in diagnosis. **Flexion burns** occur when caregivers purposefully immerse a child in hot liquids and the body part immersed is held in a flexed position so that a "zebra" pattern occurs (Monteleone, 1996). For example, a child who has hot coffee thrown on his arm may flex the arm so that only the top parts of the forearm and upper arm are burned, and the inside of the arm is protected by flexion in response to the oncoming hot liquid. **Contact burns** involve certain implements such as curling irons, steam irons, cigarette lighters, matches, hot pots, space heaters, or radiators. Old burn marks should give additional cues to nurses that an abusive pattern may exist in the family.

Most abuse deaths are the result of neurological injuries (Widner-Kolberg, 1997). Head injuries are the main cause of these deaths, and involve skull fractures and intracranial hemorrhage (Philip, Traisman, & Philip, 1995). Head injury can also lead to brain damage with developmental delays. Shaken baby syndrome, another type of head injury, first described in 1946 by Caffey, affects between 750 and 3,750 children per year (Beardsley, 1997). **Shaken baby syn-**

drome (SBS) is defined as vigorous manual shaking of a child, usually less than three years of age, that results in a subdural hematoma of the brain, occult bone fractures, and retinal hemorrhages (Kivlin, Kimmons, Lazoritz, & Ruttum, 2000; Wyszynski, 1999). The infant is usually held around the trunk, impeding venous return and causing a pooling of blood in the larger vessels, especially of the head. The shaking motion causes tearing of the large vessels within the head, and the increased blood volume because of impeded venous return contributes to rupture of the blood vessels (Kivlin, et al., 2000). One-third die from their injuries; and one-third experience permanent injury such as mental retardation, vision impairment, seizures, paralysis, developmental delays, spasticity, hearing loss, or blindness (Coody, Brown, Montgomery, Flynn, & Yetman, 1994). The development of technology, in particular, computed tomography (CT) scans and magnetic resonance imaging, has resulted in better identification and diagnosis of SBS. In the past, injuries associated with SBS may have been attributed to sudden infant death syndrome or unusual or mysterious neurological disorders (Chiocca, 1995). Shaken baby syndrome can go unattended, undetected, and unreported because there often are no outward symptoms. In addition, caregivers are not always willing to acknowledge they were responsible for shaking a baby (Butler, 1995).

Infants and children should be suspected of SBS with any signs of head injury, including poor feeding or vomiting, irritability, listlessness, lethargy, bradycardia, apnea, seizures, coma, bulging fontanels, large head circumference, hypothermia, failure to thrive, or other diffuse symptoms (Coody, et al., 1994; Locsin, 1999). An ophthalmologic examination assists in confirming a diagnosis as a classic sign is retinal hemorrhage, usually bilaterally with subdural or subarachnoid hemorrhages (Kivlin, et al., 2000). It is also important for the nurse to be alert to significant alterations in neurological symptoms of a child even when a family member claims no apparent reason for the acute neurological symptoms.

SBS should be managed by a multidisciplinary team, and includes a neurological evaluation, ophthalmologic examination, CAT scan, ultrasound, radiography, and careful history of the injury or illness. Birth trauma, meningitis, severe accidental trauma, infection, severe coagulopathy (hemophilia, von Willebrand's disease, and vitamin K deficiency), seizure disorders, and metabolic disorders should be ruled out before the diagnosis of SBS is determined (Chiocca, 1995; Kivlin, et al., 2000; Coody, et al., 1994).

Risk factors for SBS include caregivers' gender as well as those experiencing stressful life events such as social, physical, or financial problems. Men are responsible for 60% of the physical abuse and physical abuse deaths attributed to SBS. A mother's partner or boyfriend, as well as baby-sitters have been implicated (Advisory Board on Child Abuse and Neglect, 1995).

Abdominal injuries rank second to neurological injuries as the major cause of abuse-related death (Widner-Kolberg, 1997). Blunt trauma to the abdomen may cause lacerations to internal organs (liver, bladder, spleen, pancreas, bowel) resulting in distension. Bruising may be absent or minimal. If an abdominal injury is suspected, the child should also be examined for puncture wounds and the hematocrit monitored because of possible internal hemorrhage.

Clinical Manifestations: Psychological

Physically abused children may also exhibit passive behaviors such as withdrawal, depression, and/or a sad mood. Other behaviors can include anger, hostility, or being frightened when approached. Children who have been physically abused may also harm their siblings, peers, pets, and/or neighborhood animals (Cicchetti, Toth, & Lynch, 1995). Box 36-2 lists other behavioral indicators of abuse.

Diagnosis

The diagnosis of physical abuse is based on a complete nursing history and assessment, medical examination, and laboratory tests. X rays or CT scans may also be ordered to confirm the diagnosis.

Treatment

Treatment may vary depending on the severity of abuse. Extreme physical abuse including internal hemorrhage or organ injury will likely require admission to a pediatric intensive care unit. Neurological evaluation and monitoring may be necessary if a head injury is suspected. Consultation with specialists such as orthopedists or neurologists may also be required. The child will often need counseling, and the caregiver will need education related to parenting skills, anger management, and normal human development so the abuse is not repeated. Table 36-3 lists some measures of assessment of parental care. In some cases, removal of the child from the abuser's care will be mandated.

BOX 36-2 Behavioral indicators of physical abuse

- Frightened stance when adults approach
- Hyper-alert when caregivers give directions
- Anxiety and distress when hearing other children cry
- Fear of returning home
- Increased startle reflex
- Overeagerness to please
- Lack of ability to attach to caregiver
- Extremes of behavior: aggressive, or passive and withdrawn
- Frequent daydreams or staring into space
- Detached stance toward others

TABLE 36-3 Measures for Assessing Parental Care

Measure	Respondents	Authors
Adolescent Abuse Inventory	Adolescents who are parents	Sebes, 1986
Psychological Maltreatment Scale	Administered by a trained observer	Taylor, Underwood, Thomas, and Franklin, 1988
Home Observation for Measurement of The Environment (HOME) Inventory	Administered by a trained observer	Caldwell and Bradley, 1984
Family Experiences Questionnaire	Adolescents	Briere and Runtz, 1988

Nursing Management

The nursing assessment for a child suspected of being physically abused should include a comprehensive evaluation, photographs, and written documentation of the body systems affected by using a body chart and careful descriptions (Box 36-3). It is also important to obtain height and weight measurements to determine whether or not they are within the normal range for age. The integumentary system, including the skin, scalp, bottoms of the feet, and the complete trunk and genital areas should be carefully examined. All bruises, scars, burns, and discoloration of the skin should be noted and in some institutions photographs taken to document the injuries. The musculoskeletal system should be assessed for painful muscles, swollen ribs, or past fractures. The urinary/genital system will also need to be evaluated, and the presence of blood or protein in the urine, along with past urinary tract infections noted. Finally, the child's mental status should be assessed utilizing the information listed in Box 36-4 and Box 36-5.

Relevant information about a family's history of or experience with abuse can be obtained from conversations with the caregivers and the child. Because nurses are professionals perceived as helpful and caring, caregivers and children may be more open and honest in sharing information with the nurse about how discipline is practiced and how problems in the family are handled. Box 36-6 and Box 36-7 provide guidelines to use when talking with both the child and caregiver.

BOX 36-3 History and physical assessment categories—Child abuse

- Location, color, size, shape of any injury recorded on body chart
- Specific characteristics of bruise, including an outline and the depth of injury
- Pain or tenderness associated with injury
- Complete assessment of all body systems
- General level of hygiene
- Exact date, time, and place of event
- Chronological account of injury
- Witnesses present at time of injury
- Exact quotations by child and caregiver of how the injury occurred

BOX 36-4 Psychological assessment categories—Child abuse

- Appearance
- Mood (feelings, lability, fluctuations, appropriateness, ease in displaying feelings)
- Manner of relating to examiner
- Modes of thinking and intellectual skills
- Play (capacity, fantasy, amount, quality of involvement, use of materials, themes, spontaneity, and interaction with examiner)
- Sensorimotor development (fine and gross motor activities, symmetry of movement, eye-hand coordination)
- Speech and language skills; the capacity to communicate with examiner

BOX 36-5 Interpersonal assessment: Caregiver—Child abuse

- Willingness to contribute information
- Level of cooperation during interview
- Capacity to display empathy/support/care toward the child, and the child's response
- Non-verbal behaviors, affect, level of cooperation (eye contact, posture)
- Quality of child/caregiver relationship (fearful, anxious, hostile, indifferent, close)

BOX 36-6 Interviewing the child

- Interview privately without interruptions.
- Reassure child is not "in trouble" nor has done anything wrong. (Because children often assume they are to blame for the caregiver's actions, it is important to remind them the injuries are not their fault.)
- Assure child the conversation is confidential; if the information provided needs to be shared with others, inform the child.
- Consider the child's developmental level when talking about the incident. Use the child's own words when documenting the incident (they become part of the legal record).
- Allow talking at own pace; use a supportive matter-of-fact attitude.
- Encourage the child to show injuries.
- Utilize therapeutic play, drawings, puppet play, or story time to share thoughts and feelings if the child does not have verbal skills to talk openly about experiences.
- Inform child it is okay to talk to the caregiver about conversations with the nurse.
- If the authorities are to be notified, both child and caregivers need to be informed.

BOX 36-7 Interviewing the caregivers

- Allow caregivers to feel comfortable; conduct interview privately.
- Be professional, honest, direct, and avoid showing anger or hostility.
- Establish a supportive relationship.
- Be aware of the role Child Protective Services will play in the situation so accurate information needs to be provided; explain how Child Protective Services will provide support and assistance.
- Inform caregivers not to punish the child for sharing information.

Munchausen Syndrome

Asher (1951) coined the term "Munchausen syndrome" to designate patients who traveled from hospital to hospital presenting with illnesses and receiving treatments that at times included surgery. The condition was named after Baron Karl Friedrich Hieronymus Freiherr van Munchausen (1720–1797), a German cavalry officer, who was also a world-class liar.

The label **Munchausen syndrome by proxy** refers to caregivers who fabricate signs and symptoms of disease and/or expose their child to harmful medical interventions

Case Study/Care Plan

The Physically Abused Child

Peter, a six-year-old male, was admitted for whip marks and bruises that are approximately one-half inch wide on his back and legs. The caregiver is his 25-year-old mother, Holly, who also has three other children under 5 years of age. Currently she is living in a shelter because she is unemployed and has no money for rent. Ted, her partner who used to be in charge of the children's discipline, abandoned Holly and the children 6 months ago. She cried during the interview and indicated the only way to make her children behave is to hit them with a belt.

Nursing Care Plan

Nursing Diagnosis #1

Interrupted family process caused by disrupted attachment, lack of nurturing qualities, or past abusive parenting experiences.

Expected Outcomes

1. Peter will begin to feel safe with Holly.
2. Holly will begin to model appropriate nurturing behaviors toward Peter.

Interventions/*Rationales*

1. Teach nurturing behaviors to Holly. *Caregivers need to be taught normal human development and the role of nurturing in facilitating development.*

continues

continued

2. Focus on the ability to comfort Peter, provide age-appropriate discipline, engage in age-appropriate activities, and understand Peter's needs based on normal growth and development. *Positive attachment behaviors provide the foundation for nurturing caregiver roles.*

3. Explore with Holly behavior that may interfere with the ability to nurture. *Caregivers may have personal problems that impact their caregiving ability.*

4. Teach and engage in role-modeling behaviors with Peter. *Intergenerational transmission of violence is common.*

5. Provide time during hospitalization where Peter and Holly can participate in age-appropriate, nurturing activities. *Caregivers may not have had nurturing experiences during their childhood years and need support and acknowledgment for their caring efforts and information about how to nurture.*

6. Be supportive and nurturing to Holly when attempting to change her behavior. *Caregivers need opportunities to engage in play activities with their child and practice supportive behaviors.*

7. Provide referral for counseling and in-home supportive resources if needed. *Caregivers may need ongoing in-home support from community agencies.*

Evaluation

Peter is more comfortable around Holly. Holly will demonstrate nurturing attachment behaviors toward Peter. Holly will acknowledge past problems and willingness to accept support.

Nursing Diagnosis #2

Risk for trauma related to evidence of physical abuse, physical neglect, and an unsafe environment.

Expected Outcomes

1. Peter will remain safe within the family system: no evidence of physical abuse or neglect.
2. The family will be involved in ongoing counseling to eliminate abusive behaviors.
3. Holly will be open and responsive to supportive interventions.

Interventions/*Rationales*

1. Assess Peter's physical and emotional status; intervene as indicated in Nursing Diagnosis #1. Refer to appropriate counseling and support. *An emotional status assessment may reflect signs of post-traumatic stress disorder from repeated abusive episodes. Interventions listed previously will help prevent further abuse.*

2. Refer family to appropriate counseling and explain importance of obtaining ongoing counseling. *Ongoing counseling will decrease abuse and increase parenting skills.*

3. Approach Holly in a supportive and nonjudgmental manner. *The child's safety rests on ensuring that caregivers stay in the health care system and utilize services.*

4. Provide Holly education in age-appropriate and safe discipline, time-out methods; age-appropriate growth and development; Peter's need for psychological and social support; nutrition; self-care activities; care of a sick child; and enhancement of nurturing behaviors. *Teaching normal development behavior and discipline practices helps improve interactions.*

Evaluation

1. Peter and Holly will accept teaching and resources offered; Peter remains free from further injury.
2. Holly will attend counseling and integrate information into her behavior with her children.
3. Holly will understand value of attending/participating in counseling and integrate information taught into her interactions with her children.

continues

continued

Nursing Diagnosis #3

Situational low self-esteem related to past physical abuse and neglect and unsafe environment.

Expected Outcomes

Peter will express feelings related to past abuse.

Peter will regain a sense of control and positive self-regard.

Interventions/*Rationales*

1. Acknowledge to Peter that he is safe and loved; encourage talking and supporting child's attempts at talking about experiences. *Support builds trust and security.*

2. Encourage Peter to engage in self-care decisions, give praise and support to initiate the activities. *Positive experiences facilitate self-esteem and sense of control.*

Evaluation

Peter begins to feel more comfortable and begins talking about experiences related to abuse.

Peter will be able to express positive feelings toward self, engage in age-appropriate activities, and demonstrate the ability to have control through choice of several aspects of daily activities.

and painful invasive procedures. The individual parent or caregiver (usually the mother) who injures children in this manner is recognized as a child abuser. The *Diagnostic and Statistical Manual of Mental Disorders* classifies Munchausen syndrome by proxy as a Fictitious Disorder Not Otherwise Specified (APA, 1994).The criteria for a caregiver to meet the diagnosis of the Munchausen Syndrome include (a) intentional production or feigning of psychological or physical signs or symptoms in a person who is under the individual's care; (b) external incentives for the behavior causing illness or injury are absent; (c) motivation for the behavior is to assume a sick role by proxy; (d) the behavior is not accounted for by another mental disorder (APA, 1994, p.727).

The adult abuser receives this diagnosis rather than the child, and uses the disease to escape from marital, physical, and/or emotional problems, or poor self-esteem (Palmer & Yoshimura, 1984; Meadow, 1985). By attending to the supposed needs of the child, the caregiver escapes the reality of his/her problems. Many times there is also a history of psychiatric problems and treatment (Yorker & Kaham, 1990), and there usually is a poor emotional relationship between the child's parents. Frequently the caregiver has had some exposure to the medical field and is quickly accepted as competent by professionals caring for the child.

Children are often brought to the hospital or emergency room with a variety of suspected problems including infections, electrolyte imbalances, nonaccidental poisonings, apnea, hemorrhage, seizures, and/or respiratory illnesses. Assessment includes videotaping the child/caregiver interaction when Munchausen syndrome by proxy is suspected. The warning signs of the disease in a child are found in Box 36-8.

Nursing Management

Nursing management includes establishing a trusting relationship with caregivers, accurately assessing family dynamics,

BOX 36-8 Warning signs of Munchausen syndrome by proxy

- Prolonged, unexpected, or extraordinary illness; extensive history provided by mother.
- Inappropriate signs and symptoms with no relationship to the history provided.
- Several prior medical contacts and evaluations, with negative diagnostic findings.
- Appropriate treatment is poorly tolerated and ineffective.
- Past family history of serious childhood disorders and possibly unexplained sibling deaths. (Meadow, 1985)

Reflective Thinking

Beliefs and values about child abuse

1. What is your personal understanding of why child abuse occurs?
2. How can you advocate for a child in spite of caregivers' protests or denials?
3. How do you feel about disciplining a child with physical force?

REFLECTIONS FROM FAMILIES

Chad has not been doing well in preschool. He hits and punches the other children, has been having terrible temper tantrums, and is sent home from school at least once a week. The program director has advised me to place him in a therapeutic nursery program. During that time, I began to realize that the many times I have spanked and hit Chad with my belt have caused him to want to hurt other children. At first I could not believe this, because this is how my mother raised me. I know I need to discipline differently to stop Chad from hurting others. I am now seeking assistance from a nurse who works in the preschool program.

patterns of illness, and quality of relationships; carefully documenting all caregiver/child interactions and behaviors; corroborating all histories with appropriate professionals and reporting inconsistencies; reviewing suspected cases of Munchausen syndrome by proxy with the multidisciplinary teams; and following up as indicated to the appropriate child protection agencies and mental health services.

Childhood Abandonment and Neglect

Child abandonment is defined as a caregiver's intentional withholding, without just cause or excuse, of care, presence, love, protection, maintenance, and affection. According to Munkel (1989), there are six types of abandonment: a child (1) is left to die (for instance, the newborn is left in a garbage can by the mother); (2) is left with others and the caregiver does not return; (3) is locked out of the house and forced to survive on the street; (4) is left without supervision; (5) does not receive any love or affection (emotional abandonment); or (6) a parent refuses custody.

Child neglect occurs when a child experiences predictable injury or impairment because of caregiver inattention. Neglect is often suspected in children who are not of normal height and weight for age. In addition, neglectful caregivers may not have kept up with yearly child health assessments, or acted on school recommendations for such services as speech, language, or physical therapy evaluations. Other signs of child neglect appear in Box 36-9.

BOX 36-9 Signs/symptoms of neglect

Inadequate Care (General):

Inappropriate meals (serving cereal for breakfast, lunch, and nothing for dinner)
Clothing that is old, dirty, inappropriate for age, or fits poorly
Lack of personal hygiene
Lack of health care maintenance (routine immunizations, yearly examinations)
Poor supervision, inadequate limit setting (allowing a 5-year-old to play outside until 11 PM)
Child welfare endangerment caused by caregiver dependency on chemicals/drugs

Inadequate Physical Environment:

Inadequate shelter (unheated rooms, lack of running water or proper plumbing)
Inadequate sleeping conditions (having female child sleep with an older brother)
Poor sanitary conditions (garbage in the home or play area)
Structural/electrical/fire hazards (unprotected electrical outlets)
Chemicals/drugs not in locked cabinets or within child's reach
Water temperature hazards (temperature too hot)

Inadequate Parenting:

Frequent school absences
Inappropriate discipline (locked in a closet, physically punished)
Emotional abandonment (never attending school conferences, not involved in caregiver-child school-related activities)
Locked out of house
Independent decisions made without setting parent limits
Parent uncooperative when school supports child

Research Highlight

Characteristics of Troubled Youths in a Shelter

Study Purpose

To a) discover if runaway youths have experienced abuse; b) describe the characteristics of these young runaways; c) identify significant events in their life; and d) suggest interventions to help these young runaways and their families.

Methods

Seventy-eight runaway youths in central Florida completed the Codington Life Events Scale and a structured clinical interview.

Findings

Many runaway youths experienced some form of abuse from their caregivers: 46.5% reported physical abuse; 23.3% reported sexual abuse; 2.3% reported emotional abuse; and 29.9% reported a combination of physical, sexual, and emotional abuse. The young people were also exposed to drugs and alcohol, and experiencing high levels of stressful life events.

Implications

Become more involved and advocate for this disenfranchised population; provide outreach services that help connect these adolescents to multidisciplinary service providers such as counseling services, family counseling, in-home family services, and parenting education. Educate teachers to identify the early warning signs of abuse and enact appropriate services for these needy adolescents. Attention to services that intervene with the precursors of runaway behavior can prevent runaway episodes in the future.

Citation

Gary, F., Moorhead, J., & Warren, J. (1996). Characteristics of troubled youths in a shelter. *Archives of Psychiatric Nursing, X,*(1), 41–48.

Nursing Management

Nursing interventions for child neglect are similar to those of physical abuse. In addition, the nurse should understand the child's attachment to the caregiver even though the caregiver is neglectful. The nurse should provide a safe, positive, trusting, and nurturing environment, where the child is allowed to interact with other children and receive adult attention in a caring and warm manner. The child may need an explanation regarding why the caregiver may not be allowed to visit, or why the child is placed in foster care. Additional services needed for families of neglected children or foster families include visiting nurse service, homemaker services, parenting classes, parent support groups, follow-up programs with school systems, and parent hotline telephone numbers when feelings of anger or frustration are building within the family setting.

Psychological Abuse

Psychological abuse is defined as acts of omission (willfully not attending a child's graduation or award ceremony) or commission (a child is told that he/she is ugly) deemed psychologically damaging. It also involves the presence of hostile behavior as well as the absence of positive parenting behaviors. O'Hagan (1993) indicated the sustained, repetitive nature of the behavior qualifies it as psychologically damaging and abusive. Messages like "Nothing you do is of any value or good enough," or "You are no-good and worthless" have serious consequences when it comes from a significant caregiver or attachment figure during childhood (Berlin & Vondra, 1999). Caregivers can be aware or unaware of the hurt and emotional pain their words cause, and often are repeating experiences they had with their own caregivers relative to discipline and guidance, without considering the effects and meaning they have on their child's psychological growth (Youngblade & Belsky, 1990).

Lesnik-Oberstein, Koers, and Cohen (1995) believe factors affecting psychological abuse operate at many systemic levels (individual, family, community, and sub-cultural) and are related to six factors: (1) a lower level of moral reasoning that supports treating a child in hurtful ways; (2) cultural approval of certain verbal aggression; (3) lack of effect of past abuse; (4) alcohol; (5) absence of support systems resulting in frustration and harsh discipline; and (6) low levels of empathy toward a child so the effect of harmful actions or words is missing.

Egeland and Erickson (1987) believe emotionally unavailable or psychologically neglectful caregivers stem from a person's unmet emotional needs coupled with low levels of social support. Many times caregivers did not experience caring, warm, and comforting parenting styles that taught them how to nurture their children. Psychiatric illnesses such as depression or personality disorders are additional risk factors for psychological abuse. Finally, a caregiver's behavior may represent the re-creation of patterns of psychological abuse experienced as a child, or poor problem-solving ability.

Indicators suggesting psychological abuse are found in Box 36-10. Assessment scales that identify children who are abused or caregivers who are at increased risk to maltreat infants and children are listed in Table 36-4.

A multidisciplinary team, composed of a nurse, physician, and social worker needs to work collaboratively in assessing and diagnosing psychological abuse. Areas for assessment include the clinical manifestations listed earlier as well as noting if the child has school-related problems such as poor grades, or withdrawn behaviors.

Treatment may involve complete physical examination and X rays to ensure physical or sexual abuse is not present also. Professionals who work with children suspected of being abused may also have interactions with the legal system and CPS workers for coordinated, multidisciplinary efforts. Treatment will be initiated by the legal and court system to protect children and will include ongoing supervision, family counseling, and resources such as parenting and anger management classes.

BOX 36-10 Indicators of psychological abuse

Poor self-esteem
Poor academic performance
Acting-out behaviors in school and community
Fighting and hitting other children
Lack of friends or peer group
Lack of involvement in school and after-school activities
Depression
Little time spent at home
Suicidal ideation
Involvement in drugs/alcohol
Problems with personal hygiene
Self-defeating and self-mutilating behaviors
Lack of trust in adults
Speech disorder
Failure to thrive
Physical illness

Reflective Thinking

Psychological Abuse

Seven-year-old Ryan comes from an upper middle class family where both parents are employed. Ryan has developed suicidal ideation in response to ongoing verbal abuse and being either left at home alone or with neighbors most of the week. This is his father Carl's second marriage, and Carl spends most of his time with his new wife. Your nursing assessment reveals Ryan is depressed, withdrawn in school, and failing three major subjects. Ryan's teacher reports that since the divorce, he is "not the same." The teacher knows Ryan was very close to his mother but Carl was awarded custody. When you interview Ryan, he reports his father always tells him he is "worthless, just like his mother," he "always puts me down no matter what grades I bring home," and he "never allows me to leave the house to play with my friends after school."

1. What would you say to Ryan?
2. How would you handle the report of abuse from Ryan?

Sexual Abuse

Sexual abuse is defined as exploitive sexual act(s) imposed on a child who lacks the emotional, cognitive, or maturational development to deal with the actions (Helfer & Kempe, 1987). There are several forms of sexual abuse or maltreatment, including assault, incest, exploitation, exhibitionism, pedophilia, and child molestation.

TABLE 36-4 Scales to Use in Assessing Abused Children and/or Abusive Caregivers

Measure	Description
Maternal Attitude Scale (Cohler, Weiss, & Grunebaum, 1970)	Maternal beliefs about child needs and parenting practices
Family Stress Checklist (Murphy, Orkow, & Nicola, 1985)	Parental experiences of abuse, mental illness, psychological problems, and other risk factors
Home Observation for Measurement of Environment (Caldwell & Bradley, 1984)	Measures the quality and quantity of support for development available in a child's home environment

Assault is an unlawful, sudden, violent attack on another person; **rape,** considered a type of assault, is sexual intercourse with force or a threat of force, and without a person's consent. **Statutory rape** is consensual sexual relations between a minor and an adult. **Date** or **acquaintance rape** is sexual intercourse with force or threat where the victim and perpetrator know one another either socially or professionally. Teenagers and college-age students are at most risk for this type of abuse.

Incest is sexual intercourse between closely related persons. Caregivers from upper socioeconomic levels and high achievers are just as likely to abuse their children in this manner, but less likely to be detected, as those from lower socioeconomic classes (Yates, 1991). Incest by fathers, stepfathers, and siblings has increased over the past 20 years. In fact, sibling incest has been estimated to be at least five times more common than parent-child incest (Canavan, Meyer, & Higgs, 1992). Characteristics of incestuous families include power imbalances in the family; fear of authority in the children; isolation from the community; denial; blurred and inappropriate boundaries/role confusion; highly sexualized or highly repressive atmosphere; history of multigenerational sexual/physical abuse, or alcoholism; lack of empathy; poor communication patterns; inadequate limit setting; and emotional deprivation (Heiman, 1992).

Exploitation involves prostitution and child pornography. Exploitation can range from nudity, disrobing, and genital exposure by an adult in front of a child, to observing a child undress, bathe or use the toilet, intimate kissing, fondling, or masturbation. The child's emotional development is affected by this type of abuse, resulting in shame, guilt, depression, anxiety, psychosomatic disorder, substance abuse, attention deficit hyperactive disorders, and conduct/oppositional disorders (Berlin & Vondra, 1999). **Exhibitionism** is exposing one's genitals to strangers. **Pedophilia** is when an adult directs his or her sexual interests primarily or exclusively toward children. **Child molestation** is sexual involvement (oral-genital contact, genital fondling and viewing, masturbation) involving a child.

Certain factors place children at risk for sexual assault or incest (Finkelhor, 1988). Those factors include the presence of a stepfather in the home; a caregiver and child who are not emotionally connected; a caregiver who never finished high school, is sexually punitive or repressive, or has an income under $10,000; and the child has two or fewer friends.

Many times children are raised by caregivers who were sexually or physically abused themselves (Cooper, Murphy, & Haynes, 1996). These caregivers either do not believe they were sexually assaulted or kept it a secret from their family members. Therefore, the caregiver fails to protect or teach their own children how to protect themselves from potentially unsafe situations. In addition, personal safety rules may not be discussed openly in the family. For example, a twelve-year-old girl who allows a male friend of the family to visit the house while the caregiver is not present in the home and is consequently raped, should have been taught to never let anyone, even friends of the family, into the home while alone.

Finkelhor (1988) suggests four factors describe the experience of sexually abused children, and the consequent effect they have on their growth and development. The factors are traumatic sexualization, stigmatization, betrayal, and powerlessness.

First, children can be rewarded for inappropriate and unsafe sexual behavior, and learn affection and love are equated with sex. Termed **traumatic sexualization**, the child is confused and becomes preoccupied with sexual behavior, demonstrates precocious sexual behaviors or prostitution, or becomes sexually aggressive toward peers and younger children. The children may also have flashbacks of past sexual assaults.

The second factor, stigmatization, occurs when abusers blame children for their sexual behaviors by telling them they (the children) asked to be touched or did not make the abuser stop after it started. The child is perceived as "spoiled goods," feels different from other children, and has a lowered sense of self-esteem. The secret of this abuse is maintained by coercion or threats related to personal and bodily safety.

In betrayal, a close family member or family friend victimizes the child who then experiences a breach of trust, care, and protection. The child is unable to tell anyone about the abuse because of being physically threatened or fearing retaliation. Manifestations include anxiety, depression, mistrust, anger, hostility, and clinging or aggressive behaviors.

Finally, the child experiences a sense of extreme powerlessness, vulnerability, fear, violation of bodily integrity, and the inability to control the assaults. Even though the child may tell an adult about the abuse, the adult often does not believe the child because the adult may have been sexually abused, is denying this abuse, or is unable to tolerate any thoughts and feelings related to past abuse. Table 36-5 lists other manifestations of sexual abuse in children.

Assessment of the physical signs of sexual abuse requires special care and attention. In addition to the physical indicators listed in Table 36-5, any venereal disease or diagnosis of pregnancy in a young adolescent is a strong indicator of sexual abuse and may require further investigation, interviewing, or referral. Refer to Box 36-11 and Box 36-12 for more information about suspected sexual abuse.

A colopscopic examination of the genital and rectal areas by an expert in the field is often requested by law enforcement officials to determine if there is evidence of acute trauma or past injury (Burns, Barber, Brady, & Dunn, 1996). Any sexual abuse that involves oral, genital, rectal, or penile contact or penetration within 72 hours normally requires collection of appropriate forensics specimens (Burns, et al., 1996), and cultures for *Neisseria gonorrhea*, *Chlamydia trachomatis*, syphilis, HIV, hepatitis B, herpes simplex, bacterial vaginosis, human papillomavirus, and *T. vaginitis*.

TABLE 36-5 Manifestations of Sexual Abuse in Children

Inappropriate Coping Behaviors	Mood Regulation Problems	Cognitive Problems	Sexual Problems	Physical Indicators
• Substance use/abuse • Running away from home • Self-mutilation • Victimizing others • Eating disorders • Sleeping problems	• Depression • Anxiety • Hostility • Irritability • Phobias • Aggression	• Learning problems • Failing grades • Daydreaming • Dissociation • Nightmares • Low self-esteem	• Sexualized or promiscuous behaviors • Prostitution • Confusion about sexual identity • Masturbation	• A strong fear of examination • Presence of sexually transmitted diseases • Abnormal discharge or odor from genital area • Repeated urinary tract infections • Encopresis • Enuresis • Urethral irritation • Rectal/vaginal tears; bruising around the buttocks and hip areas; cuts, tears, or bleeding around the anal mucosa • A broken hymen (activity such as gymnastics or horseback riding, use of tampons or forceful wiping during diaper change may also cause a broken hymen [Estes, 2002])

The local forensic medical authority should be consulted prior to examination and a kit is often provided with written instructions regarding obtaining and preserving specimens. Specimens from the cervix, vagina, and rectum are needed to check for gonorrhea, motile sperm, acid phosphatase, or the presence of blood group antigens.

Other strategies for evaluating suspected sexual abuse in children include asking them to make a family drawing and then talking about the drawing. The child could also be asked who takes care of them, important things or activities they do together, or if family members engage in activities that scare or make the child sad. If a child begins to disclose sexual information during these conversations, be sure to seek additional staff, such as a physician or social worker, to validate and corroborate the statements.

The child and nurse may also need to use a common set of terms to talk about sexualized behaviors. Having the child or caregiver give the usual names for body parts helps improve communication as families may have special names for breasts, penis, buttock, and so forth. An easy way to learn family terms is to have the child label body parts on a human figure drawing. Then the nurse can be more sensitive in interactions and if the child talks about inappropriate touching or abuse, the nurse will know what the child means.

Another way of eliciting information is through puppet play, which can facilitate a child's ability to talk about secrets surrounding sexual abuse. The child may be more likely to share a problem, or get permission from the nurse that it is "OK" to talk about other people touching their body parts during play activities. This also supports the child's attempt to deal with the shame and potential consequences of telling and talking about their own experiences.

Children suspected of being sexually abused should be referred to specialists in child and adolescent psychiatry, a clinical social worker, or a clinical psychologist specializing in sexual abuse. The nurse and other professionals can then work collaboratively to devise more effective ways to help the child deal with the powerlessness and guilt of the abuse. The nurse must follow facility protocol when suspecting child abuse.

Many children who have been sexually abused are diagnosed with post-traumatic stress disorder (PTSD) (APA, 1994). Refer to chapter 35 for aditional information about PTSD.

Children who have experienced sexual abuse present with a wide range of symptoms and require complex intervention strategies. Immediate issues relate to ensuring a safe and protective place for the child and requiring all suspicious symptoms be reported to the proper authorities. If

BOX 36-11 When sexual abuse is suspected

Only an experienced member of the child abuse team should perform a genitalia examination. Adequate explanation, preparation, and possible sedation prior to examination are important, even though speculum examination of prepubescent females is often not required. The examination should be careful and complete, with accurate documentation of any bleeding, bruising, ligature, or teeth marks. Be sure to note the child's general appearance (including state of cleanliness) and demeanor and save all clothing in a sealed bag. Photograph any wound or injury. Use of a Wood's lamp can help in identifying semen.

(Hazinski, 1992)

BOX 36-12 Questions to ask if sexual abuse is suspected (can be asked of either caregiver or child)

- How are beds arranged; do children sleep in parents' bed?
- Who bathes the children; are the doors open or closed during this time?
- Are the bedroom doors kept open or closed at night?
- Does either parent have trouble sleeping at night and where do they go if he or she awakens?
- Do the children and a parent have secrets from the other parent?
- Does the child engage in activities that the other parent is suspicious of?
- Do the children have a method for keeping themselves safe from being sexually abused?

Kids Want To Know

Is it my fault that my daddy hurt me this way?

Seven-year-old Gwyneth was admitted with a diagnosis of gonococcal infection. While she was your client, she was evaluated by the pediatric psychologist for suspected sexual abuse. After she disclosed to the psychologist that her mother's boyfriend had sexually abused her, she states to you: "It was all my fault that he did this to me." The nurse responds: "It is never your fault for what happened. It is always the adult who is responsible for making you feel this way."

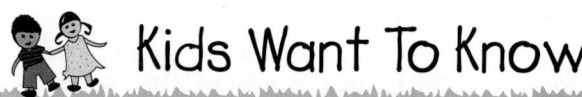

hospitalization is required, the child must be protected and all caregiver visitations supervised. During caregiver's visits, documentation of interactions as with all suspected cases of abuse is critical. If the child is depressed or anxious, the nurse should spend time alleviating fears and anxieties. Efforts to prepare the child for discharge to other family members or foster care will also need to be addressed.

Ongoing enrollment in individual and family treatment by teams specializing in sexual abuse treatment is essential. Cognitive changes in memory, academic functioning, and level of awareness are occurring. Therefore, caregivers need to understand children cannot remember what happened, may begin failing in school and appear to daydream and stare. This behavior should not be considered uncooperative or acting out and should never be punished.

Teachers may need to be informed of the possibility of academic problems, the child provided with extra positive attention, and monitored in the school setting to ensure no further victimization occurs. Children may react violently to loud noises such as fire and police sirens. In addition, the child should not be exposed to any additional traumatic movie or television programs as this may stimulate memories and result in behavior problems. The child may have frequent nightmares and sleeping problems, and may need to have a night light or medications for sleep. Eating problems (overeating) may serve to soothe the child if the caregiver is

Family Teaching

Ways for Caregivers to Protect the Child from Sexual Abuse

1. Teach child to have a name for private parts of their body, such as calling their buttock a "butt or bottom."
2. Teach child to differentiate appropriate or safe touch (hugs, kisses on the cheek) from inappropriate touch such as touching private areas of body.
3. Teach children to shake hands with others so they feel safer.
4. Teach child to tell a trusted caregiver or a teacher immediately if anyone touches them inappropriately.
5. Teach child about good secrets (birthday parties) and bad secrets (if someone were to touch them inappropriately and asks them to keep it a secret).
6. Teach child the four basic feeling states (sad, angry, mad, and scared), and help the child learn how to share feelings.
7. Empower the child to maintain personal boundaries, not approach strangers or sit on adult laps, verbalize feelings when certain children or adults touch them in ways that do not "feel" OK.
8. Supervise play, especially when children are of different ages. Do not allow children to play unsupervised or in bedrooms with the door shut.
9. Be alert to any changes in feelings or behaviors after a child returns from visiting friends or family members.
10. Become involved in school activities and support programs that teach personal safety skills.
11. Be aware of the National Committee to Prevent Child Abuse (NCPCA) materials that can be used to help caregivers and children prevent sexual abuse. Contact information can be found in the Resources section of this chapter.

Critical Thinking

Identifying Sexual Abuse

You are caring for six-year-old Onesha who has a diagnosis of chronic urinary tract infections. She has just been admitted and complains of pain in her abdomen. You go into her room to take her vital signs. She appears sad and withdrawn, and asks you to stay with her when her father visits because she does not want him to touch her "flower." You ask her to tell you what her "flower" is and she points to her vaginal area. You believe further assessment for possible sexual abuse is indicated. What interventions will need to be completed?

REFLECTIONS FROM FAMILIES

I just learned that my thirteen-year-old daughter, Ariana, was molested by her boyfriend at school today. She came home crying and initially went to her room and told me it was nothing serious. After a time, I realized she was still crying. I sat with her and she finally admitted that her new boyfriend, Ronnie, touched her breasts and would not stop so she had to hide in the girl's bathroom until he left school. I have always taught my daughters never to let anyone touch them without their permission. We are left wondering what to do. Do we bring it to the attention of the principal? Do we leave it alone? We need help in deciding our next steps.

unable to provide a safe and nurturing environment. Finally, the child may have angry and violent outbursts, which need to be acknowledged as anger directed to the perpetrator and handled within therapy.

PREVENTION OF CHILD ABUSE AND NEGLECT

Several strategies can reduce the occurrence of abuse. The first is directed at preventing maladaptive behaviors by providing help before the behavior occurs. Caregivers can assess their own family of origin and make informed choices regarding raising their children differently from how they were raised if abused. Nurses can facilitate this by providing parenting classes both in the community and health care settings where caregivers can be encouraged to teach their children respect for both genders, individual family role expectations, normal growth and development, and appropriate methods of communicating (verbal and nonverbal) that distinguish between nurturing affection and erotic contact. Children need to be able to discuss sexual issues, engage in family problem solving, receive accurate information, and have shared sexual values and attitudes (Maddock & Larson, 1995). Consequently, the family atmosphere and experiences will be sexually age-appropriate, respectful of members' personal space, and demonstrate open and honest communication concerning sexual issues. Children will know about appropriate and safe touch between caregivers and siblings and that any breach of this safe touch will immediately be reported to a responsible person for follow-up.

A second strategy focuses on high-risk communities. Even though child abuse occurs in all socioeconomic levels, identifying families that are at high risk is critical. Poverty, high community violence, substandard housing, high unemployment, and welfare-dependent communities are areas for special interventions. Support for a family's basic survival needs (economic and material) can contribute to a more stable home environment and improve the caregivers' capacity to rear children competently. Communities can assist by providing food pantries, second-hand clothing, and household supplies to supplement needy families at times of crisis.

This second strategy can also include parent competency enhancement programs developed by professionals who are knowledgeable about growth and development and share strategies for effective parenting. Local schools, community colleges, hospitals, and social service agencies normally provide these programs at low cost for caregivers. Pediatric and obstetric units can also be instrumental in combining resources to jointly offer such programs for new parents and caregivers. Formalized content can include growth and development across the life span, and specific issues related to each developmental stage, such as temper tantrums, toilet training, or assertive discipline. Other areas include how to play with your child, how to help your child learn, effective praise and encouragement, effective limit setting, and handling common misbehaviors (Institute of Medicine, 1994). In addition, caregivers may need to learn how to care for a sick child, how to take a temperature, how to deal with common childhood illnesses such as fever and colds, and when to seek medical services.

The third strategy focuses on a child's ability to recognize and resist assault. Here children are taught to (1) recognize potentially abusive situations; (2) resist by saying "no" and removing themselves from the situation or perpetrator; (3) report previous or ongoing abuse to an authority figure; and (4) learn that it is never their fault (Wurtile, 1998). The children focus on the idea that they are the "boss" of their bodies and can make rules to protect their bodies.

The fourth strategy focuses on reducing the long-term impact of physical and emotional abuse by providing a variety of support services to prevent continually abusive behaviors and situations. Specific interventions include the use of crisis hotlines and increased parent-child contact with supplemental in-home services such as a visiting nurse or parent aide. These services, often offered in conjunction with Child Protective Services as support for a family at risk help caregivers learn new strategies for child discipline, anger and stress management, and healthy parenting practices. Caregiver involvement in religious affiliations can provide additional emotional and spiritual supports.

The fifth strategy focuses on maintaining or reducing the severity of the consequences of long-term abusive situations (Davidhizar & Newman-Giger, 1996), and occur in general hospitals, psychiatric inpatient hospitals, group homes, or shelters where the person struggles with sequelae of violence. For instance, children may be referred to a day treatment facility specifically established for children experiencing serious mental illness as a result of prolonged abusive parenting. These children may be diagnosed with major depression, post-traumatic stress disorder, attachment disorders, or violent behaviors. Long-term family and individual counseling, medication management, parenting classes, social skills training, and other programs to overcome the impact of long-term abuse may be required.

LEGAL ISSUES RELATED TO CHILD ABUSE AND NEGLECT

Historically, children have experienced all types and severity of physical, psychological, and sexual abuse at the hands of their caregivers. Many children were removed from their homes and caregivers and placed in houses of refuge, or juvenile, orphan, or foundling asylums. These were religious or private organizations for abandoned or abused children. However, the twentieth century awakened awareness on the part of the states and public social service agencies to take ultimate responsibility for protecting children.

Two legal doctrines have an impact on all judicial proceedings affecting abused and neglected children: *parens patriae,* where the state is vested with the power to set standards for the care and protection of children within its borders; and the state's responsibility to ensure that its actions are in the best interest of the child (Kramer, 1996). However, not until Kempe and colleagues' (1962) landmark publication, *The Battered Child Syndrome,* did efforts occur on a state level to address legislation related to child abuse (Kempe, Silverman, Steele, Droegemueller, & Silver, 1962).

Many state laws now define the grounds, set the limits, and establish procedures for limiting or severing the caregiver-child relationship. When abuse is suspected, child abuse and neglect reporting laws and welfare codes allow child protective and law enforcement agencies to investigate and intervene in family relationships (Kramer, 1996). The state's courts systems authorize juvenile or family court involvement in such cases, and the prosecution of individuals found guilty of criminal acts against a child.

Even though caregivers do have the right of due process, their right to maintain connections with their child is not as important as a child's right to an environment that is free from physical and emotional violence. Unfortunately, the child protective system is not perfect and a child removed from the family may face many years in foster care, which in itself has serious consequences. Consequently, a critical balance must be maintained when considering removing a child from the home.

Each state has child abuse and neglect laws that require they prove "(1) one or more individuals named in the state law prohibiting child abuse, (2) have physically, sexually, mentally, or emotionally abused a child, or (3) have abandoned a child, or (4) have failed to provide a child with adequate food, clothing, shelter, or parental control or supervision, or (5) have medically or educationally neglected the child, or (6) have subjected a child to an immoral or criminal lifestyle" (Kramer, 1996, p. 13). If the caregiver was aware of the abuse but did not stop it, the state must prove that individual willfully permitted the abuse through indifference and inaction in order to prosecute the perpetrator for assault and battery (Kramer, 1996).

Many states also have laws providing a legal defense to child abuse where **corporal punishment** (physical restraint or causing pain to the body by a person in authority) is inflicted by a caregiver. However, the punishment must be appropriate and reasonable to the child's misbehavior, so the force used is limited to what is believed necessary to maintain discipline, safeguard and promote the child's welfare, prevent or punish misconduct, or restrain or correct a child (Kramer, 1996). Any act that exceeds reasonable bounds is considered child abuse.

Under the law, which may vary from state to state, the act of abandonment can also result in intervention by Child Protective Services. Abandonment occurs when a caregiver fails to visit a child who lives away from the caregiver, fails to display love or affection, or has no personal contact or concern for the child's personal welfare. If a caregiver demonstrates a reasonable degree of interest, concern, and responsibility, the child has not been abandoned.

The failure to provide food, clothing, shelter, care, or supervision is considered child neglect. These actions are often combined with failure to provide adequate medical care, education, and supervision. Some states (Delaware, Iowa, Pennsylvania) include juvenile noncriminal behaviors (such as runaways who are endangering their own safety) under their neglect laws as well. Therefore in these states, caregivers of runaways or children who are endangering their own safety are considered neglectful.

On the other hand, emotional abuse does not constitute sufficient evidence to prove child abuse unless it occurs in conjunction with physical abuse. Only a few states make any attempt to define mental or emotional injury, and caregivers who neglect the educational needs of their children can be taken to court under the contribution to the delinquency of a minor complaint. Emotional abuse can also include failure on the part of the caregiver to provide an appropriate educational environment, such as enrolling a special needs child, or a child who is deaf, in a public school system.

REPORTING CHILD ABUSE

Each state has similar legal requirements for reporting child abuse. The central tenet of the reporting law designates certain persons as **mandated reporters** (individuals who are required to report to appropriate authorities suspicions of child abuse/neglect). Most states specify who is required to report, and these individuals typically include physicians, nurses, school personnel, social workers, and law enforcement personnel. These reports are usually made by telephone to the child protective agency, and followed up by a written report. If a member of the staff at a hospital makes the report, the hospital is required to provide a medical record of the child.

According to Monteleone (1996), every state reporting law contains similar information that includes what must be reported (definitions and reportable areas), who must or may report, when a report must be made, procedures to follow, rules for protective custody, immunity for good faith reporters, privileged abrogation (to do away with) of communication rights, sanctions for failure to report, and infor-

Nursing Tip:

Legal issues and child abuse

Because nurses may be called as codefendants in lawsuits, they must practice in a professional and reasonably prudent manner at all times. Specific guidelines for the nurse to consider are:

- Document all client and caregiver interactions.
- Practice within the ethical code of nursing.
- Respect client and caregiver's confidentiality. If child abuse is suspected, confidentiality can (and must) be breached.
- Do not release information to other agencies other than protective services without specific family or caregiver permission; if a child is removed from the caregiver and the Child Protective Services has temporary custody, Child Protective Services must approve release of information.
- Respect a client's right to privacy.
- Respect a client's right to refuse treatment or assessments (document accordingly).
- Know your institution's policies and procedures related to all matters of child abuse.
- Know your state's Nurse Practice Act and practice within that scope.
- Always consult with your nurse manager, risk manager, and treatment team members when indicated. (Adapted from Estes, 2002)

False accusations of abuse

Occasionally, individuals (parent, teacher, other adult) will be falsely accused of being abusive. This occurs most commonly during custody hearings associated with divorce proceedings (Coleman & Clancy, 1990), but may also occur when a child is telling a parent or an interviewer what the child thinks the adult wants to hear. Because Child Protective Services are legally charged with investigating any and all accusations of child abuse, even if they may not be true, it is important whenever interviewing a child that care be taken not to encourage the child to remember experiences that did not occur, or lead the child into make statements that did not occur.

mation regarding the existence and operation of a central registry. Those reporting abuse in good faith are immune from any civil or criminal liability.

Each state also has a child protection system that primarily protects children and, secondarily, preserves the family unit whenever possible. Taking children from their home is the least desirable method of treating child abuse, and when children are removed, the first goal is to reunify the family. Child Protective Services receive reports of suspected abuse and neglect 24 hours per day, 7 days per week, and then must investigate and determine whether or not abuse/neglect has occurred. They also petition the court to protect children and mandate caregivers to take certain remedial steps or risk losing parental rights. Child Protective Services are also responsible for establishing resources that support families in the community including teaching and assisting caregivers with basic child rearing and household skills, and providing counseling services related to mental health, parenting, anger management, and vocational resources.

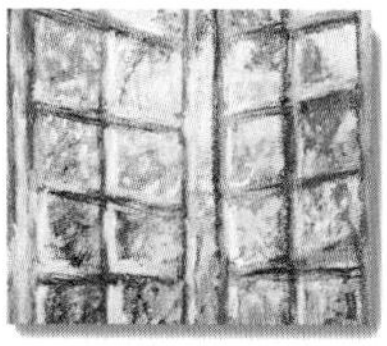

In the Real World

One of the most difficult children to care for is a child whose caregiver has been abusive or neglectful. Most people believe that a child is a special gift to be loved and cherished. Unfortunately, some caregivers do not hold similar beliefs and engage in hurtful and harmful behaviors. As nurses, we are educated to understand abuse and neglect as symptoms of some larger problem in the caregiving family. Yet, we feel anger and frustration at caregivers who can take away a child's spirit, injure them physically, or leave a child with lifetime psychological and physical scars. As nurses, we must role model caring and nurturing behaviors for abusive caregivers, coordinate resources for caregiver healing, and always be on guard to advocate and report any suspected abuse or neglect.

As professionals, nurses, physicians, police, and teachers have a legal obligation to report child abuse and neglect. In some states, any person who suspects abuse or neglect is legally required to report that abuse. Make sure you are vigilant and always aware of potential harm a child may be in. Remember, child abuse or neglect comes from all socioeconomic, ethnic, cultural, and religious backgrounds.

Key Concepts

- Child abuse includes intentional behaviors by a caregiver that can involve neglect, or physical, emotional, and/or sexual abuse. Neglect is harmful, malicious, or ignorant withholding of physical, nutrition, and health care, or emotional and eduational necessities that provide a foundation for healthy childhood development.

- Three models explaining child abuse and neglect are the Sociological Model, the Social-Interactional Systemic Model, and the Attachment Model.
- Clinical manifestations of physical abuse include bruises, fractures, burns, abdominal injuries, and neurological injuries.
- Children with an intracranial bleed (subdural or subarachnoid hemorrhages), retinal hemorrhage, and possibly long bone fractures should be suspected of having shaken baby syndrome.
- Munchausen syndrome by proxy is a pattern of behavior demonstrated by the caregiver to fabricate signs and symptoms of diseases and expose a child to harmful medical interventions and painful invasive procedures.
- Abandonment is defined as intentionally withholding from a child, without just cause or excuse, care, presence, love, protection, maintenance, and affection.
- Psychological abuse consists of acts of omission or commission (telling a child that he/she is ugly or worthless) deemed psychologically damaging, and involving hostile behavior or negative caregiving behaviors.
- Sexual abuse is an exploitive sexual act(s) imposed on a child who lacks the emotional, cognitive, or maturational development to deal with the actions.
- Nursing management of child abuse includes obtaining an accurate history and assessment, and intervening according to the type of abuse.
- The nurse is a mandatory reporter of child abuse.

Review Questions

1. Discuss the differences and similarities between child abuse and child neglect.
2. Describe the clinical manifestations of a child who has been physically abused.
3. Describe the process of transmission of violence in families.
4. Identify the nursing interventions for a child who has been abused.
5. Describe the legal issues related to reporting child abuse in your state.
6. Describe strategies for prevention for child abuse.

References

ABCAN (U.S. Advisory Board of Child Abuse and Neglect). (1995). *A nation's shame: Fatal child abuse and neglect in the United States*. Washington, DC: Government Printing Office.

American Psychiatric Association. (1994). *Diagnostic and statistical manual of mental disorders* (4th ed.). Washington, DC: Author.

Asher, R. (1951). Munchausen's syndrome. *Lancet, 1*, 339–341.

Beardsley, D. (1997). The dangers of shaking a baby. *The Wellesley TAB*, (March 18), 31–33.

Bentovin, A. (1992). Trauma—organized systems: physical and sexual abuse in families. New York: Karnac Books.

Berlin, P., & Vondra, J. (1999). Psychological maltreatment of children. In R. Ammerman & M. Hersen, *Assessment of family violence* (pp. 109–146). New York: John Wiley & Sons, Inc.

Bowlby, J. (1969). *Attachment and loss*. New York: Basic Books.

Brayden, R. M., Altemeier, W. A., Tucker, D. D., Dietrich, M. S., & Vietze, D. (1992). Antecedents of child neglect in the first two years of life. *Journal of Pediatrics, 120*, 426–429.

Briere, J., & Runtz, M. (1988). Multivariate correlates of childhood psychological and physical maltreatment among university women. *Child Abuse and Neglect, 12*, 331–341.

Burns, C., Barber, N., Brady, M., & Dunn, A. (1996). *Pediatric primary care: A handbook for nurse practitioners*. Philadelphia: W.B. Saunders.

Butler, G. (1995). Shaken baby syndrome. *Journal of Psychosocial Nursing, 33*(9), 48–50.

Caldwell, B., & Bradley, R. (1984). *Home observation for measurement of the environment*. Little Rock: University of Arkansas.

Canavan, M., Meyer, W., & Higgs, D. (1992). The female experience of sibling incest. *Journal of Marital and Family Therapy, 18*(2) 12–142.

Cicchetti, D., Toth, S. L., & Lynch, M. (1995). Bowlby's dream comes full circle: The application of attachment theory to risk and psychopathology. *Advances in Clinical Child Psychology, 17*, 1–75.

Chiocca, E. M. (1995). Shaken baby syndrome: A nursing perspective. *Pediatric Nursing, 21*(1), 33–38.

Cohler, B. J., Weiss, J. L., Grunebaum, H. U. (1970). Child-care attitudes and emotional disturbance among mothers of young children. *Genetic Psychology Monographs, 82*(1), 3–47.

Coleman, L., & Clancy, P. (1990). False allegations of child sexual abuse: Why is it happening? What can we do? *Criminal Justice* (Fall), 14.

Coody, D., Brown, M., Montgomery, D, Flynn, A., & Yetman, R. (1994). Shaken baby syndrome: Identification and prevention for nurse practitioners. *Journal of Pediatric Health Care, 8*(2), 50–56.

Cooper, C. L., Murphy, W. D., & Haynes, M. R. (1996). Characteristics of abused and nonabused adolescent sexual offenders. *Sexual Abuse: Journal of Research and Treatment, 8*(2), 105–119.

Davidhizar, R., & Newman-Giger, J. (1996). Recognizing Abuse. *International Nursing Review, 43*(5), 145–150.

Egeland, B., & Erickson, M. F. (1987). Psychologically unavailable caregiving. In M. Brasard, R. Germain, & S. Hart (Eds.), *Psychological maltreatment of children & youth* (pp. 110–120) New York: Pergamon.

Estes, M. E. Z. (2002). *Health assessment and physical examination* (2nd ed.). Albany, NY: Delmar.

Finkelhor, D. (1988). The trauma of child sexual abuse: two models. In G. Wyatt & G. Povell (Eds.), *Lasting effects of child sexual abuse* (pp. 61–84). Newbury Park: Sage.

Florsheim, P, Henry, W., & Benjamin, S. (1996). Integrating individual and interpersonal approaches to diagnosis: The structural analysis of social behavior and attachment theory. In F. Kaslow (Ed.), *Handbook of relational diagnoses* (pp. 81–101). New York: John Wiley & Sons, Inc.

Gary, F., Moorhead, J., & Warren J. (1996). Characteristics of troubled youths in a shelter. *Archives of Psychiatric Nursing, X*,(1), 41–48.

Gelles, R. J. (1987). *Family violence*. (2nd ed.). London: Sage.

Gelles, R. J. (1992). Poverty and violence toward children. *American Behavioral Scientist, 35*, 258–274.

Hazinski, M. (1992). *Nursing care of the critically ill child*. St. Louis: Mosby.

Heiman, M. (1992). Putting the puzzle together: Validating allegations of child sexual abuse. *Journal of Child Psychology and Psychiatry, 33*(2), 311–329.

Helfer, R., & Kempe, R. (1987). *The battered child*. Chicago: University of Chicago Press.

Institute of Medicine Staff. (1994). *Reducing risks for mental disorders: Frontiers for preventive intervention research*. Washington, DC: National Academy Press.

James, B. (1994). *Handbook for treatment of attachment—trauma problems on children*. New York: Lexington Books.

Kempe, C. H., Silverman, F. N., Steele, B. F., Drogemueller, W., & Silver, H. K. (1962). The battered child syndrome. *Journal of the American Medical Association, 181*, 17–24.

Kivlin, J., Simons, K., Lazoritz, S., & Ruttum, M. (2000). Shaken baby syndrome. *American Academy of Ophthalmology, 107*(7), 1246–1254.

Kotch, J., Browne, D., Ringualt, C., Stewart, P., Rvina, E., Holt, J., Lowman, B., & Jung, J. (1995). Risk of child abuse or neglect in a cohort of low-income children. *Child Abuse & Neglect, 19*(9), 1115–1130.

Kramer, D. (1996). *Legal rights of children* (Vol. 2). New York: Clark, Boardman & Callaghan.

Lesnick-Oberstein, M., Koers, A. J., & Cohen, L. (1995). Parental hostility in psychologically abusive mothers: A test of the three factor theory. *Child Abuse & Neglect, 19*, 33–49.

Locsin, A. (1999). Shaken baby syndrome: A mystery or not? *Vital Signs, 9*(4), 12–13.

Lung, C. T., & Daro, D. (1996). *Current trends in child abuse reporting and fatalities: The results of 1995 annual fifty state survey*. Chicago, IL: NCPCA.

Maddock, J., & Larson, N. (1995). *Incestuous Families*. New York: W.W. Norton & Co.

Main, M. (1996). Introduction to the special section on attachment and psychopathology: Overview of the field of attachment. *Journal of Consulting and Clinical Psychology, 64*(2), 237–243.

McClosky, L. A., Figueredo, A. J., & Koss, M. P. (1995). The effects of systemic family violence on children's mental health. *Child Development, 66*, 1239–1261.

Meadow, R. (1985). Management of Munchausen syndrome by proxy. *Archives of Disease in Childhood, 60*, 385–393.

Monteleone, Jr. (1996). *Recognition of child abuse for mandated reporter*. St. Louis, MO: G. W. Medical Publishing, Inc.

Munkel, W. I. (1989). Innocents abused. A pediatric hospital forms a team to care for sexually abused children. *Health Program 70*(7), 46–49.

Murphy, S., Orkow, B., & Nicola, R. M. (1985). Prenatal prediction of child abuse and neglect: A prospective study. *Child Abuse and Neglect*, 9(2), 225–235.

National Center on Child Abuse and Neglect. (1996). *Third national incidence study of child abuse and neglect*. Washington, DC: U.S. Dept. of Health and Human Services.

O'Hagan, K. (1993). *Emotional and psychological abuse of children*. Buffalo, NY: University of Toronto Press, 167.

Osofsky, J. (1997). *Children in a violent society*. New York: Tullford Press.

Palmer, A., & Yoshimura, G. (1984). Munchausen syndrome by proxy. *Journal of American Academy of Child Psychiatry, 23*, 503–508.

Philip, P. A., Traisman, E. S., & Philip, M. (1995). Musculoskeletal injuries in child abuse. *Physical Medicine and Rehabilitation: State of the Art Reviews*, 9(1), 251–268.

Radke-Yarrow, M., McCann, K., DeMulder, E., Belmont, B., Martinez, P., & Richardson, D. (1995). Attachment in the context of high risk. *Development & Psychopathology, 7*, 247–265.

Reid, J., Machetto, P., & Foster, S. (1999). *No safe haven: Children of substance-abusing parents*. [Online]. Available: www.casacolumbia.org/publications1456/publications_show.htm?doc_id=7167.

Sebes, J. M. (1986). Defining high risk. In J. Garbarino, C. J. Schellenbach, J. Sebes, & Associates (Eds.), *Troubled youth, troubled families* (pp. 83–120). New York: Aldine.

Sedlak, A. J., & Broadhurst, D. D. (1996). *Third national incidence study on child abuse & neglect*. Washington, DC: U.S. Department of Health and Human Services.

Straus, M. A., & Gelles, R. J. (1989). Physical violence in American families. *New Brunswick Transaction*. Piscataway, NJ.

Taylor, J., Underwood, C., Thomas, L., & Franklin, A. (1988). *Behind closed doors: Violence in the American family*. New York: Anchor Press.

U.S. Department of Health and Human Services. (1998). *Child maltreatment 1996 reports from the states to the National Child Abuse and Neglect Data System*. Washington, DC: U.S. Government Printing Office

Widner-Kolberg, M. (1997). Child abuse. *Critical care nursing of North America*, 9(2), 175–182.

Wurtile, S. (1998). School based child abuse prevention programs: Questions, answers and more questions. In J. R. Lultzker (Ed.), *Handbook of child abuse research*. New York: Plenum Press.

Wyszynski, M. (1999). Shaken baby syndrome: Identification, intervention and prevention. *Clinical Excellence for Nurse Practitioners, 3*(5), 262–267.

Yates, A. (1991). Child Sexual Abuse. In J. Wiener (Ed.), *Textbook of child & adolescent psychiatry*. Washington, DC: American Psychiatric Press.

Yorker, B., & Kaham, B. (1990). Munchausen's syndrome by proxy as a form of child abuse. *Archives of Psychiatric Nursing, 4*, 313–318.

Youngblade, L. M., & Belsky, J. (1990). The social and emotional consequences of child maltreatment. In R. Ammerman & M. Hersen (Eds.), *Children at risk: An evaluation of factors contributing to child abuse and neglect* (pp. 109–146). New York: John Wiley & Sons.

Suggested Readings

Alexander, R., & Smith, W. (1998). Shaken baby syndrome. *Infants & Young Children, 10*(3), 1–9.

Brady, M.A. (2000). Role relationship. In C. Burns, M. Brady, A. Dunn & N. Starr. *Pediatric primary care*. Philadelphia: W.B. Saunders.

Briere, J., & Runtz, M. (1990). Differential adult psychopathology associated with three types of child abuse histories. *Child Abuse and Neglect, 14*, 357–364.

Cahill, L., Kaminer, R., & Johnson, P. (1999). Developmental, cognitive and behavioral sequelae of child abuse. *Child and Adolescent Psychiatric Clinics of North America, 8*(4), 827–843.

Cappell, C., & Heiner, R. (1990). The intergenerational transmission of family aggression. *Journal of Family Violence, 5*, 135–152.

Cicchetti, D., & Greenberg, M. T. (Eds.). (1991). Special issue: Attachment and developmental psychopathology. *Development and Psychopathology*. New York: Wiley & Co.

Cicchetti, D., & Lynch, M. (1995). Failures in the expectable environment and their impact on individual development: The case of child maltreatment. In D. Cicchetti & D. Cohn. *Developmental psychopathology* (Vol. I, pp. 32–66). New York: John Wiley & Sons.

Cohen, E., Mackenzie, R. G., & Yates, G. L. (1991). HEADSS, a psychosocial risk assessment instrument: Implications for designing effective intervention programs for runaway youth. *Journal of Adolescent Health, 12*, 539–544.

Cole, P., & Putnam, F. (1992). Effect of incest on self and social functioning: A developmental psychology perspective. *Journal of Consulting and Clinical Psychology, 60*(2), 174–184.

Dozier, M., Cue, K. L., & Barnett, L. (1994). Clinicians as caregivers: Role of attachment organization in treatment. *Journal of Consulting and Clinical Psychology, 62*, 793–900.

Ewgman, B., Kevlaham, C., & Land G. (1993). The Missouri child fatality study: Under reporting of maltreatment fatalities among children younger than five years of age. *Pediatrics, 91*, 330.

Ewing-Cobbs, L., Duhaime, A., & Fletcher, J. (1995). Inflicted and noninflicted traumatic brain injury in infants and preschoolers. *Journal of Head Trauma Rehabilitation, 10*(5), 13–24.

Farrow, J. A., Deisher, R. W., & Brown, R. (1991). Introduction. *Journal of Adolescent Health, 12*, 497–499.

Finkelhor, D., Hotaling, G., Lewis, I., & Smith, C. (1990). Sexual abuse in a national survey of adult men and women: Prevalence, characteristics and risk factors. *Child Abuse & Neglect, 12*(1), 3–23.

Frank, D. (1995). Failure to thrive. In S. Parker & B. Zimmerman (Eds.), *Behavioral and developmental pediatrics: A handbook of primary care* (pp. 134–139). Boston: Little, Brown.

Friedrich, W. (1990). *Psychotherapy of sexually abused children and their families*. New York: W.W. Norton & Co.

Garbarino, J. (1995). Growing up in a socially toxic environment: Life for children and families in the 1990's. In G. B. Melton (Ed.), *Nebraska Symposium on Motivation* (Vol. 42). *The individual, the family, and the social good: Personal fulfillment in times of change* (pp. 1–20). Lincoln: NE: University of Nebraska Press.

Gil, E., & Johnson, T.C. (1993). *Sexualized children: Assessment & treatment of sexualized children and children who molest*. Rockville, Md.: Launch Press.

Green, A. (1991). Child physical abuse. In J. Wiener (Ed.), *Textbook of child & adolescent psychiatry*. Washington, DC: American Psychiatric Press.

Harris, M. J., & Kotch, J. B. (1994). Unintentional infant injuries: Sociodemographic and psychosocial factors. *Public Health Nursing, 11*(2),90–97.

Kahn-D'Angelo, L. (1989). Serious head injury during the first year of life. *Physical and Occupational Therapy in Pediatrics, 9*, 49–59.

Kaplan, S. (1996). Physical abuse of children and adolescence. In S. Kaplan. *Family violence*. Washington, DC: American Psychiatric Press, Inc.

Klebes, C., & Fay, S. (1995). Munchausen syndrome by proxy: A review, case study and nursing implications. *Journal of Pediatric Nursing, 10*(2), 93–98.

Lopez, L., & Gray, F. (1995). Logical responses to youth who run away from home. *Journal of Psychosocial Nursing, 33*(3), 9–15.

Lyons, R. (1996). Attachment relationships among children with aggressive behavior problems. The role of disorganized attachment patterns. *Journal of Consulting and Clinical Psychology, 64*(1) 64–73.

Marvin, R. S., & Stewart R. D. (1990). A family systems framework for the study of attachment. In M. T. Greenberg, D. Cicchetti, & E. M. Cummings (Eds.), *Attachment in the preschool years* (pp. 51–86). Chicago: University of Chicago Press.

North American Nursing Diagnosis Association. (2001). *Nursing diagnosis: Definitions and classifications 2001–2002*. Philadelphia: Author.

Raimondi, A. J., & Hirschauser, J. (1984). Relationship between parental socioeconomic levels and potential for child abuse. *Nurse Practitioner: American Journal of Primary Health Care, 21*(3), 144–146.

Rothbard, J., & Shaver, P. (1994). Continuity of attachment across the life span. In M. Sperling & W. Berman, (Eds.), *Attachment in adults: clinical and developmental perspective*. New York: Gilford Press.

Rutter, M. (1995). Clinical implications of attachment concepts: Retrospect and prospect. *Journal of Child Psychology and Psychiatry and Allied Disciplines, 36*, 549–571.

Sheridan, M. (1995). A proposed intergenerational model of substance abuse, family functioning & abuse/neglect. *Child Abuse & Neglect, 19*(5), 519–530.

Simons, R. L., Whitbeck, L. B., Conger, R. D., & Chyi-In, W. (1991). Intergenerational transmission of harsh parenting. *Developmental Psychology, 27*, 159–171.

U.S. Department of Health and Human Services, National Center on Child Abuse & Neglect, National Child Abuse & Neglect Data System. (1994). *Child Maltreatment—1994*. Washington, DC: U.S. Government Printing Office.

Waters, E., Vaughn, B., Posada, G., & Kondo-Ikemura, K. (1995). Caregiving, cultural and cognitive perspectives on secure-base behavior and working models: New growing points of attachment theory and research. *Society for Research in Child Development Monograph Series, 60* (Series No. 244), 2–3.

Wyatt, G. E., & Newcomb, M. (1990) Internal and external mediators of women's sexual abuse. *Journal of Consulting & Clinical Psychology, 58*, 758–767.

Resources

Organizations and Websites

American Humane Association, Children's Division
63 Inverness Drive East
Englewood, CO 80112
(303) 792-9900
(800) 227-4645
www.americanhumane.org

American Professional Society on the Abuse of Children
940 NE 13th Street, CHO 3B–3406
Oklahoma City, OK 73104
(405) 271-8202
www.apsac.org

Center for Improvement of Child Caring
11331 Ventura Blvd., Suite 103
Studio City, CA 91604-3147
(800) 325-CICC
www.ciccparenting.org

Child Welfare League of America, Inc.
440 First St., NW, Suite 310
Washington, DC 20001-2085
(202) 638-2952
www.cwla.org

Childhelp USA
15757 N. 78th St.
Scottsdale, AZ 85260
(800) 4ACHILD (800-422-4453)
www.childhelpusa.org

Effective Parenting Education for Children Every Person Influences Children (EPIC)
Buffalo State College
1000 Main Street
Buffalo, NY 14202
(716) 886-6396

Family Resources Coalition
200 South Michigan Avenue, Suite 1520
Chicago, IL 60604

Family Violence Prevention Center
383 Rhode Island Street, Suite 304
San Francisco, CA 94103
(415) 252-8900
Fax (415) 252-8991
www.endabuse.org

Kempe Children's Center
1825 Marion Street
Denver, CO 80218
(303) 864-5252
www.kempecenter.org

National Center for Education in Maternal and Child Health
2000 15th Street, North, Suite 701
Arlington, VA 22201-2617
(703) 524-7802
Fax: (703) 524-9335
www.ncemch.org

National Center on Child Abuse and Neglect (NCCAN)
Administration on Children, Youth and Families
U.S. Department of Health and Human Services
P.O. Box 1182
Washington, DC 20013
(202) 205-8586

National Clearinghouse on Child Abuse and Neglect Information
330 C Street, SW
Washington, DC 20447
(703) 385-7565
(800) FYI-3366 (800-394-3366)

National Committee for Prevention of Child Abuse
332 South Michigan Avenue, Suite 1600
Chicago, IL 60604
(312) 663-3520
Fax: (312) 939-8962

National Committee to Prevent Child Abuse (NCPCA)
200 State Road
South Deerfield, MA 01373-0200
(413) 628-7733
(800) 835-2671

Pacific Center for Violence Prevention
Building 1, Room 300
San Francisco General Hospital
San Francisco, CA 94110
(415) 285-1793
www.pcvp.org

SOS Help for Parents: A practical guide for handling common everyday behavior problems
Parent Press Online
P.O. Box 2180-T
Bowling Green, KY 42102-2180
www.sosprograms.com

APPENDIX A THE FRIEDMAN FAMILY ASSESSMENT MODEL (SHORT FORM)

Before using the following guidelines in completing family assessments, two words of caution: First, not all areas included will be germane for every family. The guidelines are comprehensive and allow depth when probing is necessary. The student should not feel that every subarea needs be covered when the broad area of inquiry poses no problems to the family or concern to the health care professional. Second, by virtue of the interdependence of the family system, one will find unavoidable redundancy. For the sake of efficiency, the assessor should try not to repeat data, but to refer the reader back to sections where this information has already been described.

IDENTIFYING DATA

1. **Family Name**
2. **Address and Phone**
3. **Family Composition**
   See Table A-1.
4. **Type of Family Form**
5. **Cultural (Ethnic) Background**
6. **Religious Identification**
7. **Social Class Status**
8. **Family's Recreational or Leisure time Activities**

DEVELOPMENTAL STAGE AND HISTORY OF FAMILY

9. **Family's Present Developmental Stage**
10. **Extent of Family Developmental Tasks Fulfillment**
11. **Nuclear Family History**
12. **History of Family of Origin of Both Parents**

ENVIRONMENTAL DATA

13. **Characteristics of Home**
14. **Characteristics of Neighborhood and Larger Community**
15. **Family's Geographic Mobility**
16. **Family's Associations and Transactions with Community**
17. **Family's Social Support System or Network**
    Ecomap
    Family genogram

FAMILY STRUCTURE

18. **Communication Patterns**
    Extent of Functional and Dysfunctional Communication (types of recurring patterns)
    Extent of Emotional (Affective) Messages and How Expressed
    Characteristics of Communication Within Family Subsystems
    Extent of Congruent and Incongruent Messages
    Types of Dysfunctional Communication
    Processes Seen in Family
    Areas of Open and Closed Communication
    Familial and Contextual Variables Affecting Communication

19. **Power Structure**
    Power Outcomes
    Decision-Making Process
    Power Bases
    Variables Affecting Family Power
    Overall Family System and Subsystem Power (family power continuum placement)

TABLE A-1 Family Composition Form

Name (Last, First)	Gender	Relationship	Date/Place of Birth	Occupation	Education
1. (Father)					
2. (Mother)					
3. (Oldest child)					
4.					
5.					
6.					
7.					
8.					

20. Role Structure

Formal Role Structure

Informal Role Structure

Analysis of Role Models (optional)

Variables Affecting Role Structure

21. Family Values

Compare the family with American or family's reference group values and/or identify important family values and their importance (priority) in family.

Congruence between the Family's Values and Values of the Family's Reference Group or Wider Community

Congruence Between the Family's Values and Family Members' Values

Variables Influencing Family Values

Values Consciously or Unconsciously Held

Presence of Value Conflicts in Family

Effect of the Above Values and Value Conflicts on Health Status of Family

FAMILY FUNCTIONS

22. Affective Function

Family Need–Response Patterns

Mutual Nurturance, Closeness, and Identification

Family attachment diagram

Separateness and Connectedness

23. Socialization Function

Family Child-Rearing Practices

Adaptability of Child-Rearing Practices for Family Form and Family's Situation

Who Is (Are) Socializing Agent(s) for Child(ren)?

Value of Children in Family

Cultural Beliefs That Influence Family's Child-Rearing Patterns

Social Class Influence on Child-Rearing Patterns

Estimation about Whether Family Is at Risk for Child-Rearing Problems and If So, Indication of High-Risk Factors

Adequacy of Home Environment for Children's Needs to Play

24. Health Care Function

Family's Health Beliefs, Values, and Behaviors

Family's Definitions of Health–Illness and Their Level of Knowledge

Family's Perceived Health Status and Illness Susceptibility

Family's Dietary Practices

Adequacy of family diet (recommended three-day food history record)

Function of mealtimes and attitudes toward food and mealtimes

Shopping (and its planning) practices

Person(s) responsible for planning, shopping, and preparation of meals

Sleep and Rest Habits

Physical Activity and Recreation Practices (not covered earlier)

Family's Drug Habits

Family's Role in Self-Care Practices

Medically Based Preventive Measures (physicals, eye and hearing tests, and immunizations)

Dental Health Practices

Family Health History (both general and specific diseases—environmentally and genetically related)

Health Care Services Received

Feelings and Perceptions Regarding Health Services

Emergency Health Services

Source of Payments for Health and Other Services

Logistics of Receiving Care

FAMILY STRESS AND COPING

25. **Short- and Long-Term Familial Stressors and Strengths**
26. **Extent of Family's Ability to Respond, Based on Objective Appraisal of Stress-Producing Situations**
27. **Coping Strategies Utilized (present/past)**
    Differences in Family Members' Ways of Coping
    Family's Inner Coping Strategies
    Family's External Coping Strategies
28. **Dysfunctional Adaptive Strategies Utilized (present/past; extent of usage)**

APPENDIX B
PHYSICAL GROWTH CHARTS

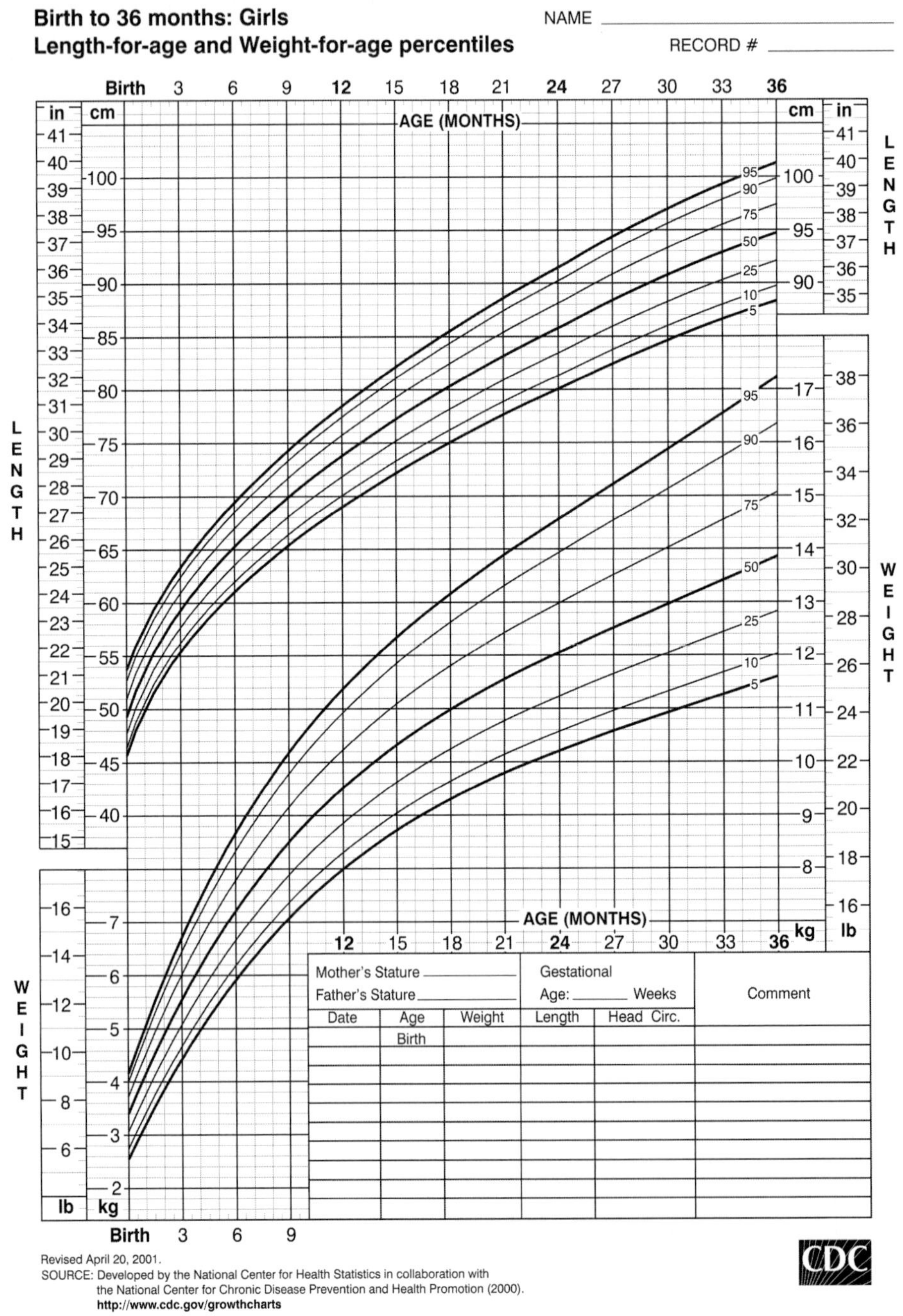

A. Girls: Birth to 36 Months (Length and Weight)

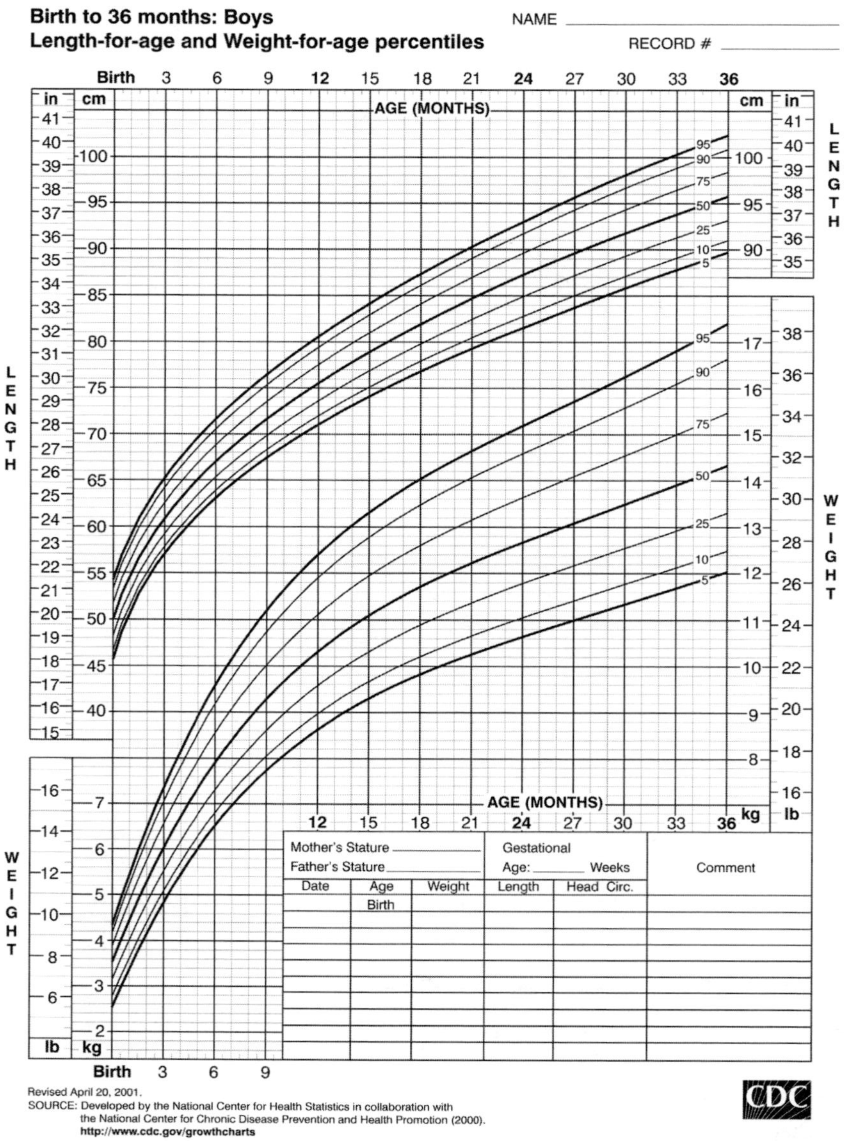

B. Boys: Birth to 36 Months (Length and Weight)

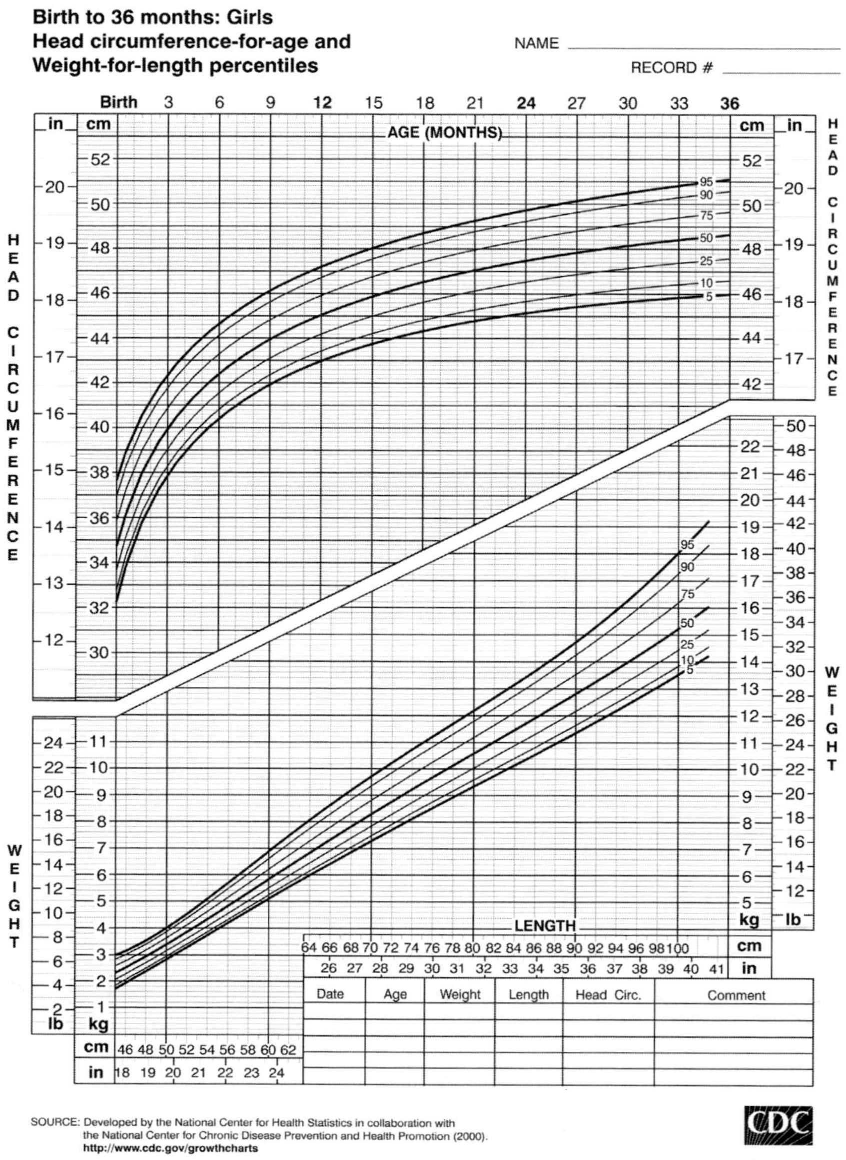

C. Girls: Birth to 36 Months (Head Circumference)

Physical Growth Charts *Continued.*

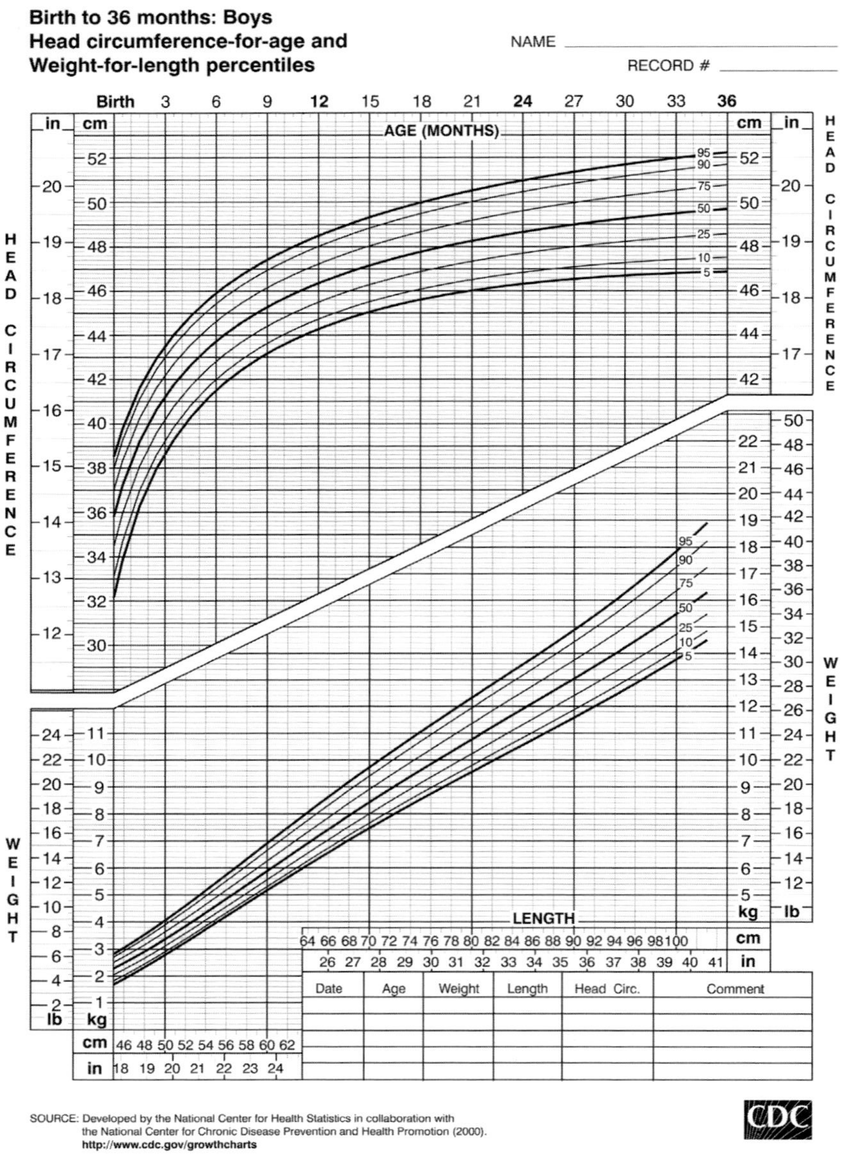

D. Boys: Birth to 36 Months (Head Circumference)

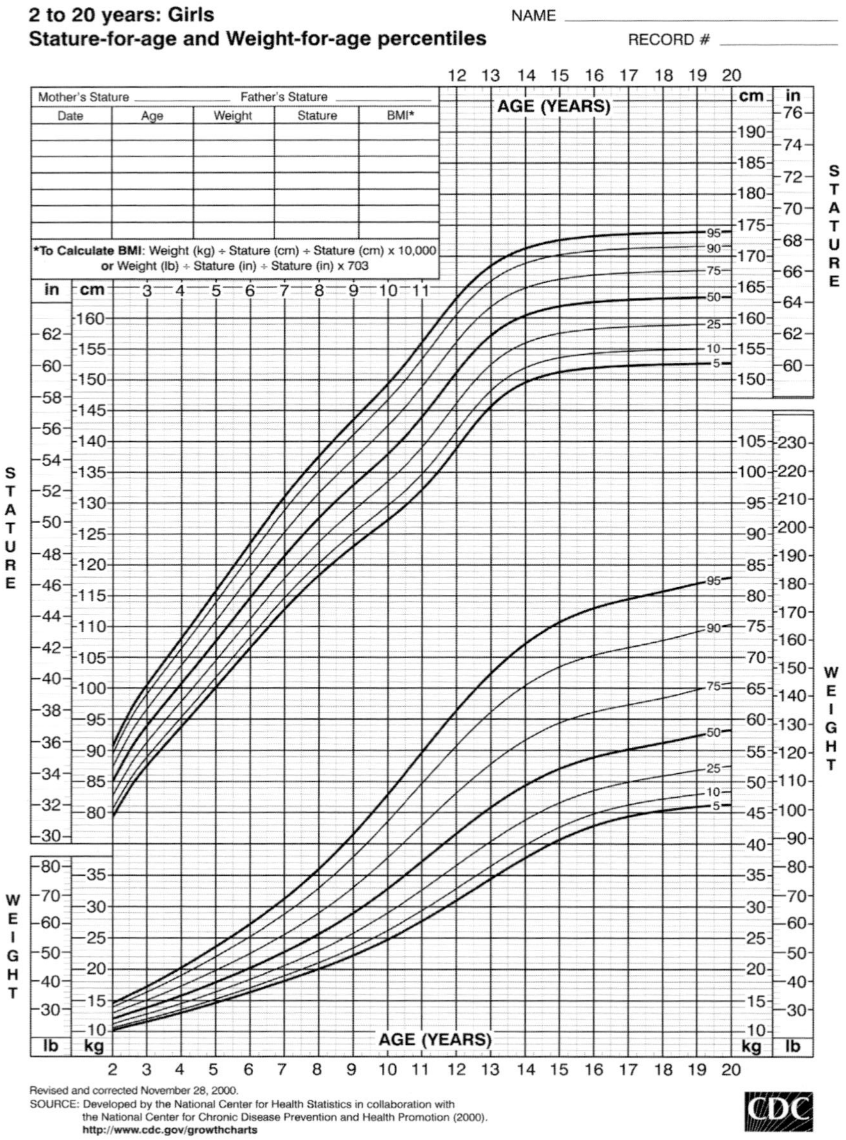

E. Girls: 2 to 20 Years (Stature and Weight)

Physical Growth Charts *Continued.*

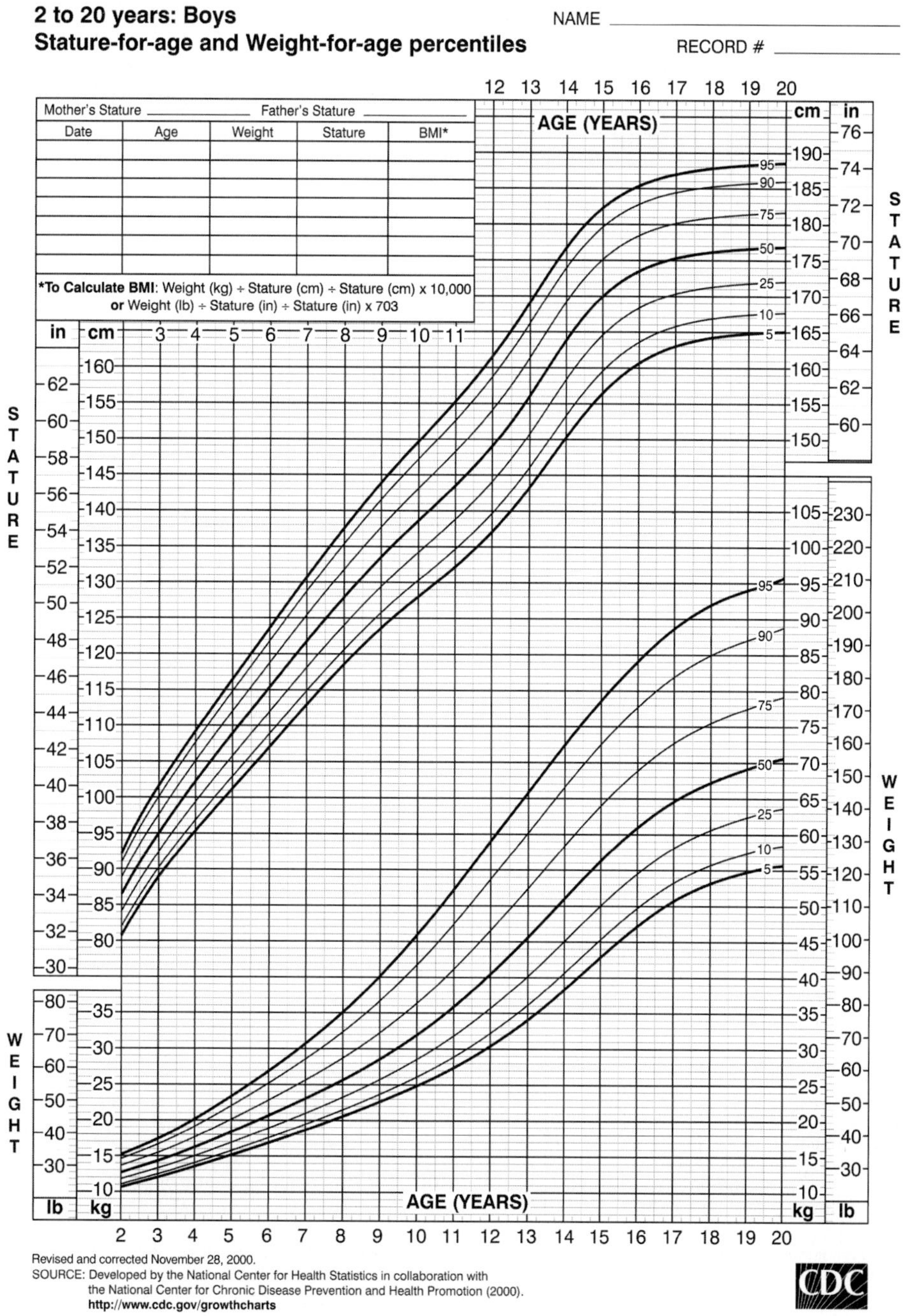

F. Boys: 2 to 20 Years (Stature and Weight)

Physical Growth Charts *Continued.*

APPENDIX C RECOMMENDED CHILDHOOD IMMUNIZATION SCHEDULE, UNITED STATES, JANUARY–DECEMBER 2001

Vaccines[1] are listed under routinely recommended ages. Bars indicate range of recommended ages for immunization. Any dose not given at the recommended age should be given as a "catch-up" immunization at any subsequent visit when indicated and feasible. Ovals indicate vaccines to be given if previously recommended doses were missed or were given earlier than the recommended minimum age.

Age ► / Vaccine ▼	Birth	1 mo	2 mo	4 mo	6 mo	12 mo	15 mo	18 mo	24 mo	4–6 yrs	11–12 yrs	14–18 yrs
Hepatitis B[2]	Hep B #1											
		Hep B #2			Hep B #3						(Hep B[2])	
Diphtheria, tetanus toxoids, and pertussis[3]			DTaP	DTaP	DTaP		DTaP[3]			DTaP	Td	
H. influenzae type b[4]			Hib	Hib	Hib	Hib						
Inactivated polio[5]			IPV	IPV	IPV[5]					IPV[5]		
Pneumococcal conjugate[6]			PCV	PCV	PCV	PCV						
Measles, Mumps, Rubella[7]						MMR				MMR[7]	(MMR[7])	
Varicella[8]						Var					(Var[8])	
Hepatitis A[9]									Hep A–in selected area[9]			

Approved by the Advisory Committee on Immunization Practices (ACIP), the American Academy of Pediatrics (AAP), and the American Academy of Family Physicians (AAFP).

1. This schedule indicates the recommended ages for routine administration of currently licensed childhood vaccines, as of 11/1/00, for children through 18 years of age. Additional vaccines may be licensed and recommended during the year. Licensed combination vaccines may be used whenever any components of the combination are indicated and its other components are not contraindicated. Providers should consult the manufacturers' package inserts for detailed recommendations.

2. *Infants born to HbsAg-negative mothers* should receive the 1st dose of hepatitis B (Hep B) vaccine by age 2 months. The 2nd dose should be at least one month after the 1st dose. The 3rd dose should be administered at least 4 months after the 1st dose and at least 2 months after the 2nd dose, but not before 6 months of age for infants.
Infants born to HbsAg-positive mothers should receive hepatitis B vaccine and 0.5 mL hepatitis B immune globulin (HBIG) within 12 hours of birth at separate sites. The 2nd dose is recommended at 1–2 months of age and the 3rd dose at 6 months of age.
Infants born to mothers whose HbsAg status is unknown should receive hepatitis B vaccine within 12 hours of birth. Maternal blood should be drawn at the time of delivery to determine the mother's HbsAg status; if the HbsAg test is positive, the infant should receive HBIG as soon as possible (no later than 1 week of age).
All children and adolescents who have not been immunized against hepatitis B should begin the series during any visit. Special efforts should be made to immunize children who were born in or whose parents were born in areas of the world with moderate or high endemicity of hepatitis B virus infection.

3. The 4th dose of DTaP (diphtheria and tetanus toxoids and acellular pertussis vaccine) may be administered as early as 12 months of age, provided 6 months have elapsed since the 3rd dose and the child is unlikely to return at age 15–18 months. Td (tetanus and diphtheria toxoids) is recommended at 11–12 years of age if at least 5 years have elapsed since the last dose of DTP, DTaP or DT. Subsequent routine Td boosters are recommended every 10 years.

4. Three *Haemophilus influenzae* type b (Hib) conjugate vaccines are licensed for infant use. If PRP-OMP (PedvaxHIB® or ComVax® [Merck]) is administered at 2 and 4 months of age, a dose at 6 months is not required. Because clinical studies in infants have demonstrated that using some combination products may induce a lower immune response to the Hib vaccine component, DTaP/Hib combination products should not be used for primary immunization in infants at 2, 4 or 6 months of age, unless FDA-approved for these ages.

5. An all-IPV schedule is recommended for routine childhood polio vaccination in the United States. All children should receive four does of IPV at 2 months, 4 months, 6–18 months, and 4–6 years of age. Oral polio vaccine (OPV) should be used only in selected circumstances.

6. The heptavalent conjugate pneumococcal vaccine (PCV) is recommended for all children 2–23 months of age. It also is recommended for certain children 24–59 months of age.

7. The 2nd dose of measles, mumps, and rubella (MMR) vaccine is recommended routinely at 4–6 years of age but may be administered during any visit, provided at least 4 weeks have elapsed since receipt of the 1st dose and that both doses are administered beginning at or after 12 months of age. Those who have not previously received the second dose should complete the schedule by the 11–12 year old visit.

8. Varicella (Var) vaccine is recommended at any visit on or after the first birthday for susceptible children, i.e. those who lack a reliable history of chickenpox (as judged by a health care provider) and who have not been immunized. Susceptible persons 13 years of age or older should receive 2 doses, given at least 4 weeks apart.

9. Hepatitis A (Hep A) is shaded to indicate its recommended use in selected states and/or regions, and for certain high risk groups; consult your local public health authority.

For additional information about the vaccines listed above, please visit the National Immunization Program Home Page at http://www.cdc.gov/nip/ or call the National Immunization Hotline at 800-232-2522 (English) or 800-232-0233 (Spanish).

APPENDIX D RECOMMENDED DIETARY ALLOWANCES

Recommended Dietary Allowances[a]

Category	Age (Yr) or Condition	Weight[b] (kg)	Weight[b] (lb)	Height[b] (cm)	Height[b] (in)	Kcal per Day	Protein (g)	Fat-Soluble Vitamins: Vitamin A (μg RE)[c]	Vitamin D (μg)[d]	Vitamin E (mg α-TE)[e]	Vitamin K (μc)
Infants	0.0–0.5	6	13	60	24	650	13	375	7.5	3	5
	0.5–1.0	9	20	71	28	850	14	375	10	4	10
Children	1–3	13	29	90	35	1300	16	400	10	6	15
	4–6	20	44	112	44	1800	24	500	10	7	20
	7–10	28	62	132	52	2000	28	700	10	7	30
Men	11–14	45	99	157	62	2500	45	1000	10	10	45
	15–18	66	145	176	69	3000	59	1000	10	10	65
Women	11–14	46	101	157	62	2200	46	800	10	8	45
	15–18	55	120	163	64	2200	44	800	10	8	55

[a] The allowances, expressed as average daily intakes over time, are intended to provide for individual variations among most normal persons as they live in the United States under usual environmental stresses. Diets should be based on a variety of common foods to provide other nutrients for which human requirements have been less well defined.

[b] Weights and heights of Reference Adults are actual medians for the U.S. population of the designated age.

[c] Retinol equivalents. 1 RE = 1 μg retinol or 6 μg β-carotene.

[d] As cholecalciferol. 10 μg cholecalciferol = 400 U of vitamin D.

[e] Tocopherol equivalents. 1 mg d-α-tocopherol = 1 α-TE.

[f] Ne Niacin equivalent = 1 mg of niacin or 60 mg of dietary tryptophan.

(From Food and Nutrition Board, National Academy of Sciences—National Research Council: *Recommended dietary allowances*, ed. 10, Washington, DC, 1989, The Council.)

Recommended Dietary Allowances[a]

Water-Soluble Vitamins							Minerals									
Vitamin C (mg)	Thiamin (mg)	Riboflavin (mg)	Niacin (mg NE)[f]	Vitamin B_6 (mg)	Folate (µg)	Vitamin B_{12} (µg)	Calcium (mg)	Phosphorus (mg)	Magnesium (mg)	Iron (mg)	Zinc (mg)	Iodine (µg)	Selenium (µg) 35			
30	0.3	0.4	5	0.3	25	0.3	400	300	40	6	5	40	10			
35	0.4	0.5	6	0.6	35	0.5	600	500	60	10	5	50	15			
40	0.7	0.8	9	1.0	50	0.7	800	800	80	10	10	70	20			
45	0.9	1.1	12	1.1	75	1.0	800	800	120	10	10	90	20			
45	1.0	1.2	13	1.4	100	1.4	800	800	170	10	10	120	20			
50	1.3	1.5	17	1.7	150	2.0	1200	1200	270	12	15	150	40			
60	1.5	1.8	20	2.0	200	2.0	1200	1200	400	12	15	150	50			
50	1.1	1.3	15	1.4	150	2.0	1200	1200	280	15	12	150	45			
60	1.1	1.3	15	1.5	180	2.0	1200	1200	300	15	12	150	50			

APPENDIX E
DENVER II

DIRECTIONS FOR ADMINISTRATION

1. Try to get child to smile by smiling, talking or waving. Do not touch him/her.
2. Child must stare at hand several seconds.
3. Parent may help guide toothbrush and put toothpaste on brush.
4. Child does not have to be able to tie shoes or button/zip in the back.
5. Move yarn slowly in an arc from one side to the other, about 8" above child's face.
6. Pass if child grasps rattle when it is touched to the backs or tips of fingers.
7. Pass if child tries to see where yarn went. Yarn should be dropped quickly from sight from tester's hand without arm movement.
8. Child must transfer cube from hand to hand without help of body, mouth, or table.
9. Pass if child picks up raisin with any part of thumb and finger.
10. Line can vary only 30 degrees or less from tester's line.
11. Make a fist with thumb pointing upward and wiggle only the thumb. Pass if child imitates and does not move any fingers other than the thumb.

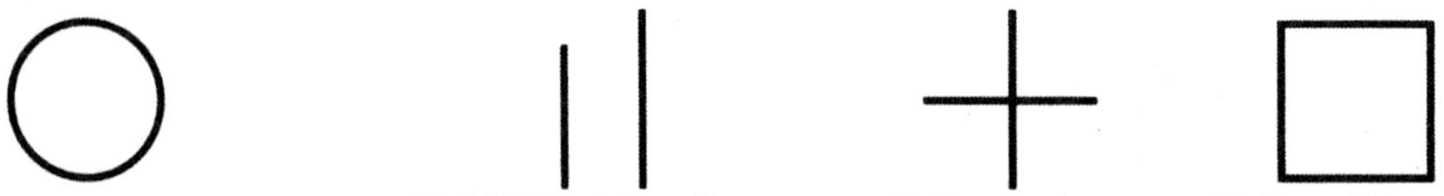

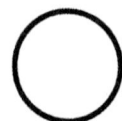

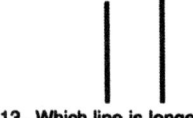

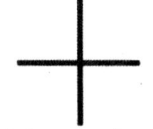

12. Pass any enclosed form. Fail continuous round motions.
13. Which line is longer? (Not bigger.) Turn paper upside down and repeat. (pass 3 of 3 or 5 of 6)
14. Pass any lines crossing near midpoint.
15. Have child copy first. If failed, demonstrate.

When giving items 12, 14, and 15, do not name the forms. Do not demonstrate 12 and 14.

16. When scoring, each pair (2 arms, 2 legs, etc.) counts as one part.
17. Place one cube in cup and shake gently near child's ear, but out of sight. Repeat for other ear.
18. Point to picture and have child name it. (No credit is given for sounds only.) If less than 4 pictures are named correctly, have child point to picture as each is named by tester.

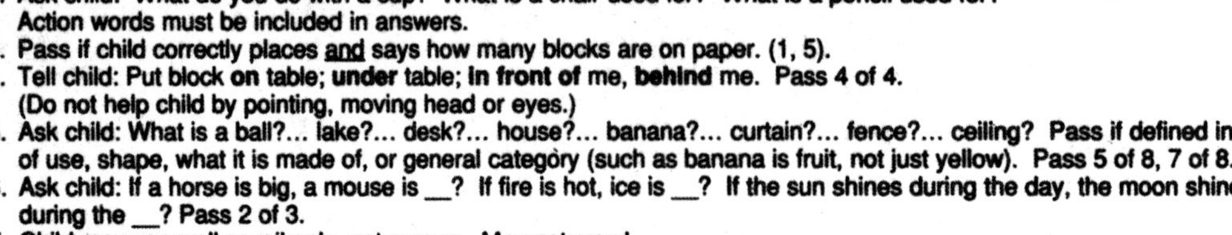

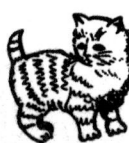

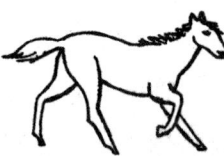

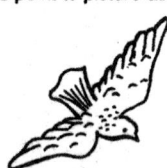

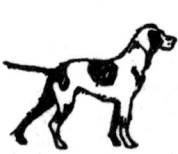

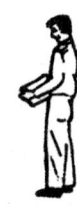

19. Using doll, tell child: Show me the nose, eyes, ears, mouth, hands, feet, tummy, hair. Pass 6 of 8.
20. Using pictures, ask child: Which one flies?... says meow?... talks?... barks?... gallops? Pass 2 of 5, 4 of 5.
21. Ask child: What do you do when you are cold?... tired?... hungry? Pass 2 of 3, 3 of 3.
22. Ask child: What do you do with a cup? What is a chair used for? What is a pencil used for? Action words must be included in answers.
23. Pass if child correctly places <u>and</u> says how many blocks are on paper. (1, 5).
24. Tell child: Put block **on** table; **under** table; **in front of** me, **behind** me. Pass 4 of 4. (Do not help child by pointing, moving head or eyes.)
25. Ask child: What is a ball?... lake?... desk?... house?... banana?... curtain?... fence?... ceiling? Pass if defined in terms of use, shape, what it is made of, or general category (such as banana is fruit, not just yellow). Pass 5 of 8, 7 of 8.
26. Ask child: If a horse is big, a mouse is __? If fire is hot, ice is __? If the sun shines during the day, the moon shines during the __? Pass 2 of 3.
27. Child may use wall or rail only, not person. May not crawl.
28. Child must throw ball overhand 3 feet to within arm's reach of tester.
29. Child must perform standing broad jump over width of test sheet (8 1/2 inches).
30. Tell child to walk forward, heel within 1 inch of toe. Tester may demonstrate. Child must walk 4 consecutive steps.
31. In the second year, half of normal children are non-compliant.

OBSERVATIONS:

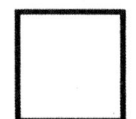

Denver II

Examiner:
Date:

Name:
Birthdate:
ID No.:

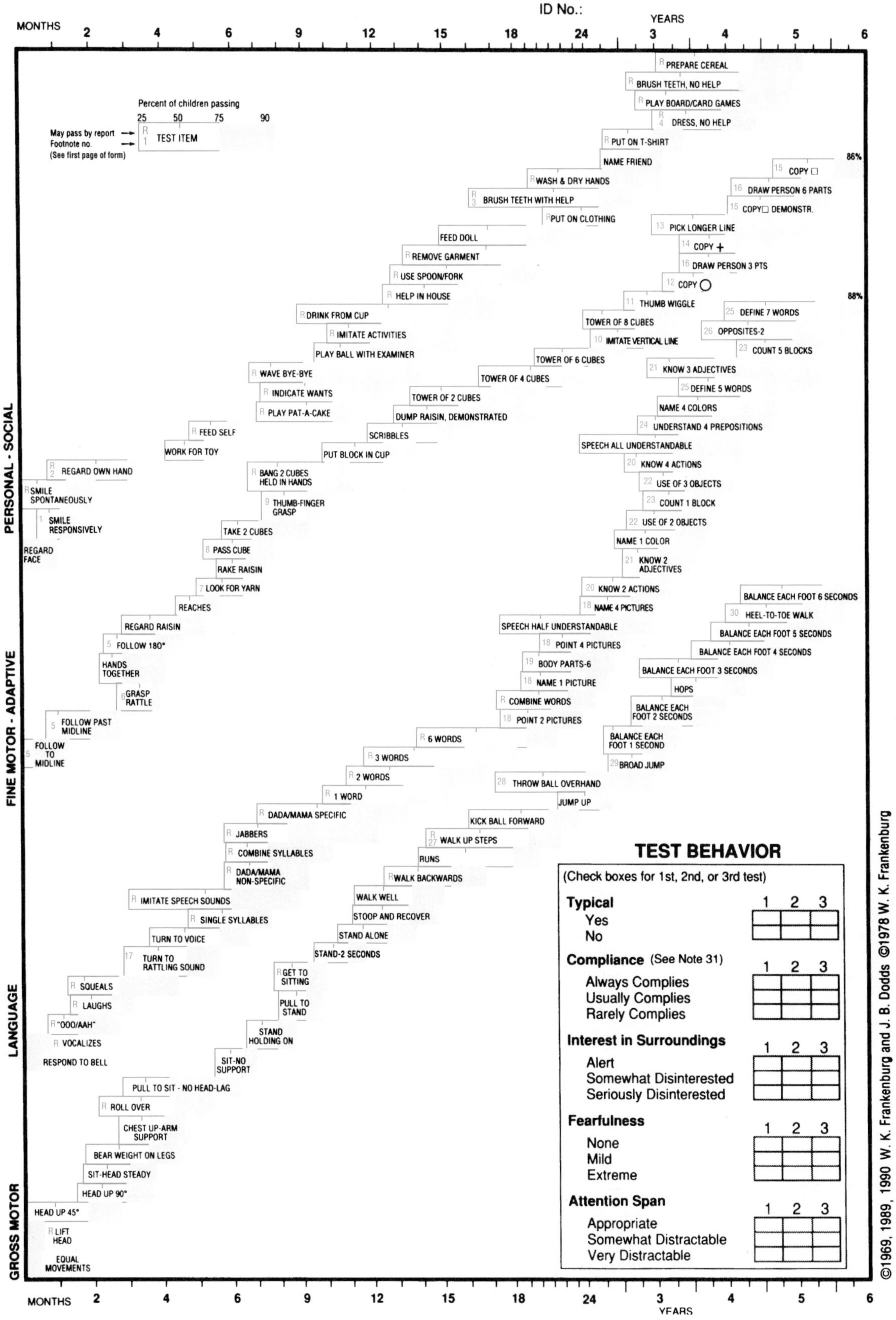

Reprinted with permission of Denver Developmental Materials, Denver, CO.

APPENDIX F SEXUAL MATURITY RATINGS (SMR)

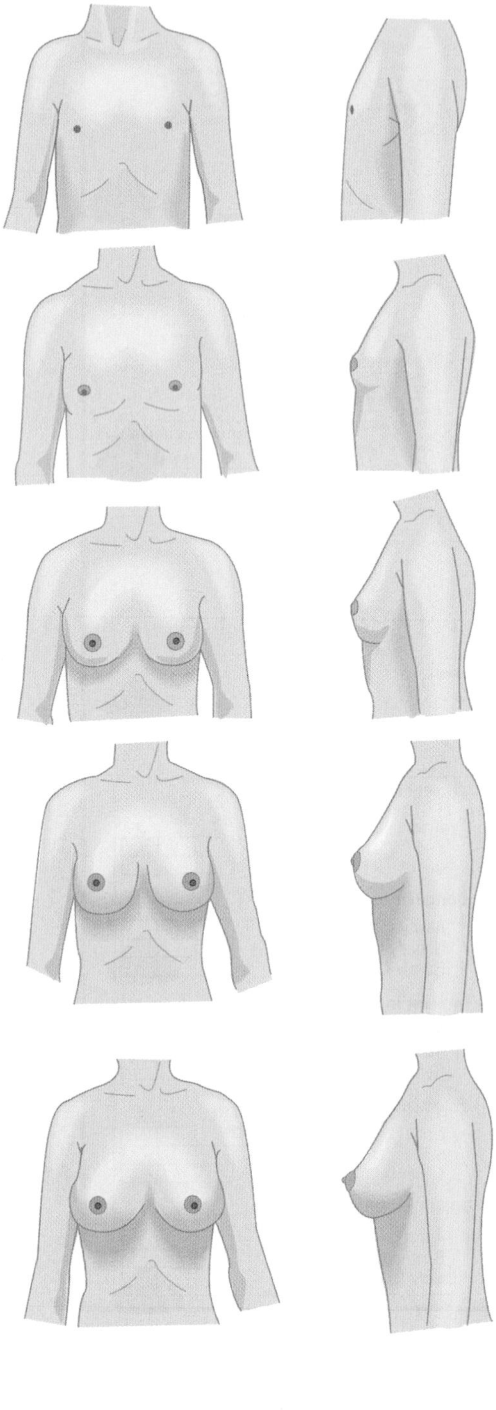

Developmental Stages

1. **Preadolescent stage** (before age 8). Nipple is small, slightly raised.
2. **Early adolescent stage.** Breast bud development (after age 8). Nipple and breast form a small mound. Areola enlarges. Height spurt begins.
3. **Adolescent stage** (10-14 years). Nipple is flush with breast shape. Breast and areola enlarge. Menses begins. Height spurt peaks.
4. **Late adolescent stage** (14–17 years). Nipple and areola form a secondary mound over the breast. Height spurt ends.
5. **Adult stage.** Nipple protrudes; areola is flush with the breast shape.

Sexual Maturity Rating for Female Breast Development

Stage 1

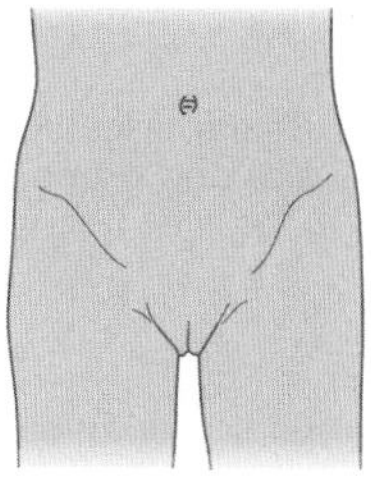

Preadolescent Stage
(before age 8)
No pubic hair, only body hair (vellus hair)

Stage 2

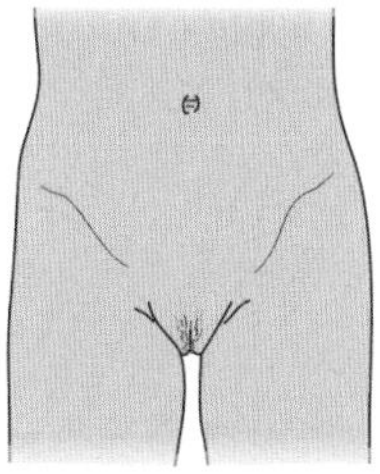

Early Adolescent Stage
(ages 8 to 12)
Sparse growth of long, slightly dark, fine pubic hair, slightly curly and located along the labia

Stage 3

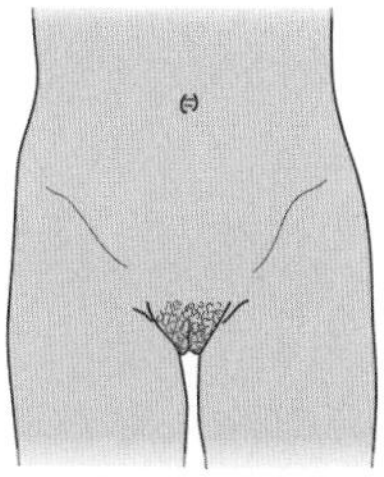

Adolescent Stage
(ages 12 to 13)
Pubic hair becomes darker, curlier, and spreads over the symphysis

Stage 4

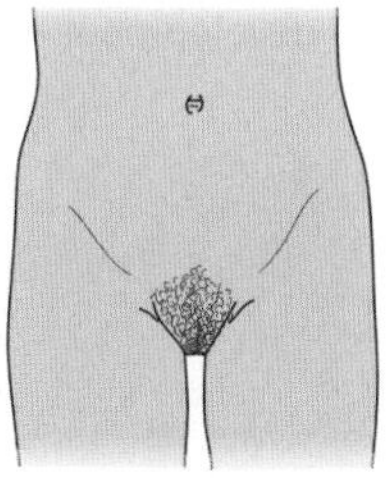

Late Adolescent Stage
(ages 13 to 15)
Texture and curl of pubic hair is similar to that of an adult but not spread to thighs

Stage 5

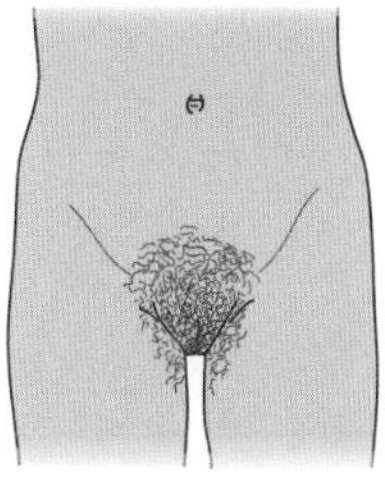

Adult Stage
Adult appearance in quality and quantity of pubic hair; growth is spread to inner aspect of thighs and abdomen

Sexual Maturity Rating (SMR) for Female Genitalia

Developmental Stage	Pubic Hair	Penis	Testes
1. 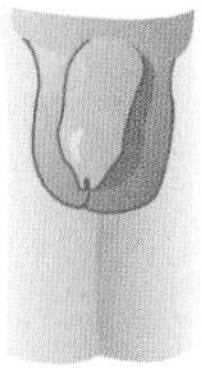	No pubic hair, only fine body hair (vellus hair)	Preadolescent; childhood size and proportion	Preadolescent; childhood size and proportion
2. 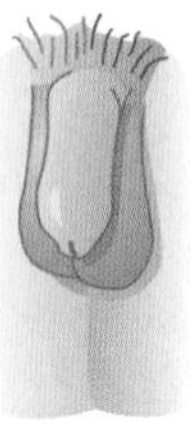	Sparse growth of long, slightly dark, straight hair	Slight or no growth	Growth in testes and scrotum; scrotum reddens and changes texture
3. 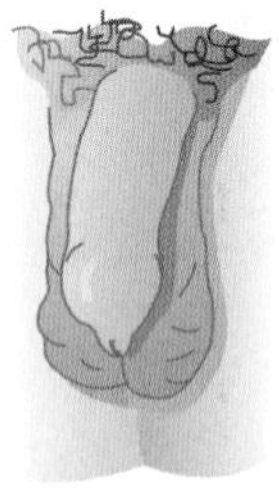	Becomes darker and coarser; slightly curled and spreads over symphysis	Growth, especially in length	Further growth
4. 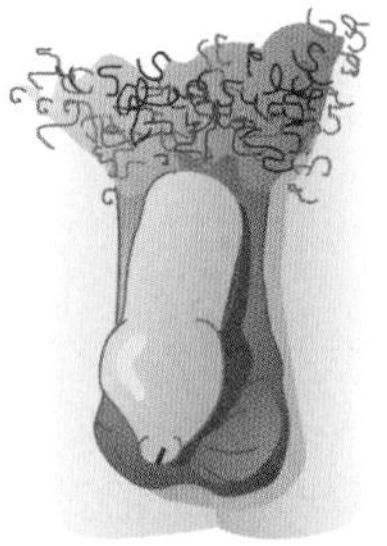	Texture and curl of pubic hair is similar to that of an adult but not spread to thighs	Further growth in length; diameter increases; development of glans	Further growth; scrotum darkens
5. 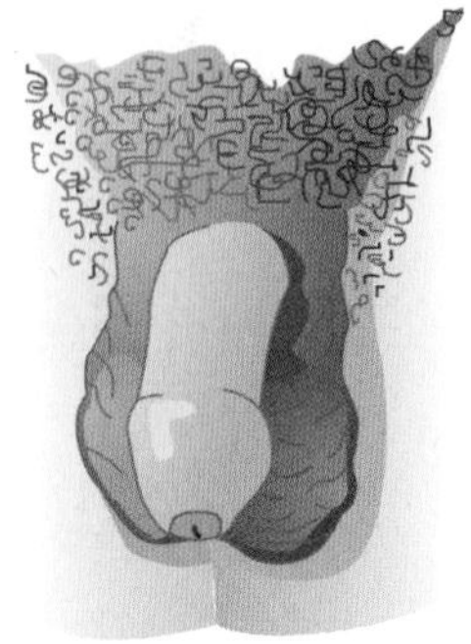	Adult appearance in quality and quantity of pubic hair; growth is spread to medial surface of thighs	Adult size and shape	Adult size and shape

Sexual Maturity Rating (SMR) for Male Genitalia

APPENDIX G CARDIOPULMONARY RESUSCITATION GUIDELINES

Summary of Differences Between Adults, Children, and Infants

CPR/Rescue Breathing	Adult and Older Child (more than 8 years old)	Child (1 to 8 years old)	Infant (less than 1 year old)
Establish that victim is unresponsive Activate emergency medical service (EMS).	Activate EMS or other emergency response number as soon as victim is found.	Activate EMS or other emergency response number after giving 1 minute of CPR.	Activate EMS or other emergency response number after giving 1 minute of CPR.
Open airway Perform head tilt–chin lift or jaw thrust.	Head tilt–chin lift (If trauma is present, use jaw thrust.)	Head tilt–chin lift (If trauma is present, use jaw thrust.)	Head tilt–chin lift (If trauma is present, use jaw thrust.)
Check for breathing (look, listen, feel) If victim is breathing, place in recovery position. If victim is not breathing normally, give 2 effective slow breaths.			
• **Initial**	2 effective breaths (2 seconds each)	2 effective breaths (1 to $1^1/_2$ seconds each)	2 effective breaths (1 to $1^1/_2$ seconds each)
• **Subsequent**	10 to 12 breaths per minute (approximate)	20 breaths per minute (approximate)	20 breaths per minute (approximate)
• **Foreign-body airway obstruction**	Abdominal thrusts	Abdominal thrusts	Back blows or chest thrusts (no abdominal thrusts)
Check for signs of circulation (breathing, coughing, movement, or pulse) If signs of circulation are present, provide airway and breathing support. If no signs of circulation are present, begin chest compressions interposed with breaths.	***Health Care Providers Only:*** • Check carotid pulse ***Lay Rescuers:*** Check for signs of circulation after giving 2 rescue breaths: • Normal breathing • Coughing • Movement If no signs of circulation are present, provide chest compressions.	***Health Care Providers Only:*** • Check carotid pulse ***Lay Rescuers:*** Check for signs of circulation after giving 2 rescue breaths: • Normal breathing • Coughing • Movement If no signs of circulation are present, provide chest compressions.	***Health Care Providers Only:*** • Check brachial pulse ***Lay Rescuers:*** Check for signs of circulation after giving 2 rescue breaths: • Normal breathing • Coughing • Movement If no signs of circulation are present, provide chest compressions.

continued

Summary of Differences Between Adults, Children, and Infants *(Continued)*

CPR/Rescue Breathing	Adult and Older Child (more than 8 years old)	Child (1 to 8 years old)	Infant (less than 1 year old)
Compression landmarks	Lower half of sternum (nipple line)	Lower half of sternum	Lower half of sternum (1 finger's width below nipple line)
Compression method	Heel of 1 hand, other hand on top	Heel of 1 hand	2 fingers
Compression depth	$1\frac{1}{2}$ to 2 inches	$\frac{1}{3}$ to $\frac{1}{2}$ the depth of the chest	$\frac{1}{3}$ to $\frac{1}{2}$ the depth of the chest
Compression rate	Approximately 100 per minute	Approximately 100 per minute	At least 100 per minute
Compression-ventilation ratio	15:2 (1 or 2 rescuers, unprotected airway)	5:1 (1 or 2 rescuers)	5:1 (1 or 2 rescuers)

Reproduced with permission. Heartsaver CPR *Copyright © 2000, American Heart Association.*

PROCEDURES

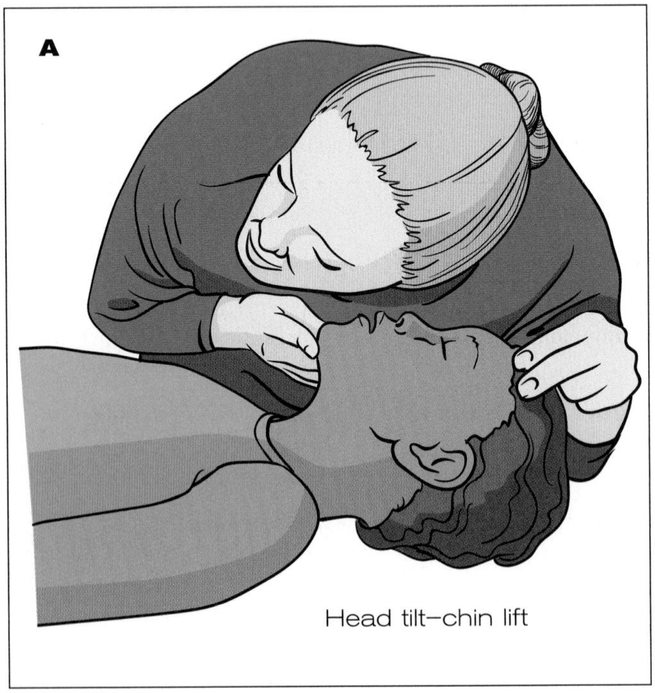

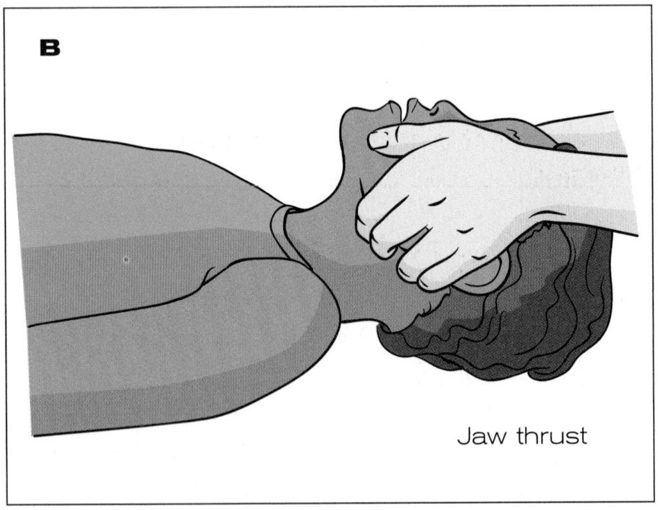

C

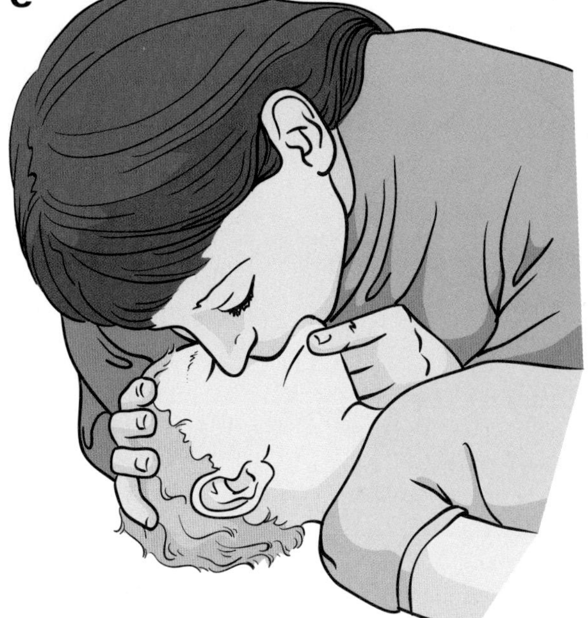

Mouth-to-nose-and-mouth rescue breathing for an infant

D

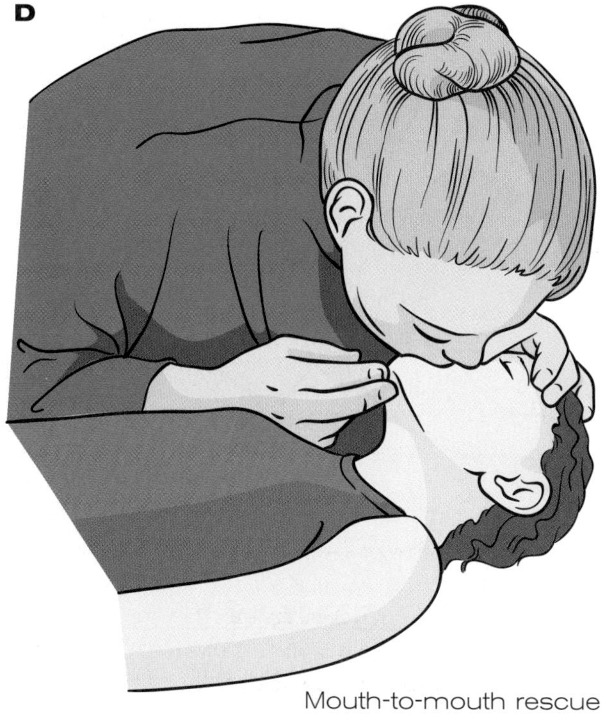

Mouth-to-mouth rescue breathing for a child

E

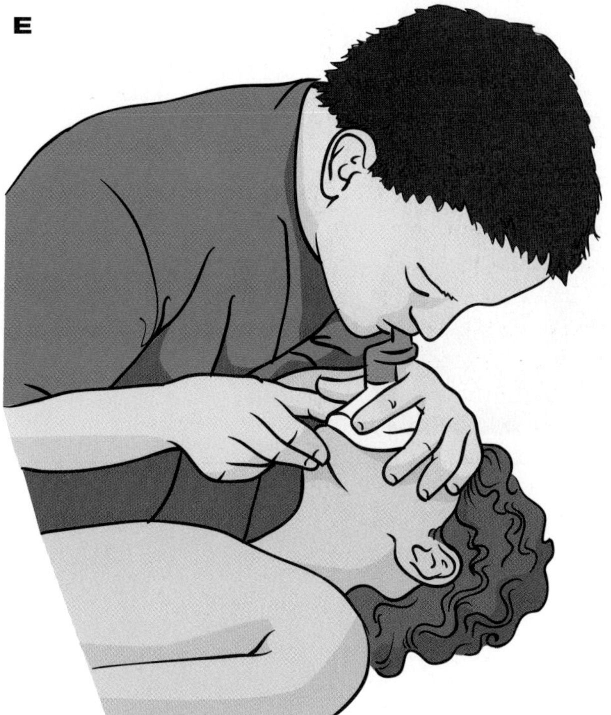

Rescue breathing with a barrier device

F

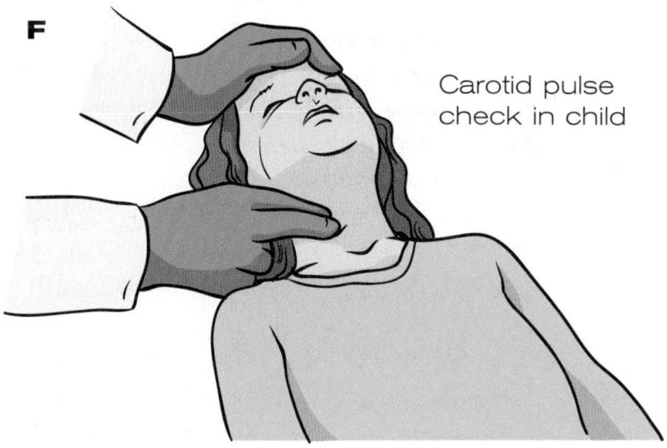

Carotid pulse check in child

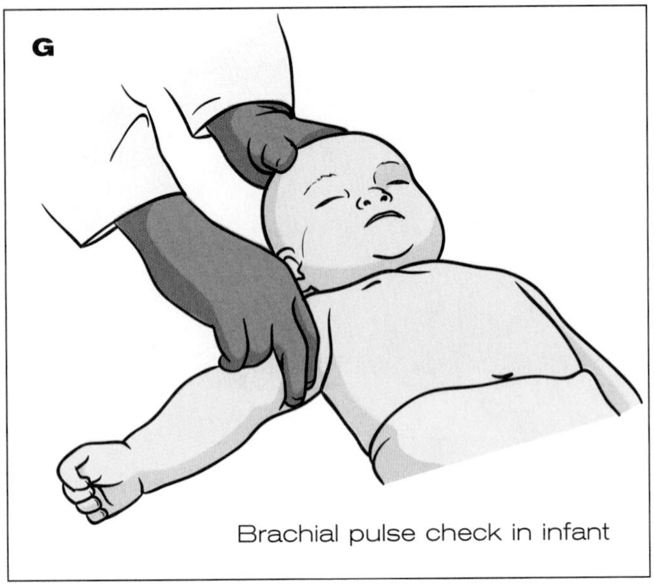

G

Brachial pulse check in infant

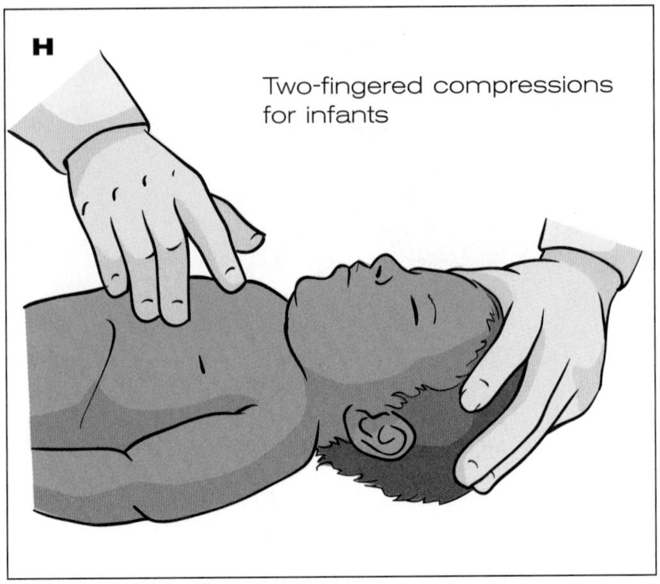

H

Two-fingered compressions for infants

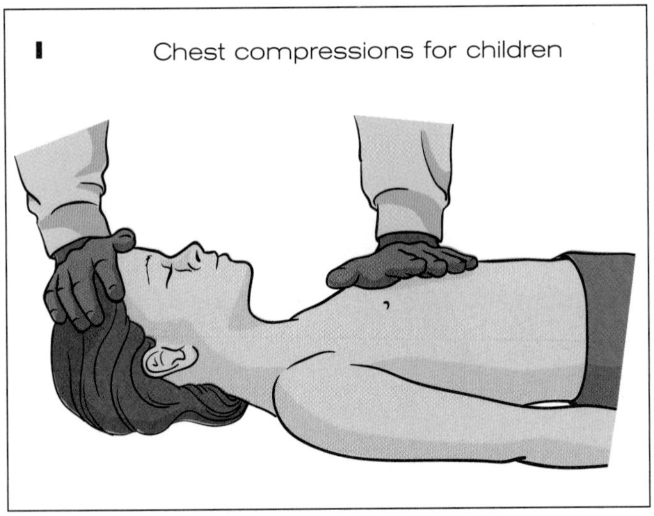

I

Chest compressions for children

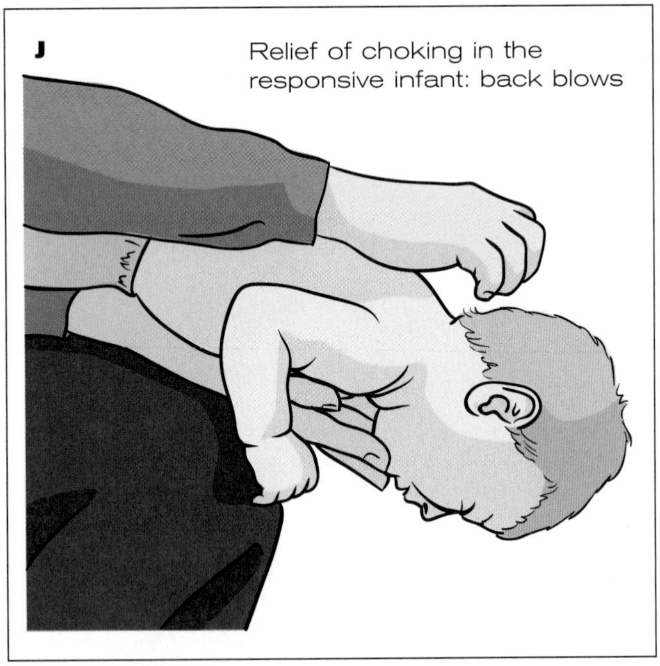

J

Relief of choking in the responsive infant: back blows

K

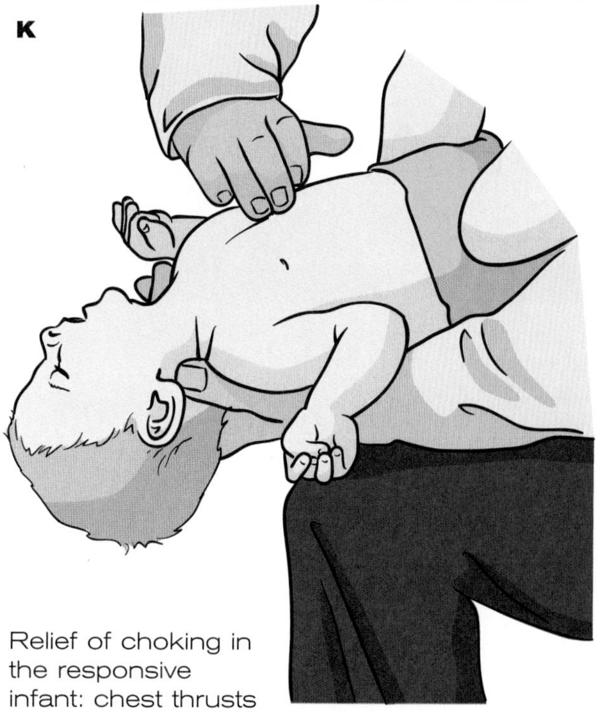

Relief of choking in the responsive infant: chest thrusts

L

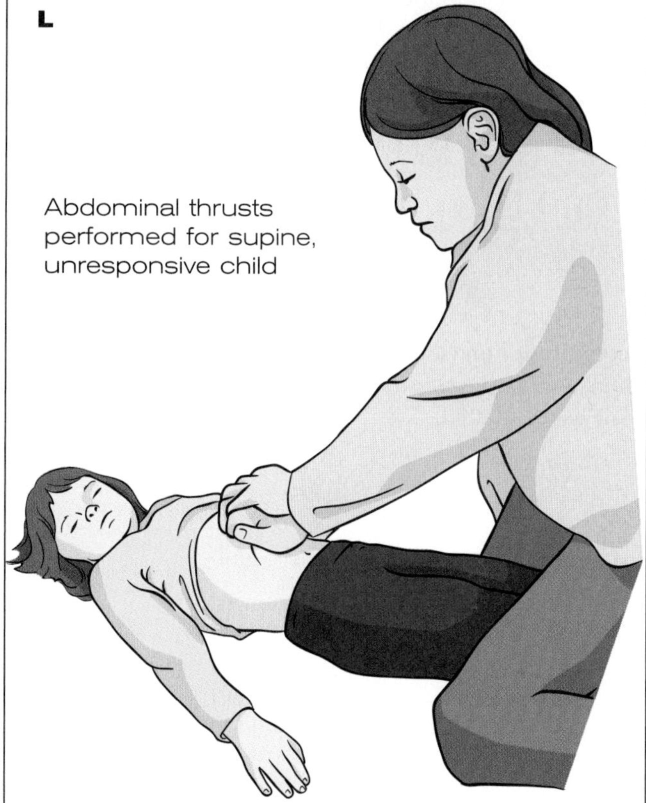

Abdominal thrusts performed for supine, unresponsive child

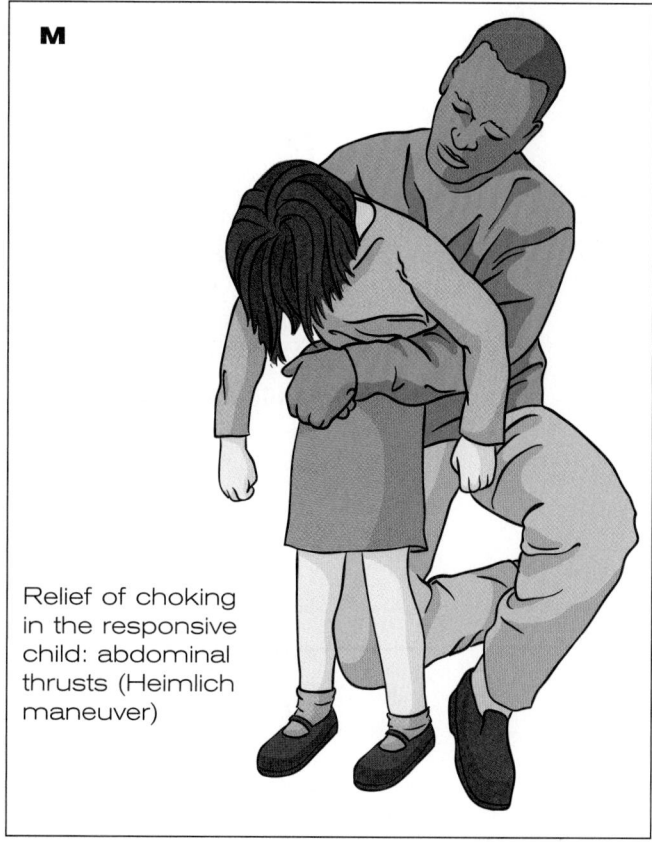

M

Relief of choking in the responsive child: abdominal thrusts (Heimlich maneuver)

APPENDIX H COMMON LABORATORY TESTS AND NORMAL VALUES

Acetaminophen (serum or plasma)

Therapeutic concentration	10–30 µg/ml
Toxic concentration	>200 µg/ml

Albumin (plasma)

Newborn	2.5–3.4 g/dl
< 5 yr	3.4–5.0 g/dl
5–19 yr	4.0–5.6 g/dl

Alkaline phosphatase (ALP) (serum)

1–9 yr	145–420 U/L
2–10 yr	100–320 U/L
11–18 yr male	100–390 U/L
11–18 yr female	100–320 U/L

Ammonia nitrogen (serum or plasma)

Newborn	90–150 mg/dl
Child	40–80 mg/dl

Amylase (serum)

1–19 yr	35–127 U/L

Antistreptolysin O titer (ASO titer) (serum)

2–4 yr	<166 Todd units
School-aged	170–330 Todd units

Bicarbonate (HCO_3) (serum)

Infant (venous)	20–24 mEq/L
>2 years (venous)	22–29 mEq/L
>2 years (arterial)	21–28 mEq/L

Bilirubin (total) (serum)

Premature Infant	
Cord blood	<2 mg/dl
0–1 day	<8 mg/dl
1–2 days	<12 mg/dl
2–5 days	<16 mg/dl
>5 days	<20 mg/dl
Full-term Infant	
Cord	<2.8 mg/dl
0–1day	<2–6 mg/dl
1–2 days	<6–8 mg/dl
2–5 days	<4–6 mg/dl
>5 days	<10 mg/dl

Bilirubin (conjugated) (serum)

0.0–0.2 mEq/L

Blood volume (whole blood)

Female	50–75 ml/Kg
Male	52–83 ml/Kg

C-reactive protein (CRP) (serum)

2–12 yr	67–1800 ng/ml

Calcium (Ca)—Total (serum)

Newborn	9.0–10.6 mg/dl
Child	8.8–10.8 mg/dl

Carbon dioxide

Partial pressure (PCO_2) (whole blood, arterial)

Newborn	27–40 mm Hg
Infant	27–41 mm Hg
Thereafter: Male	35–48 mm Hg
Female	32–45 mm Hg

Total (tCO_2) (serum or plasma)

Newborn	13–22 mmol/L
Infant	20–28 mmol/L
Child	20–28 mmol/L
Thereafter	23–30 mmol/L

Chloride (Cl) (serum)

Newborn	97–110 mmol/L
Thereafter	98–106 mmol/L

Chloride (sweat)

Normal	<40 mmol/L
Borderline	45–60 mmol/L
Cystic Fibrosis	>60 mmol/L

Cholesterol (total)

Newborn	53–135 mg/dl
Infant	70–175 mg/dl
Child	120–200 mg/dl
Adolescent	<200 mg/dl

Creatine kinase (CK, CPK) (serum)

Newborn	87–725 U/L

Creatine (serum)

Newborn	0.3–1.0 mg/dl
Infant	0.2–0.4 mg/dl
Child	0.3–0.7 mg/dl
Adolescent	0.5–1.0 mg/dl

Digoxin (serum or plasma)

Therapeutic concentration	
Congestive heart failure (CHF)	0.8–1.5 ng/ml
Arrhythmias	1.5–2.0 ng/ml
Toxic concentration	>2.5 ng/mt

Erythrocyte (RBC) count (whole blood)

Newborn	4.8–7.1 million/mm^3
3–6 mo	3.1–4.5 million/mm^3
0.5–2 yr	3.7–5.3 million/mm^3
2–6 yr	3.9–5.3 million/mm^3
6–12 yr	4.0–5.2 million/mm^3
12–18 yr: Male	4.5–5.3 million/mm^3
Female	4.1–5.1 million/mm^3

Erythrocyte sedimentation rate (ESR) (whole blood)

Westergren (modified)	
Child	0–10 mm/hr
Wintrobe	
Child	0–13 mm/hr

Fibroginogen (plasma)

Newborn	125–300 mg/dl
Thereafter	200–400 mg/dl

Glucose (serum)

Newborn	50–90 mg/dl
Child	60–100 mg/dl
Thereafter	70–105 mg/dl

Growth hormone (hGH, somatotropin) (plasma, fasting)

Newborn	5–40 ng/ml
Child	0–10 ng/ml

Hematocrit (HCT, Hct) (whole blood)

Newborn	44–72%
2 mo	28–42%
6–12 yr	35–45%
12–18 yr: Male	37–49%
Female	36–46%

Hemoglobin (Hb) (whole blood)

Newborn	14–27 g/dl
2 mo	9–14 g/dl
6–12 yr	11.5–15.5 g/dl
12–18 yr: Male	13–16 g/dl
Female	12–16 g/dl

Iron (serum)

Newborn	100–250 µg/dl
Infant	40–100 µg/dl
Child	50–120 µg/dl
Thereafter: Male	50–160 µg/dl
Female	40–150 µg/dl

Lead (whole blood)

Child	<10 µg/dl

Leukocyte (WBC) Count (whole blood)

Newborn	9–30 × 1000 cells/mm^3
1–3 yr	6.0–17.5 × 1000 cells/mm^3
4–7 yr	5.5–15.5 × 1000 cells/mm^3
8–13 yr	4.5–13.5 × 1000 cells/mm^3
Adult	4.5–11.0 × 1000 cells/mm^3

Leukocyte differential count (whole blood)

Myelocytes	0%
Neutrophils—"bands"	3–5%
Neutrophils—"segs"	54–62%
Lymphocytes	25–33%
Monocytes	3–7%
Eosinophils	1–3%
Basophils	0–0.75%

Osmolality (serum)

Child, adult	275–295 mOsmol/kg H_2O

Oxygen, partial pressure (PO_2) (whole blood, arterial)

Birth	8–24 mm Hg
1 d	54–95 mm Hg
Thereafter (decreased with age)	83–108 mm Hg

Oxygen saturation (SaO_2) (whole blood, arterial)

Newborn	85–90%
Thereafter	95–99%

Partial thromboplastin time (PTT) (whole blood) (Na citrate)

Nonactivated	60–85 seconds (Platelin)
Activated	25–35 seconds (differs with methods)

Phenylalanine (serum)

Premature	2.0–7.5 mg/dl
Newborn	1.2–3.4 mg/dl
Thereafter	0.8–1.8 mg/dl

Plasma volume (plasma)

Male	25–43 ml/kg
Female	28–45 ml/kg

Platelet count (thrombocyte count) (whole blood)

Newborn (After 1 wk. same as adult)	84–478 × 10^3 mm^3 (µl)
Adult	150–400 × 10^3 mm^3 (µl)

Potassium (serum)

<2 yr	3.0–6.0 mmol/L
2–12 yr	3.5–7.0 mmol/L
>12 yr	3.5–5.0 mmol/L

Protein (serum, total)

Premature	4.3–7.5 g/dl
Newborn	4.6–7.4 g/dl
1–7 yr	6.1–7.9 g/dl
8–12 yr	6.4–8.1 g/dl
13–19 yr	6.6–8.2 g/dl

Prothrombin time (PT)
One-stage (Quick) (whole blood)

In general	11–15 seconds (varies with type of thromboplastin)
Newborn	Prolonged by 2–3 sec

Sodium (serum or plasma)

Newborn	136–146 mmol/L
Infant	139–146 mmol/L
Child	138–145 mmol/L
Thereafter	136–146 mmol/L

Specific gravity (urine)

Newborn	1.016–1.030
Infants	1.002–1.006
Thereafter	1.016–1.030

Thyroxine (T_4, T_4 total, T_4 RIA) (serum)

Newborn	9–18 μg/dl
Infant	7–15 μg/dl
1–5 yr	7.3–15 μg/dl
5–10 yr	6.4–13.3 μg/dl
Thereafter	5–12 μg/dl

Thyrotropin (thyroid stimulating hormone [TSH])

Newborn	3–18 μIU/L by day 3 of life
Thereafter	2–10 mU/L

Triglycerides (TG) (serum) (after ≥12 hr fast)

	M	F
0–5 yr	30–86 mg/dl	32–99 mg/dl
6–11 yr	31–108 mg/dl	35–114 mg/dl
12–15 yr	36–138 mg/dl	41–138 mg/dl
16–19 yr	40–163 mg/dl	40–128 mg/dl

Triiodothyronine (T_3, T_3 total, T_3 RIA) (serum)

Newborn	72–260 ng/dl
1–5 yr	100–260 ng/dl
5–10 yr	90–240 ng/dl
10–15 yr	80–210 ng/dl
Thereafter	115–190 ng/dl

Urea nitrogen (serum or plasma)

Newborn	3–12 mg/dl
Infant/child	5–18 mg/dl
Thereafter	7–18 mg/dl

Urine volume (urine, 24 hr)

Newborn	50–300 ml/d
Infant	350–550 ml/d
Child	500–1000 ml/d
Adolescent	700–1400 ml/d
Thereafter: Male	800–1800 ml/d
Female	600–1600 ml/d (varies with intake and other factors)

Note: Normal lab values differ depending on lab used. Verify your facility's normal values.

Modified from *Delmar's Guide to Laboratory and Diagnostic Tests* by R. Daniels. (2001). Albany, NY: Delmar; *Nelson Textbook of Pediatrics* (16th ed.), by R. Behrman, R. Kliegman, and H. Jenson. (2000). Philadelphia, PA: W. B. Saunders; *A Manual of Laboratory and Diagnostic Tests* (6th ed.) by F. Fischbach. (1999). Philadelphia, PA: Lippincott.

APPENDIX I
TEMPERATURE EQUIVALENTS AND PEDIATRIC WEIGHT CONVERSION

Celsius and Fahrenheit Temperature Equivalents

Celsius	Fahrenheit	Celsius	Fahrenheit
34.0	93.2	38.4	101.1
34.2	93.6	38.6	101.4
34.4	93.9	38.8	101.8
34.6	94.3	39.0	102.2
34.8	94.6	39.2	102.5
35.0	95.0	39.4	102.9
35.2	95.4	39.6	103.2
35.4	95.7	39.8	103.6
35.6	96.1	40.0	104.0
35.8	96.4	40.2	104.3
36.0	96.8	40.4	104.7
36.2	97.1	40.6	105.1
36.4	97.5	40.8	105.4
36.6	97.8	41.0	105.8
36.8	98.2	41.2	106.1
		41.4	106.5
37.0	98.6	41.6	106.8
37.2	98.9	41.8	107.2
37.4	99.3	42.0	107.6
37.6	99.6	42.2	108.0
37.8	100.0	42.4	108.3
38.0	100.4	42.6	108.7
38.2	100.7	42.8	109.0

Conversion formulas:
Fahrenheit to Celsius (°F – 32) × (5/9) = °C
Celsius to Fahrenheit (°C) × (9/5) + 32 = °F

Pediatric Weight Conversion (Pounds to Kilograms)

Pounds	0	1	2	3	4	5	6	7	8	9
0	0.00	0.45	0.90	1.36	1.81	2.26	2.72	3.17	3.62	4.08
10	4.53	4.98	5.44	5.89	6.35	6.80	7.35	7.71	8.16	8.61
20	9.07	9.52	9.97	10.43	10.88	11.34	11.79	12.24	12.70	13.15
30	13.60	14.06	14.51	14.96	15.42	15.87	16.32	16.78	17.23	17.69
40	18.14	18.59	19.05	19.50	19.95	20.41	20.86	21.31	21.77	22.22
50	22.68	23.13	23.58	24.04	24.49	24.94	25.40	25.85	26.30	26.76
60	27.21	27.66	28.22	28.57	29.03	29.48	29.93	30.39	30.84	31.29
70	31.75	32.20	32.65	33.11	33.56	34.02	34.47	34.92	35.38	35.83
80	36.28	36.74	37.19	37.64	38.10	38.55	39.00	39.46	39.93	40.37
90	40.82	41.27	41.73	42.18	42.63	43.09	43.54	43.99	44.45	44.90
100	45.36	45.81	46.26	46.72	47.17	47.62	48.08	48.53	48.98	49.44
110	49.89	50.34	50.80	51.25	51.71	52.16	52.61	53.07	53.52	53.97
120	54.43	54.88	55.33	55.79	56.24	56.70	57.15	57.60	58.06	58.51
130	58.96	59.42	59.87	60.32	60.78	61.23	61.68	62.14	62.59	63.05
140	63.50	63.95	64.41	64.86	65.31	65.77	66.22	66.67	67.13	67.58
150	68.04	68.49	68.94	69.40	69.85	70.30	70.76	71.21	71.66	72.12
160	72.57	73.02	73.48	73.93	74.39	74.84	75.29	75.75	76.20	76.62
170	77.11	77.56	78.01	78.47	78.92	79.38	79.83	80.28	80.74	81.19
180	81.64	82.10	82.55	83.00	83.46	83.91	84.36	84.82	85.27	85.73
190	86.18	86.68	87.09	87.54	87.99	88.45	88.90	89.35	89.81	90.26
200	90.72	91.17	91.62	92.08	92.53	92.98	93.44	93.89	94.34	94.80

Example: To determine the kilogram equivalent of 43 pounds, read 40 pounds on the vertical scale, read 3 pounds on the horizontal scale, then add. 43 pounds equals 19.5 kilograms.

APPENDIX J
COMMON NANDA DIAGNOSES FOR CHILDREN AND THEIR FAMILIES

Activity intolerance
Activity intolerance, Risk for
Adaptive capacity, Decreased intracranial
Adjustment, Impaired
Airway clearance, Ineffective
Anxiety
Anxiety, Death
Aspiration, Risk for
Body image, Disturbed
Body temperature, Risk for imbalanced
Bowel incontinence
Breastfeeding, Interrupted
Breastfeeding, Effective
Breastfeeding, Ineffective
Breathing pattern, Ineffective
Cardiac output, Decreased
Caregiver role strain
Caregiver role strain, Risk for
Communication, Impaired verbal
Confusion, Acute
Confusion, Chronic
Constipation
Constipation, Perceived
Constipation, Risk for
Coping, Community, Ineffective
Coping, Community, Readiness for enhanced
Coping, Defensive
Coping, Family, Compromised
Coping, Family, Disabled
Coping, Family, Readiness for enhanced
Coping, Ineffective
Decisional conflict (specify)
Denial, Ineffective
Dentition, Impaired
Development, Risk for delayed
Diarrhea
Disuse syndrome, Risk for
Diversional activity, Deficient
Dysreflexia, Autonomic
Dysreflexia, Autonomic, Risk for
Energy field, Disturbed
Environmental interpretation syndrome, Impaired
Failure to thrive, Adult
Family processes, Dysfunctional: Alcoholism
Family processes, Interrupted
Fatigue
Fear
Fluid volume, Deficient
Fluid volume, Excess
Fluid volume, Risk for deficient
Fluid volume, Risk for imbalanced
Gas exchange, Impaired
Grieving, Anticipatory
Grieving, Dysfunctional
Growth and development, Delayed
Growth, Risk for disproportionate
Health Maintenance, Ineffective
Health-seeking behaviors (specify)
Home Maintenance, Impaired
Hopelessness
Hyperthermia
Hypothermia
Incontinence, Functional urinary
Incontinence, Reflex urinary
Incontinence, Stress urinary
Incontinence, Total urinary
Incontinence, Urge urinary
Incontinence, Urge urinary, Risk for
Infant behavior, Disorganized
Infant behavior, Readiness for enhanced
Infant behavior, Risk for disorganized
Infant feeding pattern, Ineffective
Infection, Risk for
Injury, Perioperative positioning, Risk for
Injury, Risk for
Knowledge, Deficient
Latex allergy response
Loneliness, Risk for
Memory, Impaired
Mobility, Impaired bed
Mobility, Impaired physical
Mobility, Impaired wheelchair

Nausea
Noncompliance (specify)
Nutrition, Imbalanced: Less than body requirements
Nutrition, Imbalanced: More than body requirements
Oral mucous membrane, Impaired
Pain, Acute
Pain, Chronic
Parent/infant/child attachment, Risk for impaired
Parental role conflict
Parenting, Impaired
Parenting, Impaired, Risk for
Peripheral neurovascular dysfunction, Risk for
Personal identity, Disturbed
Poisoning, Risk for
Post-trauma syndrome
Post-trauma syndrome, Risk for
Powerlessness
Protection, Ineffective
Rape-trauma syndrome
Rape-trauma syndrome, Compound reaction
Rape-trauma syndrome, Silent reaction
Relocation stress syndrome
Role performance, Ineffective
Self-care deficit, Bathing/hygiene
Self-care deficit, Dressing/grooming
Self-care deficit, Feeding
Self-care deficit, Toileting
Self-esteem, Low, Chronic
Self-esteem, Low, Situational
Self-mutilation, Risk for
Sensory perception, Disturbed (specify)
(Visual, auditory, kinesthetic, gustatory, tactile, olfactory)
Sexual Dysfunction
Sexuality Patterns, Ineffective
Skin Integrity, Impaired
Skin Integrity, Impaired, Risk for
Sleep deprivation
Sleep pattern, Disturbed
Social interaction, Impaired
Social isolation
Sorrow, Chronic
Spiritual distress, Risk for
Spiritual well-being, Readiness for enhanced
Suffocation, Risk for
Surgical recovery, Delayed
Swallowing, Impaired
Therapeutic regimen management, Effective
Therapeutic regimen management, Ineffective
Therapeutic regimen management, Ineffective community
Therapeutic regimen management, Ineffective family
Thermoregulation, Ineffective
Thought process, Disturbed
Tissue Integrity, Impaired
Tissue perfusion, Ineffective (specify type)
(Renal, cerebral, cardiopulmonary, gastrointestinal, peripheral)
Trauma, Risk for
Unilateral neglect
Urinary elimination, Impaired
Urinary retention
Ventilation, Impaired spontaneous
Ventilatory weaning response, Dysfunctional
Violence, Risk for other-directed
Violence, Risk for self-directed
Walking, Impaired
Wheelchair, Transfer Ability, Impaired

Source: North American Nursing Diagnosis Association. (2001). *Nursing Diagnoses: Definitions and Classification, 2001–2002*. Philadelphia, PA: Author.

APPENDIX K
ABBREVIATIONS

AA	Alcoholics Anonymous
AACAP	American Academy of Child and Adolescent Psychiatry
AAFP	American Academy of Family Physicians
AAMR	American Association of Mental Retardation
AAP	American Academy of Pediatrics
ABG	arterial blood gas
ACCH	Association for the Care of Children's Health
ACE	angiotensin-converting enzyme
ACHA	American College Health Association
ACIP	Advisory Committee on Immunization Practices
ACTH	adrenocorticotropic hormone
AD	atopic dermatitis
ADD	attention deficit disorder
ADH	antidiuretic hormone
ADHD	attention deficit/hyperactivity disorder
ADL	activities of daily living
AFDC	Aid for Families with Dependent Children
AGA	appropriate for gestational age
AGN	acute glomerulonephritis
AGS	adolescent growth spurt
AHA	American Heart Association
AIDS	acquired immune deficiency syndrome
AN	anorexia nervosa
ANA	American Nurses Association
ANA	antinuclear antibody
AOM	acute otitis media
APA	American Psychiatric Association
APPT	Adolescent and Pediatric Pain Tool
APSGN	acute poststreptococcal glomerulonephritis
ARDS	acute (or adult) respiratory distress syndrome
ARF	acute renal failure
ARF	acute rheumatic fever
AS	aortic stenosis
ASD	atrial septal defect
ASHA	American School Health Association
ASHA	American Speech-Language-Hearing Association
ASL	American Sign Language
ASO	antistreptolysin O
ATG	antithymocyte antibodies
A-V or AV	atrioventricular, arteriovenous
AVC	artrioventricular canal
AZT	Zidovudine, also known as ZDV
BAER	Brainstem Auditory Evoked Response
BIA	Brain Injury Association
BID	twice a day (Latin *bis in die*)
BLL	blood lead level
BMI	body mass index
BMR	basal metabolic rate
BN	bulimia nervosa
BP	blood pressure
BPD	bronchopulmonary dysplasia
BRAT diet	bananas, rice, applesauce, and toast or tea
BSE	breast self-examination
BSL	British Sign Language
BT shunt	Blalock-Taussig shunt
BUN	blood urea nitrogen
CARS	Childhood Autism Rating Scale
CAV	continuous arteriovenous
CBC	complete blood cell count
CBT	cognitive behavioral therapy
CCSC	Children's Coping Strategies Checklist
CD	Crohn's disease
CDC	U.S. Centers for Disease Control and Prevention
CDH	congenital diaphragmatic hernia
CF	cystic fibrosis
CFT	capillary filling time
CFU	colony forming units
CHB	complete heart block
CHD	congenital heart defect
CHF	congestive heart failure
CI	confidence interval
CIC	clean intermittent catheterization
CK	creatine kinase
CL	cleft lip
CMS	U.S. Centers for Medicare & Medicaid Services
CMV	cytomegalovirus
CN	cranial nerve
CNS	central nervous system
CO	cardiac output
COA	coarctation of the aorta

CP	cerebral palsy
CP	cleft palate
CPB	cardiopulmonary bypass
CPS	Child Protective Service
CPT	chest physiotherapy
CRF	chronic renal failure
CRP	C-reactive protein
CSF	cerebrospinal fluid
CSHCN	Children with Special Health Care Needs (Title V program)
CT	computerized tomography
CVA	cerebral vascular accident
CVP	central venous pressure
CXR	chest radiograph
d4T	Stavudine, also known as Zerit
DASE	Denver Articulation Screening Examinations
dB	decibel
DD	dysthymic disorder
ddC	Zalcitabine, also known as Hivid
DDH	developmental dysplasia of the hip
ddI	Didanosine, also known as Videx
DDAVP	desmopressin acetate
DDST	Denver Developmental Screening Test
DEET	diethyltoluamide
DEST	Denver Eye Screening Test
DHHS	U.S. Department of Health and Human Services
DIC	disseminated intravascular coagulopathy
DIT	Defining Issues Test
dl	deciliter
DMD	Duchenne muscular dystrophy
DMG	dimethylglycine
DNA	deoxyribonucleic acid
DRG	diagnosis-related group
DS	Down syndrome
DSM-IV	*Diagnostic and Statistical Manual of Mental Disorders*, Fourth Edition
DTaP	diphtheria, tetanus toxoid, and acellular pertussis vaccine
DTP	diphtheria, tetanus toxoid, pertussis
DTwP	DT with whole-cell pertussis
DWI	driving while intoxicated
EA	esophageal atresia
EBV	Epstein-Barr virus
ECF	extracellular fluid
ECHO	echocardiogram
ECI	early childhood intervention
ED	emergency department
EIA	enzyme immunoassay
EKG	electrocardiogram
ELISA	enzyme linked immunosorbent assay
ELM	Early Language Milestone Scale
EMG	electromyogram
EMLA	eutectic mixture of local anesthetics
EMS	emergency medical service
EPA	U.S. Environmental Protection Agency
EPSDT	early and periodic screening, diagnosis, and treatment
ESR	erythrocyte sedimentation rate
ESRF	endstage renal failure
ESSR	"enlarge, stimulate, swallow, rest"
ET	enterostomal therapist
ETT	endotracheal tube
FA	Fanconi's anemia
FAS	fetal alcohol syndrome
FDA	U.S. Food and Drug Administration
FFT	failure to thrive
FSH	follicle-stimulating hormone
GABHS	group A beta-hemolytic streptococci
GAD	generalized anxiety disorder
GER	gastroesophageal reflux
GFR	glomerular filtration rate
GH	growth hormone
GHT	gentle human touch
GI	gastrointestinal
GPA	grade point average
HAART	highly active antiretroviral therapy
HAV	hepatitis A virus
Hb A	adult hemoglobin
Hb F	fetal hemoglobin
Hb S	sickle hemoglobin (hemoglobin S)
HBV	hepatitis B virus
HCV	hepatitis C virus
HCFA	U.S. Health Care Financing Administration
HCG	human chorionic gonadotropin
HCl	hydrochloric acid
Hct	hematocrit
HD	Hirschprung's disease
HDL	high-density lipoprotein
hep B	hepatitis B vaccine
H-flu	*Haemophilus influenzae*
HIB (Hib)	*Haemophilus influenzae* type B
HIV	human immunodeficiency virus
HLHS	hypoplastic left heart syndrome
HMO	health maintenance organization
HP	Healthy People [2010]
HPS	hypertrophic pyloric stenosis
HPV	human papilloma virus
HR	heart rate
HSV-1	herpes simplex virus type I
HUD	U.S. Department of Housing and Urban Development
HUS	hemolytic uremic syndrome
Hz	hertz

IBD inflammatory bowel disease
ICF intracellular fluid
ICU intensive care unit
IDEA Individuals with Disabilities Education Act
IE infective endocarditis
IEP Individualized Educational Plan
IFSP Individual Family Service Plan
IgA immunoglobulin A
IgE immunoglobulin E
IgD immunoglobulin D
IgG immunoglobulin G
IgM immunoglobulin M
IHP Individual Health Plan
IM intramuscular
IMR infant mortality rate
INR international normalized ratio
IPV inactivated polio vaccine
IQ intelligence quotient
IRB institutional review board
ITP immune thrombocytopenic purpura
IV intravenous
IVIG intravenous immune globulin
IVP intravenous pyelogram
JA juvenile arthritis
JCA juvenile chronic arthritis
JRA juvenile rheumatoid arthritis
KD Kawasaki disease
KOH potassium hydroxide
LA left atrium
LBW low birth weight
LGMD Limb-Girdle muscular dystrophy
LCP Legg-Calve-Perthes disease
LDL low-density lipoprotein
LES lower esophageal sphincter
LGA large for gestational age
LH luteinizing hormone
LIP lymphoid interstitial pneumonia
LPD lymphoproliferative disease
LSD lysergic acid diethylamide
LTB laryngotroacheobronchitis
LV left ventricle
MCHC mean corpuscular hemoglobin concentration
MCV mean corpuscular volume
MD muscular dystrophy
MDD major depressive disorder
MDI metered dose inhaler
MDMA methylenedioxymethamphetamine
MHC mean corpuscular hemoglobin
ml milliliter
MMPI Minnesota Multiphasic Personality Inventory
MMR measles, mumps, rubella
MMWR *Morbidity and Mortality Weekly Report*
MR mental retardation
MRI magnetic resonance imaging
NA Narcotics Anonymous
NASN National Association of School Nurses
NCPCA National Committee to Prevent Child Abuse
NCV nerve conduction velocity
NEC necrotizing enterocolitis
NG nasogastric
NHANES National Health and Nutrition Examination Survey
NIAID National Institute of Allergy and Infectious Disease
NICHCY National Information Center for Children and Youth with Disabilities
NICU neonatal intensive care unit
NIS-3 Third National Incidence Study of Child Abuse and Neglect
NJ nasojejunal
NMDA N-methyl-D-aspartate
NMPMC nursing mutual participation model of care
NRTI nucleoside reverse transcriptase inhibitor
NNRTI non-nucleoside reverse transcriptase inhibitors
NOFTT non-organic failure to thrive
NPA National Pediculosis Association
NPO nothing by mouth
NS neophrotic syndrome
NS normal saline
NSAIDs nonsteroidal anti-inflammatory drugs
NVS neurovascular status
OAE otoacoustic emission test
OASPE Office of the Assistant Secretary for Planning and Evaluation
OFFT organic failure to thrive
OI osteogenesis imperfecta
OM otitis media
OME otitis media with effusion
OPV oral polio vaccine
ORS oral rehydration solution
ORT oral rehydration therapy
OSHA U.S. Occupational Safety and Health Administration
PA pulmonary artery
PCA patient-controlled analgesia
PCC Poison Control Center
PCR polymerase chain reaction
PDA patent ductus arteriosus
PERF peak expiratory flow rates
PFO patent foramen ovale
PGE prostaglandin E
PHV peak height velocity
PI protease inhibitor
PICU pediatric intensive care unit

PKU	phenylketonuria
PL	prolactin
PPD	purified protein derivative
PPI	parent-present induction
PPO	preferred provider organization
PQRST	mnemonic device for pain assessment format
PR	by rectum
prn (PRN)	as needed (pro re nata)
PS	pulmonary stenosis
PT	prothrombin time, also known as INR
PTSD	post-traumatic stress disorder
PTT	partial thromboplastin time
PVR	pulmonary vascular resistance
Q	every (quid)
QD	every day (quaque die)
RA	right atrium
RAPS	recurrent abdominal pain syndrome
RDA	recommended daily allowance
RDS	respiratory distress syndrome
REM	rapid eye movement
RF	rheumatoid factor
RICE	rest, ice, compression, elevation
RL	Ringer's lactate
RLQ	right lower quadrant
ROP	retinopathy of prematurity
RR	respiratory rate
RSV	respiratory syncytial virus
RSV-IGIV	RSV immune globulin intravenous (RespiGam)
RV	right ventricle
SA	sinoatrial
SAARDs	slow-acting anti-rheumatic drugs
SAD	separation anxiety disorder
SaO_2	oxygen saturation
SBHC	school-based health center
SBS	shaken baby syndrome
SC	subcutaneous
SCA	sickle cell anemia
SCFE	slipped capital femoral epiphysis
SCHIP	State Children's Health Insurance Program
SCT	sickle cell trait
SEE	Signed Exact English
SGA	small for gestational age
SIDS	sudden infant death syndrome
SLE	systemic lupus erythematosus
SLHC	school-linked health center
SPF	sun protection factor
SSI	Supplemental Security Income
SSRI	selective serotonin reuptake inhibitor
STAIC	State-Trait Anxiety Inventory for Children
STD	sexually transmitted disease
SUD	substance use disorder
SV	stroke volume
SVR	systemic vascular resistance
SVT	supraventricular tachycardia
TA	truncus arteriosus
TAC	tetracaine, adrenoline, cocaine
TB	tuberculosis
Td	tetanus and diphtheria
TEACCH	Treatment and Education of Autistic and Communication Handicapped Children
TEF	tracheoesophageal fistula
TEN	toxic epidermal necrolysis
TENS	transcutaneous electrical nerve stimulation
TGA	transposition of the great arteries
3TC	Lamivudine, also known as Epivir
TIBC	total iron binding capacity
TM	tympanic membrane
TOF	tetralogy of Fallot
TORCH	toxoplasmosis, other (e.g., hepatis), rubella, cytomegalovirus, and herpes simplex
TPN	total parenteral nutrition
TSH	thyroid-stimulating hormone
UA	urinalysis
UAP	unlicensed assistive personnel
UC	ulcerative colitis
UDT	undescended testis, also known as cryptorchidism
UGI	upper gastrointestinal
URI	upper respiratory infection
Urine C&S	urine culture with sensitivity
UTI	urinary tract infection
UV	ultraviolet
UVA	ultraviolet A
UVB	ultraviolet B
VCUG	voiding cystourethrogram
VLBW	very low birth weight
VSD	ventricular septal defect
VUR	vesicoureteral reflux
vWF	von Willebrand's factor
WBC	white blood cell count
WIC	Women, Infants, and Children
WPPSI	Wechsler Preschool and Primary Scale of Intelligence
WPPSI-R	Wechsler Preschool and Primary Scale of Intelligence–Revised
ZDV	Zidovudine, also known as AZT
ZPD	zone of proximal development

GLOSSARY

absence seizures—Characterized by a transient loss of consciousness that may appear as cessation of current activity; a type of generalized seizure.

absorption—Process whereby a drug moves from site of administration into the bloodstream.

acceptance—When the griever is consciously aware of what has happened or what is most likely to occur. Kubler-Ross' fifth stage of grief.

accessory muscles—Muscles used to increase ventilation in individuals with labored breathing. Accessory muscles may include muscles in the neck, back, and abdomen.

accommodation—Modification of behavior and mental structures as a result of new experiences; the process of modifying existing schema to adapt to or incorporate new experiences, Piagetian term; the ability of the eye to focus clearly on objects at all distances.

acidosis—An acid-base imbalance indicated by a blood pH below 7.35.

acoustic feedback—A whistling sound in a hearing aid caused by improper fit into ear or too high a volume.

acquired immunity—Long term protection against a new infection that forms in response to exposure to antigens in nature or vaccines.

acrocyanosis—A condition characterized by blue discoloration, coldness, and sweating of the extremities, especially the hands.

acromion process—The lateral extension of the spine of the scapula, forming the highest point of the shoulder and connecting with the clavicle at a small oval surface in the middle of the spine. It gives attachment to the deltoideus and trapezius muscles.

active euthanasia—Giving a treatment that will directly and intentionally result in the death of a person.

acute pain—Pain generally lasting 3 to 5 days and attributed to a specific injury or cause.

adaptive immune system—Produces a specific reaction to infectious agents, remembers that agent, and prevents a later infection by the same agent.

addiction—Psychological and physiological need to use a medication for nonprescribed purposes.

A-delta nerve fibers—Mylineated nerve fibers that fire rapidly.

adolescence—The time of life that begins with puberty and ends when the individual is physically and psychologically mature and able to assume adult responsibilities.

adolescent growth spurt (AGS)—Rapid acceleration in weight and height gain; lasts about 4.5 years.

adrenarche—Pubic hair development.

advocate—Nursing role involved in pleading causes for and assisting others in making informed decisions in the child and family's best interest.

affective learning—One type of learning related to feelings and emotions.

age of majority—The age, determined by state law, at which a person is considered to have all the legal rights and responsibilities of an adult.

AIDS—A term used when the immune system has become compromised enough to allow advanced HIV disease to occur.

akinetic seizures—Total lack of movement; child appears frozen in a position.

alkalosis—An acid-base imbalance indicated by a blood pH above 7.45.

allergen—Antigen responsible for clinical manifestations of allergy.

alopecia—Hair loss.

alopecia areata—The sudden onset of asymptomatic, noninflammatory, round bald patches. Traumatic alopecia, bald patches created by traction from braids, pony tails, corn rows.

amblyopia ("lazy eye")—A reduction of vision in one eye. The most common cause is strabismus; the brain suppresses the vision in the deviated eye to avoid the double image that it is receiving.

amniocentesis—The drawing out of a portion of amniotic fluid with a long aspirating needle for the purposes of direct examination, chemical testing, and cell culture.

anal stage—Anal activities become primary ways of gratifying the sexual instinct; Freud's second stage of psychosexual development.

analgesia—Pain control using medication or other interventions for relief.

anaphylaxis—An acute, life-threatening reaction to an antigen.

anastomosis—The surgical joining of two ducts, blood vessels, or bowel segments to allow flow from one to the other.

ancephaly—Absence of cranial vault with cerebral hemispheres either completely missing or greatly reduced in size.

anemia—Decrease in the hemoglobin content of the blood due to underlying disease or injury.

anencephaly—Congenital absence of major portions of the brain and malformation of the brainstem.

anergy—The inability to respond to infectious challenges.

anger—Feeling of rage, envy, and resentment. Kubler-Ross' second stage of grief.

angioedema—Swelling of the skin, subcutaneous, or submucosal tissue.

anhedonia—Markedly diminished interest or pleasure in previously enjoyed activities.

animism—Belief that inanimate objects have human qualities.

aniridia—A congenital absence of the iris.

anorexia nervosa—A potentially life-threatening disorder characterized by voluntary refusal to eat and significant weight loss.

anthracycline—Chemotherapeutic agent known to cause cardiac toxicity.

anthropometric measurements—The science of measuring the human body as to height, weight, and size of component parts, including skinfolds, to study and compare the relative proportions under normal and abnormal conditions.

antigen—A foreign substance capable of stimulating an immune response.

anuric—Without urine output.

anxiety—A subjective feeling of apprehension or uneasiness caused by uncertain, nonspecific danger or threat.

aplastic anemia—A condition in which the bone marrow fails to produce adequate numbers of erythrocytes, leukocytes, and platelets because of injury to or abnormal expression of the stem cells.

aplastic crisis—A type of sickle cell crisis characterized by a decrease in erythropoiesis.

apocrine glands—Sweat glands concentrated in the axillae, scalp, face, abdomen, and genital area.

aqueduct of Sylvius—Canal between the third and fourth ventricle through which CSF flows.

aqueductal stenosis—Stenosis of the aqueduct of Silvius; a cause of hydrocephalus.

arachnoid mater—The second meningeal membrane under which the cerebrospinal fluid flows.

Arnold-Chiari malformation (ACM) —A brain defect in the posterior fossa that allows herniation of the cerebellum, medulla, pons, and fourth ventricle into the cervical spinal canal.

arrhythmia—Abnormal heart rhythm, caused by electrical abnormalities of the heart.

art therapy—Drawings and other art objects are used to help the therapist gain information about the child, her or his behaviors, concerns, and problems.

arteriovenous malformation—A web-like tangle of vessels providing a network between the cerebral arteries and veins.

assault—An unlawful, sudden, violent attack on another person; rape is considered a type of assault.

assent—When a child is explained the process of a procedure or treatment and agrees to cooperate with it.

assimilation—Incorporating new experiences into existing mental structures; Piagetian term.

astatic-akinetic seizures (see atonic seizures).

astigmatism—Blurry vision caused by abnormal curvature of the cornea or the lens.

atelectasis—Collapse of lung tissue.

atlantoaxial deformity—A spinal deformity resulting in instability of the upper cervical spine (associated with Down syndrome).

atonic seizures—Drop attacks; sudden loss of muscle tone with the head dropping forward for a few seconds.

atopy—A heredity predisposition to develop allergic disease.

atraumatic care—A philosophy of providing therapeutic care through the use of interventions that eliminate or minimize the psychological and physical distress experienced by children and families during hospitalization.

atresia—Complete occlusion of or lack of normal opening in a body part.

atrial septostomy—A procedure to enlarge the patent foramen ovale or to create an atrial septal defect. This allows mixing of blood at the atrial level.

attachment—Reciprocal, enduring, emotional and physical affiliation behaviors between a child and a caregiver.

attention deficit hyperactive disorder (ADHD)—The presence of impaired social interaction; impaired communication, and restricted repetitive and stereotyped patterns of behavior, interests, and activities.

aura—A somatic, sensory, or psychic warning that a seizure will occur; premonition, usually lights or sounds, experienced prior to the onset of a migraine headache.

authority and social order maintaining orientation—Laws should be obeyed because they are the laws; Kohlberg's fourth stage of moral development.

autism—A genetic developmental disorder, characterized by extreme difficulty communicating with and relating to

the environment; manifested by bizarre behavior, delayed language acquisition, poor social relations, impairment of self-care skills, and altered sensory responses.
autogenous—Originating from within one's own body.
autograft—A permanent skin graft that requires transferring the child's own skin to cover the burned areas.
autoimmunity—An inability of the body to distinguish self from nonself, causing the immune system to respond against itself.
autoinoculation—Transfer of infection from one site to another on the same individual.
automatisms—Repeated nonpurposeful actions.
autonomy—The right of the client to freedom and self-determination.
autonomy versus shame and doubt—Psychosocial conflict where toddlers demonstrate independence and learn competencies related to self-care; Erikson's second stage of psychosocial development.
autopsy—Surgical and chemical analysis of the body to determine the cause of death.
average for gestational age (AGA)—Newborn lies between the 10th and 90th percentile of weight for gestational age.
avulsion—The tearing away of tissue either accidentally or surgically.
B lymphocytes—Lymphocytes produced in the bone marrow; differentiate into producers of one of five major classes of immunoglobulins
bacteremia—Bacteria in the blood.
bacteriuria—The presence of bacteria in the urine.
bad touch—Any physical contact in which the child is told "not to tell anyone."
bargaining—Attempt to postpone the occurrence of the event, by "making a deal." Kubler-Ross's third stage of grief.
barotrauma—Physical injury sustained as a result of exposure to increased environmental air pressure.
behavioral perspective—Posits that human actions and interactions come from learned responses to environmental stimuli.
behavioral therapy—Behavioral modification that uses stimulus and response to alter inappropriate behaviors. Appropriate behavior is reinforced while inappropriate behavior is extinguished and replaced with a more desirable one.
beneficence—Doing good for and to others.
bereavement—The process of mourning; an adaptation to a loss. The behavior one exhibits after a loss.
beta-thalassemia major (Cooley's anemia)—A type of thalassemia characterized by impaired beta hemoglobin synthesis that is associated with a life-threatening form of anemia.
bifid—Split into two parts.
binocularity—Fixation of two ocular images into one cerebral picture.
bioavailability—The proportion or fraction of an administered drug that reaches general circulation and is available at site of action.
bioethics—The application of moral reasoning to the life sciences, medicine, nursing, and health care.
biologic response modifiers (BRMs)—Agents and therapies used to stimulate the body's immune system to destroy cancerous cells.
biotransformation (metabolism)—Transformation or alteration of chemical structures from their original form.
blind—Vision allows only light perception; other senses are relied upon as a chief means of learning.
blindisms—Movements or behaviors that are repetitive and not purposeful, such as body rocking, eye rubbing, and head shaking. Used by blind children to compensate for inadequate stimulation.
body image—A mental conception of one's physical appearance.
bone age—Calculation of skeletal maturation utilizing an X ray of the hand and wrist or knee.
bone marrow transplantation—Replacement of hematopoietic stem cells into a person whose own bone marrow has been destroyed by disease or treatment for a malignant disease.
bottle-mouth caries (see nursing caries)
bradyarrhythmia—Abnormally slow heart rhythm.
brain death—An irreversible form of unconsciousness characterized by complete loss of brain function while the heart continues to beat.
brain stem—Area of the brain that is below the cerebellum; controls the vital centers.
bronchiectasis—A lung condition characterized by irreversible dilation and destruction of the bronchial walls.
brown fat—Increases cellular metabolic rates and oxygen consumption, resulting in heat; found primarily in the subscapular, axillary, adrenal, and mediastinal regions.
Brudzinski's sign—Sign of meningeal irritation; when child is supine, will automatically flex hips and knees if head is flexed forward.
buffer—A substance that either releases or absorbs hydrogen ions in order to maintain a stable blood pH.
bulimia nervosa—Characterized by episodes of binge eating followed by various methods purging to control weight gain.
BUN—The concentration of urea, an end-product of protein metabolism, formed in the liver and excreted by the kidney (as measured by blood urea nitrogen).
buphthalmos—Enlargement of the eyeball.

callus—Osseous material woven between the ends of a fractured bone that is ultimately replaced by new bone.
cancer—Group of diseases in which there is out-of-control growth and malignant cells.
candidiasis—Yeast infection caused by Candida species.
cao gao—Practiced by Southeast Asians; involves rubbing a coin or a spoon heated in oil on an ill child's neck, spine, and ribs; may create a burn or abrasion.
caput succedaneum—A localized pitting edema in the scalp of a fetus that may overlie sutures of the skull. It is usually formed during labor as a result of the circular pressure of the cervix on the fetal occiput.
cardiomegaly—Enlarged heart.
cardiomyopathy—Primary disease of the heart muscle caused by a multitude of etiologies (familial, infectious, ischemic) that results in poor pump function. There are three types: dilated, hypertrophic, and restrictive.
cardioversion—A process whereby an abnormal heart rhythm is converted to normal sinus rhythm. This can be accomplished by electrical cardioversion via a defibrillator, or by medication.
carditis—Inflammation of the heart.
caregiver—Nursing role involved in delivering direct nursing care to children and their families that is based on the nursing process; also a parent, guardian, or other person responsible for the child.
caregiver burden—The effect of the challenges and demands of caring for a child with a chronic condition.
care theory—A major theoretical orientation that bases ethical decision making on the individual's needs or concerns.
carriers—Persons who can harbor and spread the organism to others without becoming ill.
case management—A practice model initially developed to minimize fragmentation of services and maximize individualization of care by using a systematic approach ensuring optimal client outcomes.
cataract—Opacity (clouding) of the crystalline lens of the eye.
"catch-up" growth—A rate of growth greater than the expected rate for age.
cat's eye reflex—A whitish glow in the pupil, a sign of retinoblastoma.
causality—One of the four components of the concept of death according to Corr and Corr. The notion that death has an internal and external cause, which can be natural/unnatural or good/evil.
cavernous sinus thrombosis—A syndrome caused by an infection of the eye that results in venous congestion of the eye and paralysis of the extraocular muscles.
ceiling dose—Maximum dose of a medication thought to be effective; increasing the dose beyond this point will not increase the effectiveness.
cell mediated system—T cells; they specifically recognize antigens and interact with the B cells and other components of the innate system to inactivate the immune challenge.
cellular elements—The erythrocytes or red blood cells, the leukocytes or white blood cells, and the thrombocytes or platelets.
central hearing loss—Damage that interrupts sound transmission between the brainstem and the cerebral cortex.
cephalhematoma—Swelling caused by subcutaneous bleeding and accumulation of blood. It may begin to form in the scalp of a fetus during labor and enlarge slowly in the first few days after birth; subperiosteal bleeding over a cranial bone that is due to ruptured blood vessels from a traumatic delivery. The swelling does not cross suture lines.
cephalocaudal—Principle that growth proceeds from the head downward.
cerebellum—Found in the posterior fossa, controls motor coordination, posture, and equilibrium.
cerebral edema—An increase in intracellular fluid in the brain.
cerebral palsy (CP)—Nonprogressive motor dysfunction caused by damage in the motor areas of the brain.
cerebrum—Largest area of the brain that controls thinking, speech, vision, and hearing.
channel—The medium through which a message is transmitted; it may be visual, auditory, or kinesthetic.
chelating agent—A drug used to either prevent or reverse the toxic effects of a heavy metal or to accelerate the elimination of the metal from the body.
child abandonment—Caregiver's intentional withholding from a child, without just cause or excuse, the caregiver's care, presence, love, protection, maintenance, and opportunity for displaying affection for a child.
child abuse—A range of intentional behaviors by a parent or caregiver that can include neglect, physical, emotional, or sexual abuse.
child life program—An organized program conducted by child life staff in health care settings that are designed to promote optimum development of children and their families, to maintain normal living patterns, and to minimize psychological trauma (Child Life Council, [1995]. *Child Life Position Statement.* Rockville, MD: Author.)
child life staff—Specialists with expertise in child growth and development who provide children with opportunities in gaining a sense of mastery, for play, for learning, for self-expression, for family involvement, and for peer interaction.
child maltreatment—The intentional injury of a child.
child molestation—Sexual involvement (oral-genital contact, genital fondling and viewing, masturbation) involving a child.

child neglect—Caregiver inattention to the child's basic need for care, protection, or control, which results in the child experiencing serious injury or impairment.

chloromas—Localized collections of malignant cells.

choanal atresia—A congenital anomaly in which a bony or membraneous occlusion blocks the passageway between the nose and pharynx.

cholestasis—Interruption in the flow of bile.

chordee—Downward curvature of the penis.

chorea—Abnormal uncontrollable, involuntary, purposeless movements of extremities and the trunk.

chorionic villus sampling—A procedure for obtaining prenatal evaluation data in early pregnancy by withdrawing a chorionic villi sample from fetal membranes.

choroid plexus—Area within the ventricle that secretes cerebrospinal fluid.

chronic (cyclic) sorrow—Cyclical, never-ending grief response of caregivers of children with chronic conditions. Occurs at somewhat predictable times in the child's and family's life.

chronic condition—A physical, psychological, or cognitive condition that places limitations on day-to-day functioning or requires reliance on special treatments and is expected to last for at least several months.

chronic pain—Pain lasting for long periods of time or coming and going frequently over long periods of time.

Chvostek's sign—Twitching of the facial muscles after gently tapping over the facial nerves near the parotid gland.

circumcision—The surgical removal of the foreskin, the skin that covers the glans or head, of the penis.

classical conditioning—Learning occurs when a response that is already part of the organism's normal activities can be reproduced by an associated stimulus that previously would not have produced it.

classification—The ability to group items according to common characteristics.

clinical cure—Resolution of signs and symptoms of infection.

clinical nurse specialist—Usually a nurse with a master's degree who provides expert physical, social, and psychological support and care; consults with nursing staff and other health care personnel; educates clients and families in health care management; conducts practice outcome research; and serves as a role model for staff.

clinical pathways—Plans of care designed to achieve specific client outcomes in a defined time frame.

clinical trials—Carefully designed investigation of drug effects on human subjects.

cliques—Three to nine "buddies" or "mates" who exhibit a strong sense of cohesion.

closed adoption—An adoption where there is no contact between the birth and adoptive parents.

closed reduction—The alignment of the bone by manual manipulation or traction.

C-nerve fibers—Slow conducting, unmyelinated nerve fibers.

cognitive ability—The capacity to understand and then use phenomena in the world around us.

cognitive learning—One type of learning where describing or explaining something or answering questions occurs.

colic—Recurrent episodes of unexplained crying and inability to be consoled occurring in infant less then 3 months of age.

collaborative—Mutual sharing and working together to achieve common goals in such a way that all persons or groups are recognized and growth is enhanced.

collateral—Extra vessels that are formed to supply blood if the normal vessels are stenotic or absent.

color blindess—Color deficiency or color vision deficit.

coma—The most severe form of depressed consciousness; no response to intense painful stimuli.

comedone—Lesions associated with noninflammatory acne. Lesions may be closed (whiteheads) or open (blackheads).

commensal fungi—Fungi living on or within another organism and deriving benefit without causing harm or benefit to the host.

communicable diseases—Infectious illnesses that exhibit the potential to spread through the community.

communicating hydrocephalus—Hydrocephalus caused by an obstruction outside the ventricular system leading to decreased absorption of cerebrospinal fluid in the subarachnoid space.

communication—The process of creating common or shared meaning.

community health nursing—A synthesis of nursing and public health practice directed toward promoting, restoring, and preserving the health of a community or a total population.

compartment syndrome—Condition caused by increased pressure within a compartment, leading to impairment of circulation.

compensation—Body process used to restore blood pH to normal by changing the partial pressure of carbon dioxide (pCO_2) or the bicarbonic ion concentration.

complement—Twenty different proteins that when activated by an antigen-antibody contact respond, amplify, and "complement" antibody activity.

complex partial seizures—Partial psychomotor or temporal lobe episodes.

concrete operations—The mental ability to group objects, actions, and events.

concrete operations stage—Acquisition of logical operations and effective reasoning skills; Piaget's third stage of cognitive development; ages 7–11.

conductive hearing loss—A temporary or permanent hearing deficit that occurs when something (such as fluid) affects the progress of sound into the ear canal or across the middle ear system.

confusion—A form of depressed consciousness; although alert, disoriented to time, place, and person; unable to answer simple questions.

conjunctivitis ("pink eye")—An inflammation of the conjunctiva.

conscious sedation—Administration of central nervous system depressant drugs and/or analgesics which allows a child to be both pain-free and also sedated for a procedure.

conservation—The ability to acknowledge that a change in shape does not mean a change in amount.

consolidation phase—Second phase of leukemia therapy that aims at eradicating any residual leukemic cells.

contact burns—Burns that are the result of certain implements such as curling irons, steam irons, cigarette lighters, matches, hot pots, space heaters, or radiators.

contact dermatitis—Delayed hypersensitivity; occurs when an antigen is applied directly to the skin.

context specificity—Suggests there are differences in children related to cultural values, beliefs, and experiences.

continuity—Developmental change is orderly and built upon earlier experiences; a gradual and smooth process without abrupt shifts.

contusion—An injury resulting in damage to soft tissues, subcutaneous structures, small vessels, and muscles without disrupting the skin.

conventional level—According to Kohlberg's theory of moral development, the school-aged child is at the conventional level of moral development. During this level the child's conscience develops an internal set of "rules" that must be followed in order to "be good."

conventional morality—Societal values are internalized; moral judgments are based on a desire to uphold the law and social order or gain approval; Kohlberg's third level of moral development.

coordination of secondary schemes phase—Infant understands concepts of space and object permanence, learns to direct actions toward an intended goal, and anticipates actions of others; Piaget's fourth phase of cognitive development.

cor pulmonale—Right-sided heart failure caused by pulmonary disease.

corporal punishment—Physical restraint or infliction of pain to the body by a person in authority.

crackles—An adventitious lung sound caused when air passes over airway secretions or collapsed airways are suddenly opened.

cradle cap (seborrhea)—A dry, scaly scalp condition.

cranioschisis—Defect in the skull through which neural tissue protrudes.

craniosynostosis—Premature ossification and closing of the sutures of the skull, often associated with other skeletal defects.

craniotabes—Benign congenital thinness of the top and back of the skull of a newborn.

crawling—Pulling self forward with abdomen on the floor.

creeping—Moving on hands and knees with abdomen off floor.

cremasteric reflex—A superficial neural reflex elicited by stroking the skin of the upper thigh in a male. This action results in a brisk retraction of the testis on the side of the stimulus.

crepitus—Grating sound heard on movement of the ends of a broken bone.

cretinism—Stunted physical growth and severe mental retardation caused by untreated thyroid deficiency.

critical period—A limited time span when a child is biologically prepared to acquire certain behaviors, but needs the support of a suitably stimulating environment.

crowd—An association of two to four cliques in which relations are less intimate than in the smaller groups.

cruising—Walking sideways while holding onto furniture for support.

cryptorchidism—A developmental defect characterized by failure of one or both of the testicles to descend into the scrotum. They are retained in the abdomen or inguinal canal.

crystalluria—Crystals in the urine that may be a source of urinary irritation.

cultural relativism—Differences in children are related to cultural values, beliefs, and experiences.

cultural sensitivity—Having an awareness and appreciation of cultural influences in health care and being respectful of differences in cultural belief systems and values.

cultured epithelial autograft—Sheets of skin grown in the lab from a small skin biopsy of the client; this is a permanent skin graft that is used in children with burns covering 80% of their body.

cupping (ventosos)—Practiced by Latin American and Russian cultures; occurs by creating a vacuum under a cup or glass when a small amount of burning material is placed on the skin.

cystitis—Inflammation of the bladder with symptoms including urinary frequency and dysuria, often accompanied by urgency and tenesmus.

cystogram—Radiograph of the bladder that examines the bladder, urethra, and ureters.

cytokines—Substances secreted by cells participating in the immune response.

cytoreduction—Conditioning regimen for bone marrow transplant in which lethal doses of chemotherapy, often combined with radiation, are used to eradicate all malignant cells and to suppress the child's immune system to prevent rejection of the transplanted marrow.

cytotoxic/killer T lymphocytes—Lymphocytes that attack infected or pathogenic cells.

dacrocystitis—An infection of the lacrimal sac caused by obstruction of the nasolacrimal duct, characterized by tearing and discharge from the eye.

Dandy-Walker syndrome—An obstruction in the foramina of Luschka and Magendie causing hydrocephalus.

date or acquaintance rape—Sexual intercourse with force or threat of force where the victim and perpetrator know one another either socially or professionally.

dating scripts—What is expected of dating partners.

debridement—Removal of dead skin tissue from a burn site.

decerebrate—Rigid extensor posturing secondary to trauma to the midbrain or pons; associated with poor prognosis.

deciduous teeth—The first 20 teeth to develop and erupt in a child; also referred to as primary or baby teeth.

decontamination—Decreasing absorption of an ingested poison from the GI tract.

decorticate—Flexor posturing; associated with bilateral cerebral hemisphere injury.

deficit-orientation model—Views of chronic conditions that depict them as pathological states with major negative consequences in most, if not all, aspects of life.

delayed hypersensitivity—A cellular reaction involving T cells and macrophages; there is a longer duration between exposure and reaction.

delayed primary closure—Wound closure performed 3–5 days after the injury.

delirium—Condition where anxiety, fear, and agitation are seen.

denial—Detachment; having lost hope for permanent reunion with caregiver. Third stage in adapting to hospitalization; when the grieving person does not accept the loss or believes it is true. Kubler-Ross's first stage of grief.

deontologic theory—A major theoretical orientation focused on rules, obligation, and commitment.

depot injection—An intramuscular injection of a medication that will be absorbed over a longer period of time.

depression—A great sense of loss or sadness. Kubler-Ross's fourth stage of grief.

depressive disorder—Disturbance in mood characterized by loss of interest or pleasure in normal activities.

dermatophytes—Keratin-loving fungi that are parasitic upon the skin.

dermis—The fibrous inner layer of skin just below the epidermis.

descriptive ethics—Identification of preferences in ethical situations.

despair—Withdrawal, refusal of food, diminished communication, and general loss of interest in the environment. Second stage in adapting to hospitalization.

desquamation—Shedding of the outer layer of the epidermis.

development—Physiological, psychosocial, and cognitive changes occurring over one's life span due to growth, maturation, and learning.

developmental delay—Achievement of developmental milestones later than expected.

dextrocardia—The location of the heart in the right hemithorax, either as a result of displacement by disease or as a congenital defect.

diagnosis-related group (DRG)—A classification system used to determine Medicare payments to hospitals and providers of medical services based on client diagnosis, procedures, age, and length of hospitalization.

dialysis—Treatment that acts as a filtration system outside the body to rid the body of waste products.

diaphysis—The shaft of the long bone.

diastasis recti—The separation of the two rectus muscles along the median line of the abdominal wall.

differentiated practice—A nursing practice model being implemented in some care settings, refers to a philosophy that delineates a nurse's role and functions according to experience, competence, and education.

diffusion—The movement of a solute from an area of higher concentration to an area of lower concentration until an equilibrium is reached.

DiGeorge syndrome—A congenital syndrome associated with hypoplasia or aplasia of the thymus and parathyroid gland; it is associated with congenital heart disease. There is lack of parathyroid with hypocalcemia, and deficits of cell mediated immunity caused by hypoplasia of the thymus.

direct services—Providing nursing care to individual clients.

disability—A functional limitation that prevents or interferes with a person's ability to perform age-expected activities.

discontinuity—Development is a series of discrete steps or stages that elevate the child to more advanced or higher levels of functioning with increased age.

dislocation—A displacement of two bone ends or of a bone from its articulation with a joint.

disseminated intravascular coagulation (DIC)—A coagulation disorder in which the stimulus for coagulation overwhelms the control mechanisms that normally confine coagulation to the area of bleeding.

distribution—Process whereby a drug moves from blood to interstitial spaces of tissues and from there into cells.

diurnal cycle —Sleeping through the night alternating with daytime wakefulness.

divorce decree—Legal document approved by the court that grants divorce, divides marital property, and specifies child custody.

domestic mimicry—One way of expressing an understanding of the differentiated sex-roles observed within the family/community. In imaginative play, the child enacts the role of "mommy," "daddy," and "baby."

Down syndrome—A congenital chromosomal disorder caused by an extra chromosome 21 characterized by varying degrees of mental retardation and a characteristic appearance.

drowning—Death from a submersion incident.

dry drowning—Drowning secondary to hypoxemia resulting from intense laryngospasm; fluid has not entered the lungs.

ductus arteriosus—Fetal connection between the aorta and pulmonary artery that closes shortly after birth.

ductus venosus—A shunt in the fetus that carries oxygenated blood from the umbilical veins to the inferior vena cava.

dura mater—The first meningeal membrane that adheres to the inner surface of the skull.

dysfluency—Impaired rate, rhythm, or general flow of speech.

dyshormonogenesis—Inborn error in the synthesis of a hormone.

dysmorphic—Abnormal or unusual features, commonly associated with various genetic syndromes.

dyspnea—Shortness of breath or difficulty in breathing.

dysuria—Difficult or painful urination.

ecchymosis—Black or blue discoloration of an area of skin caused by extravasation of blood into subcutaneous tissue as a result of trauma; bruise.

eccrine glands—Sweat glands distributed across the body and responsible for thermoregulation.

echolalia—Repeating the last word or words heard; sometimes initially mistaken for true speech.

ecological theory—Bronfenbrenner's view suggesting developing individuals are embedded in a series of environmental systems.

ecomap—A visual overview of the complex ecological system of a family, showing the family's organizational patterns and relationships.

ectasia—Larger than normal.

ectoparasites—Parasites living on the surface of the host's body.

educator—Nursing role involved in providing information to clients, families, and staff as indicated and needed.

effusion—The accumulation of fluid such as in the middle ear or pleural cavity.

ego—Freud's term for the rational component of the personality.

egocentrism—View the world only from own point of view. Cannot imagine that another may have a different perspective; when children and adolescents are unable to appropriately differentiate between themselves and the objects of their attention.

Electra complex—Complex described by Freud where preschool female child has strong feelings of attraction for the caregiver of the opposite sex and thus feels that she must compete with the caregiver of the same sex.

electrolytes—Charged particles that are found in body fluid. Most important body electrolytes are sodium (Na^+), potassium (K^+), calcium (Ca^{++}), and chloride (Cl^-).

electrophysiology—Study and treatment of heart rate, rhythm, and electrical abnormalities.

elicitation phase—Phase of a hypersensitivity reaction that occurs with reexposure to the antigen.

emancipation—The legal recognition that a minor lives independently and is legally responsible for his or her own support and decision making.

emotional abuse—See psychological abuse.

empathy—The ability to put one's self in the other person's shoes—to feel as well as to intellectually know what the other person is experiencing.

empyema—An accumulation of infected fluid in a body cavity.

encephalitis—Inflammation of the brain.

encephalocele—Protrusion of the brain and meninges into a fluid-filled sac through a defect in the skull.

endocarditis—Inflammation of the endocardial lining of the heart.

endocardium—Serous inner membrane of the heart.

enterocolitis—Inflammation of the small intestine and colon.

enucleation—Surgical removal of the eye.

enuresis—Urinary incontinence.

envenomation—The poisonous effects caused by venom following a bite or sting such as that from a spider, insect, or snake.

epidermis—The outermost layer of the skin.

epidural hematomas—Space-occupying lesions in the brain usually secondary to rupture of the meningeal artery.

epilepsy—A chronic seizure disorder often associated with central nervous system pathology.

epileptogenic focus—Area in the brain where seizures originate.

epiphora—Excessive tearing.

epiphyseal growth plate—Thin layer of cartilage located between the metaphysis and the epiphysis at the end of the long bones; controls long bone growth.

epiphysis—The proximal and distal ends of the long bone.
epistaxis—Nose bleed.
Epstein's pearls—Small white pearl-like epithelial cysts that occur on both sides of the midline of the hard palate of a newborn.
equilibrium—Harmonious relationships between thought processes (assimilation, accommodation, adaptation) and the environment; Piagetian term.
erythema marginatum—Fine, pink rash.
erythema multiforme—An erythematous, maculopapular, vesicular, urticarial rash; may include target lesions; 20% are caused by drugs.
erythema toxicum—A transient newborn rash characterized by a red macular base with a white vesicular center.
erythematous—Diffuse redness over the skin.
erythrocytosis—Increase in red blood cell production in response to chronic hypoxemia.
erythropoiesis—The production of red blood cells.
erythropoietin—A hormone released by the kidneys that stimulates the bone marrow to produce red blood cells.
eschar—Thick leather-like dead skin that forms as a result of a burn.
escharotomy—Incision made into constricting eschar to restore peripheral blood circulation.
esotropia—An inward turning of one eye relative to the other fixating eye.
esotropia (convergent) strabismus—One or both eyes turn toward midline.
ethics—The study of the nature and justification of principles that guide human behaviors and that are applied when moral problems arise.
ethnocentrism—The tendency for all individuals and cultures to believe their values are the best and the most correct.
eutectic mixture of local anesthetics (EMLA)—An anesthetic cream applied for one hour or more prior to procedures such as injections and venipunctures to minimize pain.
euthanasia—Ending life by passive or active means.
euthyroid—Normal thyroid hormone levels.
evulsed tooth—Tooth that has been knocked out or removed from socket.
exancephaly—Malformation where the brain is totally exposed or herniated through a defect in the skull.
excretion—Process whereby a drug or its metabolites move from the tissues back into the circulation and then to the organs of elimination.
exhibitionism—Exposing one's genitals to strangers.
exophthalmos—Bulging of the eyeballs.
exosystem—Bronfenbrenner's term for settings influencing individuals even though not experienced directly.
exotropia—A visual disorder in which the deviating eye looks outward. The eye often is blind or has defective vision.
exotropia (divergent) strabismus—One or both eyes turn away from midline.
exploitation—A category of sexual abuse that involves prostitution and child pornography.
expressive language—The ability to use gestures, words, and written symbols to communicate with others.
extensor surfaces—Surfaces of an extremity that do not come into contact when the extremity is flexed.
extracellular fluid (ECF)—Body fluid that is outside the cells and includes interstitial, intravascular, and lymphatic fluid; ECF contains large amounts of sodium, chloride, and bicarbonate.
extracorporeal membrane oxygenator (ECMO)—A device that oxygenates the blood outside the body.
extramedullary—Outside the bone marrow.
extravasate—The leaking out of the vein of a drug that is being administered.
exudate—Fluids, cells, or other substances released from body.
family—Two or more persons who are joined by bonds of sharing and emotional closeness and who identify themselves as members of the family.
family as client—The family considered as a set of interacting parts; assessment of the dynamics among these parts renders the whole family the client.
family as context—The family considered as the context within which individuals are assessed; emphasis is placed primarily on the individual, keeping in mind that she or he is part of a larger system.
family assessment—The process of collecting data about the family structure; relationships, and interactions among individual members.
family therapy—The therapist looks at the child's symptoms or problems as a reflection of the family's problems. Family therapy may include the child, the primary caregivers, siblings, and other people from the extended family, for example, grandparents, ex-partners, and step siblings.
family-centered care—A philosophy of care that recognizes the centrality of the family in the child's life and inclusion of the family's contribution and involvement in the plan for and the delivery of care.
Fanconi's anemia—The inherited from of aplastic anemia in which the bone marrow fails to produce adequate numbers of erythrocytes, leukocytes, and platelets.
fantasy stage (of career development)—Adolescents choose careers they are most impassioned about.
febrile seizures—A type of tonic/clonic seizure usually associated with rapid rise in temperature that reaches a minimum of 39° centigrade (102.2° Fahrenheit).

fecalith—A hard, impacted mass of feces in the colon.

feedback—Information from the receiver about the message sent.

ferritin—A stored form of iron.

fibrin—The end result of the coagulation cascade and the primary protein from which clots are formed.

fibrosis—The repair and replacement of injured or infected tissue with scar tissue.

fidelity—Keeping one's promise or word.

filtration—Movement of a solute based on the force exerted by the weight of the solution.

first-pass-effect—Effect of biotransformation of a drug by the liver before reaching systemic circulation.

flaccid areflexia—Absence of response; an indication of severe brain stem injury.

flexion burns—Occur when caregivers purposefully immerse a child in hot liquids and the body part immersed is held in a flexed position so that a "zebra" pattern occurs.

flexural surfaces—Surfaces of an extremity that come into direct contact when the extremity is flexed.

fomites—Inanimate objects on which disease-causing organisms may be conveyed.

Fontan—One of three staged palliative procedures for patients with single ventricle physiology. Goal of procedure is to connect inferior vena caval blood to the pulmonary artery.

fontanels—Soft spots found at junctions of suture lines of skull bones; allow for adaptation to the pelvis shape during delivery and growth of the brain over the coming year.

foramen ovale—Normal in utero communication between the right and left atrium that normally closes after birth. A patent foramen ovale is one that has not closed.

foreclosed—Individuals who demonstrate a strong sense of commitment, but have not experienced a crisis or exploratory period to establish commitment.

forensic examination—An examination performed for the purpose of collecting medical evidence when the health care provider suspects the client may be the victim of a crime.

formal communication—Organized communication with a particular agenda.

formal operations stage—Piaget's fourth and final stage of cognitive development; individuals from 11–12 and up begin thinking systematically and rationally about hypothetical events and abstract concepts.

fragile X syndrome—A chromosomally caused syndrome that includes mental retardation, unusual behaviors, and a characteristic appearance.

friendship dyad—The most fundamental peer relation, and the one most likely to be based on similar interests and emotional support.

gastric residuals—Feeding retained in stomach following tube feeding.

gate control theory of pain—Theory which explains how pain impulses travel and are interpreted in the body.

gender identity—The way we think about ourselves as either male or female; a culmination of biological makeup, personal experiences, social expectations, and recommendations about how males and females should think and behave.

generalized seizures—Tonic/clonic movements arising from both cerebral hemispheres; usually no aura, but always loss of consciousness.

genital stage—Freud's fifth stage of psychosexual development (puberty and onward); sexual desires reemerge, but are more appropriately directed toward opposite-sex peers.

genogram—A graph outlining a family's history over a period of time, usually over three generations.

Glenn shunt—A prodecure where the superior vena cava (SVC), which normally carries unoxygenated blood back to the right atrium (RA), is disconnected from the RA and sutured directly to the right pulmonary artery.

glial cells—Cells that provide the supporting structure of the brain.

glomerular filtration rate (GFR)—The amount of fluid that is filtered by the glomeruli (a semi-permeable membrane).

gluconeogenesis—Formation of glucose in the liver from fat and protein.

glycogenolysis—Formation of glucose from glycogen.

goiter—Enlargement of the thyroid gland.

goniotomy—A surgical procedure for glaucoma. A linear incision is made into the trabecular meshwork to increase drainage of the aqueous humor from the anterior chamber of the eye, therefore controlling intraocular pressure.

good touch—Any physical contact that helps the child in getting clean or taking care of bruises or abrasions and is done by the parent or a caregiver approved by the parent.

graft versus host disease (GVHD)—An immune response that occurs after bone marrow transplant when the donor white cells perceive the client's body as foreign material to be attacked and destroyed.

grief—An individual's response to a loss. Thoughts and feelings associated with a loss.

group therapy—Involves a group of children, usually 6 to 10, with a focus on interpersonal relationships. Socialization process occurs among group members whereby feedback and support come from peers rather than from the therapist alone.

growth—A physiological increase in size through cell multiplication or differentiation.

grunting—A sound produced by the premature closure of the glottis during early expiration. Grunting increases airway pressure and preserves or increases the functional residual volume.

guarding—A rigid contraction of the abdominal wall muscles. It usually occurs as an involuntary reaction to pain such as when an examiner attempts to palpate inflamed areas or organs in the abdominal cavity.

habituation—The ability to decrease responses to disturbing stimuli.

half-life—Time required for 50% of a drug to be excreted from the body.

hand-foot syndrome—A type of vaso-occlusive crisis in the bone marrow of the hands and feet that causes severe pain.

handicap—A barrier imposed by society, the environment, or one's self in response to perceived differences.

health-orientation model—View of chronic conditions that depicts them as a common variation in life and focuses on an individual's strengths.

hearing impairment—Impairment in processing linguistic information through hearing, with or without amplification.

heave—A lifting of the cardiac area secondary to an increased workload and force of the left ventricular contraction.

helper T cells—Cells that stimulate B lymphocytes to divide and mature into plasma cells.

hemarthrosis—A condition wherein bleeding occurs in the joints, causing pain and limited movement.

hematemesis—Vomiting of blood.

hematogenous—Originating or transported in the blood.

hematomas—Pockets of blood under the skin that result from excessive bleeding into the space following trauma.

hematuria—Presence of blood in the urine.

hemihypertrophy—A relative increase in size of one half of the body as compared to the other.

hemisensory—Loss or decrease of function of a sense organ on one side of the body.

hemodialysis—A hemofiltration system that occurs outside the body. It requires an arteriovenous fistula or shunt placed in a large vessel.

hemofiltration—A continuous form of dialysis by means of an arteriovenous or venovenous shunt. These shunts, like hemodialysis, require an extracorporeal circuit through which the blood flows into a filter system.

hemoglobin (Hb)—A protein within red blood cells that enhances the cells' ability to transport oxygen to the tissues.

hemoglobin S (Hb S)—An abnormal form of hemoglobin that undergoes sickling.

hemolysis—The destruction of red blood cells.

hemophilia A—The most common type of hemophilia, caused by a deficiency of factor VIII.

hemophilia B (Christmas disease)—A type of hemophilia caused by a deficiency of factor IX (Christmas factor).

hemophilia C—A type of hemophilia caused by a deficiency of factor XI.

hemophilias—A group of bleeding disorders in which a factor in the first phase of coagulation is deficient.

hemoptysis—Coughing up blood from the respiratory tract.

hemorrhagic cystitis—An abnormal bleeding of the bladder.

hemosiderin—An iron-rich pigment that is a product of red cell hemolysis, Iron is often stored in this form.

hemosiderosis—A buildup of excess iron in the body, eventually causing organ failure and death.

hemostasis—The control of bleeding in order to maintain blood volume, pressure, and flow through injured vessels.

hepatomegaly—Liver enlargement.

herd immunity—Reduction of the number of persons susceptible to a communicable disease by immunization, preventing the spread of disease in epidemic proportions.

heterograft—Type of temporary skin graft that comes from a donor of a different species, most often pigskin.

highly active antiretroviral therapy (HAART)—Antiretroviral drugs, such as zidovudine and epivir, used to treat HIV/AIDS; administered during pregnancy and delivery or during the neonatal period.

hirsutism—Excessive body hair in a masculine distribution pattern.

HIV disease—An illness continuum, from asymptomatic to death, with an acquired immunodeficiency syndrome (AIDS) diagnosis usually occurring in the latter part of the continuum.

HIV infection—A multisystem disease known primarily for its effects on the immune system.

home health care—Skilled nursing and health-related services provided to individuals and families in their place of residence.

homeostasis—Dynamic equilibrium of the body that is maintained by dynamic processes of feedback and regulation.

homograft—Type of temporary graft of tissue that comes from a donor of the same species.

hormone—A chemical substance produced by an endocrine gland that is secreted into the bloodstream and produces a specific effect on a target organ.

humoral system—Consists of B lymphocytes.

hydrocele—A collection of fluid between the parietal and visceral layers of the tunica vaginalis.

hydrocephalus—An enlargement of the head without enlargement of the facial structures, due to an accumulation of CSF in the ventricles of the brain.

hydrolyze—To cause a substance to break down into its component parts by adding water.
hydronephrosis—Distension of the kidney caused by urine accumulating in the renal pelvis secondary to outflow obstruction.
hydrostatic pressure—Pressure of blood against the capillary walls generated by the contraction of the heart; hydrostatic pressure within the capillary bed pushes fluid across capillary membranes into the interstitial space and is balanced by osmotic pressure.
hypercapnia—An excess of carbon dioxide in the blood.
hypercyanotic spells—Spells commonly associated with tetralogy of Fallot, precipitated by agitation; result in extreme cyanosis and distress.
hyperopia (farsightedness)—Improper focusing of light on the retina; difficulty with near vision.
hyperplasia—Abnormal proliferation of normal cells.
hyperpnea—Deep, rapid respirations.
hypertonic dehydration—State in which the water loss is greater than the sodium loss.
hypertonic fluid—Fluid that is more concentrated (higher osmolality) than normal body fluid.
hypertrophy—An increase in the size of a cell or a group of cells resulting in an increase in the size of an organ.
hypertropia—Occurs when the eyes are out of vertical alignment.
hyphae—The branching outgrowths of a fungus or bacterium that invade tissue and establish an infection.
hyphema—A hemorrhage into the anterior chamber of the eye.
hypoalbuminemia—Low levels of albumin in the blood.
hypoplastic—Underdeveloped or incompletely developed organ or tissue.
hypotonic dehydration—State in which the sodium loss is greater than the water loss.
hypotonic fluid—Fluid that is less concentrated (lower osmolality) than normal body fluid.
hypoxia (hypoxic/hypoxemia)—Decreased oxygen to body tissues.
id—Freudian term for the inborn element of personality driven by selfish urges or instincts.
identity—Adolescents' definition of who they are based on their cumulative understanding of their inherent motivations, personal belief systems, and previous experiences.
identity achievement—Individuals who have experienced a crisis period and have achieved a sense of commitment to their resulting decisions.
identity diffusion—Individuals who have not experienced an identity crisis or made a commitment to any ideologic or occupational direction.
identity versus role confusion—Fifth stage of Erikson's psychosocial development whereby adolescents need to form a coherent self-definition or otherwise remain confused about life directions.
idiosyncratic—Peculiar to an individual.
imaginary audience—Adolescents' exaggerated sense that they are always on stage, the focus of others' attention.
immediate hypersensitivity—A reaction to an antigen; has a short duration between exposure and reaction.
immersion burns—Burns that are found on the arms, buttocks, or genitals that are sharply demarcated or circumferential due to either an accidental fall in hot bath water or from the child being held in hot water.
immune system—Spleen, lymph nodes, lymphoid tissue, white blood cells, phagocytes; natural killer cells; skin, mucus secretions, cilia, sebaceous gland secretions, stomach acid, normal intestinal flora that protect the human from disease.
immune thrombocytopenic purpura (ITP)—An autoimmune disorder characterized by low platelet counts and exaggerated bleeding.
immunity—Processes used by the body to protect against harmful organisms.
immunoglobulins—Chemicals that "tag" or identify an antigen or pathogen for destruction by other immune cells.
immunosuppression—The reduction or prevention of the normally occurring reaction by the immune system to respond to antigenic stimuli.
immunotherapy—The use of synthetic or natural elements to stimulate or suppress the body's immune response.
incarceration—Strangulation of a portion of the bowel leading to circulation impairment and tissue necrosis.
incest—Sexual intercourse between closely related persons.
indirect services—Consulting with school and district to deliver services to meet a child's health needs.
individual health plan (IHP)—A document, based on the health assessment of a child, that outlines special health needs, goals, and strategies necessary to improve and maintain the health of the child and allow full participation in school experiences.
individual therapy—The focus is on the child's individual behavioral, developmental, and psychological issues and problems. The age, developmental level, and psychosocial alteration of the child determine the therapeutic interventions used.
individualized educational plan (IEP)—A written plan, spelling out the type and duration of services needed for a particular child.
induction—The initial phase of chemotherapy used to reduce the tumor burden to an undetectable level.
industry—The ability to be useful and productive.
industry versus inferiority—Erikson's fourth stage of psychosocial development whereby school-aged children

learn to master important social and cognitive skills or otherwise feel incompetent.

infant mortality rate—The number of infant deaths during the first year of life per 1,000 live births.

infantile spasms—A type of seizure in which the head may suddenly drop forward while both arms and legs are flexed; eyes may roll upward or downward; infant may cry out and turn pale, cyanotic, or flushed.

infectious disease—One that can be transmitted from one person to another or from animal to human by either direct or indirect contact.

infiltrate—Exudate, blood, or other substances that pass into tissues.

inflammation—The protective response of body tissues to irritation or injury characterized by redness, heat, swelling, pain, and loss of function.

informal communication—When communication has no particular agenda or protocol.

informed consent—The duty of a health care provider to discuss the risk and benefits of a treatment or procedure with a client prior to giving care.

infratentorial—In the posterior third of the brain, primarily in the cerebellum and brain stem and below the tentorium.

initiative versus guilt—Erikson's third stage of psychosocial development whereby preschool-aged children learn to initiate new activities or otherwise become self-critical.

injury—Damage or harm to an individual resulting in destruction of health, disability, or death.

innate immune system—The first line of defense against infections; includes biochemical and physical barriers.

innate immunity—Physical barriers such as skin, mucous membranes, and cough reflex.

innate purity—Doctrine that suggests children are inherently good and born without an intuitive sense of right and wrong.

inotropes—Medications that increase the force of muscular contractions.

instrumental realistic orientation stage—Rules are obeyed to gain rewards or satisfy personal objectives; Kohlberg's second stage of moral development.

insufflation—Act of blowing air into a cavity.

intelligence quotient—The individual's functional age on the intelligence test divided by the chronologic age and multiplied by 100.

interferons—Chemicals that inhibit replication of many viruses; have anti-tumor effects; host specific rather than antigen specific; secreted by infected cells.

interleukins—Chemical mediators or messengers; also termed cytokines.

interpersonal concordance orientation—Behavior and decisions are evaluated on the basis of one's intent and concerns about others' reactions; Kohlberg's third stage of moral development.

interpersonal theory—Sullivan's view suggesting self-concept development, the key to personality development, is impacted by the home environment.

interstitial fluid—The portion of extracellular fluid that is between the cells and outside the blood and lymphatic vessels.

intertriginous—Skin surfaces that are apposing or form folds such as the interdigital, axillary, cubital, popliteal, and inguinal areas.

intertrigo—An erythematous skin eruption occurring on apposed skin surfaces.

intracellular fluid (ICF)—Body fluid that is located inside the cells; ICF contains large amounts of potassium, phosphate, sulfate, and proteins.

intracranial pressure (ICP)—The force exerted by the brain, blood, and cerebrospinal fluid within the cranial vault.

intrathecal—Administration of medication directly into the spinal canal for diffusion throughout the spinal fluid.

intravascular fluid—The portion of extracellular fluid that is in the blood vessels.

intravenous pyelogram (IVP)—Radiographic examination of the entire urinary tract; also called excretory urography.

intuitive phase—Characterized by sophisticated language, decreasing egocentrism, incessant questioning, reality-based play; Piaget's eighth phase of cognitive development.

iron deficiency anemia—An anemia caused by insufficient amounts of iron for adequate hemoglobin synthesis.

irreversibility—Knowledge that death is permanent.

isotonic dehydration—State in which the loss of sodium and water are equal.

isotonic fluid—Fluid that has the same concentration (osmolality) as normal body fluid.

Jacksonian seizures—Motor episodes beginning with tonic contractions of either the fingers of one hand, toes of one foot, or one side of the face, which then progress into tonic/clonic movements that "march" up adjacent muscles of the affected extremity or side of the body.

jaundice—The yellowish discoloration of the skin and eyes caused by excess bilirubin.

justice—Treating individuals equally or with fairness.

juvenile arthritis (JA); juvenile chronic arthritis (JCA); juvenile rheumatoid arthritis (JRA)— Term used for an inflammatory autoimmune disease causing many forms of arthritis in children.

karyotyping—Identification of the chromosomes' appearance, performed by growing cells from a blood or tissue sample, staining them during the metaphase stage of replication, and scanning them with a microscope.

kernicterus—A form of icterus neonatorum in which nuclear masses of the brain and spinal cord undergo pathologic changes accompanied by deposition of bile pigments within them.

Kernig's sign—Sign of meningeal irritation; child resists attempts to extend flexed leg or complains of pain on extension.

Kussmaul respiration—Abnormally slow, deep respiration characteristic of air hunger in acidotic states.

kyphosis—An abnormal thoracic curvature of the spine.

language—The meaningful use of words, phrases, and gestures to transmit meaning from one person to another.

large for gestational age (LGA)—An infant at greater than the 90th percentile of weight for gestational age, or >4,000 grams.

latchkey children—Children who are home alone after school for a period of time without adult supervision.

latency stage—Freud's fourth stage of psychosexual development; sexual drives are submerged, appropriate gender roles are adopted, the Oedipal/Electra conflict is resolved.

libido—Freudian term for psychic energy of basic biological instincts.

lichenification—Thickening and hardening of the skin with exaggeration of its normal markings.

limit setting—The caregiver defines boundaries and expectations for the toddler either by words, pictures, and/or role modeling. Setting boundaries requires consistency on the part of the caregiver in adhering to the limits set and following through on delivering consequences when the toddler exceeds the limits.

lipoatrophy—Indentation or atrophy of subcutaneous fat.

lipohypertrophy—Lumpiness or hypertrophy of subcutaneous fat.

lipolysis—The hydrolysis of fat.

listening—Providing verbal and nonverbal clues that communicate interest.

locomotion—The ability to move from place to place without assistance.

lordosis—Exaggerated curve of the lumbar spine, normal during the toddler years.

low birth weight—Weight of less than 2,500 grams—or 5 pounds, 8 ounces—at birth.

luxation—Complete dislocation of a joint, with no contact between articular surfaces of the joint.

lymphadenopathy—Enlargement of the lymph nodes.

lymphoblasts—Immature white cells, which when malignant are the leukemia cells that crowd out normal red cells, white cells, and platelets.

lymphokine—A substance that prevents or contains the migration of antigens.

Macewen's sign—A hollow or "cracked-pot" sound heard when percussing the head of a child with hydrocephalus.

macrosystem—Bronfenbrenner's term for the larger cultural or subcultural context of development.

maculopapular rashes—The most common form of cutaneous reactions to an antigen; symmetric, characterized by macules or papules.

mainstreaming—The placement of children with disabilities in a classroom with children without disabilities.

maintenance therapy—Phase of chemotherapy that follows consolidation in order to destroy residual cancer cells.

maldistribution—Abnormal distribution.

malignant brain edema (cerebral hyperemia)—Unique to children; a hyperemic or vascular reaction to head trauma because of the disruption in the blood-brain barrier; the mechanism to control cerebrospinal fluid absorption also is impaired.

malocclusion—An abnormality in the coming together of teeth, leaving the teeth uneven or crowded.

malpractice—Professional negligence.

managed care—A vehicle for cost-effective delivery of health care services.

manager/leader—Nursing role involved in being responsible for a group of clients or a group of staff.

mandated reporters—Individuals who are required to report to appropriate authorities suspicions of child abuse/neglect.

marginality—A situation in which a condition is less visible to others resulting in ambiguity about whether an individual is different from or like others. This results at times in inappropriate expectations.

matching hypothesis—Selection of a dating partner based on attractiveness.

maturation—Changes that are due to genetic inheritance rather than life experiences, illness, or injury.

mature minor doctrine—Some states have defined circumstances in which a child who has not reached the age of majority may make legal decisions, if that child can demonstrate adequate maturity.

meconium—First feces of a neonate, greenish black in color, tarry, and almost odorless.

medulla oblongata—Area of the brain stem that regulates the respiratory, cardiac, vasoconstrictor, sneeze, cough, and vomiting reflexes as well as cranial nerves IX, X, XI, and XII.

melanocytes—Cells within the epidermis that produce melanin, which gives pigment to the skin.

melena—Black or tarry stool indicating the presence of blood.

memory cells—T cells that remember an immune response.

menarche—The first menstrual period.

meninges—The three membranes covering the brain.

meningitis—Inflammation of the meninges.

meningocele—A sac-like herniation through the bony malformation that contains the meninges and cerebrospinal fluid.

meningomyelocele—A sac-like extrusion through the bony defect that contains the meninges, cerebrospinal fluid, and a portion of the spinal cord and/or nerve roots.

menorrhagia—Abnormally long and heavy menstrual periods.

mental combinations phase—One thinks before acting, uses memory for simple problem solving, imitates behavior of others, engages in symbolic, ritualistic play; Piaget's sixth phase of cognitive development.

mental retardation—A disorder characterized by subaverage general intellectual functioning with deficits in adaptive behavior.

mesosystem—Bronfenbrenner's term for the interrelationship between microsystems.

message—A verbal or nonverbal stimulus produced by a sender and responded to by a receiver.

metaphysis—A section of the long bone in which the diaphysis and epiphysis converge; it is responsible for growth until the child's adult height is attained.

microcephaly—A congenital anomaly characterized by a small brain with a resultant small head and a mental deficit.

microsystem—Bronfenbrenner's term for the immediate settings of a person's life (i.e., the family).

midbrain—Area of the brain stem that manages visual reflexes, tracking, and cranial nerves III and IV.

milia—A minute white cyst of the epidermis caused by obstruction of hair follicles and eccrine sweat glands. One variety is seen in newborns and disappears within a few weeks; small white papules on the nose, face, forehead, and upper torso caused by the plugging of the sebaceous gland.

minor—A person who has not yet reached the age at which he or she is considered to have the rights and responsibilities of an adult.

mixed conductive-sensorineural hearing loss—Results from interference with transmission of sound in the middle ear and along neural pathways.

modulation—The cascade of events that affect the firing of the pain nerve impulses or messages.

molding—The natural process by which a baby's head is shaped during labor as it is squeezed through the birth passage by the forces of labor.

molt—An arthropod's shedding of the exoskeleton to allow for growth.

mongolian spot—An irregularly dark pigmented area on the posterior lumbar region.

moral—Principle of right and wrong in behavior.

morality—Behavior in accordance with custom or tradition that usually reflects personal or religious beliefs.

morality of care—Gilligan's term for the dominant moral orientation of women; the individual emphasizes responsibility and concern for the welfare of others rather than abstract rights.

morality of justice—Gilligan's term for the dominant moral orientation of men; moral dilemmas are seen as inevitable conflicts between the rights of two or more parties needing to be settled by laws.

moratorium—Individuals experiencing an occupational and/or ideologic crisis that has not yet been resolved, delaying the establishment of an ideologic or occupational commitment.

mosaicism—The presence of two differing cell lines in an individual or organism.

mourning—The process an individual undergoes in order to adapt to a loss.

mucositis—An inflammation of the oral mucosa ranging from mild redness to severe painful ulceration.

Munchausen syndrome by proxy—Mental disorder that causes caregivers to fabricate signs and symptoms of disease and/or expose their child to harmful medical interventions and painful invasive procedures.

Mustard procedure—Intra-atrial baffling performed for correction of transposition of the great vessels. This procedure has almost completely been replaced by the arterial switch procedure.

mycologic cure—Cure defined as the absence of fungal species.

mycoses—Diseases caused by fungi.

myelodysplasia—Malformation of the neural tube during the first 28 days of gestation.

myelosuppression—A transient decrease in blood cell production.

myocarditis—Inflammation of the myocardium, or middle muscular layer of the heart.

myocardium—The cardiac muscle, middle layer of the heart.

myoclonic seizures—Suddden repeated contractures of muscles of the head, extremities, or torso.

myopia (nearsightedness)—Improper focusing of light on the retina; difficulty with distance vision.

nadir—The lowest point of myelosuppression.

nasal flaring—The widening of nostrils during inspiration; indicates air hunger.

natural immunity—See innate immunity.

nature—Belief that development is predetermined by genetic factors and not altered by the environment.

near-drowning—Survival for more than 24 hours after a submersion episode.

nebulized—The production of spray or mist by forcing air through a liquid.

negativism—The toddler's quest for independence leads to rejection of the wishes and ideas of others.

negligence—When a person owes a duty to another and through failure to fulfill that duty causes harm.
nephrogenesis—Development or growth of the kidney.
neutropenia—A decrease in the number of neutrophils, putting one at risk of life-threatening bacterial infections.
nevus flammeus (port wine stain)—A hemangioma or vascular tumor that does not disappear with time.
N-methyl-D-aspartate (NMDA) receptors—Chemical receptors that make spinal column nerve receptors more responsive.
nociceptors—Nerve receptors specific to pain.
noncommunicating hydrocephalus—Hydrocephalus caused by an impediment of cerebrospinal fluid flow within the ventricular system, also called obstructive hydrocephalus.
nonfunctionality—All functions that make being alive stop, and there is no longer an ability to carry out functions needed to be alive.
nonmaleficence—Doing no harm to the client.
nonverbal communication—Communicating a message without using words.
normalization—Cognitive and behavioral strategies used by a family of a child with a chronic condition in order to view itself as normal.
normative ethics—Standards of justification for moral actions and choices.
nursing caries—Dental decay that occurs from frequent and/or prolonged exposure to the sugars present in milk, formula, or juice.
nursing interview—Discussion with caregivers that provides an opportunity for the nurse to establish helping relationships while learning essential information about child and family.
nursing mutual participation model of care—A collaborative approach used in nursing practice, based on the premise that optimal therapeutic interventions result from equal partnerships between nurses and caregivers.
nurture—Belief that environmental influences affect development.
object permanence—The ability to know that an object will continue to exist even when it cannot be seen.
obstructive hydrocephalus—See noncommunicating hydrocephalus.
Oedipal/Oedipus complex—Complex described by Freud where male child has strong feelings of attraction for the caregiver of the opposite sex and thus feels that he must compete with the caregiver of the same sex.
olecranon process—A proximal projection of the ulna that forms the point of the elbow and fits into the olecranon fossa of the humerus when the forearm is extended.
oligomenorrhea—Abnormally light or a reduction in menstruation.
oliguria—A decreased ability to form and excrete urine.
oncogene—Gene that is capable of causing normal cells to transform to a malignant state.
oncotic pressure—A force within the capillary beds that holds fluids in the capillaries and is caused by the amount of plasma proteins present in the vascular system.
on-demand feeds—Feeding the newborn when hungry instead of according to a pre-arranged time schedule.
open adoption—An adoption where there is contact between the birth and adoptive parents.
open reduction—Surgical procedure for reducing a fracture or dislocation by exposing the skeletal parts involved using wires, pins, bone screws, or plates.
operation—Mental action, according to Piagetian theory.
opisthotonus—Severe spasm of back muscles, causing back to arch acutely and head to bend back on neck.
opportunistic infections—Infections that take advantage of a suppressed immune system.
oral stage—Freud's first stage of psychosexual development; children gratify the sex instinct by stimulating the lips, gums, teeth, and mouth.
ordinary model—A health orientation model of chronic conditions in which awareness of the health condition follows a developmental sequence and is not central to identity and daily activities.
original sin—Belief that children are inherently evil and selfish egotists who must be controlled by society.
orthopnea—An increase in labored breathing when lying flat.
osmolality—The concentration of solute within a solution measured by the number of moles of particles per kilogram of water; used as a measure of fluid concentration.
osmolarity—The concentration of solute within a solution measured by the number of moles per liter of water.
osmosis—Movement of water across a semipermeable membrane from a solution that has a lower solute concentration to one that has a higher solute concentration.
osmotic pressure—A force within the capillary beds that tends to pull fluid into the capillaries and serves to balance hydrostatic pressures.
osteoblastic—Bone formation by osteoblasts.
osteoblasts—Cells of mesodermal origin concerned with formation of bone.
osteoclastic—Resorption of old bony tissue by osteoclasts in periods of growth or repair.
osteotomy—Surgical procedure in which the bone is redesigned to alter the alignment or weight-bearing stress areas.
palliative—Therapies or procedures performed to relieve or reduce the intensity of uncomfortable symptoms but do not result in correction of a defect or a cure.

palpebral fissures—The opening between the margins of the upper and lower eyelids.
palpitations—Sensation of abnormal, forceful, or rapid heart beats.
pancarditis—Inflammation of the entire heart.
pancytopenia—A marked reduction in the number of RBCs, WBCs, and platelets.
papilledema—An inflammation of the optic disk, evident by edema seen on fundoscopic examination.
parallel play—The ability to play side-by-side, yet totally independent of other children. There may be close physical proximity, but seldom talking or sharing of toys.
paraverbal cues—Tone, pitch, volume, inflection, and the speed of the voice used in communication; not considered language.
parenchyma—The functional tissue of an organ as distinguished from supporting or connective tissue.
parens patrie—A legal rule that allows the state to take the place of the caregivers when the actual caregivers are unable or unwilling to provide for the best interests of the child.
parentification—The process of assuming the role of a caregiver (parent) such as caring for siblings, organizing and performing household chores.
parenting—A dynamic process that provides guidance and nurturing to a child.
paresthesia—Numbness or tingling sensation.
paroxysmal—Coughing that is severe in nature.
passive euthanasia—Allowing a person to die by not treating him or her.
passive immunity—The passing or administration of preformed antibodies to a person without that antibody.
pathogens—Organisms that invade the body and produce disease.
patient-controlled analgesia—Means of delivering pain medication by client self-administration.
peak height velocity (PHV)—The period of greatest growth in height during the adolescent growth spurt (AGS).
peak weight velocity (PWV)—The period of greatest weight gain during the AGS.
pediatric nurse practitioner—Usually a nurse with a master's degree who functions independently or under the guidance of a physician and focuses on disease prevention and minor disease management.
pedophilia—An act by an adult where the adult directs his or her sexual interests primarily or exclusively toward children.
perception—The cognitive awareness of pain experienced at the end of the physiological pain cascade.
pericardial effusion—Abnormal collection of fluid in the pericardial sac; limits filling and decreases cardiac output.
pericarditis—Inflammation of the pericardium.
pericardium—Fluid filled sac that encases the heart.
peristalsis—Coordinated, rhythmic, serial contraction of the smooth muscle of the GI tract.
peritoneal dialysis—Requires the placement of a catheter into the peritoneal cavity for the purposes of removing excess fluids, solutes, and nitrogenous wastes. This placement may or may not require an open surgical procedure.
periungual—Located around the fingernail or toenail.
personal fable—Psychological state in which adolescents have an exaggerated notion of their own uniqueness.
petechiae—Small, pinpoint, nonraised, perfectly round, purplish red spots that are a result of an intradermal or submucosal hemorrhage.
phagocytosis—The ingestion and destruction of foreign particles by cells of natural immunity.
phallic stage—Freud's third stage of psychosexual development; children gratify the sex instinct by developing an incestuous desire for the parent of the opposite gender, or fondling their own genitals.
phantom limb pain—Pain perceived to be coming from the area of an amputated limb.
pharmacodynamics—Biochemical and physiologic effects of drugs and their mechanisms of action within the body.
pharmacokinetics—Movement of drugs throughout the body by the processes of absorption, distribution, biotransformation, and excretion.
pharyngitis—Infection or inflammation of the pharynx.
photoallergies—Delayed immune responses involving previous sensitization through exposure to a chemical substance and the appearance of a skin rash following exposure to UVA radiation.
photophobia—Light sensitivity.
phototherapy—The use of special high-intensity fluorescent lights, to reduce serum bilirubin levels and prevent kernicterus.
physical abuse—Bodily injury that appears to have been inflicted by other than accidental means.
physical dependence—Physical adaptation to the presence of a drug in the bloodstream.
physiologic anorexia—A decreased appetite and ritualistic interest in limited types of food; this usually accompanies a period of slowed physiological growth and is considered a normal occurrence of toddlerhood.
pia mater—The third meningeal membrane, which is attached to the brain itself.
pilosebaceous follicle—Unit consisting of the follicle, sebaceous gland, and vellus hair. These follicles are most widely distributed across the face, chest, and upper back and contribute to the development of acne.
plasticity—The ability of neural cells in a certain area of the brain to assume the functions of a different area.

platelets—Disk-shaped cytoplasmic fragments that facilitate blood coagulation.

play therapy—The child expresses him or herself through the use of toys, dolls, blocks, cars, or other play objects. The process of being with the therapist, toy selection, and interaction during the therapy session are part of the therapeutic process.

pneumatosis intestinalis—Air within the bowel wall.

pneumoperitoneum—Free air in the peritoneal cavity.

pneumothorax—A collection of air or gas in the pleural cavity.

polyarthritis—Inflammation of many joints.

polydactyly—A congenital anomaly characterized by the presence of more than the normal number of fingers or toes.

polydipsia—Excessive thirst.

polyhydramnios—An excess of amniotic fluid.

polymorphous—Appearing in many forms.

polyphagia—Excessive hunger.

polyuria—Excretion of abnormally large quantity of urine.

pons—Area of the brainstem that controls respiratory function and cranial nerves V, VI, VII, and VIII.

postconventional morality—Kohlberg's term for the third level of moral reasoning; moral judgments are based on an abstract understanding of universal principles of justice.

postpubertal—Late adolescence.

postvoid residual urine—A measurement of the amount of urine remaining in the bladder after voiding.

preconceptual phase—Increasing use of symbols, especially language, egocentric thought, symbolic play, mental imagery; Piaget's seventh phase of cognitive development.

preconventional morality—Kohlberg's term for the first level of moral reasoning; societal rules are not yet internalized, judgments are based on reward or punishment.

preconventional or premoral stage—Initial stage of moral development described by Kohlberg where right and wrong is determined by the rules that others place upon you; impulses rule behavior; unable to differentiate right from wrong.

precordium—The part of the front of the chest that overlays the heart and the epigastrium.

preoperational stage—Piagetian term for second stage of cognitive development; children between 2 and 7 years old think symbolically and have not mastered logical operations.

prepubertal—Early adolescence.

prepuce—Skin forming a hood over the glans, which is abnormally small ventrally and may be redundant dorsally.

primary circular reaction phase—Infant performs complex, repetitive behaviors appearing to be responses to initial chance events centering on the infant's own body; Piaget's second phase of cognitive development.

primary closure—Wound closure performed shortly after the injury in which the wound edges are approximated.

primary prevention—Involves interventions that promote health and prevent disease processes from developing.

processus vaginalis—A fold of peritoneum that precedes the testicle as it descends through the inguinal canal into the scrotum.

prodrome—The earliest phase or sign of a developing condition or disease.

professional boundaries—The spaces between the nurse's power and the client's vulnerability. The power of the nurse comes from professional position and access to private knowledge about the client. Establishing boundaries allows the nurse to control this power differential and allows a safe connection to meet the client's needs.

proprioception—Awareness of posture, movement, and changes in equilibrium and knowledge of position, weight, and resistance of objects in relation to the body. (*Taber's Cyclopedic Medical Dictionary.* [2001]. Philadelphia: F.A. Davis.)

proptosis—A protrusion or forward displacement of the eyeball.

prostaglandins—A group of fatty acid substances present in many tissues. Extremely active biological substances responsible for a number of cellular interactions.

proteolysis—The hydrolysis of protein to simpler and soluble products.

proximodistal—Growth proceeds from the inside out.

pseudohermaphrodism—Ambiguous development of external genitalia.

pseudohypertrophy—Abnormal enlargement of an organ or body structure caused by an overgrowth of fatty and fibrous tissues.

pseudomenstruation—Blood observed on the diaper due to the withdrawal of the maternal hormones at the time of delivery.

pseudostrabismus—An appearance of strabismus caused by a fold of skin of the lower eyelid, which narrows the visible width of the sclera medial to the iris.

psychological abuse—Acts of omission or commission involving both the presence of hostile behavior as well as the absence of positive parenting behaviors.

psychomotor learning—One type of learning concerned with physical skills.

psychosexual theory—Freud's theoretical perspective emphasizing conflicts within the personality, unconscious motivations for behavior, and stages of development.

psychosocial theory—Theoretical perspective advocated by Erikson; stresses the complexity of interrelationships existing between emotional and physical variables during one's lifetime.

ptosis—A drooping of the eyelid.

pubertal—Middle adolescence.

puberty—The state of physical development when secondary sex characteristics begin to appear, sexual organs mature, reproduction first becomes possible, and the adolescent growth spurt starts.

pulsus paradoxus—Excessive variation in forcefulnes of arterial pulse during respiration demonstrated by a systolic reduction of more than 10 mm Hg.

punishment and obedience orientation stage—Behaviors, decisions, and conformity to rules are based on fear of punishment rather than respect for authority; Kohlberg's first stage of moral development.

pupil personnel team (service team)—A team of professionals who work together with teachers to provide interventions for students having difficulties.

purpura—Areas of blood underneath the skin or mucous membranes.

pyelonephritis—An inflammation of the kidney(s).

pyloromyotomy—Surgical procedure performed to relieve hypertrophic pyloric stenosis.

pyuria—White blood cells in the urine (a sign of bacterial or nonbacterial infection of the urinary tract).

rachischisis—Fissure in the vertebral column exposing the meninges and spinal cord.

radiation pneumonitis—Acute reaction caused by the swelling and sloughing of the endothelial cells of the small vessels of the lung, which allows fluid to accumulate in the interstitial tissues.

rape—Sexual intercourse with force or a threat of force, and without a person's consent.

rate of growth—A calculation of the amount of growth over a specific period of time.

realistic stage (of career development)—Young people begin to extensively explore and focus on available careers.

rebound tenderness—Sign of inflammation of the peritoneum elicited by a sudden release of a hand pressing on the abdomen.

receiver—The person intercepting the sender's message.

receptive language—The ability to understand spoken and written communication.

red blood cells (RBCs)—The blood cells whose primary function is to supply the tissues with oxygen.

reflexive phase—Predictable, innate survival reflexes becoming more efficient and generalized; first phase of Piaget's cognitive development.

refraction—The process by which the cornea and lens of the eye bend light rays so that they focus on the retina.

refractory seizures—Seizures lasting more than 60 minutes.

regression—Returning to a previous level of function or action. Often occurs when the toddler's routine and security are threatened (e.g., hospitalization, new baby enters family).

renal scanning—Examination of the urinary tract by ultrasound.

renal ultrasound—Radiographic examination of the kidney utilizing sound waves above the range of human hearing to formulate a two-dimensional image.

researcher—Nursing role involved in collecting, using, and evaluating evidence-based data in practice.

respiratory distress syndrome (RDS)—An inadequate production of surfactant in the lungs of premature infants, thereby reducing the surface tension of these surfaces, and interfering with the ability of the lungs to remain inflated during exhalation.

respite care—Involves having a person who relieves the usual caregiver of caregiving responsibilities for a period of time.

retractions—Inward movement of the soft tissues of the chest wall during inspiration; associated with increased respiratory effort.

retrograde—Moving backward.

reverse attention—Method of behavior management where attention is given to positive behaviors and negative behaviors are ignored.

reversibility—The ability to recognize that actions can move in reverse order.

Reye's syndrome—Acute, life-threatening, postinfectious encephalopathy.

rhizotomy—A procedure used to treat cerebral palsy, where a small secction of the spinal cord is cut.

ritualism—The repetition of sequences of occurrences, which produce structure and organization in the mind of a toddler. The repetition may involve a repeated action, phrase, and/or food/clothing choice and may continue for days or weeks.

rolandic or sylvian seizure—Tonic/clonic movements of the face with increased salivation and arrested speech; commonly occurs during sleep.

scald burns—Skin that is injured by hot water from the tap, coffee, tea, or hot cooking grease.

schema—Patterns of thought used to interpret or make sense of experiences, Piagetian term; One's own mental and/or physical structure developed through assimilation of new experiences..

school-age—The phase of development from 6 to 12 years.

school-based health clinics (SBHC)—Health centers within a school building set up and staffed by health care professionals other than the school nurse.

school-linked health clinics (SLHC)—Health centers set up and staffed by health care professionals to serve several schools, students, and other family members. May or may not be located within a school building.

scoliosis—A C-shaped or S-shaped curvature of the spine.

sebaceous glands—Glands that open into the hair follicles and secrete sebum, which helps lubricate the skin.

sebum—A complex lipid mixture produced by the sebaceous glands, which helps lubricate the skin.

secondary circular reaction phase—Infant learns from intentional behavior and begins to show some understanding of objects; Piaget's third phase of cognitive development.

secondary drowning—The rapid deterioration of respiratory function from several hours to days after successful resuscitation.

secondary intention—The natural process of wound healing that occurs when the wound edges cannot be approximated because of extensive tissue loss.

secondary prevention—Aims to detect disease in the early stages before clinical signs and symptoms manifest in order to intervene with early diagnosis and treatment.

self-competency—Adolescents' sense of how well they can function within a particular realm.

self-understanding—Adolescents' cognitive representation about themselves.

self-worth—The extent to which adolescents perceive themselves as individuals of worth.

sender—Generator of a message.

sensitive period—A time span that is optimal for certain capacities to emerge when the individual is especially receptive to environmental influences.

sensitization phase—Phase of a hypersensitivity reaction in which initial exposure to the antigen occurs.

sensorimotor stage—Piaget's first stage of cognitive development; during the first two years of life, the individual relies on motor behavior and senses to adapt to the world.

sensorineural hearing loss—Permanent hearing impairment that results from damage or malformation of the middle ear and/or auditory nerve.

separation anxiety—The behaviors demonstrated by an infant when separated from the caregiver.

sequestration crisis—A type of sickle cell crisis characterized by excessive pooling of blood in the liver and spleen.

sexual abuse—A sexual act, from fondling to vaginal or anal intercourse, imposed on a child who lacks the emotional, cognitive, or maturational development to deal with the actions.

shaken baby syndrome (SBS)—Vigorous manual shaking of a child, usually less than three years of age, that results in a subdural hematoma of the brain, occult bone fractures, and retinal hemorrhages.

sibling rivalry—Intense feelings of jealousy, envy, and stress toward a new infant sibling.

sickle cell anemia (SCA)—An anemia caused by the sickling of red blood cells caused by the presence of hemoglobin S.

simple partial seizures—Focal seizures characterized by local motor, sensory, psychic, and somatic manifestations.

sleep consolidation—Fewer periods of sleep with longer durations.

small for gestational age (SGA)—An infant who has a weight to gestational age ratio that is below the tenth percentile.

smegma—A collection of cells that shed from the outer layer of skin and gather under the foreskin of the penis.

social contract legalistic orientation—Just laws should be followed because they further human values and express the majority will; Kohlberg's fifth stage of moral development.

social learning theory—Bandura's theory; the individual learns behavior by observing behaviors of others.

social perspective taking ability—The understanding adolescents have about who they are in relation to those around them and their ability to understand the perspectives of others.

solute—A substance that is dissolved in a solution.

somnambulism—Sleepwalking.

somniloquy—Sleep talking.

somnolence syndrome—Subacute neurological toxicity seen 5–7 weeks postradiation therapy to the whole brain where drowsiness can be experienced up to 20 hours a day, and may be accompanied by fatigue, malaise, fever, dysphagia, ataxia, and transient papilledema.

span—Measurement obtained from measuring fingertip to fingertip.

speech—The physical production of sound using the oral mechanism (tongue, teeth, oral cavity, larynx).

spina bifida—A congenital, neural tube defect in the walls of the spinal cord caused by a lack of union between the laminae of the vertebrae.

spina bifida cystica—A defect in the closure of the posterior vertebral arch resulting in a protruding sac containing meninges (meningocele), spinal cord (myelocele), or both (meningomyelocele).

spina bifida occulta—A type of spina bifida where there is no herniation of the spinal cord or meninges.

splash burns—Occur when hot liquid is poured on a child; usually involves the back, lateral side of the face, or shoulder; the direction the hot liquid flows down the child's body assists in the diagnosis.

spongiosis—Inflammation of the skin's spongy layer.

sprain—A ligament that is stretched or torn from injury to a joint.

stage—The amount of spread of a malignancy, rated from stage I (1), with only local disease in one area or organ, to stage IV (4), with disseminated metastatic disease.

standard of care—Accepted action expected of an individual of a certain skill or knowledge level.

status epilepticus—A prolonged seizure or series of convulsions; loss of consciousness that may last for at least 30 minutes.

statutory rape—Consensual relations between a minor and an adult.

steatorrhea—Greater than normal amounts of fat in the feces, characterized by frothy, foul-smelling fecal matter that floats.

Stevens-Johnson syndrome—The most severe form of erythema multiforme caused by exposure to an antigen, usually a drug.

"stocking or glove" burns—Represent attempts by a child to prevent and protect himself or herself from being immersed in hot scalding tub water; burn has the appearance of a glove or stocking with an even edge.

strabismus—A condition in which each eye does not simultaneously focus on the same object in space because of lack of muscle coordination.

strain—The stretching or tearing of either a muscle or tendon from overuse, overstretching, or misuse.

stranger anxiety—The behaviors demonstrated by an infant with the appearance of a stranger and seen at approximately 8 to 12 months of age.

stratum corneum—The outermost layer of the epidermis, which is composed of several layers of dead skin cells.

stridor—A high-pitched sound produced by an obstruction of the trachea or larynx that can be heard during inspiration and/or expiration.

stupor—An unresponsive state; only responds to vigorous stimulation, and then returns to the original state once the insult is removed.

stuttering—A speech impairment in which an individual involuntarily repeats a sound or word, resulting in a loss of speech fluency.

subarachnoid villi—Area of the brain that reabsorbs CSF.

subdural hematomas—Space occupying lesions in the brain caused by rupture of the cortical veins bridging the subdural space.

subluxation—Incomplete or partial dislocation of the articular surfaces of a joint.

substance abuse—A maladaptive pattern of substance use manifested by recurrent and significant adverse consequences related to the repeated use of substance. (American Psychiatric Association. [1994]. *Diagnostic and statistical manual of mental disorders* [4th ed.]. Washington, DC: Author.)

substance P—A neuropeptide that sensitizes nerve endings to fire more rapidly.

sudden infant death syndrome (SIDS)—The sudden, unexplained death of an apparently normal and healthy infant under the age of 1 year even after a complete autopsy and review of history reveals no evidence of disease.

suicidal ideation—Thoughts about killing oneself.

suicide—The intentional or purposeful taking of one's own life. Suicide may be completed, attempted, or suicidal ideation.

sunblock—A sun protection product that reflects and scatters ultraviolet A and ultraviolet B radiation.

sunscreen—A sun protection product that absorbs the sun's rays. Protection against either or both ultraviolet A and ultraviolet B radiation may be provided.

superego—Freudian term for personality component consisting of internalized moral standards (conscience).

superior vena cava syndrome (SVC)—Syndrome caused by obstruction of the superior vena cava, resulting in edema of the face, neck, and upper trunk.

suppressor cells—T cells that reduce immunoglobulin production against a specific antigen.

suppurative—Pus forming.

supratentorial—A location in the anterior two-thirds of the brain, above the tentorium, primarily in the cerebrum.

synchronized cardioversion—Cardioversion of an abnormal rhythm to a normal rhythm using electrical shock (via a defibrillator) that senses the QRS and applies the energy in an appropriately timed manner in synchrony with the client's own rhythm. Can only be used in hemodynamically stable clients with normally upright QRS.

syncope—Fainting.

syndactylism—Congenital anomaly characterized by the fusion of the fingers or toes.

syndrome—A named condition characterized by a group of findings or attributes.

synovitis—An acute, nonpurulent inflammation of the synovial membrane of a joint; occurs most commonly in the hip joint.

T lymphocytes—The immune system's main defense against viruses; direct and regulate the immunologic response; secrete lymphokines; produced by the thymus gland.

tabula rasa—Doctrine that suggests children enter the world as a blank slate.

tachyarrhythmia—Abnormally fast heart rhythm.

tachypnea—Rapid respirations.

tamponade—An abnormal fluid collection around the heart in the mediastinal space that results in restricted filling of the heart and poor cardiac output. Can be life-threatening.

Tanner stages—The five stages of development of secondary sexual characteristics for males and females.

teething—The period of eruption of deciduous teeth.

telangiectatic nevi—A common skin condition of neonates, characterized by flat, deep-pink localized areas of capillary dilation that occur predominantly on the back of the neck, lower occiput, upper eyelids, upper lip, and bridge of the nose. The areas disappear permanently by 2 years of age.

telangiectatic nevi—Capillary hemangiomas commonly called "stork bites" that are sometimes found on the nape of the neck and the bridge of the nose.

telegraphic speech—Short sentences made up of only the key words.

teleologic theory—A major theoretical orientation that judges the rightness of actions by the ends achieved.

temper tantrums—An outward expression of the inner turmoil experienced by a toddler: openly angry and unpredictable. Usually disappears by preschool period.

temperament—The way in which a child behaviorally interacts with the surrounding environment.

tentative stage (of career development)—Adolescents begin to consider how they might fit in with the various career options they are considering.

tentorium—The dura mater located between the cerebrum and cerebellum supporting the occipital lobes.

teratogen—Any substance or process that interferes with normal prenatal development, causing developmental abnormalities in the fetus.

tertiary circular reactions phase—Characterized by interest in novelty and repetition, understanding causality, soliciting adult help, object permanence; Piaget's fifth phase of cognitive development.

tertiary prevention—Prevention directed toward children with clinically apparent disease.

thalassemias—A group of inherited autosomal recessive disorders, characterized by an impaired rate of hemoglobin chain synthesis.

therapeutic play—An intervention used by nurses and child life specialists where supervised play helps ill and hospitalized children express and understand their thoughts, feelings, and motivations.

thrill—A fine vibration, felt by an examiner's hand on a client's body over the site of an aneurysm or on the precordium, the result of turmoil in the flow of blood, indicating the presence of an organic murmur of grade 4 or greater intensity.

thrombocytopenia—A decrease in the platelet count below 150,000/ml.

tidal volume—The amount of air inhaled or exhaled with each breath.

time-out—A discipline strategy in which reinforcement for unacceptable behavior is removed to interrupt a pattern of negative behavior; a defined period of time in which the child is removed from activities and social interactions.

titration—Delivery of small doses of medication to achieve desired effect.

tolerance—Need to use increasing doses of a substance over time to achieve desired effect.

tonic/clonic seizures—Onset is usually abrupt and begins when the child loses consciousness and falls to the ground.

toxic epidermal necrolysis—An acute illness of fever, epidermal loss of more than 30% of the body surface area; 30–40% mortality rate caused by visceral involvement.

trabeculotomy—A surgical procedure for glaucoma; a direct opening between the canal of Schlemm and the anterior chamber of the eye, which controls intraocular pressure.

trajectory—The expected course of a health care alteration.

transduction—Beginning of the pain sensation when stimulus provokes electrical activity in pain receptors.

transductive reasoning—Unrelated events are linked to determine a reason for a particular event.

transferrin—An iron-transport molecule within the bloodstream.

transillumination—The use of a light to determine what structures are in the meningomyelocele.

transmission—Movement of impulses from peripheral site to terminals in spinal column dorsal horn.

trigone—A small triangular area at the base of the bladder where the ureters normally join the bladder.

trismus—Difficulty opening the mouth.

trisomy—The presence of three instead of two of a given chromosome.

tropic hormone—A hormone that causes a target organ to produce its hormone.

Trousseau's sign—Spasms of the carpals after pressure is applied to the upper arm nerves. Carpal spasms occur when the fingers contract and the individual is unable to open the hand. This is a sign of hypocalcemia.

trust versus mistrust—Erikson's first stage of psychosocial development; infants must learn to trust others to meet their needs so they learn to trust themselves.

tumor—Mass that may be either benign or malignant.

tumor lysis syndrome—Complication of initial cancer treatment; when tumor cells are killed by chemotherapy, purines are released from the lysed tumor cells, causing elevation of uric acid that can lead to renal failure.

tympanostomy—Surgical incision in the tympanic membrane for draining fluid.

uncertainty—Situations in which there is ambiguity about what can be expected. Typically results in stress.

unintentional injury—Injuries that occur without intent of harm.

universal ethical principle orientation—Right and wrong are defined on universal, comprehensive, consistent, yet personal ethical principles; Kohlberg's sixth stage of moral development.

universality—Belief that death is all inclusive, comes to every living thing; death is inevitable.

unlicensed assistive personnel (UAP)—Individuals who perform services for clients, such as first aid, medication administration, tube feedings, and catheterizations to students under the supervision of a registered nurse.

upper/lower body ratio—A ratio calculated from a measurement from the top of the head to the top of the synthesis pubis and from the synthesis pubis to the bottom of the feet.

uremia—A condition where excessive amounts of nitrogenous waste products, blood urea, and creatinine exist in the blood.

ureteropelvic obstruction—An obstruction at the junction of the ureters into the renal pelvis.

ureterovesical obstruction—An obstruction at the junction of the ureters into the bladder.

ureterovesical/vesicoureteral junction—Site where the ureter enters the bladder.

urethritis—Infection of the urethra.

urticaria—Wheal-like skin lesions seen in response to an antigen, often a drug; resolve fairly rapidly after discontinuing the drug.

values—Constructs that give meaning to our lives.

valvotomy—An incision into a cardiac valve to correct a defect.

valvulitis—Inflammation of the cardiac valves.

valvuloplasty—Procedure involving a balloon-tipped catheter used to dilate a cardiac valve.

vasculitis—Inflammation of blood vessels, including arteries or veins.

vaso-occlusive crisis—A type of sickle cell crisis characterized by the aggregation of sickled cells within a vessel, causing obstruction and infarction of the distal tissues.

vectors—Animals or insects that carry the infectious organism from one host to another.

vegetations—Abnormal growths inside body organs. In the heart they usually develop on heart valves.

vellus hair—Short, fine, often inconspicuous hair distributed across the body.

venous access device—Implanted device to facilitate the delivery of drugs, blood sampling and blood product administration, and the simultaneous administration of multiple drugs and intravenous fluids.

ventilation/perfusion (V/Q) ratio—The ratio of alveolar ventilation to capillary perfusion.

veracity—Telling the truth, particularly in health care, regarding diagnosis, treatment, or prognosis.

verbal communication—Messages using words and language.

vernix caseosa—A thick, cheesy, protective, integumentary deposit that consists of sebum and shed epithelial cells present on the newborn's skin.

verrucae—Benign epidermal tumors caused by the human papilloma virus, also known as cutaneous warts.

vertical transmission—The process of transmitting a disease from one generation to another.

vesicant—A chemotherapy agent that is a skin irritant and can cause discomfort, burning, and inflammation, if leaked outside the vein.

violent crime—Murder, forcible rape, robbery, and aggravated assault.

virilize—To develop sexual characteristics of a male. For example, a clitoris that is virilized will have the appearance of a penis.

virtue theory—A major theoretical orientation that focuses on the moral agent's intent, such as the virtue of truthfulness.

virulence—The degree or power of microorganisms to cause disease.

visual acuity—Clearness or sharpness of the image seen by the eye.

voiding cystourethrogram (VCUG)—Radiograph of bladder, urethra, and ureters during voiding.

von Willebrand's disease—A mild, congenital bleeding disorder caused by a deficiency of von Willebrand's factor.

von Willebrand's factor (vWF)—A protein that facilitates adhesion between platelets and injured vessel walls.

Waterhouse-Friderichsen syndrome—Fulminant meningococcemia.

weaning—A process of giving up one method of feeding for another.

wet drowning—Drowning caused by the aspiration of fluid into the lungs.

wheezing—A high-pitched musical sound produced by air flow through a narrowed airway.

white blood cells (WBCs)—The blood cells responsible for defending against invading microorganisms and removing debris.

windshield survey—A systematic assessment performed while the nurse travels through the community.

xanthelasma—Creamy, yellow plaque on eyelid due to hypercholesterolemia.

xanthomas—Slightly elevated yellow nodules that develop in the subcutaneous layer of skin.

xerostomia—Dryness of the mouth, which occurs from decreased or arrested production of salivary secretions.

zone of proximal development (ZPD)—Tasks that are too difficult for individuals to master alone but that can be mastered with the guidance and assistance of adults or more skilled adolescents.

INDEX

Note: Page numbers followed by "B" refer to numbered boxes. Page numbers followed by "F" refer to figures. Page numbers followed by "T" refer to tables.

A

F

G

I

O

Q

R

S

T

U

V

W

X

Z

Pediatric Nursing Skills and Student Tutorial CD-ROM

Set-Up Instructions

1. Insert disk into CD-ROM player.
2. From the Start Menu, choose *RUN*.
3. In the *Open* text box, enter **d:setup.exe** then click the *OK* button. (Substitute the letter of your CD-ROM drive for **d:**)
4. Follow the installation prompts from there.

Note: During installation, you have the opportunity to install the Pediatric Nusing Skills PDF files, the Student Tutorial (Flash!), or both. Please pay particular attention to this choice when it appears. You can always go back and reinstall other components later.

System Requirements

100 MHz Pentium with 24 MB of RAM

Microsoft Windows 95 or newer

37 megabytes of free disk space for complete installation:

Pediatric Nursing Skills PDF Files, 9 MB

Adobe Acrobat Reader (if not already installed), 20 MB

Student Tutorial (Flash!), 8 MB

CD-ROM drive, 6x or faster (8x recommended)

SVGA 24-bit color display

Netscape 4.0 (or newer) or Internet Explorer 4.0 (or newer) for PDF support

---